CW01454674

Neuro-Ophthalmology:
Diagnosis and Management

Commissioning Editor: Russell Gabbedy
Development Editor: Nani Clansey
Editorial Assistant: Poppy Garraway
Project Manager: Mahalakshmi Nithyanand
Designer: Stewart Larking
Illustration Manager: Bruce Hogarth
Illustrator: Richard Tibbitts
Marketing Manager(s) (UK/USA): Richard Jones/Helena Mutak

Neuro-Ophthalmology: Diagnosis and Management

Second Edition

Grant T. Liu, MD
Professor of Neurology and Ophthalmology

Nicholas J. Volpe, MD
Adele Niessen Professor of Ophthalmology and Neurology

Steven L. Galetta, MD
Van Meter Professor of Neurology and Ophthalmology

Division of Neuro-Ophthalmology, Departments of Neurology and Ophthalmology, Hospital of the University of Pennsylvania, Scheie Eye Institute, and the Children's Hospital of Philadelphia, University of Pennsylvania School of Medicine, Philadelphia, PA

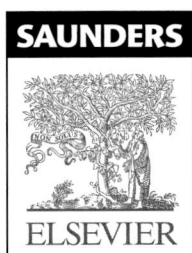

SAUNDERS

ELSEVIER

SAUNDERS
ELSEVIER

SAUNDERS is an imprint of Elsevier Inc.

© 2010, Elsevier Inc. All rights reserved.

First published 2001

13 digit ISBN here: 978-1-4160-2311-1

British Library Cataloguing in Publication Data
A catalogue record for this book is available from the British Library

Library of Congress Cataloging in Publication Data
A catalog record for this book is available from the Library of Congress

Notice
Medical knowledge is constantly changing. Standard safety precautions must be followed, but as new research and clinical experience broaden our knowledge, changes in treatment and drug therapy may become necessary or appropriate. Readers are advised to check the most current product information provided by the manufacturer of each drug to be administered to verify the recommended dose, the method and duration of administration, and contraindications. It is the responsibility of the practitioner, relying on experience and knowledge of the patient, to determine dosages and the best treatment for each individual patient. Neither the Publisher nor the author assume any liability for any injury and/or damage to persons or property arising from this publication.

The Publisher

British Library Cataloguing in Publication Data

Liu, Grant T.
  Neuro-ophthalmology : diagnosis and management.—2nd ed.
  1. Neuro-ophthalmology.   2. Neuro-ophthalmology—Diagnosis.
  I. Title   II. Volpe, Nicholas J.   III. Galetta, Steven L.
  617.7'62—dc22

  ISBN-13: 9781416023111

Printed in China
Last digit is the print number: 9 8 7 6 5 4 3

Contents

To   Alessandra and Jonathan Liu;
Nicholas, Matthew, Lena, and Tessa Volpe;
and Kristin, Michael, and Matthew Galetta

Foreword

The second edition of *Neuro-Ophthalmology: Diagnosis and Management* has arrived just in time. Ten years after the first edition appeared our copies have either been pilfered or the spines have been ripped. One of the copies has about 25 percent of the text underlined. These are clear indications of how highly the book is valued and how often it is consulted by trainees and senior staff in our neuro-ophthalmology unit. For the second edition the authors have enriched the content by seamlessly incorporating the advances in neuro-ophthalmology, ophthalmology, imaging and the pertinent neural sciences made since the first edition appeared. The scope of these advances can be inferred from the increment in the references. They constitute a major resource for readers desirous of delving into original articles. The chapter on optic neuropathies which listed 649 references in the 2000 edition now cites 1122! This despite the fact that the authors have been critical in making their selections. The illustrations have also been improved and the accompanying DVD literally animates the text. Having been co-authored by an ophthalmologist and two neurologists there is a broad perspective on neuro-ophthalmology, especially desirable since this is a specialty that crosses boundaries. Here is a book that will be as useful to experienced clinicians as it is to trainees.

Textbooks are teachers and one hopes to find in them the same qualities that make good teachers: accurate, stimulating and master of the subject. Since the authors are a team of experienced neuro-ophthalmic clinicians recognized as exceptional educators, it will come as no surprise that *Neuro-Ophthalmology: Diagnosis and Management* is a great educator. The book seems to say to the reader "Here's what you're looking for. Help yourself to whatever you need. I'll take you as far as you want to go". You will encounter no barriers between the authors and yourself. It is authoritative without being authoritarian.

Neuro-Ophthalmology: Diagnosis and Management reminds me of two neuro-ophthalmic classics: Frank Walsh's *Clinical Neuro-Ophthalmology* and David Cogan's *Neurology of the Ocular Muscles*. When you plan to only glance at a topic, the style proves so engaging and the content so engrossing that you read much further than you intended. Readers who seek a "first approximation" of a topic in this second edition will be treated to such a stimulating and inviting exposition of neuro-ophthalmic diseases and phenomena that they are apt to find themselves perusing other portions of the book.

Neuro-Ophthalmology: Diagnosis and Management has earned a place in the neuro-ophthalmic canon and should be owned by, or available to, every ophthalmologist, neurologist and neurosurgeon.

Simmons Lessell, MD
Boston, Massachusetts

Our goal with this book was to update and improve upon our successful first edition of Neuro-Ophthalmology: Diagnosis and Management. Like the first book, this one is intended to be a manageable text of well-synthesized, topically organized, and clinically relevant information, with numerous illustrations and references, which can assist clinicians with the care and understanding of patients with neuro-ophthalmic problems.

But what is the role of a medical textbook such as this one in the internet era? The three of us have discussed this question many times since the publication of our first edition. We acknowledge that our book can be neither encyclopedic, completely up to date (by the minute), nor authoritative on every subject.

On the other hand, what a one-volume neuro-ophthalmology textbook written by three seasoned clinicians (two neurologists and one ophthalmologist) can offer is even, thoughtful approaches to the diagnosis and management of disorders involving the eye and brain. We can provide helpful discourses on broad topics such as optic neuropathy, papilledema, and double vision, for instance. We can discuss disorders responsible for those problems in mild to moderate detail and provide management paradigms. Readers needing more information can go to primary sources or online. However, even in the internet and evidence-based era, many neuro-ophthalmologic conditions are still diagnosed and managed on the basis of experience and expert opinion, thus making the nuisances of clinically relevant observations and decision-making highlighted in this text so vitally important. Thus, we believe a book such as ours can still play a vital role in the education of students of neuro-ophthalmology and be an important guide for the management of their patients.

The three of us were humbled by the success of the first edition of this book. Students, residents, fellows, practitioners and reviewers have told us they find the book helpful in the diagnosis and management of their neuro-ophthalmic patients. Many professors of neuro-ophthalmology have the book on their shelf and have let us know they suggest this book first to their trainees.

We wanted to make this edition more than just an updated version of the first one by addressing the helpful criticisms of the reviewers and at the same time adding perspective gained from more years in the trenches. One of the major criticisms of the first edition was the placement of the black and white figures in the text but the corresponding color plates in a separate section. With advances in publication technology and decrease in the cost of using color figures, we are now able to place the color plates within the text. We think the readers will particularly enjoy the incorporated color fundus photos. In addition, the clinical photos are now all in color, both new ones and even the ones that were black and white in the first edition. The anatomical drawings, many of which have been redrawn, are in color as well. We think the color photographs, all highly uniform in size, color quality, and labeling, are unique compared to other texts and enhance the overall usefulness and aesthetics of the book.

Additionally, we have supplemented the text with a DVD containing videos that demonstrate critical parts of the examination and important pupillary, eyelid, and eye movement abnormalities. Some concepts, such as nystagmus and opsoclonus for example, can not be taught adequately with words alone, but are more aptly demonstrated in videos. The majority of the videos highlight relatively common entities, but we have also included examples of more rare but highly distinctive conditions such as oculomasticatory myorhythmia, cyclic oculomotor spasms, and Duane's type III. Readers can use these videos to teach their students as well.

Some reviewers suggested a radiological teaching section, but we felt that this would go beyond the scope of a book which we intend to be a reference for the diagnosis and management of neuro-ophthalmic disorders. Instead, we have provided MRI and CT images in the individual chapters where we thought imaging would be critical to the diagnosis and management of the neuro-ophthalmological condition. We still strongly believe that a good history and a "knock-out" neuro-ophthalmological examination will often trump good neuro-imaging. We did not want these critical elements of medicine to be lost in the sea of available technology, and so we placed our emphasis on the basics while presenting high quality examples of relevant neuroradiological findings. We made every effort to keep pace with technology and its profound influence on both neuro- and ophthalmic imaging.

We kept what worked. The three of us are still the only authors, and the book is only slightly larger. This book is divided into the same four parts and 19 chapters as the first edition, since many of our readers appreciated our organized topographical approach to the diagnosis and management of neuro-ophthalmological disorders. In one source, the reader can garner the wide range of neuro-ophthalmological disorders and the critical elements necessary to make a diagnosis. Likewise, we offer treatment approaches based on evidence, and where the evidence is lacking, on expert opinion. This text is a synthesis of how we think and reflects a healthy balance and compromise of our opinions in controversial areas.

While we tried to eliminate older, out-of-date references, an increase in the total number of references was unavoidable. We believe having access to extensive reference lists is the first place for the reader to go when they need more. For this reason we endeavored to maintain the classic references in the text and never hesitated to include important references of all types.

We hope you enjoy the book. We believe that students, residents, fellows, and seasoned practitioners of ophthalmology, neurology, and neuro-ophthalmology will find this well-illustrated text to be a practical guide to patient management and a source for guidelines and references. For us, there are very few professional pleasures that exceed learning and practicing neuro-ophthalmology, but surely one of them is teaching and sharing those experiences with our readers.

Grant T. Liu MD
Nicholas J. Volpe MD
Steven L. Galetta MD

Acknowledgments

For me, working on this book was a labor of love. We are extremely grateful for the positive comments we received from our first book from students, residents, fellows, reviewers, and colleagues, but our hope to improve upon it provided our inspiration to work on this second edition.

Almost ten years have passed since the first edition was published. Nick and I joined Steve at Penn in 1993, and we continue to learn from each other. This second edition reflects our ongoing friendship, mutual respect, and cooperation. It is a tribute to our second decade together.

I am also grateful to Joel Glaser and Norman Schatz for their continuing mentorship and encouragement. My parents are still always there for me. But I have many others to acknowledge in addition to those I thanked in the first edition. Our chairmen Francisco González-Scarano and Stuart Fine have been supportive of all of our efforts. Sherri Archer, my secretary, did her best to minimize the distractions while I worked on "the book."

I also truly appreciate the patience and tolerance of Nani Clansey, Russell Gabbedy, Mahalakshmi Nithyanand, and Fraser Johnston of Elsevier while guiding us through the writing and production stages of this book. Our proofreaders Lindsey Williams and Ann Grant were exceptional with their attention to detail.

The updated neuroimages and clinical photographs and videos would not have been possible without the unwavering assistance of our recent Penn Neuro-Ophthalmology fellows. I am truly indebted to Ben Osborne, Jennifer Hall, Chris Glisson, Melissa Wang Ko, Sashank Prasad, Rob Avery, Heather Moss, and Stacy Pineles who tirelessly photographed patients, downloaded MR and CT images, and tracked down fundus photos for me. Of course I have to thank our patients for allowing us to photograph them as well. I also have to thank our colleague Laura Balcer and the Penn Neurology and Ophthalmology residents for acting as patients in many of the figures for the examination and nystagmus chapters. Laura also provided us with many key figures and videos.

Most importantly, I have to express my gratitude to my wife Gerry, daughter Alessandra, and son Jonathan, from whom most of the time was taken to write this book. My family is my favorite foursome, and with them, I'm off to the first tee.

Grant T. Liu MD

There are many individuals that have contributed to my personal and professional success and, after ten more years, I have come to appreciate even more, all that so many have done for me to allow this book's second edition and many other professional dreams to come true. I am so fortunate to have (had) the parents that I do (did), Nicholas and Lydia who simply stated, "created me" and taught me to embrace learning and teaching, to work hard and to passionately pursue my dreams. I remain grateful to my early mentors, Arthur Wolintz, MD, Frederick Jakobiec, MD, Simmons Lessell, MD and Joseph Rizzo, III, MD for molding me and being my inspirations into academic ophthalmology by establishing my foundations and fueling my passions to understand, question, research and teach the art of neuro-ophthalmology. My students, residents and fellows, past present and future, remind me how much fun it really is to teach, share knowledge and why I chose a career in academic ophthalmology. My colleagues and the staff at Penn/Scheie have provided me with a rich, stimulating and high quality clinical practice and have supported me with passion as I have pursued all my dreams. Mark Moster, MD, Steve Galetta, MD and Grant Liu, MD (there would be no book without Grant) are the best partners and friends I could ever ask to have. Laura Balcer, MD, Kenneth Shindler MD, PhD and Madhura Tamhanker, MD have added another level of professional satisfaction and friendship as I have helped them to establish themselves as colleagues. Last, Stuart Fine, MD has been my most ardent supporter, trusted mentor and dearest friend, thank you Stuart for your endless commitment to me and my success.

But most of all, I wish to acknowledge my family who are my heart and soul. My brothers Russell and Robert are my best friends who I can talk to at anytime about anything. My children, Nicholas, Matthew, Lena and Tessa who everyday inspire me to achieve, remind me about how wonderful life really is and what really matters, and whose time I liberally borrow from to pursue my profession. Finally I am grateful to my wife Francesca, without her I would accomplish very little. She supports me, encourages me, makes me so much better than I could ever be on my own and makes me feel like the luckiest person in the world.

Nicholas J. Volpe MD

I would like to thank those individuals who have had a major impact in my life: My parents Louis and Winifred Galetta for their unending love. My coaches, Brother Pat Pennell, Frank McCartney, James Tuppeny, Irv Mondschein and Bill Wagner for teaching me how to win and lose. My colleagues, Grant Liu, Nicholas Volpe, Laura Balcer, Francisco Gonzalez, Robert I. Grossman, Stuart Fine, Nancy J Newman, Valerie Biousse, Eric Raps and Larry Gray for their brilliance and friendship. My mentors Norman J. Schatz, Joel Glaser and J. Lawton Smith, Donald Silberberg, Donald Gilden and Arthur K. Asbury for teaching me with untiring enthusiasm. To the residents and fellows of Penn who have taught me more than I have been able to teach them. Finally, to my family, Genie, Kristin, Michael, and Matthew for their love and support and for making it all worthwhile.

Steven L. Galetta MD

Part **One**

History and examination

CHAPTER **1**

The neuro-ophthalmic history

As in any field of medicine, the neuro-ophthalmic history guides the physician's examination and differential diagnosis. From the beginning of the history taking, the physician should attempt to categorize the patient's problem. **Table 1–1**, which mirrors the organization of this book, classifies neuro-ophthalmic disorders into three groups: afferent disorders, efferent disorders, and headache and abnormal facial sensations. It can be used as a guide in generating a differential diagnosis. Then, influenced by the patient's age, gender, underlying illnesses, and disease risk factors, the physician can narrow the list of potential diagnoses and shape the examination to confirm or eliminate each disorder.

Frequently, the correct neuro-ophthalmic disorder can be diagnosed based on the history alone. For instance, an otherwise healthy young woman with sudden vision loss in one eye with pain on eye movements probably has optic neuritis. An elderly man with hypertension, new binocular horizontal double vision worse at distance and in right gaze, and right periorbital pain most likely has a vasculopathic right sixth nerve palsy.

The various elements of the neuro-ophthalmic history (**Table 1–2**) will be reviewed in the context of neuro-ophthalmic disorders. Although important, topics such as physician demeanor, style, language use during history taking, the best environment for the interview, and the physician–patient relationship are beyond the scope of this chapter and are discussed eloquently in other text books.[1,2]

Chief complaint

The patient's age should be ascertained first. Congenital neuro-ophthalmic problems are more likely to be seen in children, and degenerative and vascular disorders are seen predominantly in adults. Neoplasms occur at all ages, although the tumor types are often age dependent. For instance, in children the most common causes of chiasmal compression are optic pathway tumors and craniopharyngiomas, while in adulthood pituitary adenomas are the most likely culprit.

The patient's gender should be noted because of the predilection of some diseases for either men or women. For example, eye complications of breast cancer are obviously more prevalent in women, but optic neuritis, giant cell arteritis, and Duane's retraction syndrome are also more common in females.

Then the patient should be asked to summarize his or her complaint in one sentence. Simple statements such as "I cannot see out of my left eye," "I have double vision," and "My left eyelid droops" are extremely helpful, and immediately allow the examiner to begin thinking about a differential diagnosis. However, when the complaint is a vague one such as "I haven't seen very well for 6 months," further historic clarification is necessary.

Table 1–1 Categorization of neuro-ophthalmic disorders

	Chapter
Visual loss and other disorders of the afferent visual pathway	
Visual loss: retinal disorders	4
Visual loss: optic neuropathies	5
Optic disc swelling: papilledema and other causes	6
Visual loss: chiasmal disorders	7
Visual loss: retrochiasmal disorders	8
Disorders of higher cortical visual function	9
Transient visual loss	10
Functional visual loss	11
Visual hallucinations and illusions	12
Efferent neuro-ophthalmic disorders	
Pupillary disorders	13
Eyelid and facial nerve disorders	14
Eye movement disorders: third, fourth, and sixth nerve palsies and other causes of diplopia and ocular misalignment	15
Eye movement disorders: gaze abnormalities	16
Eye movement disorders: nystagmus and nystagmoid eye movements	17
Orbital disease	18
Headache, facial pain, and disorders of facial sensation	19

These three major groups reflect the table of contents and organization of this book. During history taking, the examiner should attempt to categorize the patient's problem into one of these groups.

Table 1–2 The neuro-ophthalmic history

Chief complaint
Age, gender, and major complaint
History of present illness
Detailing the problem
Temporal profile of symptoms
Associated symptoms
Past neurologic and ophthalmic history
Past medical and surgical history
Review of systems
Family history
Social history

The chief complaint should be reduced to one sentence containing the patient's age, gender, and complaint: "The patient is a 45-year-old woman with left facial pain," for example.

History of present illness

The patient's chief complaint should be explored in further detail, including the temporal profile of events and any associated symptoms.

Detailing the problem

Afferent dysfunction. If the patient complains of visual loss, its pattern and degree should be explored to help localize the problem within the afferent visual pathway. The patient should be asked whether the right or left eye or both eyes are involved and whether the visual loss affects the nasal, temporal, superior, or inferior field of vision. Then the visual loss should be characterized according to its quality and degree (complete blindness, grayness, or visual distortion, for example). Defects in color perception should be noted. Higher cortical visual dysfunction should be considered when the visual complaints are vague and there is a history of dementia, stroke, or behavioral changes and no clear ocular explanation for the visual impairment.

Efferent dysfunction. The most common efferent neuro-ophthalmic complaint is double vision. Patients with diplopia should be asked whether their double vision is (1) binocular, (2) horizontal or vertical, and (3) worse in left-, right-, up-, or downgaze, or distance or near. Neurologic diplopia is almost always binocular, and the defective nerve or muscle can often be determined according to the direction in which the double vision is worse.

Blurred vision is a common complaint associated with refractive error, media opacity, and afferent dysfunction. However, the examiner should be aware that some patients complaining of blurred vision are actually found to have diplopia when questioned further. This should be suspected when the patient reports the blurred vision improves when either eye is covered.

Temporal profile of symptoms

The *chronicity, rapidity of onset,* and *pattern of symptoms* should be investigated.

Chronicity. When the symptoms first occurred should be established. This can be explored by asking, for instance, when the patient was last able to read small print. Some disorders, such as optic neuritis, usually resolve within several weeks or months. However, if visual loss has been present for several years, other diagnoses, such as a slowly growing meningioma, should be considered. Long-standing, and even intermittent, double vision implies a slowly expanding neoplasm or decompensated congenital strabismus. Old photographs of the patient, when details of the face and eyes are visible, are often extremely helpful in determining the chronicity of ptosis, pupillary abnormalities, and ocular misalignment, for example.

Rapidity of onset. A sudden onset of symptoms suggests a vascular process, such as a stroke. Inflammatory and infectious disorders may also present acutely. In contrast, symptoms associated with degenerative and compressive processes are usually more insidious, and the patient may not be able to date the exact beginning of the problem.

Pattern of symptoms. The timecourse of symptoms can be extremely helpful. Progressive symptoms suggest compressive mass lesions, while those with acute onset that plateau or improve are more consistent with vascular or inflammatory processes. Episodic visual loss could be due to migraine, carotid disease, or seizures, for instance. Fluctuating ptosis or double vision that is particularly worse in the evening is highly suggestive of myasthenia gravis.

Associated symptoms

The patient should be asked about neurologic or generalized symptoms that may not have been volunteered as they relate to the eye problem. For instance, headaches may be consistent with migraine, elevated intracranial pressure, and compressive mass lesions. Malaise, fevers, muscle aches, headaches, and jaw claudication indicate giant cell arteritis in an elderly patient with amaurosis fugax or frank visual loss. Pain is more typical of optic neuritis than ischemic optic neuropathy. Systemic weakness, dysphagia, and dyspnea suggest myasthenia gravis in a patient with ptosis or diplopia. On the other hand, in a patient with diplopia, dysarthria, and ataxia, a posterior fossa lesion is more likely.

Past neurologic and ophthalmologic history

A history of any neurologic disease, such as migraines, strokes, transient ischemic attacks, head injury, or seizures, or prior neuroimaging should be investigated. Important questions regarding past ophthalmologic problems would include those concerning previous spectacle correction, cataracts, glaucoma, strabismus, amblyopia, eye patching, or surgery.

Past medical and surgical history and review of systems

Because many neuro-ophthalmic disorders are complications of underlying medical illnesses, careful exploration and documentation of the medical and surgical history and review of systems are paramount. Inquiry regarding the presence of hypertension, diabetes, coronary artery disease, arrhythmias, cardiac valvular disease, hypercholesterolemia, and peripheral vascular disease is extremely important, but any history of cancer, rheumatologic or immunosuppressive disorders, or infectious diseases may also be highly relevant.

Special considerations in children

Diagnostic clues in children undergoing neuro-ophthalmic evaluation may be evident in the mother's pregnancy history, especially with regard to drug or alcohol exposure or infections. Details of the birth, including length of gestation, birth weight, Apgar scores, and presence of perinatal difficulties, should be noted. A developmental history, with particular attention to milestones achieved in cognitive, motor, and language function, should be taken as well. Loss of milestones suggests a degenerative disorder, while developmental delay with slow achievement of milestones suggests a static encephalopathy due to hypoxemia, for instance.

Family history

The history of any neurologic, ophthalmologic, or medical illnesses in related family members should be documented. In addition, many neuro-ophthalmic disorders, such as migraine, multiple sclerosis, and Leber's hereditary optic neuropathy, have a genetic predisposition, and so their presence in any relatives would strongly suggest their consideration.

Social history

Certain behaviors, such as illicit drug use, smoking, and alcohol consumption, may be important predisposing factors for neuro-ophthalmic disorders. For example, smoking is a risk factor for vascular disease, whereas alcohol may be associated with optic neuropathy.

Because occupational exposures may also be relevant, the examiner should inquire about the patient's job. Knowing the patient's occupation is also important in understanding how the patient's neuro-ophthalmic problem affects his or her everyday life. For instance, a dentist may be devastated by monocular visual loss and the subsequent inability to appreciate objects stereoscopically. On the other hand, an airline reservation agent, whose job likely does not require binocular vision, may not be affected as severely by a similar injury.

References

1. Bickley LS, Hoekelman RA, Bates B. Interviewing and the health history. In: Bates' Guide to Physical Examination and History Taking, 7th edn, pp 1–42. Philadelphia, Lippincott, 1999.

2. DeGowin RL, Brown DD. History and the medical record. In: DeGowin's Diagnostic Examination, 7th edn, pp 15–36. New York, McGraw-Hill, 2000.

CHAPTER **2**

The neuro-ophthalmic examination

Table 2–1 Neuro-ophthalmic examination

Afferent visual function

Visual acuity

Contrast sensitivity (optional)

Color perception

Confrontation visual fields

Amsler grid testing

Higher cortical visual function (optional)

Efferent system

Pupils

    Size
    Reactivity
    Swinging flashlight test
    Near (optional)

Eyelids

Facial nerve function

Ocular motility

    Inspection
    Ductions
    Vergences
    Assessment of ocular misalignment

External examination including orbit

**Slit-lamp examination/
  applanation tensions**

Ophthalmoscopic examination

Directed neurologic examination

Mental status

Cranial nerves

Motor function

Cerebellar function

Sensation

Gait

Reflexes

Directed general examination

The neuro-ophthalmic examination combines ophthalmic and neurologic techniques to assess the patient's vision, pupillary function, ocular motility, eyelids, orbits, fundus appearance, and neurologic status.[1-4] In most cases, after obtaining the history, the examiner should have already formed an opinion regarding the possible localization and differential diagnosis. The examination then either supports or refutes these initial impressions; examination findings may also prompt consideration of other diagnoses.

In this chapter, the major elements of the neuro-ophthalmic examination (**Table 2–1**) will be reviewed, and, in each section, disorders that affect them will be mentioned briefly. The neuro-ophthalmic examination in comatose patients will also be reviewed. The reader should then refer to the appropriate chapters for more detailed differential diagnoses and discussions of the pathologic disorders.

Afferent visual function

Measurement of afferent visual function establishes how well the patient sees. Several different aspects of vision should be evaluated, including visual acuity, color vision, and visual fields. The examiner must keep in mind that these are inherently subjective measurements and depend heavily on the patient's level of cooperation and effort.

By convention, during all tests of afferent visual function, the right eye is assessed first.

Visual acuity

Visual acuity is a measurement of the individual's capacity for visual discrimination of fine details of high contrast.[5,6] Best corrected visual acuity should be tested for each eye separately with the other eye covered by a tissue, hand, or occluding device (**Fig. 2–1A**). Distance vision is most commonly evaluated with a standard Snellen chart (**Fig. 2–2A**), and near vision with a hand-held card (**Fig. 2–2B**). Ideally, best corrected vision should be assessed using current corrective lenses or manifest refraction. If these are unavailable, a pinhole will improve most mild to moderate refractive errors in cooperative patients (**Fig. 2–1B**). In addition, patients with subnormal acuity despite best refracted correction should still be tested with pinholes, which may further improve some refractive errors (irregular astigmatism) and media opacities (cataract). When acuity cannot be corrected by a pinhole, nonrefractive causes of visual loss (see below) should be considered.

Acuity is most often recorded as *a fraction* (e.g., 20/40), where the numerator refers to the distance (in feet) from which the patient sees the letters, and the denominator refers to the distance from which a patient with normal vision sees the same letters. The normal eye can resolve a figure that

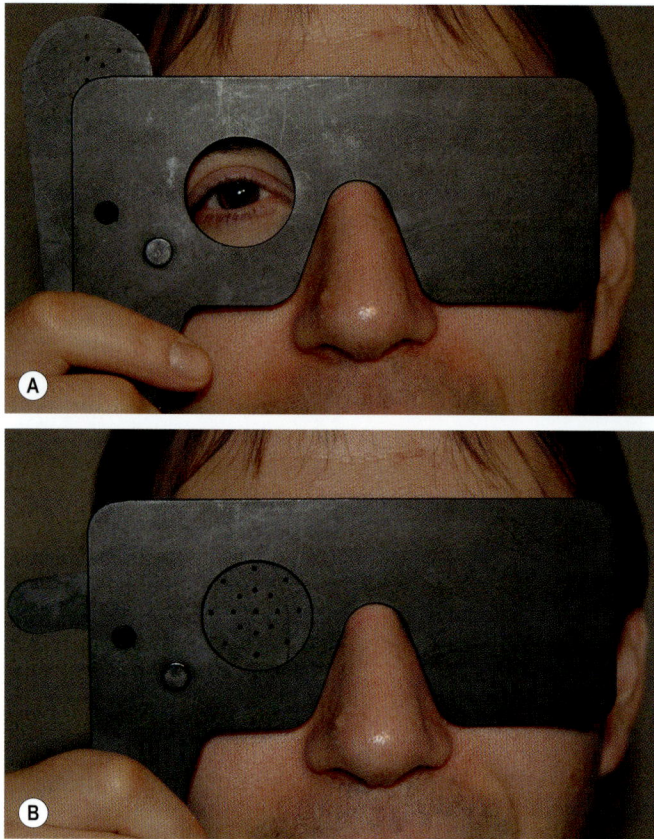

Figure 2–1. A. Occluder for testing vision one eye at a time. By convention the right eye is tested first. **B**. Occluder with pinholes. If the visual acuity is subnormal but can be improved with pinholes, refractive error or media opacities should be suspected.

subtends a visual angle of 5 minutes at a distance of 20 feet. At the distance at which a normal patient can see a line of letters on a Snellen eye chart, the widths of the lines on each letter subtend a visual angle of 1 minute, or one-fifth of the entire letter.[6] A fraction of 20/20–2 indicates the patient saw all the letters on the 20/20 line except two, while 20/20+2 means the patient was able to see the 20/20 letters plus two letters on the next (20/15) line. Usually up to two mistakes on a line or two extra letters on the next line are allowed in this notation. Most normal adults under age 40 have best corrected visual acuities of 20/20 or better in each eye.

Visual acuity at distance can also be recorded using the metric or decimal systems. When the testing is at 6 meters (close to 20 feet), the normal visual acuity is recorded as 6/6. The decimal system uses the numeric equivalent of the fractional notation: 20/20 or 6/6 is a visual acuity of 1.0. An acuity of 20/100 would be recorded as an acuity of 0.2.

If a patient is unable to read the largest Snellen letters (20/200 or 20/400), the acuity should be recorded by moving a 200-size letter toward the patient until it is seen (**Fig. 2–3**). That distance is recorded as the numerator. For example, an acuity of 4/200 means the patient was able to see the 200-size letter at 4 feet. Alternatively, the degree of vision can be recorded using the phrases "count fingers" (CF) (and at what distance), "detect hand motions" (HM), and "have light perception" (LP). An eye that is blind has "no light perception" (NLP). Criteria are used by different

agencies to determine a level of vision loss that qualifies for disability or benefits (i.e., "legal blindness") based on best corrected acuity worse than 20/200 in the better seeing eye or binocular visual field constriction to less than 20 degrees.

Unfortunately, Snellen charts have several deficiencies,[6,7] the most important of which is the nonlinear variation in the sizes of the letters from line to line. Thus, if one patient's visual acuity decreases by 20/100 to 20/200 using the chart in **Fig. 2–2A**, and another from 20/80 to 20/100, both are considered to have a decrease in visual acuity by one line. However, in the first instance the difference in letter size is 100% but in the second it is only 25%. Furthermore, a typical Snellen chart has a different number of letters on each line. The largest letters have the fewest, while the smallest letters have the most in each line. Therefore, more letters must be identified to complete smaller lines in contrast to larger lines. In addition, some letters, such as the "E," are harder to identify than the "A" or "L," for example.

To eliminate these issues and when consistency is desired among testing locations, as in multicenter clinical trials for instance, standardized Early Treatment in Diabetic Retinopathy Study (ETDRS) charts have become the gold standard (**Fig. 2–2C**).[7] Each line contains five letters, the spacing between the letters and lines is proportional to the letter sizes, the sizes of the letters decrease geometrically, and the recognizability of each letter is approximately the same.[6] Using ETDRS charts, a linear scale for visual acuity can be created by calculating the base 10 logarithm of (1/Snellen decimal notation) in what is termed the logarithm of the minimal angle of resolution (logMAR). Each line on the ETDRS chart is therefore separated by 0.1 logMAR units. So in the examples above, the logMAR score for the first patient would worsen from 0.7 to 1.0, while the second would worsen from 0.6 to 0.7, more accurately reflecting the greater fall in visual acuity for the first patient.

Visual acuity with the near card is often recorded using the Snellen fraction or the standard Jaeger notation (J1, J3, etc.). When near visual acuity is tested, presbyopic patients above 40 years of age should wear their reading glasses or bifocals. Near acuities are not as accurate as those obtained at distance, especially when the card is not held at the requisite 14 inches.

In illiterate individuals or children unable to read letters, acuity can be tested with tumbling Es[8] (**Fig. 2–4**), Allen or Lea figures[9,10] (**Fig. 2–5A**), or HOTV letters[11] (**Fig. 2–5B,C**). In younger preverbal patients, assessment of fixing on and following a light or toy by each eye separately in most instances is sufficient. Caution should be applied when examining small infants, since visual fixation normally may be inconsistent or absent until 8–16 weeks of age.[12] When quantification of visual acuities is required in very young children (for serial examinations, for instance), preferential looking tests (Teller acuities[13,14]) may be used (**Fig. 2–6**). These tests are based on the principle that a child would rather look at objects with a pattern stimulus (alternating black and white lines of specific widths) than at a homogeneous field. The frequency of the smallest pattern that the child seems to prefer is termed the grating acuity, which can be converted to Snellen equivalents. Visual acuity in a newborn is roughly 20/400 to 20/600, improves to

Based on a visual angle
of one minute

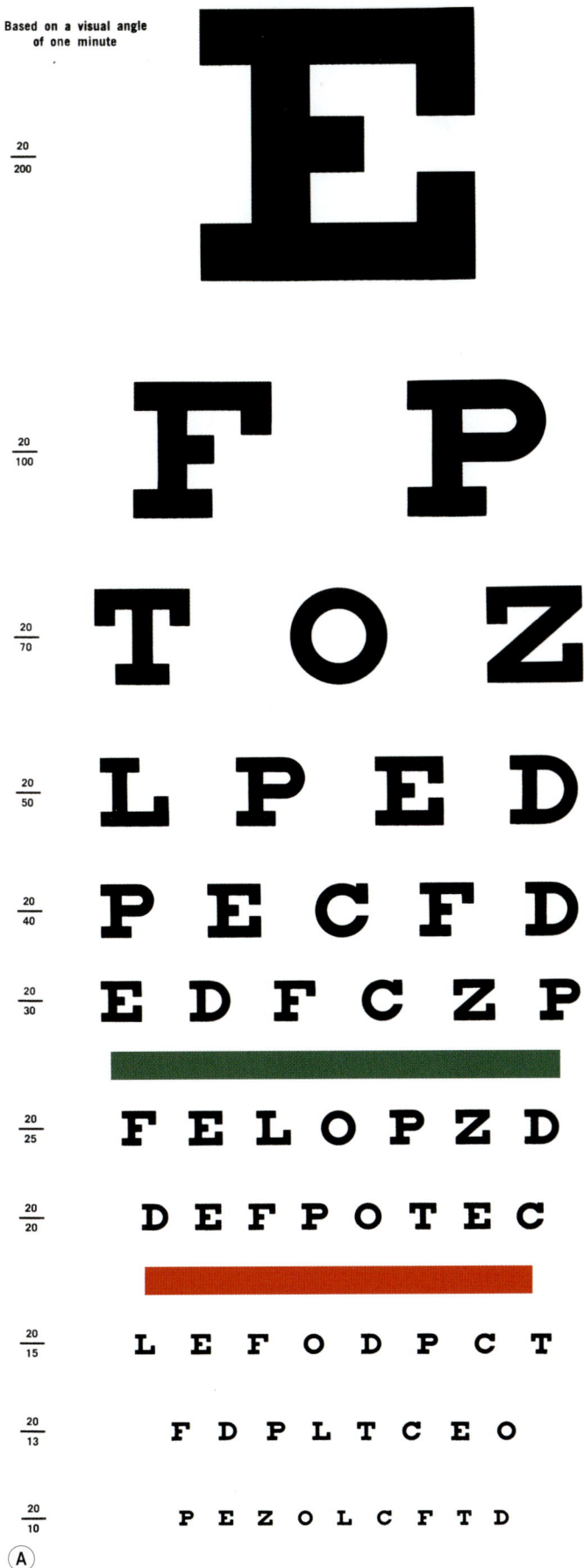

20/200

E

20/100   F P

20/70   T O Z

20/50   L P E D

20/40   P E C F D

20/30   E D F C Z P

20/25   F E L O P Z D

20/20   D E F P O T E C

20/15   L E F O D P C T

20/13   F D P L T C E O

20/10   P E Z O L C F T D

(A)

ROSENBAUM POCKET VISION SCREENER

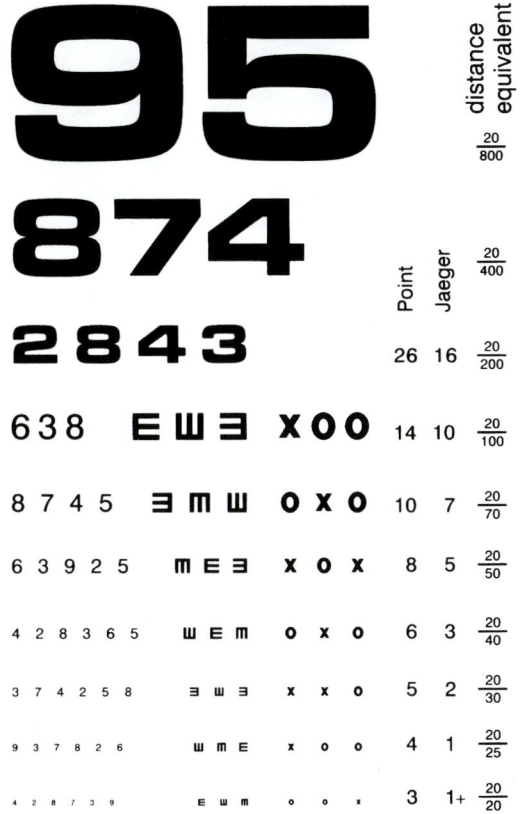

distance equivalent

95   20/800

874   20/400

			Point	Jaeger	
2843			26	16	20/200
638	E Ш Ǝ	X O O	14	10	20/100
8 7 4 5	Ǝ ᒎ Ш	O X O	10	7	20/70
6 3 9 2 5	ᒎ E Ǝ	X O X	8	5	20/50
4 2 8 3 6 5	Ш E ᒎ	o x o	6	3	20/40
3 7 4 2 5 8	Ǝ Ш Ǝ	x x o	5	2	20/30
9 3 7 8 2 6	Ш ᒎ E	x o o	4	1	20/25
4 2 8 7 3 9	E Ш ᒎ	o o x	3	1+	20/20

Card is held in good light 14 inches from eye. Record vision for each eye separately with and without glasses. Presbyopic patients should read thru bifocal segment. Check myopes with glasses only.

DESIGN COURTESY J.G. ROSENBAUM. M.D.

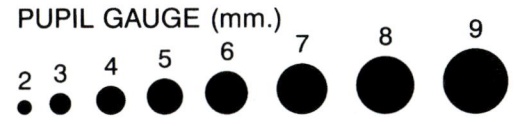

PUPIL GAUGE (mm.)
2 3 4 5 6 7 8 9

(B)

Figure 2–2. Visual acuity charts. **A**. Snellen eye chart for testing visual acuity. The largest letter at the top is the 20/200 E, while the letters at the bottom represent the 20/10 line. **B**. Near card with pupil gauge. Note that near visual acuity is often recorded using the Jaeger notation, as in "Jaeger 2" or "J2" to indicate 20/30 near acuity. **C**. Early Treatment in Diabetic Retinopathy Study (ETDRS) type chart.

PART 1 History and examination

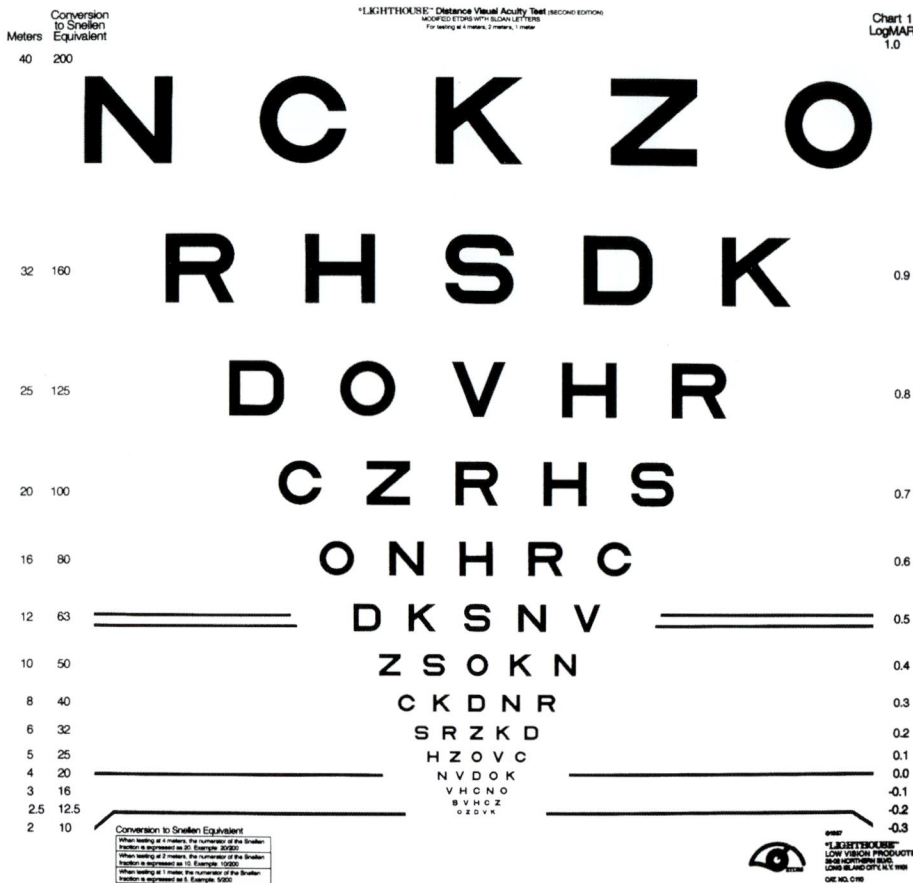

Figure 2–2. *Continued*

(C)

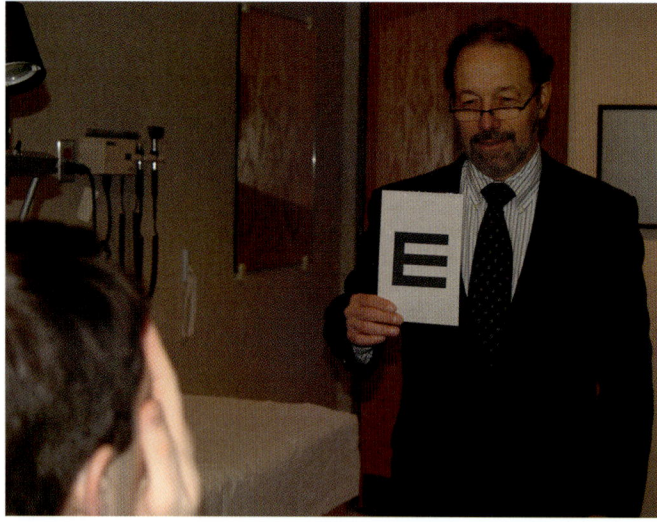

Figure 2–3. Determination of visual acuity using 200-size letters in an eye with worse than 20/200 but better than hand motions vision. The distance at which the patient can see the 20/200 E is determined. If this distance is 3 feet, then the visual acuity is recorded as "3/200."

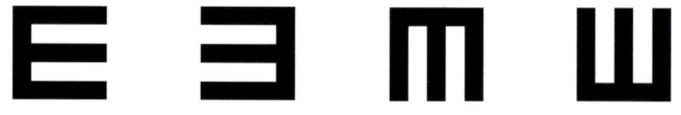

Figure 2–4. "Tumbling Es" for assessment of visual acuity in illiterate adults or children. The patient can be asked to indicate in which direction the E points (up, down, left, or right). The sizes of the Es correlate with the size of the letters on Snellen chart.

approximately 20/60 by 12 months of age, and then reaches the 20/20 level by 3–5 years of age.[15]

Ocular causes of reduced visual acuity include refractive error, amblyopia, macular lesion, or media opacity such as cataract, vitreous hemorrhage, vitritis, or corneal opacities or

irregularities. Neuro-ophthalmic processes that can decrease visual acuity are those that affect the optic nerve or chiasm. Disturbances that are posterior to the chiasm (retrochiasmal, i.e., tract, optic radiations, and occipital lobe) affect visual acuity only if they are bilateral.[16] Functional visual loss should always be considered when visual acuity is decreased without any obvious abnormality of the eye or visual pathways.

Contrast sensitivity and low-contrast letter acuity

Contrast sensitivity testing with sine-wave or square-wave gratings may be a useful adjunct in the evaluation of vision loss.[17] Conventional visual acuity measures spatial resolution at high contrast, while contrast sensitivity testing assesses spatial resolution when contrast varies. In one variation of the test, the patient is asked to identify in which

H O T V
V T H O

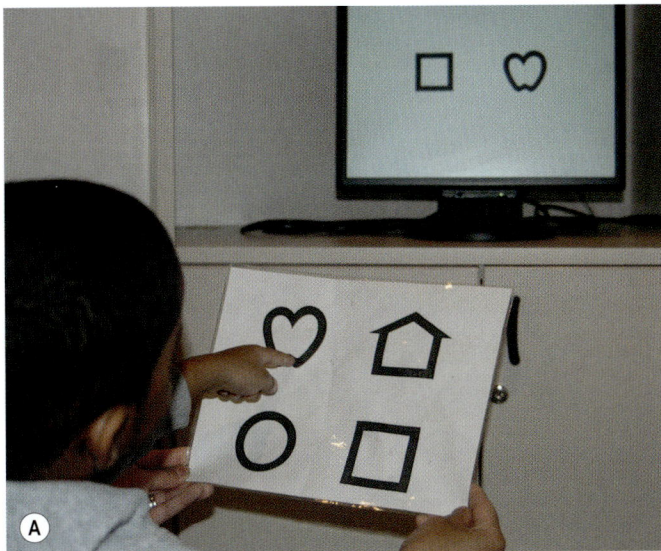

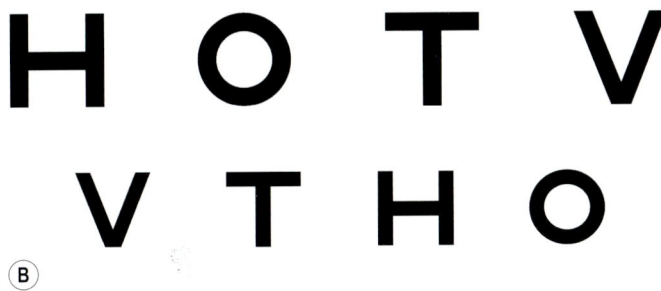

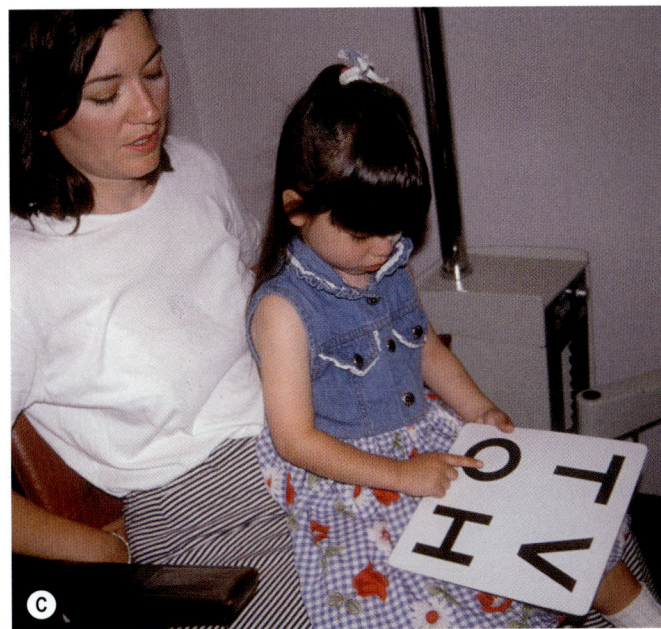

Figure 2–5. Lea and HOTV visual acuity testing in preliterate children. In both tests the child points to one of four choices to match the figure or letter he or she sees on the computer monitor or chart in the distance. The figure or letter sizes on the computer monitor or chart are varied until the best visual acuity is determined. **A.** Lea figure testing in a young child. The child matches the presented figure. **B,C.** HOTV acuity testing. In slightly older children Snellen-like H, O, T, or V letters (**B**) can be presented. **C.** As in Lea figure testing the child is asked to match the indicated letter on the chart with a hand-held card displaying the HOTV letters.

direction the gratings, which span a spectrum of spatial and temporal frequencies and are arranged in increasing difficulty, are oriented. Another version, the Pelli–Robson test,[18] is depicted in **Fig. 2–7A**. Contrast sensitivity testing should never replace acuity assessment, as its role seems limited to those situations where acuity is normal or near normal and further evaluation is desired.[19] Optic neuropathies as well as media opacities and macular disease may reduce contrast sensitivity.

Low-contrast Sloan letter acuity testing captures the minimum size at which individuals can perceive letters of a particular contrast level (shade of gray on white background). Used primarily for research at this time, Sloan charts present gray letters in ETDRS format (**Fig. 2–7B**). The testing evaluates other aspects of visual dysfunction beyond high-contrast visual acuity loss in multiple sclerosis[20] and other neurologic disorders.[21] Low-contrast acuity testing at 2.5% and 1.25% contrast levels is likely to be added to the Multiple Sclerosis Functional Composite for trials,[22] and eventually it is expected to come into clinical use.

Color perception

Color vision can be tested with standard pseudoisochromatic Ishihara or Hardy–Rand–Rittler plates, both of which contain numbers or geometric shapes that the patient is asked to identify among different colored dots (**Fig. 2–8**). Like visual acuity, color vision should be tested for each eye separately. The result is recorded as a fraction of the color plates correctly identified ("8/10" or "8 out of 10," for instance); defective color vision is termed *dyschromatopsia*, while absence of color vision is called *achromatopsia*. Their wide availability, ease of administration, and relatively low cost make the pseudoisochromatic plates a popular tool for detecting dyschromatopsias of all types, although they were originally designed to screen for congenital dyschromatopsias. Ishihara color plates (**Fig. 2–8A**) may be used, but Hardy–Rand–Rittler plates (**Fig. 2–8B**),[23] which contain blue and purple figures that screen for tritan defects (see below), may be more helpful in detecting acquired dyschromatopsia due to dominant optic neuropathy.[24,25]

For a more qualitative assessment, comparing the appearance of the color test plates or of a red bottle top, for example, with each eye can test for more subtle intereye differences in color perception. A patient with monocular "red desaturation" may state that with the affected eye the red bottle top appeared "washed out," "pink," or "orange."

Congenital dyschromatopsias are characterized by confusion between reds and greens (protan and deutan types) and blues and yellows (tritan type). Binocular, present at birth, and stable over time, they result from relative deficiencies in the red, green, and blue cone retinal photoreceptor pigments.[25] The most common inherited dyschromotopsia is an X-linked red–green defect, occurring in approximately 8–10% of males and 0.4–0.5% of females.[26] The Farnsworth D-15 (dichotomous) panel test (**Fig. 2–9**) or the larger Farnsworth–Munsell 100-hue test can be used to separate the various types. In both of these tests, patients are asked to arrange colored caps in linear sequence relative to reference caps. The D-15 is shorter and less cumbersome

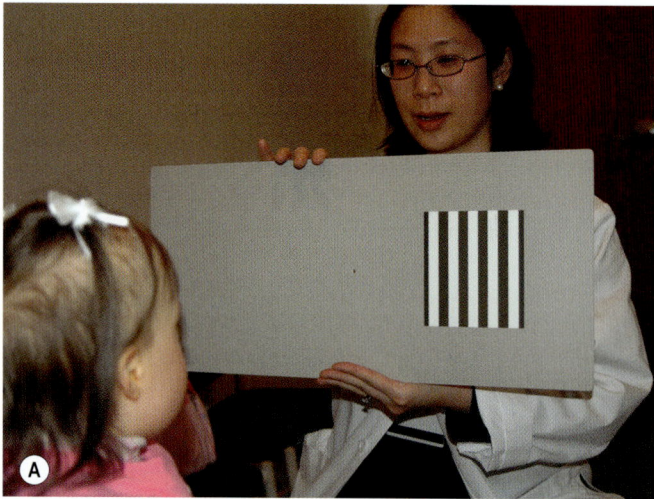

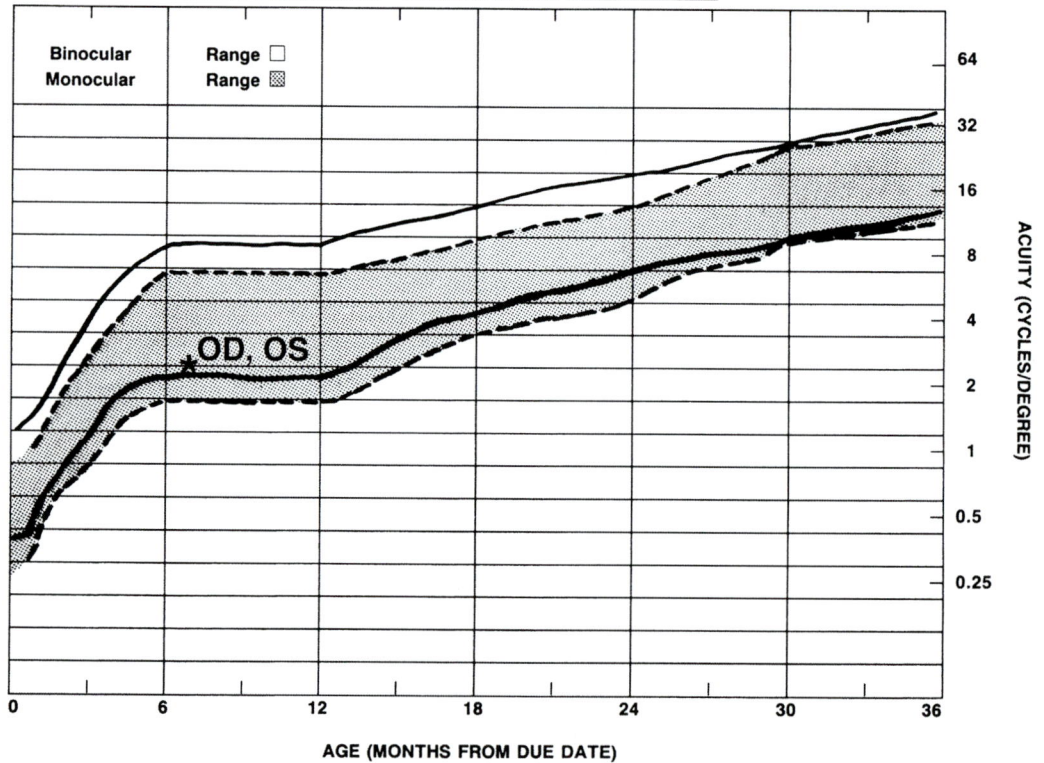

Figure 2–6. Teller acuity testing. In very young children, preferential looking tests may be used. These tests are based upon the principle that a child would rather look at objects with a pattern stimulus (alternating black and white lines of specific widths) than at a homogeneous field. The smallest pattern that the child seems to prefer is an indicator of best visual acuity ("grating acuity"). **A.** The stimuli are presented on one side of a series of rectangular hand-held cards with gray backgrounds. Visual acuity is determined by decreasing the thicknesses of the black and white stripes and presenting them to the left or right until the child no longer preferentially looks at them against the gray background on the rectangular card. The frequency difference between the stimuli on each successive card is approximately 0.5 octaves. **B.** Results are compared with age-based normal controls. The grating acuity can be converted to Snellen equivalents.

than the 100-hue test and can be performed quickly in the office under proper lighting conditions.

Acquired dyschromatopsia may result from macular, retinal, optic nerve, chiasmal, or retrochiasmal lesions. Monocular acuity loss, deficits in color vision, and a relative afferent pupillary defect (see below) are highly characteristic of an ipsilateral optic neuropathy. Acquired optic nerve diseases typically produce a red/green color deficiency, but there are several notable exceptions, such as glaucoma[27] and dominant optic atrophy as mentioned

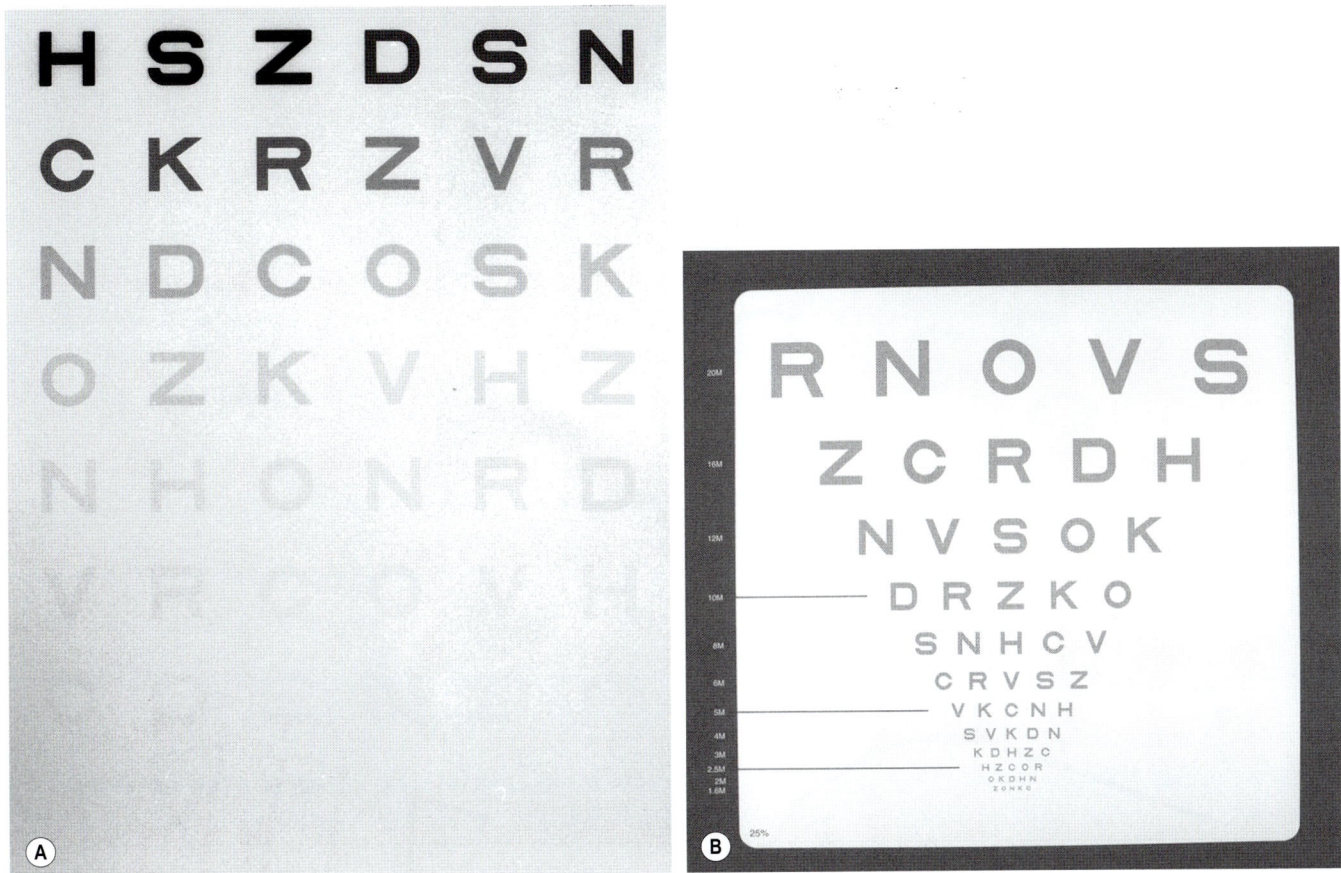

Figure 2–7. Contrast sensitivity tests. **A.** In the Pelli–Robson test, each eye is evaluated separately, and the patient is asked to identify the letters across each row, starting at the top of the chart. The level of contrast sensitivity, recorded in log units, is determined when the patient reaches a group of three letters he or she cannot identify. **B.** Low-contrast Sloan letter acuity chart (Precision Vision, LaSalle, IL). Visual acuity may be specified by Snellen notation for descriptive purposes (i.e., 20/20), by number of letters identified correctly, or by logMAR units. This photograph shows the 25% contrast level for purposes of illustrating format; the actual contrast levels used in clinical trials, 2.5% and 1.25%, have substantially lighter gray letters. The charts can be presented on hand-held cards or retroilluminated cabinets (courtesy of Dr. Laura J. Balcer).

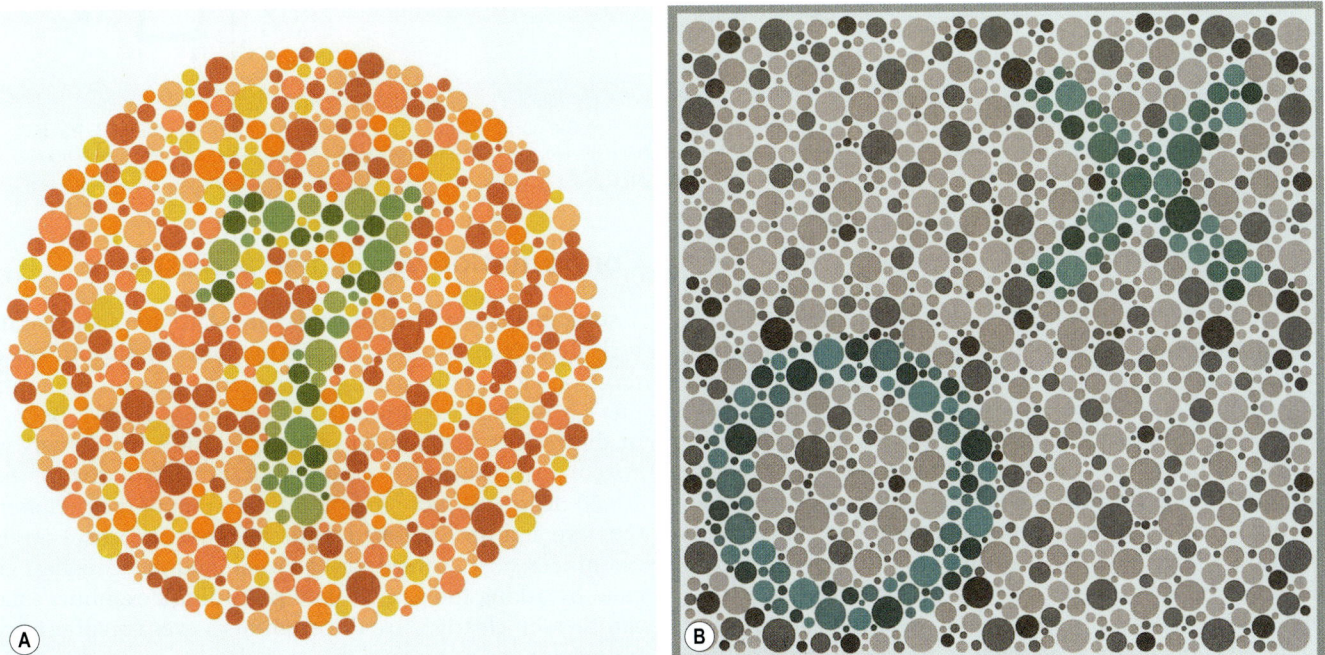

Figure 2–8. Pseudoisochromatic color plates. Each eye is tested separately. **A.** In standard pseudoisochromatic color plate testing, the patient is asked to identify the number seen within the colored dots. **B.** Hardy–Rand–Rittler color plate. In this test, the patient is asked to identify the shape or symbol seen within the dots.

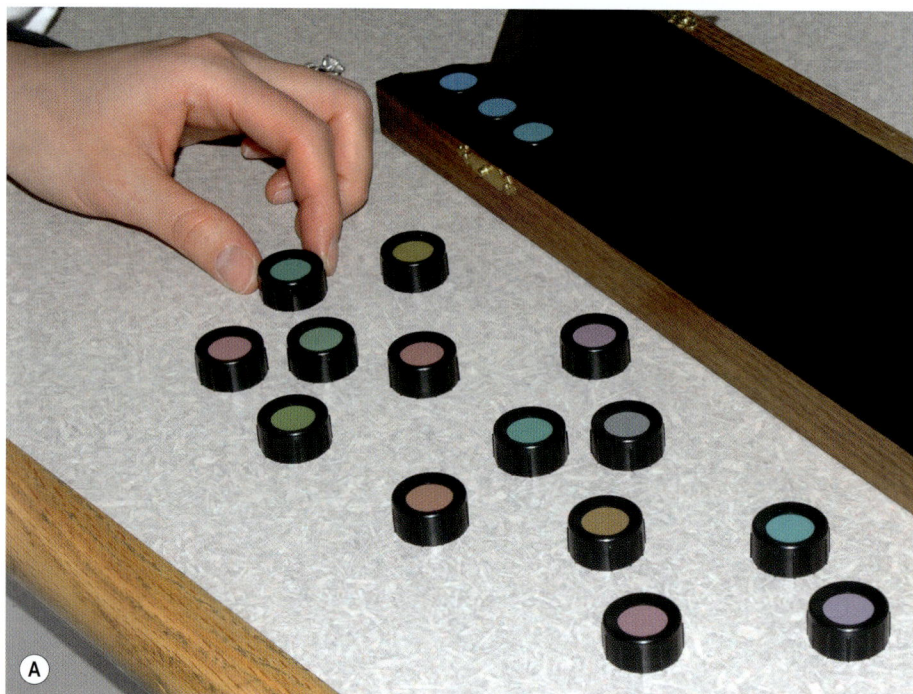

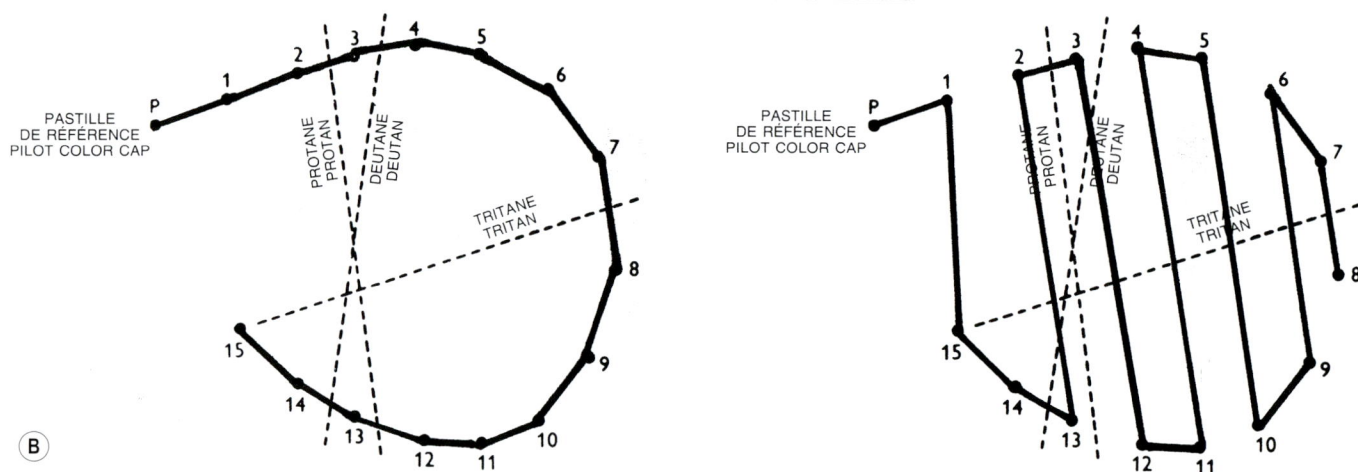

Figure 2–9. A. Farnsworth D-15 color test. The patient is asked to arrange colored discs in order of color similarity, starting with a reference disc. Each eye is tested separately. **B.** Each disc is numbered, and the results are recorded by connecting the numbers in the order in which the patient arranged the discs. Protanopes, deuteranopes, and tritanopes tend to arrange them in incorrect but characteristic, easily identifiable patterns along one of three axes. A normal response is given on the left, while a protanope's response is depicted on the right.

earlier. Dyschromatopsias occurring in the setting of retinal disease, such as cone dystrophies, Stargardt disease, and toxic retinopathies, are usually associated with pigment migration or visible disturbances of the retinal pigment epithelium on fundus examination. Color vision loss combined with only mildly reduced acuity would be more suggestive of an optic neuropathy, while color deficits due to macular disease tend to be associated with more severe acuity loss. One study demonstrated a visual acuity of worse than 20/100 due solely to visual blur is needed to affect the results of Ishihara color plate testing, and worse than 20/250 to affect Hardy–Rand–Rittler testing.[28] Retrochiasmal disturbances can produce abnormal color vision in the defective visual field. An inferior occipital lobe lesion involving the lingual and fusiform gyri can cause defective color vision in the contralateral hemifield (see Chapter 9).

Confrontation visual field assessment

Testing the patient's visual fields can be accomplished at the bedside by finger confrontation methods in all four quadrants of each eye by asking the patient to fix on the examiner's nose then to "count the fingers" (**Fig. 2–10A**). Because of the over-representation of central vision in the nervous system, assessment of each quadrant within the central 10–20 degrees is more important than that of the periphery. One eye at a time is tested while the patient focuses on the examiner's nose. Sometimes, a visual field defect is best elicited by asking the patient if all parts of the examiner's face can be seen clearly: "Are the examiner's eyes equally clear?" If the patient does not see the nose clearly, a central scotoma should be suspected. Alternatively, the examiner can hold a finger over his nose and another finger a few degrees off

Video 2.1

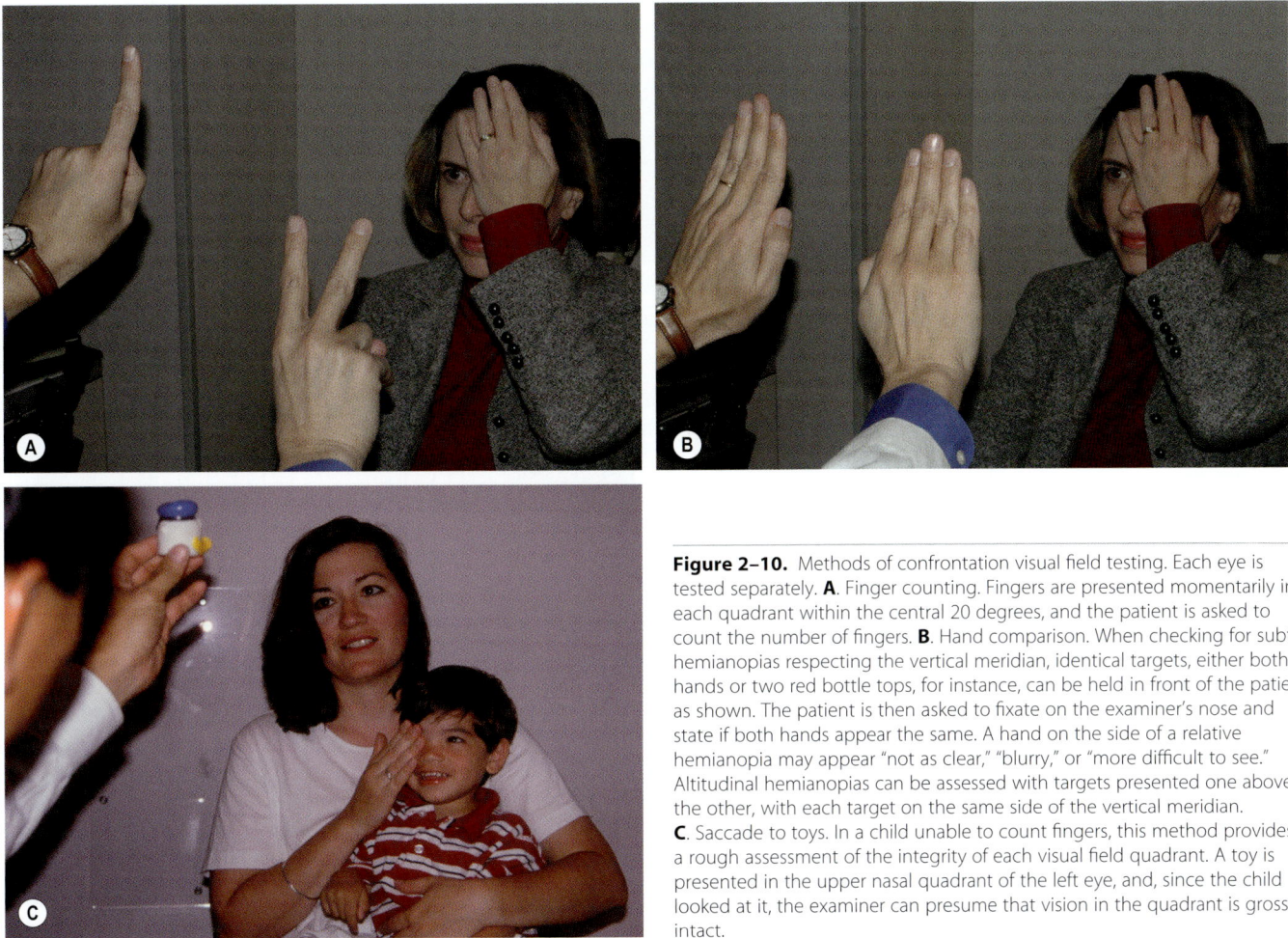

Figure 2–10. Methods of confrontation visual field testing. Each eye is tested separately. **A**. Finger counting. Fingers are presented momentarily in each quadrant within the central 20 degrees, and the patient is asked to count the number of fingers. **B**. Hand comparison. When checking for subtle hemianopias respecting the vertical meridian, identical targets, either both hands or two red bottle tops, for instance, can be held in front of the patient as shown. The patient is then asked to fixate on the examiner's nose and state if both hands appear the same. A hand on the side of a relative hemianopia may appear "not as clear," "blurry," or "more difficult to see." Altitudinal hemianopias can be assessed with targets presented one above the other, with each target on the same side of the vertical meridian. **C**. Saccade to toys. In a child unable to count fingers, this method provides a rough assessment of the integrity of each visual field quadrant. A toy is presented in the upper nasal quadrant of the left eye, and, since the child looked at it, the examiner can presume that vision in the quadrant is grossly intact.

center. If the patient sees the eccentric finger more clearly than the central one, again a central scotoma should be suspected. Testing of two separate quadrants of one eye enhances the yield of finding a field defect. Moving stimuli are almost always appreciated better than static ones, so the latter are preferable when screening for subtle field defects. Detection of finger wiggling is not as sensitive as finger counting, especially when the patient is asked to count fingers that are presented rapidly.

Red top caps can also be used in a similar fashion and enhance the sensitivity of confrontation visual field testing.[29] For example, when testing for a central scotoma, a red top cap is placed in front of the examiner's nose and another cap is held slightly off the midline. If the patient sees the cap held in the periphery as a better red, a central scotoma is suggested.

Color or subjective hand comparison is also a useful adjunct to elicit defects respecting the vertical or horizontal meridians (**Fig. 2–10B**). Caution should be applied in patients with visual inattention or neglect, as they may exhibit a field defect during double simultaneous stimulation. However, these patients will exhibit no field defect when stimulated with single targets.

Alternatively, a laser pointer can be used to screen a patient's visual field.[30] The examiner can stand behind the patient and test the various quadrants using a laser pointer projected on a tangent screen or even on a white wall. This test may be helpful as a screening tool, and may detect field defects not observed on confrontation testing.

In a patient who is aphasic, uncooperative, intubated, sedated, or very young, responses such as finger mimicry, pointing to targets presented, looking at the stimulus, or reflex blink to visual threat allow for a gross appraisal of visual field integrity. The stimulus should be silent to ensure the patient is not attending to an auditory stimulus. If the patient saccades to a visual stimulus in a given quadrant, the visual field in that area can be considered relatively intact (**Fig. 2–10C**). However, an absent reflex blink to visual threat, which depends on the intactness of the afferent visual pathway, including the occipital lobe, can be misleading. The reflex may be absent in very young normal infants and patients with Balint syndrome or neglect from right frontal and parietal lesions (see Chapter 9).[31] Care should also be taken so that the visual threat, usually a menacing hand gesture, does not move air onto the eye and elicit a corneal blink reflex (see below).

The results of confrontation visual field testing can be recorded in the chart within two circles. By convention, the visual field of the patient's right eye is drawn within the circle on the right, and the left eye's visual field in the circle on the left. Furthermore, the visual field of each eye is diagrammed from the patient's perspective. In **Fig. 2–11**, examples of documentation of normal and abnormal confrontation

Video 3.1

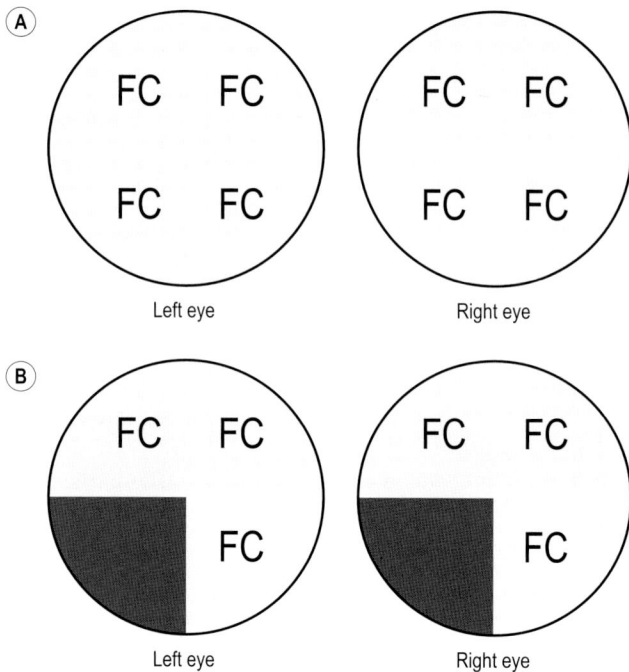

Figure 2–11. Schematic documentation of confrontation visual assessment. FC, finger counting. The fields are represented from the patient's point of view with the right eye vision recorded on the right and the left eye vision on the left. **A.** Normal confrontation visual fields. The patient is able to count fingers in all four quadrants. **B.** Left lower quadrantanopsia. The defective field is documented by black, and the patient is able to count fingers in all other quadrants.

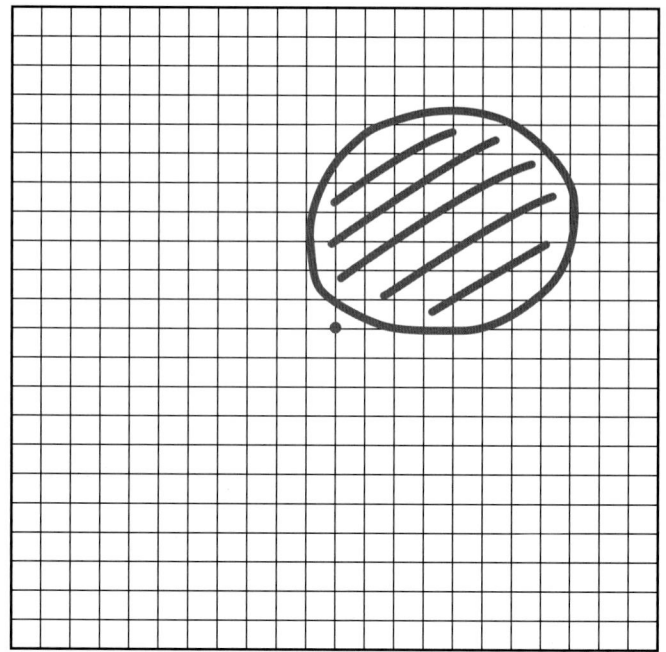

Figure 2–12. Amsler grid in a patient with central serous chorioretinopathy involving the macula inferiorly in the left eye. With the right eye covered, the patient was asked to look at the central dot and was asked if any of the lines were missing or wavy. She indicated the shaded area was blurry and distorted.

fields are given. Because confrontation techniques produce only a gross estimation of the visual fields,[29] more precise documentation requires a tangent screen, kinetic perimetry, or automated threshold perimetry. These tests and their interpretation are discussed in great detail in Chapter 3.

The visual field can be altered by lesions anywhere in the afferent visual pathway; the specific patterns of field loss and their relationship to neuroanatomic structures are also discussed in more detail in Chapter 3.

Amsler grid testing

To test central or macular vision, an Amsler grid (**Fig. 2–12**), which is similar to a piece of graph paper with a central fixation point, can be viewed by the patient at near. The patient fixates on the central dot with near correction and is asked whether all the lines are straight and whether any parts are missing, bent, or blurry.

They may perceive abnormal areas on the grid that might correspond with visual field deficits. Amsler grid testing is particularly helpful in detecting central and paracentral field defects. Small deficits (affecting only a couple of boxes) point to macular disease and may not be detected on computerized perimetry. Maculopathies also typically produce a distortion (heading of lines) in the grid pattern (*metamorphopsia*). The results of Amsler grid testing can be documented with a convention similar to that of confrontation visual field testing.

Photostress test

Also not part of the routine neuro-ophthalmic examination, the photostress test has been advocated as a method of dis-

tinguishing retinal (macular) from optic nerve causes of visual loss.[32] After best corrected visual acuity is assessed, a bright light is shone into the affected eye for 10 seconds while the other eye is covered; a penlight, halogen transilluminator, or indirect ophthalmoscope held 2–3 cm from the eye can be used. The test should be performed with undilated pupils. Once the light is removed, acuity in that eye is retested continuously until the patient can read three letters on the Snellen line just larger than the baseline acuity (i.e., 20/25 vs 20/20). The time to recovery is recorded, then the procedure is repeated with the other eye. Photostress recovery time is 27 seconds for normal eyes.[33] Optic neuropathies tend not to produce prolonged photostress recovery times, while macular disorders, such as macular edema, central serous retinopathy, and macular degeneration, may be associated with recovery times of several minutes.[33,34] The photostress recovery time is believed to be related to the amount of photopigment bleached by the light stimulus and the ability of rod and cone photoreceptors to convert photopigment back to the unbleached state.[35] Because the actual recovery time may vary according to technique and age,[36] a more useful clinical measure may be a relative photostress recovery time between the two eyes when one eye is suspected of having visual loss due to either optic nerve or macular disease.

Higher cortical visual function

Examination of visual attention, object recognition, and reading ability are important in patients with visual complaints unexplained by acuity or field loss.[37] These functions and their neuroanatomic localization are discussed in greater detail in Chapter 9.

It is often difficult to separate a dense left hemianopia from dense neglect in a patient with a large right parietal lesion. In instances where the deficits are more subtle, the examiner can screen for visual inattention by presenting visual stimuli, such as fingers, separately in each hemifield, then together on both sides of the midline (double simultaneous visual stimulation—similar to hand comparison (see **Fig. 2–10B**)). Individuals with subtle visual inattention but intact fields will see both stimuli when they are presented separately but may not see one of them when they are shown simultaneously. Other bedside tests include letter cancellation, in which the patient is asked to find a specific letter or shape within a random array.[38] Patients with left visual neglect may find the specified letter only when it appears on the right side of the page (**Fig. 2–13**). The line cancellation test, in which the individual is asked to cross lines drawn in various locations at different angles throughout the page,[39] is similar. When patients with left neglect are asked to bisect a horizontal line, they may tend to "bisect" the lines to the right of the true center.

In patients suspected of visual agnosias, informal tests of visual recognition can be performed at the bedside using common objects such as a pen, cup, or book and asking the patient to name them. An inability to recognize faces (*prosopagnosia*) can be tested with magazine or newspaper photographs containing famous faces. Standardized facial and object recognition tasks are available during more formal neuropsychologic testing. An inability to interpret complex scenes (*simultanagnosia*) can be tested with magazine pictures containing several elements or with a letter made up of smaller elements (Navon figure) (**Fig. 2–14**). Simultanagnosia may be evident when the patient is tested with Ishihara color plates and is able to recognize the colors and trace the digits but is unable to recognize the number represented among the dots.[40]

Central achromatopsia, or difficulty perceiving colors because of a cortical lesion, may be detected using the Hardy–Rand–Rittler color plates or Farnsworth D-15 tests (mentioned above), which may demonstrate complete lack of color vision. When the deficit is incomplete, as in *cerebral*

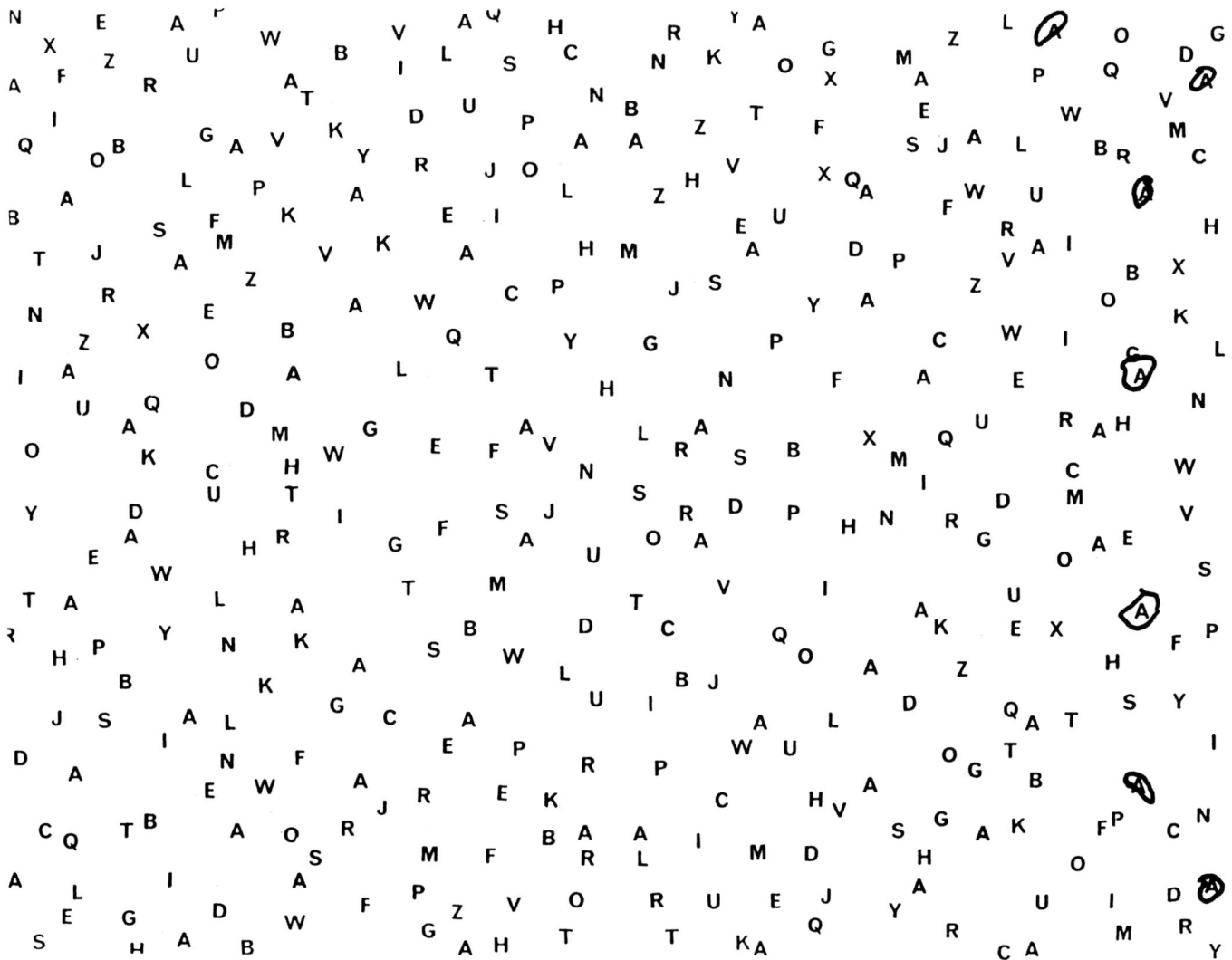

Figure 2–13. Letter cancellation. Patients are asked to identify the As within the random array. This patient with severe left neglect found only those As along the very right hand side of the page. (From Liu GT, Bolton AK, Price BH, Weintraub S. Dissociated perceptual-sensory and exploratory-motor neglect. J Neurol Neurosurg Psychiatr 1992;55:701–726, with permission.)

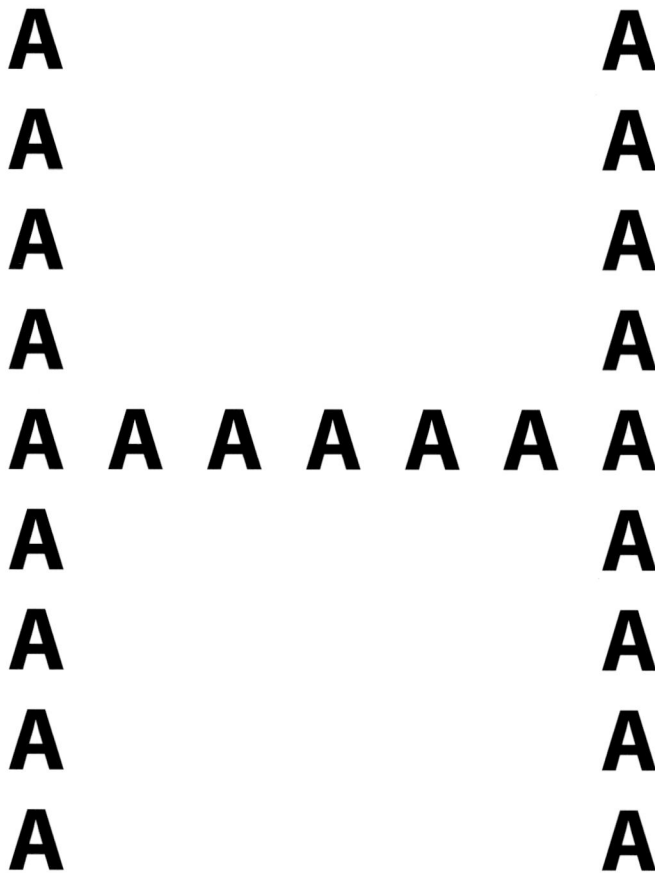

Figure 2–14. Simultanagnosia tested by a Navon figure. The letter H is drawn by arranging multiple As. A patient with simultanagnosia might be able to identify the As but will not realize that the smaller elements together make an H.

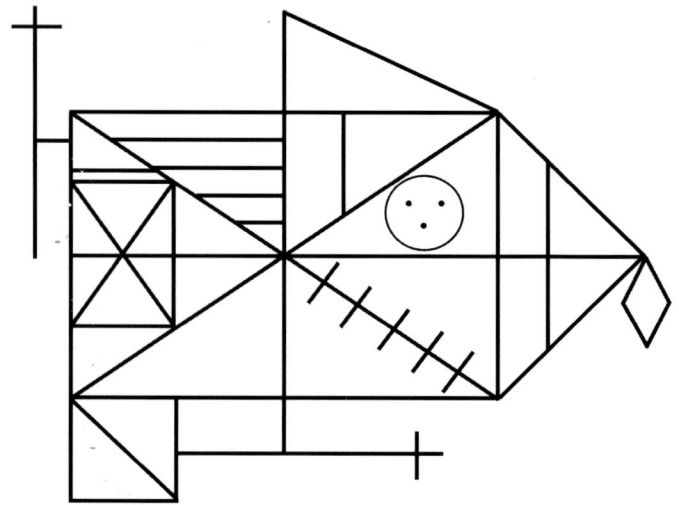

Figure 2–15. Rey–Osterrieth complex figure used for visuospatial and visual memory tasks. Patients can be asked to copy it or study the figure then redraw it from memory.

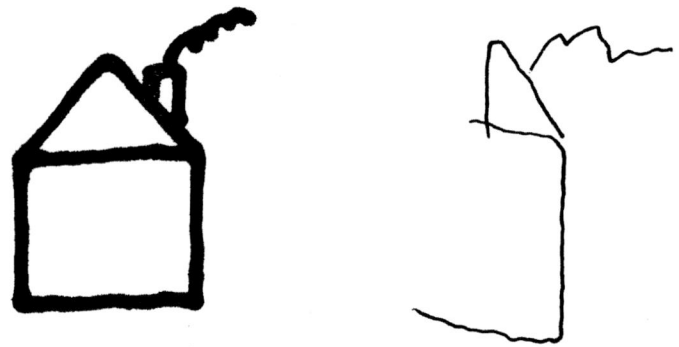

Figure 2–16. Copying a drawing. A figure of a house was drawn by the examiner (*left*), and a patient with left-sided neglect was asked to copy it. The patient's drawing (*right*) missed elements from the left side of the figure.

dyschromatopisa, a tritan (blue–yellow) defect may be demonstrated.[37]

Errors in figure or clock drawing or copying are often nonspecific. However, these tasks sometimes can provide useful information about visuospatial abilities, especially in patients with hemifield loss or hemineglect. For instance, such patients can be asked to copy a cube, house, flower, or Rey–Osterrieth complex figure (**Fig. 2–15**).[41] An individual with left hemineglect may duplicate only half of a figure (**Fig. 2–16**), whereas one with a right parietal lesion may show evidence of visuospatial difficulty. In a more difficult task, when the patient with a right parietal lesion is asked to draw a clock face, visuospatial abnormalities may be more pronounced. Errors include placing all the numbers on the right side (**Fig. 2–17**) and reversing the order of the numbers.[42] In a cautionary note, a normally drawn clock face does not exclude left unilateral spatial neglect.[43] The task can be performed with or without a predrawn circle, but, if a circle is provided, the examiner should make sure it is large enough (2–3 inches in diameter) to make the test a useful one for evaluating visuospatial function. Interested readers are referred to the informative, detailed analysis of clock drawing by Freedman et al.[44]

The ability to read should be tested along with all the other main components of language function (see Mental status evaluation, below). An individual who can see well but not read and is able to write (*alexia without agraphia*) likely has a lesion in the left occipital lobe and splenium of the corpus callosum. Pseudoalexias may be caused by hemianopias.

Efferent system

Pupils

Although pupillary dysfunction often reflects a lesion in the efferent parasympathetic pupillary pathway, abnormal pupillary reactivity also may be a sign of disorders affecting the afferent visual pathway. Some pupillary abnormalities are mentioned below in the context of the pupillary examination, but each, along with its differential diagnosis, is discussed in more detail in Chapter 13.

At a minimum, pupillary size and reactivity to light (direct responses and consensual responses during the swinging flashlight test) should be evaluated. Pupillary shape should

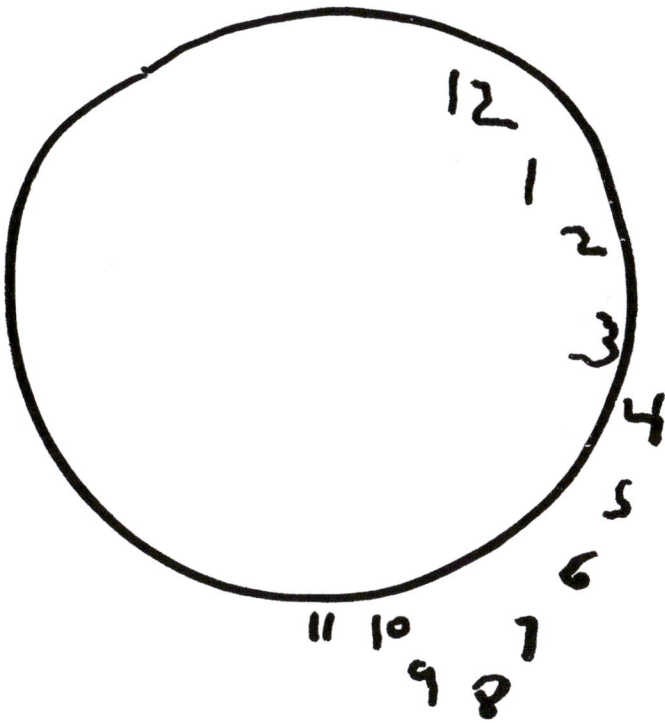

Figure 2–17. Clock drawing in a patient with a right parietal lesion. A large circle was drawn, and the patient was asked to draw in the numbers of a clock. The patient's response reflects the left-sided neglect and visuospatial difficulties.

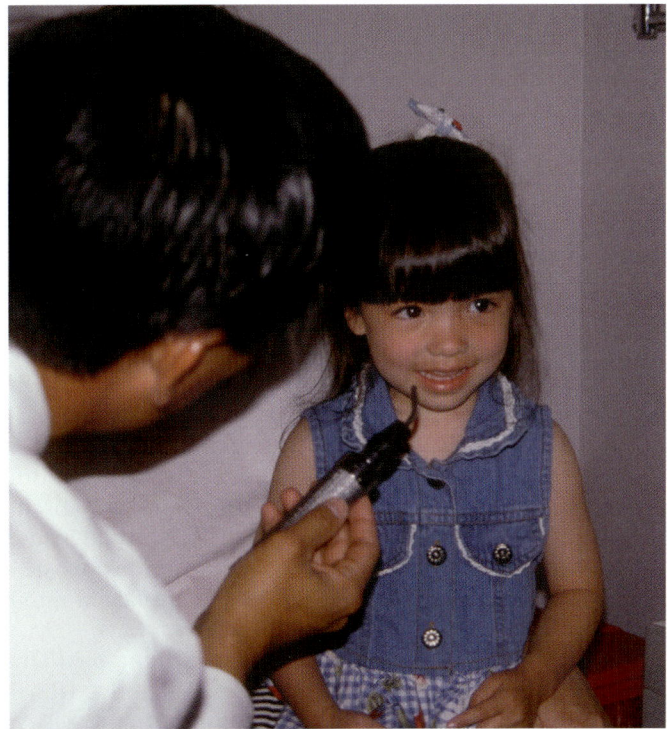

Figure 2–18. During examination of the pupils, the patient should fixate on a distance target to discourage accommodation and miosis.

be documented in those situations when it is not round; slit-lamp evaluation is helpful in these instances.

Many health professionals were taught to use the acronym "PERRLA" in the chart to document that the "*p*upils were *e*qual, *r*ound, and *r*eactive to *l*ight and *a*ccommodation." Acronyms are easier to write if one is in a rush but, as in the case of "PERRLA," do not always reflect exactly what was tested.[3] We prefer a less generic, more descriptive sentence such as "The pupils were equal in size in ambient light and reacted briskly to light without a relative afferent pupillary defect." This can also be abbreviated as "Pupils: equal and reactive. No RAPD." The roundness of the pupils is implied, and, because the pupils reacted briskly to light, it was not necessary to test their reaction while viewing a near stimulus. Alternatively, one could record the size of each pupil and their reactivity. One scale for pupil reactivity is as follows: 3+, normal brisk reaction; 2+, slightly sluggish; and 1+, sluggish. Descriptions such as "brisk," "sluggish," or "unreactive" also can be used.

Pupillary size. The most practical method of measuring pupillary size uses the pupil gauge available on most near acuity cards (see **Fig. 2–2B**). Usually, the two pupils are equal in size, and each is located slightly nasal and inferior to the center of the cornea. Transient fluctuations in pupillary diameter are normal and are termed *hippus*. In infancy the pupils are often small, but they widen as the child grows older and achieve their largest sizes in adolescence.[45] In adulthood they then become progressively more miotic.

The term *anisocoria* refers to asymmetric pupillary sizes; in cases of anisocoria the amount of pupillary inequality in ambient light and dark should be compared. In the most

common type of anisocoria, physiologic or essential, pupillary function is normal and the relative inequality is the same in light and dark (although in some instances it can be slightly worse in the dark and better in the light because of the mechanical limitations of the pupil when it is small). Long-standing pupillary inequality can be confirmed by viewing old photographs with the magnification of a slit lamp or 20-diopter lens.

Pathologic anisocoria suggests dysfunction in the efferent part of the pupillary pathway. Afferent pupillary dysfunction, due to optic nerve disease, for instance, does not produce anisocoria. In general, anisocoria greater in light implies the larger pupil has a parasympathetic abnormality, while anisocoria more prominent in the dark suggests the smaller pupil has oculosympathetic dysfunction (Horner syndrome). In the latter situation, the pupil may redilate slowly (dilation lag) when compared with the other pupil when the lights are turned down. To assess dilation lag, the examiner shines a dim light from below the patient's nose to provide minimal illumination before turning the room lights off. The size and speed of dilation are assessed for the first 2–4 seconds after the patient is placed in the dark. During this time, dilation lag should be maximal. Often, the sympathetically denervated pupils will begin to catch up in size over the next 10 seconds of observation.

Light reactivity: direct and consensual. Pupillary light reactivity (constriction) should be tested with a bright light such as a halogen transilluminator or indirect ophthalmoscope while the patient views a distant target (to prevent near-induced miosis) (**Fig. 2–18**) in a dimly lit room. We agree with Thompson et al.[46] that "it is not necessary for the room to be as dark as a coal cellar or for the light to be of xenon-arc intensity." Fixation may be difficult in smaller children or uncooperative adults who may not hold still. With the light shined in one eye, the ipsilateral pupillary light reflex is the *direct response*, while that of the contralateral is the *consensual response*. Because light from one eye will reach both Edinger–Westphal nuclei symmetrically, normally both pupils react briskly when light is shone into just one eye (i.e., the direct and consensual responses are equal) (**Fig. 2–19A**).

The direct and consensual pupillary light responses may be diminished when light is directed in an eye with optic nerve or severe retinal dysfunction. Note that in these instances both pupils still have the same resting size, which is a reflection of the total amount of light reaching the midbrain pretectum from both eyes. In unilateral blindness (no light perception) due to optic nerve or retinal injury, both direct and consensual pupillary light reactions are absent (amaurotic or deafferented) when the light is shone in the blind eye. If the direct response is defective, but the consensual response is normal, it is likely that the ipsilateral pupil is paralyzed (efferent dysfunction).

Swinging flashlight test and relative afferent pupillary defects. The *swinging flashlight test (of Levitan),*[47] during which the light is alternately directed at each eye to compare each

Video 2.2

pupil's constriction to light, is an excellent objective method for evaluating relative optic nerve function.[48,49] Testing of pupillary reactivity to light and the swinging flashlight test should be performed with a cadence. Rhythmic examination of the pupils, as well as pointing the light along the visual axis of each eye, promotes symmetric light exposure to both eyes. The light should be directed at each eye for about 1 second each ("one–one") to assess pupillary reactivity to light. Care should be taken to align the light along the visual axes, especially when the eyes are misaligned. Then the light should be alternated between each eye (without too much hesitation between eyes) for about 2 seconds each ("one–two–one–two"). Normally both pupils will exhibit symmetric constriction (**Fig. 2–19A**). Caution should be exercised in patients with anisocoria, in whom pupillary constriction may appear falsely asymmetric. In addition, testing with a light that is too bright or too dim may either mask or miss an asymmetric response.[50,51] Occasionally, asymmetric pupillary responses are best detected by rapid (less than 1 second) swings of the flashlight. In this situation, one checks for any asymmetry in the initial pupillary constriction.

An asymmetric swinging flashlight test is highly suggestive of a unilateral or asymmetric optic neuropathy or severe retinal or macular abnormality. In these instances, when

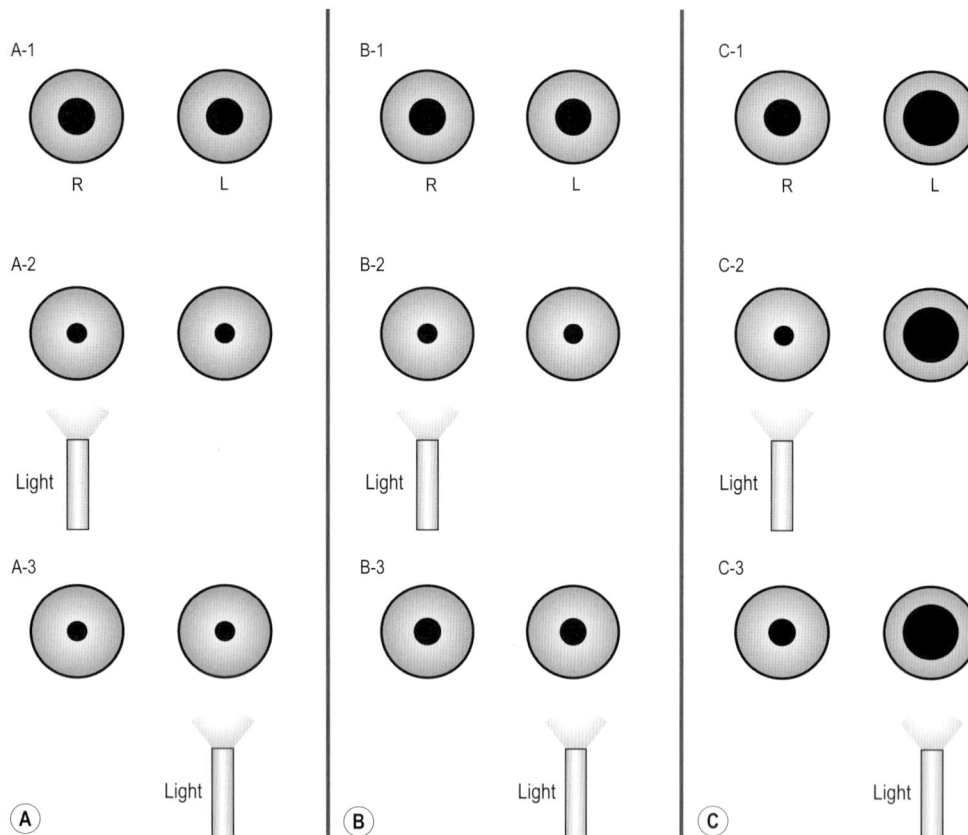

Figure 2–19. A. Normal swinging flashlight test, in which light directed in either eye elicits the same amount of pupillary constriction. **B**. Swinging flashlight test revealing a left relative afferent pupillary defect (L. RAPD) in the hypothetical setting of visual loss in the left eye due to an optic neuropathy. (*B-1*) Pupillary sizes are equal at rest in ambient lighting. (*B-2*) Light stimulation of the good right eye results in brisk bilateral pupillary constriction. (*B-3*) Light stimulation of the visually impaired left eye produces comparatively weaker pupillary constriction, and both pupils dilate. **C**. Left third nerve palsy and optic neuropathy. (*C-1*) The left pupil is fixed and dilated. (*C-2*) When the light is shone into the good right eye, the right pupil constricts normally. (*C-3*) However, when the light is shone into the left eye, the right pupil dilates because of the left optic neuropathy.

Video 2.3

light is directed in the unaffected eye, both pupils will react normally. When the light is returned to the abnormal eye, both pupils will dilate because of the comparatively weaker pupillary constriction (*relative afferent pupillary defect* (RAPD) or *Marcus Gunn pupil*) (**Fig. 2–19B**). This finding reflects the difference in the amount of afferent input reaching the pretectal region of the midbrain.[52] Even if each pupil constricts to light, but a secondary redilation (*pupillary escape*[53]) occurs in one eye, the interpretation is the same[46]—this is what Marcus Gunn originally described.[54,55] In any case, an RAPD is suggested when there is an asymmetry of the pupillary response. Although RAPDs are most suggestive of unilateral optic nerve or retinal disease, they may also be seen in asymmetric chiasmal disorders, optic tract lesions,[56] amblyopia (uncommonly),[57] and, rarely, pretectal disturbances.[58,59] The examiner should be careful not to confuse hippus with an RAPD and should not ascribe an RAPD to a media opacity. When vision is reduced in one eye and no RAPD is present, refractive error, amblyopia, media opacity, retinal disease, functional visual loss, or vision loss in the other eye should be suspected.

The swinging flashlight test requires only one working pupil. When one pupil is immobile, because of a third nerve palsy, for instance, one can still screen for an ipsilateral optic neuropathy by observing the consensual response in the fellow eye (with a second dim, obliquely directed light) during the swinging flashlight test (**Fig. 2–19C**). For example, a patient might present with a fixed and dilated pupil and poor vision in the left eye. When the light is brought back to the left eye, and the right pupil dilates, this suggests an optic neuropathy in the left eye. One should still call this a "left RAPD," but other terms include an "APD tested in a reverse fashion," "reverse Marcus Gunn pupil," or "reverse APD." With subtle APDs, observation of the reactivity of one pupil under higher magnification may be helpful. This can be accomplished while the patient is sitting at the slit lamp by watching one pupil's reaction with a dim light while performing a swinging flashlight test with a brighter transilluminator.[60] Alternatively the reactivity of both pupils may be assessed by moving the slit lamp with a bright light from one eye to the other.

Methods of grading the RAPD vary. In the "number-plus system," a "1+ RAPD OS" refers to initial constriction, but early redilation of the left pupil; "2+" indicates no initial movement of the pupil, then dilation; "3+" means immediate redilation; while a "4+ RAPD" indicates an amaurotic pupil. The "number-plus system" is inherently subjective, and responses may vary from examination to examination depending on ambient lighting and intensity of the testing light.[61] Another method, which is similar but more descriptive, assigns asymmetric responses on swinging flashlight tests into three groups: escape, amaurotic, and an "RAPD" as anything in between. Thompson et al.[46] advocate measuring the RAPD with neutral density filters, which are graded in log units. The filters are placed over the good eye during the swinging flashlight test until the pupillary responses are balanced and the RAPD is eliminated. However, again the end point is somewhat subjective. Testing with computerized pupillography is more objective and reproducible,[62] but these instruments are not widely used and are practical as

bedside tools only if portable.[63] In general, useful clinical information comes simply from the knowledge of the presence or absence of an RAPD.

A subjective quantification of the RAPD is sometimes helpful. With the transilluminator held in front of an unaffected eye, the examiner can ask, "if this amount of light is worth a dollar," then moves the light to the affected eye and asks, "then how many cents is this worth?" Reduced brightness sensation generally correlates with an RAPD.

Since an afferent pupillary defect is established by comparing the light reaction of one pupil with the other, there is no such entity as "a bilateral afferent pupillary defect."

Near. When a pupil has a sluggish reaction to light, one should see whether the pupil will constrict to a near stimulus. Pupillary constriction may be elicited by having the patient actively view a near target, such as a toy for younger children or thumb, pen, or written material for older ones (**Fig. 2–20**). The speed and amplitude of the near pupil response decreases slightly with age.[64] *Light-near dissociation* is the term applied to pupils that react poorly to light stimulation but constrict more briskly during viewing of a near target. If a pupil reacts to light, its reaction to near does not need to be tested, as pupils with intact light reactivity will also have normal constriction during viewing of a near target.

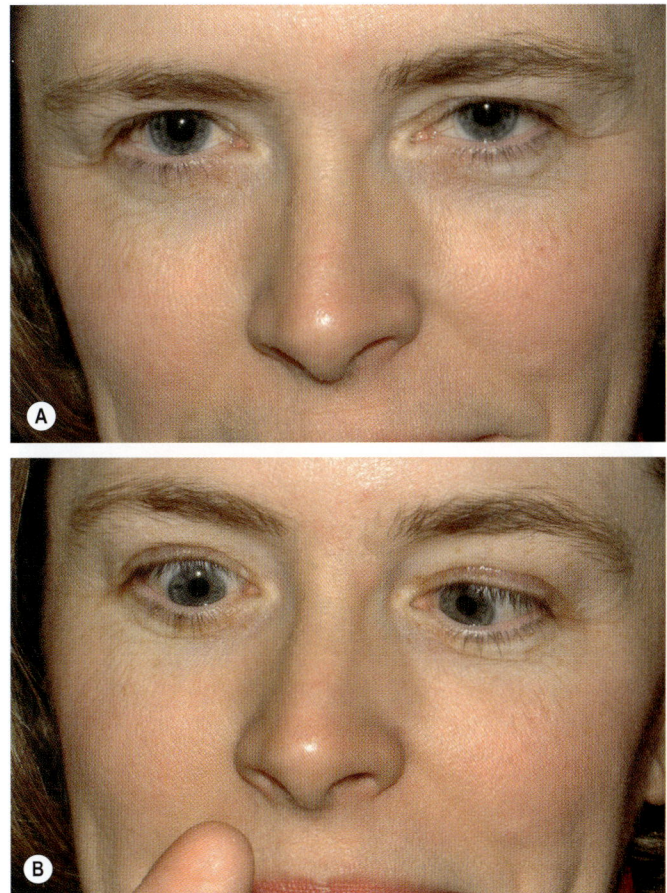

Figure 2–20. Pupillary constriction and convergence during the near response. Pupil sizes can be compared while the patient focuses at distance (**A**) versus near (**B**), using the patient's thumb or other object as a near stimulus.

Eyelids

The neuro-ophthalmic evaluation of the eyelids requires assessment of their external appearance, position, and function. Eyelid disorders are discussed in Chapter 14.

Eyelid appearance and position. First, the eyelids and their position should be observed at rest with the eyes directed straight ahead. In an adult, normally the edge of the upper eyelid lies below the limbus (junction of cornea and sclera) (**Fig. 2–21**). In a neonate, the upper eyelid may be above the limbus. Any obvious abnormalities in the shape or size of the lid should be noted. The *palpebral fissure* (**Fig. 2–21**), the opening between the upper and lower eyelids, usually meas-

ures between 9 and 12 mm in height (in the middle) when the lids are open but relaxed. An upper eyelid above the limbus ("scleral show") implies the palpebral fissure is widened, and disorders causing lid retraction or poor eyelid closure should be considered. Fissure narrowing suggests either ptosis (eyelid drooping) or excessive orbicularis contraction (see below). When evaluating a ptotic eyelid, since lower lid position may vary greatly, it is often helpful to measure the distance between the corneal light reflex and the upper lid margin. This number is referred to as the *margin reflex distance (MRD)*, which typically measures 4–5 mm.[65] A distinction between MRD1 and MRD2 is sometimes made (**Fig. 2–21**). These terms refer to the distance between the corneal light reflex and the upper and lower eyelid margins, respectively.

The examiner should also note the position of the eyelid crease (**Fig. 2–21**). It is usually approximately 10 mm from the lash margin and is formed by the skin insertion of the levator muscle. In levator dehiscence, for example, the distance from crease to lash margin increases.

Whenever possible, the chronicity of any abnormal eyelid appearance should be determined using old photographs.

Eyelid function. The levator palpebrae superioris muscle lifts the eyelid, and its function can be assessed by manually fixing the brow and asking the patient to look downward.[66] A ruler is then placed at the lid margin and the number of millimeters of lid elevation is measured as the patient looks upward (**Fig. 2–22**).[67] Normal levator function is greater than 12 mm.[65] Ptosis produced by levator dehiscence and Horner syndrome is usually associated with normal levator function. In contrast, levator function is reduced in ptosis associated with myasthenia gravis, congenital ptosis, third nerve palsies, and myopathic conditions such as chronic progressive ophthalmoparesis and myotonic dystrophy. Findings characteristic of but not specific for myasthenic ptosis include fatiguability (drooping of the eyelids after an extended period of upgaze), curtaining (elevation of a ptotic eyelid causing drooping of the other eyelid), and Cogan's lid twitch

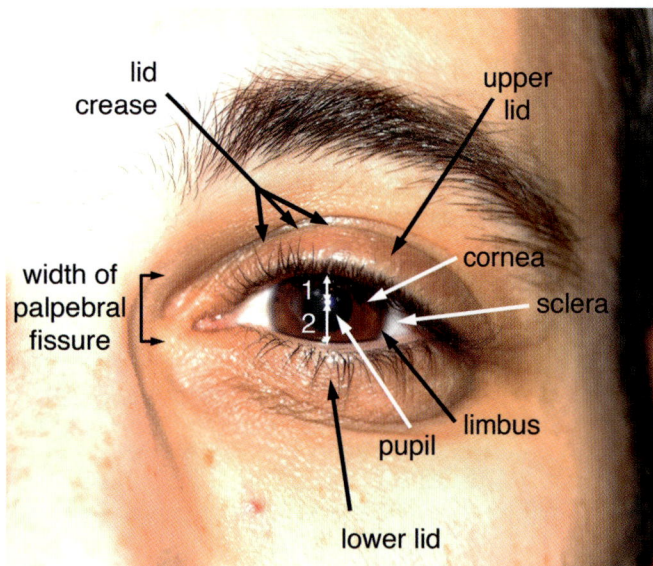

Figure 2–21. The normal left eye. 1, marginal reflex distance (MRD or MRD1), the distance between the upper eyelid edge and the corneal light reflex. 2, MRD2, the distance between the lower eyelid edge and the corneal light reflex. The lid crease (arrow) follows the curvature of the upper lid approximately 10 mm from the lash margin.

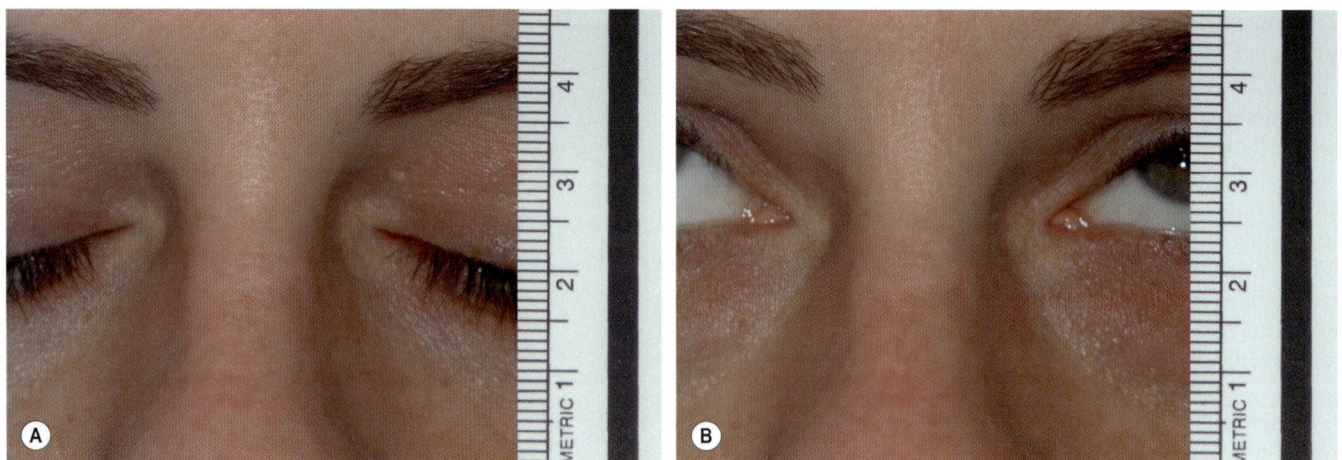

Figure 2–22. Measurement of eyelid function. **A**. To measure levator function, a ruler is placed over the center of the eyelid as the patient gazes downward. In this case, the margin of the upper lid is at the 2.0 cm mark on the ruler. **B**. Then the patient is asked to look up, and the distance the lid travelled to reach upgaze is recorded. The margin of the upper eyelid is at 3.3 cm in upgaze, so the eyelid excursion (or levator function) in this case is 13 mm, which is normal (normal greater than 12 mm). The left frontalis muscle should be neutralized by the examiner's thumb when the patient looks up.

(overshoot of the eyelid when moved from a relaxed and rested (downgaze) to primary position).

Next the lids should be examined during eye movements. During horizontal conjugate gaze, the palpebral fissure widens in the abducting eye in approximately half of normal individuals, and in about 15% the lid elevates in the adducting eye as well. During upgaze, levator tone increases to lift the upper eyelid, while, in downgaze, the eyelids should relax and follow the eyes smoothly. If the patient looks at a target moved downward and the eyelids lag behind (*lid lag*), thyroid eye disease, a dorsal midbrain lesion, or aberrant regeneration of the third nerve should be suspected.

Facial nerve

The facial nerve (VII) supplies the muscles of facial expression. In addition, it has a parasympathetic component supplying the lacrimal gland and submandibular and sublingual salivary glands, and sensory components responsible for taste and sensation of the external ear, tongue, and palate. When facial nerve dysfunction is suspected, the major goal of the examination is to establish whether the process is supra- or infranuclear. Further details regarding anatomy and disorders of the facial nerve are discussed in Chapter 14.

Motor evaluation. Assessment of facial nerve motor function begins by observing the patient at rest and noting any asymmetries of the face or blink pattern. Most supranuclear and infranuclear facial nerve palsies are associated with a flattened nasolabial fold and slightly widened palpebral fissure on the paretic side. Facial movement to emotional stimuli and voluntary command should also be assessed. A dissociation between spontaneous and voluntary movements is suggestive of supranuclear defects. Disease of the corticobulbar tracts tends to spare emotional facial responses, while those of the basal ganglia preserve voluntary movements. Preservation of forehead wrinkling and eyebrow elevation are also characteristic of supranuclear lesions.[68]

Having the patient forcefully close the eyelids while the examiner attempts to open them can test the strength of the orbicularis oculi muscles. The examiner should note asymmetries in eyelash burying or *lagophthalmos*, i.e., partial or total inability to close the lids. Having the patient smile should also be done to assess the integrity of the lower part of the facial nerve.

Excess contraction of the orbicularis oculi occurs in hemifacial spasm and blepharospasm. In subtle cases, orbicularis oculi contraction may be mistaken for eyelid ptosis (pseudoptosis), as in both the palpebral fissure may be narrowed. However, in pseudoptosis the ipsilateral eyebrow is often lower than normal. In contrast, if the palpebral fissure is narrowed because of true eyelid ptosis, the ipsilateral eyebrow is typically elevated as the patient attempts to keep the eye open by elevating the forehead.

Small contractions around the eye giving the appearance of skin rippling could be myokymia, fasciculations, or the result of aberrant reinnervation.

Taste. Taste is best tested using a cotton swab dipped in a sour, sweet, or bitter solution. Unilateral ageusia may be useful in identifying a facial lesion as peripheral, but it should be noted that bedside tests are crude and often unreliable.[68]

Tear function. Evaluation of tear function by observation alone, without actual testing, may lead to erroneous impressions (e.g., that a patient with a facial palsy is tearing excessively). Testing for tearing is of limited diagnostic or prognostic value unless tear production is drastically reduced or absent on the involved side. Further, the results of actual tear testing may be similarly misleading. Increased tear flow (*epiphora*) noted by the history can be due to exposure irritation, paralytic ectropion, obstruction of the punctum, duct or lacrimal sac, or failure of the lacrimal pump apparatus of the lower lid, and is not likely to be related to an irritative lesion of the greater superficial petrosal nerve. Similarly, decreased tearing may be due to corneal hypoesthesia rather than suggestive of a destructive process involving, for example, the greater superficial petrosal nerve.[68]

Tear testing usually involves Schirmer paper strips placed in the inferior conjunctival cul-de-sacs of each eye following topical anesthesia. To avoid erroneous results from pooled tears, the conjunctival tear lake should be dried prior to insertion of the paper strips. The length of the moistened paper is compared on the two sides after a period of 5 minutes. In the event that one of the filter strips becomes completely moistened prior to the passage of 5 minutes, both strips are removed and compared for results. Less than 5 mm of wetting is highly suggestive of tear deficiency, but this finding should be viewed in the context of the patient's clinical history and the results of the slit-lamp examination.[68]

Blink reflexes. Simulation of either cornea with a cotton wisp or tissue corner will cause a bilateral blink (*corneal blink reflex*). The absence of blinking in either eye usually suggests a lesion within the ophthalmic division of the trigeminal nerve (V1), the afferent limb of the reflex. Asymmetric blinking implies facial nerve weakness on one side.[68]

The *reflex blink to visual threat*, described above in the section Visual field testing, tests the intactness of the afferent visual pathway as well as cortical attentional mechanisms.[31] A cardinal feature of cortical blindness, for instance, is an absent blink to visual threat. On the other hand, the *reflex blink to light or dazzle* requires only intact connections from eye to brain stem.

Physiologic facial synkineses. Bell's phenomenon is discussed in more detail below in the section Eye movement. In some normal individuals, the ears will retract and flatten with conjugate lateral gaze; this is known as the *oculogyric auricular reflex* and is usually greater in the ear opposite the direction of lateral gaze. The presumed neural mechanism involves proprioceptive input from the extraocular muscles to the facial nuclear complex. In the nasolacrimal reflex, the secretion of tears may be induced by chemically stimulating the nasal mucosa with a dilute solution of ammonia or formaldehyde. The neural pathway for this reflex results from connections of the trigeminal nerve (V1) to the greater superficial petrosal nerve.

Ocular motility and alignment

The ocular motility examination consists of observation in primary gaze, evaluation of ductions and vergences, then

Video 2.4

23

detection of misalignment (strabismus). Monocular double vision is not due to an ocular motility abnormality, and when it resolves with a pinhole it is likely caused by refractive error.

Inspection. The presence of any obvious ocular misalignment or abnormal, spontaneous eye movements should be assessed first in primary gaze while the patient fixates on a distant target. *Esotropia* refers to the inward deviation of one eye relative to the other; while *exotropia* describes the outward deviation of one eye relative to the other. Any vertical misalignment is usually described by the laterality of the higher eye (e.g., a left *hypertropia* indicates the left eye is higher than the right). Adjunctive observations should include the presence or absence of head turn or tilt. When suspected but not visible with ordinary inspection, fine oscillations of the eye, such as superior oblique myokymia, may be seen more readily with the slit lamp or by witnessing movement of the optic disc during ophthalmoscopy.

Ductions. Ductions refer to monocular eye movements; rotations laterally are termed *abduction;* medially, *adduction;* upward, *elevation* (or *supraduction*); and downward, *depression* (or *infraduction*). Ductions can be tested by having the patient voluntarily direct gaze in the cardinal fields (up and right, up, up and left, right, left, down and right, down, and down and left). Ocular rotation can be recorded as a subjective percentage of normal (i.e., 70% of normal). This should be documented in the chart from the examiner's perspective (**Fig. 2–23A**). In another scheme using numbers +4 to 0 to –4, 0 indicates a normal duction, +4 means severe overaction, and –4 signifies no movement past midline (**Fig. 2–23B**).[69] The examiner should also observe the speed of the duction, which will typically be reduced with an ocular motor palsy but intact with a restrictive process.

Following instillation of a topical anesthetic, inability to move an eye despite pushing on the globe with a cotton-tip swab or pulling with forceps suggests mechanical restriction (positive forced duction test) (**Fig. 2–24**). In the forced generation test, the patient is asked to move the eye against the cotton-tip swab (**Fig. 2–24C**). Inability to do so usually indicates ocular motor nerve or muscle weakness. Patients with positive forced ductions but normal forced generations usually have a restrictive problem.

Bell's phenomenon. This is the normal upward rotation of the globe elicited during forceful eyelid closure. This palpe-bral–oculogyric reflex, likely mediated by poorly defined brain stem connections between the seventh and third nerve nuclei, is easily visible in patients with peripheral facial nerve paralysis who attempt to shut their eyes (**Fig. 2–25**). In normal patients it can be observed by having the patient try to close his or her eyes while the examiner holds the lids open. Most commonly, the eyes rotate up and out, but they may go up and in or straight up, and asymmetric left and right eye movements may be seen. However, in a study of 508 consecutive patients in an ophthalmic practice,[70] 42 (8%) had a downward response in one or both eyes, and in five (1%) the responses were horizontal.

Clinically, Bell's phenomenon can be helpful in two instances. (1) In an eye with defective voluntary supraduction, a normal Bell's phenomenon indicates a supranuclear defect with intact nuclear and infranuclear oculomotor nerve function for upgaze. For example, the reflex is preserved in upgaze paresis in Parinaud syndrome but defective in a complete third nerve palsy. (2) In patients with hemispheric defects, a stroke for example, both eyes may rotate contralateral to the lesion in a phenomenon known as *spasticity of conjugate gaze* (see Chapter 8).

Vergences. These are binocular eye movements. *Convergence* can be evaluated by having the patient look at his or her thumb or other accommodative target as it is brought toward the nose; both eyes should adduct with pupillary constriction (see **Fig. 2–20**). *Pursuit movements* should then be tested by having the patient keep his or her head still and visually track a target moved slowly horizontally or vertically (**Fig. 2–26**). The speed and accuracy of *saccades*, which are high-velocity, conjugate eye movements, should be examined by having the patient look eccentrically then quickly refixate on a target in primary gaze (the examiner's nose, for instance) (**Fig. 2–27**).

Oculocephalic responses can be evaluated by having the patient fix on a stationary target while the examiner gently rotates the head (**Fig. 2–28**) then extends and flexes the neck. The stimulus is either from proprioceptive afferents in the neck or the vestibular system, or both. Limited eye movements that are overcome by oculocephalic stimulation are likely supranuclear (see Chapter 16). In addition, with an arm extended and the chair rotated, most patients should be able to maintain visual fixation on their thumb (**Fig. 2–29**); difficulty with this task, manifesting usually as nystagmus,

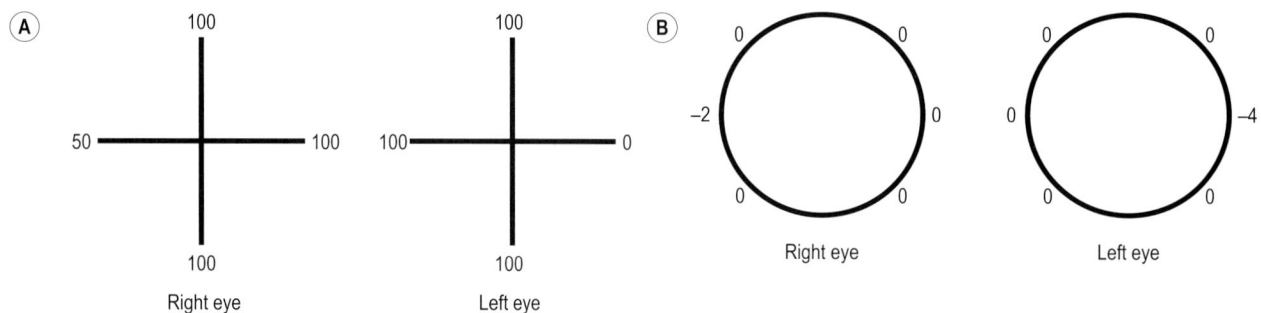

Figure 2–23. Recording ductions. **A**. In one method, the approximate percentages of the normal excursions in up, down, left, and right gazes are recorded. By convention, the diagrams are drawn from the examiner's view of the patient's eyes. In the example given, there is a partial abduction deficit of the right eye and no abduction of the left eye. **B**. In another method, ductions are graded from –4 to +4. Negative numbers indicate degrees of paralysis, while positive numbers indicate overaction. This example also shows a partial abduction deficit of the right eye and no abduction of the left eye.

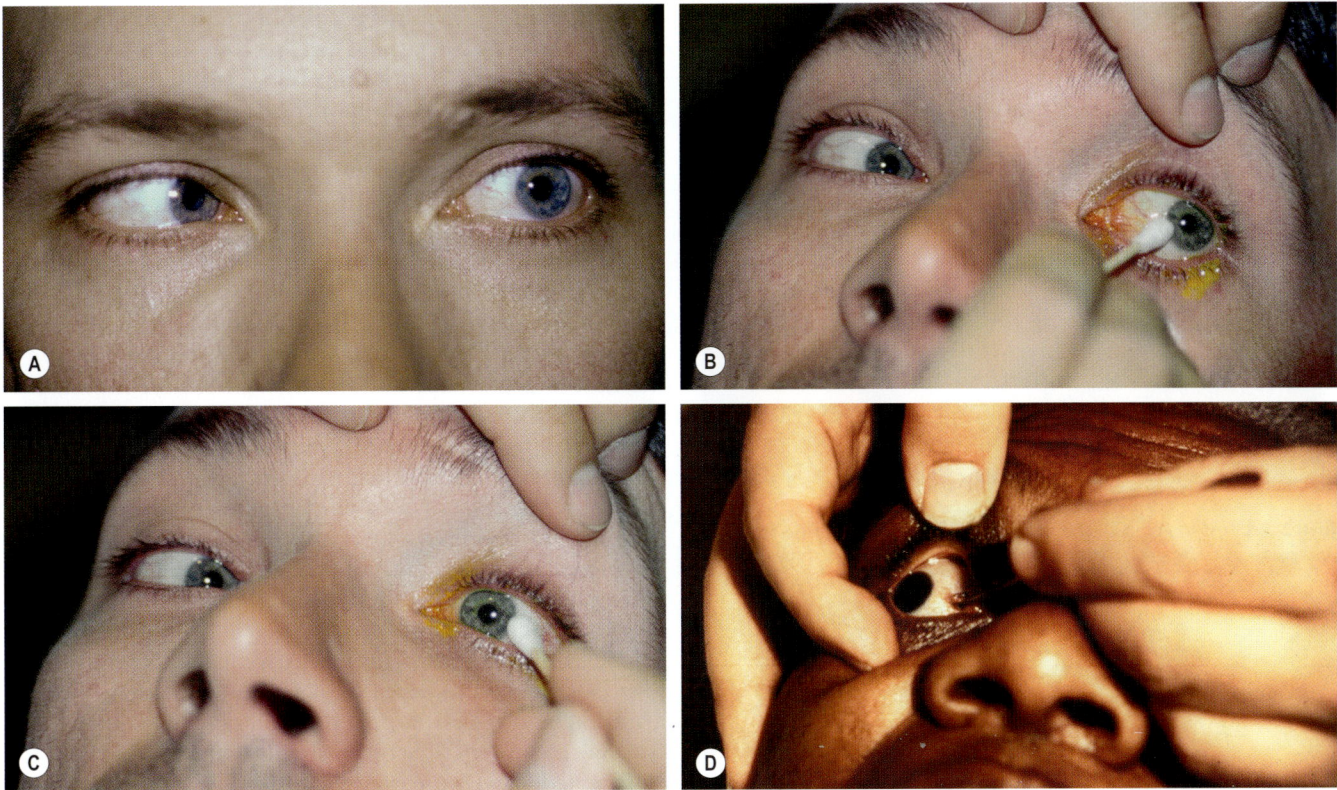

Figure 2–24. Forced ductions and generations. **A**. Left abduction deficit. **B**. Forced duction to test for muscle restriction. After instillation of topical anesthesia, an attempt is made at moving the eye laterally by pushing on it at the medial limbus with a sterile cotton swab. In this case the eye could be moved laterally, indicating the absence of restriction by the medial rectus muscle. This is *a negative forced duction test*. **C**. Forced generation to test for lateral rectus weakness. With the cotton swab on the lateral limbus, the patient is asked to abduct the eye. In this case the swab met no resistance, consistent with a lateral rectus palsy. This is a *positive forced generation test*. **D**. In an alternative method, forced ductions can be performed by pulling on the extraocular muscles with forceps. This patient had a right abduction deficit, and the medial rectus is manipulated.

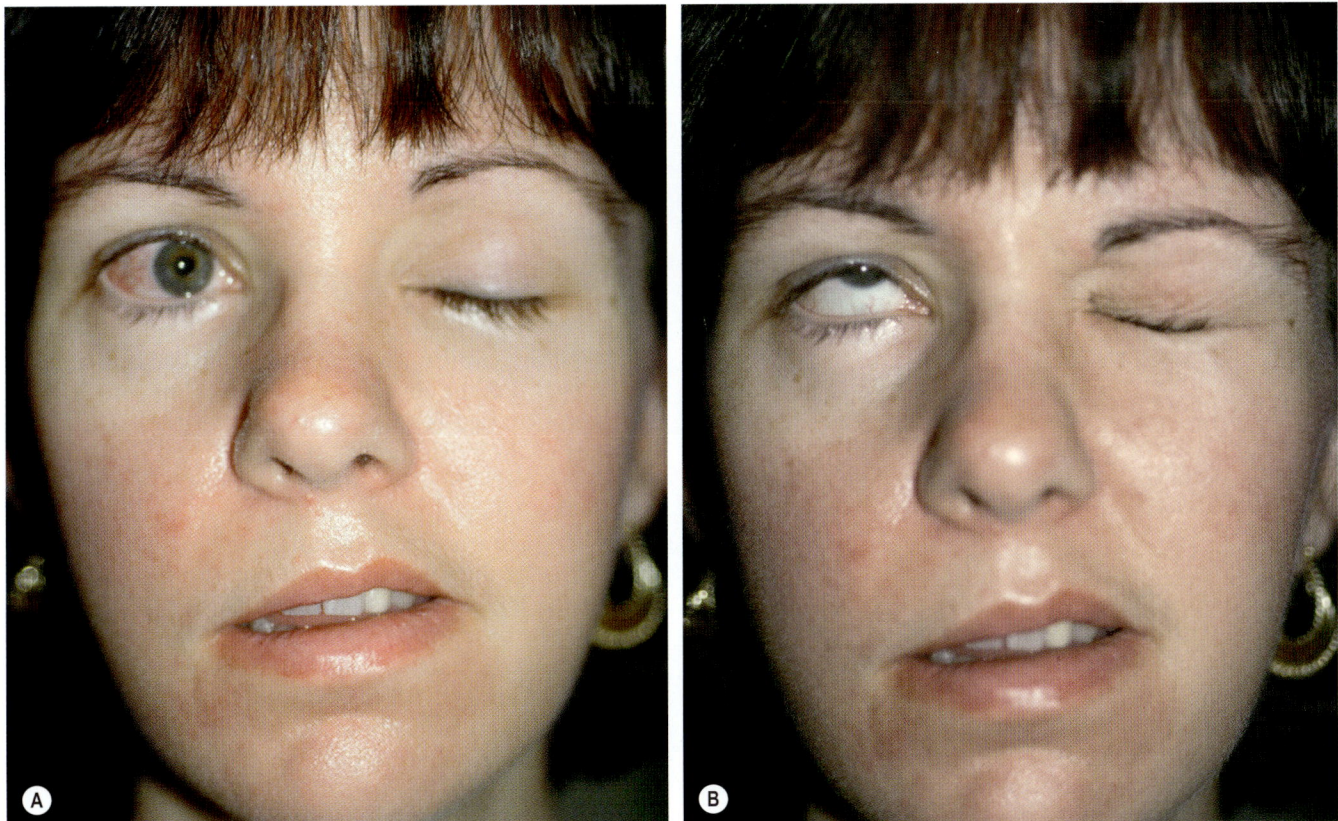

Figure 2–25. Bell's phenomenon. **A**. Traumatic right facial nerve palsy. **B**. Upon attempted eyelid closure, the right eye rotates upward.

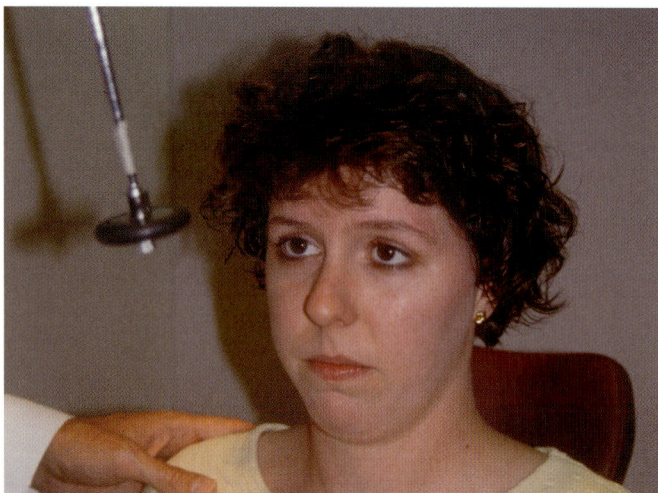

Figure 2–26. Testing pursuit. The patient is asked to fix and follow a slowly moving object, in this case, the end of a reflex hammer.

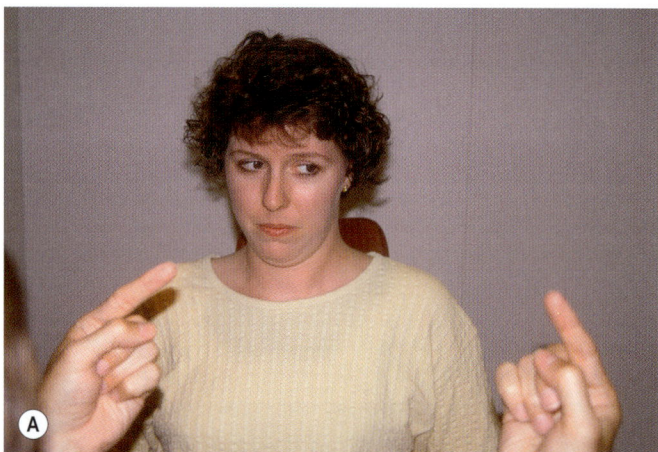

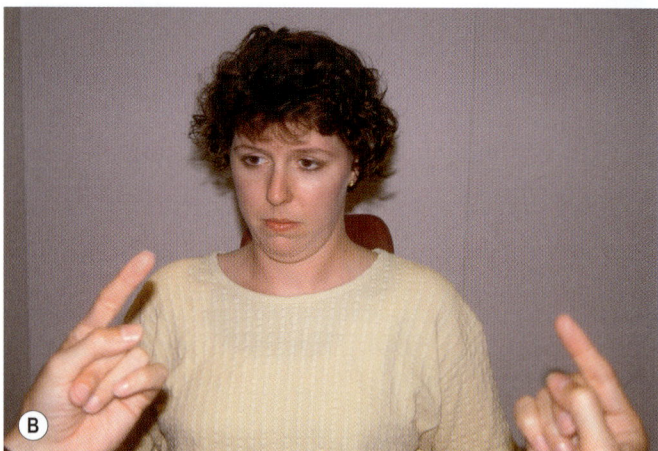

Figure 2–27. Testing saccades. **A.** The patient is asked to look at a target in the periphery. **B.** The speed and accuracy of the saccade is assessed as the patient is asked to look quickly at the target in front of her face.

suggests an inability to suppress the *vestibulo-ocular response* (VOR). This is usually a sign of cerebellar pathway dysfunction. When rotated around the examiner, infants, normally with poor fixation, manifest a VOR with tonic eye deviation in the direction of rotation followed by quick corrective jerks.

Nystagmus is a rhythmic oscillation of the eyes; two major types are seen. *Jerk nystagmus* has fast and slow phases, while *pendular nystagmus* is more sinusoidal without a fast phase. Many normal individuals have physiologic jerk nystagmus in extremes of gaze. This type of nystagmus is a low-amplitude, high-frequency nystagmus that usually fatigues with prolonged eccentric gaze. Physiologic *optokinetic nystagmus* (OKN) can be elicited by rotating a striped drum or moving a striped tape horizontally and vertically and asking the patient to "count the stripes as they go by" (**Fig. 2–30**). The slow phases of OKN are generated as the patient follows a target; the OKN fast phase is a corrective saccade to view the next target. Nystagmus and nystagmoid eye movements are discussed in Chapter 17.

Assessing ocular misalignment. Ophthalmoparesis often will be evident on evaluation of ductions alone; however, more subtle instances of misalignment may require cover or Maddox rod testing. Note both tests require sufficient vision in both eyes to view a distant target, and Maddox rod testing is not possible in the setting of visual suppression in one eye in long-standing strabismus.

The complementary cover–uncover and alternate cover tests can be used to assess ocular misalignment. A *tropia* is a misalignment that is present at all times, while a *phoria* is a misalignment that occurs only when binocularity is interrupted. Cover–uncover testing is used to detect tropias, which are manifest by any refixation movement of the fellow eye after monocular occlusion while the patient fixates on a target in the distance (**Fig. 2–31**). An outward movement of the uncovered eye signifies an *esotropia*, an inward movement implies an *exotropia*, and a downward movement indicates a *hypertropia*. Regardless of which eye is vertically impaired, the side of the higher eye denotes the deviation. For instance, a right eye that is higher is called a right hypertropia. Then the occlusion is removed and the other eye tested. During cover–uncover testing if only the covered eye deviates then only a phoria is present. Alternate cover testing, achieved by alternately occluding each eye for about a second each, breaks binocular fusion. This test reveals the full deviation: any tropia plus any latent phoria. The refixation movement of the uncovered eye is interpreted in the same manner as in cover–uncover testing.

The ocular misalignment can be neutralized and quantified by placing a prism over one eye. Each eye is then alternately covered as the amount of prism, measured in diopters, is slowly increased (prism–alternate cover test) (**Fig. 2–32**). The apex of the prism points in the direction in which the eye is deviated. Thus, if an eye is exotropic, the prism is placed over the eye with the prism base in; if an eye is esotropic, the prism is placed over the eye base out; if the eye is hypertropic, the prism is placed over the eye base down, while if the eye is hypotropic, the prism is placed over the eye with the base up. When the eyes no longer move on alternate cover testing, the deviation has been neutralized and the amount of prism required can be read off the prism bar. Deviations should be measured in the cardinal positions and at near. Vertical deviations should also be evaluated with the head tilted toward the right and left shoulders.

Video 2.5

Video 15

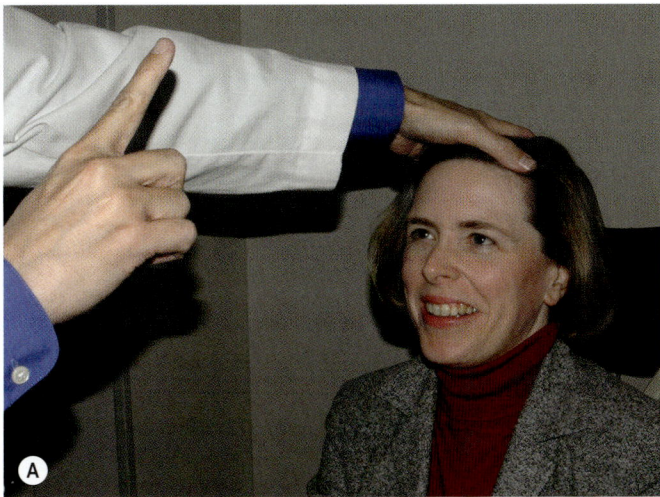

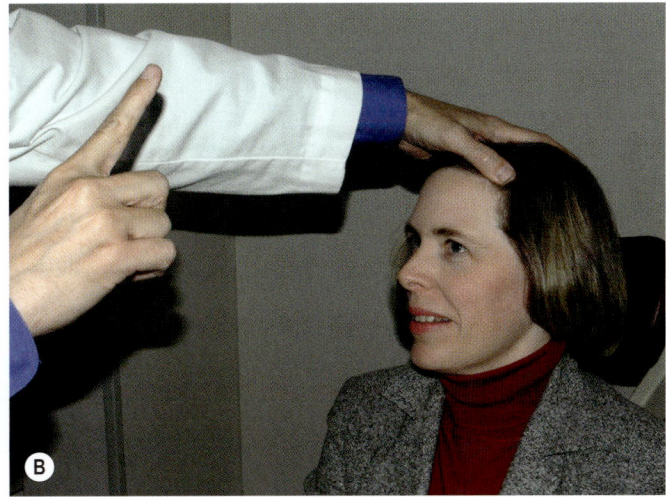

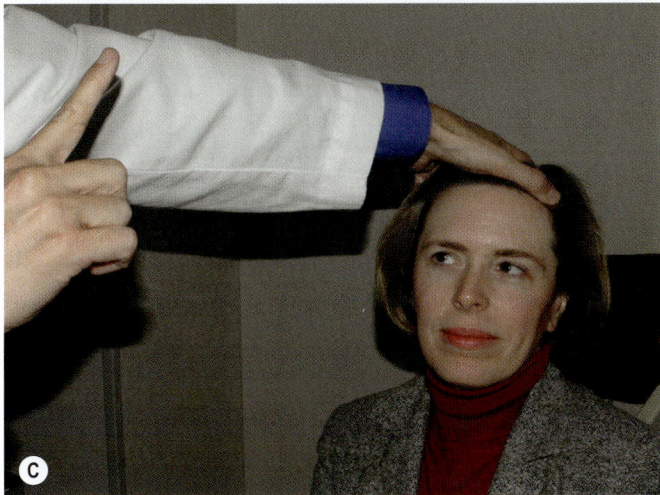

Figure 2–28. Oculocephalic eye movements. **A–C**. The patient is asked to fixate on a target in front of her face, and the head is rotated gently horizontally (shown) and vertically (not shown). Normally, the eyes rotate smoothly with full excursions in the direction opposite to the head turn.

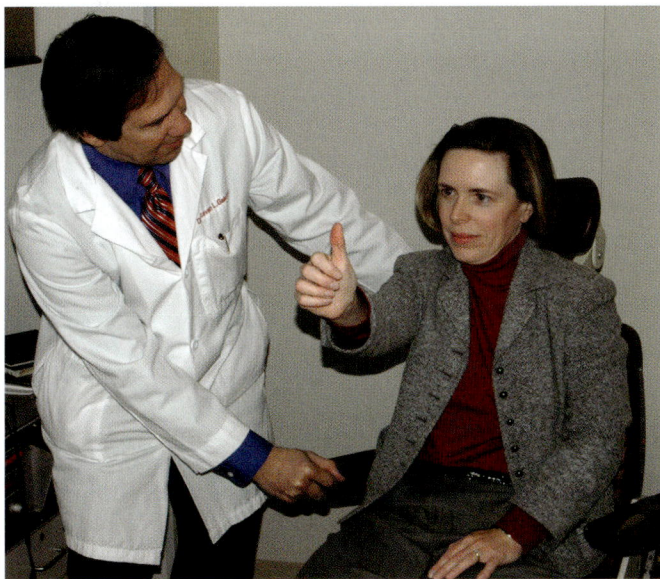

Figure 2–29. Suppressing the vestibulo-ocular response. The patient is asked to fixate on a target that will be stationary in relationship to the body, then the examination chair is rotated slowly. The eyes should remain still.

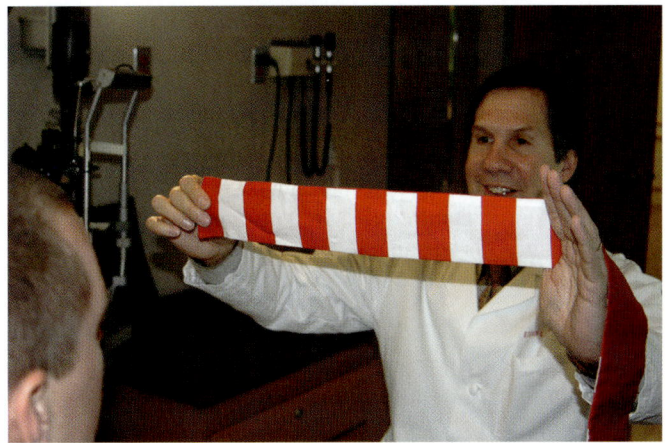

Figure 2–30. Eliciting optokinetic nystagmus. As the examiner moves a tape with red squares or other targets in the horizontal (shown) or vertical (not shown) direction, the patient is asked to "count the squares."

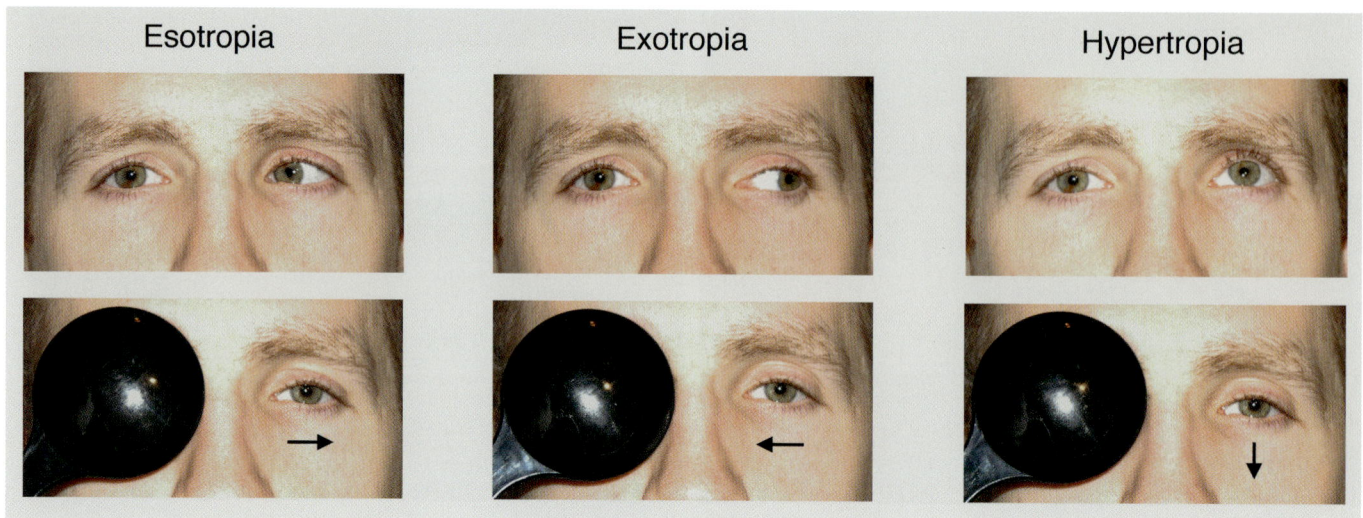

Figure 2–31. Cover testing for ocular misalignment. In each case the patient is fixing with the nonparetic right eye. Upon occlusion of the right eye, the misaligned left eye is forced to fixate. *Esotropic* eyes move laterally to fixate, while *exotropic* eyes move medially, and *hypertropic* eyes move downward to fixate. Thus, the ocular deviations can be determined by direction of the fixation movements.

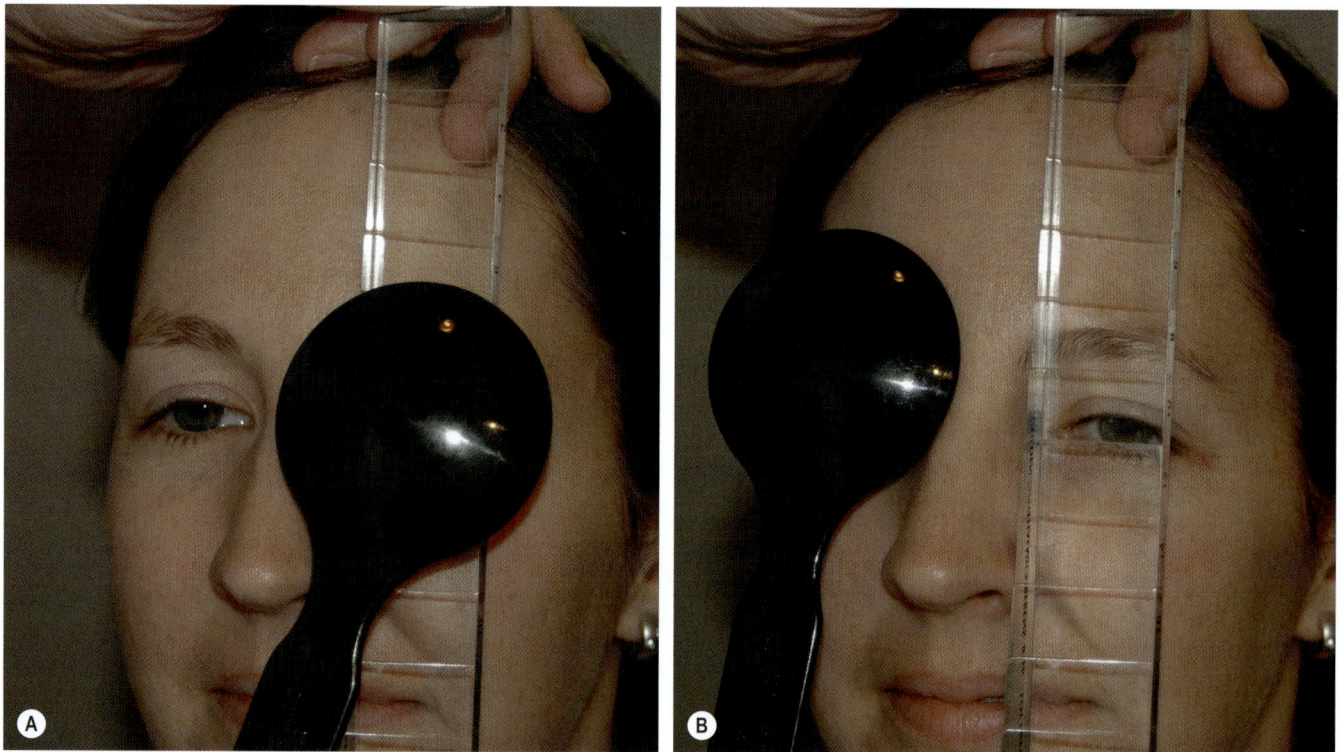

Figure 2–32. Prism–alternate cover testing for measurement of ocular misalignment. The prism bar contains a series of prisms of progressive strength (in diopters). Vertical prisms are used to measure hyperdeviations, while horizontal prisms are used in eso- and exodeviations. The patient fixates on a distant target, the eyes are alternately covered (**A,B**), and the prisms increased incrementally. The prism measurement is determined when the refixation movement, described in Figure 2–31, is neutralized.

When one eye has extraocular muscle paralysis, the primary deviation refers to measurements taken when the normal eye fixates and prisms are placed over a nonfixing paretic eye, while the secondary deviation is the measurement taken with paretic eye fixating and prisms placed over the fixing, nonparetic eye.[71] Because of Hering's Law, which states that there is equal and simultaneous innervation to yoked (synergistic muscles), the secondary deviation is always larger than the primary deviation. For example, when fixing with an eye that has a sixth nerve palsy, the esotropia will be larger than when fixing with the normal eye. This is due to the equal innervation to the nonparetic medial rectus when the paretic lateral rectus is heavily stimulated just to move the eye into the primary position.

The Maddox rod (**Fig. 2–33**), containing parallel half-cylinders, can help detect small deviations but, by itself,

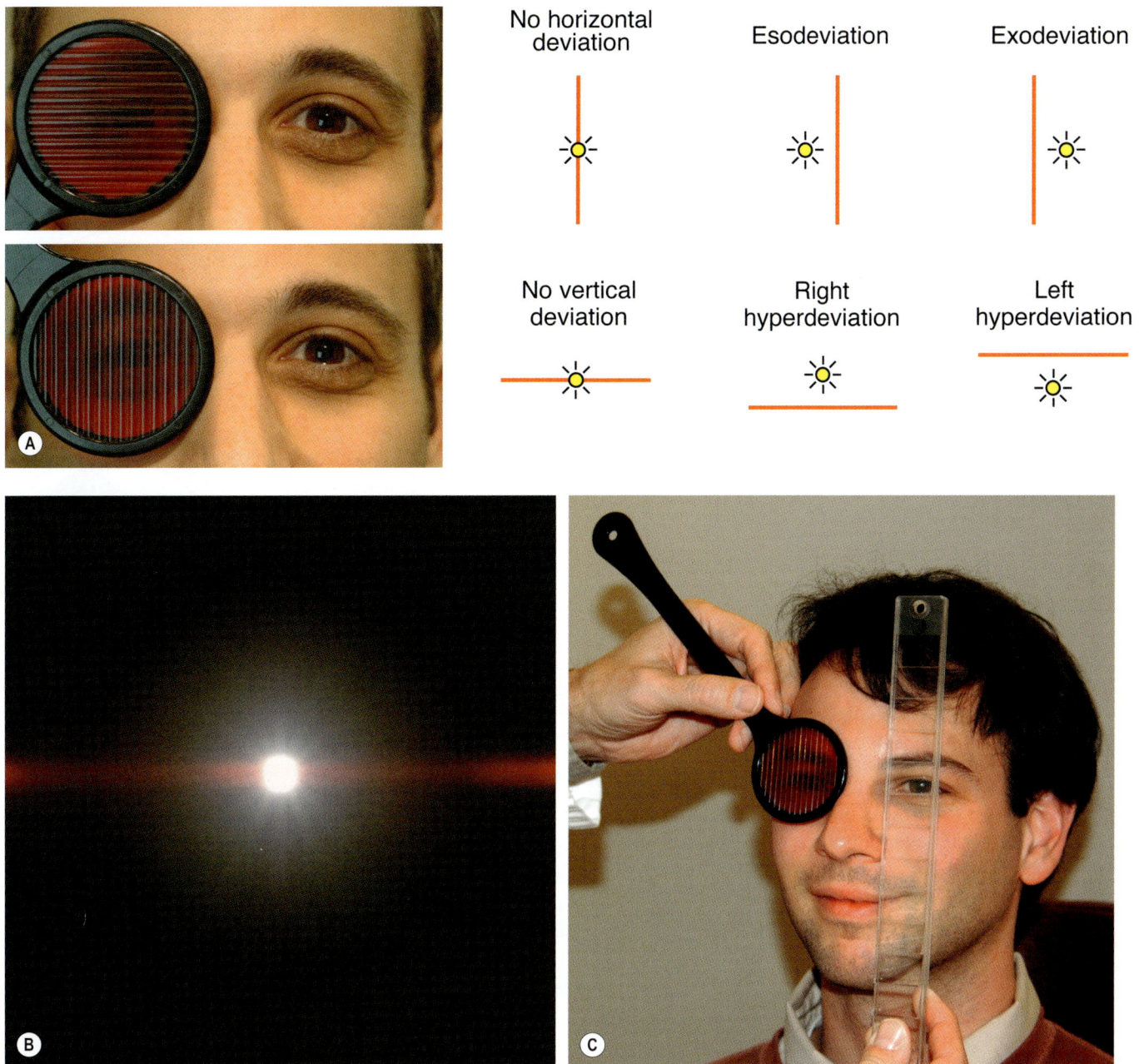

Figure 2–33. A. Maddox rod testing for ocular misalignment. By convention the Maddox rod is always placed over the right eye, and the patient is asked to fixate on a bright white light either at distance or near. A binocular patient's right eye sees a red line, while the uncovered left eye sees the white light. The illustrations on the right are drawn from the patient's perspective. *Top row*, to evaluate horizontal ocular deviations, the bars on the Maddox rod are aligned horizontally, so the patient sees a vertical red line with the right eye. If there is no horizontal deviation, the patient perceives the red line passing through the white light (depicted in yellow for illustrative purposes). If the eyes are esodeviated, the red line, whose image would abnormally fall on nasal retina, appears to the right of the white light ("uncrossed diplopia"). Exodeviated eyes would result in the red line appearing to the left of the light ("crossed diplopia") because the red image would abnormally fall on temporal retina. *Bottom row*, to evaluate vertical deviations, the bars on the Maddox rod should be oriented vertically, so the patient will see a horizontal red line with the right eye. The red line passes through the white light when there is no vertical deviation, while a red line perceived below the light implies a right hyperdeviation, and a white light perceived below the red line indicates a left hyperdeviation (i.e., the lower image corresponds to the hyperdeviated eye). Note that this test will characterize the ocular misalignment, but by itself, in the setting of paralytic or restrictive strabismus, does not indicate which eye has the abnormal motility. **B**. The horizontal red line produced by a Maddox rod superimposed on a bright light source to simulate what a patient sees during a Maddox rod test (image prepared with the assistance of Dr. Clyde Markowitz). **C**. Prisms with Maddox rod. The correct prism measurement (in diopters) is arrived at when the patient indicates the red line passes through the light.

does not identify the paretic eye. Maddox rod testing will reveal the full deviation: tropia plus latent phoria. If misalignment is detected, the direction of gaze that produces the greatest separation between images should be determined by moving the fixation light in the cardinal positions of gaze. Similar to prism/cover techniques, the ocular misalignment in each position can be measured by placing a prism over either eye until the patient sees the line passing through the light (**Fig. 2–33C**). Alternatively, the patient can express the perceived misalignment with his or her fingers or indicate in which directions of gaze the separation of the images is least and greatest. The red glass test is analogous to the Maddox

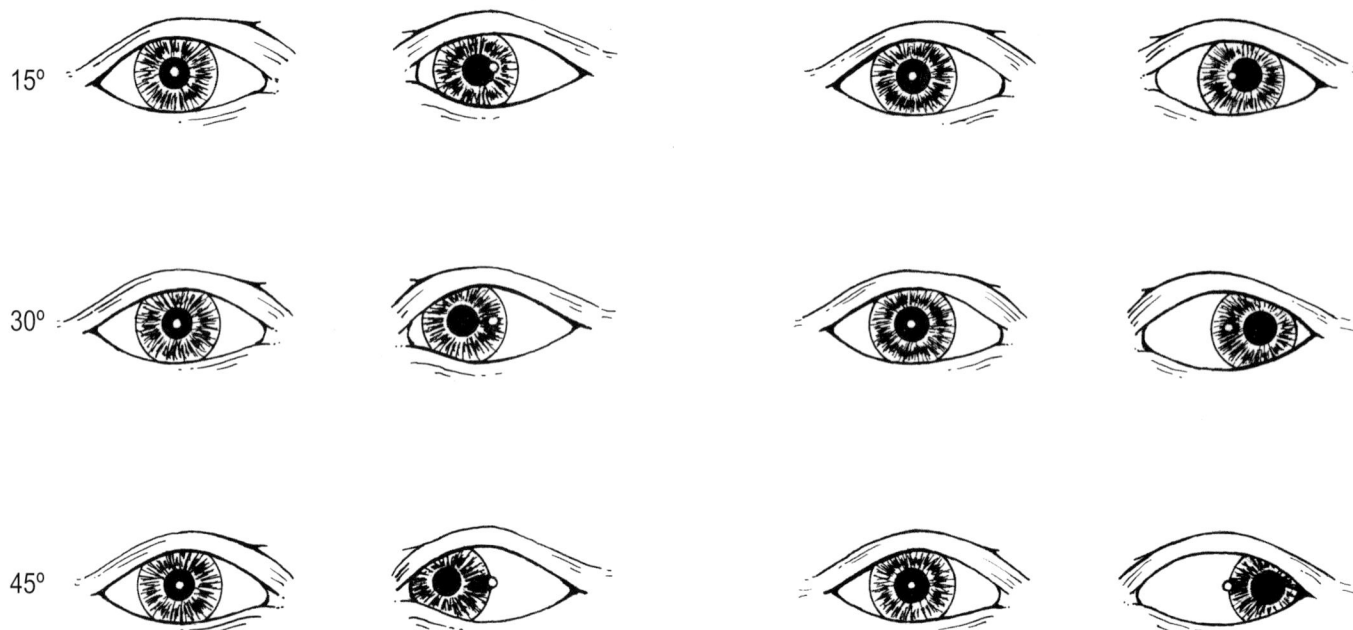

15°				
30°				
45°				

Figure 2–34. Hirschberg test. As the patient fixates on a bright light source, ocular misalignment in degrees can be estimated by observing the relationship of the corneal light reflection and the pupil and iris in the nonfixating, deviated eye. In these drawings the left eye is deviated. Light reflection at the pupillary margin, 15 degrees; in the middle of the iris, 30 degrees; and at the limbus, 45 degrees. These are approximations and obviously vary according to pupillary size.

rod test except that the patient sees a red dot rather than a red line in the red glass test.

In patients with monocular or binocular visual loss or in less cooperative patients such as children, the corneal light reflex can be used to assess ocular misalignment in the Hirschberg and Krimsky tests. In both, a bright light is directed toward the patient's face, and the patient is asked to try to look at the light; the relationship of the light's reflection and the center of the pupil is then observed. The Hirschberg test estimates the angle of misalignment (in degrees) based on the relationship of the light reflex and the iris (**Fig. 2–34**). In the Krimsky test, a variation of the Hirschberg test, a prism is placed over the nonfixating, deviated eye and increased or decreased until the light reflex is in the center of both pupils (**Fig. 2–35**). Both tests give only approximate measurements and are less accurate than prism–alternate and cover tests.[72]

Measurements that are essentially the same in all cardinal positions of gaze define comitant strabismus, while in incomitant strabismus the measurements differ. Incomitant measurements are more commonly associated with a paralyzed extraocular muscle or muscles (paralytic strabismus). On the other hand, comitant measurements are more frequently seen in long-standing, often congenital, deviations unassociated with extraocular muscle palsies (nonparalytic strabismus).

External examination

Any abnormalities of the periorbital region, such as ecchymoses or herniated fat, should be noted. When an orbital process is suspected, the eyes should be palpated and any resistance to retrodisplacement recorded. The amount of

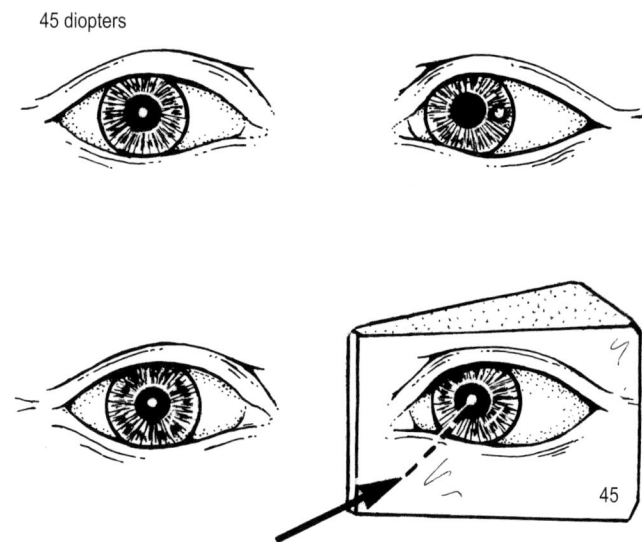

45 diopters

45

Figure 2–35. Krimsky test. As the patient fixates on a bright light source, ocular misalignment in prism diopters can be estimated when a prism moves the light reflection to the center of the cornea in the nonfixating, deviated eye.

anterior protrusion of the globe can be assessed using an exophthalmometer (Hertel, for instance (**Fig. 2–36**)), which is indispensible when following proptosis in a patient with thyroid orbitopathy, for example. Any enophthalmos, or inward displacement, can be measured relative to the fellow eye with an exophthalmometer. Any downward displacement of one globe, termed globe ptosis or dystopia, which occurs in an orbital floor fracture, for instance, can be measured relative to the normal higher eye.[73]

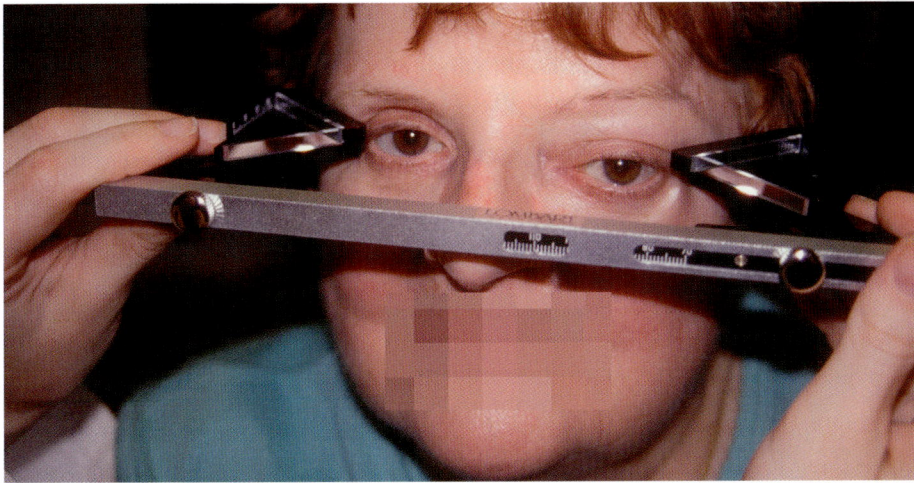

Facial sensation within the three divisions of the trigeminal nerve (V) can be tested with a finger, tissue, or cold object. The examiner should pay particular attention to left/right asymmetries in sensation and differences between the three divisions. Corneal sensation, primarily a function of the first division of the trigeminal nerve (V1), can be evaluated with a wisp of cotton. The corneal blink reflex is described above in the facial nerve section. The masseter and pterygoid muscles are innervated by the motor division of V, which is contained in V3. Jaw strength can be tested by having the patient clench his or her teeth while the examiner palpates the masseter contraction. Opening and protruding the jaw tests the pterygoids; weakness of these muscles may cause lateral jaw deviation. Trigeminal nerve anatomy and disorders of facial sensation are discussed in Chapter 19.

Slit-lamp examination

Slit-lamp examination (biomicroscopy) utilizes what essentially are a horizontally mounted microscope and a special light source to visualize directly the cornea, anterior chamber, iris, lens and vitreous. Intraocular pressures should be measured by applanation. At the bedside, a halogen transilluminator and a magnifying lens (20-diopter lens, for instance) may substitute for a portable slit lamp.

Ophthalmoscopic examination

The posterior pole of the eye can be viewed with a direct ophthalmoscope (**Fig. 2–37**) through an undilated pupil, which allows the optic disc, retinal vasculature, macula, and peripapillary retina to be carefully examined (**Fig. 2–38**). Important details of the optic disc that should be noted include its color and contour and the cup-to-disc ratio as well as the clarity of the margins. The retinal vasculature should be evaluated in detail, with particular attention to the caliber of arteries and veins, branching patterns, and, when suspected, possible emboli. The macula, best observed by asking the patient to look at the direct ophthalmoscope's light, is examined for evidence of atrophy, lipid deposition, detachment, edema, drusen, blood, or change in pigmentation.

After pharmacologic dilation of the pupil with 1% tropicamide (an anticholinergic) and 2.5% phenylephrine (a sympathomimetic) topically, the disc and fundus can be evaluated using a 78- or 90-diopter lens with the slit lamp (**Fig. 2–39**), and the retinal periphery can be examined with a 20-diopter lens via indirect ophthalmoscopy (**Fig. 2–40**). Each technique permits a stereoscopic view of the fundus, which is especially important when evaluating disc swelling, disc contour, cup-to-disc ratio, and macular thickening. In addition, both slit-lamp biomicroscopy and indirect ophthalmoscopy utilize very bright light sources, allowing greater visualization of structures in the back of the eye when there is a media opacity such as a cataract, corneal exposure, or vitritis, which may preclude direct ophthalmoscopy. The mydriatic effect of tropicamide peaks at 20–40 minutes and lasts 2–6 hours, while that of phenylephrine is maximum at 20 minutes and lasts 2–3 hours. Longer acting mydriatics, such as cyclopentolate or atropine, are unnecessary unless a cycloplegic refraction is desired. More detailed information concerning any abnormal appearance of the macula can be obtained through photography, fluorescein angiography, and ocular coherence tomography (OCT) (see Chapter 4).

Directed neurologic examination

Mental status evaluation

The level of the patient's consciousness, attention, and orientation should be documented. Verbal memory can be evaluated by requesting the patient to remember three unrelated words such as *car*, *Philadelphia*, and *honesty*, then after 5 minutes asking him or her to recite the list of items. The important components of language function (fluency, comprehension, reading, writing, repetition, and naming) should also be assessed.

Abnormalities in these "cortically based" neurologic functions often provide clues regarding neuro-ophthalmic diagnosis. For instance, hemianopias that result from lesions of the optic radiations are often associated with mental status abnormalities. Temporal lobe lesions may be accompanied by personality changes, complex partial seizures, memory deficits, fluent aphasia (if the dominant side is involved), or

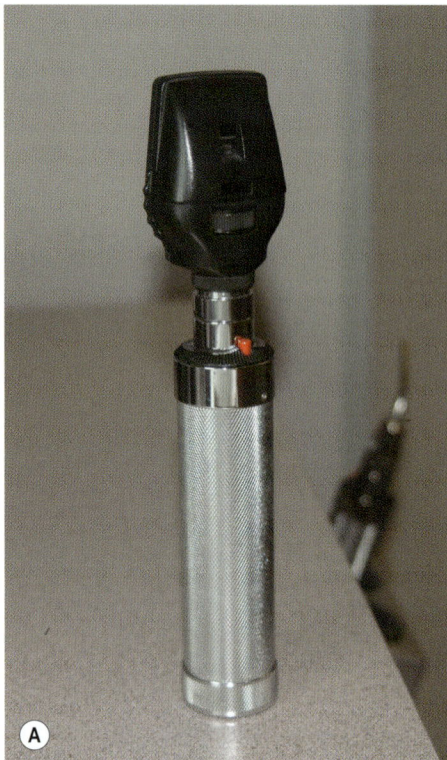

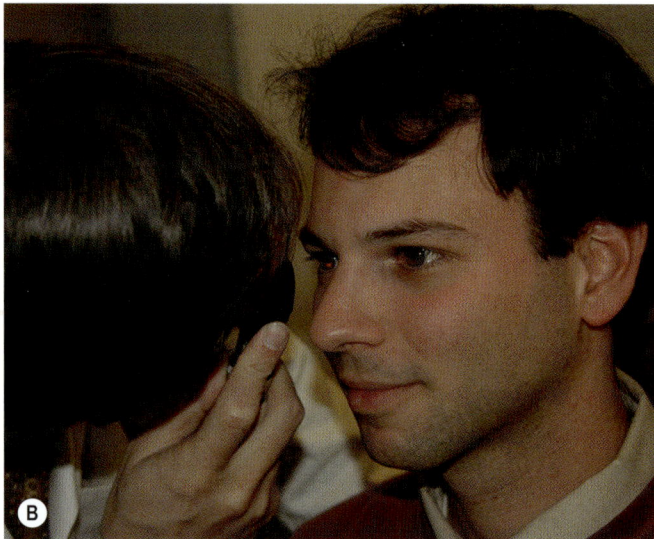

Figure 2–37. A. Direct ophthalmoscope. **B**. Direct ophthalmoscopy.

Klüver–Bucy syndrome (hypersexuality, placidity, hyperorality, visual and auditory agnosia, and apathy) with involvement of the anterior temporal lobes bilaterally. A conduction aphasia, Gerstmann syndrome (finger agnosia, agraphia, acalculia, and right–left disorientation), and tactile agnosia all suggest a dominant parietal lobe process. Left-sided neglect, topographic memory loss, and constructional and dressing apraxias, in association with a left hemianopia, suggest a nondominant, parietal lesion. More parieto-occipital or occipitally based visual disturbances such as Balint syndrome or cortical blindness may accompany dementia in Creutzfeldt–Jakob disease, progressive multifocal leukoencephalopathy, or Alzheimer's disease.

Cranial nerve evaluation

The neuro-ophthalmic examination already assessed cranial nerves II–VII in detail, so, in this part of the evaluation, the function of cranial nerves I and VIII–XII should be documented. Olfactory nerve (I) function can be tested in each nostril with coffee or perfume. The ability to discern whispers or finger rubbing is an adequate screen of acoustic nerve (VIII) function. In the Weber test, a vibrating tuning fork (preferably 128 Hz) is placed in the middle of the forehead, and normally the patient will localize the vibration to the center of the head. In sensory–neural hearing loss the patient localizes the sound to the good ear, while in conductive hearing loss the patient localizes the sound in the affected ear. In the Rinne test, the vibrating tuning fork is placed on the mastoid process (testing bone conduction) then next to the auditory meatus (testing air conduction), and the patient is asked which is heard louder. In sensory–neural hearing loss, air and bone conduction are both reduced, or bone conduction is more affected. In conductive hearing loss, air conduction is reduced.

If the voice is not hoarse, the uvula is midline, and the palate elevates symmetrically, the general somatic efferent portions of the glossopharyngeal (IX) and vagus (X) nerves should be considered intact. The sternocleidomastoid and trapezius muscles, innervated by the accessory (XI) nerve, are responsible for head turning and shoulder shrugging, respectively. Tongue protrusion, a function of the hypoglossal (XII) nerve, should be symmetric. Hypoglossal nerve dysfunction causes ipsilateral tongue deviation when the tongue is extended.

Motor function

The strength of the major muscle groups in the arms and legs should be tested; "0/5" indicates no muscle contraction, "1/5" is a flicker of contraction, "2/5" refers to movement but not against gravity, "3/5" means anti-gravity strength but not against resistance by the examiner, "4/5" refers to mild weakness, and "5/5" indicates normal strength. If present, hypotonia, rigidity, or spasticity also should be noted.

Cerebellar function

Important tests of cerebellar function include the finger–nose–finger and heel-to-knee-to-shin tasks. Difficulty with these is termed *dysmetria*. Dysdiadokinesia, an inability to perform rapid alternating movements and also an indicator of cerebellar dysfunction, may be seen during testing of fine motor movements of the fingers, for instance, or alternately tapping the palm and back of the hand against the thigh. Tandem walking also tests cerebellar function, and difficulty with this or a wide-based unsteady gait is termed *ataxia*.

Sensation

Sensory loss can accompany neuro-ophthalmic disease, especially visual loss due to cortical processes or nutritional optic neuropathies and ocular motility disorders associated with brain stem lesions. Modalities that should be tested

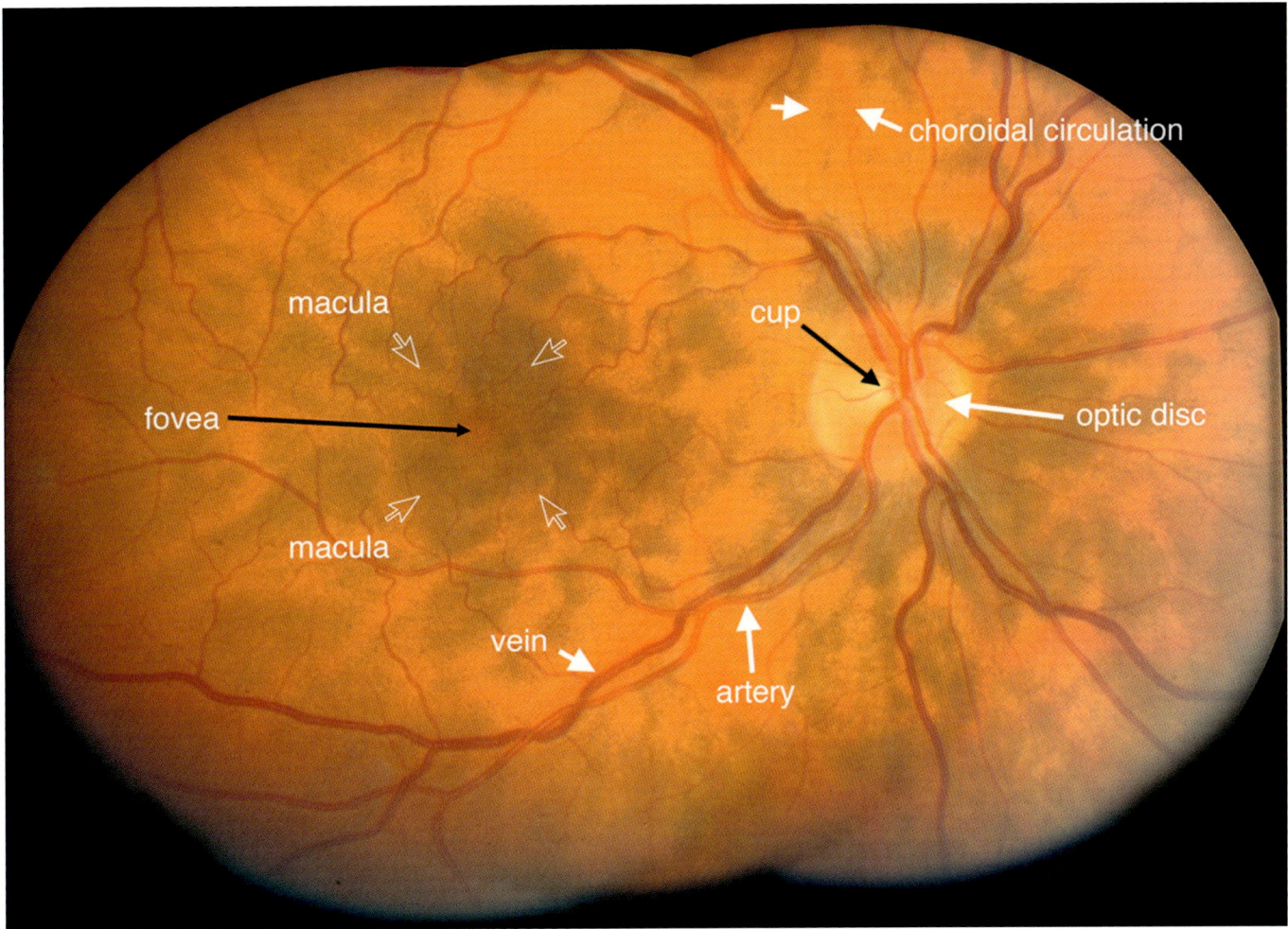

Figure 2–38. Montage of a normal right fundus, with important structures labeled. The region within the open arrows is the *macula*, the center of which is the *fovea*. The *cup* is the center of the *optic disc*. The tigroid appearance of the retina results from pigment interrupted by the *choroidal circulation* (arrows pointing to lighter color region). Retinal *veins* are darker than retinal *arteries*.

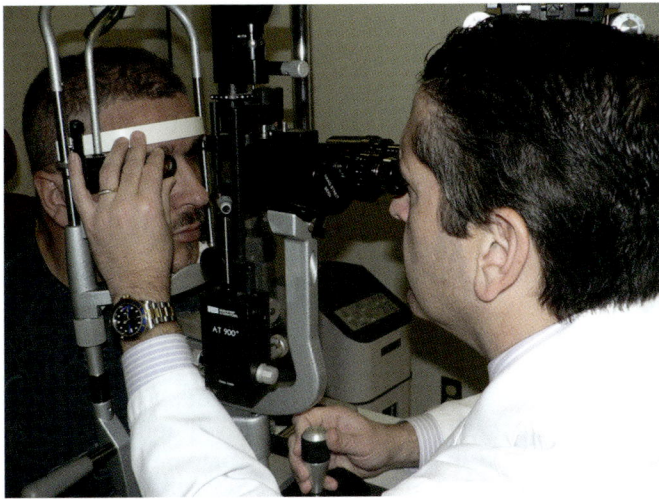

Figure 2–39. Slit-lamp biomicroscopic examination of the fundus with a 90-diopter lens.

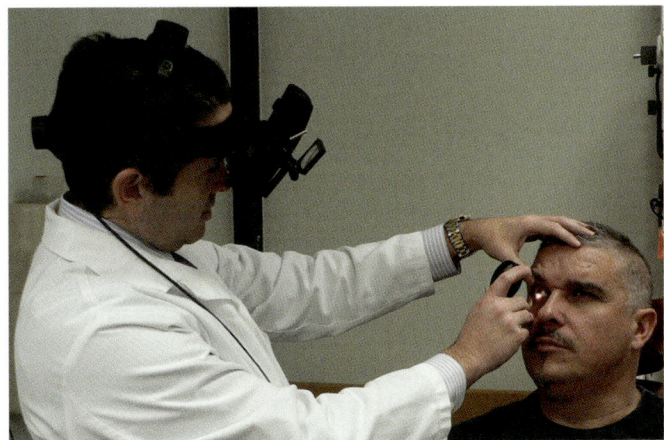

Figure 2–40. Indirect examination of the fundus with a 20-diopter lens.

include light touch, vibration, proprioception, pin prick (pain), and temperature. A homonymous field defect in combination with ipsilateral sensory loss, astereognosis (the inability to identify an object by palpation), decreased two-point discrimination, or graphesthesia (the inability to identify a number written on the hand) strongly suggests a parietal lesion. A process within the nondominant (usually right) parietal lobe can also produce a contralateral neglect syndrome or hemianopia, accompanied by contralateral sensory inattention. Pain or hemianesthesia and an ipsilateral homonymous field deficit implies coinvolvement of the thalamus and optic radiations. In a lateral medullary (Wallenberg) stroke, Horner syndrome, lateropulsion, skew deviation, and nystagmus are often accompanied by ipsilateral facial and contralateral body numbness.

Gait

The patient should be asked to walk in relaxed fashion, and the examiner should observe the patient's posture, balance, mobility, and arm swing. Gait abnormalities can suggest the presence of an extrapyramidal disorder, hemiparesis, or cerebellar dysfunction.

Reflexes

Especially in patients with ocular motor palsies, hypoactive deep tendon reflexes may suggest more widespread neuropathies such as diabetic polyneuropathy, Guillain–Barré syndrome, or mononeuritis multiplex. A tonic pupil may be associated with absent reflexes, particularly at the ankles, in Adie syndrome. Hyperactive reflexes and extensor plantar responses (Babinski sign) suggest upper motor neuron dysfunction when a cortical, brain stem, or spinal cord lesion is suspected.

Directed general examination

A thorough but directed general examination of all patients can often provide important clues to neuro-ophthalmic diagnoses. It would be impossible to list all the abnormalities one might find; however, some examples are reviewed. The patient's general appearance might suggest an underlying chromosomal, endocrinologic, or metabolic disorder. For instance, the disfiguring frontal bossing and enlargement of the mandible and hands are characteristic of acromegaly associated with a growth hormone-secreting pituitary adenoma. Patients with pseudotumor cerebri tend to be young females with obesity or a history of recent weight gain. Skin lesions, such as erythema migrans (Lyme disease) or malar rash (systemic lupus erythematosus), and abnormal discolorations, such as café au lait spots and axillary freckling (neurofibromatosis), or hypopigmented ash-leaf spots (tuberous sclerosis) also may be helpful in guiding the evaluation of patients with visual disturbances.

Evaluation of the heart rate and blood pressure and auscultation of the carotid arteries and heart are important in any patient with a possible vascular process. Amaurosis fugax due to carotid disease may be associated with carotid

Table 2–2 Neuro-ophthalmic examination in a comatose patient

Pupils
Size
Shape
Reactivity
Eye movements
Position
Spontaneous eye movements
Elicited eye movements
Oculocephalic
Cold calorics (if oculocephalic responses absent)
Corneal reflexes
Ophthalmoscopic examination

bruits, which often suggest a high-grade stenosis. A cardiac murmur might suggest an embolic source. Cranial or ocular bruits might indicate an intracranial arteriovenous malformation or carotid–cavernous fistula. In some instances of visual loss due to anterior ischemic optic neuropathy, underlying giant cell arteritis is suggested by tender, cordlike temporal arteries and scalp sensitivity.

Neuro-ophthalmic examination in comatose patients

Plum and Posner[74] emphasize the evaluation of breathing pattern, pupillary function, eye movements, and motor responses in the neurologic assessment of comatose patients, especially with regard to brain stem localization and diagnosis. Thus, neuro-ophthalmic techniques are paramount in this clinical setting (**Table 2–2**). The ocular motility examination is especially important because the pathways governing ocular motility traverse the entire brain stem, so pathology in this region often produces recognizable eye movement abnormalities. Conversely, if the eye movements are normal, it is likely the entire brain stem is intact as well.

The examiner of a comatose patient should decide, in a rostral–caudal fashion, which neuroanatomic structures have been affected by the disease process.[2,75] In general, if the brain stem is intact in a comatose patient, bilateral hemispheric or thalamic disease should be suspected. If the brain stem is injured, the dysfunction should be localized to the midbrain, pons, or medulla.

In the neuro-ophthalmic assessment, pupillary size, shape, and reactivity should be evaluated first.[2] If suspected, the absence of pupillary reaction to light should be confirmed with a magnifying lens. Unreactive pupils are suggestive of midbrain dysfunction or third nerve palsy, perhaps due to uncal herniation. Anisocoria may be due to unilateral Horner syndrome or a third nerve palsy. Bilaterally small pupils may be the result of a pontine hemorrhage or opiate toxicity. More detailed descriptions of these and other pupillary abnormalities in coma are given in Chapter 13.

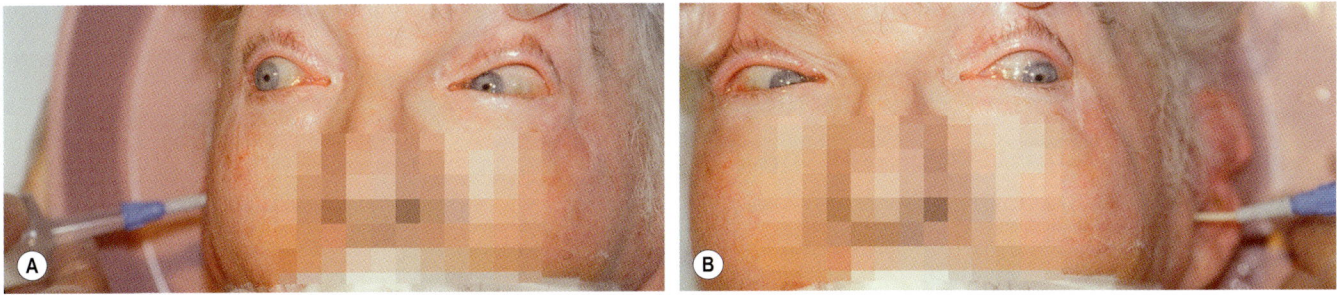

Figure 2–41. Cold caloric testing in a comatose patient. In one method a 60-ml syringe filled with ice water (from a cup of water and ice) is connected to an angiocath with the needle removed. **A.** After excluding tympanic membrane rupture, water is injected into the inner ear canal. A kidney basin is used for water runoff. In this comatose patient, cold water stimulation of the right ear resulted in tonic conjugate deviation of both eyes to the right without nystagmus to the left, suggesting intact brain stem but no cortical function. **B.** Cold water stimulation of the left ear caused tonic conjugate deviation of both eyes to the left without nystagmus to the right.

Next, eye position and spontaneous eye movements should be observed. Overt misalignment such as an esotropia may suggest a sixth nerve palsy, while vertical or oblique misalignment may imply a third nerve palsy or skew deviation (see Chapter 15). Conjugate eye deviation may signify an ipsilateral hemispheric lesion, contralateral pontine process, or contralateral irritative seizure focus (see Chapter 16). Spontaneous roving eye movements in the vertical and horizontal direction indicate normal midbrain and pontine function. Rhythmic, repetitive vertical movements such as ocular bobbing or dipping may imply a pontine lesion (see Chapter 17).

Doll's eye or oculocephalic eye movements can be elicited by turning the head horizontally then vertically. The eyes should deviate in the direction opposite to the head turn. A sixth nerve palsy, an internuclear ophthalmoplegia (see Chapter 15), or conjugate gaze paresis (see Chapter 16) may become evident this way. Oculocephalic eye movements are overly brisk in bilateral hemispheric disease, which diminishes supranuclear influences on the brain stem reflexes. In the early stages of many drug intoxications and metabolic encephalopathy, the eye movements may be abnormal, but pupillary function is preserved. Oculocephalic maneuvers should not be performed in trauma patients with possible cervical spine injury.

If there are no oculocephalic eye movements, a stronger stimulus can be provided by applying ice-cold water against the tympanic membranes, which provokes the vestibulo-ocular reflex (cold caloric test). The patient's head should be angled at 30 degrees to align the horizontal semicircular canals perpendicularly to the floor. After visual inspection to exclude rupture of the tympanic membrane, 30–60 ml of ice water can be irrigated into the external auditory canal using a large syringe and the tubing from a butterfly catheter or an angiocath without the needle (**Fig. 2–41**). A kidney basin should be placed under the ear to contain the overflow of ice water. The cold water creates convection currents in the endolymph of the horizontal semicircular canals, and inhibits the ipsilateral vestibular system. In the normal caloric response, the eyes move slowly and conjugately toward the tested ear (**Fig. 2–41**), followed by a fast corrective phase in the opposite direction to reset the eyes, then the cycle repeats. The slow phase is produced by vestibulo-ocular connections from the unopposed contralateral ear, while the fast phase

is mediated by the frontal eye fields. Warm water stimulation produces a contralateral slow phase and ipsilateral fast phase. The direction of the caloric response is named after the fast phase, and normal responses can be summarized in the mnemonic "COWS," which stands for "cold–opposite, warm–same." Caloric stimulation in the setting of a normal brain stem but bilateral hemispheric dysfunction would produce only an ipsilateral tonic slow phase. Complete brain stem injury would result in no slow or fast eye movements. The other ear can be tested after an interval of a few minutes. Bilateral caloric stimulation with cold water produces a downward slow phase, while stimulation with warm water bilaterally results in an upward slow phase.

Other important neuro-ophthalmic observations in comatose patients include testing of the corneal reflexes and examining the fundus. The corneal reflexes can be evaluated with a sterile cotton swab as described above or with drops of sterile saline. Absent corneal reflexes suggest pontine dysfunction. The ophthalmoscopic examination is often normal, but papilledema would indicate elevated intracranial pressure, for instance, while a vitreous hemorrhage (Terson syndrome) may signify an aneurysmal subarachnoid hemorrhage. Because frequent monitoring of the pupils is important in comatose patients, pharmacologic dilation of the pupils prior to ophthalmoscopic examination in general should be avoided and, if necessary, documented in the patient's record.

References

1. Galetta SL. The neuro-ophthalmologic examination. Neurosurg Clin N Am 1999;10:563–577.
2. Liu GT, Galetta SL. The neuro-ophthalmologic examination (including coma). Ophthalmol Clin North Am 2001;14:23–39.
3. Corbett JJ. The bedside and office neuro-ophthalmology examination. Semin Neurol 2003;23:63–76.
4. Lueck CJ, Gilmour DF, McIlwaine GG. Neuro-ophthalmology: examination and investigation. J Neurol Neurosurg Psychiatry 2004;75 Suppl 4:iv2–11.
5. Frisén L. Visual acuity. In: Clinical Tests of Vision, pp 24–39. New York, Raven Press, 1990.
6. Kniestedt C, Stamper RL. Visual acuity and its measurement. Ophthalmol Clin North Am 2003;16:155–170.
7. Ferris III FL, Kassoff A, Bresnick GH, et al. New visual acuity charts for clinical research. Am J Ophthalmol 1982;94:91–96.
8. Hartmann EE, Dobson V, Hainline L, et al. Preschool vision screening: summary of a task force report. Ophthalmology 2001;108:479–486.
9. Repka MX. Use of Lea symbols in young children. Br J Ophthalmol 2002;86:489–490.

10. Becker R, Hübsch S, Gräf MH, et al. Examination of young children with Lea symbols. Br J Ophthalmol 2002;86:513–516.

11. Vision in Preschoolers Study Group. Preschool visual acuity screening with HOTV and Lea symbols: testability and between-test agreement. Optom Vis Sci 2004;81:678–683.

12. Paine RS, Oppé TE. Neurological examination of children. Clin Dev Med 1966;20/21:99.

13. Mayer DL, Beiser AS, Warner AF, et al. Monocular acuity norms for the Teller Acuity Cards between ages one month and four years. Invest Ophthalmol Vis Sci 1995;36:671–685.

14. Getz LM, Dobson V, Luna B, et al. Interobserver reliability of the Teller acuity card procedure in pediatric patients. Invest Ophthalmol Vis Sci 1996;37:180–187.

15. Eustis HS. Postnatal development. In: Wright KW (ed): Pediatric Ophthalmology and Strabismus, pp 45–59. St. Louis, Mosby, 1995.

16. Frisén L. The neurology of visual acuity. Brain 1980;103:639–670.

17. Owsley C. Contrast sensitivity. Ophthalmol Clin North Am 2003;16:171–177.

18. Arditi A. Improving the design of the letter contrast sensitivity test. Invest Ophthalmol Vis Sci 2005;46:2225–2229.

19. Moseley MJ, Hill AR. Contrast sensitivity testing in clinical practice. Br J Ophthalmol 1994;78:795–797.

20. Balcer LJ, Baier ML, Pelak VS, et al. New low-contrast vision charts: reliability and test characteristics in patients with multiple sclerosis. Mult Scler 2000;6:163–171.

21. Lynch DR, Farmer JM, Rochestie D, et al. Contrast letter acuity as a measure of visual dysfunction in patients with Friedreich ataxia. J Neuroophthalmol 2002;22:270–274.

22. Balcer LJ, Baier ML, Cohen JA, et al. Contrast letter acuity as a visual component for the Multiple Sclerosis Functional Composite. Neurology 2003;61:1367–1373.

23. Cole BL, Lian KY, Lakkis C. The new Richmond HRR pseudoisochromatic test for colour vision is better than the Ishihara. Clin Exp Optom 2006;89:73–80.

24. Aroichane M, Pieramici DJ, Miller NR, et al. A comparative study of Hardy-Rand-Rittler and Ishihara colour plates for the diagnosis of nonglaucomatous optic neuropathy. Can J Ophthalmol 1996;31:350–355.

25. Melamud A, Hagstrom S, Traboulsi E. Color vision testing. Ophthalmic Genet 2004;25:159–187.

26. Swanson WH, Cohen JM. Color vision. Ophthalmol Clin North Am 2003;16:179–203.

27. Hart WM. Acquired dyschromatopsias. Surv Ophthalmol 1987;32:10–31.

28. McCulley TJ, Golnik KC, Lam BL, et al. The effect of decreased visual acuity on clinical color vision testing. Am J Ophthalmol 2006;141:194–196.

29. Pandit RJ, Gales K, Griffiths PG. Effectiveness of testing visual fields by confrontation. Lancet 2001;358:1339–1340.

30. Lee MS, Balcer LJ, Volpe NJ, et al. Laser pointer visual field screening. J Neuroophthalmol 2003;23:260–263.

31. Liu GT, Ronthal M. Reflex blink to visual threat. J Clin Neuroophthalmol 1992;12:47–56.

32. Sadun AA. Distinguishing between clinical impairments due to optic nerve or macular disease. Metab Pediatr Syst Ophthalmol 1990;13:79–84.

33. Glaser JS, Savino PJ, Sumers KD, et al. The photostress recovery test in the clinical assessment of visual function. Am J Ophthalmol 1977;83:255–260.

34. Wu G, Weiter JJ, Santos S, et al. The macular photostress test in diabetic retinopathy and age-related macular degeneration. Arch Ophthalmol 1990;108:1556–1558.

35. Zabriskie NA, Kardon RH. The pupil photostress test. Ophthalmology 1994;101:1122–1130.

36. Margrain TH, Thomson D. Sources of variability in the clinical photostress test. Ophthalmic Physiol Opt 2002;22:61–67.

37. Rizzo M. Clinical assessment of complex visual dysfunction. Semin Neurol 2000;20:75–87.

38. Weintraub S, Mesulam MM. Visual hemispatial inattention: stimulus parameters and exploratory strategies. J Neurol Neurosurg Psychiatr 1988;51:1481–1488.

39. Albert ML. A simple test of visual neglect. Neurology 1973;23:658–664.

40. Brazis PW, Graff-Radford NR, Newman NJ, et al. Ishihara color plates as a test for simultanagnosia. Am J Ophthalmol 1998;126:850–851.

41. Shin MS, Park SY, Park SR, et al. Clinical and empirical applications of the Rey-Osterrieth Complex Figure Test. Nat Protoc 2006;1:892–899.

42. Kumral E, Evyapan D. Reversed clock phenomenon. A right-hemisphere syndrome. Neurology 2000;55:151–152.

43. Ishiai S, Sugishita M, Ichikawa T, et al. Clock-drawing test and unilateral spatial neglect. Neurology 1993;43:106–110.

44. Freedman M, Leach L, Kaplan E, et al. Clock Drawing. A Neuropsychological Analysis, pp 3–8, 98–127. New York, Oxford University Press, 1994.

45. MacLachlan C, Howland HC. Normal values and standard deviations for pupil diameter and interpupillary distance in subjects aged 1 month to 19 years. Ophthalmic Physiol Opt 2002;22:175–182.

46. Thompson HS, Corbett JJ, Cox TA. How to measure the relative afferent pupillary defect. Surv Ophthalmol 1981;26:39–42.

47. Levitan P. Pupillary escape in disease of the retina or optic nerve. Arch Ophthalmol 1959;62:768–779.

48. Girkin CA. Evaluation of the pupillary light response as an objective measure of visual function. Ophthalmol Clin North Am 2003;16:143–153.

49. Bremner FD. Pupil assessment in optic nerve disorders. Eye 2004;18:1175–1181.

50. Borchert M, Sadun AA. Bright light stimuli as a mask of relative afferent pupillary defects. Am J Ophthalmol 1988;106:98–99.

51. Johnson LN. The effect of light intensity on measurement of the relative afferent pupillary defect. Am J Ophthalmol 1990;109:481–482.

52. Lagrèze W-DA, Kardon RH. Correlation of relative afferent pupillary defect and estimated retinal ganglion cell loss. Graefe's Arch Clin Exp Ophthalmol 1998;236:401–404.

53. Cox TA. Pupillary escape. Neurology 1992;42:1271–1273.

54. Burde RM, Landau WM. Clinical neuromythology. XII. Shooting backward with Marcus Gunn: a circular exercise in paralogic. Neurology 1993;43:2444–2447.

55. Enyedi LB, Dev S, Cox TA. A comparison of the Marcus Gunn and alternating light tests for afferent pupillary defects. Ophthalmology 1998;105:871–873.

56. Bell RA, Thompson HS. Relative afferent pupillary defect in optic tract hemianopsias. Am J Ophthalmol 1978;85:538–540.

57. Portnoy JZ, Thompson HS, Lennarson L, et al. Pupillary defects in amblyopia. Am J Ophthalmol 1983;96:609–614.

58. King JT, Galetta SL, Flamm ES. Relative afferent pupillary defect with normal vision in a glial brainstem tumor. Neurology 1991;41:945–946.

59. Chen CJ, Scheufele M, Sheth M, et al. Isolated relative afferent pupillary defect secondary to contralateral midbrain compression. Arch Neurol 2004;61:1451–1453.

60. Glazer-Hockstein C, Brucker AJ. The detection of a relative afferent pupillary defect. Am J Ophthalmol 2002;134:142–143.

61. Browning DJ, Tiedeman JS. The test light affects quantitation of the afferent pupillary defect. Ophthalmology 1987;94:53–55.

62. Kawasaki A, Moore P, Kardon RH. Variability of the relative afferent pupillary defect. Am J Ophthalmol 1995;120:622–633.

63. Volpe NJ, Plotkin ES, Maguire MG, et al. Portable pupillography of the swinging flashlight test to detect afferent pupillary defects. Ophthalmology 2000;107:1913–1921; discussion 1922.

64. Kasthurirangan S, Glasser A. Age related changes in the characteristics of the near pupil response. Vision Res 2006;46:1393–1403.

65. Nunery WR, Cepela M. Levator function in the evaluation and management of blepharoptosis. Ophthalmol Clin N Am 1991;4:1–16.

66. Martin TJ, Yeatts RP. Abnormalities of eyelid position and function. Semin Neurol 2000;20:31–42.

67. Galetta SL, Liu GT, Volpe NJ. Diagnostic tests in neuro-ophthalmology. Neurol Clin 1996;14:201–222.

68. May M, Galetta SL. The facial nerve and related disorders of the face. In: Glaser JS (ed): Neuro-Ophthalmology, 3rd edn, pp 239–278. Philadelphia, J. B. Lippincott, 1999.

69. Kaye SB, O'Donnell N, Holden R. Recording sensory and motor aspects of strabismus. J Pediatr Ophthalmol Strabismus 1997;34:188–190.

70. Francis I, Loughhead J. Bell's phenomena: a study of 508 patients. Aust J Ophthalmol 1984;12:15–21.

71. Wright KW. Introduction to strabismus and the ocular-motor examination. In: Wright KW (ed): Pediatric Ophthalmology and Strabismus, pp 139–158. St. Louis, Mosby, 1995.

72. Choi R, Kushner BJ. The accuracy of experienced strabismologists using the Hirschberg and Krimsky tests. Ophthalmology 1998;105:1301–1306.

73. Janecka IP. Correction of ocular dystopia. Plast Reconstr Surg 1996;97:892–899.

74. Plum F, Posner JB. The pathologic physiology of signs and symptoms of coma. In: The Diagnosis of Stupor and Coma, 3rd edn, pp 1–86. Philadelphia, F. A. Davis, 1980.

75. Liu GT. Coma. Neurosurg Clin N Am 1999;10:579–586.

Part **Two**

**Visual loss and other disorders of
the afferent visual pathway**

CHAPTER **3**

Visual loss: overview, visual field testing, and topical diagnosis

The afferent visual pathways encompass structures which perceive, relay, and process visual information: the eyes, optic nerves (cranial nerve II), chiasm, tracts, lateral geniculate nuclei, optic radiations, and striate cortex (**Fig. 3–1**). Lesions anterior to and including the chiasm may result in visual acuity (clarity) loss, color deficits, and visual field defects (abnormal central or peripheral vision). From a neuro-ophthalmic standpoint, unilateral retro-chiasmal (posterior to the chiasm) disturbances can present primarily with homonymous (both eyes involved with the same laterality) visual field defects without acuity loss. Higher order processing, instrumental in interpreting visual images, occurs in extrastriate association cortex. Abnormalities in these areas can cause, for instance, deficits in object recognition, color perception, motion detection, and visual attention (neglect of visual stimuli in left or right hemifields).

This chapter will provide an overview of these structures, detail methods of visual field testing, then describe a framework for the localization and diagnosis of disorders affecting the afferent visual pathways. Determining *where* the lesion is first, then finding out *what* it is second, is the advocated approach. Further details regarding these structures' anatomy, blood supply, organization, and neuro-ophthalmic symptoms, as well as the differential diagnosis of lesions affecting them, are detailed in Chapters 4–12.

Neuroanatomy of the afferent visual pathway: overview

The eye and retina

The eyes are the primary sensory organs of the visual system. Before reaching the retina, light travels through the ocular media, consisting of the cornea, anterior chamber, lens, and vitreous. The size of the pupil, like the aperture of a camera, regulates the amount of light reaching the retina. The cornea and lens focus light rays to produce a clear image on the retina in the absence of refractive error, and the ciliary muscle can change the lens shape to adjust for objects at different distances (*accommodation*).

Retinal photoreceptors hyperpolarize in response to light. Cone photoreceptors are more sensitive to color and are concentrated in the posterior pole of the retina, or macula, the center of which is the fovea. Rod photoreceptors, more important for night vision, predominate in the retinal periphery. Visual information is processed via horizontal, bipolar, and amacrine cells before reaching the ganglion cells, the axons of which make up the innermost portion of the retina and converge to form the optic disc and optic nerve. Temporal to the fovea, the axons are strictly oriented above and

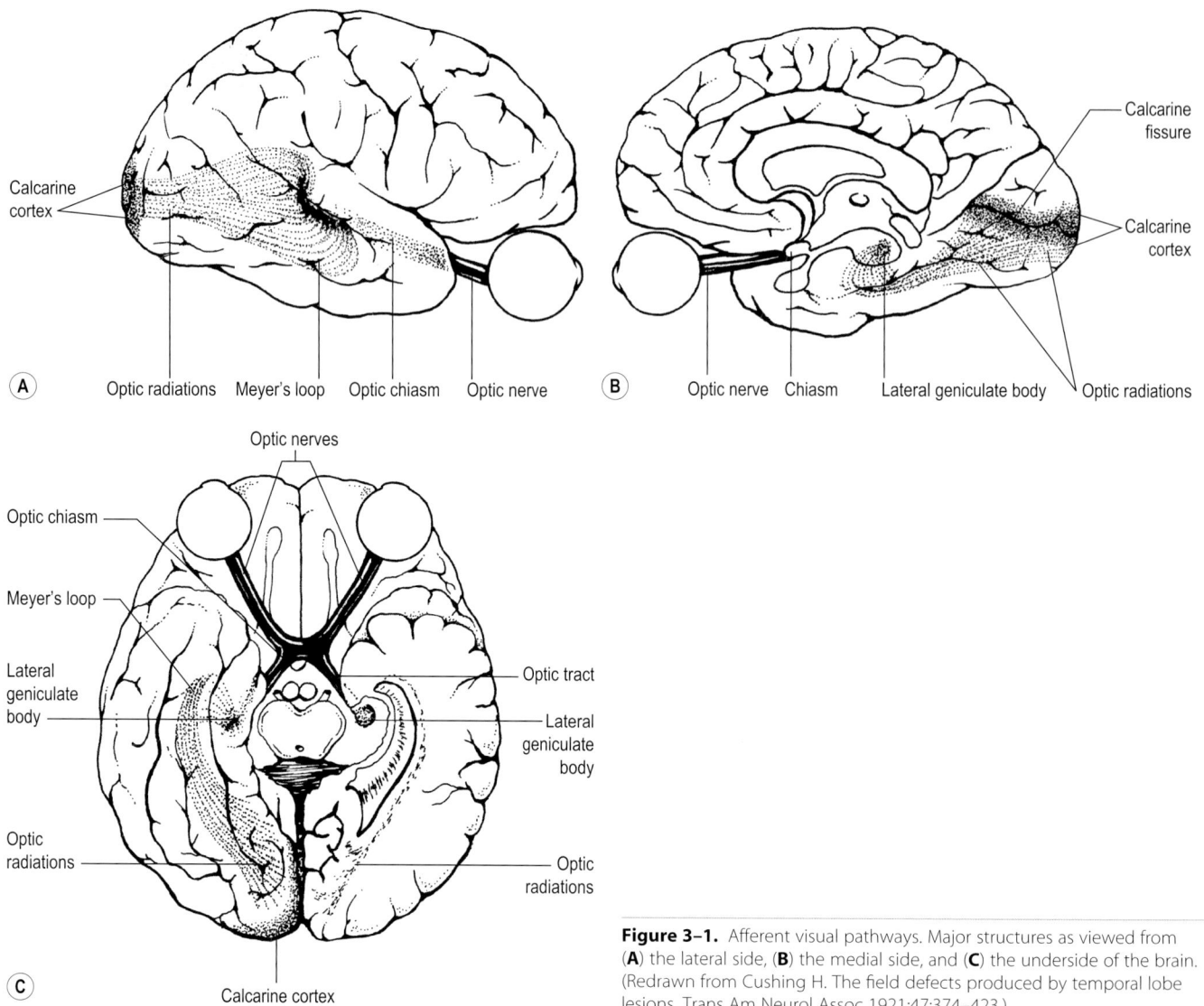

Figure 3–1. Afferent visual pathways. Major structures as viewed from (**A**) the lateral side, (**B**) the medial side, and (**C**) the underside of the brain. (Redrawn from Cushing H. The field defects produced by temporal lobe lesions. Trans Am Neurol Assoc 1921;47:374–423.)

below the horizontal raphae. For instance, ganglion cells above the raphae project their axons in an arcuate pattern to the top of the optic nerve (see **Fig. 5–1**). The optic disc represents the intraocular portion of the optic nerve anterior to the lamina cribrosa (see **Fig. 2–38**). The retina is normally transparent, and the orange-red color visible on fundus examination is due to the retinal pigment epithelium and choroidal circulation.

The retina nasal to the macula receives visual information from the temporal field, and the temporal retina from the nasal field (**Fig. 3–2**). The superior and inferior halves of the retina have a similar crossed relationship with respect to lower and upper fields of vision.

The ophthalmic artery, a branch of the internal carotid, provides most of the blood supply to the eye although there are external carotid anastomoses (see **Fig. 4–1**). The first major branch of the ophthalmic artery, the central retinal artery, pierces the dura of the optic nerve behind the globe, then travels within the nerve to emerge at the optic disc to supply the inner two-thirds of the retina. The ophthalmic

artery also gives rise to the posterior ciliary arteries, which supply the optic nerve head, choroid, and outer third of the retina.

Optic nerve, chiasm, and tract

The optic nerve has four major portions: intraocular, intraorbital, intracanalicular, and intracranial. Posterior to the lamina cribrosa, optic nerve axons are myelinated by oligodendrocytes similar to those in white matter tracts in the brain and spinal cord.

Axons from the two optic nerves join at the optic chiasm, which lies in the suprasellar region, superior to the diaphragma sella and inferior to the third ventricle and hypothalamus. At the chiasm, fibers from the nasal retina cross, and the most ventral axons from the inferior nasal retina bend into the most proximal aspect of the contralateral optic nerve (*Wilbrand's knee*), while the fibers from the temporal retina remain ipsilateral in the lateral portion of the chiasm (**Fig. 3–2**). The ratio of crossed to uncrossed fibers is 53:47.[1]

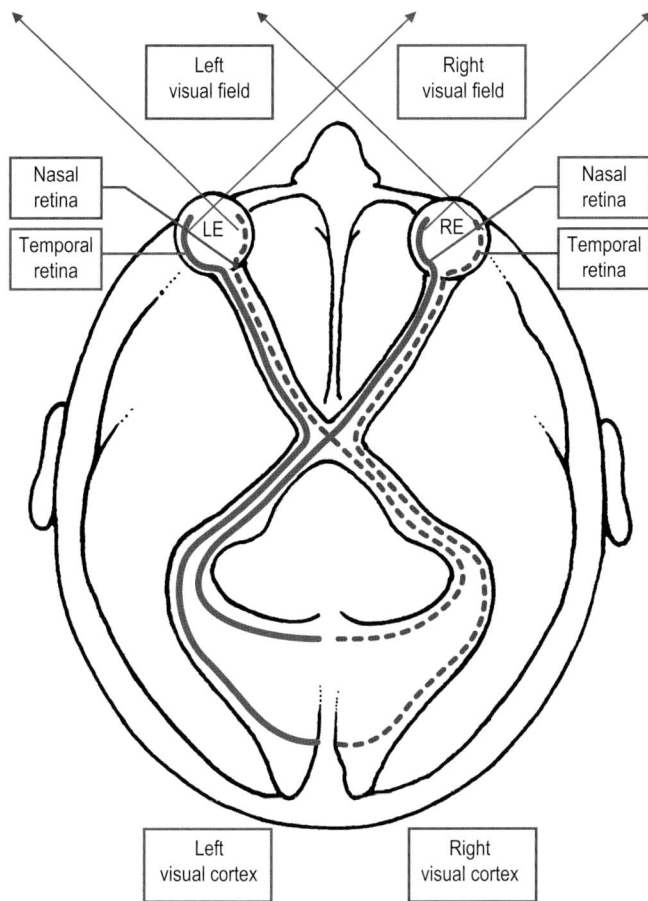

Figure 3–2. Separation of pathways for temporal and nasal visual fields. Visual information from the temporal visual field projects to the nasal retina, then via ganglion cell axons in the optic nerve crosses in the chiasm to reach the contralateral optic radiations and striate cortex anteriorly. In contrast, visual information from the nasal visual field projects to the temporal retina and the ipsilateral optic radiations and posterior striate cortex. Note that visual information from the left visual field (*dotted lines*) projects to the right cerebral hemisphere, and visual information from the right visual field (*solid lines*) projects to the left cerebral hemisphere. LE, left eye; RE, right eye. (Redrawn from Zeki S. A Vision of the Brain, p 23. Blackwell Scientific Publications, Cambridge, UK, 1993, with permission.)

Ipsilateral temporal fibers and contralateral nasal fibers join to form the optic tracts.

Geniculocalcarine pathway

At the lateral geniculate nucleus, a part of the thalamus located above the ambient cistern, the ganglion cell axons in the optic tract synapse with neurons destined to become the optic radiations. This latter structure is divided functionally and anatomically. Fibers coursing through the temporal lobe, termed *Meyer's loop*, subserve visual information from the lower retina and connect to the inferior bank of the calcarine cortex. The parietal portion of the optic radiations relays information from the upper retina to the superior bank of the calcarine cortex. Most of the optic radiations derive their blood supply from the middle cerebral artery. The medial temporal section is supplied in part by branches of the posterior cerebral artery.

Striate cortex

Brodmann area 17 (or V1, primary or striate cortex) is the end organ of the afferent visual system and is located within the calcarine cortex in the occipital lobe. Most of the striate cortex, especially the portion situated posteriorly, is devoted to macular vision. Superior and inferior banks of calcarine cortex subserve contralateral inferior and superior quadrants, respectively. The majority of the occipital lobe is supplied by the posterior cerebral artery with a contribution from the middle cerebral artery in the occipital pole region.

Visual association areas

Higher processing of visual information occurs, for example, in the lingual and fusiform gyri bordering the inferior calcarine bank in structures believed to be equivalent to area V4 in monkeys, which is responsible for color vision. In an oversimplification, temporal lobe structures govern visual recognition and memory, while parietal lobe areas are responsible for motion and spatial analysis.

Visual field testing

In patients with visual loss, the pattern of the visual field deficit can be highly localizing. Confrontation field testing, the techniques of which are detailed in Chapter 2, often provide extremely useful information. In general, the technique is specific, as field loss detected by confrontation is usually real.[2,3] However, confrontation is insensitive, as more subtle defects may be missed.[3,4]

More sensitive, reproducible, and precise visual field testing may be achieved by *automated or computerized threshold perimetry* or *kinetic testing with a Goldmann perimeter or tangent screen*. Threshold computerized perimetry of the central 30 degrees of vision, although lengthy and tedious, in many instances is a more objective and more reproducible test for patients with optic neuropathies and chiasmal disturbances and those requiring serial testing. The kinetic techniques, because they are shorter and allow interaction with the examiner, may be more appropriate for screening and for patients with significant neurologic impairment. Manual kinetic perimetry also allows the knowledgeable examiner to "search" for suspected field defects. Computerized perimetry, owing to its wide availability and ease of administration, is currently the most popular test method.

Table 3–1 summarizes the advantages, disadvantages, and most appropriate neuro-ophthalmic uses of each modality. The examiner should always keep in mind that all modalities for visual field evaluation are inherently subjective and depend on the patient's level of alertness, cooperation, ability to fixate centrally, and response rapidity. In addition, astute patients feigning visual loss can voluntarily alter their visual fields during perimetric testing (see Chapter 11).

In most cases, the visual field is tested for each eye separately. Except in patients using miotic eye drops for glaucoma, for instance, field testing should take place before pharmacologic dilation of the pupils, which tends to worsen

Table 3–1 Advantages, disadvantages, and most appropriate neuro-ophthalmic uses of computerized threshold, Goldmann kinetic, and tangent screen kinetic perimetry

	Advantages	Disadvantages	Best neuro-ophthalmic uses
Computerized threshold	Reproducible More objective More standardized Less reliance on a technician Intertechnician variability less important	Lengthy Tedious	Optic neuropathy Papilledema Chiasmal disorders Repeated follow-up
Goldmann kinetic	Short Driven by technician or doctor. Skilled perimetrist or physician can focus attention on suspected defect areas	More subjective Depends on the skills of the perimetrist	Retrochiasmal disorders Neurologically impaired patients Patients who are unable to do a computerized field test Severe visual loss Functional vision loss
Tangent screen kinetic	Short Can be performed in the examination room	Central 30° only	Central field defects Functional visual loss

performance even if accommodative dysfunction has been corrected with lenses.[5,6]

Visual fields are recorded so that the field of the right eye is on the right and the field of the left eye is on the left (see **Fig. 2–11**). The blind spot, caused by the absence of photoreceptors overlying the optic nerve, is located approximately 15 degrees temporal to and slightly below fixation and is drawn as an area without vision. As previously stated, *homonymous defects* are those present in both eyes with the same laterality. A *hemianopia* refers to loss of half of the visual field, respecting the vertical (usually) or horizontal meridian. *Congruity* refers to the symmetry of the field defect in both eyes.

Visual field testing in children. Some studies have suggested that computerized visual field testing, usually requiring several minutes per eye, can be performed reliably in young children.[7,8] However, in our experience most children less than 10 years of age have difficulty with the monotony and length of formal visual field testing, leading to high numbers of errors. Kinetic (Goldmann) visual field testing is easier for young, less cooperative children, but there is still great test–retest variability in this age group. Therefore, clinical decision-making based upon unreliable visual fields and small changes during serial visual field testing in children is problematic.

The hill of vision concept

Although the visual field is plotted on a piece of paper in two dimensions, it can be conceptualized three dimensionally as an "island or hill of vision in a sea of darkness" (**Fig. 3–3**).[9,10] The z-axis value indicates visual sensitivity, while the location within the field of vision is plotted in the x,y-plane. Foveal vision has the highest sensitivity but extends nasally and temporally only a few degrees. Thus, with increasing sensitivity (up on the z-axis), the field of vision decreases in size, and the hill peaks at fixation ($x = 0$, $y = 0$). In contrast, at low sensitivities (lower on the z-axis), the field

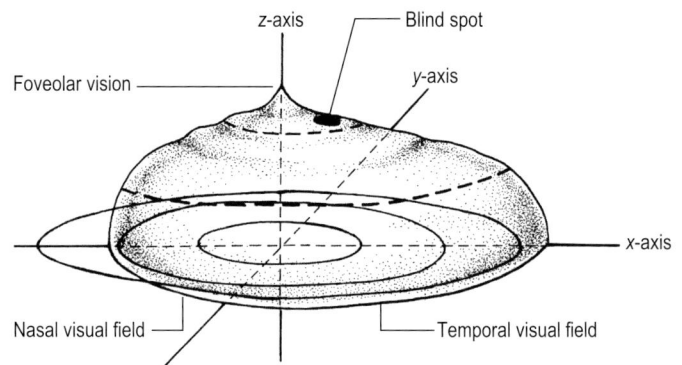

Figure 3–3. "Island of vision in a sea of blindness." This three-dimensional representation of the visual field plots visual sensitivity along the z-axis versus location within the x,y-plane.

of vision is much larger. The blind spot is depicted as an opening in the island temporal to the central peak,[11] and the opening extends all the way to the bottom of the island. Sensitivity falls more rapidly nasally than temporally. Outside of the x- and y-coordinates delimiting the bottom of the island, nothing is seen.

The major difference between threshold (static) and kinetic perimetry can be described using the hill of vision concept. Threshold perimetry determines the visual sensitivity (z-axis value) at any particular x,y point. On the other hand, kinetic perimetry plots the visual field (in the x,y-plane) for a stimulus at a given sensitivity (z-axis) level. The plot of a kinetic field can be considered to be a two-dimensional representation of the hill of vision (**Fig. 3–4**).

When visual field defects occur, the corresponding part of the island is lost (**Fig. 3–5**). Generalized visual field constriction can be conceptualized as the island of vision sinking into the sea of blindness. In these cases, the central peak occurs at a lower sensitivity level, and the field of vision at any particular sensitivity level is smaller.

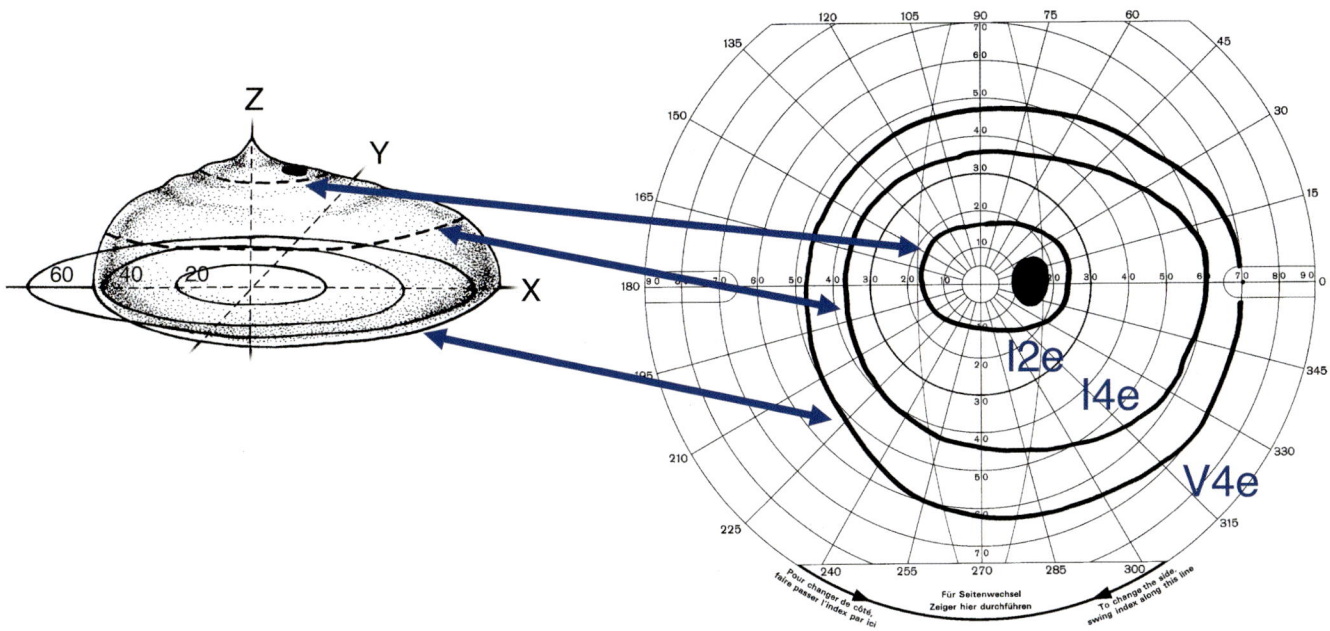

Figure 3–4. The island of vision (*left*) contains the information produced by kinetic perimetry (*right*). Kinetic perimetry plots the visual field (in the *x,y*-plane) for a stimulus at a given sensitivity (*z*-axis) level. Thus each isopter (I4e plot, for instance) on the kinetic perimetry can be translated from the island of vision.

Computerized threshold perimetry

There are many types of computerized threshold perimetry in wide use, including Humphrey (Carl Zeiss), Octopus, and Dicon.[12] The major advantages of computerized perimetry over other forms are that it permits more standardized testing procedures,[13,14] it requires less technician skill, and it is affected less by intertechnician variability.[15] Some studies have also demonstrated that automated computerized perimetry may be more sensitive to subtle field loss than Goldmann perimetry.[15] The discussion in this section will highlight the testing features of the Humphrey perimeter (**Fig. 3–6**), which is the most popular.

In the Humphrey threshold 30–2 test, the computer presents white light stimuli against a white background within the central 30 degrees of vision of each eye. Lens correction for near is provided, and the patient looks at a central target and hits a button when he or she sees the light. The stimulus size is kept the same, but the stimulus intensity is varied, and the computer records the intensity of the dimmest stimulus the patient saw at various points in the visual field. This *threshold intensity* is recorded in decibels, and the higher the number, the dimmer the stimulus and the higher the sensitivity. The computer also determines the location of the blind spot.

The test can be laborious and sometimes soporific, even for the most cooperative individuals. In the full threshold evaluation, it is not unusual for each eye to be tested with over 450 points over approximately 15 minutes. Swedish Interactive Threshold Algorithm (SITA) software programs may save up to 50–70% of test time for a Humphrey field.[16,17] Largely because the shorter test time vastly improves patient cooperation, sensitivity and reproducibility are enhanced in neuro-ophthalmic patients with these programs.[18] Thus SITA-Standard and Fast programs have become vastly preferred over standard full threshold tests in clinical practice.[19,20]

Patient reliability during a Humphrey field test is reflected in the number and proportion of fixation losses, and false-positive and false-negative responses (**Fig. 3–7**). When the patient responds to a stimulus presented in the originally plotted blind spot, a *fixation loss* is thought to have occurred. A *false-positive* response happens when the patient hits the buzzer but no light stimulus was presented. When a patient does not hit the buzzer if a stimulus of identical location and greater intensity to one that was previously detected is presented, this is considered a *false-negative* response. Either a fixation loss rate of 20% or a false-positive or a false-negative rate of 33% indicates an unreliable visual field.[21] Severe and nonorganic (see Ch. 11) visual field loss may be associated with abnormally high false-negative rates.

The printout displays the visual field data in several ways (**Fig. 3–7**),[21] including some with statistical analysis. The threshold intensities are presented in raw data form. The *gray scale* provides a graphical representation of the threshold intensities, and offers the best information for a "quick-glance" interpretation of the threshold visual field. However, the gray scale summary can be misleading and important defects may not be evident. The *total deviation map* plots the difference between each measured threshold value and those of age-matched normal values for each point in the visual field. The *pattern deviation map* accents local visual field defects in the total deviation map by correcting for the overall height of the hill of vision. This is the most accurate representation of the visual field and should be reviewed in all patients and used in comparisons for changes in examinations over time. Diffuse field loss, as might occur with a cataract, are factored out this way.

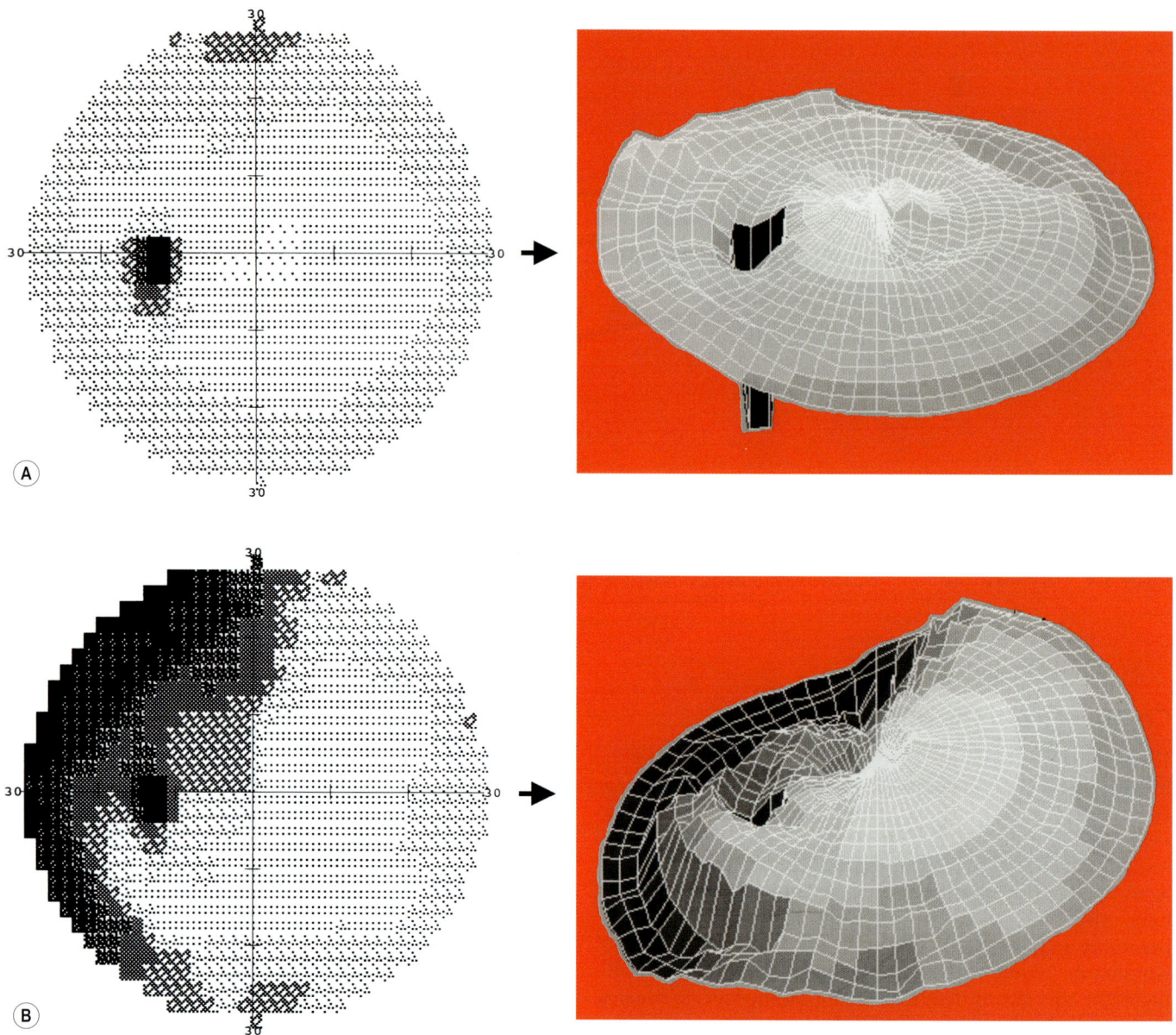

Figure 3–5. Dicon computerized threshold fields and corresponding hill of vision plots. **A.** Normal visual field of a left eye. **B.** Temporal field defect, with depression of the hill corresponding to the defective visual field. (Courtesy of Lawrence Gray, OD)

Probability displays are provided for the total deviation and pattern deviation maps. Of the global visual field indices, the *mean deviation* (MD) is the most important clinically in neuro-ophthalmic patients because it gives a "numerical equivalent" of the visual field. This figure is an average of the numbers in the total deviation plot, with each value weighted according to the normal range at that point. As a patient's visual field worsens, because of an enlarging scotoma for instance, the mean deviation becomes more negative. Serial visual fields can be compared by following the mean deviation.

Several factors may influence the patient's performance on this test. The learning curve is steep, and individuals undergoing threshold perimetry have a natural tendency to provide more reliable visual fields on subsequent testing.[22] Mild ptosis may be associated with depression of the superior visual field,[23] and cataracts, pupillary miosis,[24] and

myopia[25] may cause diffusely decreased sensitivity. The influence of age on the visual fields of normal individuals has also been studied, and a decrease in sensitivity with increasing age was found.[26,27] There may also be some variability in performance over time in different disease states.[28]

During screening full-field examinations, such as 120-point ones, the computer presents static light stimuli of fixed size and intensity, and the patient presses the button if he or she sees them. They are not typically threshold tests, and the plot depicts merely whether the light stimulus was seen or not. A "quantify defects" modification can be used to threshold test missed points. The full-field screens are helpful in detecting large field defects such as hemianopias or altitudinal field loss. However, because the points can be spread far apart, often the information provided is so vague that the test becomes uninterpretable.

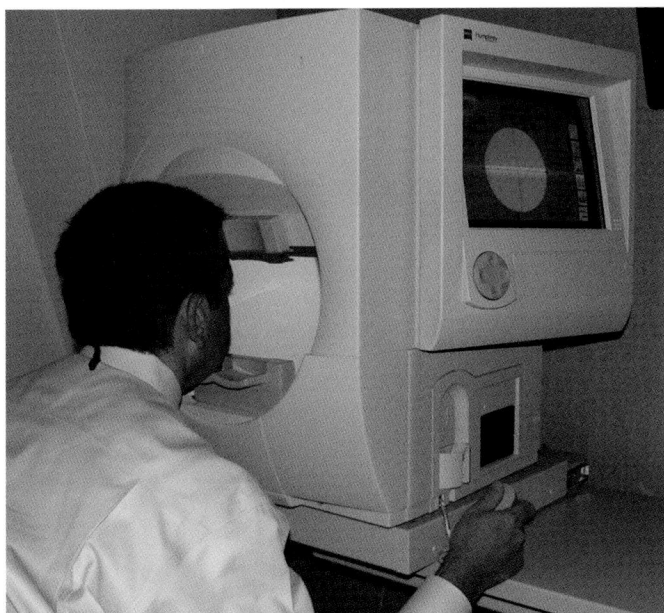

Figure 3–6. Humphrey computerized perimeter.

Other types of computerized static perimetry

Frequency doubling technology (FDT) perimetry, essentially an evaluation of contrast sensitivity throughout the central visual field, tests the patient's ability to detect sinusoidal gratings at 17 or 19 positions (**Fig. 3–8**).[16,29] Because testing takes less than 1 minute per eye, several authors have suggested frequency doubling perimetry may be better in some instances than SITA algorithms for screening in neurologic patients[30–33] and young children.[34,35] In addition, the instrument is portable and relatively inexpensive. *Short-wavelength automated perimetry (SWAP)*, which uses a blue stimulus on a yellow background, has been used primarily in glaucoma screening but with little use in neuro-ophthalmic patients.[19,36,37] Long testing time is one of the disadvantages of SWAP.

Goldmann kinetic perimetry

As the patient fixates on the central target in an illuminated bowl (**Fig. 3–9**), the perimetrist displays white dots of varying size and luminance. The stimuli are presented both centripetally and statically, and the patient hits a buzzer when he or she detects the stimulus. The perimetrist monitors the patient's fixation through a telescope, constantly encouraging the patient and reminding him or her to look straight ahead. This perimetrist–patient interaction makes the test ideal if the patient is young, has poor vision, or is neurologically impaired. Furthermore, Goldmann perimetry rarely requires more than 5–7 minutes per eye, and short breaks can be taken at the examiner's discretion. The test also can be tailored to the clinical situation: screening for chiasmal or hemianopic defects by paying particular attention to asymmetries along the vertical meridian,[38,39] arcuate field defects in glaucoma, and infranasal defects in papilledema.[40] Since the whole visual field is tested, Goldmann perimetry

will detect the rare peripheral visual field defects, due to anterior calcarine, temporal lobe, or early chiasmal compressive lesions, for instance, which may have been missed by computerized perimetry of the central 30 degrees.[41,42] Goldmann perimetry is also particularly helpful in patients with functional vision loss, in whom typical findings of spiraling, criss-crossing isopters, and nonphysiologic constriction (see Chapter 11) can often be demonstrated.

However, perimetrist bias can be a disadvantage, especially when Goldmann perimetry is used in serial follow-up. Another drawback to the technique is that the perimetrist needs a working knowledge of afferent visual pathway anatomy and related patterns of field loss.

The size of the stimulus (**Fig. 3–10**) is indicated by Roman numerals ranging from O to V, corresponding to dots measuring 0.062 mm^2 to 64 mm^2, respectively. Stimulus luminance is designated by an Arabic numeral from 1 to 4, in order of increasing brightness, together with a small letter from a to e, by convention usually held at e. The smallest, dimmest stimulus used in practice is labeled Ile, and the largest, brightest stimulus is designated by V4e. Usually the dots are white, but colored stimuli can be used in some situations, such as in the evaluation of hereditary optic neuropathies. If needed, lens correction for near is given when targets are presented within the central 30 degrees.

The results are displayed from the patient's point of view (i.e., what he or she sees). The area in which the stimulus was seen is called an *isopter*, which is labeled according to the stimulus size and luminance (**Fig. 3–10**). The normal temporal V4e field can extend at least 90 degrees, while the normal nasal V4e field can reach at least 60 degrees. In normal individuals, it is sometimes sufficient to plot only the 14e isopter, which may be suprathreshold for the entire peripheral field. The field using a test target that is either smaller or dimmer is always smaller than the field produced with a larger or brighter stimulus. *Scotomas*, circumscribed areas of visual field loss, are indicated by zones that are shaded in. The blind spot, the result of the absence of photoreceptors overlying the optic disc, is technically a scotoma and is temporal to fixation in all normal individuals.

Automated kinetic perimetry. Automated and computerized combinations of static and kinetic perimetry (**Fig. 3–11**) performed on the Octopus 101 and 900 perimeters can be used to produce results similar to Goldmann perimetry, but without the need for an experienced examiner.[43,44] Automated kinetic perimetry has been shown to be accurate and reliable in both neuro-ophthalmic disease[44] and glaucoma.[45] This technique may become increasingly more important in the future as advantages of automation are tested (reproducibility and quantification), paradigms searching for specific defects (e.g., "chiasm program") are designed, and the prevalence of manual perimeters, well-trained perimetrists, and physicians experienced with the older methods diminishes.

Tangent screen visual field testing

This test can be performed quickly in any examination room equipped with a tangent screen hung on a wall.[46] The perimetrist moves round white or colored discs or spheres over

CENTRAL 30 - 2 THRESHOLD TEST
NAME
STIMULUS   III, WHITE, BCKGND 31.5 ASB BLIND SPOT CHECK SIZE II
STRATEGY   FULL THRESHOLD

BIRTHDATE   04-09-65 DATE
FIXATION TARGET   CENTRAL   ID   TIME 01:21:31 PM
RX USED + 1.00 DS   DCX   DEG   PUPIL DIAMETER 3.0 MM   VA 20/15

RIGHT
AGE   31
FIXATION LOSSES 4/24
FALSE POS ERRORS 1/8
FALSE NEG ERRORS 0/11
QUESTIONS ASKED   453
FOVEA: 36 DB
TEST TIME 14:54

HFA S/N   640-2337

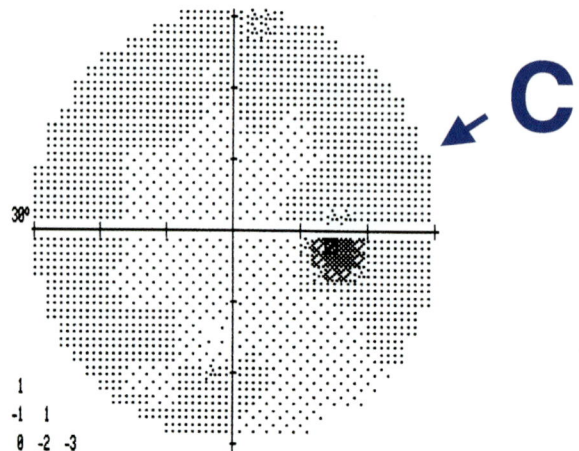

GLAUCOMA HEMIFIELD TEST (GHT)
WITHIN NORMAL LIMITS

TOTAL
DEVIATION

PATTERN
DEVIATION

PROBABILITY SYMBOLS
:: P < 5%
P < 2%
P < 1%
■ P < 0.5%

MD   - 0.43 DB
PSD   2.38 DB
SF   1.11 DB
CPSD 2.02 DB

REV 9.31

SYM		::::	:·:·:	▒	▓	▨	■	■	■	■
ASB	.8 / .1	2.5 / 1	8 / 3.2	25 / 10	79 / 32	251 / 100	794 / 316	2512 / 1000	7943 / 3162	≥ 10000
DB	41 / 50	36 / 40	31 / 35	26 / 30	21 / 25	16 / 20	11 / 15	6 / 10	1 / 5	≤ 0

SCHEIE EYE INSTITUTE556
51 N. 39TH STREET
PHILADELPHIA, PA 19104
215-662-8100

HUMPHREY INSTRUMENTS
A CARL ZEISS COMPANY

Figure 3–7. Normal Humphrey computerized 30–2 threshold visual field of the right eye. Note (**A**) the tabulation of the fixation losses and false-positive and -negative errors; (**B**) the raw data, recording the luminance, given in decibels (dB), of the dimmest stimulus the subject saw at that position in the visual field; (**C**) the gray scale, containing a conversion of the raw data using the key at the bottom of the readout; (**D**) the total deviation; (**E**) the pattern deviation; and (**F**) the statistical analysis, including the mean deviation (MD).

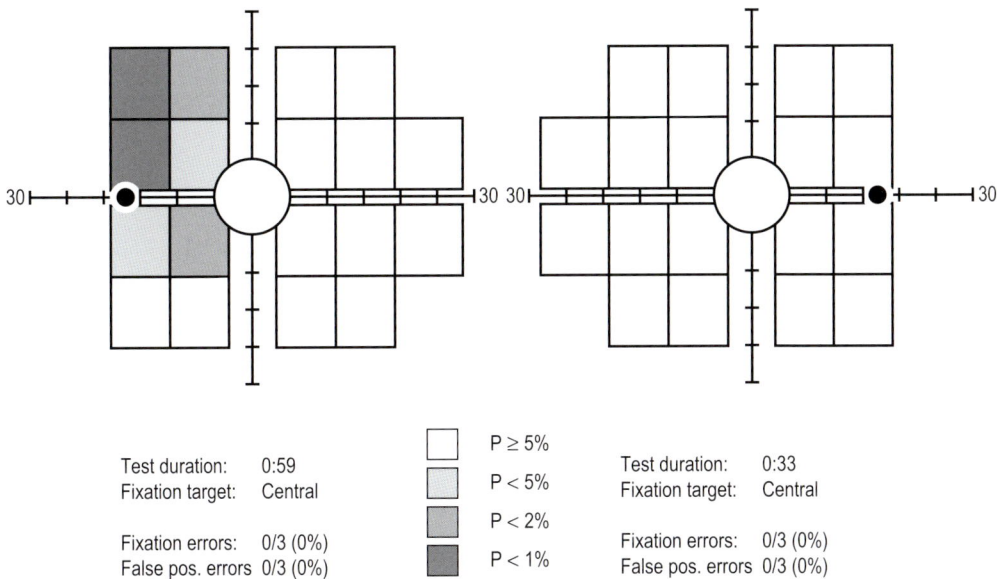

Test duration:	0:59
Fixation target:	Central
Fixation errors:	0/3 (0%)
False pos. errors	0/3 (0%)

P ≥ 5%
P < 5%
P < 2%
P < 1%

Test duration:	0:33
Fixation target:	Central
Fixation errors:	0/3 (0%)
False pos. errors	0/3 (0%)

Figure 3–8. Frequency doubling technology (FDT) perimetry in a patient with a superior temporal field defect in the left eye from a chiasmal lesion. Relative sensitivity, portability, and short test duration make FDT an effective screening tool.

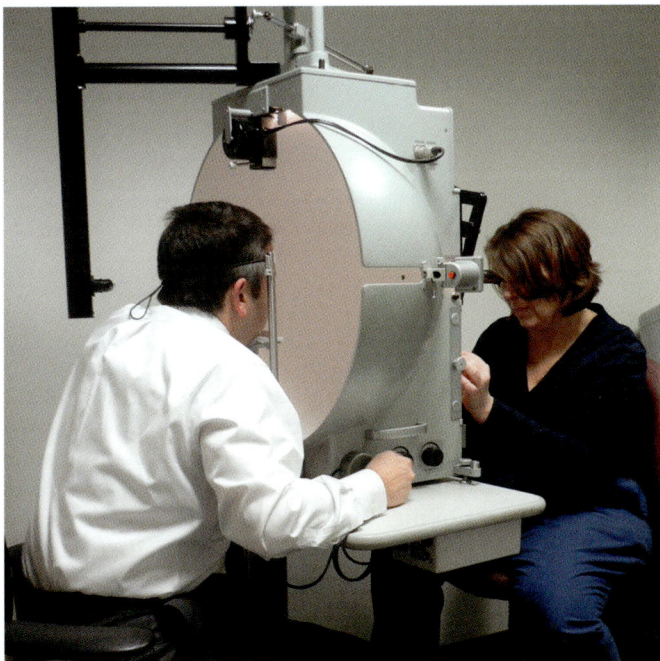

Figure 3–9. Goldmann kinetic perimetry. Note the subject (*left*) has his head in a chin-rest in the middle of the spherical bowl and presses a button in his right hand when he sees the presented stimulus. The tester administers the examination from the other side of the bowl.

a black or gray flat felt background (**Fig. 3–12A**), and, as in Goldmann perimetry, the targets are generally moved centripetally. Wearing spectacle correction, the patient usually sits 1 meter away from the screen and indicates verbally when he or she sees the visual stimulus. At this distance, on a flat surface only the central 30 degrees can be tested. The perimetrist can outline with chalk where the patient saw the target, and the results can be recorded similar to the way that

confrontation fields are drawn (see Chapter 2). The isopters are designated as a fraction, such as 3w/1000, which indicates that a 3-mm white target was used at a distance of 1000 mm (1 meter).

Small central and paracentral defects that may be missed by Goldmann perimetry or computerized field testing may be more evident with the tangent screen method. Subtle hemianopic deficits can be detected by holding two equivalent targets on both sides of fixation (**Fig. 3–12B**), and asking the patient if one appears different than the other. Perhaps the most common use of the tangent screen test is in the demonstration of nonphysiologic tubular visual fields in patients with functional visual loss (see Chapter 11).

A laser pointer with a round red or green target can also be used to present the visual stimulus during tangent screen testing in the office (**Fig. 3–13**).[47] The examiner should stand behind the patient, thereby avoiding any hints regarding the direction of the target presentation. One can also use the laser pointer during inpatient consultations for rough assessment of visual fields, substituting the tangent screen with a light-colored wall as the background.

Video 3.1

Topical diagnosis ("where" then "what")

First, the examiner should decide *where* the lesion is neuroanatomically. Based on the history, examination, and visual field testing, the examiner should be able to localize the process to retina, optic nerve, chiasm, tract, radiations, occipital lobe, or higher cortical area. Then the examiner should generate a differential diagnosis and attempt to determine *what* the lesion is. Historical features often guide the differential diagnosis, and then neuroimaging combined with other ancillary tests frequently narrow the list of possible causes.

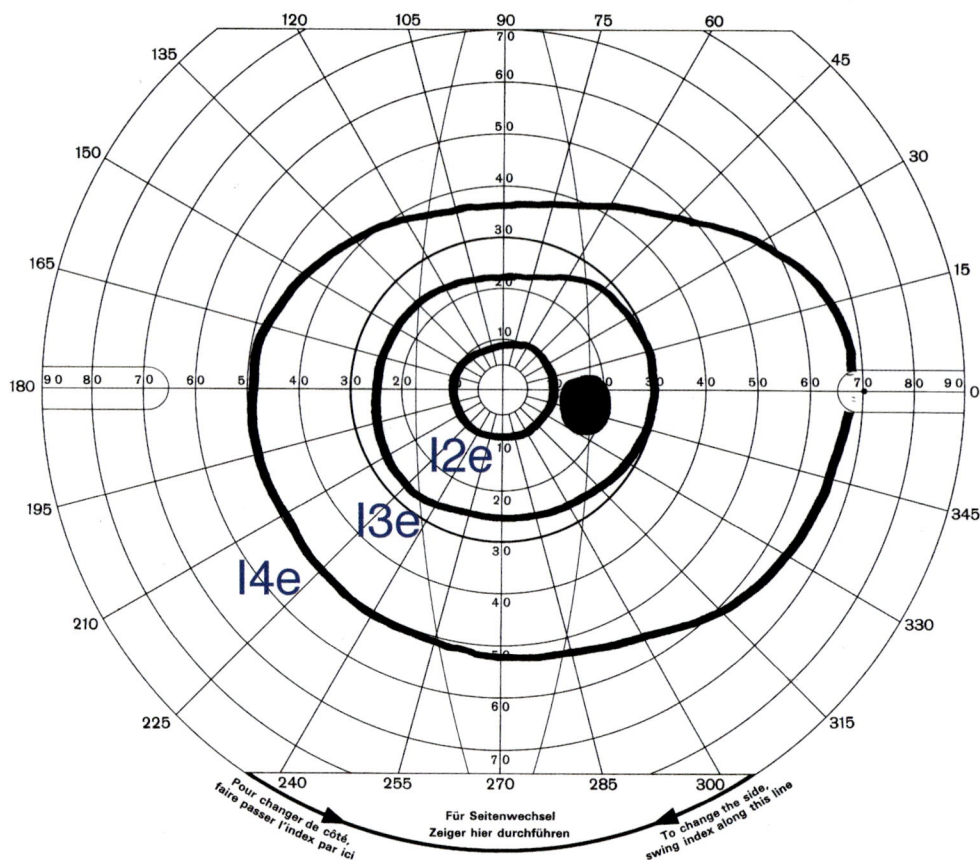

Figure 3–10. Normal Goldmann kinetic field of the right eye. The labels 14e, 13e, and 12e indicate the stimuli size and luminance (detailed in the key on bottom left-hand side of the figure). The stimuli are presented in the periphery then directed radially to the center. The dark lines indicate the point at which the subject noticed the stimulus. Note the temporal location of the blind spot and that the temporal field is larger than the right.

History

Common complaints encountered with visual loss include so-called negative phenomena such as "blurry vision" or "gray vision." Patients with higher cortical disorders may have nonspecific complaints such as "I'm having trouble seeing" or "Focusing is difficult." Patients with lesions of the afferent visual pathway may also complain of positive phenomena, such as flashing or colored lights (*phosphenes* or *photopsias*), jagged lines, or formed visual hallucinations (a false perception that a stimulus is present). The complexity of positive phenomena does not specify localization.

The temporal profile of the visual loss will suggest possible diagnoses, and its monocularity or binocularity will help in localization. As a general rule, acute or subacute visual deficits result from ischemic or inflammatory injury to the optic nerve. Vitreous hemorrhage and retinal detachment are other important considerations. Chronic or progressive visual loss, in turn, may result from a compressive, infiltrative, or degenerative process. Cataracts, refractive error, open-angle glaucoma, and retinal disorders such as age-related macular degeneration or diabetic retinopathy also need to be considered when visual symptoms are insidious.

If a patient complains of monocular visual loss, a process in one eye or optic nerve should be considered. Painless transient visual loss characterized by a "gray shade" that encroaches on vision superiorly then resolves after seconds or minutes is typical of amaurosis fugax related to carotid disease. Painful monocular visual loss occurring over days is characteristic of an inflammatory or demyelinating optic neuropathy. With binocular visual loss, a lesion of both eyes or optic nerves, or of the chiasm, tract, radiations, or occipital lobe, should be investigated. Further details regarding these specific complaints and their localizing value are provided in the respective chapters.

Associated neurologic deficits, such as motor or sensory abnormalities, will also assist in localization and often indicate a hemispheric abnormality. Medical conditions should always be investigated in the review of systems. Hypertension, diabetes, and smoking, for instance, predispose the patient to vascular disease, and a history of coronary artery disease should alert the examiner to the possibility of carotid artery insufficiency as well. Visual loss accompanied by endocrine symptoms, such as those consistent with hypopituitarism (amenorrhea, decreased libido, impotence, for example) or pituitary hypersecretion (galactorrhea, acromegaly, for example), suggests a chiasmal disorder.

Examination

Particular attention should be paid to assessment of acuity, color vision, confrontation visual fields, pupillary reactivity,

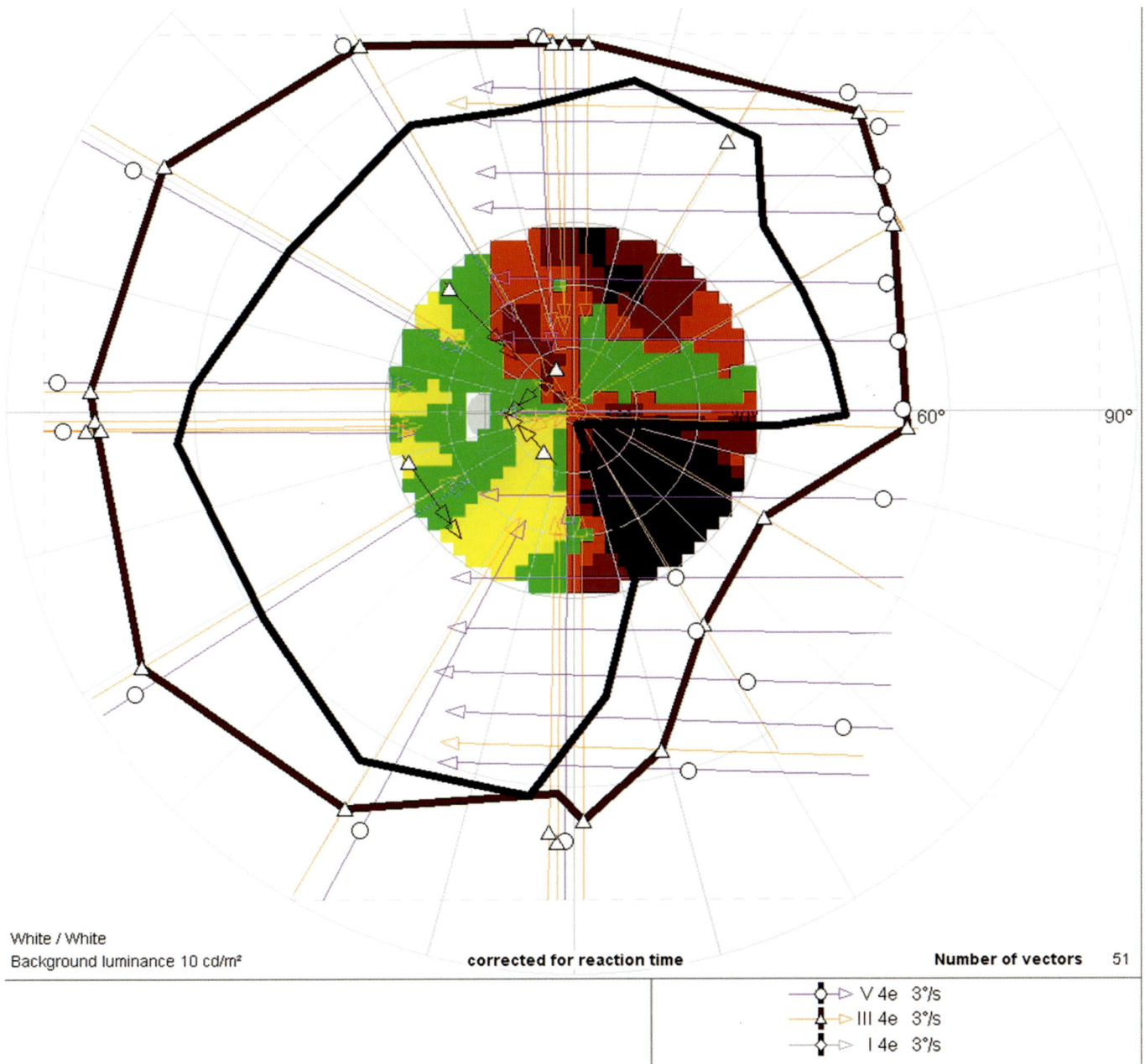

White / White
Background luminance 10 cd/m²   **corrected for reaction time**   **Number of vectors**   51

◇▷ V 4e 3°/s
△▷ III 4e 3°/s
◇▷ I 4e 3°/s

Figure 3–11. Combined static and automated Goldmann perimetry in a patient with inferior nasal quadrantic defect in the left eye. The Octopus 101 test consists of a short TOP (tendency-oriented perimetry) strategy 32 static examination followed by a series of preprogrammed kinetic vectors (arrows) using III4E (brown larger isopter) and I4E (black small isopter) stimuli. Darker areas in the static portion of the test correlated to denser defects. The vectors (arrows) used in the automated kinetic portion of the test were preprogrammed to detect defects along the vertical and horizontal meridians, and the computer corrects for reaction time.

and fundus appearance. Neuro-ophthalmic examination techniques are discussed in Chapter 2.

Monocular acuity loss, deficits in color vision, a central scotoma, a relative afferent pupillary defect, and optic disc swelling or pallor suggest an optic neuropathy. In an acute retrobulbar optic neuropathy, the optic disc may have a normal appearance. Monocular visual loss with a central scotoma, metamorphopsia, preserved color vision, and no afferent pupillary defect makes a maculopathy more likely. Bilateral loss of acuity suggests bilateral optic nerve, chiasm, or bilateral retrochiasmal lesions. Homonymous hemian-

opic field loss with normal acuity, pupillary reactivity, and fundi are normally associated with a retrogeniculate process. A hemianopia accompanied by an ipsilateral hemiparesis or sensory loss is likely to be the result of a parietal process, while an isolated hemianopia is more likely the result of an occipital lobe lesion.

When suspected, ocular causes of visual loss such as corneal or lens opacities, retinal detachments, or glaucoma should be excluded by an ophthalmologist. In general, patients with cataracts complain of blurry vision with glare, especially with automobile headlights, and those with

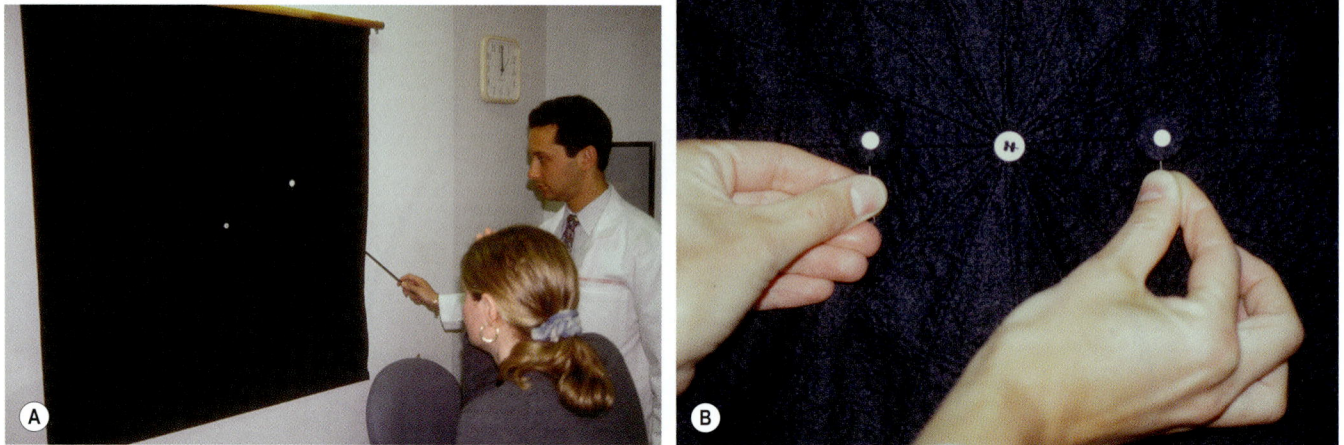

Figure 3–12. Tangent screen visual field test. Each eye is tested separately. **A.** The examiner moves a white or colored object in front of a black felt screen, and the patient points or verbalizes when he or she sees the target. The results can be recorded in white chalk on the felt, then transferred into the patient's record. **B**. Two equivalent targets can be presented while the patient fixates centrally to test for subtle central visual field defects respecting the vertical meridian.

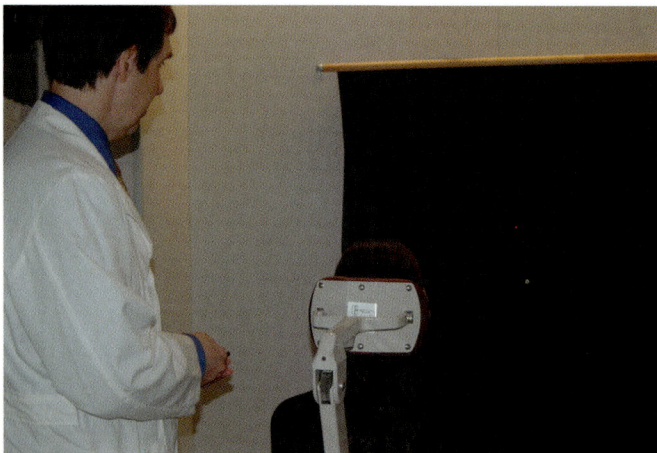

Figure 3–13. Laser pointer visual field test. The examiner stands behind the subject and tests the visual field by pointing a laser light stimulus at a wall or black tangent screen in front of the subject, who verbalizes when he or she sees the stimulus.

glaucoma have peripheral visual field loss but preserved central acuity; the visual loss associated with both of these problems is insidious. Retinal detachments may present acutely with flashes of light, floaters, or peripheral field loss.

Pattern of visual field loss

Figure 3–14 illustrates the visual field deficits characteristic of various lesions within the afferent visual pathway. As alluded to earlier, monocular visual field defects most commonly localize to the retina or optic nerve, and the patterns of field loss are typically altitudinal, central, cecocentral, or arcuate.

Monocular field defects emanating from the blind spot, as in an arcuate scotoma, for instance, are almost always related to an optic nerve lesion or a retinal vascular occlusion. A bitemporal hemianopia is very specific to the chiasm. Homonymous hemianopic deficits suggest a retrochiasmal lesion. In general, incongruous hemianopias tend to be more anterior, while congruous hemianopias, with or without macular sparing, are more characteristic of occipital disturbances. One possible explanation for this pattern is the closer grouping of retrochiasmal fibers from each eye as they proceed posteriorly. Once the homonymous hemianopia is complete, congruity can no longer be assessed, and the defect may have its origin anywhere along the retrochiasmal pathway because congruity cannot be assessed. The particular patterns of visual field loss are discussed in greater detail in Chapters 4–8.

Ancillary visual testing

Electrophysiologic testing such as a visual evoked potential (VEP) or electroretinogram (ERG) can confirm the localization to optic nerve or retina, but these tests should never replace the clinical examination. VEPs measure the cortical activity in response to flash or patterned stimuli and are abnormal in the presence of a lesion in the afferent visual pathway. A normal VEP in the setting of decreased vision and an otherwise normal examination suggests functional visual loss (see Chapter 11). Multifocal VEPs (mfVEPs) assess the response simultaneously from multiple regions throughout the visual field—the distribution is similar to areas on a dartboard.[48] Some authors have used mfVEPs as objective perimetry in the detection and follow-up of optic neuropathies and other central visual pathway disorders.[49–52]

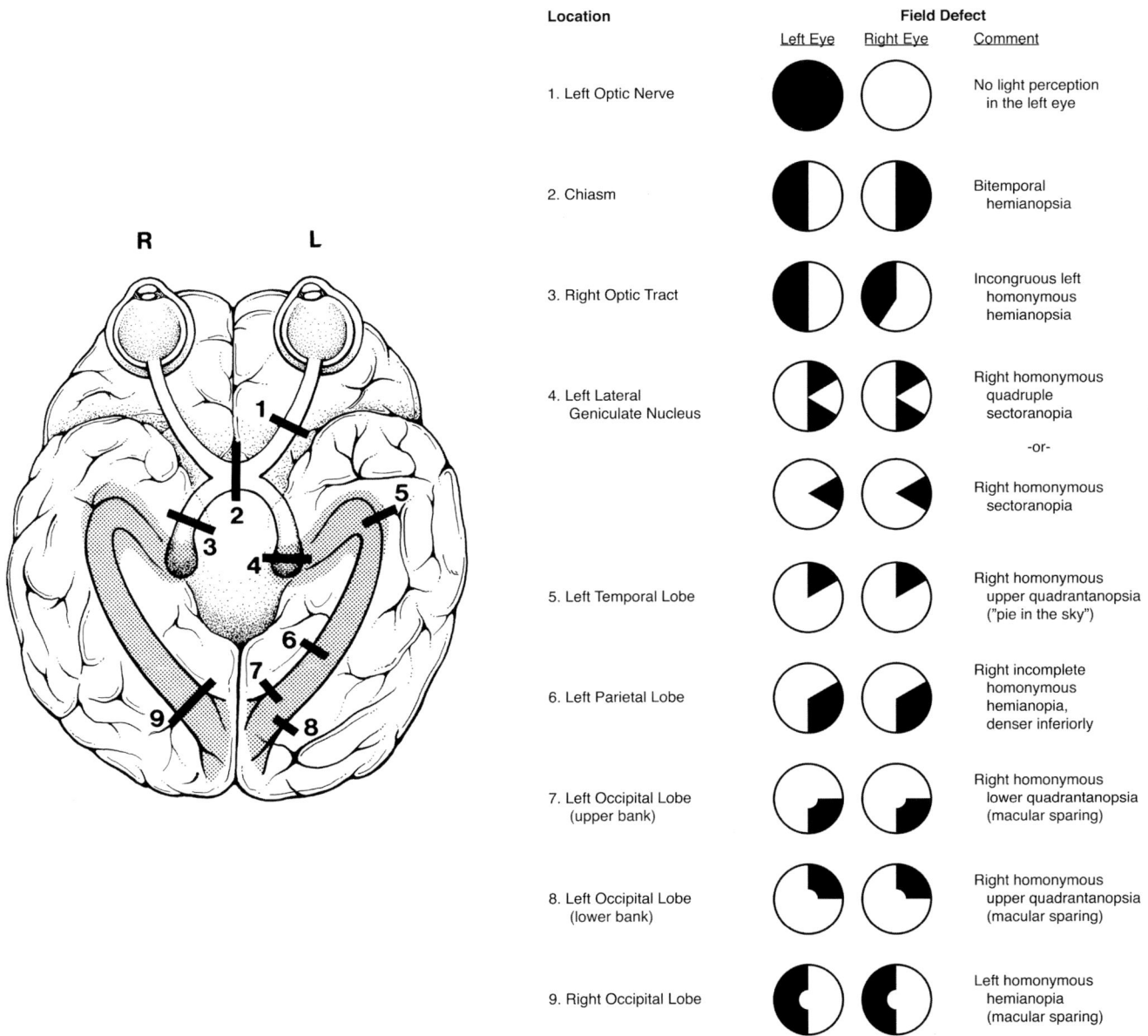

Location	Field Defect		Comment
	Left Eye	Right Eye	
1. Left Optic Nerve			No light perception in the left eye
2. Chiasm			Bitemporal hemianopsia
3. Right Optic Tract			Incongruous left homonymous hemianopsia
4. Left Lateral Geniculate Nucleus			Right homonymous quadruple sectoranopia -or- Right homonymous sectoranopia
5. Left Temporal Lobe			Right homonymous upper quadrantanopsia ("pie in the sky")
6. Left Parietal Lobe			Right incomplete homonymous hemianopia, denser inferiorly
7. Left Occipital Lobe (upper bank)			Right homonymous lower quadrantanopsia (macular sparing)
8. Left Occipital Lobe (lower bank)			Right homonymous upper quadrantanopsia (macular sparing)
9. Right Occipital Lobe			Left homonymous hemianopia (macular sparing)

Figure 3–14. Visual pathways: correlation of lesion site and field defect, view of underside of the brain. *Homonymous* refers to a defect present in both eyes with the same laterality, while a *hemianopia* refers to visual loss respecting the vertical meridian. Congruous fields are symmetric in both eyes. Note that lesions of upper or lower occipital banks produce quadrantic defects, while lesions within temporal and parietal lobes cause field defects that tend not to respect the horizontal meridian.

ERGs and multifocal ERGs, which measure rod and cone photoreceptor function, are particularly helpful in sorting out retinal dystrophies and degenerations. ERG testing is discussed in more detail in Chapter 4.

Differential diagnosis

Table 3–2 highlights examination findings, visual field abnormalities, and common causes to consider for various localizations within the afferent visual pathway. Optic neuropathies in young adults are typically inflammatory, while in older adults they are more commonly associated with vascular disease. The most common cause of a chiasmal syndrome is a compressive sellar mass. Strokes and neoplasms are the most common causes of retrochiasmal visual loss. The reader is referred to Chapters 4–8 for further details regarding the differential diagnoses and discussion of the various responsible causes.

Table 3–2 Topical diagnosis: various causes of visual loss according to lesion site within the afferent visual pathway

Lesion site	Common causes	Findings
Ocular	Refractive error, media opacities	Vision may improve with pinhole; normal pupillary reactivity
Retina	Macular degeneration, central retinal artery occlusion, central retinal vein occlusion	Visible retinal abnormality on ophthalmoscopy
Optic nerve	Inflammatory lesions (idiopathic optic neuritis, sarcoid); ischemia (atherosclerotic, vasculitic); infiltrative/infectious (neoplastic, syphilis)	Afferent pupillary defect present if unilateral; central, centrocecal, or arcuate field defect; disc swelling may be visualized if optic nerve head involved
Chiasm	Sellar mass (pituitary adenoma, craniopharyngioma, meningioma, or aneurysm)	Bitemporal hemianopia; optic atrophy if chronic
Optic tract	Sellar mass	Afferent pupillary defect variable; classically incongruous hemianopia; "bow-tie" disc atrophy if long standing
Lateral geniculate	Stroke	Incongruous hemianopia, optic atrophy late; horizontal sectoranopia or quadruple quadrantanopia suggestive of infarction
Optic radiations (parietal)	Stroke, neoplasm	Inferior contralateral quadrantanopia; normal pupillary reactivity; defective optokinetic response with targets drawn toward the lesion
Optic radiations (temporal)	Stroke, neoplasm	Superior contralateral quadrantanopia; normal pupillary reactivity
Occipital	Stroke, neoplasm	Congruous contralateral hemianopia with or without macular sparing; normal pupillary reactivity; normal optokinetic response

References

1. Kupfer C, Chumbley L, Downer JC. Quantitative histology of optic nerve, optic tract and lateral geniculate nucleus of man. J Anat 1967;101:393–401.
2. Shahinafar S, Johnson LN, Madsen RW. Confrontation visual field loss as a function of decibel sensitivity loss on automated static perimetry. Implications on the accuracy of confrontation visual field testing. Ophthalmology 1995;102:872–877.
3. Pandit RJ, Gales K, Griffiths PG. Effectiveness of testing visual fields by confrontation. Lancet 2001;358:1339–1340.
4. Trobe JD, Acosta PC, Krischer JP, et al. Confrontation visual field techniques in the detection of anterior visual pathway lesions. Ann Neurol 1981;10:28–34.
5. Lindenmuth KA, Skuta GL, Rabbani R, et al. Effects of pupillary dilation on automated perimetry in normal patients. Ophthalmology 1990;97:367–370.
6. Kudrna GR, Stanley MA, Remington LA. Pupillary dilation and its effects on automated perimetry results. J Am Optom Assoc 1995;66:675–680.
7. Donahue SP, Porter A. SITA visual field testing in children. JAAPOS 2001;5:114–117.
8. Stiebel-Kalish H, Lusky M, Yassur Y, et al. Swedish interactive thresholding algorithm fast for following visual fields in prepubertal idiopathic intracranial hypertension. Ophthalmology 2004;111:1673–1675.
9. Traquair HM. An Introduction to Clinical Perimetry, 5th edn, pp 1–16. London, Henry Kimpton, 1946.
10. Anderson DR. Introduction. In: Testing the Field of Vision, pp 1–17. St. Louis, C.V. Mosby, 1982.
11. Frisén L. The foundations of visual field testing. In: Clinical Tests of Vision, pp 55–77. New York, Raven Press, 1990.
12. Wong AY, Dodge RM, Remington LA. Comparing threshold visual fields between the Dicon TKS 4000 automated perimeter and the Humphrey Field Analyzer. J Am Optom Assoc 1995;66:706–711.
13. American Academy of Ophthalmology. Automated perimetry. Ophthalmology 1996;103:1144–1151.
14. Johnson CA. Standardizing the measurement of visual fields. Ophthalmology 1996;103:186–189.
15. Katz J, Tielsch JM, Quigley HA, et al. Automated perimetry detects visual field loss before manual Goldmann perimetry. Ophthalmology 1995;102:21–26.
16. Johnson CA. Recent developments in automated perimetry in glaucoma diagnosis and management. Curr Opin Ophthalmol 2002;13:77–84.
17. Wall M. What's new in perimetry. J Neuroophthalmol 2004;24:46–55.
18. Wall M, Punke SG, Stickney TL, et al. SITA standard in optic neuropathies and hemianopias: a comparison with full threshold testing. Invest Ophthalmol Vis Sci 2001;42:528–537.
19. Delgado MF, Nguyen NT, Cox TA, et al. Automated perimetry: a report by the American Academy of Ophthalmology. Ophthalmology 2002;109:2362–2374.
20. Szatmáry G, Biousse V, Newman NJ. Can Swedish interactive thresholding algorithm fast perimetry be used as an alternative to Goldmann perimetry in neuro-ophthalmic practice? Arch Ophthalmol 2002;120:1162–1173.
21. Anderson DR. Standard perimetry. Ophthalmol Clin North Am 2003;16:205–212, vi.
22. Heijl A, Bengtsson B. The effect of perimetric experience in patients with glaucoma. Arch Ophthalmol 1996;114:19–22.
23. Meyer DR, Stern JH, Jarvis JM, et al. Evaluating the visual field effects of blepharoptosis using automated static perimetry. Ophthalmology 1993;100:651–658.
24. Harrington DO, Drake MV. Postchiasmal visual pathway. In: The Visual Fields. Text and Atlas of Clinical Perimetry, 6th edn, pp 311–361. St. Louis, C.V. Mosby, 1990.
25. Aung T, Foster PJ, Seah SK, et al. Automated static perimetry: the influence of myopia and its method of correction. Ophthalmology 2001;108:290–295.
26. Haas A, Flammer J, Schneider U. Influence of age on the visual fields of normal subjects. Am J Ophthalmol 1986;101:199–203.
27. Jaffe GJ, Alvarado JA, Juster RP. Age-related changes of the normal visual field. Arch Ophthalmol 1986;104:1021–1025.
28. Wall M, Johnson CA, Kutzko KE, et al. Long- and short-term variability of automated perimetry result in patients with optic neuritis and healthy subjects. Arch Ophthalmol 1998;116:53–61.
29. Anderson AJ, Johnson CA. Frequency-doubling technology perimetry. Ophthalmol Clin North Am 2003;16:213–225.
30. Thomas D, Thomas R, Muliyil JP, et al. Role of frequency doubling perimetry in detecting neuro-ophthalmic visual field defects. Am J Ophthalmol 2001;131:734–741.
31. Wall M, Neahring RK, Woodward KR. Sensitivity and specificity of frequency doubling perimetry in neuro-ophthalmic disorders: a comparison with conventional automated perimetry. Invest Ophthalmol Vis Sci 2002;43:1277–1283.
32. Johnson CA. Frequency doubling technology perimetry for neuro-ophthalmological diseases. Br J Ophthalmol 2004;88:1232–1233.
33. Monteiro ML, Moura FC, Cunha LP. Frequency doubling perimetry in patients with mild and moderate pituitary tumor-associated visual field defects detected by conventional perimetry. Arq Bras Oftalmol 2007;70:323–329.
34. Blumenthal EZ, Haddad A, Horani A, et al. The reliability of frequency-doubling perimetry in young children. Ophthalmology 2004;111:435–439.
35. Quinn LM, Gardiner SK, Wheeler DT, et al. Frequency doubling technology perimetry in normal children. Am J Ophthalmol 2006;142:983–989.
36. Keltner JL, Johnson CA. Short-wavelength automated perimetry in neuro-ophthalmologic disorders. Arch Ophthalmol 1995;113:475–481.
37. Racette L, Sample PA. Short-wavelength automated perimetry. Ophthalmol Clin North Am 2003;16:227–236, vi–vii.
38. Trobe JD, Acosta PC. An algorithm for visual fields. Surv Ophthalmol 1980;24:665–670.
39. Trobe JD, Acosta PC, Krischer JP. A screening method for chiasmal visual-field defects. Arch Ophthalmol 1981;99:264–271.

40. Wall M, George D. Visual loss in pseudotumor cerebri. Incidence and defects related to visual field strategy. Arch Neurol 1987;44:170–175.

41. Wirtschafter JD, Hard-Boberg A-L, Coffman SM. Evaluating the usefulness in neuro-ophthalmology of visual field examinations peripheral to 30 degrees. Trans Am Ophthalmol Soc 1984;82:329–357.

42. Lepore FE. The preserved temporal crescent: the clinical implications of an "endangered" finding. Neurology 2001;57:1918–1921.

43. Nowomiejska K, Vonthein R, Paetzold J, et al. Comparison between semiautomated kinetic perimetry and conventional Goldmann manual kinetic perimetry in advanced visual field loss. Ophthalmology 2005;112:1343–1354.

44. Pineles SL, Volpe NJ, Miller-Ellis E, et al. Automated combined kinetic and static perimetry: an alternative to standard perimetry in patients with neuro-ophthalmic disease and glaucoma. Arch Ophthalmol 2006;124:363–369.

45. Ramirez AM, Chaya CJ, Gordon LK, et al. A comparison of semiautomated versus manual Goldmann kinetic perimetry in patients with visually significant glaucoma. J Glaucoma 2008;17:111–117.

46. Harrington DO, Drake MV. Manual perimeters: instruments and use. In: The Visual Fields. Text and Atlas of Clinical Perimetry, 6th edn, pp 13–34. St. Louis, C.V. Mosby, 1990.

47. Lee MS, Balcer LJ, Volpe NJ, et al. Laser pointer visual field screening. J Neuroophthalmol 2003;23:260–263.

48. Hood DC, Odel JG, Winn BJ. The multifocal visual evoked potential. J Neuroophthalmol 2003;23:279–289.

49. Klistorner AI, Graham SL, Grigg J, et al. Objective perimetry using the multifocal visual evoked potential in central visual pathway lesions. Br J Ophthalmol 2005;89:739–744.

50. Danesh-Meyer HV, Carroll SC, Gaskin BJ, et al. Correlation of the multifocal visual evoked potential and standard automated perimetry in compressive optic neuropathies. Invest Ophthalmol Vis Sci 2006;47:1458–1463.

51. Pakrou N, Casson R, Kaines A, et al. Multifocal objective perimetry compared with Humphrey full-threshold perimetry in patients with optic neuritis. Clin Exp Ophthalmol 2006;34:562–567.

52. Yukawa E, Matsuura T, Kim YJ, et al. Usefulness of multifocal VEP in a child requiring perimetry. Pediatr Neurol 2008;38:360–362.

53

Vision loss: retinal disorders of neuro-ophthalmic interest

While a comprehensive review of all retinal disease is beyond the scope of this text, there are several entities that are particularly important in the neuro-ophthalmic differential diagnosis of central and peripheral visual loss and positive visual phenomena. Patients with retinopathies may have symptoms and examination findings that overlap with patients with optic nerve disease and cortically based conditions. They may manifest with visual acuity loss, visual field defects, and a paucity of findings on ophthalmoscopic examination. Certain retinal disorders may also provide invaluable clues to the existence of an underlying neurologic illness or systemic disease. In this chapter, we will examine the relevant retinal anatomy, the distinction between maculopathy and optic neuropathies, maculopathies that may mimic optic neuropathy, retinal vascular emboli and insufficiency, the photoreceptor disorders important in neuro-ophthalmic differential diagnosis (big blind spot syndrome, cancer-associated retinopathies), toxic retinopathies, hereditary retinopathies of neuro-ophthalmic interest, and the retinal manifestations of neurologic and systemic diseases and phakomatoses.

Retinal anatomy

Cellular elements of the retina

The retina is a transparent structure that arises from the inner and outer layers of the embryologic optic cup. The outer layer consists of the retinal pigment epithelium (RPE) and the inner layer is a multicellular layer that makes up the neurosensory retina. The RPE consists of hexagonal cells extending from the optic nerve to the ora serata. The major functions of the RPE are to maintain the photoreceptors through vitamin A metabolism and phagocytosis of photoreceptor outer segments. Other functions include maintenance of the outer blood–retina barrier, heat and light absorption, and production of extracellular matrix. The basal sides of the RPE cells form the inner layer of Bruch's membrane separating the retina from the choroid. Separation of the RPE from the neurosensory retina is called a *retinal detachment*.

The neurosensory retina consists of neural, glial, and vascular elements. The outermost layer of the retina (furthest from the cornea and closest to the RPE) is the photoreceptor layer, consisting of rods and cones. The outer segments of the photoreceptors make contact with the RPE cells. The cell bodies of the photoreceptors make up the outer nuclear layer and are in contact with horizontal and bipolar cells through their process in the outer plexiform layer. The bipolar cells are oriented more vertically and bridge the connection to the inner plexiform layer where they synapse with ganglion cells and amacrine cells. The cell bodies of the bipolar cells, horizontal cells, and amacrine cells make up the inner nuclear layer located between the inner and outer plexiform layer. The ganglion cell axons run parallel to the surface of the retina and form the nerve fiber layer. The major glial cell of the retina is the Mueller cell, whose nucleus is in the inner nuclear layer and whose processes extend from the surface of the retina (inner limiting membrane) to the end of the outer nuclear layer (external limiting membrane). Together with some astrocytes and microglia these cells provide the nutritional and structural support to the retina.

Blood supply

The first major branch of the internal carotid artery, the ophthalmic artery, provides the blood supply of the retina. It gives rise to the central retinal artery, which supplies the inner two-thirds of the retina, and the posterior ciliary arteries, which supply the outer portions of the retina (**Fig. 4–1**). The temporal blood vessels arc above and below the macula in company with the arcuate nerve fiber bundles (ganglion cell axons). The vessels are found in the inner retinal layers and usually do not extend deeper than the inner plexiform layer. The outer retinal layers (photoreceptors and RPE) receive their oxygen and nutrients through diffusion from the vascular supply in the choroid. There is a capillary-free zone of approximately 400 μm in the fovea called the *foveal avascular zone*. The absence of vascular elements is necessary for keen visual acuity. At artery and vein crossing points, the arteries lie over the veins and a basement membrane is shared. This crossing, along with pathologic changes in the arteriole walls, may be the basis for retinal vein occlusion. The central retinal vein lies temporal to the central retinal artery in the optic nerve head and eventually drains into the superior orbital vein and cavernous sinus. The retinal blood vessels, like the cerebral blood vessels, are responsible for maintenance of the blood–retina barrier. This is accomplished through tight junctions between endothelial cells. The retinal blood vessels do not have smooth muscles or an internal elastic lamina.

A cilioretinal artery arises from the choroidal circulation and is present in about 20% of individuals (see **Fig. 4–11** for an example of a cilioretinal artery).[1] The blood supply of the choroid is from the ophthalmic artery via the branches of the anterior and posterior ciliary arteries. Branches of these arteries form discrete capillary lobules of circulation. The choroid drains through the vortex veins and then into the superior and inferior orbital veins into the cavernous sinus. The separate drainage pathway for the retina (central vein) and choroid (vortex veins) provides the anatomical basis for the development of collateral vessels in certain conditions. Pathologic processes that cause central vein obstruction (e.g., central retinal vein occlusion, papilledema, optic nerve sheath meningioma) can cause collateral or "shunt" vessels to develop between the retinal veins at the optic nerve head and the choroidal circulation.

Other details of the internal carotid and ophthalmic artery blood supply are discussed in Chapters 5 and 10.

Distinction between maculopathies and optic neuropathies

Optic neuropathies and maculopathies may manifest with similar symptoms, such as central vision loss. When optic neuropathies or maculopathies present with their classic features they are not difficult to distinguish. However, some patients with reduced acuity will have normal-appearing optic nerves and maculae. In this setting, the combination of historical information, examination findings, and laboratory studies will often aid in separating these entities (**Table 4–1**).

Symptoms

The presence of metamorphopsia or photopsia may be very helpful in localizing vision loss to the retina. Patients with metamorphopsia describe warping, bending, or crowding of the images, while those with photopsia complain of seeing sparkles of light. Both of these symptoms are very unusual in optic neuropathies. The complaint of light blindness or abnormal glare sensitivity (hemeralopia) also suggests the presence of retinal dysfunction and may be a prominent symptom in patients with cone dysfunction. In contrast, patients who detect a darkening of their vision or loss of color perception usually have optic nerve disease. Night vision loss, or nyctalopia, can commonly accompany widespread retinal photoreceptor disease. Other symptoms that accompany the vision loss may provide distinguishing features. For instance, pain in association with vision loss is exceedingly uncommon in patients with retinal problems, but may accompany optic disease, particularly inflammatory conditions such as optic neuritis.

Signs

Reduction of visual acuity is commonly encountered in both maculopathies and optic nerve disease. However, abnormalities of color vision help to distinguish macular disease from optic nerve dysfunction. For instance, when visual acuity is only mildly reduced but color vision is markedly impaired, optic nerve dysfunction is more likely. Similarly, when visual acuity is poor yet color vision is preserved, macular disease is much more likely. Two exceptions to this important clinical observation include patients with cone degenerations, who typically have very poor color vision, and patients with ischemic optic neuropathy, who may maintain excellent color vision in their intact visual field.

Photostress testing can be helpful in identifying patients with maculopathies. In macular disease there can be a prolongation of the recovery time of the photoreceptor visual pigments after prolonged bright light exposure. The test, which is described in more detail in Chapter 2, is performed by shining a bright light in the eye and finding a prolonged recovery time for visual acuity in the affected eye compared with the unaffected eye. Patients with optic neuropathy will not have a prolonged recovery time after photostress.

The presence of an afferent pupillary defect also strongly suggests the presence of optic nerve disease. Extensive and asymmetric retinal lesions are typically necessary for patients to develop a relative afferent pupil defect. In addition, visual field testing may be useful in distinguishing optic neuropathies and maculopathies. Both entities may be associated with central or centrocecal scotomas, although the presence of the latter field deficit favors optic nerve disease.

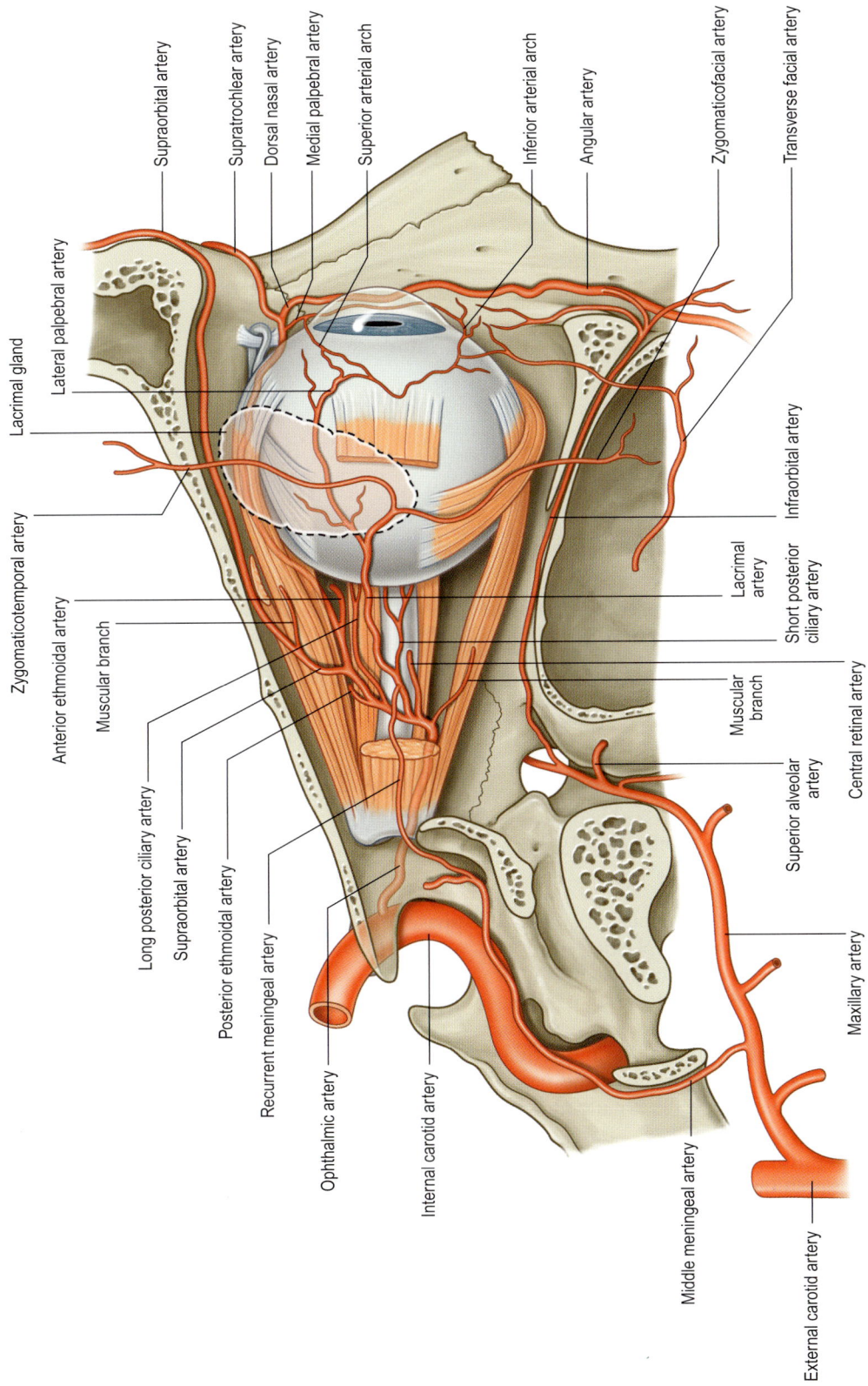

Supraorbital artery

Supratrochlear artery

Dorsal nasal artery

Medial palpebral artery

Superior arterial arch

Inferior arterial arch

Angular artery

Zygomaticofacial artery

Transverse facial artery

Lateral palpebral artery

Lacrimal gland

Zygomaticotemporal artery

Anterior ethmoidal artery

Muscular branch

Infraorbital artery

Lacrimal artery

Short posterior ciliary artery

Long posterior ciliary artery

Supraorbital artery

Posterior ethmoidal artery

Muscular branch

Central retinal artery

Recurrent meningeal artery

Superior alveolar artery

Ophthalmic artery

Internal carotid artery

Maxillary artery

Middle meningeal artery

External carotid artery

Figure 4–1. The orbit, lateral view, showing the arterial circulation, globe, and lacrimal gland. The blood supply of the retina and optic nerve derives from the ophthalmic artery, which gives rise to the central retinal artery (which enters the optic nerve about 1 cm from the nerve globe junction and travels within it to the optic nerve head and the retina) and the medial and lateral posterior ciliary arteries, which in turn supply the choriocapillaris and optic nerve head.

Table 4–1 Clinical distinction between optic neuropathy and maculopathy

Symptom, sign, or test	Optic neuropathy	Maculopathy
Symptom		
Metamorphopsia	Rare	Common
Darkening of vision	Common	Rare
Recognition of peripheral field loss by patient	Common	Rare
Transient visual obscurations	Occasionally	Rare
Photopsia	Rare	Common
Glare or light sensitivity	Rare	Sometimes
Pain	Common in optic neuritis, rare in other optic neuropathies	Rare
Sign		
Reduced acuity	Common	Common
Dyschromatopsia	Severe	Mild
Amsler grid abnormality	Missing portions or gray spots	Distorted or bent lines
Afferent pupillary defect	Common	Rare (retinal disorder needs to be severe and asymmetric)
Visual field defects	Central, arcuate, nasal, altitudinal	Central scotoma and midperipheral defects in photoreceptor disease
Ophthalmoscopy	Swollen, pale, or normal optic nerve	Occasionally pale optic nerve; macular abnormality (pigment, atrophy, edema)
Photostress recovery	Normal	Abnormal
Test		
Electroretinography (ERG)	Normal	Normal or abnormal (especially multifocal ERG)
Ocular coherence tomography	Normal macula Nerve fiber layer thinning	Abnormal, edema, thickening or thinning
Visual evoked response	Large latency delay	Small latency delay

Midperipheral, ring-type scotomas are typical of retinal degenerations, inflammatory and paraneoplastic retinopathies. Optic nerve-type field defects are reviewed in Chapter 5, and they usually assume characteristic patterns that respect the organization of the nerve fiber bundles. However, on automated visual field testing, both optic nerve and retinal disease may produce generalized depression of the visual field. This nonspecific type of field defect is usually unhelpful in distinguishing the two conditions.

Ophthalmoscopy is critical when distinguishing optic neuropathies from maculopathies. In general, abnormalities will be identified in almost all patients with significant macular or optic nerve disease, and it is only at the earliest stage of these visual problems that an abnormality may not be observed. Macular lesions that produce pigmentary changes, atrophy, or hemorrhage are usually observable on ophthalmoscopy. Optic nerve atrophy with or without nerve fiber layer dropout may be recognized on ophthalmoscopy, particularly when using the green filter light, or can be detected with ocular coherence tomography (OCT). Significant overlap may exist in the early phases of an optic neuropathy when pallor has not yet developed or in the later phases of retinal disease when mild optic disc pallor may be associated with widespread retinal disease.

Ancillary testing

Ultimately, the examiner may need to rely on other diagnostic tests to identify and localize the cause of vision loss. Evaluation of the cross-sectional anatomy of the macula has been revolutionized by OCT. This noninvasive technique relies on imaging of reflected light, much like echography images rely on reflected sound. With OCT, exquisitely detailed cross-sectional images of the retina can be obtained, and the various layers of the retina can be resolved (**Fig. 4–2**). The cross-sectional image of the retina is particularly helpful in identifying fluid and retinal edema, macula holes, choroidal neovascularization, vitreo-retinal interface abnormalities, and abnormal retinal thinning or thickening. These tomographic images can be resolved to 0.01 mm.

Fluorescein angiography (FA) may be helpful in identifying occult macular problems. For instance, patients with diabetic macular ischemia might exhibit capillary nonperfusion on FA with minimal findings on fundus examination.

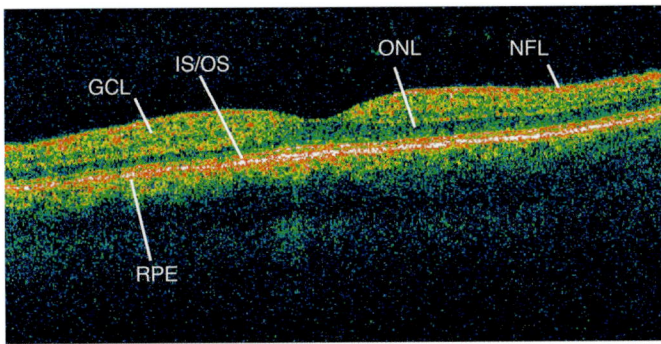

Figure 4–2. Ocular coherence tomography (3 Stratus System) section of a normal human retina. The layers of the retina can be indentified: GCL, ganglion cell layer; IS/OS, photoreceptor inner and outer segments; NFL, nerve fiber layer; ONL, outer nuclear layer; and RPE, retinal pigment epithelium.

Ophthalmoscopically occult cystoid macula edema or leakage from choroidal neovascularization can usually be easily identified with FA. The technique may also be helpful in highlighting the pigmentary abnormalities that can occur with inherited retinal degenerations such as Stargardt disease or the bull's eye pigmentary pattern common in toxic retinopathies.

Electroretinography (ERG) is another useful diagnostic tool, particularly for patients with retinal degeneration, paraneoplastic retinopathy, or acute zonal occult outer retinopathy (see below). The ERG is usually recorded using a corneal contact lens, and the signal is evoked from the retina using a flash of light. The ERG is characterized by a negative waveform (a-wave) that represents the response of the photoreceptors and a positive waveform (b-wave) that is generated by a combination of cells including the Mueller and bipolar cells. The entire response lasts less than 250 milliseconds. The ERG can be recorded under scotopic and photopic conditions to isolate the rod and cone responses. The cone-mediated response (photopic) is obtained by keeping the patient light-adapted and using a bright flash to evoke the response. In this setting the rods are bleached out and do not contribute to the waveform. The rod-mediated response (scotopic) is recorded after a prolonged period of dark adaptation and evoked with a dim light that is below the threshold of the cones. The a-wave is greatly reduced in scotopic conditions. Cone responses can also be isolated using a flickering light (30 cycles/second) since the rods cannot respond at that rate. When available, focal or multifocal ERG may provide additional information in subtle cases by examining a localized retinal flicker response from many regions of the retina.[2,3] Multifocal ERGs are very helpful in creating a "topographic" representation of retinal sensitivity across the macula and are useful in patients in whom occult macular disease is considered. Multifocal ERG may be helpful in following patients with outer retinopathies and to confirm normal function in suspected cases of nonorganic vision loss. To avoid false-positive results, testing is best performed by experienced electrophysiologists in laboratories that do the testing often.[2]

Electro-oculography is another test of retinal function and is based on the existence of an electrical potential across the retina. This potential seems to be dependent on the metabolic activity of the *pigment epithelium*, not the neurosensory retina. The oscillations in this potential can be increased by varying the levels of illumination. A reduction in the ratio of light-adapted to dark-adapted potentials represents an abnormal electro-oculogram (EOG). The EOG generally parallels the ERG but certain exceptions exist, such as vitelliform macular dystrophy, in which the ERG is normal and the EOG is abnormal.

Despite extensive evaluation, it may be impossible to localize the cause of the patient's vision loss. In this setting it is important to consider the possibility of nonorganic or functional vision loss. When doubt exists about the cause of the visual loss, one should consider screening the patient for the treatable causes of optic nerve dysfunction, including mass lesions, infections, and nutritional processes.

Maculopathies that may mimic optic neuropathy

The vast majority of patients with macular disease have findings on examination to make the diagnosis sufficiently easy if careful ophthalmoscopy is performed. For instance, a patient with age-related macular degeneration and vision loss will almost always have abnormalities that can be seen in the macula (drusen, swelling, bleeding, or atrophy) to explain the symptoms.

However, there are several macular conditions that are not well-visualized, and therefore the distinction from optic neuropathy may be difficult. These conditions are listed in **Table 4–2** and summarized below. They are often missed because the findings on clinical examination may be subtle or the clinical suspicion is not high enough. OCT has proven very helpful in identifying many of these subtle macular disorders (**Fig. 4–3**).

Central serous chorioretinopathy

Central serous chorioretinopathy results from abnormal leakage of fluid from the choroid into the subretinal spaces. It is a disorder that often affects young men, classically those with "type A" personalities, and women during pregnancy.[4-12] Other factors associated with central serous retinopathy include use of corticosteroids or psychopharmacologic

Table 4–2 Common maculopathies that may mimic optic neuropathies

Central serous maculopathy
Cystoid macular edema
Diabetic macular ischemia
Acute macular neuroretinopathy
Cone dystrophy
Toxic maculopathies
Idiopathic blind spot enlargement syndrome
Choroidal ischemia

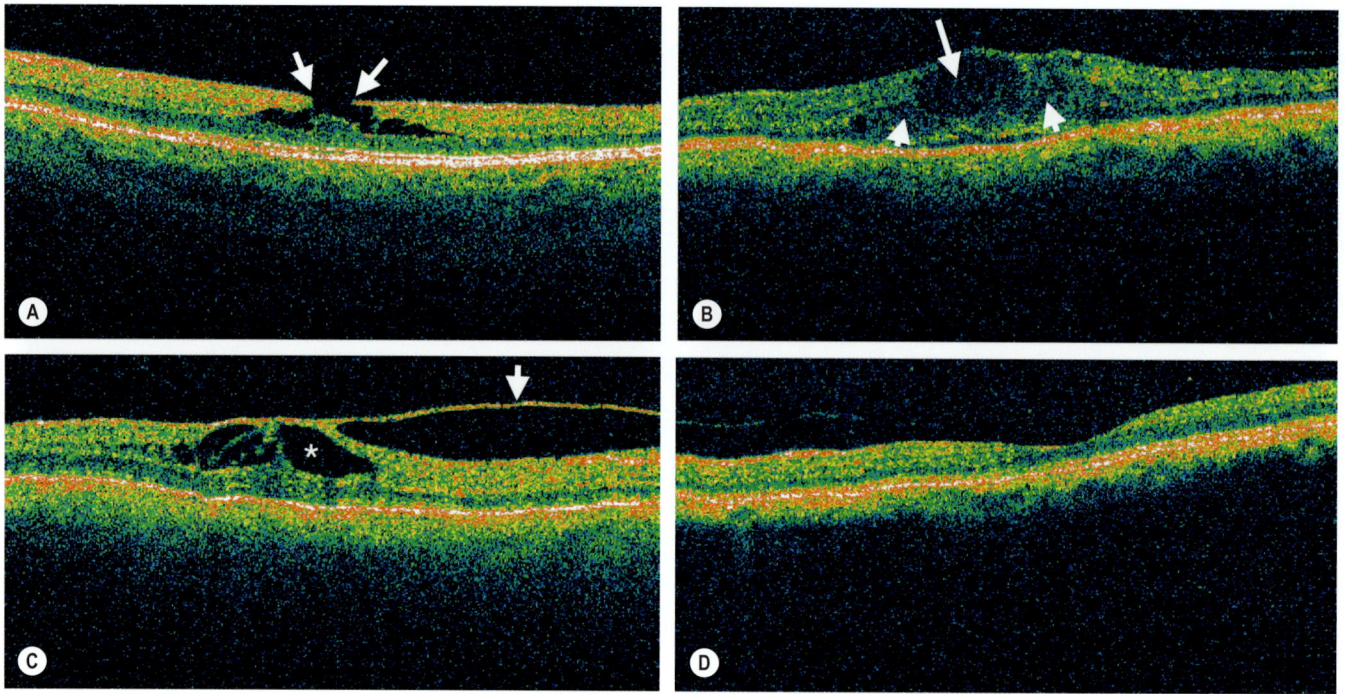

Figure 4–3. Ocular coherence tomography of common maculopathies encountered in the differential diagnosis of central vision loss. **A.** Macular hole; arrows denote the edges of the hole in the sensory retina. **B.** Macular edema, fluid spaces (arrows) are seen throughout the thickening of the retina. **C.** Cystic macular edema (asterisk) and thickening resulting from traction from an epiretinal membrane and vitreoretinal attachment (arrow). **D.** Generalized retinal thinning in a patient with cone dystrophy. Also see Figs 4–4 and 4–5.

medications, systemic hypertension, and immune suppression in organ transplantation.[13-17]

The patient may complain of sudden central visual loss and distortion. On examination, there is reduced visual acuity and a central scotoma on visual field testing. Metamorphopsia is typically present on Amsler's grid testing. An afferent pupil defect is usually not seen. The diagnosis is established best by slit-lamp biomicroscopy examination of the fundus, OCT, and FA, during which subretinal fluid in the macula will be evident (**Fig. 4–4**). The retinal elevation may be subtle and easily missed through an undilated pupil. Retrobulbar optic neuritis is the main alternative diagnosis, although pain on eye movements is usually present in that condition.

Cystoid macular edema

Cystoid macular edema (CME) most commonly occurs after cataract surgery but may occur in association with ocular inflammatory disease, macular degeneration, and diabetic retinopathy. Metamorphopsia is a common complaint. Small, shallow central visual field defects are frequently encountered and some patients will struggle with the color plates, although they do not have true dyschromatopsia. CME may be "ophthalmoscopically occult." In these cases, the thickening or elevation of the macula may be very subtle, and the typical cysts may be either absent or difficult to see.

FA and OCT are usually very helpful in identifying patients with CME not recognized by ophthalmoscopy (**Fig. 4–5**). However, patients with resolved CME may be difficult to diagnose because only mild pigmentary changes may be

evident. FA may be unhelpful in such cases. It is important to recognize CME because of the potential for effective treatment with anti-inflammatory agents.

Diabetic ischemic maculopathy

Ophthalmoscopically apparent macular edema is responsible for central vision loss in most patients with diabetic retinopathy. However, diabetic maculopathy, which may be associated with either nonproliferative or proliferative retinopathy, can take other forms including exudative or ischemic types. Closure of retinal capillaries is actually an early microvascular manifestation of diabetic retinopathy. Fortunately, this is usually not associated with significant vision loss. However, if the closure involves the arterioles, and the foveal avascular zone increases to 1000 μm, then acuity loss is common.[18] Although this type of vessel closure is easily seen on FA, other ophthalmoscopic clues include large dark retinal hemorrhages, multiple cotton-wool spots, and narrowed vessels.

However, the degree to which vision loss can be ascribed to this disorder may not correspond to the degree of ophthalmoscopic findings, and there are frequently confounding factors. Patients with advanced diabetic retinopathy and vision loss may exhibit mild optic atrophy and pigmentary changes. The visual field loss that may occur following pan-retinal photocoagulation also complicates the clinical picture. The full-field and multifocal ERG may be useful in identifying retinal dysfunction in patients with diabetic retinopathy.[19,20] When the unusual types of visual field defects are encountered, such as altitudinal defects or those respecting the vertical midline, then it is mandatory that

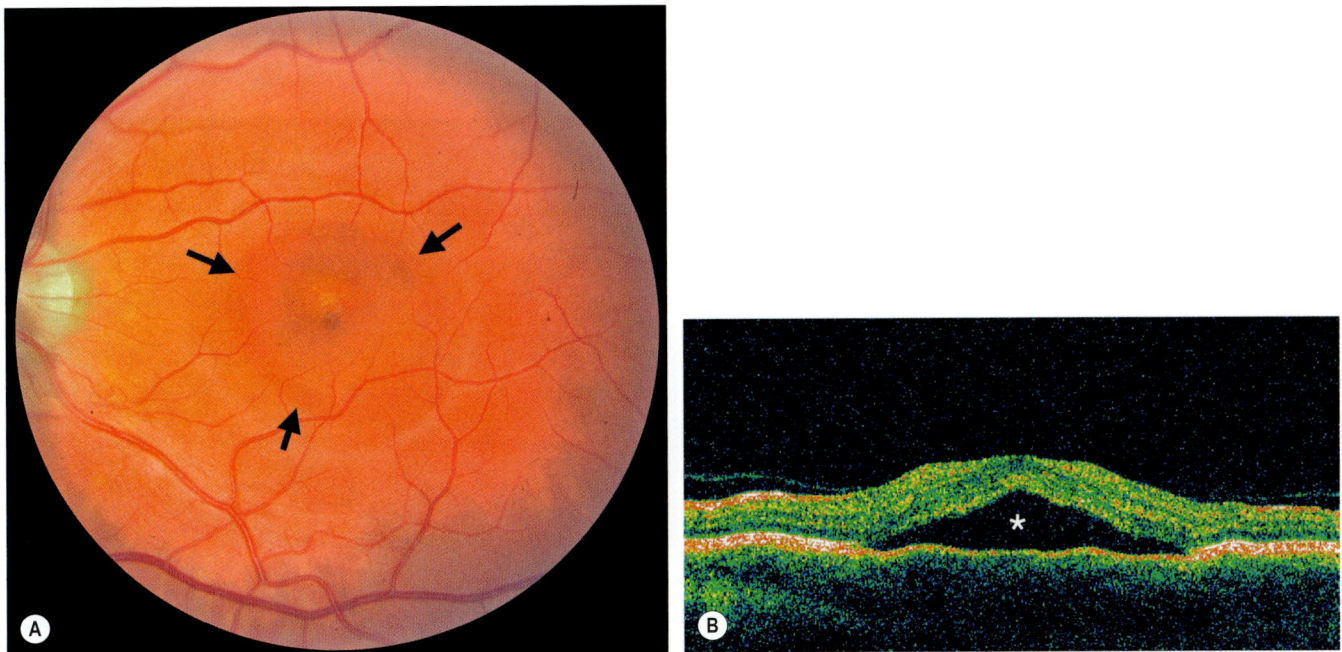

Figure 4–4. A. Fundus photograph of the left eye of a patient with central serous retinopathy. The black arrows delineate the edge of the small collection of fluid under the neurosensory retina. This view emphasizes how easily this condition can be missed when the fundus is examined with only a direct ophthalmoscope in the area of the optic nerve. **B**. OCT image of the same patient demonstrating fluid (asterisk) between the neurosensory retina and the retinal pigment epithelium (courtesy of Alexander J. Brucker, MD).

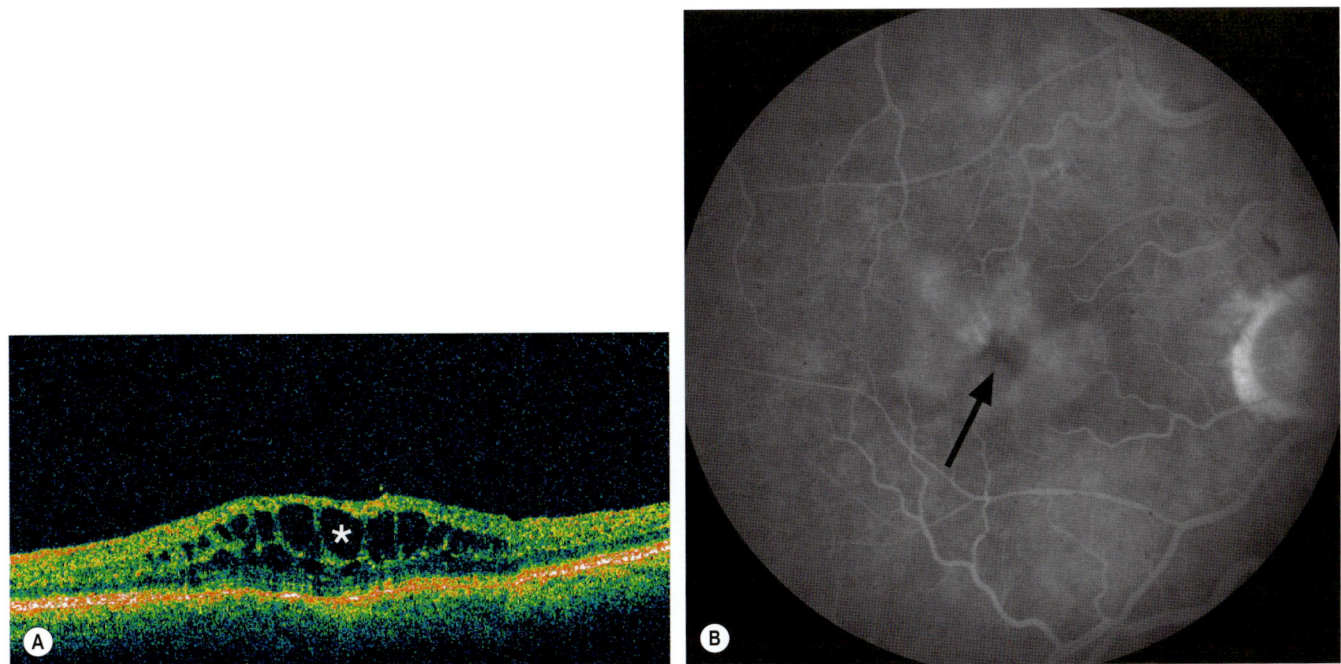

Figure 4–5. A. Ocular coherence tomography of cystoid macular edema with intraretinal cystic spaces seen (asterisk). **B**. Late-phase fluorescein angiography of cystoid macular edema demonstrating typical hyperfluorescent cyst-like spaces in the macula in petaloid pattern (black arrow).

alternative causes be considered, especially compressive optic nerve or chiasmal lesions.

Acute macular neuroretinopathy

This rare entity is also discussed below along with the big blind spot syndromes. It may be very difficult clinically to distinguish from optic neuritis because of the tendency for it to cause central vision loss in young women. A recent review identified fewer than 50 reported cases in the literature.[21] Classically, these patients have tiny, often multifocal, discrete central transient or permanent visual field defects, which are apparent only on Amsler grid testing. Scotomas correlate with an orange-brown, wedge-shaped, petalloid

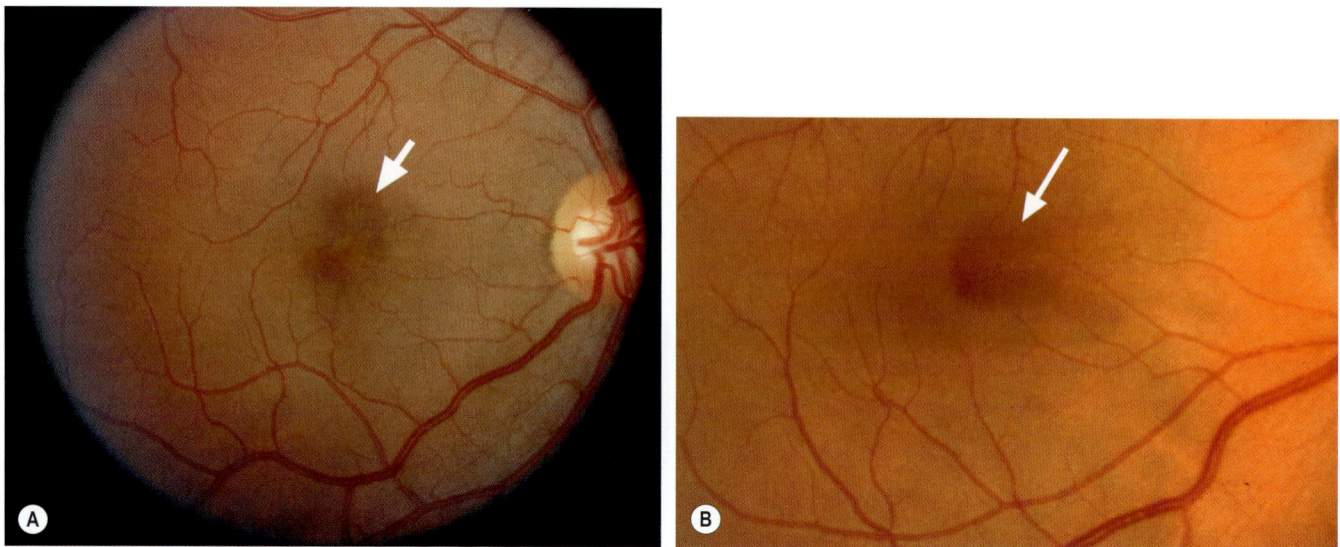

Figure 4–6. Fundus photographs of acute macular neuroretinopathy demonstrating subtle brownish discoloration of the retina. **A**. A "comma"-shaped area in the nasal parafoveal area (arrow) is seen. **B**. In another patient, a more striking petaloid, orange-brown lesion (arrow) is seen in the nasal parafoveal retina.

retinal lesion seen on ophthalmoscopy (**Fig. 4–6**). Again, this is another retinal diagnosis that is difficult to make without a careful dilated fundus examination. The pathologic process occurs in the outer retinal layers but the cause is uncertain. OCT can be very helpful in the diagnosis of acute macular neuroretinopathy (AMN).[22-24] Findings include an extra band of high reflectivity in front of the normal highly reflective band of the outer retinal complex.

Two other maculopathies commonly encountered in neuro-ophthalmic differential diagnosis, cone dystrophies and toxic maculopathies, are also discussed below.

Retinal vascular emboli and insufficiency

Retinal vascular insufficiency should be considered in the differential diagnosis of transient or permanent monocular visual loss. Emboli to the retinal vasculature, typically from the carotid artery bifurcation, are often the cause. On the other hand, asymptomatic retinal emboli are also frequently detected during ophthalmoscopy. In patients with either transient or permanent vision loss suspected to be the result of retinal vascular insufficiency or visible emboli on examination, a workup for either a carotid or a cardiac source of emboli must be pursued. This testing is detailed in Chapter 10, and usually includes a noninvasive carotid evaluation with ultrasound or magnetic resonance imaging–angiography and echocardiography. In younger patients or patients with unexplained recurrent symptoms or findings the workup can be expanded to include transesophageal echocardiography, a hematologic workup for hypercoagulable state, and occasionally conventional angiography.

Emboli

Types. There are three distinct types of retinal emboli: cholesterol, calcific, and platelet–fibrin.[25-28] The ophthalmo-

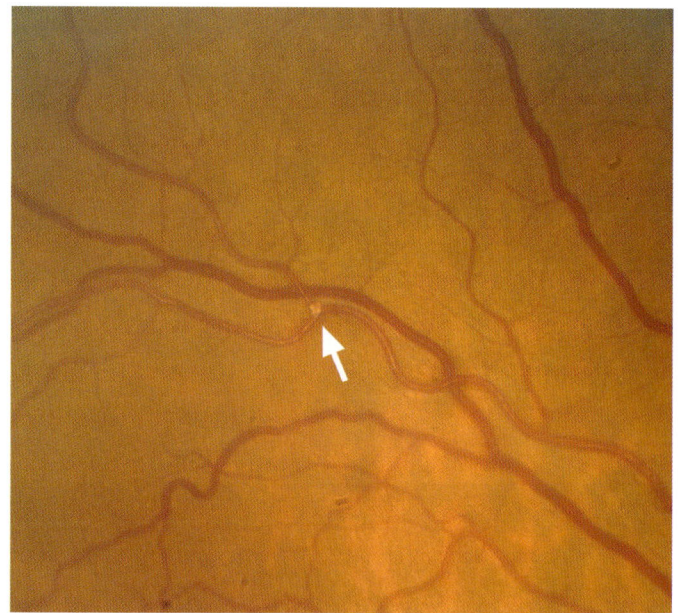

Figure 4–7. Hollenhorst plaque (arrow) at a bifurcation of a temporal retinal artery. These emboli typically have a shiny, yellow, refractile appearance and are often seen without any evidence of retinal infarction.

scopic differentiation of these types of emboli may be difficult. Sharma et al.[27] found poor intra- and interobserver reliability in differentiating retinal emboli. The authors of this study cautioned against making decisions about workup based solely on the clinical impression of the embolus type. Other more rare types of emboli include those composed of amniotic fluid, bacteria, parasites, metastatic tumors, fat, air, and talc. These types of emboli are recognized within their specific settings (i.e., talc with intravenous drug abuse, bacterial with endocarditis).

Cholesterol emboli (Hollenhorst plaques[29]), seen as gold-colored refractile bodies (**Fig. 4–7**), are the most common.

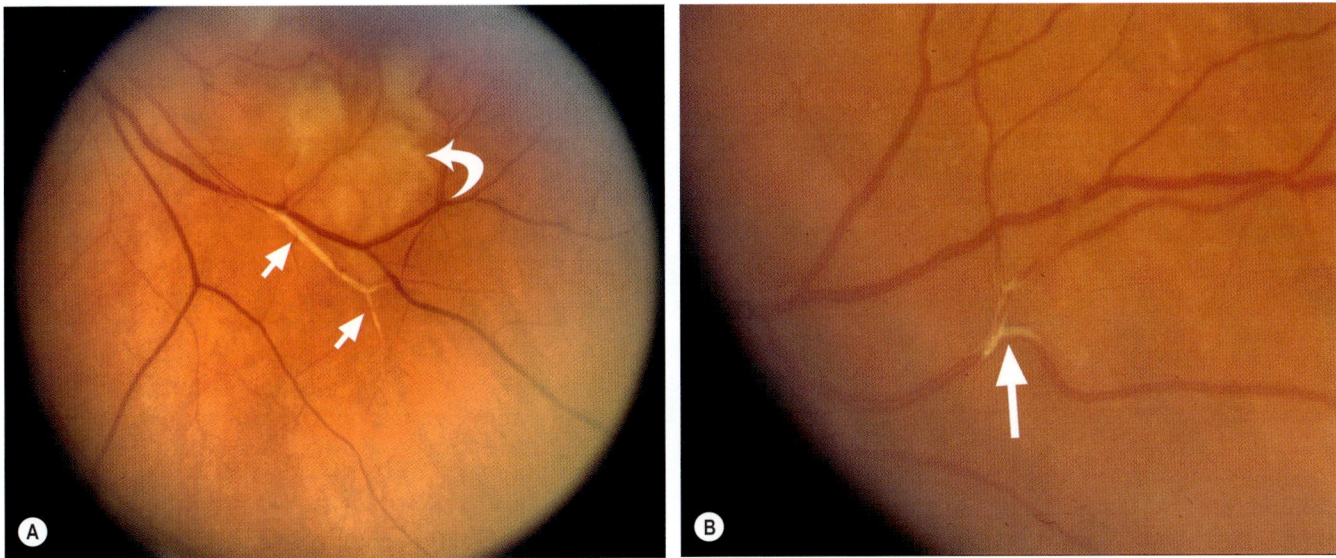

Figure 4–8. Platelet–fibrin emboli in retinal arteries. **A**. Note the yellow-gray, elongated, cast-like nature of the emboli (straight arrows) within the retinal arteries. A twig branch retinal artery occlusion (curved arrow) is seen distal to the involved artery. **B**. A platelet–fibrin embolus (arrow) without associated retinal infarction.

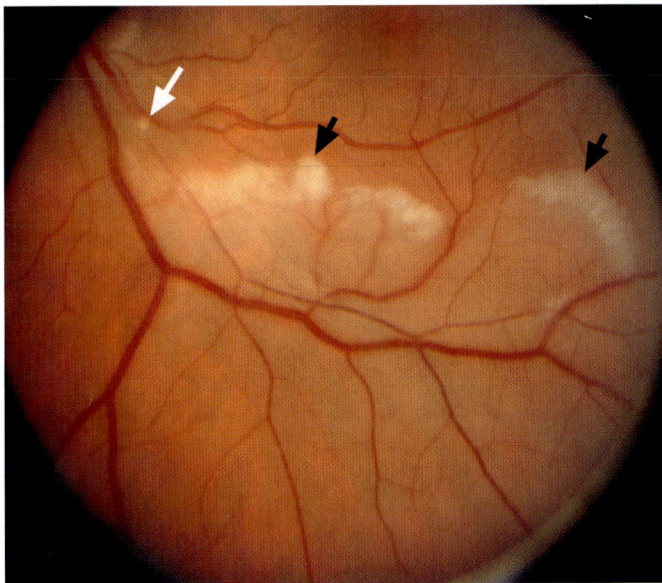

Figure 4–9. Calcific embolus of the inferotemporal retinal artery in a patient with a bicuspid aortic valve. The embolus (white arrow), which has a large globoid, gray appearance, caused a branch retinal artery occlusion with retinal whitening (black arrows).

Most cholesterol emboli lodge at bifurcations in the temporal retinal circulation. Platelet–fibrin emboli are gray and form cast-like elongated opacifications in retinal vessels (**Fig. 4–8**). These emboli may follow acute carotid thrombosis or more rarely myocardial infarction. Calcific emboli are large, globoid, and white (**Fig. 4–9**). They tend to occur in the setting of cardiac valvular disease,[30] but may also originate from a carotid source.

Prevalence and associations. The prevalence of retinal emboli in various populations has been reported to be approximately 0.9–3%.[31–36] The 5-year incidence is 0.9%.[33]

The prevalence increases with age, and they are more common in men. Emboli are associated with hypertension, smoking, vascular disease, and previous surgery.[31,32,34–38] In one study emboli were not found in association with diabetes or obesity.[35]

Carotid disease. In one series of patients with retinal emboli, 74 out of 207 underwent formal carotid angiography, and 18% of the asymptomatic patients were found to have significant stenosis (>75%).[39] The percentage was only slightly higher in symptomatic patients (21% with high-grade stenosis).[39] The stenosis was worse on the side of the embolus in 70% of patients. In another study of patients with either retinal emboli or retinal occlusion, significant carotid stenosis was found in 22% of patients and was the most common etiologic factor identified.[40] A population study agreed that approximately one-quarter of patients with retinal emboli had a carotid artery plaque.[38] In patients with retinal arterial occlusion, the presence of a retinal embolus did not predict a higher degree of stenosis in one study.[41] Asymptomatic patients with retinal emboli and carotid stenosis may in some cases benefit from carotid endarterectomy.[42] However, the decision for surgery should be made on an individual basis, as surgery for asymptomatic carotid stenosis is controversial (see Chapter 10).

Cardiac disease. Furthermore, finding an embolus also does not necessarily correlate with the presence of a structural cardiac lesion requiring intervention.[43] In patients with emboli or vessel occlusions, echocardiography may identify a cardiac source,[44] and transesophageal echocardiography is superior to transthoracic echocardiography.[45]

Associated morbidity and mortality. As recognized for decades,[46,47] cholesterol and platelet–fibrin emboli are associated with an increased risk for stroke,[33,36,40,48,49] myocardial infarction,[50] and, as a result, reduced life expectancy.[26]

Events associated with retinal vascular insufficiency

Amaurosis fugax. Amaurosis fugax (AF), or "fleeting" or transient monocular blindness, is usually sudden and is often described as a shade or curtain that obscures vision in one eye (see further discussion in Chapter 10). Visual loss may be altitudinal, peripheral, central, or even vertical. As opposed to migrainous episodes of transient vision loss, there usually are no photopsia or positive visual phenomena. Most episodes last 10 minutes or less and are painless. Transient migrainous monocular blindness can occur, but whether these events can be truly classified as migraine and whether they are separate and distinct from vasospastic AF are controversial.[51,52]

Emboli from the carotid to the retinal vasculature are a common cause of AF. These emboli may arise from internal carotid artery stenosis, dissection, or from common carotid artery disease.[53] A nasal defect may suggest an embolic mechanism because of the tendency of these particles to lodge in the temporal retinal circulation. Some emboli lodge behind the lamina cribrosa and are not visible. Others that enter the retinal circulation break up and pass distally.

AF is associated with an increased risk of a large-vessel stroke on the ipsilateral side.[54] Other causes of AF include the antiphospholipid antibody syndrome (APS; see below).[55] APS is most common in patients with lupus and can lead to AF even in children.[56] Heritable thrombophilia (factor V Leiden mutation), low protein S, high factor VIII, resistance to activated protein C, and the methylenetetrahydrofolate reductase (MTHFR) mutation may be identified in patients with AF and no other identifiable etiology (carotid or cardiac source).[57]

Retinal artery occlusion. Permanent vascular disruption may cause a central retinal artery occlusion (CRAO) or branch retinal artery occlusion (BRAO). Interestingly, for unclear reasons CRAO is associated with visible emboli in up to 20% of patients,[58] but BRAO has a higher rate, approaching 60–70%.[59] Other mechanisms of retinal vascular occlusion are possible besides emboli, including local thrombosis, hypercoagulability,[60] vasculitis, (especially temporal arteritis), vasospasm, and hypoperfusion. Although the frequency of operable carotid stenosis ipsilateral to a CRAO or BRAO varies from series to series, approximately 30–40% of patients will have >60% ipsilateral carotid stenosis.[61]

Central retinal artery occlusion. An acute CRAO is a true emergency because the potential to restore vision may exist for the first 12–24 hours. Because there are no ganglion cell axons overlying the macula, ophthalmoscopy reveals a macular cherry-red spot that results from the deep reddish color of the choroid showing through the surrounding, whitened retina (**Fig. 4–10**). In a study of 285 patients seen by a single ophthalmologist, Hayreh and Zimmerman[62] found the prevalence of ophthalmoscopic findings to be: retinal opacity in the posterior pole (58%), cherry-red spot (90%), box-carring in retinal vessels (19%), retinal arterial attenuation (32%), visible emboli (20%), optic disc edema (22%), and pallor (39%). Acutely, OCT demonstrates increased reflectivity and thickening of the inner retina and

a decreased reflectivity in the outer retina and retinal pigment epithelium/choriocapillaris layers.[63,64]

Aggressive therapies should be considered to improve the delivery of oxygen to the retina. Although some patients spontaneously improve, the prognosis for visual improvement after CRAO is poor even with heroic measures such as paracentesis, inhalation of carbogen (95% oxygen, 5% carbon dioxide) for vasodilation and increased blood flow, lowering intraocular pressure with various drugs, and ocular massage. The efficacy of these measures has never been proven, and one retrospective study suggested that the prognosis for visual recovery is not improved with these therapies.[65] Hayreh and Zimmerman[66] emphasized that the prognosis varies significantly depending on whether there was cilioretinal artery sparing, and whether reperfusion occurs, noting that, in Hayreh's personal series of 244 patients, only 50% had a residual peripheral island of vision while two-thirds of patients (particularly those with cilioretinal arteries and transient CRAO) had significant improvement. Approximately 20% of patients develop iris neovascularization.[67]

Intra-arterial fibrinolysis has been successfully used in patients with CRAO,[68] but multicenter prospective data demonstrating its efficacy are lacking.[69,70] Arnold et al.[71] reported improvement in 8 of 37 patients treated with fibrinolysis compared with none of 19 treated conventionally and noted a better prognosis in younger patients. In the USA the procedure has not yet been widely adopted and has been used in only a few academic medical centers.[72] Hayreh et al.[73] have shown, in an experimental monkey model, that the retina may survive for as long as 97 minutes with CRAO, but after that damage increases with time; after 4 hours there is profound irreversible damage.[73] This suggests a narrow but realistic time frame for intervention with clot lysis.

Branch retinal artery occlusion. Patients with BRAO similarly represent a heterogeneous group. Most patients present with and maintain better than 20/40 visual acuity.[74] Ophthalmoscopy reveals retinal whitening involving a section of retina with a partial cherry-red spot (**Fig. 4–10**). Nearly all BRAOs involve the temporal retinal arteries.[59] In the majority of cases, they occur in the setting of carotid artery disease,[75] and the workup for carotid and cardiac sources of emboli should be pursued as in patients with CRAO. BRAO has also been described in a variety of other conditions, including infectious retinopathies (toxoplasmosis, cat scratch disease), antiphospholipid antibody syndrome, protein S deficiency,[76] Susac syndrome,[77–79] temporal arteritis,[80] and the presence of anticardiolipin antibody[81] and lupus anticoagulants.[82] One study suggested that the presence of a visible embolus and BRAO were factors correlated with a significantly worse survival than age-matched controls.[83] As in the management of CRAO, aggressive maneuvers to move the embolus by lowering intraocular pressure and using vasodilators have no proven benefit.[59]

Cilioretinal artery occlusions. Similar embolic events can lead to the obstruction of the cilioretinal artery. If present, a cilioretinal artery can protect macular vision when CRAO occurs. Isolated cilioretinal artery occlusions can occur as well with loss of central vision and preservation of peripheral vision.[84–86] Cilioretinal artery occlusions have also

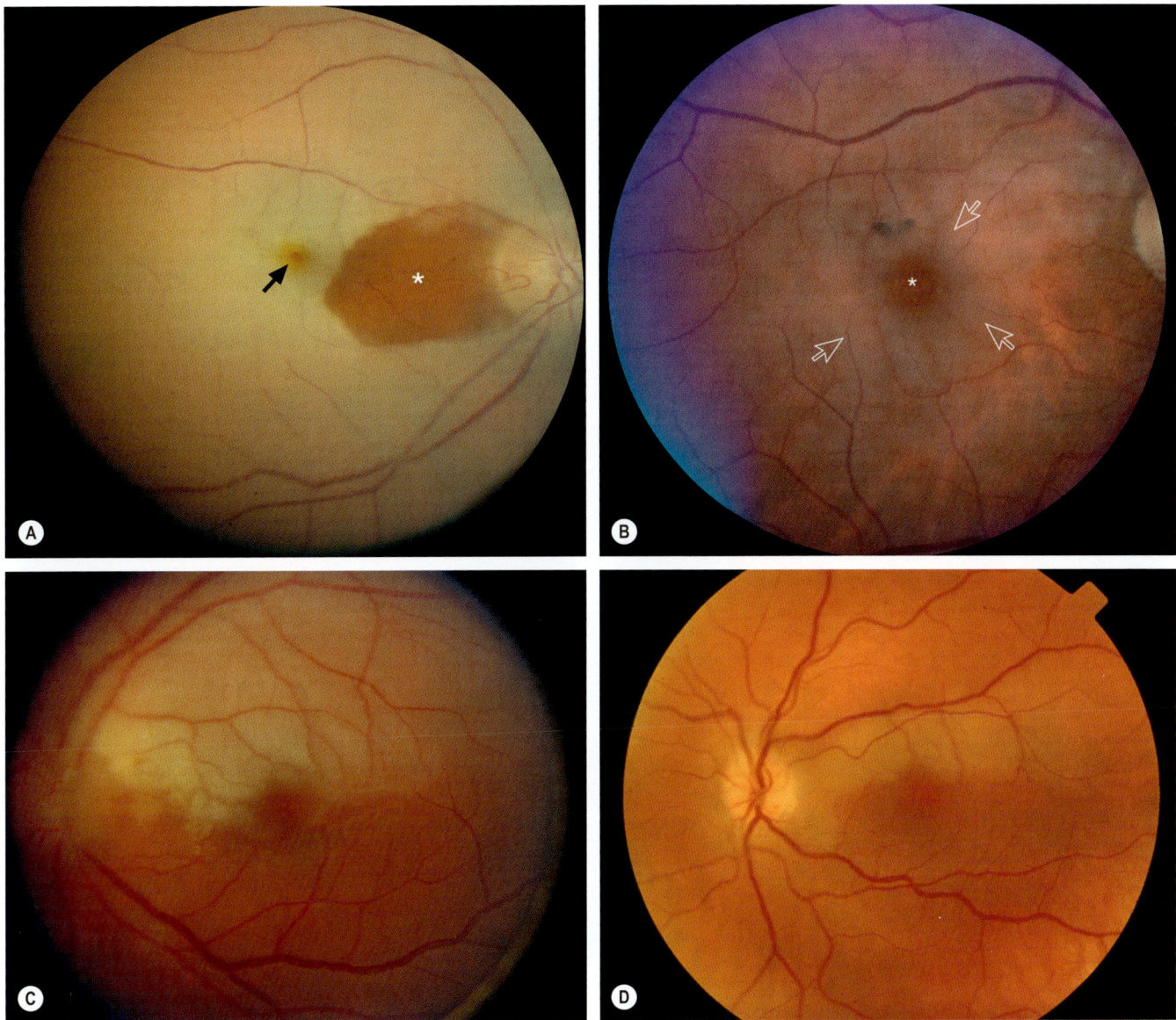

Figure 4–10. Central and branch retinal artery occlusions. Cherry-red spots from a central retinal artery occlusion can have a varied appearance depending on the time elapsed from the occlusion and the patient's pigmentation. **A**. A cherry-red spot (arrow) with extensive area of whitening around an area of cilioretinal sparing (asterisk) . **B**. Cherry-red spot (asterisk) surrounded by diffuse retinal whitening (arrows). The deep pigmentation superior to the macula is incidental. **C**. Superior branch retinal artery occlusion in a 14-year-old boy. There is a partial cherry-red spot. Extensive retinal whitening and swelling is seen, and the optic nerve also appears slightly swollen. **D**. Superior branch retinal artery occlusion with retinal whitening along the affected artery. This patient had temporal arteritis, and there is simultaneous swelling of the disc from ischemic optic neuropathy.

been described in systemic lupus erythematosus,[87] temporal arteritis,[88] carotid artery dissection,[89] antiphospholipid syndromes,[90,91] as a complication of embolization of central nervous system (CNS) lesions[92] and laser refractive surgery,[93] sickle cell disease,[94] and in association with central retinal vein occlusions in young patients (**Fig. 4–11**).[95,96]

Ocular ischemic syndrome. Hypoperfusion and subsequent ischemia of the globe associated with severe carotid disease may produce a variety of signs involving the posterior and anterior segments of the eye.[97–99] Patients may present with AF or gradual or sudden loss of vision.[99] A venous stasis retinopathy characterized by midperipheral dot and blot hemorrhages may be evident (see **Fig. 10–3**).[97–99] Optic nerve disc swelling is typically not seen until the very late stages of posterior segment ischemia. FA may reveal delayed retinal and choroidal perfusion.[97] The vascular occlusion is typically either in the ipsilateral internal carotid[100–102] or a more distal occlusion in the ophthalmic artery. Severe ocular ischemia may be caused by a carotid dissection or temporal or Takayasu arteritis.[103–106] Other manifestations of this condition are discussed in more detail in Chapter 10.

Retinal microvascular disease and associations

The presence of other retinal vascular abnormalities may be predictive of or associated with neurologic disease. Population-based studies have demonstrated that even nondiabetic individuals with retinal microaneurysms and

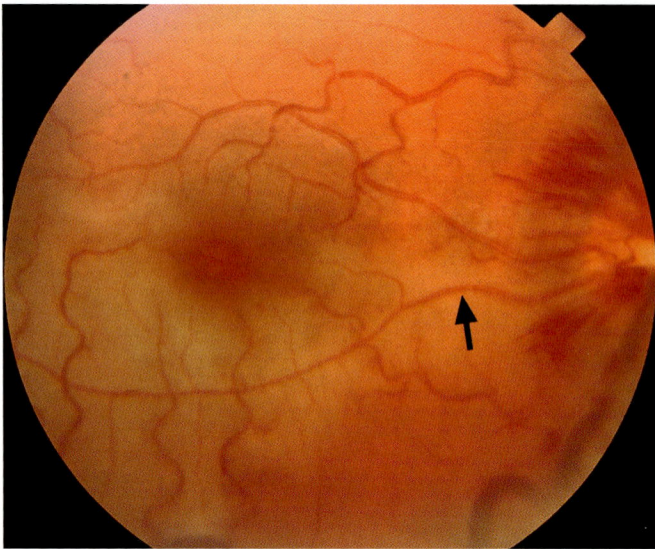

Figure 4–11. Nonischemic central retinal vein occlusion in a young man complicated by cilioretinal artery (arrow) occlusion. Retinal whitening is seen extending around the affected cilioretinal artery. Visual acuity was normal but there was a dense superior paracentral scotoma.

hemorrhages are at risk for stroke and stroke-related death.[107] Retinal arterial narrowing is associated with CNS signs of small-vessel disease such as lacunar infarcts and white matter lesions, in both hypertensive and normotensive patients.[108] For unclear reasons, narrowed retinal arteriolar diameters have,[109] and have not,[110] been shown to be associated with a higher risk of stroke. In addition, migraine and other headache patients are more likely to have retinal microvascular abnormalities such as narrowing and arteriovenous nicking.[111]

Retinal venous occlusion

Occlusive disease of the retinal venous system (branch and central retinal vein occlusion) does not result from carotid disease and is not usually associated with optic neuropathy or other neurologic disease. However, retinal vein occlusion is a common cause of acute vision loss, photopsia, optic nerve swelling, cotton-wool spots, and retinal hemorrhages, and therefore is an important neuro-ophthalmic condition to consider. Retinal vein occlusion may also be associated with systemic disorders including hypertension, connective tissue abnormalities, and hypercoagulability. Retinal venous occlusive disorders are among the most common retinal disorders encountered in practice, occurring with an incidence of 0.5%[112] to 1.6%.[113]

Central retinal vein occlusion. Acute central retinal vein occlusion (CRVO) has a characteristic and dramatic appearance characterized by tortuosity and dilation of retinal veins, retinal edema, and intraretinal hemorrhages extending away from the disc into all four quadrants. CRVO can present with and without disc edema, depending on the position of the occlusion (**Fig. 4–12**). The presence of disc edema is associated with younger age, better visual function, and less severe vascular nonperfusion, suggesting occlusion behind the lamina cribrosa.[114] Clinical distinction from primary disor-

ders of the optic nerve associated with swelling and retinal vasculitis can be difficult. In milder and incomplete forms there may be only a limited number of hemorrhages, mild venous dilation, and slight hyperemia of the disc.

CRVOs are divided into two categories, ischemic and nonischemic, based on the degree of vision loss and the amount of capillary nonperfusion on FA. Nonischemic vein occlusions have prolonged circulation time and capillary permeability breakdown on FA. Patients with ischemic CRVO are more likely to have poor vision at presentation (including an afferent pupillary defect), develop rubeosis, and require treatment with panretinal photocoagulation. FA will reveal severe capillary nonperfusion, and electroretinography will show a reduced b-/a-wave ratio.

The mechanism of CRVO is believed to be thrombosis of the central retinal vein although the actual cause of the thrombosis, and its relationship to atherosclerotic disease of the central retinal artery, is unknown.[115] Both ocular and systemic conditions have been associated with CRVO. Most studies find a high incidence of systemic hypertension and cardiovascular disease.[116] Elevated lipoprotein levels have been found in patients with retinal vein occlusion.[117] In a small number of patients, carotid disease may be a risk for the condition with a worse prognosis.[118] In younger patients collagen vascular disease may be a consideration.[119] The association of vein occlusions with thrombotic states is discussed later in this chapter.

About half of patients with CRVO resolve the occlusion without significant vision loss, but 20% go on to complete occlusion.[120] Novel treatments for CRVO include creation of retinal choroidal shunt vessels with a laser and radial optic neurotomy, which has been shown to improve the congested fundus and central vision but has not been studied prospectively.[121] Many patients with CRVO present with or develop open-angle glaucoma.

Branch retinal vein occlusion. In branch retinal vein occlusion (BRVO) the findings of venous insufficiency develop in just a portion of the retina. Such occlusions tend to occur at the point where a retinal artery and vein cross. The retinal findings typically occur in the superotemporal quadrant in an arcuate pattern of hemorrhages, cotton-wool spots, and retinal edema. The events leading to occlusion remain obscure but presumably include thrombosis of the vein perhaps caused by turbulent flow in the overlying artery, which shares the same adventitia as the vein. Fresh and recanalized thrombus has been identified in patients with BRVO.[122] Hypertension, male gender, hyperopia, diabetes, and glaucoma may all be risk factors for BRVO.[123] BRVOs are commonly complicated by macular edema, which may result in central vision loss and may be treated by macular photocoagulation.[124] Neovascularization occurs in 20–30% of patients and may be prevented or treated with scatter photocoagulation.[125,126]

Photoreceptor disorders important in neuro-ophthalmology

Paraneoplastic retinopathy (PR) and the big blind spot syndromes are two subacute retinal disorders with a normal

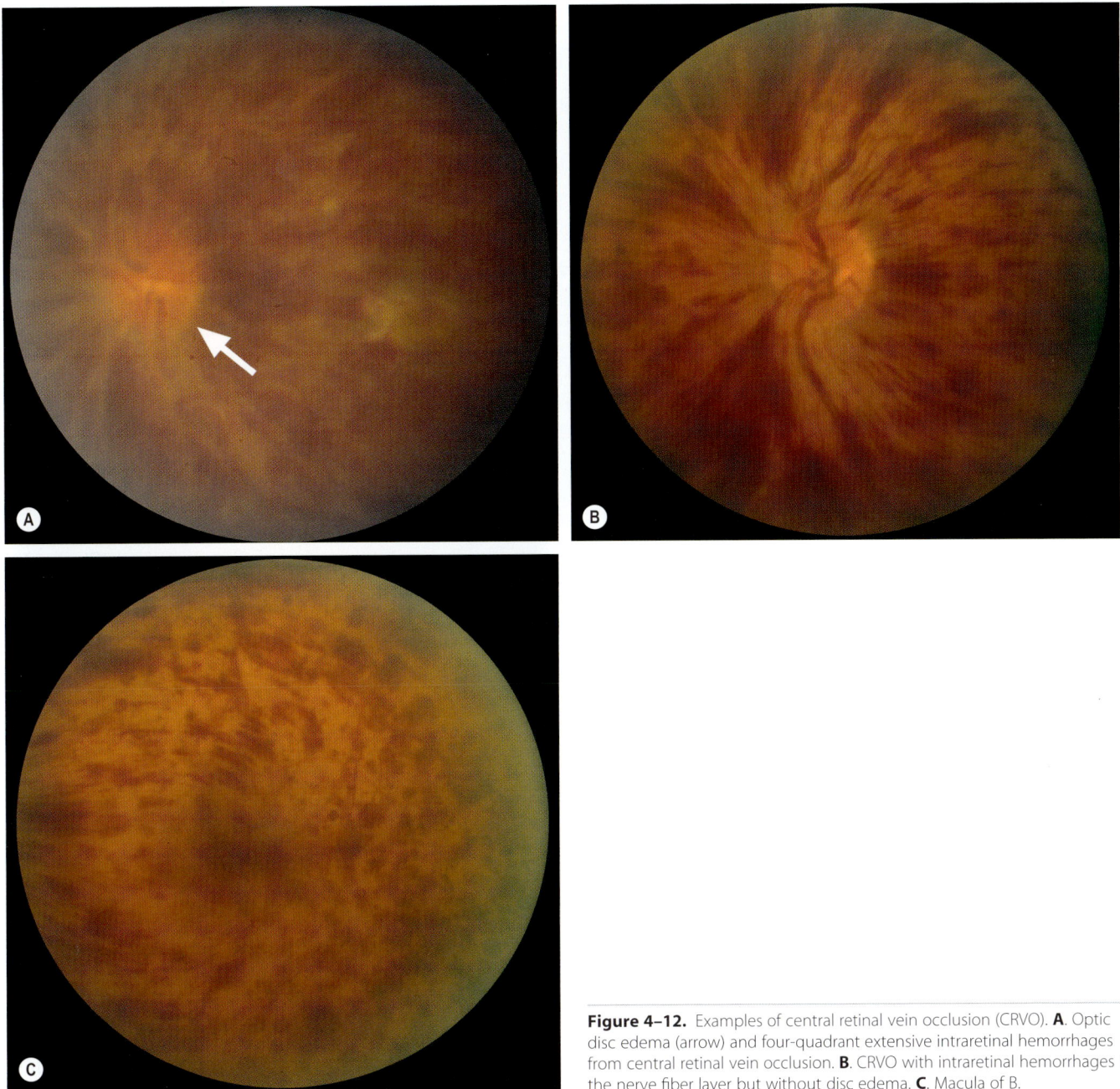

Figure 4–12. Examples of central retinal vein occlusion (CRVO). **A**. Optic disc edema (arrow) and four-quadrant extensive intraretinal hemorrhages from central retinal vein occlusion. **B**. CRVO with intraretinal hemorrhages in the nerve fiber layer but without disc edema. **C**. Macula of B.

or minimally abnormal ophthalmoscopic appearance. Although these conditions are unrelated, they are both outer retinopathies (photoreceptor dysfunction) that are important in neuro-ophthalmic differential diagnosis because their presentation may mimic that of optic neuropathies. Retinal symptoms (photopsia) and retinal signs (midperipheral field defects or enlargement of the blind spot) occur in PR and the big blind spot syndromes and are important clues to their diagnosis.

Paraneoplastic retinopathy

Primary malignancies and secondary tumors (metastatic and direct extension from adjacent structures) may produce vision loss by displacement, invasion, or compression of ocular tissues. However, ocular and neurologic dysfunction may develop in patients with cancer without direct tumor involvement. These disorders are collectively termed *paraneoplastic syndromes*. They not only present a diagnostic challenge but may provide insight into the biologic behavior of tumors and their effect on the host immune system.[127–129]

Sawyer et al.[130] were the first to recognize the unusual features of a retinopathy occurring as a remote effect of cancer. *Paraneoplastic retinopathy* refers to a syndrome of subacute deterioration of vision and retinal function resulting from a nonmetastatic, remote effect of a malignancy. The clinical features of the paraneoplastic retinopathies are summarized in **Table 4–3**. This broader term encompasses several distinct entities, including cancer-associated retinopathy

Table 4–3 Clinical features of paraneoplastic syndromes

Disorder	Pathogenesis	Clinical manifestations and course
Cancer-associated retinopathy (CAR)	Antibodies to 23-kDa antigen believed to be recoverin; other antibodies found, sometimes unknown	Subacute onset of photopsia and progressive visual field loss beginning as midperipheral scotoma
		Mild vitritis, narrowed retinal vessels
		Relentlessly progressive
		Diffuse loss of ERG
		Steroids may be helpful
Melanoma-associated retinopathy (MAR)	Antibodies to retinal bipolar cells in patients with metastatic melanoma	Onset of night blindness and dark adaption difficulties
		May have fixed nonprogressive defect
		ERG shows rod dysfunction (scotopic b-wave) and normal cone function
		ERG similar to congenital stationary night blindness
Paraneoplastic ganglion cell neuronopathy (PGCN)	Antibodies to retinal ganglion cells	Bilateral progressive loss of vision
	Immune deposits in the retina	May have optic disc swelling
		Abnormal immunoglobulin levels in CSF
		Optic nerve demyelination may occur
Cancer-associated cone dysfunction (CACD)	Antibodies to CAR antigen and 50-kDa protein	Subacute onset of glare or photosensitivity
	Loss of cones in macula	ERG shows cone dysfunction with preservation of rod function
	Infiltration by macrophages	Loss of color vision; central scotomas
Diffuse uveal melanocytic proliferation (DUMP)	Develops in women with reproductive tract cancers and men with cancers in retroperitoneal area	Bilateral subacute vision loss
		Primary tumor may not be known
		Subretinal proliferation of pigmentary cells and yellow-orange lesions at level of retinal pigmented epithelium (RPE)

CSF, cerebrospinal fluid; ERG, electroretinogram.

(CAR), which is the most common, cancer-associated cone dysfunction (CACD), melanoma-associated retinopathy (MAR), diffuse uveal melanocytic proliferation (DUMP), and paraneoplastic ganglion cell neuronopathy (PGCN). The exact prevalence of paraneoplastic retinal disorders is unknown.

Despite some fairly characteristic complaints and examination findings, the diagnosis of PR is rarely made at presentation. In addition, it is common for the syndrome to develop prior to recognition and diagnosis of the systemic malignancy.

Symptoms, signs, and electroretinography. Patients usually report the subacute onset of decreased vision or a halo of missing peripheral vision. Common complaints also include the acute onset of photopsia (flashing lights) or other positive visual phenomena. Differences in symptoms among the various entities correlate with the degree to which the rods versus cones are affected.

Visual acuity ranges from normal to markedly reduced. Other features on examination include abnormal color vision and prolonged photostress recovery time. An afferent pupil defect may be evident in cases with asymmetric retinal involvement. Goldmann visual fields may be more useful than automated perimetry since the scotomas usually begin in the midperiphery (**Fig. 4–13**). As the retinal degeneration evolves, the paracentral defects eventually connect to form a classic ring scotoma. Since the visual field defects result from retinal dysfunction, the "arcuate-type" defects typically do not respect the horizontal meridian. The outer retina does not have an anatomic demarcation along the horizontal meridian like the nerve fiber layer.

In general, there is usually a paucity of ocular findings compared with the symptoms and level of visual dysfunction. However, ocular examination may reveal a mild vitritis[131] and vascular attenuation.[131-136] Other findings described in these patients include optic disc pallor, granularity of the retinal pigment, and peripheral retinal pigmentation.

The diagnosis of PR is strongly suggested when an ERG shows evidence of diffuse retinal dysfunction in a patient with relatively precipitous visual loss. Most abnormal ERGs

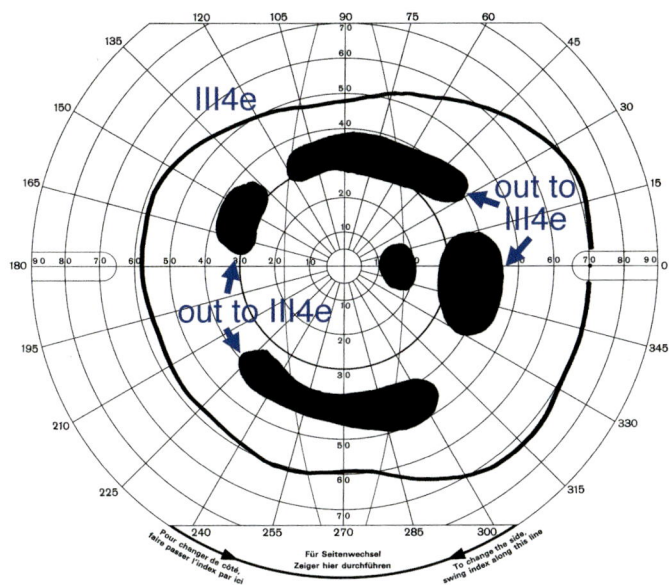

Figure 4–13. Goldmann visual field of the left eye of a patient with cancer-associated retinopathy. Photoreceptor dysfunction is manifested by midperipheral scotomas that do not respect the vertical or horizontal meridians. The scotomas are beyond 15 degrees of eccentricity.

are found in patients with chronic retinal degenerations such as retinitis pigmentosa. The ERG varies in PR depending on the particular syndrome.

Each subtype has several distinguishing signs and symptoms, ERG features, and systemic associations (**Table 4–3**).

Cancer-associated retinopathy. CAR patients, in whom rods are primarily affected, typically manifest with vision loss and night blindness (nyctalopia).[131,135,137] An abnormal scotopic ERG is usually found.

Several reports have described the histopathologic findings in CAR.[130,132,135,138–141] As expected, loss of photoreceptor inner and outer segments was present in each case. The degree of macular involvement was variable, and in general there was more rod than cone involvement.[135] Outer nuclear cell loss and the presence of inflammatory infiltrates were other notable features. Except in one case with phlebitis,[141] the retinal vasculature was typically reported as normal. The inner nuclear layer (ganglion cells) was always spared. In areas of photoreceptor loss, scattered melanophages and disruption of the retinal pigment epithelium have been observed.

Keltner and associates[140,142] were the first to propose an autoimmune pathogenesis in CAR.[57,58] They demonstrated antiretinal antibodies in a patient with cervical carcinoma in 1983.[140] These antibodies reacted with photoreceptors from normal human retina. Subsequently they performed enzyme-linked immunosorbent assay and western blot testing in four patients with CAR and found a serum antibody that bound a 23-kDa retinal antigen, which they termed the CAR *antigen*.[142] Most patients with CAR have antibodies to the 23-kDa antigen, which has subsequently been identified as recoverin (see below). Over 20 other antigens have also been identified, including enolase,[143–145] 65-kDa heat shock cognate (hsc) protein,[146] the photoreceptor nuclear receptor,[147] and neurofilaments,[148] suggesting that CAR is a hetero-

geneous group of autoimmune conditions rather than a single entity. The specific circulating antibody responsible for CACD is unknown, but, in one patient with CACD, 23-kDa and 50-kDa antibodies were identified.[149] The involved retinal antigen in patients with MAR appears to be distinct.[150] It is likely that several different antigens may elicit an immune response capable of causing retinal damage.

CAR is now thought to result from an antibody-mediated loss of photoreceptors. Presumably, antibodies are formed as part of an autoimmune reaction to tumor antigens. These antigens cross-react with retinal antigens because of shared epitopes (antigenic mimicry). Tumor necrosis can expose antigens to immunologic surveillance and result in antibody production. It is possible that the tumor cells themselves aberrantly express the retinal antigen (e.g., recoverin, see below), which becomes exposed to immune surveillance.[138] The components of the activated immune response must then cross the blood–retina barrier (presumably altered by focal or general cellular inflammation) and react with a photoreceptor antigen. Antirecoverin antibodies have been identified in the aqueous humor[151] and serum[152] of patients with CAR. However, these antibodies are also present in the blood of some who do not develop PR,[153] suggesting that other pathologic processes must occur to allow antibodies access to the retina.

Finally, the tissue-bound antibody–antigen complex must result in cell death or apoptosis.[154] The exact mechanism by which the antibody–recoverin molecule complex causes cell death is unknown. An effect on energy production seems likely since the classic immune-mediated form of destruction that includes lymphocytic cellular infiltration is not observed in most cases. Polans et al.[155] found that antibodies in patients with CAR reacted with recoverin, a calcium channel photoreceptor protein (in the calmodulin family). In addition, serum antibodies from CAR patients have been used to isolate the gene that encodes the CAR antigen from a cDNA library of human retina. The resultant nucleotide sequence was shown to have been 90% homologous to the published sequence of bovine recoverin.[156] Recoverin is the CAR antigen in most patients.

Immunohistochemistry has been used to demonstrate that the serum antiretinal antibodies affect the outer retina.[131] The pattern observed respected the anatomic boundary between the outer plexiform and inner nuclear layers. A similar immunohistochemical staining pattern occurs with antibodies directed against recoverin. Outer retinal involvement on both histopathology and immunohistochemistry supports the theory that these antibodies have a role in the pathogenesis of the disease.

Cancer-associated cone dysfunction. In contrast, CACD patients may complain of decreased acuity, dyschromatopsia, glare, photosensitivity, or reduced vision in bright light (hemeralopia), more suggestive of cone dysfunction. CACD is characterized by an abnormal cone ERG. Patients typically have color vision loss and central scotomas. Signs and symptoms are caused by loss of cones in the macula.[132] A patient with PR and isolated cone dysfunction was reported to have antibodies to a 40-kDa retinal protein that was within the outer segment, where the retinal photoreceptors lie.[157]

Melanoma-associated retinopathy. Most patients with MAR have an established diagnosis of cutaneous melanoma and present uniformly with photopsia, night blindness, and floaters.[136,158–162] A recent report described a patient with MAR and a primary melanoma in the maxillary sinus.[162] In some instances of MAR, at presentation metastatic melanoma is found.[136,150,158,163,164] Patients usually have better than 20/40 acuity at presentation, with dyschromatopsia and visual field defects (central scotomas, arcuate defects, and generalized constriction). The fundus appears normal in 50% of patients, but optic disc pallor, retinal vessel attenuation, and vitritis may be evident in other patients.[160] Unlike patients with CAR, patients with MAR typically do not experience the relentless progression to blindness.

Patients with MAR have a highly specific ERG with absent b-waves under dark-adapted conditions and normal cone amplitudes, suggesting bipolar cell dysfunction.[136,150,158,162,163] The serum from patients with MAR can be shown by immunocytochemical techniques to react with retinal bipolar cells.[165] In most cases the a- and b-wave amplitudes are markedly reduced. Progressive visual loss has been correlated with progressive reduction of ERG amplitudes. Abnormal EOGs have also been reported.[134,140] MAR antiretinal antibodies have been found in the serum of patients with melanoma but no clinical evidence of MAR, similarly to some patients who harbor CAR antibodies without retinal disease.[166] Other patients with MAR may be asymptomatic despite abnormal perimetry and ERGs.[161]

Bilateral diffuse uveal melanocytic proliferation. Bilateral DUMP manifests with subacute loss of vision that often develops prior to diagnosis of the primary neoplasm.[167–170] The most common primary tumors associated with this syndrome are carcinoma of the reproductive tract in women and cancers of the retroperitoneal area and the lungs in men. Ophthalmoscopic examination reveals bilateral proliferation of subretinal pigment and yellow-orange lesions at the level of the retinal pigment epithelium. The former retinal change may appear similar to choroidal nevi. There may be serous detachments of the retina. Early-phase FA shows a pattern of hyperfluorescence, corresponding to the abnormalities observed at the level of the retinal pigment epithelium. Uveitis and a rapidly progressive cataract may occur.

Proliferation of nonmalignant cells has been shown on histopathology, and metastases have not been reported.[167,168] The serous retinal detachments may respond to systemic corticosteroids or radiation. Treatment of the primary tumor may not alter the course of the progressive visual loss.

Paraneoplastic ganglion cell neuronopathy. PGCN is essentially a form of paraneoplastic optic neuropathy. These conditions are discussed in Chapter 5. Suffice it to say that there have been scattered reports of patients with cancer presenting with demyelinating optic neuropathies without any evidence of cancer spread to the optic nerve or meninges. One report noted the presence of immune deposits in the retina and diffuse ganglion cell loss on histopathologic evaluation.[171]

Laboratory findings. FA occasionally shows periphlebitis.[141,172] Standard laboratory testing (i.e., blood chemistries and serum immunoglobulin levels) have no role in the diagnosis of PR. However, identification of serum antiretinal antibodies is an important diagnostic aid and can now be obtained commercially.

Systemic evaluation. In individuals with suspected PR, a careful review of the patient's medical history and laboratory investigations should be undertaken to identify the underlying systemic malignancy. Approximately one-half of the cases of PR are diagnosed prior to the discovery of the malignancy.[130,135,137,140,142] Like many of the other paraneoplastic syndromes, two-thirds of patients with PR will have small cell carcinoma of the lung. Other associated tumors include melanoma in MAR,[136,158,164] breast carcinoma,[173] uterine carcinoma,[132,139,174] cervical carcinoma,[140] thymoma,[175] and lymphoma.[176] In one reported patient there were three primary tumors (prostate, bladder, larynx).[134] PR has not been reported to occur with other paraneoplastic neurologic diseases.

Differential diagnosis. PR must be distinguished from four broad categories of anterior visual pathway disease which may occur in this setting, including conditions that appear clinically similar but are not associated with systemic malignancy, conditions secondary to direct spread of tumor, toxic effects of chemotherapy, and other paraneoplastic conditions.[127,129] Compressive or inflammatory lesions of the anterior visual pathway must be considered in all instances of subacute visual loss. Optic neuritis is a common misdiagnosis in patients ultimately shown to have PR.[134,135] However, optic neuritis and ischemic optic neuropathy can usually be excluded on clinical grounds. Nearly all reported cases underwent neuroimaging of the anterior visual pathway to rule out a compressive lesion prior to diagnosis. Less common causes of subacute visual loss such as toxic, hereditary, and nutritional optic neuropathies should be considered and excluded based on historical and laboratory information. Ultimately, an abnormal ERG will distinguish PR from optic neuropathy.

The rapid rate of visual deterioration distinguishes PR from other retinal degenerations such as retinitis pigmentosa. The two conditions otherwise may mimic each other since both conditions result from photoreceptor dysfunction. In contrast to PR patients, most individuals with retinitis pigmentosa have abnormal fundi with pigmentary deposition.

Alternatively, vision loss may develop by a variety of mechanisms in the cancer patient. Carcinomatous meningitis may produce an optic neuropathy. In this situation, the neuroimaging of the optic nerve and meninges and/or spinal fluid chemistry and cytology will typically be abnormal. Visual loss may also occur as a result of the toxic effects of chemotherapy. Chemotherapeutic agents including 1,3-bis(2-chloroethyl)-l-nitrosurea (BCNU), vincristine, and cis-platinum have been reported to cause optic neuropathy. Radiation therapy may cause retrobulbar optic neuropathy months to years after treatment. The optic nerves or chiasm may show enhancement and enlargement on magnetic resonance imaging (MRI). Paraneoplastic optic neuropathy (PON) has also been observed in patients with small cell carcinoma of the lung (see also Chapter 5).[177–180]

Treatment. To reduce systemic levels of antiretinal antibody, the therapy most often suggested has been immunosuppression. Treatment of the primary malignancy usually does not seem to alter the course of visual loss, although one reported patient had mild improvement.[172]

The mainstay of therapy is systemic corticosteroids.[181] Other systemic immunosuppressive drugs have not been tried systematically. Visual acuity and fields in PR patients have been reported to improve with steroids.[141,172,173,181] In one patient, visual acuity decreased each time the steroids were tapered and improved when they were reinstated.[140] Keltner et al.[181] reported a patient with elevated levels of serum antibodies that could be reduced with steroids. The elevated antibody titers were associated with visual deterioration. Some patients fail to improve with corticosteroids.[130,174] Plasmapheresis has been tried unsuccessfully in one case.[182] Espandar et al.[183] reported a patient with CAR who did not respond to plasma exchange, cyclosporine, and steroids, but improved with treatment with alemtuzumab, a monoclonal antibody against the cell surface glycoprotein CD52 expressed on B and T lymphocytes and monocytes. Patients with MAR often respond to intravenous immunoglobulin and metastasectomy.[160]

Course. Patients with PR should be followed closely with serial acuities, visual fields, ERGs, and antiretinal antibody titers. The clinical course of PR is variable although rapid progression of CAR is the rule. Some MAR patients may remain stable. Development then worsening of a ring scotoma is characteristic of CAR. Patients are usually significantly visually impaired and progression to profound bilateral loss of vision occurs within weeks to months. Many patients die before they become totally blind. Retinal arterioles typically become more attenuated over time, and the ERG responses progressively decline. The serum level of serum antiretinal antibodies may correlate with success of treatment and severity of the disease.

Big blind spot syndromes

The term *big blind spot syndrome* has been used to describe several different entities, all of which present with enlargement of the physiologic blind spot. These disorders include acute idiopathic blind spot enlargement (AIBSE) and multiple evanescent white dot syndrome (MEWDS). Enlargement of the blind spot is due either to optic nerve head swelling with displacement of the peripapillary retina or to dysfunction of the peripapillary retina when the optic nerve is ophthalmoscopically normal. Patients reported with AIBSE and MEWDS have a fairly uniform presentation, with the acute onset of a visual field defect around the physiologic blind spot accompanied by photopsia. Visual acuity is usually normal,[184–187] and the visual field defects typically have steep borders. These disorders all likely affect the outer retina and therefore may lie within the spectrum of a single disease. These diseases are more common in women.[187,188]

Acute idiopathic blind spot enlargement. In 1988 Fletcher et al.[185] described seven patients, age 25–39, with the acute onset of photopsia and enlargement of the blind spot without optic disc swelling. Two patients had abnormal multifocal ERGs, and the authors concluded that the syndrome resulted from peripapillary retinal dysfunction. Their patients had no abnormalities on FA, although two patients had peripapillary retinal pigment abnormalities. Two patients had recurrences, and three had recovery of their visual fields.

The term AIBSE syndrome is now used to describe patients with the acute onset of positive visual phenomena and an enlarged blind spot occasionally associated with mild disc swelling (**Fig. 4–14**). Peripapillary pigmentary changes are common (**Fig. 4–14**).[187] The field defects, which may be more easily detected with blue on white perimetry,[189] generally have steep borders and can mimic the temporal visual field defects of chiasmal disease (**Fig. 4–15**). Retinal pigment epithelial or choroidal abnormalities and disc staining on FA may be seen.[190,191] Full-field ERGs are often normal but focal and multifocal ERGs directed at the peripapillary retina are abnormal (**Fig. 4–16**).[185,191–193] Photopsia tends to resolve over time, although in most patients the visual field defect persists.[187]

Multiple evanescent white dot syndrome. In 1984, Jampol et al.[194] and Takeda et al.[195] described the MEWDS. Jampol et al.[194] reported 11 patients (10 women) with acute unilateral vision loss, scotomas, and multiple evanescent white lesions at the level of the retinal pigment epithelium (**Fig. 4–17**). Many of these and subsequently reported cases of MEWDS have had blind spot enlargement.[194,196–199] Full-field ERG abnormalities in patients with MEWDS have also been recognized.[194,196–201] FA can confirm the retinal pigment epithelial defects (**Fig. 4–18**) and sometimes reveal disc staining as well. No treatment is known, and patients often have persistence of the visual field defect and recurrences.

The optic nerve may occasionally be involved in MEWDS. Dodwell et al.[202] emphasized the importance of MEWDS in the neuro-ophthalmic differential diagnosis of vision loss. The optic nerve may be involved by the presumed inflammatory process either directly or secondarily, from contiguous spread of retinal or vascular inflammation. Although an afferent pupil defect and dyschromatopsia suggests optic nerve involvement, the possibility of simultaneous retinal ganglion cell and photoreceptor dysfunction needs to be considered. The white dots in MEWDS tend to extend centripetally away from the disc.

Differential diagnosis. The high prevalence of initial misdiagnoses, the overlap with other common neuro-ophthalmic entities, and the variability of clinical findings make the big blind spot syndromes an important consideration in the neuro-ophthalmic differential diagnosis of vision loss. Photopsia may be incorrectly ascribed to migraine. The abrupt onset of a visual field defect in a young patient might suggest optic neuritis. The presence of the enlarged blind spot and disc hyperemia might suggest papilledema or a temporal defect from a chiasmal lesion.

Pathogenesis. Inflammatory changes, predisposition in women, sporadic occurrence, and relatively acute onset of symptoms suggest an autoimmune or infectious cause. Chung et al.[203] have reported elevated levels of serum immunoglobulins in patients with MEWDS, although Jacobson et al.[201] were unable to demonstrate histochemical evidence of retinal antibodies. Another variant of this group of conditions, termed *acute annular outer retinopathy*, has been described in which patients develop a visible grayish annular

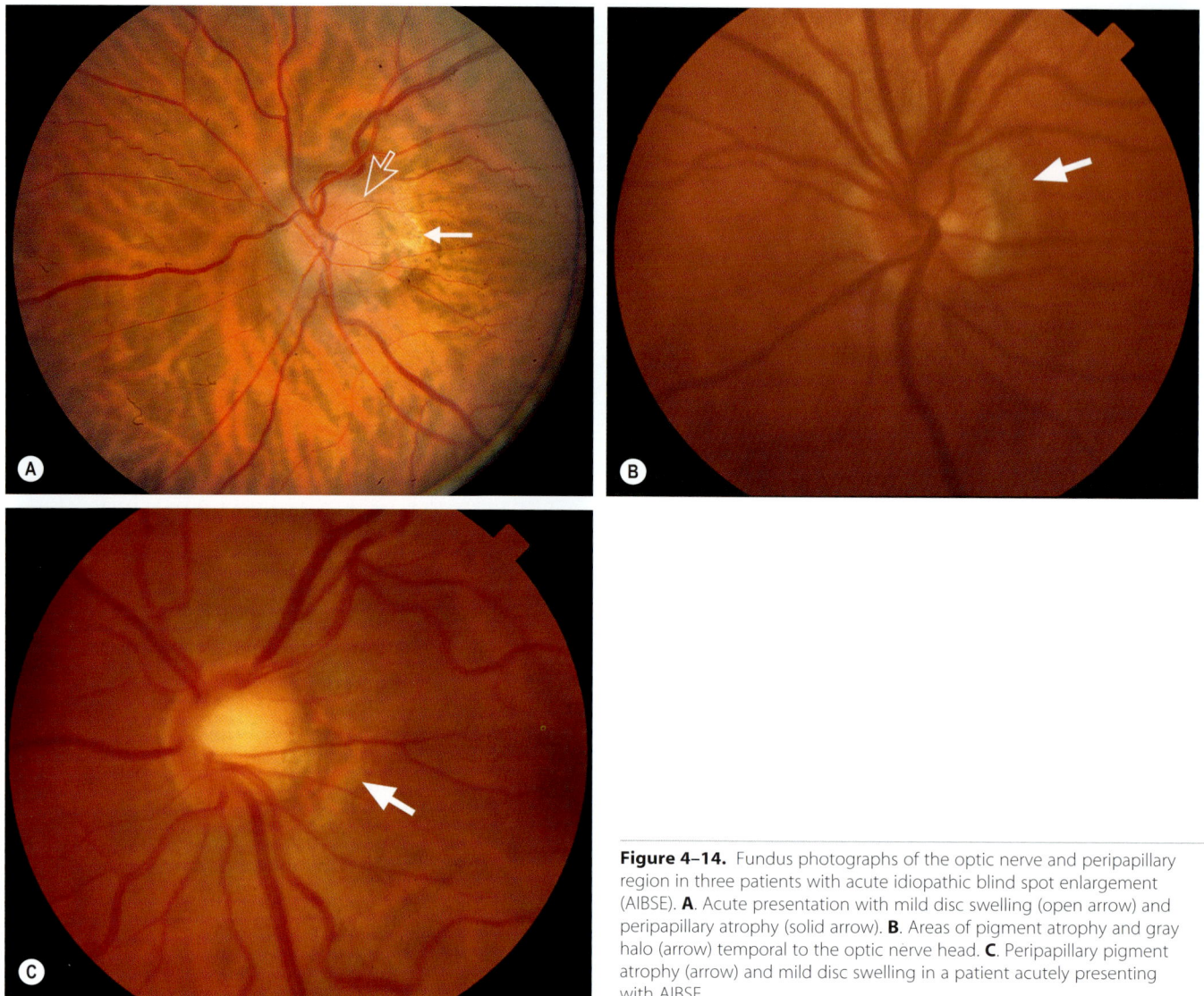

Figure 4–14. Fundus photographs of the optic nerve and peripapillary region in three patients with acute idiopathic blind spot enlargement (AIBSE). **A**. Acute presentation with mild disc swelling (open arrow) and peripapillary atrophy (solid arrow). **B**. Areas of pigment atrophy and gray halo (arrow) temporal to the optic nerve head. **C**. Peripapillary pigment atrophy (arrow) and mild disc swelling in a patient acutely presenting with AIBSE.

ring in the retina.[204,205] Gass and Stern[204] speculated that the grayish ring represented an immune ring at the leading edge of the inflammation. The patient described by Luckie et al.[205] seemed to respond to acyclovir, and they concluded that this implicated a herpesvirus as the cause.

To date there have been no histopathologic studies of eyes of patients with AIBSE. No abnormal laboratory value has been consistently identified in patients with any of these syndromes. Members of the same family have been affected although there is no information to suggest a specific heritable pattern.

Overlapping clinical profiles. Since AIBSE shares many features with MEWDS, these conditions may lie within the spectrum of a single genetic or autoimmune disease.[206,207] In fact, Gass and colleagues[184,186,208] suggested the term *acute zonal occult outer retinopathy* (AZOOR) as an umbrella term for AIBSE, MEWDS, acute macular neuroretinopathy (AMN), and multifocal choroiditis. All four conditions are frequently characterized by acute focal loss of outer retinal function associated with photopsia, occurrence predominantly in young women, minimal or no initial fundus changes, and

ERG abnormalities.[209] As with patients with PR, the presence of photopsia suggests photoreceptor dysfunction.

In a subsequent publication, Gass et al.[188] followed a single subset of 51 patients with AZOOR that included patients initially labeled as AIBSE but in whom a more widespread, relapsing bilateral condition diagnosed as AZOOR developed. These patients are distinct from the isolated, unilateral nonrecurrent nature of AIBSE as reported by Volpe et al.[187] He concluded that AZOOR is characterized by photopsia with acute loss of one or more zones of visual function, usually normal fundi initially, and ERG changes in one or both eyes. AZOOR, like AIBSE, occurs more frequently in women and more frequently in patients with other autoimmune diseases. Visual acuity is usually normal, but recovery of visual field occurs only infrequently. The cause of AZOOR is unknown, and there is no known treatment. Francis et al.[210] emphasized the importance of an ERG and EOG early in the course to make the diagnosis. They identified a consistent pattern of abnormality that also suggests in addition to photoreceptor dysfunction, inner retinal abnormalities.[210]

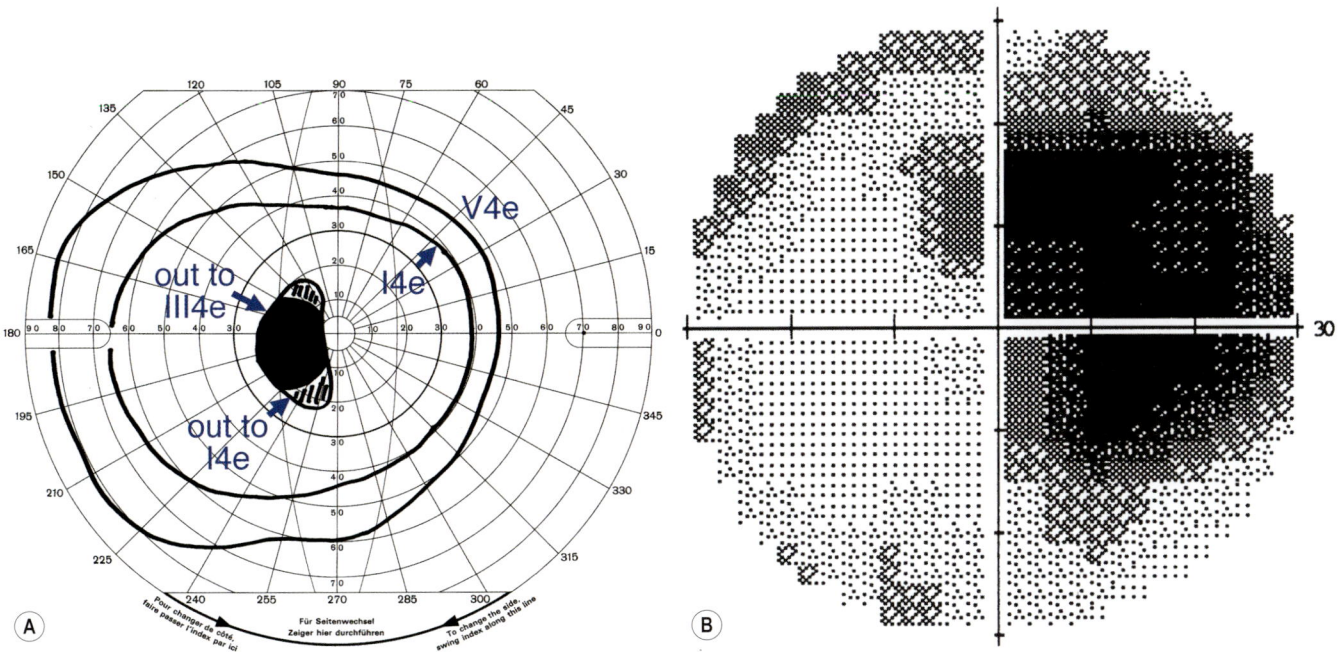

Figure 4–15. Visual field defects in acute idiopathic blind spot enlargement syndrome (AIBSE). **A.** Goldmann visual field of the left eye in a patient with AIBSE. The defect is dense and centered on the blind spot. **B.** Grayscale output of the threshold computerized visual field of the right eye in a patient with AIBSE. A dense, steeply bordered temporal visual field defect attached to the blind spot is seen.

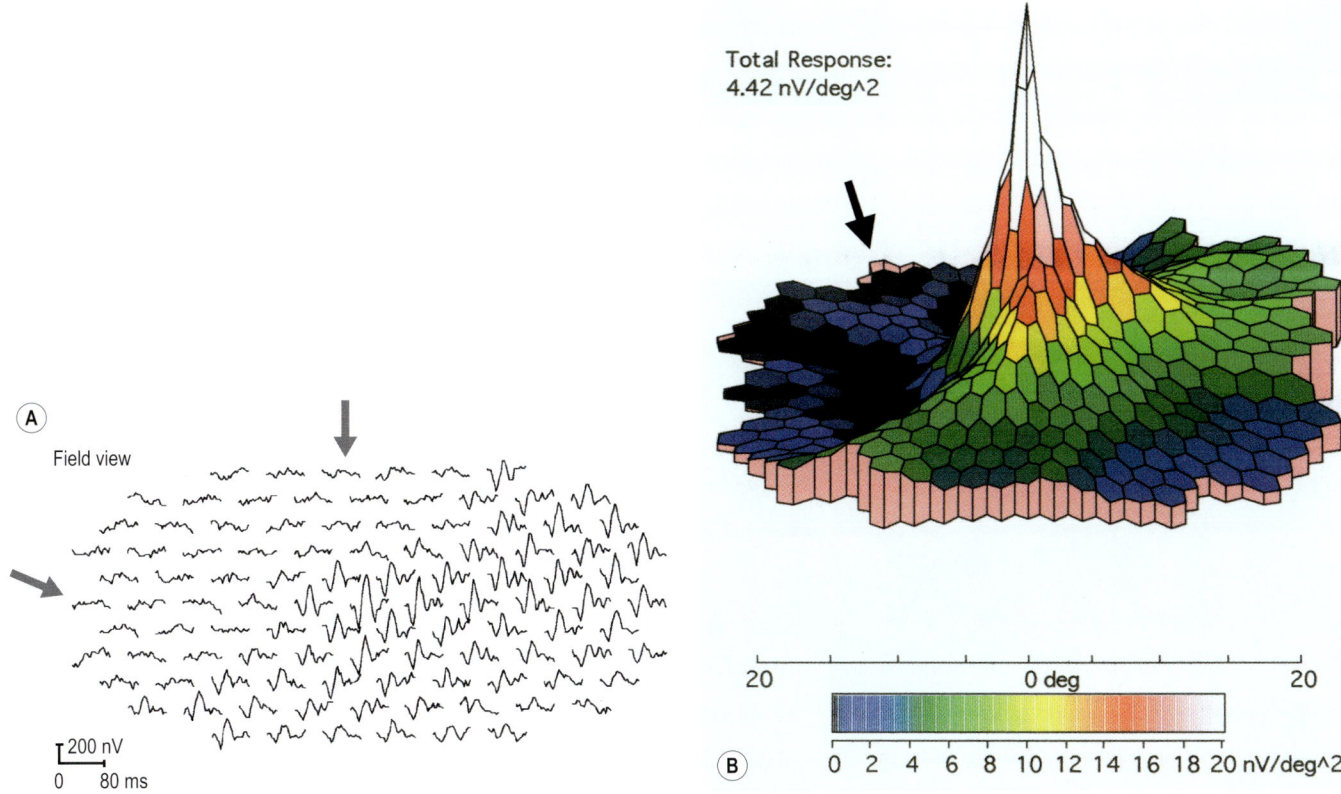

Figure 4–16. Multifocal ERG in AIBSE affecting the left eye. **A.** Patient tracings (field view) demonstrating reduced amplitudes of wave forms (arrows) temporal to fixation. **B.** Graphic representation demonstrating preservation of foveal peak and then sharp drop off (arrow) in the temporal area around the blind spot.

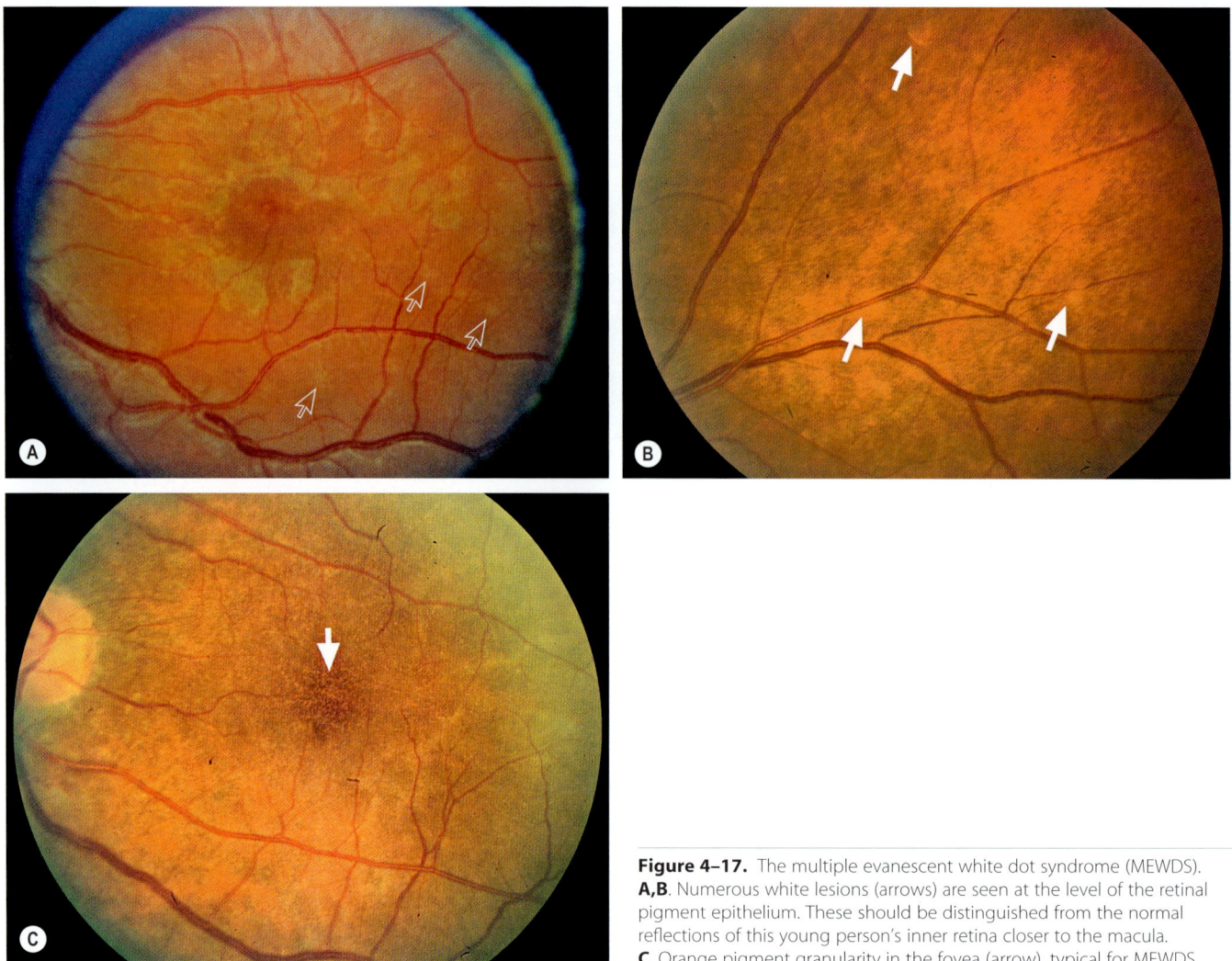

Figure 4–17. The multiple evanescent white dot syndrome (MEWDS). **A,B**. Numerous white lesions (arrows) are seen at the level of the retinal pigment epithelium. These should be distinguished from the normal reflections of this young person's inner retina closer to the macula. **C**. Orange pigment granularity in the fovea (arrow), typical for MEWDS.

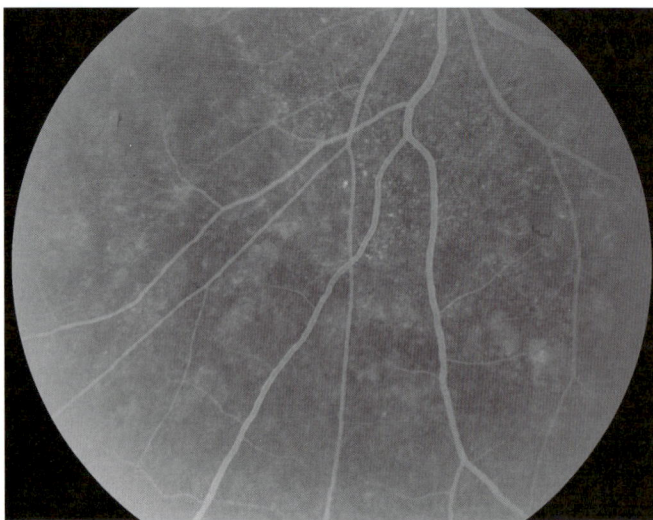

Toxic retinopathy

Because numerous systemic diseases and their treatment are encountered in neuro-ophthalmic practice, it is worthwhile to be aware of the toxic effects that some medications can have on the retina. These are summarized in **Table 4–4**. The best known retinal toxin is digoxin. Patients typically develop xanthopsia (yellow vision), scintillating scotomas, and paracentral scotomas.[211–213] Patients may have abnormalities in the cone (photopic) b-wave implicit times.[214] Color vision defects may be the earliest manifestation, and screening for digoxin toxicity with color vision testing has been suggested.[215] Patients may develop visual symptoms even when the serum digoxin level is in the therapeutic range.[216] Digoxin retinal toxicity is also discussed in Chapter 12.

Several different drugs such as tamoxifen,[217–220] canthaxanthine,[221,222] and methoxyflurane can cause a crystalline retinopathy.[223] The deposits in the case of tamoxifen appear to be products of axonal degeneration.[219] The complication is sufficiently rare and has minimal affect on vision, so widespread screening is not recommended.[218] In the case of methoxyflurane, oxalosis results from metabolism of the

Figure 4–18. Late-phase fluorescein angiogram in a patient with multiple evanescent white dot syndrome. There are numerous late-staining lesions at the level of the retinal pigment epithelium.

drug. Various diuretics, nicotinic acid, and epinephrine can cause CME. Isotretinoin has been reported to affect retinal function and result in abnormal night vision.[224–227]

Quinine, used primarily in the treatment of malaria, is toxic to the retinal photoreceptors and ganglion cells. Chloroquine and hydroxychloroquine, used to treat malaria

Table 4–4 Ophthalmic manifestations of drugs causing retinal toxicity

Drug	Ophthalmic manifestations
Digoxin	Xanthopsia (yellow vision)
	Positive visual phenomena
	Decreased color vision
Tamoxifen	Crystalline deposits in the macula
Canthaxanthine	Crystalline deposits in the macula
Thioridazine	Pigmentary deposits on corneal and anterior lens capsule
	Pigmentary retinopathy
Isotretinoin	Decreased night vision
Chloroquine and hydroxychloroquine	Corneal whirl
	Bull's eye maculopathy
Nicotinic acid	Cystoid macular edema
Quinine	Retinal photoreceptor and ganglion cell toxicity
Vigabatrin	ERG abnormalities
	Visual field constriction
Sildenafil	Halos and blue vision

and collagen vascular disorders, cause a dose-related pigmentary retinopathy.[228–235] Other ocular findings include corneal whirl-type deposits and poliosis (patch of white hair). The macular changes begin as a pigment mottling but then become a horizontally elongated bull's eye (**Fig. 4–19**). Patients slowly develop reduced central acuity, central visual field defects, and dyschromatopsia. Abnormalities in the perifoveal photoreceptor inner segment/outer segment junction can be demonstrated in symptomatic patients with high-resolution OCT. Patients may also have abnormalities on mERG[236,237] (which may precede any clinical symptoms or perimetric findings[238]) and demonstrate fundus autofluorescence.[239] It appears that the toxicity is dose related, and hydroxychloroquine dosages less than 6.5 mg/kg/day appear to be safe.[234] The drug is excreted very slowly; therefore, toxicity can progress even after the drug is discontinued. Although it has been a subject of some debate, many experts feel that screening for retinopathy in patients taking hydroxychloroquine is unnecessary unless the daily dose exceeds 6.5 mg/kg/day or the patient has been on the drug for more than 5 years.[228,231,233] The American Academy of Ophthalmology has offered guidelines for screening and has established criteria for low- and high-risk patients.[240] In terms of retinal toxicity, hydroxychloroquine seems to be the safer of the two drugs.[230]

Vigabatrin, an anticonvulsant, can cause ERG abnormalities and concentric visual field constriction in as many as half of patients taking the drug.[241–243] This selective irreversible inhibitor of gamma-aminobutyric acid (GABA)-transaminase increases GABA available in CNS synapses. Cone dysfunction is most common,[244–246] but Mueller cell abnormalities have also been suggested.[247] A clinical pattern of peripheral retinal atrophy and nasal disc atrophy has been reported.[248] Although visual acuity, color vision, and ERG amplitude may recover after stopping the drug if visual field

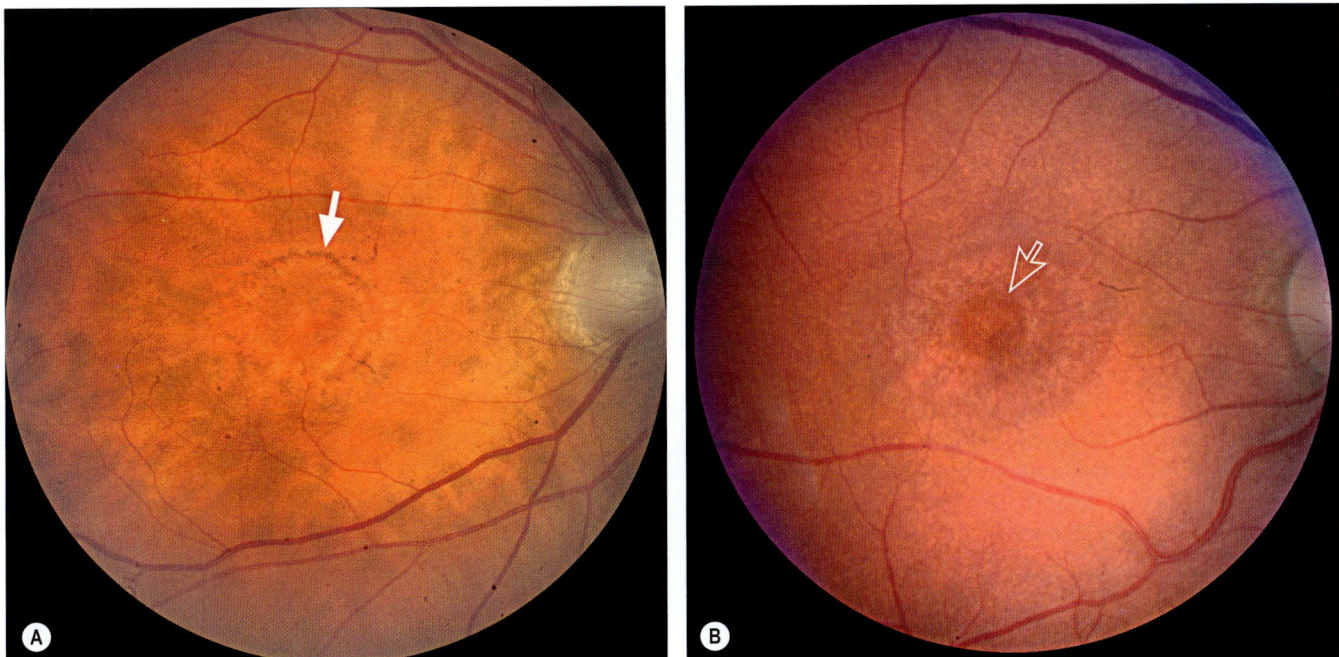

Figure 4–19. "Bull's eye" pigmentary abnormalities (arrows) in patients with (**A**) chloroquine and (**B**) hydroxychloroquine retinal toxicity.

Table 4–5 Common hereditary macular disorders with a recognizable fundus appearance

Disease	Fundus appearance
Best disease (vitelliform dystrophy)	Egg yolk appearance; may develop scarring and neovascularization
Adult foveomacular dystrophy	Symmetric, oval, yellow subretinal lesion
Familial drusen	Numerous drusen may coalesce; choroidal neovascularization
Central areolar choroidal dystrophy	Early: pigment granularity
	Late: circular zone of RPE and choriocapillary atrophy
Myopic degeneration	Peripapillary atrophy, staphyloma, lacquer cracks
Stargardt disease (atrophic macular dystrophy with flecks) (fundus flavimaculatus)	Angulated flecks and atrophy in retina, "beaten bronze" appearance, dark "silent choroid" on fluorescein angiography
Juvenile retinoschisis	Foveal retinoschisis
Butterfly-shaped pattern dystrophy	Reticular butterfly-shaped pattern of pigmentation in macula

RPE, retinal pigment epithelium.

loss is mild or minimal, vigabatrin-associated visual field deficits tend not to improve.[249,250] In patients electing to continue the drug despite visual field loss, the visual deficits usually do not progress.[251] Patients on vigabatrin should undergo ERGs and visual examinations including confrontation or formal perimetry, if able, every 6 months while on the drug. Because children on vigabatrin are often moderately or severely neurologically impaired and unable to provide useful visual field assessments, the ERGs in such patients become the only way to detect and monitor the retinal toxicity.[252]

Sildenafil, also mentioned in Chapter 12, can cause subjective halos and blue vision, perhaps due to phosphodiesterase-6 inhibition by the drug at the level of the rod and cone photoreceptors.[253,254]

Hereditary retinal dystrophies in neuro-ophthalmic differential diagnosis

The clinical spectrum of hereditary retinal degenerations includes a variety of presentations that overlap with common neuro-ophthalmic conditions. In particular, patients with hereditary retinal degenerations may present with insidious central vision loss, dyschromatopsia, and visual field defects. The vast majority of patients with typical retinitis pigmentosa present with a rod-dominated picture characterized by nyctalopia (night blindness), peripheral vision loss, and a characteristic bone spicule pigmentation of the peripheral retina. Rarely patients present without any abnormal pigment accumulation. A subset of patients with heritable retinal degenerations have cone-dominated presentations that are characterized by light- or glare-induced blindness (hemeralopia), central vision loss, and dyschromatopsia. Prominent macular changes may be evident on ophthalmoscopy.

Cone or cone-rod dystrophies

Cone dystrophies or cone-rod dystrophies usually present in middle age and have a variable inheritance pattern.

The visual acuity and color vision may be moderately reduced at a time when the macular changes are subtle or absent on ophthalmoscopy. These disorders should be considered in all patients with bilateral subnormal acuity and color vision. In many cases the family history is not helpful. Perhaps these represent the existence of spontaneous mutations or the variable clinical expressivity of the disorder.

Classification. We use the term *cone dystrophy* to describe patients with progressive and heritable central vision loss who do not have an ophthalmoscopic appearance suggesting an alternative dystrophy (**Table 4–5**). Cone dystrophies are a heterogeneous group of inherited disorders that result in dysfunction of the cone photoreceptors and their postreceptoral pathways. These disorders have been classified on the basis of their relative involvement of cones or rods and central versus peripheral photoreceptors.[255] According to their natural history, the cone dystrophies may also be divided into two groups: "stationary" and "progressive."[256] Based on careful study of several pedigrees, the genes responsible for some of these conditions have been elucidated.[257–262] Identification of the genotypes will ultimately lead to a proper classification system and better understanding of the phenotypic variability.

Clinical features. Patients present with abnormal light sensitivity (photophobia or hemeralopia), photopsia, and reduced vision. Identifying the symptom of abnormal light sensitivity is critical in making the diagnosis. This light sensitivity may be erroneously interpreted as optical glare and lead to unnecessary cataract surgery. Symptoms typically develop over many years. Examination reveals reduced central acuity (20/30 to 20/400), dyschromatopsia, central scotomas on visual field testing, and pigmentary alterations in the macula (**Fig. 4–20**). Changes in color vision may be the first sign of the disease.[263] These patients have an abnormal ERG with cones affected more than rods, or only cones affected. Nonrecordable or abnormal (reduced b-wave amplitude or oscillatory potential), photopic (recorded in light, cone-mediated) responses on the ERG are likely to be detected. However, more specific information might be obtained from a focal or multifocal ERG that evaluates

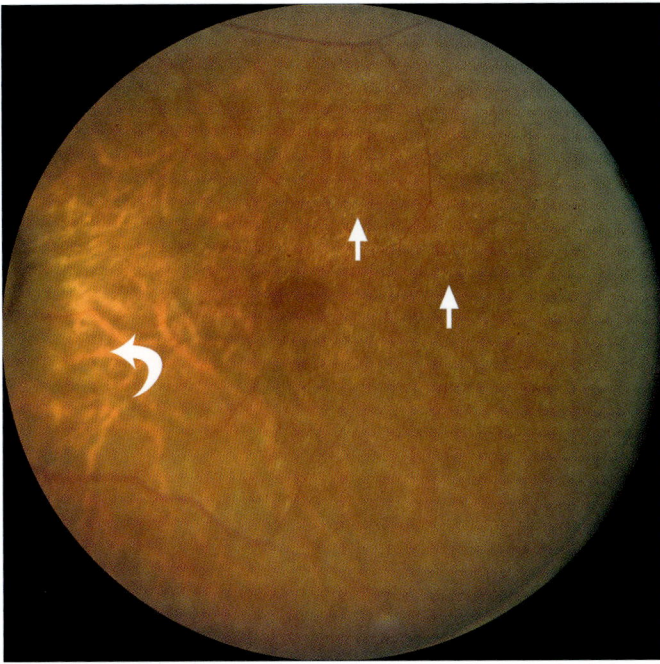

Figure 4–20. Fundus of the left eye of a patient with cone dystrophy. In addition to granular macular pigmentation (straight arrows) there is peripapillary pigment atrophy (curved arrow).

central retinal function (**Fig. 4–21**).[264] An ERG may be used to follow these patients to determine the rate of disease progression.[265] OCT may reveal thinning of the outer retina–choroid complex (ORCC)[266] (**Fig. 4–3**). Optic disc pallor may also develop.[267]

Hereditary maculopathies with ophthalmoscopic abnormalities

Several heritable conditions affect the macula and result in a diagnostic fundus appearance. Some of the more common maculopathies are summarized in **Table 4–5**. Each has a characteristic fundus appearance and therefore would not be confused with an optic neuropathy. For instance, a patient with Stargardt disease (**Fig. 4–22**) would be recognized based on the abnormal fundus appearance and FA.[268] However, early in their course these conditions may be hard to recognize since symptoms of decreased central vision may precede the development of the typical fundus lesion.

Mitochondrial diseases

Kearns–Sayre syndrome. Retinal dystrophy or degeneration may be associated with chronic progressive external ophthalmoplegia (CPEO). Onset of retinopathy before age 20 combined with heart block,[269–272] ataxia, and/or cerebrospinal fluid protein above 100 mg/dl is termed *Kearns–Sayre syndrome* (KSS).[273] This condition is caused by mitochondrial

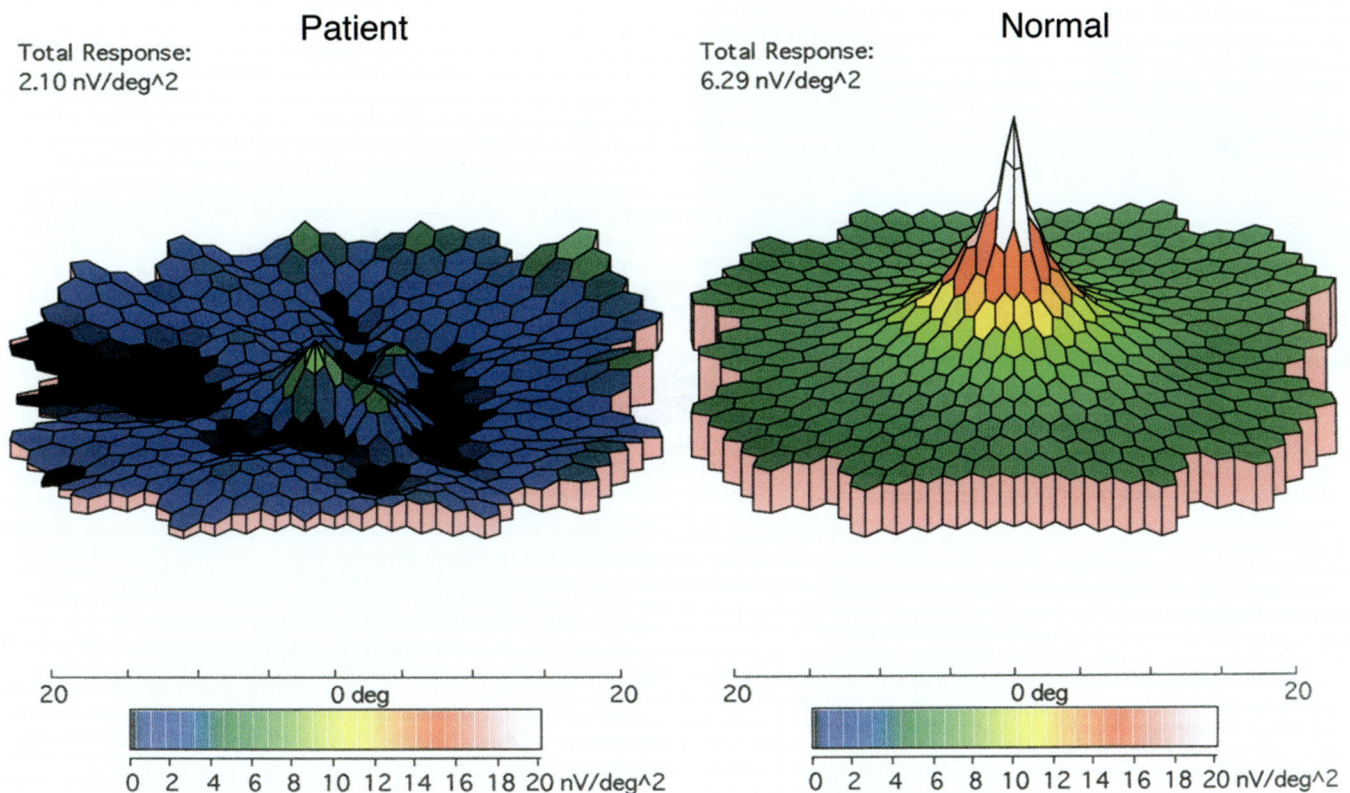

Figure 4–21. Multifocal electroretinogram in a patient with cone dystrophy. A diffuse loss of responses (nV/deg2) and absent foveal peak is seen on the patient's tracings on the left compared with normal responses seen on the right.

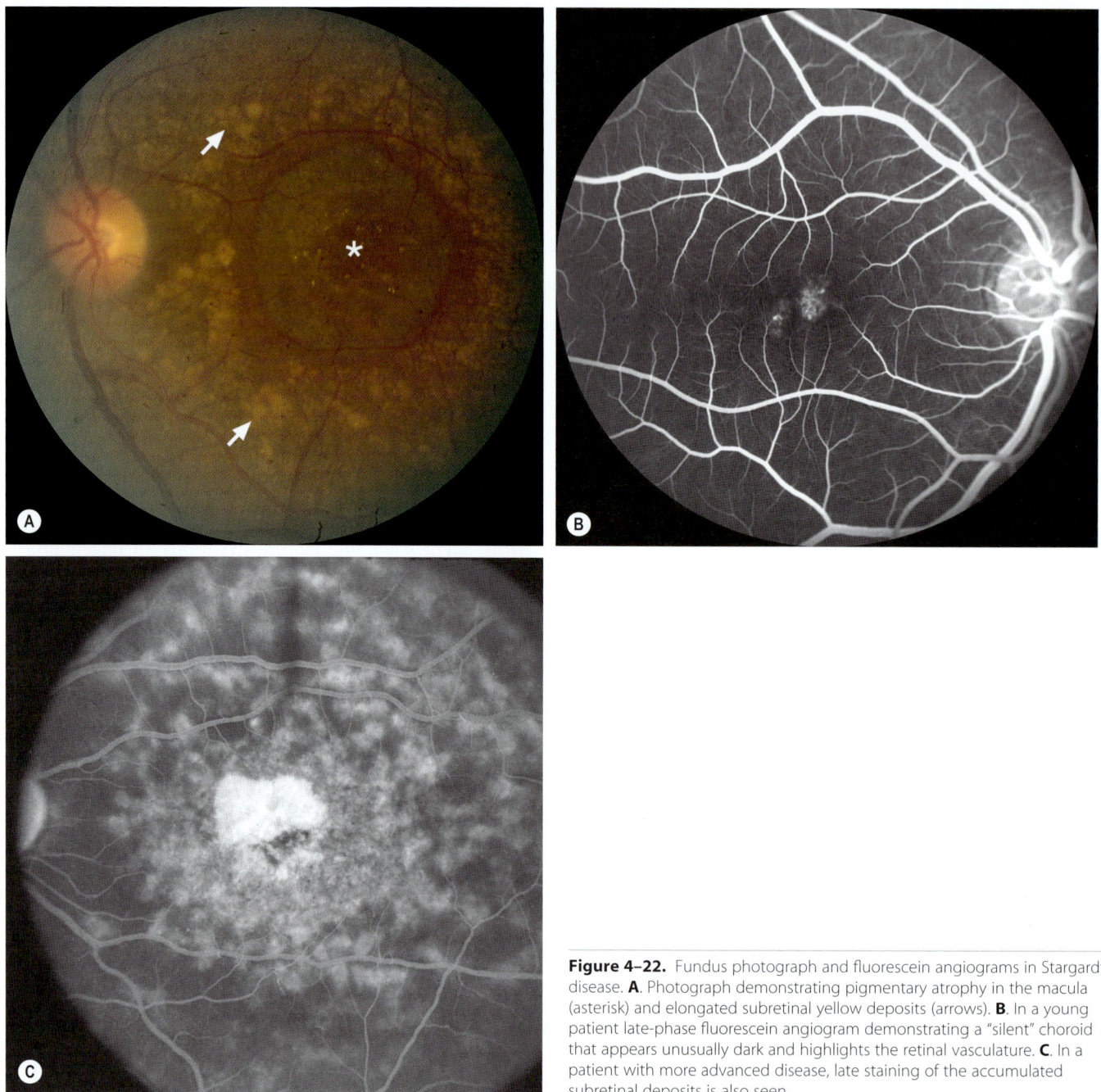

Figure 4–22. Fundus photograph and fluorescein angiograms in Stargardt disease. **A**. Photograph demonstrating pigmentary atrophy in the macula (asterisk) and elongated subretinal yellow deposits (arrows). **B**. In a young patient late-phase fluorescein angiogram demonstrating a "silent" choroid that appears unusually dark and highlights the retinal vasculature. **C**. In a patient with more advanced disease, late staining of the accumulated subretinal deposits is also seen.

DNA deletions.[274–281] Approximately one-third of patients will have some type of pigmentary retinopathy.[282] Many patients have salt-and-pepper type retinopathy with some macular dysfunction and ERG abnormalities. Other patients develop more widespread and progressive retinal dysfunction.[282,283] CPEO and KSS are detailed in Chapter 14.

MELAS. Another important mitochondrial disorder is mitochondrial encephalopathy with lactic acidosis and stroke-like episodes (MELAS). This condition frequently presents with stroke-like episodes that may cause retrochiasmal visual loss. The condition usually results from a mutation at position 3243 of the mitochondrial DNA.[284] Like those with KSS, patients with MELAS can have a pigmentary abnormality in the retina. Visual symptoms related to the retina are usually absent or mild. Also, the pigmentary changes identified are subtle and occur primarily in the macula.[285,286] Histopathologically, degeneration of photoreceptor outer segments in the macula has been identified.[287] MELAS is discussed further in Chapter 8.

NARP. This rare mitochondrial disorder is characterized by *n*europathy, *a*taxia, and *r*etinitis *p*igmentosa.[288] Other clinical features include proximal muscle weakness, developmental delay, ataxia, seizures, and dementia.[289] The disease is maternally inherited, and a responsible mutation at position 8993 of the ATPase 6 gene has been identified.[290] This is the same gene identified in some patients with Leigh disease (see Chapter 16).

Other diseases with retinal and neurologic manifestations

Microangiopathy of the brain, retina, and inner ear (Susac syndrome). This disorder predominantly affects young women.[291–296] It is also known as Susac syndrome to honor the man who recognized its characteristic features.[295,297–299] Ninety percent of patients present with retinal arterial occlusions, and in 60% they are bilateral.[297–299] Yellow retinal wall plaques can be seen in midarteriolar segments of involved vessels, in contrast to Hollenhorst plaques which occur at vascular bifurcations.[300] Mean age of onset is 30 years.[297] Although it resembles primary angiitis of the nervous system, it is the sensorineural hearing loss and retinal ischemic changes that mark it as a distinct entity. Hearing loss occurs in two-thirds of patients.[297–299] Like primary CNS angiitis, the disorder is confined to the CNS. Global encephalopathy is common, occurring in 44% of patients.[297]

Involved areas of the brain demonstrate microinfarction of the gray and white matter.[301–303] Central corpus callosum black holes, highly suggestive of Susac syndrome, develop on brain MRI as the active lesions resolve. Linear defects (spokes) and rather large characteristic round lesions (snowballs) are seen on MRI as well as cortical, deep gray, and leptomeningeal involvement.[79] The lesions may enhance and may also be observed on diffusion-weighted imaging.[301–303] Pathologically, involved segments have demonstrated vessel thickening or sclerosis.[294] Although the pathogenesis of this disorder is unknown, evidence points to autoimmune-related endothelial damage. In this regard, Notis et al.[304] have demonstrated multifocal retinal vessel hyperfluorescence on FA 5 days prior to retinal infarction.

Treatment with variable success has been achieved in Susac syndrome with corticosteroids and other immunosuppressive agents.[79,294,305,306] Anticoagulation has not been effective although aspirin may be a useful adjunct. One patient apparently responded to the combination of antiplatelet and calcium channel blocker therapy.[296] Vision loss in Susac syndrome has been successfully treated with hyperbaric oxygen.[307] Intravenous gamma globulin has also been anecdotally successful in treating this disorder and may be the most efficacious therapy. The prognosis is generally good as the disease tends to be self-limited.[297]

Acute posterior multifocal placoid pigment epitheliopathy. Acute posterior multifocal placoid pigment epitheliopathy (APMPPE) is a disorder first recognized by Gass in 1968.[308] This acute, but self-limiting, disorder produces characteristic multifocal gray-white flat lesions at the level of the retinal pigment epithelium.[308] Pigment epithelial abnormalities seem to result from dysfunction of the choroidal vasculature.[309,310] Neurologic manifestations have included headache, transient ischemic attacks, dysacusis, tinnitus, cerebral vasculitis, and stroke.[311–317] Stroke and aseptic meningitis are the two major pathologic substrates for the neurologic dysfunction seen in APMPPE. In a review of nine previously reported cases of stroke with APMPPE,[318] five patients had angiographic changes suggesting vasculitis. Only two cases had histologic proof of vasculitis. One patient had a positive muscle biopsy[314] and the other a brain biopsy that revealed

granulomatosis inflammation of medium-sized arteries.[317] The infarcts have a tendency to involve the posterior circulation and the basal ganglia region. The strokes usually occur at the time of the visual loss, but may precede or follow the ocular manifestations.[318] One patient with APMPPE had a more widespread systemic necrotizing vasculitis with features suggesting both Wegener's granulomatosis and polyarteritis nodosa.[319] These observations suggest that the choroid is primarily involved by a diffuse vasculitic process that interrupts choroidal perfusion and causes the characteristic fundus lesion. Although cerebral vasculitis may remit spontaneously, aggressive immunosuppressive therapy has been suggested. Corticosteroids in combination with cyclophosphamide for 6–12 months is one proposed regimen.[318] The visual prognosis is generally good although initial involvement of the fovea and older age portend a worse visual outcome.[320]

Eale disease and Cogan syndrome. Eale disease and Cogan syndrome are primary vasculitic disorders of the eye but are infrequently associated with cerebral vasculitis. Both are distinguished from isolated CNS angiitis by their associated eye findings. Eale disease is a disorder of young, healthy men who develop retinal vasculitis, vitreous hemorrhage, and peripheral nonperfusion of the retina with subsequent neovascularization.[321] Treatment is with laser photocoagulation. Besides the ocular manifestations, the CNS may rarely be affected. Patients have been reported with stroke,[322,323] myelopathy, and vasculitis.[324–328] Pathologically, both demyelinating and vasculitic changes have been noted within the CNS of patients with Eale disease.[317] The prognosis for maintenance of good visual recovery is usually good but some patients have severe vision loss secondary to the neovascular complications.

Cogan syndrome is characterized by the presence of nonsyphilitic interstitial keratitis and vestibulo-auditory dysfunction (hearing loss).[329] Again the CNS may occasionally be affected. Reported neurologic manifestations include headaches, seizures, ataxia, cranial nerve palsies, stroke, and meningoencephalitis.[330]

CADASIL. Cerebral autosomal dominant arteriopathy with subcortical infarcts and leukoencephalopathy (CADASIL) is an arteriopathy affecting the small arteries and arterioles of the brain. CADASIL presents in young or middle adulthood with mood disorders, migraine with aura, transient ischemic attacks, or stroke.[331] Patients develop recurrent subcortical ischemic strokes, with characteristic diffuse white matter signal abnormalities on MRI, leading to a stepwise decline and dementia with frontal lobe features.

Retinal abnormalities in CADASIL have become well recognized. These include thickening or narrowing of the retinal arterioles, peripapillary arteriolar sheathing, arteriovenous nicking, cotton-wool spots, and nerve fiber loss.[332–335] Iris atrophy, lens opacities,[305] and ischemic optic neuropathy in association with CADASIL have also been reported.[336]

The histopathologic hallmark of CADASIL is a characteristic granular alternation of the arterial media that corresponds to the accumulation of electron-dense material surrounding the smooth muscle cells.[337] The thickening or narrowing of retinal vessels is likely as a result of similar deposition of granular material.[338] The presence of this granular material was originally described in brain vessels but identical electron microscopic studies have demonstrated similar findings in the media of peripheral tissue arteries. This allows for a pathologic diagnosis of the disease by a simple skin, muscle, or nerve biopsy. The defective gene in CADASIL is Notch3 (chromosome 19), which encodes a cell surface receptor expressed in vascular smooth muscle cells and pericytes.[339] There is no effective treatment.

Spinocerebellar ataxias

The spinocerebellar ataxias (SCAs) are a group of conditions characterized by loss of neurons in the cerebellar cortex, basis pontis, and inferior olivary nucleus. Clinically, patients develop progressive ataxia with pyramidal and brain stem signs, and many patients develop supranuclear ophthalmoparesis (see Chapter 16 for further discussion). Patients with SCAs may have either optic atrophy or a pigmentary retinal degeneration.

In particular, patients with SCA-7 (autosomal dominant cerebellar ataxia (ADCA) type II) manifest with progressive ataxia and vision loss secondary to retinal degeneration. The genetic defect has been mapped to chromosome 3p.[340–342] The gene appears to be an abnormal CAG repeat that has been identified in pedigrees from around the world.[343–345] The onset of symptoms is usually in the second or third decade. Two-thirds of patients will manifest with ataxia while one-third present with ataxia with visual loss.[346] Vision loss may precede the development of ataxia but is often not recognized by the patient because of its insidious onset. The visual deficits are typically bilateral, symmetric, and mostly central.[347] Patients maintain relatively normal peripheral fields but develop reduced acuity, dyschromatopsia, and central scotomas with macular atrophy similar to other cone rod dystrophies.[348,349] Pigmentary changes in the macula may have a bull's eye appearance (**Fig. 4–23**),[350,351] and a pigmentary retinopathy similar to Kearns–Sayre syndrome has been reported.[352] These pigmentary changes can extend into the periphery, and over time optic atrophy may develop. The cone-derived, photopic, full-field ERG, or focal ERG or PERG (pattern electroretinogram) is reduced.[350] The rod responses are not affected until late in the disease. Severe

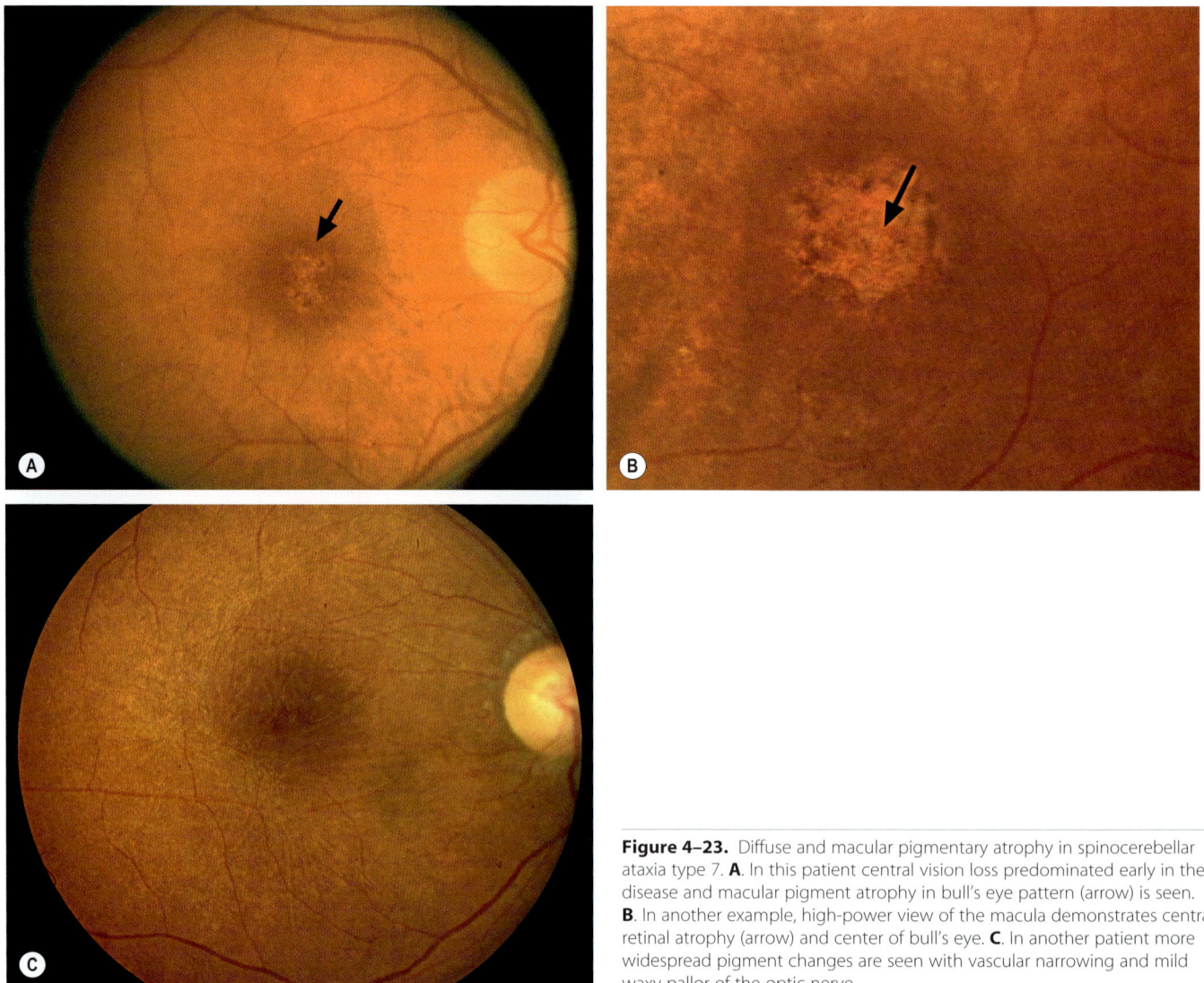

Figure 4–23. Diffuse and macular pigmentary atrophy in spinocerebellar ataxia type 7. **A.** In this patient central vision loss predominated early in the disease and macular pigment atrophy in bull's eye pattern (arrow) is seen. **B.** In another example, high-power view of the macula demonstrates central retinal atrophy (arrow) and center of bull's eye. **C.** In another patient more widespread pigment changes are seen with vascular narrowing and mild waxy pallor of the optic nerve.

atrophy of the retina has been demonstrated at autopsy.[353] About half of the patients develop supranuclear ophthalmoplegia (see Chapter 16).

Metabolic diseases

Ophthalmologists and neurologists must be aware of the various metabolic storage diseases that have retinal manifestations, as these eye abnormalities may allow for early, accurate diagnoses. These are summarized in **Table 4–6**. These findings are present only in some of the patients and therefore the absence of a cherry-red spot or abnormal pigmentation in the neurologically impaired child or adult does not exclude these diagnoses.

Table 4–6 Retinal posterior segment manifestations of metabolic disorders

Storage disorders with cherry-red spot[354,533]
Tay–Sachs disease
Niemann–Pick disease (types A, B, C, and D)
Metachromatic leukodystrophy
Sialidosis (types I and II)
Infantile GM$_2$ gangliosidosis (Sandhoff disease)
Farber disease (lipogranulomatosis)
Retinal pigmentary degeneration
Mucopolysaccharidoses
Gaucher disease
Refsum disease (phytanic acid lipidosis)
Neuronal ceroid lipofuscinosis
Mucolipidosis
Cystinuria
Abetalipoproteinemia
Kearns–Sayre syndrome
Hallervorden–Spatz syndrome (pantothenate kinase-associated neurodegeneration (PKAN))
Spinocerebellar ataxia type 7 (and occasionally type 1)
Usher syndrome
Cockayne disease
Aicardi syndrome
Optic atrophy
Krabbe disease
Metachromatic leukodystrophy
Adrenoleukodystrophy
Alexander disease
Spinocerebellar ataxia type 1 and Friedreich's ataxia
Spongy degeneration
Pelizaeus–Merzbacher disease
Alpers disease

Macular cherry-red spot. This finding is the result of lipid, sphingolipid, or oligosaccharide deposition in the retinal ganglion cell axons surrounding the macula.[354,355] Because overlying retinal ganglion cell axons border but do not overlie it, the red choroidal circulation in the fovea is visible. Vision loss, a cherry-red spot, and loss of motor function in infancy is highly suggestive of Tay–Sachs disease due to hexosaminodase A deficiency.

Abnormal retinal pigmentation. Of the disorders listed in Table 4–6, the most common conditions to present with prominent neurologic and retinal pigmentary abnormalities are neuronal ceroid lipofuscinosis, abetalipoproteinemia, Aicardi syndrome, Kearns–Sayre syndrome, and spinocerebellar ataxia type 7. The last two are discussed earlier in this chapter. In the juvenile form of neuronal ceroid lipofuscinosis (Batten disease), children exhibit motor and cognitive decline, progressive visual loss, a bull's eye maculopathy, and a flat ERG reflecting widespread rod and cone dysfunction.[356] In abetalipoproteinemia (Bassen–Kornzweig syndrome), abnormal betalipoprotein results in defective absorption of fat-soluble vitamins, including vitamin E. Prominent neuro-ophthalmic manifestations include widespread pigmentary retinal changes and ataxia. Aicardi syndrome is characterized by absence of the corpus callosum, infantile spasms, and chorioretinal lacunae,[357] which look like white punched out holes in the retina.

Optic atrophy. Most of the neurologic conditions listed in Table 4–6 which present with optic atrophy are discussed elsewhere in this book.

Thrombotic disorders (hypercoagulable states)

These conditions include a variety of disorders that are characterized by abnormal clotting and ischemic events. They are generally more common in woman and in addition may be associated with a number of systemic conditions, particularly autoimmune disorders. Their ophthalmic presentations are characterized by amaurosis fugax from retinal ischemia, retinopathy associated with cotton-wool spots and intraretinal hemorrhages, and occasionally permanent deficits from choroidal ischemia, retinal artery occlusions, and ischemic optic neuropathy.

Antiphospholipid antibody syndrome. Caused by antibodies such as the lupus anticoagulants and anticardiolipin antibodies, this is the best known of the thrombotic syndromes. Patients with antiphospholipid antibodies are more commonly women under age 50. There may be a history of lupus and repeated fetal loss. Many have a history of transient ischemic attack, or arterial or venous thrombosis that is otherwise unexplained. Patients may be thrombocytopenic and the partial thromboplastin time may be prolonged. A variety of ocular symptoms and findings, 15–88% in various series,[358] have been reported in patients with antiphospholipid syndrome.[82,91,359–364] Transient changes in vision are common.[82,363] Occlusions of both retinal veins and arteries (**Fig. 4–24**) have been reported.[91,363,364] However, in one prospective series,[365] only a minority of patients with visual disturbances were found to have retinopathy. The authors concluded that the majority of transient visual symptoms described could be attributed to a central neurologic problem. Neurologic findings in these patients can be grouped into three clinical patterns: encephalopathy, multiple cerebral infarctions, and migraine-like headaches.[366-368]

Other thrombotic disorders. Other disorders of the clotting pathway that may lead to visual symptoms and signs include deficiencies of protein C, protein S, and antithrombin III[369] and hyperhomocysteinemia. Finally, activated protein C resistance can be seen with the factor V Leiden mutation, which has been reported in association with both retinal vein and retinal artery occlusions.[370-375] Until there is a more definitive understanding of the roles these factors play in retinal vascular occlusion, we recommend screening for these disorders in all patients under age 50 with amaurosis fugax or retinal arterial or venous occlusion.

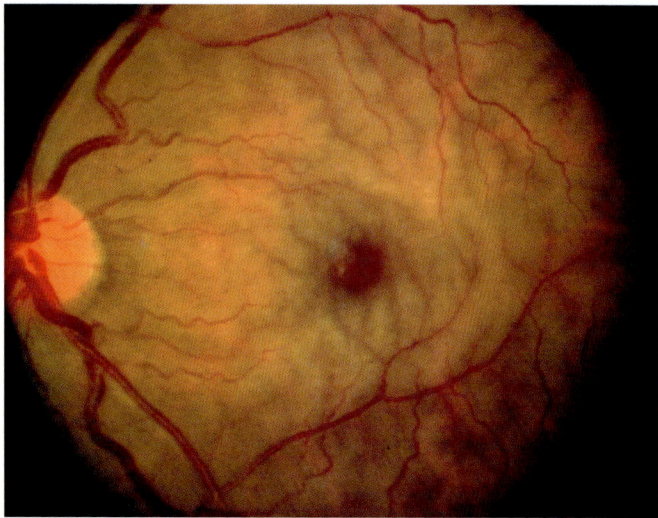

Figure 4–24. Fundus photograph demonstrating retinal whitening and ischemia in a patient with hypercoagulable state due to systemic lupus erythematosus and antiphospholipid antibodies.

Vogt–Koyanagi–Harada syndrome

Vogt–Koyanagi–Harada (VKH) syndrome, the best-known uveomeningeal syndrome, is a systemic disorder involving many organ systems, including the eye, skin, meninges, and ear. It is most common in Japan[376,377] and parts of Latin America but is uncommon in the USA (except in American Indians) and in individuals of northern European ancestry.[378] There are many theories concerning the etiology of VKH syndrome that have focused on infectious and immune-mediated diseases. It seems most likely to result from deranged T-cell function.[379-381] Recently several patients have been reported to develop VKH in association with interferon alpha-2b/ribavirin therapy for hepatitis C and multiple sclerosis.[382-386]

Patients usually present in the second to fourth decade, although it has been described in children as young as 4 years old.[387-389] The disease usually develops in stages initially characterized by a flu-like syndrome associated with headache, aseptic meningitis (meningismus), dysacusis, and tinnitus. These symptoms may be present for several weeks. This is followed by the ocular symptoms of anterior and posterior uveitis, inferior exudative retinal detachments,[378] and disc swelling (**Fig. 4–25**). The uveitis is usually bilateral and granulomatous in nature. Synechiae and cataract formation are common.[390] The anterior chamber may become shallow secondary to swelling of the ciliary processes.[391] About 40% of patients develop glaucoma, which may be open or closed angle.[392] The retinal pigmented epithelium (RPE) eventually becomes severely depigmented as the serous retinal detachments resolve. Ultimately pigmentary changes in the retina lead to an appearance which has been termed the "sunset glow fundus," a finding which in one study was correlated with the degree of cerebrospinal fluid pleocytosis.[393] Subretinal yellow-white lesions may be seen in the peripheral retina. Neovascularization of the disc and retina with vitreous hemorrhage may also develop.[394] Sensorineural hearing loss is common,[395] and patients complain

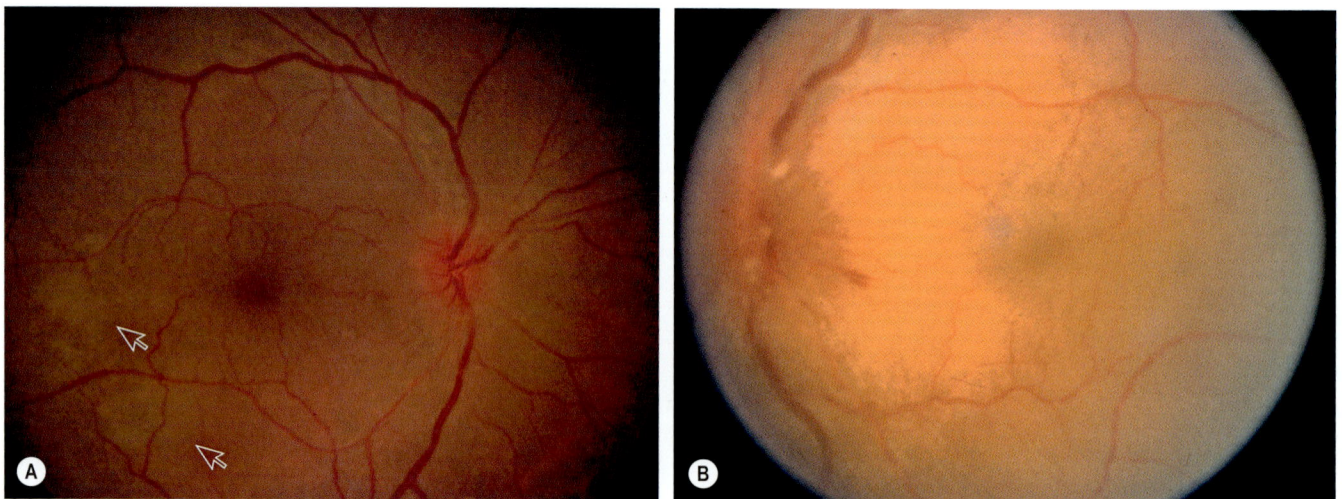

Figure 4–25. Fundus photograph of the right (**A**) and left (**B**) eye of a patient with Vogt–Koyanagi–Harada syndrome. Bilateral optic disc swelling and diffuse, yellow, subretinal infiltrates (arrows in A point to discrete lesions). There are areas of retinal thickening in the right eye and extensive exudative retinal detachment in the left eye.

of a peculiar sensitivity to touch of the hair and skin. In the later stages, patients develop depigmentation of the skin (vitiligo) and hair (poliosis) of any part of the body.

In the early stages, FA will reveal multiple pinpoint sources of leakage.[396] Indocyanine green angiography may reveal patchy infiltrates, suggesting an inflammatory disorder of the choroid with subsequent circulatory compromise.[397] Echography reveals diffuse, low to medium reflective thickening of the choroid and serous retinal detachment.[398] MRI may demonstrate a similar thickening and enhancement of the choroid and retina.[399] During the early stages lumbar puncture will reveal a pleocytosis with lymphocytes and monocytes although the necessity of spinal fluid examination in typical cases has been questioned.[400] Later in the course the spinal fluid may return to normal, and therefore if performed the lumbar puncture should be done early.

VKH syndrome is typically treated with corticosteroids,[401,402] However, the early use of other immunomodulatory (i.e., mycophenolate mofetil and cyclosporine) therapies may provide a superior visual outcome.[403] Incomplete responses and steroid dependency are commonly encountered.[404] Most patients require treatment for at least a year. Successful therapy with intravenous immunoglobulin has also been reported.[405] About 60% of patients maintain 20/30 or better vision.[378]

Retinal manifestations of systemic inflammatory and infectious diseases

A variety of systemic infectious and inflammatory conditions may be associated with retinal manifestations. Retinal findings may take many different forms, including retinal phlebitis, retinal and choroidal granulomas, cotton-wool spots, and optic nerve head swelling. Patients may be asymptomatic with abnormalities detected on initial screening examinations. In other patients, ophthalmic symptoms and retinal abnormalities are the initial manifestations of the systemic disease.

Sarcoidosis

Sarcoidosis, a multisystem granulomatous disorder of unknown etiology, is the third most common cause of uveitis after idiopathic cases and those associated with HLA B-27.[406] Population studies suggest the HLA-DPB1*0101 type is a significant risk factor, and that there is a strong genetic component to disease development.[407] The incidence is estimated at 1/100 000 with a female preponderance.[408] Most studies find about 30–50% of sarcoidosis patients have ophthalmic involvement.[408,409] However, in one series as many as 79% of sarcoidosis patients had ocular manifestations, and the most common was granulomatous anterior uveitis (**Fig. 4–26**).[410] Ophthalmic manifestations of sarcoidosis are listed in **Table 4–7**.[411] Presentations of sarcoidosis differ across different populations and races. For example, African Americans tend to present at younger ages,[412] and, in India, posterior segment manifestations are more common.[413] Vitritis and retinal perivasculitis (seen in

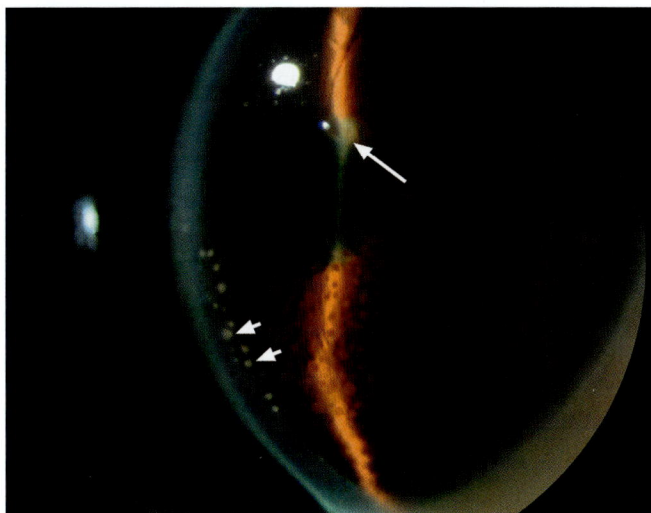

Figure 4–26. Anterior segment slit-beam photograph of a patient with granulomatous uveitis secondary to sarcoidosis. Keratic precipitates (short arrows) on the corneal endothelium and iris posterior synechia (adhesions of the iris to the lens; long arrow) are seen.

Table 4–7 Ophthalmic manifestations of sarcoidosis

Anterior segment
Anterior uveitis
Iris nodules
Conjunctival granulomas
Nodules on trabecular meshwork
Interstitial keratitis
Band keratopathy
Posterior segment/retinal
Vitritis
Periphlebitis
Chorioretinitis
Choroidal nodules
Retinal neovascularization
Retinal vein occlusion
Optic nerve/chiasm
Optic perineuritis (see Chapter 5)
Optic disc edema (see Chapter 5)
Optic neuropathy (see Chapter 5)
Chiasmal/hypothalamic involvement (see Chapter 7)
Orbit/external
Lacrimal gland enlargement
Keratoconjunctivitis sicca
Orbital granuloma
Enlarged extraocular muscles

about two-thirds of patients) and spotty retinochoroidal exudates (seen in about half of patients) are the most common posterior segment manifestations of sarcoidosis.[410,414–416] Vitreous inflammation may appear as a simple cellular infiltrate. Other patients will demonstrate the classic "snowballs" or "string of pearls" appearance (**Fig. 4–26**). Midperipheral phlebitis is seen and characterized by perivascular sheathing (**Fig. 4–27**). Periphlebitis may be more posterior and associated with disc edema.[416] FA will highlight vessel wall and disc staining (**Fig. 4–28**). More severe cases of periphlebitis are associated with the classic appearance of candle wax drippings. Retinal vein occlusion rarely complicates the periphlebitis.[417] Chorioretinal lesions or granulomas may manifest as discrete infiltrates or nodules,[418–420] "punched-out" chorioretinal scars, or as a large choroidal nodular lesion simulating a metastatic tumor (**Fig. 4–29**).[421] Indocyanine green angiography may show choroidal abnormalities before any lesions can be detected ophthalmoscopi-

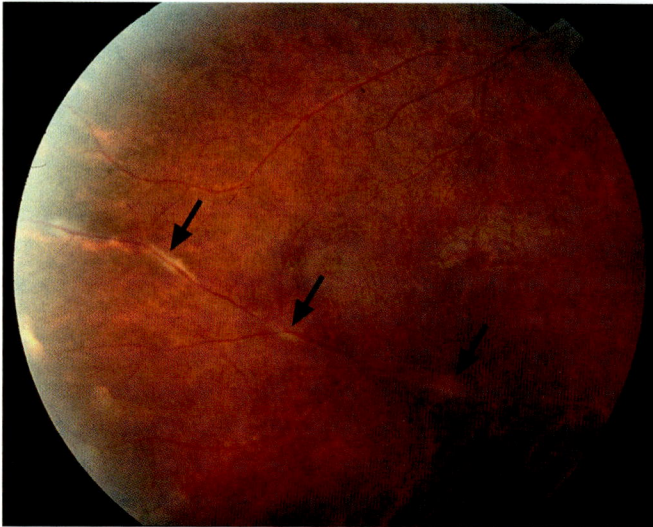

Figure 4–27. Perivascular cuffing (arrows) and phlebitis in a patient with sarcoidosis.

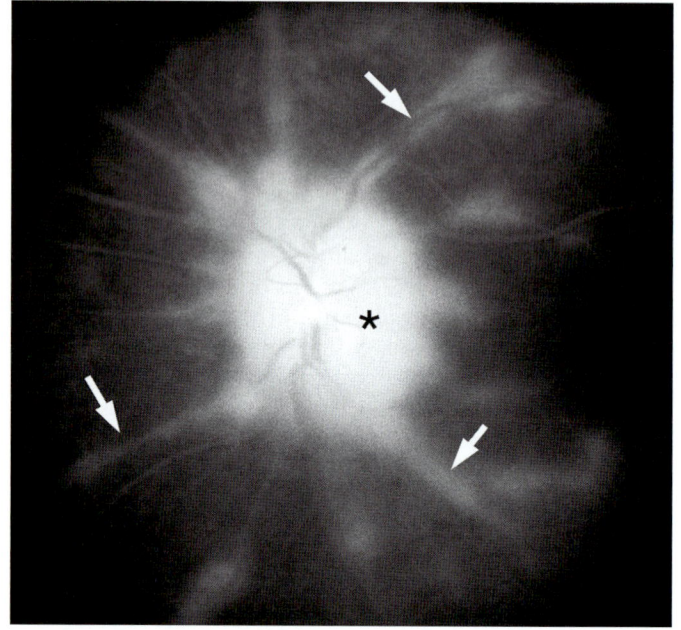

Figure 4–28. Optic disc edema and phlebitis in a patient with sarcoidosis. Vessel wall staining (arrows) and optic disc staining (asterisk) are seen on fluorescein angiography.

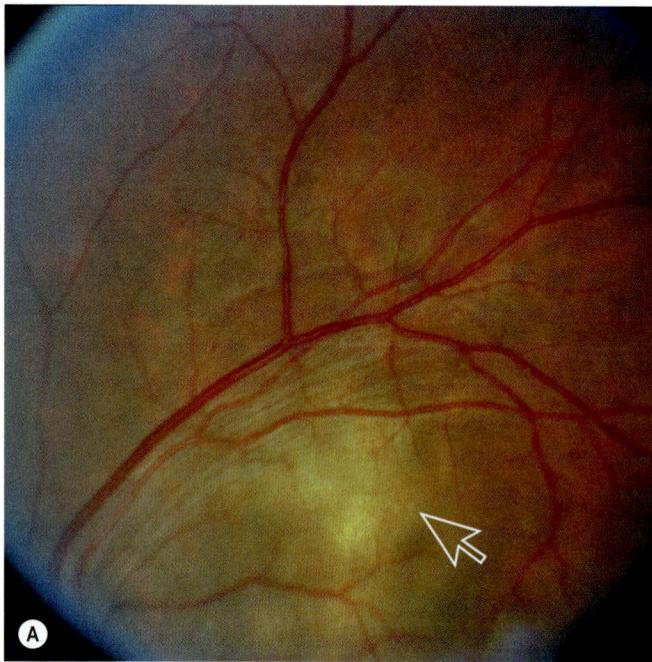

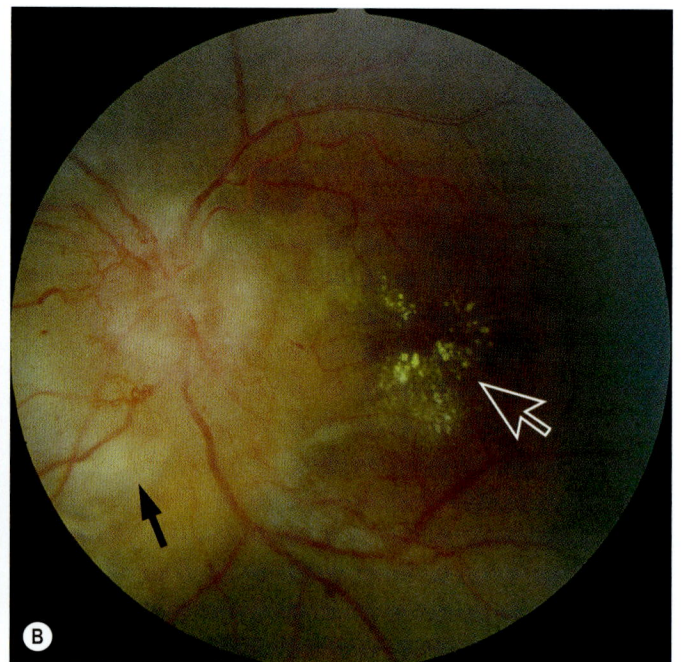

Figure 4–29. Retinal findings in sarcoidosis in two patients. **A.** Large subretinal, yellow mass (arrow) typical of a sarcoid granuloma is seen in the superotemporal macula. **B.** Optic disc edema, intraretinal exudates in stellate pattern (open arrow) and large confluent, yellow, peripapillary subretinal mass (black arrow) are seen (courtesy of Alexander J. Brucker, MD).

cally.[422] Arterial macroaneurysms have also been described.[423] Neovascularization of the retina or optic nerve head is a rare complication of sarcoidosis. Optic nerve head involvement is discussed in Chapter 5.

Patients with suspected ocular sarcoidosis should be screened with chest roentgenography (or chest computed tomography (CT)), angiotensin I-converting enzyme (ACE) levels, and occasionally gallium scanning. In many medical centers, gallium scanning has been replaced by body positron emission tomography (PET) to search for a biopsy site. The diagnosis is often established by transbronchial biopsy.[424,425] If there is an abnormal conjunctival appearance then conjunctival biopsy may be used to confirm the diagnosis.[426] Further details regarding diagnosing sarcoidosis are discussed in Chapter 5.

Treatment of the ocular complications of sarcoidosis is accomplished with topical steroids, injectable depot steroids, and systemic immunosuppression with steroids or steroid-sparing agents. Posterior segment manifestations usually require oral steroids. However, if there are no symptoms and only peripheral chorioretinitis is present, it is reasonable to observe the patient without treatment. Karma and associates[427] classified the course of ocular sarcoidosis into three categories: monophasic, relapsing, or chronic. The prognosis was poor for patients with the chronic form of the disease, with no patients retaining 20/30 vision or better. In contrast, 88% of patients in the monophasic group retained 20/30 vision or better.[427]

Systemic lupus erythematosus

In addition to the development of lupus anticoagulants (see above), patients with systemic lupus erythematosus (SLE) may develop a primary retinal vasculitis. Retinal findings were present in about 30% of patients in one series.[428] Retinal phlebitis may be most likely to occur when CNS lupus is present.[429] This manifests as perivascular cuffing by white blood cells or discrete focal leakage on FA.[428] Patients may develop retinal hemorrhage, exudates, choroiditis,[430] and cotton-wool spots. Vasculitis affects arteries and veins and eventually leads to vaso-occlusive phenomena, including retinal infarction[431,432] (see **Fig. 4-24**) and subsequent neovascularization. A choroidopathy similar to that seen in eclampsia and characterized by serous retinal detachments has been described in patients with SLE.[433,434]

Cat scratch disease

Cat scratch disease is a self-limited systemic illness caused by a Gram-negative bacillus, *Bartonella henselae*. The organism is inoculated by the bite or scratch of an infected animal. However, animal fleas may also transmit the disease, and exposures can often be difficult to identify in suspected cases. Patients can subsequently develop lymphadenopathy, fever, and malaise. The most recognized ophthalmic manifestation of cat scratch disease is optic nerve head swelling and macular star formation (i.e., neuroretinitis; see Chapter 5). However, other patients with *Bartonella* infection manifest with vision loss as a result of uveitis and retinal infiltrates.[435] Discrete white retinal or choroidal lesions are the most common posterior-segment manifestation of cat scratch

disease and may be observed in over 80% of patients.[435] Disc swelling and macular star formation were found in 63% of patients in the same series. Other findings may include arterial and venous occlusions. A unique presentation in patients with human immunodeficiency virus (HIV) has been described with a subretinal mass and an associated unusual vascular network.[436] Because malignant hypertension (see below) may produce a similar ophthalmoscopic picture, blood pressure should be carefully checked in all patients thought to have neuroretinitis from cat scratch disease. Diagnosis can be confirmed by testing for *Bartonella* antibodies in the peripheral blood or by polymerase chain reaction testing of ocular tissue.[437-439]

Subacute sclerosing panencephalitis (SSPE)

Optic atrophy and macular pigmentary changes can be seen in SSPE,[440,441] a progressive infection of the CNS by a defective measles virus. Often heralded by personality changes, SSPE leads typically to seizures, mental deterioration, and myoclonus.

Acute retinal necrosis (ARN)

This visually devastating retinitis, characterized by retinal vasculitis, hemorrhages, detachments, and necrosis in addition to vitreal and aqueous inflammation and optic neuritis, is primarily caused by herpesvirus infections (herpes simplex virus (HSV), varicella zoster virus (VZV), cytomegalovirus (CMV), and Epstein–Barr (EBV) virus).[442,443] Several cases of ARN have been reported in association with HSV and VZV encephalitis.[443] Prompt therapy with antiviral agents such as acyclovir, steroids to reduce inflammation, and laser and surgical management of the retinal complications are the best options for improving visual outcome.[442]

Malignant hypertension and eclampsia

Chronic hypertension can be associated with a typical retinopathy characterized by cotton-wool spots and vascular abnormalities (**Fig. 4-30**). However, severe (malignant) hypertension leads to a breakdown of the blood–retina barrier, with resultant optic disc edema, flame-shaped hemorrhages, cotton-wool spots, and lipid exudation into the retina (**Fig. 4-30**). Hayreh and colleagues[444-448] studied hypertensive retinopathy in monkeys. The earliest ophthalmic manifestations were cotton-wool spots as a result of terminal retinal arteriole ischemia.[446] Lipid exudates may accumulate in Henle's layer, creating a picture similar to neuroretinitis.[449,450] Disc edema may result from local optic nerve head ischemia and disrupted axonal transport or from elevated intracranial pressure that may accompany hypertensive encephalopathy. Malignant hypertension may also be associated with choroidopathy as a result of choriocapillaris occlusion.[451] These patients have focal areas of opaque retinal pigment epithelium known as Elsching spots, which may demonstrate leakage on FA.[444] Occasionally, patients with malignant hypertension develop exudative retinal detachments. Similar areas of focal fluid leakage and sensory retinal detachment may be seen as a manifestation of eclampsia even without other hypertension-related retinal

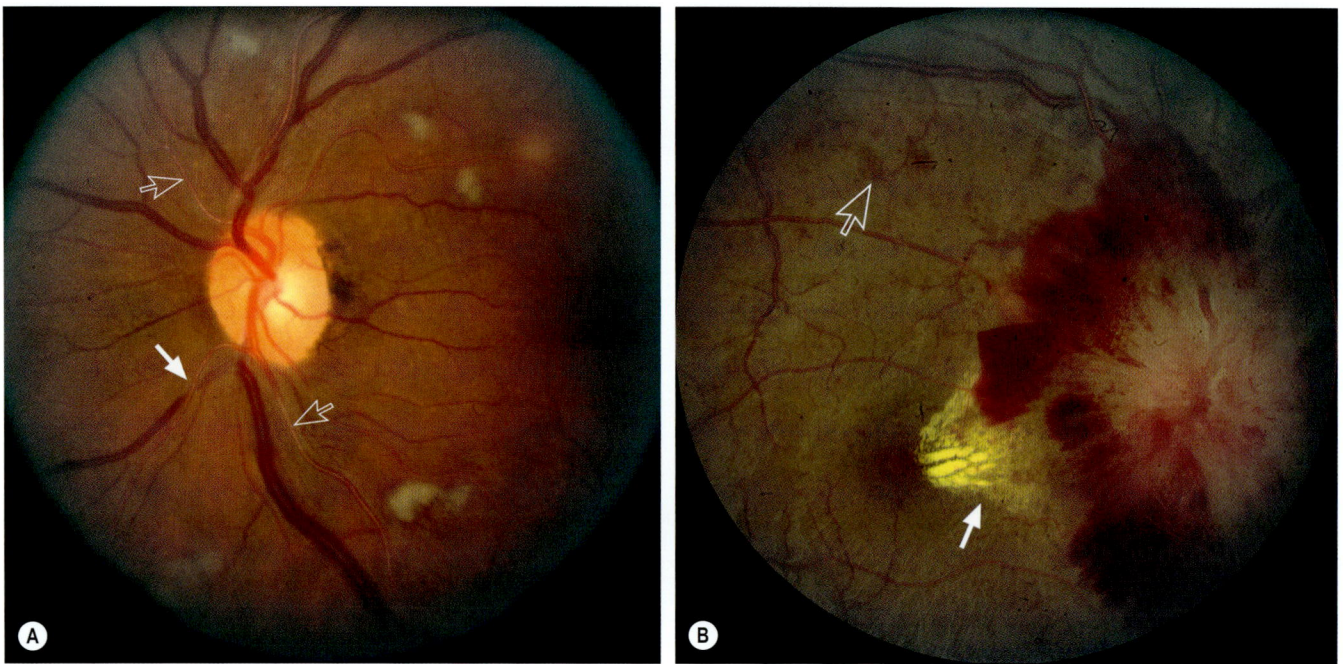

Figure 4–30. Fundus findings in systemic hypertension. **A**. Hypertensive retinopathy with cotton-wool spots, arterior–venous nicking (solid arrow) and "silver wiring of vessels"(open arrows). **B**. Optic disc swelling in malignant hypertension. Mild engorgement of the retinal veins is seen, as well as intraretinal hemorrhage (open arrow) and lipid exudate into the macula in a partial macular star (solid arrow).

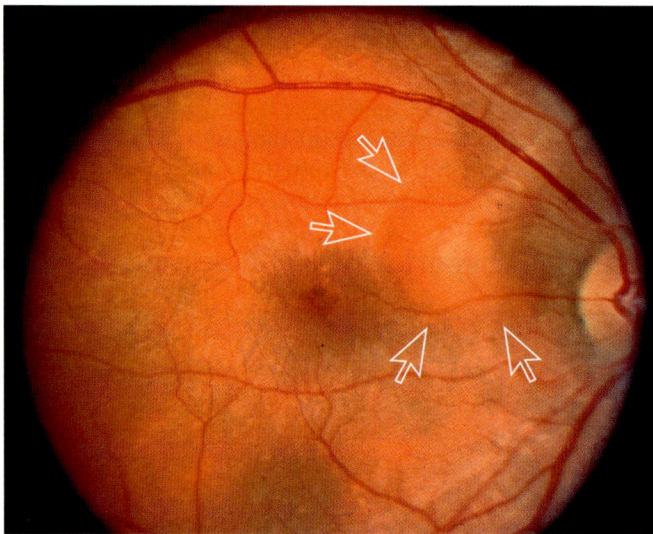

Figure 4–31. Serous detachment of the retina (arrows) in a patient with vision loss and eclampsia.

changes (**Fig. 4–31**).[451] These can be confirmed by mERG abnormalities and OCT.[452–454]

Blood dyscrasias

In anemic patients, an ophthalmoscopic picture very similar to malignant hypertension may be observed. Anemia produces retinal ischemia only when it is sudden or severe. In the setting of acute, severe anemia the oxygen-carrying capacity of the blood is severely compromised and autoregulatory mechanisms have not yet compensated for the change. Patients may develop disc swelling, cotton-wool spots, and

intraretinal hemorrhages concentrated in the peripapillary region (**Fig. 4–32**).

Homozygous sickle cell anemia is the most common hemoglobinopathy to cause retinal manifestations. In this condition the abnormal shape of the red blood cells causes vascular occlusion in the retinal periphery. More posterior areas develop neovascularization, heralded by arteriovenous anastomoses that become shunt vessels with a characteristic fan-shaped appearance.

The leukemias may also present with retinal findings by causing retinal ischemia. The retinal ischemia may develop as a consequence of the associated anemia, the increased viscosity of the blood, or the occlusion of vessels by large clumps of white cells. Patients with leukemia may also have intraretinal hemorrhages (some with white centers Roth spots), preretinal hemorrhages, vitreous hemorrhage, and cotton-wool spots[455–457] (**Fig. 4–33**).

Phakomatoses

The phakomatoses are a group of hereditary conditions characterized by the presence of hamartomas of the skin, blood vessels, and nervous system (**Table 4–8**), and several have prominent retinal manifestations. The more common phakomatoses are neurofibromatosis types I and II, tuberous sclerosis (Bourneville disease), encephalotrigeminal angiomatosis (Sturge–Weber syndrome), angiomatosis of the retina and cerebellum (von Hippel–Lindau disease), racemose angioma of the midbrain and retina (Wyburn–Mason syndrome), and ataxia telangiectasia (Louis–Bar syndrome). Except for the telangiectasia of the conjunctiva in Louis–Bar syndrome, all of these growths represent hamartomas

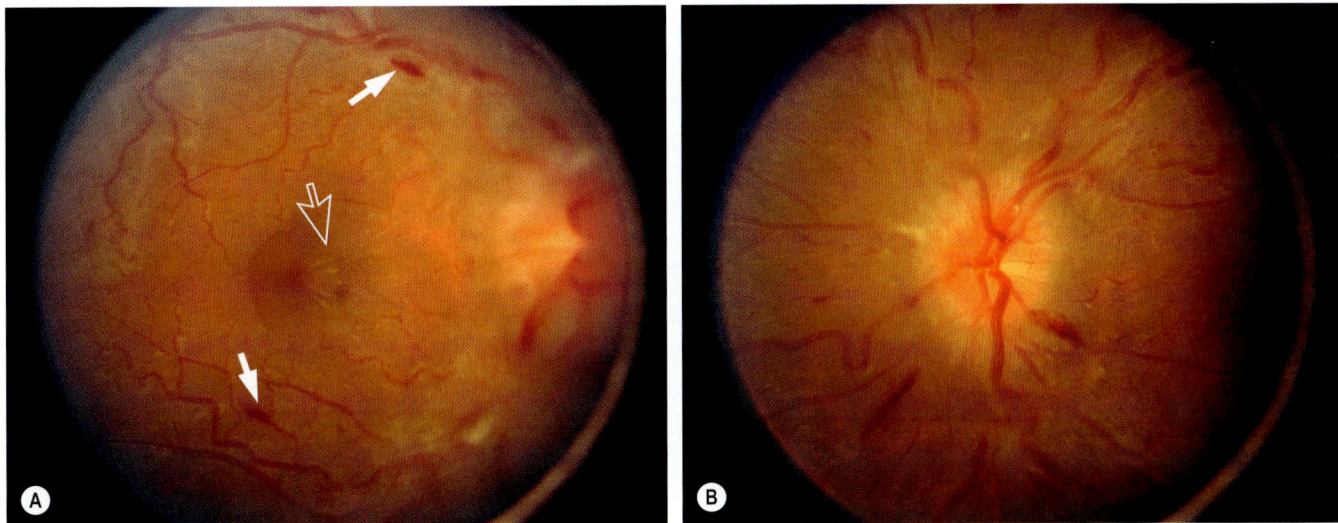

Figure 4–32. Fundus photographs of a patient with the acute onset of profound anemia. **A**. Macular edema and partial star formation (open arrow) with intraretinal hemorrhages (solid arrows) (right eye). **B**. Disc swelling and retinal vein engorgement (right eye).

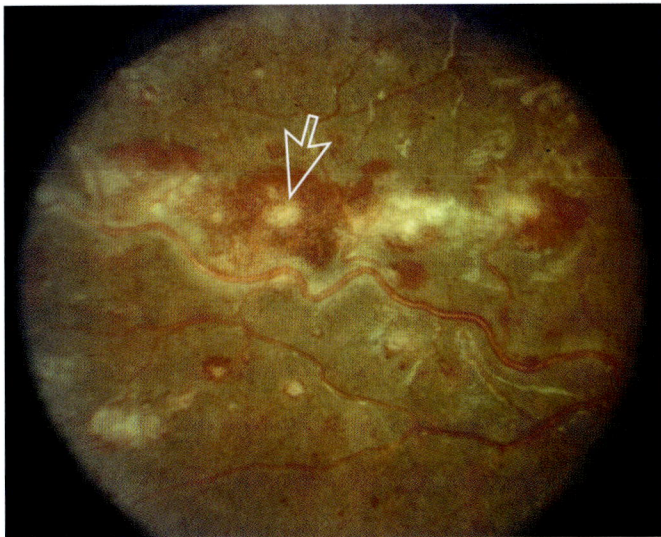

Figure 4–33. Intraretinal and white centered hemorrhages (Roth spots; arrow) in a patient with acute leukemia.

(abnormal growth of mature cells). Telangiectasias of the conjunctiva are hamartias. Hamartias result from developmental abnormalities of the cells in the normal area of growth.

The phakomatoses with salient retinal manifestations will be discussed here. Neurofibromatosis type I is discussed in detail in Chapter 7, while ataxia telangiectasia is reviewed in Chapter 16.

Neurofibromatosis type II

Neurofibromatosis type II (NF-2) was formerly called central NF, but is now known to be a distinct disorder inherited in an autosomal dominant fashion. Unlike NF-1, which has been localized to chromosome 17, the gene for NF-2 is a tumor suppressor on chromosome 22 that encodes for the protein neurofibromin.[458,459] The diagnosis of NF-2 can be satisfied by bilateral acoustic neuromas or a unilateral acous-

tic neuroma and a first-degree relative with bilateral acoustic neuromas.[460] NF-2 is associated with other intracranial and intraspinal tumors, especially meningiomas.[461] Prominent ocular findings are posterior subcapsular cataracts,[462,463] retinal hamartomata,[464–467] epiretinal membranes,[463–467] and bilateral optic nerve sheath meningiomas (**Fig. 4–34**).[469] Early ophthalmologic evaluation looking for typical lens and retinal findings is extremely helpful in establishing the diagnosis.[470,471] Choroidal hyperfluorescence in the macular region on FA has been shown to present in asymptomatic NF2 patients without vision loss.[472] Lisch nodules are a rare finding in NF-2[468] and are much more commonly seen in NF-1.

Tuberous sclerosis

The classic triad of tuberous sclerosis (TS) includes facial angioma (adenoma sebaceum), mental retardation, and seizures, but frequently there are also ocular, renal, pulmonary, and cardiac manifestations.[473–475] The condition is dominantly inherited with a high rate of new mutations.[476] We have seen several children with TS whose parents were unknowingly affected as well. Responsible defects in two tumor suppressor genes, TSC1 (on chromosome 9q34, coding for hamartin) and TSC2 (on chromosome 16p13, coding for tuberin), have been identified, and either may cause TS.[477–482] Although there is a tendency for patients with TSC2 mutations to be more neurologically affected, for the most part there is considerable overlap, making their clinical phenotypes virtually indistinguishable.[483]

The most characteristic eye finding is a retinal astrocytic hamartoma, found in 44–90% of patients.[484] Astrocytic hamartomas, of which there are two major types, may occur anywhere in the fundus. The multinodular lesions reside in the posterior pole and are typically elevated, yellowish-white, and mulberry-like in appearance. These are often near the optic nerve (**Fig. 4–35**) and therefore may resemble giant optic disc drusen. Unlike drusen, however, they tend to obscure the underlying retinal vessels. These retinal lesions are similar in appearance to those observed in NF-2 and

Table 4-8 Clinical features of the major phakomatoses

Disease	Inheritance	CNS findings	Major eye findings	Skin findings	Systemic findings	Further discussion
Neurofibromatosis type 1	Sporadic and dominant	Optic pathway gliomas	Iris Lisch nodules	Café au lait spots	Pheochromocytoma	Chapter 7
		T2-weighted gray and white matter hyperintensities on MRI	Optic pathway glioma	Axillary/inguinal freckling	Neurofibromas	
		Secondary neoplasms	Enlarged corneal nerves	Neurofibromas	Scoliosis	
		Attention deficit and learning disorders	Eyelid neurofibromas		Bony dysplasias	
			Glaucoma			
			Sphenoid wing dysplasia			
			Retinal nevi and hypopigmentation			
Neurofibromatosis type 2	Dominant	Acoustic neuromas	Posterior subcapsular cataracts	Café au lait spots	None	Chapter 4
		Gliomas	Epiretinal membranes			
		Ependymomas	Retinal hamartomas			
		Meningiomas				
		Schwannomas				
Tuberous sclerosis	Dominant	Seizures	Retinal astrocytomas	Facial angioma (adenoma sebacium)	Renal angiomyolipoma	Chapter 4
		Cortical tubers		Periungual fibromas	Cardiac rhabdomyoma	
		Developmental delay				

Syndrome	Inheritance	CNS manifestations	Ocular manifestations	Skin manifestations	Systemic manifestations	Reference
(Tuberous sclerosis — continued)		Subependymal nodules and giant cell astrocytomas		Shagreen patch, Hypopigmented nodules		
von Hippel–Lindau disease	Dominant	Cerebellar hemangioblastoma	Retinal angiomas	None	Pheochromocytoma, renal cysts, renal carcinoma, hemangioblastoma of pancreas, liver, lung	Chapter 4
Ataxia–telangiectasia	Recessive	Cerebellar atrophy, ataxia, developmental delay	Telangiectasia of conjunctiva, ocular motor apraxia	None	Sinopulmonary infections, leukemia	Chapter 16
Sturge–Weber	Sporadic	Seizures, Meningeal angiomas, intracranial calcifications, Homonymous hemianopia, Transient visual loss	Choroidal hemangioma, glaucoma	Facial angioma	None	Chapter 4, Chapter 8
Wyburn–Mason syndrome	Sporadic	Intracranial (midbrain) arteriovenous malformations	Retinal arteriovenous malformations	Cutaneous hemangiomata	Bone and soft-tissue hypertrophy	Chapter 4

CNS, central nervous system; MRI, magnetic resonance imaging.

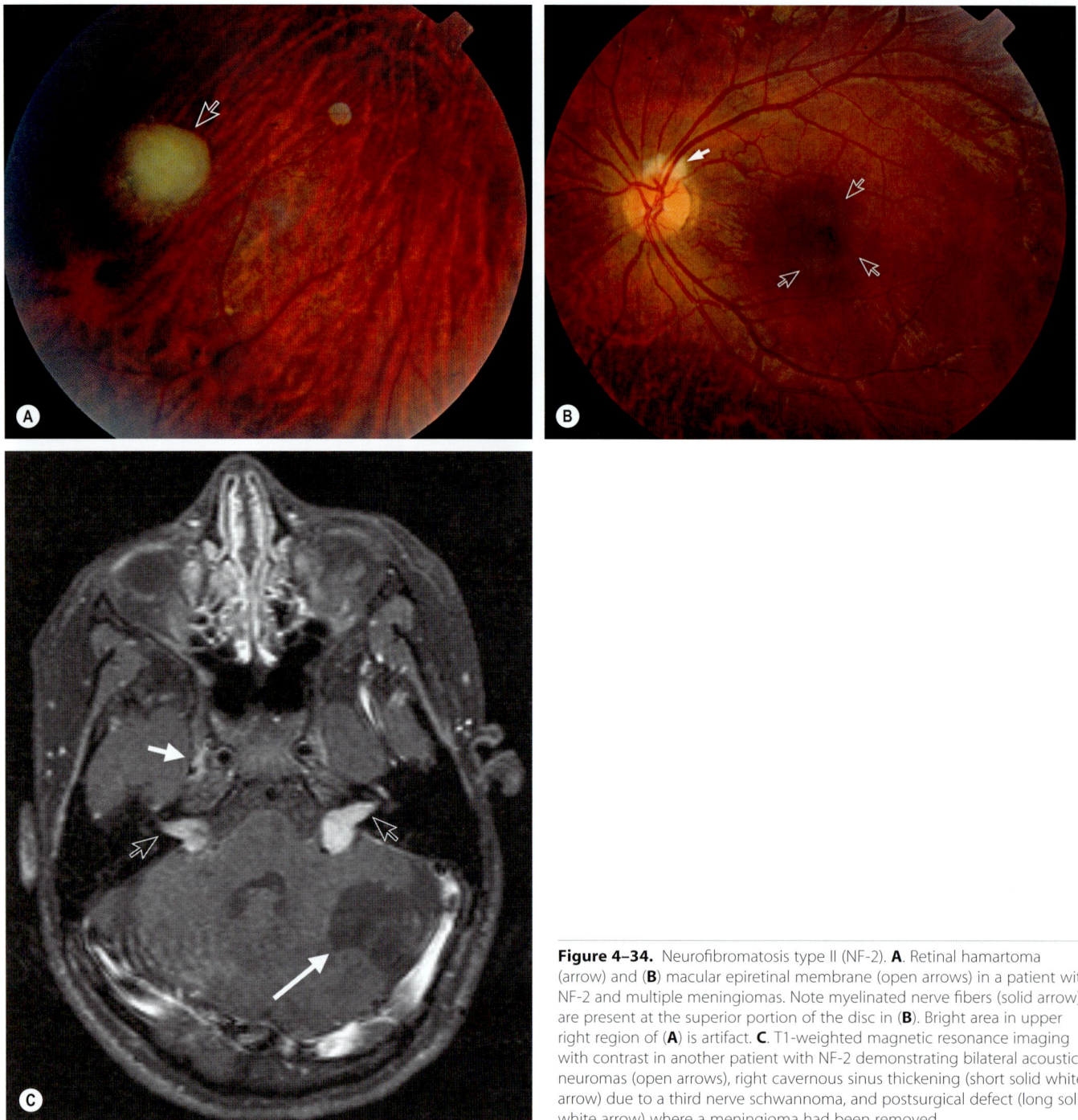

Figure 4–34. Neurofibromatosis type II (NF-2). **A**. Retinal hamartoma (arrow) and (**B**) macular epiretinal membrane (open arrows) in a patient with NF-2 and multiple meningiomas. Note myelinated nerve fibers (solid arrow) are present at the superior portion of the disc in (**B**). Bright area in upper right region of (**A**) is artifact. **C**. T1-weighted magnetic resonance imaging with contrast in another patient with NF-2 demonstrating bilateral acoustic neuromas (open arrows), right cavernous sinus thickening (short solid white arrow) due to a third nerve schwannoma, and postsurgical defect (long solid white arrow) where a meningioma had been removed.

sarcoidosis of the optic nerve head. Astrocytic hamartomas of the second type (**Fig. 4–35**) are smaller, flatter, whiter, and more translucent, and may mimic cotton-wool spots as they lie along the nerve fiber layer. Although these are also found in the posterior pole, they are more likely than the first type to be found further in the periphery. There is also an inter-mediary type,[485] and we have seen a rarely described exo-phytic retinal hamartoma.[486] In one series of 100 patients,[484] retinal hamartomas were seen in 44%. The multinodular "mulberry" lesion was seen in 24 (55%), the flat, translucent lesion was observed in 31 (70%), and the transitional type lesion was seen in four of the 44 patients (9%).[484]

The hamartomas arise from the retinal ganglion cell layer and are composed of astrocytes. Eventually they may involve all layers of retina. They contain large blood vessels and are not malignant. Autofluorescence and FA can be helpful in identifying astrocytic hamartomas.[487] Retinal lesions in TS usually require no treatment as they rarely produce vision loss. However, we have seen large lesions involve the macula causing visual loss and leukocoria. The classic teaching is that most children have their full complement of mature retinal hamartomas by age 1 year, but rarely lesions arising,[488] enlarging,[489] calcifying, and even regressing[490] later in life have been well documented. In addition to the retinal

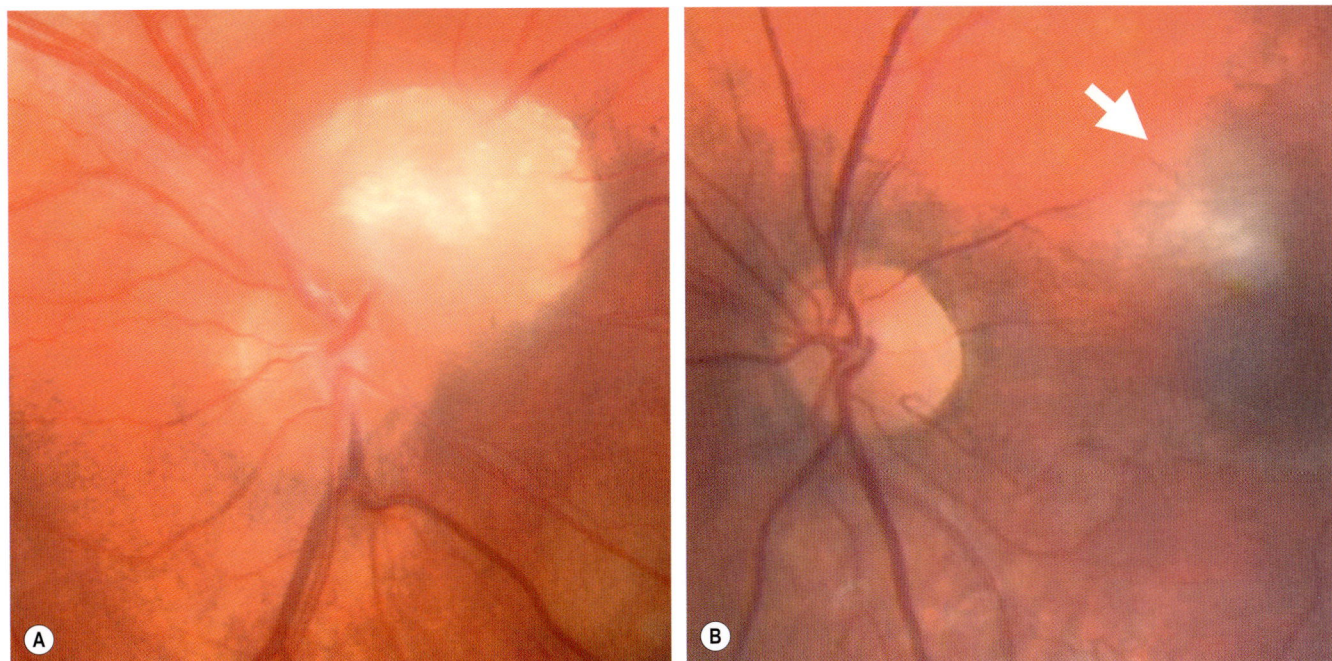

Figure 4–35. Retinal hamartomas in tuberous sclerosis. **A**. The first patient has a round, elevated, yellowish-white lesion above the optic disc. The irregular surface resembles drusen or tapioca. **B**. Another patient has a nerve fiber layer hamartoma (arrow) that is less elevated and is located above the macula. In both patients the hamartomas were visually asymptomatic.

hamartomas, other retinal findings include depigmented, punched out lesions of the retina, colobomas, and optic atrophy. Papilledema, sometimes with associated visual loss,[491] can occur when there is hydrocephalus caused by obstruction of the foramen of Monro (see below). External findings are primarily eyelid angiofibromas.

CNS manifestations include seizures, which eventually occur in 70–90% of patients, and are the most common presenting neurologic symptom in TS.[492,493] The onset of seizures occurs in infancy, usually manifesting as infantile spasms. Tonic–clonic seizures may occur after the first year of life. Mental retardation, sometimes severe, is common, occurring in 50–60% of patients.

Neuroimaging techniques are helpful in identifying the typical cortical tubers, which produce high signal on T2-weighted MRI (**Fig. 4–36**).[494] They may also be seen as calcific opacities on CT. Subependymal nodules may lie along the ventricular surface. These nodules may continue to proliferate, at which point they are classified as subependymal giant cell astrocytomas. These are often found in patients between 5 and 18 years of age and rarely become malignant. They occur commonly near the foramen of Monro and can grow sufficiently large to obstruct cerebrospinal fluid and cause hydrocephalus.[491]

The skin manifestations (**Fig. 4–37**) of TS occur in almost all patients.[495] Hypomelanotic macules (ash-leaf patches, hypopigmented macules) are found in up to 90% of patients and can be single or multiple. They are usually 1–2 cm in diameter, but they may vary in size. Use of an ultraviolet light (Wood's lamp) in a dark room may help locate these macules, especially in lightly pigmented individuals. Facial angiomas are present in about 50% of patients and are usually first noted when the patient is between 3 and 5 years

of age. Often confused with acne, they are small, but often confluent, pink or light brown, raised nodules typically located in the malar area and nasolabial folds. They may have a prominent vascular component and can cause recurrent bleeding. Other dermatologic manifestations include shagreen patches (leathery areas), ungual fibromas, and forehead plaques.

Other systemic findings include cardiac rhabdomyomas, kidney angiomyolipomas, renal cell carcinomas, pulmonary lymphangiomatosis, and dental enamel pits. Thus, all patients with TS should undergo neuro-ophthalmologic and dermatologic examinations, head MRI, echocardiography, and ultrasound of the kidneys. Unless there is a specific reason, after the initial eye screening annual eye examinations are unnecessary.[496] If an infant with TS is examined, we typically schedule to see the child back just one more time at age 4 or 5 years since there is a small chance retinal hamartomas might arise anew or change.

von Hippel–Lindau disease

von Hippel–Lindau (VHL) disease, or retinal angiomatosis, is an autosomal dominant condition with incomplete penetrance and variable expressivity. The defect is caused by mutations in VHL, a tumor suppressor gene located on chromosome 3p25–26.[497–499] The eponym of von Hippel disease is used when just the retina is involved. VHL disease is the term used for those cases with both CNS and retinal involvement. The condition represents a dysgenesis of neuroectoderm and mesoderm, but the basic defect is not known. Features of the condition include angiomatosis of the retina, capillary hemangioblastomas of the CNS, and cysts or tumors of the viscera. The disease may be lethal and careful

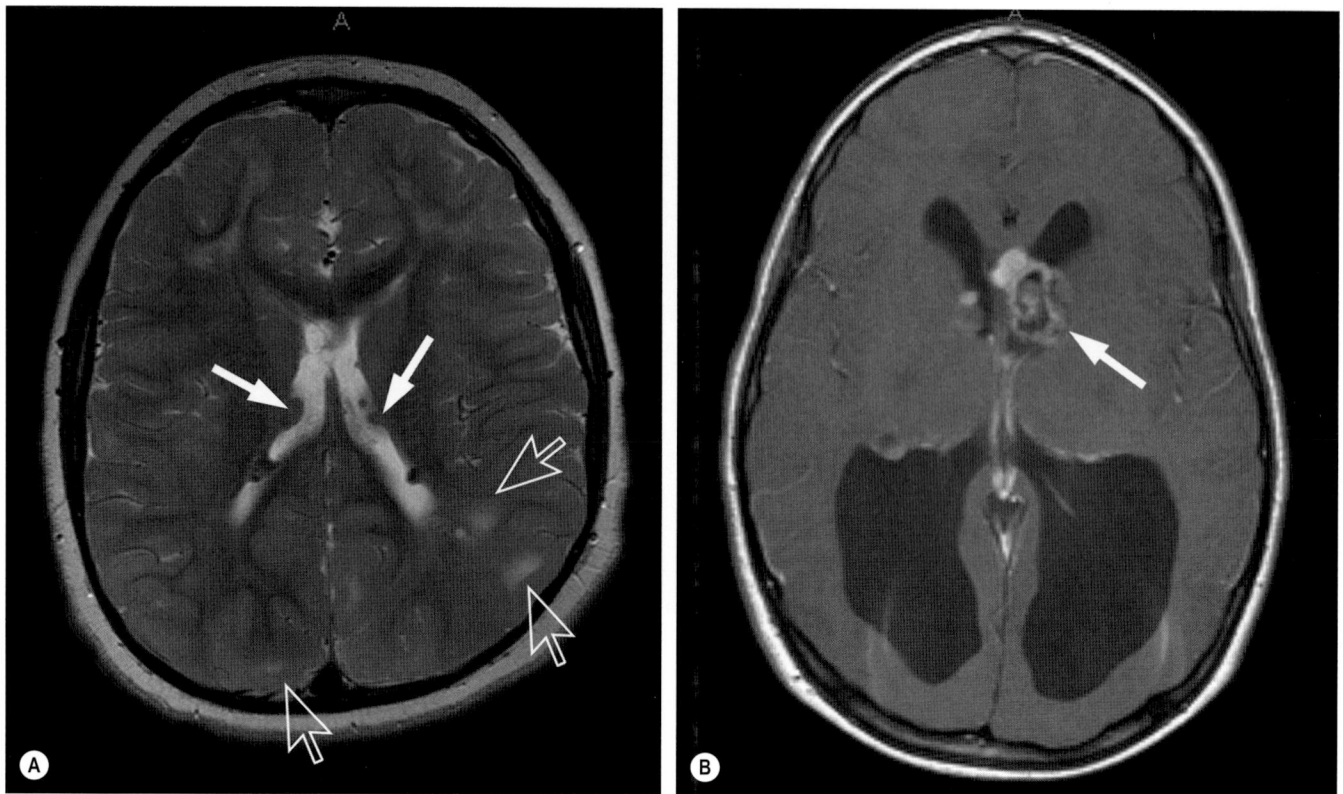

Figure 4–36. Magnetic resonance imaging (MRI) scans in tuberous sclerosis. **A**. T2-weighted axial MRI. Cortical tubers, characterized by abnormal architecture of the cortex and underlying white matter, may be seen (open arrows). Subependymal nodules (solid arrows) can be seen along the lining of the lateral ventricles. **B**. T1-weighted axial MRI with gadolinium. Large subependymal giant astrocytoma (arrow) obstructing the third ventricle, leading to hydrocephalus (manifested by ventricular enlargement).

monitoring is necessary to detect the associated renal cell carcinoma and pheochromocytoma. Cysts and angiomatous tumors involving the visceral organs are usually asymptomatic.

Retinal angiomatosis, found in approximately one-half of patients, is usually the first observed manifestation of the condition.[500–502] These tumors are usually in a midperipheral location,[503] but occasionally are in the posterior pole or rarely in the intraorbital portion of the optic nerve. The lesions are bilateral in about one-half of the patients, and multiple lesions are seen in one eye in one-third of patients.[500,503,504] The earliest lesion is a small capillary cluster the size and configuration of a diabetic microaneurysm. The fully developed classic lesions consist of an elevated, globular, pink retinal tumor that is often fed by a dilated tortuous retinal artery. Abnormal vessels on the disc may point to the anteriorly located tumor. Tumor enlargement is associated with lipid exudation and retinal detachment. Vision loss occurs in more than half of the patients with angiomatoses.[500,503,504] Therapy for these lesions includes photocoagulation, cryotherapy, and diathermy. Because these procedures are usually successful in obliterating small VHL angiomas, early treatment is recommended.[505] Argon laser can be used with small lesions and applied directly to the surface of the small angioma, with good long-term preservation of vision.[506] Cryotherapy and brachytherapy are useful in patients with larger tumors that are more anteriorly located and in eyes with media opacity.[507] Occasionally

treatment of larger tumors can be followed by massive exudation and retinal detachment.

Cerebellar hemangioblastomas, occurring in about half of patients, are the most common CNS finding. A typical hemangioblastoma consists of a small, highly vascular nodule within a much larger fluid-filled cyst. There can be striking hypertrophy of the feeding and draining vessels. Microscopically a hemangioblastoma is composed of fine capillaries within a matrix of lipid-laden foam cells. Mitotic figures are not present. The retinal angioma has a similar histologic appearance but lacks the cystic component. The tumor has usually become symptomatic at the time of diagnosis and presents in the second to fourth decades of life with signs of hydrocephalus or cerebellar dysfunction. Medullary and spinal hemangioblastomas are relatively less common, but a medullary lesion may be lethal if it compresses vital brain stem structures. The spinal lesions most often appear in the upper cervical cord. Hemangioblastomas may rarely involve the optic nerve and chiasm.[508,509]

Renal cell carcinoma is recognized clinically in one-third of patients and presents as hematuria, obstructive nephropathy, or an abdominal mass. Pheochromocytomas are usually asymptomatic and occur in less than 10% of patients.[510] These lesions tend to cluster in certain predisposed families. VHL without pheochromocytomas has been labeled type 1, while types 2A and 2B refer to those with pheochromocytomas and sometimes with or usually without renal cell

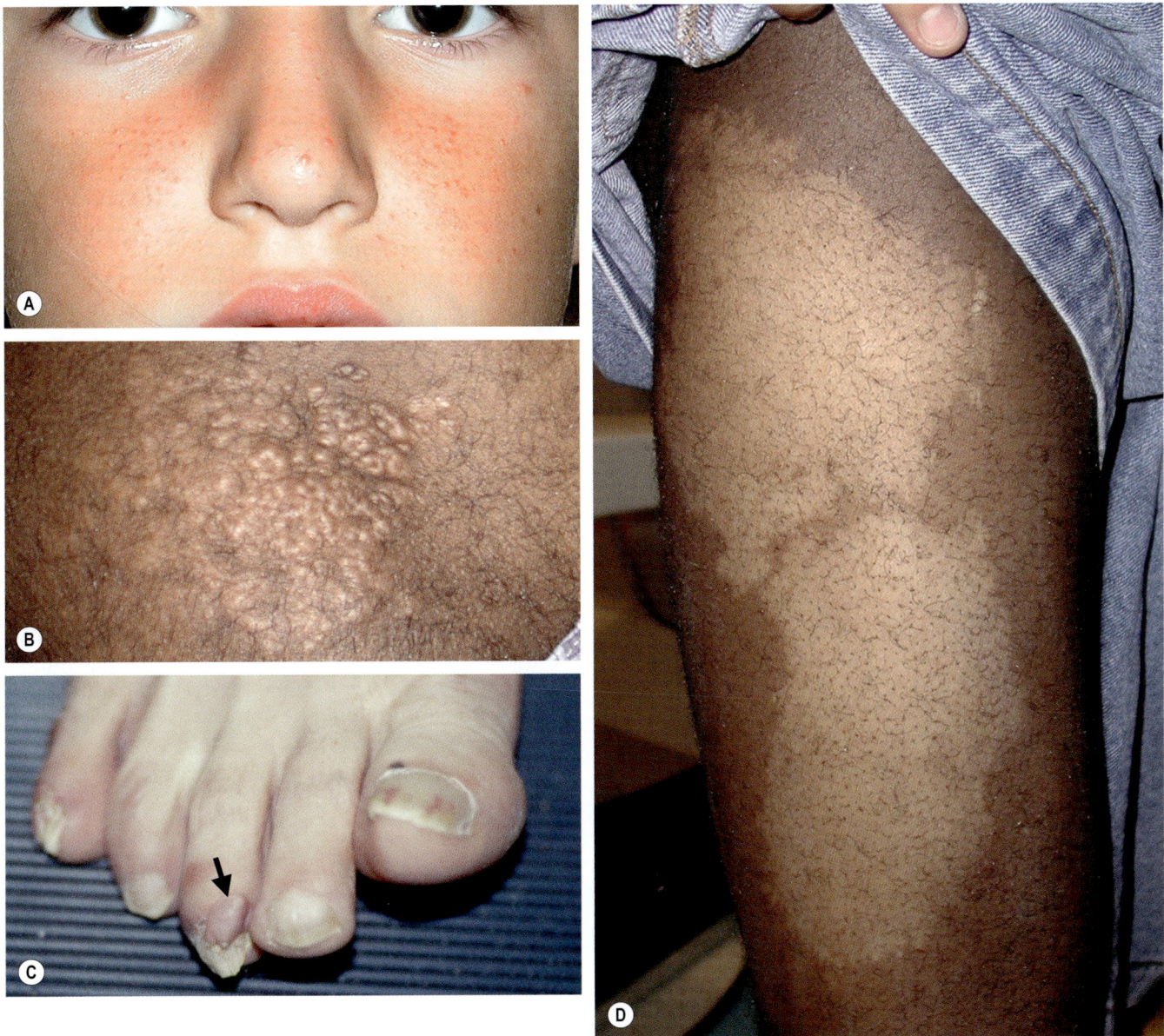

Figure 4–37. Common dermatologic manifestations of tuberous sclerosis. **A.** Facial angiofibromas (adenoma sebacium). **B.** Shagreen patch, an area of thick, leathery skin, on the patient's lower back. **C.** Ungual fibroma (arrow). **D.** Hypopigmented macules in a darkly pigmented individual (same patient as B).

carcinomas, respectively.[511] Renal and pancreatic cysts, pancreatic islet cell tumors, epididymal papillary cystadenomas, and endolymphatic sac papillary adenocarcinomas may also be seen.[512] Polycythemia has been reported in up to 25% of VHL patients and particularly in those with cerebellar hemangioblastoma.

Encephalotrigeminal angiomatosis (Sturge–Weber syndrome)

Sturge–Weber syndrome (SWS) is characterized by the triad of skin, CNS, and ocular findings. Although the nevus flammeus (cutaneous hemifacial hemangioma) of the face is the most obvious sign, the major symptomatic manifestations are due to CNS involvement. The facial port wine stain (see **Fig. 8–33**) may occur with or without one of the other major manifestations: leptomeningeal angiomatosis, cerebral gyriform calcifications, and glaucoma. These are usually unilateral and ipsilateral. The syndrome shows no well-established genetic, sexual, or racial predilection.

The ocular manifestations of SWS are choroidal hemangioma and glaucoma. Sixty percent of SWS patients develop glaucoma.[513] Of these patients, 60% have the disease prior to age 2 years and can develop buphthalmos. Congenital glaucoma is most often associated with involvement of the upper lid by the facial hemangioma present at birth.[514] The actual cause of the glaucoma is not certain and several mechanisms may play a role. These include (1) outflow obstruction by an angle malformation and associated increased vascularity of the iris, (2) occlusion of the angle from anterior synechiae as a secondary phenomenon in patients with choroidal hemangioma and retinal detachment, (3) elevation of episcleral pressure, reducing outflow, (4) hypersecretion of aqueous, and (5) elevation of the intraocular pressure that results from increased permeability of the thin-walled vessels of the choroidal hemangioma. In general, patients with SWS have prominent iris processes that adhere to the trabecular meshwork on gonioscopy. This indicates a primary defect in the development of the angle. Trabeculotomy in infants and trabeculectomy in older patients are effective surgical therapies for patients with SWS and glaucoma.[515–517] Latanoprost may be very effective in these patients.[518]

Choroidal hemangioma occurs in 55% of patients with SWS.[519] These hemangiomas are relatively flat, isolated lesions usually up to several millimeters in diameter and located in the posterior portion of the fundus. Occasionally, they may be diffuse and involve larger areas of choroid and, in such cases, appear similar to red velvet or ketchup. Choroidal hemangiomas are usually situated temporal to the optic disc, have their greatest height in the macular region, and are surrounded by dilated choroidal and retinal vessels. Choroidal hemangiomas demonstrate a characteristic pattern of extratumoral hyperfluorescent spots on indocyanine green angiography. This technique can be used to identify these lesions when they are not visible clinically or not seen on conventional FA.[520,521] The lesions may be visible on MRI with gadolinium enhancement.[522] Typically choroidal hemangiomas cause no visual disturbances until early adulthood. During this slow-growth phase, they may be associated with cystoid degeneration of the overlying sensory retina, and they may eventually produce an exudative retinal detachment. Rarely calcifications occur in the angiomatous choroid. The hemangiomas have been successfully treated with irradiation,[523–526] but usually they are observed. Other ocular findings in SWS include heterochromia iridis, conjunctival angioma and dilation of episcleral vessels, tortuosity of retinal vessels, bilateral lens subluxation, anisocoria, and coloboma of the iris and optic nerve head.

The dermatologic manifestations include the nevus flammeus, which usually corresponds to the distribution of the ophthalmic, maxillary, and, more rarely, mandibular divisions of the trigeminal nerve. The lesion may extend to the region of the upper cervical nerves. Histopathologically, the skin vessels appear normal until late childhood, at which time they become widely dilated ectatic blood-filled capillaries. The deep dermal and subcutaneous vessels are affected in the more nodular lesions. The nevi do not regress and usually do not respond to local sclerosing agents or steroids.

The pathognomonic feature of the SWS is the CNS angioma of the pia and arachnoid mater (see discussion in Chapter 8). As a result of this angioma, the vascular circulation of the underlying cerebral cortex is often altered, leading to superficial calcification. The majority of patients will have intracranial calcifications on CT. On plain roentgenograms the calcifications appear as double curvilinear densities (tramlines). These cortical abnormalities result in focal or generalized seizures, contralateral hemiplegia, and mental retardation. The lesions can be identified in the first or second decade of life and may increase in size up until the second decade of life, at which point they remain stable.

Ataxia telangiectasia (Louis–Bar syndrome)

Louis–Bar syndrome (LBS) is characterized by progressive cerebellar ataxia, cutaneous and conjunctival telangiectasias, and recurrent sinopulmonary infections. Unlike the other phakomatoses, it appears to be inherited in a recessive fashion, and the genetic defect has been localized to chromosome 11. The conjunctival telangiectasias are similar to those seen in SWS but are bilateral and not associated with lesions of the choroid or the skin.

This phakomatosis is discussed in detail in Chapter 16.

Wyburn–Mason syndrome

Patients with Wyburn–Mason syndrome (WMS) develop retinal, brain, and occasionally facial arteriovenous malformations (AVMs).[527–529] AVMs are direct communications between arteries and veins and involve the CNS, the ocular adnexa, and the nasopharynx. In WMS, AVMs have a predilection for the midbrain. Cerebral AVMs are discussed in detail in Chapter 8, and dural AVMs in Chapter 15.

Retinal AVMs in Wyburn–Mason syndrome are congenital, unilateral malformations that have a predilection for involvement of the vessels of the posterior pole.[530] These lesions appear as arterial and venous dilations with marked tortuosity of a sector of the retinal circulation. Although most retinal AVMs are stable, several complications have been reported, including hemorrhage, vein occlusion, and neovascular glaucoma.[531,532]

References

1. Nipken LH, Schmidt D. Incidence, localization, length and course of the cilioretinal artery. Is there an effect on the course of temporal renal arteries? Klin Monatsbl Augenheilkd 1996;208:229–234.
2. Hood DC, Odel JG, Chen CS, et al. The multifocal electroretinogram. J Neuroophthalmol 2003;23:225–235.
3. Lai TY, Chan WM, Lai RY, et al. The clinical applications of multifocal electroretinography: a systematic review. Surv Ophthalmol 2007;52:61–96.
4. Jampol LM, Weinreb R, Yannuzzi L. Involvement of corticosteroids and catecholamines in the pathogenesis of central serous chorioretinopathy: a rationale for new treatment strategies. Ophthalmology 2002;109:1765–1766.
5. Haimovici R, Koh S, Gagnon DR, et al. Risk factors for central serous chorioretinopathy: a case-control study. Ophthalmology 2004;111:244–249.
6. Ko W. Central serous chorioretinopathy associated with pregnancy. J Ophthalmic Nurs Technol 1992;11:203–205.
7. Schultz KL, Birnbaum AD, Goldstein DA. Ocular disease in pregnancy. Curr Opin Ophthalmol 2005;16:308–314.
8. Sheth BP, Mieler WF. Ocular complications of pregnancy. Curr Opin Ophthalmol 2001;12:455–463.
9. Sunness JS. The pregnant woman's eye. Surv Ophthalmol 1988;32:219–238.
10. Sunness JS, Haller JA, Fine SL. Central serous chorioretinopathy and pregnancy. Arch Ophthalmol 1993;111:360–364.
11. Wynn PA. Idiopathic central serous chorioretinopathy: a physical complication of stress? Occup Med (Lond) 2001;51:139–140.
12. Yannuzzi LA. Type-A behavior and central serous chorioretinopathy. Retina 1987;7:111–131.
13. Tittl MK, Spaide RF, Wong D, et al. Systemic findings associated with central serous chorioretinopathy. Am J Ophthalmol 1999;128:63–68.
14. Bouzas EA, Karadimas P, Pournaras CJ. Central serous chorioretinopathy and glucocorticoids. Surv Ophthalmol 2002;47:431–448.
15. Chung H, Kim KH, Kim JG, et al. Retinal complications in patients with solid organ or bone marrow transplantations. Transplantation 2007;83:694–699.
16. Fawzi AA, Holland GN, Kreiger AE, et al. Central serous chorioretinopathy after solid organ transplantation. Ophthalmology 2006;113:805–813.
17. Moon SJ, Mieler WF. Retinal complications of bone marrow and solid organ transplantation. Curr Opin Ophthalmol 2003;14:433–442.
18. Bresnick GH, Condit R, Syrjala S, et al. Abnormalities of the foveal avascular zone in diabetic retinopathy. Arch Ophthalmol 1984;102:1286–1293.
19. Fortune B, Schneck ME, Adams AJ. Multifocal electroretinogram delays reveal local retinal dysfunction in early diabetic retinopathy. Invest Oph Vis Sci 1999;40:2638–2651.

20. Tzekov R, Arden GB. The electroretinogram in diabetic retinopathy. Surv Ophthalmol 1999;44:53–60.

21. Turbeville SD, Cowan LD, Gass JD. Acute macular neuroretinopathy: a review of the literature. Surv Ophthalmol 2003;48:1–11.

22. Feigl B, Haas A. Optical coherence tomography (OCT) in acute macular neuroretinopathy. Acta Ophthalmol Scand 2000;78:714–716.

23. Monson BK, Greenberg PB, Greenberg E, et al. High-speed, ultra-high-resolution optical coherence tomography of acute macular neuroretinopathy. Br J Ophthalmol 2007;91:119–120.

24. Shukla D, Arora A, Ambatkar S, et al. Optical coherence tomography findings in acute macular neuroretinopathy. Eye 2005;19:107–108.

25. Arruga J, Sanders MD. Ophthalmologic findings in 70 patients with evidence of retinal embolism. Ophthalmology 1982;89:1336–1347.

26. Howard RS, Russell RW. Prognosis of patients with retinal embolism. J Neurol Neurosurg Psychiatry 1987;50:1142–1147.

27. Sharma S, Pater JL, Lam M, et al. Can different types of retinal emboli be reliably differentiated from one another? An inter- and intraobserver agreement study. Can J Ophthalmol 1998;33:144–148.

28. Younge BR. The significance of retinal emboli. J Clin Neuroophthalmol 1989;9: 190–194.

29. Hollenhorst RW. Significance of bright plaques in the retinal arterioles. JAMA 1961;178:23–29.

30. Ramakrishna G, Malouf JF, Younge BR, et al. Calcific retinal embolism as an indicator of severe unrecognised cardiovascular disease. Heart 2005;91:1154–1157.

31. Cugati S, Wang JJ, Rochtchina E, et al. Ten-year incidence of retinal emboli in an older population. Stroke 2006;37:908–910.

32. Hoki SL, Varma R, Lai MY, et al. Prevalence and associations of asymptomatic retinal emboli in Latinos: The Los Angeles Latino Eye Study (LALES). Am J Ophthalmol 2008;145:143–148.

33. Klein R, Klein BE, Jensen SC, et al. Retinal emboli and stroke. The Beaver Dam Eye Study. Arch Ophthalmol 1999;117:1063–1068.

34. Klein R, Klein BE, Moss SE, et al. Retinal emboli and cardiovascular disease: the Beaver Dam Eye Study. Arch Ophthalmol 2003;121:1446–1451.

35. Mitchell P, Wang JJ, Li W, et al. Prevalence of asymptomatic retinal emboli in an Australian urban community. Stroke 1997;28:63–66.

36. Wang JJ, Cugati S, Knudtson MD, et al. Retinal arteriolar emboli and long-term mortality: pooled data analysis from two older populations. Stroke 2006;37:1833–1836.

37. Bruno A, Russell PW, Jones WL, et al. Concomitants of asymptomatic retinal cholesterol emboli. Stroke 1992;23:900–902.

38. Wong TY, Larsen EKM, Klein R, et al. Cardiovascular risk factors for retinal vein occlusion and arteriolar emboli. The Atherosclerosis Risk in Communities & Cardiovascular Health Studies. Ophthalmology 2005;112:540–547.

39. O'Donnell BA, Mitchell P. The clinical features and associations of retinal emboli. Aust N Z J Ophthalmol 1992;20:11–17.

40. Babikian V, Wijman CA, Koleini B, et al. Retinal ischemia and embolism. Etiologies and outcomes based on a prospective study. Cerebrovasc Dis 2001;12:108–113.

41. Sharma S, Brown GC, Pater JL, et al. Does a visible retinal embolus increase the likelihood of hemodynamically significant carotid artery stenosis in patients with acute retinal arterial occlusion? Arch Ophthalmol 1998;116:1602–1606.

42. Executive Committee for the Asymptomatic Carotid Atherosclerosis Study. Endarterectomy for asymptomatic carotid artery stenosis. JAMA 1995;273:1421–1428.

43. Sharma S, Brown GC, Cruess AF. Accuracy of visible retinal emboli for the detection of cardioembolic lesions requiring anticoagulation or cardiac surgery. Retinal Emboli of Cardiac Origin Study Group. Br J Ophthalmol 1998;82:655–658.

44. Mouradian M, Wijman CA, Tomasian D, et al. Echocardiographic findings of patients with retinal ischemia or embolism. J Neuroimaging 2002;12:219–223.

45. Kramer M, Goldenberg-Cohen N, Shapira Y, et al. Role of transesophageal echocardiography in the evaluation of patients with retinal artery occlusion. Ophthalmology 2001;108:1461–1464.

46. Pfaffenbach DD, Hollenhorst RW. Morbidity and survivorship of patients with emboli crystals in the ocular fundus. Am J Ophthalmol 1973;75:66–72.

47. Savino PJ, Glaser JS, Cassidy J. Retinal stroke: is the patient at risk? Arch Ophthalmol 1977;95:1185–1189.

48. Wong TY, Klein R. Retinal arteriolar emboli: epidemiology and risk of stroke. Curr Opin Ophthalmol 2002;13:142–146.

49. Klein R, Klein BE, Moss SE, et al. Retinal emboli and cardiovascular disease: the Beaver Dam Eye Study. Trans Am Ophthalmol Soc 2003;101:173–180; discussion 180–172.

50. Bruno A, Jones WL, Austin JK, et al. Vascular outcome in men with asymptomatic retinal cholesterol emboli. A cohort study. Ann Intern Med 1995;122:249–253.

51. Grosberg BM, Solomon S, Friedman DI, et al. Retinal migraine reappraised. Cephalalgia 2006;26:1275–1286.

52. Hill DL, Daroff RB, Ducros A, et al. Most cases labeled as "retinal migraine" are not migraine. J Neuroophthalmol 2007;27:3–8.

53. Hoya K, Morikawa E, Tamura A, et al. Common carotid artery stenosis and amaurosis fugax. J Stroke Cerebrovasc Dis 2008;17:1–4.

54. De Schryver EL, Algra A, Donders RC, et al. Type of stroke after transient monocular blindness or retinal infarction of presumed arterial origin. J Neurol Neurosurg Psychiatry 2006;77:734–738.

55. Suvajac G, Stojanovich L, Milenkovich S. Ocular manifestations in antiphospholipid syndrome. Autoimmun Rev 2007;6:409–414.

56. Campos LM, Kiss MH, D'Amico EA, et al. Antiphospholipid antibodies and antiphospholipid syndrome in 57 children and adolescents with systemic lupus erythematosus. Lupus 2003;12:820–826.

57. Glueck CJ, Goldenberg N, Bell H, et al. Amaurosis fugax: associations with heritable thrombophilia. Clin Appl Thromb Hemost 2005;11:235–241.

58. Brown GC, Magargal LE. Central retinal artery obstruction and visual acuity. Ophthalmology 1982;89:14–19.

59. Ros MA, Magargal LE, Uram M. Branch retinal-artery obstruction: a review of 201 eyes. Ann Ophthalmol 1989;21:103–107.

60. Glueck CJ, Wang P, Hutchins R, et al. Ocular vascular thrombotic events: central retinal vein and central retinal artery occlusions. Clin Appl Thromb Hemost 2008;14:286–294.

61. Merchut MP, Gupta SR, Naheedy MH. The relation of retinal artery occlusion and carotid artery stenosis. Stroke 1988;19:1239–1242.

62. Hayreh SS, Zimmerman MB. Fundus changes in central retinal artery occlusion. Retina 2007;27:276–289.

63. Falkenberry SM, Ip MS, Blodi BA, et al. Optical coherence tomography findings in central retinal artery occlusion. Ophthalmic Surg Lasers Imaging 2006;37:502–505.

64. Ozdemir H, Karacorlu S, Karacorlu M. Optical coherence tomography findings in central retinal artery occlusion. Retina 2006;26:110–112.

65. Atebara NH, Brown GC, Cater J. Efficacy of anterior chamber paracentesis and carbogen in treating acute nonarteritic central retinal artery occlusion. Ophthalmology 1995;102:2029–2034.

66. Hayreh SS, Zimmerman MB. Central retinal artery occlusion: visual outcome. Am J Ophthalmol 2005;140:376–391.

67. Duker JS, Sivalingam A, Brown GC, et al. A prospective study of acute central retinal artery obstruction. The incidence of secondary ocular neovascularization. Arch Ophthalmol 1991;109:339–342.

68. Schmidt D, Schumacher M, Wakhloo AK. Microcatheter urokinase infusion in central retinal artery occlusion. Am J Ophthalmol 1992;113:429–434.

69. Biousse V, Calvetti O, Bruce BB, et al. Thrombolysis for central retinal artery occlusion. J Neuroophthalmol 2007;27:215–230.

70. Feltgen N, Neubauer A, Jurklies B, et al. Multicenter study of the European Assessment Group for Lysis in the Eye (EAGLE) for the treatment of central retinal artery occlusion: design issues and implications. EAGLE Study report no. 1. Graefes Arch Clin Exp Ophthalmol 2006;244:950–956.

71. Arnold M, Koerner U, Remonda L, et al. Comparison of intra-arterial thrombolysis with conventional treatment in patients with acute central retinal artery occlusion. J Neurol Neurosurg Psychiatry 2005;76:196–199.

72. Suri MF, Nasar A, Hussein HM, et al. Intra-arterial thrombolysis for central retinal artery occlusion in United States: Nationwide In-patient Survey 2001–2003. J Neuroimaging 2007;17:339–343.

73. Hayreh SS, Zimmerman MB, Kimura A, et al. Central retinal artery occlusion. Retinal survival time. Exp Eye Res 2004;78:723–736.

74. Yuzurihara D, Iijima H. Visual outcome in central retinal and branch retinal artery occlusion. Jpn J Ophthalmol 2004;48:490–492.

75. McDonough RL, Forteza AM, Flynn HW, Jr. Internal carotid artery dissection causing a branch retinal artery occlusion in a young adult. Am J Ophthalmol 1998;125:706–708.

76. Greven CM, Weaver RG, Owen J, et al. Protein S deficiency and bilateral branch retinal artery occlusion. Ophthalmology 1991;98:33–34.

77. Gross M, Eliashar R. Update on Susac's syndrome. Curr Opin Neurol 2005;18:311–314.

78. Susac JO, Calabrese LH, Baylin E, et al. Branch retinal artery occlusions as the presenting feature of primary central nervous system vasculitis. Clin Exp Rheumatol 2004;22:S70–74.

79. Susac JO, Egan RA, Rennebohm RM, et al. Susac's syndrome: 1975–2005 microangiopathy/autoimmune endotheliopathy. J Neurol Sci 2007;257:270–272.

80. Fineman MS, Savino PJ, Federman JL, et al. Branch retinal artery occlusion as the initial sign of giant cell arteritis. Am J Ophthalmol 1996;122:428–430.

81. Crofts JW, Nussbaum JJ, Levine SR, et al. Retinitis pigmentosa and branch retinal artery occlusion with anticardiolipin antibody. Case report. Arch Ophthalmol 1989;107:324.

82. Levine SR, Crofts JW, Lesser GR, et al. Visual symptoms associated with the presence of a lupus anticoagulant. Ophthalmology 1988;95:686–692.

83. De Potter P, Zografos L. Survival prognosis of patients with retinal artery occlusion and associated carotid artery disease. Graefes Arch Clin Exp Ophthalmol 1993;231:212–216.

84. Brown GC, Moffat K, Cruess A, et al. Cilioretinal artery obstruction. Retina 1983;3: 182–187.

85. Gangwar DN, Grewal SP, Jain IS, et al. Cilioretinal artery occlusion: a case report. Ann Ophthalmol 1984;16:1022–1024.

86. Horton JC. Embolic cilioretinal artery occlusion with atherosclerosis of the ipsilateral carotid artery. Retina 1995;15:441–444.

87. el Asrar AM, Naddaf HO, al Momen AK, et al. Systemic lupus erythematosus flare-up manifesting as a cilioretinal artery occlusion. Lupus 1995;4:158–160.

88. Hayreh SS, Podhajsky PA, Zimmerman B. Ocular manifestations of giant cell arteritis. Am J Ophthalmol 1998;125:509–520.

89. Hwang JF, Chen SN, Chiu SL, et al. Embolic cilioretinal artery occlusion due to carotid artery dissection. Am J Ophthalmol 2004;138:496–498.

90. Carrero JL, Sanjurjo FJ. Bilateral cilioretinal artery occlusion in antiphospholipid syndrome. Retina 2006;26:104–106.

91. Dori D, Gelfand YA, Brenner B, et al. Cilioretinal artery occlusion: an ocular complication of primary antiphospholipid syndrome. Retina 1997;17:555–557.

92. Kunikata H, Tamai M. Cilioretinal artery occlusions following embolization of an artery to an intracranial meningioma. Graefes Arch Clin Exp Ophthalmol 2006;244:401–403.

93. Ahmadieh H, Javadi MA. Cilioretinal artery occlusion following laser in situ keratomileusis. Retina 2005;25:533–537.

94. Kachmaryk MM, Trimble SN, Gieser RG. Cilioretinal artery occlusion in sickle cell trait and rheumatoid arthritis. Retina 1995;15:501–504.

95. Noble KG. Central retinal vein occlusion and cilioretinal artery infarction. Am J Ophthalmol 1994;118:811–813.

96. Schatz H, Fong AC, McDonald HR, et al. Cilioretinal artery occlusion in young adults with central retinal vein occlusion. Ophthalmology 1991;98:594–601.

97. Brown GC, Magargal LE. The ocular ischemic syndrome. Clinical, fluorescein angiographic and carotid angiographic features. Int Ophthalmol 1988;11:239–251.

98. Costa VP, Kuzniec S, Molnar LJ, et al. Clinical findings and hemodynamic changes associated with severe occlusive carotid artery disease. Ophthalmology 1997;104:1994–2002.

99. Mizener JB, Podhajsky P, Hayreh SS. Ocular ischemic syndrome. Ophthalmology 1997;104:859–864.

100. Baumgartner RW, Bogousslavsky J. Clinical manifestations of carotid dissection. Front Neurol Neurosci 2005;20:70–76.

101. Shah Q, Messe SR. Cervicocranial arterial dissection. Curr Treat Options Neurol 2007;9:55–62.

102. Takaki Y, Nagata M, Shinoda K, et al. Severe acute ocular ischemia associated with spontaneous internal carotid artery dissection. Int Ophthalmol 2008;28:447–449.

103. Casson RJ, Fleming FK, Shaikh A, et al. Bilateral ocular ischemic syndrome secondary to giant cell arteritis. Arch Ophthalmol 2001;119:306–307.

104. Koz OG, Ates A, Numan Alp M, et al. Bilateral ocular ischemic syndrome as an initial manifestation of Takayasu's arteritis associated with carotid steal syndrome. Rheumatol Int 2007;27:299–302.

105. Schmidt D. Ocular ichemia syndrome: a malignant course of giant cell arteritis. Eur J Med Res 2005;10:233–242.

106. Worrall M, Atebara N, Meredith T, et al. Bilateral ocular ischemic syndrome in Takayasu disease. Retina 2001;21:75–76.

107. Mitchell P, Wang JJ, Wong TY, et al. Retinal microvascular signs and risk of stroke and stroke mortality. Neurology 2005;65:1005–1009.

108. Kwa VI, van der Sande JJ, Stam J, et al. Retinal arterial changes correlate with cerebral small-vessel disease. Neurology 2002;59:1536–1540.

109. Wong TY, Klein R, Couper DJ, et al. Retinal microvascular abnormalities and incident stroke: the Atherosclerosis Risk in Communities Study. Lancet 2001;358:1134–1140.

110. Ikram MK, de Jong FJ, Bos MJ, et al. Retinal vessel diameters and risk of stroke: the Rotterdam Study. Neurology 2006;66:1339–1343.

111. Rose KM, Wong TY, Carson AP, et al. Migraine and retinal microvascular abnormalities. The Atherosclerosis Risk in Communities Study. Neurology 2007;68:1694–1700.

112. David R, Zangwill L, Badarna M, et al. Epidemiology of retinal vein occlusion and its association with glaucoma and increased intraocular pressure. Ophthalmologica 1988;197:69–74.

113. Cugati S, Wang JJ, Rochtchina E, et al. Ten-year incidence of retinal vein occlusion in an older population: the Blue Mountains Eye Study. Arch Ophthalmol 2006;124:726–732.

114. Beaumont PE, Kang HK. Pattern of vascular nonperfusion in retinal venous occlusions occurring within the optic nerve with and without optic nerve head swelling. Arch Ophthalmol 2000;118:1357–1363.

115. Green WR, Chan CC, Hutchins GM, et al. Central retinal vein occlusion: a prospective histopathologic study of 29 eyes in 28 cases. Trans Am Ophthalmol Soc 1981;79:371–422.

116. Rath EZ, Frank RN, Shin DH, et al. Risk factors for retinal vein occlusions. A case-control study. Ophthalmology 1992;99:509–514.

117. Dodson PM, Galton DJ, Hamilton AM, et al. Retinal vein occlusion and the prevalence of lipoprotein abnormalities. Br J Ophthalmol 1982;66:161–164.

118. Matsushima C, Wakabayashi Y, Iwamoto T, et al. Relationship between retinal vein occlusion and carotid artery lesions. Retina 2007;27:1038–1043.

119. Quinlan PM, Elman MJ, Bhatt AK, et al. The natural course of central retinal vein occlusion [see comments]. Am J Ophthalmol 1990;110:118–123.

120. Zegarra H, Gutman FA, Zakov N, et al. Partial occlusion of the central retinal vein. Am J Ophthalmol 1983;96:330–337.

121. Hasselbach HC, Ruefer F, Feltgen N, et al. Treatment of central retinal vein occlusion by radial optic neurotomy in 107 cases. Graefes Arch Clin Exp Ophthalmol 2007;245:1145–1156.

122. Frangieh GT, Green WR, Barraquer Somers E, et al. Histopathologic study of nine branch retinal vein occlusions. Arch Ophthalmol 1982;100:1132–1140.

123. Johnston RL, Brucker AJ, Steinmann W, et al. Risk factors of branch retinal vein occlusion. Arch Ophthalmol 1985;103:1831–1832.

124. Finkelstein D. Argon laser photocoagulation for macular edema in branch vein occlusion. Ophthalmology 1986;93:975–977.

125. Branch Vein Occlusion Study Group. Argon laser scatter photocoagulation for prevention of neovascularization and vitreous hemorrhage in branch vein occlusion. A randomized clinical trial. Arch Ophthalmol 1986;104:34–41.

126. Hayreh SS, Rojas P, Podhajsky P, et al. Ocular neovascularization with retinal vascular occlusion. III. Incidence of ocular neovascularization with retinal vein occlusion. Ophthalmology 1983;90:488–506.

127. Rizzo JF, Volpe NJ. Cancer-associated retinopathy. In: Pepose JS, Holland G, Wilheimus K (eds): Ocular Infection and Immunity, pp 585–599. St. Louis, Mosby-Year Book, 1996.

128. Chan JW. Paraneoplastic retinopathies and optic neuropathies. Surv Ophthalmol 2003;48:12–38.

129. Volpe NJ, Rizzo JF. Retinal disease in neuro-ophthalmology: paraneoplastic retinopathy and the big blindspot syndrome. Semin Ophthalmol 1995;10:234–241.

130. Sawyer RA, Selhorst JB, Zimmerman LE, et al. Blindness caused by photoreceptor degeneration as a remote effect of cancer. Am J Ophthalmol 1976;81:606–613.

131. Jacobson DM, Thirkill CE, Tipping SJ. A clinical triad to diagnose paraneoplastic retinopathy. Ann Neurol 1990;28:162–167.

132. Cogan DG, Kuwabara T, Currie J, et al. Paraneoplastic retinopathy simulating cone dystrophy with achromatopsia. Klin Monatsbl Augenheilkd 1990;197:156–158.

133. Hammerstein W, Jurgens H, Gobel U. Retinal degeneration and embryonal rhabdomyosarcoma of the thorax. Fortschr Ophthalmol 1991;88:463–465.

134. Matsui Y, Mehta MC, Katsumi O, et al. Electrophysiological findings in paraneoplastic retinopathy. Graefes Arch Clin Exp Oph 1992;230:324–328.

135. Rizzo JF, Gittinger JW. Selective immunohistochemical staining in the paraneoplastic retinopathy syndrome. Ophthalmology 1992;99:1286–1295.

136. Rush JA. Paraneoplastic retinopathy in malignant melanoma. Am J Ophthalmol 1993;115:390–391.

137. Chung SM, Selhorst JB. Cancer-associated retinopathy. Ophthal Clin N A 1992;5:587–596.

138. Adamus G, Guy J, Schmied JL, et al. Role of anti-recoverin autoantibodies in cancer-associated retinopathy. Invest Ophthalmol Vis Sci 1993;34:2626–2633.

139. Campo E, Brunier MN, Merino MJ. Small cell carcinoma of the endometrium with associated ocular paraneoplastic syndrome. Cancer 1992;69:2283–2288.

140. Keltner JL, Roth AM, Chang RS. Photoreceptor degeneration: possible autoimmune disorder. Arch Ophthalmol 1983;101:564–569.

141. Ohnishi Y, Ohara S, Sakamoto T, et al. Cancer-associated retinopathy with retinal phlebitis. Br J Ophthalmol 1993;77:795–798.

142. Thirkill CE, Roth AM, Keltner JL. Cancer-associated retinopathy. Arch Ophthalmol 1987;105:372–375.

143. Adamus G, Amundson D, Seigel GM, et al. Anti-enolase-alpha autoantibodies in cancer-associated retinopathy: epitope mapping and cytotoxicity on retinal cells. J Autoimmun 1998;11:671–677.

144. Dot C, Guigay J, Adamus G. Anti-alpha-enolase antibodies in cancer-associated retinopathy with small cell carcinoma of the lung. Am J Ophthalmol 2005;139:746–747.

145. Ejma M, Misiuk-Hojlo M, Gorczyca WA, et al. Antibodies to 46-kDa retinal antigen in a patient with breast carcinoma and cancer-associated retinopathy. Breast Cancer Res Treat 2008;110:269–271.

146. Ohguro H, Ogawa K, Nakagawa T. Recoverin and Hsc 70 are found as autoantigens in patients with cancer-associated retinopathy. Invest Ophthalmol Vis Sci 1999;40:82–89.

147. Eichen JG, Dalmau J, Demopoulos A, et al. The photoreceptor cell-specific nuclear receptor is an autoantigen of paraneoplastic retinopathy. J Neuroophthalmol 2001;21:168–172.

148. Kornguth SE, Kalinke T, Grunwald GB, et al. Anti-neurofilament antibodies in the sera of patients with small cell carcinoma of the lung and with visual paraneoplastic syndrome. Cancer Res 1986;46:2588–2595.

149. Jacobson DM, Thirkill CE. Paraneoplastic cone dysfunction: an unusual visual remote effect of cancer [letter]. Arch Ophthalmol 1995;113:1580–1582.

150. Milam AH, Saari JC, Jacobson SG, et al. Autoantibodies against retinal bipolar cells in cutaneous melanoma-associated retinopathy. Invest Ophthalmol Vis Sci 1993;34:91–100.

151. Ohguro H, Maruyama I, Nakazawa M, et al. Antirecoverin antibody in the aqueous humor of a patient with cancer-associated retinopathy. Am J Ophthalmol 2002;134:605–607.

152. Ohguro H, Yokoi Y, Ohguro I, et al. Clinical and immunologic aspects of cancer-associated retinopathy. Am J Ophthalmol 2004;137:1117–1119.

153. Bazhin AV, Shifrina ON, Savchenko MS, et al. Low titre autoantibodies against recoverin in sera of patients with small cell lung cancer but without a loss of vision. Lung Cancer 2001;34:99–104.

154. Adamus G. Autoantibody-induced apoptosis as a possible mechanism of autoimmune retinopathy. Autoimmun Rev 2003;2:63–68.

155. Polans AS, Burton MD, Haley TL, et al. Recoverin, but not visinin, is an autoantigen in the human retina identified with a cancer-associated retinopathy. Invest Ophthalmol Vis Sci 1993;34:81–90.

156. Thirkill CE, Tait RC, Tyler NK, et al. The cancer-associated retinopathy antigen is a recoverin-like protein. Invest Ophthalmol Vis Sci 1992;33:2768–2772.

157. Parc CE, Azan E, Bonnel S, et al. Cone dysfunction as a paraneoplastic syndrome associated with retinal antigens approximating 40 kiloDalton. Ophthalmic Genet 2006;27:57–61.

158. Berson EL, Lessell S. Paraneoplastic night blindness with malignant melanoma. Am J Ophthalmol 1988;106:307–311.

159. Borkowski LM, Grover S, Fishman GA, et al. Retinal findings in melanoma-associated retinopathy. Am J Ophthalmol 2001;132:273–275.

160. Keltner JL, Thirkill CE, Yip PT. Clinical and immunologic characteristics of melanoma-associated retinopathy syndrome: eleven new cases and a review of 51 previously published cases. J Neuroophthalmol 2001;21:173–187.

161. Pfohler C, Haus A, Palmowski A, et al. Melanoma-associated retinopathy: high frequency of subclinical findings in patients with melanoma. Br J Dermatol 2003;149:74–78.

162. Singh AD, Milam AH, Shields CL, et al. Melanoma associated retinopathy. Am J Ophthalmol 1995;119:369–370.

163. Alexander KR, Fishman GA, Peachy NS, et al. "On" response defect in paraneoplastic night blindness with cutaneous malignant melanoma. Invest Ophthalmol Vis Sci 1992;33:477–483.

164. Andreasson S, Ponjavic V, Ehinger B. Full-field electroretinogram in a patient with cutaneous melanoma-associated retinopathy. Acta Ophthalmol 1993;71:487–490.

165. Potter MJ, Thirkill CE, Dam OM, et al. Clinical and immunocytochemical findings in a case of melanoma-associated retinopathy. Ophthalmology 1999;106:2121–2125.

166. Ladewig G, Reinhold U, Thirkill CE, et al. Incidence of antiretinal antibodies in melanoma: screening of 77 serum samples from 51 patients with American Joint Committee on Cancer stage I-IV. Br J Dermatol 2005;152:931–938.

167. Borruat FX, Othenin-Girard P, Uffer S, et al. Natural history of diffuse uveal melanocytic proliferation. Ophthalmology 1992;99:1698–1704.

168. Leys AM, Dierick HG. RMS: early lesions of bilateral diffuse melanocytic proliferation. Arch Ophthalmol 1991;109:1590–1594.

169. Margo CE, Pavan PR, Gendelman D, et al. Bilateral melanocytic uveal tumors associated with systemic nonocular malignancy: malignant melanomas or benign paraneoplastic syndrome. Retina 1987;7:137–141.

170. Ryll DL, Campbell RJ, Robertson DM, et al. Pseudometastatic lesions of the choroid. Ophthalmology 1980;87:1181–1186.

171. Grunwald GB, Kornguth SE, Towfighi J, et al. Autoimmune basis for visual paraneoplastic syndrome in patients with small cell lung carcinoma. Retinal immune deposits and ablation of retinal ganglion cells. Cancer 1987;60:780–786.

172. Oohira A, Tamaki Y, Nagahara K, et al. A case of paraneoplastic retinopathy. Jpn J Ophthalmol 1993;37:28–31.

173. Klingele TG, Burde RM, Rappazzo JA, et al. Paraneoplastic retinopathy. J Clin Neuroophthalmol 1984;4:239–245.

174. Crofts JW, Bachynski BN, Odel JG. Visual paraneoplastic syndrome associated with undifferentiated endometrial carcinoma. Can J Ophthalmol 1988;23:128–132.

175. Yamada G, Ohguro H, Aketa K, et al. Invasive thymoma with paraneoplastic retinopathy. Hum Pathol 2003;34:717–719.

176. Alexander KR, Barnes CS, Fishman GA, et al. Nature of the cone ON-pathway dysfunction in melanoma-associated retinopathy. Invest Ophthalmol Vis Sci 2002;43:1189–1197.

177. Boghen D, Sebag M, Michaud J. Paraneoplastic optic neuritis and encephalomyelitis. Report of a case. Arch Neurol 1988;45:353–356.

178. Malik S, Furlan AJ, Sweeney PJ, et al. Optic neuropathy: a rare paraneoplastic syndrome. J Clin Neuroophthalmol 1992;12:137–141.

179. Pillay N, Gilbert JJ, Ebers GC, et al. Internuclear ophthalmoplegia and "optic neuritis": paraneoplastic effects of bronchial carcinoma. Neurology 1984;34:788–791.

180. Waterston JA, Gilligan BS. Paraneoplastic optic neuritis and external ophthalmoplegia. Aust NZ J Med 1986;16:703–704.

181. Keltner JL, Thirkill CE, Tyler NK, et al. Management and monitoring of cancer-associated retinopathy. Arch Ophthalmol 1992;110:48–53.

182. Thirkill CE, Fitzgerald P, Sergott RC, et al. Cancer-associated retinopathy (CAR syndrome) with antibodies reacting with retinal, optic-nerve, and cancer cells. N Engl J Med 1989;321:1589–1594.

183. Espandar L, O'Brien S, Thirkill C, et al. Successful treatment of cancer-associated retinopathy with alemtuzumab. J Neurooncol 2007;83:295–302.

184. Callanan D, Gass JD. Multifocal choroiditis and choroidal neovascularization associated with the multiple evanescent white dot and acute idiopathic blind spot enlargement syndrome. Ophthalmology 1992;99:1678–1685.

185. Fletcher WA, Imes RK, Goodman D, et al. Acute idiopathic blindspot enlargement. A big blindspot syndrome without optic disc edema. Arch Ophthalmol 1988;106:44–49.

186. Gass JDM, Hamed LM. Acute macular neuroretinopathy and multiple evanescent white dot syndrome occurring in the same patients. Arch Ophthalmol 1989;107:189–193.

187. Volpe NJ, Rizzo JF, Lessell S. Acute idiopathic blindspot enlargement syndrome: a report of 27 new cases. Arch Ophthalmol 2001;119:59–63.

188. Gass JD, Agarwal A, Scott IU. Acute zonal occult outer retinopathy: a long-term follow-up study. Am J Ophthalmol 2002;134:329–339.

189. Machida S, Haga-Sano M, Ishibe T, et al. Decrease of blue cone sensitivity in acute idiopathic blind spot enlargement syndrome. Am J Ophthalmol 2004;138:296–299.

190. Khorram KD, Jampol LM, Rosenberg MA. Blind spot enlargement as a manifestation of multifocal choroiditis. Arch Ophthalmol 1991;109:1403–1407.

191. Singh K, deFrank MP, Shults WT, et al. Acute idiopathic blind spot enlargement. A spectrum of disease. Ophthalmology 1991;98:497–502.

192. Kondo N, Kondo M, Miyake Y. Acute idiopathic blind spot enlargement syndrome: prolonged retinal dysfunction revealed by multifocal electroretinogram technique. Am J Ophthalmol 2001;132:126–128.

193. Watzke RC, Shults WT. Clinical features and natural history of the acute idiopathic enlarged blind spot syndrome. Ophthalmology 2002;109:1326–1335.

194. Jampol LM, Sieving PA, Pugh D, et al. Multiple evanescent white dot syndrome. I. Clinical findings. Arch Ophthalmol 1984;102:671–674.

195. Takeda M, Kimura S, Tamiya M. Acute disseminated retinal pigment epitheliopathy. Folia Ophthalmol Japan 1984;35:2613–2620.

196. Aaberg TM, Campo RV, Joffe L. Recurrences and bilaterality in the multiple evanescent white-dot syndrome. Am J Ophthalmol 1985;100:29–37.

197. Hamed LM, Glaser JS, Gass JDM, et al. Protracted enlargement of the blind spot in the multiple evanescent white dot syndrome. Arch Ophthalmol 1989;107:194–198.

198. Leys A, Leys M, Jonckheere P, et al. Multiple evanescent white dot syndrome (MEWDS). Bull Soc Belge Ophtalmol 1990;236:97–108.

199. Nakao K, Isashiki M. Multiple evanescent white dot syndrome. Jpn J Ophthalmol 1986;30:376–384.

200. Borruat FX, Othenin Girard P, Safran AB. Multiple evanescent white dot syndrome. Klin Monatsbl Augenheilkd 1991;198:453–456.

201. Jacobson SG, Morales DS, Sun XK, et al. Pattern of retinal dysfunction in acute zonal occult outer retinopathy. Ophthalmology 1995;102:1187–1198.

202. Dodwell DG, Jampol LM, Rosenberg M, et al. Optic nerve involvement associated with the multiple evanescent white-dot syndrome. Ophthalmology 1990;97:862–868.

203. Chung YM, Yeh TS, Liu JH. Increased serum IgM and IgG in the multiple evanescent white dot syndrome. Am J Ophthalmol 1987;104:187–188.

204. Gass JDM, Stern C. Acute annular outer retinopathy as a variant of acute zonal occult outer retinopathy. Am J Ophthalmol 1995;119:330–334.

205. Luckie A, Ai E, Piero ED. Progressive zonal outer retinitis. Am J Ophthalmol 1994;118:583–588.

206. Gass JD. Are acute zonal occult outer retinopathy and the white spot syndromes (AZOOR complex) specific autoimmune diseases? Am J Ophthalmol 2003;135:380–381.

207. Jampol LM, Becker KG. White spot syndromes of the retina: a hypothesis based on the common genetic hypothesis of autoimmune/inflammatory disease. Am J Ophthalmol 2003;135:376–379.

208. Gass JD. Acute zonal occult outer retinopathy. Donders Lecture: The Netherlands Ophthalmological Society, Maastricht, Holland, June 19, 1992. J Clin Neuroophthalmol 1993;13:79–97.

209. Jacobson DM. Acute zonal occult outer retinopathy and central nervous system inflammation. J Neuroophthalmol 1996;16:172–177.

210. Francis PJ, Marinescu A, Fitzke FW, et al. Acute zonal occult outer retinopathy: towards a set of diagnostic criteria. Br J Ophthalmol 2005;89:70–73.

211. Closson RG. Visual hallucinations as the earliest symptom of digoxin intoxication. Arch Neurol 1983;40:386.

212. Johnson LN. Digoxin toxicity presenting with visual disturbance and trigeminal neuralgia. Neurology 1990;40:1469–1470.

213. Piltz JR, Wertenbaker C, Lance SE, et al. Digoxin toxicity. Recognizing the varied visual presentations. J Clin Neuroophthalmol 1993;13:275–280.

214. Weleber RG, Shults WT. Digoxin retinal toxicity. Clinical and electrophysiological evaluation of a cone dysfunction syndrome. Arch Ophthalmol 1981;99:1568–1572.

215. Chuman MA, LeSage J. Color vision deficiencies in two cases of digoxin toxicity. Am J Ophthalmol 1985;100:682–685.

216. Wolin MJ. Digoxin visual toxicity with therapeutic blood levels of digoxin. Am J Ophthalmol 1998;125:406–407.

217. Ah Song R, Sasco AJ. Tamoxifen and ocular toxicity. Cancer Detect Prev 1997;21:522–531.

218. Heier JS, Dragoo RA, Enzenauer RW, et al. Screening for ocular toxicity in asymptomatic patients treated with tamoxifen. Am J Ophthalmol 1994;117:772–775.

219. Kaiser Kupfer MI, Kupfer C, Rodrigues MM. Tamoxifen retinopathy. A clinicopathologic report. Ophthalmology 1981;88:89–93.

220. Lee AG. Tamoxifen retinopathy. J Neuroophthalmol 1998;18:276.

221. Espaillat A, Aiello LP, Arrigg PG, et al. Canthaxanthine retinopathy. Arch Ophthalmol 1999;117:412–413.

222. Sharkey JA. Idiopathic canthaxanthine retinopathy. Eur J Ophthalmol 1993;3:226–228.

223. Novak MA, Roth AS, Levine MR. Calcium oxalate retinopathy associated with methoxyflurane abuse. Retina 1988;8:230–236.

224. Denman S, Weleber R, Hanifin JM, et al. Abnormal night vision and altered dark adaptometry in patients treated with isotretinoin for acne [letter]. J Am Acad Dermatol 1986;14:692–693.

225. Lerman S. Ocular side effects of accutane therapy. Lens Eye Toxic Res 1992;9:429–438.

226. Maclean H, Wright M, Choi D, et al. Abnormal night vision with isotretinoin therapy for acne [letter]. Clin Exp Dermatol 1995;20:86.

227. Weleber RG, Denman ST, Hanifin JM, et al. Abnormal retinal function associated with isotretinoin therapy for acne. Arch Ophthalmol 1986;104:831–837.

228. Block JA. Hydroxychloroquine and retinal safety. Lancet 1998;351:771.

229. Easterbrook M. Chloroquine retinopathy. Arch Ophthalmol 1991;109:1362.

230. Finbloom DS, Silver K, Newsome DA, et al. Comparison of hydroxychloroquine and chloroquine use and the development of retinal toxicity. J Rheumatol 1985;12:692–694.

231. Levy GD, Munz SJ, Paschal J, et al. Incidence of hydroxychloroquine retinopathy in 1,207 patients in a large multicenter outpatient practice. Arthritis Rheum 1997;40:1482–1486.

232. Mavrikakis M, Papazoglou S, Sfikakis PP, et al. Retinal toxicity in long term hydroxychloroquine treatment. Ann Rheum Dis 1996;55:187–189.

233. Mazzuca SA, Yung R, Brandt KD, et al. Current practices for monitoring ocular toxicity related to hydroxychloroquine (Plaquenil) therapy. J Rheumatol 1994;21:59–63.

234. Spalton DJ, Verdon Roe GM, Hughes GR. Hydroxychloroquine, dosage parameters and retinopathy. Lupus 1993;2:355–358.

235. Weiner A, Sandberg MA, Gaudio AR, et al. Hydroxychloroquine retinopathy. Am J Ophthalmol 1991;112:528–534.

236. Lyons JS, Severns ML. Detection of early hydroxychloroquine retinal toxicity enhanced by ring ratio analysis of multifocal electroretinography. Am J Ophthalmol 2007;143:801–809.

237. Rodriguez-Padilla JA, Hedges TR, 3rd, Monson B, et al. High-speed ultra-high-resolution optical coherence tomography findings in hydroxychloroquine retinopathy. Arch Ophthalmol 2007;125:775–780.

238. Maturi RK, Yu M, Weleber RG. Multifocal electroretinographic evaluation of long-term hydroxychloroquine users. Arch Ophthalmol 2004;122:973–981.

239. Kellner U, Renner AB, Tillack H. Fundus autofluorescence and mfERG for early detection of retinal alterations in patients using chloroquine/hydroxychloroquine. Invest Ophthalmol Vis Sci 2006;47:3531–3538.

240. Marmor MF, Carr RE, Easterbrook M, et al. Recommendations on screening for chloroquine and hydroxychloroquine retinopathy: a report by the American Academy of Ophthalmology. Ophthalmology 2002;109:1377–1382.

241. Kälviäinen R, Nousiainen I, Mäntyjärvi M, et al. Vigabatrin, a gabaergic antiepileptic drug, causes concentric visual field defects. Neurology 1999;53:922–926.

242. Verrotti A, Manco R, Matricardi S, et al. Antiepileptic drugs and visual function. Pediatr Neurol 2007;36:353–360.

243. Miller NR, Johnson MA, Paul SR, et al. Visual dysfunction in patients receiving vigabatrin. Clinical and electrophysiologic findings. Neurology 1999;53:2082–2087.

244. Banin E, Shalev RS, Obolensky A, et al. Retinal function abnormalities in patients treated with vigabatrin. Arch Ophthalmol 2003;121:811–816.

245. Harding GF, Wild JM, Robertson KA, et al. Separating the retinal electrophysiologic effects of vigabatrin: treatment versus field loss. Neurology 2000;55:347–352.

246. Westall CA, Logan WJ, Smith K, et al. The Hospital for Sick Children, Toronto, Longitudinal ERG study of children on vigabatrin. Doc Ophthalmol 2002;104:133–149.

247. Coupland SG, Zackon DH, Leonard BC, et al. Vigabatrin effect on inner retinal function. Ophthalmology 2001;108:1493–1496; discussion 1497–1498.

248. Buncic JR, Westall CA, Panton CM, et al. Characteristic retinal atrophy with secondary "inverse" optic atrophy identifies vigabatrin toxicity in children. Ophthalmology 2004;111:1935–1942.

249. Johnson MA, Krauss GL, Miller NR, et al. Visual function loss from vigabatrin: effect of stopping the drug. Neurology 2000;55:40–45.

250. Nousiainen I, Mäntyjärvi M, Kälviäinen R. No reversion in vigabatrin-associated visual field defects. Neurology 2001;57:1916–1917.

251. Best JL, Acheson JF. The natural history of Vigabatrin associated visual field defects in patients electing to continue their medication. Eye 2005;19:41–44.

252. Miller NR. Using the electroretinogram to detect and monitor the retinal toxicity of anticonvulsants. Neurology 2000;55:333–334.

253. Gabrieli CB, Regine F, Vingolo EM, et al. Subjective visual halos after sildenafil (Viagra) administration: electroretinographic evaluation. Ophthalmology 2001;108:877–881.

254. Laties A, Zrenner E. Viagra (sildenafil citrate) and ophthalmology. Prog Retin Eye Res 2002;21:485–506.

255. Szlyk JP, Fishman GA, Alexander KR, et al. Clinical subtypes of cone-rod dystrophy. Arch Ophthalmol 1993;111:781–788.

256. Simunovic MP, Moore AT. The cone dystrophies. Eye 1998;12:553–565.

257. Balciuniene J, Johansson K, Sandgren O, et al. A gene for autosomal dominant progressive cone dystrophy (CORD5) maps to chromosome 17p12-p13. Genomics 1995;30:281–286.

258. Kelsell RE, Gregory Evans K, Payne AM, et al. Mutations in the retinal guanylate cyclase (RETGC-1) gene in dominant cone-rod dystrophy. Hum Mol Genet 1998;7:1179–1184.

259. Meire FM, Bergen AA, De Rouck A, et al. X linked progressive cone dystrophy. Localisation of the gene locus to Xp21-p11.1 by linkage analysis. Br J Ophthalmol 1994;78:103–108.

260. Nakazawa M, Kikawa E, Chida Y, et al. Autosomal dominant cone-rod dystrophy associated with mutations in codon 244 (Asn244His) and codon 184 (Tyr184Ser) of the peripherin/RDS gene. Arch Ophthalmol 1996;114:72–78.

261. Smith M, Whittock N, Searle A, et al. Phenotype of autosomal dominant cone-rod dystrophy due to the R838C mutation of the GUCY2D gene encoding retinal guanylate cyclase-1. Eye 2007;21:1220–1225.

262. Paunescu K, Preising MN, Janke B, et al. Genotype-phenotype correlation in a German family with a novel complex CRX mutation extending the open reading frame. Ophthalmology 2007;114:1348–1357.

263. Mantyjarvi MI. Color vision defect as first symptom of progressive cone-rod dystrophy. J Clin Neuroophthalmol 1990;10:266–270.

264. Kretschmann U, Seeliger M, Ruether K, et al. Spatial cone activity distribution in diseases of the posterior pole determined by multifocal electroretinography. Vision Res 1998;38:3817–3828.

265. Birch DG, Anderson JL, Fish GE. Yearly rates of rod and cone functional loss in retinitis pigmentosa and cone-rod dystrophy. Ophthalmology 1999;106:258–268.

266. Huang Y, Cideciyan AV, Papastergiou GI, et al. Relation of optical coherence tomography to microanatomy in normal and rd chickens. Invest Ophthalmol Vis Sci 1998;39:2405–2416.

267. Krauss HR, Heckenlively JR. Visual field changes in cone-rod degenerations. Arch Ophthalmol 1982;100:1784–1790.

268. Rotenstreich Y, Fishman GA, Anderson RJ. Visual acuity loss and clinical observations in a large series of patients with Stargardt disease. Ophthalmology 2003;110:1151–1158.

269. Berio A, Oliaro E, Piazzi A. Three cases of Kearns-Sayre syndrome with cardiac blocks. Panminerva Med 2007;49:45–46.

270. Chawla S, Coku J, Forbes T, et al. Kearns-Sayre syndrome presenting as complete heart block. Pediatr Cardiol 2008;29:659–662.

271. Skinner JR, Yang T, Purvis D, et al. Coinheritance of long QT syndrome and Kearns-Sayre syndrome. Heart Rhythm 2007;4:1568–1572.

272. Young TJ, Shah AK, Lee MH, et al. Kearns-Sayre syndrome: a case report and review of cardiovascular complications. Pacing Clin Electrophysiol 2005;28:454–457.

273. Kearns TP, Sayre GP. Retinitis pigmentosa, external ophthalmoplegia and complete heart block. Arch Ophthalmol 1958;60:280–289.

274. Brockington M, Alsanjari N, Sweeney MG, et al. Kearns-Sayre syndrome associated with mitochondrial DNA deletion or duplication: a molecular genetic and pathological study. J Neurol Sci 1995;131:78–87.

275. Alemi M, Prigione A, Wong A, et al. Mitochondrial DNA deletions inhibit proteasomal activity and stimulate an autophagic transcript. Free Radic Biol Med 2007;42:32–43.

276. Chae JH, Hwang H, Lim BC, et al. Clinical features of A3243G mitochondrial tRNA mutation. Brain Dev 2004;26:459–462.

277. Vazquez-Acevedo M, Vazquez-Memije ME, Mutchinick OM, et al. A case of Kearns-Sayre syndrome with the 4,977-bp common deletion associated with a novel 7,704-bp deletion. Neurol Sci 2002;23:247–250.

278. Mita S, Schmidt B, Schon EA, et al. Detection of "deleted" mitochondrial genomes in cytochrome-c oxidase-deficient muscle fibers of a patient with Kearns-Sayre syndrome. Proc Natl Acad Sci USA 1989;86:9509–9513.

279. Schon EA, Rizzuto R, Moraes CT, et al. A direct repeat is a hotspot for large-scale deletion of human mitochondrial DNA. Science 1989;244:346–349.

280. Vazquez Acevedo M, Coria R, Gonzalez Astiazaran A, et al. Characterization of a 5025 base pair mitochondrial DNA deletion in Kearns-Sayre syndrome. Biochim Biophys Acta 1995;1271:363–368.

281. Zeviani M, Moraes CT, DiMauro S, et al. Deletions of mitochondrial DNA in Kearns-Sayre syndrome. 1988 [classical article]. Neurology 1998;51:1525 and 1528 pages following.

282. Mullie MA, Harding AE, Petty RK, et al. The retinal manifestations of mitochondrial myopathy. A study of 22 cases. Arch Ophthalmol 1985;103:1825–1830.

283. Francois J. Metabolic tapetoretinal degenerations. Surv Ophthalmol 1982;26:293–333.

284. Fang W, Huang CC, Lee CC, et al. Ophthalmologic manifestations in MELAS syndrome. Arch Neurol 1993;50:977–980.

285. Isashiki Y, Nakagawa M, Ohba N, et al. Retinal manifestations in mitochondrial diseases associated with mitochondrial DNA mutation. Acta Ophthalmol Scand 1998;76:6–13.

286. Sue CM, Mitchell P, Crimmins DS, et al. Pigmentary retinopathy associated with the mitochondrial DNA 3243 point mutation. Neurology 1997;49:1013–1017.

287. Rummelt V, Folberg R, Ionasescu V, et al. Ocular pathology of MELAS syndrome with mitochondrial DNA nucleotide 3243 point mutation. Ophthalmology 1993;100:1757–1766.

288. Kerrison JB, Biousse V, Newman NJ. Retinopathy of NARP syndrome. Arch Ophthalmol 2000;118:298–299.

289. Johns DR. Mitochondrial DNA and disease. N Engl J Med 1995;333:638–644.

290. Holt IJ, Harding AE, Petty RKH, et al. A new mitochondrial disease associated with mitochondrial DNA heteroplasmy. Am J Hum Genet 1990;46:428–433.

291. Bogousslavsky J, Gaio JM, Caplan LR, et al. Encephalopathy, deafness and blindness in young women: a distinct retinocochleocerebral arteriolopathy? J Neurol Neurosurg Psychiatry 1989;52:43–46.

292. Coppeto JR, Currie JN, Monteiro ML, et al. A syndrome of arterial-occlusive retinopathy and encephalopathy. Am J Ophthalmol 1984;98:189–202.

293. Monteiro ML, Swanson RA, Coppeto JR, et al. A microangiopathic syndrome of encephalopathy, hearing loss, and retinal arteriolar occlusions. Neurology 1985;35:1113–1121.

294. Susac JO. Susac's syndrome: the triad of microangiopathy of the brain and retina with hearing loss in young women. Neurology 1994;44:591–593.

295. Susac JO, Hardman JM, Selhorst JB. Microangiopathy of the brain and retina. Neurology 1979;29:313–316.

296. Wildemann B, Schulin C, Storch Hagenlocher B, et al. Susac's syndrome: improvement with combined antiplatelet and calcium antagonist therapy [letter]. Stroke 1996;27:149–151.

297. O'Halloran HS, Pearson PA, Lee WB, et al. Microangiopathy of the brain, retina, and cochlea (Susac syndrome). A report of five cases and a review of the literature. Ophthalmology 1998;105:1038–1044.

298. Petty GW, Engel AG, Younge BR, et al. Retinocochleocerebral vasculopathy. Medicine Baltimore 1998;77:12–40.

299. Papo T, Biousse V, Lehoang P, et al. Susac syndrome. Medicine Baltimore 1998;77:3–11.

300. Egan RA, Ha Nguyen T, Gass JD, et al. Retinal arterial wall plaques in Susac syndrome. Am J Ophthalmol 2003;135:483–486.

301. Susac JO, Murtagh FR, Egan RA, et al. MRI findings in Susac's syndrome. Neurology 2003;61:1783–1787.

302. White ML, Zhang Y, Smoker WR. Evolution of lesions in Susac syndrome at serial MR imaging with diffusion-weighted imaging and apparent diffusion coefficient values. AJNR Am J Neuroradiol 2004;25:706–713.

303. Xu MS, Tan CB, Umapathi T, et al. Susac syndrome: serial diffusion-weighted MR imaging. Magn Reson Imaging 2004;22:1295–1298.

304. Notis CM, Kitei RA, Cafferty MS, et al. Microangiopathy of brain, retina, and inner ear. J Neuroophthalmol 1995;15:1–8.

305. Fox RJ, Costello F, Judkins AR, et al. Treatment of Susac syndrome with gamma globulin and corticosteroids. J Neurol Sci 2006;251:17–22.

306. Rennebohm RM, Susac JO. Treatment of Susac's syndrome. J Neurol Sci 2007;257:215–220.

307. Li HK, Dejean BJ, Tang RA. Reversal of visual loss with hyperbaric oxygen treatment in a patient with Susac syndrome. Ophthalmology 1996;103:2091–2098.

308. Gass JD. Acute posterior multifocal placoid pigment epitheliopathy. Arch Ophthalmol 1968;80:177–185.

309. Howe LJ, Woon H, Graham EM, et al. Choroidal hypoperfusion in acute posterior multifocal placoid pigment epitheliopathy. An indocyanine green angiography study. Ophthalmology 1995;102:790–798.

310. Park D, Schatz H, McDonald HR, et al. Acute multifocal posterior placoid pigment epitheliopathy: a theory of pathogenesis. Retina 1995;15:351–352.

311. Althaus C, Unsold R, Figge C, et al. Cerebral complications in acute posterior multifocal placoid pigment epitheliopathy. Ger J Ophthalmol 1993;2:150–154.

312. O'Halloran HS, Berger JR, Lee WB, et al. Acute multifocal placoid pigment epitheliopathy and central nervous system involvement. Nine new cases and a review of the literature. Ophthalmology 2001;108:861–868.

313. de Vries JJ, den Dunnen WFA, Kruithof IG, et al. Acute posterior multifocal placoid pigment epitheliopathy with cerebral vasculitis: a multisystem granulomatous disease. Arch Ophthalmol 2006;124:910–913.

314. Bewermeyer H, Nelles G, Huber M, et al. Pontine infarction in acute posterior multifocal placoid pigment epitheliopathy. J Neurol 1993;241:22–26.

315. Kersten DH, Lessell S, Carlow TJ. Acute posterior multifocal placoid pigment epitheliopathy and late-onset meningo-encephalitis. Ophthalmology 1987;94:393–396.

316. Weinstein JM, Bresnick GH, Bell CL, et al. Acute posterior multifocal placoid pigment epitheliopathy associated with cerebral vasculitis. J Clin Neuroophthalmol 1988;8:195–201.

317. Wilson CA, Choromokos EA, Sheppard R. Acute posterior multifocal placoid pigment epitheliopathy and cerebral vasculitis. Arch Ophthalmol 1988;106:796–800.

318. Comu S, Verstraeten T, Rinkoff JS, et al. Neurological manifestations of acute posterior multifocal placoid pigment epitheliopathy. Stroke 1996;27:996–1001.

319. Hsu CT, Harlan JB, Goldberg MF, et al. Acute posterior multifocal placoid pigment epitheliopathy associated with a systemic necrotizing vasculitis. Retina 2003;23:64–68.

320. Roberts TV, Mitchell P. Acute posterior multifocal placoid pigment epitheliopathy: a long-term study. Aust N Z J Ophthalmol 1997;25:277–281.

321. Moyenin P, Grange JD. Eales' syndrome. Clinical aspects, therapeutic indications and course of 29 cases. J Fr Ophtalmol 1987;10:123–128.

322. Biswas J, Raghavendran R, Pinakin G, et al. Presumed Eales' disease with neurologic involvement: report of three cases. Retina 2001;21:141–145.

323. Misra UK, Jha S, Kalita J, et al. Stroke: a rare presentation of Eales' disease. A case report. Angiology 1996;47:73–76.

324. Atabay C, Erdem E, Kansu T, et al. Eales disease with internuclear ophthalmoplegia. Ann Ophthalmol 1992;24:267–269.

325. Gordon MF, Coyle PK, Golub B. Eales' disease presenting as stroke in the young adult. Ann Neurol 1988;24:264–266.

326. Katz B, Wheeler D, Weinreb RN, et al. Eales' disease with central nervous system infarction. Ann Ophthalmol 1991;23:460–463.

327. Kutsal YG, Altioklar K, Atasu S, et al. Eales' disease with hemiplegia. Clin Neurol Neurosurg 1987;89:283–286.

328. Phanthumchinda K. Eales' disease with myelopathy. J Med Assoc Thai 1992;75:255–258.

329. Gluth MB, Baratz KH, Matteson EL, et al. Cogan syndrome: a retrospective review of 60 patients throughout a half century. Mayo Clin Proc 2006;81:483–488.

330. Bicknell JM, Holland JV. Neurologic manifestations of Cogan's syndrome. Neurology 1978;28:278–281.

331. Bousser MG, Biousse V. Small vessel vasculopathies affecting the central nervous system. J Neuroophthalmol 2004;24:56–61.

332. Cumurciuc R, Massin P, Paques M, et al. Retinal abnormalities in CADASIL: a retrospective study of 18 patients. J Neurol Neurosurg Psychiatry 2004;75:1058–1060.

333. Robinson W, Galetta SL, McCluskey L, et al. Retinal findings in cerebral autosomal dominant arteriopathy with subcortical infarcts and leukoencephalopathy (CADASIL). Surv Ophthalmol 2001;45:445–448.

334. Haritoglou C, Rudolph G, Hoops JP, et al. Retinal vascular abnormalities in CADASIL. Neurology 2004;62:1202–1205.

335. Roine S, Harju M, Kivela TT, et al. Ophthalmologic findings in cerebral autosomal dominant arteriopathy with subcortical infarcts and leukoencephalopathy: a cross-sectional study. Ophthalmology 2006;113:1411–1417.

336. Rufa A, De Stefano N, Dotti MT, et al. Acute unilateral visual loss as the first symptom of cerebral autosomal dominant arteriopathy with subcortical infarcts and leukoencephalopathy. Arch Neurol 2004;61:577–580.

337. Rubio A, Rifkin D, Powers JM, et al. Phenotypic variability of CADASIL and novel morphologic findings. Acta Neuropathol Berl 1997;94:247–254.

338. Haritoglou C, Hoops JP, Stefani FH, et al. Histologic abnormalities in ocular blood vessels of CADASIL patients. Am J Ophthalmol 2004;138:302–305.

339. Joutel A, Vahedi K, Corpechot C, et al. Strong clustering and stereotyped nature of Notch3 mutations in CADASIL patients. Lancet 1997;350:1511–1515.

340. Gouw LG, Kaplan CD, Haines JH, et al. Retinal degeneration characterizes a spinocerebellar ataxia mapping to chromosome 3p. Nat Genet 1995;10:89–93.

341. Holmberg M, Johansson J, Forsgren L, et al. Localization of autosomal dominant cerebellar ataxia associated with retinal degeneration and anticipation to chromosome 3p12-p21.1. Hum Mol Genet 1995;4:1441–1445.

342. Jobsis GJ, Weber JW, Barth PG, et al. Autosomal dominant cerebellar ataxia with retinal degeneration (ADCA II): clinical and neuropathological findings in two pedigrees and genetic linkage to 3p12-p21.1. J Neurol Neurosurg Psychiatry 1997;62:367–371.

343. David G, Abbas N, Stevanin G, et al. Cloning of the SCA7 gene reveals a highly unstable CAG repeat expansion. Nat Genet 1997;17:65–70.

344. David G, Durr A, Stevanin G, et al. Molecular and clinical correlations in autosomal dominant cerebellar ataxia with progressive macular dystrophy (SCA7). Hum Mol Genet 1998;7:165–170.

345. Johansson J, Forsgren L, Sandgren O, et al. Expanded CAG repeats in Swedish spinocerebellar ataxia type 7 (SCA7) patients: effect of CAG repeat length on the clinical manifestation. Hum Mol Genet 1998;7:171–176.

346. Enevoldson TP, Sanders MD, Harding AE. Autosomal dominant cerebellar ataxia with pigmentary macular dystrophy. A clinical and genetic study of eight families. Brain 1994;117:445–460.

347. Hamilton SR, Chatrian GE, Mills RP, et al. Cone dysfunction in a subgroup of patients with autosomal dominant cerebellar ataxia. Arch Ophthalmol 1990;108:551–556.

348. Aleman TS, Cideciyan AV, Volpe NJ, et al. Spinocerebellar ataxia type 7 (SCA7) shows a cone-rod dystrophy phenotype. Exp Eye Res 2002;74:737–745.

349. Michalik A, Martin JJ, Van Broeckhoven C. Spinocerebellar ataxia type 7 associated with pigmentary retinal dystrophy. Eur J Hum Genet 2004;12:2–15.

350. Duinkerke Eerola KU, Cruysberg JR, Deutman AF. Atrophic maculopathy associated with hereditary ataxia. Am J Ophthalmol 1980;90:597–603.

351. Ahn JK, Seo JM, Chung H, et al. Anatomical and functional characteristics in atrophic maculopathy associated with spinocerebellar ataxia type 7. Am J Ophthalmol 2005;139:923–925.

352. Gupta SN, Marks HG. Spinocerebellar ataxia type 7 mimicking Kearns-Sayre syndrome: a clinical diagnosis is desirable. J Neurol Sci 2008;264:173–176.

353. Martin JJ, Van Regemorter N, Krols L, et al. On an autosomal dominant form of retinal-cerebellar degeneration: an autopsy study of five patients in one family. Acta Neuropathol Berl 1994;88:277–286.

354. Leavitt JA, Kotagal S. The "cherry red" spot. Pediatr Neurol 2007;37:74–75.

355. Heroman JW, Rychwalski P, Barr CC. Cherry red spot in sialidosis (mucolipidosis type I). Arch Ophthalmol 2008;126:270–271.

356. Boustany RM, Britton JW, Parisi JE, et al. A 23-year-old man with seizures and visual deficit. Neurology 2008;70:73–78.

357. Rosser T. Aicardi syndrome. Arch Neurol 2003;60:1471–1473.

358. Durrani OM, Gordon C, Murray PI. Primary anti-phospholipid antibody syndrome (APS): current concepts. Surv Ophthalmol 2002;47:215–238.

359. Asherson RA, Merry P, Acheson JF, et al. Antiphospholipid antibodies: a risk factor for occlusive ocular vascular disease in systemic lupus erythematosus and the "primary" antiphospholipid syndrome. Ann Rheum Dis 1989;48:358–361.

360. Coroi M, Bontas E, Defranceschi M, et al. Ocular manifestations of antiphospholipid (Hughes) syndrome: minor features? Oftalmologia 2007;51:16–22.

361. Maaroufi RM, Hamdi R, Jmili N, et al. Antiphospholipid syndrome and retinal vein occlusion in adults. East Mediterr Health J 2004;10:627–632.

362. Miserocchi E, Baltatzis S, Foster CS. Ocular features associated with anticardiolipin antibodies: a descriptive study. Am J Ophthalmol 2001;131:451–456.

363. Castanon C, Amigo MC, Banales JL, et al. Ocular vaso-occlusive disease in primary antiphospholipid syndrome. Ophthalmology 1995;102:256–262.

364. Kleiner RC, Najarian LV, Schatten S, et al. Vaso-occlusive retinopathy associated with antiphospholipid antibodies (lupus anticoagulant retinopathy). Ophthalmology 1989;96:896–904.

365. Gelfand YA, Dori D, Miller B, et al. Visual disturbances and pathologic ocular findings in primary antiphospholipid syndrome. Ophthalmology 1999;106:1537–1540.

366. Briley DP, Coull BM, Goodnight SH, Jr. Neurological disease associated with antiphospholipid antibodies. Ann Neurol 1989;25:221–227.

367. Dafer RM, Biller J. Antiphospholipid syndrome: role of antiphospholipid antibodies in neurology. Hematol Oncol Clin North Am 2008;22:95–105, vii.

368. Levine SR, Welch KM. The spectrum of neurologic disease associated with antiphospholipid antibodies. Lupus anticoagulants and anticardiolipin antibodies. Arch Neurol 1987;44:876–883.

369. Iijima H, Gohdo T, Imai M, et al. Thrombin-antithrombin III complex in acute retinal vein occlusion. Am J Ophthalmol 1998;126:677–682.

370. Gottlieb JL, Blice JP, Mestichelli B, et al. Activated protein C resistance, factor V Leiden, and central retinal vein occlusion in young adults. Arch Ophthalmol 1998;116:577–579.

371. Tekeli O, Gursel E, Buyurgan H. Protein C, protein S and antithrombin III deficiencies in retinal vein occlusion. Acta Ophthalmol Scand 1999;77:628–630.

372. Price DT, Ridker PM. Factor V Leiden mutation and the risks for thromboembolic disease: a clinical perspective [see comments]. Ann Intern Med 1997;127:895–903.

373. Spagnolo BV, Nasrallah FP. Bilateral retinal vein occlusion associated with factor V Leiden mutation. Retina 1998;18:377–378.

374. Talmon T, Scharf J, Mayer E, et al. Retinal arterial occlusion in a child with factor V Leiden and thermolabile methylene tetrahydrofolate reductase mutations [see comments]. Am J Ophthalmol 1997;124:689–691.

375. Tayyanipour R, Pulido JS, Postel EA, et al. Arterial vascular occlusion associated with factor V Leiden gene mutation. Retina 1998;18:376–377.

376. Kotake S, Furudate N, Sasamoto Y, et al. Characteristics of endogenous uveitis in Hokkaido, Japan. Graefes Arch Clin Exp Ophthalmol 1996;234:599–603.

377. Murakami S, Inaba Y, Mochizuki M, et al. A nationwide survey on the occurrence of Vogt-Koyanagi-Harada disease in Japan. Jpn J Ophthalmol 1994;38:208–213.

378. Moorthy RS, Inomata H, Rao NA. Vogt-Koyanagi-Harada syndrome. Surv Ophthalmol 1995;39:265–292.

379. Maezawa N, Yano A. Two distinct cytotoxic T lymphocyte subpopulations in patients with Vogt-Koyanagi-Harada disease that recognize human melanoma cells. Microbiol Immunol 1984;28:219–231.

380. Maezawa N, Yano A, Taniguchi M, et al. The role of cytotoxic T lymphocytes in the pathogenesis of Vogt-Koyanagi-Harada disease. Ophthalmologica 1982;185:179–186.

381. Norose K, Yano A, Wang XC, et al. Dominance of activated T cells and interleukin-6 in aqueous humor in Vogt-Koyanagi-Harada disease. Invest Ophthalmol Vis Sci 1994;35:33–39.

382. Kasahara A, Hiraide A, Tomita N, et al. Vogt-Koyanagi-Harada disease occurring during interferon alpha therapy for chronic hepatitis C. J Gastroenterol 2004;39:1106–1109.

383. Montero JA, Sanchis ME, Fernandez-Munoz M. Vogt-Koyanagi-Harada syndrome in a case of multiple sclerosis. J Neuroophthalmol 2007;27:36–40.

384. Papastathopoulos K, Bouzas E, Naoum G, et al. Vogt-Koyanagi-Harada disease associated with interferon-A and ribavirin therapy for chronic hepatitis C infection. J Infect 2006;52:e59–61.

385. Sene D, Touitou V, Bodaghi B, et al. Intraocular complications of IFN-alpha and ribavirin therapy in patients with chronic viral hepatitis C. World J Gastroenterol 2007;13:3137–3140.

386. Sylvestre DL, Disston AR, Bui DP. Vogt-Koyanagi-Harada disease associated with interferon alpha-2b/ribavirin combination therapy. J Viral Hepat 2003;10:467–470.

387. Cunningham ET, Jr., Demetrius R, Frieden IJ, et al. Vogt-Koyanagi-Harada syndrome in a 4-year old child. Am J Ophthalmol 1995;120:675–677.

388. Gruich MJ, Evans OB, Storey JM, et al. Vogt-Koyanagi-Harada syndrome in a 4-year-old child. Pediatr Neurol 1995;13:50–51.

389. Rathinam SR, Vijayalakshmi P, Namperumalsamy P, et al. Vogt-Koyanagi-Harada syndrome in children. Ocul Immunol Inflamm 1998;6:155–161.

390. Moorthy RS, Rajeev B, Smith RE, et al. Incidence and management of cataracts in Vogt-Koyanagi-Harada syndrome. Am J Ophthalmol 1994;118:197–204.

391. Kawano Y, Tawara A, Nishioka Y, et al. Ultrasound biomicroscopic analysis of transient shallow anterior chamber in Vogt-Koyanagi-Harada syndrome. Am J Ophthalmol 1996;121:720–723.

392. Forster DJ, Rao NA, Hill RA, et al. Incidence and management of glaucoma in Vogt-Koyanagi-Harada syndrome. Ophthalmology 1993;100:613–618.

393. Keino H, Goto H, Mori H, et al. Association between severity of inflammation in CNS and development of sunset glow fundus in Vogt-Koyanagi-Harada disease. Am J Ophthalmol 2006;141:1140–1142.

394. Moorthy RS, Chong LP, Smith RE, et al. Subretinal neovascular membranes in Vogt-Koyanagi-Harada syndrome. Am J Ophthalmol 1993;116:164–170.

395. Ondrey FG, Moldestad E, Mastroianni MA, et al. Sensorineural hearing loss in Vogt-Koyanagi-Harada syndrome. Laryngoscope 2006;116:1873–1876.

396. Fardeau C, Tran TH, Gharbi B, et al. Retinal fluorescein and indocyanine green angiography and optical coherence tomography in successive stages of Vogt-Koyanagi-Harada disease. Int Ophthalmol 2007;27:163–172.

397. Oshima Y, Harino S, Hara Y, et al. Indocyanine green angiographic findings in Vogt-Koyanagi-Harada disease. Am J Ophthalmol 1996;122:58–66.

398. Forster DJ, Cano MR, Green RL, et al. Echographic features of the Vogt-Koyanagi-Harada syndrome. Arch Ophthalmol 1990;108:1421–1426.

399. Ibanez HE, Grand MG, Meredith TA, et al. Magnetic resonance imaging findings in Vogt-Koyanagi-Harada syndrome. Retina 1994;14:164–168.

400. Tsai JH, Sukavatcharin S, Rao NA. Utility of lumbar puncture in diagnosis of Vogt-Koyanagi-Harada disease. Int Ophthalmol 2007;27:189–194.

401. Hayasaka S, Okabe H, Takahashi J. Systemic corticosteroid treatment in Vogt-Koyanagi-Harada disease. Graefes Arch Clin Exp Ophthalmol 1982;218:9–13.

402. Sasamoto Y, Ohno S, Matsuda H. Studies on corticosteroid therapy in Vogt-Koyanagi-Harada disease. Ophthalmologica 1990;201:162–167.

403. Paredes I, Ahmed M, Foster CS. Immunomodulatory therapy for Vogt-Koyanagi-Harada patients as first-line therapy. Ocul Immunol Inflamm 2006;14:87–90.

404. Limon S, Girard P, Bloch Michel E, et al. Current aspects of the Vogt-Koyanagi-Harada syndrome. Apropos of 9 cases. J Fr Ophtalmol 1985;8:29–35.

405. Helveston WR, Gilmore R. Treatment of Vogt-Koyanagi-Harada syndrome with intravenous immunoglobulin. Neurology 1996;46:584–585.

406. Rodriguez A, Calonge M, Pedroza Seres M, et al. Referral patterns of uveitis in a tertiary eye care center. Arch Ophthalmol 1996;114:593–599.

407. Rossman MD, Thompson B, Frederick M, et al. HLA-DRB1*1101: a significant risk factor for sarcoidosis in blacks and whites. Am J Hum Genet 2003;73:720–735.

408. Morimoto T, Azuma A, Abe S, et al. Epidemiology of sarcoidosis in Japan. Eur Respir J 2007.

409. Jabs DA, Johns CJ. Ocular involvement in chronic sarcoidosis. Am J Ophthalmol 1986;102:297–301.

410. Ohara K, Okubo A, Sasaki H, et al. Intraocular manifestations of systemic sarcoidosis. Jpn J Ophthalmol 1992;36:452–457.

411. Matsuo T, Fujiwara N, Nakata Y. First presenting signs or symptoms of sarcoidosis in a Japanese population. Jpn J Ophthalmol 2005;49:149–152.

412. Evans M, Sharma O, LaBree L, et al. Differences in clinical findings between Caucasians and African Americans with biopsy-proven sarcoidosis. Ophthalmology 2007;114:325–333.

413. Khanna A, Sidhu U, Bajwa G, et al. Pattern of ocular manifestations in patients with sarcoidosis in developing countries. Acta Ophthalmol Scand 2007;85:609–612.

414. Brinkman CJ, Rothova A. Fundus pathology in neurosarcoidosis. Int Ophthalmol 1993;17:23–26.

415. Spalton DJ, Sanders MD. Fundus changes in histologically confirmed sarcoidosis. Br J Ophthalmol 1981;65:348–358.

416. Thorne JE, Galetta SL. Disc edema and retinal periphlebitis as the initial manifestation of sarcoidosis. Arch Neurol 1998;55:862–863.

417. Kimmel AS, McCarthy MJ, Blodi CF, et al. Branch retinal vein occlusion in sarcoidosis. Am J Ophthalmol 1989;107:561–562.

418. Cook BE, Jr., Robertson DM. Confluent choroidal infiltrates with sarcoidosis. Retina 2000;20:1–7.

419. Desai UR, Tawansy KA, Joondeph BC, et al. Choroidal granulomas in systemic sarcoidosis. Retina 2001;21:40–47.

420. Thorne JE, Brucker AJ. Choroidal white lesions as an early manifestation of sarcoidosis. Retina 2000;20:8–15.

421. Tingey DP, Gonder JR. Ocular sarcoidosis presenting as a solitary choroidal mass. Can J Ophthalmol 1992;27:25–29.

422. Wolfensberger TJ, Herbort CP. Indocyanine green angiographic features in ocular sarcoidosis. Ophthalmology 1999;106:285–289.

423. Rothova A, Lardenoye C. Arterial macroaneurysms in peripheral multifocal chorioretinitis associated with sarcoidosis. Ophthalmology 1998;105:1393–1397.

424. Kosmorsky GS, Meisler DM, Rice TW, et al. Chest computed tomography and mediastinoscopy in the diagnosis of sarcoidosis-associated uveitis. Am J Ophthalmol 1998;126:132–134.

425. Ohara K, Okubo A, Kamata K, et al. Transbronchial lung biopsy in the diagnosis of suspected ocular sarcoidosis. Arch Ophthalmol 1993;111:642–644.

426. Nichols CW, Eagle RC, Jr., Yanoff M, et al. Conjunctival biopsy as an aid in the evaluation of the patient with suspected sarcoidosis. Ophthalmology 1980;87:287–291.

427. Karma A, Huhti E, Poukkula A. Course and outcome of ocular sarcoidosis. Am J Ophthalmol 1988;106:467–472.

428. Lanham JG, Barrie T, Kohner EM, et al. SLE retinopathy: evaluation by fluorescein angiography. Ann Rheum Dis 1982;41:473–478.

429. Jabs DA, Fine SL, Hochberg MC, et al. Severe retinal vaso-occlusive disease in systemic lupus erythematous. Arch Ophthalmol 1986;104:558–563.

430. Shimura M, Tatehana Y, Yasuda K, et al. Choroiditis in systemic lupus erythematosus: systemic steroid therapy and focal laser treatment. Jpn J Ophthalmol 2003;47:312–315.

431. Hall S, Buettner H, Luthra HS. Occlusive retinal vascular disease in systemic lupus erythematosus. J Rheumatol 1984;11:846–850.

432. Au A, O'Day J. Review of severe vaso-occlusive retinopathy in systemic lupus erythematosus and the antiphospholipid syndrome: associations, visual outcomes, complications and treatment. Clin Exp Ophthalmol 2004;32:87–100.

433. Abu el Asrar AM, Naddaf HO, Mitwali A. Choroidopathy in a case of systemic lupus erythematosus. Lupus 1995;4:496–497.

434. Benitez del Castillo JM, Castillo A, Fernandez Cruz A, et al. Persistent choroidopathy in systemic lupus erythematosus. Doc Ophthalmol 1994;88:175–178.

435. Solley WA, Martin DF, Newman NJ, et al. Cat scratch disease. Posterior segment manifestations. Ophthalmology 1999;106:1546–1553.

436. Curi AL, Machado DO, Heringer G, et al. Ocular manifestation of cat-scratch disease in HIV-positive patients. Am J Ophthalmol 2006;141:400–401.

437. Fukushima A, Yasuoka M, Tsukahara M, et al. A case of cat scratch disease neuroretinitis confirmed by polymerase chain reaction. Jpn J Ophthalmol 2003;47:405–408.

438. Labalette P, Bermond D, Dedes V, et al. Cat-scratch disease neuroretinitis diagnosed by a polymerase chain reaction approach. Am J Ophthalmol 2001;132:575–576.

439. Starck T, Madsen BW. Positive polymerase chain reaction and histology with borderline serology in Parinaud's oculoglandular syndrome. Cornea 2002;21:625–627.

440. Berker N, Batman C, Guven A, et al. Optic atrophy and macular degeneration as initial presentations of subacute sclerosing panencephalitis. Am J Ophthalmol 2004;138:879–881.

441. Babu RB, Biswas J. Bilateral macular retinitis as the presenting feature of subacute sclerosing panencephalitis. J Neuroophthalmol 2007;27:288–291.

442. Lau CH, Missotten T, Salzmann J, et al. Acute retinal necrosis features, management, and outcomes. Ophthalmology 2007;114:756–762.

443. Vandercam T, Hintzen RQ, de Boer JH, et al. Herpetic encephalitis is a risk factor for acute retinal necrosis. Neurology 2008;71:1268–1274.

444. Hayreh SS, Servais GE, Virdi PS. Fundus lesions in malignant hypertension. VI. Hypertensive choroidopathy. Ophthalmology 1986;93:1383–1400.

445. Hayreh SS, Servais GE, Virdi PS. Fundus lesions in malignant hypertension. IV. Focal intraretinal periarteriolar transudates. Ophthalmology 1986;93:60–73.

446. Hayreh SS, Servais GE, Virdi PS. Cotton-wool spots (inner retinal ischemic spots) in malignant arterial hypertension. Ophthalmologica 1989;198:197–215.

447. Hayreh SS, Servais GE, Virdi PS. Retinal arteriolar changes in malignant arterial hypertension. Ophthalmologica 1989;198:178–196.

448. Hayreh SS, Servais GE, Virdi PS, et al. Fundus lesions in malignant hypertension. III. Arterial blood pressure, biochemical, and fundus changes. Ophthalmology 1986;93:45–59.

449. Leavitt JA, Pruthi S, Morgenstern BZ. Hypertensive retinopathy mimicking neuroretinitis in a twelve-year-old girl. Surv Ophthalmol 1997;41:477–480.

450. Noble KG. Hypertensive retinopathy simulating Leber idiopathic stellate neuroretinitis [letter]. Arch Ophthalmol 1997;115:1594–1595.

451. Oliver M, Uchenik D. Bilateral exudative retinal detachment in eclampsia without hypertensive retinopathy. Am J Ophthalmol 1980;90:792–796.

452. Androudi S, Ekonomidis P, Kump L, et al. OCT-3 study of serous retinal detachment in a preeclamptic patient. Semin Ophthalmol 2007;22:189–191.

453. Kwok AK, Li JZ, Lai TY, et al. Multifocal electroretinographic and angiographic changes in pre-eclampsia. Br J Ophthalmol 2001;85:111–112.

454. Somfai GM, Mihaltz K, Tulassay E, et al. Diagnosis of serous neuroretinal detachments of the macula in severe preeclamptic patients with optical coherence tomography. Hypertens Pregnancy 2006;25:11–20.

455. Karesh JW, Goldman EJ, Reck K, et al. A prospective ophthalmic evaluation of patients with acute myeloid leukemia: correlation of ocular and hematologic findings. J Clin Oncol 1989;7:1528–1532.

456. Perazella MA, Magaldi J. Images in clinical medicine. Retinopathy in leukemia. N Engl J Med 1994;331:922.

457. Wiznia RA, Rose A, Levy AL. Occlusive microvascular retinopathy with optic disc and retinal neovascularization in acute lymphocytic leukemia. Retina 1994;14:253–255.

458. Rouleau GA, Merel P, Lutchman M, et al. Alteration in a new gene encoding a putative membrane-organizing protein causes neuro-fibromatosis type 2. Nature 1993;363:515–521.

459. Trofatter JA, MacCollin MM, Rutter JL, et al. A novel moesin-, ezrin-, radixin-like gene is a candidate for the neurofibromatosis 2 tumor suppressor. Cell 1993;72:791–800.

460. Ferner RE. Neurofibromatosis 1 and neurofibromatosis 2: a twenty first century perspective. Lancet Neurol 2007;6:340–351.

461. Nunes F, MacCollin M. Neurofibromatosis 2 in the pediatric population. J Child Neurol 2003;18:718–724.

462. Kaiser Kupfer MI, Freidlin V, Datiles MB, et al. The association of posterior capsular lens opacities with bilateral acoustic neuromas in patients with neurofibromatosis type 2. Arch Ophthalmol 1989;107:541–544.

463. Kaye LD, Rothner AD, Beauchamp GR, et al. Ocular findings associated with neurofibromatosis type II. Ophthalmology 1992;99:1424–1429.

464. Landau K, Yasargil GM. Ocular fundus in neurofibromatosis type 2. Br J Ophthalmol 1993;77:646–649.

465. Mautner VF, Hazim W, Pohlmann K, et al. Ophthalmologic spectrum of neurofibromatosis type 2 in childhood. Klin Monatsbl Augenheilkd 1996;208:58–62.

466. Meyers SM, Gutman FA, Kaye LD, et al. Retinal changes associated with neurofibromatosis 2. Trans Am Ophthalmol Soc 1995;93:245–252; discussion 252–247.

467. Sivalingam A, Augsburger J, Perilongo G, et al. Combined hamartoma of the retina and retinal pigment epithelium in a patient with neurofibromatosis type 2. J Pediatr Ophthalmol Strabismus 1991;28:320–322.

468. Garretto NS, Ameriso S, Molina HA, et al. Type 2 neurofibromatosis with Lisch nodules. Neurofibromatosis 1989;2:315–321.

469. Cunliffe IA, Moffat DA, Hardy DG, et al. Bilateral optic nerve sheath meningiomas in a patient with neurofibromatosis type 2. Br J Ophthalmol 1992;76:310–312.

470. Evans DG, Huson SM, Donnai D, et al. A genetic study of type 2 neurofibromatosis in the United Kingdom. II. Guidelines for genetic counselling. J Med Genet 1992;29:847–852.

471. Bosch MM, Boltshauser E, Harpes P, et al. Ophthalmologic findings and long-term course in patients with neurofibromatosis type 2. Am J Ophthalmol 2006;141:1068–1077.

472. Feucht M, Richard G, Mautner VF. Neurofibromatosis 2 leads to choroidal hyperfluorescence in fluorescein angiography. Graefes Arch Clin Exp Ophthalmol 2007;245:949–953.

473. Crino PB, Nathanson KL, Henske EP. The tuberous sclerosis complex. N Engl J Med 2006;355:1345–1356.

474. Hyman MH, Whittemore VH. National Institutes of Health consensus conference: tuberous sclerosis complex. Arch Neurol 2000;57:662–665.

475. Roach ES, Sparagana SP. Diagnosis of tuberous sclerosis complex. J Child Neurol 2004;19:643–649.

476. Au KS, Williams AT, Roach ES, et al. Genotype/phenotype correlation in 325 individuals referred for a diagnosis of tuberous sclerosis complex in the United States. Genet Med 2007;9:88–100.

477. Crino PB, Henske EP. New developments in the neurobiology of the tuberous sclerosis complex. Neurology 1999;53:1384–1390.

478. Fahsold R, Rott HD, Lorenz P. A third gene locus for tuberous sclerosis is closely linked to the phenylalanine hydroxylase gene locus. Hum Genet 1991;88:85–90.

479. Fryer AE, Chalmers A, Connor JM, et al. Evidence that the gene for tuberous sclerosis is on chromosome 9. Lancet 1987;1:659–661.

480. Haines JL, Short MP, Kwiatkowski DJ, et al. Localization of one gene for tuberous sclerosis within 9q32–9q34, and further evidence for heterogeneity. Am J Hum Genet 1991;49:764–772.

481. Kandt RS, Haines JL, Smith M, et al. Linkage of an important gene locus for tuberous sclerosis to a chromosome 16 marker for polycystic kidney disease. Nat Genet 1992;2:37–41.

482. Smith M, Smalley S, Cantor R, et al. Mapping of a gene determining tuberous sclerosis to human chromosome 11q14–11q23. Genomics 1990;6:105–114.

483. Jansen FE, Braams O, Vincken KL, et al. Overlapping neurologic and cognitive phenotypes in patients with TSC1 or TSC2 mutations. Neurology 2008;70:908–915.

484. Rowley SA, O'Callaghan FJ, Osborne JP. Ophthalmic manifestations of tuberous sclerosis: a population based study. Br J Ophthalmol 2001;85:420–423.

485. Williams R, Taylor D. Tuberous sclerosis. Surv Ophthalmol 1985;30:143–154.

486. Wolter JR, Mertus JM. Exophytic retinal astrocytoma in tuberous sclerosis. J Ped Ophthalmol 1969;6:186–190.

487. Mennel S, Meyer CH, Eggarter F, et al. Autofluorescence and angiographic findings of retinal astrocytic hamartomas in tuberous sclerosis. Ophthalmologica 2005;219:350–356.

488. Zimmer Galler IE, Robertson DM. Long-term observation of retinal lesions in tuberous sclerosis. Am J Ophthalmol 1995;119:318–324.

489. Shields JA, Eagle RC, Jr., Shields CL, et al. Aggressive retinal astrocytomas in 4 patients with tuberous sclerosis complex. Arch Ophthalmol 2005;123:856–863

490. Kiratli H, Bilgic S. Spontaneous regression of retinal astrocytic hamartoma in a patient with tuberous sclerosis. Am J Ophthalmol 2002;133:715–716.

491. Dotan SA, Trobe JD, Gebarski SS. Visual loss in tuberous sclerosis. Neurology 1991;41:1915–1917.

492. Webb DW, Fryer AE, Osborne JP. Morbidity associated with tuberous sclerosis: a population study. Dev Med Child Neurol 1996;38:146–155.

493. Datta AN, Hahn CD, Sahin M. Clinical presentation and diagnosis of tuberous sclerosis complex in infancy. J Child Neurol 2008;23:268–273.

494. DiMario FJ, Jr. Brain abnormalities in tuberous sclerosis complex. J Child Neurol 2004;19:650–657.

495. Webb DW, Clarke A, Fryer A, et al. The cutaneous features of tuberous sclerosis: a population study. Br J Dermatol 1996;135:1–5.

496. Roach ES, DiMario FJ, Kandt RS, et al. Tuberous Sclerosis Consensus Conference: recommendations for diagnostic evaluation. National Tuberous Sclerosis Association. J Child Neurol 1999;14:401–407.

497. Latif F, Tory K, Gnarra J, et al. Identification of the von Hippel-Lindau disease tumor suppressor gene. Science 1993;260:1317–1320.

498. Maher ER, Bentley E, Yates JR, et al. Mapping of von Hippel-Lindau disease to chromosome 3p confirmed by genetic linkage analysis. J Neurol Sci 1990;100:27–30.

499. Maher ER, Bentley E, Yates JR, et al. Mapping of the von Hippel-Lindau disease locus to a small region of chromosome 3p by genetic linkage analysis. Genomics 1991;10:957–960.

500. Webster AR, Maher ER, Moore AT. Clinical characteristics of ocular angiomatosis in von Hippel-Lindau disease and correlation with germline mutation. Arch Ophthalmol 1999;117:371–378.

501. Singh AD, Shields CL, Shields JA. von Hippel-Lindau disease. Surv Ophthalmol 2001;46:117–142.

502. Kreusel KM, Bechrakis NE, Krause L, et al. Retinal angiomatosis in von Hippel-Lindau disease: a longitudinal ophthalmologic study. Ophthalmology 2006;113:1418–1424.

503. Wong WT, Agron E, Coleman HR, et al. Clinical characterization of retinal capillary hemangioblastomas in a large population of patients with von Hippel-Lindau disease. Ophthalmology 2008;115:181–188.

504. Moore AT, Maher ER, Rosen P, et al. Ophthalmological screening for von Hippel-Lindau disease. Eye 1991;5:723–728.

505. Singh AD, Nouri M, Shields CL, et al. Treatment of retinal capillary hemangioma. Ophthalmology 2002;109:1799–1806.

506. Rosa RH, Jr., Goldberg MF, Green WR. Clinicopathologic correlation of argon laser photocoagulation of retinal angiomas in a patient with von Hippel-Lindau disease followed for more than 20 years. Retina 1996;16:145–156.

507. Kreusel KM, Bornfeld N, Lommatzsch A, et al. Ruthenium-106 brachytherapy for peripheral retinal capillary hemangioma. Ophthalmology 1998;105:1386–1392.

508. Balcer LJ, Galetta SL, Curtis M, et al. von Hippel-Lindau disease manifesting as a chiasmal syndrome. Surv Ophthalmol 1995;39:302–306.

509. Meyerle CB, Dahr SS, Wetjen NM, et al. Clinical course of retrobulbar hemangioblastomas in von Hippel-Lindau disease. Ophthalmology 2008;115:1382–1389.

510. Atuk NO, Stolle C, Owen JA, Jr., et al. Pheochromocytoma in von Hippel-Lindau disease: clinical presentation and mutation analysis in a large, multigenerational kindred. J Clin Endocrinol Metab 1998;83:117–120.

511. Allen RC, Webster AR, Sui R, et al. Molecular characterization and ophthalmic investigation of a large family with type 2A von Hippel-Lindau disease. Arch Ophthalmol 2001;119:1659–1665.

512. Couch V, Lindor NM, Karnes PS, et al. von Hippel-Lindau disease. Mayo Clin Proc 2000;75:265–272.

513. Sujansky E, Conradi S. Outcome of Sturge-Weber syndrome in 52 adults. Am J Med Genet 1995;57:35–45.

514. Phelps CD. The pathogenesis of glaucoma in Sturge-Weber syndrome. Ophthalmology 1978;85:276–286.

515. Agarwal HC, Sihota R, et al. Sturge-Weber syndrome: management of glaucoma with combined trabeculotomy-trabeculectomy. Ophthalmic Surg 1993;24:399–402.

516. Awad AH, Mullaney PB, Al Mesfer S, et al. Glaucoma in Sturge-Weber syndrome. JAAOS 1999;3:40–45.

517. Iwach AG, Hoskins HD, Jr., Hetherington J, Jr., et al. Analysis of surgical and medical management of glaucoma in Sturge-Weber syndrome. Ophthalmology 1990;97:904–909.

518. Yang CB, Freedman SF, Myers JS, et al. Use of latanoprost in the treatment of glaucoma associated with Sturge-Weber syndrome. Am J Ophthalmol 1998;126:600–602.

519. Sullivan TJ, Clarke MP, Morin JD. The ocular manifestations of the Sturge-Weber syndrome. J Pediatr Ophthalmol Strabismus 1992;29:349–356.

520. Schalenbourg A, Piguet B, Zografos L. Indocyanine green angiographic findings in choroidal hemangiomas: a study of 75 cases. Ophthalmologica 2000;214:246–252.

521. Wen F, Wu D. Indocyanine green angiographic findings in diffuse choroidal hemangioma associated with Sturge-Weber syndrome. Graefes Arch Clin Exp Ophthalmol 2000;238:625–627.

522. Griffiths PD, Boodram MB, Blaser S, et al. Abnormal ocular enhancement in Sturge-Weber syndrome: correlation of ocular MR and CT findings with clinical and intracranial imaging findings. AJNR: Am J Neuroradiol 1996;17:749–754.

523. Gottlieb JL, Murray TG, Gass JD. Low-dose external beam irradiation for bilateral diffuse choroidal hemangioma [letter]. Arch Ophthalmol 1998;116:815–817.

524. Schilling H, Sauerwein W, Lommatzsch A, et al. Long-term results after low dose ocular irradiation for choroidal haemangiomas. Br J Ophthalmol 1997;81:267–273.

525. Zografos L, Bercher L, Chamot L, et al. Cobalt-60 treatment of choroidal hemangiomas. Am J Ophthalmol 1996;121:190–199.

526. Zografos L, Egger E, Bercher L, et al. Proton beam irradiation of choroidal hemangiomas. Am J Ophthalmol 1998;126:261–268.

527. Rizzo R, Pavone L, Pero G, et al. A neurocutaneous disorder with a severe course: Wyburn-Mason's syndrome. J Child Neurol 2004;19:908–911.

528. Reck SD, Zacks DN, Eibschitz-Tsimhoni M. Retinal and intracranial arteriovenous malformations: Wyburn-Mason syndrome. J Neuroophthalmol 2005;25:205–208.

529. Schmidt D, Pache M, Schumacher M. The congenital unilateral retinocephalic vascular malformation syndrome (Bonnet-Dechaume-Blanc syndrome or Wyburn-Mason syndrome): review of the literature. Surv Ophthalmol 2008;53:227–249.

530. Dayani PN, Sadun AA. A case report of Wyburn-Mason syndrome and review of the literature. Neuroradiology 2007;49:445–456.

531. Effron L, Zakov ZN, Tomsak RL. Neovascular glaucoma as a complication of the Wyburn-Mason syndrome. J Clin Neuroophthalmol 1985;5:95–98.

532. Shah GK, Shields JA, Lanning RC. Branch retinal vein obstruction secondary to retinal arteriovenous communication. Am J Ophthalmol 1998;126:446–448.

533. Kivlin JD, Sanborn GE, Myers GG. The cherry-red spot in Tay-Sachs and other storage diseases. Ann Neurol 1985;17:356–360.

Visual loss: optic neuropathies

The diagnosis of optic neuropathy is usually considered under two circumstances: (1) when visual loss is associated with an anomalous, swollen, or pale optic disc, or (2) when the fundus examination is normal but deficits in acuity, color, and visual field are accompanied by an afferent pupillary defect. In each of these situations the examiner must rely upon historical information, examination findings, and diagnostic testing first to confirm the presence of optic nerve dysfunction, then to determine its etiology.

An understanding of optic nerve anatomy and physiology is important when approaching patients with optic nerve dysfunction, and this chapter will review these topics. Typical clinical features of optic neuropathies will then be detailed. The subsequent discussion will suggest an approach to the patient with an optic neuropathy and then outline a strategy used to distinguish between the various optic neuropathies. The features (presentation, examination, and management) of the different causes of optic nerve dysfunction will then be addressed.

Optic nerve anatomy and physiology

The optic nerve is composed of 1.2 million retinal ganglion cell axons.[1-3] The axons form the nerve fiber layer and eventually synapse in the lateral geniculate body, the pretectum, the superior colliculus, the accessory optic nuclei, and the suprachiasmatic nuclei in the hypothalamus. The supporting cells and blood supply of the optic nerve change throughout its course, which is generally divided into four sections: intraocular, intraorbital, intracanalicular, and intracranial. In fact, the optic nerve is more like a brain tract and less like the other cranial nerves. The optic nerve, like all other parts of the central nervous system, is invested by meninges including the dura (which blends into the sclera) and the arachnoidal and pial membranes. It is myelinated by oligodendrocytes beyond the lamina cribosa and is supported by astrocytes like the white matter in the brain and spinal cord. This is unlike peripheral nerves, which are myelinated by Schwann cells. In addition, the optic nerve has virtually no capacity for regeneration.

Ganglion cells and the intraocular optic nerve

The cell bodies of retinal ganglion cells and dendrites synapse with amacrine and bipolar cells in the inner plexiform layer of the retina. There are different types of retinal ganglion cells and each type may have a specific visual function. There is currently no agreed upon classification. The concept of parallel processing was introduced to recognize that different types of visual information are processed in parallel streams throughout the pre- and postgeniculate visual pathways.[4-7] Two broad pathways are generally thought to exist. The first is largely responsible for high spatial resolution, color vision, and fine stereopsis and is referred to as the parvocellular or P

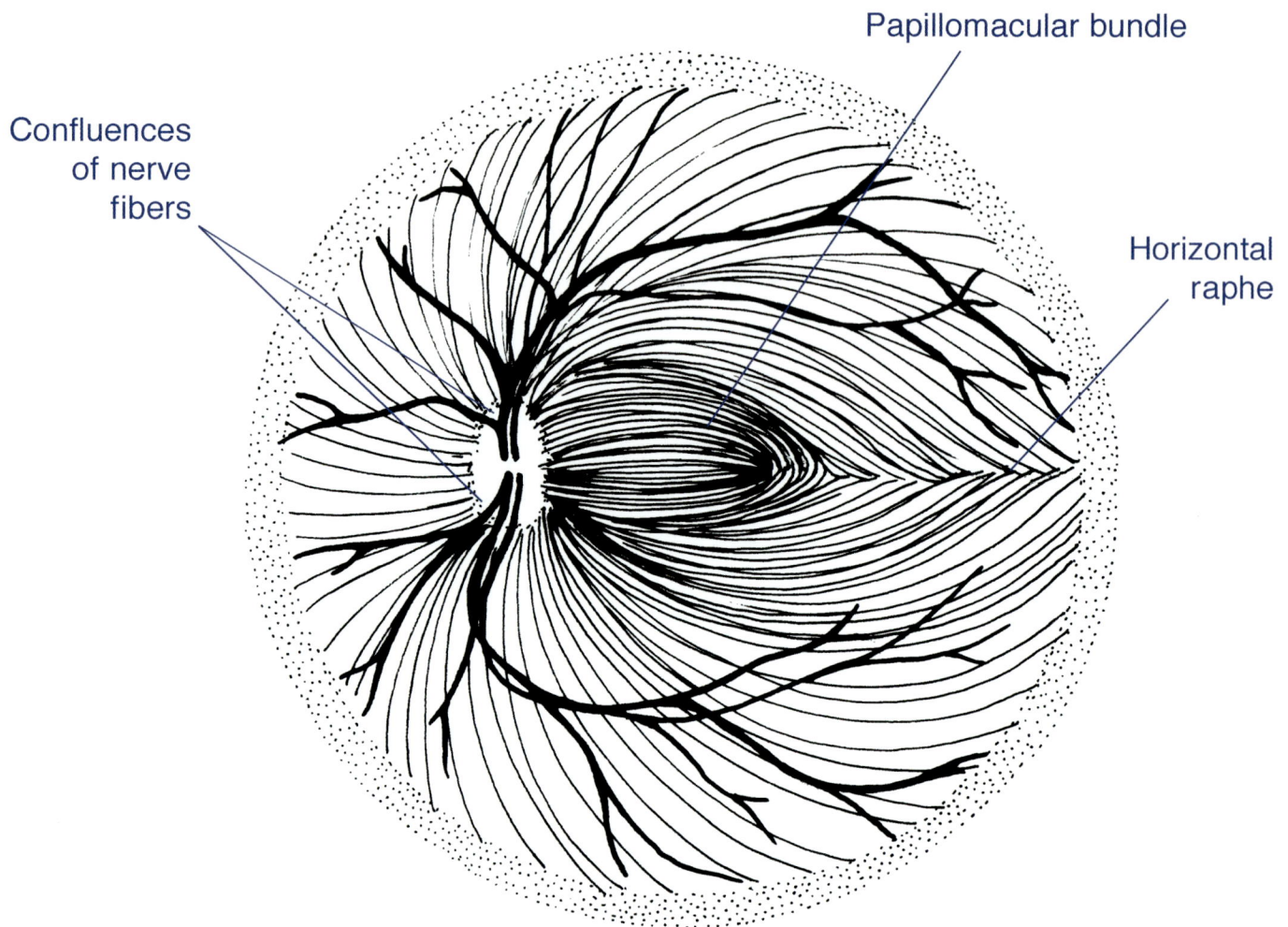

Figure 5–1. Distribution of retinal ganglion cell axons as they travel to the optic nerve. Fibers from the nasal, superonasal, and inferonasal retinal travel directly to the disc with the thickest nerve fiber layer at the superior and inferior poles of the disc. Fibers from the nasal half of the macula extend directly to the temporal portion of the optic nerve in the papillomacular bundle. Fibers from the temporal macula are separated by the horizontal raphe, above and below which they originate and arch around the fovea to enter the superior and inferior portions of the disc. These nerve fiber bundles are the basis for the different types of visual field defects that result from optic nerve disease.

pathway based on the layers in the lateral geniculate body (LGB) to which they project. The second (magnocellular, M or luminance) pathways are responsible for low spatial resolution, motion, and coarse stereopsis. For the purposes of understanding retinal neurophysiology, ganglion cell types generally can be divided into these two different broad categories, M (large) and P (small) cells.[8] M cells project to the magnocellular layer and P cells project to the parvocellular layer of the LGB. As would be expected, the macula (fine spatial resolution) contains mostly P cells; in the peripheral retina the difference in numbers of each type of cell is much less. These two distinct populations of cells persist throughout the retrogeniculate pathways into the ocular dominance columns of the striate cortex, at which there are probably extensive interactions between the various pathways. The relationship between magnocellular and parvocellular pathways and higher cortical areas is discussed in Chapter 9.

Each of the retinal ganglion cells projects to a specific portion of the striate cortex to preserve the strict point-to-point correspondence (retinotopy). Temporal retinal nerve fibers are arranged on either side of the horizontal raphe and arch around the fovea (arcuate bundles) to divert the

retinal elements, except the photoreceptors, away from the fovea (**Fig. 5–1**). These fibers enter the superior and inferior poles of the disc. Immediately adjacent to the disc, the nerve fiber layer reaches its maximal thickness of 200 μm. The horizontal raphe divides the superior and inferior retinal fibers and is the anatomic basis for several types of visual field defects (e.g., nasal steps, altitudinal defects). Nasal macular ganglion cells travel directly to the temporal portion of the disc in the papillomacular bundle. Ganglion cells from the central 5 degrees of visual field constitute approximately one-third of the total number of axons at the disc. Fibers from the retina nasal to the disc enter the nasal portion of the optic nerve. As they enter the optic nerve head, ganglion cell axons reorganize so that the axons from peripheral ganglion cells are most superficial in the nerve fiber layer and form the more peripheral portions of the optic nerve and macular ganglion cell axons form the center of the nerve.[9]

As they turn to exit the eye at the scleral canal, the optic nerve fibers are supported by the lamina choroidalis. Astrocytes make up a large portion of these supporting cells, and they are intertwined, creating a basket-like structure through

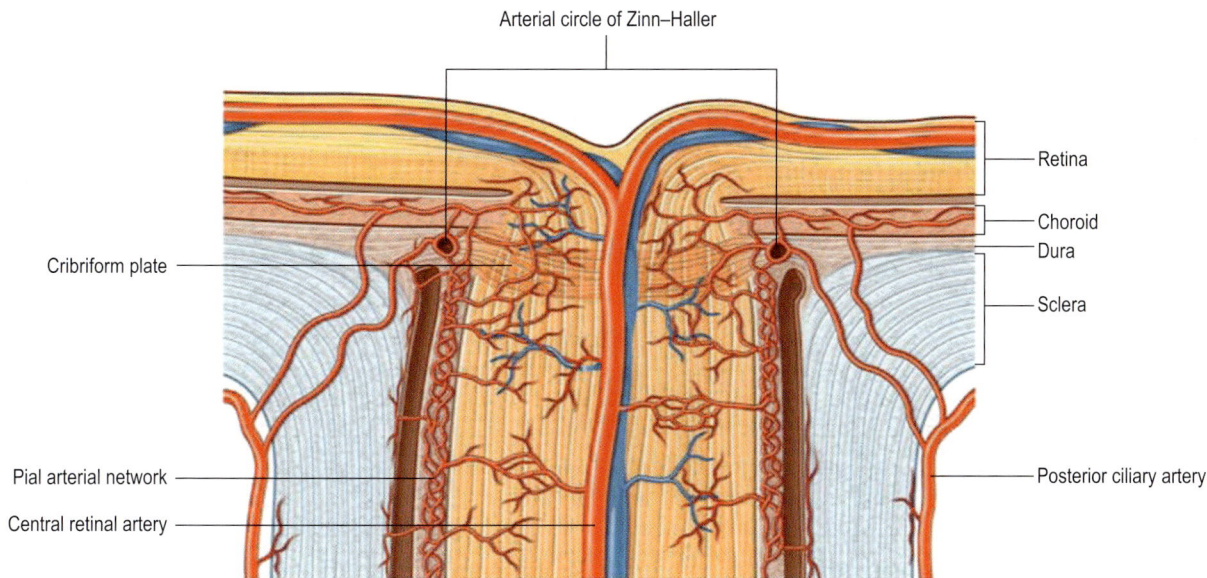

Figure 5–2. The circulation of the optic nerve head. The blood is derived primarily from the arteriolar anastomotic circle of Zinn–Haller, which is supplied by the posterior ciliary arteries, the pial arteriole plexus, and the peripapillary choroid. (Redrawn from Hayreh SS. Br J Ophthalmol 1963:47, with permission.)

which the optic nerve axons pass. The astrocytes extend from the lamina cribosa, the main structural support of the optic nerve as it exits the globe, and their processes are in intimate contact with the axons. Presumably they maintain the axons physiologically, providing glycogen stores, clearing excess potassium, and providing nutrient transport from capillaries in this area. The glial cells may also play a critical role in regulating blood flow.[10-12] The lamina cribrosa contains plates or beams of collagen (types I, III, V, and VI) with interspersed elastin fibers creating a basket-like configuration.[13-16] This combination provides both structure and elastic resiliency along the laminar beams and, along with the astrocytes, provides metabolic support to the axons. Differences exist in the size and thickness of the laminar beams. The largest holes in the lamina cribrosa (most axons, least structural support) are in the superior and inferior portions of the disc (arcuate bundles), and this may be one explanation why these fibers might be the most vulnerable to changes in intraocular pressure.[17] Once the axons pass the lamina cribrosa, oligodendrocytes assume the major supportive role.

All of the blood supply to the optic nerve is ultimately derived from the ophthalmic artery. The nerve fiber layer of the retina receives its blood supply from branches of the central retinal artery, and, when present, cilioretinal arteries also contribute to the peripapillary nerve fiber layer. A capillary bed from the central retinal artery provides the blood flow to the superficial optic nerve head. Branches of the short posterior ciliary arteries are the major blood supply to the optic nerve head below its surface. The area of the nerve served by each posterior ciliary artery is variable and segmental. Since anastomoses between the posterior ciliary arteries are scant, the optic nerve head can be a watershed area. The nature of the blood supply by the posterior ciliary arteries to the optic nerve head is the likely explanation for the segmental disc swelling and/or atrophy that often accompanies ischemic processes. Twigs of the posterior ciliary arteries reach the capillary plexus in the area of the

lamina choroidalis and lamina cribrosa through branches of the intrascleral circle of Zinn–Haller and from branches of choroidal vessels that supply the choriocapillaris (**Fig. 5–2**).[18,19] Capillaries in the region of the lamina cribrosa are within the laminar beams and surround the nerve fiber bundles.[20]

Intraorbital optic nerve

Several environmental changes occur as the axons pass through the lamina cribrosa, which is essentially at the level of the sclera. Optic nerve myelination begins (oligodendrocytes) and the pressure gradient on the axons increases as they are subjected first to intraocular pressure then to the intracranial pressure, which is transmitted through the subarachnoid space all the way up to the nerve globe junction. The intraorbital optic nerve is between 20 and 30 mm in length and is always longer than the distance from the globe to the orbital apex. Therefore there is always slack (the nerve usually takes on an S shape) to allow for unrestricted eye movements. Each axon is surrounded by myelin and glial cells, which provide metabolic support at the nodes of Ranvier. The entire nerve is surrounded by closely adherent pia mater. Arachnoid trabeculae connect the pia to the surrounding dura, which at the apex of the orbit is contiguous with the annulus of Zinn. The optic nerve is divided into septae by collagenous connective tissue which also contains the centripetally penetrating capillaries from the pia. These are supplied largely by recurrent branches of the short posterior ciliary arteries and capillary branches of the ophthalmic artery. Capillaries are also supplied anteriorly by branches from the central retinal artery, which pierces the optic nerve 10–15 mm from the nerve–globe junction. There may also be collateral circulation to the intraorbital optic nerve through anastomotic branches from the external carotid artery. These branches can be supplied from the middle meningeal, superficial temporal, and transverse facial arteries.

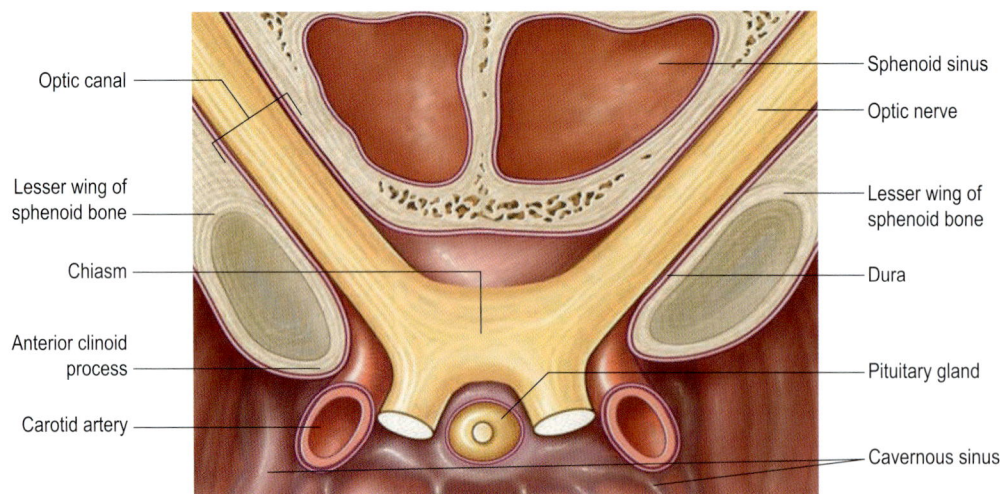

Figure 5–3. The optic canal sits between the two bases of the lesser wing of the sphenoid bone and contains the optic nerve, meninges, sympathetic plexus, and ophthalmic artery. Anteriorly the dura coalesces to form the annulus of Zinn. The space is tight and the dura is fixed to the bone. The sphenoid sinus forms the medial wall of the canal. The chiasm sits behind the sphenoid sinus and the intracranial opening of the canal is formed by the anterior clinoid process. Lateral to the chiasm is the cavernous sinus which contains the carotid artery.

Nerve fiber orientation within the optic nerve is highly specific. In the first third of the optic nerve, macular fibers lie temporally and then move to occupy the central portion of the optic nerve. Nasal retinal fibers remain in the nasal portion of the intraorbital optic nerve. The superior temporal fibers are located above the temporally located macular fibers and the inferior fibers are located below the macular fibers.

Intracanalicular optic nerve

After leaving the orbit, the optic nerve enters the optic canal, which sits within the two bases of the lesser wing of the sphenoid bone (**Fig. 5–3**). The medial wall of the canal forms the lateral wall of the sphenoid sinus and in some patients is absent, causing the meninges to contact the sinus mucosa directly.[21] The thickest bones of the canal are located at the orbital apex. The orbital plate of the frontal bone separates the canal from the overlying frontal lobe. Contained within the canal are also the ophthalmic artery, the meninges, and the sympathetic plexus. The dura and therefore the optic nerve are fixed to the periosteum throughout the canal, which is usually around 10 mm in length. This tight space makes the optic nerve particularly vulnerable to trauma and small space-occupying lesions in this area. The two optic canals run medially toward each other and rise at a 45 degree angle. In the optic canal, the blood vessels of the pial plexus are usually supplied by the internal carotid artery.

Intracranial optic nerve

The length of the intracranial optic nerve is variable (4–15 mm), depending on the position of the chiasm in relation to the sella turcica (above the sella, prefixed, or postfixed; see Chapter 7). The course of the intracranial optic nerve is upward at a 45 degree angle to reach the chiasm. Immediately above the nerves lie the anterior cerebral and anterior communicating arteries, and above these lie the olfactory nerves and frontal lobes. Just lateral to each nerve lies the internal carotid artery, and the ophthalmic artery arises from the internal carotid just below the optic nerve. Just under each optic nerve and above the pituitary gland lies the planum sphenoidale. The blood supply to the pial plexus of vessels supplying the optic nerve can arise from branches of the internal carotid artery, the anterior cerebral arteries, or from the anterior communicating artery.

Optic nerve physiology

Maintenance of the ganglion cell axons' structure, clearance of expired organelles, and energy supply to the synapse is accomplished through axoplasmic transport. Axoplasmic flow disruption has been demonstrated in experimental papilledema[22] and secondary to acute elevation of intraocular pressure.[23–26] In addition, many pathological processes (ischemia, compression, inflammation, and toxins) can result in impaired axoplasmic transport. Therefore, some believe that impaired axoplasmic transport may be the final common pathway for optic nerve damage in most disease processes.[27]

The diameter of a ganglion cell axon is approximately 100 times larger than the cell body, and the maintenance of axonal health is dependent on effective axonal transport. Orthograde axonal transport refers to movement away from the cell body (towards the lateral geniculate body) and retrograde transport occurs toward the cell body. Orthograde transport occurs at both slow and fast speeds and is dependent upon the cytoskeleton of the axon (microtubules, neurofilaments, and microfilaments). Transported materials include proteins and transmitters, and these are transported in smooth surface vesicles at a rate of about 400 mm/day (5 hours to LGB). The elements of the cytoskeleton (microtubules, neurofilaments) are transported at a slower rate of 1–4 mm/day.[28] Retrograde transport (towards the cell body) of pinocytic vesicles and lysosomes occurs at a rate of about 200 mm/day. Movement of vesicles along the cytoskeleton is dependent upon actin, kinesin, and dynein. How these motor proteins accomplish transport along the microtubule is not clear, but it may occur in a fashion similar to the sliding filament system seen in muscles. The transport process is dependent upon availability of oxygen and energy (ATP), which is delivered by mitochondria moving constantly in orthograde and retrograde fashions. Disruption of axonal transport by energy deprivation, by anoxia, or by compression will therefore result in optic nerve dysfunction.

Information from ganglion cells to the LGB is provided by varying the rate of action potentials. Light stimulates the retinal photoreceptors, and in turn signals are modified by the horizontal, bipolar, and amacrine cells before reaching the ganglion cells. There are many more photoreceptors than ganglion cells (approximately 130 : 1) and the input to an individual ganglion cell is thought to be organized in a center/surround fashion. This is the initial coding system for visual information. Some ganglion cells have on-center receptive fields, and increase their action potential firing rate when the visual stimulus is a circle of light in the middle, surrounded by darkness. Off-center ganglion cells prefer stimuli with darkness in the middle, surrounded by light. The various rates (for example sustained firing versus transient firing) at which ganglion cells produce action potentials in response to stimulation is the basis for the distinction between cells believed to be responsible for fine spatial resolution and those responsible for motion detection and initiation of visual reflexes.[29]

History

The cause of many optic neuropathies can be correctly identified after reviewing the patient's history. The temporal profile of the visual loss is most important, including the rapidity of the visual loss and the time to visual nadir. Next, attention should be given to associated symptoms, both ocular and nonocular. Some related ocular symptoms that should be considered include pain (in particular pain worsened by eye movements); bulging, fullness, or proptosis of the globe; redness; photophobia; and positive visual phenomena. Nonocular neurologic symptoms would include headache, anosmia, facial paresthesias or numbness, facial weakness, bladder incontinence, transient weakness or numbness, hearing loss, and audible intracranial noises. Clues to any underlying systemic illness should be sought, as well as evidence of recent infection or ongoing rheumatologic symptoms. Risk factors for vasculopathic disease should be identified in addition to systemic medications which may have secondary effects on the optic nerve. A careful family history should attempt to identify relatives with decreased vision or with degenerative neurologic illness, glaucoma, or migraine.

Examination

Most patients with optic neuropathy can be identified by the characteristic combination of acuity loss, color deficiency, visual field defect, an afferent pupillary defect, and an abnormal-appearing optic nerve on ophthalmoscopy (anomalous, swollen, or pale). Along with the historical review, the different features of each of these abnormal parameters are often helpful in identifying the particular cause of optic nerve dysfunction. Specific examination techniques are detailed in Chapter 2.

Systemic evaluation

The examination of the patient with suspected optic neuropathy begins with the general evaluation of the patient's physical health, mental status, and vital signs. Markedly elevated blood pressure in a patient with swollen discs suggests the presence of malignant hypertension. An irregular pulse from atrial fibrillation suggests that an acutely acquired visual field defect might be the result of an embolic arterial occlusion. A rapid pulse might suggest hyperthyroidism, and obesity and recent weight gain would point to idiopathic intracranial hypertension. Profound cachexia might suggest cancer spread, temporal arteritis, or nutritional amblyopia. Odd behavior might suggest early on the possibility of nonorganic or functional visual loss.

Visual acuity

Although visual acuity is commonly reduced in optic neuropathies, the finding is highly variable. In fact, visual acuity is the least sensitive of all the tested functions and is not always helpful in identifying the presence of optic neuropathy or its cause. For instance, profound optic nerve dysfunction with an afferent pupillary defect, dyschromatopsia, and visual field loss may be present with 20/15 visual acuity. Furthermore, virtually any of the causes of optic nerve dysfunction can be associated with any level of visual acuity loss.

Color vision

Dyschromatopsia and, in particular, the mismatch of good acuity and poor color vision are very important and sensitive indicators of optic nerve dysfunction. The basis for this mismatch is not completely understood. It may reflect the fact that the optic nerve is largely composed of ganglion cell axons arising in the macular region, and these axons have a one-to-one relationship with the high density of cones in this region. However, there are many patients with profound optic nerve dysfunction that may do relatively well with color plate testing and notice only a mild difference in color saturation between the two eyes.

Contrast sensitivity

Abnormal contrast sensitivity is another sign of optic nerve dysfunction. Some patients with optic neuropathy have good acuity but may have reduced contrast sensitivity thresholds. It is also helpful in patients with congenital dyschromatopsia who are suspected of having an optic nerve problem, and color plate testing cannot be used. Less commonly, it can be used to document recovery in optic neuritis, which is almost always associated with a reduction in contrast sensitivity. Recently, low-contrast sensitivity testing has been incorporated in the evaluation of new drugs for the treatment of multiple sclerosis and optic neuritis.

Video 2.3

Pupils

The identification of a relative afferent pupil defect (RAPD) is very helpful in localizing vision loss to the optic nerve and is the hallmark of asymmetric disease of the anterior visual pathway. The swinging flashlight test is described in detail in Chapter 2.

Pulfrich phenomenon

Pulfrich described a phenomenon that is occasionally reported as a symptom in patients with optic neuropathy. It can be tested for in the office. The Pulfrich phenomenon is a stereo-illusion in which a to-and-fro motion in the plane facing the subject is seen as an elliptical movement by an individual with a unilateral optic neuropathy.[30] An object (ball on a string or pen) is swung in front of both eyes.[31] For example, from the eye with a unilateral optic neuropathy, the information is delayed in reaching the cortex, relative to the normal eye. This delay in time between the two eyes is interpreted by the cortex as a separation in space, creating the stereo-illusion. The movement is always perceived as toward the diseased eye, i.e., right eye, counterclockwise and left eye, clockwise. Affected patients may report difficulty with driving, walking, or tasks in the household utilizing stereopsis.[32] Treatment may consist of placing a filter in front of the normal eye.[32] The Pulfrich phenomenon is only infrequently seen in patients with decreased vision due to media opacities or retinal disease.

Visual fields

The hallmark of an optic neuropathy is an abnormal visual field. Concepts of visual field testing and the various types and their advantages and disadvantages are discussed in Chapter 3. Patients with optic neuropathy have visual field defects that generally fall into three different categories. These are (1) generalized constriction, (2) central defects, and (3) nerve fiber bundle defects:

Generalized constriction. This type of field defect (**Fig. 5–4**) is the least specific and the hardest to localize. In these patients, kinetic perimetry shows reduced size of the peripheral isopters, and on automated perimetry peripheral rim defects are seen with a general reduction in sensitivity. The examiner must be careful in interpreting fields with generalized constriction as there are many non-neuro-ophthalmic causes of this type of defect including media opacities, small pupils, poor patient cooperation, retinal degenerations, and non-organic visual loss. However, diffuse suppression of the visual field on automated perimetry is in fact the most common defect in patients with optic neuritis.[33]

Central defects. These include central scotomas, paracentral defects, and centrocecal scotomas (**Fig. 5–4**). These three types of visual fields are related and imply involvement of the central portion of the optic nerve. Centrocecal scotomas are common defects in patients with hereditary, nutritional, and toxic optic neuropathies, but can be seen in any of the optic neuropathies. Any patient who has reduced central visual acuity must have a central scotoma by definition, although such defects are not always measurable on perimetry. Central field defects are also the rule in patients with macular disease.

Nerve fiber bundle defects. The third category includes arcuate defects, altitudinal defects, and nasal steps (**Fig. 5–4**). These defects, as they are so named, imply a localization to a particular group of nerve fibers. In general, they respect the horizontal meridian because of the anatomic boundary of the horizontal raphe. These field defects occasionally may also respect the vertical meridian, but this finding should be considered atypical, and patients with such fields should be investigated for the possibility of intracranial disease (see Chapter 7). The nerve fiber bundle types of visual field defects can be seen in all of the different optic neuropathies, but certain patterns are more frequent. For instance, altitudinal defects are the most common defects in ischemic optic neuropathy. In general, visual field defects will help to confirm the presence of an optic neuropathy but will not be diagnostic of a specific etiology.

Ophthalmoscopy

Optic disc appearance. The normal optic nerve (**Fig. 5–5**) has a pinkish, orange color with sharp margins.[34] The nerve fiber layer is best seen at the 6 and 12 o'clock position where it is thickest. A central cup is identifiable and the vessels can be seen clearly as they cross the margin of the disc. The normal optic disc area varies between 2.1 and 2.8 mm^2.[34] Highly myopic eyes (> −8.00) may have abnormally large discs, while highly hyperopic eyes (> +4.00) may have abnormally small discs.[35]

Disc swelling. Optic neuropathies are frequently associated with disc swelling or edema. The term papilledema is used only for discs that are swollen from elevated intracranial pressure. Ophthalmoscopic features of a swollen optic nerve include hyperemia, elevation of the optic nerve head, and edema of the nerve fiber layer blurring the disc margins. The cup may be obliterated, and there may be associated retinal or choroidal folds. There may be venous dilation, associated splinter hemorrhages, dilated capillaries, exudates, or cotton-wool spots. Swollen optic nerves resulting from anterior visual pathway compressive lesions may have features that suggest chronicity (absence of hemorrhages, pseudodrusen from axoplasmic stasis, pallor) or collateral vessels from retinal to ciliary circulation ("shunt vessels").

Disc atrophy or pallor. Although this technically implies a histopathologic diagnosis, the term optic atrophy is often substituted for the ophthalmoscopic observation of optic nerve head pallor or loss of pinkness which commonly accompanies permanent damage to the optic nerve. A combination of the loss of the superficial capillary bed along with the loss of tissue volume and astrocytic proliferation is responsible for this change in optic nerve head color. Reduced blood flow to the optic nerve head has been demonstrated by fluorescein angiography[36] and direct blood flow measurements.[37] When using the term optic atrophy, the examiner is identifying ganglion cell death, not reduction or involution of function as the term atrophy applies in other conditions. Atrophy can be graded as mild to severe and may

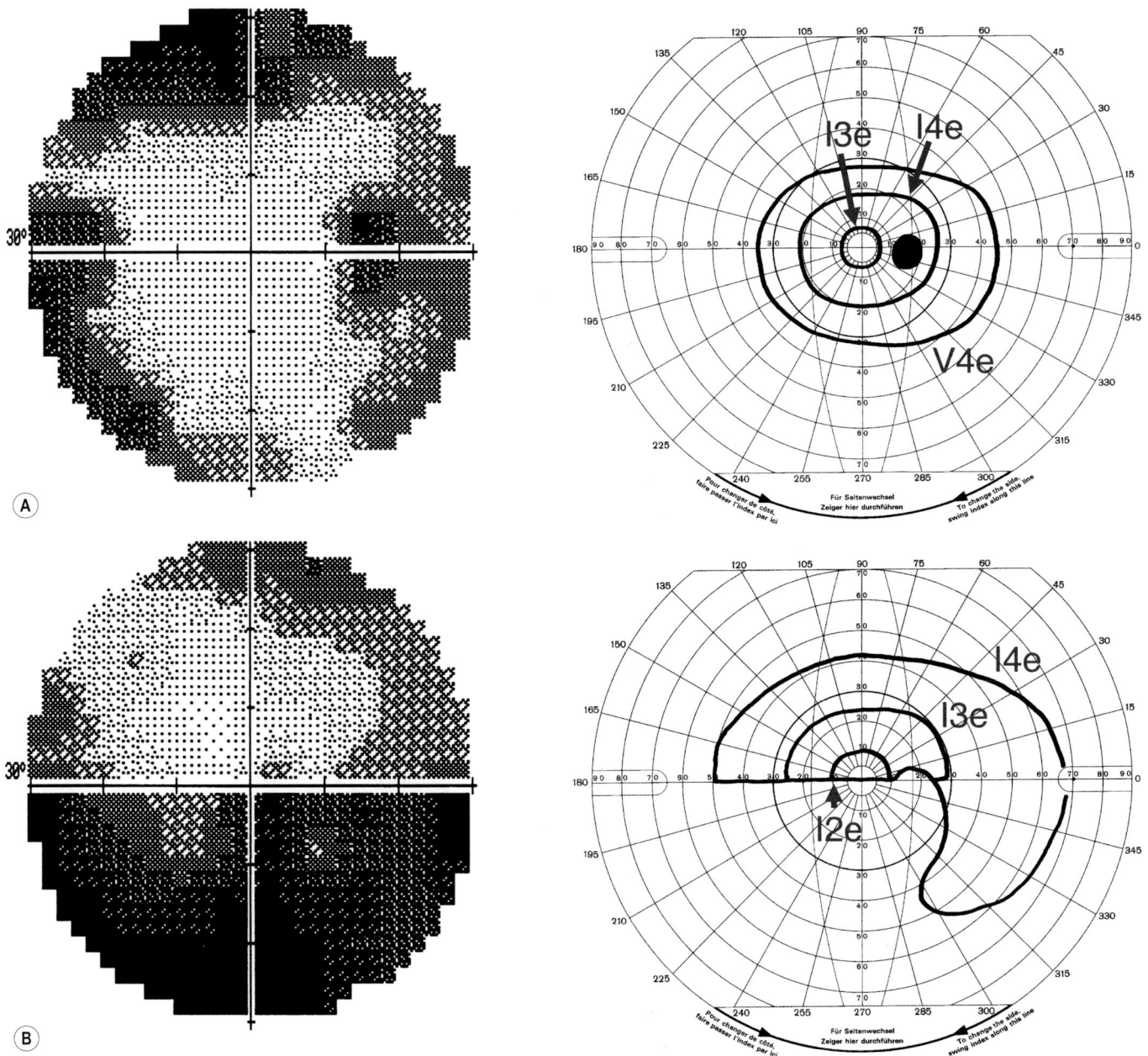

Figure 5–4. Paired examples of static threshold perimetry gray-scale (left) and kinetic perimetry visual fields (right) seen in optic neuropathies. Note the threshold and kinetic perimeters have different scales. The first pair of fields (**A**) demonstrate generalized constriction which is the least specific, and hardest to localize, type of visual field defect. It can also be seen with media opacities or retinal disease or simply from slow reactions during testing. Altitudinal (**B**), nasal step (**C**, note the incomplete connection to the blind spot), and arcuate (**D**) defects are characteristic of optic neuropathies and represent nerve fiber bundle defects. Central scotomas (**E**) and centrocecal defects (**F**, central defects attached to the blindspot) are also commonly seen with optic neuropathies.

take on a characteristic pattern (altitudinal, sectoral, bow tie, or temporal), which can be a clue to disease pathogenesis or localization. For instance, superior sectoral atrophy might be associated with inferior field loss. Not infrequently, optic atrophy is accompanied by cupping. This may simply be a normal evolution of appearance or may reflect a defective structural integrity of the optic nerve in the setting of atrophy.[26,38]

Primary optic atrophy occurs without significant swelling or reactive gliosis. Secondary atrophy implies previous swelling and subsequent gliotic reaction which accompanies the nerve atrophy. In the former (primary optic atrophy) the disc pallor is associated with sharp disc margins and easily visible details on the disc surface and vasculature (**Fig. 5–6**). Most patients (even those with some swelling initially) with acute optic neuropathies later develop primary optic atrophy. In the latter case (secondary optic atrophy) there is a haze to the disc surface or overlying nerve fiber layer which obscures the disc margin and the ophthalmoscopic view of the disc's surface details (**Fig. 5–7**). The typical setting for secondary optic atrophy is atrophic papilledema (see Chapter 6), compressive optic neuropathy with prior disc edema, or severe

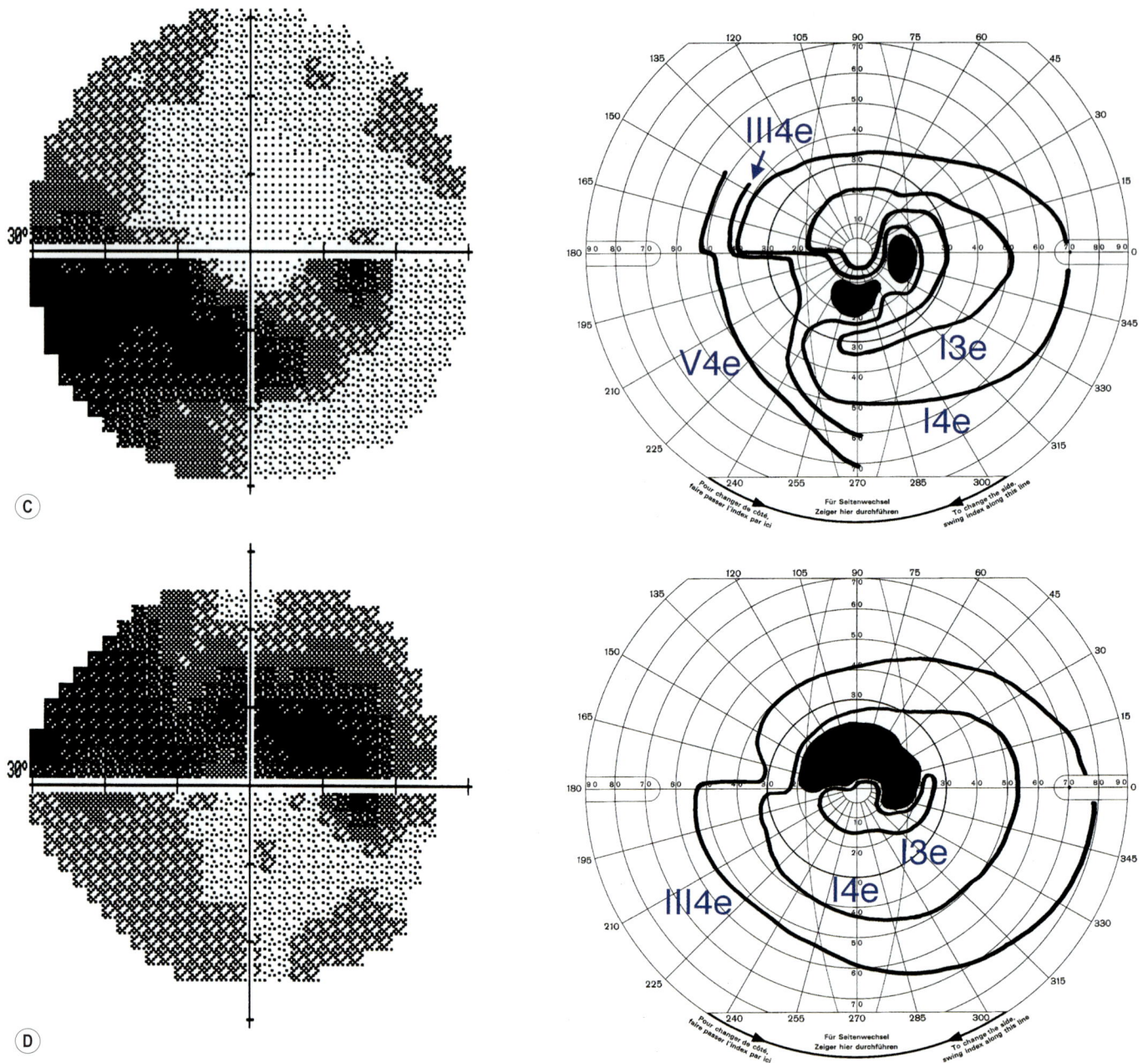

Figure 5–4. *Continued*

inflammatory disc edema. In some cases, pallor of the disc might not yet be evident but the examiner can identify defects in the nerve fiber layer. In this setting there is a sharp cut-off from the normal-appearing nerve fibers to an area with an absence of fibers (**Fig. 5–8**). These defects can be more easily seen with red free light (**Fig. 5–8**), and an alternating "rake-like" pattern of normal and defective nerve fibers may be observed.

Related retinal lesions. When the disc is swollen, other fundus findings may aid in the diagnosis. For instance, dilated and tortuous retinal veins accompanied by retinal hemorrhages suggests a retinal vein occlusion, while macular lipid deposition suggests neuroretinitis. When the disc is normal, the examiner should be absolutely certain a macular lesion is not mimicking an optic neuropathy.

Slit-lamp examination

Other causes of visual acuity loss, such as corneal, lens, or vitreous opacities, should be excluded. The presence of iritis or uveitis would suggest an inflammatory disorder.

Nerve fiber layer imaging

Recently, various imaging modalities have become popular to evaluate the nerve fiber layer in patients with optic neuropathy. These techniques include (1) ocular coherence tomography (OCT), which is based on imaging of reflected light; (2) scanning laser tomography (SLT, e.g., Heidelberg retina tomograph), which is based on confocal scanning illumina-

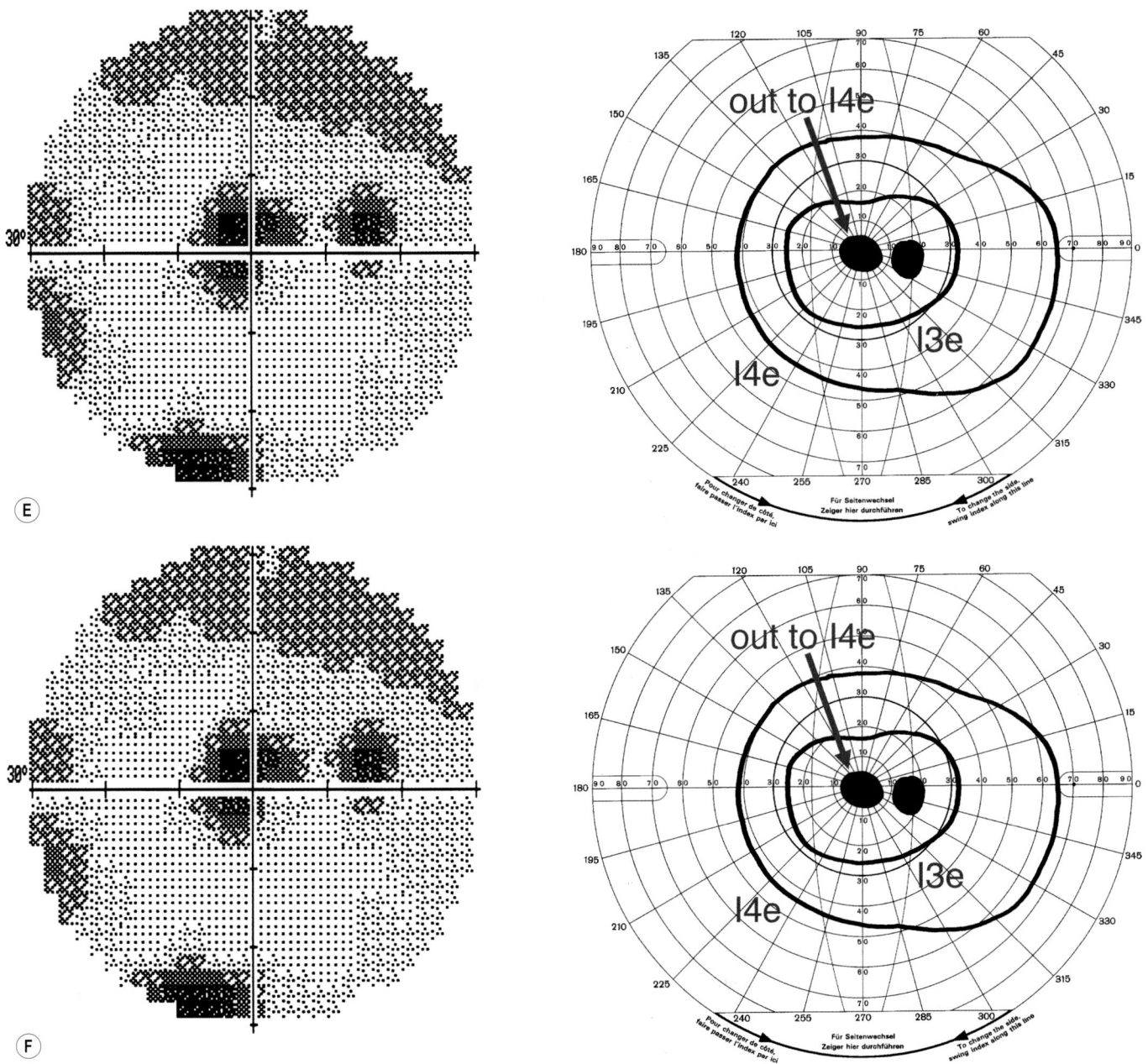

Figure 5–4. *Continued*

tion using near infrared diode laser and imaging; and (3) scanning laser polarimetry (GDx nerve fiber layer analyzer), in which a confocal scanning laser ophthalmoscope and integrated polarimeter quantitatively evaluate the retinal nerve fiber layer based on the birefringence of the microtubules in the retinal ganglion cell axons. These methodologies have been firmly established in the field of glaucoma to follow the thickness of the nerve fiber layer around the disc. Recently, the use of these instruments, particularly OCT, has become popular in neuro-ophthalmic practice to identify and localize disease to the optic nerve head (**Fig. 5–9**) and follow patients with various progressive optic neuropathies. OCT can also be very helpful in evaluating patients with unexplained central vision loss and possible maculopathy (see Chapter 4).

Approach to patients with optic neuropathy

When the history and examination are typical of optic neuropathy (visual acuity and color vision loss, decreased contrast sensitivity, afferent pupillary defect, and typical visual field defect), four different diagnostic groups should be considered, based upon the ophthalmoscopic appearance of the disc: *anomalous, swollen, normal,* and *pale.* Clinically, there is considerable overlap among these four groups of patients although we believe distinguishing between them serves as a useful framework when considering the differential diagnoses of an optic neuropathy. For instance, patients with anterior ischemic optic neuropathy always have abnormally

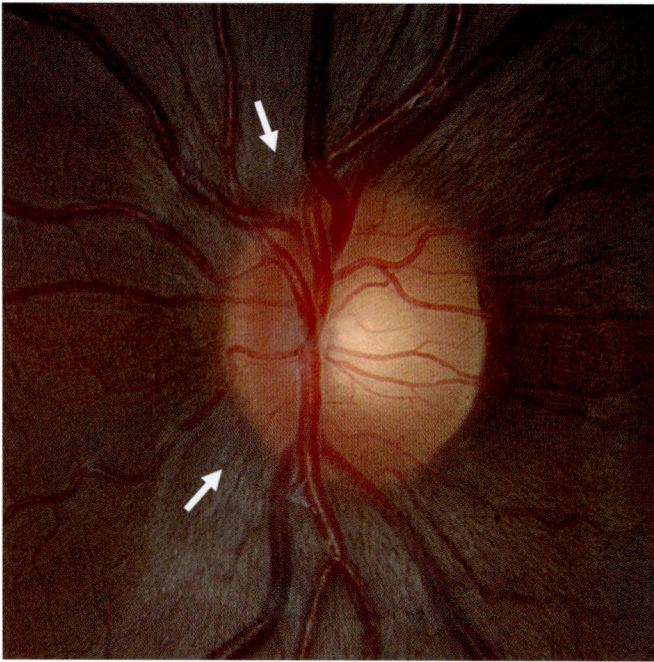

Figure 5–5. The normal-appearing optic nerve. Margins are sharp and color is diffusely pink. Nerve fiber striations are seen best at the 10 to 12 o'clock and 6 to 8 o'clock positions just beyond the disc edge (arrows). Despite this, the vessels are clearly seen traversing the nerve fiber layer and are not obscured by these fibers.

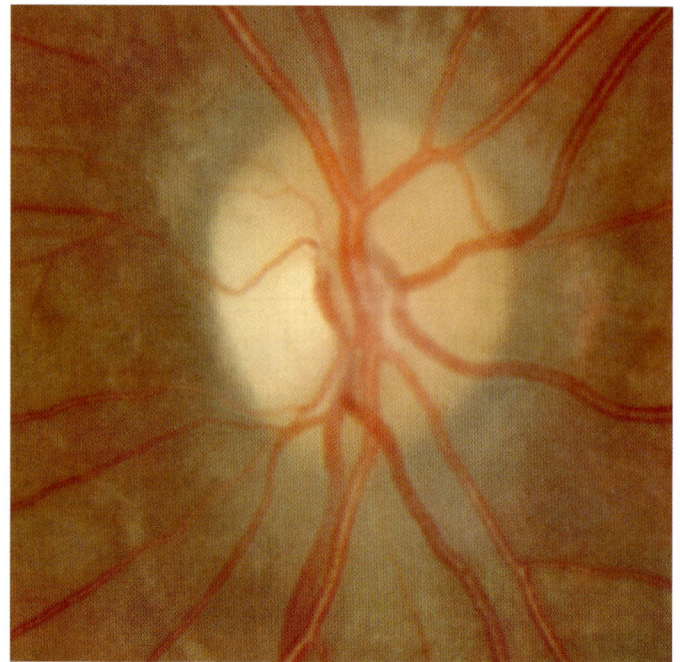

Figure 5–7. Secondary optic atrophy (developing after disc swelling). As with primary atrophy, the disc is pale but there is haziness to the area of the disc margin from previous swelling and reactive gliosis.

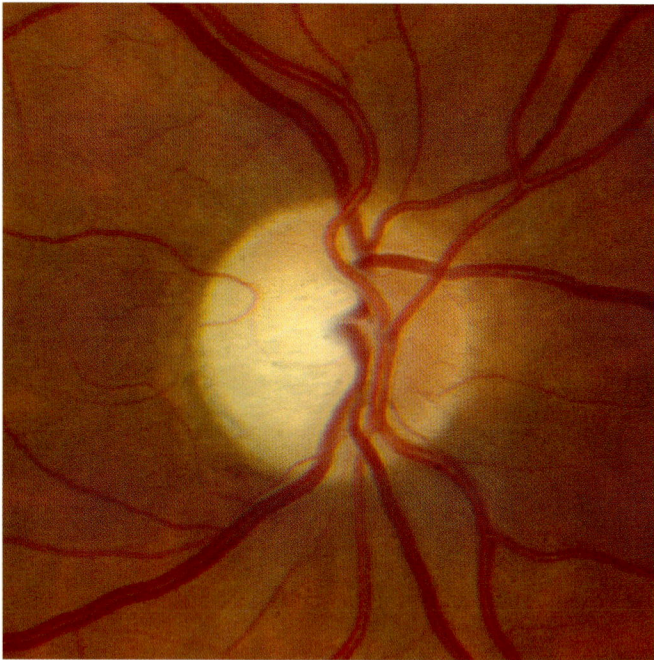

Figure 5–6. Primary optic atrophy. The disc shows temporal pallor and has sharp, distinct margins.

Table 5–1 Congenital disc anomalies

Optic nerve hypoplasia
Tilted discs
Optic pits
Optic disc colobomas
Morning glory disc anomaly
Staphyloma
Pseudopapilledema
Optic disc drusen
Myelinated retinal nerve fibers

and the rest of the examination to make the correct diagnosis.

Anomalous discs

These are due to congenital anomalies, and they are listed in **Table 5–1**.

Swollen optic nerves

Table 5–2 lists optic neuropathies that may present with disc swelling. The most common diagnoses to consider here are anterior ischemic optic neuropathy and optic neuritis. Patients with anterior ischemic optic neuropathy will generally be older with vasculopathic risk factors such as diabetes and hypertension. Those with optic neuritis are typically younger and often have periocular pain exacerbated by eye movements.

Papilledema or disc edema from elevated intracranial pressure is discussed elsewhere (Chapter 6) but it is important to note the relative mismatch between the amount of

appearing (swollen) optic nerves, and occult compressive lesions are important to consider in the setting of visual loss and a normal fundus. The appearance of congenital disc anomalies are usually distinct. However, when the disc is swollen, normal, or atrophic, usually the examiner will have to rely heavily on the clinical presentation, historical details,

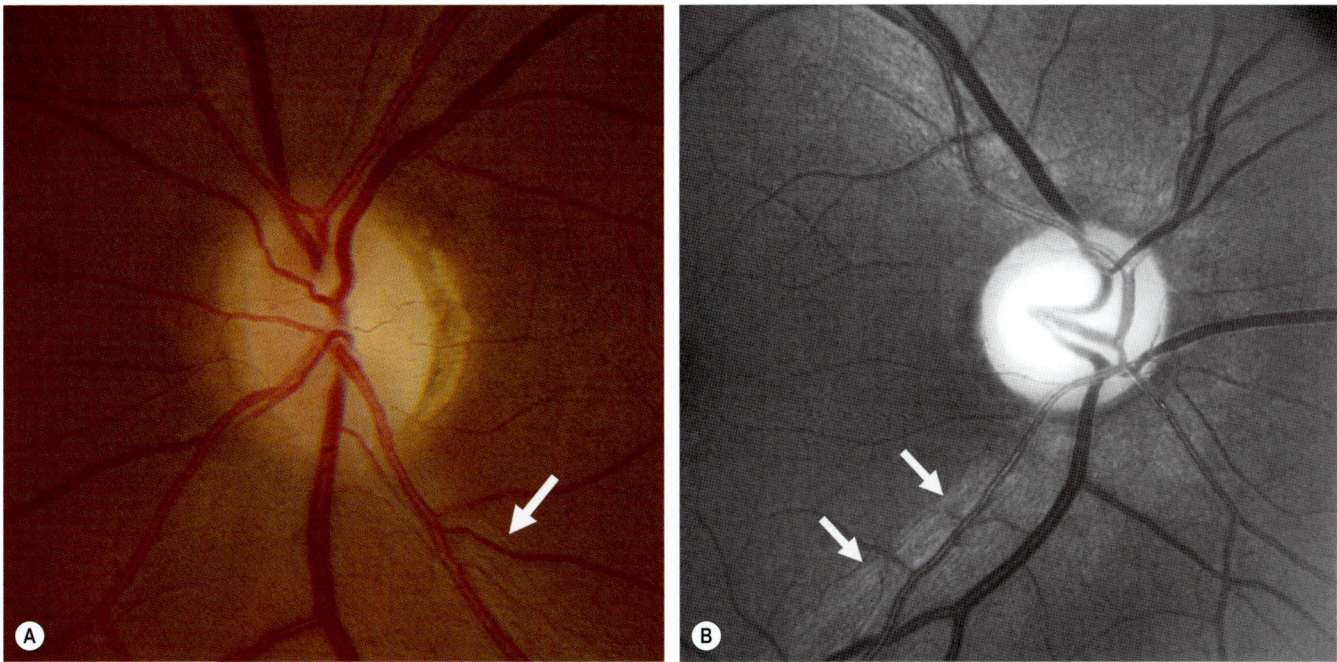

Figure 5–8. A. Left optic nerve with minimal temporal pallor and a sharp cut-off in the nerve fiber layer demarcating corresponding loss of ganglion cell axons entering the temporal aspect of the disc. The arrow delineates the beginning of the normal nerve fibers. **B**. Red free photograph of right eye of a different patient demonstrates optic disc pallor with nerve fiber layer defect (arrows). The area of normal striations of the nerve fibers abruptly begins (arrows).

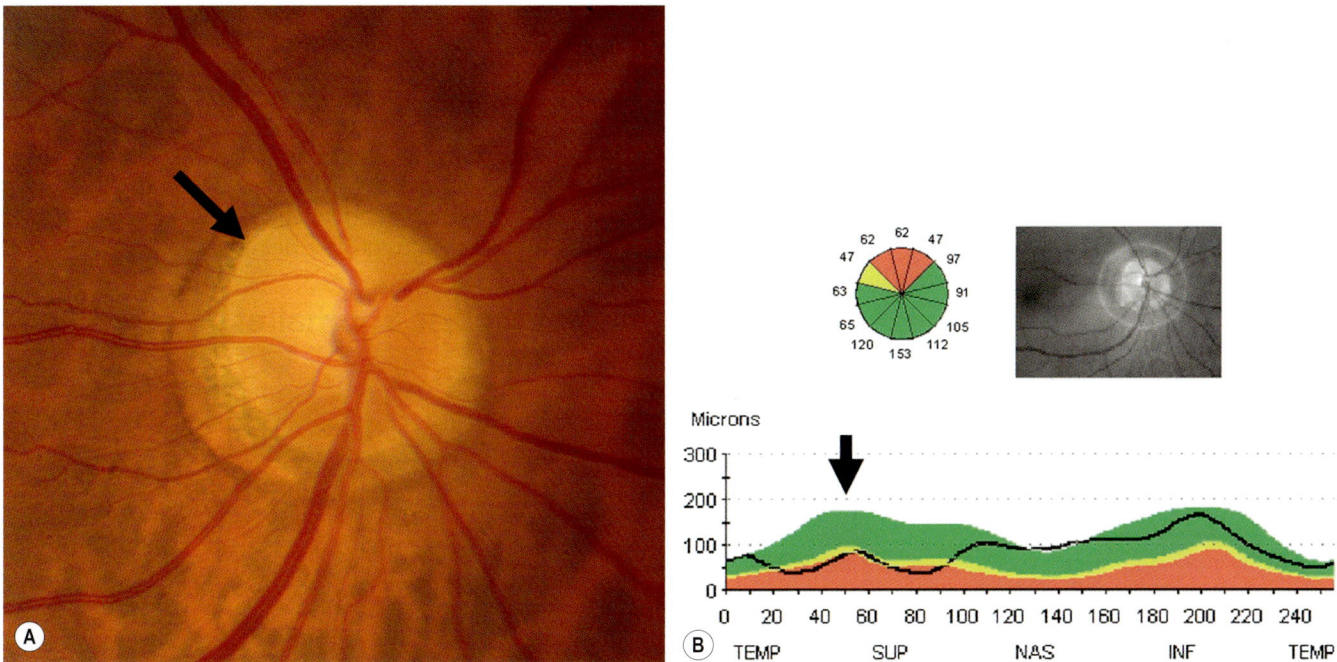

Figure 5–9. Ocular coherence tomography (OCT) in the evaluation of the nerve fiber layer (NFL). This patient had a history of ischemic optic neuropathy with inferior field loss. **A**. Photo of the disc shows only mild pallor (arrow) but (**B**) OCT nicely demonstrates NFL thinning superiorly (black arrow).

disc swelling and visual function in papilledema. A markedly swollen optic nerve with relatively preserved visual acuity is the hallmark of papilledema in its early stages. Acuity loss and central field defects would be more characteristic of optic neuropathy.

In more rare circumstances other features of the examination will help to identify the cause of the swollen disc with vision loss. The presence of vitritis would suggest the possibility of infectious disc swelling as in syphilitic uveitis with optic neuropathy. The presence of a macular star makes neuroretinitis the most likely diagnosis. Other infiltrative conditions such as leukemia might be associated with retinal hemorrhages or a distinct mass in the optic nerve head.

Table 5–2 Common causes of optic neuropathies that can present with disc swelling

Idiopathic optic neuritis
Anterior ischemic optic neuropathy
Diabetic papillopathy
Optic nerve tumors
  Optic nerve glioma
  Optic nerve sheath meningioma
Inflammatory optic neuropathies
  Sarcoidosis
  Optic perineuritis
Infectious optic neuropathies
  Syphilitic optic neuropathy
  Lyme-associated optic neuropathy
Radiation optic neuropathy
Toxic optic neuropathy
  Amiodarone associated, e.g., infiltrative optic neuropathy
  Lymphoma/leukemia
  Metastatic tumor
Uveitis-associated optic neuropathy
Acute and chronic papilledema

Table 5–3 Acute optic neuropathies that commonly present with normal-appearing optic nerves (retrobulbar optic neuropathies)

Optic neuritis
Traumatic optic neuropathy
Compressive optic neuropathy (early)
Posterior ischemic optic neuropathy
Radiation optic neuropathy

Normal-appearing optic nerves

In retrobulbar optic neuropathies, the normal fundus appearance acutely implies that the disease process is occurring in the optic nerve behind the lamina cribrosa in its intraorbital, intracanalicular, or intracranial portions. Entities that can commonly present with a normal-appearing fundus are listed in **Table 5–3**. The examiner should be aware of overlap in certain conditions, such as optic neuritis, in which one-third of patients will have a swollen optic nerve head; Leber's hereditary optic neuropathy, in which the nerve can have a pseudoswollen appearance; or radiation-induced optic neuropathy, in which stigmata of radiation retinopathy may be present and/or the optic nerve may be acutely swollen. Whenever the optic nerve appears normal in a suspected optic neuropathy the macular region should be carefully examined. Chapter 4 contains a discussion of the differentiation between optic neuropathy and maculopathy.

Optic disc pallor

Optic atrophy (disc pallor) may be evident on the initial examination or can evolve on subsequent evaluations. All of the conditions listed in **Tables 5–2** and **5–3**, when associated with permanent visual dysfunction, will be accompanied ultimately by the development of optic atrophy. In this setting the examiner will identify a history of a previous episode consistent with the clinical picture; for example, a

Table 5–4 Optic neuropathies commonly presenting with optic disc pallor at initial evaluation

Compressive optic neuropathy
Toxic/nutritional optic neuropathy
Infectious (syphilitic) optic neuropathy
Hereditary (dominant) optic atrophy

previous inflammatory, ischemic, or traumatic injury to the optic nerve. In some instances, patients become suddenly aware of their visual loss at a time after the process began (pseudosudden onset), and their initial examination will reveal optic atrophy. Entities which commonly present in this fashion are listed in **Table 5–4**. Most importantly, chronic progressive visual loss accompanied by disc pallor strongly suggests a compressive lesion. Thus, in patients with unexplained optic atrophy, neuroimaging is the most important diagnostic test. Other laboratory testing, such as serologies, vitamin levels, or genetic evaluation, should be guided by historical and examination findings.[39]

Rarely, some individuals with long-standing, "stable" visual loss from a distant history of optic atrophy due to a childhood neoplasm, for instance, may later in adulthood experience gradual visual loss not due to tumor recurrence or any other obvious cause. This phenomenon has been attributed to normal age-related axonal loss in an individual with an already compromised optic nerve.[40] Similar observations have been made in patients with congenital disc anomalies.[41]

In summary, in most cases of suspected optic neuropathy, careful consideration of historical details, general examination, and the ophthalmoscopic appearance of the optic nerve head will lead to the correct diagnosis long before any ancillary tests are ordered. The specific optic neuropathies will now be discussed in greater detail.

Congenital disc anomalies

In this category are included a variety of disorders (**Table 5–1**) whose hallmark is an abnormal-appearing optic nerve, each with a pathognomonic or distinct "diagnostic appearance." These anomalies take many different forms, and generally for the congenital condition represent an embryologic mishap with resulting malformation. Congenital optic disc anomalies account for about 15% of severe visual impairment in children.[42] Occasionally, systemic associations will be identified to point the examiner to the correct optic nerve anomaly. The importance of treating superimposed amblyopia and the high prevalence of systemic abnormalities in these patients make it critically important to identify these patients.[43]

The level of visual loss associated with congenital disc anomalies ranges from minimal visual dysfunction to total blindness. In children, the most common ophthalmic presentation of a unilateral disc anomaly is strabismus (usually sensory eso- or exotropia), while those with bilateral disc anomalies more frequently present at a young age with poor vision or nystagmus.[43,44] In some adults, a routine eye examination may demonstrate acuity or visual field abnormalities, and the fundus examination will disclose the previously unrecognized disc anomaly. Many such patients are unaware of long-standing defects or arbitrarily ascribe visual problems to a childhood "lazy eye," for example. Some patients with congenital anomalies will become acutely aware of their visual deficit, confusing the examiner since the visual field defect, by its nature, must have predated the onset of the symptomatic awareness of reduced vision. Usually the visual deficit is static. However, it is important to recognize that some congenital or developmental abnormalities rarely may be associated with newly acquired vision loss. For example, macular detachment may complicate a congenital optic pit or optic disc drusen may be associated with anterior ischemic optic neuropathy.

Hypoplasia

Characterized ophthalmoscopically by an optic disc with a small diameter (**Fig. 5–10**), optic nerve hypoplasia (ONH) is a variable condition that can be associated with either minimal or marked visual dysfunction. Hypoplasia can be unilateral or bilateral, and may or may not be associated with a more widespread neurologic developmental disorder.[45] This is the most common congenital optic nerve abnormality, representing 47% of patients with congenital disc abnormalities in one series.[43] Embryologically, the reduced number of functioning axons may result from the exaggeration of a normal developmental process. That is, early on, at 16–17 weeks, there are approximately 3 million optic nerve axons which ultimately are reduced to approximately one million at the time of birth. Hypoplasia may

therefore be an overdone, but normal, process of involution.[46]

Affected patients can have any level of visual function ranging from minimal acuity or field loss to no light perception (NLP), and bilateral ONH is more common than unilateral cases.[43,45,47] Severe reduction in disc diameter on the fundus examination is often simple to identify, particularly when unilateral and comparison with the normal eye can be made. However, when mild this finding may be subtle and hard to recognize, and sometimes the loss of nerve fiber layer is best viewed using red-free light during ophthalmoscopy.[48] Because the examination in young infants may be difficult, the diagnosis of a mild degree of hypoplasia in this age group can be extremely problematic and can often be made only subjectively. The appearance of hypoplastic nerves can be quite variable, and the key to making the diagnosis is identifying the true edge of the optic nerve (**Fig. 5–10**). In general, more severely hypoplastic nerves are associated with poorer vision,[49] because a smaller disc has fewer ganglion cell axons passing through it. Classically, but seen only in a minority of cases, there is a ring of visible sclera and pigmentation surrounding the optic nerve. This creates a peripapillary halo, or the so-called "double-ring sign" (**Fig. 5–10**).[50] One study[51] suggested that ONH associated with tortuosity of the retinal veins might be a marker of endocrinopathy (see below). Magnetic resonance (MR) imaging frequently demonstrates reduced cross-sectional area of the optic nerves[52] and chiasm. In addition, rarely, the optic nerves fail to form at all in a condition known as *optic nerve aplasia*[53,54] (**Fig. 5–11**). Aplasia may be uni- or bilateral, and in monocular cases is often associated in the

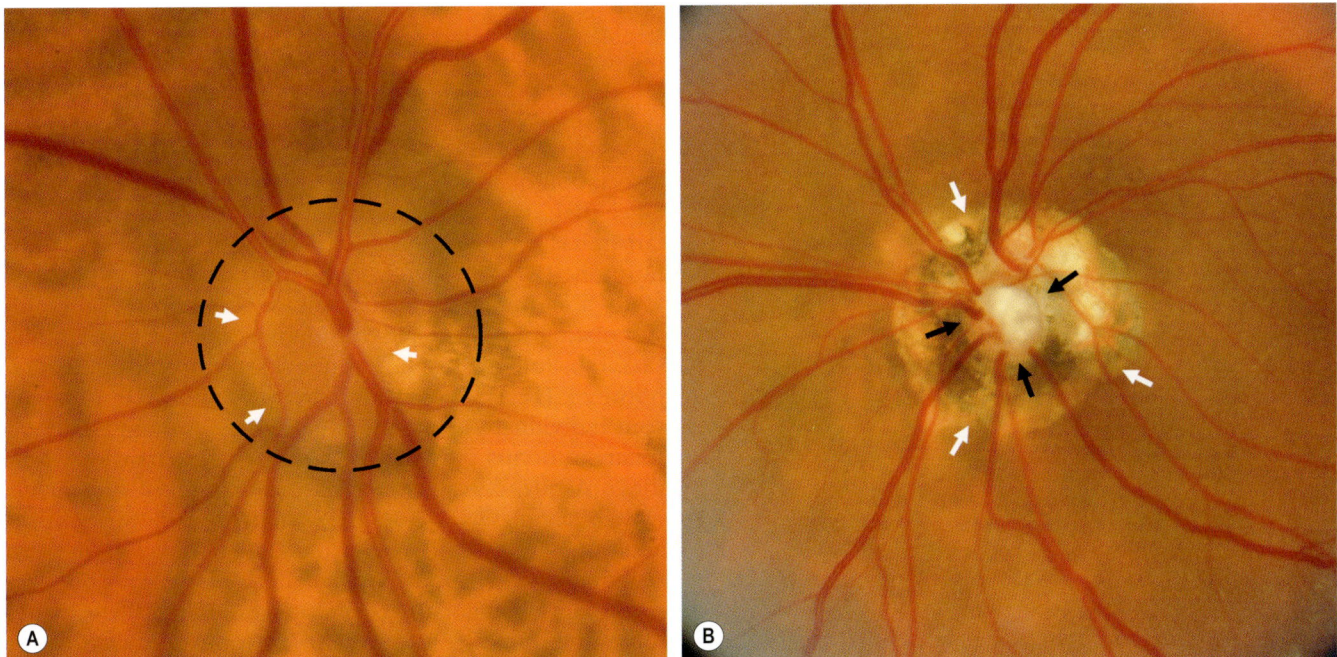

Figure 5–10. The optic nerve hypoplasia spectrum. **A**. Mild hypoplasia appreciated when comparing the size of the optic nerve head with the caliber of the retinal vessels (see Fig. 5–5 for normal ratio). The edge of the hypoplastic nerve is marked by the small arrows. The black dashed line approximates the size of a normal optic nerve. The nerve is about one-half of the normal size when judged by the vessels, which are of normal caliber. **B**. More severe optic nerve hypoplasia (black arrows on nerve edge) accompanied by peripapillary pigmentary abnormalities and anomalous "spoke-like" take-off of the retinal vessels. The classic double ring sign is present and is the result of the white ring of visible bare sclera (white arrows) bordered by the pigment epithelium that surrounds the optic nerve.

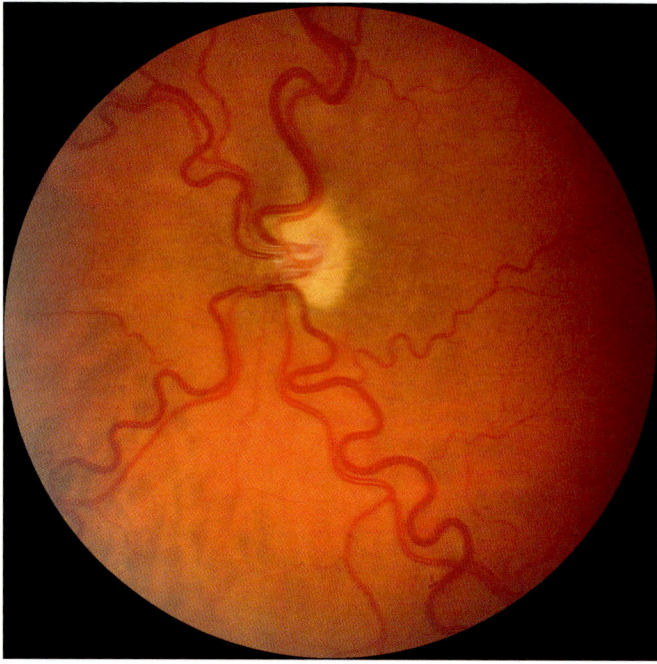

Figure 5–11. Aplasia of the optic nerve with no normal disc tissue seen, and only retinal vessels pass through small scleral opening. Marked tortuosity of the retinal veins and arteries is seen.

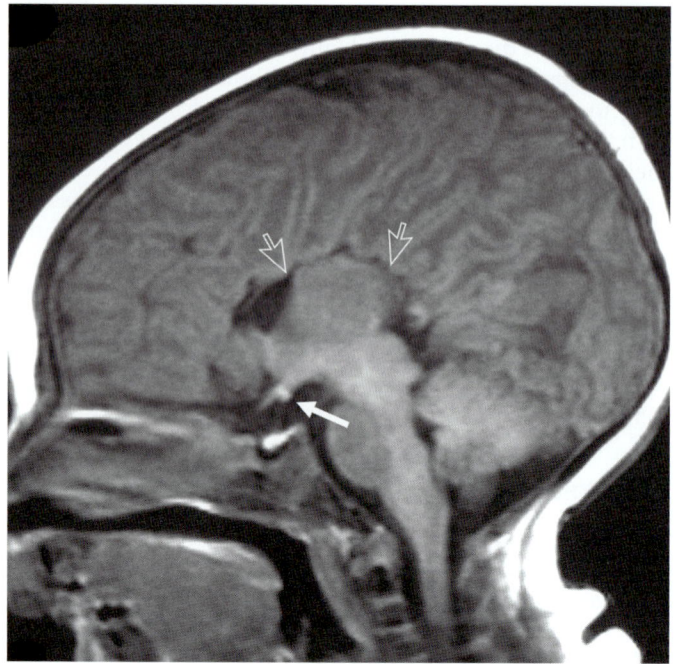

Figure 5–12. Absence of the septum pellucidum (asterisk in single midline ventricle) in septo-optic dysplasia demonstrated on a coronal T1-weighted MRI. Also note the chiasm (arrow) is extremely thin. For comparison with figures of normal suprasellar structures see Chapter 7.

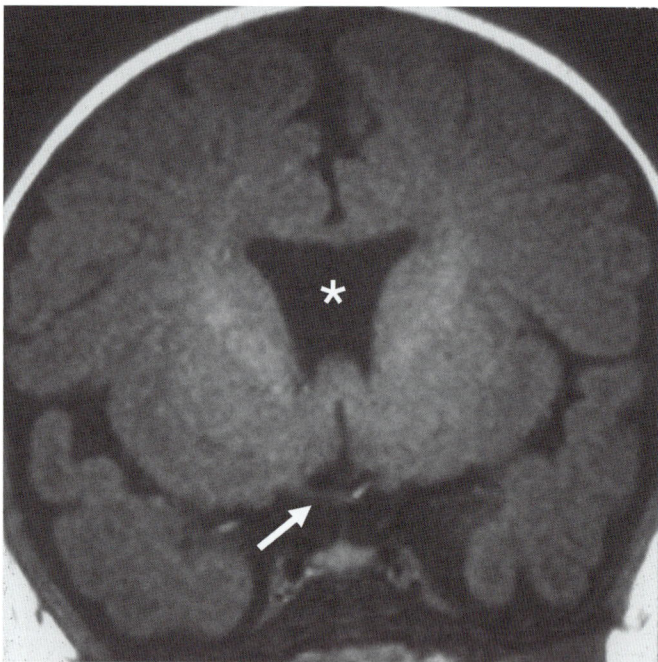

Figure 5–13. Ectopic pituitary (solid arrow), at the area of increased signal intensity at the tuber cinereum, and agenesis of the corpus callosum (open arrows point to the area where the corpus callosum is normally situated) in septo-optic dysplasia demonstrated on a sagittal T1-weighted unenhanced MRI. For comparison with figures of normal suprasellar structures see Chapter 7.

same eye with microphthalmos in an otherwise healthy individual.[55]

Associated features. ONH may occur in isolation or in combination with other midline developmental abnormalities which share the same embryologic forebrain derivation. In *deMorsier syndrome*, or septo-optic dysplasia, ONH is associated with absence of the septum pellucidum (**Fig. 5–12**).

In one series of 68 patients with ONH, 30 were found to have an absent or abnormal septum pellucidum.[56] A dysgenetic, thin, or absent corpus callosum may also be seen in this disorder. The condition likely has a genetic etiology with environmental factors altering the penetrance and phenotype. Abnormalities in the developmental genes, HEX1 and SOX2 and SOX3, have been identified in several pedigrees.[57–65]

In addition, in 1970 Hoyt and colleagues[66] reported the association of septo-optic dysplasia and pituitary dwarfism. Since then, the symptom complex of ONH and hypopituitarism has been well recognized and well studied.[67] Growth hormone (GH) deficiency is the most common endocrinologic abnormality, but decreased secretion of thyroid-stimulating hormone (TSH), adrenocorticotropic hormone (ACTH), luteinizing hormone (LH), follicle-stimulating hormone (FSH), and antidiuretic hormone (ADH) may be seen individually or in combination.[68,69] Although hypopituitarism occurs only in a minority of patients with ONH, the consequences can be devastating. In one series of patients with bilateral ONH,[70] 11.5% had panhypopituitarism. In addition, at least five cases of sudden death have been reported,[71] each attributed to the effects of corticotropin deficiency, thermoregulatory disturbances, and diabetes insipidus. The presence of posterior ectopic pituitary tissue, usually seen as an abnormal area of hyperintensity at or near the tuber cinereum on T1-weighted magnetic resonance imaging (MRI) (**Fig. 5–13**)[72] or absence of the normal posterior pituitary bright spot, correlates highly with hypopituitarism.[73] In one purported mechanism,[44] posterior pituitary ectopia is attributed to a perinatal insult to the hypophyseal portal system, resulting in necrosis of the infundibulum. However, other authors have suggested an earlier dysembryogenesis of the developing optic nerves and pituitary stalk.[74]

Septo-optic dysplasia is also associated with schizencephaly, a cortical migrational abnormality producing cerebral clefts extending from and including the ventricular lining to the cortical surface (**Fig. 5–14**). Schizencephaly may manifest clinically with developmental delay, contralateral hemiparesis, and seizures.[75] Kuban et al.[76] have suggested that the combination of septo-optic dysplasia and schizencephaly may result from a perinatal insult at or around the sixth week of embryogenesis, at which time cerebral morphogenesis, development of the eye, and delineation of the lamina terminalis, which forms the septum pellucidum, take place.

Other associated cortical migrational abnormalities seen in association with ONH include cortical heterotopias, polymicrogyria, and pachygyria.[72,77] Cortical migrational and corpus callosum abnormalities tend to correlate with developmental delay and neurological symptoms such as seizures.[56,78–80] Olfactory tract and bulb hypoplasia also have been reported with ONH.[81]

A wide variety of congenital ocular syndromes have been recognized to occur with ONH.[43,47] These include: persistent hyperplastic primary vitreous (PHPV),[82] colobomas, Duane syndrome, albinism, aniridia, Goldenhar syndrome, Aicardi syndrome, hemifacial atrophy, Klippel–Trenauney–Weber syndrome, microphthalmos, and blepharophimosis.[83] ONH may also occur in association with congenital suprasellar

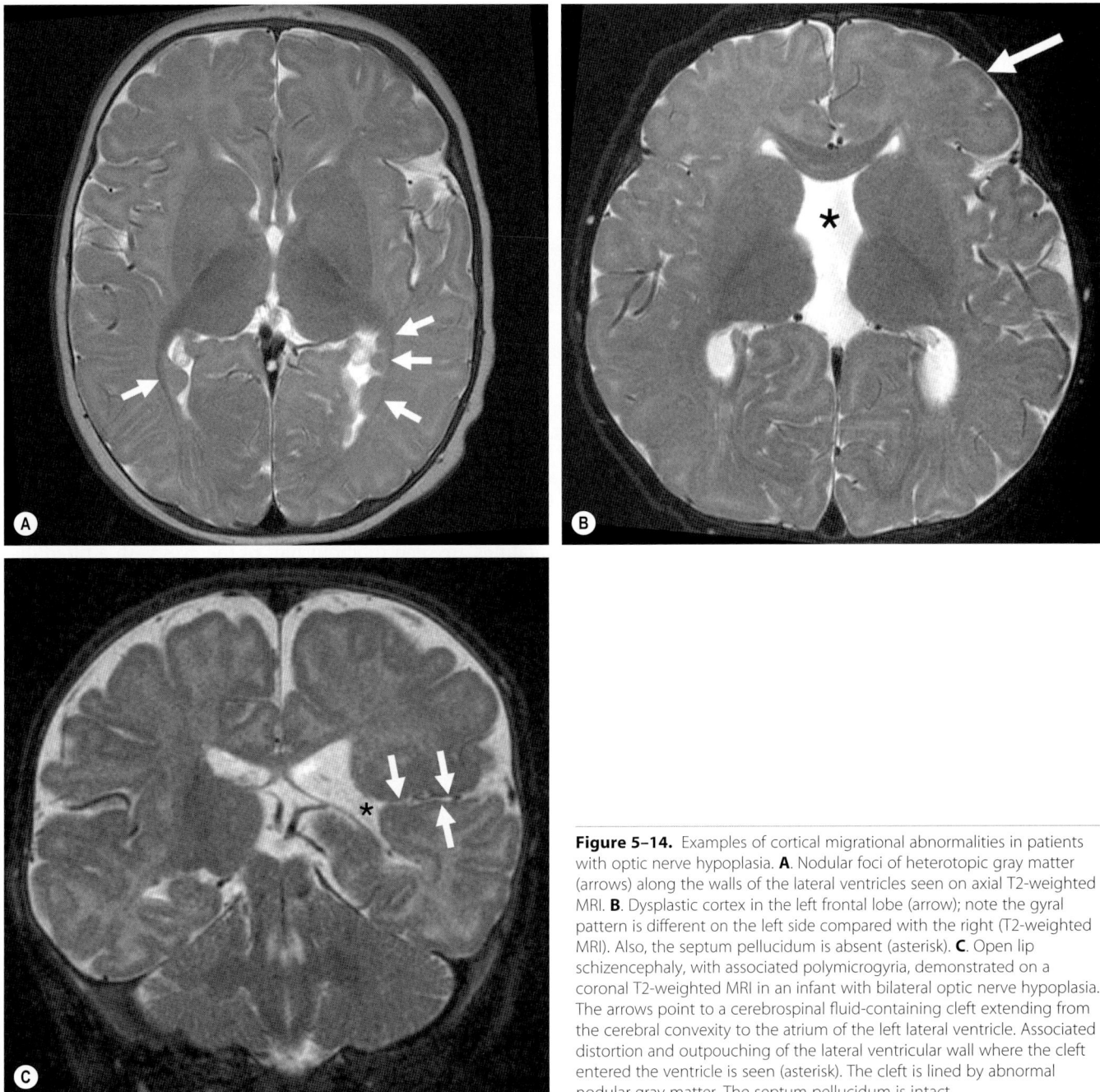

Figure 5–14. Examples of cortical migrational abnormalities in patients with optic nerve hypoplasia. **A**. Nodular foci of heterotopic gray matter (arrows) along the walls of the lateral ventricles seen on axial T2-weighted MRI. **B**. Dysplastic cortex in the left frontal lobe (arrow); note the gyral pattern is different on the left side compared with the right (T2-weighted MRI). Also, the septum pellucidum is absent (asterisk). **C**. Open lip schizencephaly, with associated polymicrogyria, demonstrated on a coronal T2-weighted MRI in an infant with bilateral optic nerve hypoplasia. The arrows point to a cerebrospinal fluid-containing cleft extending from the cerebral convexity to the atrium of the left lateral ventricle. Associated distortion and outpouching of the lateral ventricular wall where the cleft entered the ventricle is seen (asterisk). The cleft is lined by abnormal nodular gray matter. The septum pellucidum is intact.

tumors such as craniopharyngiomas, chiasmal/hypothalamic gliomas,[84] and teratomas.[85] The mechanism in these cases is thought to be tumor compression of the visual pathways early in life, precluding normal optic nerve development. ONH has also been recognized as a consequence of maternal use of alcohol (fetal alcohol syndrome), cocaine, phenytoin, and lysergic acid diethylamide (LSD), and reported in association with mitochondrial disorders.[86]

Evaluation. In all young children, because the new diagnosis of ONH has several potential ophthalmologic, neurologic, developmental, and endocrinologic implications, a thorough clinical and radiological assessment is mandated. Pediatric ophthalmologic evaluations are necessary for assessment and management of possible visual impairment, amblyopia, refractive error, nystagmus, and strabismus. Some authors[87] have previously suggested neuroradiologic and endocrinologic evaluations only in children with bilateral ONH and poor vision. However, Brodsky and Glasier's[72] careful clinical–radiologic study demonstrated that some children with unilateral ONH, who seem normal otherwise, may have absence of the septum pellucidum or posterior pituitary ectopia evident on MRI.

Which children should undergo endocrinological evaluation is less clear. Phillips et al.[88] concluded all their endocrinologically normal children with ONH had normal MRIs, while those with hypopituitarism had posterior pituitary ectopia, absence of the pituitary infundibulum, or posterior pituitary bright spot. On the other hand, more recent studies have suggested that a normal pituitary on MRI does not rule out pituitary insufficiency.[89,90]

Therefore, in our approach, all young children with ONH, whether uni- or bilateral, should undergo (1) MRI with attention to the pituitary region and cortex and (2) a complete evaluation and hormone screen by a pediatric endocrinologist, independent of MRI findings. Radiographic demonstration of cortical migrational or corpus callosum abnormalities should prompt an evaluation by a pediatric neurologist. Otherwise normal older children or adults with newly detected ONH without historical evidence of endocrinologic (e.g., normal growth), neurologic, or developmental abnormalities usually need no further workup because any radiographic anomalies will be incidental.

Segmental hypoplasia. A peculiar variant is superior segmental ONH, which can occur for unclear reasons, most commonly in children of diabetic mothers.[91–95] One study[96] found 8.8% of offspring of diabetic mothers at risk had this condition, but it may also occur without a history of maternal diabetes.[91,97] Inferior visual field defects are detected in patients who are usually asymptomatic or perhaps have a long history of tripping or bumping into objects at their feet. The field defect corresponds to the segmental superior hypoplasia of the optic nerve (**Fig. 5–15**). Typically the superior rim of the disc is thin and the central retinal artery appears to arise out of the superior portion of the disc (**Fig. 5–15**). OCT can be helpful in securing the diagnosis in cases that are ophthalmoscopically unclear.[93] There may also be abnormal peripapillary pigment superiorly.[98] Another variant of the segmental hypoplasia of the disc has been described by Yamamoto et al.[99] in a review of fundus photographs in a

large series of patients. The findings were present in 0.3% of photographs but there was no clinical correlation with visual field loss. Patients generally had larger cups and more segmental areas of disc hypoplasia seemingly distinct from the "topless" disc of diabetic mothers. In another form of segmental optic nerve hypoplasia, the nasal portion of the disc is poorly formed. Nasal hypoplasia (**Fig. 5–16**) is often associated with dense visual field defects which attach to the blindspot and extend to the periphery.[100]

Hemiopic hypoplasia. Finally, the term hypoplasia has also been applied to the entity of homonymous hemiopic hypoplasia. This condition results from transsynaptic atrophy of the optic nerve in patients with congenital hemispheric lesions (often also associated with hemiplegia). The disc classically takes on a pattern of bow-tie atrophy in the eye contralateral to the hemispheric lesion and of subtle hypoplasia on the side of the hemispheric lesion.[101] Transsynaptic degeneration of ganglion cell axons is probably also responsible for ONH or pallor associated with periventricular leukomalacia[102] or more severe encephalomalacia due to in utero or perinatal injury (see Chapter 8).[72]

Tilted disc anomaly

Tilted discs arise when the optic nerve enters the sclera at an oblique angle, and the typical crescent creates a disparity in the opening of the retina compared with the sclera. In the Beijing eye study, tilted optic discs were present in about 0.4% of eyes of adult Chinese and were associated with medium myopia, astigmatism, decreased visual acuity, and visual field defects.[103] A tilted disc is more common in high myopes and those with astigmatism,[104] and associated temporal visual field defects do not respect the vertical meridian. The discs typically appear tilted and turned, and the vessels arise anomalously from the disc (**Fig. 5–17**). The corresponding temporal visual field defects (**Fig. 5–18**), which do not respect the vertical meridian, are important to distinguish from acquired bitemporal hemianopias. Color vision abnormalities are seen in about half of the eyes with a tilted disc anomaly.[105] Nerve fiber layer measurement and multifocal ERG most commonly show abnormalities in the superior nerve fiber layer.[106–108]

Optic colobomas and pits

Faulty closure of the inferonasal quadrant of the embryonic fetal fissure of the optic stalk and cup may cause incomplete formation, termed a coloboma, of the iris, optic nerve, retina, and choroid.[109] The anatomic defects are usually located inferiorly. Children with colobomas may present with microphthalmos, microcornea, iris defects, visual loss, and strabismus.[110] Colobomatous involvement of the optic disc is highly variable but can affect a portion of, or the entire, nerve head.[111] Alternatively, only the peripapillary retinal pigment epithelium and choroid may be involved. Ophthalmoscopically, the typical finding is a large excavated disc with visible nerve tissue at the superior rim and a white egg-shaped defect inferiorly (**Fig. 5–19**).[50] Optic disc colobomas are frequently associated with fundus colobomas.[112] Acuity and visual field loss, often superiorly, may be evident. On neuroimaging, misshapen globes and enlargement of the

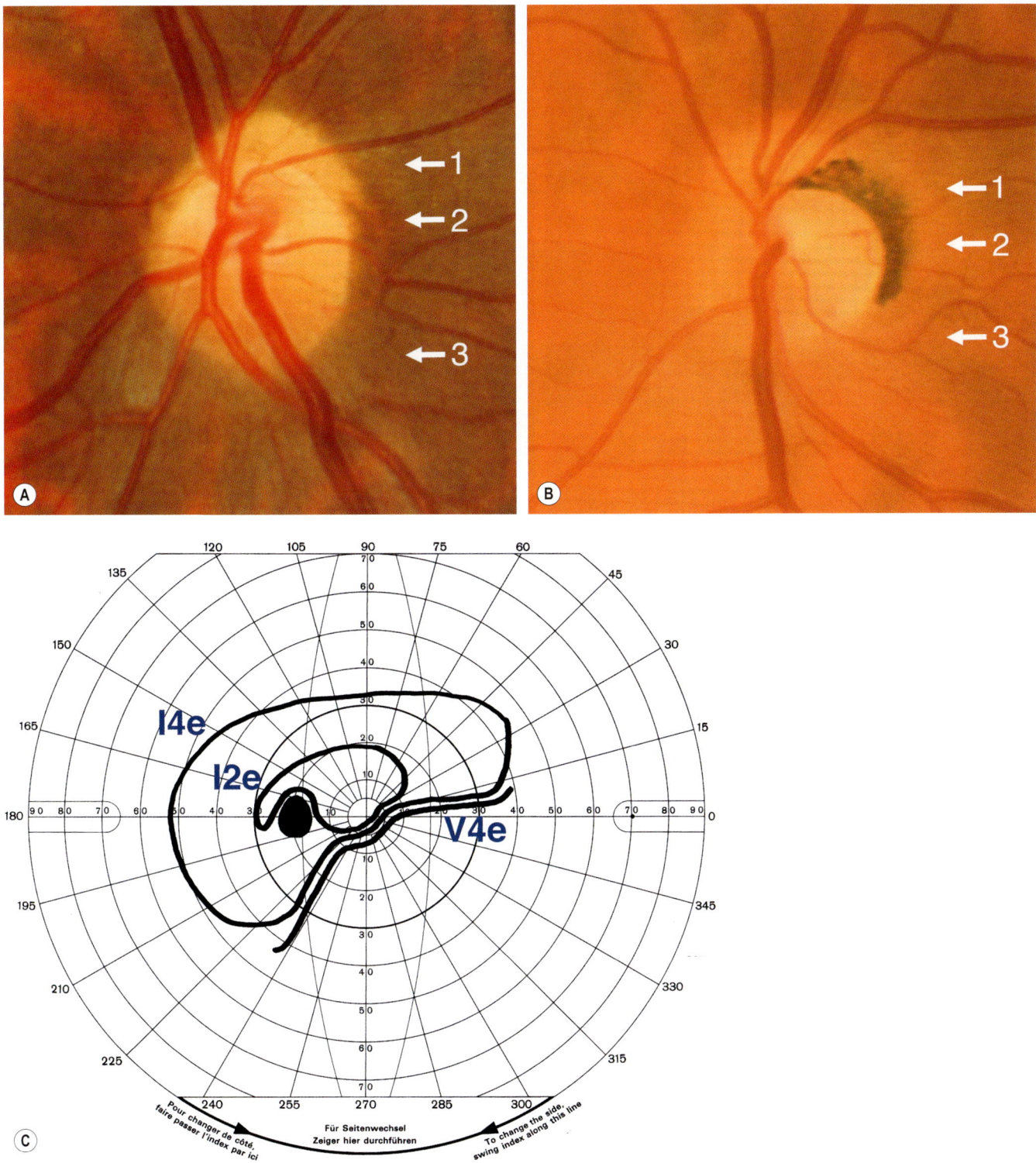

Figure 5–15. Superior segmental optic nerve hypoplasia in two patients. **A**. Optic nerve in a patient with superior segmental hypoplasia of the optic disc demonstrating only a small thin area of nerve tissue superiorly (between numbers 1 (top of disc) and 2 (center of cup)) compared with the distance between 2 and 3 (bottom of disc). The retinal vessels seem to arise out of the superior portion of the disc. **B**. Similar appearance and asymmetry of nerve substance above the center of the cup (between 1 and 2) compared with below the center of the cup (2 and 3) in another patient with superior segmental optic nerve hypoplasia. **C**. Goldmann visual field from the left eye of a patient whose optic nerve is pictured in (**B**) demonstrating characteristic inferior visual field loss. The patient's mother was diabetic.

Left eye

Right eye

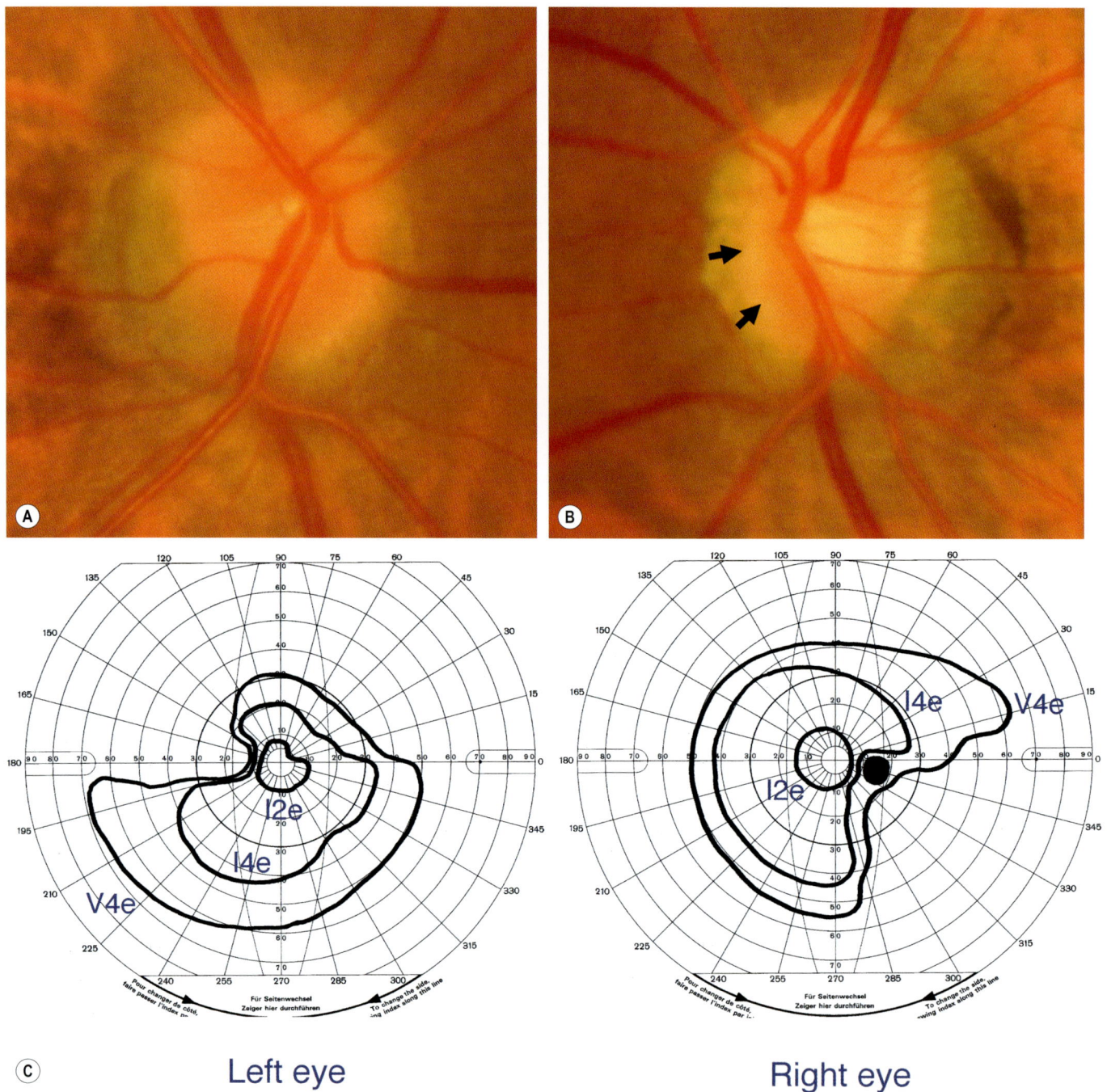

Figure 5–16. Right (**A**) and left (**B**) optic nerves of a patient with bilateral nasal disc hypoplasia. The discs appear tilted, and the vessels seem to originate from the nasal portion of the disc. There is peripapillary atrophy, and the nasal neuroretinal rim (arrows in (**B**)) is very thin compared with the temporal rim. **C**. Goldmann visual fields of the same patient. There is a "bitemporal hemianopia," as the field defects break to the periphery from the blindspot. However, the defects do not respect the vertical meridian, as seen best in the superior aspect of the left eye visual field.

optic nerve near the globe may be seen (**Fig. 5–20**). Patients with colobomas also should be investigated radiographically for the possibility of other forebrain abnormalities, especially basal encephaloceles (see Morning glory disc associations below).[113,114]

Colobomas may occur in association with other systemic abnormalities and chromosomal syndromes.[109] The CHARGE syndrome consists of *c*oloboma, *h*eart defect, *a*tresia choane, *r*etarded growth and development, *g*enital anomalies, *e*ar deformities and deafness. In patients with this syndrome,

the colobomas are most often bilateral and associated with chorioretinal colobomas, and affected individuals should be screened for the CHD7 gene.[115,116] The *renal–coloboma syndrome* is an autosomal dominant disorder associated with renal abnormalities and optic nerve defects, caused by mutations of the PAX2 gene.[117-121] The term *papillorenal* syndrome has also been used and may be more appropriate for this condition, as other disc anomalies such as optic pits, morning glory discs, and dysplastic discs can be seen.[122] Furthermore, some authors[123,124] have argued that the anomalous discs in

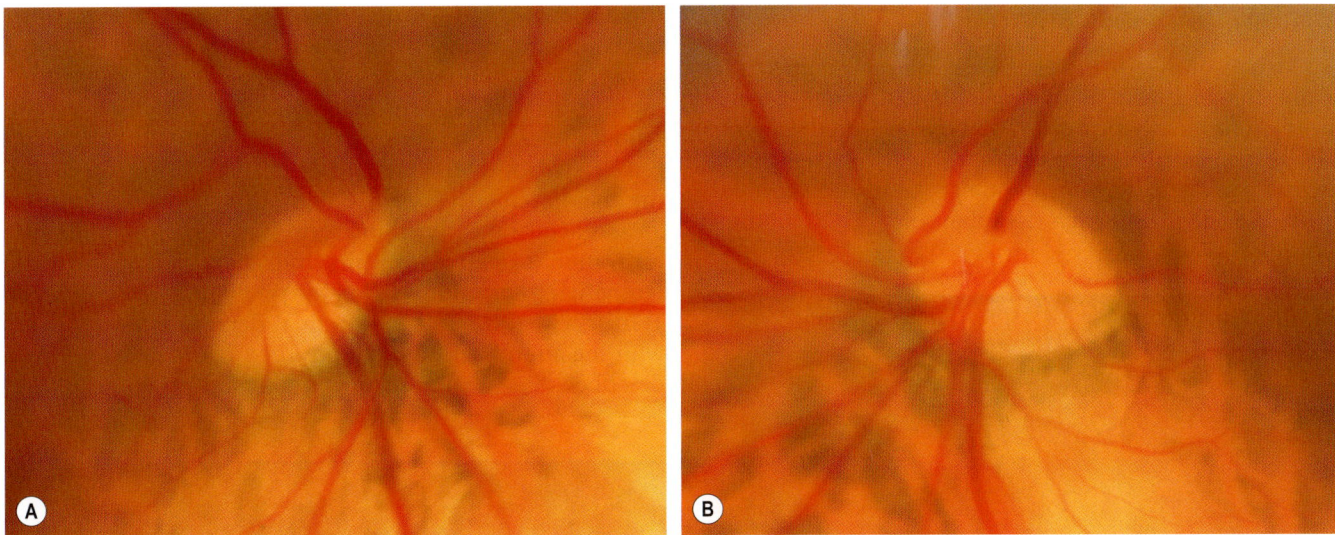

Figure 5–17. Optic nerve appearance of the (**A**) right and (**B**) left eye of a patient with severe tilted disc anomaly. The optic nerves enter the sclera at an oblique angle, and the normal disc architecture is difficult to identify.

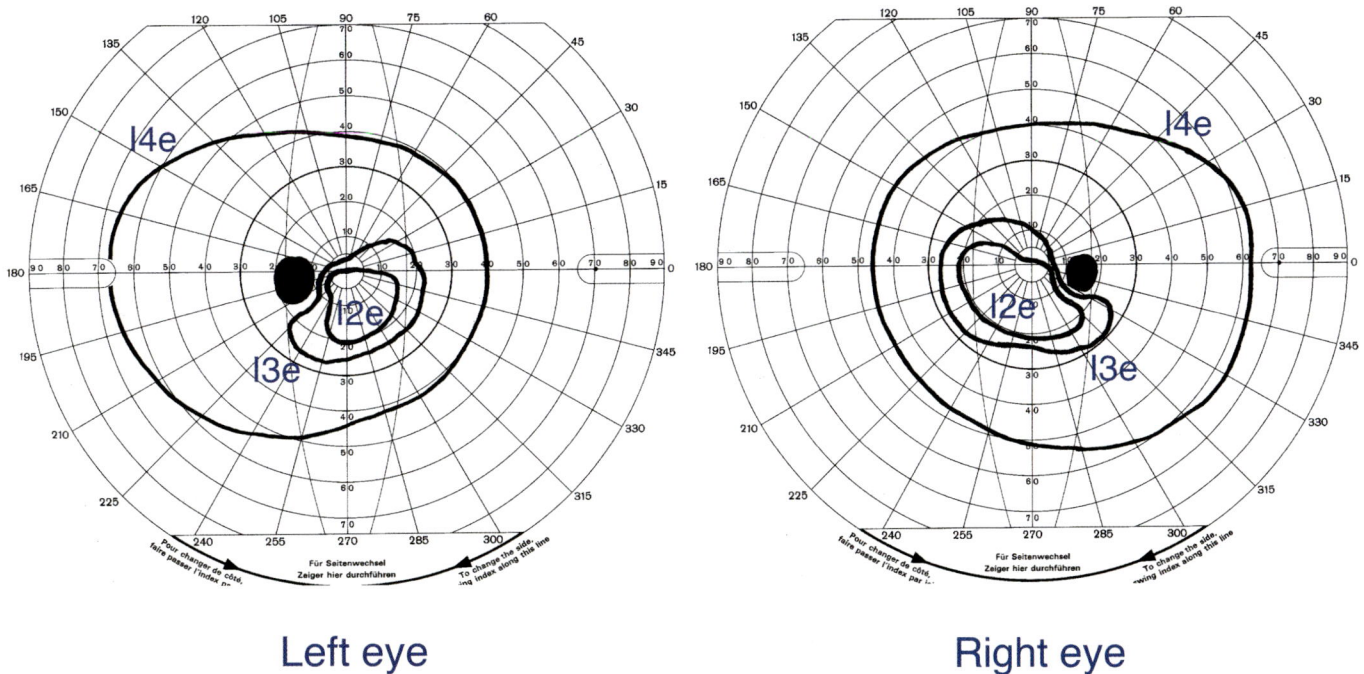

Left eye

Right eye

Figure 5–18. Goldmann visual field of a patient with tilted discs. The defects appear in the smaller isopters and are worse superiorly. Notice the defects slant across the temporal field and do not respect the vertical meridian, distinguishing them from the bitemporal hemianopia of chiasmal disease.

this disorder are characterized by central excavation, attenuation of the central retinal artery and vein, and multiple cilioretinal vessels, and that these abnormalities are the result of a vascular dysgenesis and not caused by incomplete closure of the embryonic fissure as in classic colobomas.

Optic pits (**Fig. 5–21**) are small excavations of the neural retinal rim of the optic disc, usually involving the inferotemporal portion of the optic nerve. In the Beijing eye study, in which fundus photographs were examined, one patient out of 4000 was found to have an optic pit, suggesting the prevalence is less than 0.1%.[125] The area of the "missing" disc is often associated with a corresponding superior arcuate field defect.[126] These temporal disc abnormalities can lead to serous detachment of the macula[127] and macula retinal schisis.[128,129] Serous detachments are thought to occur from fluid flowing from the vitreous cavity through the pit and elevating the sensory retina. Membranes demonstrated on OCT spanning the optic cup may protect against the development of maculopathy.[130] Acquired "pit"-like defects have been described involving the temporal disc rim with a population prevalence of 0.19%[131] and are found most commonly in patients with glaucoma.[131,132] It has been suggested that optic pits and colobomas share the same embryologic mechanism, and the former represents a milder variant of the latter.[50]

Morning glory disc anomaly

The morning glory disc is a congenital anomaly named after the flower which it resembles (**Figs 5–22A** and **5–23A**). A congenital funnel-shaped excavation of the posterior fundus typically incorporates the optic disc. Other characteristic features include disc enlargement, orange color, and surrounding choroidal pigmentary disturbances.[50] OCT findings include enlargement of the nerve head, a thick nerve fiber layer, and thinning of the retina in the macula.[133] The retinal vessels curve from the disc edge and travel radially, producing a "spoke-like" vessel configuration.[134] The normal central retinal vasculature is conspicuously absent ophthalmoscopically. Arteriovenous connections may branch between the major retinal vessels, sometimes creating a rosette or arcade appearance on fluorescein angiography.[135] The disc excavation is often filled with white glial tissue and vascular remnants. The vision is usually poor in the affected eye. Transient vision loss[136] and retinal detachments associated with the anomaly leading to acquired visual loss have been described.[50]

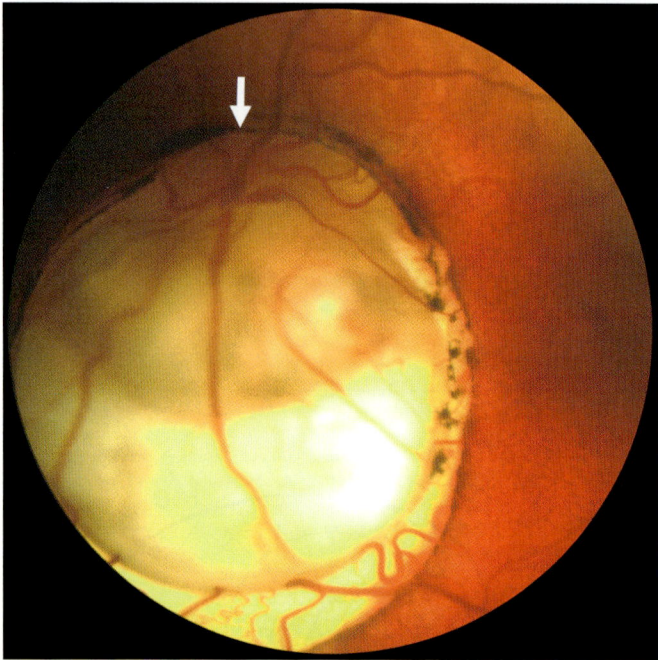

Figure 5–19. Extensive coloboma involving the peripapillary posterior pole. The optic nerve (arrow) is seen at the superior edge of the coloboma within the excavated area.

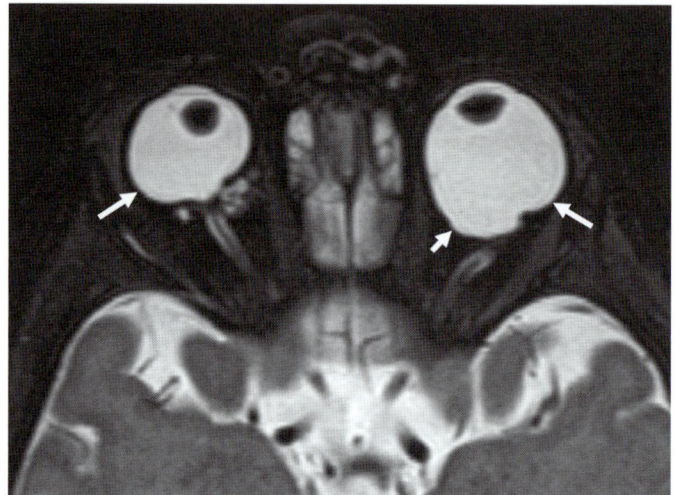

Figure 5–20. Axial T2-weighted MRI in a patient with bilateral colobomas demonstrating irregular outpouching and globe contour changes posteriorly in both eyes (arrows).

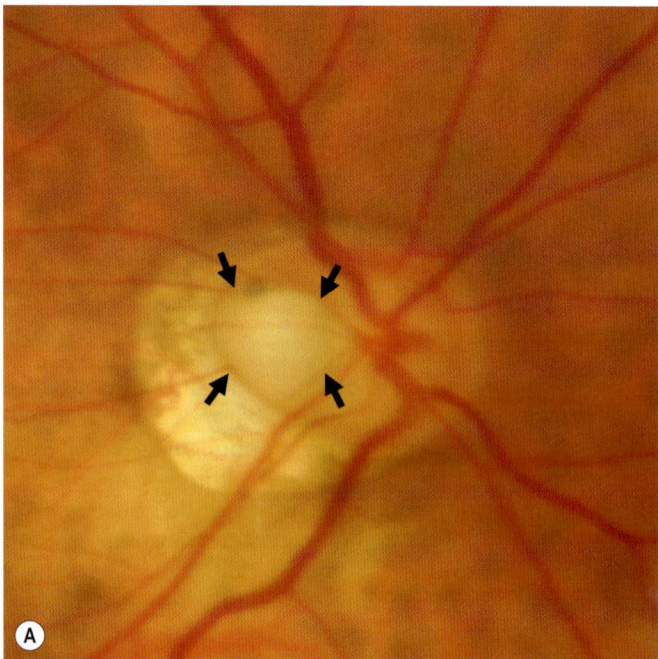

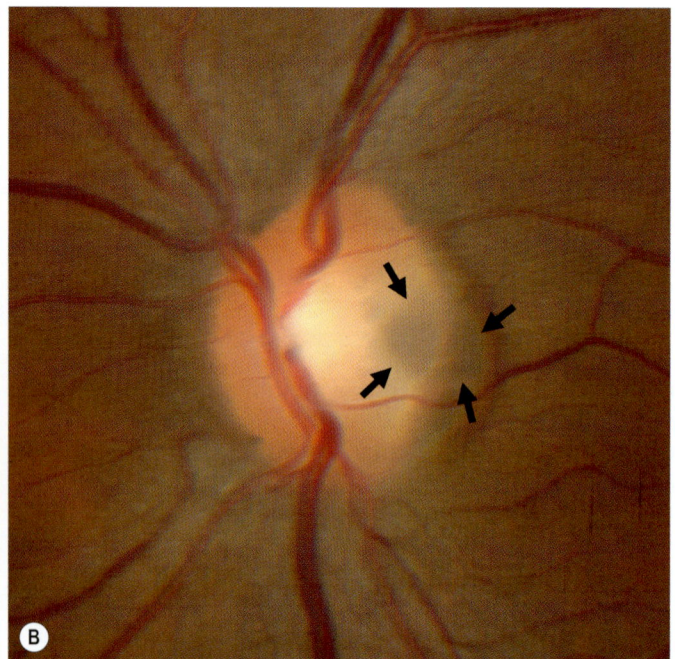

Figure 5–21. Optic pits in two different patients (**A**, **B**). The pits appear as focal gray excavations (outlined by arrows) in the temporal portion of the optic nerve head and can extend into the retina (**B**).

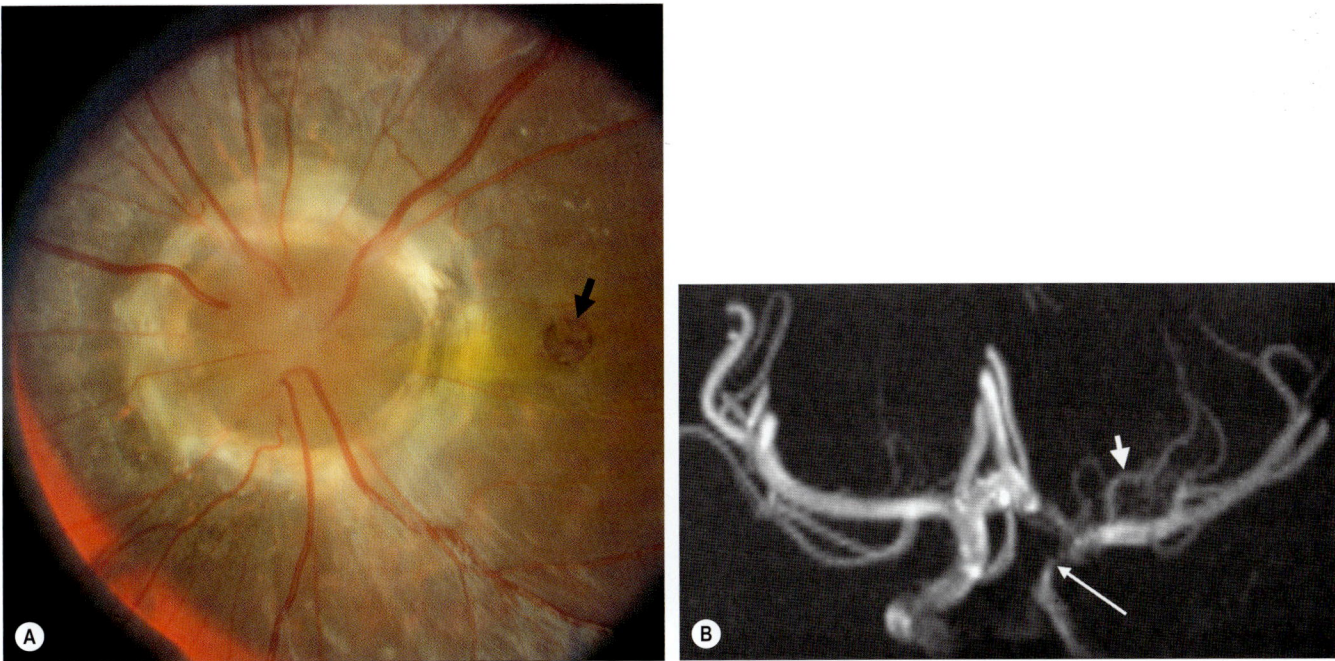

Figure 5–22. Morning glory disc and moya-moya vessels. **A.** Fundus photograph of the left eye demonstrating morning glory disc and macular hole (arrow). The macular hole appears closer to the disc than normal due to the enlargement of the optic disc rim. **B.** Coronal reconstruction of three-dimensional time-of-flight magnetic resonance angiography, with segmentation to show the anterior circulation of the carotid arteries, demonstrating a decrease in size of the caliber of the left internal carotid artery relative to the normal-sized right internal carotid artery with more focal marked narrowing of the distal portion (long white arrow). The bifurcation into the middle and anterior cerebral artery is also involved and markedly narrowed. There is an increase in the size of the lenticulo-striate vessels (short white arrow) producing a moya-moya appearance at this site.[141]

The anomaly is likely related to defective closure of the embryonic fissure, similar to a coloboma, but others purport a mesenchymal abnormality.[50,137] The glial and vascular abnormalities are felt to result from primary neuroectodermal dysgenesis.[50,137]

In addition, there have been several reports[138–143] of patients with morning glory disc anomaly and moya-moya disease (**Fig. 5–22**), which is a rare idiopathic cerebrovascular disorder characterized by progressive bilateral stenosis or occlusion of the distal internal carotid arteries and formation of a collateral vascular network in the basal ganglia region. The term moya-moya refers to the Japanese term for "puff of smoke," which describes the angiographic appearance of the abnormal vessels. Other similar intracranial vascular anomalies of the have been reported.[144] The association of morning glory disc and these blood vessel anomalies suggests the disc anomaly may in some cases result from intracranial vascular dysgenesis.

Morning glory disc anomaly is also associated with transsphenoidal basal encephalocele (**Fig. 5–23**),[145] a condition which encompasses a complex series of malformations characterized by herniation of the chiasm, hypothalamus, pituitary, and anterior cerebral arteries through a bony defect in the anterior skull base.[143,146,147] Other abnormalities include hypertelorism (**Fig. 5–23**), depressed nasal bridge, midline upper lid notch, cleft palate, panhypopituitarism, and callosal agenesis. Herniated tissue may present as a pulsatile posterior nasal mass, and surgical removal, because of potential disastrous vascular, endocrine, and visual consequences, is for the most part contraindicated.[50] Morning

glory discs have also been described in neurofibromatosis type 2.[148]

Evaluation. Patients with morning glory disc should undergo an MRI to exclude a basal encephalocele, and MRI angiography should also be considered to exclude moya-moya vessels and other intracranial vascular anomalies which may place the individual at risk for cerebrovascular ischemia. Neuroimaging often demonstrates the widened, excavated nature of the optic nerve head and distal optic nerve.[149]

Staphyloma

In addition to disc colobomas and morning glory disc anomaly, staphylomas should also be considered in the differential diagnosis of excavated disc anomalies. The entire disc lies within a deep peripapillary excavation, but features which distinguish it from the other two related anomalies include a relatively normal disc, preservation of the normal retinal vasculature, and absence of a central glial tuft.[50] There are no commonly associated central nervous system abnormalities. Staphylomas are most often unilateral and associated with high myopia, poor vision, and amblyopia.[150]

Optic neuropathy associated with optic disc drusen

Pseudopapilledema, optic nerve head drusen, and their distinction from true papilledema are discussed in detail in Chapter 6. However, because visual loss associated with disc

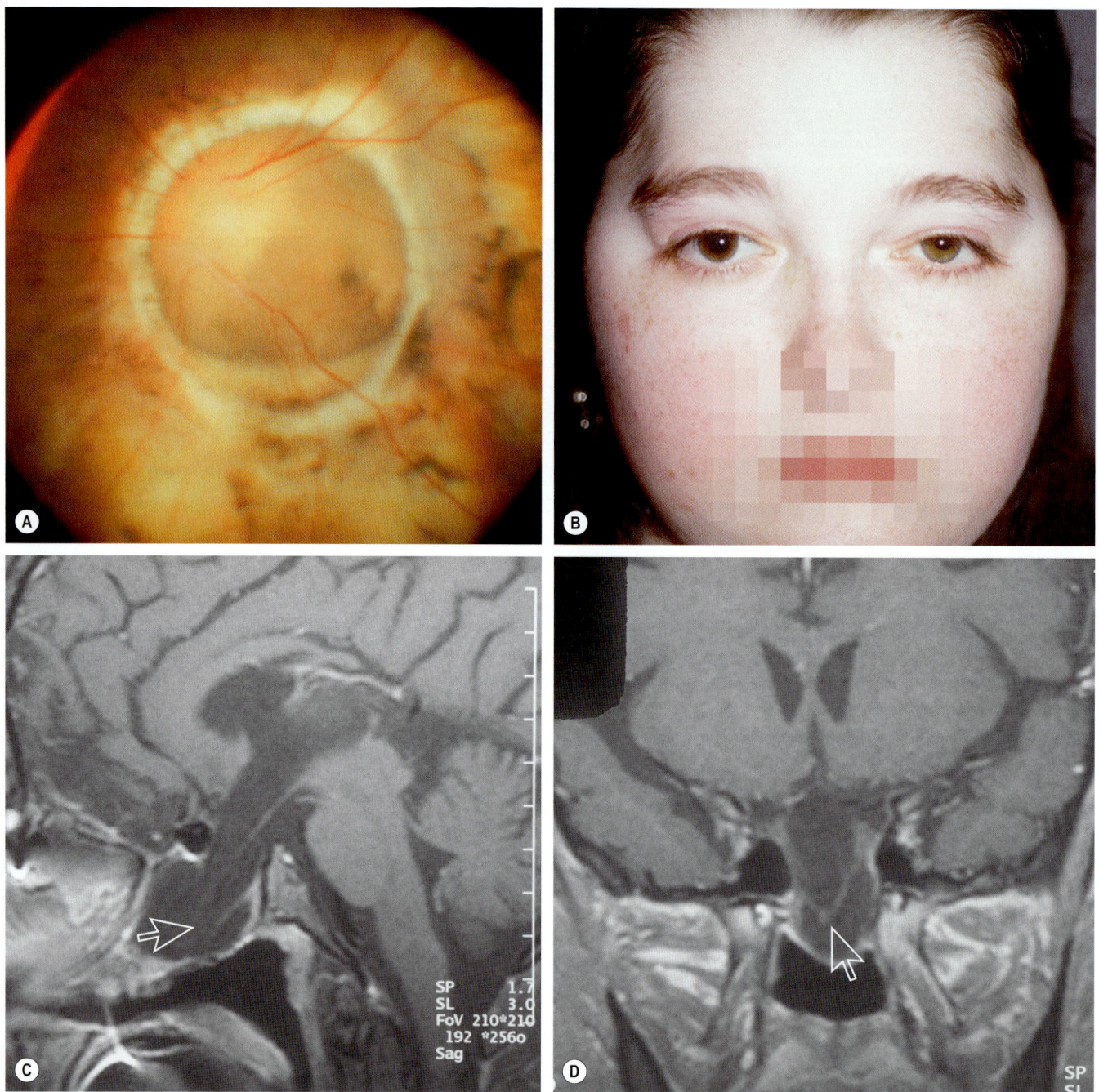

Figure 5–23. Morning glory disc and transsphenoidal encephalocele. **A**. Morning glory disc. **B**. The patient has hypertelorism (increased distance between the two orbits), and the right pupil is pharmacologically dilated. Sagittal (**C**) and (**D**) coronal T1-weighted gadolinium-enhanced MRI demonstrating a transsphenoidal encephalocele, with herniation of the chiasm (arrow) into the sella.

drusen is truly an optic neuropathy, it will be reviewed here. Drusen occur in 3–24/1000 people.[151]

Many patients with disc drusen are completely asymptomatic, although between 50% and 70% will have visual field defects.[152–154] Although most patients will be identified during a routine fundus examination (**Fig. 5–24**), some are detected after an abnormal visual field test is obtained in the setting of vague, progressive (insidious) vision loss. Others are identified when elevated optic nerves are evaluated for possible papilledema (drusen are visible in only about 50% of patients).[154] Contact between disc drusen and nearby nerve fibers presumably results in nerve fiber layer thin-

ning[155] and axonal dysfunction. Optic nerve-type visual field defects are produced that may be progressive and are more common in patients with visible as opposed to buried drusen.[154,156] Drusen are almost never associated with central vision loss unless erosion of a blood vessel leads to a hemorrhage in the macular region. In the absence of macular injury, all patients with central visual acuity loss and optic nerve head drusen should be investigated. Typical nerve fiber bundle-type defects are seen including arcuate defects and nasal steps (**Fig. 5–25**), and optic disc pallor may develop (**Fig. 5–24**). OCT can be used to follow the peripapillary nerve fiber layer thickness.[157]

On rare occasions patients present with sudden and more catastrophic vision loss. This is most often on the basis of a superimposed ischemic optic neuropathy, which may or may not be associated with true disc edema and splinter hemorrhages (**Fig. 5–26**).[158–163] Patients with drusen-associated ischemic optic neuropathy tend to be younger, but otherwise have a similar prevalence of vasculopathic risk factors to non-drusen-associated cases.[164] Transient vision loss prior to the fixed deficit and a reasonably favorable visual prognosis have been noted with drusen-associated ischemic optic neuropathy.[164] Other ocular ischemic conditions have been observed in association with optic nerve head drusen, including central retinal artery, branch retinal artery, and central vein occlusions.

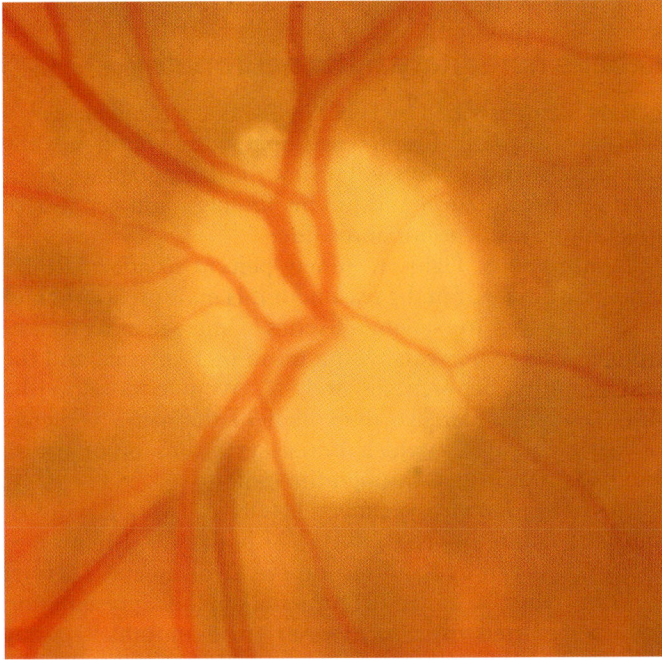

Figure 5–24. Optic disc drusen associated with visual loss. Drusen are evident as translucent crystalline deposits, and significant optic disc pallor has developed.

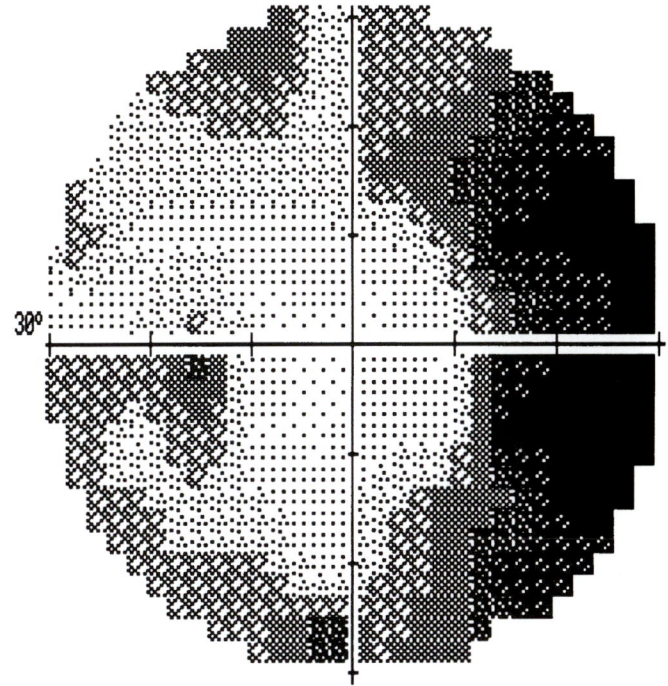

Figure 5–25. Static perimetry demonstrates typical nasal visual field constriction in a patient with optic disc drusen.

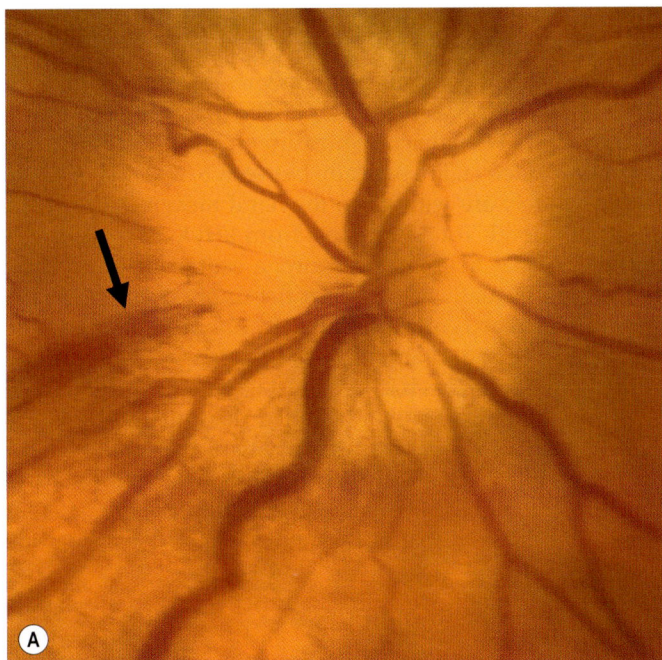

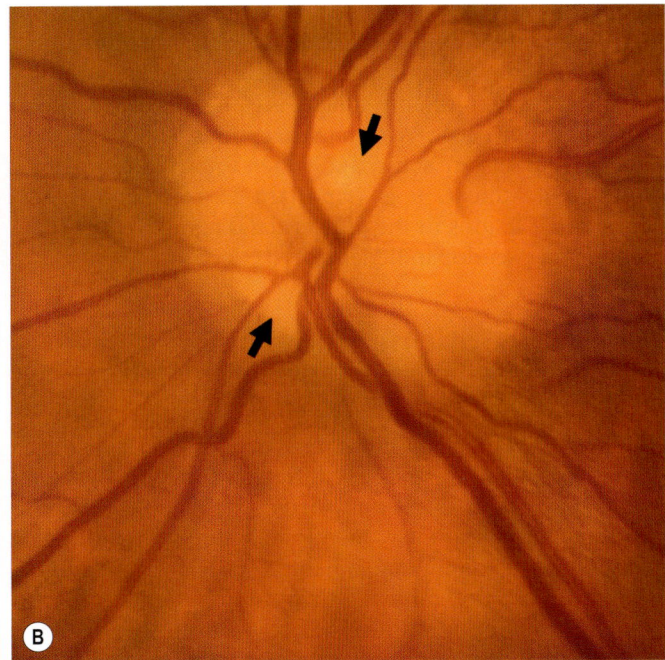

Figure 5–26. Optic disc drusen with associated anterior ischemic optic neuropathy in the right eye. **A.** The right optic nerve is hyperemic with nerve fiber layer edema and associated splinter hemorrhage (arrow). **B.** Buried disc drusen (yellow spots under disc surface, see arrows) can be seen in the patient's uninvolved left eye.

Vision loss associated with optic disc drusen can also be caused by peripapillary neovascularization, which can be identified by its characteristic yellow or gray appearance. There may be an associated hemorrhage or serous detachment of the retina. Best identified with fluorescein angiography, neovascularization is thought to result from chronic optic disc ischemia.[165]

Treatment. There is no known treatment for visual loss associated with optic disc drusen. Repeat computerized visual fields over years will generally show only slight changes, and therefore can be done to comfort and reassure the patient on an annual basis. However, serial visual fields in asymptomatic patients with optic disc drusen is unnecessary. Some have suggested that a lower threshold for treatment of intraocular pressure should be considered in patients with optic disc drusen, deteriorating visual fields, and borderline intraocular pressures.[151] Some neuro-ophthalmologists have advocated the use of intraocular pressure-lowering agents even in the presence of a normal intraocular pressure. Optic nerve sheath fenestration appears to convey no benefit in the treatment of this disorder, but experience has been limited. Neovascularization may be observed or treated with laser photocoagulation or surgery.[165]

Myelinated retinal nerve fibers

Lacking oligodendrocytes, the retina is usually unmyelinated. Myelinated retinal nerve fibers are anomalous white patches of myelin which are often contiguous with the optic disc and typically contained within the nerve fiber layer (see Fig. 4–34B).[166] When viewed with high magnification, the edges appear serrated or feathery as the myelination aligns along the nerve fibers. This feature distinguishes these lesions from cotton-wool spots. Occasionally the myelinated nerve fibers are large, extending along the temporal vascular arcades. They can also be located away from the disc in the retinal periphery. Although usually asymptomatic, some involved eyes are myopic with associated anisometropic amblyopia.[167] When the myelinated area is extensive, visual field defects may occur. With rare exceptions,[168] myelinated retinal nerve fibers are static, and, when found incidentally, require no treatment. It is important to recognize these benign retinal lesions in the differential diagnosis of retinal ischemia and pseudopapilledema.

Hereditary optic neuropathies

These represent a heterogeneous group of diseases characterized by an inheritance pattern that may be spontaneous, recessive, dominant, or mitochondrial, and in which vision loss occurs as the result of optic nerve dysfunction. Hereditary optic neuropathies may manifest as monosymptomatic lesions or may accompany other central nervous system disease. They can present as subtle fixed deficits in early life (Kjer's dominant optic atrophy) or as catastrophic sequential vision loss in adolescence or early adulthood (Leber's hereditary optic neuropathy (LHON)). They will be recognized in the setting of the appropriate family history, the highly suggestive clinical presentations, and, in some cases, by specific

genetic testing. A variation on this theme includes patients who develop optic atrophy in association with heritable neuronal lipid storage diseases. The examiner is best served by working within a framework that defines these entities on a clinical basis. Their modes of presentation and examination findings are unique. As molecular genetics continues to evolve, we will have a better understanding of the pathogenesis of these conditions, more accurate classifications, and ultimately effective gene-directed therapy.[169]

Leber's hereditary optic neuropathy

LHON, first described by Leber in 1871,[170] typically causes a subacute, sequential optic neuropathy in young healthy individuals. This section will review the demographics, characteristic presentation and fundus findings, and genetics of this unique mitochondrial disorder.

Demographics. Eighty to ninety percent of affected individuals are males, but the reason for this male predominance is unclear.[171–174] In Newman's series,[171] the age at onset was from 8 years to 60 years with a mean of 27.6 years and the vast majority between 26 and 37. Women develop the disease at an older age than men in the same pedigree; however, the age at which initial symptoms occur varies. LHON is transmitted through the mother.

Neuro-ophthalmic symptoms. LHON causes an acute or subacute failure of vision in one or both eyes. The average interval between first and second eye involvement is several months, with a range from simultaneous presentation (which occurred in 55% of cases) to 9 months.[171] Many simultaneous cases may represent sequential involvement of the eyes in which the attack in the first eye went unrecognized. The vision loss is usually painless although headache occasionally occurs. Uhthoff's symptom[171,175] (worsening of vision associated with elevation of body temperature; see Optic neuritis, below) and recurrent visual loss[176] have been reported in LHON.

Neuro-ophthalmic signs. Patients present with signs of an acute optic neuropathy, with loss of central vision, and dyschromatopsia. Visual acuity measurements reflect the dense central field defect, are typically between 5/200 and 20/200, but only rarely are reduced to the hand movements or light perception level. Total blindness from LHON is exceedingly unusual. Visual field testing shows a central or centrocecal scotoma in virtually all cases. In the uninvolved fellow eye mild subclinical central visual field abnormalities can be found before more dramatic visual loss ensues.[177] Although pupillary light reflexes had been thought to be normal, more definitive studies have demonstrated that afferent pupillary defects are typically present when visual loss is unilateral or asymmetric.[178,179] This issue is still controversial, however, as some investigators have suggested that pupillary afferent fibers are relatively spared compared with those mediating vision.

The classic disc appearance in patients with acute LHON was emphasized by Smith et al. in 1973.[175] Characteristic findings include "circumpapillary telangiectatic microangiopathy" and "pseudoedema" or swelling with hyperemia of the nerve fiber layer around the disc (**Fig. 5–27**), and the absence of true edema or staining of the disc on fluorescein

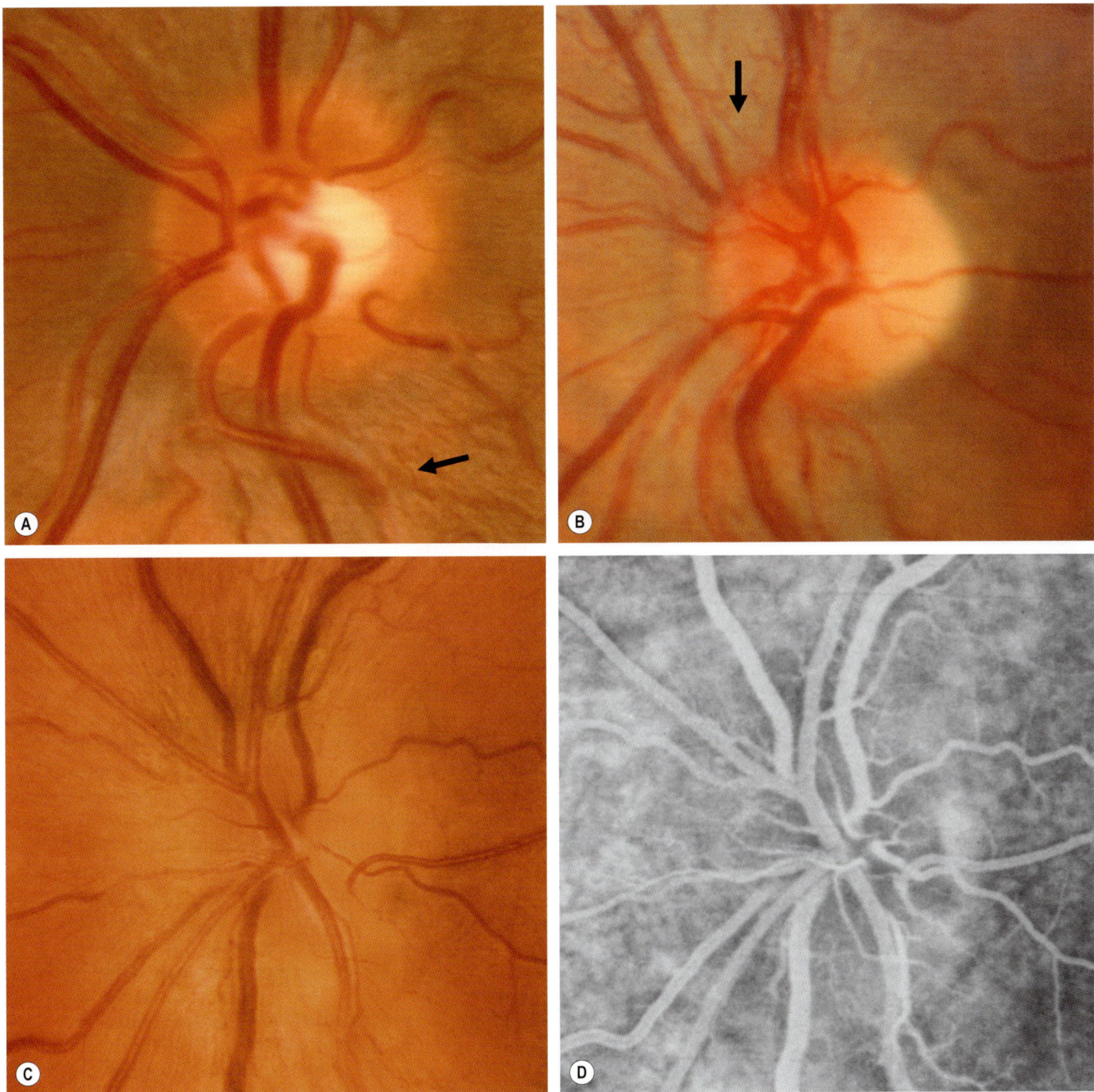

Figure 5–27. Spectrum of optic nerve abnormalities in acute Leber's hereditary optic neuropathy. **A.** Patient 1. Mild nerve fiber elevation inferiorly with dilated capillaries (arrow). **B.** Patient 2. This disc appears more hyperemic with dilated surface capillaries and swelling and haziness to the nerve fiber layer best seen superiorly (arrow). **C.** Patient 3. More extensive pseudoswelling with obscuration of the disc margin. However on fluorescein angiography (**D**) in the same patient there is no disc leakage or staining.

angiography. If these fundus features are identified, genetic testing should be performed without additional testing for other acute causes of optic neuropathy. These findings can also be used to identify patients within a family at risk for developing the disease, as they are present in a subset of patients who are in the preclinical phase of the disease.[172,174,180] About two-thirds of the male and one-third of the female asymptomatic descendants of affected females have the characteristic fundus changes. OCT initially shows thickening of the nerve fiber layer followed by thinning in the atrophic phase.[181]

However, there are many cases in which the acute nerve fiber layer and vascular changes are absent, and the disc may have a normal appearance. Patients with LHON subsequently develop optic atrophy regardless of the fundus appearance acutely. After the onset of optic atrophy, it is difficult to identify patients with LHON ophthalmoscopically because the acute findings of pseudopapilledema and telangiectasias have resolved (**Fig. 5–28**).[38] Fortunately, spontaneous visual recovery may occur in 4–32% of cases, depending upon the specific mutation (see below).[171,172,182–185]

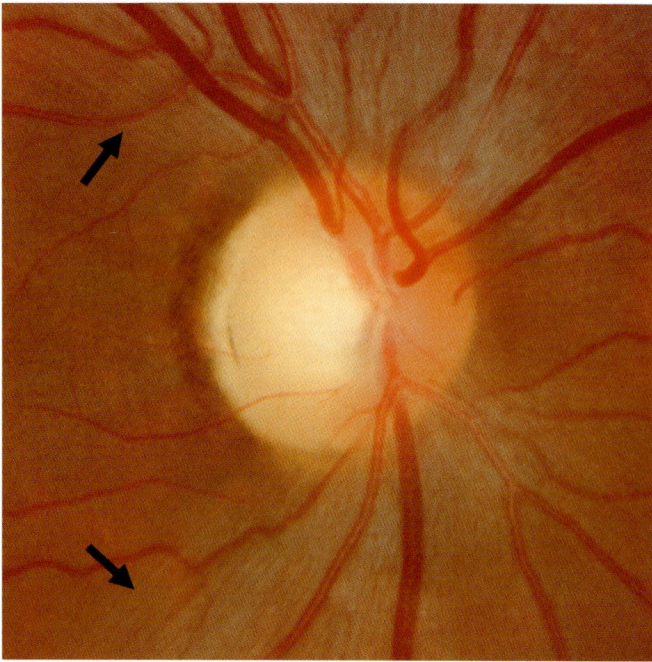

Figure 5–28. Subacute appearance of the right optic nerve of a patient with Leber's hereditary optic neuropathy who had presented months earlier. There is still nerve fiber layer prominence but temporal pallor with loss of nerve fibers in the papillomacular bundle has developed, as evidenced by the sharp cut-off from the normal nerve fibers (arrows) with rake-like defects.

Cerebrospinal fluid analysis and electroretinography are not helpful. Visual-evoked responses showed prolonged latency and reduced amplitude and have been reported to also be abnormal in some asymptomatic relatives of patients with LHON.[174] MRI, particularly with short time inversion recovery (STIR) sequences, may demonstrate optic nerve high signal abnormalities,[186] and optic nerve enhancement and chiasm enlargement have also been reported.[187,188]

Other associations. The ophthalmoscopically visible local changes have led many to conclude that there are unique features that place the intraocular optic nerve and perhaps only the papillomacular bundle ganglion cells at greatest risk for damage in LHON. However, central and peripheral nervous system and systemic abnormalities have also been reported. For instance, nonspecific white matter lesions have been observed on MRI scans of some affected individuals.[187,188] In addition a disease resembling multiple sclerosis has also been reported to occur with LHON.[180,189–195] In Newman's series,[171] three out of 72 patients with LHON also had a peripheral neuropathy.

Cardiac conduction defects and arrhythmias and skeletal deformities have been associated with LHON. Abnormal electrocardiograms (ECGs), specifically conduction abnormalities, have been convincingly demonstrated in various pedigrees.[196–199] Wolff–Parkinson–White and Lown–Ganong–Levine were the most common abnormalities found. Other ECG abnormalities included Q waves, atrial fibrillation, bundle branch blocks, ventricular hypertrophy, supraventricular tachycardia, premature ventricular contractions, and short QT interval.[171] The cardiac disease is often asymptomatic and can be found in patients with no evi-

dence of optic neuropathy. Patients with LHON have also been found to have skeletal deformities including congenital hip dislocation, arachnodactyly, pes cavus, talipes equinovarus, kyphoscoliosis, arched palate, and spondyloepiphyseal dysplasia.

Mitochondrial genetics. Because mothers transmit LHON vertically to their offspring, and males do not pass on the disease, mitochondrial inheritance became the most plausible explanation. In their seminal studies, Wallace and colleagues[200,201] demonstrated a mitochondrial DNA point mutation in which a nucleotide substitution occurred at position 11778 in nine out of 11 families with LHON. A guanine to adenine substitution causes a change of the basic amino acid arginine to histidine. The result is an abnormal subunit 4 (ND4) of the NADH dehydrogenase:coenzyme Q1 reductase subunit (complex I), which is the first enzyme in the pathway of oxidative phosphorylation. The 11 778 mutation has been identified in pedigrees and spontaneous singleton cases. In addition, other causative mutations at position 3460 and 14484 have been identified.[202–207] These mutations affect the ND1 and ND6 subunit genes of complex I, respectively.[208–210]

Alone, these mutations do not explain the variable occurrence of the disease within the same pedigree, its wide spectrum of phenotypic expression, and the susceptibility of male offspring. Variable phenotypic expression of the mtDNA mutation is, as of now, unexplained. The three theories that have been advanced to explain this are (1) heteroplasmy (coexistence of mutant and normal mtDNA), (2) a second genetic factor possibly on the X chromosome, and, finally, (3) environmental factors. Although it is most likely that all of these factors contribute to the phenotypic expression of the disease, there is increasing evidence to suggest that either a nuclear and or an X-linked factor contribute to the development of the disease.[211–215] Recently large optic disc size has been shown in individuals harboring the LHON mutation to be protective against vision loss and associated with increased recovery rates if vision loss occurs.[216] External factors capable of damaging oxidative phosphorylation, such as cyanide poisoning (cigarette smoking), alcohol, and environmental toxins, may also contribute to the onset of visual loss. None of these predictably accompany the acute visual deterioration in affected individuals, but it seems feasible that they can alter "genetically programmed" cell death.

Genetic testing. Patients with suspected LHON should be tested for one of the three primary mutations: 11778 (69% of cases), 3460 (13% of cases), 14484 (14% of cases).[169] The rate of spontaneous recovery is highest in patients with the 14484 mutation and lowest with the 11778 and 3460 mutations.[217] Genetic counseling can be offered if a mutation is identified.

Treatment. There is no known effective treatment or prophylaxis for the visual loss that occurs with LHON. Steroids, cyanide antagonists, and hydroxycobalamin have been tried without effect. Some physicians recommend that family members in LHON pedigrees and patients affected in one eye with LHON avoid tobacco and heavy alcohol use. Some success has been reported in other diseases that affect mitochondrial energy production with the use of cofactors such as succinate and coenzyme Q.[218–220] However, their value in treating or preventing LHON remains to be proven. In the future it may be possible to treat LHON with allotypic gene therapy using an adenovirus vector carrying the nuclear encoded version of the gene normally made by mitochondria. The missing protein can then be synthesized in the cytoplasm and transported to the mitochondria. The superficially located ganglion cells of the eye may prove uniquely amenable to this type of treatment.[213,221]

Dominant optic atrophy

In his description of 19 affected families, Kjer[222] reported the details of a dominantly inherited optic neuropathy that now bears his name. Dominant optic atrophy (DOA) is the most common hereditary optic neuropathy, affecting about 1 in 50 000 people.[223]

Patients typically present before the end of the first decade of life with the insidious onset of bilateral (although often asymmetric) vision loss. Acuities range from 20/20 to 20/200, and patients typically have central and centrocecal visual field defects with intact peripheral isopters.[224] Forty percent of patients retain acuity of 20/60 or better.[222] Presentation with nystagmus is uncommon. Progression of vision loss is very variable with many patients remaining stable after the second decade and others losing vision very slowly over decades.[225,226] Color vision loss typically occurs along the blue–yellow or tritanopic axis (see Chapter 2).[227,228] The associated optic disc pallor often takes on a striking wedge-like appearance with temporal excavation of the neuroretinal rim (**Fig. 5–29**), although the whole disc sometimes is pale.[229] The condition is usually neurologically isolated except for a few clusters of cases with associated sensorineural hearing loss.[230,231] OCT studies have demonstrated isolated involvement of the nerve fiber and ganglion cell layer with normal outer retina and photoreceptor layers.[232]

Since the disease is dominantly inherited, examination of first-degree relatives often aids in the diagnosis of patients suspected of having dominant optic atrophy. Because of the highly variable degree of visual dysfunction, seemingly asymptomatic adult and child relatives can often be identified if visual acuity or color loss or optic atrophy are present.

Recently pedigree analysis has identified the gene implicated in Kjer's dominant optic atrophy. First linkage analyses mapped the defect to the chromosome 3q region.[233] More recently it has been confirmed that most families with DOA have deletions and insertions (over 70 mutations have been reported) in this region termed the OPA1 gene at the 3q27–3q28 chromosome.[234–240] This has allowed for more accurate identification of symptomatic and asymptomatic carriers.[224,241,242] A much less common locus on 18q12.2–12.3 has also been identified.[243] It may be reasonable to screen for OPA1 gene abnormalities in patients with sporadic otherwise unexplained optic atrophy.[244] Cohn and associates[245] have emphasized, however, that the OPA1 mutations are found in only about two-thirds of patients, and that there are likely to be other genetic and environmental factors that contribute to the disease development and presentation. The OPA1 gene product, a dynamin-related GTPase, is believed to be involved in mitochondrial fusion, cristae organization, and control of apoptosis, and OPA1 mutations may lead to mitochondrial DNA dysfunction.[246–248]

Histopathologic studies have demonstrated diffuse loss of retinal ganglion cells, suggesting primary ganglion cell death as the mechanism of disease.[249] Spontaneous improvement has not been reported.

Management. There is no known effective treatment at this time. When dominant optic atrophy is considered in children without affected family members, compressive lesions and other causes of optic neuropathy with pallor should be excluded. Patients should be screened for sensory neural hearing loss as this occurs with increased frequency in this subgroup of patients.[228]

Recessive optic atrophy

Both simple (isolated) and complex (associated defects) forms of recessively inherited optic neuropathy exist. As is typical of most genetic conditions, the recessive form of hereditary optic atrophy is generally much more severe than the dominant form. Patients present in early childhood (age 2–4 years) with more profound visual acuity loss and searching nystagmus.[250] There is often a history of parental consanguinity. Visual acuity is usually stable, and whether this occurs congenitally is unknown. There is usually diffuse disc pallor and attenuation of retinal vessels. Distinction from photoreceptor dysfunction in Leber's congenital amaurosis can be accomplished with electroretinography, which should be normal in recessive optic atrophy. Complicated, recessive optic atrophy, when associated with spinocerebellar degeneration, cerebellar ataxia, pyramidal tract dysfunction, and mental retardation is termed Behr syndrome.[251] Some regard this as part of the continuum of optic atrophy associated with hereditary ataxias.[252]

DIDMOAD (Wolfram syndrome)

Wolfram or DIDMOAD (*d*iabetes *i*nsipidus, *d*iabetes *m*ellitus, *o*ptic *a*trophy, and *d*eafness) syndrome encompasses the above findings and presents in childhood or adolescence.[253,254] There is a great degree of variability in presentation but the hallmark is optic atrophy with progressive vision and hearing loss in a juvenile-onset diabetic.[255] Vision is usually worse than 20/200.[256] Other reported abnormalities include ptosis, ataxia, seizures, mental retardation, nystagmus, abnormal ERG, abnormal cerebrospinal fluid (CSF) protein, and short stature. Most patients die as young adults in their thirties and forties. Neuropathological studies have demonstrated atrophy of the optic nerve, chiasm, brain stem, and cerebellum.[256,257] The inheritance pattern is autosomal recessive and there is now extensive evidence to suggest localization to chromosome 4p and the WFS1 gene.[255,258–266] While there is extensive evidence linking the disorder to the WFS1 gene and the production of a protein "Wolframin," the function of this protein is unknown. The significance of the numerous mutations that have been identified in various pedigrees and how they correlate with the highly variable nature of the disease presentation is also unclear.

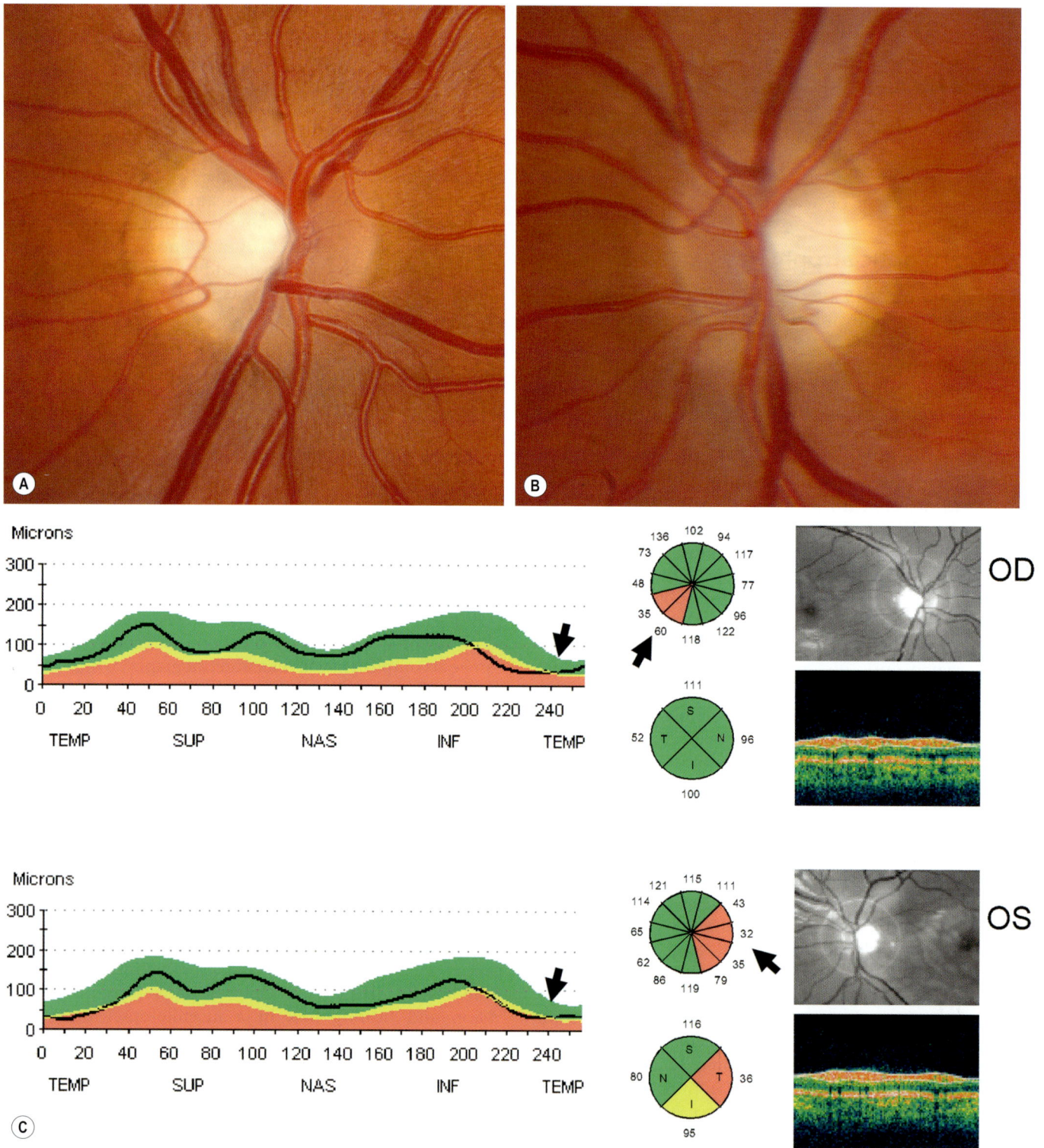

Figure 5–29. Optic nerve appearance of the right (**A**) and left (**B**) eye of a patient with dominantly inherited optic neuropathy (Kjer's) demonstrating a wedge of pallor and excavation involving the temporal portion of the optic nerve as well as nerve fiber layer (NFL) loss. (**C**) Ocular coherence tomography in the same patient demonstrates the NFL loss is limited to the temporal portion of the disc (arrows) and is greater in the left eye than the right eye.

Optic atrophy associated with neurologic and metabolic disease

Optic atrophy and progressive visual dysfunction frequently accompanies a variety of other inherited, degenerative neurologic conditions (**Table 5–5**). In each of these conditions

progressive visual loss occurs with dyschromatopsia, central or centrocecal field defects, and optic atrophy. Visual loss progresses along with systemic neurologic syndrome but vision loss usually remains moderate. Optic atrophy occurs in conjunction with spinocerebellar degenerations (see Chapter 16), ataxias, and sensory motor peripheral

Table 5–5 Metabolic and degenerative neurologic diseases associated with optic atrophy

Ataxias[1109]
  Spinocerebellar degenerations (SCAs— see Chapter 15)[1110]
  Friedreich's ataxia
  Charcot–Marie–Tooth
  Olivopontocerebellar atrophy

Mucopolysaccharidoses
  Hurler
  Scheie
  Hunter A,B
  Sanfilippo A, B
  Morquio
  Maroteaux–Lamy A

Lipidoses
  Tay–Sachs
  Adrenoleukodystrophy
  Metachromatic leukodystrophy
  Generalized gangliosidosis
  Juvenile gangliosidosis
  Niemann–Pick A
  Krabbe disease
  Pelizaeus–Merzbacher disease

Others
  Myotonic dystrophy[1111,1112]
  Pantothenate kinase-associated neurodegeneration
    (Hallervorden–Spatz syndrome)[1113]

neuropathies. Friedreich's ataxia[267–269] and Charcot–Marie–Tooth[270–272] are classic neurologic syndromes associated with optic atrophy. In Harding's series[273] of 90 patients with Friedrich's ataxia, most patients presented before age 25 with limb and truncal ataxia and absent decreased deep tendon reflexes. Visual acuity was usually not affected but 25% of patients had optic atrophy and two-thirds had abnormal visual-evoked potentials. The condition is autosomal recessive caused by a gene mutation on chromosome 9 and is characterized by an excessive number of GAA repeat sequences.[274,275] Progressive optic atrophy is also recognized in patients with congenital deafness.[276,277] More recently primary retinal degenerations have been recognized to occur in conjunction with these inherited ataxias (see Chapter 4) The spinocerebellar ataxias, particularly SCA1 and less so for SCA3, are associated with primary optic atrophy.[278,279] Recognizing vision loss localized to the optic nerve or retina can be very helpful in the characterization and evaluation of patients with hereditary ataxia.[280]

Lysosomal storage diseases (inherited deficiency of an enzyme required for normal metabolism of lysosomal macromolecules) are associated with a variety of ocular manifestations. In particular, optic atrophy results from ganglion cell damage from these accumulated materials. The conditions most commonly associated with optic atrophy are the mucopolysaccharidoses (Hurler and Scheie syndromes) and the lipidoses (gangliosidosis, Tay–Sachs disease, Neimann–Pick disease (see Chapter 16), adrenoleukodystrophy (see Chapter 8), and metachromatic leukodystrophy). Storage disorders with retinal manifestations are also discussed in Chapter 4.

Inflammatory optic neuropathies

Inflammatory optic neuropathies are characterized by acute or subacute, often painful, vision loss that results from inflammation of the optic nerve. They are the most common causes of optic neuropathy in young adults. The term idiopathic *optic neuritis* has come to have an even more specific implication: inflammatory optic neuropathy that usually accompanies demyelinating disease. Other inflammatory optic neuropathies include contiguous spread of inflammation from meninges, sinuses, and orbital soft tissues. These processes may be immune mediated, granulomatous, or infectious. Some patients may be labeled as having papillitis (a nonspecific term) when the inflammatory process leads to optic nerve-head swelling.

Optic neuritis

The vast majority of patients with inflammatory optic neuropathy have optic neuritis, a nerve inflammation secondary to demyelination. In many patients optic neuritis is the heralding manifestation of multiple sclerosis (MS).[281]

The Optic Neuritis Treatment Trial (ONTT)[282] has provided the best prospective data regarding the clinical presentation, visual outcome, and development of multiple sclerosis in patients with optic neuritis. The profound and far-reaching implications of the ONTT have been reviewed.[283,284]

The study was multicentered and entered 448 patients who were treated with an oral placebo, with intravenous steroids followed by an oral steroids taper, or with oral steroids alone. Each patient had a detailed history and ophthalmic and neurologic examinations. Visual acuity, color vision, contrast sensitivity, and Humphrey and Goldmann visual fields were recorded for each patient. Every patient had blood work for syphilis and lupus, and a fraction who consented underwent lumbar puncture. Patients were followed for all four of the measurable visual parameters and for the development of clinically definite multiple sclerosis.

Demographics. Patients with optic neuritis are typically young, with a peak incidence in the third and fourth decades (9–60), and more women than men are affected.[285] In the ONTT, 77% of the patients were women, 85% were white, and the mean age was 32. The prevalence of optic neuritis varies to some extent based on geography and race. Several studies have examined the incidence of optic neuritis, and in general the range is between 1 and 6.4 new cases per year per 100,000 population.[286,287] It is clear that rates vary with race, geography, and latitude, with whites of northern European ancestry at latitudes distant from the equator being most susceptible. Whites of Mediterranean ancestry are less commonly affected, and in African Americans and Asians the condition is relatively uncommon. Some studies have demonstrated a seasonal pattern to its incidence.[288] South African blacks tend to have bilateral optic neuropathy with a poorer

Table 5–6 Common symptoms in optic neuritis

Decreased vision
Visual field defects
Reduced color vision
Uhthoff's symptom
Decreased depth perception
Pain
Phosphenes
  Movement-induced
  Sound-induced

Table 5–7 Common examination findings in optic neuritis

Visual acuity loss
Dyschromatopsia
Reduced contrast sensitivity
Reduced stereoacuity
Visual field loss
  Global reduced sensitivity
  Central or centrocecal defects
  Altitudinal defects
Afferent pupillary defect
Normal or swollen optic nerve

visual prognosis and a lower association with multiple sclerosis.[289]

Neuro-ophthalmic symptoms. Vision loss is rapid in onset, usually over a period of hours to a few days. Symptoms commonly reported by optic neuritis patients are summarized in **Table 5–6**. Vision loss can progress for up to 1–2 weeks. Reduced color vision invariably accompanies the vision loss in optic neuritis. Patients frequently report a darkening or reduced vividness of color. Red objects may be described as either pinker or browner in patients with dyschromatopsia.

Characteristic pain precedes the vision loss by a few days and is present in the majority of patients (92% in the ONTT).[285] Globe tenderness and worsening of pain on eye movements are typical. The exact origin of the pain is unknown but presumably is the result of the pulling on the dura (in contact with the inflamed nerve) by the eye muscle origin from the annulus of Zinn.[290,291] Because this pain characteristically disappears after 3–5 days, pain persisting for longer than 7 days should be considered atypical and prompt an investigation for other causes of pain and optic neuropathy such as a systemic inflammatory condition, scleritis, malignant glioma, orbital inflammatory syndrome, aneurysm, or a sinus mucocele.

Phosphenes or flashing lights described by patients with optic neuritis generally take a variety of forms, including lights, sparkles, and shifting squares. They may be exacerbated by eye movements or loud noises.[292–294] These symptoms were present in 30% of patients in the ONTT.[285] These phosphenes can accompany the acute loss of vision and can also persist for months after resolution. They are not unique to inflammatory optic neuropathies but can occur in the setting of compressive lesions as well. The presence of phosphenes should also raise the possibility of concomitant retinal disease, as in neuroretinitis.

Uhthoff's symptom is a transient visual obscuration associated with elevation in body temperature.[295,296] The symptom can be provoked by as little as hot food or cooking but most typically is brought on by physical exertion or a hot shower.[296] Vision loss generally takes the form of blurring, graying, or reduced color vision and begins minutes after exposure to heat. Minutes to 1 hour later, vision returns to baseline without residual deficits. This symptom is not unique to optic neuritis patients and has been described in hereditary, toxic, compressive,[297] and sarcoid[298] optic neuropathies. Uhthoff's symptom tends to relapse and remit, and return of the symptom after a period of time does not necessarily

herald the onset of recurrent inflammation. For unclear reasons, the presence of Uhthoff's symptom may be a poor prognostic indicator as it correlates with white matter lesions on MRI and with the subsequent development of multiple sclerosis and recurrent optic neuritis.[296]

Neuro-ophthalmic signs (**Table 5–7**). Patients typically have reduced visual acuity ranging from nearly normal to NLP. In the ONTT,[282,285] 10% of patients had 20/20 vision, 25% had between 20/25 and 20/40 acuity, 29% had 20/50 to 20/190, and 36% had between 20/200 and NLP.

Dyschromatopsia can usually be easily identified by testing with pseudoisochromatic color plates and noting asymmetry between the eyes. More sensitive and extensive testing can be done with the Farnsworth–Munsell 100-hue test, but in clinical practice this is unnecessary. In the ONTT the 100-hue test was only modestly more sensitive than the Ishihara plates in detecting dyschromatopsia (88% abnormal by plates and 94% abnormal by the 100-hue test).[285] Further analysis of these data identified certain trends concerning the type of color vision loss (blue–yellow versus red–green at presentation and then after recovery). Ultimately Katz[299] concluded that no specific type of color defect was predictably associated with optic neuritis, and that the type of defect can change during the course of recovery. Subjective inter-eye differences can usually be brought out by asking patients to describe their perception of these plates or a red test object.

Contrast sensitivity was measurably abnormal in 98% of patients in the ONTT when compared with age-matched controls.[285] In fact, contrast sensitivity in optic neuritis was found to be the most sensitive indicator of visual dysfunction in acute and recovered optic neuritis.[300]

Patients with optic neuritis almost always have some visual field loss. On manual kinetic perimetry and tangent screen testing, the most common visual field defects in optic neuritis are central scotomas. The ONTT used computer static threshold perimetry as their standard and found 45% of the patients had diffuse field loss and 55% had local defects.[33] Of these localized visual field defects, the most common were altitudinal defects (29%) and "three-quadrant defects" (14%). Combined, central, and centrocecal defects occurred in 16% of patients. Overall these patterns of visual field loss represent the full spectrum of "optic nerve"-type field defects and do not aid the examiner in distinguishing optic neuritis from other causes of optic nerve dysfunction.[301]

The ONTT carefully studied fellow eye abnormalities in patients with acute unilateral optic neuritis.[302] Visual field defects were the most common (48% of patients) although abnormalities in acuity, color vision, and contrast sensitivity were also identified. Most of these deficits resolved over several months. Because all of the abnormal visual function parameters tended to improve with time, they were not thought to be false positives or spurious results. The question remains as to whether these represent subtle simultaneous bilateral attacks or unrecognized previous attacks. Also, whether these patients with bilateral findings are at increased risk of developing multiple sclerosis is uncertain.

On the fundus examination about one-third of patients have mild optic nerve-head swelling[285] (**Fig. 5–30**). This finding is generally much less marked than the swelling in papilledema, and it is less sectoral and unassociated with the capillary dilation and splinter hemorrhages typical of anterior ischemic optic neuropathy.[285] Less than 5% of patients have retinal exudates, phlebitis, or vitreous cells.[285] Extensive vitritis and retinal vein sheathing (**Fig. 5–30**) is unusual in optic neuritis and in this setting alternative diagnoses such as sarcoidosis and syphilis should be considered. Patients with typical optic neuritis do not later develop a macular "star." Such stars are more consistent with neuroretinitis (see below), a condition that is believed not to be a precursor of MS. Atypical findings of acute demyelinating optic neuritis include (1) no light perception vision, (2) optic disc or retinal hemorrhages, (3) severe optic disc swelling,

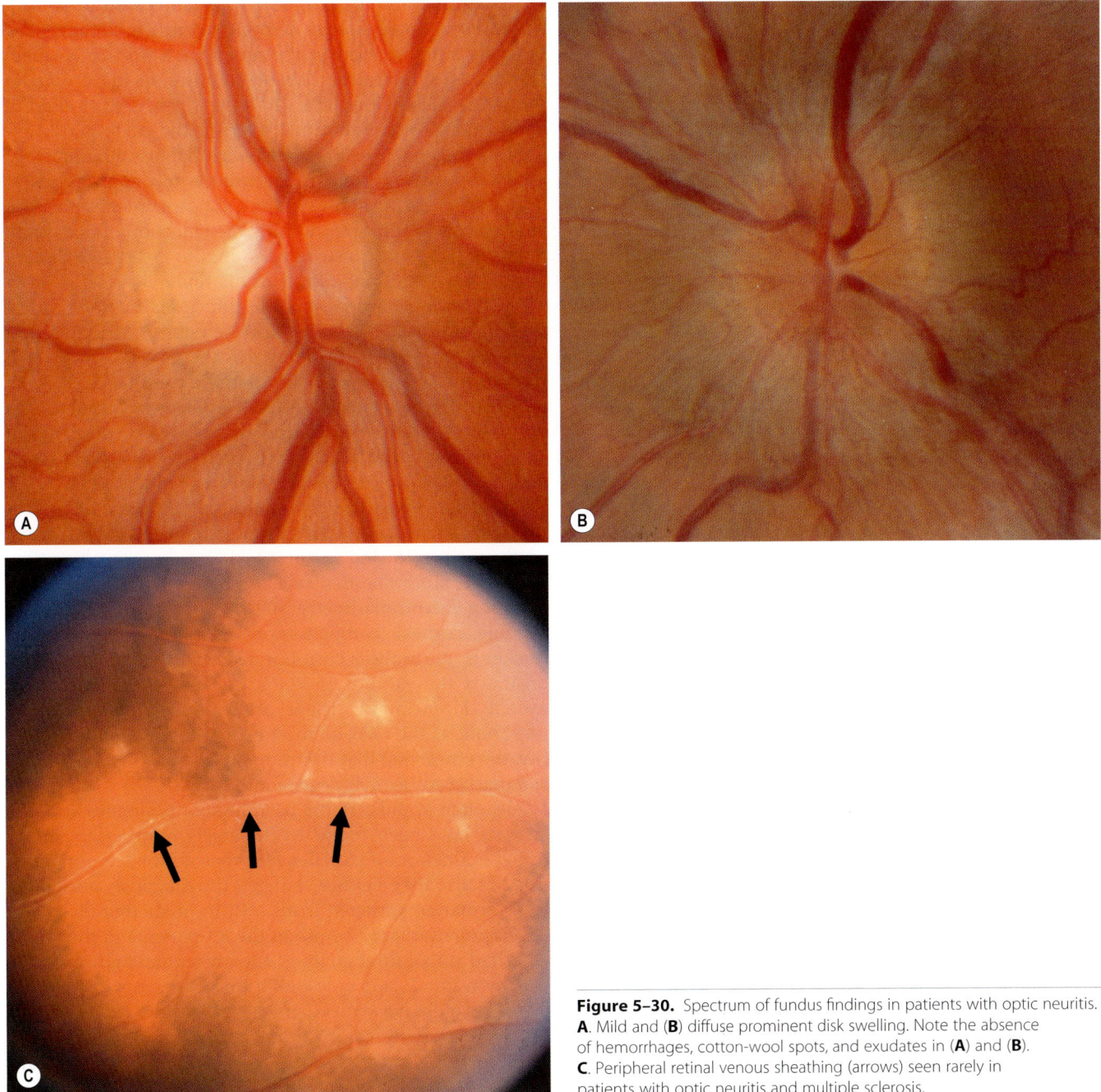

Figure 5–30. Spectrum of fundus findings in patients with optic neuritis. **A**. Mild and (**B**) diffuse prominent disk swelling. Note the absence of hemorrhages, cotton-wool spots, and exudates in (**A**) and (**B**). **C**. Peripheral retinal venous sheathing (arrows) seen rarely in patients with optic neuritis and multiple sclerosis.

(4) macular exudates, (5) absence of pain, (6) uveitis, and (7) bilateral visual loss. Although bilateral simultaneous optic neuritis is unusual in adults and requires a full evaluation, the majority of cases are still demyelinating.[303,304]

Diagnostic studies. The ONTT demonstrated that in typical patients (young patients with subacute vision loss and pain on eye movements), no laboratory test (blood studies, lumbar puncture, or MRI) aided in the diagnosis of idiopathic optic neuritis. These tests were done on patients entering the study, and they did not alter the course, treatment, or ultimate visual outcome of any of the patients.[285] However, the study did demonstrate a potential value for MRI in identifying patients at increased risk of developing MS.

MRI abnormalities consistent with plaques in the white matter of patients with optic neuritis are well recognized (**Fig. 5–31**). Abnormalities and enhancement are the result of breakdown of the blood–brain barrier. In the ONTT, 59% of patients with a previous normal neurologic history had clinically silent white matter lesions.[305] The most typical findings are >3 mm in diameter, T2 hyperintense lesions in the periventricular white matter, subcortical white matter, and pons.[306] These findings may be nonspecific and have been seen in "normal" patients and patients with other systemic inflammatory conditions. Enhancement of the lesions on T1 images indicates active plaques. To some extent, the presence and number of white matter lesions depends on the MR technique used. The use of STIR and FLAIR (fluid level attenuated inversion recovery) sequences increases the sensitivity of detecting these white matter lesions. In the ONTT,[305] patients' MRI scans were graded from 0 to IV depending on the number of typical white matter signal abnormalities. Only 41% of patients had normal studies. The significance of the baseline MRI scans is discussed below in the section on the relationship of optic neuritis to MS.

Over 90% of patients with optic neuritis have demonstrable lesions in the affected optic nerve using STIR sequences with fat-suppressed views of the orbit and an orbital surface coil[307] (**Fig. 5–32**). It has been shown that poor visual function may correlate with optic nerve lesion size and location in the optic canal. The lesions in the canal may be the most damaging because the tight bony canal causes secondary compression as the nerve swells.[308,309] This site is relatively uncommon, as the anterior and mid-orbital portions of the optic nerve are most frequently involved. Enhancement with gadolinium indicates an active process. Eye pain is more common when the orbital portion of the optic nerve or >10 mm of the nerve enhances.[290] When recovery occurs with the restoration of the blood–brain barrier, the nerve no longer enhances with gadolinium.

Visual-evoked potentials (VEPs) are only an extension of the neuro-ophthalmic examination and should not be used to make a diagnosis of optic neuritis in the setting of unexplained vision loss. Although changes in the VEPs can provide objective information to help confirm the diagnosis of optic neuritis, the diagnosis will always be a clinical one. In general, the occipital pattern VEPs will show marked latency changes with amplitude changes that generally correlate with the level of acuity loss. Usually the hallmark of optic neuritis would be markedly prolonged latency (p100) with relative preservation of amplitude. The development of

multifocal VEPs (mVEPs), which measure the conduction from multiple segments of the visual field (see Chapter 3), may be a more sensitive instrument than conventional VEP. In one study, 97.3% of eyes with optic neuritis had an abnormal mVEP; abnormalities included decreased amplitude in 96% of patients and increased latency in 68.4%.[310] Other optic neuropathies (presumably with more direct axonal injury) generally have lower amplitudes with less effect on latency. Despite these generalizations there is significant overlap and variability, and, therefore, we almost never use or recommend VEPs or mVEPs in the routine diagnosis or management of acute optic neuropathies. Recovery of the latency and improved conduction speed reflect recovery of the blockade owing to inflammatory changes and edema.

Originally developed to monitor patients with macular pathology (see Chapter 4) and glaucoma, OCT is now being recognized for its emerging role in patients with optic neuritis. The pathophysiology of optic neuritis is characterized by acute inflammation of the optic nerve with consequent loss of axons. Over time, degeneration results in thinning of the retinal nerve fiber layer (RNFL), which is composed of ganglion cell axons destined to form the optic nerve.[311,312] OCT has made it possible to assess axonal loss quantitatively and noninvasively, and this technique has applications to both optic neuritis and MS. The OCT technology functions analogously to ultrasound, using the reflection of near infrared light (820 nm), instead of sound, to create two-dimensional, cross-sectional images of the retina.

OCT studies have confirmed reductions in RNFL thickness in eyes with a history of optic neuritis.[313] One recent study demonstrated thinning of the RNFL within 3–6 months of an acute episode of optic neuritis in 74% of patients.[313] Such reductions in RNFL thickness correlate with decreases in visual function, as represented by measures of high-contrast visual acuity, computerized visual field mean deviation, and color vision.[314] Greater reductions in RNFL also correlated with less complete visual recovery, suggesting that OCT may have utility in predicting persistent visual dysfunction following an episode of optic neuritis.[313] Retinal nerve fiber abnormalities have also been demonstrated using scanning laser polarimetry (GDx).[315] In this study, using variable corneal compensation measurements of RNFL thickness, the authors corroborated OCT findings and demonstrated the validity of RNFL thickness as a marker for axonal degeneration. These observations are particularly important as the GDx method measures microtubule integrity, thus implying that thinning of the NFL on GDx studies is a marker for axonal degeneration in MS.[315]

Although popular in the past, lumbar punctures and CSF analysis have been found to be largely unnecessary in the initial evaluation of patients with typical isolated optic neuritis because they neither changed the diagnosis nor added to information garnered from MRI in predicting the future development of MS.[316] Among the 83 patients in the ONTT who had spinal fluid analysis, the protein and glucose were usually normal, and only one-third of patients had a pleocytosis usually between 6 and 27 WBC/mm³. Myelin basic protein was detected in about one-fifth of patients, and immunoglobulin (Ig)G synthesis in about two-fifths. Oligoclonal banding occurred in approximately half of the patients

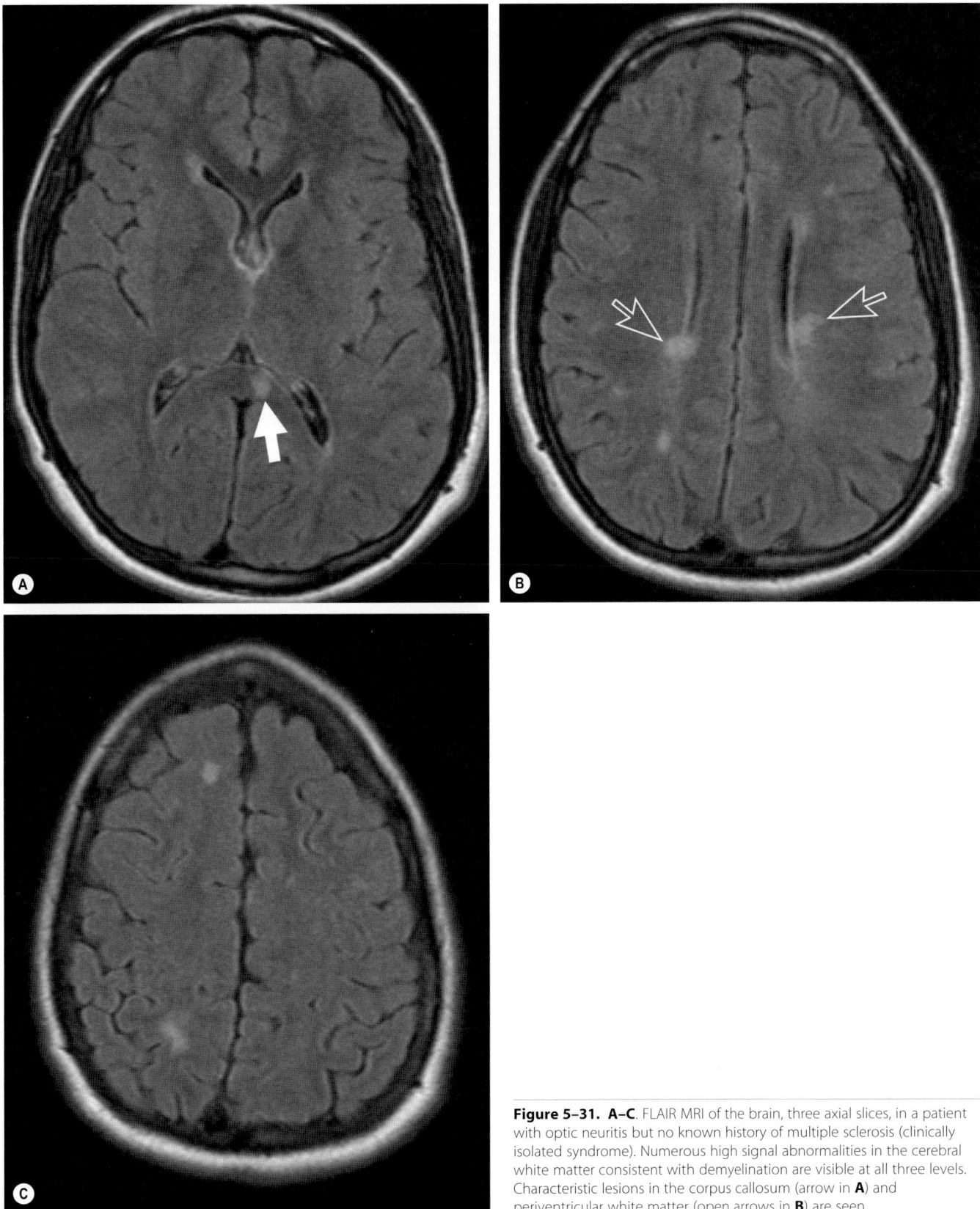

Figure 5–31. A–C. FLAIR MRI of the brain, three axial slices, in a patient with optic neuritis but no known history of multiple sclerosis (clinically isolated syndrome). Numerous high signal abnormalities in the cerebral white matter consistent with demyelination are visible at all three levels. Characteristic lesions in the corpus callosum (arrow in **A**) and periventricular white matter (open arrows in **B**) are seen.

and was associated with the future development of clinically definite MS. However, oligoclonal banding usually occurred in the presence of white matter lesions on MRI, which is less invasive and had a greater predictive value. Other studies have found the combination of an abnormal MRI scan and the presence of oligoclonal banding to be strongly associated with the development of MS.[317–320] In general, we would recommend CSF examination only for those patients with atypical optic neuritis or in those with unusual brain MRI findings.

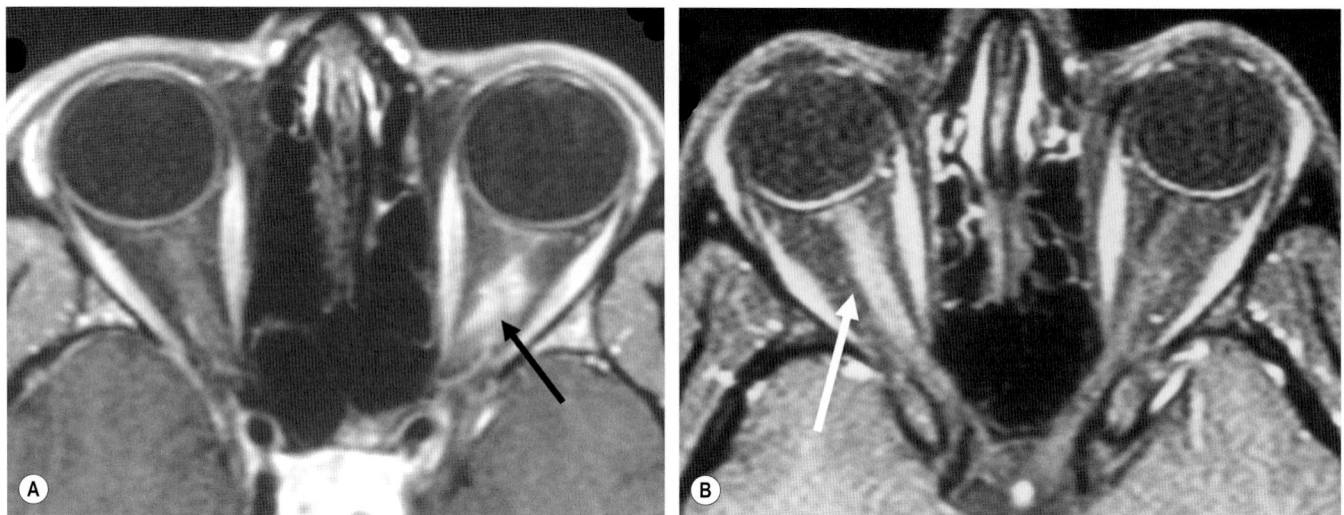

Figure 5–32. Axial T1-weighted, fat-suppressed, gadolinium-enhanced orbital MRIs in patients with acute optic neuritis. **A**. The MRI demonstrates focal enhancement (arrow) of the left optic nerve, and in another patient (**B**) more diffuse enhancement of the right optic nerve (arrow) is seen.

Course and recovery. The ONTT clearly demonstrated that the long-term visual prognosis in optic neuritis without treatment was the same as when either oral or intravenous steroids were given.[321] The same study demonstrated that intravenous steroids increased the rate at which vision recovered, but at 1 year all treatment groups tested similarly. This finding was confirmed in another study[322] which compared intravenous methylprednisolone with placebo in patients with either short or long segments of optic nerve enhancement on MRI. In the ONTT, oral prednisone increased the rate of recurrent optic neuritis, particularly at the 2 and 5 year follow-up periods.[282,323] At 10 years, the risk of recurrence remained higher in the oral prednisone group (44%) than in the placebo (31%, p = 0.07) and methylprednisolone groups (29%, p = 0.03), although these differences were not as robust as those seen earlier in the study.[324] At 15 years,[325] 72% of the eyes in the ONTT had visual acuity of at least 20/20 and 66% of patients had better than 20/20 acuity in both eyes demonstrating that long-term prognosis is excellent. Vision was worse in patients with MS than in those without MS. Quality-of-life scores were lower in patients with decreased vision and neurologic disability.

Recovery from optic neuritis is fairly prompt and usually nearly complete. In almost all of the patients in the ONTT (regardless of treatment type), recovery began within 1 month.[326] The ONTT[327] and other reports[328] have shown that patients with initial poor acuity (20/400 to NLP), more severe visual field loss, and more profound reduction of contrast sensitivity have a poorer prognosis, although most still improve to better than 20/40 vision. Furthermore, those patients with a visual acuity of 20/50 or worse at 1 month will usually have moderate to severe residual visual impairment.[327]

However, there is great variability in the quality of the "20/20" vision that remains. Recovery to 20/20 vision does not truly capture the types of visual dysfunction and the symptomatology that many patients report following recovery from optic neuritis. In the ONTT,[329] 63% of patients thought that their vision had not recovered to normal, although only a few reported any difficulty carrying on daily activities. Among 215 patients who reported their vision to be somewhat or much worse than it was before their optic neuritis, 43% had either normal results or only one abnormal result on all four measures of visual function tested (acuity, color, contrast, field).[329] Stereoacuity (despite normal Snellen acuity) was found to be abnormal in 85% of 27 patients in an earlier study.[330] In addition, patients with MS reported significant reduction in vision quality-of-life issues despite having normal visual acuity.[331,332]

One study suggested that visual loss in optic neuritis in African Americans was more severe at onset and after 1 year of follow-up than that in Caucasians.[333]

Multiple sclerosis. Because of the close association between optic neuritis and MS, the features and treatment of MS will be summarized before their relationship is discussed below.

MS is characterized by transient neurologic dysfunction, lasting days or weeks, owing to focal demyelination in the central nervous system (CNS). In addition to optic neuritis, other common clinical manifestations include double vision owing to involvement of the medial longitudinal fasciculus (internuclear ophthalmoplegia (INO)) (see Chapter 15), ataxia and nystagmus due to cerebellar white matter tract involvement (see Chapter 17), extremity weakness, bladder difficulty, and sensory abnormalities. Rarely, patients may also have uveitis (pars planitis and panuveitis).[334] MS primarily affects young adults, most often women, but children and older adults may also develop the disease.

In most individuals the initial course of MS is relapsing–remitting, with neurologic exacerbations separated by weeks, months, or years. Spontaneous recovery or near-recovery is the rule at this stage. Unfortunately, more severely affected patients may exhibit a progressive form of the disorder. This is manifested by a continuous decline in neurologic function that may have a profound effect on vision, ambulation, and cognition. Although the observations have been inconsistent and the reasons unclear, there may be an increased risk of attacks in the initial 6 month postpartum period in women with relapsing–remitting disease.[335]

Pathologically, new demyelinative plaques are characterized by perivascular inflammatory cell infiltration by CD4+ T cells.[336] Chronically, the plaques typically exhibit myelin destruction, disappearance of oligodendrocytes, and astrocyte proliferation. It is also now well recognized that axonal transection may be seen in many instances,[311] perhaps explaining the irreversibility of some neurologic deficits. Radiographically, the white matter lesions are typically periventricular and often project perpendicularly from the ventricular surface. However, recent attention has been directed at MRI demonstration of brain atrophy and spectographic evidence of neuronal cell loss in MS.[337]

The cause is unclear, but MS is likely an autoimmune process that occurs in genetically susceptible individuals following an environmental exposure.[338] An immune cross-reaction to viral antigens has been implicated.[339] A greater incidence of MS in Caucasians and first-degree relatives of affected individuals, and single-nucleotide polymorphisms found in families with MS,[340] support the notion that genetic factors may also play a role. The possibility of an environmental factor is also supported by the preponderance of cases in northern latitudes.

The diagnosis of MS is primarily a clinical one and can be formally established when a patient has an idiopathic syndrome consistent with inflammatory demyelination of the optic nerve, brain, and spinal cord. However, MRI abnormalities are playing a larger role in making the diagnosis of MS.[341,342] The McDonald criteria were established to enable the diagnosis of MS when a patient has had one or more clinical events consistent with demyelination and then has MRI evidence of disease dissemination in time and space (**Table 5–8**).[343,344]

Treatment options in MS may be classified as symptomatic or preventative. Although most exacerbations are self-limited, those causing weakness or incoordination are usually treated with a short course of high-dose intravenous methylprednisolone. Other treatment options that are rarely used for acute attacks in relapsing–remitting disease include intramuscular adrenocorticotropic hormone (ACTH) and intravenous immune globulin. Plasma exchange may be used in patients with severe neurologic dysfunction poorly responsive to corticosteroids.

The immunomodulatory medications interferon-β1a, interferon-β1b, and glatiramer acetate have been approved for use in patients with relapsing–remitting multiple sclerosis and are the mainstays of MS therapy.[345] In large controlled studies, each decreased the frequency of exacerbations and slowed the rate of appearance of new white matter lesions on MRI.[346-355] Interferon-β1a medications also delay the progression of sustained neurologic disability.[347,356]

The chemotherapeutic agent mitoxantrone is approved for patients with more advanced forms of multiple sclerosis. This drug is limited by the potential side-effects of cardiotoxicity and secondary leukemia. The medication natalizumab is also approved by the Federal Drug Administration (FDA) for the treatment of the relapsing forms of multiple sclerosis. Natalizumab demonstrated a robust effect on MS relapses, disability progression, and MRI changes when compared with patients receiving placebo.[357] However, the use of natalizumab has been associated with progressive multifocal leukoencephalopathy (PML; see Chapter 8), and thus natalizumab is primarily used as a second-line therapy for multiple sclerosis.[358]

With the development of preventative therapy options for MS, some debate exists whether it is reasonable to begin immunomodulatory therapy for patients with their initial demyelinating event and a brain MRI that shows white matter change typical of MS. Some experts advocate an initial observation period to better determine the patient's disease progression before initiating therapy. They argue that many patients could avoid long-term therapy—and the financial expense and adverse effects that accompany it—without affecting the patient's long-term prognosis. Other physicians argue that such patients cannot be consistently identified, and that delaying treatment risks long-term, irreversible disability.[359,360] Until we can reliably determine which patients can safely defer treatment, we recommend offering long-term therapy to all patients with a first demyelinating event whose MRI suggests high risk for MS.

The relationship between optic neuritis and multiple sclerosis. Optic neuritis can occur in patients who have already developed MS, or it can be the first manifestation. Many patients with MS will have optic neuritis at some time during the course of their illness (**Table 5–9**). The clinical features of optic neuritis are indistinguishable in patients with or without MS.

In previously normal patients with optic neuritis and other clinically isolated syndromes (CIS) such as an INO or transverse myelitis, the most reliable predictor for the future development of MS is the presence of white matter lesions on MRI. In long-term follow-up, the risk of clinically definite MS is approximately 60–90% with a positive MRI and 20–25% when the baseline MRI scan is normal (**Table 5–9**).[303,357,361,362] Other clinical and demographic features are also predictive. In the 15 year follow-up in the ONTT, MS did not develop in any patient with a normal MRI scan who had (1) painless visual loss, (2) severe optic disc edema, (3) disc or peripapillary hemorrhage, (4) macular exudates, or (5) no light perception vision.[303] In patients with a normal baseline MRI scan, male gender and the presence of disc swelling were associated with a smaller risk of converting to MS. Fifteen years after a bout of optic neuritis, 50% of

Table 5–8 McDonald criteria to diagnose multiple sclerosis (MS) based on MRI evidence of disease dissemination in space or time in a patient who has had one or more clinical events consistent with demyelination.[343] The diagnosis of MS can also be established based upon clinical criteria, e.g., two events separated in space and time

Dissemination in space
3 or 4 of the following:
1) 9 T2 lesions or positive gadolinium enhancement
2) >3 periventricular lesions
3) >1 juxtacortical lesions
4) >1 infratentorial lesions (includes spinal cord or brain stem)

Dissemination in time
Established if a new T2 lesion appears 30 days from disease onset

Table 5–9 Prospective studies examining the risk of developing multiple sclerosis (MS) after a first attack of optic neuritis (not clinically isolated syndromes per se)

Study	Location	Follow-up (years)	Proportion developing MS	Comments
Landy (1983)[1114]	Australia	Range 1–29	71%	
Francis et al. (1987)[1115]	UK	Mean 11.6	57%	By life-table analysis, probability of MS by 15 years was 75%
Rizzo & Lessell (1988)[281]	New England (USA)	Mean 14.9	58%	By life-table analysis, probability of MS by 15 years was 74% for women and 34% for men
Sandberg-Wollheim et al. (1990)[1116]	Sweden	Mean 12.9	38%	By life-table analysis, probability of MS by 15 years was 45%
Morrissey et al. (1993)[306]	UK	Mean 5.3	Normal MRI: 6%; abnormal MRI: 82%	MRI white matter lesions were associated with development of MS
Jacobs et al. (1997)[366]	New York (USA)	Range 4 months to 19 years	Normal MRI: 16%; abnormal MRI: 38%	MRI white matter lesions were associated with development of MS
Optic Neuritis Study Group (ONTT) (1997)[1117]	USA and Canada	5	Normal MRI: 16%; abnormal MRI: 51%	MRI white matter lesions were associated with development of MS
Söderström et al. (1998)[319]	Sweden	Mean 2.1	3 or more lesions on MRI: 62.5%; less than 3 lesions on MRI: 13%	
Ghezzi et al. (1999)[1118]	Italy	Mean 6.3	Normal MRI: 0%; abnormal MRI: 51%	
Optic Neuritis Study Group (ONTT) (2003)[303]	USA and Canada	10	Normal MRI: 22%; abnormal MRI: 56%	MRI white matter lesions were associated with development of MS
Tintore et al. (2005)[364]	Barcelona	Median follow-up 39 months	Abnormal MRI 67%	Baseline MRI abnormal in 50.8% of ON vs 76% of brain stem and spinal cord patients with a clinically isolated syndrome. Risk of MS is similar when baseline MRI is abnormal
Optic Neuritis Study Group (ONTT) (2008)[363]	USA and Canada	15	Normal MRI 25%; abnormal MRI 72%	MRI white matter lesions were associated with development of MS

patients had developed MS; 72% of those with one or more brain MRI lesions at presentation and 25% of those with no lesions.[363]

In a prospective study of 320 patients with clinically isolated syndromes,[364] the rates of conversion to MS were the same regardless of the type of CIS. After a median follow-up period of 39 months, approximately 70% of patients with clinically isolated syndromes and abnormal baseline MRI had developed MS. Of note, only 49% of the patients with optic neuritis had a positive MRI at baseline compared with 76% with brain stem and spinal cord syndromes. The authors emphasize that those patients with a positive baseline MRI and a clinically isolated syndrome act similarly in their conversion to MS. Patients with optic neuritis as a first demyelinating event tend to have brain MRI lesions less frequently than do those with spinal cord or brain stem presentations.[364]

Although less predictive, the following other tests are also associated with the development of MS if positive at the time of the first attack of optic neuritis: CSF oligoclonal bands,[317,320,365] increased CSF IgG synthesis,[366] HLA-DR2 antigen,[319,367] and somatosensory-evoked potentials.

Several OCT studies have also supported the notion that subclinical axon loss and visual abnormalities occur in MS patients (**Fig. 5–33**), even in eyes without a clinical history of acute optic neuritis.[313,314,368,369] Fisher et al.[368] demonstrated that, among MS patients and disease-free controls, the greatest decreases in RNFL thickness occurred in eyes affected by optic neuritis; however, the unaffected eyes of patients with MS also showed reductions in RNFL thickness,

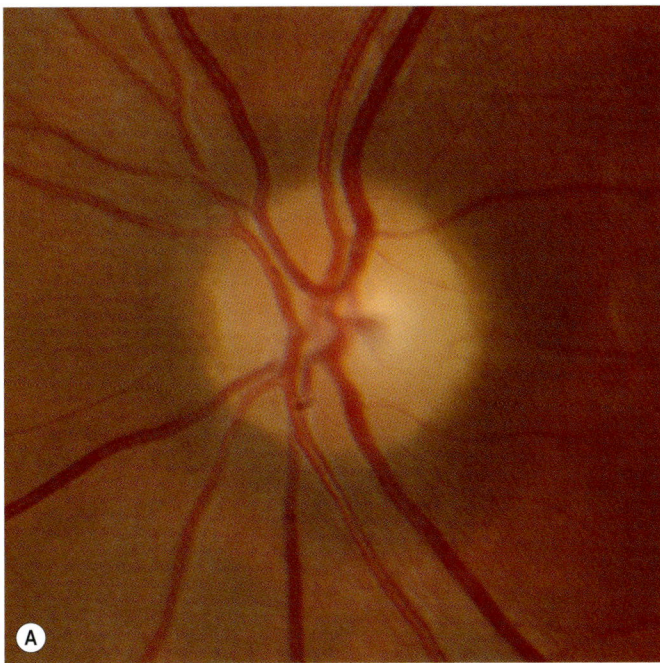

Figure 5–33. A. Left optic nerve appearance in a patient with multiple sclerosis but no known history of optic neuritis showing mild temporal pallor, which correlated on ocular coherence tomography (**B**) with nerve fiber layer (NFL) thinning (arrows). The average NFL thickness was 88.01 μm, which is significantly reduced.

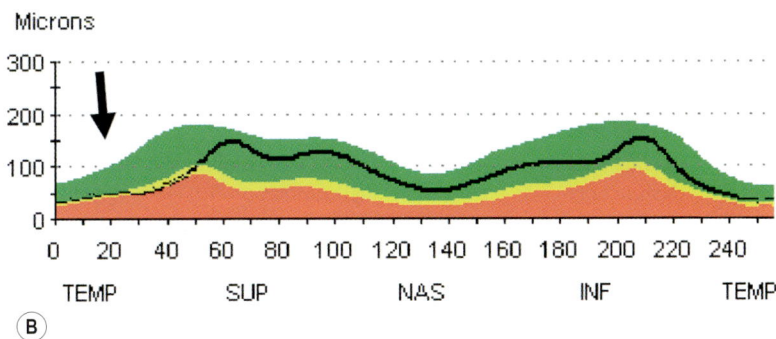

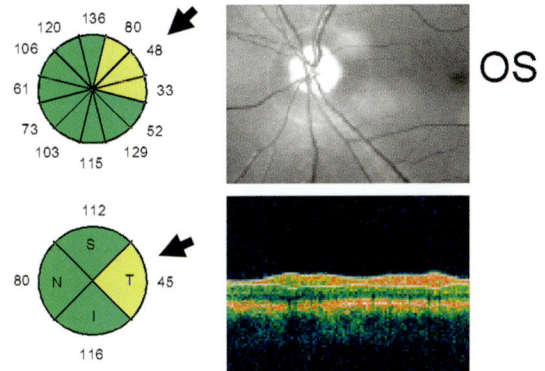

relative to disease-free controls (p = 0.03). This capacity of OCT to identify subclinical axon loss may facilitate early intervention and better long-term visual outcomes.[369] These data suggest that OCT may serve an important future role in monitoring patients with optic neuritis and MS, both clinically and in the setting of treatment trials.

Evaluation of optic neuritis in typical cases. In typical cases of optic neuritis (acute or subacute monocular visual loss with pain on eye movements in a young adult), MRI scanning of the brain is the only requisite test. The predictive value of MRI is important in patient counseling, and some patients with abnormal MRI scans may desire treatment to reduce the relative risk of early conversion to MS (see below). Serum serologies, lumbar punctures, and evoked potentials are unnecessary. Typical patients should be followed within the first week or two to document the visual nadir, then at 4 weeks to insure that vision starts to recover spontaneously. Those with disc swelling should be observed for development of a macular star (see neuroretinitis).

Treatment in typical cases. Many patients, especially those with normal MRI scans, will not require any treatment and vision usually improves spontaneously. However, intrave-

nous corticosteroids followed by a short course of oral steroids may be considered in two instances:

1. In patients with white matter lesions on MRI, steroid treatment should be offered to reduce the risk of developing MS for the first 2 years. The ONTT demonstrated that a course of intravenous steroids given at the time of an acute attack of optic neuritis, particularly in patients with abnormal MRI scans, reduced the rate of development of clinically definite MS in the first 2 years (**Table 5–10**).[370] Although controversial, and potentially affected by reanalysis bias,[284,371–373] these findings led to the broad recommendation that patients with optic neuritis and abnormal MRI scans should be treated with steroids to reduce the risk of developing MS.[312,374,375] Subsequently, after 3 years that beneficial effect disappeared.[376]

2. We have a low threshold to use intravenous corticosteroid treatment in patients with severe unilateral or bilateral visual loss because of their slightly poorer visual prognosis and because steroids may hasten recovery. The protocol established by the

Table 5–10 Treatment options for acute demyelinating optic neuritis in monosymptomatic patients at high risk for multiple sclerosis (MS)

Study	Medications (standard dosage)	Potential side-effects	Potential benefits of therapy
Short-term therapy:			
Optic Neuritis Treatment Trial (ONTT, n = 457)[282,370]	Intravenous (IV) methylprednisolone (250 mg every 6 hours × 3 days) + oral prednisone taper (1 mg/kg/day × 11 days, 4 day taper (20 mg day 1; 10 mg days 2 and 4))	Sleep disturbances, mild mood changes, stomach upset, weight gain, hyperglycemia, worsening hypertension	Hastens visual recovery but does not affect long-term visual outcome Reduced rate of MS development within first 2 years Oral prednisone alone at dose of 1 mg/kg may increase risk of recurrent optic neuritis and should be avoided
Long-term therapy:			
Controlled High Risk Avonex MS Prevention Trial (CHAMPS, n = 383)[361]	Interferon β-1a (30 μg intramuscularly (IM) weekly)	Flu-like symptoms (fever, chills, myalgias: may be treated symptomatically), depression, anemia, hepatic dysfunction	Reduced 3-year probability of MS (2nd demyelinating event) vs placebo (35% vs 50%) Lower rates of new but clinically silent MRI lesion accumulation (T2, T1-enhancing)
Early Treatment of MS Study (ETOMS, n = 308)[383]	Interferon β-1a (22 μg subcutaneously (SC) weekly)*	Injection site inflammation, flu-like symptoms (fever, chills, myalgias: may be treated symptomatically), anemia, hepatic dysfunction	Reduced 2-year probability of MS (2nd demyelinating event) vs placebo (34% vs 45%) Increased time to 2nd demyelinating event (569 vs 252 days) Lower rates of new MRI lesion accumulation (T2) (16% vs 6%)
Betaferon in Newly Emerging MS for Initial Treatment (BENEFIT, n = 468)[385]	Interferon β-1b (250 μg subcutaneously (SC) every other day)	Injection site inflammation, flu-like symptoms (fever, chills, myalgias: may be treated symptomatically), hepatic dysfunction	1) Reduced 2-year probability of MS (2nd demyelinating event) vs placebo (28% vs 85%) 2) Reduced 2-year probability of McDonald MS (69% vs 85%) 3) Increased time to 2nd demyelinating event (618 vs 255 days) 4) Lower cumulative number of newly active MRI lesions (3.7 vs 8.5)
Glatiramer Acetate in Clinically Isolated Syndrome PRECISE (n = 481)[1122]	Glatiramer acetate 20 mg subcutaneously every day	Injection site inflammation, lipoatrophy, postinjection palpitations, anxiety, chest pain	1) Reduced probability of 2nd demyelinating event by 45% 2) Increased time to 2nd demyelinating event (722 vs 336 days) 3) Reduced number of new T2 lesions by 61%

*Note that the ETOMS study used 22 μg interferon β-1a, while standard therapy for relapsing–remitting MS is 44 μg.
Modified from Burkholder BM, Galetta SL, Balcer LJ. Acute demyelinating optic neuritis. Expert Rev Ophthalmol 2006;1:159–170.

ONTT is methylprednisolone 250 mg intravenously q.i.d. for 3 days, followed by prednisone 1 mg/kg q.d. for days 4–14, then 20 mg of prednisone on day 15, and 10 mg on days 16 and 18. At home, intravenous steroids (1 g methylprednisolone every day for 3 days) can be administered safely in relatively young healthy individuals, and, if there are no relative contraindications such as diabetes, peptic ulcer disease, or coronary artery disease, the risk is small.[377] Hospitalization may be required in older individuals and in those with the aforementioned medical illnesses. Because of the increased risk of recurrent episodes, patients with optic neuritis should not be given oral prednisone alone.[378] Despite the abundance of class I clinical trial evidence, disappointingly ophthalmologists and neurologists around the world have not universally adopted the protocol outlined above.[379-382] There are still many practitioners who prescribe oral steroids and others who prescribe steroids with the false notion that they improve final visual outcome.

Therapy for the patient with the clinically isolated syndrome. In patients with a CIS and a brain MRI with typical white matter lesions, interferon-β or glatiramer acetate can be given to reduce the risk of developing MS. Supportive evidence comes from several large clinical trials (**Table 5–10**).[383-385]

Other therapies for optic neuritis. Although the use of oral high-dose methylprednisolone in one study was not associated with an increased risk of recurrent attacks,[386] the small size of this study precluded any definite conclusions regarding its use in acute optic neuritis. Small studies have suggested that intravenous immunoglobulin (IVIg) may have some benefit in patients with substantial visual deficits following optic neuritis.[387] However, subsequent randomized trials in which the outcome measure was either visual acuity or contrast sensitivity failed to demonstrate a significant benefit with this treatment.[388-390] Furthermore, the routine use of IVIg in optic neuritis and MS remains limited by cost and availability.

Plasma exchange, used successfully in other inflammatory and demyelinating disorders, may have a role in treating patients with optic neuritis who are unresponsive to other therapies. In a retrospective review of 10 patients with steroid-refractory optic neuritis, plasma exchange was associated with short-term improvement in visual acuity in seven of these patients.[391] However, a large prospective controlled trial is necessary to better understand the role of plasma exchange in this refractory patient population.

Evaluation of optic neuritis in atypical cases. Criteria for atypical optic neuritis include (1) marked disc swelling, (2) vitritis, (3) progression of visual loss after 1 week, (4) lack of partial recovery within 4 weeks of onset of visual loss, and (5) persistent pain. A suggested workup with diagnostic considerations in these cases is given in **Table 5–11**. Compressive lesions will have been excluded by MRI.

Neuromyelitis optica (Devic disease)

Neuromyelitis optica (NMO) is classically described as a severe demyelinating disease that preferentially targets the optic nerves and spinal cord; however, more recent observations suggest that occasional patients may have a more benign course resembling that of MS.[392] Patients typically present with acute-onset optic neuritis, closely preceded or followed by paraparesis or paraplegia. It tends to occur in young adults, but is also well recognized in children. Both monophasic illnesses and recurrent attacks have been described.[393] Patients tend to present with visual loss and evidence of spinal cord dysfunction within 8 weeks of each other.

Table 5–11 Suggested diagnostic considerations, laboratory evaluation, and distinguishing features in *atypical* cases of optic neuritis

Entity	Laboratory test	Comment
Optic nerve compression	MRI	Progressive loss of vision beyond 10 days
Carcinomatous meningitis	CSF cytology	Systemic tumor almost always present
Syphilis	MHATP	Papillitis with hemorrhage Optic perineuritis Uveitis
Lyme	Serum Lyme titer	Endemic area Erythema chronicum migrans Optic perineuritis
Sarcoid	ACE CXR	Optic nerve granuloma Uveitis Periphlebitis
Anterior ischemic optic neuropathy	ESR	Age > 50 Segmental disc swelling Disc hemorrhage
Lupus	ANA	Arthritis Antiphospholipid antibody syndrome
Nutritional	B_{12} level serum copper	Progressive optic atrophy Pernicious anemia Ileum dysfunction Gastric surgery
Leber's hereditary optic neuropathy	Mitochondrial analysis	Males > females Pseudo-disc edema Telangiectasias

ACE, angiotensin converting enzyme; ANA, antinuclear antibody; CSF, cerebrospinal fluid; CXR, chest radiograph; ESR, erythrocyte sedimentation rate; MHATP, microhemagglutination–*Treponema pallidum*; MRI, magnetic resonance imaging.

In contrast to typical demyelinating optic neuritis, the vision loss observed in NMO is often bilateral and severe, occasionally progressing to blindness.[394] Some patients may have frequent recurrent episodes of optic neuritis. Periorbital pain, an almost universal feature in typical demyelinating optic neuritis, is not as common in NMO. The optic disc may appear normal or swollen, and varying degrees of visual recovery can occur. Like idiopathic optic neuritis, NMO-associated optic neuritis is associated with significant thinning of the nerve fiber layer on OCT, which correlates with visual function and quality of life.[395]

MR imaging typically demonstrates scattered areas of demyelination, concentrated in the optic nerves, chiasm, and spinal cord. Lesions of the spinal cord are longitudinally extensive, involving at least three vertebral segments.[396] Although diagnostic criteria for NMO originally excluded patients with brain lesions on MRI, it is now believed that brain lesions may be seen in as many of 60% of patients with NMO. However, these lesions are typically non-specific, and only about 10% have the typical MS morphology.[359,396]

Spinal fluid abnormalities may include a pleocytosis of greater than 50 cells/mm³ and oligoclonal bands may be observed in 20–30% of patients. This contrasts with established MS in which a moderate pleocytosis is rare, and oligoclonal banding is seen in 70–90% of patients.

Autopsy studies have demonstrated typical demyelinating plaques (like MS) in some patients, while in others a necrotizing myelitis (unlike MS) with thickened blood vessel walls was found.[397,398] Astrocytosis, reactive gliosis, and microcavitation may be seen pathologically in the optic nerves.[398] Because of the necrotizing nature of the lesions, the prognosis for recovery may be worse from both a visual and neurologic standpoint, especially in elderly patients. In a review of the literature,[399] 22% of the reported cases developed respiratory failure, 16% died in the acute stages, 14% had a poor neurologic outcome, and 70% of patients improved neurologically. Older age was a poor prognostic factor along with CSF pleocytosis and more severe myelitis. In this same study, 42% of the patients had a recurrence of a demyelinating event suggestive of multiple sclerosis with the other 58% having a monophasic illness without recurrence.[399] Many patients in the latter group had prodromal symptoms suggestive of a viral illness and a course suggestive of a post-infectious encephalomyelitis.

There is no definitive diagnostic test for NMO. A recently discovered serum IgG autoantibody is associated with NMO, with reported 73% sensitivity and 94% specificity.[400,401] The antibody targets an aquaporin channel, located in the astrocytic foot processes of the blood–brain barrier, that functions in fluid homeostasis.[402] The antibody has also been detected in patients with NMO without optic nerve involvement.[403]

It is still uncertain whether NMO is a variant of MS or a unique entity. There is considerable overlap between NMO and MS,[392] as reflected by the new diagnostic criteria proposed by the Mayo Clinic for NMO.[401] These criteria eliminate the requirement that symptoms must be referable to the optic nerves and spinal cord exclusively; similarly, brain lesions on MRI no longer preclude a diagnosis of NMO.

Currently, the diagnosis of NMO is best established when a patient has had at least one episode of optic neuritis, transverse myelitis, and a longitudinally extensive spinal cord lesion on MRI (>3 segments long). The diagnosis is bolstered by detecting the NMO antibodies and by having a normal or nondiagnostic baseline brain MRI.

There is no standard treatment for optic neuritis in the context of NMO, although high-dose intravenous corticosteroids may be beneficial in lessening the severity of the attack and speeding recovery of visual function. One small case series suggested that the combination of long-term prednisone and azathioprine may decrease disability and prevent relapses in patients with NMO.[404] This study led to a recent case series by Cree et al.[405] and Jacob et al.[406] which demonstrated the potential benefit of rituximab as a treatment for NMO. In patients with refractory disease, plasmapheresis followed by IVIg may be useful in treating an acute demyelinating attack.

Neuromyelitis optica is also well recognized in children.[407–411] In one study,[409] all patients had a preceding viral syndrome, 90% had bilateral visual loss, and all patients had disc swelling. In this same study,[409] vision in all patients recovered to 20/20 (some with optic atrophy), and no patients had recurrences of neurologic illness. However, our experience is less sanguine, and we have treated some children with multiple exacerbations and permanent visual loss

Other systemic conditions may be associated with Devic disease. These include systemic lupus erythematosus,[412] other connective tissue diseases such as Sjogren syndrome,[413] and pulmonary tuberculosis.[414,415]

Pediatric optic neuritis and multiple sclerosis

For many reasons, inflammatory disease of the optic nerve in children is quite different from that in adults. While there are some children and adolescents who have unilateral attacks of demyelinating optic neuritis and later develop MS, there are many others with an illness that seems to be quite distinct from the adult variety of the disease. Like adults, most children experience acute loss of vision associated with an afferent pupil defect and visual field defects. Unlike adults, however, children have a much higher likelihood of having bilateral involvement (50–75%) and disc swelling (50–75%).[416–420]

There have been no formal studies evaluating the optimal treatment of childhood optic neuritis. However, because of the patients' young ages, we favor more aggressive evaluation and treatment when visual loss is unilateral and severe or bilateral at any level. Workup includes MRI scanning, serologies, and lumbar puncture to exclude other causes. Hospitalization and 3–5 days of intravenous methylprednisolone (4 mg/kg q.i.d.) therapy is initiated, followed by an oral prednisone taper (starting at 1 mg/kg, then reduced over 2–4 weeks). Prognosis for recovery in children is generally excellent, with more than 80% of children returning to 20/20 or better,[418,420,421] and 96% returning to 20/40 or better.[416] Good et al.,[423] however, reported a series of 10 children, seven of whom remained at 20/200 or worse.

Etiologic considerations in childhood optic neuritis suggest that there may be three distinct subsets of patients. First, one group has their neurologic event (immune mediated) in the setting of postinfectious acute disseminated encephalomyelitis (ADEM), with or without radiographically demonstrable white matter lesions.[424,425] Typically following a febrile illness or vaccination, this group of patients has a monophasic demyelinating illness with recovery and without recurrence.[426] The second group may present with "idiopathic" (genetic predisposition with environmental trigger) demyelination, recover, but later develop recurrent a neurologic illness suggestive of MS or neuromyelitis optica.[477] The possibility that these two groups are linked and that viral illness or vaccinations are important triggers of multiple sclerosis has also been proposed.[427] For instance, cases of childhood optic neuritis and multiple sclerosis have been reported after viral illnesses and varicella.[427-430] A third group of pediatric patients have a benign condition characterized by isolated optic neuritis, typically with bilateral involvement and with disc swelling, and a normal brain MRI. Although recurrences of optic neuritis may occur in this group, patients in this category tend not to develop MS.

Overall, between 10% and 50% of children with optic neuritis eventually develop MS.[416,420,421,423,431-436] In one series of children with optic neuritis and an average follow-up of 7.3 years, brain MRI scanning was found to be a very important prognostic factor as three out of seven children with white matter lesions developed MS, while none of 11 patients without white matter lesions developed MS.[416]

MS in children is recognized in patients as young as 2 years old.[437-439] When compared with adult MS patients, children with MS take longer to convert to the secondary progressive form (median 28 years), but do so at a relatively younger age (median 41 years old).[440] Many of the same disease-modifying therapies used in adults are being used in younger patients as well.[441-443]

Sarcoidosis

This disease is a multisystem disorder of unknown etiology, characterized pathologically by noncaseating epithelioid cell granulomas.[444] It is much more common in African Americans and slightly more common in women than in men. The initial onset of the systemic illness may be an isolated visual or neurologic presentation, or there may be systemic symptoms including rash, fevers, night sweats, diarrhea, pulmonary symptoms, and lymphadenopathy. Most patients will have hilar adenopathy detectable on chest radiograph, as extrapulmonary sarcoidosis without hilar adenopathy is rare. Central nervous system involvement in sarcoidosis occurs in about 5% of cases.[445,446] The most common neurologic complication is seventh nerve palsy (see Chapter 14), followed by involvement of other cranial nerves, aseptic meningitis, and peripheral neuropathy.

On the other hand, ocular involvement in sarcoidosis occurs in about 25% of patients.[447] In the vast majority this takes the form of a relapsing and remitting anterior uveitis, often associated with ocular hypertension. In patients with posterior segment involvement, sarcoidosis most commonly

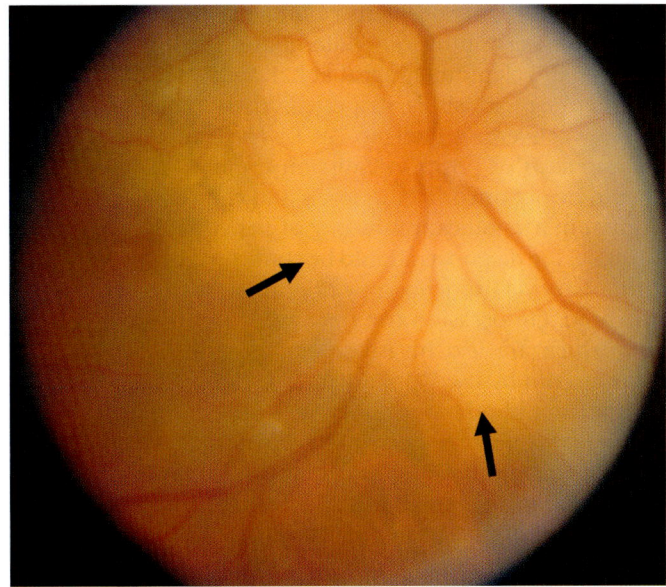

Figure 5–34. Optic nerve head appearance in a patient with sarcoidosis and swelling of the optic nerve head and peripapillary subretinal granulomas (arrows).

presents with retinal vasculitis, vitreous infiltrates, and choroidal lesions, often with associated disc swelling (see Chapter 4).

Optic nerve involvement in the setting of sarcoidosis can taken many different forms.[448,449] Some patients present with a syndrome similar to idiopathic optic neuritis. Other patients have an optic nerve head or subretinal granuloma (**Fig. 5–34**), while others may have a swollen nerve (due to either optic nerve or optic nerve sheath infiltration).[450] Also common is a pure retrobulbar presentation with a normal-appearing optic nerve head.[448,449] Sarcoidosis is also a well-recognized cause of perineuritis (see below) and can cause gaze-evoked amaurosis.[451]

Patients can present with progressive vision loss, and in general have less pain than patients with idiopathic optic neuritis. No light perception vision is common and should heighten the suspicion for sarcoid in patients with optic neuropathies.[449] Vision loss initially may be steroid responsive. Other patients have a relentless downhill course, despite the use of steroids, and develop profound visual impairment. Cases with spontaneous improvement and isolated disc swelling without optic nerve dysfunction have been reported.[452] Sarcoidosis with optic nerve involvement must be considered in all patients thought to have inflammatory or compressive disease of the anterior visual pathway (also see Chapter 7). Important clues are the presence of a steroid-responsive optic neuropathy and findings atypical for ordinary optic neuritis such as vitritis, retinal vasculitis, or enlargement of the optic nerve on MRI scanning.[448,449] Sarcoidosis can also present as an orbital inflammatory syndrome (see Chapter 18).

Diagnostic studies/evaluation. Sarcoidosis presenting with a markedly thickened optic nerve sheath on MRI scan, mimicking optic nerve sheath meningioma, is well recognized.[453-456] Imaging of the orbit will often reveal a "mass lesion," lacrimal gland enlargement, or optic nerve and/or sheath enhancement.[457] MRI may also demonstrate periventricular multifocal white matter lesions in CNS sarcoidosis[458] or leptomeningeal enhancement.[449]

When sarcoidosis is suspected, chest radiograph, angiotensin converting enzyme (ACE) level and, if necessary, gallium scan or positron emission tomography (PET) scan should be obtained.[459] ACE levels and chest imaging may be normal in a significant minority of patients.[448,449] Whenever possible, the diagnosis should be confirmed by biopsy (often pulmonary via bronchoscopy or of hilar nodes via mediastinoscopy). On occasion conjunctival or lacrimal gland biopsies, which are less invasive than the pulmonary or hilar biopsies, can be used and are diagnostic.[460,461] In general we do not favor blind biopsies of any organ but prefer to biopsy tissue that is visibly affected or is abnormal on radiograph, imaging, or gallium scan. Finally, it is reasonable to consider sarcoidosis in all cases of unexplained optic neuropathy, and screening with chest radiograph and ACE levels will occasionally suggest the diagnosis.[448,449]

Treatment. Treatment with systemic steroids is likely to be required for a protracted time (weeks to months).[462] Other patients require chronic immunosuppression with alternative cytotoxic drugs.[462,463] Treatment is generally with systemic steroids and cyclosporine.[464,465] Infliximab[466,467] has been reported to be effective as well.

Optic perineuritis and orbital inflammatory syndromes

Optic perineuritis is a term used to describe an optic neuropathy presumably due to inflammation of the optic nerve sheath. In many cases the etiology is unknown. The clinical constellation of bilateral optic neuropathy (often with relative central vision sparing), associated with pain, typical MRI findings of sheath enhancement, and steroid responsiveness is highly suggestive of this condition.[468] Histopathologically, these patients have been shown to have nonspecific chronic inflammation, occasionally granulomatous and often associated with varying degrees of fibroplasia and collagen deposition.[469–472]

In our experience, patients with this condition fall into three broad categories. The first are patients with optic neuropathy but with other evidence of an acute orbital inflammatory syndrome (orbital pseudotumor) such as proptosis, eyelid swelling, eye muscle involvement, and posterior scleritis. Neuroimaging reveals orbital inflammatory changes as well as optic nerve sheath enhancement. This entity is discussed in more detail in Chapter 18. The second group of patients have optic perineuritis in the setting of a systemic condition, most commonly sarcoidosis, syphilis, Lyme disease or tuberculosis. In the final group the condition is idiopathic with no evidence of orbital disease or systemic infection.

The distinction of optic neuritis from optic perineuritis is based largely on clinical presentation and radiographic demonstration of optic nerve sheath thickening or enhancement in the latter. Patients tend to be older and the disease is often bilateral in perineuritis.[468] Vision loss may be mild initially, and the optic nerve head is often swollen with secondary retinal venous stasis changes, dilation of vessels, and peripheral retinal hemorrhages (**Fig. 5–35**). Clinically it must be distinguished from papilledema since both share the clinical features of bilateral disc swelling and relatively good visual function. In most patients with perineuritis, the CSF exhibits a normal opening pressure with a mild pleocytosis. Patients may also have an acute presentation that mimics optic neuritis, or they may present with an insidiously progressive optic neuropathy.

Diagnostic studies/evaluation. The presence of associated vitreous cells and infiltrates is suggestive of a systemic condition associated with the perineuritis, and extensive workup for sarcoidosis, syphilis, Lyme disease, and tuberculosis should be initiated in such cases. Optic nerve sheath thickening can be documented with orbital ultrasound and either CT or MRI scanning. Contrast enhancement of the sheath is more prominent than enhancement of the nerve itself (**Fig. 5–35**). Radiographically, perineuritis can be difficult to distinguish from optic nerve sheath meningioma.[471] If there is more widespread evidence of meningeal involvement then syphilitic, cryptococcal, tuberculous, and carcinomatous meningitis are more likely. If papilledema is considered, patients with headache should undergo lumbar puncture to rule out elevated intracranial pressure.

Treatment. Treatment for perineuritis is directed either at the systemic infection or with systemic steroids.[468] In our experience, patients with infectious perineuritis are often successfully treated, with good recovery of vision. However, the idiopathic variety, or that associated with orbital inflammation, can take a chronic form that is resistant to steroid treatment and is associated with significant fibrosis of the optic nerve sheath.

Uveitis-associated disc swelling

Patients with uveitis, particularly with posterior segment involvement, can have disc swelling. A nonspecific process resulting from simple breakdown of the blood–retina barrier in posterior uveitis should be distinguished from an inflammatory process involving the optic nerve itself. The former is more common as for instance in pars planitis, where disc swelling may be accompanied by cystoid macular edema. In this setting, there is usually only enlargement of the blindspot without evidence of optic neuropathy. In the second group of patients, an inflammatory or infectious process, often granulomatous (commonly sarcoid or syphilis), involves the nerve itself, and significant visual dysfunction with optic neuropathy is often present. Optic disc swelling can also accompany hypotony, which may occur with chronic uveitis.

Optic neuropathy related to systemic lupus erythematosus

Optic neuropathy is an important but uncommon neuro-ophthalmic complication of systemic lupus erythematosus.[473] Optic neuropathy was found in only 2/150 (1.3%) of patients with lupus in the Johns Hopkins series.[474] Jabs et al.[474] reported seven such cases and reviewed 24 other cases reported in the literature. Interestingly, 13 of the 24 (54%) of the cases of lupus-related optic neuropathy were

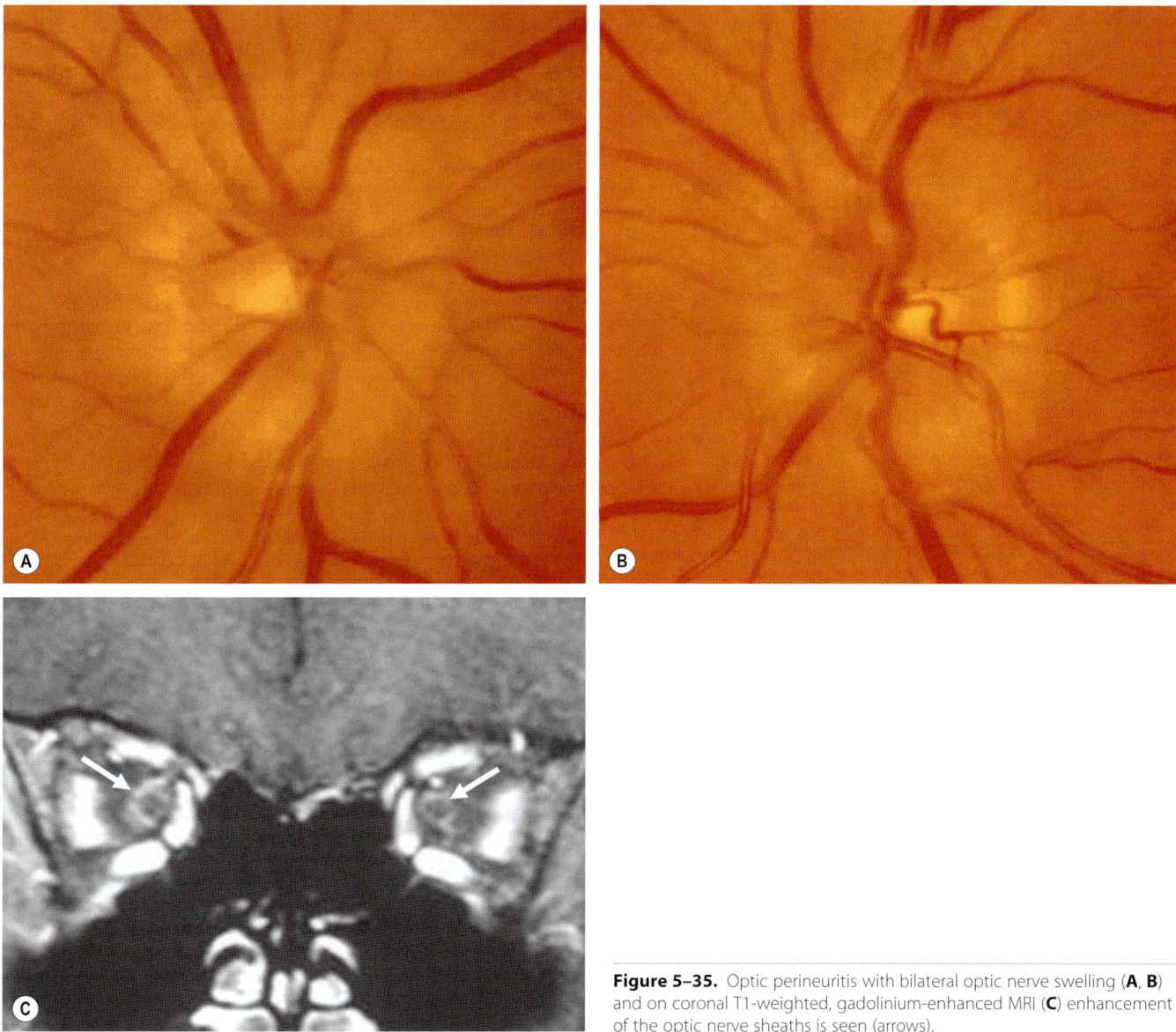

Figure 5–35. Optic perineuritis with bilateral optic nerve swelling (**A**, **B**) and on coronal T1-weighted, gadolinium-enhanced MRI (**C**) enhancement of the optic nerve sheaths is seen (arrows).

associated with transverse myelitis. This pattern of optic neuropathy with transverse myelitis mimics Devic neuromyelitis optica (see above).[412]

Optic nerve dysfunction can take different forms including optic neuritis, papillitis, and anterior or posterior ischemic optic neuropathy (AION, see below).[475] The disc swelling may be associated with exudates (**Fig. 5–36**). It is unclear, but the pathogenesis is related to either demyelination or varying degrees of small vessel vaso-occlusive disease. Vision loss is often profound and when suspected should be treated promptly with steroids. MRI scanning may show enhancement of the optic nerve.[475,476] These patients require initial treatment with high-dose intravenous methylprednisolone, and many require chronic steroids. Retinal vasculitis may manifest with painless retinal ischemic changes. In this situation, an associated hypercoagulable state should be excluded and anticoagulation considered.

Other neuro-ophthalmic complications of lupus are detailed in Chapters 4 and 8.

Autoimmune (or relapsing or recurrent) optic neuropathy

This distinct variety of optic nerve inflammation is similar to lupus optic neuropathy. This likely represents a heterogeneous group of conditions, some with recognized systemic autoimmune disease, with isolated, recurrent, often bilateral, steroid-responsive optic neuropathy and various autoimmune markers on serologic testing including NMO antibodies.[477–481] In many of these patients no specific connective tissue diagnosis can be made using strict clinical or serologic criteria, despite extensive searching.[482] The entity of autoimmune optic neuropathy is believed to be a chronic autoimmune condition characterized by recurrences of visual loss and steroid dependency.[483,484] Its similarity to lupus optic neuropathy suggests that an optic nerve antigen may be susceptible to an autoimmune attack. An alternative possibility is that optic nerve dysfunction arises in the setting of autoimmune disease as a result of small vessel occlusion

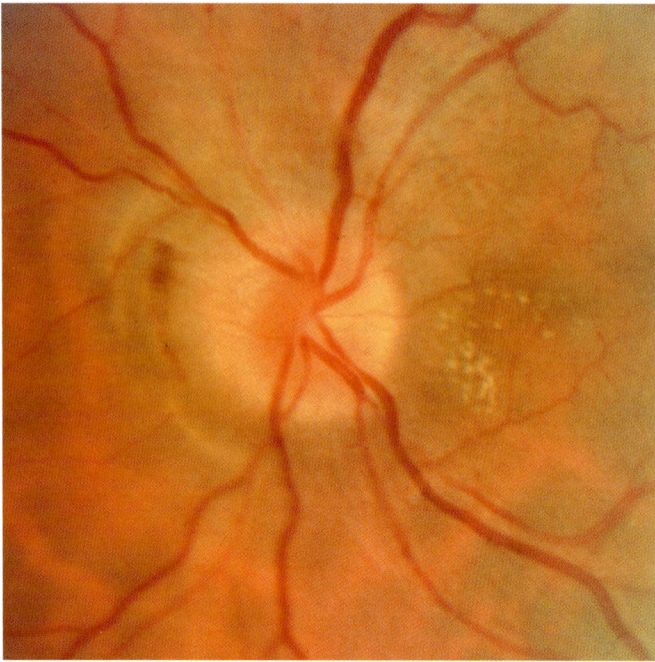

Figure 5–36. Optic nerve appearance in a patient with systemic lupus erythematosus and optic neuritis. Chronic disc swelling and retinal exudates are present.

from immune complex deposition or a hypercoagulable state. Some cases have had abnormal skin biopsies, with perivascular infiltrate and immune complex deposition within the dermis.[484,485] Affected patients are generally adults aged 25–55, but the condition probably occurs at any age. Bee sting optic neuropathy is felt to be a unique autoimmune-type optic neuropathy.[486,487]

Evaluation and treatment. We recommend a search for an autoimmune condition in any patient who has "optic neuritis," which worsens for more than 1 week after initial steroid therapy, or in any patient who fails to begin to improve by the third week after onset of visual loss (see atypical optic neuritis, above). In suspected cases, ANA testing, NMO antibodies, and skin biopsy should be considered.[484] Rheumatologic consultation, consideration of a skin biopsy to exclude vasculitis, and serologies should be considered in these patients to identify a possible systemic autoimmune condition. Early recognition can lead to successful treatment with high doses of steroids. Other immunosuppressive therapies are often required to supplement steroid therapy in this chronic and relapsing condition.[484,488–490] In most patients the optic neuropathy remains isolated without development of another systemic autoimmune disease or specific syndrome.[484]

Idiopathic hypertrophic pachymeningitis

This condition is characterized by localized or diffuse thickening of the meninges.[491] Affected patients present with headache, optic neuropathy, or other cranial neuropathies. MRI may demonstrate dural thickening and enhancement, and lumbar puncture often shows a lymphocytic pleocytosis and elevated protein. When unclear, the diagnosis may depend on a biopsy of the leptomeninges, which typically

reveals nonspecific inflammation without evidence of sarcoidosis, infection, or neoplasm. Most patients are treated effectively with corticosteroids, but many additionally require steroid-sparing immunosuppressive agents.

Infectious optic neuropathies

Sinusitis and mucoceles

For decades it was believed that the vast majority of cases of optic neuritis resulted from contiguous disease and inflammation in the paranasal sinuses. Subsequently it has been shown that the radiographic presence of sinus inflammation and mucosal thickening is fairly ubiquitous, and that most cases of optic neuritis result from demyelination. Nevertheless, it is clear that paranasal sinus disease (sinusitis and mucoceles) may cause (1) a condition not dissimilar in presentation to optic neuritis (acute optic neuropathy plus pain on eye movements) or (2) progressive optic neuropathy from chronic compression.

In many cases the optic neuropathy results from compression or inflammation from a nearby mucocele.[492–494] In other cases contiguous inflammation in the posterior ethmoid and sphenoid sinus causes optic nerve dysfunction without mass effect.[495–497] This may occur more commonly in patients with no medial wall of the optic canal (meninges in direct contact with sinus mucosa), an anatomic variant which occurs in about 4% of normal patients.[21]

Evaluation and treatment. This diagnosis should be entertained in all cases of acute optic neuropathy that are atypical for optic neuritis in any way. In particular, it should be suspected in elderly patients, patients with a history of severe sinus disease, when there are associated fevers or ophthalmoplegia, or when progression of optic neuritis occurs beyond 2 weeks.

When significant sinusitis is identified on MRI scanning in these patients (**Fig. 5–37**), particularly in the posterior ethmoid and sphenoid sinuses, or when a mucocele is present, prompt otolaryngologic consultation should be sought. Antibiotic and often surgical therapy can be considered. In this setting, visual loss can often be totally reversed unless it was chronic or associated with optic atrophy at presentation.[496]

Neuroretinitis

The term neuroretinitis refers to the combination of optic neuropathy and retinal "inflammation" characterized ophthalmoscopically with the unique association of disc edema and peripapillary or macular hard exudates, which form a "star" or sunburst pattern around the fovea (**Fig. 5–38**). The condition was first described by Leber and is therefore frequently referred to as Leber's stellate neuroretinitis.[498] Subsequently several series have described this heterogeneous disorder.[499,500] Neuroretinitis is frequently a manifestation of a systemic infection, so an etiology should be sought when the diagnosis is made. Although the initial presentation can be very similar to idiopathic (demyelinating) optic neuritis, a macular star associated with optic neuritis is not associated with an increased risk of developing MS.

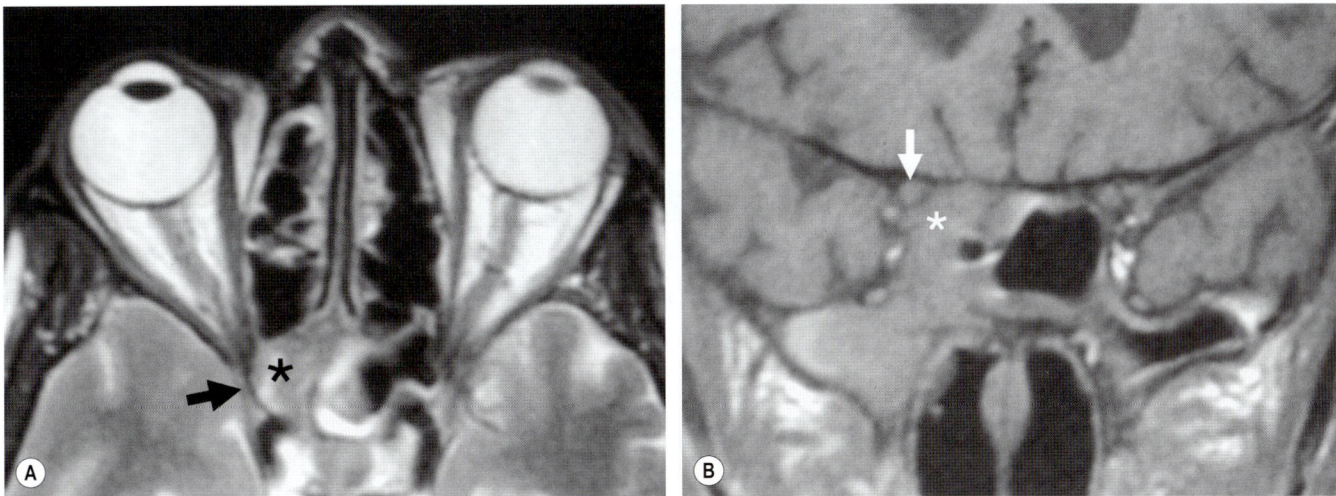

Figure 5–37. Sphenoid sinusitis causing optic nerve dysfunction. Axial T2-weighted MRI (**A**) showing extensive ethmoid and sphenoid sinusitis (asterisk) adjacent to the optic canal (arrow). **B**. On coronal T1-weighted MRI the optic nerve (arrow) is seen adjacent to the area of infection and inflammation (asterisk).

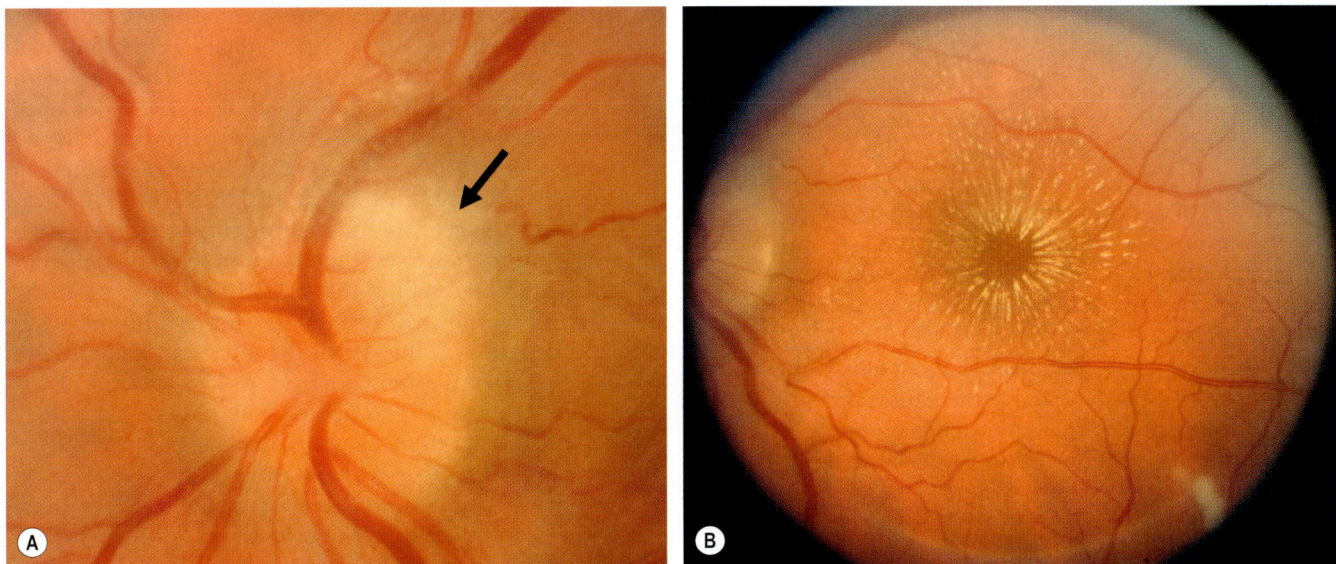

Figure 5–38. Fundus appearance in a patient with neuroretinitis. **A**. Acutely there is focal pale disc swelling superiorly. **B**. Within 1 week the classic macular star developed.

The macular star results from fluid leakage from optic disc capillaries into Henle's layer (outer plexiform), which retains the lipid precipitates and can be seen on OCT (**Fig. 5–39**). All of the leakage is believed to be from the disc since the retinal vasculature does not leak on fluorescein angiography. In fact, the presence of these exudates can be a nonspecific finding in any patient with disc swelling.[501–503] For instance, at least a partial star can occasionally be seen in patients with a variety of different causes of optic disc swelling, such as ischemic optic neuropathy or papilledema (see Chapter 6).

Therefore, we group patients with the finding of optic disc edema with a macular lipid star into two groups:

1. *Idiopathic or infectious neuroretinitis.* Patients in this group present with decreased vision and a swollen optic nerve, and initially a diagnosis of optic neuritis may be made, but within 1–2 weeks the macular star is

evident. Patients in this group are generally aged 10–50 with no sex predilection. Occasionally they have pain around the eye or bilateral involvement.[499,500] Neuroretinitis has been reported in children and behaves similarly to the disease in adults.[504] In up to 50% of patients with neuroretinitis, a preceding viral illness is reported.

The examination is notable for moderate acuity loss (usually 20/40–20/200) but can be as poor as light perception. Typical features of optic nerve dysfunction are present with decreased color vision, nerve fiber defects on visual field testing, and afferent pupil defects. Vitreous cells are present in about 90%.[499,500] The disc swelling can either be focal or diffuse, and sometimes it has a pale quality. Development of the lipid star is often preceded by serous detachment of the

147

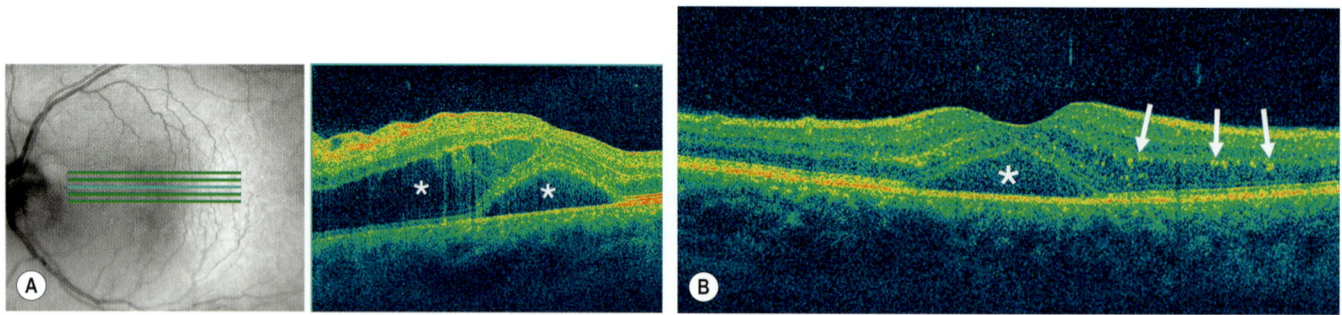

Figure 5–39. Ocular coherence tomography findings in neuroretinitis. **A**. Acutely there is an extensive area of subretinal fluid (asterisks) extending to the macula. **B**. Discrete areas of high reflectivity (arrows) are seen in the nerve fiber layer of Henle and correspond to the retinal exudates.

macula or evidence of inflammation in the peripheral retina. The prognosis for visual recovery is excellent although recurrent neuroretinitis with poor visual outcome has been reported.[505] Bilateral cases occur rarely.[506]

Important infectious causes of neuroretinitis include cat scratch disease (*Bartonella henselae* bacillus),[507,508] syphilis,[509,510] Lyme disease,[511,512] and toxoplasmosis.[513,514] Patients with *Bartonella* infection frequently will describe cat scratches and a recent viral illness with fever and adenopathy.[515] The diagnosis can be confirmed by detecting positive antibody titers or by finding *Bartonella* DNA by polymerase chain reaction (PCR).[516–518] Endocarditis has been reported as a complication of *B. henselae* infection, and encephalopathy and meningitis in patients with concurrent human immunodeficiency virus infection have been described.[507,519]

2. *Macular star due to other causes of disc swelling.* These patients have a fairly typical presentation of an optic neuropathy associated with disc edema (e.g., ischemic optic neuropathy[520]) and curiously, usually delayed a few weeks from presentation, develop a macular star. In these patients the original diagnosis may be rethought and consideration should be given to papilledema associated with increased intracranial pressure or malignant hypertension as the cause of the swelling and exudates. As in the first group of patients, development of a macular star is often preceded by serous macular detachment.

Evaluation and treatment. At the time of diagnosis of neuroretinitis, appropriate historical review and laboratory tests should be ordered to rule out the infectious etiologies listed above. Many cases of neuroretinitis will be titer negative and presumably idiopathic. Appropriate antibiotic therapy is indicated when syphilis, Lyme disease, or toxoplasmosis is diagnosed.

However, the most frequent diagnosis confirmed in patients with neuroretinitis will be *Bartonella* species infection (cat scratch disease).[521–523] Bartonella infection is considered to be self-limited and no treatment has been proven to be beneficial in cat scratch-associated neuroretinitis. Reed and associates[523] reported that treatment with doxycycline and rifampin seemed to shorten the course when compared with historic controls. We consider using doxycycline if

visual loss is severe or disc swelling persists beyond 3 weeks. Most patients recover, but some are left with residual visual symptoms secondary to optic nerve dysfunction.

Syphilis

After a steady decrease in cases, ophthalmic presentations of syphilis have become more common over the last several years, particularly in individuals coinfected with human immunodeficiency virus (HIV).[524,525] Therefore syphilis should always be in the differential diagnosis of unexplained optic nerve disease.[526] Optic neuropathy is not uncommon in patients with secondary syphilis. Patients can develop retrobulbar optic neuritis, papillitis with retinal vasculitis,[527] and perineuritis and neuroretinitis in the setting of secondary lues.[528] Disc swelling, hemorrhages, dilated veins (phlebitis), and subretinal infiltrates (**Fig. 5–40**) are highly suggestive of syphilis. The severity of visual symptoms is variable and depends on the site of the infection. Patients with syphilitic perineuritis tend to have more mild visual loss (sometimes none at all) compared with patients with direct optic nerve involvement. Bilateral disease is almost always present, often with other evidence of secondary syphilis such as rash, uveitis, and mild signs of meningeal inflammation.[529] MRI scanning in perineuritis shows diffuse thickening and enhancement of the optic nerve sheath.[530] In contrast, progressive vision loss with optic atrophy can also been seen as a manifestation of tertiary syphilis. This is a slowly progressive (generally not episodic) visual deterioration not associated with other active inflammation of the eye.

Diagnostic studies/evaluation. Syphilitic optic neuropathy can almost always be diagnosed with appropriate serum and CSF serologies except in the setting of HIV infection, which can alter test results with seronegative disease.[531] In the non-HIV-infected individual, the serum microhemagluttin assay for *Treponema pallidum* (MHA-TP) or the FTA-ABS should almost always be positive in the patient with neuroophthalmic signs and symptoms suggestive of syphilis. The serum VDRL and RPR are also useful screening tests, but they may be negative in neurosyphilis. Although a positive CSF VDRL is confirmatory of a diagnosis of neurosyphilis, it is often negative and therefore cannot be used solely to exclude this diagnosis. Often, one relies on the presence of a positive serum test and the presence of elevated CSF white blood cell count or protein concentration to determine disease activity. Since the presentation of syphilitic optic neuropathy is quite

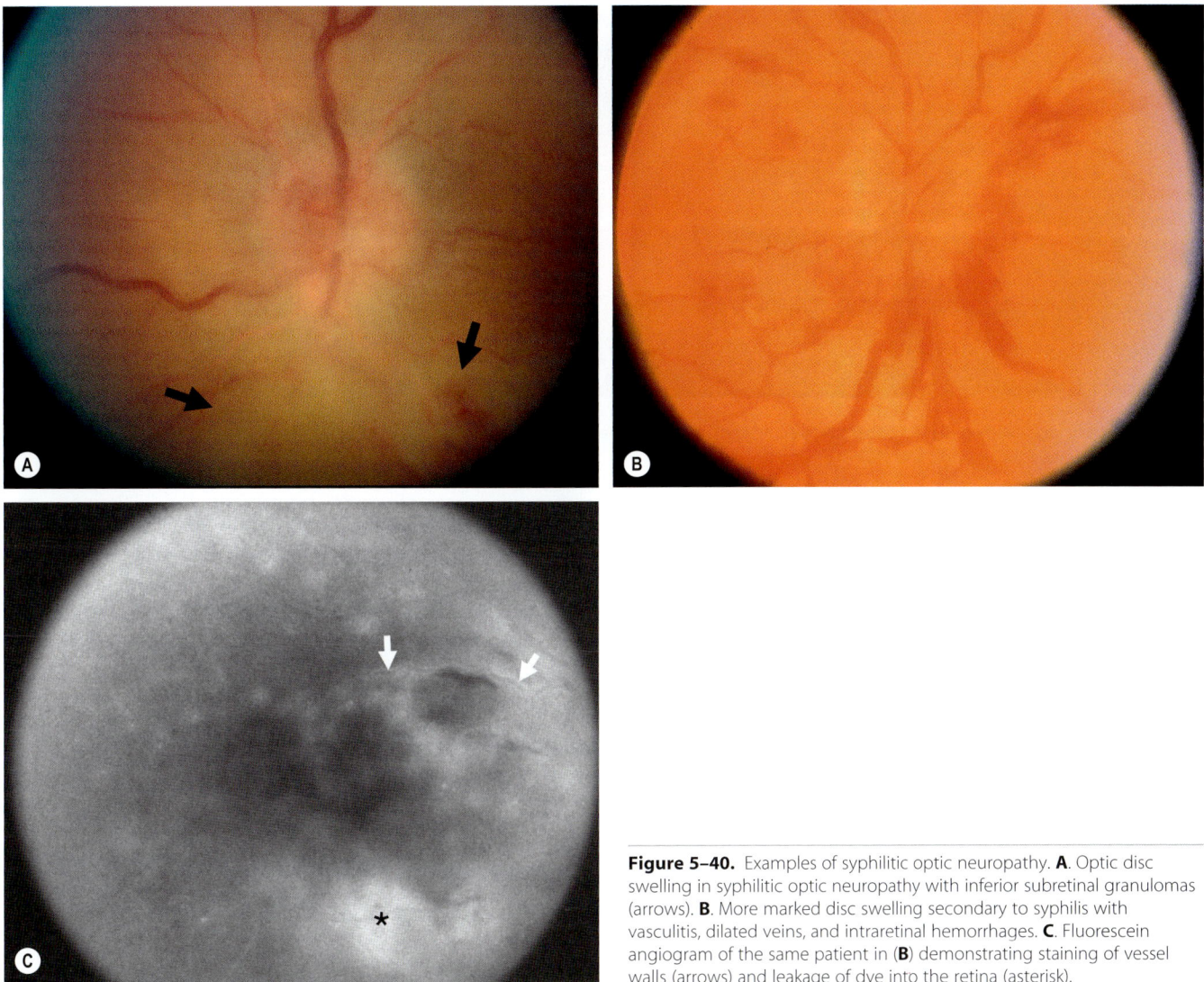

Figure 5–40. Examples of syphilitic optic neuropathy. **A**. Optic disc swelling in syphilitic optic neuropathy with inferior subretinal granulomas (arrows). **B**. More marked disc swelling secondary to syphilis with vasculitis, dilated veins, and intraretinal hemorrhages. **C**. Fluorescein angiogram of the same patient in (**B**) demonstrating staining of vessel walls (arrows) and leakage of dye into the retina (asterisk).

variable, the clinical suspicion for this condition must exist in all cases of atypical inflammatory optic neuropathy and unexplained progressive optic atrophy. A postinfectious illness similar to NMO has been described in patients with syphilis.[532]

Treatment. Treatment of syphilitic optic neuropathy with positive CSF VDRL and presumed tertiary syphilis must be with intravenous aqueous penicillin.[509,510] Secondary syphilis with perineuritis and normal CSF has been treated successfully with intramuscular procaine penicillin.[510] Sometimes after successful treatment with antibiotics, steroids can be used to treat persisting inflammation.[533] The disease in patients with HIV virus is similar. Syphilitic optic nerve involvement has been reported as an initial manifestation of HIV infection and tends to have an excellent prognosis with appropriate treatment.[534]

Lyme disease

The neurologic manifestations of Lyme disease are protean,[535] and the neuro-ophthalmic manifestations have been reviewed.[536,537] Lyme associated optic neuritis and perineuri-

tis are rare,[538] and the diagnosis should be made primarily in patients who have a history of erythema migrans, a bout of arthritis, and positive titers in serum and CSF whenever possible. We recommend that a positive serum Lyme titer be confirmed by western blot testing since there is a relatively high rate of false positives seen with conventional serum antibody titer level testing. In a series of 28 patients with optic neuritis and a positive Lyme titer, only one patient with papillitis and posterior uveitis had convincing evidence of Lyme disease; there were no definite cases of Lyme-associated retrobulbar neuritis or neuroretinitis in this study.[537] Many of the reported cases of Lyme-associated optic neuritis and ischemic optic neuropathy are circumspect. They were based simply on recent exposure and presence of serum titers, neither of which is adequate to implicate Lyme as the definite cause of optic nerve dysfunction.[536] For instance, Jacobson[539] performed follow-up on four of his previously reported patients[540] with optic neuritis and Lyme seropositivity. Two were found to have developed multiple sclerosis, suggesting the seropositivity was coincidental.

Lyme is also an important cause of low-grade meningitis associated with elevated intracranial pressure and a

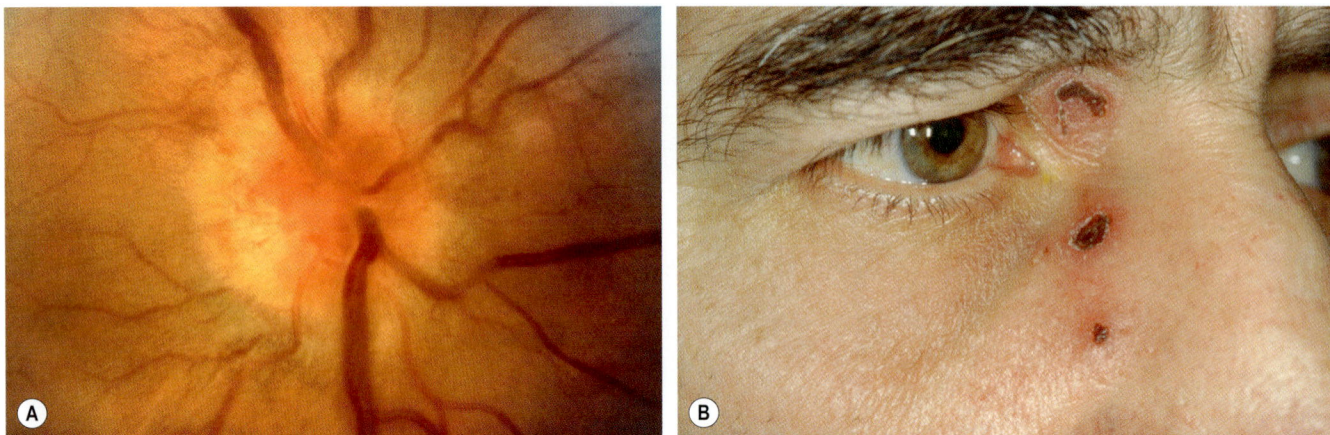

Figure 5–41. Optic disc swelling (**A**) in a patient with acute optic neuritis in the setting of a typical V1 distribution herpes zoster eruption (**B**).

pseudotumor cerebri-like presentation (see Chapter 6).[511,536] When the optic nerve is involved, the picture is usually one with uveitis-associated neuroretinitis and unusual fluorescein angiographic criteria including neuroretinal edema and patchy and diffuse hyperfluorescence.[512] In some patients, neuroretinitis can be resistant to antibiotic treatment.[512]

HIV-associated optic neuropathies

Systemic immunosuppression is an important risk factor for primary infection of the optic nerve from a variety of pathogens.[541] In the acquired immunodeficiency syndrome (AIDS), infectious optic neuropathy may result from primary HIV infection of the nerve, cytomegalovirus infection, or acute retinal necrosis associated with herpesvirus. In addition optic neuropathy can develop in the setting of granulomatous inflammation of the meninges associated with cryptococcus, toxoplasmosis, tuberculosis, aspergillus, or syphilis. These can also cause elevated intracranial pressure with papilledema and associated progressive visual loss. Primary HIV optic neuropathy can present as an acute retrobulbar optic neuritis with pain on eye movements or a slowly progressive condition.[542] Treatment with steroids or antivirals may be effective. The condition likely results from direct HIV infection of the optic nerve, or alternatively nerve damage can result from the immune reaction directed against the infected optic nerve.

Cytomegalovirus (CMV) infection is the most common opportunistic infection to involve the posterior segment of the eye. The majority of patients develop retinitis with associated hemorrhagic necrosis. This herpesvirus can primarily infect the optic nerve and cause a papillitis or the optic nerve can be involved secondarily by contiguous spread from adjacent retina.[543–545] Papillitis occurs in about 4% of patients with CMV retinitis. Patients require management with high and prolonged doses of intravenous foscarnet or ganciclovir, and the prognosis for visual recovery is very variable.[543,546–548] CMV papillitis has also been described in an immunocompetent individual.[546]

Fungal disease can involve the optic nerves through granulomatous inflammation of the meninges. Cryptococcus is the most common fungal infection of the CNS and most common cause of optic neuropathy.[549,550] Patients can present with either sudden vision loss or progressive vision loss from papilledema associated with elevated intracranial pressure. The mechanisms for vision loss include direct fungal invasion and adhesive arachnoiditis along with elevated intracranial pressure. Optic nerve sheath fenestration may be beneficial in some patients along with systemic treatment with amphotericin B (see Chapter 6).

Herpes zoster

Optic neuropathy can occur in patients with recent herpes zoster ophthalmicus. It must be very rare given the paucity of reported cases compared with the prevalence of this infection. Vision loss can take the form of a catastrophic ischemic event, perhaps from an angiitis, or behave more like an inflammatory optic neuropathy related to zoster infection of the nerve.[551] This condition is well recognized in both immune-competent and -incompetent patients.[552–554] In immunocompromised patients varicella zoster optic neuritis can be precede retinitis and result in severe permanent vision loss.[554–556] The visual loss may occur soon after the onset of the rash but may also be delayed by weeks, and in immunocompromised patients may occur without the characteristic rash.[557] The vision loss is usually unilateral and severe. There maybe papillitis (**Fig. 5–41**) with a macular star or the fundus may be normal. MRI scan may show optic nerve or nerve sheath enhancement.[558] Treatment with acyclovir and steroids can be attempted with variable results.[558] An optic neuritis-like illness has also been described after primary varicella (chicken pox) infection.[559]

Ischemic optic neuropathies

Ischemic optic neuropathy (ION) is an acute, presumably vascular optic neuropathy. Sudden, often catastrophic, "stroke-like" vision loss in elderly patients with vasculopathic risk factors is typical of this condition. ION essentially occurs in two broad settings: non-arteritic vs arteritic.

The non-arteritic variety is almost always anterior with optic nerve head swelling, by definition. Thus the term non-arteritic, anterior ION (AION) is applied to this group. The

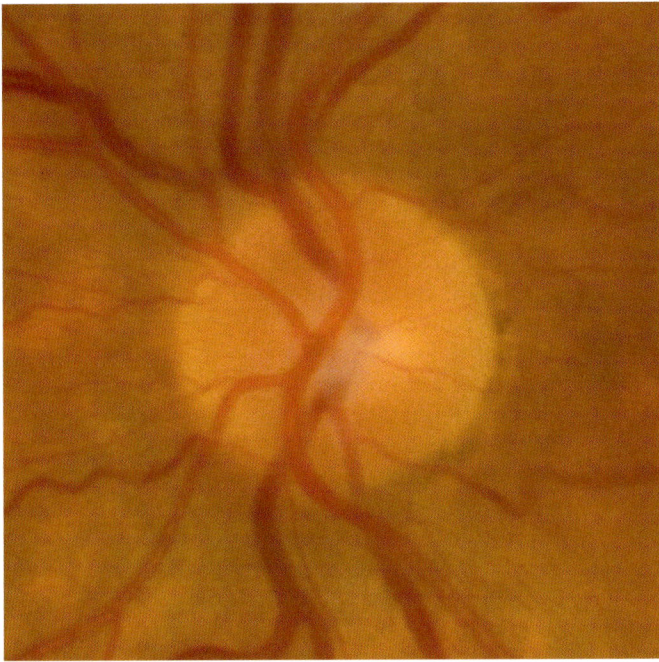

Figure 5–42. The typical appearance of the "disc at risk" for development of anterior ischemic optic neuropathy. The nerve is small and there is no cup.

majority of these patients are elderly, have diabetes and/or hypertension, and are particularly at risk if they have a small, crowded optic nerve head (**Fig. 5–42**). Other systemic conditions which have been reported in association with AION include antiphospholipid antibody syndrome, previous radiation therapy, juvenile diabetes, shock, severe hypertension, and migraine.

Arteritic ION is usually due to temporal arteritis. Patients in this group can present either with disc swelling (arteritic AION) or without disc swelling. The latter presentation is termed arteritic posterior ischemic optic neuropathy (PION) and is sufficiently rare as an idiopathic condition that in an elderly patient temporal arteritis should always be excluded. When arteritic ION is a heralding manifestation of temporal arteritis, other generalized symptoms are usually present.

The remainder of this section will discuss the diagnosis and management of non-arteritic and arteritic ION in detail and also highlight some of the other less common varieties.

Non-arteritic ischemic optic neuropathy

AION is the most common cause of unilateral optic nerve swelling and optic neuropathy in adults over age 50.[560] The term ischemic optic neuropathy was used in 1966 to describe 11 patients with the characteristic triad of vision loss, afferent pupil defect, and a swollen optic nerve.[561]

Demographics. The majority of patients are 60–70 years of age, but there is no absolute age range. In the Bascom Palmer series, Boghen and Glaser[562] described 37 patients with non-arteritic AION, and the age range was 40–80. Although there was a minimum age requirement of 50 for eligibility, the Ischemic Optic Neuropathy Decompression Trial (IONDT) found a mean age of 66 ± 8.7.[563] This study

randomized patients with AION and visual acuity worse than 20/64 to either optic nerve sheath decompression or observation.

Population studies of patients 50 years or older suggest an annual incidence rate of 2.3–10/100 000 population/year and a increased rate in Caucasians compared with African Americans or Hispanic individuals.[560,564] The condition is less common but well reported in individuals less than age 50 although many such patients are referred to tertiary centers because of their atypical age (23% in one series).[565] There is an increased risk in patients with diabetes mellitus, hypercholesterolemia, ischemic heart disease, and systemic hypertension.[566,567] In the IONDT 47% of the patients had hypertension and 24% had diabetes mellitus.[563] The prevalence of these systemic risk factors was lower in patients who were not randomized because their affected eye had vision better than 20/64. This suggests hypertension and diabetes may be risk factors for more significant vision loss. Diabetic patients with ION may have a higher prevalence of hypertension and heart disease than nondiabetic patients.[568] Familial ION has been described and it tends to affect individuals at a younger age and is more often bilateral.[569] Younger patients with ION still have a high prevalence of vasculopathic risk factors (especially hypertension and hyperlipidemia) or underlying conditions such as vaculitis or hypercoaguability.[565,570]

Nocturnal hypotension, in some cases due to the treatment of arterial hypertension, may be a separate and distinct risk factor which may explain the high rate of vision loss which occurs upon awakening.[571,572] Decreased blood pressure at night has been demonstrated in patients with progressive vision loss.[573,574] Another important risk factor is the disc at risk or crowded optic nerve head.[575–578] The fellow eye is often found to have a small or absent cup. The high prevalence of small cupless disc as a risk factor for ION has been confirmed with modern optic nerve head imaging methods.[579–581] Studies have shown hyperopic refractive errors and smoking to be possible risk factors[582,583] although a different study found no increased risk from smoking.[584] Patients with non-arteritic ION do not have an increased incidence of carotid disease on the affected side compared with age-matched controls.[585]

Sleep apnea may be a separate and distinct risk factor for development of non-arteritic ION.[586–591] In the series reported by Mojon et al.[589] 71% of 17 patients with ION had sleep apnea compared with 17% of matched controls. Palombi et al.[591] found sleep apnea in 89% of 27 patients with ION, and ION patients were more likely to report symptoms of sleep apnea than matched controls.[588] The possible mechanisms of sleep apnea contributing to the development of ION include effects on optic nerve head blood flow autoregulation and prolonged hypoxia.

Erectile dysfunction drugs and ION. In 2002, Pomeranz et al.[592] reported a series of patients who developed ION in the hours after taking erectile dysfunction drugs (phosphodiesterase-5 (PDE-5) inhibitors). Since then there have been numerous similar case reports,[593–601] and much debate as to whether the relationship is causal or a coincidence given that both the use of these drugs and ION tend to occur in the same vasculopathic population.[602–608] Thurtell and Tomsak[609] provide a thorough review of the topic. Most compelling are the cases associated with repeated episodes of transient, permanent, or sequential vision loss with repeated doses of PDE-5 inhibitors.[593,610,611] Currently there are only case reports describing the possible association. McGwin et al.[612] did not find a higher incidence of erectile dysfunction drug use in men with a history of ION compared with age-matched controls. Gorkin et al.[613] reviewed the data from over 100 clinical trials of sildenafil and found only one case of ION and estimated the annual incidence to be 2.8/100 000, which is not different from the reported incidence of ION in population studies. The PDE-5 inhibitor does lower systemic blood pressure slightly. Since the medications are often taken at night (and PDE-5 inhibitor-associated ION is most often noted in the morning), it is possible they contribute to nocturnal hypotension. Much deliberation will continue on this topic until it is studied prospectively. Most experts agree, however, that patients who have had ION in one eye should be cautioned against the use of PDE-5 inhibitors, particularly if they have systemic risk factors and a "disc at risk."

Neuro-ophthalmic symptoms. Most patients with ION describe a sudden onset of monocular visual loss, often upon awakening (40% in IONDT study[563]). It usually is maximal when noted, and often does not progress. There are usually no prodromal ocular symptoms and no associated systemic symptoms. The presence of prodromal amaurosis fugax or diplopia should increase the suspicion for temporal arteritis. Pain is rare in idiopathic ION but can occur in about 10% of patients.[614]

Neuro-ophthalmic signs. Examination findings are typical of an optic neuropathy with reduced acuity (at any level), dyschromatopsia, an afferent pupil defect, visual field loss which is most often inferior altitudinal,[301,562,615] and (again by definition) disc edema which is often pale and sectoral with splinter hemorrhages and dilated capillaries on the disc surface (**Fig. 5–43**). In the IONDT, 49% of patients had better than 20/64 visual acuity at the time of presentation and 34% had worse than 20/200.[563] Patients typically have dyschromatopsia. However, many patients will identify color plates correctly, and the dyschromatopsia is detected only by subjective comparison between the eyes. An afferent pupillary defect should be present unless the other eye had a similar previous problem. Visual field defects comprise any "optic nerve" type in addition to the classic altitudinal field loss. Up to one-quarter of patients will have central scotomas.[301] Vitritis is absent, so its presence should increase the clinical suspicion for alternative inflammatory and infectious diagnoses.

The characteristic disc appearance (**Fig. 5–43**) has sectoral swelling and splinter hemorrhages, often with attenuation of the peripapillar arterioles.[616] If a previous attack in the other eye resulted in a pale disc, the term pseudo-Foster Kennedy syndrome applies with ischemic swelling in the newly affected eye and old atrophy in the other eye (**Fig. 5–44**; see also Chapter 6).[617] Sequential attacks of ischemic optic neuropathy are distinguished from the true Foster Kennedy syndrome by inferior field loss and visual acuity reduction in the eye with the swollen optic nerve in consecutive ION.

Diagnostic studies/evaluation. Usually no further diagnostic studies need be obtained although the erythrocyte sedimentation rate (ESR) and C-reactive protein levels should be checked to screen for temporal arteritis (see below). However, carefully timed fluorescein angiography may also be able to distinguish ION disc swelling from other causes of disc swelling by demonstrating delayed optic nerve head filling.[618,619] OCT studies have demonstrated a mild amount of subretinal fluid in some patients with ION. This observation might explain some of the visual acuity recovery that occurs in certain patients.[620]

MRI scanning does not have a role in the diagnosis of acute anterior ION but on occasion is necessary to exclude compressive and infiltrative conditions mimicking simple ION. Gadolinium enhancement of the optic nerve may occur but is rare and more common in arteritic ION. Patients with non-arteritic ION have been shown to have an increased number of white matter ischemic changes compared with age- and disease-matched controls.[621] This likely reflects the presence of vasculopathic risk factors. Both pattern ERG and VEP (amplitude and latency) have been shown to be abnormal in patients with ION.[622]

Clinical course. The majority of patients have a fixed deficit, but either progressive vision loss in the first month or alternatively spontaneous recovery can occur.[623–625] One of the surprising outcomes of IONDT was the high rate of spontaneous improvement. Forty-three percent of the patients who received no treatment recovered three or more lines of vision.[626] In addition to proving surgery to be unhelpful, much was learned about the clinical profile and natural history of ION in the IONDT.[627,628] Other studies have also demonstrated spontaneous visual improvement.[623,629] Hayreh and Zimmerman[568] showed no difference in the degree of acuity and field improvement between diabetic and nondiabetic patients. OCT can be used to follow the initial retinal nerve fiber layer swelling associated with ION and the subsequent thinning that usually correlates well with the area of visual field loss.[630–632] Optic atrophy, often with altitudinal disc pallor (**Fig. 5–45**), develops as the disc edema resolves and there may be "luxury perfusion" or presumed upregulated capillaries on the surface of the ischemic disc.[633] Disc edema may resolve faster in patients with more prominent vision loss perhaps because more severely diseased axons die more quickly.[634]

Some patients will be examined during a peculiar asymptomatic phase of the disease in which no visual dysfunction is measured, but the disc is swollen. This premonitory phase of disc swelling often progresses to cause visual loss but may also resolve spontaneously.[635–637] Development of symptomatic ION with vision loss in these patients occurs in about 45% of patients, on average 6 weeks after the disc swelling is noted.[638]

One study suggested a lifetime risk of 30–40% of second eye involvement;[639] however, in the cohort of patients in the IONDT the 5 year risk was only 14.7%.[640] The cumulative incidence rates are even higher in older patients and patients with diabetes[568] and hypertension. Although one study suggested an increased risk of cerebrovascular and cardiovascular disease in ION patients,[641] this study has been criticized, and many feel that there is probably no increased risk for

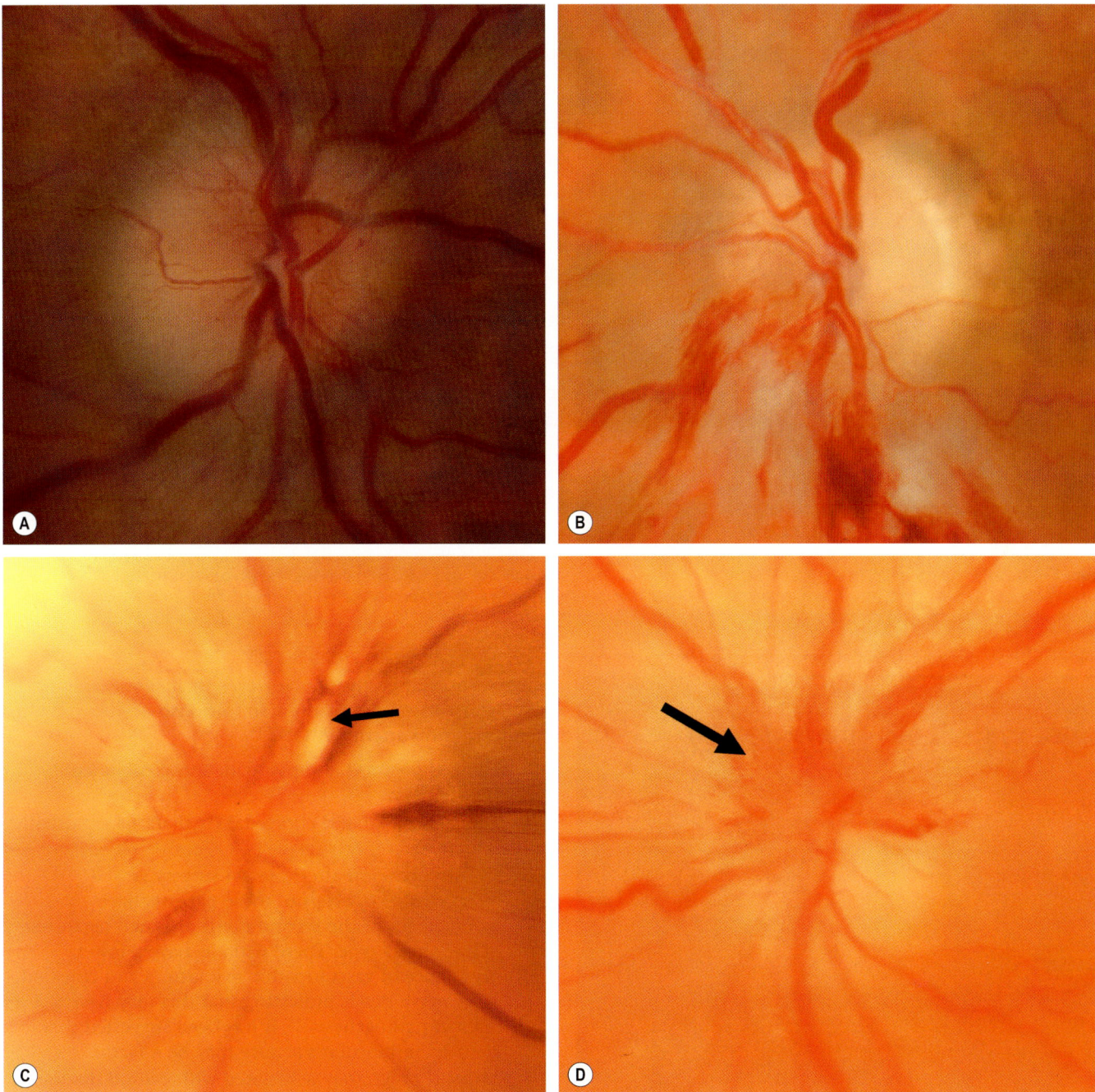

Figure 5–43. Typical appearances of the optic nerve in acute anterior ischemic optic neuropathy. In each case there is disc edema. Initially swelling may only be mild (**A**) and can be confused with the appearance of optic neuritis. Other commonly associated findings are (**B**) segmental swelling and splinter hemorrhages, (**C**) more diffuse swelling with a cotton-wool spot (arrow), and (**D**) dilated capillaries or luxury perfusion (arrow) on the disc surface.

these conditions in patients with ION. Two recent studies examined the correlation between the visual dysfunction between the two eyes to determine whether the result in one predicted the outcome of the other.[642,643] In one study there was high correlation and in the other there was not.

Pathogenesis. The pathogenesis of non-arteritic ION remains obscure.[644,645] Hayreh[646] has provided much of the information concerning factors contributing to the pathogenesis of ION. AION may result from insufficiency in the posterior ciliary artery circulation and branches of the peripapillary choroidal artery system. They may occlude with subsequent infarction of the ganglion cell axons where they

coalesce to form the optic nerve head.[647] How systemic microvascular disease, a crowded optic nerve head, and possibly nocturnal hypotension ultimately lead to optic nerve head infarction is not certain.[644] Intuitively it is postulated that microvascular, atherosclerotic capillary disease compromises already narrowed lumens (from the crowded disc). Ultimately relative poor perfusion and catastrophic infarction occurs when perfusion pressure is reduced below a critical level. Experimental occlusion of the posterior ciliary arteries in monkeys results in a similar clinical appearance to ION with pale disc swelling.[648] It is also possible that axons within a small crowded optic nerve which swells are

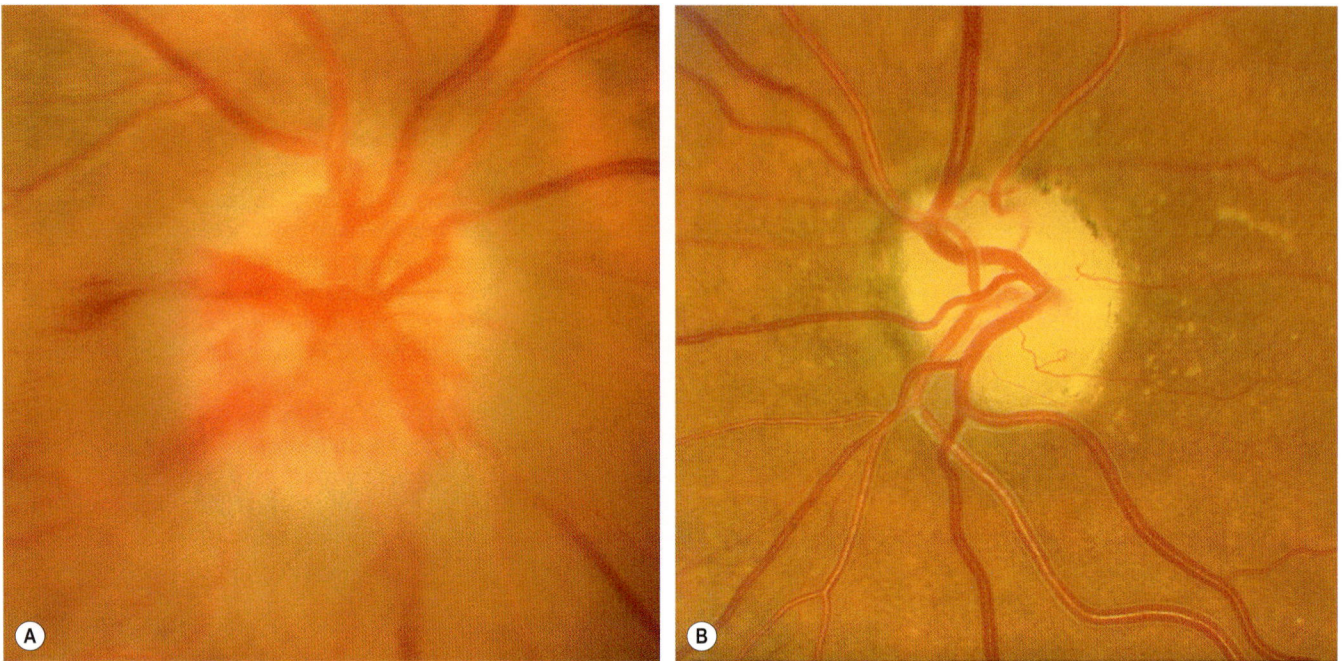

Figure 5–44. Right and left optic nerves of a patient with acute vision loss in the right eye associated with disc swelling (**A**) and disc pallor in the left eye (**B**) from preexisting optic neuropathy. This appearance of pallor in one eye and swelling in the other most commonly results from sequential attacks of ischemic optic neuropathy, as in this case, and is termed the pseudo-Foster Kennedy syndrome.

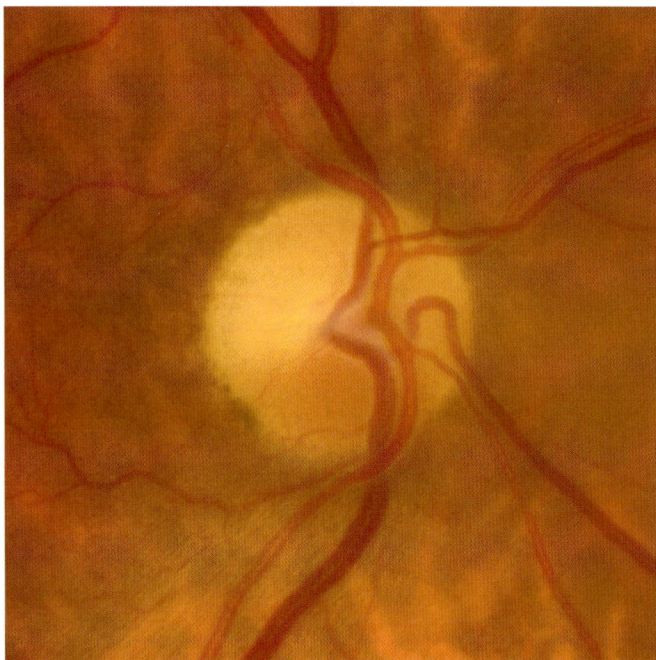

Figure 5–45. Superior segmental atrophy in a patient with inferior vision loss after a previous attack of anterior ischemic optic neuropathy.

more vulnerable to tissue ischemia, as in a compartment syndrome.[649,650] There is little evidence to suggest that an embolic event may cause non-arteritic ION.[651]

Several other factors support a vascular occlusive etiology: sudden onset, association with diabetes, hypercholesterolemia, and hypertension, lack of evidence of inflammation, similarities in presentation to the arteritic variety, and a similar syndrome can be created in animals with an experi-

mental vascular occlusion. However, there are several factors which cast some doubt on a simple vaso-occlusive pathogenesis in non-arteritic AION:[644]

1. There is no good autopsy evidence of occluded vessels.
2. The cilioretinal and choroidal circulations are usually spared.
3. Occurrence soon after cataract surgery is well recognized.[652–660] Half of these patients have involvement of the second eye if operated regardless of anesthesia type. These patients have a lower prevalence of vasculopathic risk factors and crowded optic nerve heads indicating that this may have a distinct pathogenesis.[660] It has been suggested that elevated intraocular pressure may be a factor.
4. AION is only rarely associated with carotid disease.
5. Sequential attacks in two eyes are separated by months or years without intervening evidence of vascular occlusion affecting other organs.
6. Patients may have months of premonitory disc edema prior to visual loss.[635,636]
7. One cause for ION is major blood loss (see below). In this setting there may be a delay of hours to days before vision loss occurs.[661]
8. There are well recognized cases of progression over weeks.[623–625]
9. Cases of embolic ION are only rarely reported and are distinctly different from the typical presentation.[662]
10. Repeated attacks in the same eye are unusual.[663] A protective effect from the first attack is certainly atypical for other kinds of vaso-occlusive disease such as stroke or myocardial infarction.

Recently some authors have hypothesized that the pathogenesis of ION may be related to venous obstruction in the nerve head.[645] In this scheme, venous occlusion leads to the development of a compartment syndrome and disc swelling. Ultimately, the pathogenesis and treatment of ION may be aided by a newly described rodent model of ION.[664,665]

Other systemic associations with non-arteritic AION. In addition to the general atherosclerotic risk factors of diabetes and hypertension, ION has been reported in the setting of other systemic afflictions. A hypercoagulable state secondary to antiphospholipid antibodies has been reported to occur in patients with AION, thus "young" patients with ION should be investigated for this possibility.[666-668] However, prothrombotic states in general are not associated with AION.[669] Homocysteine has been implicated in some series as a risk factor for ION, but other studies' levels have not confirmed this association.[670-672] Patients with uremia have been described with vision loss and optic nerve swelling presumably on an ischemic basis.[673,674] Visual loss is bilateral and improvement with hemodialysis has been reported. A possible component to the disc swelling from elevated intracranial pressure has been postulated.[673] Other patients with acute hypertensive crisis, as in the setting of preeclampsia, have been reported to develop ION.[675] Although perhaps an example of two common, unrelated conditions occurring in the same patient, typical migrainous episodes followed by AION have been reported.[676,677]

Treatment. There is no known effective therapy. Although steroids are usually thought to be ineffective, a controversial retrospective study showed better vision and quicker resolution of disc swelling with the use of steroids.[678] The significance of these findings is uncertain and there has not been widespread adaptation of steroid treatment in ION although they are occasionally used in practice. Optic nerve sheath fenestration or decompression was used and seemed to improve vision in some progressive cases.[679-681] Other series did not support the findings of these authors,[682,683] and ultimately the IONDT was undertaken to answer the question definitively. The study concluded that the surgery was not beneficial and may be harmful since the group receiving surgery had a lower rate of visual recovery and a higher rate of loss of three or more lines of acuity.[626,684]

Hyperbaric oxygen[685] and aspirin[686] have also been shown to be ineffective in altering the early course of ischemic optic neuropathy. Heparin and warfarin are also unhelpful. Interestingly, levodopa and carbidopa have been shown to improve visual acuity in patients with even long-standing vision loss from ischemic optic neuropathy.[687] In this prospective, double-masked trial with 20 subjects, however, no effect on color vision or mean deviation of visual field was observed. This treatment effect has not been confirmed in other studies, and therefore the use of levodopa has not been widely adopted.[688] Small groups or single patients have been reported to improve with transvitreal optic neurotomy[689] or intravitreal bevacizumab[690] and triamcinolone.[691] Finally, the protective effect of a previous attack of ION is powerful, as recurrence within a previously affected eye is rare.[663] This has led Burde[578] to suggest prophylactic pan retinal photocoagulation to produce controlled optic atrophy, a treatment that has not yet been pursued or tested.

There is also no effective prophylaxis for second-eye involvement. For this purpose we often place patients with non-arteritic AION on daily low-dose aspirin therapy, but there is no prospective proof of its efficacy.[692,693]

Clinical distinction between optic neuritis and ION. The clinical profile of these two groups of patients can overlap significantly, particularly in adults between the ages of 30 and 50, when they present with disc swelling but without pain on eye movements.[301] There are no laboratory tests to distinguish the two entities. However, in most instances the distinction is easily made based on consideration of the patient's age, associated symptoms, and examination findings. Patients under age 40 almost never get ION. The presence of pain is common in ON, while it is present in less than 10% of ION patients, and generally is not exacerbated by eye movements.[614] Also, a normal-appearing nerve is common in ON and by definition not seen in AION. Warner et al.[616] found that altitudinal swelling, pallor, arterial attenuation, and hemorrhage were more common in AION than in ON. Factors which are not helpful in distinguishing the two entities are sex, presenting visual acuity, and laboratory tests. Depending on the type of defect, the visual fields may be helpful in identifying typical ION from ON, as patients with ION typically have inferior altitudinal field loss.[694] However, there is enough overlap to make the distinction based on field criteria alone impossible. Maximal visual loss within 24 hours is not uncommon in optic neuritis and progression for up to 10 days can occur with ION.

Temporal arteritis and ION

Visual symptoms due to temporal (giant cell, cranial, granulomatous, Horton's) arteritis are a neuro-ophthalmic emergency. Acute vision loss, the most feared complication of this disorder, occurs in between 7% and 60% of patients.[695] The most common mechanism is arteritic ION, referring to sudden optic nerve infarction due to vessel lumens narrowed by vasculitis. A non-ocular cause of visual loss in temporal arteritis, occipital lobe infarction, is reviewed in Chapter 8. Since many cases of blindness in giant cell arteritis are preventable with immediate administration of corticosteroids, suspected patients require emergent diagnosis and intervention.

Demographics. There is an increased incidence in women (3 : 1). Most affected individuals are Caucasian, but patients in other racial groups may be affected.[696] The prevalence of giant cell arteritis increases with age, affecting about 12–20/100 000 over age 50[697,698] but 100/100 000 patients over age 80.[699-702] Most patients are over age 70, and cases below age 50 are exceedingly rare,[703] making patients with AION due to giant cell arteritis on average older than patients with non-arteritic AION.

Pathology. The vasculitis involves large and mid-sized arteries containing an elastic lamina. For the most part, these vessels tend to be extradural. The arteritis has a predilection for the superficial temporal, vertebral, ophthalmic, and posterior ciliary arteries.[704] This distribution explains the high frequency of blindness and the occasional cerebellar, brain stem, and occipital lobe strokes observed in this disorder.

Optic nerve infarction typically occurs at a retrolaminar or prelaminar/retrolaminar watershed zone supplied by branches of the short ciliary arteries and branches of the ophthalmic artery.[705] Other vessels less commonly involved include the internal carotid, external carotid and central retinal arteries. In addition, dissection due to involvement of the proximal aorta and myocardial infarction from vasculitis in the coronary arteries have both been reported.[706]

Histologically, early cases are characterized by lymphocytes limited to the internal or external elastic lamina or adventitia of the vessel wall, with destruction of those layers. More marked involvement is typified by involvement of all vascular layers. Necrosis and granulomas containing multinucleated histiocytic and foreign body giant cells, histiocytes, and lymphocytes may be seen.[707] Inflammation of the arterial wall narrows the vessel lumen and causes thrombosis and vascular occlusion.[708]

Pathogenesis. The greater incidence in Caucasians and an association with HLA antigens DR3, DR4, DR5, DRB1, and Cw3 suggest giant cell arteritis may have a genetic component.[707,709] Immunologic studies have demonstrated involvement of humoral and cellular immunity, particularly of T-cell function.[709,710] Tissue and T-cell production of interferons and macrophage secretion of interleukins are also likely important.[711] The simultaneous occurrence of giant cell arteritis in a husband and wife,[712] and demonstration of varicella virus DNA in arteries of some patients with giant cell arteritis,[713] supports a possible environmental exposure or infectious etiology.

Neuro-ophthalmic symptoms. Patients may have premonitory episodes of transient monocular blindness prior to visual loss (sometimes when rising from a supine position) related to impaired ocular blood flow.[714] Another complaint may be bright-light amaurosis, caused by the increased metabolic demands of photoreceptors for which blood supply is unavailable.[715] Transient episodes of binocular diplopia[716] and formed visual hallucinations[717] may occur as well.

Visual loss is usually sudden and severe, and sometimes there is accompanying pain. Simultaneous bilateral vision loss occurs in between 20% and 62% of patients with temporal arteritis.[716,718–722] In untreated patients, one study found second eye involvement occurs in approximately 75% of patients within days, and usually within a week.[719]

In contrast, simultaneous presentation with non-arteritic ION is rare and usually occurs only as a complication of surgery or with significant blood loss. **Table 5–12** contrasts the clinical presentations of arteritic and non-arteritic ischemic optic neuropathy.

Neuro-ophthalmic signs. The neuro-ophthalmic complications of giant cell arteritis have been the topic of several reviews.[709,723–726] Visual complications of giant cell arteritis develop in about 30% of patients with biopsy-proven disease.[727] Anterior ischemic optic neuropathy is the most common (80–90%) cause of vision loss in temporal arteritis (**Table 5–13**).[716,719–721,728,729] Visual loss is usually profound and in general is more severe than in non-arteritic ION.[562,716,722] Hand motion and no light perception vision, which are uncommon in the non-arteritic version, occurred in 24% of eyes in one series.[716]

The disc edema of arteritic AION is classically described as chalky white and may extend away from the disc (**Fig. 5–46**). Alternatively the infarction may be posterior or retro-

Table 5–12 The clinical distinction between and non-arteritic and arteritic ischemic optic neuropathy

Criteria	Non-arteritic	Arteritic
Age	Any, usually 60–70	Rare under 50, most over 70
Race	No difference	More common in Caucasians, less common in African Americans
Sex	No difference	More common in women
Preceding systemic symptoms	None	Common
Preceding ocular symptoms	None	Common, transient visual loss or diplopia
Pain	Rare	Common
Vision loss	Minimal to severe	Usually severe
Simultaneous involvement of eyes	Extremely rare	Occasional
Second eye involvement	15–30% in months or years	75% within days or weeks
Disc appearance	Sectoral edema	Normal or chalky white swelling
Sedimentation rate	Less than 40	Any; usually greater than 90
Fluorescein angiogram	Normal; can have delayed optic nerve head filling	Choroidal filling defects
Anatomic predisposition	Small crowded optic nerve head	None
Other signs of ocular ischemia	Never	Occasional
Late optic atrophy	Simple pallor	Can have cupping
Response to steroids	None proven	Systemically—definite Vision—sometimes

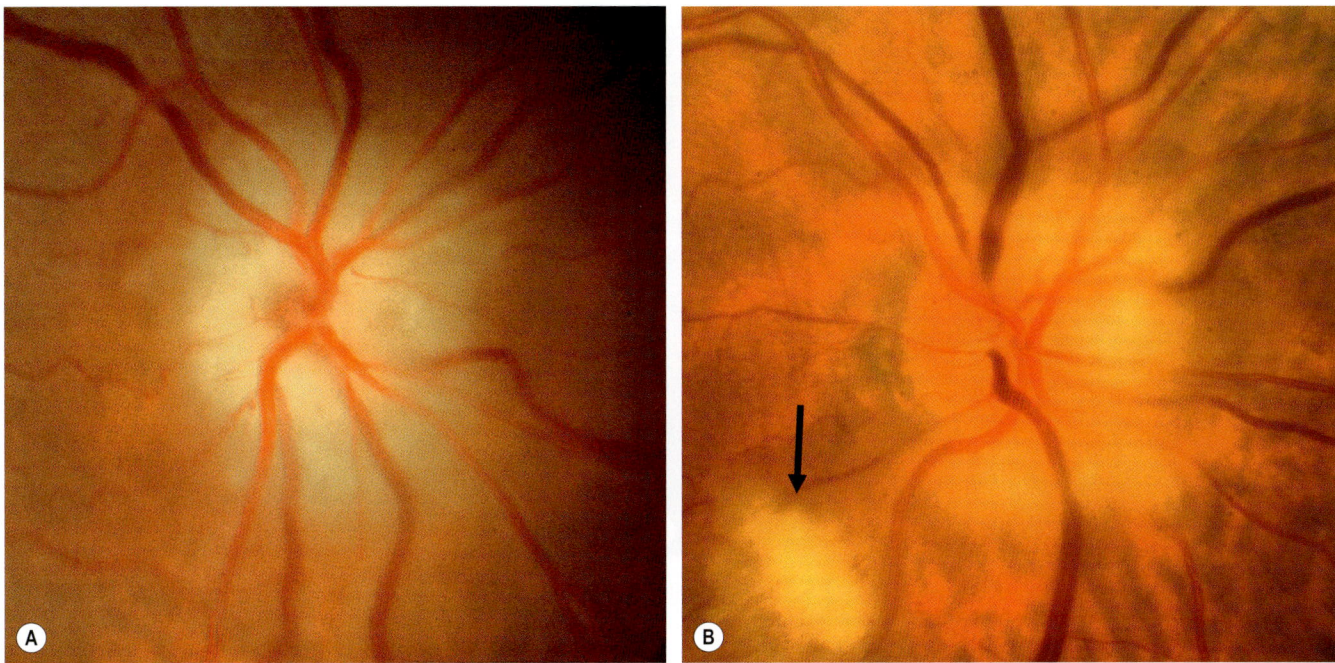

Figure 5–46. Acutely swollen optic nerves in arteritic ischemic optic neuropathy. The swelling may have a diffuse chalky white appearance (**A**) or be more focal and white with a cotton-wool spot (arrow) away from the disc (**B**).

Table 5–13 Etiology of visual loss (n = 63 eyes) in one study of 45 patients with biopsy-proven giant cell arteritis

Anterior ischemic optic neuropathy (AION)*	55 (88%)
Posterior ischemic optic neuropathy (PION)	2 (3%)
Central retinal artery occlusion (CRAO)	3 (5%)
Branch retinal artery occlusion (BRAO)	3 (5%)
Choroidal infarction	4 (6%)
Optic atrophy (exact etiology unclear)	3 (5%)

AION, anterior ischemic optic neuropathy; PION, posterior ischemic optic neuropathy; CRAO, central retinal artery occlusion; BRAO, branch retinal artery occlusion.
*AION and CRAO, one eye; AION and BRAO, two eyes; AION and choroidal infarct, four eyes.
From Liu GT et al.,[716] with permission.

bulbar without disc swelling (posterior ischemic optic neuropathy (PION), see below). Cotton-wool spots may be an early sign (**Fig. 5–47**).[730] Vision loss may also occur on the basis of choroidal ischemia[731] or branch or central retinal artery occlusion (**Fig. 5–48**). The simultaneous presence of AION and retinal arterial occlusion indicates ophthalmic artery involvement. Since few other disorders cause both of these together in the same eye, this combination makes the diagnosis arteritis until proven otherwise. Later in the course when optic atrophy supervenes, it is often associated with cupping[732–734] (**Fig. 5–49**). In contrast, cupping is only rarely found after non-arteritic AION.[735]

There may also be signs of ocular ischemia.[736,737] Even without ocular ischemia, intraocular pressure may be low.[738] Motility disturbances may also occur and result from ischemia of the extraocular muscles, ischemic ocular motor

nerve palsies, or brain stem stroke (see Chapter 15).[739] Orbital inflammatory masses due to giant cell arteritis also have been reported.[740]

Systemic symptoms and signs. Most patients with visual complications due to giant cell arteritis will have premonitory systemic symptoms (**Table 5–14**) for days or years prior to or accompanying their visual symptoms. Patients may have polymyalgia rheumatica (proximal muscle ache, stiffness, and arthralgias), headache, scalp tenderness, jaw claudication when chewing or talking, fever, malaise, or weight loss.[741] Most of these symptoms are due to end-organ ischemia. Headaches and jaw claudication are the most common symptoms, and jaw claudication may predict a higher risk for vision loss.[716,718,742] In fact the new onset of headache in any elderly patient should raise the possibility of giant cell arteritis. Less common systemic complications include scalp and tongue necrosis[743,744] (**Fig. 5–50**) and tongue or swallowing claudication. Between 16% and 26% of patients with visual complications due to giant cell arteritis will have an "occult" form[719,729,745,746] with ophthalmic complaints but no systemic symptoms.

Physical examination will generally show an ill-appearing patient. Cachexia and pallor may be evident. The temporal artery may be tender, prominent, cord-like, and pulseless.

The major neurologic complications of giant cell arteritis,[747] such as cerebrovascular symptoms[748] and other cranial nerve palsies,[749] are discussed further in Chapters 8 and 15. Aseptic meningoradiculitis[750] and dural enhancement[751] may also occur. As alluded to earlier, cardiovascular manifestations include aortic aneurysm, dissection, or rupture, coronary artery disease, and aortic valve insufficiency.[752]

Establishing the diagnosis. In our experience, patients with AION or CRAO due to giant cell arteritis can be identified by any combination of (1) age over 50, (2) typical fundus

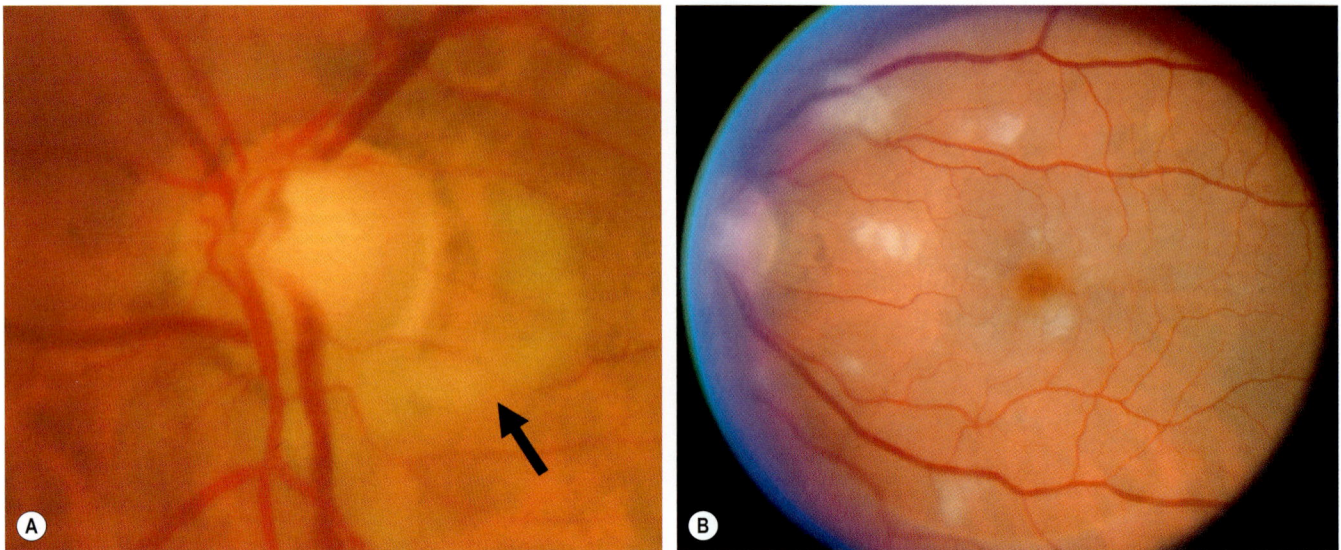

Figure 5–47. Ophthalmoscopic appearance of the left eye of two different patients who presented with severe vision loss due to temporal arteritis. **A**. A large cotton-wool spot (temporal to the disc) is the only visible abnormality, and in the second patient (**B**) more extensive, scattered cotton-wool spots are seen. In these patients vision loss was presumably on the basis of choroidal ischemia or posterior ischemic optic neuropathy.

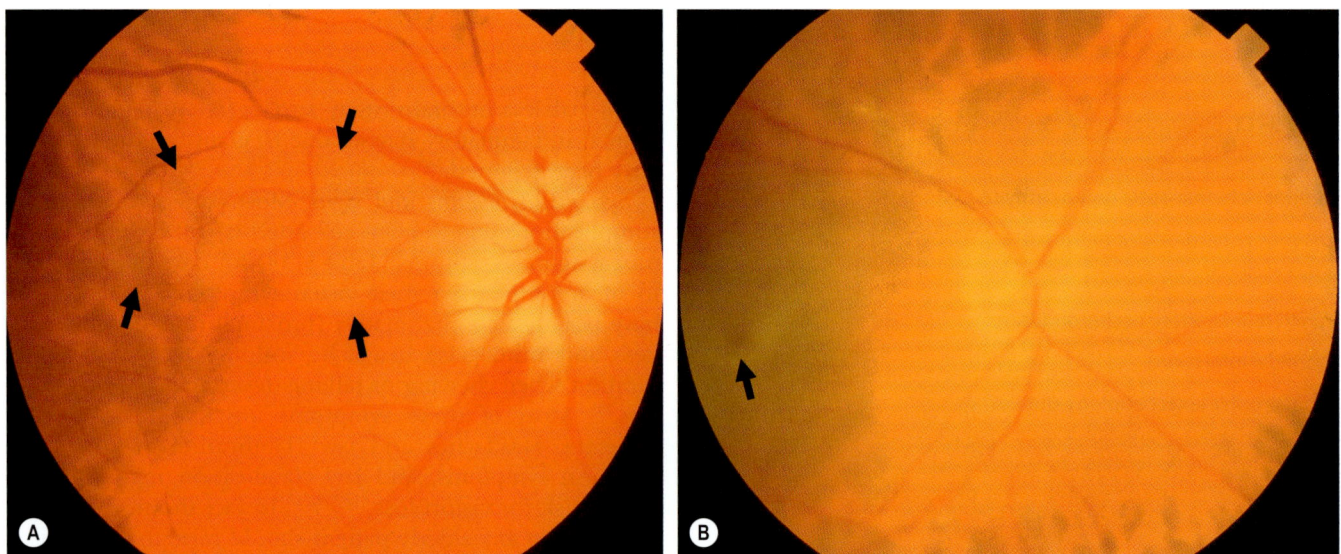

Figure 5–48. Retinal ischemia in temporal arteritis. **A**. Combined ischemic optic neuropathy with chalky white disc swelling and retinal whitening (arrows) secondary to branch retinal artery occlusion. **B**. Central retinal artery occlusion from temporal arteritis. A macular cherry red spot (arrow) is present, but there is no visible occlusive embolus.

appearance (disc swelling with or without retinal infarction), (3) typical systemic symptoms, (4) high erythrocyte sedimentation rate, (5) positive temporal artery biopsy, (6) high C-reactive protein (CRP), or (7) abnormal fluorescein angiography. When systemic symptoms are absent in so-called "occult" temporal arteritis,[746] almost always the ESR is elevated.[716] If the ESR is normal, alternatively almost always systemic symptoms are present. In other words, visual loss due to giant cell arteritis with a normal ESR and without systemic symptoms would be unusual. Although more strict criteria for the diagnosis of giant cell arteritis have been published,[753] we have found the above guidelines to be extremely helpful in clinical practice.

The discussion below details the various laboratory tests.

Blood tests. Normal ESRs can be estimated by the following formula: (age × 0.5) for men and ((age + 10) × 0.5) for women. The ESR is usually elevated in giant cell arteritis and often is above 90 mm/h. However, elevated ESRs are nonspecific, since a number of normal elderly patients have increased ESRs and half of the people with ESRs over 50 have no explanation found.[754,755] In addition, as many as 22% of patients with temporal arteritis and visual symptoms can have normal ESRs.[699,716,756] Permanent vision loss is more likely to occur in patients with a relatively low ESR[727] and in patients with thrombocytosis.[757]

In a recent study, an elevated CRP (>2.45 mg/dl), another acute phase reactant, was more sensitive (100%) than the ESR (>47 mm/h) for the diagnosis of giant cell arteritis.[742]

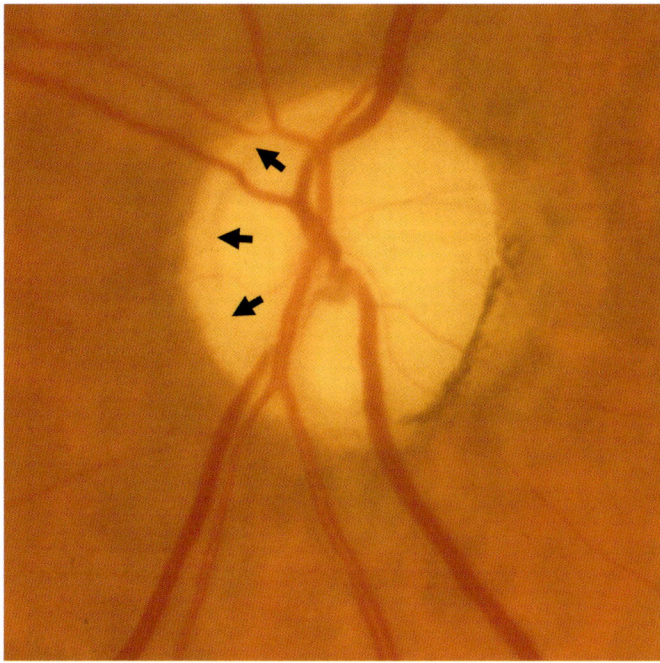

Figure 5–49. Optic atrophy with cupping after ischemic optic neuropathy secondary to temporal arteritis. The arrows highlight the edge of the cup, seen best nasally.

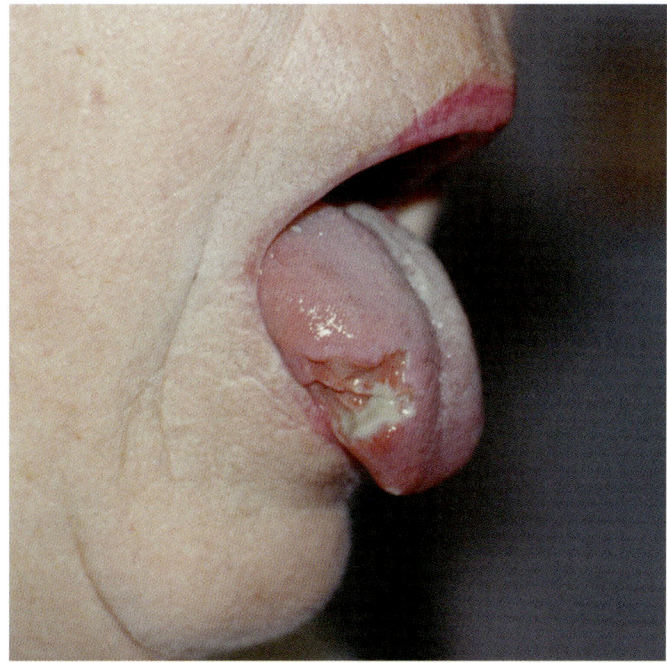

Figure 5–50. Necrosis of the tongue in a patient with temporal arteritis.

Table 5–14 Systemic symptoms prior to ophthalmic presentation in one study of 45 patients with biopsy-proven giant cell arteritis and visual symptoms

Headache	58%
Jaw claudication	53%
Weight loss	31%
Malaise	22%
Polymyalgia rheumatica	22%
Anorexia	20%
Fever	11%
Neck pain	11%
Scalp tenderness	11%
Anemia	9%
Dementia	4%
Swallowing claudication	4%
Confusion, facial pain, periorbital edema, somnolence, tinnitus, vertigo	Each 2%

From Liu GT et al.,[716] with permission.

The combination of an elevated sedimentation rate and CRP yielded a specificity of 97% for the diagnosis of giant cell arteritis.[758] Thrombocytosis is also commonly found in GCA patients and can be used to supplement the ESR and CRP results when distinguishing arteritic and non-arteritic ION.[759–761] Chronic mild to moderate normochromic anemia also may be evident.[707]

Fluorescein angiography. Fluorescein or indocyanine angiography may show delayed choroidal filling and focal, patchy perfusion defects (**Fig. 5–51**).[762–765] We have found this test to be extremely useful because of its relative sensitivity and specificity for giant cell arteritis when those angiographic features are demonstrated.

Temporal artery biopsy. If temporal arteritis is clinically suspected, a temporal artery biopsy should almost always be performed (**Fig. 5–52**). The procedure rarely results in significant complications, and therefore the threshold to perform a biopsy should be low. A high ratio of negative to positive results is acceptable. Skip lesions are often present, so generally long segments (greater than 3 cm) are recommended.[766–768] Grossly at the time of surgery, arterial abnormalities are often present and consist of irregular thickening, stiffness, and a mottled gray appearance (**Fig. 5–53**). Multiple transverse sections should be made of each segment. Histopathologic evaluation (**Fig. 5–54**) reveals transmural inflammation, with destruction of the internal elastic lamina, obliteration of the lumen, and characteristic epithelioid cell and giant cells. False-positive temporal artery biopsies are rare, but have been seen in Wegener's granulomatosis[769] and sarcoidosis,[770] for example. Rarely necessary, alternative biopsy sites include the occipital artery.[771]

The issue of whether to obtain a bilateral or unilateral temporal artery biopsy remains controversial.[772,773] In many cases the initial biopsy can be seen to be grossly abnormal at the time of surgery (**Fig. 5–53**), and only a unilateral biopsy needs to be performed. We obtain bilateral biopsies when the initial biopsy is negative or equivocal, and the clinical suspicion for GCA remains high. We analyzed our series of 88 unilateral biopsies and found a one-sided procedure adequately excluded GCA when the pretest suspicion was low.[774] Only one patient subsequently went on to have a positive biopsy. Therefore, for experienced physicians, a unilateral TAB is sufficient in populations for which clinical

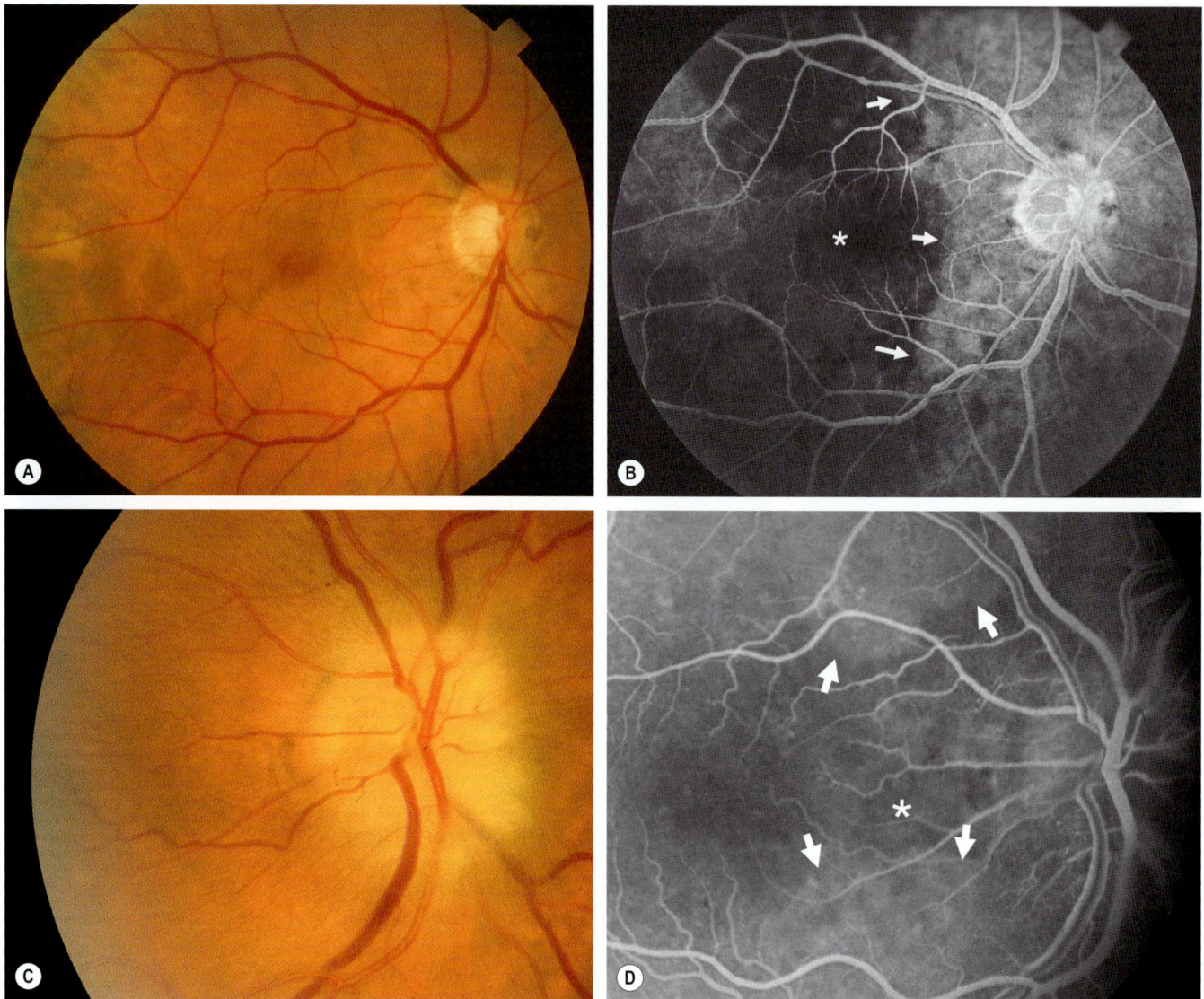

Figure 5–51. Fundus photographs and fluorescein angiograms in two patients (**A–B**, **C–D**) with temporal arteritis and vision loss. **A**. Color fundus photograph of a patient with multiple episode of transient vision loss. **B**. The area of normal choroidal perfusion around the disc is seen to end abruptly (arrows), and more temporally there is a large patchy area of nonperfusion (asterisk). **C**. Ischemic disc edema in temporal arteritis and (**D**) fluorescein angiography demonstrates normal choroidal perfusion ending abruptly (arrows) with an area of choroidal nonperfusion (asterisk) between the disc and macula.

suspicion is low. In one study, fever, jaw claudication, pale optic disc edema, or any systemic symptom other than headache were found more commonly in patients found to have arteritis.[774] In another report the combination of jaw claudication and double vision was highly predictive of a positive biopsy.[775] Danesh-Meyer et al.[776] also found a relatively low yield from a second biopsy (only 1% discordance rate),[776] whereas Pless et al.[777] and Boyev et al.[778] found discordance rates of 3% and 5% in their series. In the Boyev study of 186 patients who had bilateral biopsies, only six (3%) had a different pathology between the two sides.[778] In three cases, the findings were consistent with healed arteritis and in the other three cases early arteritis was suggested. Thus, the added value of a second contralateral temporal biopsy is relatively low.

There is no reason to withhold treatment while waiting to do a biopsy. Histopathologic evidence of arteritis can be seen at least 1 week after treatment with steroids.[779] It is also now well established that biopsies in some chronic cases can still reflect diagnostic pathology several weeks and maybe even years after steroid therapy has begun.[716,780–783]

Only rarely, based on clinical grounds is a diagnosis of biopsy-negative temporal arteritis made. We caution against making this diagnosis either routinely or without biopsy on a presumptive basis. Too often, months later during steroid treatment, which can often lead to devastating side-effects for the patient,[784] the clinician is left in a quandary whether steroids can be discontinued or should be replaced because no tissue diagnosis was made.

Noninvasive vascular studies. Color Doppler may demonstrate abnormal flow within the ophthalmic, central retinal, and short posterior ciliary arteries,[785] and temporal artery wall abnormalities may also be seen with this modality.[786,787] Currently these tests are not part of our usual workup.

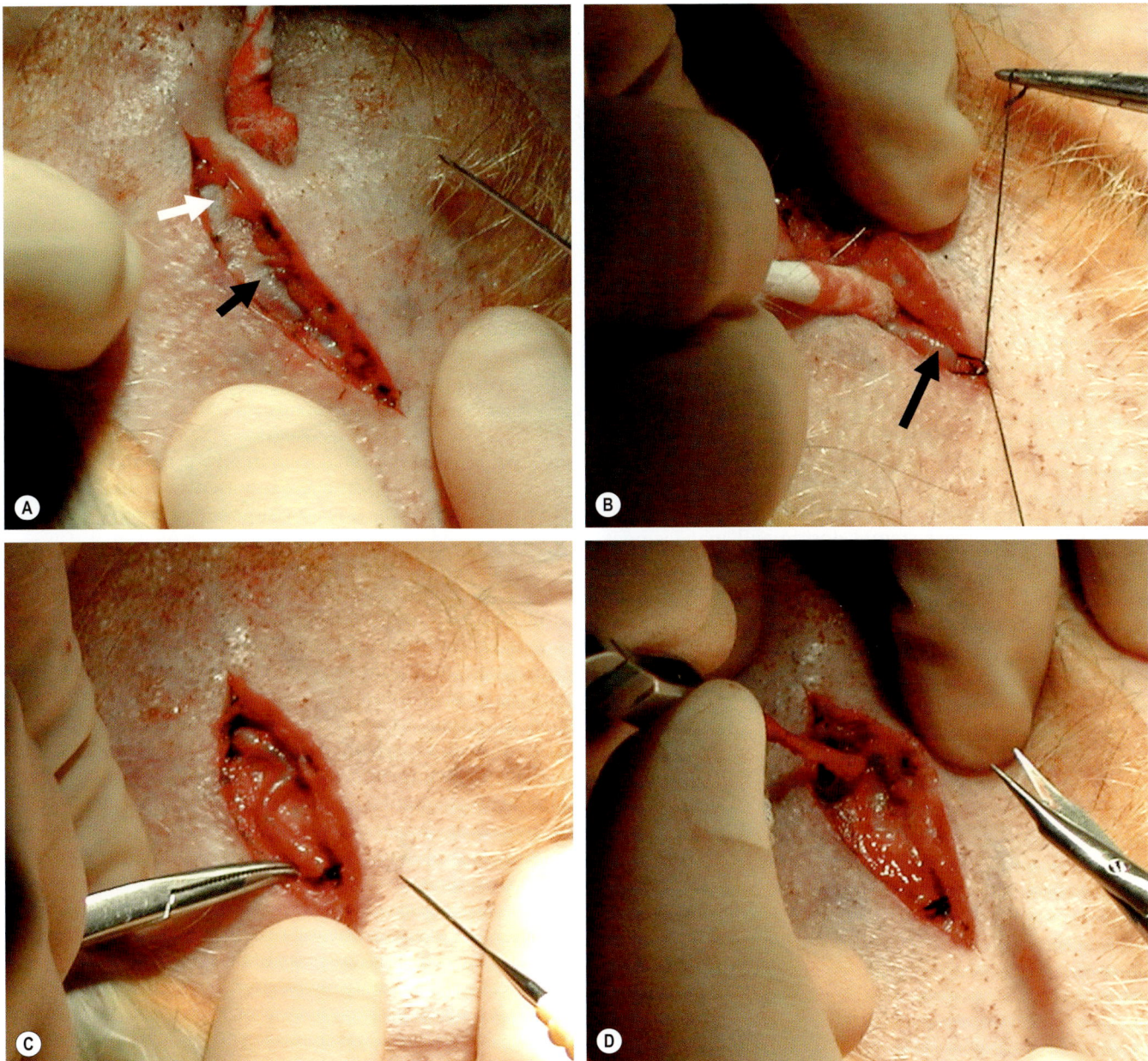

Figure 5–52. Sequence of steps used to perform temporal artery biopsy, which can be performed in the office under local anesthesia. Location of the artery either by palpation of the pulse or with Doppler is critical. An incision is made directly over the artery through the skin and subcuticular layers. **A.** The dissection is carried through the subcutaneous fat with cautery down to the superficial temporal fascia (white arrow). The artery (black arrow) can be seen as a purplish ridge in the fascia. Blunt dissection is used to separate the artery from the surrounding fascia. **B.** A silk suture ligature is tied around both ends of the artery (arrow). **C.** The artery is separated completely from the surrounding fascia with blunt dissection. **D.** The segment of artery between the two sutures is then removed with sharp dissection.

Management/treatment. When patients present with vision loss, successful prevention of second eye involvement is the goal of prompt and accurate diagnosis. There is also a risk for neurologic and cardiac complications in untreated patients. Evidence from anecdotal and retrospective studies suggest that (1) corticosteroids retard the progression of visual loss, (2) corticosteroids may diminish the risk of fellow-eye involvement, (3) on occasion (15–34%) steroids may restore some vision, sometimes dramatically, and (4) intravenous steroids may be more effective than oral steroids in protecting the fellow-eye and enhancing visual prognosis, in part because of a higher intravenous corticosteroid dose

and greater bioavailability.[716,718,788–795] In Chan et al.'s series,[796] vision improved in 40% of intravenous treated compared with 13% of orally treated patients. Alternatively some authors have argued that intravenous steroids are no more effective than oral regimens.[797,798] However, it is our impression that while systemic symptoms may respond to oral doses, patients with visual symptoms due to giant cell arteritis require larger doses of corticosteroids given intravenously.

Therefore, in the absence of prospective data, in cases in which diagnosis is strongly suspected and visual symptoms or signs are present, we recommend emergent intravenous steroid therapy (methylprednisolone 250 mg q.i.d. intravenously) for 3–5 days with ulcer prophylaxis. Because affected patients are typically elderly and therefore more prone to steroid-related cardiac and gastrointestinal side-effects, patients should be hospitalized while receiving intravenous steroids. To improve blood flow to the orbit, patients should lie flat for 24 hours, and aspirin can be given, but antiplatelet therapy has not become standard in our practice.

The high ESR and systemic symptoms usually improve rapidly with steroids, often after the first dose. Following the intravenous treatment, prednisone 1 mg/kg per day is given orally. The steroid dose should remain high for the first month, then the dose can be tapered slowly over 6–12 months, as long as it is confirmed that the ESR stays normal and systemic symptoms are absent before each drop in dose. Many individuals require a small daily or every other day maintenance dose of prednisone beyond this period. Side-effects from chronic steroid usage such as osteoporosis and skin breakdown are common in this age group,[799] so a physician knowledgeable and experienced in the use of steroids should supervise steroid dosing and management of side-effects.

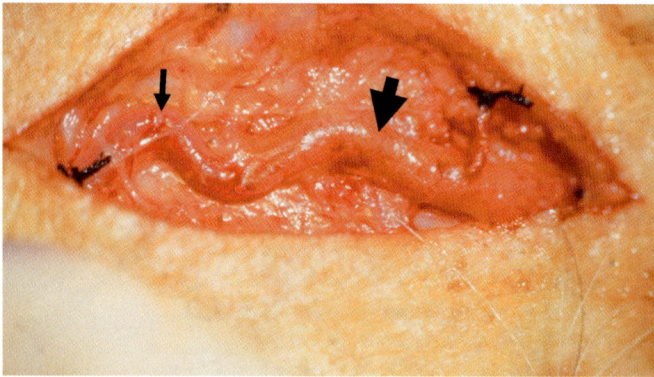

Figure 5–53. Gross abnormalities in the appearance of the superficial temporal artery at the time of biopsy in a patient with temporal arteritis. The thinner, more normal-appearing artery is seen to the left (thin arrow) and the thickened, gray, more mottled artery is seen in the middle (thick arrow).

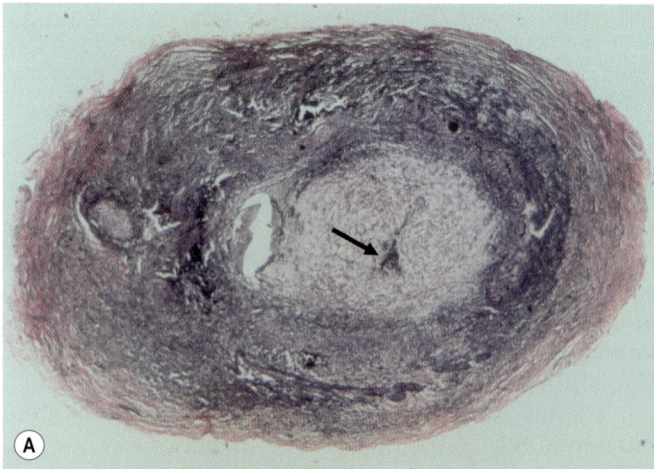

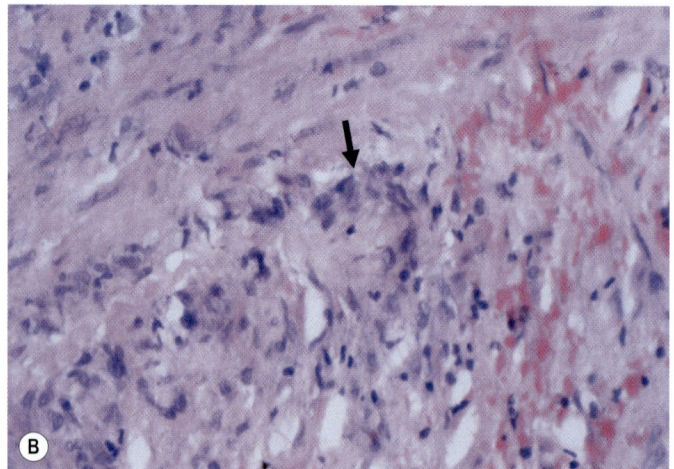

Cases of giant cell arteritis refractory to corticosteroids are extremely challenging.[737,800] Some patients demonstrate flow-related ophthalmologic and neurologic phenomena, requiring Trendelenburg positioning or heparinization.[715,801] In addition, some patients' symptoms recur many months or even years following initial corticosteroid treatment.[716,802] Repeat temporal artery biopsies can demonstrate persistent or recurrent arteritis in these cases.[803] In these instances, steroid sparing, antiinflammatory and immunomodulating therapy such as methotrexate[804] or dapsone[805,806] can be considered, but side-effects may limit the use of these medications. A prospective recent study tested the addition of infliximab to the early steroid regimen in patients with polymyalgia rheumatica and found no benefit and even a possible harmful effect.[807]

Visual prognosis. The prognosis for visual improvement in giant cell arteritis is relatively poor.[719,808] Many studies[721,808,809] reported absolutely no recovery in NLP eyes, an observation the Bascom Palmer series[716] supported with the exception of one case. Progressive vision loss can also occur despite steroid therapy, oral or intravenous, in 9–14% of patients.[716,718,810,811] In one series, vision loss occurred in the first week in approximately 27% of eyes despite high-dose intravenous steroids.[812] Late recurrences of ION while on treatment are often associated with recurrence of systemic symptoms and abnormal laboratory testing (ESR), so patients must be followed closely to identify these important clues to disease activity.[813] Sometimes, however, recurrences arise unpredictably without warning.[814]

Nonetheless, there are there several anecdotal reports of patients with giant cell arteritis and AION[705,788,793–795] or central retinal artery occlusion[792] who enjoyed remarkable visual improvement. Literature reviews and institutional series demonstrate that as few as 5%,[815] and many as 15–34%, of patients may experience some recovery of vision.[716,718,816] When recovery occurs it is mostly manifested with improved acuity and less often with significant visual field recovery.[817] Relatively higher rates of improvement have been attributed to the use of intravenous versus oral corticosteroids, as a greater percentage of patients (9/23

Figure 5–54. Histopathology of superficial temporal artery biopsy. **A**. Low-power view, elastin stain, demonstrating transmural inflammation and obliteration of the arterial lumen (arrow). **B**. Higher power (hematoxylin and eosin stain) demonstrating a giant cell (arrow).

(39%) vs 5/18 (28%)) improved after intravenous treatment in the Bascom Palmer series.[716] However, this difference was not statistically significant, and as alluded to earlier, the advantages of intravenous over oral treatment are controversial.[797,798] Visual recovery without steroid treatment is rare.[816]

Relationship between polymyalgia rheumatica and temporal arteritis. It is possible they represent the same rheumatologic disorder, except the term temporal arteritis is used to describe cases with involvement of the arteries of the head. Patients with polymyalgia rheumatica may develop temporal arteritis and visual loss despite years of corticosteroid treatment.[716] The best treatment regimen, i.e., low-dose versus high-dose corticosteroids or some alternative medication, for preventing ophthalmic complications in polymyalgia rheumatica and in cases of temporal arteritis without previous ocular symptoms has not been established.[818-822] Patients without cranial symptoms can develop them at any time in the course of their polymyalgia rheumatica.[823]

Posterior ischemic optic neuropathy (PION)

Posterior ION, presumably due to infarction of the retrolaminar optic nerve, should prompt a thorough systemic workup. Sadda et al.[824] have suggested dividing patients with posterior ION into three groups: those with giant cell arteritis, those with perioperative vision loss, and finally those with only vasculopathic risk factors. In contrast to non-arteritic AION, non-arteritic PION is unusual. The diagnosis of a retrobulbar ischemic optic neuropathy in an elderly patient demands immediate investigation for temporal arteritis, inflammatory causes, compressive lesions, and an infiltrative process associated with carcinomatous meningitis or CNS infection, for example. Hayreh[825] reported a series of patients and emphasized the importance of excluding giant cell arteritis, the high prevalence of central field defect and the potential benefit of steroid treatment. In eyes with non-arteritic PION, 34% experienced improvement in vision, 28% remained stable, and 38% worsened. Carotid artery disease and stroke history were both associated with increased risk of poor final visual outcome.[824] Inflammatory conditions, such as lupus and polyarteritis nodosa, and infectious causes, including herpes and varicella zoster, have been reported in association with PION.[826,827] Sickle cell disease has also been reported as a cause.[828] Neuroimaging is also required to exclude the sudden presentation of a compressive mass lesion such as pituitary apoplexy or an ophthalmic artery aneurysm.

Migraine has also been reported as a cause of posterior ischemic optic neuropathy.[829] One series identified diabetes, hypertension, and carotid stenosis as risk factors for PION,[830] but in our experience such cases are exceedingly rare.

Ischemic optic neuropathy associated with surgery or blood loss

In so-called "shock"-associated ischemic optic neuropathy, additional risk factors of anemia, atherosclerosis, or severe blood loss are often present with low blood pressure to produce infarction of the optic nerve.[831-839] Cases of perioperative vision loss particularly in association with spine and cardiac surgery have been increasingly recognized.[840-842] This devastating complication of surgery is relatively rare but is a common cause of postoperative vision loss. The disorder may occur in anterior (disc swelling) or posterior (normal disc) forms. Sometimes the disc swelling can be minimal despite very poor vision suggesting that the majority of the optic nerve injury is retrolaminar. In addition to spine and cardiac surgery,[843-853] it has most often been reported in association with radical neck dissection.[854-858] The incidence of perioperative ION in the relatively high-risk situations of cardiac and spine surgery is less than 0.1%.[842,844,850,853] Perioperative vision loss is often bilateral and severe, and the presentation may be delayed by hours or days after the surgery. When disc swelling occurs, it tends to be pallid. Risk factors include arterial hypotension, anemia, hypoxia, pressor support, long operative time, preexisting vascular risk factors, and a small cup to disc ratio. No definite blood pressure threshold has been identified, and it is likely a combination of several risk factors. Head position with the face down and elevation of orbital venous pressure may be a factor in some cases. Similar events have been reported after dialysis.[859-864] Once recognized, correction of severe anemia (hemoglobin less than 8 mg/dl) should be considered. However, no treatment protocol is established, and the prognosis for recovery is poor.

Diabetic papillopathy

The spectrum of disc swelling in diabetic patients ranges from the typical older patient with diabetes and common AION to the young juvenile diabetic with benign disc swelling that resolves without residua. This is a continuum, as some young patients can develop mild optic neuropathy and some older diabetics can have transient optic nerve swelling without vision loss.

Benign diabetic papillopathy or papillophlebitis occurs usually in type I or juvenile-onset, insulin-dependent diabetic patients.[865-867] The onset is usually between age 20 and 40, and patients have generally had diabetes for years. Mild visual loss to approximately 20/40 is not uncommon, and there is often corresponding enlargement of the blind spot with occasional arcuate or central field defects. Typically prominent telangiectactic vascular dilation (**Fig. 5-55**) is evident on the disc surface, and contiguous swelling may extend into the macula.[866] Disc edema may be bilateral and may be prolonged with a highly variable course. Patients have an increased risk for subsequent disc neovascularization.[866,868] Visual recovery begins weeks to months after onset and may precede the resolution of the disc swelling. Intravitreal and periocular steroid injection may aid resolution of disc swelling and improve vision.[869,870] Mild optic atrophy can develop. The pathogenesis of this condition is poorly understood but most likely is disruption of blood flow to the optic disc surface, sufficient to cause swelling and interfere with axoplasmic transport but insufficient to cause impaired nerve function. In the setting of bilateral disc swelling, it is important to distinguish this condition from papilledema.

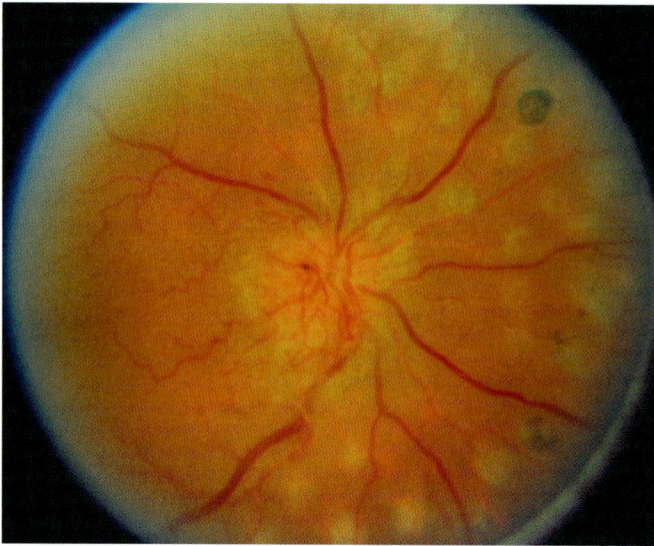

Figure 5–55. Appearance of the optic nerve in acute diabetic papillopathy. In addition to the swelling there are dilated vessels on the disc surface. These vessels often resolve as the disc swelling abates or can progress to disc neovascularization. Round atrophic lesions in the retinal periphery are the result of previous pan-retinal photocoagulation.

Compressive optic neuropathies

Compressive lesions can be predicted by their typical presentation with slowly progressive visual loss and optic nerve atrophy. Although less common, compressive optic neuropathy should still be considered in patients with acute vision loss, and in addition most individuals with unexplained vision loss should undergo MRI scanning to exclude this potentially treatable cause.

Etiology. Compressive optic neuropathy can result in the setting of benign or malignant neoplasms, contiguous sinus (mucocele) lesions or osseous process (fibrous dysplasia), enlarged extraocular muscles or abnormal vascular structures such as aneurysms. This condition can develop intrinsically from the nerve substance or from adjacent structures. More rarely they are the result of infiltrative processes or from tumor metastases. **Table 5–15** summarizes the important causes of compressive optic neuropathy.

Symptoms. Ophthalmic and non-ophthalmic symptoms generally evolve subacutely or insidiously (**Table 5–16**). Sudden vision loss can be superimposed on a chronic compressive problem such as: hemorrhage into a lymphangioma (chocolate cyst) or in a pituitary tumor (apoplexy), expansion of a cystic lesion as with craniopharyngioma, rapid enlargement of a parainfectious lesion such as a mucocele, and, finally, rapid expansion of an aneurysm. Other associated symptoms are outlined in **Table 5–16**.

Neuro-ophthalmic signs. Patients usually present with reduced acuity and color vision and visual field defects typical of an optic neuropathy (central, centrocecal or nerve fiber bundle). The optic nerve may appear normal, pale (**Fig. 5–56**), or swollen. Nerve fiber loss can be detected and monitored using OCT (**Fig. 5–56**). Optic disc swelling can result from compression and axoplasmic stasis, elevated intracranial pressure or direct nerve infiltration. Compression will

Table 5–15 Compressive lesions of the optic nerve

Intraorbital
  Primary orbital tumors (see Chapter 18)
    Cavernous hemangioma
    Schwannoma
  Secondary orbital tumors (see Chapter 18)
    Sinus tumor
    Metastatic tumors
Enlarged extraocular muscles (see Chapter 18)

Intraorbital/intracanalicular/intracranial
  Optic nerve neoplasms (primary)
    Optic nerve glioma (juvenile benign)
    Malignant optic nerve glioma
    Optic nerve sheath meningioma
  Optic nerve neoplasms (metastatic)
    Carcinomatous meningitis
    Optic nerve metastasis
    Lymphoma
    Leukemia
    Myeloma

Intracanalicular/intracranial
  Nontumor sinus causes
    Mucocele
  Paraclinoid tumors
    Meningioma
  Vascular causes
    Aneurysm
    Ectatic carotid arteries
  "Chiasmal" lesions (see Chapter 7)
    Pituitary adenoma
    Craniopharyngioma
    Suprasellar meningioma
  Other causes
    Fibrous dysplasia

Table 5–16 Common ophthalmic and non-ophthalmic symptoms associated with compressive optic neuropathy

Ophthalmic
  Reduced vision
    Subacute progression
    "Pseudosudden" onset from unrecognized disease
  Decreased color vision
  Gaze-evoked amaurosis
  Pain on eye movement
  Orbital fullness
  Proptosis
  Ptosis

Non-ophthalmic
  Headache (mass effect or dural involvement)
  Facial numbness or paresthesias (trigeminal nerve involvement)
  Reduced sense of smell (olfactory nerve involvement)
  Endocrine abnormalities (hypothalamic/pituitary axis involvement)

result in optic nerve head swelling only when the lesion is intraorbital. It is not a consequence of an intracanalicular or intracranial lesion, which more typically result directly in optic atrophy. Papilledema is an unusual cause for disc swelling in the setting of compressive optic neuropathy

RNFL thickness map

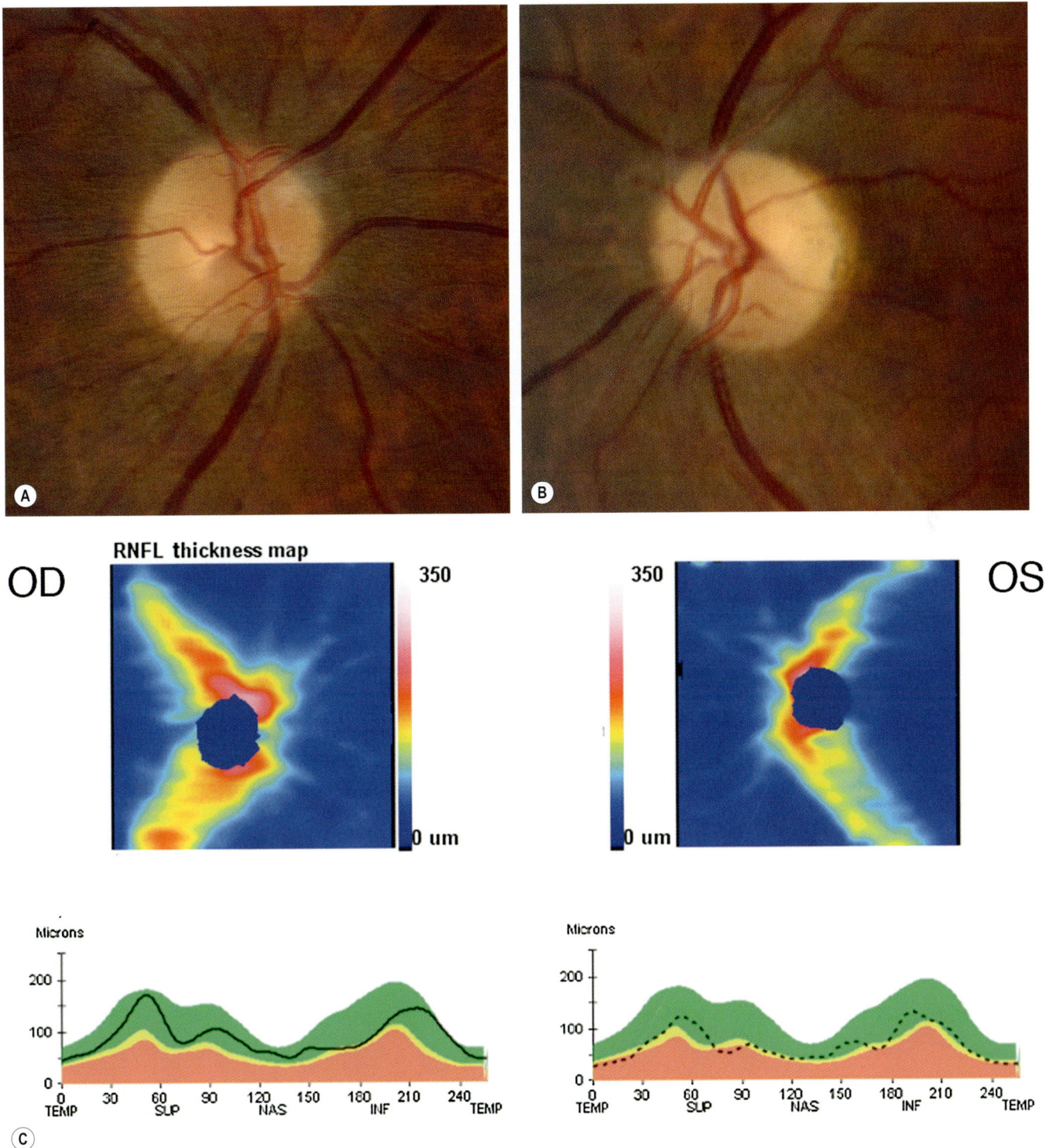

Figure 5–56. A,B. Optic nerve appearances in compressive optic neuropathy from a paraclinoid meningioma. The patient had symptoms and visual field loss in the left eye only. Disc pallor is mild OD (**A**) but more prominent OS (**B**). **C**. Ocular coherence tomography (OCT) demonstrates nerve fiber layer (NFL) thinning (OS) on both a thickness plot (top row) and the line graph (bottom row). Note the thinner (less red and pink) NFL of the left eye compared with the right eye (top row). In the line graph of the left eye, the NFL thickness (dashed line) dips into the red and yellow zones. OCT can be used to confirm and follow NFL loss in patients with compressive lesions.

except with large subfrontal meningiomas and with massive lesions that compress the third ventricle and cause obstructive hydrocephalus. When a large frontal lobe lesion compresses one optic nerve with resultant ipsilateral optic atrophy and elevates intracranial pressure to cause contral-

ateral papilledema, this is the Foster Kennedy syndrome (see Chapter 6).[871] Swelling may be accompanied by collateral ("shunt") vessels (**Fig. 5–57**) which bypass the central retinal vein and allow blood to flow from the retinal circulation directly into the ciliary circulation. They are common with optic nerve sheath meningioma but also occur with gliomas and chronic papilledema. Visual loss in the setting of extrinsic compression of the optic nerve results from a combination of Wallerian (ascending or beginning at the cell body) axonal degeneration, demyelination, and axonal dysfunction.

Diagnostic studies/neuroimaging. The diagnosis of compressive lesions of the anterior visual pathways requires neuroimaging. The best modality for the orbits and brain is an MRI scan with fat saturated orbital views and gadolinium enhancement. This technique offers excellent views of the globe, optic nerve head, optic nerve, optic nerve sheath, extraocular muscles, and orbital apex. It is far superior to CT scanning in the evaluation of the intracranial portion of the optic nerve, the chiasm, and the cavernous sinus. CT scanning serves an ancillary role and is helpful in evaluating bony changes, tumor calcification, and paranasal sinus disease.

The remaining discussion highlights the various compressive etiologies. However, primarily orbital processes, such as Graves or thyroid eye disease, are covered in Chapter 18; metastatic lesions are summarized later in this chapter in the section discussing cancer; and sellar processes which can cause intracranial compression of the optic nerve are discussed in Chapter 7.

Primary optic nerve neoplasms: optic nerve glioma (juvenile, benign)

Primary gliomas of the anterior visual pathways are of two different varieties. The first is the juvenile, benign, pilocytic astrocytoma. The second is the rare malignant glioblastoma of adulthood.

The benign optic gliomas of childhood generally present in the first decade of life with proptosis and slowly progressive painless vision loss (**Fig. 5–58**).[872] The disc may be swollen or pale and secondary strabismus often accompanies the vision loss. Visual field defects are generally central scotomas but temporal or bitemporal field defects may occur if the prechiasmatic portion of the nerve is involved.[873] Rare ophthalmic complications include congenital glaucoma with buphthalmos ("ox eye"), central retinal vein occlusion, iris rubeosis with neovascular glaucoma, and ocular ischemic syndrome.

Demographics. Most patients present in childhood, before age 10. About one-quarter (range 10–70%, depending on series) of the patients with optic nerve and chiasmal gliomas have neurofibromatosis (NF) type 1.[874] In contrast, about 8–30% of patients with NF-1 develop anterior visual pathway

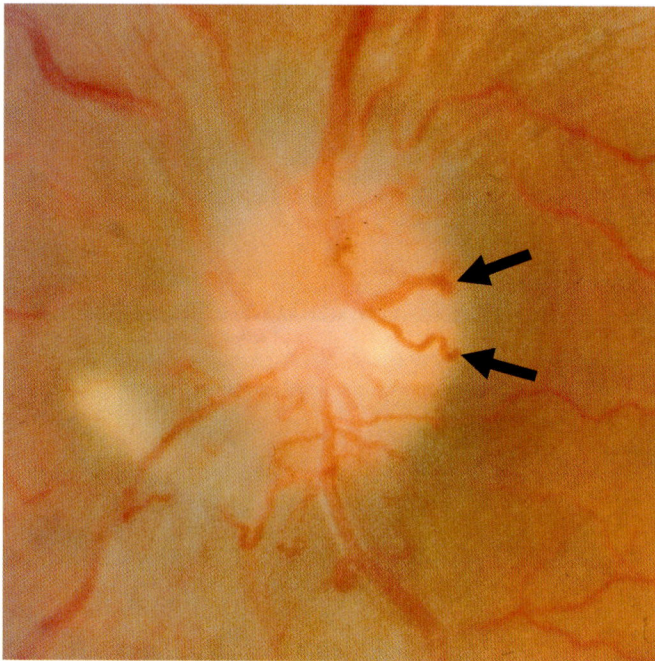

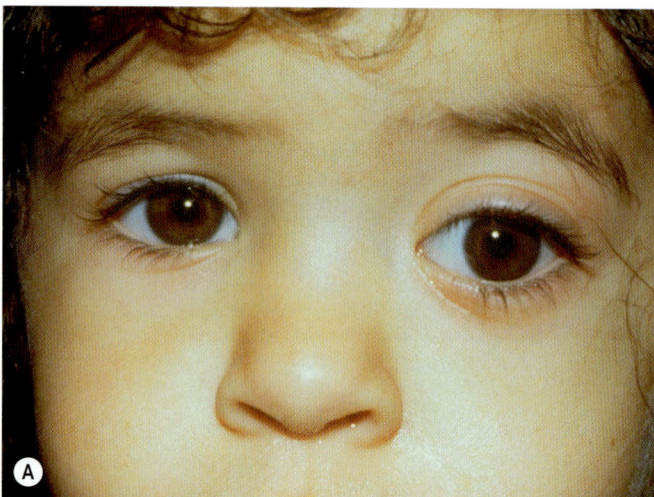

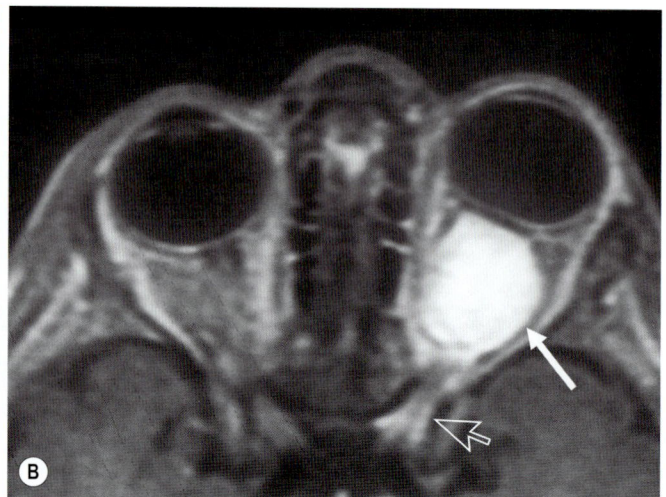

Figure 5–57. Chronic disc swelling from a subfrontal meningioma with disc collateral vessels (arrows) which connect the retinal venous system to the choroid, thereby bypassing the central retinal vein. In this setting, the disc swelling and collateral vessels could develop from either chronically elevated intracranial pressure or direct nerve compression.

Figure 5–58. Optic nerve glioma. **A**. Proptosis and inferior globe displacement (OS) in a young girl with decreased vision from an optic nerve glioma. **B**. Axial T1-weighted, fat saturated, gadolinium-enhanced MRI scan of the orbits demonstrating an optic nerve glioma in the left orbit. The intraorbital portion (solid white arrow) of the left optic nerve exhibits fusiform enlargement and enhancement, while the intracranial portion (white open arrow) is only slightly thickened, but also enhances.

gliomas,[875,876] and in approximately half of this subset, there is no associated visual loss.[877,878] The relationship between NF-1 and optic pathway gliomas is discussed in more detail in the section on chiasmal/hypothalamic gliomas in Chapter 7.

Diagnostic studies/neuroimaging. Neuroimaging typically reveals fusiform enlargement, kinking, and enhancement of the optic nerve (**Fig. 5–58**).[879,880] MRI is preferred over CT in this setting because of its superiority in evaluating the possibility of intracranial extension. At the time of detection about half of the tumors already exhibit chiasmal involvement.[881] The diagnosis is generally a clinical and radiographic one, and biopsy of a suspected optic nerve glioma is almost never needed, especially in the setting of NF-1. Certain radiographic features including a cystic appearance of "pseudo CSF" sign are typical of NF-1-associated gliomas.[882,883] In our experience, bilateral optic nerve enlargement without chiasmal involvement is virtually pathognomonic of NF-1.

Pathology. Histologically the tumors are generally juvenile pilocytic astrocytomas. They are intrinsic optic nerve tumors which only rarely extend outside the optic nerve sheath, and they appear benign without mitosis, cellular atypia, or necrosis. Occasionally proliferation of arachnoid around the tumor may simulate a meningioma.

Clinical course. The clinical course is highly variable. Most tumors grow only very slowly and may have self-limited growth. Many patients with tumors confined to the orbit will maintain good vision and in some rare instances even improve spontaneously.[872] Alvord and Lofton[881] projected, however, that all tumors eventually grow, with 70% showing progression within 3 years. Some believe that the prognosis is worse in non-NF cases, and this has been our impression as well.

Optic nerve glioma presenting without radiographic demonstration of chiasmal or hypothalamic involvement, which subsequently extended posteriorly, are uncommon. To our knowledge, there have been only two published, well-documented reports.[884,885] However, the first case was examined with CT scanning only, and it is possible that microscopic infiltration of the chiasm in the initial study was missed. Using modern generation gadolinium-enhanced MRI, with thin, high-resolution sections through the chiasm and proximal optic nerve, we have yet to see any patient with an optic nerve glioma with unequivocal sparing of the chiasm at presentation who later developed chiasmal involvement. Visual-evoked responses correlate with MRI findings and may be a reasonable noninvasive adjunct for following these patients.[886]

Treatment. It cannot be overemphasized that, in younger children, an optic nerve tumor is amblyogenic. Therefore, in children under age 8 with monocular vision loss from an optic pathway tumor, part-time occlusion therapy (patching) of the unaffected eye is recommended under the direction of a pediatric ophthalmologist.[887] This is an attempt to reverse any possible amblyopic component of visual loss complicating that due to optic neuropathy. In many patients we have been able to regain several lines of visual acuity within weeks of diagnosis. Thus, in terms of visual recovery, we consider patching the most effective therapy.

Usually serial neuro-ophthalmic examinations and MRI scanning are performed to exclude clinical or radiographic progression, and treatment is usually not given in patients with NF-1 unless radiographic progression or visual loss has occurred.[888] Either is an indication for more aggressive treatment, and options include chemotherapy, radiation, or surgical removal of the tumor. Chemotherapy with vincristine and carboplatin would be first-line treatment in any child, while radiation of the optic nerve tumor would be the option only if this or other chemotherapeutic regimens were ineffective. In some instances tumor bulk and proptosis may improve with chemotherapy. Although the long-term prognosis for maintaining vision is good when radiation is given, there may be unacceptable associated endocrinologic and neurologic side-effects.[888] These complications are discussed in more detail in the glioma section in Chapter 7. Therefore radiation is now rarely used as a first-line treatment.

Surgical removal of the prechiasmatic portion of the optic nerve is a better option than chemotherapy or radiation when the eye is almost blind and (1) the proptosis is severe and cosmetically unacceptable or (2) when the tumor appears on serial scanning to be encroaching upon a previously uninvolved chiasm.[889,890] The procedure requires a combined approach by an orbital surgeon to excise the intraorbital portion, and a neurosurgeon, via craniotomy, to remove the intracanalicular and intracranial portion. The extraocular muscles and the nerves supplying them are spared.

Primary optic nerve neoplasms: malignant optic nerve glioma (glioblastoma)

Malignant optic nerve glioblastoma, a high-grade glial neoplasm of the anterior visual pathway, is a much rarer, distinct condition which affects middle older age adults. The presentation with unilateral or bilateral visual loss, headache, and pain on eye movements is similar to that of inflammatory conditions such as optic neuritis or sarcoidosis.[891,892] Patients often have disc swelling (**Fig. 5–59**), and the fundus appearance may mimic that of venous stasis retinopathy.[893,894] Patients can progress to bilateral blindness within weeks. With intraorbital involvement there is proptosis and conjunctival chemosis, and there can be progression to neovascular glaucoma. MRI shows enlargement and enhancement of the optic nerve, and the tumor can spread intracranially via the chiasm and tracts, later often involving the diencephalon (**Fig. 5–59**). Death usually occurs within months. Radiation and chemotherapy may be associated with some preservation of vision and prolongation of life. Early in the course, transient visual improvement may occur when steroids are used empirically before the correct diagnosis is made.

Involvement of the chiasm is discussed in Chapter 7.

Meningiomas of the optic nerve sheath

Compressive optic neuropathy may result from primary optic nerve sheath meningiomas (ONSM). These occur primarily in middle-aged women (2 : 1 men) and are usually unilateral. Bilateral and multifocal cases occur in

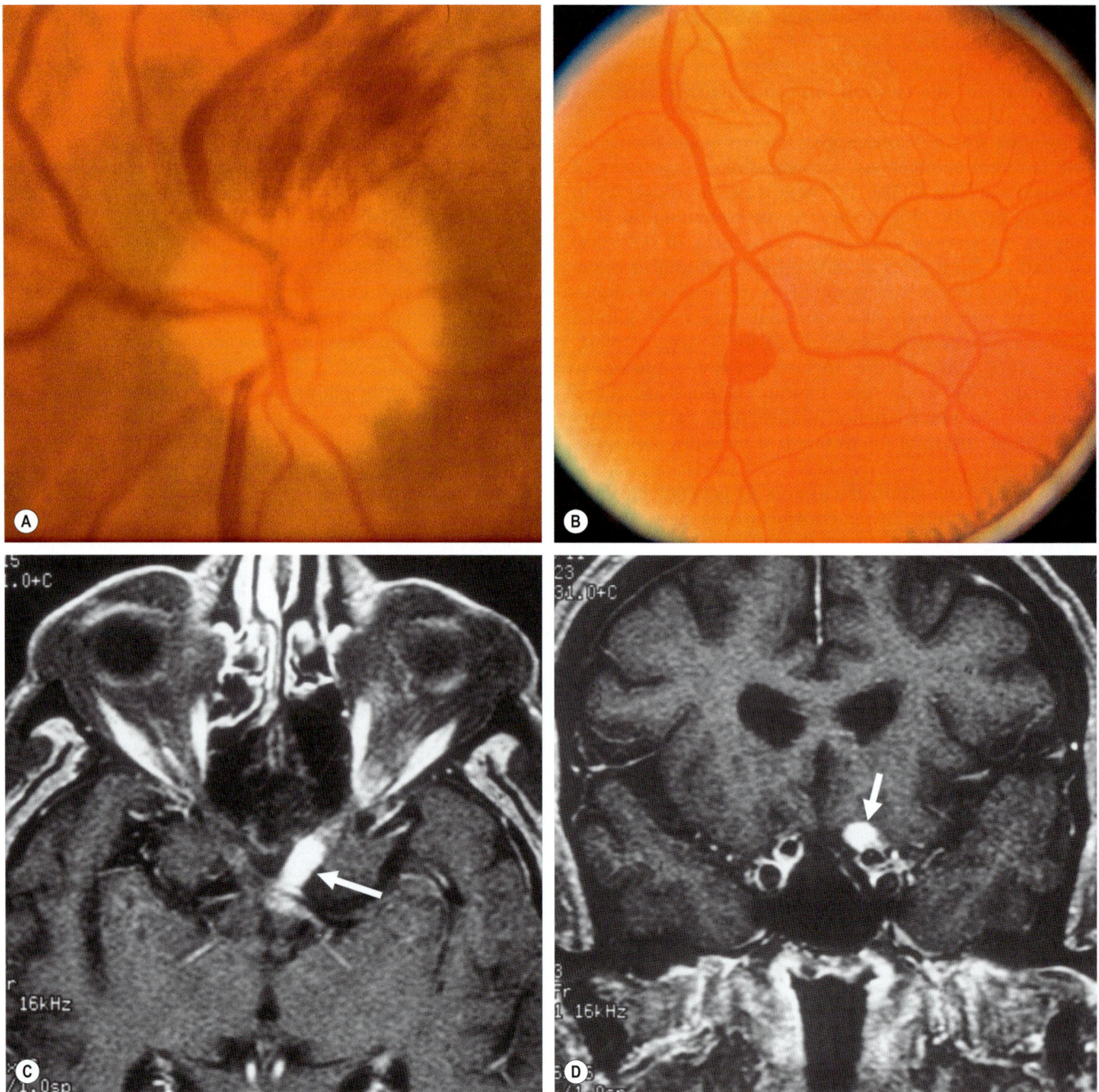

Figure 5–59. Glioblastoma of the optic nerve presenting with (**A**) disc swelling and (**B**) peripheral retinal hemorrhage secondary to central retinal vein compression and subsequent venous stasis. Axial (**C**) and coronal (**D**) T1-weighted MRI with gadolinium shows thickening and enhancement of the optic nerve (white arrows). Three months later there is extensive growth of the tumor seen on axial (**E**) and coronal (**F**) T1-weighted MRI scan with enhancing tissue (arrows) extending into the surrounding brain parenchyma.

neurofibromatosis type 2 (NF-2).[895,896] In children the condition is rare and often associated with a more malignant tumor and NF-2.[897]

Pathology and growth characteristics. The tumors arise from meningothelial cells in the arachnoid villi. Optic nerve sheath meningiomas surround the optic nerve and result in impaired axonal transport and interfere with the pial blood supply to the optic nerve. Growth of these tumors is usually indolent over many years but the rate may increase with pregnancy.[898]

Neuro-ophthalmic symptoms and signs. Patients usually present with slowly progressive vision loss, and other visual complaints include double vision, transient visual obscurations, and gaze-evoked amaurosis.[899–901] On occasion they are aware of headache or notice proptosis.

Patients have moderate to severe acuity loss with 15–50% having better than 20/40, and 20–60% having less than 20/200 acuity.[899–901] Dyschromatopsia is usually present, and visual field defects commonly seen include central scotomas, enlarged blind spots, and generalized constric-

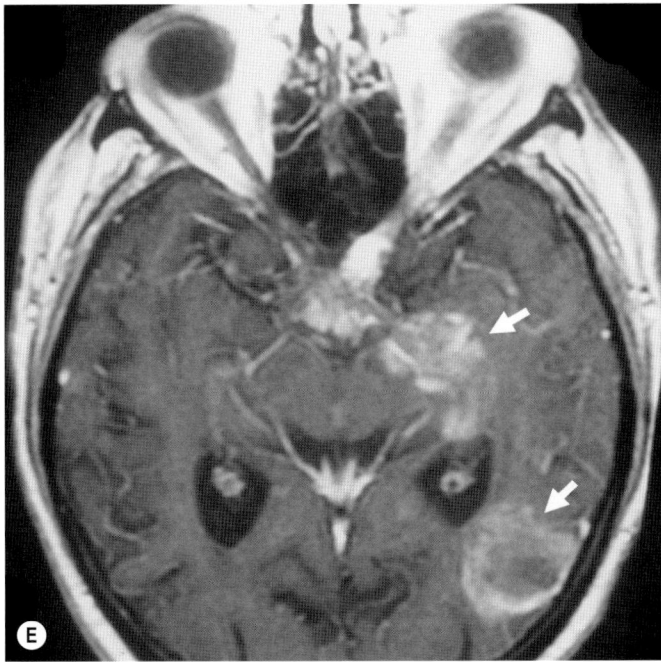

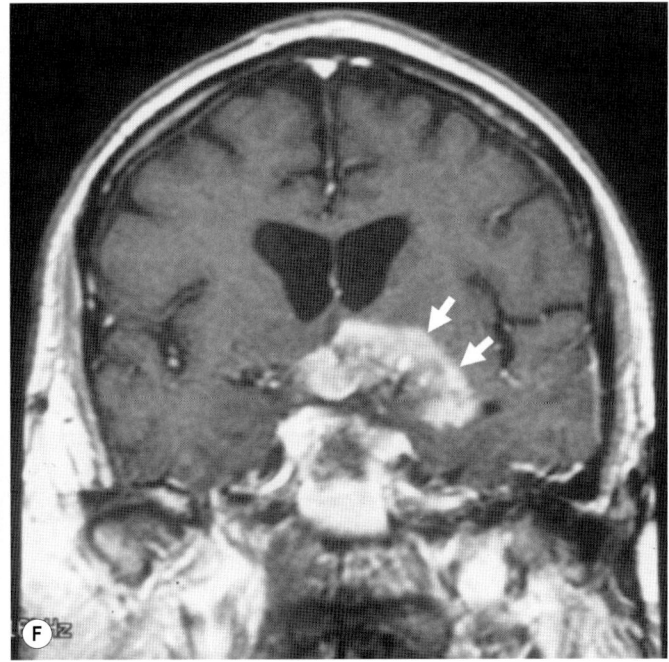

Figure 5–59. *Continued*

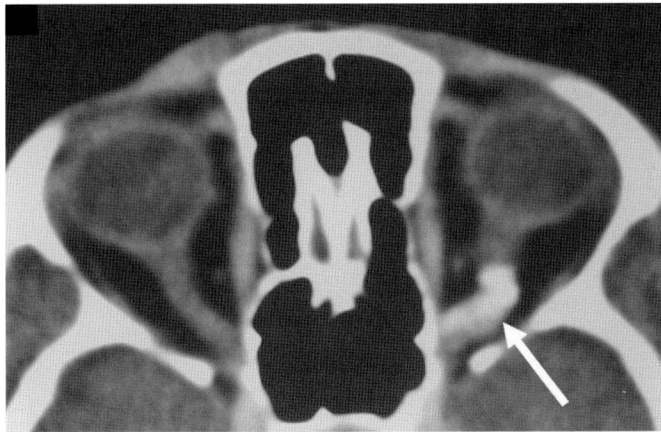

Figure 5–60. CT scan of optic nerve sheath meningioma. Axial CT scan without contrast shows thickening and calcification of the left optic nerve (arrow).

tion. The optic disc almost always appears abnormal as about half the patients have optic atrophy and half have disc swelling.[899-901] Optociliary collateral vessels are present in 15–33% of patients and are commonly seen in both swollen and atrophic nerves.[645] Most patients have measurable proptosis.

Diagnostic studies/neuroimaging. Neuroimaging is usually diagnostic, showing diffuse, tubular optic nerve enlargement (**Figs 5–60** and **5–61**). On CT, calcification (**Fig. 5–60**) or a "tram track sign," referring to two parallel lines along the length of the nerve, are often seen.[880,900] MRI is now the procedure of choice to identify and determine the extent of ONSM (**Fig. 5–61**).[902,903] The tumor is isointense with brain on T1 and T2 images and smoothly enhances with gadolinium.[904] Often the MRI will show the tumor to be separate from the optic nerve proper on coronal views, and exquisite

demonstration of the details of the intracanalicular optic nerve helps to identify intracranial extension. Given the tight confines of the optic canal, ONSM arising in this region may be visually symptomatic despite being subtle radiographically (**Fig. 5–62**).

The pattern of fusiform enlargement overlaps with optic nerve glioma, but kinking is not seen with meningioma. The diagnosis is therefore established on clinical and radiographic grounds, and, like glioma, tumor biopsy is almost never needed. The radiographic appearance of ONSM also can be simulated by orbital pseudotumor (particularly the sclerosing variety), optic perineuritis,[530] sarcoid infiltration, and lymphomatous and carcinomatous meningitis. All of these conditions present much more rapidly than ONSM and are more likely to be associated with pain.

Clinical course. The natural history of these tumors is characterized by insidious progression, sometimes to complete blindness of the eye. Visual function has been reported to remain unchanged for many years in some patients with ONSM, and rarely spontaneous improvement of vision can occur.[905] Fortunately, intracranial extension of optic nerve sheath meningioma is quite rare.

Treatment. In the rare equivocal case, biopsy is required to establish the diagnosis. This is recommended only in an eye with poor vision after serial lumbar punctures to exclude inflammation and neoplasm were normal, and after steroids failed to improve vision.

The mainstay of management for optic nerve sheath meningioma is radiation therapy.[901,906-908] This modality is generally reserved for adult patients with salvageable vision. Several reports over the last several years have uniformly demonstrated the benefit of radiation in either improving vision, visual fields, and disc swelling or at least halting visual loss.[909-922] If visual function is good, better than 20/40 with mild field loss, for example, then observation alone can

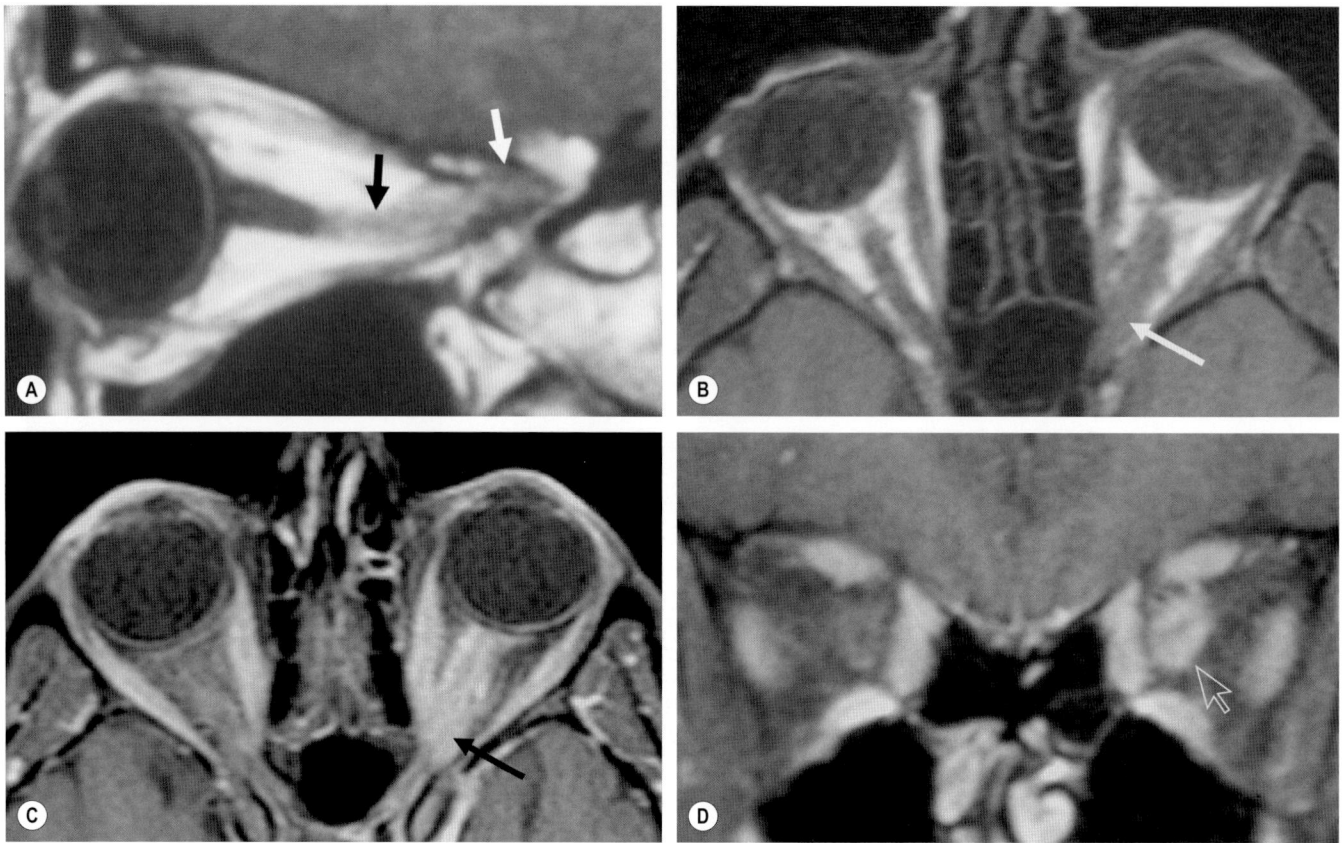

Figure 5–61. Magnetic resonance (MR) imaging of optic nerve sheath meningioma. **A**. Sagittal T1-weighted MR image showing diffuse sheath enlargement. Enhancement is clearly seen (black arrow), and the nerve widens (white arrow) toward the orbital apex. **B**. Axial, T1-weighted MR image with left optic nerve sheath meningioma with diffuse enlargement of the intraorbital optic nerve (arrow). T1-weighted, fat-suppressed gadolinium-enhanced imaging, axial (**C**) and coronal (**D**) views, demonstrates enhancement and thickening (arrows) of the nerve sheath.

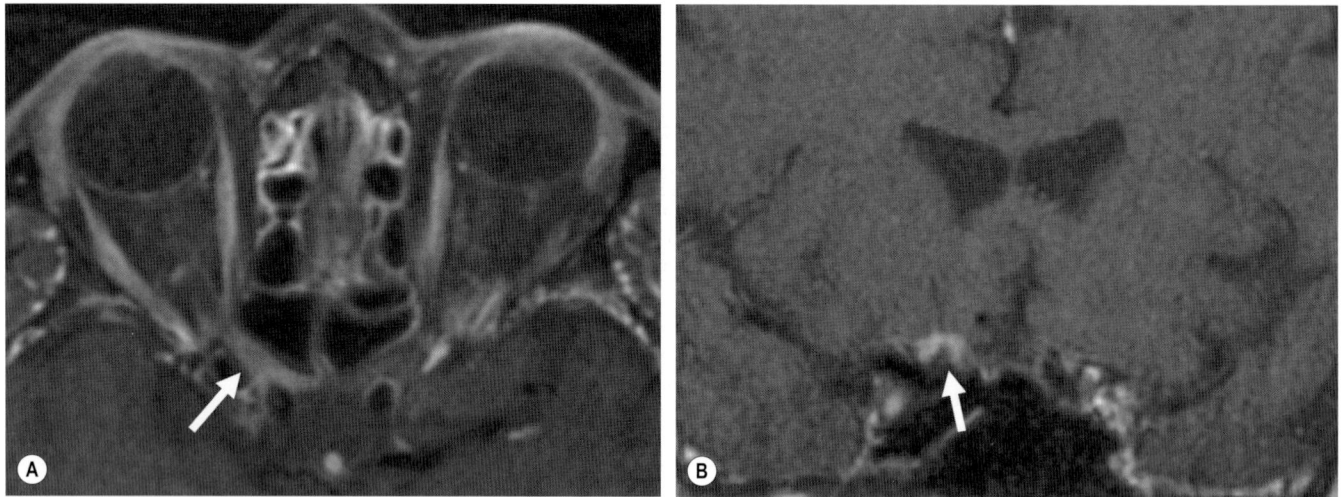

Figure 5–62. Magnetic resonance (MR) imaging of optic canal meningioma. Diffuse enhancement (arrow) is seen on the axial (**A**) and coronal (**B**) T1-weighted MR images with gadolinium.

be used until progression is documented. Radiation therapy can be offered when vision loss progresses.

Surgical excision is not recommended as a method for improving vision but is used to treat blind, uncomfortable, or unsightly eyes or to reduce the risk of intracranial extension. In patients with intracranial extension, surgery and radiation have been tried. Surgical results are poor,[899] although radiation has been shown to be of some benefit in these instances.[923] The potential benefit of surgery, however, is much greater in ONSM than in surgical decompression (not necessarily excision) of meningiomas arising secondarily from sphenoid wing and paraclinoid meningiomas.[924,925]

Table 5-17 Specific neuro-ophthalmic presentations in meningiomas at the base of skull[1119]

Tumor location	Neuro-ophthalmic findings
Planum sphenoidale and olfactory groove	Optic neuropathy, Foster Kennedy syndrome
Tuberculum sellae	Unilateral or bilateral vision loss often with chiasmal involvement
Optic canal and anterior clinoid process	Unilateral or chiasmal vision loss, orbital extension
Medial sphenoid wing	Optic neuropathy and ophthalmoplegia
Lateral sphenoid wing	Proptosis and ophthalmoplegia without optic neuropathy
Diaphragma sellae	Chiasmal syndrome

Meningiomas of the skull base

Alternatively, meningiomas arising from the planum sphenoidale or olfactory groove may involve the optic nerve in its intraorbital or intracanalicular portions (**Table 5-17**). Suprasellar, tuberculum sellae, parasellar, and sphenoid wing meningiomas can also cause optic neuropathy, but because suprasellar and tuberculum sellae meningiomas more commonly cause chiasmal compression, and the other two more likely lead to eye movement disorders, they are discussed in more detail in Chapters 7 and 15, respectively. The section on meningiomas in Chapter 7 also provides an overview of the pathology, associations, and neuroimaging characteristics of skull base meningiomas.

Planum sphenoidale and olfactory groove meningiomas. Tumors that involve only the olfactory groove do not cause vision loss as they are not in contact with the optic nerve or chiasm. However, tumors from this site can grow sufficiently large without causing many other neurologic symptoms. Patients may present with papilledema from mass effect and further historical review may reveal anosmia and behavior suggestive of frontal lobe dysfunction. The tumors can grow posteriorly over the planum sphenoidale to reach the superior aspect of the intracranial optic nerves and cause direct compression and symptoms of decreased vision. In this setting, with compression of one optic nerve as well as intracranial pressure elevation, presentation with the Foster Kennedy syndrome is possible.

Visual symptoms most often develop insidiously and are sometimes isolated. Patients are generally found to have moderate to severe vision loss and either a normal-appearing optic nerve or optic atrophy. Neuroimaging is usually sufficient to make the diagnosis of skull based meningiomas (**Fig. 5-63**) and therefore biopsy is rarely needed. MRI features include isointense, smoothly enhancing masses (**Figs 5-63 and 5-64**) with dural tails (**Fig. 5-64**).

Treatment and visual outcome. The clinical course is usually one of chronic progression. Older patients with only mild to moderate symptoms, who are not necessarily good surgical candidates, can be observed with serial visual fields and MRI scans. Patients who are found to have an intact nerve fiber layer (NFL) on OCT have a more favorable prognosis for vision recovery than those with demonstrable pretreatment thinning of the NFL.[926] Currently chemotherapy is not generally used to treat meningiomas although previous reports suggested that progesterone receptor antagonists may be useful.[927,928] The mainstays of management of these basal meningiomas are surgery and radiation, which are often used in combination. With microsurgical techniques patients have an excellent chance (44–62%) for improvement of vision, and this is the procedure of choice in patients well enough to undergo craniotomy.[924,925,929-936] Unfortunately in these same series up to 25% of patients worsen after surgery, and mortality rates are as high as 10%. Unroofing and decompressing the optic canal may be particularly important in restoring vision.[934,937] Radiation has been shown in one series to improve vision,[923] and should be used in patients who are poor surgical risks or in whom there is significant residual tumor. Less than 45 cGy should be used to avoid the late complication of radiation-induced damage to the chiasm or optic nerves.[938]

Aneurysms

The intracranial optic nerve is closely related to the anterior cerebral artery, the anterior communicating artery, the ophthalmic artery, and the supraclinoid portion of the internal carotid artery in the anterior aspect of the circle of Willis (see **Fig. 7-2**). Both saccular (berry) aneurysms and fusiform (atherosclerotic) aneurysms are well-known causes of compressive optic neuropathy. Berry aneurysms typically arise from pre-existing defects in the media and elastica of arteries at the site of arterial bifurcations. They are rare in children but develop with increasing frequency related to age. They range in size from a few millimeters up to 5 or 6 cm. The very small and very large aneurysms have a very low risk for rupture and bleeding.[939] It is the large or giant aneurysms that are generally associated with compression of the anterior visual pathways.

Giant aneurysms arising from the ophthalmic artery, the carotid ophthalmic junction and the supraclinoid carotid artery can all present with unilateral compressive optic neuropathy or chiasmal syndrome (see Chapter 7). In particular, aneurysms in the supraclinoid region characteristically present with a nasal scotoma.[940] Patients with compressive optic neuropathy from aneurysms may have fluctuating vision perhaps related to vascular spasm or spontaneous changes in aneurysm size. Alternatively, acute vision loss due to an aneurysm may mimic optic neuritis.[941] MRI (**Fig. 5-65**), magnetic resonance angiography, or computed tomography angiography are the initial procedures of choice in patients suspected of having an aneurysm, but the gold standard for diagnosis is formal cerebral angiography. Radiographic features of aneurysms in this area are reviewed in Chapter 7.

Clinical course/treatment. The natural history of these lesions is generally unfavorable, as many untreated patients later develop subarachnoid hemorrhage, blindness,

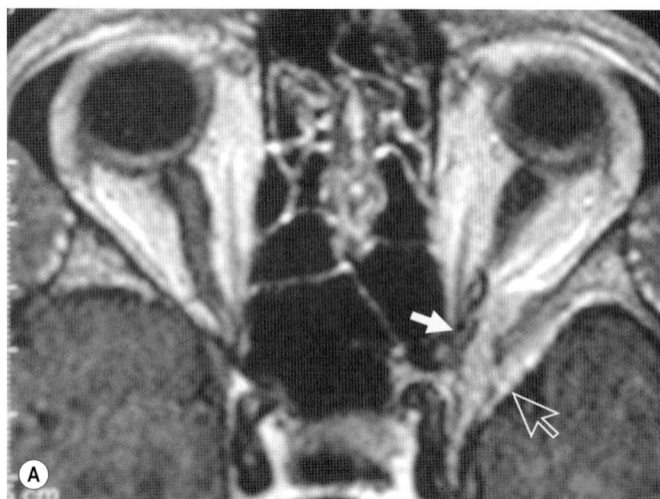

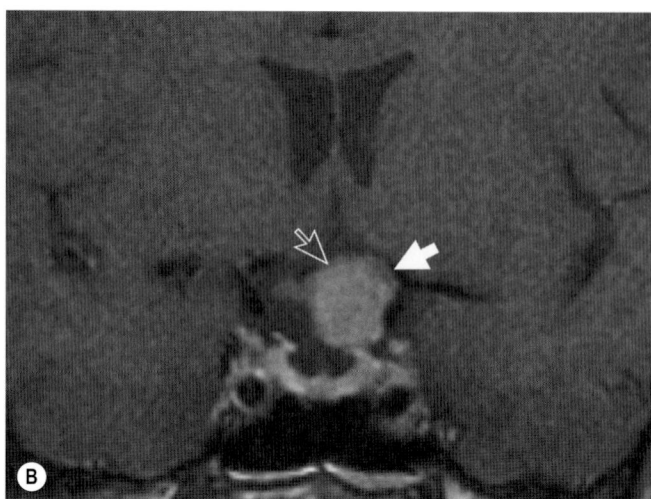

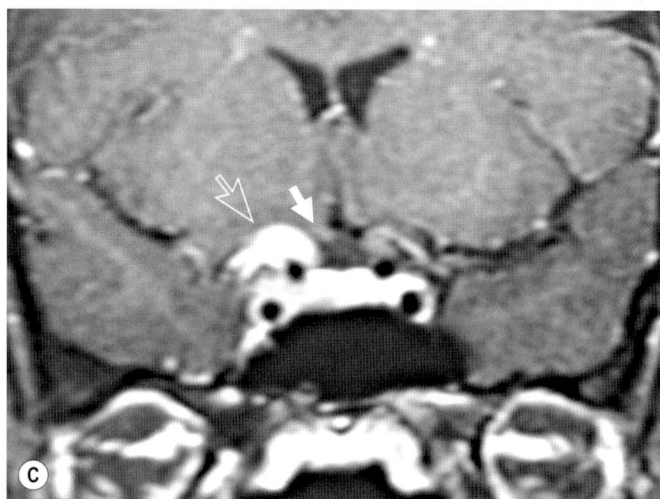

Figure 5–63. Meningiomas of the anterior visual pathway causing compressive optic neuropathy. **A**. Axial T1-weighted gadolinium-enhanced magnetic resonance imaging (MRI) showing left sphenoid wing meningioma (open arrow at the lateral edge) involving the orbital apex and causing compression of the optic nerve (solid arrow). **B**. Coronal, T1-weighted, gadolinium-enhanced MRI of a planum sphenoidale meningioma. A smoothly enhancing mass (open arrow) contacts the chiasm-left optic nerve junction (solid arrow). **C**. Coronal, T1-weighted, gadolinium-enhanced MRI of paraclinoid meningioma (open arrow) encroaches upon the optic nerve (solid arrow).

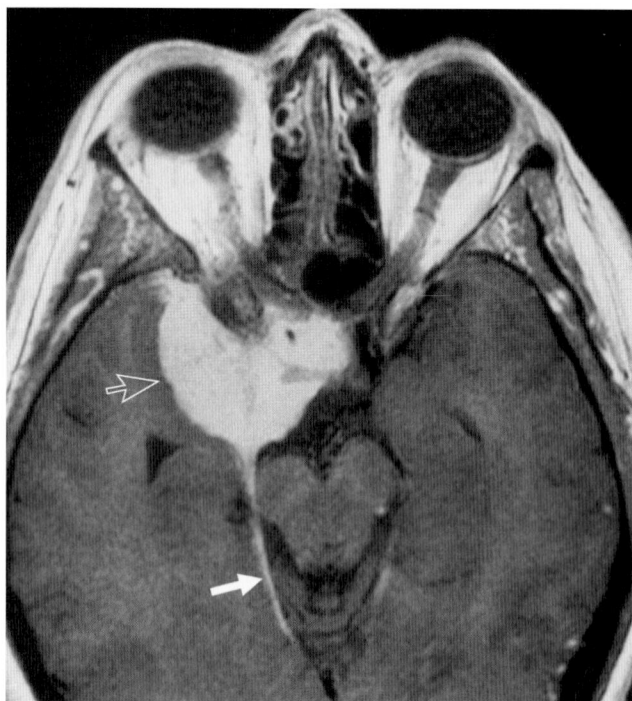

Figure 5–65. Coronal, T1-weighted magnetic resonance imaging demonstrating an aneurysm (solid arrow) in contact with the left optic nerve (open arrow).

Figure 5–64. Contrast-enhanced, axial, T1-weighted magnetic resonance imaging of a smoothly enhancing sphenoid wing meningioma (open arrow) with a dural tail (solid arrow).

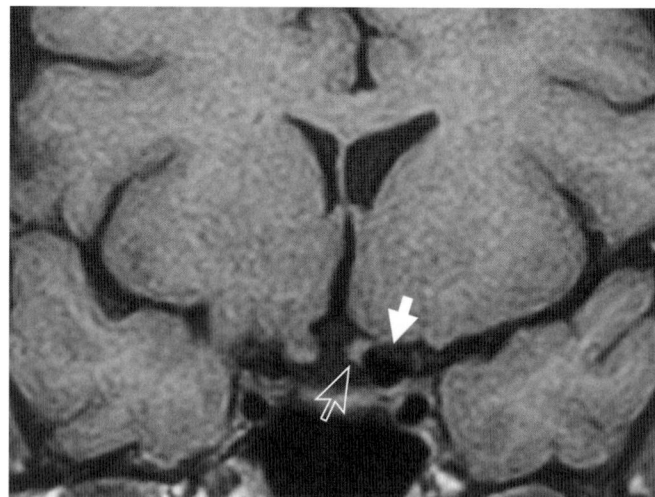

dementia, or homonymous hemianopia.[942] Treatment of aneurysms in this area is either surgical or endovascular,[942–944] and is reviewed in more detail in Chapter 7. Vision loss as a complication of surgery for these aneurysms has been reported.[945]

Fusiform aneurysms or ectatic dilation of the carotid artery may also compress the intracranial optic nerve or chiasm. They have been postulated as some of the causes of optic neuropathy in elderly patients, and in particular they may have a role in the pathogenesis of some cases of low tension glaucoma.[946,947] However, Jacobson demonstrated that contact between the carotid artery and optic nerve or chiasm is seen in 70% of asymptomatic patients.[948] True compression by a dolichoectatic artery significant enough to produce vision loss is relatively rare.[646]

Osseous disorders of the optic canal

Insidiously progressive optic neuropathy due to stenosis of the optic canal is a common sequela of cranial osseous disorders such as fibrous dysplasia and osteopetrosis.[949] Fibrous dysplasia is discussed in detail in Chapter 18. Metastases to this region, which may also cause compressive optic neuropathy, would more likely cause acute or subacute visual loss.

The optic atrophy seen in craniosynostoses, disorders characterized by premature closure of the cranial sutures such as Apert's[950] and Crouzon's[951] syndrome, is believed to result not from bony compression but from elevated intracranial pressure. Because not all cases develop papilledema prior to optic atrophy, the exact mechanism is unclear.[952]

Low-tension glaucoma and optic nerve cupping

The distinction between glaucomatous optic neuropathy and alternative causes of optic neuropathy is rarely difficult. Patients with glaucoma are usually easily identified by their high intraocular pressures. However, in glaucoma with low or normal pressures or in optic neuropathies with optic nerve cupping, the clinical distinction may be very complicated. Since making this separation is critical in order to avoid missed diagnoses and unnecessary treatment, these two common scenarios will be reviewed.

Low or normal tension glaucoma (LTG)

LTG is a condition in which glaucoma-like field defects, optic nerve head cupping, and normal intraocular pressures are present. The prevalence of LTG varies in large series of glaucoma patients from 7–70%.[953] In the Baltimore Eye Survey, 16.7% of glaucomatous eyes never had a recorded IOP greater than 21 mmHg, the usual upper limit of normal.[954] There is now ample evidence that central corneal thickness affects pressures as measured by applanation. Before intraocular pressures are declared normal, the central corneal thickness should be measured with ultrasonographic pachymetry. Eyes with thin corneas may have artifactually low pressures. LTG probably includes several different subsets of patients. Some patients have unrecognized (undocumented) elevated intraocular pressure or have secondary causes of glaucoma that are currently inactive such as uveitis, intermittent narrow angle or traumatic angle recession. Some patients have normal pressures with visual

field progression but had higher pressures in the past. The term "burned-out" glaucoma has often been applied to these patients. Finally, perhaps the most interesting subset of patients have a progressive optic neuropathy characterized by cupping of the optic nerve head (Fig. 5–66) without ever having elevated intraocular pressures. Many believe that these patients have a truly unique disease, perhaps of an ischemic or vascular nature.

Studies have shown an increase in both the incidence of migraine and ischemic white matter disease on MRI scan in patients with LTG.[955,956] While this observation supports a vascular, non-intraocular-pressure-related theory for the etiology of low tension glaucoma, most patients studied with LTG behave much more like patients with primary open angle glaucoma and elevated intraocular pressure than patients with "vascular optic neuropathies" such as ION. Slow and relentless progression over years (non-episodic visual loss) is the rule with relatively symmetric disease between the eyes, along with preservation of central and color vision. LTG patients tend to have more focal atrophy and cupping of the disc, disc hemorrhages and more dense visual field defects extending closer to fixation than in high tension glaucoma. There is still sufficient overlap with high pressure glaucoma to make the two entities, in most situations, clinically indistinguishable except for the absence of elevated intraocular pressure.

Other causes of optic neuropathy with optic nerve cupping

Several common scenarios occur in which optic nerve cupping due to high or normal tension glaucoma is considered, but alternative causes of optic neuropathy are more likely. These situations are: (1) progressive vision loss in the setting of an established diagnosis of glaucoma and normal pressure; (2) visual field loss, optic nerve head cupping, and pallor of the neuroretinal rim without elevated intraocular pressure, and (3) glaucoma complicated by episodic or rapidly progressive vision loss.

Alternative causes of *acquired cupping of the optic nerve* include anterior visual pathway compression by meningiomas, craniopharyngiomas, pituitary adenomas and aneurysms.[38,957] Cupping has also been described in previous anterior (particularly arteritic) and posterior ischemic optic neuropathy, optic neuritis, shock- or hypotension-induced optic neuropathy, syphilitic optic neuropathy, traumatic optic neuropathy, dominantly inherited optic atrophy, Leber's hereditary optic neuropathy, and methanol-induced optic neuropathy.[958]

Based on careful review of historical information, the examiner should be able to identify most patients with these alternative diagnoses. However, on historical features alone, compressive lesions may be less obvious.

We suggest four criteria that in our experience are positive predictors of these other causes of optic neuropathy. These include (1) the presence of headache or other neurologic symptoms, (2) atypical visual field defects (those respecting the vertical meridian, central or centrocecal scotomas), (3) atypical rate of progression of visual field loss, and, finally, (4) pallor beyond the cupping of the optic nerve, i.e., the

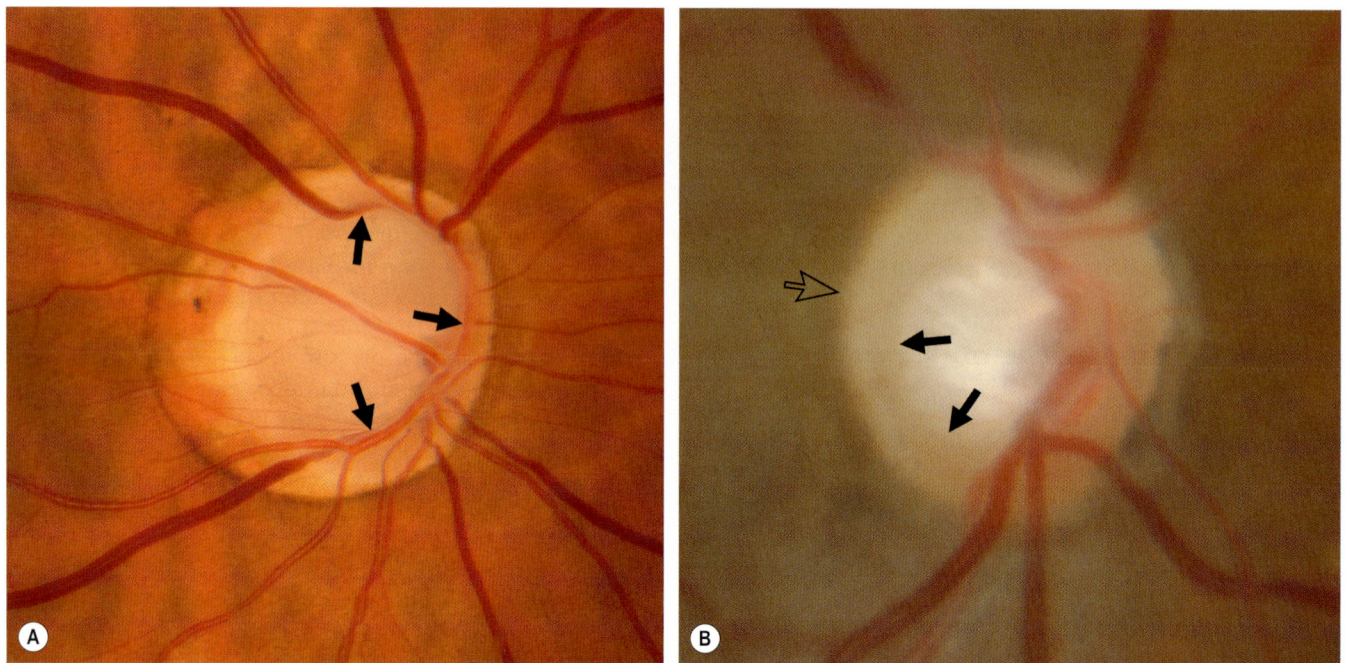

Figure 5–66. Glaucomatous (**A**) vs nonglaucomatous (**B**) cupping. **A**. Typical appearance of advanced glaucomatous cupping. The cup (arrows) extends nearly to the disc rim. Regions where the vessels bend (e.g., arrow at the top of the disc) are clues to determine the size of the cup. **B**. Although the nerve has a significant cup (arrows), the intact neuroretinal rim is pale (open arrow) (pallor beyond cupping) in a patient with nonglaucomatous optic neuropathy.

nerve rim is pale, especially nasally (**Fig. 5–66**). In Bianchi-Marzoli et al.'s series[957] of 29 patients with cupping from compressive anterior visual pathway lesions, only one had cupping and field loss as an isolated manifestation of their optic neuropathy. All others had reduced acuity, dyschromatopsia, or an afferent pupillary defect. Other clinical features more commonly seen in compressive lesions, for instance, and less frequently associated with LTG include presentation under age 50, symptoms of decreased vision, and fluctuating vision. In another series,[959] acuity worse than 20/40 was another feature more associated with cupping due to an intracranial mass lesion.

Evaluation. Our workup of atypical patients would include an MRI scan of the brain and orbits with gadolinium, syphilis serology, and, in patients with central field defects, B_{12} and folate levels. In some situations additional testing for sarcoidosis and other autoimmune conditions is indicated based on patient history and demographics.

Episodic or rapidly progressive vision loss may occur in some patients with a well-established history of glaucoma. Some of these patients have a subtype of LTG in which abrupt loss of vision mimics ischemic optic neuropathy. However, optic nerve head swelling is absent and there is often a splinter hemorrhage at the disc margin (**Fig. 5–67**). This area of the disc often develops focally atrophy and cupping. Workup of these patients is generally unrevealing, but screening for vasculitis (ESR, ANA, RF) is indicated as well as careful blood pressure monitoring for episodes of systemic hypotension. These patients may have a true vascular optic neuropathy. A second subtype of patients in this group has both glaucoma and a superimposed distinct cause of vision loss such as ischemic optic neuropathy or a compressive lesion. Any patient who reliably describes sudden or rapidly progressive

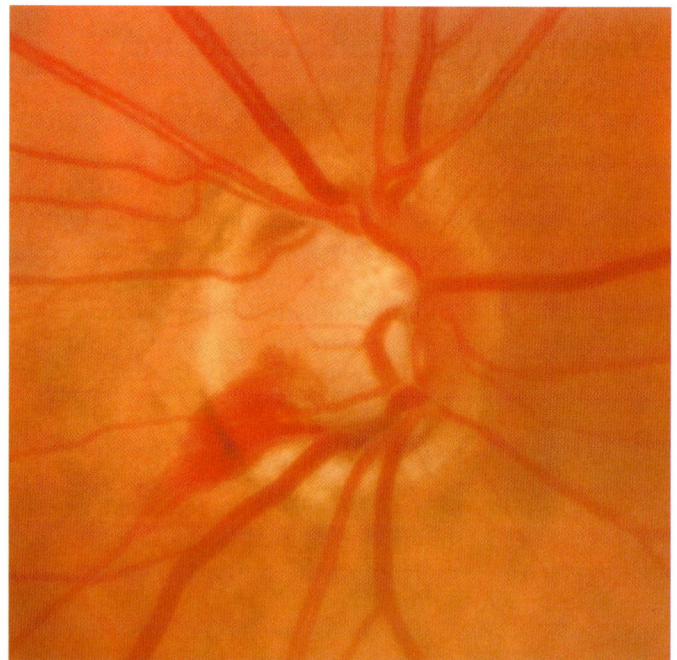

Figure 5–67. Cupping of the optic nerve associated with a splinter hemorrhage at the disc margin.

vision loss in the setting of glaucoma should also be evaluated for other causes of optic neuropathy.

LASIK-induced optic neuropathy

The rare occurrence of optic neuropathy following laser-assisted in situ keratomileusis (LASIK) refractive surgery has been reported.[960,961] The proposed mechanisms include

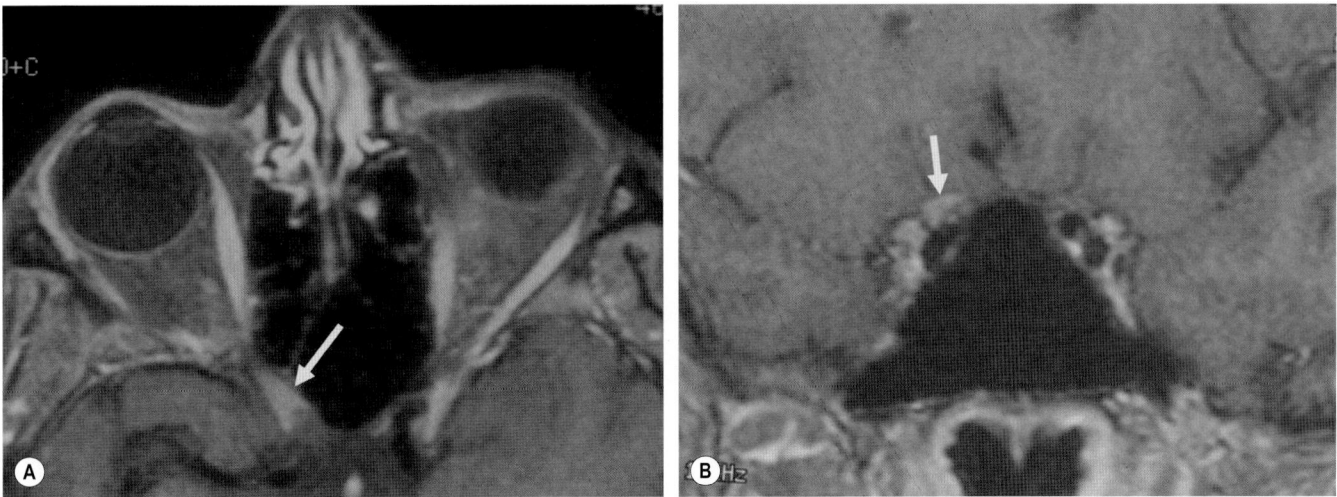

Figure 5–68. Axial (**A**) and coronal (**B**) T1-weighted gadolinium enhanced magnetic resonance imaging of a patient with carcinomatous meningitis and right optic nerve involvement. Abnormal enhancement (arrow) of the intracranial right optic nerve can be seen.

barotrauma and ischemia related to transient elevation in intraocular pressure during the procedure.

Optic neuropathies associated with cancer

A history of cancer in a patient with neuro-ophthalmic symptoms raises important diagnostic considerations. Several important entities must be considered in patients with vision loss or eye movement problems. The secondary effects of cancer are typically the result of local invasion, metastases, or the consequences of asthenia. The direct effects of cancer on the eye, its adnexa, and the central nervous system are well known. Primary ocular malignancies, secondary tumors (metastatic and direct extension from adjacent structures) as well as parasellar tumors (primary and secondary) cause vision loss because of displacement or compression of the eye or optic nerve. In the past two decades, unusual instances of organ failure, not resulting from the direct affect of cancer on the organ, have been recognized in patients with cancer and have been collectively termed paraneoplastic syndromes. These syndromes not only present diagnostic challenges but also provide insight into the biological behavior of tumors and their effect on the host immune system. Finally, toxicity of antineoplastic drugs and previous irradiation can result in vision loss.

Carcinomatous meningitis

Carcinomatous meningitis is a common cause of multiple cranial neuropathies secondary to multifocal seeding of the leptomeninges. It is typically a late manifestation of cancer, and the third and sixth nerves are the most commonly involved. Next most commonly involved are the facial, trigeminal, and acoustic nerves. Common primary tumors metastasizing to the meninges include breast and lung. Optic neuropathy in these patients can mimic posterior

ischemic neuropathy with acute or subacute vision loss with a normal fundus. Alternatively, the nerve may be swollen as in ischemic optic neuropathy. The mechanism of optic nerve dysfunction may be infiltrative, ischemic, demyelinative, or compressive.[962–965] The diagnosis must be suspected and usually can be made based on the presence of abnormal CSF with increased protein and neoplastic cells. It may require three to six CSF cytological examinations to make the diagnosis. Although MRI scanning (**Fig. 5–68**) might reveal thickening of the optic nerve or abnormal meningeal enhancement, it may also have been normal initially.

Optic nerve metastases

Isolated metastases to the optic nerve are uncommon but well-recognized, representing about 5% of all intraocular metastases.[966] Reported primary neoplasms include breast, lung, stomach, and pancreas.[967,968] In 20% of patients the primary site is unknown.[966] Ophthalmoscopically there may be a visible mass invading the optic nerve head (**Fig. 5–69**). Vascular compression may result in a central retinal vein or artery occlusion.[969] Alternatively, the fundus acutely may be normal if the metastasis is situated more posteriorly, and the clinical scenario may mimic retrobulbar optic neuritis. Radiographically the optic nerve may exhibit fusiform enlargement, like an intraorbital optic nerve meningioma or glioma.[969–971] Corticosteroids, radiation, and chemotherapy may be indicated. The overall associated mortality is high.

The choroid and orbit are more common sites for metastasis to the eye, and the optic nerve may be involved from secondary extension from these structures. Compressive optic neuropathy may result from metastases to the bony optic canal.[972]

Other neoplasms of the optic disc

Capillary angiomas are fleshy appearing lesions of the optic nerve head (**Fig. 5–70**). These benign vascular tumors can present de novo or in patients with von Hippel–Lindau

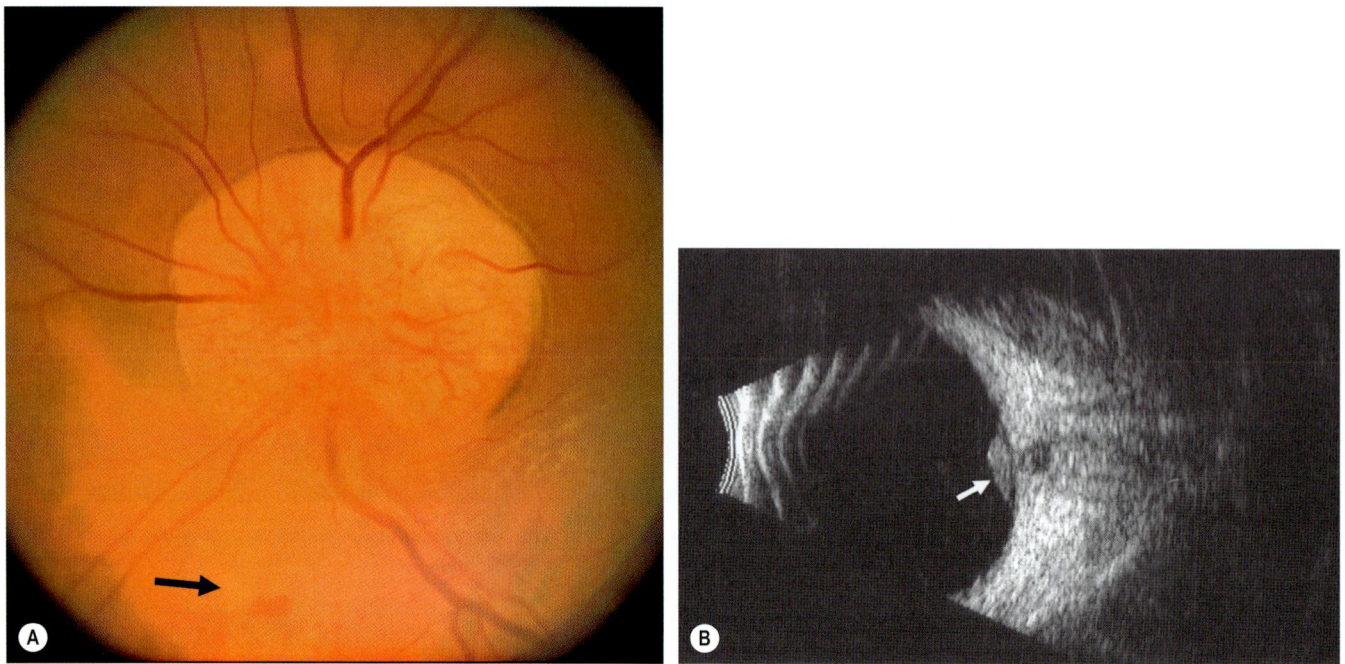

Figure 5–69. Optic nerve head metastasis from breast cancer. **A**. Fundus photography revealing massive infiltration and swelling of the optic nerve and subretinal space (arrow). **B**. B-scan orbital echography demonstrating substantial enlargement of the optic nerve head (arrow).

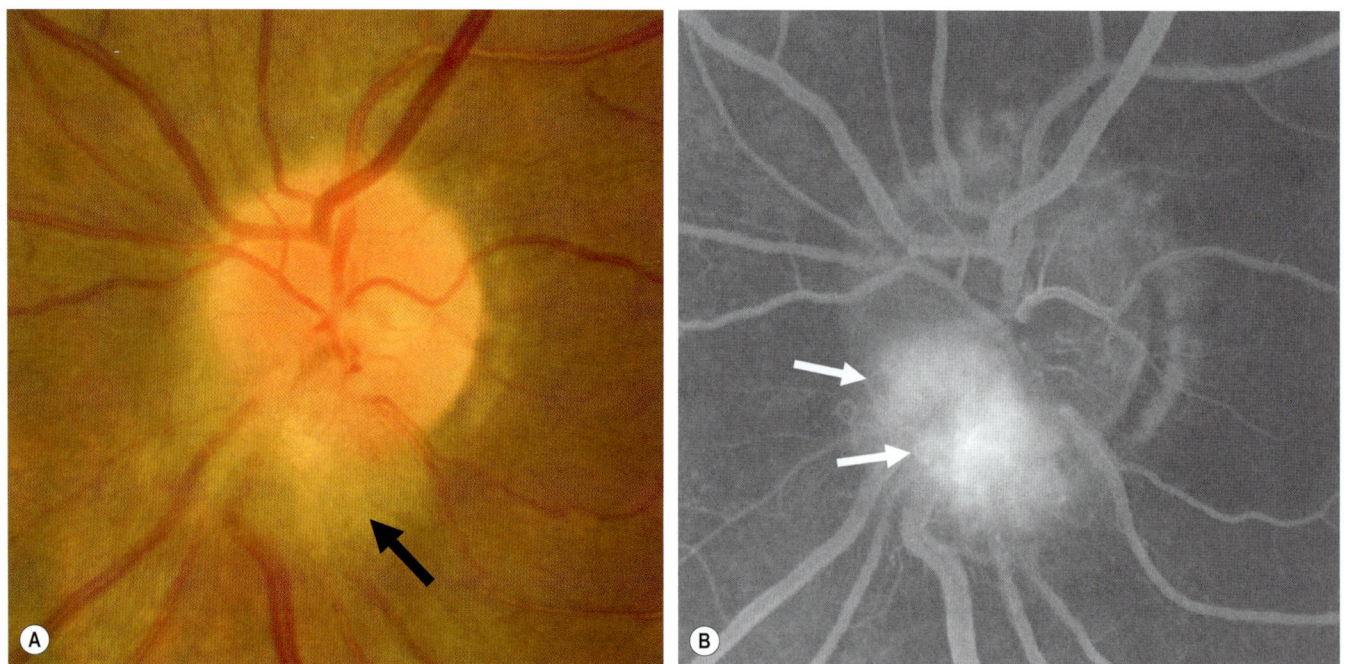

Figure 5–70. Capillary angioma of the disc. **A**. Color fundus photograph of the left shows a fleshy focal grayish lesion (arrow) with a few small dilated capillaries on the surface. **B**. Late phase fluorescein angiogram of the same patient details the fine vascular nature (arrows) of the lesion but shows no leakage. The patient did not have von Hippel–Lindau disease.

disease. They generally cause minimal symptoms, but vision loss can occur in association with fluid exudation or bleeding.

Melanocytomas of the optic disc are benign pigmented tumors composed of nevus cells. More common in dark-skinned individuals, they are usually asymptomatic and static.[973,974] Severe visual loss and malignant transformation can occur but are uncommon.[975,976]

Lymphoma and leukemia

Optic neuropathies associated with lymphoma or leukemia are rare but can result from a variety of different causes. Cases of direct infiltration of the optic nerve head in both diseases have been reported. In addition, optic neuropathy can be part of the presentation of lymphomatous meningitis.[977,978] In this setting lymphoma causes vision loss by direct

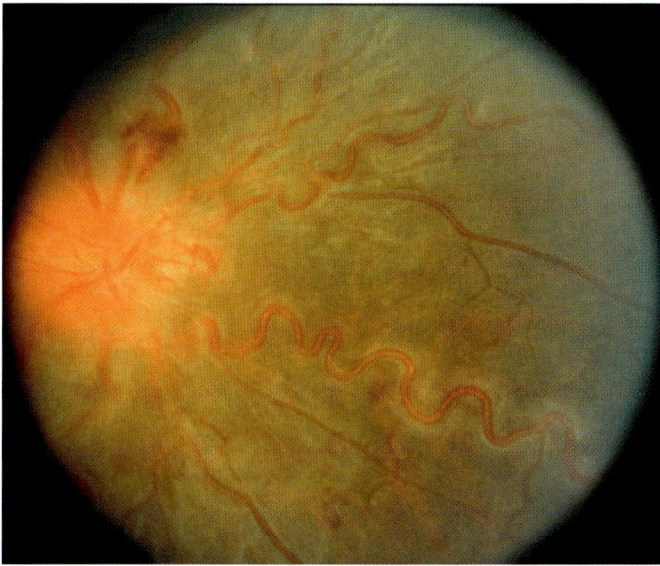

Figure 5–71. Leukemic optic neuropathy as evidenced by massive disc swelling, a peripapillary hemorrhage, and venous distension and tortuosity. Retinal infiltration in the same patient is depicted in Fig. 4–33.

invasion via the pial septae.[979] Lymphoma can also present as a mass lesion in the orbit,[980] and MRI can demonstrate abnormal optic nerve enhancement.[977] In some instances it is impossible to determine whether the optic neuropathy results from tumor infiltration or as a side-effect of treatment with radiation or chemotherapy. Optic neuropathy has been reported as a manifestation of lymphoma thought to be in remission.[981]

A similar spectrum exists in patients with leukemic optic neuropathy. Direct infiltration of the optic nerve head can cause massive swelling, and there may be associated retinal infiltration with hemorrhages (**Figs 5–71 and 4–33**).[982] Optic neuropathy usually accompanies other manifestations of central nervous system involvement. MRI scans typically demonstrate optic nerve enhancement, but they may be normal so a high clinical suspicion must exist.[983] Histopathologic studies reveal direct infiltration of the optic nerve via pial septae.[984,985] Vision loss results from vascular compromise or chronic axoplasmic stasis from swelling. Patients with chronic lymphocytic leukemia have been reported to have a more insidious course with progressive visual field loss associated with optic atrophy.[986] Careful consideration should be given to the possibility that vision loss is a consequence of chemotherapy as opposed to leukemic infiltration, particularly in patients treated with vincristine.[987] Radiation is the mainstay of treatment for patients with progressive vision loss and optic nerve involvement from leukemia and lymphoma.

Paraneoplastic optic neuropathy

In paraneoplastic conditions, distant organ failure develops in the setting of cancer but not as a result of direct invasion, metastatic spread, or treatment. The process is mediated by an antibody directed against a tumor antigen which then crossreacts with a host (nontumor) antigen. Although paraneoplastic retinopathy (photoreceptor dysfunction, see

Chapter 4) is the most common type of paraneoplastic process causing vision loss, rare cases of paraneoplastic optic neuropathy have been described.

Paraneoplastic optic neuropathy (PON) has been reported in patients with carcinoma of the lung.[988–994] Patients develop visual loss and commonly have optic nerve swelling. Vision loss can precede the presentation of the systemic malignancy and generally progresses over a period of weeks. Spontaneous visual recovery and improvement on steroids have been observed. Many patients have a concurrent paraneoplastic cerebellar syndrome characterized by dysarthria and ataxia.[992,993] Neuropathologic examinations have demonstrated simultaneous involvement of the brain stem with findings typical of paraneoplastic encephalomyelitis. Based on histopathologic demonstration of perivascular lymphocytic infiltration, gliosis, and demyelination of the optic nerves, the condition is thought to be inflammatory and might be more accurately termed paraneoplastic optic neuritis.[989–993]

The most frequently identified paraneoplastic antibody is CV2/CRMP-5.[995–1000] In the paraneoplastic syndrome associated with this antibody, an optic neuropathy with disc swelling, retinitis, and vitreous cells may occur. Associated neurologic symptoms include peripheral neuropathy, ataxia, and limbic encephalitis with dementia. Rarely, this paraneoplastic disorder can present as an isolated optic neuropathy without other neurologic symptoms.[999] The most frequent tumors identified include small cell carcinoma of the lung and thymoma. The syndrome sometimes responds to treatment of the underlying malignancy along with corticosteroids or intravenous gamma globulin.

Radiation optic neuropathy (RON)

Delayed radiation damage to the anterior visual pathways has been reported in association with radiation for ocular, sinus, intracranial, and intraorbital malignancies.[1001–1003] It is believed to result from cumulative damage to glial cells and vascular endothelial cells[1004] and typically occurs 18–36 months after a total dose of 50 Gy. Optic nerve dysfunction results from microvasculopathy and occlusive endarteritis with subsequent optic nerve ischemia. There may also be a component of direct neuronal demyelination and degeneration before vascular changes are seen.

When radiation is likely to include the anterior visual pathways in the field, a maximum total dose of 5000–6000 cGy in fractions under 200 cGy is considered to be associated with an acceptable low risk. RON occurs most frequently with irradiation of pituitary adenoma (incidence less than 0.5%),[1005] but has been documented with treatment of parasellar meningioma, craniopharyngioma, sinus carcinoma, nasopharyngeal carcinoma, skull base tumors such as chordoma, and intraocular tumors. It has been described with gamma knife stereotactic radiosurgery in addition to conventional external beam irradiation.[1006,1007] Gamma knife radiation doses of up to 8 Gy to the optic nerve are associated with an approximately 2% risk of radiation optic neuropathy.[1008]

The differential diagnosis of RON includes recurrent tumor, secondary empty sella syndrome with sagging of the chiasm, optic nerve and chiasmal arachnoiditis, and radiation-induced parasellar tumors. In fact, tumor recurrence is the most common cause of late visual deterioration after CNS tumor excision and radiation.

Neuro-ophthalmic signs. RON typically presents with acute, painless visual loss in one or both eyes. There is no correlation with patient age, and the vision loss is often severe. The majority of cases occur within 3 years after completion of radiation therapy with a peak incidence at 1–1.5 years. Vision loss from optic neuropathy can either include disc swelling (**Fig. 5–72**) or can be retrobulbar. Disc swelling can be nonspecific but may also be accompanied by stigmata of radiation retinopathy including cotton-wool spots, intraretinal vascular abnormalities, and hemorrhages. Unfortunately, progression of visual loss over weeks to months is common. Spontaneous recovery is extremely rare. Chiasmal

syndromes from radiation optic neuropathy are discussed in Chapter 7.

Evaluation. CT images of CNS radionecrosis may show regions of decreased attenuation in white matter and slight enhancement with contrast. With MRI scanning the optic nerves may appear slightly swollen but otherwise normal on unenhanced studies, and usually demonstrate focal contrast enhancement with T1-weighted Gd-DTPA images (**Fig. 5–73**). The enhancement may resolve after the acute phase of visual loss.[1009] MRI is the study of choice to distinguish radiation optic neuropathy from recurrent tumor.

Treatment. There is no proven effective treatment for RON, but occasionally systemic corticosteroids are successful. Their mechanism of action is not clear, but steroids may reduce overall tissue edema and retard demyelination. Hyperbaric oxygen has been used in the treatment of radiation optic neuropathy with mixed results.[1010–1016] Heparin followed by prolonged coumadinization has been used successfully in the treatment of cerebral radionecrosis, myelopathy, and plexopathy.[1017] Although there are some anecdotal reports of its success in treating RON,[1018] the role of anticoagulation is uncertain.

Nutritional and toxic optic neuropathies

Toxic and nutritional optic neuropathies are often described together because they both frequently present with slowly progressive, bilateral vision loss with dyschromatopsia, and central or centrocecal scotomas. Diagnostic criteria proposed by Lessell[1019] are summarized in **Table 5–18**. These entities are uncommon but are considered frequently in the differential diagnosis of unexplained vision loss. Care must be taken to distinguish these conditions from hereditary optic neuropathies, retinopathies, and nonorganic visual loss.

Toxic optic neuropathies are usually recognized by the patient's exposure history. Patients commonly encounter these substances either through therapy with antibiotics or

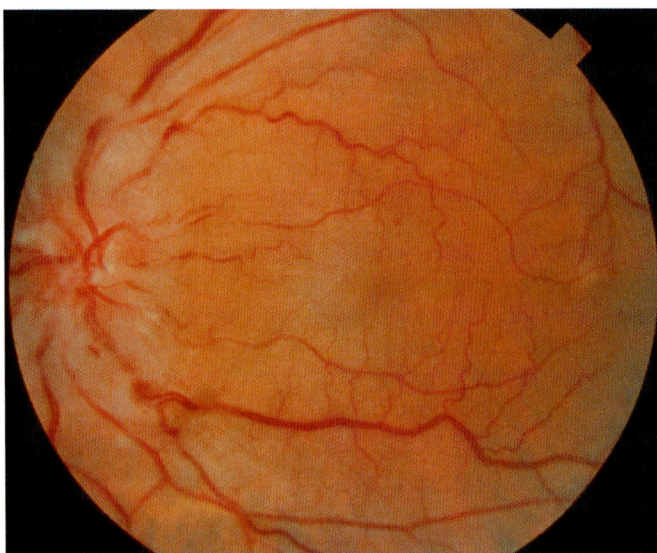

Figure 5–72. Fundus appearance in acute radiation optic neuropathy associated with disc swelling.

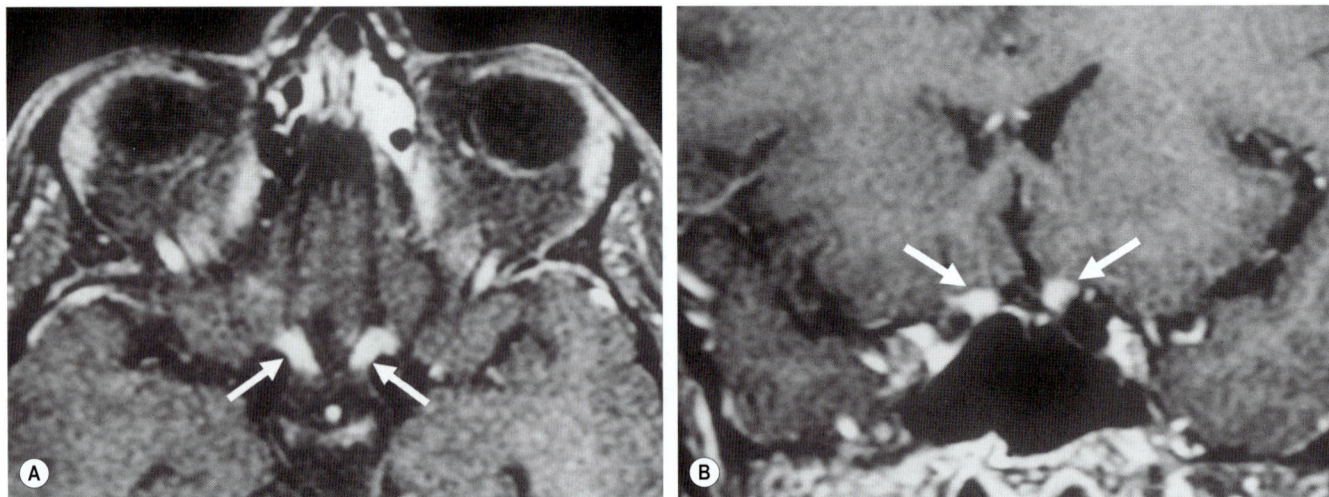

Figure 5–73. Axial (**A**) and coronal (**B**), T1-weighted, gadolinium-enhanced magnetic resonance imaging of the optic nerves in a patient with bilateral radiation induced optic neuropathy following radiation treatment of a sinus tumor. Both optic nerves (arrows) in their intracranial portions enhance with gadolinium. Visual loss progressed over weeks, and ultimately the patient had no light perception in both eyes despite hyperbaric oxygen and anticoagulation.

Table 5–18 Diagnostic criteria for toxic and nutritional optic neuropathies[1019]

Gradual painless progression
Bilateral
Dyschromatopsia
Centrocecal field defects
Vision better than hand movements
Optic disc appearance normal initially
Absence of metamorphopsia
Absence of hallucinations
Improvement with treatment or removal of offending toxin

chemotherapeutic agents, recreational drug abuse, or industrial exposure. Therefore toxic optic neuropathy might limit the usefulness of a drug or cause a substance to be hazardous in the work place. Deficiency or nutritional optic neuropathies typically arise in individuals who are malnourished, have a malabsorption problem, or are involved in a widespread epidemic limiting adequate nutrition.[1020]

B₁₂ deficiency

Vitamin B_{12} is found in milk, eggs, meat, and cheese and must be ingested. Vitamin B_{12} deficiency, which takes years to develop, generally arises in several different clinical settings. The first and most common is pernicious anemia. This autoimmune condition, characterized in most cases by antiparietal cell antibodies, results in gastric atrophy, reduced intrinsic factor production by gastric parietal cells, and B_{12} malabsorption. It affects middle-aged individuals and can cause a megaloblastic anemia. An associated neurologic condition, subacute combined degeneration of the spinal cord, can develop. In this setting, patients develop both a peripheral neuropathy with numbness, tingling, and decreased deep tendon reflexes, and leg weakness with extensor plantar responses from myelopathy. The second setting is in patients with a previous history of partial or complete removal of the stomach or ileum, rendering them unable to absorb B_{12}. The third setting, simple lack of B_{12} in the diet as might occur with a strict vegan or an extremely finicky eater, is the rarest. Finally, repeat exposure to nitrous oxide may produce vitamin B_{12} deficiency by inactivating cobalamin.

A 1959 review identified 29 cases of B_{12} optic neuropathy in the world literature, suggesting the condition is very rare.[1021] Although several cases have been added, the modern literature still contains few such cases.[1022] Patients present as outlined above with slowly progressive vision loss with dyschromatopsia and centrocecal scotomas. The optic nerve may be normal or may demonstrate pallor and nerve fiber defects (**Fig. 5–74**). Vision loss may precede the recognition of the anemia or the other neurologic symptoms.[1021] Visual-evoked response abnormalities have been found in patients without visual symptoms.[1023] MRI scan may show focal demyelination of the optic nerve.[1024] The diagnosis is confirmed by low serum B_{12} levels or elevated methylmalonic acid or homocysteine,[1025] both of which require B_{12} for their metabolism. Treatment is with parenteral hydroxycobalamin, and with prompt therapy, vision loss may be reversible.

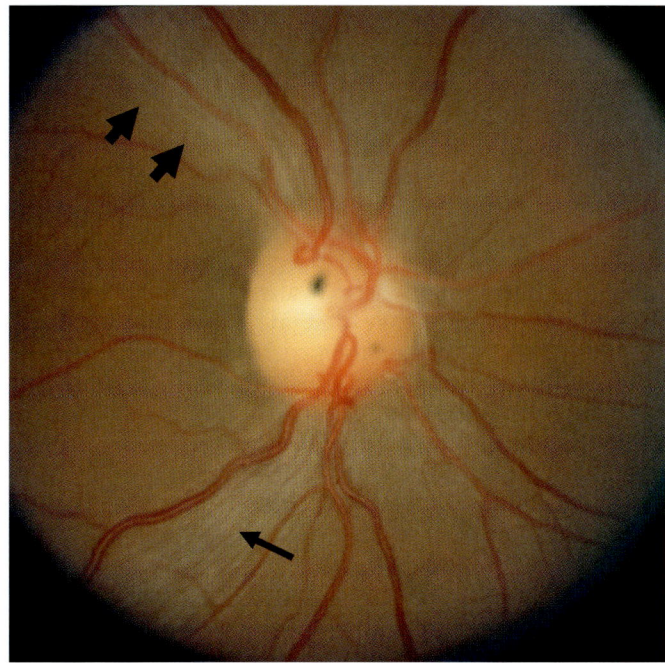

Figure 5–74. Ophthalmoscopic appearance in B_{12} deficiency. There is temporal pallor of the optic nerve head, nerve fiber drop-out in the papillomacular bundle (short thick arrows), and rake-like defects in the nerve fiber layer (single thin arrow).

Optic neuropathy has been shown in primate studies to be the result of demyelination involving the papillomacular bundle.[1026,1027] The pathogenesis remains unclear, but may result from build-up of toxic levels of cyanide (especially in cigarette smokers) or improper fatty acid synthesis leading to myelin dysfunction. Rizzo[1022] proposed that adenosine triphosphate deficiency may be a final common pathway for B_{12} optic neuropathy, Leber's hereditary optic neuropathy, and tobacco–alcohol amblyopia.

Other vitamin deficiencies. Deficiencies in thiamine (B_1), pyridoxine (B_6), folic acid, niacin, and riboflavin (B_2) have all been suggested causes of optic neuropathy. Deficiency in thiamine typically results in beri beri or Wernicke's encephalopathy. Vision loss in prisoners of war is one purported example of thiamine optic neuropathy, as their visual deficits improved with thiamine supplementation.[1028] Ketogenic and high-protein, low-carbohydrate diets may also put a patient at risk for developing thiamine deficiency. In the case of pyridoxine there has not been a causal relationship established between the deficiency state and optic neuropathy. However, certain drugs like isoniazid bind pyridoxine, and the toxicity of this drug has been attributed to altered pyridoxine availability. For riboflavin, niacin, and folic acid, cases of deficiency associated optic neuropathy were reported in the first half of the century but were largely speculative. These are not important causes of nutritional amblyopia, and their causative role in the development of optic neuropathy remains suspect.

Tobacco–alcohol amblyopia

The most commonly recognized nutritional or toxic optic neuropathy may actually be a combination of both a nutritional deficiency state and a toxic effect from tobacco smoking. Small series of patients with this so called tobacco–alcohol amblyopia or optic neuropathy have been reported.[1029-1032] Patients typically complain of an insidiously progressive loss of central vision and dyschromatopsia. Acute changes in the appearance of the fundus have been described and include peripapillary dilated vessels and hemorrhages.[1033,1034]

The exact role of the nutritional component and the toxic effects of alcohol are debated. Patients often under-report their daily alcohol intake and are malnourished. Since neither ethyl alcohol nor tobacco have been found to be directly toxic to the anterior visual pathways, it is generally felt that poor nutrition is central to the development of decreased vision. Cyanide intoxication may play a role as well. Similar conditions can occur in patients who abuse either alcohol or tobacco. Histopathologic evaluation has shown prominent loss of both papillomacular bundle nerve fibers as well as diffuse nerve fiber loss.[1035]

Specific vitamin deficiencies are infrequently identified, but testing for B_{12} and folate levels should be performed. All attempts should be made to convince the patient to reduce alcohol intake. Even if they are unsuccessful, recovery may result if a nutritious diet with B vitamin supplementation (including hydroxycobalamin parenterally) is instituted.[1029,1031] Since tobacco–alcohol amblyopia is a diagnosis of exclusion, mimickers such as compressive and Leber's hereditary optic neuropathy[1036] should be ruled out.

Cuban and tropical optic neuropathies

An epidemic of optic neuropathy with features similar to toxic and nutritional optic neuropathy occurred in Cuba. Numerous reports characterized these patients, who developed optic and peripheral neuropathies.[1037-1044] Between 1991 and 1993, epidemic optic and peripheral neuropathy affected more than 51 000 people in Cuba. A study by Cuban and US investigators characterized and identified risk factors for the optic neuropathy.[1041] In 123 patients with severe optic neuropathy, prominent clinical features included subacute loss of vision with field defects, dyschromatopsia, optic-nerve pallor, and decreased vibratory and temperature sense in the legs. Tobacco use, particularly cigar smoking, increased the risk of optic neuropathy. High dietary intakes of methionine, vitamin B_{12}, and riboflavin reduced the risk. They concluded that the epidemic of optic and peripheral neuropathies in Cuba between 1991 and 1993 appeared to be linked to tobacco use and the malnutrition caused by Cuba's economic situation. Some have suggested a role for mitochondrial mutations, in particular the mutations associated with Leber's hereditary optic neuropathy, but this remains controversial.[1038-1040,1044] Improvement in visual symptoms occurred with the initiation of vitamin supplementation in the population.[1043]

Other groupings of possible toxic and/or nutritional optic neuropathies include tropical amblyopia and Jamaican optic neuropathy. The pathogenesis of these conditions remains unproven, and they may be the same condition or even a hereditary optic neuropathy. The largest series of patients

with tropical amblyopia was reported by Osuntokun and Osuntokon.[1045] Two hundred and eighty-eight patients with ataxia and optic neuropathy were examined. Other features included peripheral neuropathy and decreased hearing. An unusual feature was the presence of peripheral field constriction without central defects in most patients. The role of poor nutrition and the ingestion of cassava (cyanide source) was unclear. Jamaican optic neuropathy is similar although the condition tends to affect teenagers and is unaccompanied by other neurologic symptoms.[1046] Similar pathogenic mechanisms have been considered including a genetic defect, treponemal infection, nutritional defects, and toxic by-products in homemade "bush teas." A similar syndrome has been described in patients in Tanzania.[1047]

Specific toxic optic neuropathies

Methanol. Methanol is a well-recognized optic nerve toxin and can cause profound vision loss even in small doses. The presentation is quite different from other toxic optic neuropathies because patients may develop sudden vision loss with disc swelling, and they may be comatose with metabolic acidosis. Patients are typically inebriated, then within 18–48 hours develop headache, dyspnea, vomiting, abdominal pain, and bilateral visual blurring. Visual symptoms initially may be transient. Patients may have ingested methanol in a suicide attempt or as an inadvertent contaminant in homemade alcohols. Benton and Calhoun[1048] reported the largest series of patients (n = 320) who ingested methanol as a contaminant of bootleg whiskey.

The acute optic disc edema is indistinguishable from papilledema. Disc swelling has been demonstrated in experimental methanol poisoning in monkeys,[1049] and results from axoplasmic stasis secondary to demyelination and axoplasmic obstruction.[1050] The pathogenesis of these changes is presumed to be a histotoxic anoxia occurring in a vascular watershed.[1050] Although the majority of the damage is believed to result from demyelination of the retrolaminar optic nerve,[1050,1051] electrophysiologic studies suggest additional widespread photoreceptor and Mueller cell dysfunction.[1052] Treatment is aimed at the acidosis and includes dialysis and intravenous ethyl alcohol, which interferes with methanol metabolism. Morbidity is high, and the prognosis for visual recovery is poor. Optic atrophy develops and can be accompanied by cupping.[958]

Ethambutol. Ethambutol causes a dose-related optic neuropathy and was recognized as an optic nerve toxin soon after its introduction as a treatment for tuberculosis. In one large series of 800 patients taking ethambutol, 1.5% developed a toxic optic neuropathy.[1053] The toxicity is thought to result from its chelating properties. A typical presentation includes either central field defects with loss of acuity and dyschromatopsia or well-preserved central visual function with peripheral visual field loss.[1054] Chiasmal-type central bitemporal field loss may also occur. Vision loss is not accompanied by other neurologic symptoms. Doses less than 15 mg/kg/day are thought to be safe, but in patients taking between 15 and 25 mg/kg/day visual symptoms generally develop over a period of months.[1054,1055] More severe and irreversible vision loss has been reported in patients treated with ethambutol for renal tuberculosis.[1056] Dyschromatopsia (particularly for green) and loss of contrast sensitivity are reported to be early signs of visual loss.[1057] OCT measurements of the nerve fiber layer can be used to follow patients and may predict recovery in the setting of normal measurements.[1058,1059] Some visual improvement typically occurs with discontinuation of the drug but abnormalities in the visual fields and contrast sensitivity may persist.[1060] Older patients may be less likely to recover.[1061]

Amiodarone. An optic neuropathy with disc swelling very similar to anterior ischemic optic neuropathy has been reported in patients taking the anti-arrhythmia drug amiodarone.[1062–1071] Debate still exists as to whether this is a true toxic optic neuropathy caused by amiodarone versus ordinary ischemic optic neuropathy. Most evidence for the condition comes only from case reports, and the only prospective study of over 800 patients taking amiodarone suggested the incidence of the condition to be at most 0.1%.[1072] The patient population taking the drug is likely to be vasculopathic and at risk for ordinary ION, further clouding the issue. However, some clinical features may distinguish amiodarone-associated optic neuropathy from ION.[1070] For instance, visual loss may be insidious over months, often with bilateral simultaneous involvement of the eyes, and is usually less severe than in ordinary ION.[1062,1064,1073,1074] The disc swelling may last for months, and some recovery can be associated with discontinuation of the drug.[1066] Abnormal lamellar inclusions in optic nerve axons have been identified on histopathologic study.[1063]

Halogenated hydroxyquinolines. Halogenated hydroxyquinolines have been implicated in the development of myelopathy and optic neuropathy (subacute myelo-optic neuropathy; SMON). The drug was used to prevent diarrhea when traveling and for other gastrointestinal symptoms. The condition has largely been reported in Japan.[1075] Patients develop optic atrophy with severe vision loss which may be partially reversible with discontinuation of the drug.

Tumor necrosis factor-α inhibitors. Optic neuritis has been reported as a complication of TNF-α inhibitors used to treat juvenile idiopathic[1076] and rheumatoid arthritis.[1077] It is not certain whether the optic neuritis was caused by the drugs or whether the vision loss occurred as a result of the underlying disease.

Other toxic optic neuropathies. As more drugs are developed to treat neoplasms, an increasing number of optic nerve toxins have been identified. In some instances multiple drug regimens for chemotherapy and bone marrow transplantation are associated with optic neuropathy, and the specific cause cannot be identified.[1078] Interferon-α used to treat hepatitis as well as certain cancers may be associated with an ION-like optic neuropathy. The optic neuropathy is often bilateral and may recur after the drug is restarted.[1079–1083] The list of other drugs reported to cause toxic optic neuropathy is long and is summarized in **Table 5–19**. The table does not describe every reported optic nerve toxin but supplements the discussion above with some of the more commonly encountered ones.

Table 5–19 Other drugs (not discussed in detail in the text) which can cause toxic optic neuropathy[1019–1121]

Drug	Clinical features
Arsenicals	Irreversible
Busulfan	Also causes cataract
Carmustine (BCNU)	Also retinal degeneration
Chloramphenicol	Disc swelling, associated peripheral neuropathy
Cisplatin	May have disc swelling, associated peripheral neuropathy and ototoxicity
Cytosine arabanoside	Optic nerve toxicity when given intrathecally
Digitalis	Likely more prominent effect is on the retina
Disulfiram	Rapid vision loss and recovery when discontinued, acetaldehyde may cause optic neuropathy
Ethylene glycol	Acute vision loss, disc swelling, similar course to methanol-induced optic neuropathy
Fludarabine	Encephalopathy
Hydrogen sulfide	Blindness and reduced hearing
Interferon	Disc edema and decreased vision
Isoniazid	Sensory neuropathy reversible with pyridoxine, disc swelling, retinal hemorrhages
Lead	Disc edema, retinal pigment epithelium changes
Linezolid	Reversible optic neuropathy and irreversible peripheral neuropathy
Methotrexate	Disc edema, idiosyncratic, reversible
Organophosphates	Chronic exposure, ganglion cells reduced
Quinine	Ganglion cell damage
Toluene	Industrial exposure, reversible
Vincristine	Demyelination, also ophthalmoplegia and cortical blindness

Traumatic optic neuropathy

Of the various forms of vision loss due to trauma, optic nerve injuries are some of the most difficult to diagnose and treat. Hippocrates may have been the first to recognize this condition when he identified the phenomenon of acute and delayed vision loss after injuries placed to and slightly above the brow. In truth he may have identified patients with traumatic glaucoma or cataracts, but he clearly highlighted the brow as the point of impact. It is now recognized that the brow and other facial eminences are most frequently the

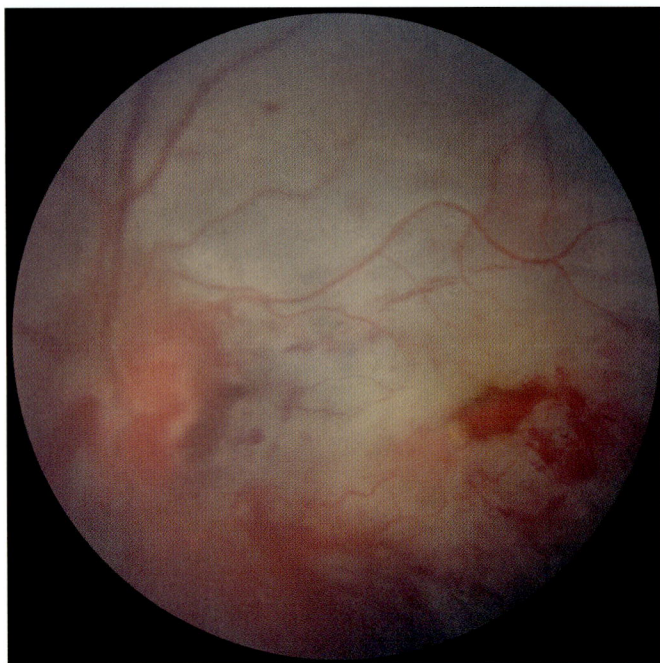

Figure 5–75. Fundus appearance of acute optic nerve avulsion after penetrating orbital trauma. Hemorrhage and retinal whitening secondary to disruption of blood flow to the eye are seen. (Courtesy of Nicholas Mahoney, MD, and Alexander Brucker, MD).

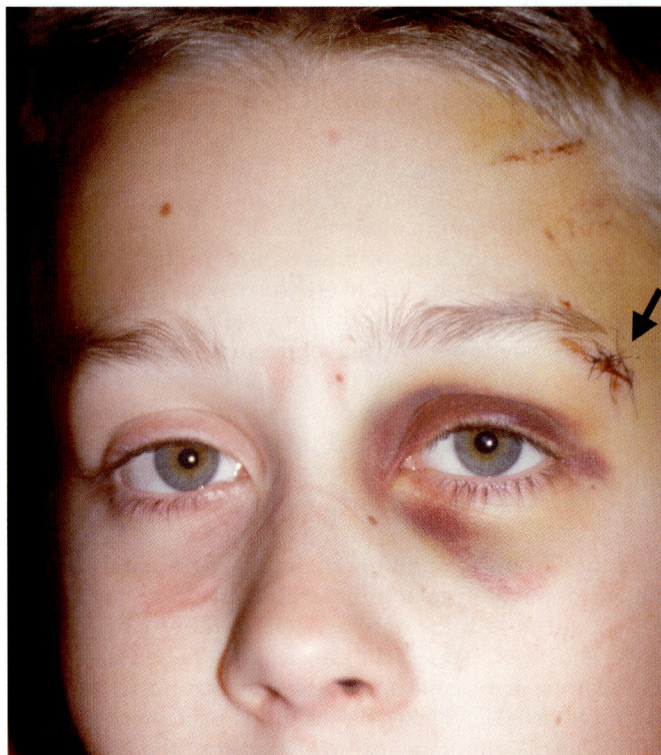

Figure 5–76. Location of typical trauma near the brow in indirect traumatic optic neuropathy. While riding his bicycle, this boy fell and hit the left side of his head on a cement wall, leading to an optic neuropathy in the left eye. Note the point of impact near his eyebrow at the sutured laceration (arrow) and the orbital ecchymoses, both typical for patients with this condition.

site of impact in patients with posterior indirect traumatic optic neuropathy (TON) (see below).

Traumatic optic neuropathy can take many forms. *Direct* injuries are caused by projectiles or penetrating objects that enter the orbit. Self-inflicted optic nerve trauma can also occur.[1084,1085] *Indirect* injuries are caused by forces that are transmitted to the optic nerve from the globe and orbit. Examples of this type include posterior indirect traumatic optic neuropathy, which is discussed in more detail below, and optic nerve avulsion. The latter may occur with only minor damage to the front of the eye if it is rotated forcefully, causing separation of the optic nerve as it exits the globe.[1086] Ophthalmoscopically, avulsion is often accompanied by intraocular hemorrhages, which may preclude viewing the nerve head (**Fig. 5–75**).[1087,1088] The visual prognosis following optic nerve avulsion is poor.[1089] Also recognized are a traumatic form of ischemic optic neuropathy and optic nerve dysfunction due to optic nerve sheath or orbital hemorrhages.

Posterior indirect traumatic optic neuropathy

Posterior indirect traumatic optic neuropathy is traumatic loss of vision that occurs without external or initial ophthalmoscopic evidence of injury to the eye or the nerve. This condition occurs in patients of all ages, and, as with any traumatic condition, it is most common in young men. It is estimated that 2–5% of patients with head injuries have TON, and therefore, based on the incidence of head injuries, there are four or five cases of TON/100 000 population per year. Frontal blows are most common and one study showed a high rate in patients involved in falls from bicycles

(**Fig. 5–76**).[1090] Patients need not have loss of consciousness, and the entity certainly occurs in situations of relatively minor head trauma.

Neuro-ophthalmic signs. As with any optic neuropathy, there is loss of acuity and color vision, an afferent pupil defect, and visual field defects of any type although central scotomas and altitudinal defects are most common. The fundus is initially normal.

Mechanism. The mechanism of injury in posterior indirect traumatic optic neuropathy is uncertain but likely multifactorial. In part, the injury to the optic nerve probably occurs as the head hits a hard surface and suddenly decelerates, but the eyeball continues forward. This creates shearing forces that damage the optic nerve's canalicular portion, which is tightly fixed by dural attachments. In addition, holographic interferometric studies performed by Anderson and Panje Gross[1091] have shown that forces to the facial eminences are focally manifested around the optic foramen. The combination of these two factors leads to compressing, stretching, and contusing of the optic nerve. These injuries may than cause the nerve to swell, and in the tight bony optic canal there is no room for expansion. Therefore, delayed visual loss may result from further compression from edema within the optic canal.

Diagnostic studies/neuroimaging. Optic canal fractures are identified in only approximately one-third of patients (**Fig. 5–77**), and therefore identification of a fracture is *not* necessary for the diagnosis.[1090] Coronal CT images are best

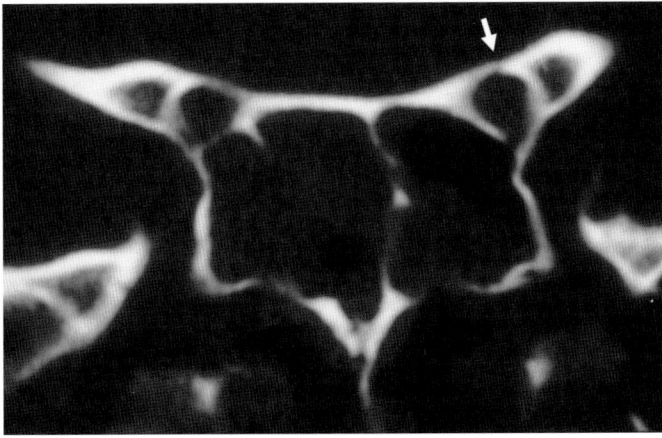

Figure 5–77. Coronal bone window computed tomography scan demonstrating a fracture (arrow) of the left optic canal.

for identifying these fractures. The optic canal is located in the superior posterior lateral aspect of the sphenoid sinus.

Differential diagnosis. Admittedly, ophthalmoscopic evaluation is difficult in patients with altered consciousness, as their pupils cannot be dilated while pupillary status is monitored in acute hospital settings. Important entities that need to be considered in the differential diagnosis include pre-existing optic neuropathy, traumatic retinal injury, and factitious visual loss since many patients are seeking secondary gain in the setting of the injury. The absence of an afferent pupillary defect would support nonphysiologic visual loss.

Treatment. Review of several series reveals that one-quarter to one-half of patients improve spontaneously.[1090–1095] There are two available options for treatment. Corticosteroids can be used to treat optic nerve swelling and inflammation. Alternatively, since the nerve is swollen within the confines of a tight bony canal, removal of those bones to decompress the canal and prevent compression may also improve the condition. In a comparative, nonrandomized study[1096] comparing observation with treatment with corticosteroids or optic canal decompression, no clear benefit was found for either of these modalities. Vision improved by three Snellen lines in 57% of the untreated group, 32% of the surgery group, and 52% of the steroid group. Based on careful review of the literature (Cochrane database), no treatment has been shown to be convincingly effective.[1097,1098] Therefore, there is no standard of care for the treatment of TON, and observation alone is reasonable.

The use of megadose steroids is extrapolated from traumatic spinal cord injury studies. Bracken et al.[1099] and Braughler and Hall[1100] in the National Acute Spinal Cord Injury Trial showed that megadose steroids were effective in reducing permanent deficits in patients with spinal cord injury. Glucocorticoid activity is less important in the purported mechanism than the ability of these agents in high doses to scavenge free radicals and prevent lipid peroxidation, perhaps a final pathway in white matter injury.

Importantly, however, there is some recent evidence that steroids may be detrimental in patients with head injuries. Experimental work in rats suggests that methylprednisolone may exacerbate axonal loss following crush injury in the

optic nerve.[1101] Results from the Corticosteroid Randomization after Significant Head Injury (CRASH) Study suggest that high-dose steroids are associated with increased mortality when given in the context of head injury.[1102,1103] The mortality rate following the injury was 21.1% in the steroid group and 17.9% in the placebo group, refuting previous smaller studies that reported improved survival following steroid treatment for head injury.

Experimental work is currently being conducted to examine the ability of *N*-methyl-D-aspartate receptor antagonists, lazaroids, or 21-aminosteroids with and without vitamin E analogs, calcium channel blockers, and GM1 gangliosides to prevent lipid peroxidation and free radical damage in nerve tissue. These compounds may some day prove to be effective medical treatments of TON.

Both transcranial and extracranial surgical decompression of the optic canal have also shown promise. Uncontrolled and retrospective studies have demonstrated an approximately 70% improvement rate in patients who have extracranial surgery performed via a transethmoidal transsphenoidal route.[1093,1104–1107] Endoscopic approaches are also available. The complication rate is very low with no major morbidity or death. However, since the carotid canal sits next to the optic canal, this procedure should not be performed by inexperienced surgeons. Optic canal decompression is indicated when there is radiologic evidence of a bony fragment or hematoma impinging on the optic nerve. It can also be considered in patients in whom surgery is being performed to repair other facial fractures, or in patients with vision loss that deteriorates while on steroids. It should only be considered in patients who are conscious and can understand the potential risks and benefits of this procedure that has unproven efficacy.

In general, we often choose observation and discourage any treatment beyond moderate doses of steroids in most cases.[1108] This is particularly true in any patient in whom diagnostic ambiguity exists (simultaneous globe injury or limited examination secondary to cooperation). Each institution should try to identify a team including a (neuro-) ophthalmologist, neuroradiologist, and otolaryngologist to care for patients with traumatic optic neuropathy.

References

1. Kupfer C, Chumbley L, Downer JC. Quantitative histology of optic nerve optic tract and lateral geniculate nucleus of man. J Anat 1967;101:393–401.
2. Potts AM, Hodges D, Sherman CB, et al. Morphology of the primate optic nerve: I-III. Invest Ophthalmol Vis Sci 1972;11:980–1016.
3. Oppel O. Mikroskopische untersuchungen uber die anzahl und kaliber der markhaltigen nervenfasern im fasciculus opticus des menshen. Arch Ophthalmol 1963;166:19–27.
4. Maunsell JHR. Functional visual streams. Curr Opin Neurobiol 1992;2:506–510.
5. Merigan WH, Maunsell JHR. How parallel are the primate visual pathways? Annu Rev Neurosci 1993;16:369–402.
6. Shapley R. Visual sensitivity and parallel retinocortical channels. Annu Rev Psychol 1990;41:635–658.
7. Sadun AA. Parallel processing in the human visual system: a new perspective. Neuro-ophthalmology 1986;6:351–352.
8. Kaplan E, Shapley RM. The primate retina contains two types of ganglion cells with high and low contrast sensitivity. Proc Natl Acad Sci USA 1986;83:2755–2757.
9. Ogden TE. Nerve fiber layer of the macaque retina: retinotopic organization. Invest Ophthalmol Vis Sci 1983;24:85–98.
10. Gordon GR, Mulligan SJ, MacVicar BA. Astrocyte control of the cerebrovasculature. Glia 2007;55:1214–1221.

11. Iadecola C, Nedergaard M. Glial regulation of the cerebral microvasculature. Nat Neurosci 2007;10:1369–1376.

12. Ransom B, Behar T, Nedergaard M. New roles for astrocytes (stars at last). Trends Neurosci 2003;26:520–522.

13. Hernandez MR, Luo XX, Igoe F, et al. Extracellular matrix of the human lamina cribrosa. Am J Ophthalmol 1987;104:567–576.

14. Hernandez MR, Igoe F, Neufeld AH. Extracellular matrix of the human optic nerve head. Am J Ophthalmol 1986;102:139–148.

15. Morrison JC, Jerdan JA, L'Hernault NL, et al. The extracellular matrix composition of the monkey optic nerve head. Invest Ophthalmol Vis Sci 1988;29:1141–1150.

16. Morrison JC, Jerdan JA, Dorman ME, et al. Structural proteins of the neonatal and adult lamina cribrosa. Arch Ophthalmol 1989;107:1220–1224.

17. Quigley HA. Regional differences in the structure of the lamina cribrosa and their relationship to glaucomatous visual field loss. Arch Ophthalmol 1981;99:137–143.

18. Hayreh SS. The 1994 Von Sallman Lecture: the optic nerve head circulation in health and disease. Exp Eye Res 1995;61:259–272.

19. Onda E, Cioffi GA, Bacon DR, et al. Microvasculature of the human optic nerve. Am J Ophthalmol 1995;120:92–102.

20. Mackenzie PJ, Cioffi GA. Vascular anatomy of the optic nerve head. Can J Ophthalmol 2008;43:308–312.

21. Maniscalo JE, Habal MB. Microanatomy of the optic canal. J Neurosurg 1978;48:402–406.

22. Minckler DS, Tso MO. Experimental papilledema produced by cyclocryotherapy. Am J Ophthalmol 1976;82:577–589.

23. Minckler DS, Bunt AH, Johanson GW. Orthograde and retrograde axoplasmic transport during ocular hypertension in the monkey. Invest Ophthalmol Vis Sci 1977;16:426–441.

24. Quigley HA, Anderson DR. The dynamics and location of axonal transport blockade by acute intraocular pressure elevation in primate optic nerve. Invest Ophthalmol Vis Sci 1976;15:606–616.

25. Quigley HA, Guy J, Anderson DR. Blockade of rapid axonal transport: effect of intraocular pressure elevation in primate optic nerve. Arch Ophthalmol 1979;97:525–531.

26. Quigley HA, Flower RW, Addicks EM, et al. The mechanism of optic nerve damage in experimental acute intraocular pressure elevation. Invest Ophthalmol Vis Sci 1980;19:505–517.

27. Morrison JC. Anatomy and physiology of the optic nerve. In: Kline LB (ed): Optic Nerve Disorders. San Francisco, American Academy of Ophthalmology and Palace Press, 1996: 1–20.

28. Hoffman PN, Lasek RJ. The slow component of axonal transport: identification of major structural polypeptides of the axon and their generality among mammalian neurons. J Cell Biol 1975;66:351–366.

29. Ikeda H, Wright MJ. Receptive field organization of "sustained" and "transient" retinal ganglion cells which subserve different functional roles. J Physiol (Lond) 1972;222:769–800.

30. Diaper CJM. Pulfrich revisited. Surv Ophthalmol 1997;41:493–499.

31. Mojon DS, Rosler KM, Oetliker H. A bedside test to determine motion stereopsis using the Pulfrich phenomenon. Ophthalmology 1998;105:1337–1344.

32. Diaper CJM, Dutton GN, Heron G. The Pulfrich phenomenon: its symptoms and their management. J Neuroophthalmol 1999;12:12.

33. Keltner JL, Johnson CA, Spurr JO, et al. Baseline visual field profile of optic neuritis. The experience of the optic neuritis treatment trial. Optic Neuritis Study Group. Arch Ophthalmol 1993;111:231–234.

34. Jonas JB, Budde WM, Panda-Jonas S. Ophthalmoscopic evaluation of the optic nerve head. Surv Ophthalmol 1999;43:293–320.

35. Jonas JB. Optic disk size correlated with refractive error. Am J Ophthalmol 2005;139:346–348.

36. Frisén L, Claesson M. Narrowing of the retinal arterioles in descending optic atrophy: a quantitative clinical study. Ophthalmology 1984;91:1342–1346.

37. Sebag J, Delori FC, Feke GT, et al. Anterior optic nerve blood flow decreases in clinical neurogenic optic atrophy. Ophthalmology 1986;93:858–865.

38. Trobe JD, Glaser JS, Cassady JC. Optic atrophy: differential diagnosis by fundus observation alone. Arch Ophthalmol 1986;98:1040–1045.

39. Lee AG, Chau FY, Golnik KC, et al. The diagnostic yield of the evaluation for isolated unexplained optic atrophy. Ophthalmology 2005;112:757–759.

40. Kim JW, Rizzo JF, Lessell S. Delayed visual decline in patients with "stable" optic neuropathy. Arch Ophthalmol 2005;123:785–788.

41. Spandau UH, Jonas JB, Gass A. Progressive visual loss in optic nerve hypoplasia and bilateral microdiscs. Arch Neurol 2002;59:1829–1830.

42. Rahi JS, Cable N. Severe visual impairment and blindness in children in the UK. Lancet 2003;362:1359–1365.

43. Kim MR, Park SE, Oh SY. Clinical feature analysis of congenital optic nerve abnormalities. Jpn J Ophthalmol 2006;50:250–255.

44. Brodsky MC, Baker RS, Hamed LM. Congenital optic disc anomalies. In: Pediatric Neuro-ophthalmology. New York, Springer-Verlag, 1996.

45. Garcia ML, Ty EB, Taban M, et al. Systemic and ocular findings in 100 patients with optic nerve hypoplasia. J Child Neurol 2006;21:949–956.

46. Hoyt CS, Good WV. Do we really understand the difference between optic nerve hypoplasia and optic atrophy? Eye 1992;6:201–204.

47. Hellstrom A, Wiklund LM, Svensson E. The clinical and morphologic spectrum of optic nerve hypoplasia. J AAPOS 1999;3:212–220.

48. Manor RS, Korczyn AD. Retinal red-free light photographs in two congenital conditions: a case of optic hypoplasia and a case of congenital hemianopia. Ophthalmologica 1976;173:119–127.

49. Borchert M, McCulloch D, Rother C, et al. Clinical assessment, optic disk measurements, and visual-evoked potential in optic nerve hypoplasia. Am J Ophthalmol 1995;120:605–612.

50. Brodsky MC. Congenital optic disk anomalies. Surv Ophthalmol 1994;39:89–112.

51. Hellström A, Wiklund L-M, Svensson E, et al. Optic nerve hypoplasia with isolated tortuosity of the retinal veins. Arch Ophthalmol 1999;117:880–884.

52. Birkebaek NH, Patel L, Wright NB, et al. Optic nerve size evaluated by magnetic resonance imaging in children with optic nerve hypoplasia, multiple pituitary hormone deficiency, isolated growth hormone deficiency, and idiopathic short stature. J Pediatr 2004;145:536–541.

53. Scott IU, Warman R, Altman N. Bilateral aplasia of the optic nerves, chiasm, and tracts. Am J Ophthalmol 1997;124:409–410.

54. Brodsky MC, Atreides SP, Fowlkes JL, et al. Optic nerve aplasia in an infant with congenital hypopituitarism and posterior pituitary ectopia. Arch Ophthalmol 2004;122:125–126.

55. Margo CE, Hamed LM, Fang E, et al. Optic nerve aplasia. Arch Ophthalmol 1992;110:1610–1613.

56. Riedl S, Vosahlo J, Battelino T, et al. Refining clinical phenotypes in septo-optic dysplasia based on MRI findings. Eur J Pediatr 2008;167:1269–1276.

57. Brickman JM, Clements M, Tyrell R, et al. Molecular effects of novel mutations in Hesx1/HESX1 associated with human pituitary disorders. Development 2001;128:5189–5199.

58. Dattani ML, Martinez-Barbera J, Thomas PQ, et al. Molecular genetics of septo-optic dysplasia. Horm Res 2000;53 Suppl 1:26–33.

59. Dattani MT, Martinez-Barbera JP, Thomas PQ, et al. HESX1: a novel gene implicated in a familial form of septo-optic dysplasia. Acta Paediatr Suppl 1999;88:49–54.

60. Dattani MT, Robinson IC. HESX1 and septo-optic dysplasia. Rev Endocr Metab Disord 2002;3:289–300.

61. Kelberman D, Dattani MT. Genetics of septo-optic dysplasia. Pituitary 2007;10:393–407.

62. Kelberman D, Dattani MT. Septo-optic dysplasia: novel insights into the aetiology. Horm Res 2008;69:257–265.

63. McNay DE, Turton JP, Kelberman D, et al. HESX1 mutations are an uncommon cause of septooptic dysplasia and hypopituitarism. J Clin Endocrinol Metab 2007;92:691–697.

64. Sajedi E, Gaston-Massuet C, Signore M, et al. Analysis of mouse models carrying the I26T and R160C substitutions in the transcriptional repressor HESX1 as models for septo-optic dysplasia and hypopituitarism. Dis Model Mech 2008;1:241–254.

65. Schuelke M, Krude H, Finckh B, et al. Septo-optic dysplasia associated with a new mitochondrial cytochrome b mutation. Ann Neurol 2002;51:388–392.

66. Hoyt WF, Kaplan SL, Grumbach MM, et al. Septo-optic dysplasia and pituitary dwarfism. Lancet 1970;1:893–894.

67. Morishima A, Aranoff GS. Syndrome of septo-optic pituitary dysplasia: the clinical spectrum. Brain Dev 1986;8:233–239.

68. Margalith D, Tze WJ, Jan JE. Congenital optic nerve hypoplasia with hypothalamic-pituitary dysplasia. Am J Dis Child 1985;139:361–366.

69. Costin G, Murphree AL. Hypothalamic-pituitary function in children with optic nerve hypoplasia. Am J Dis Child 1985;139:249–254.

70. Siatkowski RM, Sanchez JC, Andrade R, et al. The clinical, neuroradiographic, and endocrinologic profile of patients with bilateral optic nerve hypoplasia. Ophthalmology 1997;104:493–496.

71. Brodsky MC, Conte FA, Taylor D, et al. Sudden death in septo-optic dysplasia. Report of 5 cases. Arch Ophthalmol 1997;115:66–70.

72. Brodsky MC, Glasier CM. Optic nerve hypoplasia: clinical significance of associated central nervous system abnormalities on magnetic resonance imaging. Arch Ophthalmol 1993;111:66–74.

73. Sorkin JA, Davis PC, Meacham LR, et al. Optic nerve hypoplasia: absence of posterior pituitary bright signal on magnetic resonance imaging correlates with diabetes insipidus. Am J Ophthalmol 1996;122:717–723.

74. Brodsky MC. Optic nerve hypoplasia with posterior pituitary ectopia: male predominance and nonassociation with breech delivery. Am J Ophthalmol 1999;127:238–239.

75. Maeda T, Akaishi M, Shimizu M, et al. The subclassification of schizencephaly and its clinical characterization. Brain Dev 2009;31:694–701.

76. Kuban KCK, Teele RL, Wallman J. Septo-optic-dysplasia-schizencephaly. Radiographic and clinical features. Pediatr Radiol 1989;19:145–150.

77. Miller SP, Shevell MI, Patenaude Y, et al. Septo-optic dysplasia plus: a spectrum of malformations of cortical development. Neurology 2000;54:1701–1703.

78. Polizzi A, Pavone P, Iannetti P, et al. Septo-optic dysplasia complex: a heterogeneous malformation syndrome. Pediatr Neurol 2006;34:66–71.

79. Lubinsky MS. Hypothesis: septo-optic dysplasia is a vascular disruption sequence. Am J Med Genet 1997;69:235–236.

80. Garcia-Filion P, Epport K, Nelson M, et al. Neuroradiographic, endocrinologic, and ophthalmic correlates of adverse developmental outcomes in children with optic nerve hypoplasia: a prospective study. Pediatrics 2008;121:e653–659.

81. Levine LM, Bhatti MT, Mancuso AA. Septo-optic dysplasia with olfactory tract and bulb hypoplasia. J AAPOS 2001;5:398–399.

82. Katsuya Lauer A, Balish MJ, Palmer EA. Persistent hyperplastic primary vitreous associated with septo-optic-pituitary dysplasia and schizencephaly. Arch Ophthalmol 2000;118:578–580.

83. Frisén L, Holmegaard L. Spectrum of optic nerve hypoplasia. Br J Ophthalmol 1978;62:7–15.

84. Taylor D. Congenital tumours of the anterior visual system with dysplasia of the optic disc. Br J Ophthalmol 1982;66:455–463.

85. Lee JT, Hall TR, Bateman JB. Optic nerve hypoplasia secondary to intracranial teratoma. Am J Ophthalmol 1997;124:705–706.

86. Taban M, Cohen BH, David Rothner A, et al. Association of optic nerve hypoplasia with mitochondrial cytopathies. J Child Neurol 2006;21:956–960.

87. Lambert SR, Hoyt CS, Narahara MH. Optic nerve hypoplasia. Surv Ophthalmol 1987;32:1–9.

88. Phillips PH, Spear C, Brodsky MC. Magnetic resonance diagnosis of congenital hypopituitarism in children with optic nerve hypoplasia. J AAPOS 2001;5:275–280.

89. Haddad NG, Eugster EA. Hypopituitarism and neurodevelopmental abnormalities in relation to central nervous system structural defects in children with optic nerve hypoplasia. J Pediatr Endocrinol Metab 2005;18:853–858.

90. Ahmad T, Garcia-Filion P, Borchert M, et al. Endocrinological and auxological abnormalities in young children with optic nerve hypoplasia: a prospective study. J Pediatr 2006;148:78–84.

91. Takagi M, Abe H, Hatase T, et al. Superior segmental optic nerve hypoplasia in youth. Jpn J Ophthalmol 2008;52:468–474.

92. Foroozan R. Superior segmental optic nerve hypoplasia and diabetes mellitus. J Diabetes Complications 2005;19:165–167.

93. Unoki K, Ohba N, Hoyt WF. Optical coherence tomography of superior segmental optic hypoplasia. Br J Ophthalmol 2002;86:910–914.

94. Purvin VA. Superior segmental optic nerve hypoplasia. J Neuroophthalmol 2002;22:116–117.

95. Kim RY, Hoyt WF, Lessell S, et al. Superior segmental optic hypoplasia: a sign of maternal diabetes. Arch Ophthalmol 1989;107:1312–1315.

96. Landau K, Bajka JD, Kirchschläger BM. Topless optic disks in children of mothers with type I diabetes mellitus. Am J Ophthalmol 1998;125:605–611.

97. Hashimoto M, Ohtsuka K, Nakagawa T, et al. Topless optic disk syndrome without maternal diabetes mellitus. Am J Ophthalmol 1999;128:111–112.

98. Nelson M, Lessell S, Sadun AA. Optic nerve hypoplasia and maternal diabetes mellitus. Arch Neurol 1986;43:20–25.

99. Yamamoto T, Sato M, Iwase A. Superior segmental optic hypoplasia found in Tajimi Eye Health Care Project participants. Jpn J Ophthalmol 2004;48:578–583.

100. Buchanan TAS, Hoyt WF. Temporal visual field defects associated with nasal hypoplasia of the optic disc. Br J Ophthalmol 1981;65:636–640.

101. Hoyt WF, Rios-Montenegro EN, Behrens MM, et al. Homonymous hemioptic hypoplasia. Br J Ophthalmol 1972;56:537–545.

102. Jacobson L, Hellström A, Flodmark O. Large cups in normal-sized optic discs. A variant of optic nerve hypoplasia in children with periventricular leukomalacia. Arch Ophthalmol 1997;115:1263–1269.

103. You QS, Xu L, Jonas JB. Tilted optic discs: The Beijing Eye Study. Eye 2008;22:728–729.

104. Vongphanit J, Mitchell P, Wang JJ. Population prevalence of tilted optic disks and the relationship of this sign to refractive error. Am J Ophthalmol 2002;133:679–685.

105. Vuori ML, Mantyjarvi M. Tilted disc syndrome and colour vision. Acta Ophthalmol Scand 2007;85:648–652.

106. Bozkurt B, Irkec M, Tatlipinar S, et al. Retinal nerve fiber layer analysis and interpretation of GDx parameters in patients with tilted disc syndrome. Int Ophthalmol 2001;24:27–31.

107. Gurlu VP, Alymgyl ML. Retinal nerve fiber analysis and tomography of the optic disc in eyes with tilted disc syndrome. Ophthalmic Surg Lasers Imaging 2005;36:494–502.

108. Moschos MM, Triglianos A, Rotsos T, et al. Tilted disc syndrome: an OCT and mfERG study. Doc Ophthalmol 2009;119:23–28.

109. Onwochei BC, Simon JW, Bateman JB, et al. Ocular colobomata. Surv Ophthalmol 2000;45:175–194.

110. Hornby SJ, Adolph S, Gilbert CE, et al. Visual acuity in children with coloboma: clinical features and a new phenotypic classification system. Ophthalmology 2000;107:511–520.

111. Berk AT, Yaman A, Saatci AO. Ocular and systemic findings associated with optic disc colobomas. J Pediatr Ophthalmol Strabismus 2003;40:272–278.

112. Gopal L, Badrinath SS, Kuma KS, et al. Optic disc in fundus coloboma. Ophthalmology 1996;103:2120–2127.

113. Apple DJ, Rabb MF, Walsh PM. Congenital anomalies of the optic disc. Surv Ophthalmol 1982;27:3–41.

114. Pagen RA. Ocular colobomas. Surv Ophthalmol 1981;25:223–236.

115. Lalani SR, Safiullah AM, Fernbach SD, et al. Spectrum of CHD7 mutations in 110 individuals with CHARGE syndrome and genotype-phenotype correlation. Am J Hum Genet 2006;78:303–314.

116. McMain K, Robitaille J, Smith I, et al. Ocular features of CHARGE syndrome. J AAPOS 2008;12:460–465.

117. Chung GW, Edwards AO, Schimmenti LA, et al. Renal-coloboma syndrome: report of a novel PAX2 gene mutation. Am J Ophthalmol 2001;132:910–914.

118. Dureau P, Attie-Bitach T, Salomon R, et al. Renal coloboma syndrome. Ophthalmology 2001;108:1912–1916.

119. Schimmenti LA, Manligas GS, Sieving PA. Optic nerve dysplasia and renal insufficiency in a family with a novel PAX2 mutation, Arg115X: further ophthalmologic delineation of the renal-coloboma syndrome. Ophthalmic Genet 2003;24:191–202.

120. Taranta A, Palma A, De Luca V, et al. Renal-coloboma syndrome: a single nucleotide deletion in the PAX2 gene at exon 8 is associated with a highly variable phenotype. Clin Nephrol 2007;67:1–4.

121. Yoshimura K, Yoshida S, Yamaji Y, et al. De novo insG619 mutation in PAX2 gene in a Japanese patient with papillorenal syndrome. Am J Ophthalmol 2005;139:733–735.

122. Khan AO, Nowilaty SR. Early diagnosis of the papillorenal syndrome by optic disc morphology. J Neuroophthalmol 2005;25:209–211.

123. Parsa CF, Goldberg MF, Hunter DG. No colobomas in "renal coloboma" syndrome [letter]. Ophthalmology 2003;110:251; author reply 251–252.

124. Parsa CF, Silva ED, Sundin OH, et al. Redefining papillorenal syndrome: an underdiagnosed cause of ocular and renal morbidity. Ophthalmology 2001;108:738–749.

125. Wang Y, Xu L, Jonas JB. Prevalence of congenital optic disc pits in adult Chinese: The Beijing Eye Study. Eur J Ophthalmol 2006;16:863–864.

126. Brown GC, Shields JA, Goldberg RE. Congenital pits of the optic nerve head. II. Clinical studies in humans. Ophthalmology 1980;87:51–65.

127. Kranenburg EW. Crater-like holes in the optic disc and central serous retinopathy. Arch Ophthalmol 1960;64:912–924.

128. Hirakata A, Hida T, Ogasawara A, et al. Multilayered retinoschisis associated with optic disc pit. Jpn J Ophthalmol 2005;49:414–416.

129. Karacorlu SA, Karacorlu M, Ozdemir H, et al. Optical coherence tomography in optic pit maculopathy. Int Ophthalmol 2007;27:293–297.

130. Doyle E, Trivedi D, Good P, et al. High resolution optical coherence tomography demonstration of membranes spanning optic disc pits and colobomas. Br J Ophthalmol 2009;93:360–365.

131. Healey PR, Mitchell P. The prevalence of optic disc pits and their relationship to glaucoma. J Glaucoma 2008;17:11–14.

132. Cashwell LF, Ford JG. Central visual field changes associated with acquired pits of the optic nerve. Ophthalmology 1995;102:1270–1278.

133. Srinivasan G, Venkatesh P, Garg S. Optical coherence tomographic characteristics in morning glory disc anomaly. Can J Ophthalmol 2007;42:307–309.

134. Kinder P. Morning glory syndrome: unusual congenital optic disk anomaly. Am J Ophthalmol 1970;69:376–384.

135. Brodsky MC, Wilson RS. Retinal arteriovenous communications in the morning glory disc anomaly. Ophthalmol 1995;113:410–411.

136. Brodsky MC. Contractile morning glory disc causing transient monocular blindness in a child. Arch Ophthalmol 2006;124:1199–1201.

137. Pollock S. The morning glory disc anomaly: contractile movement, classification, and embryogenesis. Doc Ophthalmol 1987;65:439–460.

138. Bakri SJ, Siker D, Masaryk T, et al. Ocular malformations, moyamoya disease, and midline cranial defects: a distinct syndrome. Am J Ophthalmol 1999;127:356–357.

139. Hanson RR, Price RL, Rothner AD, et al. Developmental anomalies of the optic disc and carotid circulation: a new association. J Clin Neuroophthalmol 1985;5:3–8.

140. Loddenkemper T, Friedman NR, Ruggieri PM, et al. Pituitary stalk duplication in association with moya moya disease and bilateral morning glory disc anomaly: broadening the clinical spectrum of midline defects. J Neurol 2008;255:885–890.

141. Massaro M, Thorarensen O, Liu GT, et al. Morning glory disc anomaly and moyamoya vessels. Arch Ophthalmol 1998;116:253–254.

142. Murphy MA, Perlman EM, Rogg JM, et al. Reversible carotid artery narrowing in morning glory disc anomaly. J Neuroophthalmol 2005;25:198–201.

143. Quah BL, Hamilton J, Blaser S, et al. Morning glory disc anomaly, midline cranial defects and abnormal carotid circulation: an association worth looking for. Pediatr Radiol 2005;35:525–528.

144. Lenhart PD, Lambert SR, Newman NJ, et al. Intracranial vascular anomalies in patients with morning glory disk anomaly. Am J Ophthalmol 2006;142:644–650.

145. Goldhammer Y, Smith JL. Optic nerve anomalies in basal encephalocele. Arch Ophthalmol 1975;93:115–118.

146. Chen CS, David D, Hanieh A. Morning glory syndrome and basal encephalocele. Childs Nerv Syst 2004;20:87–90.

147. Komiyama M, Yasui T, Sakamoto H, et al. Basal meningoencephalocele, anomaly of optic disc and panhypopituitarism in association with moyamoya disease. Pediatr Neurosurg 2000;33:100–104.

148. Brodsky MC, Landau K, Wilson RS, et al. Morning glory disc anomaly in neurofibromatosis type 2. Arch Ophthalmol 1999;117:839–841.

149. Murphy BL. Optic nerve coloboma (morning glory syndrome): CT findings. Radiology 1994;91:59–61.

150. Kim SH, Choi MY, Yu YS, et al. Peripapillary staphyloma: clinical features and visual outcome in 19 cases. Arch Ophthalmol 2005;123:1371–1376.

151. Auw-Haedrich C, Staubach F, Witschel H. Optic disk drusen. Surv Ophthalmol 2002;47:515–532.

152. Lorentzen SE. Drusen of the optic disc. A clinical and genetic study. Acta Ophthalmol 1966;Suppl 90:1–180.

153. Savino PJ, Glaser JS, Rosenberg MA. A clinical analysis of pseudopapilledema. II. Visual field defects. Arch Ophthalmol 1979;97:71–75.

154. Wilkins JM, Pomeranz HD. Visual manifestations of visible and buried optic disc drusen. J Neuroophthalmol 2004;24:125–129.

155. Roh S, Noecker RJ, Schuman JS, et al. Effect of optic nerve head drusen on nerve fiber layer thickness. Ophthalmology 1998;105:878–885.

156. Katz BJ, Pomeranz HD. Visual field defects and retinal nerve fiber layer defects in eyes with buried optic nerve drusen. Am J Ophthalmol 2006;141:248–253.

157. Ocakoglu O, Ustundag C, Koyluoglu N, et al. Long term follow-up of retinal nerve fiber layer thickness in eyes with optic nerve head drusen. Curr Eye Res 2003;26:277–280.

158. Gittinger JW, Lessell S, Bondar RL. Ischemic optic neuropathy associated with disc drusen. J Clin Neuroophthalmol 1984;4:79–84.

159. Michaelson C, Behrens M, Odel J. Bilateral anterior ischemic optic neuropathy associated with optic disc drusen and systemic hypotension. Br J Ophthalmol 1989;73:762–764.

160. Moody TA, Irvine AR, Cahn PH, et al. Sudden visual field constriction associated with optic disc drusen. J Clin Neuroophthalmol 1993;13:8–13.

161. Sarkies NJ, Sanders MD. Optic disc drusen and episodic visual loss. Br J Ophthalmol 1987;71:537–539.

162. Beck RW, Corbett JJ, Thompson HS, et al. Decreased visual acuity from optic disc drusen. Arch Ophthalmol 1985;103:1155–1159.

163. Newman WD, Dorrell ED. Anterior ischemic optic neuropathy associated with disc drusen. J Neuroophthalmol 1996;16:7–8.

164. Purvin V, King R, Kawasaki A, et al. Anterior ischemic optic neuropathy in eyes with optic disc drusen. Arch Ophthalmol 2004;122:48–53.

165. Sullu Y, Yildiz L, Erkan D. Submacular surgery for choroidal neovascularization secondary to optic disc drusen. Am J Ophthalmol 2003;136:367–370.

166. Straatsma BR, Foos RY, Heckenlively JR, et al. Myelinated retinal nerve fibers. Am J Ophthalmol 1981;91:25–38.

167. Kee C, Hwang JM. Visual prognosis of amblyopia associated with myelinated retinal nerve fibers. Am J Ophthalmol 2005;139:259–265.

168. Jean-Louis G, Katz BJ, Digre KB, et al. Acquired and progressive retinal nerve fiber layer myelination in an adolescent. Am J Ophthalmol 2000;130:361–362.

169. Newman NJ. Hereditary optic neuropathies: from the mitochondria to the optic nerve. Am J Ophthalmol 2005;140:517–523.

170. Leber T. Ueber hereditare und congenital angelegte Sehnervenleiden. Albrecht von Graefes Arch Klin Exp Ophthalmol 1871;17:249–291.

171. Newman NJ, Lott MT, Wallace DC. The clinical characteristics of pedigrees of Leber's hereditary optic neuropathy with the 11778 mutation. Am J Ophthalmol 1991;111:750–762.

172. Nikoskelainen E, Hoyt WF, Nummelin K. Ophthalmoscopic findings in Leber's hereditary optic neuropathy. I. Fundus findings in asymptomatic family members. Arch Ophthalmol 1982;100:1597–1602.

173. Nikoskelainen EK, Savontaus ML, Wanne OP. Leber's hereditary optic neuroretinopathy, a maternally inherited disease: a genealogical study in four pedigrees. Arch Ophthalmol 1987;105:665–671.

174. Carroll WM, Mastaglia FL. Leber's optic neuropathy: a clinical and visual evoked potential study of affected and asymptomatic members of a six generation family. Brain 1979;102:559–580.

175. Smith JL, Hoyt WF, Susac JO. Ocular fundus in acute Leber optic neuropathy. Arch Ophthalmol 1973;90:349–354.

176. Newman-Toker DE, Horton JC, Lessell S. Recurrent visual loss in Leber hereditary optic neuropathy. Arch Ophthalmol 2003;121:288–291.

177. Newman NJ, Biousse V, Newman SA, et al. Progression of visual field defects in leber hereditary optic neuropathy: experience of the LHON treatment trial. Am J Ophthalmol 2006;141:1061–1067.

178. Jacobson DM, Stone EM, Miller NR, et al. Relative afferent pupillary defects in patients with Leber hereditary optic neuropathy and unilateral visual loss. Am J Ophthalmol 1998;126:291–295.

179. Lüdtke H, Kriegbaum C, Leo-Kottler B, et al. Pupillary light reflexes in patients with Leber's hereditary optic neuropathy. Graefes Arch Clin Exp Ophthalmol 1999;237:207–211.

180. Nikoskelainen E, Sogg RL, Rosenthal AR, et al. The early phase in Leber hereditary optic atrophy. Arch Ophthalmol 1977;95:969–978.

181. Barboni P, Savini G, Valentino ML, et al. Retinal nerve fiber layer evaluation by optical coherence tomography in Leber's hereditary optic neuropathy. Ophthalmology 2005;112:120–126.

182. Acaroglu G, Kansu T, Dogulu CF. Visual recovery patterns in children with Leber's hereditary optic neuropathy. Int Ophthalmol 2001;24:349–355.

183. Lessell S, Gise RL, Krohel GB. Bilateral optic neuropathy with remission in young men: variation on a theme by Leber? Arch Neurol 1983;40:2–6.

184. Nakamura M, Yamamoto M. Variable pattern of visual recovery of Leber's hereditary optic neuropathy. Br J Ophthalmol 2000;84:534–535.

185. Yamada K, Mashima Y, Kigasawa K, et al. High incidence of visual recovery among four Japanese patients with Leber's hereditary optic neuropathy with the 14484 mutation. J Neuroophthalmol 1997;17:103–107.

186. Kermode AG, Moseley IF, Kendall BE, et al. Magnetic resonance imaging in Leber's optic neuropathy. J Neurol Neurosurg Psychiat 1989;52:671–674.

187. Phillips PH, Vaphiades M, Glasier CM, et al. Chiasmal enlargement and optic nerve enhancement on magnetic resonance imaging in leber hereditary optic neuropathy. Arch Ophthalmol 2003;121:577–579.

188. Vaphiades MS, Phillips PH, Turbin RE. Optic nerve and chiasmal enhancement in Leber hereditary optic neuropathy. J Neuroophthalmol 2003;23:104–105.

189. Bhatti MT, Newman NJ. A multiple sclerosis-like illness in a man harboring the mtDNA 14484 mutation. J Neuroophthalmol 1999;19:28–33.

190. Kuker W, Weir A, Quaghebeur G, et al. White matter changes in Leber's hereditary optic neuropathy: MRI findings. Eur J Neurol 2007;14:591–593.

191. Olsen NK, Hansen AW, Norby S, et al. Leber's hereditary optic neuropathy associated with a disorder indistinguishable from multiple sclerosis in a male harbouring the mitochondrial DNA 11778 mutation. Acta Neurol Scand 1995;91:326–329.

192. Palan A, Stehouwer A, Went LN. Studies on Leber's optic neuropathy III. Doc Ophthalmol 1989;71:77–87.

193. Parry-Jones AR, Mitchell JD, Gunarwardena WJ, et al. Leber's hereditary optic neuropathy associated with multiple sclerosis: Harding's syndrome. Pract Neurol 2008;8:118–121.

194. Perez F, Anne O, Debruxelles S, et al. Leber's optic neuropathy associated with disseminated white matter disease: a case report and review. Clin Neurol Neurosurg 2009;111:83–86.

195. Vanopdenbosch L, Dubois B, D'Hooghe MB, et al. Mitochondrial mutations of Leber's hereditary optic neuropathy: a risk factor for multiple sclerosis. J Neurol 2000;247:535–543.

196. Nikoskelainen E, Wanne O, Dahl M. Pre-excitation syndrome and Leber's hereditary optic neuropathy. Lancet 1985;1:696.

197. Ortiz RG, Newman NJ, Manoukian SV, et al. Optic disk cupping and electrocardiographic abnormalities in an American pedigree with Leber's hereditary optic neuropathy. Am J Ophthalmol 1992;113:561–566.

198. Rose FC, Bowden AN, Bowden P. The heart in Leber's optic atrophy. Br J Ophthalmol 1970;54:388–393.

199. Sorajja P, Sweeney MG, Chalmers R, et al. Cardiac abnormalities in patients with Leber's hereditary optic neuropathy. Heart 2003;89:791–792.

200. Singh G, Lott MT, Wallace DC. A mitochondrial DNA mutation as a cause of Leber's hereditary optic neuropathy. N Engl J Med 1989;320:1300–1305.

201. Wallace DC, Singh G, Lott MT, et al. Mitochondrial DNA mutation associated with Leber's hereditary optic neuropathy. Science 1988;242:1427–1430.

202. Howell N, Kubacka I, Xu M, et al. Leber hereditary optic neuropathy: involvement of the mitochondrial ND1 gene and evidence for an intragenic suppressor mutation. Am J Hum Genet 1991;48:935–942.

203. Johns DR, Heher KL, Miller NR, et al. Leber's hereditary optic neuropathy: clinical characteristics of the 14484 mutation. Arch Ophthalmol 1993;111:495–498.

204. Johns DR, Neufield MJ. An ND-6 mitochondrial DNA mutation associated with Leber's hereditary optic neropathy. Biochem Biophys Res Commun 1992;187:1551–1557.

205. Johns DR, Smith KH, Miller NR. Leber's hereditary optic neuropathy: clinical characteristics of the 3460 mutation. Arch Ophthalmol 1992;110:1577–1581.

206. Johns DR, Smith KH, Savino PJ, et al. Leber's hereditary optic neuropathy: clinical characteristics of the 15257 mutation. Ophthalmology 1993;100:981–986.

207. Zhang S, Wang L, Hao Y, et al. T14484C and T14502C in the mitochondrial ND6 gene are associated with Leber's hereditary optic neuropathy in a Chinese family. Mitochondrion 2008;8:205–210.

208. Pezzi PP, De Negri AM, Sadun F, et al. Childhood Leber's hereditary optic neuropathy (ND1/3460) with visual recovery. Pediatr Neurol 1998;19:308–312.

209. Cock HR, Tabrizi SJ, Cooper JM, et al. The influence of nuclear background on the biochemical expression of 3460 Leber's hereditary optic neuropathy. Ann Neurol 1998;44:187–193.

210. Carelli V, Ghelli A, Bucchi L, et al. Biochemical features of mtDNA 14484 (ND6/M64V) point mutation associated with Leber's hereditary optic neuropathy. Ann Neurol 1999;45:320–328.

211. Hudson G, Keers S, Yu Wai Man P, et al. Identification of an X-chromosomal locus and haplotype modulating the phenotype of a mitochondrial DNA disorder. Am J Hum Genet 2005;77:1086–1091.

212. Ishikawa K, Funayama T, Ohde H, et al. Genetic variants of TP53 and EPHX1 in Leber's hereditary optic neuropathy and their relationship to age at onset. Jpn J Ophthalmol 2005;49:121–126.

213. Larsson NG. Leber hereditary optic neuropathy: a nuclear solution of a mitochondrial problem. Ann Neurol 2002;52:529–530.

214. Shankar SP, Fingert JH, Carelli V, et al. Evidence for a novel x-linked modifier locus for Leber's hereditary optic neuropathy. Ophthalmic Genet 2008;29:17–24.

215. Yen MY, Wang AG, Wei YH. Leber's hereditary optic neuropathy: a multifactorial disease. Prog Retin Eye Res 2006;25:381–396.

216. Ramos Cdo V, Bellusci C, Savini G, et al. Association of optic disc size with development and prognosis of Leber's hereditary optic neuropathy. Invest Ophthalmol Vis Sci 2009;50:1666–1674.

217. Spruijt L, Kolbach DN, de Coo RF, et al. Influence of mutation type on clinical expression of Leber hereditary optic neuropathy. Am J Ophthalmol 2006;141:676–682.

218. Bresolin N, Bet L, Binda A, et al. Clinical and biochemical correlations in mitochondrial myopathies treated with coenzyme Q10. Neurology 1988;38:892–899.

219. Shoffner JM, Lott MT, Voljavec AS, et al. Spontaneous Kearns-Sayre/chronic external ophthalmoplegia plus syndrome associated with a mitochondrial DNA deletion: a slip-replication model and metabolic therapy. Proc Natl Acad Sci USA 1989;86:7952–7956.

220. Wallace DC. Mitochondrial DNA mutations and neuromuscular disease. Trends Genet 1989;5:9–13.

221. Guy J, Qi X, Pallotti F, et al. Rescue of a mitochondrial deficiency causing Leber hereditary optic neuropathy. Ann Neurol 2002;52:534–542.

222. Kjer P. Infantile optic atrophy with dominant mode of inheritance: a clinical and genetic study of 19 Danish families. Acta Ophthalmol (Suppl 54):1–46.

223. Kjer B, Eiberg H, Kjer P, et al. Dominant optic atrophy mapped to chromosome 3q region. II. Clinical and epidemiological aspects. Acta Ophthalmol Scand 1996;74:3–7.

224. Votruba M, Fitzke FW, Holder GE, et al. Clinical features in affected individuals from 21 pedigrees with dominant optic atrophy. Arch Ophthalmol 1998;116:793–800.

225. Cohn AC, Toomes C, Hewitt AW, et al. The natural history of OPA1-related autosomal dominant optic atrophy. Br J Ophthalmol 2008;92:1333–1336.

226. Elliot D, Traboulsi EI, Maumenee IH. Visual prognosis in autosomal dominant optic atrophy. Am J Ophthalmol 1993;115:360–367.

227. Kline LB, Glaser JS. Dominant optic atrophy: the clinical profile. Arch Ophthalmol 1979;97:1680–1686.

228. Hoyt CS. Autosomal dominant optic atrophy: a spectrum of disability. Ophthalmology 1980;87:245–251.

229. Votruba M, Thiselton D, Bhattacharya SS. Optic disc morphology of patients with OPA1 autosomal dominant optic atrophy. Br J Ophthalmol 2003;87:48–53.

230. Amati-Bonneau P, Guichet A, Olichon A, et al. OPA1 R445H mutation in optic atrophy associated with sensorineural deafness. Ann Neurol 2005;58:958–963.

231. Amati-Bonneau P, Odent S, Derrien C, et al. The association of autosomal dominant optic atrophy and moderate deafness may be due to the R445H mutation in the OPA1 gene. Am J Ophthalmol 2003;136:1170–1171.

232. Ito Y, Nakamura M, Yamakoshi T, et al. Reduction of inner retinal thickness in patients with autosomal dominant optic atrophy associated with OPA1 mutations. Invest Ophthalmol Vis Sci 2007;48:4079–4086.

233. Eiberg H, Kjer B, Kjer P, et al. Dominant optic atrophy (OPA1) mapped to chromosome 3q region. I. Linkage analysis. Hum Mol Genet 1994;3:977–980.

234. Brown J, Finger JH, Taylor CM, et al. Clinical and genetic analysis of a family affected with dominant optic atrophy (OPA1). Arch Ophthalmol 1997;115:95–103.

235. Delettre C, Griffoin JM, Kaplan J, et al. Mutation spectrum and splicing variants in the OPA1 gene. Hum Genet 2001;109:584–591.

236. Delettre C, Lenaers G, Belenguer P, et al. Gene structure and chromosomal localization of mouse Opa1: its exclusion from the Bst locus. BMC Genet 2003;4:8.

237. Delettre C, Lenaers G, Griffoin JM, et al. Nuclear gene OPA1, encoding a mitochondrial dynamin-related protein, is mutated in dominant optic atrophy. Nat Genet 2000;26:207–210.

238. Delettre C, Lenaers G, Pelloquin L, et al. OPA1 (Kjer type) dominant optic atrophy: a novel mitochondrial disease. Mol Genet Metab 2002;75:97–107.

239. Johnston RL, Burdon MA, Spalton DJ, et al. Dominant optic atrophy, Kjer type. Linkage analysis and clinical features in a large British pedigree. Arch Ophthalmol 1997;117:100–103.

240. Kerrison JB, Arnould VJ, Ferraz Sallum JM, et al. Genetic heterogeneity of dominant optic atrophy, Kjer type: identification of a second locus on chromosome 18q12.2–12.3. Arch Ophthalmol 1999;117:805–810.

241. Wiggs JL. Genomic mapping of Kjer dominant optic atrophy. Arch Ophthalmol 1997;115:115–116.

242. Johnston RL, Seller MJ, Behnam JT, et al. Dominant optic atrophy. Refining the clinical diagnostic criteria in light of genetic linkage studies. Ophthalmology 1999;106:123–128.

243. Votruba M, Moore AT, Bhattacharya SS. Clinical features, molecular genetics, and pathophysiology of dominant optic atrophy. J Med Genet 1998;35:793–800.

244. Nakamura M, Lin J, Ueno S, et al. Novel mutations in the OPA1 gene and associated clinical features in Japanese patients with optic atrophy. Ophthalmology 2006;113:483–488.

245. Cohn AC, Toomes C, Potter C, et al. Autosomal dominant optic atrophy: penetrance and expressivity in patients with OPA1 mutations. Am J Ophthalmol 2007;143:656–662.

246. Amati-Bonneau P, Valentino ML, Reynier P, et al. OPA1 mutations induce mitochondrial DNA instability and optic atrophy "plus" phenotypes. Brain 2008;131:338–351.

247. Chinnery PF, Griffiths PG. Optic mitochondriopathies. Neurology 2005;64:940–941.

248. Kim JY, Hwang JM, Ko HS, et al. Mitochondrial DNA content is decreased in autosomal dominant optic atrophy. Neurology 2005;64:966–972.

249. Johnston PB, Glaser RN, Smith VC, et al. A clinicopathologic study of autosomal dominant optic atrophy. Am J Ophthalmol 1979;88:868–875.

250. Waardenburg PJ. Different types of hereditary optic atrophy. Acta Genet Statist Med 1957;7:287–290.

251. Behr C. Die Komplizierte, Hereditar-familare optikusatrophie des kindesalters: Ein bisher nicht beschriebener symptomkomplex. Klin Monatsbl Augenheilkd 1909;47:138–160.

252. Horoupian DS, Zuker DK, Moshe S, et al. Behr syndrome: a clinicopathologic report. Neurology 1979;29:323.

253. Wolfram DJ. Diabetes mellitus and simple optic atrophy among siblings. Mayo Clin Proc 1938;13:715–717.

254. Lessell S, Rosman NP. Juvenile diabetes mellitus and atrophy. Arch Neurol 1977;34:759–765.

255. Hardy C, Khanim F, Torres R, et al. Clinical and molecular genetic analysis of 19 Wolfram syndrome kindreds demonstrating a wide spectrum of mutations in WFS1. Am J Hum Genet 1999;65:1279–1290.

256. Barrett TG, Bundey SE, Fielder AR, et al. Optic atrophy in Wolfram (DIDMOAD) syndrome. Eye 1997;11:882–888.

257. Genís D, Dávalos A, Molins A, et al. Wolfram syndrome: a neuropathological study. Acta Neuropathologica 1997;93:426–429.

258. Bespalova IN, Van Camp G, Bom SJ, et al. Mutations in the Wolfram syndrome 1 gene (WFS1) are a common cause of low frequency sensorineural hearing loss. Hum Mol Genet 2001;10:2501–2508.

259. Colosimo A, Guida V, Rigoli L, et al. Molecular detection of novel WFS1 mutations in patients with Wolfram syndrome by a DHPLC-based assay. Hum Mutat 2003;21:622–629.

260. Domenech E, Gomez-Zaera M, Nunes V. WFS1 mutations in Spanish patients with diabetes mellitus and deafness. Eur J Hum Genet 2002;10:421–426.

261. Evans KL, Lawson D, Meitinger T, et al. Mutational analysis of the Wolfram syndrome gene in two families with chromosome 4p-linked bipolar affective disorder. Am J Med Genet 2000;96:158–160.

262. Hofmann S, Bauer MF. Wolfram syndrome-associated mutations lead to instability and proteasomal degradation of wolframin. FEBS Lett 2006;580:4000–4004.

263. Inoue H, Tanizawa Y, Wasson J, et al. A gene encoding a transmembrane protein is mutated in patients with diabetes mellitus and optic atrophy (Wolfram syndrome). Nat Genet 1998;20:143–148.

264. Inukai K, Awata T, Inoue K, et al. Identification of a novel WFS1 mutation (AFF344–345ins) in Japanese patients with Wolfram syndrome. Diabetes Res Clin Pract 2005;69:136–141.

265. Lesperance MM, Hall JW, 3rd, San Agustin TB, et al. Mutations in the Wolfram syndrome type 1 gene (WFS1) define a clinical entity of dominant low-frequency sensorineural hearing loss. Arch Otolaryngol Head Neck Surg 2003;129:411–420.

266. Wasson J, Permutt MA. Candidate gene studies reveal that the WFS1 gene joins the expanding list of novel type 2 diabetes genes. Diabetologia 2008;51:391–393.

267. Alldredge CD, Schlieve CR, Miller NR, et al. Pathophysiology of the optic neuropathy associated with Friedreich ataxia. Arch Ophthalmol 2003;121:1582–1585.

268. Carroll WM, Kriss A, Baraitser M, et al. The incidence and nature of visual pathway involvement in Friedreich's ataxia: a clinical and visual evoked potential study of 22 patients. Brain 1980;103:413–434.

269. Livingstone IR, Mastaglia FL, Edis R, et al. Visual involvement in Friedreich's ataxia and hereditary spastic ataxia: a clinical and visual evoked response study. Arch Neurol 1981;38:75–79.

270. Hoyt WF. Charcot-Marie-Tooth disease with primary optic atrophy. Arch Ophthlamol 1960;64:925–928.

271. Kuhlenbaumer G, Young P, Hunermund G, et al. Clinical features and molecular genetics of hereditary peripheral neuropathies. J Neurol 2002;249:1629–1650.

272. Voo I, Allf BE, Udar N, et al. Hereditary motor and sensory neuropathy type VI with optic atrophy. Am J Ophthalmol 2003;136:670–677.

273. Harding AE. Friedreich's ataxia: a clinical and genetic study of 90 families with an analysis of early diagnostic criteria and intrafamilial clustering of clinical features. Brain 1981;104:589–620.

274. Chamberlain S, Shaw J, Rowland A, et al. Mapping of mutation causing Friedreich's ataxia to human chromosome 9. Nature 1988;334:248–250.

275. Fujita R, Agid Y, Trouillas P, et al. Confirmation of linkage of Friedreich ataxia to chromosome 9 and identification of a new closely linked marker. Genomics 1989;4:110–111.

276. Konigsmark BW, Knox DL, Hussels IE, et al. Dominant congenital deafness and progressive optic nerve atrophy. Occurrence in four generations of a family. Arch Ophthalmol 1974;91:99–103.

277. Kollarits CR, Pinheiro ML, Swann ER, et al. The autosomal dominant syndrome of progressive optic atrophy and congenital deafness. Am J Ophthalmol 1979;87:789–792.

278. Burk K, Abele M, Fetter M, et al. Autosomal dominant cerebellar ataxia type I clinical features and MRI in families with SCA1, SCA2 and SCA3. Brain 1996;119 (Pt 5):1497–1505.

279. Lee WY, Jin DK, Oh MR, et al. Frequency analysis and clinical characterization of spinocerebellar ataxia types 1, 2, 3, 6, and 7 in Korean patients. Arch Neurol 2003;60:858–863.

280. Paulson H, Ammache Z. Ataxia and hereditary disorders. Neurol Clin 2001;19:759–782, viii.

281. Rizzo JF, Lessell S. Risk of developing multiple sclerosis after uncomplicated optic neuritis. Neurology 1988;38:185–190.

282. Beck RW, Cleary PA, Anderson MM, et al. A randomized, controlled trial of corticosteroids in the treatment of acute optic neuritis. N Engl J Med 1992;326:581–588.

283. Beck RW, Gal RL. Treatment of acute optic neuritis: a summary of findings from the optic neuritis treatment trial. Arch Ophthalmol 2008;126:994–995.

284. Volpe NJ. The optic neuritis treatment trial: a definitive answer and profound impact with unexpected results. Arch Ophthalmol 2008;126:996–999.

285. Optic Neuritis Study Group. The clinical profile of optic neuritis. Experience of the Optic Neuritis Treatment Trial. Arch Ophthalmol 1991;109:1673–1678.

286. Percy AK, Nobrega FT, Kurland LT. Optic neuritis and multiple sclerosis. An epidemiologic study. Arch Ophthalmol 1972;87:135–139.

287. Wikstrom J. The epidemiology of optic neuritis in Finland. Acta Neurol Scand 1975;52:196–206.

288. Jin Y-P, de Pedro-Cuesta J, Söderström M, et al. Incidence of optic neuritis in Stockholm, Sweden, 1990–1995. Arch Neurol 1999;56:975–980.

289. Pokroy R, Modi G, Saffer D. Optic neuritis in an urban black African community. Eye 2001;15:469–473.

290. Fazzone HE, Lefton DR, Kupersmith MJ. Optic neuritis: correlation of pain and magnetic resonance imaging. Ophthalmology 2003;110:1646–1649.

291. Lepore FE. The origin of pain in optic neuritis. Arch Neurol 1991;48:748–749.

292. Davis FA, Bergen D, Schauf C, et al. Movement phosphenes in optic neuritis: a new clinical sign. Neurology 1976;26:1100–1104.

293. Lessell S, Cohen MM. Phosphenes induced by sound. Neurology 1979;29:1524–1526.

294. Swerdloff MA, Zieker AW, Krohel GB. Movement phosphenes in optic neuritis. J Clin Neuroophthalmol 1981;1:279–282.

295. Uhthoff W. Untersuchungen uber die bei der multiplen Herdsklerose vorkommenden Augenstorungen. Arch Psychiatry 1889;21:303.

296. Scholl GB, Song HS, Wray SH. Uhthoff's symptom in optic neuritis: relationship to magnetic resonance imaging and development of multiple sclerosis. Ann Neurol 1991;30:180–184.

297. Lepore FE. Uhthoff's symptom in disorders of the anterior visual pathways. Neurology 1994;44:1036–1038.

298. Haupert CL, Newman NJ. Prolonged Uhthoff phenomenon in sarcoidosis. Am J Ophthalmol 1997;124:564–566.

299. Katz B. The dyschromatopsia of optic neuritis: a descriptive analysis of data from the optic neuritis treatment trial. Trans Am Ophthalmol Soc 1995;93:685–708.

300. Trobe JD, Beck RW, Moke PS, et al. Contrast sensitivity and other vision tests in the optic neuritis treatment trial. Am J Ophthalmol 1996;121:547–553.

301. Rizzo JF, Lessell S. Optic neuritis and ischemic optic neuropathy: overlapping clinical profiles. Arch Ophthalmol 1991;100:1668–1672.

302. Beck RW, Kupersmith MJ, Cleary PA, et al. Fellow eye abnormalities in acute unilateral optic neuritis. Experience of the optic neuritis treatment trial. Ophthalmology 1993;100:691–697.

303. Beck RW, Trobe JD, Moke PS, et al. High- and low-risk profiles for the development of multiple sclerosis within 10 years after optic neuritis: experience of the optic neuritis treatment trial. Arch Ophthalmol 2003;121:944–949.

304. de la Cruz J, Kupersmith MJ. Clinical profile of simultaneous bilateral optic neuritis in adults. Br J Ophthalmol 2006;90:551–554.

305. Beck RW, Arrington J, Murtagh FR. Brain MRI in acute optic neuritis. Experience of the Optic Neuritis Study Group. Arch Neurol 1993;8:841–846.

306. Morrissey SP, Miller DH, Kendall BE, et al. The significance of brain magnetic resonance imaging abnormalities at presentation with clinically isolated syndromes suggestive of multiple sclerosis. Brain 1993;116:135–146.

307. Rizzo IIIrd JF, Andreoli CM, Rabinov JD. Use of magnetic resonance imaging to differentiate optic neuritis and nonarteritic anterior ischemic optic neuropathy. Ophthalmology 2002;109:1679–1684.

308. Dunker S, Wiegand W. Prognostic value of magnetic resonance imaging in monosymptomatic optic neuritis. Ophthalmology 1996;103:1768–1773.

309. Kupersmith MJ, Alban T, Zeiffer B, et al. Contrast-enhanced MRI in acute optic neuritis: relationship to visual performance. Brain 2002;125:812–822.

310. Fraser CL, Klistorner A, Graham SL, et al. Multifocal visual evoked potential analysis of inflammatory or demyelinating optic neuritis. Ophthalmology 2006;113:323. e321–323.

311. Trapp BD, Peterson J, Ransohoff RM, et al. Axonal transection in the lesions of multiple sclerosis. N Engl J Med 1998;338:278–285.

312. Frohman EM, Frohman TC, Zee DS, et al. The neuro-ophthalmology of multiple sclerosis. Lancet Neurol 2005;4:111–121.

313. Costello F, Coupland S, Hodge W, et al. Quantifying axonal loss after optic neuritis with optical coherence tomography. Ann Neurol 2006;59:963–969.

314. Trip SA, Schlottmann PG, Jones SJ, et al. Retinal nerve fiber layer axonal loss and visual dysfunction in optic neuritis. Ann Neurol 2005;58:383–391.

315. Zaveri MS, Conger A, Salter A, et al. Retinal imaging by laser polarimetry and optical coherence tomography evidence of axonal degeneration in multiple sclerosis. Arch Neurol 2008;65:924–928.

316. Rolak LA, Beck RW, Paty DW, et al. Cerebrospinal fluid in acute optic neuritis: experience of the optic neuritis treatment trial. Neurology 1996;46:368–372.

317. Cole SR, Beck RW, Moke PS, et al. The predictive value of CSF oligoclonal banding for MS 5 years after optic neuritis. Optic Neuritis Study Group. Neurology 1998;51:885–887.

318. Masjuan J, Alvarez-Cermeno JC, Garcia-Barragan N, et al. Clinically isolated syndromes: a new oligoclonal band test accurately predicts conversion to MS. Neurology 2006;66:576–578.

319. Söderström M, Ya-Ping J, Hillert J, et al. Optic neuritis. Prognosis for multiple sclerosis from MRI, CSF, and HLA findings. Neurology 1998;50:708–714.

320. Tumani H, Tourtellotte WW, Peter JB, et al. Acute optic neuritis: combined immunological markers and magnetic resonance imaging predict subsequent development of multiple sclerosis. The Optic Neuritis Study Group. J Neurol Sci 1998;155:44–49.

321. Beck RW, Cleary PA, the Optic Neuritis Study Group. Optic neuritis treatment trial. One year follow-up results. Arch Ophthalmol 1993;111:773–775.

322. Kapoor R, Miller DH, Jones SJ, et al. Effects of intravenous methylprednisolone on outcome in MRI-based prognostic subgroups in acute optic neuritis. Neurology 1998;50:230–237.

323. Optic Neuritis Study Group. Visual function five years after optic neuritis: experience of the Optic Neuritis Treatment Trial. Arch Ophthalmol 1997;115:1545–1552.

324. Beck RW, Gal RL, Bhatti MT, et al. Visual function more than 10 years after optic neuritis: experience of the optic neuritis treatment trial. Am J Ophthalmol 2004;137:77–83.

325. Visual function 15 years after optic neuritis: a final follow-up report from the Optic Neuritis Treatment Trial. Ophthalmology 2008;115:1079–1082.

326. Beck RW, Cleary PA, Backlund JC, et al. The course of visual recovery after optic neuritis. Experience of the optic neuritis treatment trial. Ophthalmology 1994;101:1771–1778.

327. Kupersmith MJ, Gal RL, Beck RW, et al. Visual function at baseline and 1 month in acute optic neuritis: predictors of visual outcome. Neurology 2007;69:508–514.

328. Slamovits TL, Rosen CE, Cheng KP, et al. Visual recovery in patients with optic neuritis and visual loss to no light perception. Am J Ophthalmol 1991;111:209–214.

329. Cleary PA, Beck RW, Bourque LB, et al. Visual symptoms after optic neuritis. Results from the Optic Neuritis Treatment Trial. J Neuroophthalmol 1997;17:18–23.

330. Fleishman JA, Beck RW, Linares OA, et al. Deficits in visual function after resolution of optic neuritis. Ophthalmology 1987;94:1029–1035.

331. Ma SL, Shea JA, Galetta SL, et al. Self-reported visual dysfunction in multiple sclerosis: new data from the VFQ-25 and development of an MS-specific vision questionnaire. Am J Ophthalmol 2002;133:686–692.

332. Raphael BA, Galetta KM, Jacobs DA, et al. Validation and test characteristics of a 10-item neuro-ophthalmic supplement to the NEI-VFQ-25. Am J Ophthalmol 2006;142:1026–1035.

333. Phillips PH, Newman NJ, Lynn MJ. Optic neuritis in African Americans. Arch Neurol 1998;55:186–192.

334. Biousse V, Trichet C, Bloch-Michel E, et al. Multiple sclerosis associated with uveitis in two large clinic-based series. Neurology 1999;52:179–181.

335. Confavreux C, Hutchinson M, Hours MM, et al. Rate of pregnancy-related relapse in multiple sclerosis. N Engl J Med 1998;339:285–291.

336. Lucchinetti CF, Rodriguez M. The controversy surrounding the pathogenesis of the multiple sclerosis lesion. Mayo Clin Proc 1997;72:665–678.

337. Gonen O, Catalaa I, Babb JS, et al. Total brain N-acetylaspartate. A new measure of disease load in MS. Neurology 2000;54:15–19.

338. Rudick RA, Cohen JA, Weinstock-Guttman B, et al. Management of multiple sclerosis. N Engl J Med 1997;337:1604–1611.

339. Arnason BGW. Pathophysiology of multiple sclerosis: finding the mechanisms of demyelination. Adv Neuroimmunol 1996;3:13–18.

340. Hafler DA, Compston A, Sawcer S, et al. Risk alleles for multiple sclerosis identified by a genomewide study. N Engl J Med 2007;357:851–862.

341. Barkhof F, Filippi M, Miller DH, et al. Comparison of MRI criteria at first presentation to predict conversion to clinically definite multiple sclerosis. Brain 1997;120:2059–2069.

342. Tintore M, Rovira A, Martinez MJ, et al. Isolated demyelinating syndromes: comparison of different MR imaging criteria to predict conversion to clinically definite multiple sclerosis. AJNR Am J Neuroradiol 2000;21:702–706.

343. McDonald WI, Compston A, Edan G, et al. Recommended diagnostic criteria for multiple sclerosis: guidelines from the International Panel on the diagnosis of multiple sclerosis. Ann Neurol 2001;50:121–127.

344. Polman CH, Reingold SC, Edan G, et al. Diagnostic criteria for multiple sclerosis: 2005 revisions to the "McDonald Criteria." Ann Neurol 2005;58:840–846.

345. Rudick RA. Disease-modifying drugs for relapsing-remitting multiple sclerosis and future directions for multiple sclerosis therapeutics. Arch Neurol 1999;56:1079–1084.

346. Comi G, Filippi M, Wolinsky JS. European/Canadian multicenter, double-blind, randomized, placebo-controlled study of the effects of glatiramer acetate on magnetic resonance imaging: measured disease activity and burden in patients with relapsing multiple sclerosis. European/Canadian Glatiramer Acetate Study Group. Ann Neurol 2001;49:290–297.

347. Jacobs LD, Cookfair DL, Rudick RA, et al. Intramuscular interferon beta-1a for disease progression in relapsing multiple sclerosis. Ann Neurol 1996;39:285–294.

348. Johnson KP, Brooks BR, Cohen JA, et al. Copolymer 1 reduces relapse rate and improves disability in relapsing-remitting multiple sclerosis: results of a phase III multicenter, double-blind, placebo-controlled trial. Neurology 1995;45:1268–1276.

349. Johnson KP, Brooks BR, Cohen JA, et al. Extended use of glatiramer acetate (Copaxone) is well tolerated and maintains its clinical effect on multiple sclerosis relapse rate and degree of disability. Neurology 1998;50:701–708.

350. Li DKB, Paty DW, et al., UBC MS/MRI Analysis Research Group. Magnetic resonance imaging results of the PRISMS trial: a randomized, double-blind, placebo-controlled study of interferon-beta 1a in relapsing-remitting multiple sclerosis. Ann Neurol 1999;46:197–206.

351. Paty DW, Li DKB, et al., the UBC MS/MRI Study Group. Interferon beta-1b is effective in relapsing-remitting multiple sclerosis. II. MRI analysis results of a multicenter, randomized, double-blind, placebo-controlled trial. Neurology 1993;43:662–667.

352. Simon JH, Jacobs LD, Campion M, et al. Magnetic resonance studies of intramuscular interferon beta-1a for relapsing multiple sclerosis. Ann Neurol 1998;43:79–87.

353. The IFNB Multiple Sclerosis Study Group. Interferon beta-1b is effective in relapsing-remitting multiple sclerosis. I. Clinical results of a multicenter, randomized, double-blind, placebo-controlled trial. Neurology 1993;43:655–661.

354. The IFNB Multiple Sclerosis Study Group and the University of British Columbia MS/MRI Analysis Group. Interferon beta-1b in the treatment of multiple sclerosis. Final outcome of the randomized controlled trial. Neurology 1995;45:1277–1285.

355. Zhao GJ, Koopmans RA, Li DKB, et al. Effect of interferon beta-1b in MS. Assessment of annual accumulation of PD/T2 activity on MRI. Neurology 2000;54:200–206.

356. Rudick RA, Goodkin DE, Jacobs LD, et al. Impact of interferon beta-1a on neurologic disability in relapsing multiple sclerosis. Neurology 1997;49:358–363.

357. Polman CH, O'Connor PW, Havrdova E, et al. A randomized, placebo-controlled trial of natalizumab for relapsing multiple sclerosis. N Engl J Med 2006;354:899–910.

358. Yousry TA, Major EO, Ryschkewitsch C, et al. Evaluation of patients treated with natalizumab for progressive multifocal leukoencephalopathy. N Engl J Med 2006;354:924–933.

359. Pittock SJ, Lennon VA, Krecke K, et al. Brain abnormalities in neuromyelitis optica. Arch Neurol 2006;63:390–396.

360. Frohman EM, Havrdova E, Lublin F, et al. Most patients with multiple sclerosis or a clinically isolated demyelinating syndrome should be treated at the time of diagnosis. Arch Neurol 2006;63:614–619.

361. Jacobs LD, Beck RW, Simon JH, et al. Intramuscular interferon beta-1a therapy initiated during a first demyelinating event in multiple sclerosis. CHAMPS Study Group. N Engl J Med 2000;343:898–904.

362. Brex PA, Ciccarelli O, O'Riordan JI, et al. A longitudinal study of abnormalities on MRI and disability from multiple sclerosis. N Engl J Med 2002;346:158–164.

363. Optic Neuritis Study Group. Multiple sclerosis risk after optic neuritis: final optic neuritis treatment trial follow-up. Arch Neurol 2008;65:727–732.

364. Tintore M, Rovira A, Rio J, et al. Is optic neuritis more benign than other first attacks in multiple sclerosis? Ann Neurol 2005;57:210–215.

365. Tintore M, Rovira A, Rio J, et al. Do oligoclonal bands add information to MRI in first attacks of multiple sclerosis? Neurology 2008;70:1079–1083.

366. Jacobs LD, Kaba SE, Miller CM, et al. Correlation of clinical, magnetic resonance imaging, and cerebrospinal fluid findings in optic neuritis. Ann Neurol 1997;41:392–398.

367. Frederiksen JL, Madsen HO, Ryder LP, et al. HLA typing in acute optic neuritis. Relation to multiple sclerosis and magnetic resonance imaging findings. Arch Neurol 1996;54:76–80.

368. Fisher JB, Jacobs DA, Markowitz CE, et al. Relation of visual function to retinal nerve fiber layer thickness in multiple sclerosis. Ophthalmology 2006;113:324–332.

369. Rebolleda G, Munoz-Negrete FJ, Noval S, et al. New ways to look at an old problem. Surv Ophthalmol 2006;51:169–173.

370. Beck RW, Cleary PA, Trobe JD, et al. The effect of corticosteroids for acute optic neuritis on the subsequent development of multiple sclerosis. N Engl J Med 1993;329:1764–1769.

371. Goodin DS. Treatment of optic neuritis. Neurology 1993;43:2731–2732.

372. Goodin DS. Corticosteroids and optic neuritis. Neurology 1993;43:632–633; author reply 633–634.

373. Goodin DS. Perils and pitfalls in the interpretation of clinical trials: a reflection on the recent experience in multiple sclerosis. Neuroepidemiology 1999;18:53–63.

374. Kaufman DI, Trobe JD, Eggenberger ER, et al. Practice parameter: the role of corticosteroids in the management of acute monosymptomatic optic neuritis. Report of the Quality Standards Subcommittee of the American Academy of Neurology. Neurology 2000;54:2039–2044.

375. Balcer LJ. Clinical practice. Optic neuritis. N Engl J Med 2006;354:1273–1280.

376. Beck RW. The optic neuritis treatment trial. Three year follow up results. Arch Ophthalmol 1995;113:136–137.

377. Chrousos GA, Kattah JC, Beck RW, et al. Side effects of glucocorticoid treatment. Experience in the optic neuritis treatment trial. JAMA 1993;269:2110–2112.

378. Trobe JD, Sieving PC, Guire KE, et al. The impact of the Optic Neuritis Treatment Trial on the practices of ophthalmologists and neurologists. Ophthalmology 1999;106:2047–2053.

379. Trobe JD, Sieving PC, Guire KE, et al. The impact of the optic neuritis treatment trial on the practices of ophthalmologists and neurologists. Ophthalmology 1999;106:2047–2053.

380. Lueck CJ, Danesh-Meyer HV, Margrie FJ, et al. Management of acute optic neuritis: a survey of neurologists and ophthalmologists in Australia and New Zealand. J Clin Neurosci 2008;15:1340–1345.

381. Biousse V, Calvetti O, Drews-Botsch CD, et al. Management of optic neuritis and impact of clinical trials: an international survey. J Neurol Sci 2009;276:69–74.

382. Atkins EJ, Drews-Botsch CD, Newman NJ, et al. Management of optic neuritis in Canada: survey of ophthalmologists and neurologists. Can J Neurol Sci 2008;35:179–184.

383. Comi G, Filippi M, Barkhof F, et al. Effect of early interferon treatment on conversion to definite multiple sclerosis: a randomised study. Lancet 2001;357:1576–1582.

384. Filippi M, Rovaris M, Inglese M, et al. Interferon beta-1a for brain tissue loss in patients at presentation with syndromes suggestive of multiple sclerosis: a randomised, double-blind, placebo-controlled trial. Lancet 2004;364:1489–1496.

385. Kappos L, Polman CH, Freedman MS, et al. Treatment with interferon beta-1b delays conversion to clinically definite and McDonald MS in patients with clinically isolated syndromes. Neurology 2006;67:1242–1249.

386. Sellebjerg F, Nielsen HS, Frederiksen JL, et al. A randomized, controlled trial of oral high-dose methylprednisolone in acute optic neuritis. Neurology 1999;52:1479–1484.

387. van Engelen BGM, Hommes OR, Pinkers A, et al. Improved vision after intravenous immunoglobulin in stable demyelinating optic neuritis [letter]. Ann Neurol 1992;32:834–835.

388. Noseworthy JH, O'Brien PC, Petterson TM, et al. A randomized trial of intravenous immunoglobulin in inflammatory demyelinating optic neuritis. Neurology 2001;56:1514–1522.

389. Achiron A, Kishner I, Sarova-Pinhas I, et al. Intravenous immunoglobulin treatment following the first demyelinating event suggestive of multiple sclerosis: a randomized, double-blind, placebo-controlled trial. Arch Neurol 2004;61:1515–1520.

390. Roed HG, Langkilde A, Sellebjerg F, et al. A double-blind, randomized trial of IV immunoglobulin treatment in acute optic neuritis. Neurology 2005;64:804–810.

391. Ruprecht K, Klinker E, Dintelmann T, et al. Plasma exchange for severe optic neuritis: treatment of 10 patients. Neurology 2004;63:1081–1083.

392. Galetta SL, Bennett J. Neuromyelitis optica is a variant of multiple sclerosis. Arch Neurol 2007;64:901–903.

393. Wingerchuk DM, Hogancamp WF, O'Brien PC, et al. The clinical course of neuromyelitis optica (Devic's syndrome). Neurology 1999;53:1107–1114.

394. Merle H, Olindo S, Bonnan M, et al. Natural history of the visual impairment of relapsing neuromyelitis optica. Ophthalmology 2007;114:810–815.

395. de Seze J, Blanc F, Jeanjean L, et al. Optical coherence tomography in neuromyelitis optica. Arch Neurol 2008;65:920–923.

396. Filippi M, Rocca MA. MR imaging of Devic's neuromyelitis optica. Neurol Sci 2004;25 Suppl 4:S371–373.

397. Lefkowitz D, Angelo JN. Neuromyelitis optica with unusual vascular changes. Arch Neurol 1984;41:1103–1105.

398. Mandler RN, Davis LE, Jeffrey DR, et al. Devic's neuromyelitis optica: a clinicopathological study of 8 patients. Ann Neurol 1993;34:162–168.

399. Whitham RH, Brey RL. Neuromyelitis optica: two new cases and review of the literature. J Clin Neuroophthalmol 1985;5(4):263–269.

400. Lennon VA, Wingerchuk DM, Kryzer TJ, et al. A serum autoantibody marker of neuromyelitis optica: distinction from multiple sclerosis. Lancet 2004;364:2106–2112.

401. Wingerchuk DM, Lennon VA, Pittock SJ, et al. Revised diagnostic criteria for neuromyelitis optica. Neurology 2006;66:1485–1489.

402. Lennon VA, Kryzer TJ, Pittock SJ, et al. IgG marker of optic-spinal multiple sclerosis binds to the aquaporin-4 water channel. J Exp Med 2005;202:473–477.

403. Hamnik SE, Hacein-Bey L, Biller J, et al. Neuromyelitis optica (NMO) antibody positivity in patients with transverse myelitis and no visual manifestations. Semin Ophthalmol 2008;23:191–200.

404. Mandler RN, Ahmed W, Dencoff JE. Devic's neuromyelitis optica: a prospective study of seven patients treated with prednisone and azathioprine. Neurology 1998;51:1219–1220.

405. Cree BA, Lamb S, Morgan K, et al. An open label study of the effects of rituximab in neuromyelitis optica. Neurology 2005;64:1270–1272.

406. Jacob A, Weinshenker BG, Violich I, et al. Treatment of neuromyelitis optica with rituximab: retrospective analysis of 25 patients. Arch Neurol 2008;65:1443–1448.

407. Banwell B, Tenembaum S, Lennon VA, et al. Neuromyelitis optica-IgG in childhood inflammatory demyelinating CNS disorders. Neurology 2008;70:344–352.

408. Hudson LA, Bernard TJ, Tseng BS, et al. Neuromyelitis optica immunoglobulin G in a child. Pediatr Neurol 2006;35:370–372.

409. Jeffery AR, Buncic JR. Pediatric Devic's neuromyelitis optica. J Pediatr Ophthalmol Strabismus 1996;33:223–229.

410. Loma IP, Asato MR, Filipink RA, et al. Neuromyelitis optica in a young child with positive serum autoantibody. Pediatr Neurol 2008;39:209–212.

411. McKeon A, Lennon VA, Lotze T, et al. CNS aquaporin-4 autoimmunity in children. Neurology 2008;71:93–100.

412. April RS, Vansonnenberg E. A case of neuromyelitis optica (Devic's syndrome) in systemic lupus erythematosus. Neurology 1976;26:1066–1070.

413. Arabshahi B, Pollock AN, Sherry DD, et al. Devic disease in a child with primary Sjögren syndrome. J Child Neurol 2006;21:285–286.

414. Silber MH, Willcox PA, Bowen RM, et al. Neuromyelitis optica (Devic's syndrome) and pulmonary tuberculosis. Neurology 1990;40:934–938.

415. O'Riordan JI, Gallagher HL, Thompson AJ, et al. Clinical, CSF, and MRI findings in Devic's neuromelitis optica. J Neurol Neurosurg Psychiatry 1996;60:382–387.

416. Bonhomme GR, Waldman AT, Balcer LJ, et al. Pediatric optic neuritis: brain MRI abnormalities and risk of multiple sclerosis. Neurology 2009;72:881–885.

417. Kennedy C, Carter S. Relation of optic neuritis to multiple sclerosis in children. Pediatrics 1961;28:1253–1258.

418. Kriss A, Francis DA, Cuendet B. Recovery of optic neuritis in childhood. J Neurol Neurosurg Psychiatry 1988;51:1253–1258.

419. Mizota A, Niimura M, Adachi-Usami E. Clinical characteristics of Japanese children with optic neuritis. Pediatr Neurol 2004;31:42–45.

420. Riikonen R, Donner M, Erkkila H. Optic neuritis in children and its relationship to multiple sclerosis: a clinical study of 21 children. Dev Med Child Neurol 1988;30(3):349–359.

421. Kennedy C, Carroll FD. Optic neuritis in children. Arch Ophthalmol 1960;63:747–755.

422. Waldman AT, Balcer LJ. Pediatric optic neuritis. In: Chabas D, Waubant E, eds., Demyelinating disorders of the CNS in childhood. Cambridge University Press, Cambridge (in press).

423. Good WV, Muci-Mendoza R, Berg BO, et al. Optic neuritis in children with poor recovery of vision. Aust N Z J Ophthalmol 1992;20:319–323.

424. Kotlus BS, Slavin ML, Guthrie DS, et al. Ophthalmologic manifestations in pediatric patients with acute disseminated encephalomyelitis. J AAPOS 2005;9:179–183.

425. Tenembaum S, Chitnis T, Ness J, et al. Acute disseminated encephalomyelitis. Neurology 2007;68:S23–36.

426. Menge T, Hemmer B, Nessler S, et al. Acute disseminated encephalomyelitis: an update. Arch Neurol 2005;62:1673–1680.

427. Riikonen R. The role of infection and vaccination in the genesis of optic neuritis and multiple sclerosis in children. Acta Neurol Scand 1989;80:425–431.

428. Farris BK, Pickard DJ. Bilateral postinfectious optic neuritis and intravenous steroid therapy in children. Ophthalmology 1990;97:339–345.

429. Stevenson VL, Acheson JF, Ball J, et al. Optic neuritis following measles/rubella vaccination in two 13-year-old children [letter]. Br J Ophthalmol 1996;80:1110–1111.

430. Purvin V, Hrisomalos N, Dunn D. Varicella optic neuritis. Neurology 1988;38:501–503.

431. Brady KM, Brar AS, Lee AG, et al. Optic neuritis in children: clinical features and visual outcome. J AAPOS 1999;3:98–103.

432. Cakmakli G, Kurne A, Guven A, et al. Childhood optic neuritis: the pediatric neurologist's perspective. Eur J Paediatr Neurol 2009;13:452–457.

433. Lana-Peixoto MA, Andrade GC. The clinical profile of childhood optic neuritis. Arq Neuropsiquiatr 2001;59:311–317.

434. Lucchinetti CF, Kiers L, O'Duffy A, et al. Risk factors for developing multiple sclerosis after childhood optic neuritis. Neurology 1997;49:1413–1418.

435. Visudhiphan P, Chiemchanya S, Santadusit S. Optic neuritis in children: recurrence and subsequent development of multiple sclerosis. Pediatr Neurol 1995;13:293–295.

436. Wilejto M, Shroff M, Buncic JR, et al. The clinical features, MRI findings, and outcome of optic neuritis in children. Neurology 2006;67:258–262.

437. Belopitova L, Guergueltcheva PV, Bojinova V. Definite and suspected multiple sclerosis in children: long-term follow-up and magnetic resonance imaging findings. J Child Neurol 2001;16:317–324.

438. Ness JM, Chabas D, Sadovnick AD, et al. Clinical features of children and adolescents with multiple sclerosis. Neurology 2007;68:S37–45.

439. Weng WC, Yang CC, Yu TW, et al. Multiple sclerosis with childhood onset: report of 21 cases in Taiwan. Pediatr Neurol 2006;35:327–334.

440. Renoux C, Vukusic S, Mikaeloff Y, et al. Natural history of multiple sclerosis with childhood onset. N Engl J Med 2007;356:2603–2613.

441. Banwell B, Ghezzi A, Bar-Or A, et al. Multiple sclerosis in children: clinical diagnosis, therapeutic strategies, and future directions. Lancet Neurol 2007;6:887–902.

442. Pohl D, Waubant E, Banwell B, et al. Treatment of pediatric multiple sclerosis and variants. Neurology 2007;68:S54–65.

443. Tenembaum SN, Segura MJ. Interferon beta-1a treatment in childhood and juvenile-onset multiple sclerosis. Neurology 2006;67:511–513.

444. Iannuzzi MC, Rybicki BA, Teirstein AS. Sarcoidosis. N Engl J Med 2007;357:2153–2165.

445. Stern BJ, Krumholz A, Johns C, et al. Sarcoidosis and its neurological manifestations. Arch Neurol 1985;42:909–917.

446. Delaney P. Neurologic manifestations in sarcoidosis. Review of the literature with a report of 23 cases. Ann Intern Med 1977;87:336–345.

447. Jabs DA, Johns CJ. Ocular involvement in chronic sarcoidosis. Am J Ophthalmol 1986;102:297–301.

448. Frohman LP, Guirgis M, Turbin RE, et al. Sarcoidosis of the anterior visual pathway: 24 new cases. J Neuroophthalmol 2003;23:190–197.

449. Koczman JJ, Rouleau J, Gaunt M, et al. Neuro-ophthalmic sarcoidosis: the University of Iowa experience. Semin Ophthalmol 2008;23:157–168.

450. Beardsley TL, Brown SVL, Sydnor CF, et al. Eleven cases of sarcoidosis of the optic nerve. Am J Ophthalmol 1984;97:62–77.

451. Sheth HG, O'Sullivan EP, Graham EM, et al. Gaze-evoked amaurosis in optic neuropathy due to probable sarcoidosis. Eye 2006;20:1078–1080.

452. Galetta SL, Schatz NJ, Glaser JS. Acute sarcoid optic neuropathy with spontaneous recovery. J Clin Neuroophthalmol 1989;9:27–32.

453. Ing EB, Garrity JA, Cross SA, et al. Sarcoid masquerading as optic nerve sheath meningioma. Mayo Clin Proc 1997;72:38–43.

454. Graham EM, Ellis CJ, Sanders MD, et al. Optic neuropathy in sarcoidosis. J Neurol Neurosurg Psychiatry 1986;49:756–763.

455. Beck AD, Newman NJ, Grossniklaus HE, et al. Optic nerve enlargement and chronic visual loss. Surv Ophthalmol 1994;38:555–556.

456. Carmody RF, Mafee MF, Goodwin JA, et al. Orbital and optic pathway sarcoidosis: MR findings. AJNR Am J Neuroradiol 1994;15:775–783.

457. Mavrikakis I, Rootman J. Diverse clinical presentations of orbital sarcoid. Am J Ophthalmol 2007;144:769–775.

458. Miller DH, Kendall BE, Barter S, et al. Magnetic resonance imaging in central nervous system sarcoidosis. Neurology 1988;38:378–383.

459. Lynch 3rd JP. Neurosarcoidosis: how good are the diagnostic tests? J Neuroophthalmol 2003;23:187–189.

460. Weinreb RN. Diagnosing sarcoidosis by transconjunctival biopsy of the lacrimal gland. Am J Ophthalmol 1984;97:573–576.

461. Nichols CW, Eagle RC, Yanoff M, et al. Conjunctival biopsy as an aid in the evaluation of the patient with suspected sarcoidosis. Ophthalmology 1980;87:287–291.

462. Gelwan MJ, Kellen RI, Burde RM, et al. Sarcoidosis of the anterior visual pathway: successes and failures. J Neurol Neurosurg Psychiatry 1988;51:1473–1480.

463. Maust HA, Foroozan R, Sergott RC, et al. Use of methotrexate in sarcoid-associated optic neuropathy. Ophthalmology 2003;110:559–563.

464. Bielory L, Frohman LP. Low-dose cyclosporine therapy of granulomatous optic neuropathy and orbitopathy. Ophthalmology 1991;98:1732–1736.

465. Frohman LP, Grigorian R, Bielory L. Neuro-ophthalmic manifestations of sarcoidosis: clinical spectrum, evaluation, and management. J Neuroophthalmol 2001;21:132–137.

466. Carter JD, Valeriano J, Vasey FB, et al. Refractory neurosarcoidosis: a dramatic response to infliximab. Am J Med 2004;117:277–279.

467. Salama B, Gicquel JJ, Lenoble P, et al. Optic neuropathy in refractory neurosarcoidosis treated with TNF-alpha antagonist. Can J Ophthalmol 2006;41:766–768.

468. Purvin V, Kawasaki A, Jacobson DM. Optic perineuritis: clinical and radiographic features. Arch Ophthalmol 2001;119:1299–1306.

469. Krohel GB, Charles H, Smith RS. Granulomatous optic neuropathy. Arch Ophthalmol 1981;99:1053–1055.

470. Kennerdell JS, Dresner SC. The non specific orbital inflammatory syndromes. Surv Ophthalmol 1984;29:93–103.

471. Dutton JJ, Anderson RL. Idiopathic inflammatory optic neuritis simulating optic nerve sheath meningioma. Am J Ophthalmol 1985;100:424–430.

472. Margo CE, Levy MH, Beck RW. Bilateral idiopathic inflammation of the optic nerve sheaths. Ophthalmology 1989;96:200–206.

473. Lessell S. The neuro-ophthalmology of systemic lupus erythematosus. Doc Ophthalmol 1979;47:13–42.

474. Jabs DA, Miller NR, Newman SA, et al. Optic neuropathy in systemic lupus erythematosus. Arch Ophthalmol 1986;104:564–568.

475. Lin YC, Wang AG, Yen MY. Systemic lupus erythematosus-associated optic neuritis: clinical experience and literature review. Acta Ophthalmol 2009;87:204–210.

476. Sato T, Unno S, Hagiwara K, et al. Magnetic resonance imaging of optic neuritis in a patient with systemic lupus erythematosus. Intern Med 2006;45:121.

477. Bejot Y, Osseby GV, Ben Salem D, et al. Bilateral optic neuropathy revealing Sjogren's syndrome. Rev Neurol (Paris) 2008;164:1044–1047.

478. Frohman L, Turbin R, Bielory L, et al. Autoimmune optic neuropathy with anticardiolipin antibody mimicking multiple sclerosis in a child. Am J Ophthalmol 2003;136:358–360.

479. Goodwin J. Autoimmune optic neuropathy. Curr Neurol Neurosci Rep 2006;6:396–402.

480. Hirunwiwatkul P, Trobe JD. Optic neuropathy associated with periostitis in relapsing polychondritis. J Neuroophthalmol 2007;27:16–21.

481. Pirko I, Blauwet LK, Lesnick TG, et al. The natural history of recurrent optic neuritis. Arch Neurol 2004;61:1401–1405.

482. Kidd D, Burton B, Plant GT, et al. Chronic relapsing inflammatory optic neuropathy (CRION). Brain 2003;126:276–284.

483. Dutton JJ, Burde RM, Klingele TG. Autoimmune retrobulbar optic neuritis. Am J Ophthalmol 1982;94:11–17.

484. Kupersmith MJ, Burde RM, Warren FA, et al. Autoimmune optic neuropathy: evaluation and treatment. J Neurol Neurosurg Psychiatry 1988;51:1381–1386.

485. Riedel P, Wall M, Grey A, et al. Autoimmune optic neuropathy [letter]. Arch Ophthalmol 1998;116:1121–1124.

486. Song HS, Wray SH. Bee sting optic neuritis. A case report with visual evoked potentials. J Clin Neuroophthalmol 1991;11:45–49.

487. Berrios RR, Serrano LA. Bilateral optic neuritis after a bee sting. Am J Ophthalmol 1994;117:677–678.

488. Kurz D, Egan RA, Rosenbaum JT. Treatment of corticosteroid dependent optic neuropathy with intravenous immunoglobulin. Am J Ophthalmol 2005;140:1132–1133.

489. Myers TD, Smith JR, Wertheim MS, et al. Use of corticosteroid sparing systemic immunosuppression for treatment of corticosteroid dependent optic neuritis not associated with demyelinating disease. Br J Ophthalmol 2004;88:673–680.

490. Unsold R. Neuropathies of the optic nerve in inflammatory systemic diseases and vasculitis. A frequently misdiagnosed early symptom. Ophthalmology 1994;91:251–262.

491. Kupersmith MJ, Martin V, Heller G, et al. Idiopathic hypertrophic pachymeningitis. Neurology 2004;62:686–694.

492. Slavin ML, Liebergall DA. Acute unilateral visual loss in the elderly due to retrobulbar optic neuropathy. Surv Ophthalmol 1996;41:261–267.

493. Johnson LN, Hepler RS, Yee RD, et al. Sphenoid sinus mucocele (anterior clinoid variant) mimicking diabetic ophthalmoplegia and retrobulbar neuritis. Am J Ophthalmol 1986;102:111–115.

494. Dunya IM, Frangieh GT, Heilman CB, et al. Anterior clinoid mucocele masquerading as a retrobulbar neuritis. Ophthal Plast Reconstr Surg 1996;12:171–173.

495. Galati LT, Baredes S, Mauriello J, et al. Visual loss reversed after treatment of acute bacterial sinusitis. Laryngoscope 1996;106:148–151.

496. Lee LA, Huang CC, Lee TJ. Prolonged visual disturbance secondary to isolated sphenoid sinus disease. Laryngoscope 2004;114:986–990.

497. Rothstein J, Maisel RH, Berlinger NT, et al. Relationship of optic neuritis to disease of the paranasal sinuses. Laryngoscope 1984;94:1501–1508.

498. Casson RJ, O'Day J, Crompton JL. Leber's idiopathic stellate neuroretinitis: differential diagnosis and approach to management. Aust N Z J Ophthalmol 1999;27:65–69.

499. Dreyer RF, Hopen G, Gass JD, et al. Leber's idiopathic stellate neuroretinitis. Arch Ophthalmol 1984;102:1140–1145.

500. Maitland CG, Miller NR. Neuroretinitis. Arch Ophthalmol 1984;102:1146–1150.

501. Leavitt JA, Pruthi S, Morgenstern BZ. Hypertensive retinopathy mimicking neuroretinitis in a twelve year old girl. Surv Ophthalmol 1997;41:477–480.

502. Brazis PW, Lee AG. Optic disc edema with a macular star. Mayo Clin Proc 1996;71:1162–1166.

503. Verm A, Lee AG. Bilateral optic disc edema with macular exudates as the manifesting sign of a cerebral arteriovenous malformation. Am J Ophthalmol 1997;123:422–424.

504. Weiss AH, Beck RW. Neuroretinitis in childhood. J Pediatr Ophthalmol Strab 1989;26:198–203.

505. Purvin VA, Chioran G. Recurrent neuroretinitis. Arch Ophthalmol 1994;112:365–371.

506. Wade NK, Po S, Wong IG, et al. Bilateral Bartonella-associated neuroretinitis. Retina 1999;19:355–356.

507. Drancourt M, Birtles R, Chaumentin G, et al. New serotype of Bartonella henselae in endocarditis and cat scratch disease. Lancet 1996;347:441–443.

508. Wong MT, Dolan MJ, Lattuada CP, et al. Neuroretinitis, aseptic meningitis, and lymphadenitis associate with Bartonella (Rochalimaea) henselae infection in immunocompetent patients and patients infected with human immunodeficiency virus type 1. Clin Infect Dis 1995;21:352–360.

509. Folk JC, Weingeist TA, Corbett JJ, et al. Syphilitic neuroretinitis. Am J Ophthalmol 1983;95:480–486.

510. Arruga J, Valentines J, Mauri F, et al. Neuroretinitis in acquired syphilis. Ophthalmology 1985;92:262–270.

511. Lesser RS, Kornmehl EW, Pachner AR, et al. Neuro-ophthalmologic manifestations of Lyme disease. Ophthalmology 1990;97:699–706.

512. Karma A, Stenborg T, Summanen P, et al. Long-term follow-up of chronic Lyme neuroretinitis. Retina 1996;16:505–509.

513. Fish RH, Hoskins JC, Kline LB. Toxoplasmosis neuroretinitis. Ophthalmology 1993;100:1177–1182.

514. Burnett AJ, Shortt SG, Isaac-Renton J, et al. Multiple cases of acquired toxoplasmosis retinitis presenting in an outbreak. Ophthalmology 1998;105:1032–1037.

515. Guauri RR, Lee AG, Purvin V. Optic disk edema with a macular star. Surv Ophthalmol 1998;43:270–274.

516. Cunningham ET, Koehler JE. Ocular bartonellosis. Am J Ophthalmol 2000;130:340–349.

517. Fukushima A, Yasuoka M, Tsukahara M, et al. A case of cat scratch disease neuroretinitis confirmed by polymerase chain reaction. Jpn J Ophthalmol 2003;47:405–408.

518. Labalette P, Bermond D, Dedes V, et al. Cat-scratch disease neuroretinitis diagnosed by a polymerase chain reaction approach. Am J Ophthalmol 2001;132:575–576.

519. Marra CM. Neurologic complications of Bartonella henselae infection. Curr Opin Neurol 1995;8:164–169.

520. Tomsak RL, Zakov ZN. Nonarteritic anterior ischemic optic neuropathy with macular edema: visual improvement and fluorescein angiographic characteristics. J Neuroophthalmol 1998;18:166–168.

521. Suhler EB, Lauer AK, Rosenbaum JT. Prevalence of serologic evidence of cat scratch disease in patients with neuroretinitis. Ophthalmology 2000;107:871–876.

522. Wear DJ, Marglieth AM, Hadfield TL, et al. Cat scratch disease. A bacterial infection. Science 1983;221:1403–1405.

523. Reed JB, Scales DK, Wong MT, et al. Bartonella henselae neuroretinitis in cat scratch disease. Diagnosis, management and sequelae. Ophthalmology 1998;105:459–466.

524. Browning DJ. Posterior segment manifestations of active ocular syphilis, their response to a neurosyphilis regimen of penicillin therapy, and the influence of human immunodeficiency virus status on response. Ophthalmology 2000;107:2015–2023.

525. Zetola NM, Engelman J, Jensen TP, et al. Syphilis in the United States: an update for clinicians with an emphasis on HIV coinfection. Mayo Clin Proc 2007;82:1091–1102.

526. Chao JR, Khurana RN, Fawzi AA, et al. Syphilis: reemergence of an old adversary. Ophthalmology 2006;113:2074–2079.

527. Yokoi M, Kase M. Retinal vasculitis due to secondary syphilis. Jpn J Ophthalmol 2004;48:65–67.

528. Kiss S, Damico FM, Young LH. Ocular manifestations and treatment of syphilis. Semin Ophthalmol 2005;20:161–167.

529. Weinstein JM, Lexow SS, Ho P, et al. Acute syphilitic optic neuritis. Arch Ophthalmol 1981;99:1392–1395.

530. Frohman L, Wolansky L. Magnetic resonance imaging of syphilitic optic neuritis/perineuritis. J Neuroophthalmol 1997;17:57–59.

531. Johns BR, Tierney M, Felsustein D. Alteration in the natural history of neurosyphilis by the concurrent infection with the human immunodeficiency virus. N Engl J Med 1987;316:1569–1572.

532. Wilcox RA, Burrow J, Slee M, et al. Neuromyelitis optica (Devic's disease) in a patient with syphilis. Mult Scler 2008;14:268–271.

533. Solebo AL, Westcott M. Corticosteroids in ocular syphilis. Ophthalmology 2007;114:1593.

534. Mcleish WM, Pulido JS, Holland S, et al. The ocular manifestations of syphilis in the human immunodeficiency virus type-1 infected host. Ophthalmology 1990;97:196–203.

535. Finkel M. Lyme disease and its neurologic complications. Arch Neurol 1988;45:99–104.

536. Balcer LJ, Winterkorn JM, Galetta SL. Neuro-ophthalmic manifestations of Lyme disease. J Neuroophthalmol 1997;108:108–121.

537. Sibony P, Halperin J, Coyle PK, et al. Reactive Lyme serology in optic neuritis. J Neuroophthalmol 2005;25:71–82.

538. Rothermel H, Hedges 3rd TR, Steere AC. Optic neuropathy in children with Lyme disease. Pediatrics 2001;108:477–481.

539. Jacobson DM. Lyme disease and optic neuritis: long-term follow-up of seropositive patients. Neurology 2003;60:881–882.

540. Jacobson DM, Marx JJ, Dlesk A. Frequency and clinical significance of Lyme seropositivity in patients with isolated optic neuritis. Neurology 1991;41:706–711.

541. Winward KE, Hamed LM, Glaser JS. The spectrum of optic nerve disease in human immunodeficiency virus infection. Am J Ophthalmol 1989;107:373–380.

542. Newman NJ, Lessell S. Bilateral optic neuropathies with remission in two HIV positive men. J Clin Neuroophthalmol 1992;12:1–5.

543. Patel SS, Rutzen AR, Marx JL, et al. Cytomegalovirus papillitis in patients with acquired immune deficiency syndrome. Visual prognosis of patients treated with ganciclovir and/or foscarnet. Ophthalmology 1996;103:1476–1482.

544. Baglivo E, Leuenberger PM, Kraus KH. Presumed bilateral cytomegalovirus-induced optic neuropathy in an immunocompetent person. A case report. J Neuroophthalmol 1996;16:14–17.

545. Mansor AM, Li HK. Cytomegalovirus optic neuritis: characteristics, therapy and survival. Ophthalmologica 1995;209:260–266.

546. De Silva SR, Chohan G, Jones D, et al. Cytomegalovirus papillitis in an immunocompetent patient. J Neuroophthalmol 2008;28:126–127.

547. Ioannidis AS, Bacon J, Frith P. Juxtapapillary cytomegalovirus retinitis with optic neuritis. J Neuroophthalmol 2008;28:128–130.

548. Mansour AM. Cytomegalovirus optic neuritis. Curr Opin Ophthalmol 1997;8:55–58.

549. Cohen DB, Glasgow BJ. Bilateral optic nerve cryptococcosis in sudden blindness in patients with acquired immune deficiency syndrome. Ophthalmology 1993;100:1689–1694.

550. Lipson BK, Freeman WR, Beniz J. Optic neuropathy associated with cryptococcal arachnoiditis in AIDS patients. Am J Ophthalmol 1989;107:523–527.

551. Gunduz K, Ozdemir O. Bilateral retrobulbar optic neuritis following unilateral herpes zoster ophthalmicus. Ophthalmologica 1994;208:61–64.

552. Deane JS, Bibby K. Bilateral optic neuritis following herpes zoster. Arch Ophthalmol 1995;113:972–973.

553. Litoff D, Catalano RA. Herpes zoster optic neuritis in human immunodeficiency virus infection. Arch Ophthalmol 1990;108:782–783.

554. Shayegani A, Odel JG, Kazim M, et al. Varicella zoster virus retrobulbar optic neuritis in a patient with human immunodeficiency virus. Am J Ophthalmol 1996;122:586–588.

555. Lee MS, Cooney EL, Stoessel KM, et al. Varicella zoster virus retrobulbar optic neuritis preceding retinitis in patients with acquired immune deficiency syndrome. Ophthalmology 1998;105:467–471.

556. Meenken C, van den Horn GJ, de Smet MD, et al. Optic neuritis heralding varicella zoster virus retinitis in a patient with acquired immunodeficiency syndrome. Ann Neurol 1998;43:534–536.

557. Liu JZ, Brown P, Tselis A. Unilateral retrobulbar optic neuritis due to varicella zoster virus in a patient with AIDS: a case report and review of the literature. J Neurol Sci 2005;237:97–101.

558. Wang AG, Liu JH, Hsu WM, et al. Optic neuritis in herpes zoster ophthalmicus. Jpn J Ophthalmol 2000;44:550–554.

559. Selbst RG, Selhorst JB, Harbison JW, et al. Parainfectious optic neuritis. Report and review following varicella. Arch Neurol 1983;40:347–350.

560. Johnson LN, Arnold AC. Incidence of nonarteritic and arteritic anterior ischemic optic neuropathy. Population-based study in the state of Missouri and Los Angeles County, California. J Neuroophthalmol 1994;14:38–44.

561. Miller GR, Smith JL. Ischemic optic neuropathy. Am J Ophthalmol 1966;62:103–115.

562. Boghen DR, Glaser JS. Ischaemic optic neuropathy. The clinical profile and natural history. Brain 1975;98:689–708.

563. Ischemic Optic Neuropathy Decompression Trial Study Group. Characteristics of patients with nonarteritic anterior ischemic optic neuropathy eligible for the Ischemic Optic Neuropathy Decompression Trial. Arch Ophthalmol 1996;114:1366–1374.

564. Hattenhauer MG, Leavitt JA, Hodge DO, et al. Incidence of nonarteritic anterior ischemic optic neuropathy. Am J Ophthalmol 1997;123:103–107.

565. Preechawat P, Bruce BB, Newman NJ, et al. Anterior ischemic optic neuropathy in patients younger than 50 years. Am J Ophthalmol 2007;144:953–960.

566. Hayreh SS, Joos KM, Podhajsky PA, et al. Systemic diseases associated with nonarteritic anterior ischemic optic neuropathy. Am J Ophthalmol 1994;118:766–780.

567. Jacobson DM, Vierkant RA, Belongia EA. Nonarteritic anterior ischemic optic neuropathy. A case-control study of potential risk factors. Arch Ophthalmol 1997;115:1403–1407.

568. Hayreh SS, Zimmerman MB. Nonarteritic anterior ischemic optic neuropathy: clinical characteristics in diabetic patients versus nondiabetic patients. Ophthalmology 2008;115:1818–1825.

569. Hayreh SS, Fingert JH, Stone E, et al. Familial non-arteritic anterior ischemic optic neuropathy. Graefes Arch Clin Exp Ophthalmol 2008;246:1295–1305.

570. Deramo VA, Sergott RC, Augsburger JJ, et al. Ischemic optic neuropathy as the first manifestation of elevated cholesterol levels in young patients. Ophthalmology 2003;110:1041–1046.

571. Hayreh SS, Podhajsky PA, Zimmerman B. Nonarteritic anterior ischemic optic neuropathy: time of onset of visual loss. Am J Ophthalmol 1997;124:641–647.

572. Hayreh SS, Podhajsky P, Zimmerman MB. Role of nocturnal arterial hypotension in optic nerve head ischemic disorders. Ophthalmologica 1999;213:76–96.

573. Landau K, Winterkorn JM, Mailloux LU, et al. 24 hour blood pressure monitoring in patients with anterior ischemic optic neuropathy. Arch Ophthalmol 1996;114:570–575.

574. Hayreh SS, Zimmerman MB, Podhajsky P, et al. Nocturnal arterial hypotension and its role in optic nerve head and ocular ischemic disorders. Am J Ophthalmol 1994;117:603–624.

575. Doro S, Lessell S. Cup disc ratio and ischemic optic neuropathy. Arch Ophthalmol 1993;103:1143–1144.

576. Beck RW, Servais GE, Hayreh SS. Anterior ischemic optic neuropathy. IX. Cup-to-disc ratio and its role in pathogenesis. Ophthalmology 1987;94:1502–1508.

577. Beck RW, Savino PJ, Repka MX, et al. Optic disc structure in anterior ischemic optic neuropathy. Ophthalmology 1984;91:1334–1337.

578. Burde RM. Optic disc risk factors for non arteritic ischemic optic neuropathy. Am J Ophthalmol 1993;115:759–763.

579. Contreras I, Rebolleda G, Noval S, et al. Optic disc evaluation by optical coherence tomography in nonarteritic anterior ischemic optic neuropathy. Invest Ophthalmol Vis Sci 2007;48:4087–4092.

580. Saito H, Tomidokoro A, Sugimoto E, et al. Optic disc topography and peripapillary retinal nerve fiber layer thickness in nonarteritic ischemic optic neuropathy and open-angle glaucoma. Ophthalmology 2006;113:1340–1344.

581. Saito H, Tomidokoro A, Tomita G, et al. Optic disc and peripapillary morphology in unilateral nonarteritic anterior ischemic optic neuropathy and age- and refraction-matched normals. Ophthalmology 2008;115:1585–1590.

582. Katz B, Spencer WH. Hyperopia as a risk factor for nonarteritic anterior ischemic optic neuropathy. Am J Ophthalmol 1993;15:754–758.

583. Chung SM, Gay CA, McCrary JA. Nonarteritic ischemic optic neuropathy. The impact of tobacco use. Ophthalmology 1994;101:779–782.

584. Hayreh SS, Jonas JB, Zimmerman MB. Nonarteritic anterior ischemic optic neuropathy and tobacco smoking. Ophthalmology 2007;114:804–809.

585. Fry CL, Carter JE, Kanter MC, et al. Anterior ischemic optic neuropathy is not associated with carotid artery atherosclerosis. Stroke 1993;24:539–542.

586. Behbehani R, Mathews MK, Sergott RC, et al. Nonarteritic anterior ischemic optic neuropathy in patients with sleep apnea while being treated with continuous positive airway pressure. Am J Ophthalmol 2005;139:518–521.

587. Lee AG. Three questions on the role of sleep apnea syndrome in optic disc edema. Arch Ophthalmol 2001;119:1225.

588. Li J, McGwin Jr. G, Vaphiades MS, et al. Non-arteritic anterior ischaemic optic neuropathy and presumed sleep apnoea syndrome screened by the Sleep Apnea scale of the Sleep Disorders Questionnaire (SA-SDQ). Br J Ophthalmol 2007;91:1524–1527.

589. Mojon DS, Hedges 3rd TR, Ehrenberg B, et al. Association between sleep apnea syndrome and nonarteritic anterior ischemic optic neuropathy. Arch Ophthalmol 2002;120:601–605.

590. Mojon DS, Mathis J, Zulauf M, et al. Optic neuropathy associated with sleep apnea syndrome. Ophthalmology 1998;105:874–877.

591. Palombi K, Renard E, Levy P, et al. Non-arteritic anterior ischaemic optic neuropathy is nearly systematically associated with obstructive sleep apnoea. Br J Ophthalmol 2006;90:879–882.

592. Pomeranz HD, Smith KH, Hart Jr. WM, et al. Sildenafil-associated nonarteritic anterior ischemic optic neuropathy. Ophthalmology 2002;109:584–587.

593. Bollinger K, Lee MS. Recurrent visual field defect and ischemic optic neuropathy associated with tadalafil rechallenge. Arch Ophthalmol 2005;123:400–401.

594. Boshier A, Pambakian N, Shakir SA. A case of nonarteritic ischemic optic neuropathy (NAION) in a male patient taking sildenafil. Int J Clin Pharmacol Ther 2002;40:422–423.

595. Carter JE. Anterior ischemic optic neuropathy and stroke with use of PDE-5 inhibitors for erectile dysfunction: cause or coincidence? J Neurol Sci 2007;262:89–97.

596. Escaravage Jr. GK, Wright Jr. JD, Givre SJ. Tadalafil associated with anterior ischemic optic neuropathy. Arch Ophthalmol 2005;123:399–400.

597. Lee AG, Newman NJ. Erectile dysfunction drugs and nonarteritic anterior ischemic optic neuropathy. Am J Ophthalmol 2005;140:707–708.

598. Margo CE, French DD. Ischemic optic neuropathy in male veterans prescribed phosphodiesterase-5 inhibitors. Am J Ophthalmol 2007;143:538–539.

599. Peter NM, Singh MV, Fox PD. Tadalafil-associated anterior ischaemic optic neuropathy. Eye 2005;19:715–717.

600. Pomeranz HD, Bhavsar AR. Nonarteritic ischemic optic neuropathy developing soon after use of sildenafil (viagra): a report of seven new cases. J Neuroophthalmol 2005;25:9–13.

601. Wooltorton E. Visual loss with erectile dysfunction medications. CMAJ 2006;175:355.

602. FDA updates labeling for erectile dysfunction drugs. FDA Consum 2005;39:3.

603. Viagra and loss of vision. Med Lett Drugs Ther 2005;47:49.

604. Dundar SO. Visual loss associated with erectile dysfunction drugs. Can J Ophthalmol 2007;42:10–12.

605. Hayreh SS. Erectile dysfunction drugs and non-arteritic anterior ischemic optic neuropathy: is there a cause and effect relationship? J Neuroophthalmol 2005;25:295–298.

606. Pomeranz HD. Can erectile dysfunction drug use lead to ischaemic optic neuropathy? Br J Ophthalmol 2006;90:127–128.

607. Sobel RE, Cappelleri JC. NAION and treatment of erectile dysfunction: reply from Pfizer. Br J Ophthalmol 2006;90:927.

608. Verit A, Oguz H. Ophthalmic aspects of erectile dysfunction drugs. Am J Ophthalmol 2006;141:598; author reply 599.

609. Thurtell MJ, Tomsak RL. Nonarteritic anterior ischemic optic neuropathy with PDE-5 inhibitors for erectile dysfunction. Int J Impot Res 2008;20:537–543.

610. Gedik S, Yilmaz G, Akova YA. Sildenafil-associated consecutive nonarteritic anterior ischaemic optic neuropathy, cilioretinal artery occlusion, and central retinal vein occlusion in a haemodialysis patient. Eye 2007;21:129–130.

611. Pepin S, Pitha-Rowe I. Stepwise decline in visual field after serial sildenafil use. J Neuroophthalmol 2008;28:76–77.

612. McGwin Jr. G, Vaphiades MS, Hall TA, et al. Non-arteritic anterior ischaemic optic neuropathy and the treatment of erectile dysfunction. Br J Ophthalmol 2006;90:154–157.

613. Gorkin L, Hvidsten K, Sobel RE, et al. Sildenafil citrate use and the incidence of nonarteritic anterior ischemic optic neuropathy. Int J Clin Pract 2006;60:500–503.

614. Swartz NG, Beck RW, Savino PJ, et al. Pain in anterior ischemic optic neuropathy. J Neuroophthalmol 1995;15:9–10.

615. Repka MX, Savino PJ, Schatz NJ, et al. Clinical profile and long-term implications of anterior ischemic optic neuropathy. Am J Ophthalmol 1983;96:478–483.

616. Warner JEA, Lessell S, Rizzo JF, et al. Does optic disc appearance distinguish ischemic optic neuropathy from optic neuritis. Arch Ophthalmol 1997;115:1408–1410.

617. Schatz NJ, Smith JL. Non-tumor causes of the Foster Kennedy syndrome. J Neurosurg 1967;27:37–44.

618. Arnold AC, Hepler RS. Fluorescein angiography in acute nonarteritic anterior ischemic optic neuropathy. Am J Ophthalmol 1994;117:222–230.

619. Arnold AC, Badr MA, Hepler RS. Fluorescein angiography in nonischemic optic disc edema. Arch Ophthalmol 1996;114:293–298.

620. Hedges 3rd TR, Vuong LN, Gonzalez-Garcia AO, et al. Subretinal fluid from anterior ischemic optic neuropathy demonstrated by optical coherence tomography. Arch Ophthalmol 2008;126:812–815.

621. Arnold AC, Hepler RS, Hamilton DR, et al. Magnetic resonance imaging of the brain in nonarteritic ischemic optic neuropathy. J Neuroophthalmol 1995;15:158–160.

622. Parisi V, Gallinaro G, Ziccardi L, et al. Electrophysiological assessment of visual function in patients with non-arteritic ischaemic optic neuropathy. Eur J Neurol 2008;15:839–845.

623. Arnold AC, Hepler RS. Natural history of non arteritic ischemic optic neuropathy. J Neuroophthalmol 1994;14:66–69.

624. Borchert M, Lessell S. Progressive and recurrent nonarteritic anterior ischemic optic neuropathy. Am J Ophthalmol 1988;106:433–449.

625. Kline LB. Progression of visual field defects in ischemic optic neuropathy. Am J Ophthalmol 1988;106:199–203.

626. The Ischemic Optic Neuropathy Decompression Trial Research Group. Optic nerve decompression surgery for nonarteritic ischemic optic neuropathy (NAION) is not effective and may be harmful. JAMA 1995;273:625–632.

627. Levin LA. Lessons from the ischemic optic neuropathy decompression trial: a decade later. Arch Ophthalmol 2007;125:1570–1571.

628. Newman NJ. The ischemic optic neuropathy decompression trial. Arch Ophthalmol 2007;125:1568–1570.

629. Barrett DA, Glaser JS, Schatz NJ, et al. Spontaneous recovery of vision in progressive anterior ischaemic optic neuropathy. J Clin Neuroophthalmol 1992;12:219–225.

630. Alasil T, Tan O, Lu AT, et al. Correlation of Fourier domain optical coherence tomography retinal nerve fiber layer maps with visual fields in nonarteritic ischemic optic neuropathy. Ophthalmic Surg Lasers Imaging 2008;39:S71–79.

631. Contreras I, Noval S, Rebolleda G, et al. Follow-up of nonarteritic anterior ischemic optic neuropathy with optical coherence tomography. Ophthalmology 2007;114:2338–2344.

632. Deleon-Ortega J, Carroll KE, Arthur SN, et al. Correlations between retinal nerve fiber layer and visual field in eyes with nonarteritic anterior ischemic optic neuropathy. Am J Ophthalmol 2007;143:288–294.

633. Friedland S, Winterkorn JM, Burde RM. Luxury perfusion following anterior ischemic optic neuropathy. J Neuroophthalmol 1996;16:163–171.

634. Hayreh SS, Zimmerman MB. Optic disc edema in non-arteritic anterior ischemic optic neuropathy. Graefes Arch Clin Exp Ophthalmol 2007;245:1107–1121.

635. Gordon RN, Burde RM, Slamovits T. Asymptomatic optic disc edema. J Neuroophthalmol 1997;17:29–32.

636. Hayreh SS. Anterior ischemic optic neuropathy. V. Optic disc edema an early sign. Arch Ophthalmol 1981;99:1030–1040.

637. Prenner JL, Sharma A, Ibarra MS, et al. Prolonged premonitory optic disc signs in anterior ischemic optic neuropathy. J Neuroophthalmol 2002;22:110–112.

638. Hayreh SS, Zimmerman MB. Incipient nonarteritic anterior ischemic optic neuropathy. Ophthalmology 2007;114:1763–1772.

639. Beri M, Klugman MR, Kohler JA, et al. Anterior ischemic optic neuropathy. VII. Incidence of bilaterality and various influencing factors. Ophthalmology 1987;94:1020–1028.

640. Newman NJ, Scherer R, Langenberg P, et al. The fellow eye in NAION: report from the ischemic optic neuropathy decompression trial follow-up study. Am J Ophthalmol 2002;134:317–328.

641. Guyer DR, Miller NR, Auer CL, et al. The risk of cerebrovascular disease in patients with anterior ischemic optic neuropathy. Arch Ophthalmol 1985;103:1136–1142.

642. WuDunn D, Zimmerman K, Sadun AA, et al. Comparison of visual function in fellow eyes after bilateral nonarteritic anterior ischemic optic neuropathy. Ophthalmology 1997;104:104–111.

643. Boone MI, Massry GG, Frankel RA, et al. Visual outcome in bilateral nonarteritic ischemic optic neuropathy. Ophthalmology 1996;103:1223–1228.

644. Lessell S. Nonarteritic anterior ischemic optic neuropathy: enigma variations [editorial]. Arch Ophthalmol 1999;117:386–388.

645. Levin LA, Danesh-Meyer HV. Hypothesis: a venous etiology for nonarteritic anterior ischemic optic neuropathy. Arch Ophthalmol 2008;126:1582–1585.

646. Hayreh SS. Anterior ischemic optic neuropathy. I. Terminology and pathogenesis. Br J Ophthalmol 1974;58:955–963.

647. Hayreh SS. Anterior ischaemic optic neuropathy. Differentiation of arteritic from non-arteritic type and its management. Eye 1990;4:25–41.

648. McLeod D, Marshall J, Kohner EM. Role of axoplasmic transport in the pathophysiology of ischaemic disc swelling. Br J Ophthalmol 1980;64:247–261.

649. Arnold AC. Pathogenesis of nonarteritic anterior ischemic optic neuropathy. J Neuroophthalmol 2003;23:157–163.

650. Tesser RA, Niendorf ER, Levin LA. The morphology of an infarct in nonarteritic anterior ischemic optic neuropathy. Ophthalmology 2003;110:2031–2035.

651. Liebermann MF, Shahi A, Green WR. Embolic ischemic optic neuropathy. Am J Ophthalmol 1978;86:206–210.

652. Cullen JF. Ischaemic optic neuropathy. Trans Ophthalmol Soc UK 1967;87:759–774.

653. Elston J. Non-arteritic anterior ischaemic optic neuropathy and cataract surgery. Br J Ophthalmol 2007;91:563.

654. Fontes BM, Jung LS, Soriano ES, et al. Nonarteritic anterior ischemic optic neuropathy after uneventful phacoemulsification: case report. Arq Bras Oftalmol 2007;70:544–546.

655. Harris MJ. Incidence of NAION with cataract extraction. Ophthalmology 2002;109:630; author reply 630.

656. Hayreh SS. Anterior ischemic optic neuropathy. IV. Occurrence after cataract extraction. Arch Ophthalmol 1980;98:1410–1416.

657. Lam BL, Jabaly-Habib H, Al-Sheikh N, et al. Risk of non-arteritic anterior ischaemic optic neuropathy (NAION) after cataract extraction in the fellow eye of patients with prior unilateral NAION. Br J Ophthalmol 2007;91:585–587.

658. Luscavage LE, Volpe NJ, Liss R. Posterior ischemic optic neuropathy after uncomplicated cataract extraction. Am J Ophthalmol 2001;132:408–409.

659. McCulley TJ, Lam BL, Feuer WJ. Nonarteritic anterior ischemic optic neuropathy and surgery of the anterior segment: temporal relationship analysis. Am J Ophthalmol 2003;136:1171–1172.

660. McCulley TJ, Lam BL, Feuer WJ. A comparison of risk factors for postoperative and spontaneous nonarteritic anterior ischemic optic neuropathy. J Neuroophthalmol 2005;25:22–24.

661. Hayreh SS. Anterior ischemic optic neuropathy. VIII. Clinical features and pathogenesis of post-hemorrhagic amaurosis. Ophthalmology 1987;94:1488–1502.

662. Kim SK, Volpe NJ, Stoltz RA. Contemporaneous retinal and optic nerve infarcts, choroidal non-perfusion, and Hollenhorst plaque: are these all embolic events? J Neuroophthalmol 2006;26:113–116.

663. Hayreh SS, Podhajsky PA, Zimmerman B. Ipsilateral recurrence of nonarteritic anterior ischemic optic neuropathy. Am J Ophthalmol 2001;132:734–742.

664. Bernstein SL, Guo Y, Kelman SE, et al. Functional and cellular responses in a novel rodent model of anterior ischemic optic neuropathy. Invest Ophthalmol Vis Sci 2003;44:4153–4162.

665. Slater BJ, Mehrabian Z, Guo Y, et al. Rodent anterior ischemic optic neuropathy (rAION) induces regional retinal ganglion cell apoptosis with a unique temporal pattern. Invest Ophthalmol Vis Sci 2008;49:3671–3676.

666. Galetta SL, Plock GL, Kushner MJ, et al. Ocular thrombosis associated with antiphospholipid antibodies. Ann Ophthalmol 1991;23:207–212.

667. Bertram B, Remky A, Arend O, et al. Protein C, protein S, and antithrombin III in acute ocular occlusive diseases. Ger J Ophthalmol 1995;4:332–335.

668. Rosler DH, Conway MD, Anaya JM, et al. Ischemic optic neuropathy and high-level anticardiolipin antibodies in primary Sjogren's syndrome. Lupus 1995;4:155–157.

669. Salomon O, Huna-Baron R, Kurtz S, et al. Analysis of prothrombotic and vascular risk factors in patients with nonarteritic anterior ischemic optic neuropathy. Ophthalmology 1999;106:739–742.

670. Biousse V, Kerrison JB, Newman NJ. Is non-arteritic anterior ischaemic optic neuropathy related to homocysteine? Br J Ophthalmol 2000;84:555.

671. Kawasaki A, Purvin VA, Burgett RA. Hyperhomocysteinaemia in young patients with non-arteritic anterior ischaemic optic neuropathy. Br J Ophthalmol 1999;83:1287–1290.

672. Pianka P, Almog Y, Man O, et al. Hyperhomocystinemia in patients with nonarteritic anterior ischemic optic neuropathy, central retinal artery occlusion, and central retinal vein occlusion. Ophthalmology 2000;107:1588–1592.

673. Hamed LM, Winward KE, Glaser JS, et al. Optic neuropathy in uremia. Am J Ophthalmol 1989;108:30–35.

674. Knox DL, Hanneken AM, Hollows FC. Uremic optic neuropathy. Arch Ophthalmol 1988;106:50–54.

675. Beck RW, Gamel JW, Willcourt RJ, et al. Acute ischemic optic neuropathy in severe preeclampsia. Am J Ophthalmol 1980;90:342–346.

676. Katz B. Bilateral sequential migrainous ischemic optic neuropathy. Am J Ophthalmol 1985;99:489.

677. O'Hara M, O'Connor PS. Migrainous optic neuropathy. J Clin Neuroophthalmol 1984;4:85–90.

678. Hayreh SS, Zimmerman MB. Non-arteritic anterior ischemic optic neuropathy: role of systemic corticosteroid therapy. Graefes Arch Clin Exp Ophthalmol 2008;246: 1029–1046.

679. Sergott RC, Cohen MS, Bosley TM, et al. Optic nerve decompression may improve the progressive form of non arteritic ischemic optic neuropathy. Arch Ophthalmol 1989;107:1743–1754.

680. Spoor TC, McHenry JG, Lau-Sickon L. Progressive and static nonarteritic ischemic optic neuropathy treated by optic nerve sheath decompression. Ophthalmology 1993;100:306–311.

681. Kelman SE, Elman MJ. Optic nerve sheath decompression for nonarteritic ischemic optic neuropathy improves multiple visual function measurements. Arch Ophthalmol 1991;109:667–671.

682. Glaser JS, Teimory M, Schatz NJ. Optic nerve sheath fenestration for progressive ischemic optic neuropathy. Results in second series consisting of 21 eyes. Arch Ophthalmol 1994;112:1047–1050.

683. Yee RD, Selky AK, Purvin VA. Outcomes of optic nerve sheath decompression for nonarteritic ischemic optic neuropathy. J Neuroophthalmol 1994;14:70–76.

684. Ischemic Optic Neuropathy Decompression Trial Research Group. Ischemic optic neuropathy decompression trial. Twenty-fourth-month update. Arch Ophthalmol 2000;118:793–798.

685. Arnold AC, Hepler RS, Lieber M, et al. Hyperbaric oxygen therapy for nonarteritic anterior ischemic optic neuropathy. Am J Ophthalmol 1996;122:535–541.

686. Botelho PJ, Johnson LN, Arnold AC. The effect of aspirin on the visual outcome of nonarteritic anterior ischemic optic neuropathy. Am J Ophthalmol 1996;121:450–451.

687. Johnson LN, Gould TJ, Krohel GB. Effect of levodopa and carbidopa on recovery of visual function in patients with nonarteritic anterior ischemic optic neuropathy of longer than six months' duration. Am J Ophthalmol 1996;121:77–83.

688. Simsek T, Eryilmaz T, Acaroglu G. Efficacy of levodopa and carbidopa on visual function in patients with non-arteritic anterior ischaemic optic neuropathy. Int J Clin Pract 2005;59:287–290.

689. Soheilian M, Yazdani S, Alizadeh-Ghavidel L, et al. Surgery for optic neuropathy [letter]. Ophthalmology 2008;115:1099.

690. Bennett JL, Thomas S, Olson JL, et al. Treatment of nonarteritic anterior ischemic optic neuropathy with intravitreal bevacizumab. J Neuroophthalmol 2007;27:238–240.

691. Kaderli B, Avci R, Yucel A, et al. Intravitreal triamcinolone improves recovery of visual acuity in nonarteritic anterior ischemic optic neuropathy. J Neuroophthalmol 2007;27:164–168.

692. Beck RW, Hayreh SS, Podhajsky P, et al. Aspirin therapy in nonarteritic anterior ischemic optic neuropathy. Am J Ophthalmol 1997;123:212–217.

693. Kupersmith MJ, Frohman L, Sanderson M, et al. Aspirin reduces the incidence of second eye NAION: a retrospective study. J Neuroophthalmol 1997;17:250–253.

694. Gerling J, Meyer JH, Kommerell G. Visual field defects in optic neuritis and anterior ischemic optic neuropathy: distinctive features. Graefes Arch Clin Exp Ophthalmol 1998;236:188–192.

695. Goodman BW. Temporal arteritis. Am J Med 1979;67:839–852.

696. Lam BL, Wirthlin RS, Gonzalez A, et al. Giant cell arteritis among Hispanic Americans. Am J Ophthalmol 2007;143:161–163.

697. Gonzalez-Gay MA, Miranda-Filloy JA, Lopez-Diaz MJ, et al. Giant cell arteritis in northwestern Spain: a 25-year epidemiologic study. Medicine (Baltimore) 2007;86: 61–68.

698. Liu NH, LaBree LD, Feldon SE, et al. The epidemiology of giant cell arteritis: a 12-year retrospective study. Ophthalmology 2001;108:1145–1149.

699. Biller J, Asconape J, Weinblatt ME, et al. Temporal arteritis associated with a normal sedimentation rate. JAMA 1982;247:486–487.

700. Bengtsson B-A, Malmvall B-E. The epidemiology of giant cell arteritis including temporal arteritis and polymyalgia rheumatica. Incidences of different clinical presentations and eye complications. Arthritis Rheum 1981;24:899–904.

701. Hauser WA, Ferguson RH, Holley KE, et al. Temporal arteritis in Rochester, Minnesota, 1951 to 1967. Mayo Clin Proc 1971;46:597–602.

702. Huston KA, Hunder GG, Lie JT, et al. Temporal arteritis: a 25-year epidemiologic, clinical, and pathologic study. Ann Intern Med 1978;88:162–167.

703. Shah P, Murray PI, Harry J. An unusual case of giant cell arteritis. Am J Ophthalmol 1993;115:393–394.

704. Wilkinson IMS, Russell RWR. Arteries of the head and neck in giant cell arteritis. A pathological study to show the pattern of arterial involvement. Arch Neurol 1972;27:378–391.

705. Kattah JC, Mejico L, Chrousos GA, et al. Pathologic findings in a steroid-responsive optic nerve infarct in giant-cell arteritis. Neurology 1999;53:177–180.

706. Säve-Söderbergh J, Malmvall B-E, Andersson R, et al. Giant cell arteritis as a cause of death. JAMA 1986;255:493–496.

707. Hunder GG. Giant cell arteritis and polymyalgia rheumatica. In: Kelley WN, Harris ED, Ruddy S, et al. (eds): Textbook of Rheumatology, 3rd edn. Philadelphia, W. B. Saunders, 1989: 1200–1208.

708. McDonnell PJ, Moore GW, Miller NR, et al. Temporal arteritis. A clinicopathologic study. Ophthalmology 1986;93:518–530.

709. Ghanchi FD, Dutton GN. Current concepts in giant cell (temporal) arteritis. Surv Ophthalmol 1997;42:99–123.

710. Weyand CM, Goronzy JJ. Medium- and large-vessel vasculitis. N Engl J Med 2003;349:160–169.

711. Weyand CM, Bartley GB. Giant cell arteritis: new concepts in pathogenesis and implications for management. Am J Ophthalmol 1997;123:392–395.

712. Galetta SL, Raps EC, Wulc AE, et al. Conjugal temporal arteritis. Neurology 1990;40:1839–1842.

713. Mitchell BM, Font RL. Detection of varicella zoster virus DNA in some patients with giant cell arteritis. Invest Ophthalmol Vis Sci 2001;42:2572–2577.

714. Finelli P. Alternating amaurosis fugax and temporal arteritis. Am J Ophthalmol 1997;123:850–851.

715. Galetta SL, Balcer LJ, Liu GT. Giant cell arteritis with unusual flow related neuro-ophthalmologic manifestations. Neurology 1997;49:1463–1465.

716. Liu GT, Glaser JS, Schatz NJ, et al. Visual morbidity in giant cell arteritis: clinical characteristics and prognosis for vision. Ophthalmology 1994;101: 1779–1785.

717. Hart CT. Formed visual hallucinations: a symptom of cranial arteritis. BMJ 1967;3:643–644.

718. Aiello PD, Trautmann JC, McPhee TJ, et al. Visual prognosis in giant cell arteritis. Ophthalmology 1993;100:550–555.

719. Jonasson F, Cullen JF, Elton RA. Temporal arteritis. A 14-year epidemiological, clinical and prognostic study. Scot Med J 1979;24:111–117.

720. Graham E. Survival in temporal arteritis. Trans Ophthalmol Soc UK 1980;100: 108–110.

721. Wagener HP, Hollenhorst RW. The ocular lesions of temporal arteritis. Am J Ophthalmol 1958;45:617–630.

722. Eshaghian J. Controversies regarding giant cell (temporal, cranial) arteritis. Doc Ophthalmol 1979;47:43–67.

723. Cullen JF, Coleiro JA. Ophthalmic complications of giant cell arteritis. Surv Ophthalmol 1976;20:247–260.

724. Keltner JL. Giant-cell arteritis. Signs and symptoms. Ophthalmology 1982;89: 1101–1110.

725. Mehler MF, Rabinowich L. The clinical neuro-ophthalmologic spectrum of temporal arteritis. Am J Med 1988;85:839–843.

726. Rahman W, Rahman FZ. Giant cell (temporal) arteritis: an overview and update. Surv Ophthalmol 2005;50:415–428.

727. Salvarani C, Cimino L, Macchioni P, et al. Risk factors for visual loss in an Italian population-based cohort of patients with giant cell arteritis. Arthritis Rheum 2005;53:293–297.

728. Gonzalez-Gay MA, Garcia-Porrua C, Llorca J, et al. Visual manifestations of giant cell arteritis. Trends and clinical spectrum in 161 patients. Medicine (Baltimore) 2000;79: 283–292.

729. Hayreh SS, Podhajsky PA, Zimmerman B. Occult giant cell arteritis: ocular manifestations. Am J Ophthalmol 1998;125:521–526.

730. Melberg MS, Grand MG, Dieckert JP, et al. Cotton wool spots and the early diagnosis of giant cell arteritis. Ophthalmology 1995;102:1611–1614.

731. Slavin ML, Barondes MJ. Visual loss caused by choroidal ischemia preceding anterior ischemic optic neuropathy in giant cell arteritis. Am J Ophthalmol 1994;117:81–86.

732. Sebag J, Thomas JV, Epstein DL, et al. Optic disc cupping in arteritic anterior ischemic optic neuropathy resembles glaucomatous cupping. Ophthalmology 1986;93:357–361.

733. Hayreh SS, Jonas JB. Optic disc morphology after arteritic anterior ischemic optic neuropathy. Ophthalmology 2001;108:1586–1594.

734. Danesh-Meyer H, Savino PJ, Spaeth GL, et al. Comparison of arteritis and nonarteritic anterior ischemic optic neuropathies with the Heidelberg Retina Tomograph. Ophthalmology 2005;112:1104–1112.

735. Danesh-Meyer HV, Savino PJ, Sergott RC. The prevalence of cupping in end-stage arteritic and nonarteritic anterior ischemic optic neuropathy. Ophthalmology 2001;108:593–598.

736. Hamed LM, Guy JR, Moster ML, et al. Giant cell arteritis in the ocular ischemic syndrome. Am J Ophthalmol 1992;113:702–705.

737. Hwang JM, Girkin CA, Perry JD, et al. Bilateral ocular ischemic syndrome secondary to giant cell arteritis progressing despite corticosteroid treatment. Am J Ophthalmol 1999;127:102–104.

738. Huna-Baron R, Mizrachi IB, Glovinsky Y. Intraocular pressure is low in eyes with giant cell arteritis. J Neuroophthalmol 2006;26:273–275.

739. Barricks ME, Traviesa DB, Glaser JS, et al. Ophthalmoplegia in cranial arteritis. Brain 1977;100:209–221.

740. Cockerham KP, Cockerham GC, Brown HG, et al. Radiosensitive orbital inflammation associated with temporal arteritis. J Neuroophthalmol 2003;23:117–121.

741. Salvarani C, Cantini F, Boiardi L, et al. Polymyalgia rheumatica and giant-cell arteritis. N Engl J Med 2002;347:261–271.

742. Hayreh SS, Podhajsky PA, Raman R, et al. Giant cell arteritis: validity and reliability of various diagnostic criteria. Am J Ophthalmol 1997;123:285–296.

743. Dudenhoefer EJ, Cornblath WT, Schatz MP. Scalp necrosis with giant cell arteritis. Ophthalmology 1998;105:1875–1878.

744. Rudd JC, Fineman MS, Sergott RC. Ischemic scalp necrosis preceding loss of visual acuity in giant cell arteritis. Arch Ophthalmol 1998;116:1690–1691.

745. Simmons RJ, Cogan DG. Occult temporal arteritis. Arch Ophthalmol 1962;68:8–18.

746. Cullen JF. Occult temporal arteritis. A common cause of blindness in old age. Br J Ophthalmol 1967;51:513–525.

747. Caselli RJ, Hunder GG, Whisnant JP. Neurologic disease in biopsy proven giant cell (temporal) arteritis. Neurology 1988;38:352–359.

748. Thielen KR, Wijdicks EFM, Nichols DA. Giant cell (temporal arteritis): involvement of the vertebral and internal carotid arteries. Mayo Clin Proc 1998;73:444–446.

749. Gout O, Viala K, Lyon-Caen O. Giant cell arteritis and Vernet's syndrome. Neurology 1998;50:1862–1864.

750. Roelcke U, Eschle D, Kappos L, et al. Meningoradiculitis associated with giant cell arteritis. Neurology 2002;59:1811–1812.

751. Joelson E, Ruthrauff B, Ali F, et al. Multifocal dural enhancement associated with temporal arteritis. Arch Neurol 2000;57:119–122.

752. Eberhardt RT, Dhadly M. Giant cell arteritis: diagnosis, management, and cardiovascular implications. Cardiol Rev 2007;15:55–61.

753. Hunder GG, Bloch DA, Michel BA, et al. The American College of Rheumatology 1990 criteria for the classification of giant cell arteritis. Arthritis Rheum 1990;33:1122–1128.

754. Milne JS, Williamson J. The ESR in older people. Gerontol Clin 1972;14:36–42.

755. Miller A, Green M, Robinson D. Simple rule for calculating normal erythrocyte sedimentation rate. BMJ (Clin Res Ed) 1983;286:266.

756. Jacobson DM, Slamovitz TL. Erythrocyte sedimentation rate and its relationship to hematocrit in giant cell arteritis. Arch Ophthalmol 1987;105:965–967.

757. Liozon E, Herrmann F, Ly K, et al. Risk factors for visual loss in giant cell (temporal) arteritis: a prospective study of 174 patients. Am J Med 2001;111:211–217.

758. Parikh M, Miller NR, Lee AG, et al. Prevalence of a normal C-reactive protein with an elevated erythrocyte sedimentation rate in biopsy-proven giant cell arteritis. Ophthalmology 2006;113:1842–1845.

759. Costello F, Zimmerman MB, Podhajsky PA, et al. Role of thrombocytosis in diagnosis of giant cell arteritis and differentiation of arteritic from non-arteritic anterior ischemic optic neuropathy. Eur J Ophthalmol 2004;14:245–257.

760. Foroozan R, Danesh-Meyer H, Savino PJ, et al. Thrombocytosis in patients with biopsy-proven giant cell arteritis. Ophthalmology 2002;109:1267–1271.

761. Lincoff NS, Erlich PD, Brass LS. Thrombocytosis in temporal arteritis rising platelet counts: a red flag for giant cell arteritis. J Neuroophthalmol 2000;20:67–72.

762. Mack HG, O'Day J, Currie JN. Delayed choroidal perfusion in giant cell arteritis. J Clin Neuroophthalmol 1991;11:221–227.

763. Quillen DA, Cantore WA, Schwartz SR, et al. Choroidal non perfusion in giant cell arteritis. Am J Ophthalmol 1993;116:171–175.

764. Siatkowski RM, Gass JDM, Glaser JS, et al. Fluorescein angiography in the diagnosis of giant cell arteritis. Am J Ophthalmol 1993;115:57–63.

765. Sadun F, Pece A, Brancato R. Fluorescein and indocyanine green angiography in arteritic anterior ischaemic optic neuropathy [letter]. Br J Ophthalmol 1998;82:1344–1345.

766. Klein RG, Campbell RJ, Hunder GG, et al. Skip lesions in temporal arteritis. Mayo Clin Proc 1976;51:504–510.

767. Chambers WA, Bernadino VB. Specimen length in temporal artery biopsies. J Clin Neuroophthalmol 1988;8:121–125.

768. Albert DM, Ruchman ML, Keltner JL. Skip areas in temporal arteritis. Arch Ophthalmol 1976;94:2072–2077.

769. Nishino H, DeRemee RA, Rubino FA, et al. Wegener's granulomatosis associated with vasculitis of the temporal artery: report of five cases. Mayo Clin Proc 1993;68:115–121.

770. Levy MH, Margo CE. Temporal artery biopsy and sarcoidosis. Am J Ophthalmol 1994;117:409–410.

771. Kattah JC, Cupps T, Manz HJ, et al. Occipital artery biopsy: a diagnostic alternative in giant cell arteritis. Neurology 1991;41:949–950.

772. Lessell S. Bilateral temporal artery biopsies in giant cell arteritis. J Neuroophthalmol 2000;20:220–221.

773. Lee AG. Efficacy of unilateral versus bilateral temporal artery biopsies for the diagnosis of giant cell arteritis. Am J Ophthalmol 2000;129:118–119.

774. Hall JK, Volpe NJ, Galetta SL, et al. The role of unilateral temporal artery biopsy. Ophthalmology 2003;110:543–548.

775. Younge BR, Cook Jr. BE, Bartley GB, et al. Initiation of glucocorticoid therapy: before or after temporal artery biopsy? Mayo Clin Proc 2004;79:483–491.

776. Danesh-Meyer HV, Savino PJ, Eagle Jr. RC, et al. Low diagnostic yield with second biopsies in suspected giant cell arteritis. J Neuroophthalmol 2000;20:213–215.

777. Pless M, Rizzo 3rd JF, Lamkin JC, et al. Concordance of bilateral temporal artery biopsy in giant cell arteritis. J Neuroophthalmol 2000;20:216–218.

778. Boyev LR, Miller NR, Green WR. Efficacy of unilateral versus bilateral temporal artery biopsies for the diagnosis of giant cell arteritis. Am J Ophthalmol 1999;128:211–215.

779. Allison MC, Gallagher PJ. Temporal artery biopsy and corticosteroid treatment. Ann Rheum Dis 1984;43:416–417.

780. Achkar AA, Lie JT, Hunder GG, et al. How does previous corticosteroid therapy affect the biopsy findings in giant cell (temporal) arteritis? Ann Intern Med 1994;120:987–992.

781. Guevara RA, Newman NJ, Grossniklaus HE. Positive temporal artery biopsy 6 months after prednisone treatment. Arch Ophthalmol 1998;116:1252–1253.

782. Ray-Chaudhuri N, Kine DA, Tijani SO, et al. Effect of prior steroid treatment on temporal artery biopsy findings in giant cell arteritis. Br J Ophthalmol 2002;86:530–532.

783. To KW, Enzer YR, Tsiaras WG. Temporal artery biopsy after one month of corticosteroid therapy. Am J Ophthalmol 1994;117:265–267.

784. Wiggins RE. Invasive aspergillosis. A complication of treatment of temporal arteritis. J Neuroophthalmol 1995;15:36–38.

785. Ho AC, Sergott RC, Regillo CD, et al. Color Doppler hemodynamics of giant cell arteritis. Arch Ophthalmol 1994;112:938–945.

786. Schmidt D, Hetzel A, Reinhard M, et al. Comparison between color duplex ultrasonography and histology of the temporal artery in cranial arteritis (giant cell arteritis). Eur J Med Res 2003;8:1–7.

787. Schmidt WA, Kraft HE, Vorpahl K, et al. Color duplex ultrasonography in the diagnosis of temporal arteritis. N Engl J Med 1997;337:1336–1342.

788. Diamond JP. Treatable blindness in temporal arteritis. Br J Ophthalmol 1991;75:432.

789. Diamond JP. IV steroid treatment in giant cell arteritis [letter]. Ophthalmology 1993;100:291–292.

790. Fraser JA, Weyand CM, Newman NJ, et al. The treatment of giant cell arteritis. Rev Neurol Dis 2008;5:140–152.

791. Lipton RB, Solomon S, Wertenbaker C. Gradual loss and recovery of vision in temporal arteritis. Arch Intern Med 1985;145:2252–2253.

792. Matzkin DC, Slamovits TL, Sachs R, et al. Visual recovery in two patients after intravenous methylprednisolone treatment of central retinal artery occlusion secondary to giant-cell arteritis. Ophthalmology 1992;99:68–71.

793. Model DG. Reversal of blindness in temporal arteritis with methylprednisolone [letter]. Lancet 1978;1:340.

794. Postel EA, Pollock SC. Recovery of vision in a 47-year-old man with fulminant giant cell arteritis. J Clin Neuroophthalmol 1993;13:262–270.

795. Rosenfeld SI, Kosmorsky GS, Klingele TG, et al. Treatment of temporal arteritis with ocular involvement. Am J Med 1986;80:143–145.

796. Chan CC, Paine M, O'Day J. Steroid management in giant cell arteritis. Br J Ophthalmol 2001;85:1061–1064.

797. Cornblath WT, Eggenberger ER. Progressive vision loss from giant cell arteritis despite high dose intravenous methylprednisolone. Ophthalmology 1997;104:854–858.

798. Clearkin LG. IV steroids for central retinal artery occlusion in giant-cell arteritis [letter]. Ophthalmology 1992;99:1482–1483.

799. Rubinow A, Brandt KD, Cohen AS, et al. Iatrogenic morbidity accompanying suppression of temporal arteritis by adrenal corticosteroids. Ann Ophthalmol 1984;16:258–265.

800. Hayreh SS, Zimmerman B. Visual deterioration in giant cell arteritis patients while on high doses of corticosteroid therapy. Ophthalmology 2003;110:1204–1215.

801. Diego M, Margo CE. Postural vision loss in giant cell arteritis. J Neuroophthalmol 1998;18:124–126.

802. Cullen JF. Temporal arteritis. Occurrence of ocular complications 7 years after diagnosis. Br J Ophthalmol 1972;56:584–588.

803. Evans JM, Batts KP, Hunder GG. Persistent giant cell arteritis despite corticosteroid treatment. Mayo Clin Proc 1994;69:1060–1061.

804. Jover JA, Hernandez-Garcia C, Morado IC, et al. Combined treatment of giant-cell arteritis with methotrexate and prednisone: a randomized, double-blind, placebo-controlled trial. Ann Intern Med 2001;134:106–114.

805. Boesen P, Dideriksen K, Stentoft J, et al. Dapsone in temporal arteritis and polymyalgia rheumatica [letter]. J Rheumatol 1988;15:879–880.

806. Reinitz E, Aversa A. Long-term treatment of temporal arteritis with dapsone. Am J Med 1988;85:456–457.

807. Salvarani C, Macchioni P, Manzini C, et al. Infliximab plus prednisone or placebo plus prednisone for the initial treatment of polymyalgia rheumatica: a randomized trial. Ann Intern Med 2007;146:631–639.

808. Meadows SP. Temporal or giant cell arteritis. Proc R Soc Med 1966;59:329–333.

809. Birkhead NC, Wagener HP, Shick RM. Treatment of temporal arteritis with adrenal corticosteroids. Results in fifty-five cases in which lesion was proved at biopsy. JAMA 1957;163:821–827.

810. Slavin ML, Margolis AJ. Progressive anterior ischemic optic neuropathy due to giant cell arteritis despite high-dose intravenous corticosteroids [letter]. Arch Ophthalmol 1988;106:1167.

811. Rauser M, Rismondo V. Ischemic optic neuropathy during corticosteroid therapy for giant cell arteritis. Arch Ophthalmol 1995;113:707–708.

812. Danesh-Meyer H, Savino PJ, Gamble GG. Poor prognosis of visual outcome after visual loss from giant cell arteritis. Ophthalmology 2005;112:1098–1103.

813. Chan CC, Paine M, O'Day J. Predictors of recurrent ischemic optic neuropathy in giant cell arteritis. J Neuroophthalmol 2005;25:14–17.

814. Kim N, Trobe JD, Flint A, et al. Late ipsilateral recurrence of ischemic optic neuropathy in giant cell arteritis. J Neuroophthalmol 2003;23:122–126.

815. Hayreh SS, Zimmerman B, Kardon RH. Visual improvement with corticosteroid therapy in giant cell arteritis. Report of a large study and review of literature. Acta Ophthalmol Scand 2002;80:355–367.

816. Schneider HA, Weber AA, Ballen PH. The visual prognosis in temporal arteritis. Ann Ophthalmol 1971;3:1215–1230.

817. Foroozan R, Deramo VA, Buono LM, et al. Recovery of visual function in patients with biopsy-proven giant cell arteritis. Ophthalmology 2003;110:539–542.

818. Soelberg Sørensen P, Lorenzen I. Giant-cell arteritis, temporal arteritis and polymyalgia rheumatica. A retrospective study of 63 patients. Acta Med Scand 1977;201:207–213.

819. Hugod C, Scheibel M. Temporal arteritis: progressive affection of vision during high-level corticosteroid therapy. A case report. Acta Med Scand 1979;205:445–446.

820. Delecoeuillerie G, Joly P, Cohen De Lara A, et al. Polymyalgia rheumatica and temporal arteritis: a retrospective analysis of prognostic features and different corticosteroid regimens (11 year survey of 210 patients). Ann Rheum Dis 1988;47:733–739.

821. Faarvang KL, Pontoppidan Thyssen E. Giant cell arteritis: loss of vision during corticosteroid treatment. J Intern Med 1989;225:215–216.

822. Myles AB, Perera T, Ridley MG. Prevention of blindness in giant cell arteritis by corticosteroid treatment. Br J Rheumatol 1992;31:103–105.

823. Hernandez-Rodriguez J, Font C, Garcia-Martinez A, et al. Development of ischemic complications in patients with giant cell arteritis presenting with apparently isolated polymyalgia rheumatica: study of a series of 100 patients. Medicine (Baltimore) 2007;86:233–241.

824. Sadda SR, Nee M, Miller NR, et al. Clinical spectrum of posterior ischemic optic neuropathy. Am J Ophthalmol 2001;132:743–750.

825. Hayreh SS. Posterior ischaemic optic neuropathy: clinical features, pathogenesis, and management. Eye 2004;18:1188–1206.

826. Gilden DH, Lipton HL, Wolf JS, et al. Two patients with unusual forms of varicella-zoster virus vasculopathy. N Engl J Med 2002;347:1500–1503.

827. Harrison EQ. Complications of herpes zoster ophthalmicus. Am J Ophthalmol 1965;60:1111–1114.

828. Perlman JI, Forman S, Gonzalez ER. Retrobulbar ischemic optic neuropathy associated with sickle cell disease. J Neuroophthalmol 1994;14:45–48.

829. Lee AG, Brazis PW, Miller NR. Posterior ischemic optic neuropathy associated with migraine. Headache 1996;36:506–510.

830. Isayama Y, Takahashi T, Inoue M, et al. Posterior ischemic optic neuropathy. III. Clinical diagnosis. Ophthalmologica 1983;187:141–147.

831. Johnson MW, Kincaid MC, Trobe JD. Bilateral retrobulbar optic nerve infarctions after blood loss and hypotension. A clinicopathologic case study. Ophthalmology 1987;94:1577–1584.

832. Shaked G, Gavriel A, Roy-Shapira A. Anterior ischemic optic neuropathy after hemorrhagic shock. J Trauma 1998;44:923–925.

833. Katz DM, Trobe JD, Cornblath WT, et al. Ischemic optic neuropathy after lumbar spine surgery. Arch Ophthalmol 1994;112:925–931.

834. Lee AG. Ischemic optic neuropathy following lumbar spine surgery. Case report. J Neurosurg 1995;83:348–349.

835. Rizzo JF, Lessell S. Posterior ischemic optic neuropathy during general surgery. Am J Ophthalmol 1987;103:808–811.

836. Schobel GA, Schmidbauer M, Millesi W, et al. Posterior ischemic optic neuropathy following bilateral radical neck dissection. Int J Oral Maxillofac Surg 1995;24: 283–287.

837. Shapira OM, Kimmel WA, Lindsey PS, et al. Anterior ischemic optic neuropathy after open heart operations. Ann Thorac Surg 1996;61:660–666.

838. Sweeney PJ, Breuer AC, Selhorst JB, et al. Ischemic optic neuropathy: a complication of cardiopulmonary bypass surgery. Neurology 1982;32:560–562.

839. Alexandrakis G, Lam B. Bilateral posterior ischemic optic neuropathy after spinal surgery. Am J Ophthalmol 1999;127:354–355.

840. Buono LM, Foroozan R. Perioperative posterior ischemic optic neuropathy: review of the literature. Surv Ophthalmol 2005;50:15–26.

841. Moster ML. Visual loss after coronary artery bypass surgery. Surv Ophthalmol 1998;42:453–457.

842. Newman NJ. Perioperative visual loss after nonocular surgeries. Am J Ophthalmol 2008;145:604–610.

843. Bennett HL, Origlieri C, Sakamuri S. Perioperative ischemic optic neuropathy (POION). Spine 2005;30:2706; author reply 2707.

844. Chang SH, Miller NR. The incidence of vision loss due to perioperative ischemic optic neuropathy associated with spine surgery: the Johns Hopkins Hospital Experience. Spine 2005;30:1299–1302.

845. Dunker S, Hsu HY, Sebag J, et al. Perioperative risk factors for posterior ischemic optic neuropathy. J Am Coll Surg 2002;194:705–710.

846. Ho VT, Newman NJ, Song S, et al. Ischemic optic neuropathy following spine surgery. J Neurosurg Anesthesiol 2005;17:38–44.

847. Kalyani SD, Miller NR, Dong LM, et al. Incidence of and risk factors for perioperative optic neuropathy after cardiac surgery. Ann Thorac Surg 2004;78:34–37.

848. Lee LA, Roth S, Posner KL, et al. The American Society of Anesthesiologists Postoperative Visual Loss Registry: analysis of 93 spine surgery cases with postoperative visual loss. Anesthesiology 2006;105:652–659; quiz 867–658.

849. Myers MA, Hamilton SR, Bogosian AJ, et al. Visual loss as a complication of spine surgery. A review of 37 cases. Spine 1997;22:1325–1329.

850. Nuttall GA, Garrity JA, Dearani JA, et al. Risk factors for ischemic optic neuropathy after cardiopulmonary bypass: a matched case/control study. Anesth Analg 2001;93:1410–1416.

851. Patil CG, Lad EM, Lad SP, et al. Visual loss after spine surgery: a population-based study. Spine 2008;33:1491–1496.

852. Stambough JL, Dolan D, Werner R, et al. Ophthalmologic complications associated with prone positioning in spine surgery. J Am Acad Orthop Surg 2007;15:156–165.

853. Stevens WR, Glazer PA, Kelley SD, et al. Ophthalmic complications after spinal surgery. Spine 1997;22:1319–1324.

854. Aydin O, Memisoglu I, Ozturk M, et al. Anterior ischemic optic neuropathy after unilateral radical neck dissection: case report and review. Auris Nasus Larynx 2008;35:308–312.

855. Marks SC, Jaques DA, Hirata RM, et al. Blindness following bilateral radical neck dissection. Head Neck 1990;12:342–345.

856. Nawa Y, Jaques JD, Miller NR, et al. Bilateral posterior optic neuropathy after bilateral radical neck dissection and hypotension. Graefes Arch Clin Exp Ophthalmol 1992;230:301–308.

857. Pazos GA, Leonard DW, Blice J, et al. Blindness after bilateral neck dissection: case report and review. Am J Otolaryngol 1999;20:340–345.

858. Worrell L, Rowe M, Petti G. Amaurosis: a complication of bilateral radical neck dissection. Am J Otolaryngol 2002;23:56–59.

859. Basile C, Addabbo G, Montanaro A. Anterior ischemic optic neuropathy and dialysis: role of hypotension and anemia. J Nephrol 2001;14:420–423.

860. Buono LM, Foroozan R, Savino PJ, et al. Posterior ischemic optic neuropathy after hemodialysis. Ophthalmology 2003;110:1216–1218.

861. Chutorian AM, Winterkorn JM, Geffner M. Anterior ischemic optic neuropathy in children: case reports and review of the literature. Pediatr Neurol 2002;26:358–364.

862. Kirmizis D, Belechri AM, Trigoudis D, et al. Anterior ischemic optic neuropathy in an extreme dipper dialysis patient. Hemodial Int 2005;9:143–146.

863. Korzets A, Marashek I, Schwartz A, et al. Ischemic optic neuropathy in dialyzed patients: a previously unrecognized manifestation of calcific uremic arteriolopathy. Am J Kidney Dis 2004;44:e93–97.

864. Servilla KS, Groggel GC. Anterior ischemic optic neuropathy as a complication of hemodialysis. Am J Kidney Dis 1986;8:61–63.

865. Barr CG, Glaser JS, Blankenship G. Acute disc swelling in juvenile diabetes: clinical profile and natural history in 12 cases. Arch Ophthalmol 1980;98:2185–2192.

866. Regillo CD, Brown GC, Savino PJ, et al. Diabetic papillopathy. Patient characteristics and fundus findings. Arch Ophthalmol 1995;113:889–895.

867. Skillern PG, Lokhart G. Optic neuritis and uncontrolled diabetes mellitus in 14 patients. Ann Intern Med 1959;51:468–475.

868. Ho AC, Maguire AM, Yanuzzi LA, et al. Rapidly progressive optic disc neovascularization after diabetic papillopathy. Am J Ophthalmol 1995;120: 673–675.

869. Mansour AM, El-Dairi MA, Shehab MA, et al. Periocular corticosteroids in diabetic papillopathy. Eye 2005;19:45–51.

870. Al-Haddad CE, Jurdi FA, Bashshur ZF. Intravitreal triamcinolone acetonide for the management of diabetic papillopathy. Am J Ophthalmol 2004;137:1151–1153.

871. Kennedy F. Retrobulbar neuritis as an exact diagnostic sign of certain tumors and abscesses in the frontal lobes. Am J Med Sci 1911;142:355–368.

872. Wright JE, McNab AA, McDonald WI. Optic nerve glioma and the management of optic nerve tumours in the young. Br J Ophthalmol 1989;73:967–974.

873. Trobe JD, Glaser JS. Quantitative perimetry in compressive optic neuropathy and optic neuritis. Arch Ophthalmol 1978;96:1210–1216.

874. Dutton JJ. Gliomas of the anterior visual pathways. Surv Ophthalmol 1994;38: 427–452.

875. Listernick R, Louis DN, Packer RJ, et al. Optic pathway gliomas in children with neurofibromatosis 1: consensus statement from the NF1 Optic Pathway Glioma Task Force. Ann Neurol 1997;41:143–149.

876. Listernick R, Charrow J, Greenwald M, et al. Natural history of optic pathway tumors in children with neurofibromatosis type 1: a longitudinal study. J Pediatr 1994;125: 63–66.

877. Balcer LJ, Liu GT, Heller G, et al. Visual loss in children with neurofibromatosis type 1 and optic pathway gliomas: relation to tumor location by magnetic resonance imaging. Am J Ophthalmol 2001;131:442–445.

878. Lewis RA, Gerson LP, Axelson KA, et al. von Recklinghausen neurofibromatosis. II. Incidence of optic gliomata. Ophthalmology 1984;91:929–935.

879. Haik BG, Louis LS, Bierly J, et al. Magnetic resonance imaging in the evaluation of optic nerve gliomas. Ophthalmology 1987;94:709–717.

880. Jakobiec FA, Depot MJ, Kennerdell JS, et al. Combined clinical and computed tomographic diagnosis of orbital glioma and meningioma. Ophthalmology 1984;91:137–155.

881. Alvord EC, Lofton S. Gliomas of the optic nerve or chiasm: outcome by patients' age, tumor site, and treatment. J Neurosurg 1988;68:85–98.

882. Seiff SR, Brodsky MC, MacDonald G, et al. Orbital optic glioma in neurofibromatosis. Magnetic resonance diagnosis of perineural arachnoidal gliomatosis. Arch Ophthalmol 1987;105:1689–1692.

883. Brodsky MC. The "pseudo-CSF" signal of orbital optic glioma on magnetic resonance imaging: a signature of neurofibromatosis. Surv Ophthalmol 1993;38:213–218.

884. McDonnell P, Miller NR. Chiasmatic and hypothalamic extension of optic nerve glioma. Arch Ophthalmol 1983;101:1412–1415.

885. Walrath JD, Engelbert M, Kazim M. Magnetic resonance imaging evidence of optic nerve glioma progression into and beyond the optic chiasm. Ophthal Plast Reconstr Surg 2008;24:473–475.

886. Falsini B, Ziccardi L, Lazzareschi I, et al. Longitudinal assessment of childhood optic gliomas: relationship between flicker visual evoked potentials and magnetic resonance imaging findings. J Neurooncol 2008;88:87–96.

887. Kushner BJ. Functional amblyopia associated with abnormalities of the optic nerve. Arch Ophthalmol 1984;102:683–685.

888. Tow SL, Chandela S, Miller NR, et al. Long-term outcome in children with gliomas of the anterior visual pathway. Pediatr Neurol 2003;28:262–270.

889. Gaini SM, Tomei G, Arienta C, et al. Optic nerve and chiasmal gliomas in children. J Neurosurg Sci 1982;26:33–39.

890. Redfern RM, Scholtz CL. Long term survival with optic nerve glioma. Surg Neurol 1980;14:371–375.

891. Pollock JM, Greiner FG, Crowder JB, et al. Neurosarcoidosis mimicking a malignant optic glioma. J Neuroophthalmol 2008;28:214–216.

892. Chacko JG, Lam BL, Adusumilli J, et al. Multicentric malignant glioma of adulthood masquerading as optic neuritis. Br J Ophthalmol 2008;Oct 31.

893. Spoor TC, Kennerdell JS, Martinez AJ, et al. Malignant gliomas of the optic nerve pathways. Am J Ophthalmol 1980;89:284–292.

894. Hoyt WF, Meshel LG, Lessell S, et al. Malignant optic glioma of adulthood. Brain 1973;96:121–132.

895. Bosch MM, Wichmann WW, Boltshauser E, et al. Optic nerve sheath meningiomas in patients with neurofibromatosis type 2. Arch Ophthalmol 2006;124:379–385.

896. Cunliffe IA, Moffat DA, Hardy DG, et al. Bilateral optic nerve sheath meningiomas in a patient with neurofibromatosis type 2. Br J Ophthalmol 1992;76:310–312.

897. Harold Lee HB, Garrity JA, Cameron JD, et al. Primary optic nerve sheath meningioma in children. Surv Ophthalmol 2008;53:543–558.

898. Bickerstaff ER, Small JM, Guest IA. The relapsing course of certain meningiomas in relation to pregnancy and menstruation. J Neurol Neurosurg Psychiatry 1958;21: 89–91.

899. Sarkies NJ. Optic nerve sheath meningiomas: diagnostic features and therapeutic alternatives. Eye 1987;1:597–602.

900. Sibony PA, Krauss HR, Kennerdell JS, et al. Optic nerve sheath meningiomas: clinical manifestations. Ophthalmology 1984;91:1313–1326.

901. Wright JE, Call NB, Liaricos S. Primary optic nerve meningiomas. Br J Ophthalmol 1980;64:553–558.

902. Zimmerman CF, Schatz NJ, Glaser JS. Magnetic resonance imaging of optic nerve meningiomas: enhancement with gadolinium-DTPA. Ophthalmology 1990;97:585–591.

903. Lindblom B, Truwit CL, Hoyt WF. Optic nerve sheath meningioma. Definition of intraorbital, intracanalicular, and intracranial components with magnetic resonance imaging. Ophthalmology 1992;99:560–566.

904. Mafee MF, Goodwin J, Dorodi S. Optic nerve sheath meningiomas. Role of MR imaging. Radiol Clin North Am 1999;37:37–58.

905. Egan RA, Lessell S. A contribution to the natural history of optic nerve sheath meningiomas. Arch Ophthalmol 2002;120:1505–1508.

906. Smith JL, Vuksanovic MM, Yates BM, et al. Radiation therapy for primary optic nerve meningiomas. J Clin Neuroophthalmol 1981;1:85–99.

907. Kennerdell JS, Maroon JC, Malton M, et al. The management of optic nerve sheath meningiomas. Am J Ophthalmol 1988;106:450–457.

908. Klink DF, Miller NR, Williams J. Preservation of residual vision 2 years after stereotactic radiosurgery for a presumed optic nerve sheath meningioma. J Neuroophthalmol 1998;18:117–120.

909. Andrews DW, Faroozan R, Yang BP, et al. Fractionated stereotactic radiotherapy for the treatment of optic nerve sheath meningiomas: preliminary observations of 33 optic nerves in 30 patients with historical comparison to observation with or without prior surgery. Neurosurg 2002;51:890–902.

910. Baumert BG, Villa S, Studer G, et al. Early improvements in vision after fractionated stereotactic radiotherapy for primary optic nerve sheath meningioma. Radiother Oncol 2004;72:169–174.

911. Carrasco JR, Penne RB. Optic nerve sheath meningiomas and advanced treatment options. Curr Opin Ophthalmol 2004;15:406–410.

912. Jeremic B, Pitz S. Primary optic nerve sheath meningioma: stereotactic fractionated radiation therapy as an emerging treatment of choice. Cancer 2007;110:714–722.

913. Landert M, Baumert BG, Bosch MM, et al. The visual impact of fractionated stereotactic conformal radiotherapy on seven eyes with optic nerve sheath meningiomas. J Neuroophthalmol 2005;25:86–91.

914. Liu JK, Forman S, Hershewe GL, et al. Optic nerve sheath meningiomas: visual improvement after stereotactic radiotherapy. Neurosurg 2002;50:950–955.

915. Melian E, Jay WM. Primary radiotherapy for optic nerve sheath meningioma. Semin Ophthalmol 2004;19:130–140.

916. Miller NR. Radiation for optic nerve meningiomas: is this the answer? Ophthalmology 2002;109:833–834.

917. Moyer PD, Golnik KC, Breneman J. Treatment of optic nerve sheath meningioma with three-dimensional conformal radiation. Am J Ophthalmol 2000;129:694–696.

918. Pitz S, Becker G, Schiefer U, et al. Stereotactic fractionated irradiation of optic nerve sheath meningioma: a new treatment alternative. Br J Ophthalmol 2002;86:1265–1268.

919. Saeed P, Rootman J, Nugent RA, et al. Optic nerve sheath meningioma. Ophthalmology 2003;110:2019–2030.

920. Sitathanee C, Dhanachai M, Poonyathalang A, et al. Stereotactic radiation therapy for optic nerve sheath meningioma; an experience at Ramathibodi Hospital. J Med Assoc Thai 2006;89:1665–1669.

921. Turbin RE, Thompson CR, Kennerdell JS, et al. A long-term visual outcome comparison in patients with optic nerve sheath meningioma managed with observation, surgery, radiotherapy, or surgery and radiotherapy. Ophthalmology 2002;109:890–899.

922. Vagefi MR, Larson DA, Horton JC. Optic nerve sheath meningioma: visual improvement during radiation treatment. Am J Ophthalmol 2006;142:343–344.

923. Kupersmith MJ, Warren FA, Newell J, et al. Irradiation of meningiomas of the intracranial anterior visual pathway. Ann Neurol 1987;21:131–137.

924. Rosenstein J, Symon L. Surgical management of suprasellar meningioma. 2. Prognosis for visual function following craniotomy. J Neurosurg 1984;61:642–648.

925. Andrews BT, Wilson CB. Suprasellar meningiomas: the effect of tumor location on postoperative visual outcome. J Neurosurg 1988;69:523–528.

926. Danesh-Meyer HV, Papchenko T, Savino PJ, et al. In vivo retinal nerve fiber layer thickness measured by optical coherence tomography predicts visual recovery after surgery for parachiasmal tumors. Invest Ophthalmol Vis Sci 2008;49:1879–1885.

927. Grunberg SM, Weiss MH, Russell CA, et al. Long-term administration of mifepristone (RU486): clinical tolerance during extended treatment of meningioma. Cancer Invest 2006;24:727–733.

928. Grunberg SM, Weiss MH, Spitz IM, et al. Treatment of unresectable meningiomas with the antiprogesterone agent mifepristone. J Neurosurg 1991;74:861–866.

929. Rosenberg LF, Miller NR. Visual results after microsurgical removal of meningiomas involving the anterior visual system. Arch Ophthalmol 1984;102:1019–1023.

930. Margalit N, Kesler A, Ezer H, et al. Tuberculum and diaphragma sella meningioma: surgical technique and visual outcome in a series of 20 cases operated over a 2.5-year period. Acta Neurochir (Wien) 2007;149:1199–1204.

931. Kitano M, Taneda M, Nakao Y. Postoperative improvement in visual function in patients with tuberculum sellae meningiomas: results of the extended transsphenoidal and transcranial approaches. J Neurosurg 2007;107:337–346.

932. Grisoli F, Vincentelli F, Raybaud C, et al. Intrasellar meningioma. Surg Neurol 1983;20:36–41.

933. Bassiouni H, Asgari S, Stolke D. Tuberculum sellae meningiomas: functional outcome in a consecutive series treated microsurgically. Surg Neurol 2006;66:37–44.

934. Schick U, Hassler W. Surgical management of tuberculum sellae meningiomas: involvement of the optic canal and visual outcome. J Neurol Neurosurg Psychiatry 2005;76:977–983.

935. Schick U, Bleyen J, Bani A, et al. Management of meningiomas en plaque of the sphenoid wing. J Neurosurg 2006;104:208–214.

936. Chicani CF, Miller NR. Visual outcome in surgically treated suprasellar meningiomas. J Neuroophthalmol 2003;23:3–10.

937. Nozaki K, Kikuta K, Takagi Y, et al. Effect of early optic canal unroofing on the outcome of visual functions in surgery for meningiomas of the tuberculum sellae and planum sphenoidale. Neurosurg 2008;62:839–844.

938. Kline LB, Kim JY, Ceballos R. Radiation optic neuropathy. Ophthalmology 1985;92:1118–1126.

939. Wiebers DO, Whisnant JP, O'Fallon WM. The natural history of unruptured intracranial aneurysms. N Engl J Med 1981;304:696–698.

940. Farris BK, Smith JL, David NJ. The nasal junction scotoma in giant aneurysms. Ophthalmology 1986;93:895–905.

941. Craenen G, Brown SM, Freedman KA, et al. Rapid, painless unilateral vision loss in a 37-year-old healthy woman. Surv Ophthalmol 2004;49:343–348.

942. Vargas ME, Kupersmith MJ, Setton A, et al. Endovascular treatment of giant aneurysms which cause visual loss. Ophthalmology 1994;101:1091–1098.

943. Ferguson GG, Drake CG. Carotid-ophthalmic aneurysms: the surgical management of those cases presenting with compression of the optic nerves and chiasm alone. Clin Neurosurg 1980;27:263–307.

944. Kupersmith MJ, Berenstein A, Choi IS, et al. Percutaneous transvascular treatment of giant carotid aneurysms: neuro-ophthalmologic findings. Neurology 1984;34:328–335.

945. Rizzo 3rd JF. Visual loss after neurosurgical repair of paraclinoid aneurysms. Ophthalmology 1995;102:905–910.

946. Gutman I, Melamed S, Askenazi I, et al. Optic nerve compression by carotid arteries in low tension glaucoma. Graefes Arch Clin Exp Ophthalmol 1993;231:711–717.

947. Kalenak JW, Kosmorsky GS, Hassenbusch SJ. Compression of the intracranial optic nerve mimicking unilateral normal pressure glaucoma. J Clin Neuroophthalmol 1992;12:230–235.

948. Jacobson DM, Warner JJ, Broste SK. Optic nerve contact and compression by the carotid artery in asymptomatic patients. Am J Ophthalmol 1997;123:677–683.

949. Kerr NC, Wang WC, Mohadjer Y, et al. Reversal of optic canal stenosis in osteopetrosis after bone marrow transplant. Am J Ophthalmol 2000;130:370–372.

950. Khong JJ, Anderson P, Gray TL, et al. Ophthalmic findings in Apert's syndrome after craniofacial surgery: twenty-nine years' experience. Ophthalmology 2006;113:347–352.

951. Gray TL, Casey T, Selva D, et al. Ophthalmic sequelae of Crouzon syndrome. Ophthalmology 2005;112:1129–1134.

952. Liasis A, Nischal KK, Walters B, et al. Monitoring visual function in children with syndromic craniosynostosis: a comparison of 3 methods. Arch Ophthalmol 2006;124:1119–1126.

953. Grosskreutz C, Netland PA. Low-tension glaucoma. Int Ophthalmol Clin 1994;34:173–185.

954. Sommer A, Tielsch JM, Katz J, et al. Relationship between intraocular pressure and primary open angle glaucoma among white and black Americans. The Baltimore Eye Survey. Arch Ophthalmol 1991;109:1090–1095.

955. Stroman GA, Stewart WC, Golnik KC, et al. Magnetic resonance imaging in patients with low tension glaucoma. Arch Ophthalmol 1995;113:168–172.

956. Corbett JJ, Phelps CD, Eslinger P, et al. The neurologic evaluation of patients with low-tension glaucoma. Invest Ophthalmol Vis Sci 1985;26:1101–1104.

957. Bianchi-Marzoli S, Rizzo JF, Brancato R, et al. Quantitative analysis of optic disc cupping in compressive optic neuropathy. Ophthalmology 1995;102:436–440.

958. Sharma M, Volpe NJ, Dreyer EB. Methanol-induced optic nerve cupping. Arch Ophthalmol 1999;117:286.

959. Greenfield DS, Siatkowski RM, Glaser JS, et al. The cupped disc. Who needs neuroimaging? Ophthalmology 1998;105:1866–1874.

960. Bushley DM, Parmley VC, Paglen P. Visual field defect associated with laser in situ keratomileusis. Am J Ophthalmol 2000;129:668–671.

961. Cameron BD, Saffra NA, Strominger MB. Laser in situ keratomileusis-induced optic neuropathy. Ophthalmology 2001;108:660–665.

962. Wasserstrom WF, Glass JP, Posner JB. Diagnosis and treatment of leptomeningeal metastases from solid tumors: experience with 90 patients. Cancer 1982;49:759–769.

963. Katz J, Valsamis M, Jampel R. Ocular signs in diffuse carcinomatous meningitis. Am J Ophthalmol 1961;52:681–690.

964. Altrocchi P, Eckman P. Meningeal carcinomatosis and blindness. J Neurol Neurosurg Psychiatry 1973;36:206–210.

965. Case records of the Massachusetts General Hospital. Weekly clinicopathological exercises. Case 14-1988. A 40-year-old man with rapidly progressive blindness and multiple cranial-nerve deficits. N Engl J Med 1988;318:903–915.

966. Shields JA, Shields CL, Singh AD. Metastatic neoplasms in the optic disc: the 1999 Bjerrum Lecture: part 2. Arch Ophthalmol 2000;118:217–224.

967. Arnold AC, Hepler RS, Foos RY. Isolated metastasis to the optic nerve. Surv Ophthalmol 1981;26:75–83.

968. Sung JU, Lam BL, Curtin VT, et al. Metastatic gastric carcinoma to the optic nerve. Arch Ophthalmol 1998;116:692–693.

969. Backhouse O, Simmons I, Frank A, et al. Optic nerve breast metastasis mimicking meningioma. Aust N Z J Ophthalmol 1998;26:247–249.

970. Mansour AM, Dinowitz K, Chaljub G, et al. Metastatic lesion of the optic nerve. J Clin Neuroophthalmol 1993;13:102–104.

971. Newman NJ, Grossniklaus HE, Wojno TH. Breast carcinoma metastatic to the optic nerve. Arch Ophthalmol 1996;114:102–103.

972. Kattah JC, Chrousos GC, Roberts J, et al. Metastatic prostate cancer to the optic canal. Ophthalmology 1993;100:1711–1715.

973. Shields JA, Demirci H, Mashayekhi A, et al. Melanocytoma of the optic disk: a review. Surv Ophthalmol 2006;51:93–104.

974. Zografos L, Othenin-Girard CB, Desjardins L, et al. Melanocytomas of the optic disk. Am J Ophthalmol 2004;138:964–969.

975. Kim IK, Dryja TP, Lessell S, et al. Melanocytoma of the optic nerve associated with sound-induced phosphenes. Arch Ophthalmol 2006;124:273–277.

976. Shields JA, Shields CL, Ehya H, et al. Total blindness from presumed optic nerve melanocytoma. Am J Ophthalmol 2005;139:1113–1114.

977. Strominger MB, Schatz NJ, Glaser JS. Lymphomatous optic neuropathy. Am J Ophthalmol 1993;116:774–776.

978. Coppeto JR, Monteiro ML, Cannarozzi DB. Optic neuropathy associated with chronic lymphomatous meningitis. J Clin Neuroophthalmol 1988;8:39–45.

979. Donoso LA, Magargal LE, Eiferman RA. Meningeal carcinomatosis secondary to malignant lymphoma (Burkitt's pattern). J Pediatr Ophthalmol Strabismus 1981;18:48–50.

980. Kline LB, Garcia JH, Harsh GR. Lymphomatous optic neuropathy. Arch Ophthalmol 1984;102:1655–1657.

981. Kay MC. Optic neuropathy secondary to lymphoma. J Clin Neuroophthalmol 1986;6:31–34.

982. Ko MW, Tamhankar MA, Volpe NJ, et al. Acute promyelocytic leukemic involvement of the optic nerves following mitoxantrone treatment for multiple sclerosis. J Neurol Sci 2008;273:144–147.

983. Schockket LS, Massaro-Giordano M, Volpe NJ, et al. Bilateral optic nerve infiltration in central nervous system leukemia. Am J Ophthalmol 2003;135:94–96.

984. Takahashi T, Oda Y, Isayama Y. Leukemic optic neuropathy. Ophthalmologica 1982;185:37–45.

985. Brown GC, Shields JA, Augsburger JJ, et al. Leukemic optic neuropathy. Int Ophthalmol 1981;3:111–116.

986. Currie JN, Lessell S, Lessell IM, et al. Optic neuropathy in chronic lymphocytic leukemia. Arch Ophthalmol 1988;106:654–660.

987. Norton SW, Stockman JA. Unilateral optic neuropathy following vincristine chemotherapy. J Pediatr Ophthalmol Strabismus 1979;16:190–193.

988. Waterston JA, Gilligan BS. Paraneoplastic optic neuritis and external ophthalmoplegia. Aust N Z J Med 1986;16:703–704.

989. Pillay N, Gilbert JJ, Ebers GC, et al. Internuclear ophthalmoplegia and "optic neuritis": paraneoplastic effects of bronchial carcinoma. Neurology 1984;34:788–791.

990. Boghen D, Sebag M, Michaud J. Paraneoplastic optic neuritis and encephalomyelitis. Report of a case. Arch Neurol 1988;45:353–356.

991. Malik S, Furlan AJ, Sweeney PJ, et al. Optic neuropathy: a rare paraneoplastic syndrome. J Clin Neuroophthalmol 1992;12:137–141.

992. Luiz JE, Lee AG, Keltner JL, et al. Paraneoplastic optic neuropathy and autoantibody production in small-cell carcinoma of the lung. J Neuroophthalmol 1998;18:178–181.

993. de la Sayette V, Bertran F, Honnorat J, et al. Paraneoplastic cerebellar syndrome and optic neuritis with anti-CV2 antibodies: clinical response to excision of the primary tumor. Arch Neurol 1998;55:405–408.

994. Blumenthal D, Schochet Jr. S, Gutmann L, et al. Small-cell carcinoma of the lung presenting with paraneoplastic peripheral nerve microvasculitis and optic neuropathy [letter]. Muscle & Nerve 1998;21:1358–1359.

995. Yu Z, Kryzer TJ, Griesmann GE, et al. CRMP-5 neuronal autoantibody: marker of lung cancer and thymoma-related autoimmunity. Ann Neurol 2001;49:146–154.

996. Thambisetty MR, Scherzer CR, Yu Z, et al. Paraneoplastic optic neuropathy and cerebellar ataxia with small cell carcinoma of the lung. J Neuroophthalmol 2001;21:164–167.

997. Sheorajpanday R, Slabbynck H, Van De Sompel W, et al. Small cell lung carcinoma presenting as collapsin response-mediating protein (CRMP)-5 paraneoplastic optic neuropathy. J Neuroophthalmol 2006;26:168–172.

998. Pulido J, Cross SA, Lennon VA, et al. Bilateral autoimmune optic neuritis and vitreitis related to CRMP-5-IgG: intravitreal triamcinolone acetonide therapy of four eyes. Eye 2008;22:1191–1193.

999. Margolin E, Flint A, Trobe JD. High-titer collapsin response-mediating protein-associated (CRMP-5) paraneoplastic optic neuropathy and vitritis as the only clinical manifestations in a patient with small cell lung carcinoma. J Neuroophthalmol 2008;28:17–22.

1000. Cross SA, Salomao DR, Parisi JE, et al. Paraneoplastic autoimmune optic neuritis with retinitis defined by CRMP-5-IgG. Ann Neurol 2003;54:38–50.

1001. Schatz NJ, Lichtenstein S, Corbett JJ. Delayed radiation necrosis of the optic nerves and chiasm. In: Glaser JS, Smith JL (eds): Neuro-ophthalmology Symposium of the University of Miami and the Bascom Palmer Eye Institute, vol. VIII. St. Louis, C.V. Mosby, 1975:131–139.

1002. Lessell S. Friendly fire: neurogenic visual loss from radiation therapy. J Neuroophthalmol 2004;24:243–250.

1003. Danesh-Meyer HV. Radiation-induced optic neuropathy. J Clin Neurosci 2008;15:95–100.

1004. Levin LA, Gragoudas ES, Lessell S. Endothelial cell loss in irradiated optic nerves. Ophthalmology 2000;107:370–374.

1005. van den Bergh AC, Schoorl MA, Dullaart RP, et al. Lack of radiation optic neuropathy in 72 patients treated for pituitary adenoma. J Neuroophthalmol 2004;24:200–205.

1006. Girkin CA, Comey CH, Lunsford LD, et al. Radiation optic neuropathy after stereotactic radiosurgery. Ophthalmology 1997;104:1634–1643.

1007. Leber KA, Berglöff J, Pendl G. Dose-response tolerance of the visual pathways and cranial nerves of the cavernous sinus to stereotactic radiosurgery. J Neurosurg 1998;88:43–50.

1008. Stafford SL, Pollock BE, Leavitt JA, et al. A study on the radiation tolerance of the optic nerves and chiasm after stereotactic radiosurgery. Int J Radiat Oncol Biol Phys 2003;55:1177–1181.

1009. Zimmerman CF, Schatz NJ, Glaser GS. Magnetic resonance imaging in radiation optic neuropathy. Am J Ophthalmol 1990;110:389–394.

1010. Roden D, Bosley TM, Fowble B, et al. Delayed radiation injury to the retrobulbar optic nerves and chiasm. Clinical syndrome and treatment with hyperbaric oxygen and corticosteroids. Ophthalmology 1990;97:346–351.

1011. Levy RL, Miller NR. Hyperbaric oxygen therapy for radiation-induced optic neuropathy. Ann Acad Med Singapore 2006;35:151–157.

1012. Guy J, Schatz NJ. Hyperbaric oxygen in the treatment of radiation optic neuropathy. Ophthalmology 1986;93:1083–1090.

1013. Butler Jr. FK, Hagan C, Murphy-Lavoie H. Hyperbaric oxygen therapy and the eye. Undersea Hyperb Med 2008;35:333–387.

1014. Boschetti M, De Lucchi M, Giusti M, et al. Partial visual recovery from radiation-induced optic neuropathy after hyperbaric oxygen therapy in a patient with Cushing disease. Eur J Endocrinol 2006;154:813–818.

1015. Borruat FX, Schatz NJ, Glaser JS, et al. Visual recovery from radiation induced optic neuropathy: the role of hyperbaric oxygen therapy. J Clin Neuroophthalmol 1993;13:98–101.

1016. Al-Waili NS, Butler GJ, Beale J, et al. Hyperbaric oxygen and malignancies: a potential role in radiotherapy, chemotherapy, tumor surgery and phototherapy. Med Sci Monit 2005;11:RA279–289.

1017. Glantz MJ, Burger PC, Friedman AH, et al. Treatment of radiation-induced nervous system injury with heparin and warfarin. Neurology 1994;44:2020–2027.

1018. Landau K, Killer HE. Radiation damage [letter]. Neurology 1996;46:889.

1019. Lessell S. Toxic and deficiency optic neuropathies. In: Smith JL, Glaser JS (eds). Neuro-ophthalmology; Symposium of the University of Miami and the Bascom Palmer Eye Institute, pp 21–37. St. Louis, C.V. Mosby, 1973.

1020. Lessell S. Nutritional amblyopia. J Neuroophthalmol 1998;18:106–111.

1021. Hamilton HE, Ellis PE, Sheets RF. Visual impairment due to optic neuropathy in pernicious anemia: report of a case and review of the literature. Blood 1959;14:378–385.

1022. Rizzo JF. Adenosine triphosphate deficiency: a genre of optic neuropathy. Neurology 1995;45:11–16.

1023. Troncoso J, Mancall EL, Schatz NJ. Visual evoked responses in pernicious anemia. Arch Neurol 1979;36:168–169.

1024. Misra UK, Kalita J, Das A. Vitamin B12 deficiency neurological syndromes: a clinical, MRI and electrodiagnostic study. Electromyogr Clin Neurophysiol 2003;43:57–64.

1025. Lindenbaum J, Healton EB, Savage DG, et al. Neuropsychiatric disorders caused by cobalamin deficiency in the absence of anemia or macrocytosis. N Engl J Med 1988;318:1720–1728.

1026. Chester EM, Agamanopolis DP, Harris JW, et al. Optic atrophy in experimental vitamin B12 deficiency in monkeys. Acta Neurol Scand 1980;61:9–26.

1027. Hind VMD. Degeneration in the peripheral visual pathway of B12-deficient monkeys. Trans Ophthalmol Soc UK 1970;90:839–846.

1028. Bloom SM, Merz EH, Taylor WW. Nutritional amblyopia in American prisoners of war liberated from the Japanese. Am J Ophthalmol 1946;29:1248–1257.

1029. Samples JR, Younge BR. Tobacco-alcohol amblyopia. J Clin Neuroophthalmol 1981;1:213–218.

1030. Wokes F. Tobacco amblyopia. Lancet 1958;2:526–527.

1031. Rizzo JF, Lessell S. Tobacco amblyopia. Am J Ophthalmol 1993;116:84–87.

1032. Heaton JM, McCormick AJA, Freeman AG. Tobacco amblyopia: clinical manifestations of vitamin B12 deficiency. Lancet 1958;2:286–290.

1033. Frisén L. Fundus changes in acute malnutritional optic neuropathy. Arch Ophthalmol 1983;101:577–579.

1034. Carroll FD. Nutritional amblyopia. Arch Ophthalmol 1966;76:406–411.

1035. Quigley HA, Addicks EM, Green WR. Optic nerve damage in human glaucoma. III. Quantitative correlation of nerve fiber loss and visual field defect in glaucoma, ischemic neuropathy, papilledema, and toxic neuropathy. Arch Ophthalmol 1982;100:135–146.

1036. Cullom ME, Heher KL, Miller NR, et al. Leber's hereditary optic neuropathy masquerading as tobacco-alcohol amblyopia. Arch Ophthalmol 1993;111:1482–1485.

1037. Roman GC. An epidemic in Cuba of optic neuropathy, sensorineural deafness, peripheral sensory neuropathy and dorsolateral myeloneuropathy. J Neurol Sci 1994;127:11–28.

1038. Newman NJ, Torroni A, Brown MD, et al. Epidemic neuropathy in Cuba not associated with mitochondrial DNA mutations found in Leber's hereditary optic neuropathy patients. Cuban Neuropathy Field Investigation Team. Am J Ophthalmol 1994;118:158–168.

1039. Johns DR, Neufeld MJ, Hedges TR. Mitochondrial DNA mutations in Cuban optic and peripheral neuropathy. J Neuroophthalmol 1994;14:135–140.

1040. Johns DR, Sadun AA. Cuban epidemic optic neuropathy. Mitochondrial DNA analysis. J Neuroophthalmol 1994;14:130–134.

1041. The Cuba Neuropathy Field Investigation Team. Epidemic optic neuropathy in Cuba: clinical characterization and risk factors. N Engl J Med 1995;333:1176–1182.

1042. Sadun AA, Martone JF, Muci-Mendoza R, et al. Epidemic optic neuropathy in Cuba. Eye findings. Arch Ophthalmol 1994;112:691–699.

1043. Mojon DS, Kaufmann P, Odel JG, et al. Clinical course of a cohort in the Cuban epidemic optic and peripheral neuropathy. Neurology 1997;48:19–22.

1044. Hirano M, Cleary JM, Stewart AM, et al. Mitochondrial DNA mutations in an outbreak of optic neuropathy in Cuba. Neurology 1994;44:843–845.

1045. Osuntokun BO, Osuntokun O. Tropical amblyopia in Nigerians. Am J Ophthalmol 1971;72:708–716.

1046. Carroll FD. Jamaican optic neuropathy in immigrants to the United States. Am J Ophthalmol 1971;71:261–265.

1047. Plant GT, Mtanda AT, Arden GB, et al. An epidemic of optic neuropathy in Tanzania: characterization of the visual disorder and associated peripheral neuropathy. J Neurol Sci 1997;145:127–140.

1048. Benton CD, Calhoun FP. The ocular effects of methyl alcohol poisoning. Report of a catastrophe involving three hundred and twenty persons. Trans Am Acad Ophthalmol Otolaryngol 1952;56:875–885.

1049. Hayreh MS, Hayreh S, Baumbach GL, et al. Methyl alcohol poisoning. III. Ocular toxicity. Arch Ophthalmol 1977;95:1851–1858.

1050. Sharpe JA, Hostovsky M, Bilbao JM, et al. Methanol optic neuropathy: a histopathological study. Neurology 1982;32:1093–1100.

1051. Naeser P. Optic nerve involvement in a case of methanol poisoning. Br J Ophthalmol 1988;72:778–781.

1052. McKellar MJ, Hidajat RR, Elder MJ. Acute ocular methanol toxicity: clinical and electrophysiological features. Aust N Z J Ophthalmol 1997;25:225–230.

1053. Lee EJ, Kim SJ, Choung HK, et al. Incidence and clinical features of ethambutol-induced optic neuropathy in Korea. J Neuroophthalmol 2008;28:269–277.

1054. Leibold JE. The ocular toxicity of ethambutol and its relation to dose. N Y Acad Sci 1966;135:904–909.

1055. Barron GJ, Tepper L, Iovine G. Ocular toxicity from ethambutol. Am J Ophthalmol 1974;77:256–260.

1056. DeVita EG, Miao M, Sadun AA. Optic neuropathy in ethambutol-treated renal tuberculosis. J Clin Neuroophthalmol 1987;7:77–86.

1057. Salmon JF, Carmichael TR, Welsh NH. Use of contrast sensitivity measurement in the detection of subclinical ethambutol toxic optic neuropathy. Br J Ophthalmol 1987;71:192–196.

1058. Zoumalan CI, Sadun AA. Optical coherence tomography can monitor reversible nerve-fibre layer changes in a patient with ethambutol-induced optic neuropathy. Br J Ophthalmol 2007;91:839–840.

1059. Chai SJ, Foroozan R. Decreased retinal nerve fibre layer thickness detected by optical coherence tomography in patients with ethambutol-induced optic neuropathy. Br J Ophthalmol 2007;91:895–897.

1060. Woung LC, Jou JR, Liaw SL. Visual function in recovered ethambutol optic neuropathy. J Ocul Pharmacol Ther 1995;11:411–419.

1061. Tsai RK, Lee YH. Reversibility of ethambutol optic neuropathy. J Ocul Pharmacol Ther 1997;13:473–477.

1062. Garett SN, Kearney JJ, Schiffman JS. Amiodarone optic neuropathy. J Clin Neuroophthalmol 1988;8:105–110.

1063. Mansour AM, Puklin JE, O'Grady R. Optic nerve ultrastructure following amiodarone therapy. J Clin Neuroophthalmol 1988;8:231–237.

1064. Nazarian SM, Jay WM. Bilateral optic neuropathy associated with amiodarone therapy. J Clin Neuroophthalmol 1988;8:25–28.

1065. Gittinger JW, Asdourian GK. Papillopathy caused by amiodarone. Arch Ophthalmol 1987;105:349–351.

1066. Feiner LA, Younge BR, Kazmier FJ, et al. Optic neuropathy and amiodarone therapy. Mayo Clin Proc 1987;62:702–717.

1067. Chen D, Hedges TR. Amiodarone optic neuropathy: review. Semin Ophthalmol 2003;18:169–173.

1068. Macaluso DC, Shults WT, Fraunfelder FT. Features of amiodarone-induced optic neuropathy. Am J Ophthalmol 1999;127:610–612.

1069. Murphy MA, Murphy JF. Amiodarone and optic neuropathy: the heart of the matter. J Neuroophthalmol 2005;25:232–236.

1070. Purvin V, Kawasaki A, Borruat FX. Optic neuropathy in patients using amiodarone. Arch Ophthalmol 2006;124:696–701.

1071. Younge BR. Amiodarone and ischemic optic neuropathy. J Neuroophthalmol 2007;27:85–86.

1072. Mindel JS, Anderson J, Hellkamp A, et al. Absence of bilateral vision loss from amiodarone: a randomized trial. Am Heart J 2007;153:837–842.

1073. Palimar P, Cota N. Bilateral anterior ischaemic optic neuropathy following amiodarone [letter]. Eye 1998;12:894–896.

1074. Macaluso DC, Shults WT, Fraunfelder FT. Features of amiodarone-induced optic neuropathy. Am J Ophthalmol 1999;127:610–612.

1075. Kono R. Subacute myelo-optico neuropathy, a new neurological disease prevailing in Japan. Jpn J Med Sci Biol 1971;24:195–216.

1076. Tauber T, Turetz J, Barash J, et al. Optic neuritis associated with etanercept therapy for juvenile arthritis. J AAPOS 2006;10:26–29.

1077. Foroozan R, Buono LM, Sergott RC, et al. Retrobulbar optic neuritis associated with infliximab. Arch Ophthalmol 2002;120:985–987.

1078. Khawly JA, Rubin P, Petros W, et al. Retinopathy and optic neuropathy in bone marrow transplantation for breast cancer. Ophthalmology 1996;103:87–95.

1079. Chan JW. Bilateral non-arteritic ischemic optic neuropathy associated with pegylated interferon for chronic hepatitis C. Eye 2007;21:877–878.

1080. Gupta R, Singh S, Tang R, et al. Anterior ischemic optic neuropathy caused by interferon alpha therapy. Am J Med 2002;112:683–684.

1081. Lohmann CP, Kroher G, Bogenrieder T, et al. Severe loss of vision during adjuvant interferon alfa-2b treatment for malignant melanoma. Lancet 1999;353:1326.

1082. Purvin VA. Anterior ischemic optic neuropathy secondary to interferon alfa. Arch Ophthalmol 1995;113:1041–1044.

1083. Vardizer Y, Linhart Y, Loewenstein A, et al. Interferon-alpha-associated bilateral simultaneous ischemic optic neuropathy. J Neuroophthalmol 2003;23:256–259.

1084. Borruat FX, Kawasaki A. Optic nerve massaging: an extremely rare cause of self-inflicted blindness. Am J Ophthalmol 2005;139:715–716.

1085. Leibovitch I, Pietris G, Casson R, et al. Oedipism: bilateral self-enucleation. Am J Emerg Med 2006;24:127–128.

1086. Fard AK, Merbs SL, Pieramici DJ. Optic nerve avulsion from a diving injury. Am J Ophthalmol 1997;124:562–564.

1087. Tsopelas NV, Arvanitis PG. Avulsion of the optic nerve head after orbital trauma. Arch Ophthalmol 1998;116:394.

1088. Espaillat A, To K. Optic nerve avulsion. Arch Ophthalmol 1998;116:540–541.

1089. Foster BS, March GA, Lucarelli MJ, et al. Optic nerve avulsion. Arch Ophthalmol 1997;115:623–630.

1090. Lessell S. Indirect optic nerve trauma. Arch Ophthalmol 1989;107:382–386.

1091. Anderson RL, Panje Gross CE. Optic nerve blindness following blunt forehead trauma. Ophthalmology 1982;89:445–455.

1092. Kline LB, Morawetz RB, Swaid SN. Indirect injury of the optic nerve. Neurosurgery 1984;14:756–764.

1093. Joseph MP, Lessell S, Rizzo J, et al. Extracranial optic nerve decompression for traumatic optic neuropathy. Arch Ophthalmol 1990;108:1091–1093.

1094. Seiff SR. High dose corticosteroids for treatment of vision loss due to indirect injury to the optic nerve. Ophthalmic Surg 1990;21:389–395.

1095. Steinsapir KD, Goldberg RA. Traumatic optic neuropathy. Surv Ophthalmol 1994;38:487–518.

1096. Levin LA, Beck RW, Joseph MP, et al. The treatment of traumatic optic neuropathy. The International Optic Nerve Trauma Study. Ophthalmology 1999;106:1268–1277.

1097. Yu-Wai-Man P, Griffiths PG. Steroids for traumatic optic neuropathy. Cochrane Database Syst Rev 2007:CD006032.

1098. Yu Wai Man P, Griffiths PG. Surgery for traumatic optic neuropathy. Cochrane Database Syst Rev 2005:CD005024.

1099. Bracken MB, Collins WF, Freeman DF, et al. A randomized, controlled trial of methylprednisolone or naloxone in the treatment of acute spinal-cord injury: results of the second national Acute Spinal Cord Injury Study. N Engl J Med 1990;322: 1405–1411.

1100. Braughler JM, Hall ED. Current applications of "high dose" steroid therapy for CNS injury. J Neurosurg 1985;62:806–810.

1101. Steinsapir KD, Goldberg RA, Sinha S, et al. Methylprednisolone exacerbates axonal loss following optic nerve trauma in rats. Restor Neurol Neurosci 2000;17:157–163.

1102. Edwards P, Arango M, Balica L, et al. Final results of MRC CRASH, a randomised placebo-controlled trial of intravenous corticosteroid in adults with head injury: outcomes at 6 months. Lancet 2005;365:1957–1959.

1103. Roberts I, Yates D, Sandercock P, et al. Effect of intravenous corticosteroids on death within 14 days in 10008 adults with clinically significant head injury (MRC CRASH trial): randomised placebo-controlled trial. Lancet 2004;364:1321–1328.

1104. Wu N, Yin ZQ, Wang Y. Traumatic optic neuropathy therapy: an update of clinical and experimental studies. J Int Med Res 2008;36:883–889.

1105. Li KK, Teknos TN, Lai A, et al. Traumatic optic neuropathy: result in 45 consecutive surgically treated patients. Otolaryngol Head Neck Surg 1999;120:5–11.

1106. Chen CT, Huang F, Tsay PK, et al. Endoscopically assisted transconjunctival decompression of traumatic optic neuropathy. J Craniofac Surg 2007;18:19–26.

1107. Acheson JF. Optic nerve disorders: role of canal and nerve sheath decompression surgery. Eye 2004;18:1169–1174.

1108. Steinsapir KD. Treatment of traumatic optic neuropathy with high-dose corticosteroid. J Neuroophthalmol 2006;26:65–67.

1109. Rabiah PK, Bateman JB, Demer JL, et al. Ophthalmologic findings in patients with ataxia. Am J Ophthalmol 1997;123:108–117.

1110. Abe T, Abe K, Aoki M, et al. Ocular changes in patients with spinocerebellar degeneration and repeated trinucleotide expansion of spinocerebellar ataxia type 1 gene. Am J Ophthalmol 1997;115:231–236.

1111. Gamez J, Montane D, Martorell L, et al. Bilateral optic nerve atrophy in myotonic dystrophy. Am J Ophthalmol 2001;131:398–400.

1112. Nystuen A, Costeff H, Elpeleg ON, et al. Iraqi-Jewish kindreds with optic atrophy plus (3-methylglutaconic aciduria type 3) demonstrate linkage disequilibrium with the CTG repeat in the 3′ untranslated region of the myotonic dystrophy protein kinase gene. Hum Mol Genet 1997;6:563–569.

1113. Hayflick SJ, Westaway SK, Levinson B, et al. Genetic, clinical, and radiographic delineation of Hallervorden-Spatz syndrome. N Engl J Med 2003;348:33–40.

1114. Landy PJ. A prospective study of the risk of developing multiple sclerosis in optic neuritis in a tropical and subtropical area. J Neurol Neurosurg Psychiatry 1983;46: 659–661.

1115. Francis DA, Compston DAS, Batchelor JR, et al. A reassessment of the risk of multiple sclerosis developing in patients with optic neuritis after extended follow up. J Neurol Neurosurg Psychiatry 1987;50:758–765.

1116. Sandberg-Wollheim M, Bynke H, Cronqvist S, et al. A long-term prospective study of optic neuritis: evaluation of risk factors. Ann Neurol 1990;27:386–393.

1117. Optic Neuritis Study Group. The 5-year risk of MS after optic neuritis: experience of the Optic Neuritis Treatment Trial. Neurology 1997;49:1404–1413.

1118. Ghezzi A, Martinelli V, Torri V, et al. Long-term follow-up of isolated optic neuritis: the risk of developing multiple sclerosis, its outcome, and the prognostic role of paraclinical tests. J Neurol 1999;246:770–775.

1119. Slavin ML. Compression of the anterior visual pathways. In: Kline LB (ed): Optic Nerve Disorders. San Francisco, American Academy of Ophthalmology, Palace Press, 1996: 91–137.

1120. Imperia PS, Lazarus HM, Lass JH. Ocular complications of systemic cancer chemotherapy. Surv Ophthalmol 1989;34:209–230.

1121. Lessell S. Toxic and deficiency optic neuropathies. In: Miller NR, Newman NJ (eds): Walsh and Hoyt's Clinical Neuro-ophthalmology, 5th edn. Baltimore, Williams & Wilkins, 1998: 663–680.

1122. Comi G. PreCISe study. Presented at the 60th Annual Meeting of the American Academy of Neurology (AAN). Chicago, IL, April 16, 2008.

CHAPTER 6

Optic disc swelling: papilledema and other causes

The distinction between papilledema (disc swelling secondary to increased intracranial pressure), disc swelling associated with optic neuropathy, and disc elevation due to pseudopapilledema will be reviewed first. Then, the fundus appearance of papilledema, the associated visual loss and its mechanisms, and the differential diagnosis in and evaluation of patients with papilledema will be discussed. Conditions associated with papilledema will then be covered, with the greatest emphasis placed on diagnosis and management of a relatively common non-tumor cause of papilledema, pseudotumor cerebri.

Distinction of papilledema from optic neuropathy, pseudopapilledema, and other causes of disc swelling

Table 6-1 outlines the differential diagnosis of a swollen disc. The term papilledema refers to optic disc swelling due to increased intracranial pressure, and the two conditions most commonly mistaken for it are disc swelling due to optic neuropathy and pseudopapilledema (disc elevation without nerve fiber layer edema). The distinction between these three major causes of disc swelling is aided by review of the history, evaluation of visual function, ophthalmoscopic appearance of the disc, and ancillary testing. At times the diagnosis may be difficult, but there are some useful, general guidelines.[1-3]

Signs and symptoms of elevated intracranial pressure, such as headache, nausea, vomiting, and abducens paresis, should suggest the diagnosis of papilledema. However, caution should be applied in this regard, as patients may present with headache unrelated to their disc swelling. For instance, we have seen patients with migraine headaches and pseudopapilledema, and others with headache associated with optic neuritis.

Ophthalmoscopically, the disc swelling due to optic neuropathy and that due to papilledema may be similar **(Fig. 6-1)**. However, optic neuropathies such as optic neuritis or ischemic optic neuropathy typically lead to more severe visual loss which is usually sudden in onset, unilateral, and associated with an afferent pupillary defect and impaired color vision.[4] Papilledema, on the other hand, is more frequently bilateral and more commonly leads initially to visual deficits such as enlarged blind spots and peripheral field constriction, about which the patient may not be aware. The various optic neuropathies are discussed in more detail in Chapter 5.

Pseudopapilledema

Pseudopapilledema (or pseudo-disc edema) is the term used to describe optic nerve variants or abnormalities that mimic papilledema

Table 6–1 Differential diagnosis of a swollen optic disc: causes according to frequency

Most common	Common	Uncommon
Papilledema	Central retinal vein occlusion	Ocular hypotony
Optic neuritis	Diabetic papillopathy	Intraocular inflammation (uveitis)
Anterior ischemic optic neuropathy		Malignant hypertension
Pseudopapilledema		Optic perineuritis
		Papillitis
		Intrinsic optic disc tumors
		Leber's hereditary optic neuropathy
		Optic nerve infiltration sarcoidosis lymphoma leukemia plasma cell dyscrasia

ophthalmoscopically, including congenital anomolies,[5] tilting, hypoplasia, crowded hyperopic disc, optic disc hamartoma, myelinated nerve fibers, and optic nerve head drusen (**Figs. 6–2** and **6–3**). Visual loss, which may occur in some cases, is longstanding, painless, and frequently unnoticed by the patient. The diagnosis may be aided by serial dilated fundus examinations and review of stereo disc photographs; pseudopapilledema will be stable over time, while untreated papilledema might change. Ophthalmoscopic hallmarks of pseudopapilledema include anomalous retinal vasculature (abnormal branching pattern, for instance), absence of a central cup, irregular disc margins, and vessels which pass over the disc normally without being obscured by the nerve fiber layer. They also tend to be less elevated without swelling of the nerve fiber layer, hemorrhages, or exudates, in contrast to discs with true disc edema. The presence of spontaneous venous pulsations obviously favors pseudopapilledema although their absence does not always indicate true papilledema. In addition, discs with true papilledema will leak during fluorescein angiography, in contrast to those with pseudopapilledema, which tend not to leak or show only late staining.[1] Discs with pseudopapilledema often have nerve fiber-related field defects, so visual field testing cannot be used to separate pseudopapilledema from true papilledema.

Disc drusen

Optic disc drusen (hyaline bodies) are calcium deposits within the nerve head.[6] In general, they are not visible at birth or in infancy but become more noticeable by the end of the first decade of life.[7] When on the surface of the disc, they appear as refractile, tapioca-like bodies that are easily identified ophthalmoscopically (**Fig. 6–2**). If they are buried

(between the surface and the lamina cribrosa), as they usually are in childhood, they may simple elevate the optic nerve head. Drusen are often associated with an anomalous retinal artery branching pattern which includes a spoke-like appearance secondary to trifurcations of the first order vessels.[8] The disc generally takes on a yellowish appearance.

On occasion suspected drusen can be more easily seen if the disc is retroilluminated. To perform this technique a spot or beam of light from the direct ophthalmoscope or slit lamp is focused on the nasal peripapillary retina. The disc is then observed in the darkened field next to the light. Drusen may give the disc a translucent appearance with the disc drusen highlighted.

Various types of hemorrhages can also be associated with disc drusen. The most typical is a peripapillary subretinal hemorrhage, which may ultimately cause peripapillary pigmentary disruption or hyperpigmentation. On occasion drusen-associated hemorrhages are related to a peripapillary subretinal neovascular membrane.[9] In rare instances, papilledema may be superimposed upon underlying pseudopapilledema due to optic nerve head drusen.[10]

Optic disc drusen are thought to consist of intracellular axonal debris which accumulate throughout life because of a defect in axonal metabolism.[11,12] A small scleral canal is thought to cause this defect,[13] but this is uncertain.[14] They are present in approximately 0.3–2.0% of the population, and in about two-thirds of cases are bilateral.[15] Some instances are familial, inherited presumably in an autosomal dominant fashion with incomplete penetrance.[16,17] Rarely they are associated with angioid streaks and retinitis pigmentosa,[16,18] but there are no other established systemic associations.[6]

If optic disc drusen are suspected but cannot be definitively identified ophthalmoscopically, then a diagnostic workup may confirm their presence. They may autofluoresce when photographed through a fluorescein filter (without dye injection) (**Fig. 6–2**).[19,20] The most predictable way to confirm a diagnosis of disc drusen is combined A and B scan ultrasonography.[6,15,21,22] This technique may demonstrate disc elevation secondary to highly reflective material. Computed tomography (CT) scan with axial sections through the nerve globe junction may also reveal calcifications secondary to drusen (**Fig. 6–2**).

Other causes

Other causes of disc swelling that should be contrasted from papilledema include (1) central retinal vein occlusion, which is characterized additionally by dilated, tortuous veins and intra- and peripheral retinal hemorrhages; (2) ocular hypotony;[23] (3) intraocular inflammation (e.g. uveitis); (4) diabetic papillopathy; (5) optic perineuritis (idiopathic or due to syphilis, for instance); (6) intrinsic optic disc tumors,[24] such as hemangiomas (in von Hippel–Lindau, for example), astrocytic hamartomas (in tuberous sclerosis), and optic disc gliomas; (7) Leber's hereditary optic neuropathy; (8) optic nerve infiltration by neoplasms, antibodies in plasma

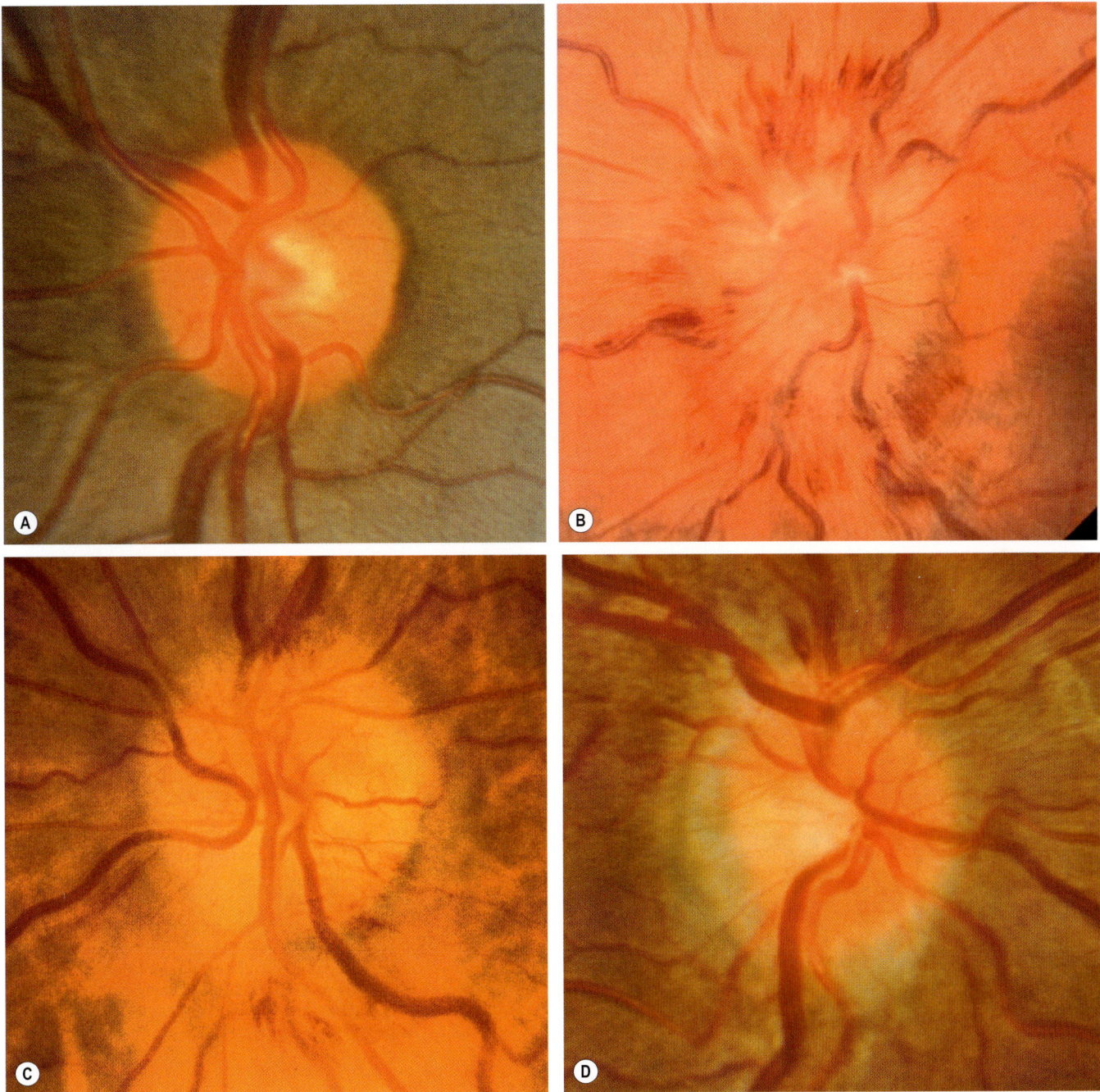

Figure 6–1. A. Normal optic disc. Disc swelling associated with (**B**) elevated intracranial pressure (papilledema), (**C**) anterior ischemic optic neuropathy, and (**D**) optic neuritis.

cell dyscrasia,[25] or sarcoidosis, for instance; (9) high altitudes;[26] and (10) malignant hypertension—the associated disc swelling had been previously related to elevated cerebrospinal fluid (CSF) pressure; however, more recent experimental and clinical observations have suggested that an ischemic optic neuropathy may also be responsible.[27–29] Disc swelling due to malignant hypertension is frequently accompanied by cotton-wool spots in the retina, and macular serous retinal detachment and lipid star formation.[30] Many of these entities are discussed in more detail in the chapters on retinal disorders and optic neuropathies (Chapters 4 and 5).

Fundus appearance of papilledema

Mechanism

The force of elevated CSF is transmitted to tissue fluid between axons in the optic nerve head, leading to axoplas-

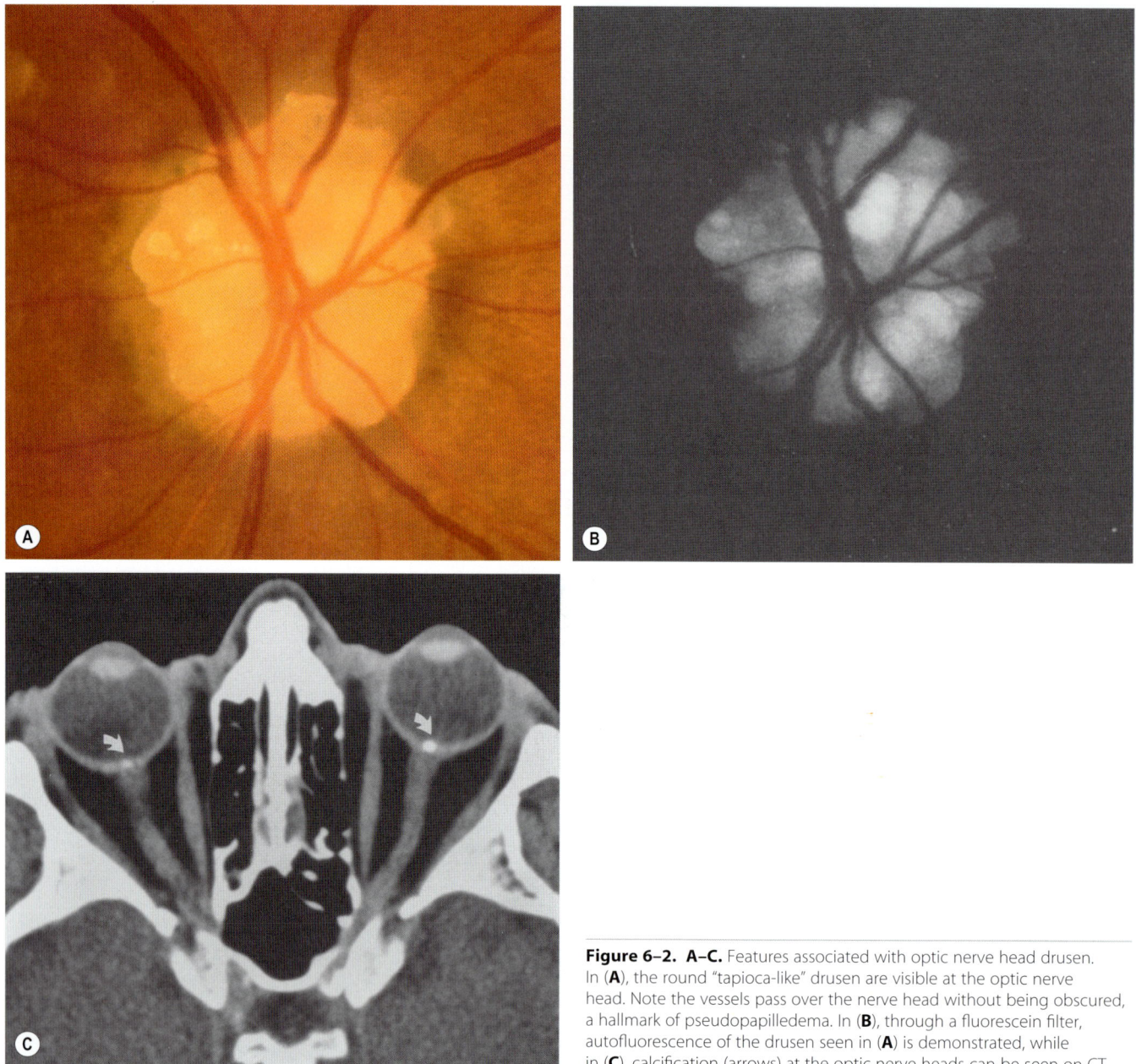

Figure 6–2. A–C. Features associated with optic nerve head drusen. In (**A**), the round "tapioca-like" drusen are visible at the optic nerve head. Note the vessels pass over the nerve head without being obscured, a hallmark of pseudopapilledema. In (**B**), through a fluorescein filter, autofluorescence of the drusen seen in (**A**) is demonstrated, while in (**C**), calcification (arrows) at the optic nerve heads can be seen on CT.

mic stasis in the prelaminar portion of the optic nerve (**Fig. 6–4**).[31] This causes axonal swelling which is observable ophthalmoscopically as a swollen optic disc.[32]

Early and acute papilledema

Early disc swelling associated with elevated intracranial pressure appears first superiorly and inferiorly, then nasally, and finally temporally (**Fig. 6–5**). This pattern follows the relative thickness of the nerve fiber layer, in descending order, at different locations around the optic disc.[27] Elevation of the nerve fiber layer obscures the underlying vessels and blurs the disc margins (**Fig. 6–5c–e**).

Usually, the development of papilledema requires at least 1–5 days of persistently elevated intracranial pressure.[27] However, sudden rises in intracranial pressure, caused by

an acute subarachnoid or intraparenchymal hemorrhage for instance, occasionally may result in papilledema that develops rapidly within hours.[33] Selhorst et al.[34] witnessed the development of papilledema within 1 hour in a patient with acute aneurysmal rupture. Because axoplasmic stasis could not develop so quickly, they surmised that a sudden, severe rise in intracranial pressure could force axoplasm retrogradely from the intraorbital optic nerve into the optic nerve head.

The vascular changes associated with papilledema are secondary to the nerve fiber swelling. Compression of capillaries and venules on the disc cause venous stasis and dilation, formation of microaneurysms, and disc and peripapillary radial hemorrhages. The disc becomes hyperemic because of the capillary dilation. Cotton wool spots represent ischemic areas within the nerve fiber layer (**Fig. 6–5**). Compression

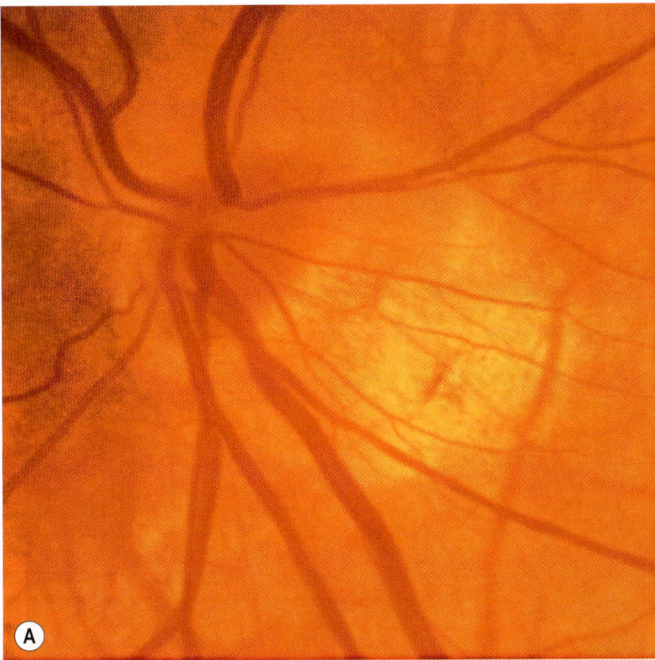

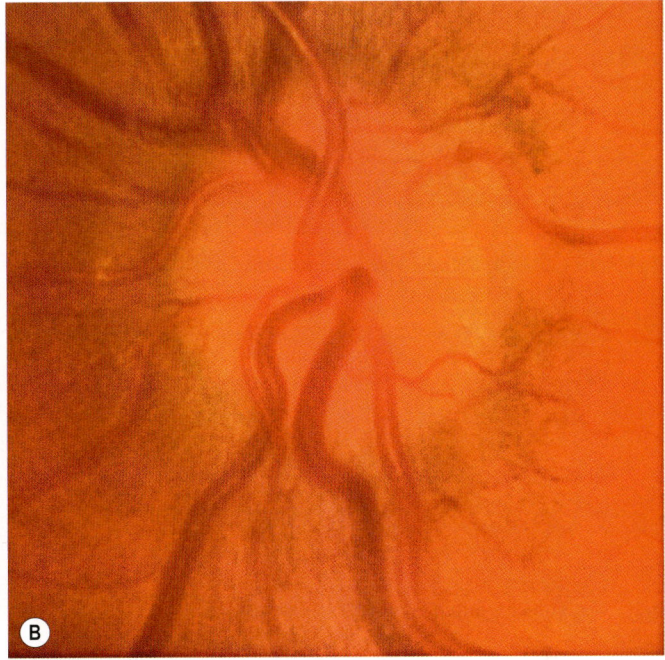

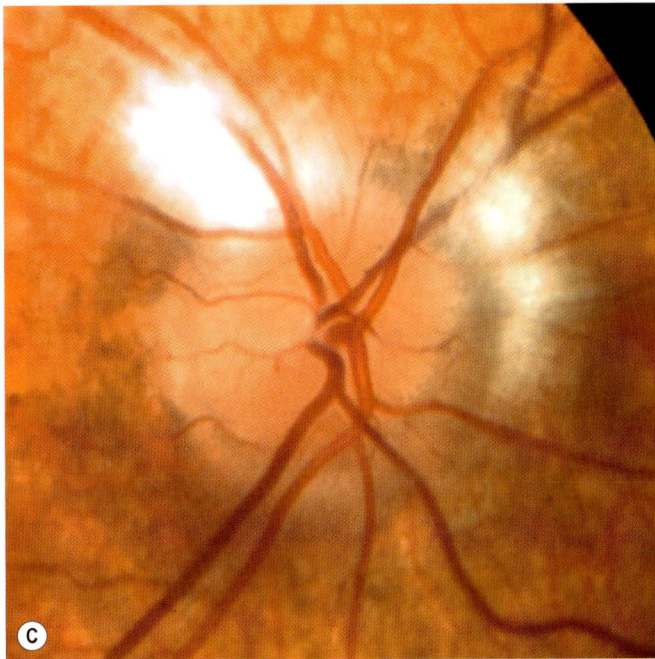

Figure 6–3. Other examples of pseudopapilledema include (**A**) a tilted disc, (**B**) a congenitally small, crowded disc with anomalous vessels and absence of a central cup, and (**C**) a disc with myelinated nerve fibers.

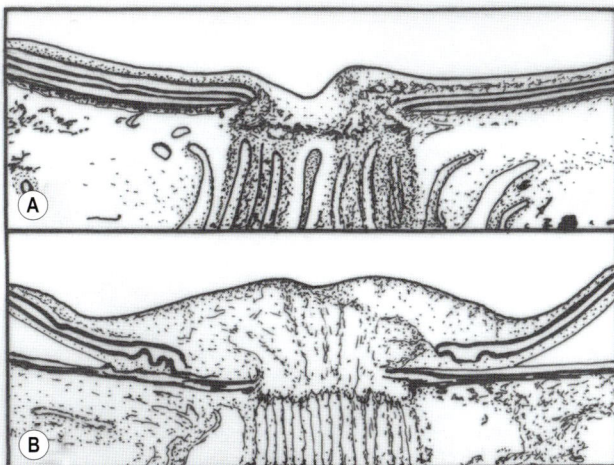

Figure 6–4. Drawing depicting histologic sections of normal optic nerve (**A**) and papilledema (**B**). Note the papilledema is characterized by axoplasmic stasis in the prelaminar portion of the optic nerve.

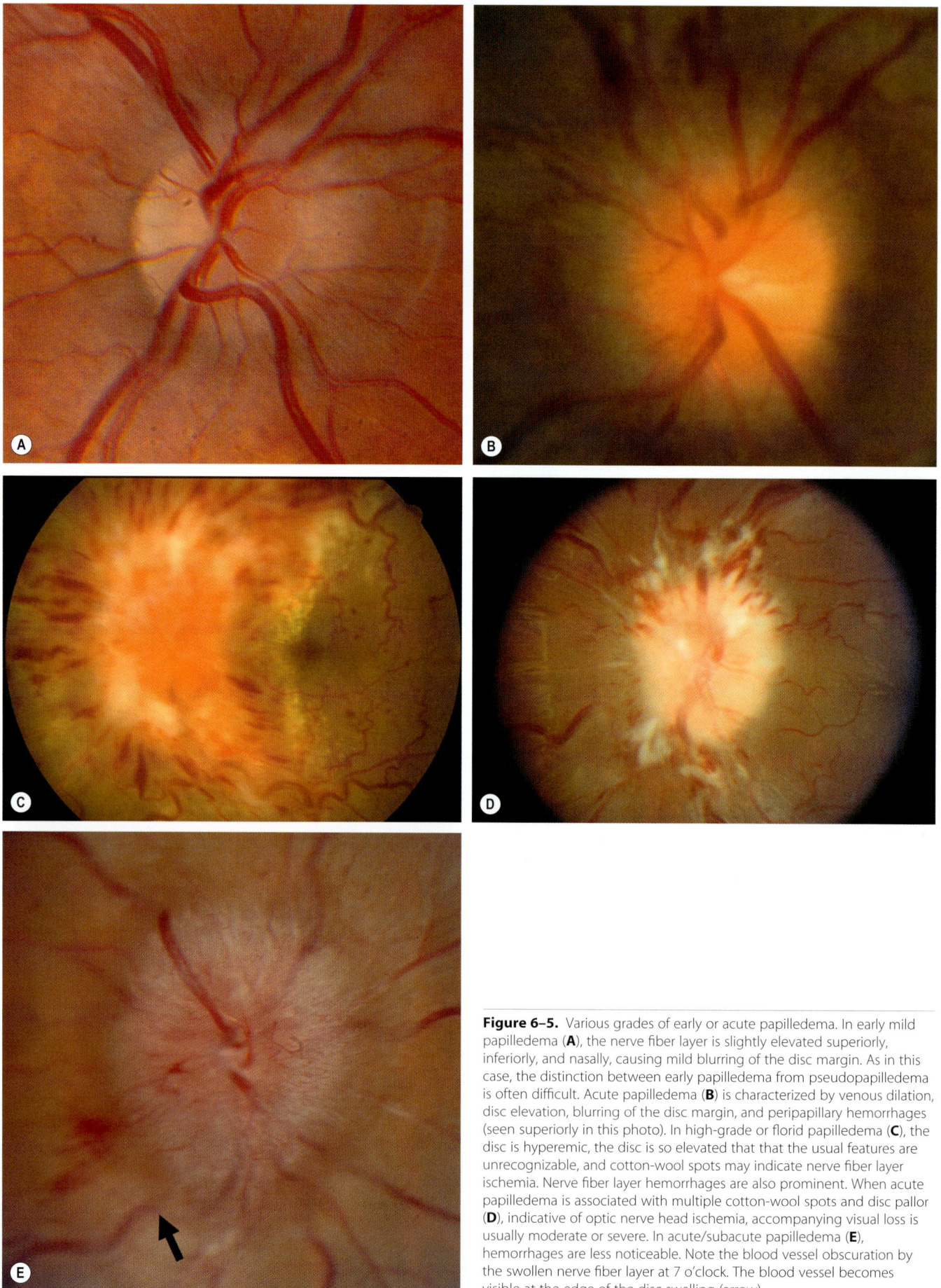

Figure 6–5. Various grades of early or acute papilledema. In early mild papilledema (**A**), the nerve fiber layer is slightly elevated superiorly, inferiorly, and nasally, causing mild blurring of the disc margin. As in this case, the distinction between early papilledema from pseudopapilledema is often difficult. Acute papilledema (**B**) is characterized by venous dilation, disc elevation, blurring of the disc margin, and peripapillary hemorrhages (seen superiorly in this photo). In high-grade or florid papilledema (**C**), the disc is hyperemic, the disc is so elevated that that the usual features are unrecognizable, and cotton-wool spots may indicate nerve fiber layer ischemia. Nerve fiber layer hemorrhages are also prominent. When acute papilledema is associated with multiple cotton-wool spots and disc pallor (**D**), indicative of optic nerve head ischemia, accompanying visual loss is usually moderate or severe. In acute/subacute papilledema (**E**), hemorrhages are less noticeable. Note the blood vessel obscuration by the swollen nerve fiber layer at 7 o'clock. The blood vessel becomes visible at the edge of the disc swelling (arrow).

of the central retinal vein can lead to retinal venous engorgement and tortuosity[28] and disappearance of spontaneous venous pulsations, which are pulse-related dilations and contractions of large venous branches in or overlying the disc. The best place to look for spontaneous venous pulsations is within the central cup of the disc and where the veins bend. Spontaneous venous pulsations are most evident in patients with deep and large cups. The presence of spontaneous venous pulsations implies the intracranial pressure is less than 180 mm H_2O at the time of viewing.[35] However, the absence of spontaneous venous pulsations does not imply elevated intracranial pressure, for as many as 10% of the normal population may not have them in either eye.[35,36]

Grading systems for papilledema have been devised,[37] but more commonly descriptive terminology is used.[38] The term mild papilledema refers to slight disc elevation with some or no peripapillary hemorrhages. High-grade or florid papilledema is characterized by severe disc elevation with cotton-wool spots, peripapillary hemorrhages, and venous engorgement **(Fig. 6–5)**. The degree of papilledema is usually symmetric in both eyes, but asymmetric[39] and even unilateral[40–43] papilledema may occur. A subarachnoidal meshwork within the optic canal can act as an incomplete barrier to transmission of CSF pressure between the intracranial vault and anterior optic nerve.[44,45] Anatomic differences in this meshwork may account for asymmetric papilledema as well as interpersonal variation in disc swelling with the same CSF pressure. Alternatively, Lepore[39] proposed age-related changes in the lamina cribosa due to increased collagen and decreased elasticity might protect the optic nerve head from elevated intracranial pressure. Atrophic portions of an optic nerve head cannot develop disc swelling, but intact portions can[46,47] (see Foster Kennedy syndrome, below).

Chronic papilledema

Table 6–2 compares the features of acute and chronic papilledema. The disc takes on a "champagne-cork" appearance **(Fig. 6–6)** when papilledema has been present for weeks or months. Typically, peripapillary hemorrhages are conspicuously absent. White exudates, representing extruded axoplasm, commonly overlie the disc (pseudodrusen). Chronic papilledema may also be associated with venous collateral vessels **(Fig. 6–7)** and peripapillary subretinal neovascularization.[48,49] The collateral vessels form when decreased flow through the central retinal vein causes compensatory dilation of pre-existing communications between retinal and ciliary venous circulations.[48]

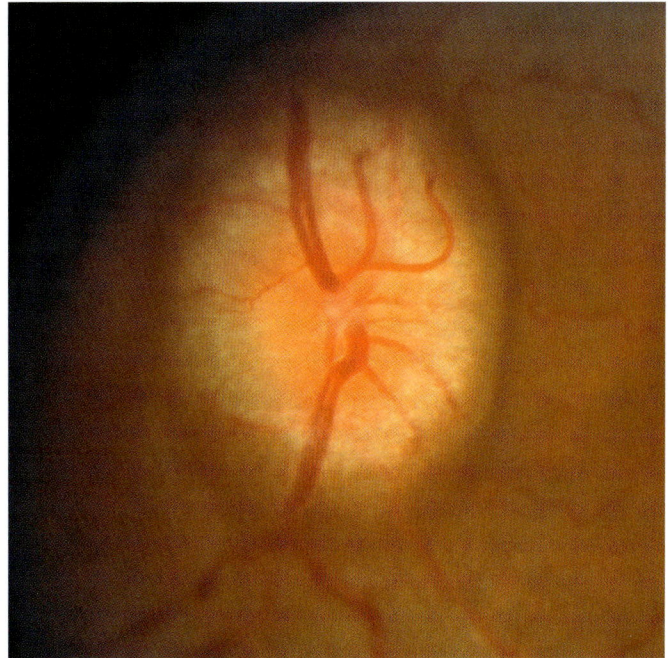

Figure 6–6. "Champagne-cork" appearance of chronic papilledema. The whitish, glistening areas on the optic disc head represent gliosis and extruded axoplasm. Note conspicuous absence of peripapillary hemorrhages.

Table 6–2 Fundus characteristics of acute and chronic papilledema

Common to both *acute* and *chronic* papilledema
Disc elevation
Venous distention and tortuosity
Obscuration of the normal disc margin and overlying retinal vessels
Absence of spontaneous venous pulsations

Characteristic typical of *acute* papilledema
Disc hyperemia
Cotton wool spots
Peripapillary hemorrhages

Characteristics typical of *chronic* papilledema
"Champagne-cork" appearance
Overlying gliosis and extruded axoplasm (pseudodrusen)
Disc atrophy
Venous collateral vessels
Peripapillary subretinal neovascularization

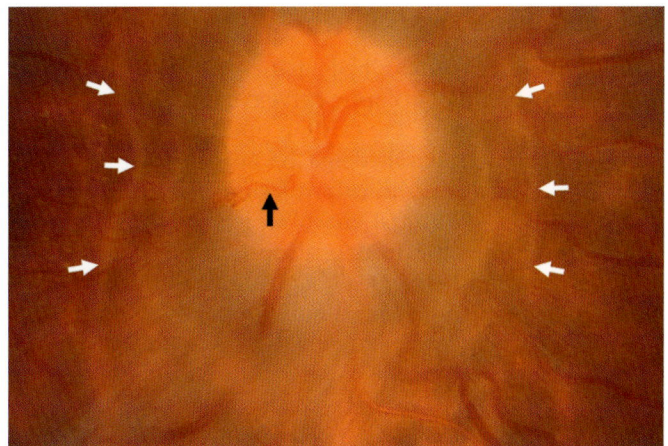

Figure 6–7. Peripapillary "high-water marks" (white arrows) indicative of previous retinal elevation associated with papilledema. Lipid exudate is visible near the white arrows on the left side of the photograph. The black arrow at 8 o'clock at the optic disc points to a venous collateral vessel.

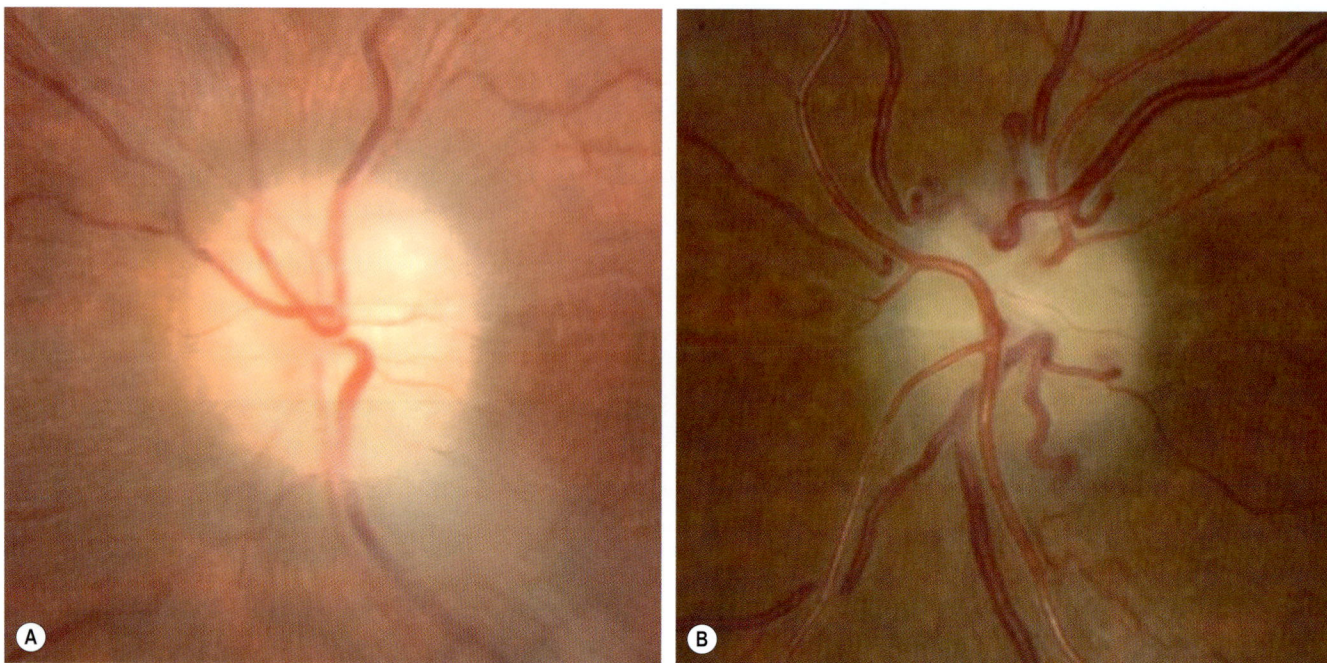

Figure 6–8. Examples of chronic atrophic papilledema. **A.** Pale swollen disc due to long-standing, untreated obstructive hydrocephalus (see corresponding MRI in Fig. 6–15E). Note blood vessel narrowing. **B.** Gliotic, pale, swollen disc with collateral ("shunt") vessels due to pseudotumor cerebri and non-compliance with treatment and follow-up.

Atrophic papilledema

When swollen nerve fibers die, the disc atrophies and swelling becomes pale and less prominent (**Fig. 6–8**). Arterial branches, especially peripapillary, become attenuated.

Treated papilledema

If the elevated intracranial pressure is treated prior to atrophy of nerve fibers, papilledema usually resolves completely over the ensuing weeks or months (**Fig. 6–9**). However, some patients, particularly those with permanent visual loss, are left with some degree of disc pallor and residual disc elevation because of gliosis (secondary disc pallor) (**Fig. 6–10**).[50]

Foster Kennedy syndrome

Foster Kennedy[51] described patients with ipsilateral disc pallor, secondary to optic nerve compression, and contralateral papilledema. Pre-existing optic atrophy precludes the development of papilledema, because there are no fibers to swell.[31] Classically, the culprit lesion in Foster Kennedy syndrome is a subfrontal mass, typically a meningioma, which compresses the ipsilateral optic nerve, causing disc atrophy. If the lesion is large enough to cause elevated intracranial pressure, papilledema results in the contralateral eye only, owing to the ipsilateral nerve atrophy (**Fig. 6–11**). Bilateral optic nerve compression is another possible mechanism.[52] Non-tumor causes, resulting in pseudo-Foster Kennedy syndrome, are actually more common.[53] One example is consecutive anterior ischemic optic neuropathy, characterized by new ischemic disc swelling in one eye accompanied by longstanding disc atrophy resulting from a previous ischemic event in the other eye (see **Fig. 5–44**).

Unlike the true Foster Kennedy syndrome, the eye with the disc swelling will usually have impaired visual acuity.

Retinal findings associated with papilledema

Secondary effects on the macula are common causes of acute reduction in visual acuity and metamorphopsia in papilledema (**Table 6–3**). For instance, in severe disc swelling, fluid may extend to the macula by dissecting between the axons of the nerve fiber layer.[31,54] Macular edema is difficult to see with a direct ophthalmoscope but is more readily visible using biomicroscopy and best demonstrated with optical coherence tomography (see below).[55] Retinal or choroidal folds,[56] lipid (hard exudate) stars,[57] hemorrhages,[58] and pigment epithelial and photoreceptor disturbances in the macula may also be associated with papilledema (**Fig. 6–12**). Indentation or flattening of the posterior globe by a rigid optic nerve sheath is one proposed mechanism for choroidal folds in papilledema.[59,60] Shortening of the globe's axial length or flattening of the posterior pole may also account

Table 6–3 Retinal findings associated with papilledema

Common	Uncommon
Macular changes	Subretinal neovascular
Edema	membrane
Lipid (hard exudate) stars	Venous stasis retinopathy
Pigment epithelial disturbances	Retinal artery occlusion
Retinal or choroidal folds	
Hemorrhages	
Peripapillary "high-water" mark	

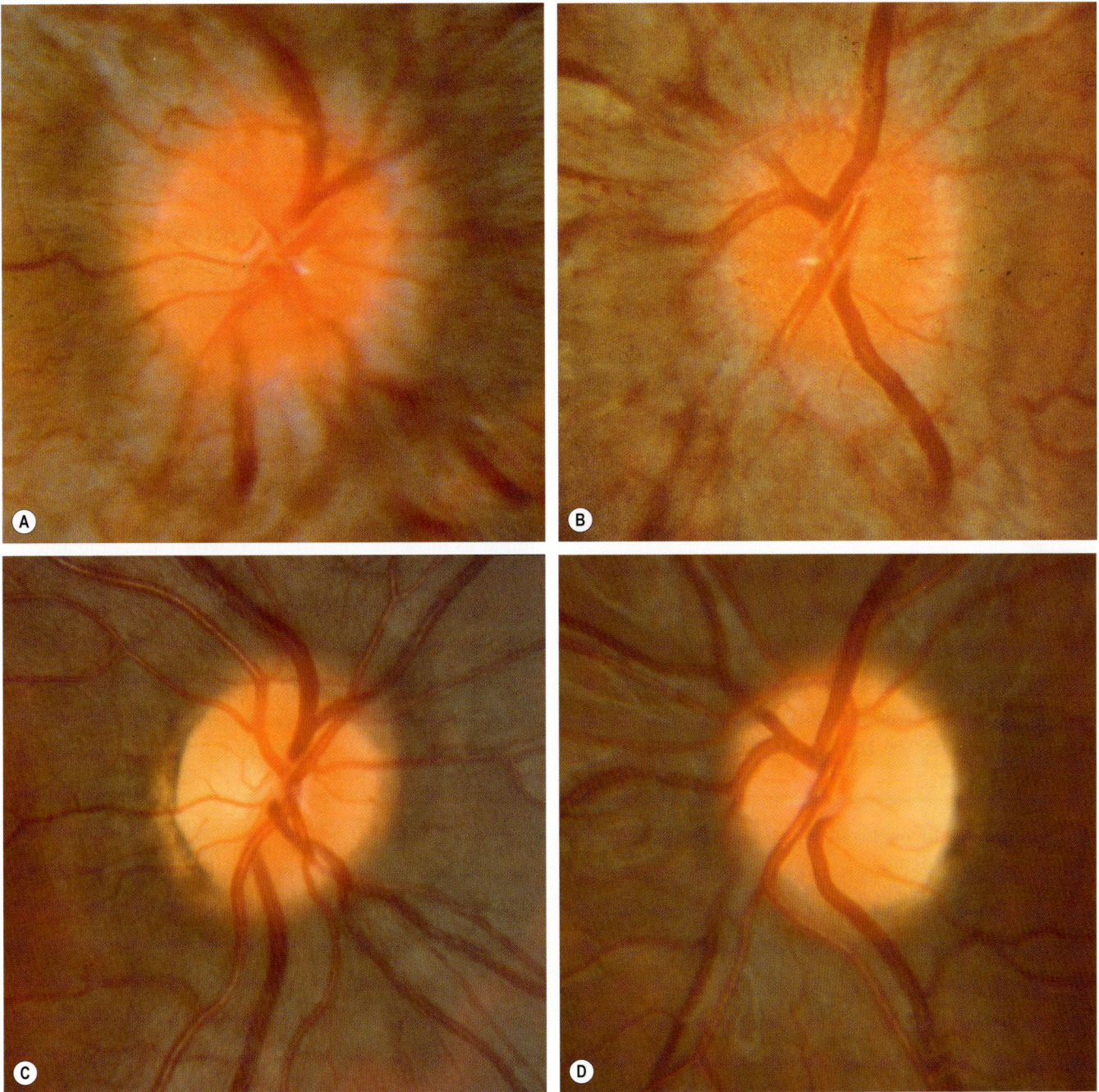

Figure 6–9. Papilledema associated with pseudotumor cerebri: **A.** right eye; **B.** left eye. Six months after medical treatment the disc swelling has completely resolved: **C.** right eye; **D.** left eye.

for the association between intracranial hypertension, papilledema, folds, and acquired hyperopia.[61,62] Choroidal folds actually occur in Bruch's membrane.[63]

Hemorrhages associated with papilledema are usually peripapillary and retinal (within the nerve fiber layer), but occasionally can be found more than one or two disc diameters away from the optic nerve head or in the sub-hyaloid and vitreous spaces.[64] Rarely, hemorrhages are due to peripapillary subretinal neovascular membranes, seen best on fluorescein angiography.[65,66] When these membranes extend towards the fovea, photocoagulation may be indicated.[67] Venous stasis retinopathy[68] and central[69] or branch[70] retinal artery occlusion, due to compression of vascular

structures in the optic nerve, are rare but have been documented.

Once the papilledema improves with the appropriate treatment, hemorrhages, folds, macular edema, and lipid stars tend to resolve over weeks as well. One may see residual macular pigment epithelial disturbances if lipid, folds, or edema had been present,[71] or circumpapillary "high-water" marks delineating the prior extent of peripapillary retinal elevation caused by disc swelling **(Figs. 6–7 and 6–12c);** in contrast these retinal abnormalities may require months or years to resolve. Unfortunately subretinal neovascular membranes and associated subretinal hemorrhages may cause irreversible visual loss.[72]

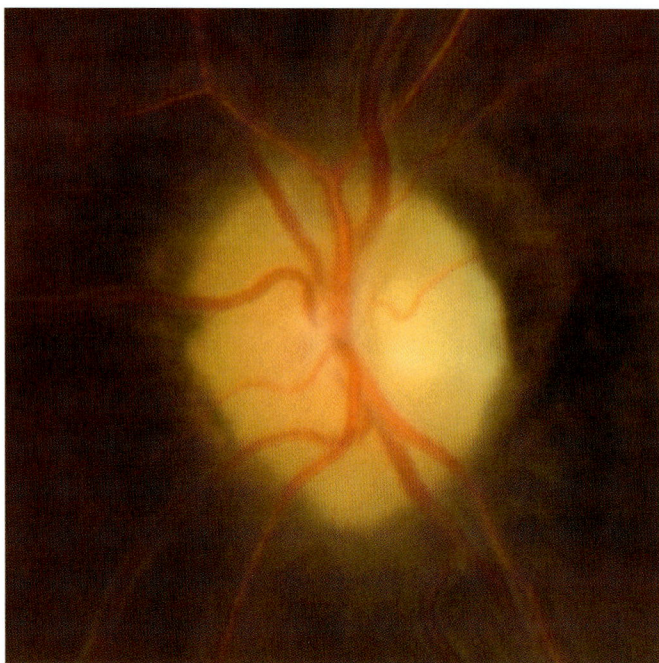

Figure 6–10. Papilledema has resolved, but the disc is pale and gliotic, in a patient with permanent vision loss. The edge of the disc is still slightly elevated in a "heaped-up" fashion (secondary disc pallor).

Fluorescein angiography, echography, optical coherence tomography and other optic nerve imaging techniques in papilledema

These modalities aid in the diagnosis and sometimes the follow-up of papilledema.

Fluorescein angiography. Hayreh[27] has detailed the typical fluorescein angiographic findings associated with papilledema. In the retinal arterial phase, fluorescence may be absent when disc swelling is severe enough to delay the prelaminar circulation. During the retinal arteriovenous phase, dilated capillaries, microaneurysms, and flame-shaped hemorrhages may be demonstrated on the surface of the disc and peripapillary retina. Fluorescein may leak from superficial dilated capillaries during the retinal venous phase. During the late phase, classically there is hyperfluorescence of the superficial and deep portions of the optic disc.

Ultrasound. Ultrasonography is used frequently in our practice to help distinguish papilledema from pseudo-papilledema, particularly when optic disc drusen are suspected. In patients with papilledema, A-scan echography of the optic nerve can suggest increased subarachnoid fluid within the nerve sheath by demonstrating a reduction in nerve sheath diameter by 10% when the eye rotates laterally 30 degrees ("positive 30 degree test").[73] However, increased subarachnoid fluid is non-specific and may be seen in optic neuritis, optic nerve trauma, and compressive optic neuropathy. Furthermore, caution in its interpretation must be applied, as echography is extremely operator dependent.

Optic nerve and retinal imaging. Optical coherence tomography (OCT) may demonstrate increased retinal nerve

fiber layer thickness in papilledema.[74,75] This finding on OCT has been shown to correlate with mean deviation on computerized perimetry, and its resolution with visual field improvement.[76] Whether OCT can readily distinguish papilledema from pseudopapilledema is uncertain.[77] Johnson et al.,[78] however, demonstrated thickening of the nasal nerve fiber layer and an increased subretinal hypo-reflective space in optic disc edema extending further from the disc than in pseudopapilledema.

Laser scanning tomography, using the Heidelberg retinal tomograph (HRT), can quantify the degree of change in papilledema.[79–81] It has been suggested that tomography measurements correlate with CSF opening pressures[81] and visual field deficits.[82]

Visual deficits associated with papilledema and their mechanism

Visual loss due to papilledema is for the most part related to optic nerve head dysfunction.[83] The field deficits are similar to those in other disorders which affect the anterior optic nerve, such as glaucoma, and they do not align along the vertical meridian, as in chiasmal or retrochiasmal lesions.[84] It is less certain whether ischemia or axoplasmic stasis causes axonal dysfunction. Rapid improvement in vision following optic nerve sheath decompression suggests axoplasmic stasis plays at least some part,[85] but cases with frank optic nerve ischemia have been documented as well.[86] Pre-existing anemia or hypertension may be associated with more severe visual loss, perhaps by aggravating optic nerve head ischemia.[48,87]

Blind spot enlargement is commonly associated with papilledema **(Fig. 6–13)**. The etiology is either mechanical displacement and folding of the peripapillary retina or a refractive scotoma caused by relative hyperopia due to peripapillary retinal elevation.[88] Nasal defects (especially inferiorly[89]) are also common initially, in part because the temporal arcuate bundles are densest, and hence more susceptible to axoplasmic stasis and compression.[84] Further involvement of nerve fibers leads to arcuate defects then field constriction **(Fig. 6–13)**.[48,90] Once sufficient nerve fiber layer loss develops, central visual acuity loss results.[48] Central visual defects and metamorphopsia in acute papilledema are uncommon, but when they occur are almost always due to retinal processes affecting the macula (see above).

Visual field testing

Computerized threshold perimetry of the central 30 degrees of vision (static targets, Humphrey 30-2 program), although lengthy and tedious, in most instances is a good objective and reproducible test for patients with papilledema.[91] Each field can be quantified using the average of all the threshold values (in decibels (dB)) for each measured area, allowing for objective, numerical comparison of serial fields. Kinetic Goldmann perimetry[92] is more appropriate for patients with significant visual loss and those who are less cooperative, such as children. However, automated perimeters are more widely available, and because of the advantages outlined

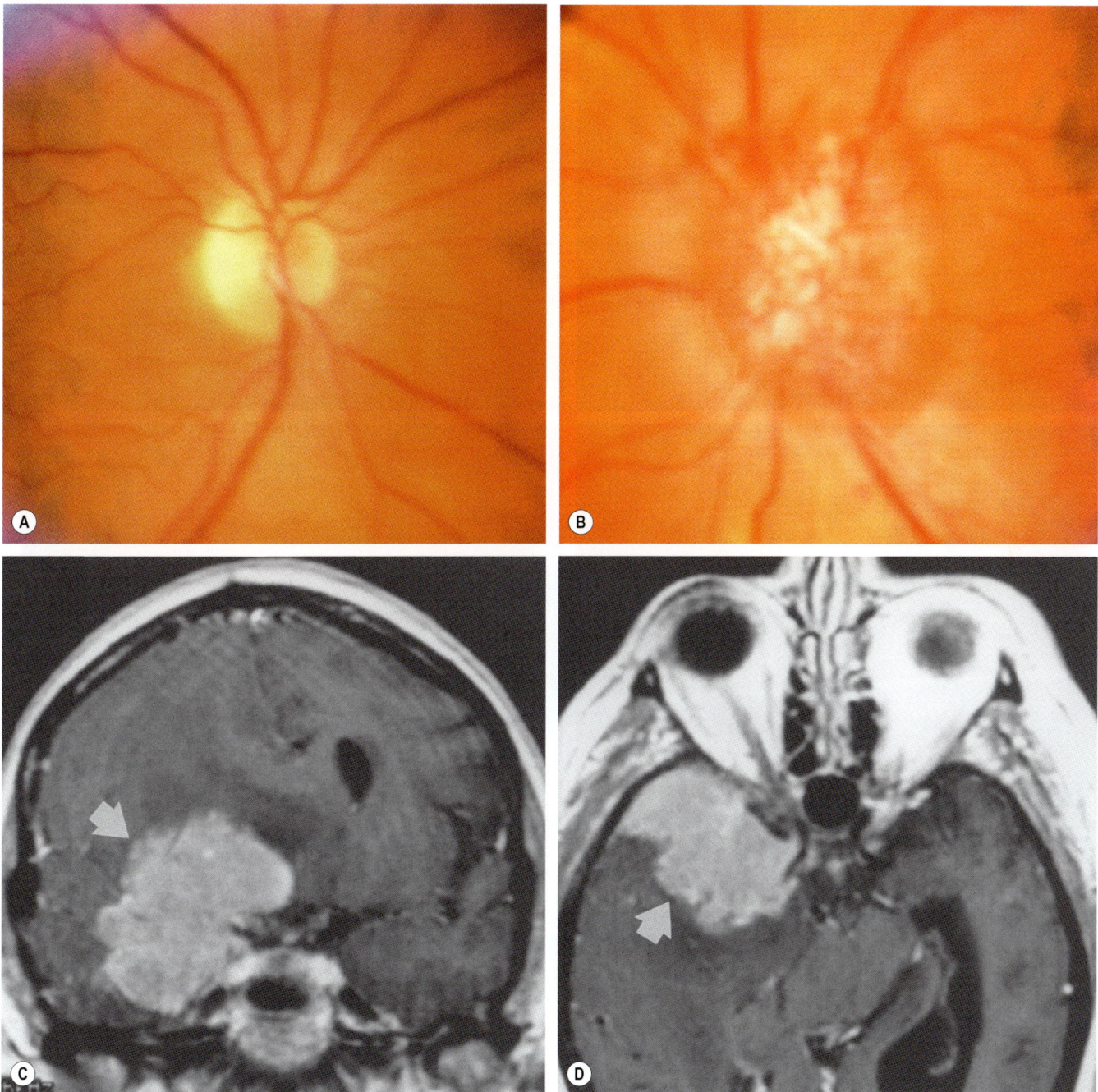

Figure 6–11. Foster Kennedy syndrome. This patient presented with progressive behavioral changes, headaches, and counting fingers vision in the right eye. Fundus examination revealed optic atrophy in the right eye (**A**) and papilledema in the left eye (**B**). Gadolinium-enhanced coronal magnetic resonance imaging (MRI) (**C**) demonstrates a large meningioma (arrow) compressing the right frontal and temporal lobes, right optic nerve, and third ventricle. The axial MRI scan (**D**) shows dilation of the left lateral ventricle consistent with noncommunicating hydrocephalus.

above, most patients with papilledema should be tested, and, if necessary, followed with serial threshold field examinations. Finger confrontation methods and tangent screen examinations are too insensitive to detect subtle visual loss.[93]

It is often difficult to correlate the severity of disc swelling with the amount of visual loss. As the papilledema becomes more chronic, nerve fibers atrophy, reducing the amount of disc swelling. Hence chronically atrophic swollen discs, likely associated with severe visual loss, tend not to be grossly elevated. However, in the acute setting it may be useful to generalize that mild disc elevation is usually associ-

ated with more minor field deficits than high-grade, florid papilledema.[48,94] Furthermore, at presentation, a normally shaped and colored disc without swelling should be associated with a normal visual field.

Transient visual obscurations

These are uni- or bilateral episodes of visual loss lasting for seconds. They can occur rarely or several times per day, and are associated with changes in posture such as standing or bending over. Patients may describe a gray cloud or "puff of

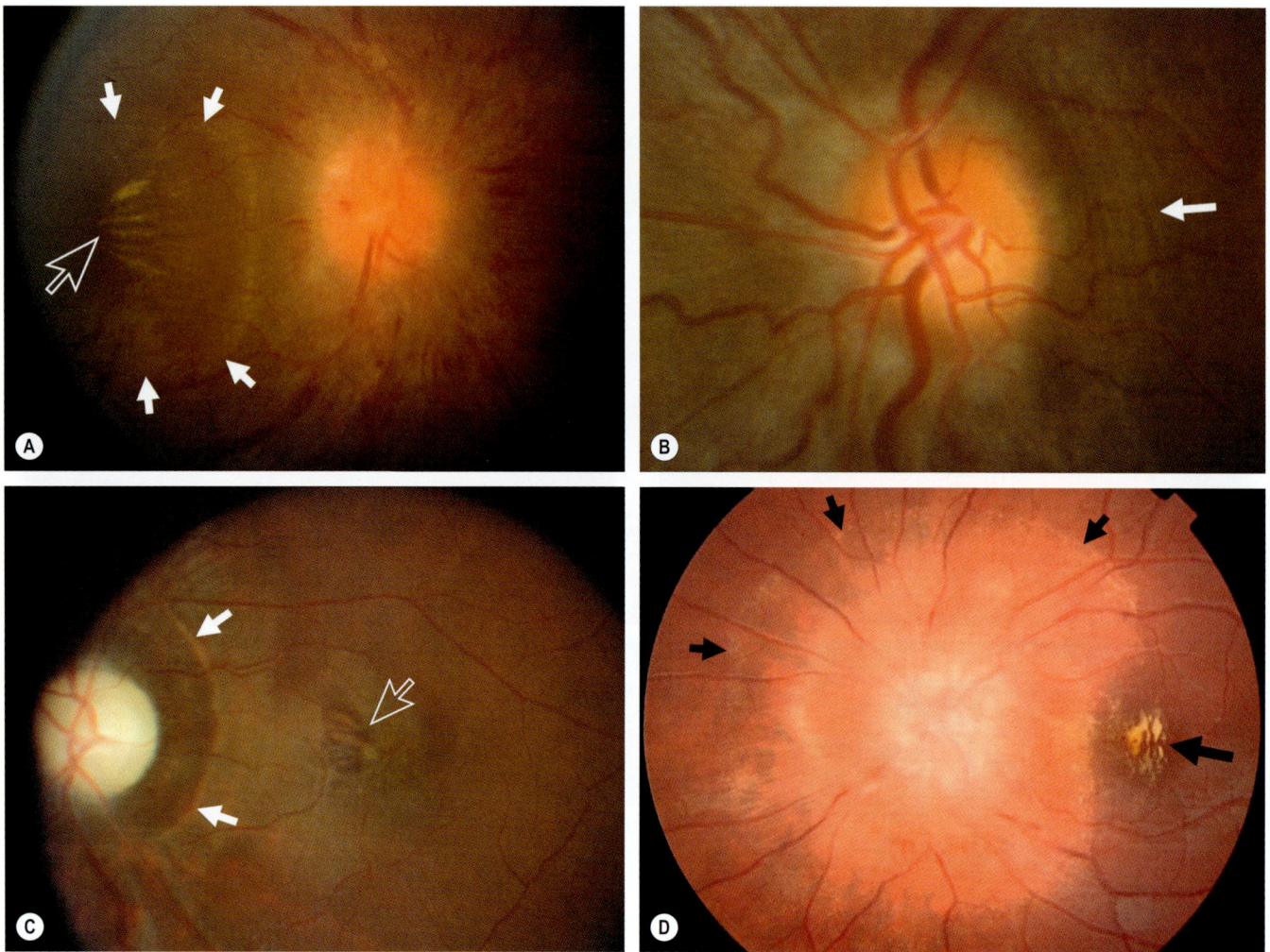

Figure 6–12. Retinal abnormalities associated with papilledema. **A.** Disc swelling is associated with macular edema (delineated by small arrows) and a lipid star (large open arrow). **B.** Circumferential folds (arrow). **C.** The left fundus in an individual with pseudotumor cerebri who had had severe visual loss associated with florid papilledema with macular edema and a lipid star similar to **A.** One year after optic nerve sheath fenestration, the vision improved, but optic nerve pallor, a residual "high-water mark" (solid arrows), and macular retinal pigment epithelial disturbances (large open arrow) are demonstrated in **C.** **D.** Papilledema and macular (large arrow) and peripapillary (small arrows) lipid deposition due to Lyme meningitis.

smoke"-like phenomenon that lasts for a few seconds. Likely they result from transient ischemia at the optic nerve head.[95] Transient visual obscurations do not correlate with intracranial pressure, extent of visual loss, or severity of disc edema.[96] They have also been reported in patients with other conditions causing optic nerve swelling or elevation.[95]

Differential diagnosis in patients with papilledema

Table 6–4 outlines causes of papilledema, and groups them according to frequency. A history of seizures, unilateral motor or sensory findings on examination, reflex asymmetry, or extensor plantar reflexes suggests a mass or other focal lesion. A sudden onset of severe headache, altered mentation, and neurologic deficits would be consistent with an acute intracranial hemorrhage. In a young female who is overweight or has a history of recent weight gain, and who has papilledema and a normal neurological examination, pseudotumor cerebri is a likely possibility. Limb weakness

might suggest a spinal tumor or demyelinating polyneuropathy. Hypertension should be excluded. Special considerations in children are discussed below.

Evaluation of the patient with papilledema

In patients with papilledema, we recommend urgent neurological evaluation and neuroimaging (magnetic resonance imaging (MRI) or computed tomography (CT) with contrast) to rule out an intracranial mass lesion, hemorrhage, hydrocephalus, or venous thrombosis **(Table 6–5)**. MR venography[97] should be requested as well when venous clot is suspected. MR angiography may be ordered if a dural arteriovenous malformation is considered as a possible cause of elevated intracranial pressure. If neuroimaging is normal, a lumbar puncture (LP) is necessary to rule out meningitis and to document the CSF opening pressure.[91] If neuroimaging reveals a venous thrombosis, it is still helpful to measure the opening pressure, and in these patients, as

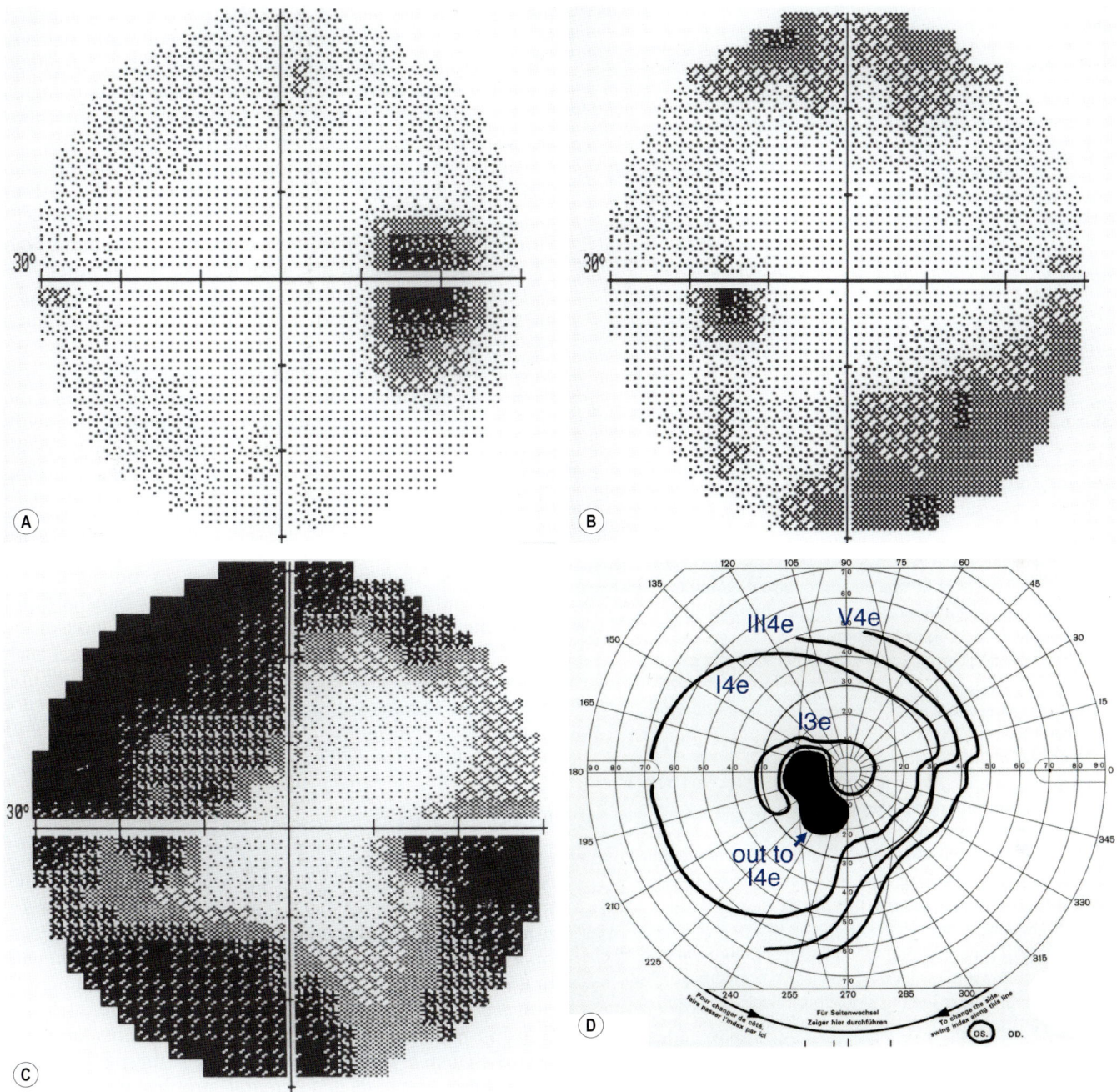

Figure 6–13. Examples of Humphrey (threshold) 30-2 computerized perimetry demonstrating (**A**) typical enlarged blind spot, (**B**) infranasal constriction, and (**C**) diffuse constriction due to papilledema associated with pseudotumor cerebri. The grayscale plots the central 30 degrees of vision. **D.** Goldmann (kinetic) visual field typical for visual loss associated with papilledema due to pseudotumor cerebri. Enlarged blind spot, inferior nerve fiber bundle defect, and infranasal constriction are present. (A, B, and D from Galetta SL et al. Neurol Clin 1996;14:201–222, with permission.)

well as those with pseudotumor cerebri, the LP often alleviates the headache. The LP should be performed with the patient relaxed in a lateral decubitus position, with the head and spine at the same level and the neck and knees slightly flexed. Normal CSF opening pressure in an adult is less than 250 mm H_2O.[98] In children the range for a normal CSF pressure is less certain,[99] but a pressure above 280 mm H_2O should be considered abnormal.[466] CSF measurements should also include at least those for protein, glucose, cell count and differential, gram stain, culture, cryptococcal antigen, and India ink. Papilledema, normal neuroimaging, elevated CSF opening pressure but normal CSF constituents

strongly suggests pseudotumor cerebri. CSF pleocytosis with or without elevated protein suggests meningitis. Bloody CSF or xanthochromia implies an intracranial hemorrhage, even if the neuroimaging is normal.

In the emergency setting, the presence of papilledema may alter management in patients with fever, stiff neck, and decreased mentation suggestive of bacterial meningitis.[100] Papilledema, indicative of elevated intracranial pressure, may reflect an abscess or hydrocephalus in these patients and a tendency to herniate. In one approach, emergent empiric intravenous antibiotics can be given, then neuroimaging performed prior to a lumbar puncture. However, the

Table 6–4 Causes of papilledema, according to frequency

Common	Uncommon
Intracranial mass lesion	Dural sinus
Pseudotumor cerebri	arteriovenous
Hydrocephalus	malformation
Intracranial hemorrhage	Obstructive sleep apnea
Venous thrombosis/obstruction	Guillain-Barré syndrome
Meningitis	Chronic inflammatory
	demyelinating
	polyneuropathy
	Spinal cord tumors
	Craniosynostoses
	Non-accidental injury

Table 6–5 Evaluation of patients with papilledema. See text for details

I. Distinguish from other causes of disc swelling (see Table 6–1), based upon clinical, fundus, and adjunctive laboratory features.

II. Clinical history
Rapidity of onset of headache and/or visual symptoms which might suggest a hemorrhage, venous thrombosis, or quickly expanding mass lesion
Other neurologic symptoms such as hemiparesis, sensory loss, or ataxia, e.g. to suggest a mass lesion
Body habitus (overweight female suggests pseudotumor cerebri)

III. Neuro-ophthalmic examination
Including careful visual field testing looking for field defects associated with papilledema

IV. Neurological examination
Evidence of mental status abnormalities, focal neurological abnormalities, or long tract signs suggest a mass lesion
Fever and stiff neck suggest meningitis

V. Neuroimaging
Magnetic resonance imaging (MRI) or computed tomography with contrast to exclude a mass lesion or hydrocephalus
MRI-venography, if venous sinus thrombosis suspected

VI. Lumbar puncture
Measurement of opening pressure when neuroimaging is unrevealing or if a venous sinus thrombosis is detected
Cerebrospinal fluid tests to exclude meningitis, e.g.: protein, glucose, cell count with differential, gram stain, culture, Cryptococcal antigen, and India ink.
When the clinical scenario requires the consideration of other entities: syphilis serologies, acid fast staining, cytology for malignant cells, angiotensin converting enzyme, Lyme titers

absence of papilledema should not be used to rule out elevated intracranial pressure.

Papilledema in children

Much of the differential diagnosis of papilledema in children overlaps that of adults, but there are some special considerations in younger age groups. Of the patients seen by the neuro-ophthalmology service at the Children's Hospital of Philadelphia, the most common cause of papilledema is a brain neoplasm, and pseudotumor cerebri is the next most frequent. Other commonly seen etiologies are meningitis (particularly Lyme), aqueductal stenosis, venous thrombosis, craniosynostoses, and non-accidental injury.

Papilledema may be less frequent in infants because the cranial sutures have not closed, allowing the cranial vault to expand in response to elevated intracranial pressure.[101] However, in cases where the pressure is exceedingly high or when it elevates rapidly, papilledema is still possible.[24] A bulging anterior fontanelle and enlarging head size are better indications of elevated intracranial pressure in this age group.

Craniosynostosis associated with Crouzon or Apert syndrome, for instance, refers to the premature closure of the cranial sutures. If brain growth exceeds that of the skull, elevated intracranial pressure and papilledema may result. Serial fundus examinations are important in the monitoring of these patients before or after craniofacial procedures.[102] The papilledema is usually chronic, and untreated cases can suffer from blindness.[103]

The most common ocular finding in non-accidental injury (child abuse, shaken-baby syndrome, battered-child syndrome, etc.[104]) is retinal hemorrhages in any layer of the retina.[105,106] While papilledema is seen in only 5% of such cases,[107] it usually indicates an accompanying subdural hematoma.[24] In these unfortunate instances, other evidence of non-accidental trauma, such as ecchymoses, fractures, or burns, should be sought.[108]

Mass lesions

Although papilledema is an excellent sign of elevated intracranial pressure, the absence of disc swelling does not necessarily rule out an intracranial mass lesion such as a neoplasm or abscess. In a series of patients (age range 0–90 years) with brain tumors presenting to an emergency department,[109] only 28% had papilledema. Van Crevel[110] studied the relationship between papilledema and brain tumors, and suggested that disc swelling is less likely if the patients were older, because age-related cerebral atrophy may allow for greater tumor expansion without causing elevated intracranial pressure, and also if the tumor were located in the parietal lobe. In his study, tumor size correlated poorly with the presence of papilledema. In contrast, childhood brain tumors, which are more commonly located in the posterior fossa and frequently cause fourth ventricular compression and non-communicating hydrocephalus, may be more likely to present with papilledema (65% in one pediatric series[101]).

Two types of cerebral neoplasms, gliomatosis cerebri and leptomeningeal primitive neuroectodermal tumors, deserve particular mention, as they may mimic pseudotumor cerebri (see below). Affected patients may present initially with papilledema, elevated CSF opening pressure with normal constituents, and normal neuroimaging. However, subsequent mental status changes and neurologic deterioration are inevitable with these tumors, and MRI at this point will likely demonstrate the characteristic infiltrative lesions of the cerebral hemispheres, brainstem, or leptomeninges.[111,112]

Cerebral hemorrhage

The types of intracranial hemorrhages associated with papilledema include aneurysmal or arteriovenous malformation (AVM)-related subarachnoid hemorrhage, acute subdural hematoma, and intraparenchymal hemorrhage. CT scanning is better than MRI at identifying the presence and location of acute blood. Hemorrhagic or xanthochromic CSF can confirm a subarachnoid hemorrhage, and formal angiography should be performed when an aneurysm or AVM is suspected. CT or MR angiography can be used as a screening tool, but they do not have the sensitivity of conventional angiography in excluding aneurysms. Elevated intracranial pressure results from mass effect produced by a hematoma or obstructive hydrocephalus from subarachnoid blood. As discussed above, acute rises in intracranial pressure associated with intracranial hemorrhages may result in the development of papilledema within hours. However, for unclear reasons, papilledema due to subarachnoid or intraparenchymal hemorrhage occurs only in a minority of patients, despite the presence of elevated intracranial pressure. Papilledema occurred in only 16% in one series of patients with ruptured aneurysms.[113] Therefore, normal optic nerve appearance should not be the sole criterion to exclude the presence of elevated intracranial pressure.[114]

In Terson syndrome, acute subarachnoid bleeding (more typically) or an acute subdural hematoma causes intraocular hemorrhage in the vitreous, preretinal (subhyaloid), intraretinal, or subretinal spaces **(Fig. 6–14)**.[115] In prospective series,[116–119] intraocular hemorrhages occurred in 17–28% of adults with subarachnoid hemorrhages, but it was inconsistent as to whether the presence of Terson syndrome was related to the severity of the subarachnoid hemorrhage. Terson syndrome is uncommon (8%) in children with intracranial hemorrhages not related to abuse.[120]

Preretinal hemorrhages in Terson syndrome usually occur between the temporal vascular arcades and can characteristically layer out. When present, vitreous hemorrhages can prevent adequate visualization of retinal hemorrhages. Severe, sudden rises in intracranial pressure can be transmitted to the optic nerve,[121,122] and Garfinkle et al.[116] suggested subsequent compression of both the central retinal vein and retinochoroidal anastomoses could result in an acute decrease in venous drainage from the retina and cause stasis and intraocular hemorrhage. Tracking of blood within the optic nerve sheath subarachnoid space and into the vitreous has been proposed, but similar ocular hemorrhages may be seen in patients with sudden elevations in intracranial pressure without subarachnoid hemorrhage **(Fig. 6–14)**.

In Schultz et al.'s study,[115] affected eyes in Terson syndrome had visual acuities ranging from 20/20 to light perception, and the natural history was for spontaneous resorption of the blood and moderate to good spontaneous recovery in vision within 9 months. Epiretinal membranes developed commonly, but their etiology was unclear. Vitrectomy allowed faster recovery, but the visual prognosis was

no different. Thus, vitreous surgery[123] might be reserved for young children with immature visual systems at risk for amblyopia and adults with bilateral involvement.

Trauma

In one study,[34] papilledema was identified in only 3.5% of patients with acute head injury. Its presence had little correlation with the degree of elevated intracranial pressure, and its absence did not rule out increased intracranial pressure. On the other hand, papilledema is much more common (approximately 50%) in patients with chronic subdural hematomas.[34]

Meningitis

Patients with infectious meningitis can develop papilledema and sixth nerve palsies associated with elevated intracranial pressure. Infectious etiologies include bacteria (e.g. pneumococcus), Lyme borrelia, tuberculosis,[124] and cryptococcus, for instance. When basilar meningitis causes obstructive hydrocephalus, shunting is usually required.[125]

Of the patients with Lyme meningitis, papilledema and sixth nerve palsies seem more common in children affected with the disorder.[126,127] In fact, the most common mimicker of pseudotumor cerebri (see below) in children with normal imaging in our experience is Lyme meningitis. Almost all patients do extremely well with resolution of symptoms within weeks following treatment with intravenous antibiotics such as ceftriaxone, and some evidence suggests oral doxycycline may be effective in Lyme meningitis as well.[128] We have added acetazolamide in affected patients until disc swelling resolves, but there is no evidence that this is necessary. Several authors[129,130] have used the term "pseudotumor cerebri due to Lyme disease" in these cases; however, that is inappropriate because these patients have abnormal CSF contents.

Cryptococcal meningitis is notorious for causing catastrophic visual loss associated with disc swelling.[131,132] The mechanism is due either to the effects of high intracranial pressure or to direct optic nerve invasion by the cryptococci.[133] In addition to antifungal agents,[134] acetazolamide can be used in cases with mild visual loss secondary to disc swelling.[135] However, optic nerve sheath decompression has become the treatment of choice for severe visual loss in this infection, particularly when there is elevated intracranial pressure.[136]

Papilledema due to viral or other causes of aseptic meningitis, such as chemical or drug-induced,[137] is much less common and was seen in only 2% of patients in one series.[138] Papilledema may occur in patients with elevated intracranial pressure due to carcinomatous or sarcoid meningitis, and hydrocephalus is the usual cause in these instances.[139]

Papilledema in association with elevated intracranial pressure and idiopathic CSF lymphocytic pleocytosis is well recognized[140,141] but is a diagnosis of exclusion. In most cases the condition is self-limited, but we have treated such patients with acetazolamide.

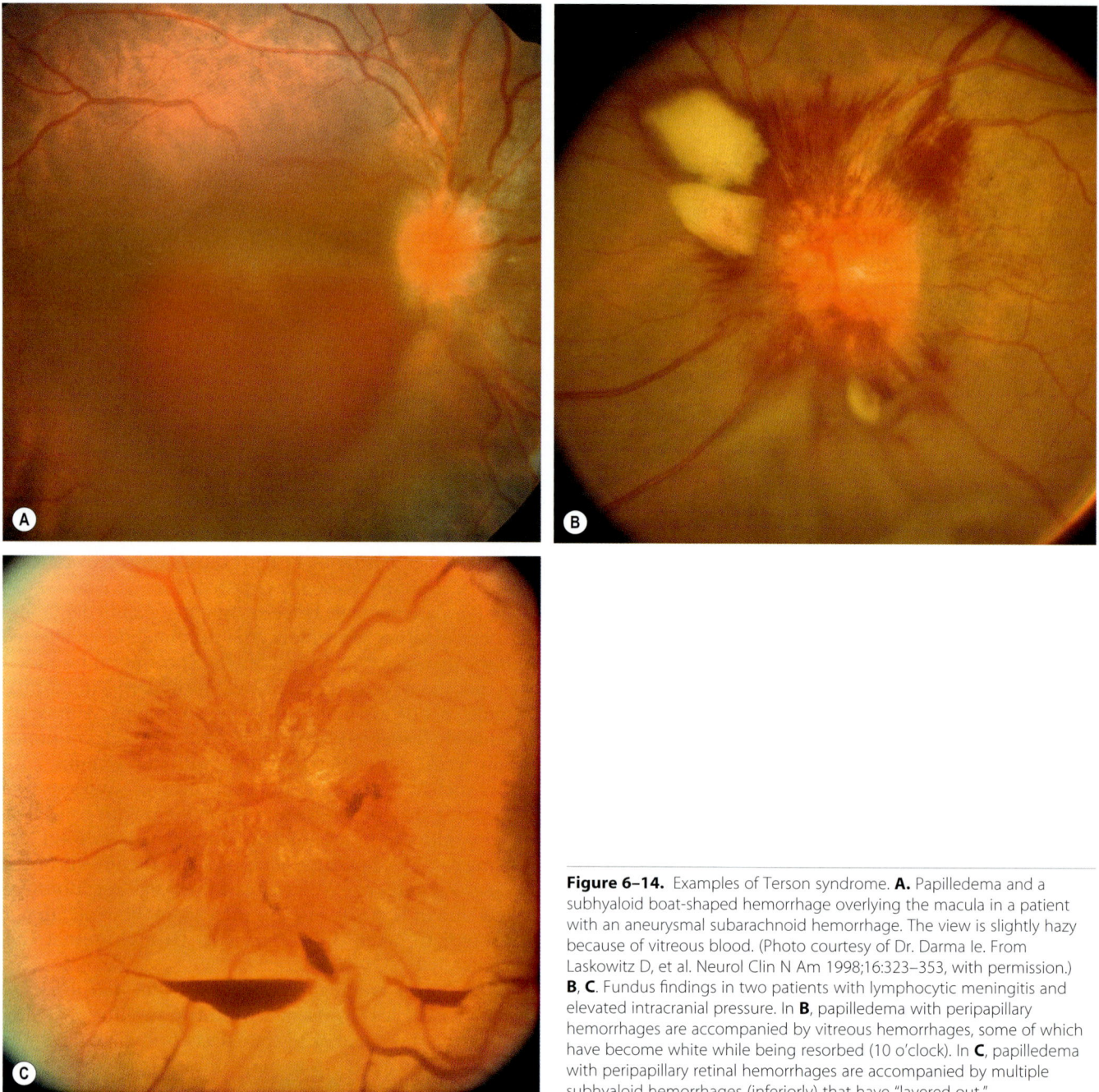

Figure 6–14. Examples of Terson syndrome. **A.** Papilledema and a subhyaloid boat-shaped hemorrhage overlying the macula in a patient with an aneurysmal subarachnoid hemorrhage. The view is slightly hazy because of vitreous blood. (Photo courtesy of Dr. Darma Ie. From Laskowitz D, et al. Neurol Clin N Am 1998;16:323–353, with permission.) **B, C.** Fundus findings in two patients with lymphocytic meningitis and elevated intracranial pressure. In **B**, papilledema with peripapillary hemorrhages are accompanied by vitreous hemorrhages, some of which have become white while being resorbed (10 o'clock). In **C**, papilledema with peripapillary retinal hemorrhages are accompanied by multiple subhyaloid hemorrhages (inferiorly) that have "layered out."

Hydrocephalus

Obstructive (non-communicating) hydrocephalus results from compression of the ventricular system or its associated foramina (e.g. Monroe, sylvian aqueduct) **(Fig. 6–15)**. As outlined above, common causes included neoplasms, intraventricular or subarachnoid blood, and meningitis. Other etiologies which should be considered include congenital aqueductal stenosis, myelomeningocele, and in endemic areas, cysticercosis.[142]

In addition to treatment of the primary problem, many patients with obstructive hydrocephalus will require a shunting procedure. Endoscopic procedures, including third ven-triculostomy, may also be considered in some instances.[143] Papilledema, if present preoperatively, usually resolves following successful CSF diversion.[144] However, some require periodic ophthalmic or neuro-ophthalmic examinations because ocular signs may signify shunt failure even in the absence of headache, nausea, vomiting, or ventriculo-megaly.[145–148] We treated a girl with a lumboperitoneal shunt who complained only of transient visual obscurations. Disc swelling and nerve fiber-related visual field defects had recurred, and the shunt was found to have malfunctioned.

A post-decompression optic neuropathy has been described, in which patients with papilledema develop acute visual loss following rapid decreases in CSF pressure due to shunting or decompressive craniotomy.[149] The postulated

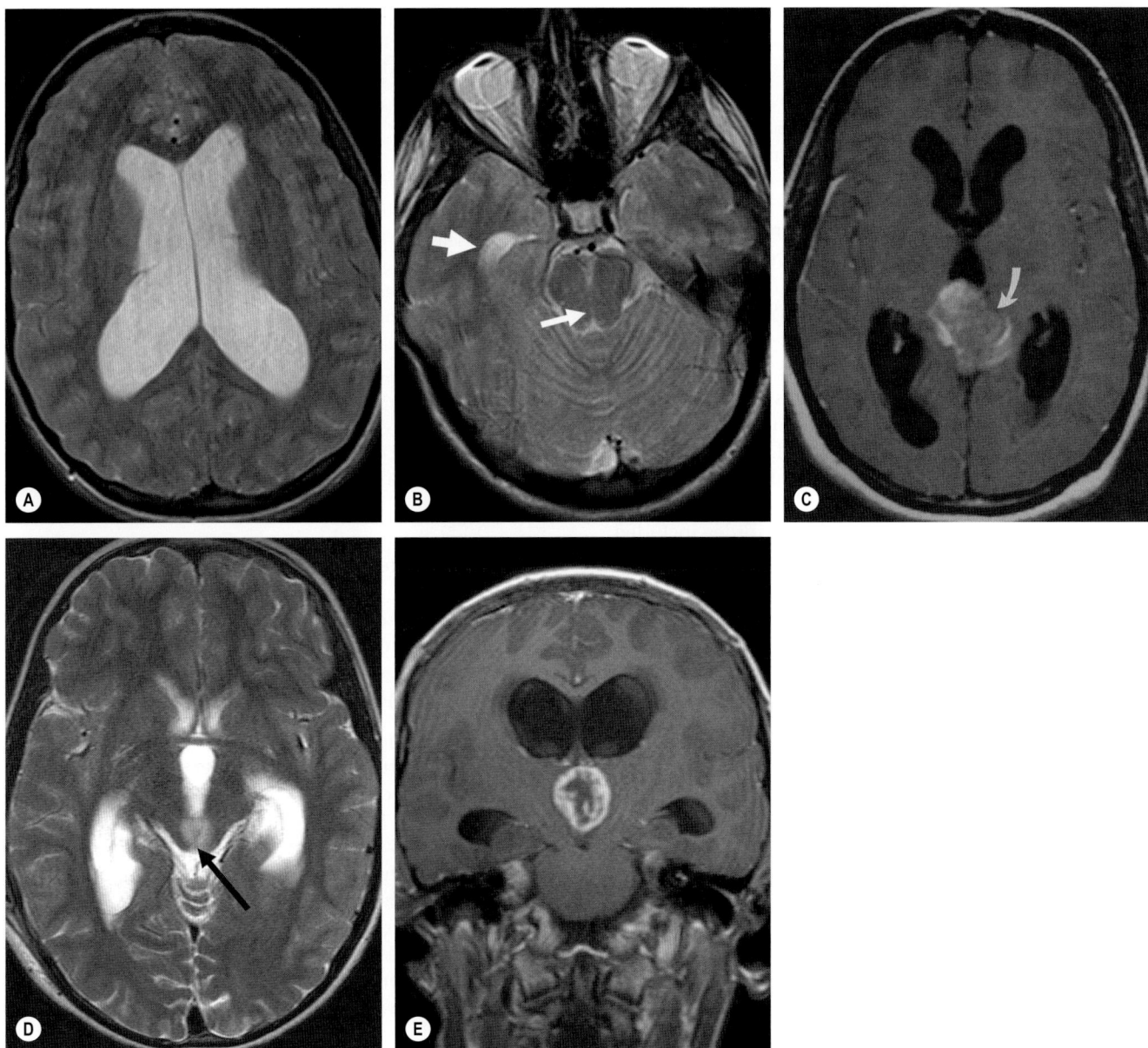

Figure 6–15. MRI demonstration of causes of hydrocephalus associated with papilledema. Note the enlarged ventricles in all images. **A, B.** Axial images demonstrating (**A**) hydrocephalus in an 18 year old with (**B**) previously unrecognized aqueductal stenosis (smaller arrow points to absence of the normally more prominent signal of a patent cerebral aqueduct; the larger arrow points to the abnormally dilated temporal horn of the lateral ventricle). **C.** T1-weighted gadolinium-enhanced image showing noncommunicating hydrocephalus in a young woman who presented with headaches, a sixth nerve palsy, and papilledema due to a pinealblastoma (arrow). **D.** Tectal glioma (arrow), which obstructed the cerebral aqueduct as seen on a T2-weighted image. **E.** Third ventricular astrocytoma (arrow). See Fig. 6–8A for corresponding fundus photo.

mechanism is hypoperfusion to the prelaminar portion of the optic nerve, and the visual prognosis is poor.[150] Fortunately, we have found this complication to be an uncommon one.

In addition, children who are shunted for hydrocephalus early in life may later develop slit-ventricle syndrome, an uncommon condition characterized by headaches and subnormal ventricular sizes.[151,152] Some affected patients we have followed developed elevated intracranial pressure and papilledema, in part due to skull non-compliance, despite normal shunt function. Treatment in these cases consisted of either acetazolamide or neurosurgical cranial vault expansion. In other reports, lumboperitoneal[153] and cisterna

magna-ventricular[154] shunting were used. In another subset of patients, the ventricles are normal or subnormal in size during asymptomatic periods, but when symptomatic with headaches, mild ventriculomegaly is evident. Intermittent proximal shunt malfunction is the cause in these cases, and these individuals respond to proximal shunt revision.[155]

Pseudotumor cerebri (idiopathic intracranial hypertension)

Features common to all patients with pseudotumor cerebri are elevated intracranial pressure measured during a lumbar

Table 6–6 Modified-modified Dandy criteria[156,157] for the diagnosis of pseudotumor cerebri

1. If symptoms or signs present, they may only reflect those of generalized intracranial hypertension or papilledema.
2. Documented elevated intracranial pressure measured in the lateral decubitus position.
3. Normal CSF composition.
4. No evidence of hydrocephalus, mass, structural, or vascular lesion on MRI or contrast-enhanced CT for typical patients, and MRI and MR venography for all others.
5. No other cause of intracranial hypertension identified.

Table 6–7 Conditions and drugs associated with pseudotumor cerebri. Only those which have been proven or are highly likely to be associated are listed.

Weight-related
Obesity
Recent weight gain

Medical conditions
Addison's disease
Anemia
Systemic lupus erythematosus
Withdrawal from chronic corticosteroids

Drugs
Synthetic growth hormone
Tetracycline and related derivatives
Vitamin A related
    All trans-retinoic acid (ATRA)
    Hypervitaminosis A (vitamin, liver, or isotretinoin intake)

puncture, normal spinal fluid constituents, and neuroimaging which excludes a mass lesion or venous thrombosis. The diagnosis is formally established when the modified-modified Dandy criteria[156,157] are satisfied **(Table 6–6)**. The greatest morbidity from this disorder is visual loss related to optic disc swelling.

Historically, other terms used for this disorder included "otitic hydrocephalus," because many cases in the pre-antibiotic era were associated with mastoiditis and venous thrombosis (see below). Foley[158,159] coined the term "benign intracranial hypertension," which was also advocated by Weisberg[160] and even used by more recent authors.[161–163] This designation should be eschewed, however, because the condition may be associated with severe debilitating visual loss in as many as 25% of patients,[87,164] and therefore it is not always "benign." Instead, many experts today advocate the use of the term "idiopathic intracranial hypertension."[96,165,166] However, we have found "pseudotumor cerebri," "pseudotumor," or "pseudotumor cerebri syndrome"[167] more descriptive terms and therefore easier for patients (and many physicians) to remember. Furthermore, the term "pseudotumor cerebri" is still applicable in situations in which a cause is identified (i.e. not idiopathic).

Demographics

In cases which are idiopathic, the patients are almost uniformly females in early adulthood and are overweight or have a history of recent weight gain. In four large series, approximately 90% were women and the mean age was 27.8–34 years.[87,96,168,169] The approximate annual incidence of pseudotumor cerebri is 0.9–1.7/100 000 in the general population.[170–172] However, among females 15–44 years of age the incidence is 3.3–12.0/100 000, and among obese females in this age group the incidence climbs to 7.9–21.4/100 000.[170–172] Case–control studies[168,173,174] confirm that obesity and recent weight gain of as little as 5% are more common among patients with pseudotumor cerebri than among controls. It is uncertain whether there is a racial predilection for this disorder, as the racial distribution in each reported series reflects the makeup of the local population.

When men develop pseudotumor cerebri, they tend to be either in a similar age distribution to affected women, or slightly older, and they are also usually obese.[175–177] However, when pseudotumor cerebri in a man is suspected, the treating physician should be overly meticulous in excluding other responsible etiologies (see below). Sleep apnea may be more prevalent in men with pseudotumor cerebri.[177–180]

Pseudotumor in children is discussed in more detail at the end of this section.

Associated conditions and drugs

Table 6–7 lists the most notable conditions and drugs which according to the literature and our experience are associated with pseudotumor cerebri, and affected patients satisfy the modified-modified Dandy criteria for its diagnosis. More comprehensive lists have been published elsewhere.[96,157,181]

Anemia. Pseudotumor cerebri has been associated with several forms of acquired anemia including iron deficiency,[182–184] aplastic anemia,[185,186] hemolytic anemia,[187,188] and sickle cell disease.[189] The mechanism by which anemia causes pseudotumor is unclear, but has been theorized to result from tissue hypoxia leading to increased capillary permeability or abnormalities in hemodynamics leading to increased cerebral blood flow (high-flow state).

Steroid withdrawal. Steroid withdrawal (not steroid use) is a well-recognized, but infrequently well-documented, risk factor,[190] most commonly occurring in children on chronic corticosteroids for respiratory, renal, or dermatologic disorders.[164,191] Discontinuation of a short course of steroids taken for a few days or weeks is not a risk factor. In a related condition, we have seen a patient who developed pseudotumor cerebri following removal of a longstanding adrenocorticotrophic hormone (ACTH)-secreting pituitary tumor (Cushing disease, see Chapter 7).

Synthetic growth hormone. First reported in 1993, there have been multiple cases of pseudotumor in children treated with recombinant (biosynthetic) human growth hormone (GH).[99,192] In a large database analysis, the prevalence of pseudotumor in the GH-treated population was approximately 100 times greater than in the normal population.[193] It appears that risk factors such as obesity, Turner syndrome, chronic renal failure, Prader–Willi syndrome, and delayed puberty can increase the risk of developing pseudotumor in this setting.[194]

It has been proposed that growth hormone passes the blood–brain barrier, acts locally to increase levels of IGF-1, which in turn increases CSF production from the choroid plexus.[195] Furthermore, it seems as though aggressive GH dosing places a child at a higher risk of developing pseudotumor; thus, starting hormone therapy at the lowest recommended dose, with prudent gradual titration to higher doses if needed has been advised.[196] Caution must be applied when diagnosing papilledema in a patient with GH deficiency as congenital disk anomalies (hypoplasia or small crowded discs) may be seen in children with hypopituitarism.[197]

Tetracycline derivatives. The evidence regarding their role in pseudotumor cerebri is convincing.[198–203] They are commonly prescribed drugs, especially for acne. Gardner et al.[198] reviewed the literature regarding the relationship between pseudotumor and tetracycline, and its synthetic relative, minocycline. A true association was suggested in many affected patients who improved following removal of the drug and recurrence in some who then restarted the medication. The authors also suggested a combination of other factors, including genetic susceptibility. Female gender and obesity may predispose some to developing pseudotumor when these medications are used.[200] Additionally, there have been several cases of pseudotumor occurring in twins treated with tetracyclines, and thus it is possible that genetic susceptibility may also predispose certain individuals to pseudotumor.[198]

Vitamin A, ATRA, and related compounds. Vitamin A intoxication may produce signs and symptoms consistent with pseudotumor cerebri. In a prospective study on adults, hypervitaminosis, either secondary to increased levels, altered metabolism, or hypersensitivity to vitamin A, was shown to be associated with pseudotumor.[204] Additionally, in a double-blind, randomized, placebo-controlled trial, infants given vitamin A supplementation were more likely to develop bulging fontanelles than those who did not.[205] There have been several reports of cases of pseudotumor after acne treatment with isotretinoin (13-cis retinoic acid), a vitamin A derivative,[206] with or without tetracyclines (discussed above).[207,208] Combination therapy seems to increase the risk.

In addition, there have also been several reports on the development of pseudotumor in patients with acute promyelocytic leukemia (APML) treated with all-trans retinoic acid (ATRA), a vitamin A derivative.[209–216] Several studies have shown that children, especially those under 8, are more sensitive to the effects of ATRA on the central nervous system than adults.[209,217] Therefore, it has been suggested that lower dose regimens of ATRA should be considered in children to avoid potential side-effects such as the development of pseudotumor.[218]

Addison disease. A possible association between papilledema and Addison disease (adrenal insufficiency in spite of elevated ACTH levels) has been suggested.[219,220] Glucocorticoid and mineralocorticoid replacement resulted in resolution of symptoms in two reports,[219,220] with one patient requiring additional treatment with acetazolamide.[219]

Systemic lupus erythematosus. Lupus has been described as causing pseudotumor cerebri.[221,222] The mechanism is unclear, but patients may be predisposed because of renal insufficiency or a hypercoagulable state.

Questionable and mistaken associations

The literature is replete with purported disease and drug associations, but many reported cases must be reviewed skeptically because they fail to satisfy the modified Dandy criteria. Several authors incorrectly diagnosed pseudotumor cerebri, as their patients had abnormal neurologic findings including decreased mental status, ataxia, hemiparesis, third-nerve palsy, asymmetric reflexes, and extensor plantar responses. In some, the CSF profile is abnormal due to pleocytosis or elevated protein. Other reported patients lacked either CSF examinations or adequate neuroradiologic studies. In others, hypercoagulable states leading to undetected intracranial venous thromboses may have been present, and in some reports, the diagnosis of pseudotumor was likely to be purely coincidental as no plausible explanation for the association between pseudotumor and the described condition could be provided. We mention some of the more prominent supposed associations here to emphasize that these conditions have not been convincingly shown to cause pseudotumor.

Lyme meningitis. Papilledema and elevated intracranial pressure can develop in Lyme meningitis, discussed elsewhere in this chapter. However, by definition pseudotumor cannot be caused by Lyme meningitis, as there are cells in the spinal fluid.

Renal failure and transplantation. Purportedly, children with *impaired renal function* may be at higher risk of developing idiopathic intracranial hypertension.[223] It has also been suggested that those who undergo *renal transplantation* may also be at greater risk post transplantation.[224] In one retrospective analysis of children undergoing renal transplant in the United Kingdom over an 11- year period, it was claimed that 4.4% developed pseudotumor cerebri post transplantation.[225] However, it must be noted that almost all of the reported patients were treated with chronic immunosuppressive medication, including corticosteroids, and many had other risk factors, including obesity and treatment with growth hormone, that could have also increased their risk of developing pseudotumor.[224,226]

Mechanism

The cause of pseudotumor cerebri is unclear, but any explanation must account for elevated intracranial pressure with normal neuroimaging (without hydrocephalus), CSF constituents, and neurological examinations. *Decreased CSF absorption by the arachnoid villi* is the most likely explanation suggested by radioisotope cisternography and other observations.[227–230] However, it is possible that decreased CSF absorption is a secondary phenomenon, resulting from compression of the arachnoid villi by elevated intracranial pressure from any cause.[231]

Abnormal CSF pressure gradients caused by *increased intracranial venous pressure* may also account for decreased absorption.[161] *Elevated intra-abdominal pressure* secondary to obesity may increase pleural pressure and cardiac filling pressure, thereby leading to increased intracranial venous pressure and elevated intracranial pressure.[232] King et al.[233] performed cerebral venography and manometry in patients with pseudotumor cerebri, and they found consistently elevated venous pressures. In addition, narrowing of the transverse (lateral) sinuses has been demonstrated in many patients with pseudotumor cerebri (**Fig. 6–16**),[234] suggesting possible abnormalities in venous blood flow. It is unclear whether these pressure and anatomical abnormalities are the cause or the consequences of pseudotumor, but the latter is more likely. Previously, it was thought that unrecognized thrombi may be the cause of tapered stenoses and filling defects in transverse sinuses in patients with pseudotumor.[235] However, the elevated venous pressures[236] and sinus narrowing[237–239] often, but not always,[240] resolve with lowering of CSF pressure. This implies that increased intracranial pressure caused the elevated venous pressures[241,242] and collapse of the walls of transverse sinuses.[243]

Elevated brain volume secondary to cerebral edema or increased cerebral blood volume has also been proposed,[244–247] but the histologic evidence is less supportive.[248] Studies using MRI of brain water self-diffusion also suggested increased water mobility caused interstitial and intracellular fluid accumulation.[249,250] More recent pathologic studies by Wall et al.[251] failed to reveal cerebral edema in two patients, although the autopsies were performed 1–2.5 years after presentation. Wall et al.[251] also reviewed three of the biopsies reported by Sahs and Joynt,[245] and the authors found no convincing evidence of cerebral edema. *Increased rate of CSF formation* is also unlikely,[252,253] as choroid plexus papillomas tend to cause hydrocephalus.

The association between pseudotumor cerebri and female gender and obesity suggests an *endocrine basis* for the disorder. The previously mentioned reports of pseudotumor cerebri occurring in corticosteroid-deficient states such as Addison disease,[220] ACTH deficiency, and following removal of an ACTH-secreting pituitary adenoma,[254,255] imply an abnormality in the adrenal–pituitary axis. Furthermore, corticosteroids in many instances effectively treat pseudotumor cerebri,[96] and corticosteroid withdrawal is associated with pseudotumor cerebri,[190] suggesting that corticosteroids have an effect on CSF dynamics. In addition, one study[256] suggested patients with pseudotumor cerebri and orthostatic edema may have elevated vasopressin levels, leading to fluid retention. However, Soelberg Sørensen et al.[257] screened a series of patients with pseudotumor cerebri and found no consistent abnormality in pituitary, gonadal, thyroid, or adrenal function.

Hypercoagulable states without obvious dural sinus thromboses have been reported in association with and in some cases used to explain the mechanism for pseudotumor cerebri.[258–261] For instance, it has been proposed that patients with pseudotumor may have genetic thrombotic risk factors that predispose them to microvascular occlusion in the arachnoid villi.[259] In published cohorts of patients with pseudotumor, several individuals were found to have antiphospholipid antibodies, hyperfibrinogenemia, or other conditions related to thrombosis.[258,260,262]

Recent studies have shown that both serum retinol binding protein (RBP)[263] and levels of retinol[264,265] and vitamin A[266] in the cerebrospinal fluid are elevated in those with pseudotumor cerebri, as compared to normal controls. It has been proposed that excess retinol and RBP in the serum are transported to the cerebrospinal fluid where retinol is toxic to arachnoid granulations, thereby disrupting CSF absorption.[264,266] Alternatively RBP could alter aquaporin expression[267] or act as a signaling molecule,[268] in either case leading to abnormal CSF secretion by the choroid plexus or CSF absorption by the arachnoid villi.

In summary, the mechanism is likely to be decreased CSF absorption due either to dysfunction at the level of the arachnoid villi or to elevated intracranial venous pressures. The association of pseudotumor cerebri and so many other conditions suggests that these purported mechanisms may be the final common pathway, but the inciting factors may be multiple.

Presenting signs and symptoms

The frequency of presenting symptoms is likely underestimated in the various retrospective series,[48,87,160,169,269] and the best data come from a prospective study by Wall and George.[84] Headache was the most common complaint, occurring in 94% of patients in their study. Many had related neck stiffness or retrobulbar pain, the latter sometimes exacerbated by eye movements. Seventy-two percent reported transient visual obscurations (TVOs). Photopsias (54%), diplopia (38%), and visual loss (26%) were less frequent ophthalmic complaints. Sixty percent of patients complained of a pulsatile intracranial noise, characterized either by tinnitus or a "whooshing." The bruit sounds are usually subjective (internal), but occasionally they can be auscultated or externally audible.[270] The cause of the noise is likely transmission of systolic pulsations of high-pressure CSF against the exposed walls of the dural venous sinuses, leading to turbulent blood flow through the venous sinuses.[271] Mentation and level of alertness was normal in all patients. There have also been reports of patients presenting with gaze-evoked amaurosis (see Chapter 9).[272]

Eye movement abnormalities other than abducens palsies are unusual, but third[273,274] and fourth nerve dysfunction,[275] internuclear ophthalmoplegia, bilateral ophthalmoplegia,[276] skew deviation, and nystagmus have been reported. Seventh nerve dysfunction is also commonly recognized.[277] Selky et al.[278] hypothesized that facial palsies associated with elevated intracranial pressure resulted from brainstem shifts leading to stretching and compression of the extra-axial facial nerve in the bony facial canal. Cases with hemifacial spasm have also been reported.[279,280] In addition, trigeminal[281,282] and acoustic neuropathies[283] have been observed. Technically, such patients with ophthalmoplegia and cranial nerve dysfunction other than abducens palsies do not satisfy the modified Dandy criteria, but in well-documented cases no other cause for the elevated intracranial pressure could be found.[276]

Round and Keane[284] reviewed the "minor" symptoms of elevated intracranial pressure in their patients with pseudotumor cerebri. Neck stiffness, distal extremity paresthesias, and low back pain were not uncommon. They hypothesized that these symptoms were related to nerve root irritation or spinal root pouch enlargement. Joint pains of unclear etiology was another complaint described.

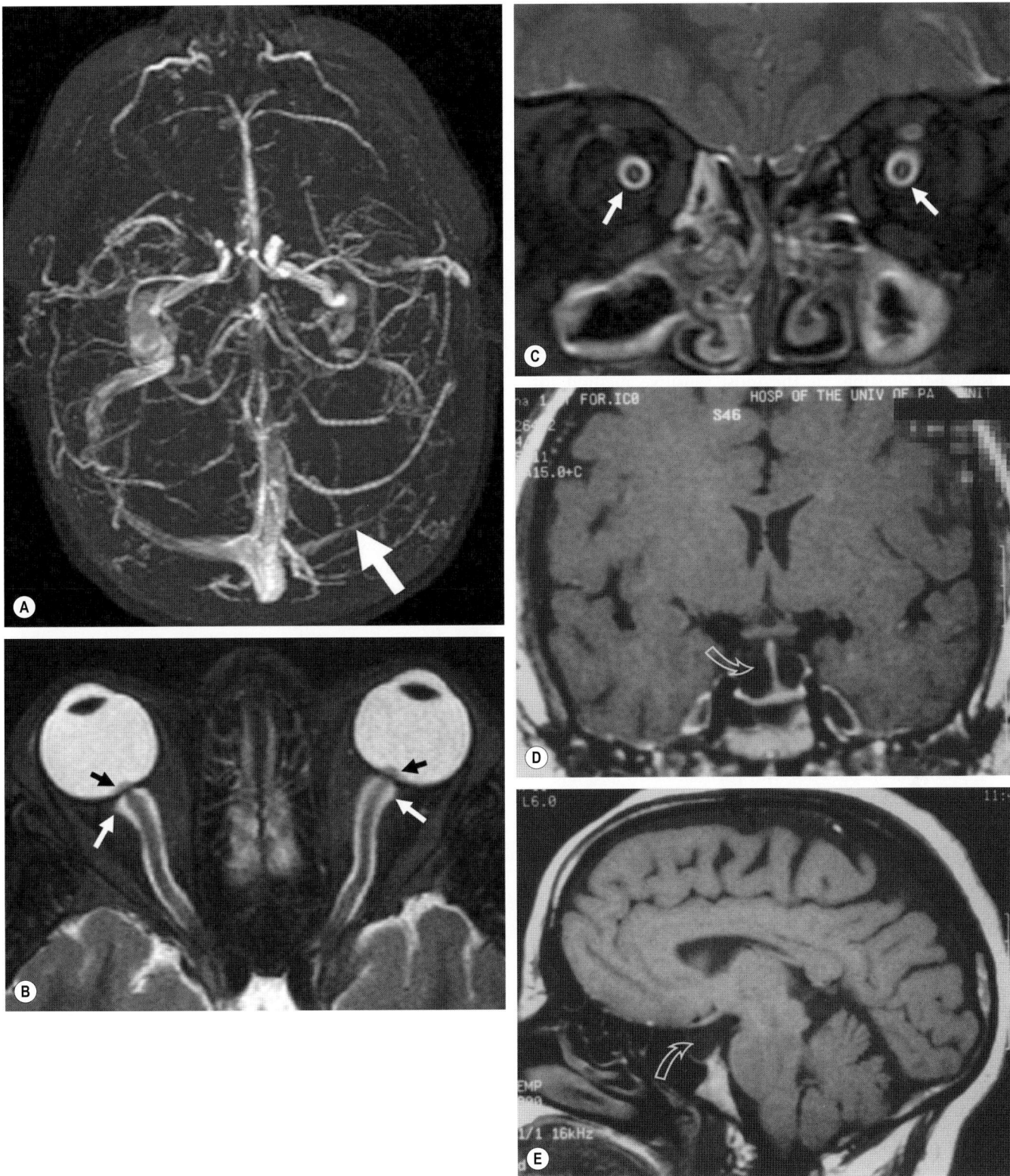

Figure 6–16. Magnetic resonance imaging (MRI) venogram and MRI findings associated with pseudotumor cerebri. **A.** MRI venogram, axial view, demonstrating narrowing of the left transverse sinus (arrow). **B.** T2-weighted image shows optic disc elevation (black arrows), dilated optic nerve sheaths (white arrows), tortuous optic nerves, and indentation of the globes posteriorly. **C.** T2-weighted coronal image in another patient shows dilated optic nerve sheaths (arrows). **D and E.** Empty sella (open white arrow) is demonstrated in sagittal T1-weighted sagittal (**D**) and coronal (**E**) images. Note the absence of the normal pituitary contents, which seem pushed to the bottom of the sella.

Neuro-ophthalmic findings

Visual loss. When it occurs, visual loss is typically insidious, and most patients are unaware of minor deficits because central vision is usually spared. Severe loss of visual acuity in pseudotumor cerebri is uncommon,[85] except when the papilledema is chronic or when there is retinal involvement,[285] such as a neurosensory retinal detachment, macular lipid exudate, or hemorrhage.[58] Most likely, the extent of visual loss does not correlate with the frequency of TVOs,[84] but conflicting opinions exist.[48] Sudden visual loss can occur although oftentimes it seems to be the result of sudden awareness, or rarely from acute optic nerve ischemia[86] or retinal artery occlusion.[66,69,70] An uncommon but well-recognized fulminant presentation can occur, in which patients develop acute and severe visual loss over days.[85,286]

Visual field testing[91] is the most sensitive method for detecting visual loss in these patients, and the most common abnormalities are blind spot enlargement, generalized constriction of isopters, and inferior nasal field loss (see **Fig. 6–13**).[96] Because of reasons outlined above, we prefer to test and follow patients with computerized threshold visual fields, which tend to be more objective and reproducible. In Wall and George's prospective study,[84] 96% of patients had some abnormality detected on Goldmann perimetry, while 92% had deficits on computerized testing. As a cautionary note, we have encountered many patients with pseudotumor cerebri with advanced vision loss who have had a component of functional visual loss.[287] Often in these individuals, there are confounding psychiatric, medical, and psychosocial issues. Tangent screen visual field examination may be necessary to document nonphysiologic field constriction.

Visual acuity, color vision, and pupillary reactivity are typically normal in patients with pseudotumor, and about one-half have abnormal contrast sensitivity,[84] in comparison with the higher incidence of visual field deficits. Sixth nerve palsies occur also in just a minority (approximately one-fifth).[84] Therefore, these parameters are felt to be insensitive measures of alteration in visual function when compared to visual field testing.[96] Most experienced clinicians do not use contrast sensitivity or visual evoked potentials in the evaluation or follow-up of patients with pseudotumor cerebri.[288]

Risk factors for more severe visual loss at presentation include male gender[177] and black race.[177]

Papilledema. Papilledema is uniformly present, can be asymmetric, and in uncommon instances is unilateral.[39,40] In asymmetric cases, the vision loss is usually worse in the eye with the more severe swelling.[289] There are also patients in whom intracranial pressure is elevated but papilledema does not develop (see below).

Neuroimaging.[91] Although either is acceptable, MRI of the brain with gadolinium is preferred over CT scanning with contrast to exclude hydrocephalus or any cause of elevated intracranial pressure such as a mass lesion, venous sinus thrombosis, or dural arteriovenous malformation. Common radiographic findings in pseudotumor cerebri include an empty sella,[290] dilation of the optic nerve sheaths,[291] and elevation of the optic disc (**Fig. 6–16**).[292] Occasionally on MR images the swollen optic disc will enhance.[293,294] The empty sella is thought to result from chronically elevated intracranial pressure associated with a congenitally incompetent diaphragma sella.[295,296] Many patients will have "slit-like" ventricles,[297] but in at least two studies[292,298] age-matched controls had similar ventricular sizes. Some studies[299] have suggested sulci effacement on CT scanning is a helpful radiologic sign, but we have found this to be an inconsistent feature.

Others[233,235] have employed venography in the workup of their patients with pseudotumor cerebri. Because of the risks of the procedure, we have not done so. We prefer to use less invasive, albeit less sensitive, MR venograms in addition to regular MR sequences as a better screen for patients suspected of having a venous sinus thrombosis (see below). Such individuals might include thin females or those with mastoiditis, for instance. Commonly seen narrowing of the transverse sinuses demonstrated on MR venography was discussed above.

Cerebrospinal fluid.[91] Following normal neuroimaging, a lumbar puncture is necessary to rule out meningitis, e.g., and to document the CSF opening pressure. When bedside LPs are difficult due to patient obesity, fluoroscopically guided LPs may be necessary. LPs should not be performed in patients with low-lying cerebellar tonsils because of the risk of fatal herniation.[300]

To establish the diagnosis of pseudotumor cerebri, the CSF opening pressure should exceed 250 mm H_2O, the upper limit of normal for most obese and non-obese adults.[98,301] Approximately 20–30 cc of CSF can be removed although the optimal amount has not been studied. It is not necessary to measure the closing pressure. In suspected cases with a normal CSF opening pressure, monitoring for 1 hour with an epidural transducer or subarachnoid bolt may be considered,[231] but this is rarely done in clinical practice. The cell count and glucose should be normal, and the protein normal or low. One study[302] found an inverse relationship between CSF opening pressure and CSF protein, while another[303] refuted this and documented CSF protein <20 mg/dl in only 26% of patients. Many patients will enjoy relief of their headache after the first LP. Serial LPs, either to withdraw more fluid or follow the CSF pressures, have a limited role in the management of this disorder (see below).[304]

Other imaging modalities. Some authors have advocated the use of ultrasonography of the optic nerve[305] and confocal scanning laser tomography of the optic disc.[79–82,306,307] However, other than confirmation of papilledema, we have not found these modalities to add to the clinical examination, visual field testing, fundus exam, neuroimaging, and CSF examination in the diagnosis and management of patients with pseudotumor.

Management

While the diagnosis requires a neurologist, the management of patient with pseudotumor cerebri also requires the skills of an ophthalmologist or neuro-ophthalmologist to assess the vision and fundi.[165] The initial evaluation of a patient with suspected pseudotumor cerebri should include complete ophthalmic and neurologic examinations and computerized visual field testing. The MRI and LP, in that order, should then be performed. Follow-up examinations should include assessment of visual fields, visual acuity, color vision, pupillary reactivity, ocular motility and alignment, and fundus appearance. Patients should be followed either weekly or biweekly initially, then, if vision stabilizes or improves, the intervals between examinations can be lengthened. To monitor disc swelling, stereo fundus photographs can be taken at presentation, then again once the papilledema resolves. The latter serves as future reference should the patient's symptoms recur. All non-pregnant obese patients are strongly encouraged to lose weight, and often they are referred to a nutritionist. Improvement in pseudotumor cerebri has been documented anecdotally following a rice/reduction diet[308] and gastric bypass surgery[309] and in retrospective studies.[310,311] Potentially inciting risk factors, such as systemic lupus erythematosus or Addison disease, should be treated, and offending medications such as tetracycline or vitamin A should be discontinued.

Treatment modalities which are no longer routinely recommended include subtemporal decompression, chronic corticosteroids, and serial lumbar punctures. The role of subtemporal or suboccipital cranial decompression (removing part of the skull to relieve elevated intracranial pressure), because of severe side-effects such as subdural hematomas and seizures, is mostly of historical interest.[312,313] Chronic steroid treatment is complicated by elevated intraocular pressures, weight gain, and difficulty weaning off the medication.[87]

Following intracranial pressures with repeated lumbar punctures is unnecessary, impractical, invasive, and punitive.[165] They are poorly tolerated, and serial lumbar punctures are ineffective as a long-term treatment.[304] It is impossible for serial LPs alone to remove enough fluid to relieve elevated intracranial pressure as CSF is produced at a rate of 0.35 ml/min, allowing the entire CSF circulation to be replenished in just 2 hours.[231] In fact, we believe most patients require just one (the first) spinal tap, which is both diagnostic and sometimes therapeutic, without the need of repeating the procedure. Its long-lasting effects are likely due to a persistent CSF leak at the LP site, or decompression of the arachnoid villi, allowing improved CSF absorption.[231] In general, there is no need for chronic monitoring of CSF pressure.[314,315]

Corbett and Thompson[165] have emphasized that treatment decisions should not rest on the frequency of TVOs, presence of diplopia, severity of the papilledema, or CSF opening or closing pressure. Instead, the modern management of pseudotumor cerebri is based largely upon the level of visual loss, as additional therapeutic strategies should be guided by visual fields and visual acuity **(Table 6–8)**.[94,316] Thus, in addition to the measures such as weight loss mentioned above, treatment suggestions according to level of visual loss are as follows:

1. *For patients with no visual loss.* Patients with no visual loss, headache, or other symptoms can be observed. Those with headache may be treated with acetaminophen, nonsteroidal anti-inflammatory agents, tricyclic antidepressants, or beta-blockers, for instance

Table 6–8 Management of pseudotumor cerebri, based upon the severity and progression of visual deficits

1. No visual loss	Symptomatic headache (migraine) therapy Weight reduction, if necessary Acetazolamide
2. Mild visual loss	Acetazolamide Furosemide Weight reduction, if necessary
3. Severe, or progression of visual loss	Optic nerve sheath decompression (ONSD) High-dose IV steroids and acetazolamide Lumbo-peritoneal shunt for failed ONSD or intractable headache

(but not steroids). Weight loss is highly recommended. Acetazolamide (see below) may be used in these instances as well but may not be necessary.

2. *For patients with mild to moderate visual loss.* Most patients with pseudotumor cerebri fall into this group. Visual deficits include enlarged blind spots, arcuate defects, mild peripheral constriction, and visual acuity of 20/30 or better. Acetazolamide, a carbonic anhydrase inhibitor which decreases CSF production, is the first-line medication in these instances, although its efficacy has been documented only anecdotally[317,318] and has not been proven by a prospective trial. We prefer acetazolamide 500 mg sequels, orally two or three times per day, as a starting dose, and will increase the total dosage to 3 grams if necessary. The drug is not contraindicated in those with sulfa allergies, as cross-reactivity is likely to be more theoretical than real.[319] Its major side-effects include paresthesias of the lips, fingers, and toes (which most patients tolerate), abnormal taste (particularly a metallic taste with carbonated beverages), nausea, vomiting, malaise, sedation, renal calculi, and metabolic acidosis.[231,320] In our practices, we typically do not routinely monitor electrolytes or blood counts in patients taking acetazolamide as the metabolic abnormalities are usually inconsequential, and aplastic anemia associated with acetazolamide is extraordinarily rare.[321] The dose can be lowered in individuals not tolerating the drug.[322] Most individuals in this group will do extremely well with acetazolamide, with resolution of the field defects and papilledema within 3–6 months, after which the medication can be tapered. When acetazolamide is not tolerated, we switch the patient to furosemide (20–40 mg) and monitor the potassium carefully.

If acetazolamide or furosemide fail, topiramate (1.5–3.0 mg/kg per day in two divided doses, and no more than 400 mg/day) may be used, particularly when the patient is obese or headache is a major issue. Topiramate, an antiepileptic medication, has secondary carbonic anhydrase activity. The use of this medication in pseudotumor is relatively new,[323,324] and it is unclear whether it is superior to acetazolamide in reducing CSF pressure. However, topiramate has the added benefit of appetite suppression and weight loss in many patients, it is excellent for treatment of chronic daily headache, and it has been used safely for years in patients with epilepsy. The dosage should be built up slowly over weeks (25 mg/week) to reduce the risk of cognitive side-effects, which are more likely to occur with rapid dose escalations and at doses higher than 200 mg/day.[325] Topiramate can be added to acetazolamide. Zonisamide, another drug with secondary carbonic anhydrase activity and appetite suppression, may be used in similar doses if the side-effects of topiramate are not tolerated.[326]

3. *For patients with severe or progressive visual loss despite medical management.* Optic nerve sheath fenestration surgery is the primary option for these patients,[327] which fortunately make up only a minority of those with pseudotumor cerebri. Other indications for optic nerve surgery are severe visual loss at presentation, inability to comply with medications, poor follow-up, or inability to cooperate with visual field testing.[165] As stated previously, nonorganic visual loss should be excluded since nonphysiologic tubular visual fields may be mistaken for field loss associated with papilledema.[287]

During optic nerve sheath fenestration, windows or slits are created through the dura and arachnoid surrounding the optic nerve (**Fig. 6–17**), allowing CSF egress, local relief of CSF pressure, and improvement in papilledema. Although the procedure had previously been suggested for this condition,[328] three series[329–331] provided the impetus for more widespread use of this technique in patients with visual loss due to pseudotumor cerebri. Acuity or fields improved in 85–100% of patients in these three reports. Interestingly, of the 33 patients who had only one eye operated upon, 24 patients (73%) experienced improvement in disc swelling bilaterally, and of the patients who had headache, two-thirds had some relief postoperatively.[165] Others[327,332,333] have subsequently published similar results.

When both eyes are affected by acuity or field loss, the eye with the worse vision should be operated upon first. If the fellow eye does not improve and also requires surgery, that can be performed a few days later. Simultaneous bilateral surgery is ill-advised. The lateral orbitotomy approach has been used,[334] but the medial approach (transconjunctival and under the medial rectus muscle) is less complicated and more popular. The medial approach also avoids the temporal posterior ciliary artery, and therefore makes a catastrophic vascular event involving the blood supply to the submacular choroid less likely. At the time of surgery, either three longitudinal slits in the dura are made with blunt lysis of subarachnoid adhesions or a window of dura can be excised. The latter approach is more technically demanding and there has never been a study to show that it is superior to simply incising the sheath. The surgery can easily be performed with retrobulbar or subtenon's local anesthesia; however, these techniques do not allow monitoring of pupil size during the surgery and or assessment of the vision immediately postoperatively.[335] While this information is

not critical to the successful intraoperative or postoperative management of the patient, they do provide assurance of a good outcome to the operating surgeon. Since most of the patients are young and otherwise healthy, our preference is for general anesthesia. Admission to the hospital postoperatively affords the best management of postoperative pain and allows the staff to monitor the patient for postoperative bleeding.

Complication rates in various series are as low as 4.9%[336] and as high as 40%.[337] Minor complications include temporary motility dysfunction, usually an adduction deficit owing to the temporary disinsertion of the medial rectus muscle, and a transient tonic pupil, resulting from damage to the short ciliary nerves or their blood supply.[337] Uncommon major complications include branch and central retinal artery occlusions,[337] choroidal infarction,[338] and worsening optic neuropathy.[339,340]

While instantaneous decompression of the optic nerve is essentially guaranteed by this procedure, whether this type of surgery provides a long-term fistula or drain is uncertain. Improvement of disc swelling in the fellow eye and resolution of headache suggests sheath decompression acts as a filtering procedure.[341,342] Postoperative MRI may demonstrate a decrease in intrasheath fluid and collections of fluid within the orbit.[343] Pathologic studies of eyes following sheath decompression suggest CSF exits either via intact open fistulas in the dura or via enclosed blebs of fibrosis.[344] Transient cyst-like structures, contiguous to the fenestration site, have been imaged and may also act as filters.[345,346] However, evidence against the filtration hypothesis is (1) an inability to demonstrate extravasation of iopamidol dye into the orbit following intrathecal injection, despite its visualization in the subarachnoid space by CT scanning, and (2) inconsistent CSF pressure measurements, both lowered and persistently elevated,[347,348] following the procedure. Alternatively, fat and Tenon's capsule may attach to the openings or fenestrations, and extensive scarring and adhesions are almost always seen on reoperations. Chronic adhesion of the dura to the retrolaminar portion of the optic nerve may prevent the transmission of high CSF pressure to the optic nerve head.[341] Another possible mechanism for the effectiveness of sheath decompression is improved blood flow in the short posterior ciliary arteries.

Optic nerve sheath decompression is more effective in reversing visual loss due to acute papilledema, in contrast to that due to chronic disc swelling.[349] In the long term, vision stabilizes or improves in the majority, but as many as 32% of operated eyes may experience deterioration following initially successful surgery.[350] A reoperation can be performed,[349] but we prefer a CSF shunting procedure in these instances.

If the severe visual loss is sudden, if central visual loss is caused by macular edema, or if optic nerve sheath fenestration is not immediately available, then high-dose IV steroids combined with acetazolamide is another treatment option.[351] IV methylprednisolone, 250 mg four times per day for 5 days can be given in combination with acetazolamide sequels 500 mg three times per day and ranitidine. Lack of immediate improvement is an indication for optic nerve sheath decompression. The IV steroids are followed by 80 mg

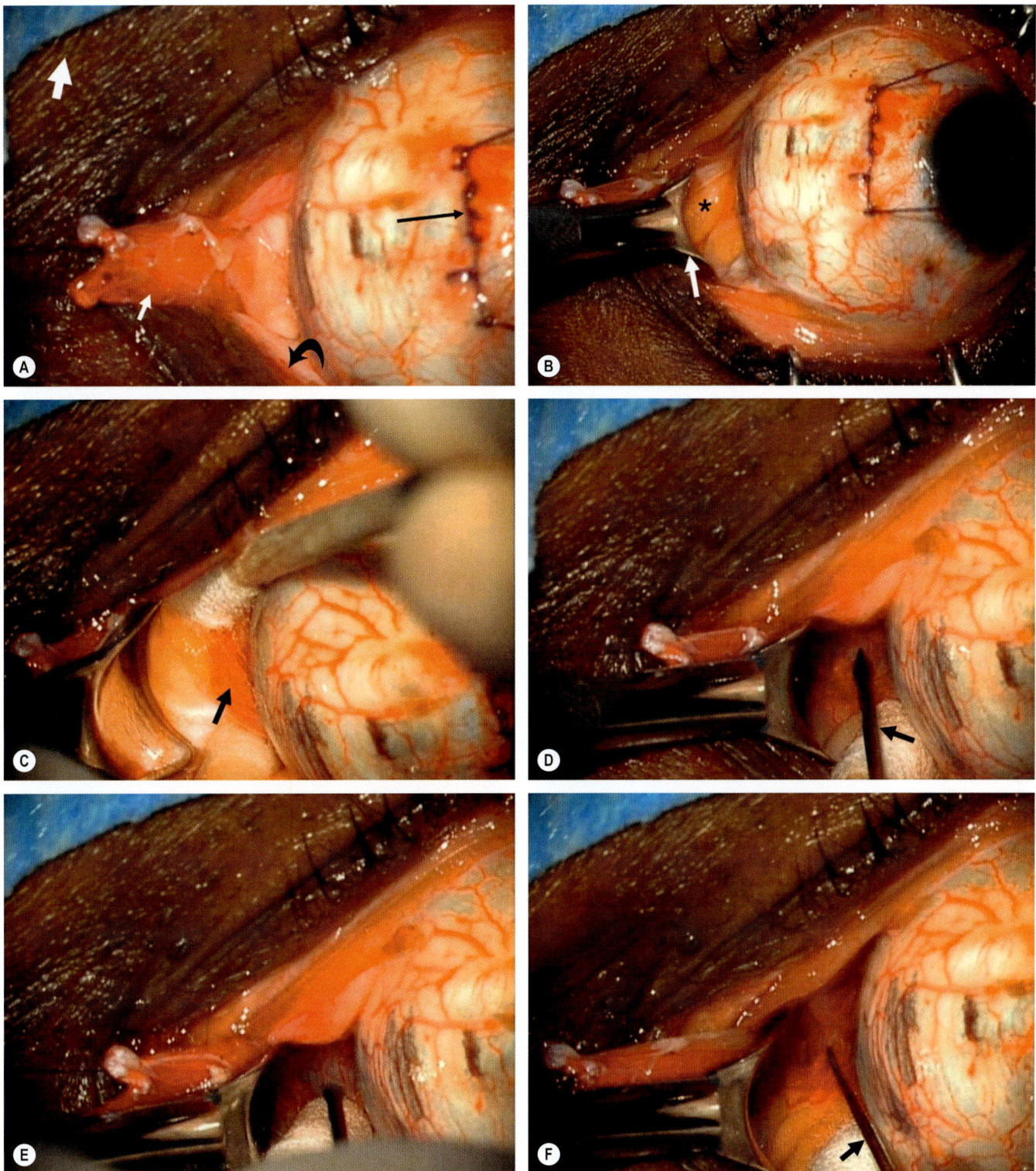

Figure 6–17. Surgeon's view of the right eye for optic nerve sheath fenestration (ONSF) in pseudotumor cerebri. **A.** The solid arrow head is on the patient's skin between the lower eyelid and nose and points to the patient's feet. A medial conjunctival peritomy was performed and the conjunctiva (curved arrow) was reflected medially. The medial rectus (short closed arrowhead) then was isolated on a Vicryl suture in a standard fashion and detached from the globe. During the procedure it was reflected medially. A 5-0 Vicryl suture was then sutured into the medial rectus insertion site (straight arrow) in a running locking fashion. **B.** The globe was retracted upward and laterally. A medial orbital retractor (straight arrow) was used to retract the medial rectus and medial orbital tissue toward the nose. Orbital fat (asterisks) is seen. **C.** The fat was dissected bluntly using cotton tip applicators exposing the posterior medial orbit and the optic nerve sheath (longer straight arrow). Ciliary vessels are visible around the optic nerve sheath. **D.** Next, an MVR blade (arrow) which has a spade-like shape is brought to the sheath. **E.** The width of the blade is used to create a slit in the optic nerve sheath through which spinal fluid egressed. The process was repeated three times. **F.** A curved tenotomy hook (arrow) was then passed from one previously made slit to the next within the subarachnoid space. Gentle movements were used to lyse subarachnoid adhesions.

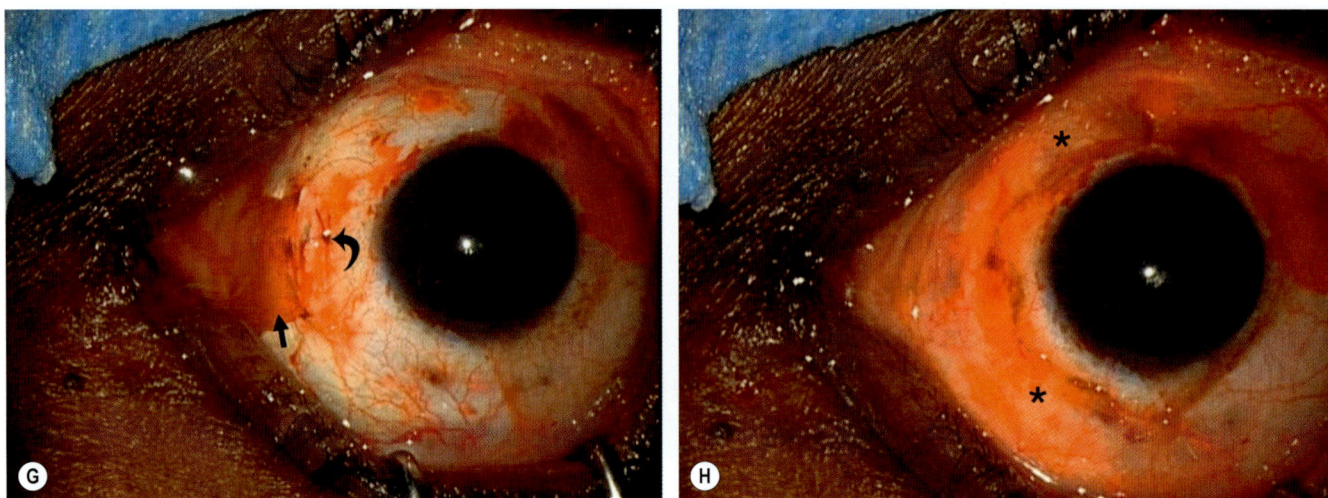

Figure 6–17. cont'd G. After hemostasis was achieved, the previously placed Vicryl sutures (curved arrowhead) were used to reattach the medial rectus muscle (straight arrow) to the sclera. **H.** Lastly, the conjunctiva (asterisks) is closed over the muscle.

prednisone orally, tapered over 4 weeks in order to avoid the side-effects of chronic use, and the acetazolamide is continued until the disc swelling resolves.

We reserve lumboperitoneal or ventriculoperitoneal (VP) shunting for patients in whom headache is the major problem or in whom visual loss progresses despite optic nerve sheath fenestration.[352] Although lumboperitoneal shunting is effective in treating visual loss,[353-355] shunt failure and low-pressure headaches are common enough in our opinion not to make it a first-line therapy.[356] Sometimes within the same patient, shunts fail several times, requiring multiple shunt revisions. Relatively small or normal ventricle sizes make VP difficult.[357] However, because VP shunting may have higher patency rates than lumboperitoneal shunting and the technology for inserting VP shunts is improving, its use in pseudotumor may become more popular.[358,359]

Bariatric surgery. These surgeries, including gastric banding, gastric bypass, and gastroplasty, because they are so highly effective in reducing weight,[360] may be recommended in morbidly obese patients with pseudotumor cerebri.[309] As the population has become more overweight over the past three decades, the number of shunting procedures and bariatric surgeries for pseudotumor cerebri has increased.[361]

Endovascular treatment. Based upon the frequent finding on MRI venography of narrowed transverse sinuses, endovascular stenting of the venous sinuses has been advocated by some authors.[362] However, because it is so highly controversial whether the venous sinus narrowing is the cause or result of the elevated intracranial pressure, and stenting is invasive, at this time we are not recommending this procedure for our patients with pseudotumor.[242]

Special considerations in associated conditions. When pseudotumor is due to a medication, stopping the drug is often sufficient to resolve headaches, papilledema, and elevated CSF pressure. However, other causes of intracranial hypertension should still be excluded with neuroimaging and CSF examination. We have used acetazolamide when headaches and vision loss are present. If desired, restarting the medica-

tion later, such as growth hormone, at a lower dose typically prevents symptom recurrence.

In patients with pseudotumor cerebri related to withdrawal from chronic steroids, our approach has been to restart the steroids at the dose maintained prior to the withdrawal, along with treating with acetazolamide. Once the disc swelling resolves, then the acetazolamide can be tapered. Subsequently the steroid dose can be decreased at a rate slower than that which leads to the pseudotumor.

Pregnant patients. Digre et al.[363] compared pregnant patients with pseudotumor cerebri and those without, and they found that those with pseudotumor tended to be obese. Women who are pregnant and develop pseudotumor cerebri can be treated similarly to non-pregnant patients except for the following three caveats: (1) because of a single case report of a sacrococcygeal teratoma in an infant following the mother's use of acetazolamide in the first trimester, the drug should be reserved for use only in the last two trimesters; furthermore, despite anecdotal evidence that acetazolamide may have no adverse effects in pregnancy,[364] its safety has not yet been proven in pregnancy; (2) stronger diuretics should not be used; and (3) weight reduction should not be recommended.[231,363] Therapeutic abortions are also unnecessary, and vaginal deliveries are allowed.[365]

Outcome

Most patients with mild to moderate visual loss tend to recover vision following medical therapy.[366] Papilledema usually resolves completely over weeks or months, but many patients are left with some residual disc elevation, especially nasally, macular pigment epithelial changes if lipid or edema had been present, or circumferential "high-water" marks delineating the prior extent of peripapillary retinal elevation associated with disc swelling. Thus, for future reference we often obtain disc photographs following resolution of disc swelling. In general, follow-up need not extend past 6 or 12 months past tapering of medication.

Among those with severe visual loss requiring surgery, residual acuity and field deficits are not uncommon and are occasionally debilitating.[87,164] In Wall and George's series,[84] approximately 3% of eyes had visual acuity worse than 20/100. The rare malignant or fulminant cases often seem recalcitrant to medications, optic nerve sheath fenestration, and lumboperitoneal shunting. We agree with Spoor et al.[350] that recurrences are more frequent in this group. Therefore, follow-up in these patients should include semi-annual examinations for at least 2–3 years following surgery. In addition to the aforementioned residual fundus changes, most patients in this group are left with some degree of optic atrophy.

Large studies suggest that men[177] and black people[367] have a worse visual prognosis than women and non-black people, respectively, with pseudotumor cerebri. Other underlying conditions which may predispose to a worse visual outcome may include older age, high myopia, anemia,[48] hypertension,[87] and uremia.[368]

Recurrence has been reported in 8–40% of patients.[87,269,369,370] In our experience recurrence is frequently associated with weight gain. Rarely some patients with pseudotumor develop a chronic form requiring years of treatment with acetazolamide.[371]

Pseudotumor cerebri without papilledema

Pseudotumor cerebri without papilledema has also been reported.[372–374] The diagnosis in these patients is suggested by chronic daily headache, pulsatile tinnitus, obesity, female sex,[375] and bilateral transverse sinus narrowing on MRI venography,[376] and is confirmed by lumbar puncture. In patients without papilledema, in general there should be no threat of vision loss, and treatment is usually geared towards symptomatic headache management. In our experience and that of others,[376–378] patients with this condition tend to have CSF opening pressures which are only slightly elevated (250–300 mm H_2O), compared to higher pressures in those with papilledema. Furthermore, patients with pseudotumor cerebri without papilledema also tend to have headaches which are more severe, chronic, refractory to medical treatment, and associated with functional features. Some authors recommend performing spinal taps and checking CSF pressures to screen for this condition in patients with unexplained chronic headaches, particularly those who are overweight.[373,377]

Pediatric pseudotumor cerebri

Although pseudotumor cerebri occurs more frequently in adults, its occurrence in pediatric patients, even infants and young children, is not uncommon.[99,379] Rampant obesity in childhood[380,381] is one reason. However, disparities from the condition in adults include more heterogeneous demographic features and asymptomatic presentations, suggesting that at least in the youngest age groups there may be a different underlying mechanism.

Several series have been reported,[382–391] and in contrast to the female predominance among adults and adolescents, males constitute approximately 50% of prepubertal pediatric patients with pseudotumor cerebri. Like adults, affected adolescents tend to be overweight, but obesity and weight gain are not associated risk factors in patients under 11 years of age.[388] Thus, we have seen several young thin boys with pseudotumor cerebri, most without an obvious cause for their disorder. Pseudotumor associated with synthetic growth hormone and ATRA are more commonly seen in children rather than adults because these medications are typically used in younger age groups. Reports of pseudotumor cerebri associated with Down syndrome have also been published.[392]

Asymptomatic idiopathic intracranial hypertension, diagnosed when papilledema is incidentally noticed during a routine physical exam, is a well-recognized entity in children.[388,390,393–398] This type of presentation is more common in younger age groups. These children have no headache or visual complaints. It is unclear why this occurs; one plausible explanation is that preschool and young school age children often undergo routine eye exams.

Unfortunately, children are not immune from the severe visual loss which may affect adults.[164,383] One report suggested puberty was a risk factor for less favorable visual outcome.[399] We tend not to follow younger children with computerized visual field testing because they have difficulty producing dependable, repeatable results. Sixth nerve palsies are more common (approximately one-third) in children.[388] As in adults, management principles are based upon the level of visual loss in children. First-line treatment is medical with acetazolamide (15 mg/day divided into three equal doses), but severe or progressive visual loss may be require optic nerve sheath fenestration[400,401] or shunting.[402]

Venous thrombosis/obstruction

Elevated intracranial pressure and papilledema can result from thrombosis or obstruction of the cerebral dural venous sinuses, which drain blood from the brain (**Fig. 6–18**). The superior sagittal sinus runs along the superior portion of the falx cerebri, while the inferior sagittal sinus, which lies along the inferior portion of the falx, joins the great vein of Galen to drain into the straight sinus. The superior sagittal sinus, straight sinus, and two transverse sinuses frequently join posteriorly at the confluence of sinuses (or torcular herophili), but in many instances the superior sagittal sinus drains into the right transverse sinus and the straight sinus directly into the left transverse sinus. In turn, the transverse sinuses drain into the sigmoid sinuses, each of which empties into the internal jugular veins.[403] Impaired flow in any of these sinuses can cause venous hypertension and subsequently decrease CSF absorption.

The causes of clot formation within the sinuses are multiple, but fall largely into three categories:

1. *Hypercoagulable states.* These include Behçet disease,[404,405] the presence of antiphospholipid antibodies[406] or lupus anticoagulant, protein C or S deficiency,[407] antithrombin III deficiency, factor V Leiden mutation, elevated factor VIII levels,[408] homozygosity for thermolabile methylene tetrahydrofolate reductase polymorphisms,[409] oral contraceptive use, pregnancy, cancer, and thrombocytosis.[410] Venous thrombosis due

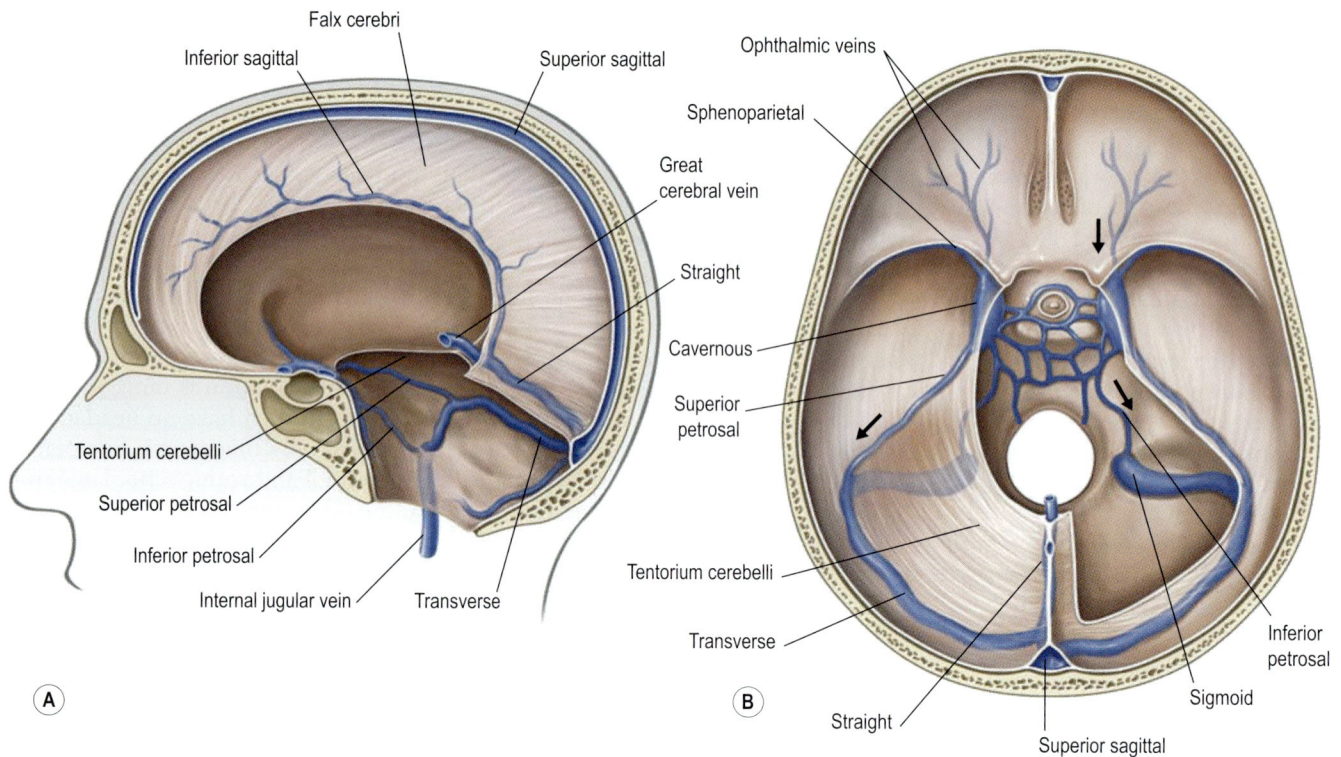

Figure 6–18. Major venous sinuses of the dura mater in (**A**) sagittal and (**B**) axial views. The arrows indicate the direction of blood flow.

to hypercoagulability may be a mechanism for many of the pseudotumor-like presentations in patients with systemic lupus erythematosus.[411–415] L-Asparaginase predisposes to clot formation by decreasing antithrombin III levels. Cerebral venous thrombosis is also a recognized complication of paroxysmal nocturnal hemoglobinuria.[416,417]

2. *Contiguous infection.* Although antibiotics have made lateral sinus thrombosis secondary to adjoining mastoiditis or middle-ear infections uncommon,[418] such cases are still seen (**Fig. 6–19**).[410,419] The mechanism is likely contiguous vessel wall inflammation and thrombophlebitis. The term "otitic hydrocephalus"[158] has been applied to these cases, but the designation is a misnomer because affected patients do not have hydrocephalus. When an abducens palsy is present, it tends to be ipsilateral to the involved ear.[158] Surgical excision of infected mastoid tissue may be required.

3. *Contiguous neoplasm.* Neoplasms may compress the venous sinuses, impeding venous drainage and leading to clot formation (**Fig. 6–20**). Reported examples include medulloblastoma, sarcoma, melanoma,[405] meningioma,[420] and metastases.[421]

Radical neck dissection or iatrogenic ligation of one of the draining veins or sinuses can result in outflow obstruction.[410,422] Venous catheterization (jugular or subclavian, for instance) may be associated with local clot formation and venous hypertension. Outflow obstruction without clot can result from direct tumor compression by a parasagittal meningioma (superior sagittal sinus)[410,423] or glomus jugulare[424] or other base of skull[425] tumors (jugular veins). We have also

seen venous thromboses associated with epidural hematomas due to head trauma.

Presenting signs and symptoms

In most instances the neuro-ophthalmic features are similar to those with pseudotumor cerebri: i.e., headache, nausea and vomiting, papilledema, optic nerve-related visual loss, and sixth nerve palsies.[410,426] The signs and symptoms often develop more rapidly in patients with venous sinus thrombosis than in those with pseudotumor cerebri. Many authors[427,428] have stressed that without venography, the two conditions may be mistaken for one another. However, patients with venous thrombosis may develop altered mentation, and cortical vein thrombosis and cerebral infarction can, for instance, lead to hemiparesis, hemisensory loss, and seizures.[429,430] Thrombosis of the transverse and sigmoid sinuses may also lead to seventh and eighth nerve dysfunction.[431]

Thromboses of the dural venous sinuses, as described above, should be distinguished from those of the deep venous drainage (e.g., internal cerebral veins, and the vein of Galen). Patients with the latter tend to present more acutely with altered consciousness and long tract signs. The signs and symptoms of elevated intracranial pressure, although present, are less prominent.[432]

Neuroimaging

A safe and effective method for visualizing cerebral venous thrombosis combines MRI with gadolinium, with sagittal images especially, and MR venography.[97,422] The clot tends to enhance on T1-weighted enhanced MR images. Axial CT

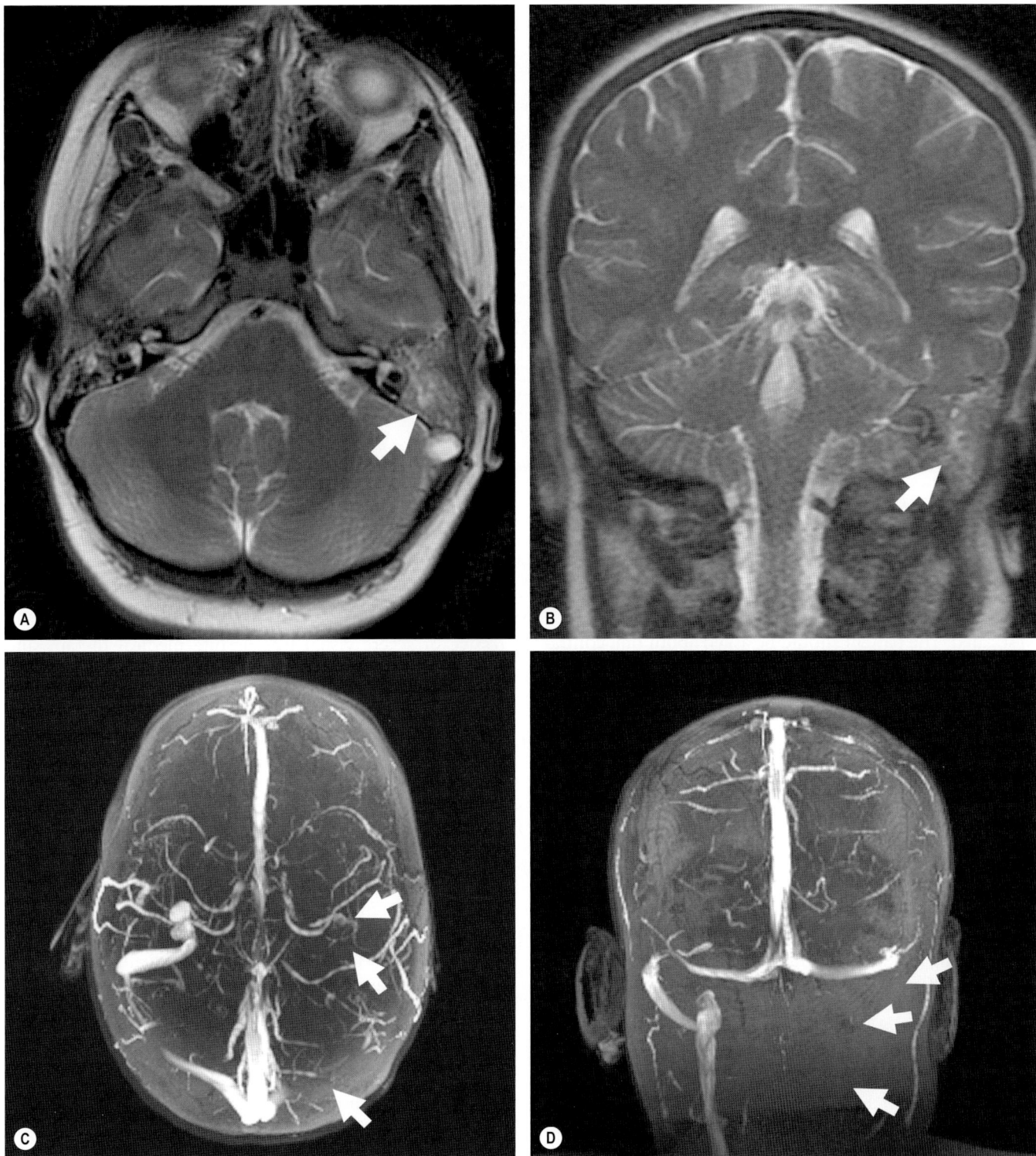

Figure 6–19. Venous sinus thrombosis due to mastoiditis in a 7-year-old boy who presented with papilledema and double vision. Axial (**A**) and coronal (**B**) T2-weighted MRIs demonstrating mastoiditis, left (arrow) worse than right. Axial (**C**) and coronal (**D**) MRI venogram showing absence of flow (arrows) in the left transverse and sigmoid sinuses and left internal jugular vein, consistent with venous thrombosis.

scans with contrast may demonstrate the characteristic "empty delta sign" at the intersection of the straight sinus and distal superior sagittal sinus.[422] Characteristically the ventricles are small on neuroimaging. We have found MRI and MR venography sufficient for managing these patients, without requiring the use of formal venography.

Workup

If a clot is demonstrated radiologically, then prior ear infections, neck surgery, and intravenous catheters as a source should be excluded. Clinical evidence for Behçet's (oral and genital ulcers) or lupus (rashes or joint aches) should be

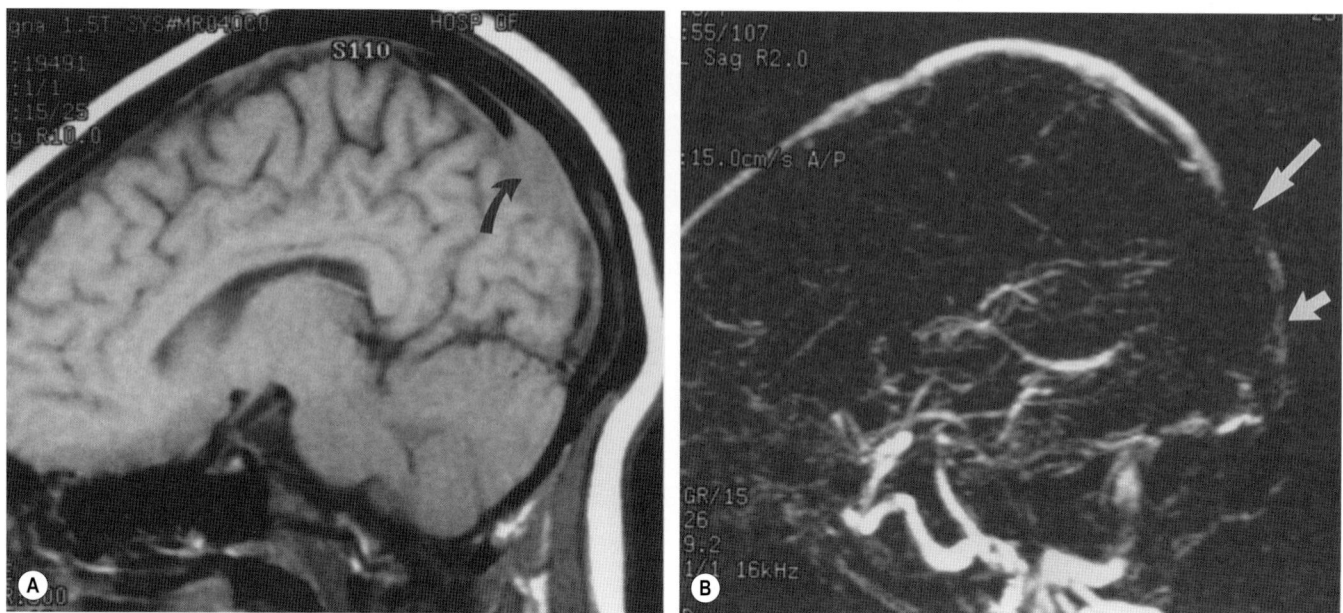

Figure 6–20. Venous thrombosis secondary to tumor compression by presumed lymphoma. This thin woman presented with bilateral papilledema and headaches, and the sagittal T1-weighted MRI (**A**) demonstrated a mass (arrow) compressing the posterior portion of the superior sagittal sinus. **B.** The MR venogram (TR 26, TE 9.2) shows occlusion of the sinus (large arrow) and poor venous flow (small arrow). A parotid mass was biopsied and disclosed B-cell lymphoma. The patient also had splenic and bone marrow involvement and a pleural effusion. Venous sinus compression, headaches, and disc swelling resolved following chemotherapy and whole-brain and focal radiation.

investigated. The patient should be asked about oral contraceptive use or personal and family history of clotting disorders or miscarriages. In unclear cases, laboratory investigation should include screening for antiphospholipid antibodies, lupus anticoagulant, protein C or S or antithrombin III deficiency, factor V Leiden mutation, antinuclear antibodies, high levels of factor VIII, and thrombocytosis. In cases without mass effect, lumbar puncture should be performed to document the opening pressure, and the vision should be assessed carefully, including visual field testing.

Treatment

If identifiable, the offending drug should be discontinued, or underlying medical condition or mass lesion treated. Because dehydration and hypotension can aggravate cerebral thromboses, and overhydration can worsen elevated intracranial pressure, patients should be kept euvolemic with judicious use of intravenous fluids. Anticoagulation is recommended to reduce the risk of clot propagation with intravenous or low-molecular-weight heparin for 5–7 days followed by warfarin for 6 months,[433,434] especially in cases due to primary hypercoagulable states, and even in patients with evidence of hemorrhage.[435] Selective catheterization and urokinase infusion have been used in some centers,[436] but its safety and efficacy need to be confirmed. Depending on clinical status and follow-up radiologic studies, oral anticoagulation should be continued for at least 3 months.[403]

As in pseudotumor cerebri, acetazolamide can be used to treat elevated intracranial pressure and mild field loss.[437] Any diuretic, however, should be used with caution with monitoring of fluid status and blood pressure because of the potential for worsening the thrombosis. Patients with pro-

gressive or severe visual loss despite medical therapy and treatment of the offending source should undergo optic nerve sheath fenestration.[423,438] The visual outcome is favorable in most instances.[410] Lumboperitoneal shunting should be used in patients in whom headache or nausea and vomiting are refractory to acetazolamide, anticoagulation, and conservative medical therapy.

Arteriovenous malformations of the dural sinuses

Prehemorrhagic dural arteriovenous malformations (AVMs) which drain into the venous sinuses (AV fistulas) can cause elevated intracranial pressure and papilledema without ventriculomegaly by increasing blood flow within the sinuses (**Fig. 6–21**) or by causing venous thrombosis.[439,440] Both mechanisms can lead to decreased CSF absorption. Less commonly, unruptured cerebral AVMs can drain into the superior sagittal sinus and cause similar symptoms.[441] If a dural AVM drains into the transverse sinus, a cranial bruit may be audible, and the patient may complain of tinnitus.[442] The dural AVM may be evident on MRI or CT with contrast. However, formal angiography is usually required to outline the vascular anatomy including feeding and draining vessels.[443] Treatment options include surgical excision of the AVM or embolization. However, some larger AVMs are incurable, and elevated intracranial pressure and papilledema may require further management with acetazolamide, optic nerve sheath fenestration, or lumboperitoneal shunting.[444] Cerebral AVMs, which are much more common, are discussed in Chapter 8, while dural AVMs are reviewed in more detail in Chapter 15.

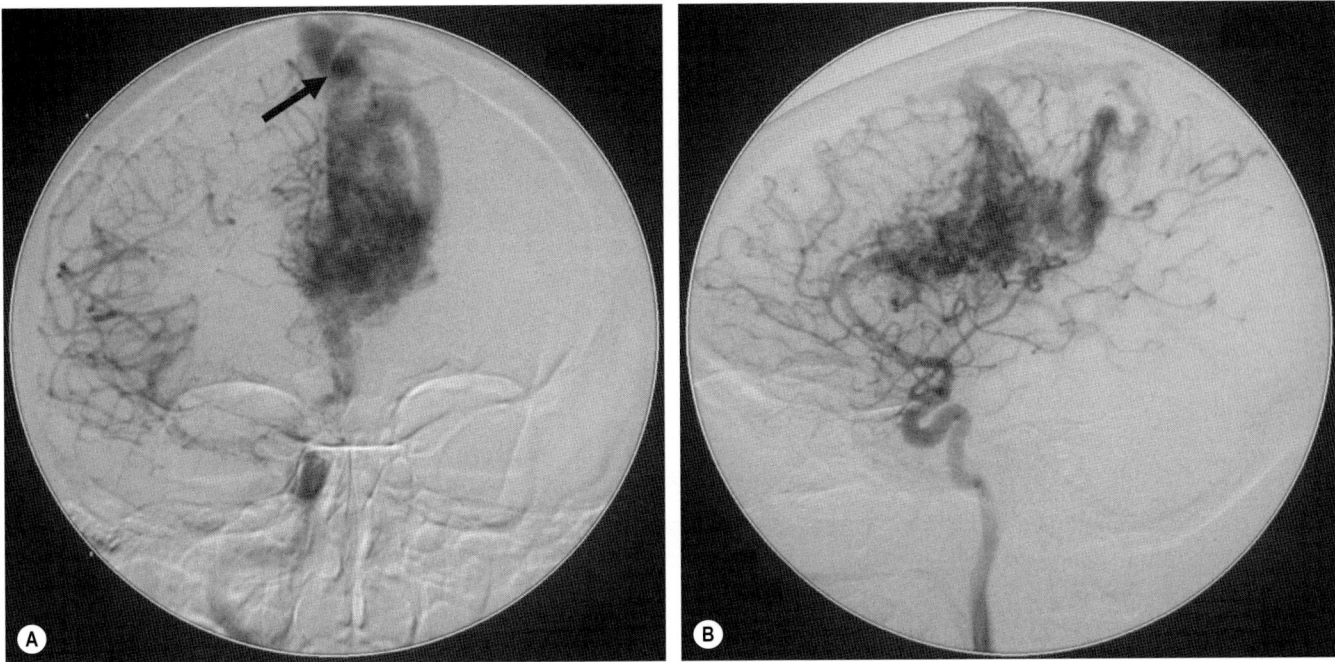

Figure 6–21. Arteriovenous malformation (AVM) associated with papilledema due to shunting into the venous sinuses. Contrast angiography, right internal carotid injection, demonstrating a AVM in the pericallosal region at the level of the body of corpus callosum involving bilateral medial frontal lobe regions (**A**. coronal; **B**. sagittal). The predominant feeders are bilateral anterior cerebral arteries, lenticulostriate branches off M1 segment of the left middle cerebral artery and splenial branch off the left posterior cerebral artery. Elevated intracranial pressure was due to superficial venous drainage into the superior sagittal sinus (arrow) and deep venous drainage via the internal cerebral vein into the straight sinus (not shown).

Pulmonary disease

Elevated intracranial pressure and papilledema may develop in the setting of respiratory insufficiency as a result of hypercapnea-induced cerebral vasodilation.[445-447] These patients can be distinguished by their lethargy, peripheral retinal hemorrhages (due to the venous hypertension), arterial blood gas results, and high serum bicarbonate.[448]

Obese patients with the Pickwickian syndrome (sleep apnea/obesity hypoventilation syndrome) may develop papilledema,[448,449] and it is easy to mistakenly diagnose them with pseudotumor cerebri. Excess fat in the hypopharynx leads to obstructive sleep apnea, chronic hypoxemia and hypercapnea, pulmonary hypertension, right-sided heart failure, and venous hypertension. The papilledema tends to respond to treatment of the lung abnormalities including oxygenation, positive airway pressure, and weight reduction, under the direction of a pulmonologist.[448] If there is mild visual field loss associated with the disc swelling, acetazolamide can be added.

Guillain–Barré syndrome and chronic inflammatory demyelinating polyneuropathy

These conditions, discussed in more detail in Chapter 14, are characterized by muscle weakness and areflexia due to inflammatory demyelinating polyneuropathy. Chronic inflammatory demyelinating polyneuropathy (CIDP) has a slowly progressive or relapsing–remitting course, and rare cases with papilledema have been reported.[450,451] In Guillain–Barré syndrome (GBS), typified by acute to subacute weakness, papilledema may be seen in approximately 1–3% of cases.[452] According to Ropper et al.,[452] disc swelling, when it occurs, generally develops during the third week of this illness. However, papilledema may go unnoticed because daily fundus exams may not be performed in these patients, and they may be paralyzed, intubated, and unable to complain about headache or abnormal vision. We have seen one patient with GBS[453] who received respiratory support for 3 months and upon discontinuation of ventilatory assistance, told us she had had blurry vision in the left eye for weeks. Only then was chronic papilledema detected, and the CSF pressure was measured and found to be elevated. Abducens palsies are unreliable as a sign of elevated intracranial pressure in this setting because the sixth nerves are commonly affected in GBS.

The combination of papilledema, elevated intracranial pressure, and GBS is generally associated with high CSF protein levels (above 200 mg/dl). Decreased CSF resorption by the arachnoid villi due to elevated protein concentrations is one proposed mechanism for the papilledema, but other possibilities include increased CSF outflow resistance, hydrocephalus,[454] and increased venous pressure.[450,452] Several authors[452,453,455,456] have used the term pseudotumor cerebri in these situations; however, the designation is technically incorrect if the CSF protein or neuroimaging is abnormal.

Neuro-ophthalmic management may be difficult in these instances because their poor medical condition may preclude careful assessment of visual acuity and fields. However, as in pseudotumor cerebri, acetazolamide,[450] corticosteroids,[453] and optic nerve sheath fenestration[450,451] may be used to treat documentable visual loss, based upon the level of its severity.

Spinal cord tumors

Papilledema and elevated intracranial pressure are well-established but uncommon complications of spinal cord tumors.[457–462] Approximately 40% involve spinal cord ependymomas.[457] Elevated CSF protein causing decreased CSF absorption by the arachnoid villi has also been a purported mechanism in these instances, but abnormal CSF dynamics caused by tumor cell dissemination, tumor mucin production, recurrent subarachnoid hemorrhages, compression of the lumbar spinal sac, and tumor production of a chemical that leads to defective CSF absorption have been considered as well.[457,460,461,463] We have also seen a lumbar subdural abscess that produced a very elevated CSF protein associated with papilledema.[464] *Froin syndrome* is used to describe CSF with yellow color and high protein due to spinal block.

An MRI of the spine with and without gadolinium is recommended when paraparesis or quadriparesis, lumbar pain, a sensory level, hyperreflexia, extensor plantar responses, or bladder dysfunction are present. Neuroimaging of the brain in these instances may reveal associated communicating hydrocephalus. Treatment would include neurosurgical removal or biopsy of the spinal cord tumor as well as a ventriculostomy or ventriculoperitoneal shunt, if necessary.

Chiari malformation

Uncommonly, Chiari malformation type 1, in which the cerebellar tonsils extend below the foramen magnum, can lead to elevated intracranial pressure and papilledema.[465] The cause is not clear but may be due to disrupted CSF flow dynamics, and neurosurgical suboccipital decompression is the best treatment option.

References

1. Corbett JJ. Problems in the diagnosis and treatment of pseudotumor cerebri. Can J Neurol Sci 1983;10:221–229.
2. Sergott RC. Diagnosis and management of vision-threatening papilledema. Semin Neurol 1986;6:176–184.
3. Whiting AS, Johnson LN. Papilledema. Clinical clues and differential diagnosis. Am Fam Physician 1992;45:1125–1134.
4. Stammen J, Unsold R, Arendt G, et al. Etiology and pathogenetic mechanisms of optic disc swelling with visual loss. An interdisciplinary prospective pilot study of 102 cases. Ophthalmologica 1999;213:40–47.
5. Brodsky MC. Congenital optic disk anomalies. Surv Ophthalmol 1994;39:89–112.
6. Kheterpal S, Good PA, Beale DJ, et al. Imaging of optic disc drusen: a comparative study. Eye 1995;9:67–69.
7. Hoover DL, Robb RM, Peterson RA. Optic disc drusen in childhood. J Ped Ophthalmol Strab 1988;25:191–195.
8. Rosenberg MA, Savino PJ, Glaser JS. A clinical analysis of pseudopapilledema. I. Population, laterality, acuity, refractive error, ophthalmoscopic characteristics and coincident disease. Arch Ophthalmol 1979;97:65–70.
9. Rubinstein K, Ali M. Retinal complications of optic disc drusen. Br J Ophthalmol 1982;66:83–95.
10. Rossiter JD, Lockwood AJ, Evans AR. Coexistence of optic disc drusen and idiopathic intracranial hypertension in a child. Eye 2005;19:234–235.
11. Apple DJ, Rabb MF, Walsh PM. Congenital anomalies of the optic disc. Surv Ophthalmol 1982;27:3–41.
12. Tso MO. Pathology and pathogenesis of drusen of the optic nerve head. Ophthalmology 1981;88:1066–1080.
13. Auw-Haedrich C, Staubach F, Witschel H. Optic disk drusen. Surv Ophthalmol 2002;47:515–532.
14. Floyd MS, Katz BJ, Digre KB. Measurement of the scleral canal using optical coherence tomography in patients with optic nerve drusen. Am J Ophthalmol 2005;139:664–669.
15. Boldt HC, Byrne SF, DiBernardo C. Echographic evaluation of optic disc drusen. J Clin Neuroophthalmol 1991;11:85–91.
16. Lorentzen SE. Drusen of the optic disc. A clinical and genetic study. Acta Ophthalmol 1966;Suppl 90:1–180.
17. Antcliff RJ, Spalton DJ. Are optic disc drusen inherited? Ophthalmology 1999;106:1278–1281.
18. Buys YM, Pavlin CJ. Retinitis pigmentosa, nanophthalmos, and optic disc drusen: a case report. Ophthalmology 1999;106:619–622.
19. Mustonen E, Nieminen H. Optic disc drusen: a photographic study. I: Autofluorescence pictures and fluorescein angiography. Acta Ophthalmol 1982;60:849–858.
20. Froula PD, Bartley GB, Garrity JA, et al. The differential diagnosis of orbital calcification as detected on computed tomography scans. Mayo Clinic Proc 1993;68:256–261.
21. McNicholas MM, Power WJ, Griffin JF. Sonography in optic disk drusen. Imaging findings and role in diagnosis when funduscopic findings are normal. AJR Am J Roentgenol 1994;162:161–163.
22. Kurz-Levin MM, Landau K. A comparison of imaging techniques for diagnosing drusen of the optic nerve head. Arch Ophthalmol 1999;117:1045–1049.
23. Kawasaki A, Purvin V. Unilateral optic disc edema following trabeculectomy. J Neuroophthalmol 1998;18:121–123.
24. Brodsky MC, Baker RS, Hamed LM. The swollen optic disc in childhood. In: Pediatric Neuro-ophthalmology, pp 76–124. New York, Springer-Verlag, 1996.
25. Wong VA, Wade NK. POEMS syndrome: an unusual cause of bilateral optic disk swelling. Am J Ophthalmol 1998;126:452–454.
26. Bosch MM, Barthelmes D, Merz TM, et al. High incidence of optic disc swelling at very high altitudes. Arch Ophthalmol 2008;126:644–650.
27. Hayreh SS. Optic disc edema in raised intracranial pressure. V. Pathogenesis. Arch Ophthalmol 1977;95:1553–1565.
28. Hayreh SS. Pathogenesis of optic disc oedema. In: Kennard C, Rose FC (eds). Physiological Aspects of Clinical neuro-ophthalmology, pp 431–447. Chicago, Year Book, 1988.
29. Lee AG, Beaver HA. Acute bilateral optic disk edema with a macular star figure in a 12-year-old girl. Surv Ophthalmol 2002;47:42–49.
30. Wall M. Optic disk edema with cotton-wool spots. Surv Ophthalmol 1995;39:502–508.
31. Wirtschafter JD, Rizzo FJ, Smiley BC. Optic nerve axoplasm and papilledema. Surv Ophthalmol 1975;20:157–189.
32. Tso MOM, Hayreh SS. Optic disc edema in raised intracranial pressure. III. A pathologic study of experimental papilledema. Arch Ophthalmol 1977;95:1448–1457.
33. Pagani LF. The rapid appearance of papilledema. J Neurosurg 1969;30:247–249.
34. Selhorst JB, Gudeman SK, Butterworth JF, et al. Papilledema after acute head injury. Neurosurgery 1985;16:357–363.
35. Levin BE. The clinical significance of spontaneous pulsations of the retinal vein. Arch Neurol 1978;35:37–40.
36. Lorentzen SE. Incidence of spontaneous venous pulsations in the retina. Acta Ophthalmol 1970;48:765–770.
37. Frisén L. Swelling of the optic nerve head. A staging scheme. J Neurol Neurosurg Psychiatr 1982;45:13–18.
38. Sanders M. The Bowman Lecture. Papilloedema. "The pendulum of progress". Eye 1997;11:267–294.
39. Lepore FE. Unilateral and highly asymmetric papilledema in pseudotumor cerebri. Neurology 1992;42:676–678.
40. Strominger MB, Weiss GB, Mehler MF. Asymptomatic unilateral papilledema in pseudotumor cerebri. J Clin Neuroophthalmol 1992;12:238–241.
41. Yohai RA, Bullock JD, Margolis JH. Unilateral optic disk edema and a contralateral temporal fossa mass. Am J Ophthalmol 1993;115:261–262.
42. Moster ML. Unilateral disk edema in a young woman. Surv Ophthalmol 1995;39:409–416.
43. Huna-Baron R, Landau K, Rosenberg M, et al. Unilateral swollen disc due to increased intracranial pressure. Neurology 2001;56:1588–1590.
44. Kardon RH. The pathogenesis of visual field loss in idiopathic intracranial hypertension. North American Neuro-ophthalmology Society meeting 1992.
45. Hayreh SS. Pathogenesis of oedema of the optic disc (papilloedema). Br J Ophthalmol 1964;48:522–543.
46. Ing EB, Leavitt JA, Younge BR. Papilledema following bowtie optic atrophy. Arch Ophthalmol 1996;114:356–357.
47. Mehta JS, Plant GT, Acheson JF. Twin and triple peaks papilledema. Ophthalmology 2005;112:1299–1301.
48. Orcutt JC, Page NGR, Sanders MD. Factors affecting visual loss in benign intracranial hypertension. Ophthalmology 1984;91:1303–1312.
49. Wendel L, Lee AG, Boldt HC, et al. Subretinal neovascular membrane in idiopathic intracranial hypertension. Am J Ophthalmol 2006;141:573–574.
50. Soelberg Sørensen P, Krogsaa B, Gjerris F. Clinical course and prognosis of pseudotumor cerebri. A prospective study of 24 patients. Acta Neurol Scand 1988;77:164–172.

51. Kennedy F. A further note on the diagnostic value of retrobulbar neuritis in expanding lesions of the frontal lobes. With a report of this syndrome in a case of aneurysm of the right internal carotid artery. JAMA 1916;67:1361–1363.

52. Watnick RL, Trobe JD. Bilateral optic nerve compression as a mechanism for the Foster Kennedy syndrome. Ophthalmology 1989;96:1793–1798.

53. Schatz NJ, Smith JL. Non-tumor causes of the Foster Kennedy syndrome. J Neurosurg 1967;27:37–44.

54. Pollock SC. Acute papilledema and visual loss in a patient with pseudotumor cerebri [letter]. Arch Ophthalmol 1987;105:752–753.

55. Hoye VJ, Berrocal AM, Hedges TR, 3rd, et al. Optical coherence tomography demonstrates subretinal macular edema from papilledema. Arch Ophthalmol 2001;119:1287–1290.

56. Mitchell DJ, Steahly LP. Pseudotumor cerebri and macular disease. Retina 1989;9: 115–117.

57. Verm A, Lee AG. Bilateral optic disk edema with macular exudates as the manifesting sign of a cerebral arteriovenous malformation. Am J Ophthalmol 1997;123:422–424.

58. Talks SJ, Mossa F, Elston JS. The contribution of macular changes to visual loss in benign intracranial hypertension. Eye 1998;12:806–808.

59. Morris AT, Sanders MD. Macular changes resulting from papilloedema. Br J Ophthalmol 1980;64:211–216.

60. Griebel SR, Kosmorsky GS. Choroidal folds associated with increased intracranial pressure. Am J Ophthalmol 2000;129:513–516.

61. Bird AC, Sanders MD. Choroidal folds in association with papilloedema. Br J Ophthalmol 1973;57:89–97.

62. Jacobson DM. Intracranial hypertension and the syndrome of acquired hyperopia with choroidal folds. J Neuroophthalmol 1995;15:178–185.

63. Bullock JD, Egbert PR. The origin of choroidal folds. A clinical, histopathological, and experimental study. Doc Ophthalmol 1974;37:261–293.

64. Keane JR. Papilledema with unusual ocular hemorrhages. Arch Ophthalmol 1981;99: 262–263.

65. Jamison RR. Subretinal neovascularization and papilledema associated with pseudotumor cerebri. Am J Ophthalmol 1978;85:78–81.

66. Troost BT, Sufit RL, Grand MG. Sudden monocular visual loss in pseudotumor cerebri. Arch Neurol 1979;36:440–442.

67. Akova YA, Kansu T, Yazar Z, et al. Macular subretinal neovascular membrane associated with pseudotumor cerebri. J Neuroophthalmol 1994;14:193–195.

68. Galvin R, Sanders MD. Peripheral retinal haemorrhages with papilledema. Br J Ophthalmol 1980;64:262–266.

69. Baker RS, Buncic JR. Sudden visual loss in pseudotumor cerebri due to central retinal artery occlusion. Arch Neurol 1984;41:1274–1276.

70. Lam BL, Siatkowski RM, Fox GM, et al. Visual loss in pseudotumor cerebri from branch retinal artery occlusion. Am J Ophthalmol 1992;113:334–336.

71. Gittinger JW, Asdourian GK. Macular abnormalities in papilledema from pseudotumor cerebri. Ophthalmology 1989;96:192–194.

72. Carter SR, Seiff SR. Macular changes in pseudotumor cerebri before and after optic nerve sheath fenestration. Ophthalmology 1995;102:937–941.

73. Galetta SL, Byrne SF, Smith JL. Echographic correlation of optic nerve sheath size and cerebrospinal fluid pressure. J Clin Neuroophthalmol 1989;9:79–82.

74. Ophir A, Karatas M, Ramirez JA, et al. OCT and chronic papilledema [letter]. Ophthalmology 2005;112:2238.

75. Savini G, Bellusci C, Carbonelli M, et al. Detection and quantification of retinal nerve fiber layer thickness in optic disc edema using stratus OCT. Arch Ophthalmol 2006;124:1111–1117.

76. Rebolleda G, Munoz-Negrete FJ. Follow-up of mild papilledema in idiopathic intracranial hypertension with optical coherence tomography. Invest Ophthalmol Vis Sci 2008;ePub ahead of print.

77. Karam EZ, Hedges TR. Optical coherence tomography of the retinal nerve fibre layer in mild papilloedema and pseudopapilledema. Br J Ophthalmol 2005;89:294–298.

78. Johnson LN, Diehl ML, Hamm CW, et al. Differentiating optic disc edema from optic nerve head drusen on optical coherence tomography. Arch Ophthalmol 2009;127: 45–49.

79. Trick GL, Vesti E, Tawansy K, et al. Quantitative evaluation of papilledema in pseudotumor cerebri. Invest Ophthalmol Vis Sci 1998;39:1964–1971.

80. Trick GL, Bhatt SS, Dahl D, et al. Optic disc topography in pseudopapilledema. A comparison to pseudotumor cerebri. J Neuroophthalmol 2001;21:240–244.

81. Heckmann JG, Weber M, Junemann AG, et al. Laser scanning tomography of the optic nerve vs CSF opening pressure in idiopathic intracranial hypertension. Neurology 2004;62:1221–1223.

82. Salgarello T, Falsini B, Tedesco S, et al. Correlation of optic nerve head tomography with visual field sensitivity in papilledema. Invest Ophthalmol Vis Sci 2001;42: 1487–1494.

83. Hayreh SS. Optic disc edema in raised intracranial pressure. VI. Associated visual disturbances and their pathogenesis. Arch Ophthalmol 1977;95:1566–1579.

84. Wall M, George D. Idiopathic intracranial hypertension. A prospective study of 50 patients. Brain 1991;114:155–180.

85. Liu GT, Volpe NJ, Schatz NJ, et al. Severe acute visual loss caused by pseudotumor cerebri and lumboperitoneal shunt failure. Am J Ophthalmol 1996;122: 129–131.

86. Green GJ, Lessell S, Loewenstein JI. Ischemic optic neuropathy in chronic papilledema. Arch Ophthalmol 1980;98:502–504.

87. Corbett JJ, Savino PJ, Thompson HS, et al. Visual loss in pseudotumor cerebri. Follow-up of 57 patients from five to 41 years and a profile of 14 patients with permanent severe visual loss. Arch Neurol 1982;39:461–474.

88. Corbett JJ, Jacobson DM, Mauer RC, et al. Enlargement of the blind spot caused by papilledema. Am J Ophthalmol 1988;105:261–265.

89. Hedges TR, Legge RH, Peli E, et al. Retinal nerve fiber layer changes and visual field loss in idopathic intracranial hypertension. Ophthalmology 1995;102:1242–1247.

90. Gu XZ, Tsai JC, Wurdeman A, et al. Pattern of axonal loss in longstanding papilledema due to idiopathic intracranial hypertension. Curr Eye Res 1995;14:173–180.

91. Galetta SL, Liu GT, Volpe NJ. Diagnostic testing in neurology. Neuro-ophthalmology. Neurol Clin 1996;14:201–222.

92. Wall M, George D. Visual loss in pseudotumor cerebri. Incidence and defects related to visual field strategy. Arch Neurol 1987;44:170–175.

93. Wall M. Sensory visual testing in idiopathic intracranial hypertension. Measures sensitive to change. Neurology 1990;40:1859–1864.

94. Wall M. Idiopathic intracranial hypertension: mechanisms of visual loss and disease management. Semin Neurol 2000;20:89–95.

95. Sadun AA, Currie JN, Lessell S. Transient visual obscurations with elevated optic discs. Ann Neurol 1984;16:489–494.

96. Wall M. Idiopathic intracranial hypertension. Neurol Clinics 1991;9:73–95.

97. Mattle HP, Wentz KU, Edelman RR, et al. Cerebral venography with MR. Radiology 1991;178:453–458.

98. Corbett JJ, Mehta MP. Cerebrospinal fluid pressure in normal obese subjects and patients with pseudotumor cerebri. Neurology 1983;33:1386–1388.

99. Rangwala LM, Liu GT. Pediatric idiopathic intracranial hypertension. Surv Ophthalmol 2007;52:597–617.

100. Archer BD. Computed tomography before lumbar puncture in acute meningitis. A review of the risks and benefits. Can Med Assoc J 1993;148:961–965.

101. Allen ED, Byrd SE, Darling CF. The clinical and radiological evaluation of primary brain tumors in children, Part I. Clinical evaluation. J Natl Med Assoc 1993;85:445–451.

102. Siddiqi SN, Posnick JC, Buncic R, et al. The detection and management of intracranial hypertension after initial suture release and decompression for craniofacial dysostosis syndromes. Neurosurgery 1995;36:703–709.

103. Billson FA, Hudson RL. Surgical treatment of chronic papilloedema in children. Br J Ophthalmol 1975;59:92–95.

104. Wissow LS. Child abuse and neglect. N Engl J Med 1995;332:1425–1431.

105. Kaur B, Taylor D. Fundus hemorrhages in infancy. Surv Ophthalmol 1992;37:1–17.

106. Kivlin JD, Simons KB, Lazoritz S, et al. Shaken baby syndrome. Ophthalmology 2000;107:1246–1254.

107. Morad Y, Kim YM, Armstrong DC, et al. Correlation between retinal abnormalities and intracranial abnormalities in the shaken baby syndrome. Am J Ophthalmol 2002;134: 354–359.

108. Duhaime A-C, Christian CW, Rorke LB, et al. Nonaccidental head injury in infants - the "shaken-baby syndrome". N Engl J Med 1998;338:1822–1829.

109. Snyder H, Robinson K, Shah D, et al. Signs and symptoms of patients with brain tumors presenting to the emergency department. J Emerg Med 1993;11:253–258.

110. Van Crevel H. Papilloedema, CSF pressure, and CSF flow in cerebral tumours. J Neurol Neurosurg Psychiatr 1979;42:493–500.

111. Weston P, Lear J. Gliomatosis cerebri or benign intracranial hypertension? Postgrad Med J 1995;71:380–381.

112. Ebinger F, Bruhl K, Gutjahr P. Early diffuse leptomeningeal primitive neuroectodermal tumors can escape detection by magnetic resonance imaging. Childs Nerv Syst 2000;16:398–401.

113. Fahmy JA. Papilloedema associated with ruptured intracranial aneurysms. Acta Ophthalmol 1972;50:793–802.

114. Steffen H, Eifert B, Aschoff A, et al. The diagnostic value of optic disc evaluation in acute elevated intracranial pressure. Ophthalmology 1996;103:1229–1232.

115. Schultz PN, Sobol WM, Weingeist TA. Long-term visual outcome in Terson syndrome. Ophthalmology 1991;98:1814–1819.

116. Garfinkle AM, Danys IR, Nicolle DA, et al. Terson's syndrome: a reversible cause of blindness following subarachnoid hemorrhage. J Neurosurg 1992;76:766–771.

117. Frizzell RT, Kuhn F, Morris R, et al. Screening for ocular hemorrhages in patients with ruptured cerebral aneurysms. A prospective study of 99 patients. Neurosurgery 1997;41:529–534.

118. Kuhn F, Morris R, Witherspoon CD, et al. Terson syndrome. Results of vitrectomy and the significance of vitreous hemorrhage in patients with subarachnoid hemorrhage. Ophthalmology 1998;105:472–477.

119. Ness T, Janknecht P, Berghorn C. Frequency of ocular hemorrhages in patients with subarachnoidal hemorrhage. Graefes Arch Clin Exp Ophthalmol 2005;243:859–862.

120. Schloff S, Mullaney PB, Armstrong DC, et al. Retinal findings in children with intracranial hemorrhage. Ophthalmology 2002;109:1472–1476.

121. Velikay M, Datlinger P, Stolba U, et al. Retinal detachment with severe proliferative vitreoretinopathy in Terson syndrome. Ophthalmology 1994;101:35–37.

122. Ogawa T, Kitaoka T, Dake Y, et al. Terson syndrome. A case report suggesting the mechanism of vitreous hemorrhage. Ophthalmology 2001;108:1654–1656.

123. Garweg JG, Koerner F. Outcome indicators for vitrectomy in Terson syndrome. Acta Ophthalmol 2009;87:222–226.

124. Molavi A, LeFrock JL. Tuberculous meningitis. Med Clin N Am 1985;69:315–331.

125. Tang LM. Ventriculoperitoneal shunt in cryptococcal meningitis with hydrocephalus. Surg Neurol 1990;33:314–319.

126. Lesser RL, Kornmehl EW, Pachner AR, et al. Neuro-ophthalmologic manifestations of Lyme disease. Ophthalmology 1990;97:699–706.

127. Belman AL, Iyer M, Coyle PK, et al. Neurologic manifestations in children with North American Lyme disease. Neurology 1993;43:2609–2614.

128. Halperin JJ, Shapiro ED, Logigian E, et al. Practice parameter. Treatment of nervous system Lyme disease (an evidence-based review). Report of the Quality Standards Subcommittee of the American Academy of Neurology. Neurology 2007;69:91–102.

129. Kan L, Sood SK, Maytal J. Pseudotumor cerebri in Lyme disease. A case report and literature review. Pediatr Neurol 1998;18:439–441.

130. Härtel C, Schilling S, Neppert B, et al. Intracranial hypertension in neuroborreliosis. Dev Med Child Neurol 2002;44:641–642.

131. Kestelyn P, Taelman H, Bogaerts J, et al. Ophthalmic manifestations of infections with Cryptococcus neoformans in patients with the acquired immunodeficiency syndrome. Am J Ophthalmol 1993;116:721–727.

132. Rex JH, Larsen RA, Dismukes WE, et al. Catastrophic visual loss due to Cryptococcus neoformans meningitis. Medicine 1993;72:207–224.

133. Cohen DB, Glasgow BJ. Bilateral optic nerve cryptococcosis in sudden blindness in patients with acquired immune deficiency syndrome. Ophthalmology 1993;100: 1689–1694.

134. van der Horst CM, Saag MS, Cloud GA, et al. Treatment of cryptococcal meningitis associated with the acquired immunodeficiency syndrome. N Engl J Med 1997;337: 15–21.

135. Johnston SR, Corbett EL, Foster O, et al. Raised intracranial pressure and visual complications in AIDS patients with cryptococcal meningitis. J Infect 1992;24:185–189.

136. Garrity JA, Herman DC, Imes R, et al. Optic nerve sheath decompression for visual loss in patients with acquired immunodeficiency syndrome and cryptococcal meningitis with papilledema. Am J Ophthalmol 1993;116:472–478.

137. Strominger MB, Liu GT, Schatz NJ. Optic disk swelling and abducens palsies associated with OKT3. Am J Ophthalmol 1995;119:664–665.

138. Lamonte M, Silberstein SD, Marcelis JF. Headache associated with aseptic meningitis. Headache 1995;35:520–526.

139. Balm M, Hammack J. Leptomeningeal carcinomatosis. Arch Neurol 1996;53:626–632.

140. Morrison DG, Phuah HK, Reddy AT, et al. Ophthalmologic involvement in the syndrome of headache, neurologic deficits, and cerebrospinal fluid lymphocytosis. Ophthalmology 2003;110:115–118.

141. Barkana Y, Levin N, Goldhammer Y, et al. Chronic intracranial hypertension with unexplained cerebrospinal fluid pleocytosis. J Neuroophthalmol 2004;24:106–108.

142. Wallin MT, Kurtzke JF. Neurocysticercosis in the United States. Review of an important emerging infection. Neurology 2004;63:1559–1564.

143. Sandberg DI. Endoscopic management of hydrocephalus in pediatric patients. A review of indications, techniques, and outcomes. J Child Neurol 2008;23:550–560.

144. Corbett JJ. Neuro-ophthalmologic complications of hydrocephalus and shunting procedures. Semin Neurol 1986;6:111–123.

145. Arroyo HA, Jan LE, McCormick AQ, et al. Permanent visual loss after shunt malfunction. Neurology 1985;35:25–29.

146. Katz DM, Trobe JD, Muraszko KM, et al. Shunt failure without ventriculomegaly proclaimed by ophthalmic findings. J Neurosurg 1994;81:721–725.

147. Lee AG. Visual loss as the manifesting symptom of ventriculoperitoneal shunt malfunction. Am J Ophthalmol 1996;122:127–129.

148. Mizrachi IB, Trobe JD, Gebarski SS, et al. Papilledema in the assessment of ventriculomegaly. J Neuroophthalmol 2006;26:260–263.

149. Newman NJ. Bilateral visual loss and disc edema in a 15-year-old girl. Surv Ophthalmol 1994;38:365–370.

150. Beck RW, Greenberg HS. Post-decompression optic neuropathy. J Neurosurg 1985;63: 196–199.

151. Obana WG, Raskin NH, Cogen PH, et al. Antimigraine treatment for slit-ventricle syndrome. Neurosurgery 1990;27:760–763.

152. Nguyen TN, Polomeno RC, Farmer JP, et al. Ophthalmic complications of slit-ventricle syndrome in children. Ophthalmology 2002;109:520–524; discussion 524–525.

153. Le H, Yamini B, Frim DM. Lumboperitoneal shunting as a treatment for slit ventricle syndrome. Pediatr Neurosurg 2002;36:178–182.

154. Rekate HL, Nadkarni T, Wallace D. Severe intracranial hypertension in slit ventricle syndrome managed using a cisterna magna-ventricle-peritoneum shunt. J Neurosurg 2006;104:240–244.

155. Epstein F, Lapras C, Wisoff JH. "Slit-ventricle syndrome": etiology and treatment. Pediatr Neurosci 1988;14:5–10.

156. Smith JL. Whence pseudotumor cerebri? [editorial]. J Clin Neuroophthalmol 1985;5:55–56.

157. Friedman DI, Jacobson DM. Diagnostic criteria for idiopathic intracranial hypertension. Neurology 2002;59:1492–1495.

158. Foley J I. Benign forms of intracranial hypertension—"toxic" and "otitic" hydrocephalus. Brain 1955;78:1–13.

159. Bandyopadhyay S. Pseudotumor cerebri. Arch Neurol 2001;58:1699–1701.

160. Weisberg LA. Benign intracranial hypertension. Medicine 1975;54:197–207.

161. Greitz D, Hannerz J, Rähn T, et al. MR imaging of cerebrospinal fluid dynamics in health and disease. On the vascular pathogenesis of communicating hydrocephalus and benign intracranial hypertension. Acta Radiol 1994;35:204–211.

162. Malozowski S, Tanner LA, Wysowski DK, et al. Benign intracranial hypertension in children with growth hormone deficiency treated with growth hormone. J Pediatr 1995;126:996–999.

163. Schwarz S, Husstedt IW, Georgiadis D, et al. Benign intracranial hypertension in an HIV-infected patient: headache as the only presenting sign [letter]. AIDS 1995;9: 657–658.

164. Lessell S, Rosman NP. Permanent visual impairment in childhood pseudotumor cerebri. Arch Neurol 1986;43:801–804.

165. Corbett JJ, Thompson HS. The rational management of idiopathic intracranial hypertension. Arch Neurol 1989;46:1049–1051.

166. Corbett JJ. "Pseudotumor cerebri" by any other name [editorial]. Arch Ophthalmol 2000;118:1685.

167. Johnston I, Owler B, Pickard J. The Pseudotumor Cerebri Syndrome. Pseudotumor Cerebri, Idiopathic Intracranial Hypertension, Benign Intracranial Hypertension and Related Conditions, pp 1–356. Cambridge, Cambridge University Press, 2007.

168. Giuseffi V, Wall M, Siegel PZ, et al. Symptoms and disease associations in idiopathic intracranial hypertension (pseudotumor cerebri). A case-control study. Neurology 1991;41:239–244.

169. Galvin JA, Van Stavern GP. Clinical characterization of idiopathic intracranial hypertension at the Detroit Medical Center. J Neurol Sci 2004;223:157–160.

170. Durcan FJ, Corbett JJ, Wall M. The incidence of pseudotumor cerebri. Population studies in Iowa and Louisiana. Arch Neurol 1988;45:875–877.

171. Radhakrishnan K, Ahlskog JE, Cross SA, et al. Idiopathic intracranial hypertension (pseudotumor cerebri). Descriptive epidemiology in Rochester, Minn, 1976 to 1990. Arch Neurol 1993;50:78–80.

172. Radhakrishnan K, Thacker AK, Bohlaga NH, et al. Epidemiology of idiopathic intracranial hypertension. A prospective and case-control study. J Neurol Sci 1993;116:18–28.

173. Ireland B, Corbett JJ, Wallace RB. The search for causes of idiopathic intracranial hypertension. A preliminary case-control study. Arch Neurol 1990;47:315–320.

174. Daniels AB, Liu GT, Volpe NJ, et al. Profiles of obesity, weight gain, and quality of life in idiopathic intracranial hypertension (pseudotumor cerebri). Am J Ophthalmol 2007;143:635–641.

175. Digre KB, Corbett JJ. Pseudotumor cerebri in men. Arch Neurol 1988;45:866–872.

176. Kesler A, Goldhammer Y, Gadoth N. Do men with pseudomotor cerebri share the same characteristics as women? A retrospective review of 141 cases. J Neuroophthalmol 2001;21:15–17.

177. Bruce BB, Kedar S, Van Stavern GP, et al. Idiopathic intracranial hypertension in men. Neurology 2009;72:304–309.

178. Marcus DM, Lynn J, Miller JJ, et al. Sleep disorders. A risk factor for pseudotumor cerebri? J Neuroophthalmol 2001;21:121–123.

179. Lee AG, Golnik K, Kardon R, et al. Sleep apnea and intracranial hypertension in men. Ophthalmology 2002;109:482–485.

180. Wall M, Purvin V. Idiopathic intracranial hypertension in men and the relationship to sleep apnea [editorial]. Neurology 2009;72:300–301.

181. Friedman DI. A practical approach to intracranial hypertension. Headache Currents 2005;2:1–10.

182. Yager JY, Hartfield DS. Neurologic manifestations of iron deficiency in childhood. Pediatr Neurol 2002;27:85–92.

183. Tugal O, Jacobson R, Berezin S, et al. Recurrent benign intracranial hypertension due to iron deficiency anemia. Case report and review of the literature. Am J Pediatr Hematol Oncol 1994;16:266–270.

184. Biousse V, Rucker JC, Vignal C, et al. Anemia and papilledema. Am J Ophthalmol 2003;135:437–446.

185. Jeng MR, Rieman M, Bhakta M, et al. Pseudotumor cerebri in two adolescents with acquired aplastic anemia. J Pediatr Hematol Oncol 2002;24:765–768.

186. Nazir SA, Siatkowski RM. Pseudotumor cerebri in idiopathic aplastic anemia. J AAPOS 2003;7:71–74.

187. Taylor JP, Galetta SL, Asbury AK, et al. Hemolytic anemia presenting as idiopathic intracranial hypertension. Neurology 2002;59:960–961.

188. Vargiami E, Zafeiriou DI, Gombakis NP, et al. Hemolytic anemia presenting with idiopathic intracranial hypertension. Pediatr Neurol 2008;38:53–54.

189. Henry M, Driscoll MC, Miller M, et al. Pseudotumor cerebri in children with sickle cell disease. A case series. Pediatrics 2004;113:e265–e269.

190. Liu GT, Kay MD, Bienfang DC, et al. Pseudotumor cerebri associated with corticosteroid withdrawal in inflammatory bowel disease. Am J Ophthalmol 1994;117:352–357.

191. Weisberg LA, Chutorian AM. Pseudotumor cerebri of childhood. Am J Dis Child 1977;131:1243–1248.

192. Malozowski S, Tanner LA, Wysowski D, et al. Growth hormone, insulin-like growth factor I, and benign intracranial hypertension [letter]. N Engl J Med 1993;329:665–666.

193. Reeves GD, Doyle DA. Growth hormone treatment and pseudotumor cerebri. Coincidence or close relationship? J Pediatr Endocrinol Metab 2002;15 Suppl 2: 723–730.

194. Blethen SL. Complications of growth hormone therapy in children. Curr Opin Pediatr 1995;7:466–471.

195. Johansson JO, Larson G, Andersson M, et al. Treatment of growth hormone-deficient adults with recombinant human growth hormone increases the concentration of growth hormone in the cerebrospinal fluid and affects neurotransmitters. Neuroendocrinology 1995;61:57–66.

196. Crock PA, McKenzie JD, Nicoll AM, et al. Benign intracranial hypertension and recombinant growth hormone therapy in Australia and New Zealand. Acta Paediatr 1998;87:381–386.

197. Collett-Solberg PF, Liu GT, Satin-Smith M, et al. Pseudopapilledema and congenital disc anomalies in growth hormone deficiency. J Pediatr Endocrinol Metab 1998;11: 261–265.

198. Gardner K, Cox T, Digre KB. Idiopathic intracranial hypertension associated with tetracycline use in fraternal twins. Case reports and review. Neurology 1995; 45:6–10.

199. Chiu AM, Chuenkongkaew WL, Cornblath WT, et al. Minocycline treatment and pseudotumor cerebri syndrome. Am J Ophthalmol 1998;126:116–121.

200. Quinn AG, Singer SB, Buncic JR. Pediatric tetracycline-induced pseudotumor cerebri. J AAPOS 1999;3:53–57.

201. Weese-Mayer DE, Yang RJ, Mayer JR, et al. Minocycline and pseudotumor cerebri. The well-known but well-kept secret [letter]. Pediatrics 2001;108:519–520.

202. Friedman DI, Gordon LK, Egan RA, et al. Doxycycline and intracranial hypertension. Neurology 2004;62:2297–2299.

203. Kesler A, Goldhammer Y, Hadayer A, et al. The outcome of pseudotumor cerebri induced by tetracycline therapy. Acta Neurol Scand 2004;110:408–411.

204. Jacobson DM, Berg R, Wall M, et al. Serum vitamin A concentration is elevated in idiopathic intracranial hypertension. Neurology 1999;53:1114–1118.

205. Baqui AH, de Francisco A, Arifeen SE, et al. Bulging fontanelle after supplementation with 25,000 IU of vitamin A in infancy using immunization contacts. Acta Paediatr 1995;84:863–866.

206. Fraunfelder FW, Fraunfelder FT, Corbett JJ. Isotretinoin-associated intracranial hypertension. Ophthalmology 2004;111:1248–1250.

207. Lee AG. Pseudotumor cerebri after treatment with tetracycline and isotretinoin for acne. Cutis 1995;55:165–168.

208. Moskowitz Y, Leibowitz E, Ronen M, et al. Pseudotumor cerebri induced by vitamin A combined with minocycline. Ann Ophthalmol 1993;25:306–308.

209. Mahmoud HH, Hurwitz CA, Roberts WM, et al. Tretinoin toxicity in children with acute promyelocytic leukaemia. Lancet 1993;342:1394–1395.

210. Frankel SR, Eardley A, Heller G, et al. All-trans retinoic acid for acute promyelocytic leukemia. Results of the New York Study. Ann Intern Med 1994;120:278–286.

211. Varadi G, Lossos A, Or R, et al. Successful allogeneic bone marrow transplantation in a patient with ATRA-induced pseudotumor cerebri [letter]. Am J Hematol 1995;50:147–148.

212. Visani G, Bontempo G, Manfroi S, et al. All-trans-retinoic acid and pseudotumor cerebri in a young adult with acute promyelocytic leukemia: a possible disease association. Haematologica 1996;81:152–154.

213. Sano F, Tsuji K, Kunika N, et al. Pseudotumor cerebri in a patient with acute promyelocytic leukemia during treatment with all-trans retinoic acid. Intern Med 1998;37:546–549.

214. Schroeter T, Lanvers C, Herding H, et al. Pseudotumor cerebri induced by all-trans-retinoic acid in a child treated for acute promyelocytic leukemia. Med Pediatr Oncol 2000;34:284–286.

215. Guirgis MF, Lueder GT. Intracranial hypertension secondary to all-trans retinoic acid treatment for leukemia. Diagnosis and management. J AAPOS 2003;7:432–434.

216. Colucciello M. Pseudotumor cerebri induced by all-trans retinoic acid treatment of acute promyelocytic leukemia. Arch Ophthalmol 2003;121:1064–1065.

217. Smith MA, Adamson PC, Balis FM, et al. Phase I and pharmacokinetic evaluation of all-trans-retinoic acid in pediatric patients with cancer. J Clin Oncol 1992;10:1666–1673.

218. Degos L, Dombret H, Chomienne C, et al. All-trans-retinoic acid as a differentiating agent in the treatment of acute promyelocytic leukemia. Blood 1995;85:2643–2653.

219. Condulis N, Germain G, Charest N, et al. Pseudotumor cerebri: a presenting manifestation of Addison's disease. Clin Pediatr 1997;36:711–713.

220. Alexandrakis G, Filatov V, Walsh T. Pseudotumor cerebri in a 12-year old boy with Addison's disease. Am J Ophthalmol 1993;116:650–651.

221. Vachvanichsanong P, Dissaneewate P, Vasikananont P. Pseudotumor cerebri in a boy with systemic lupus erythematosus. Am J Dis Child 1992;146:1417–1419.

222. Green L, Vinker S, Amital H, et al. Pseudotumor cerebri in systemic lupus erythematosus. Semin Arthritis Rheum 1995;25:103–108.

223. Mourani CC, Mallat SG, Moukarzel MY, et al. Kidney transplantation after a severe form of pseudotumor cerebri. Pediatr Nephrol 1998;12:709–711.

224. Chamberlain CE, Fitzgibbon E, Wassermann EM, et al. Idiopathic intracranial hypertension following kidney transplantation. A case report and review of the literature. Pediatr Transplant 2005;9:545–550.

225. Francis PJ, Haywood S, Rigden S, et al. Benign intracranial hypertension in children following renal transplantation. Pediatr Nephrol 2003;18:1265–1269.

226. Katz B, Moster ML, Slavin ML. Disk edema subsequent to renal transplantation. Surv Ophthalmol 1997;41:315–320.

227. Johnston I. The reduced CSF absorption syndrome. A reappraisal of benign intracranial hypertension and related conditions. Lancet 1973;2:418–420.

228. Gjerris F, Sørensen PS, Vorstrup S, et al. Intracranial pressure, conductance to cerebrospinal fluid outflow and cerebral blood flow in patients with benign intracranial hypertension. Ann Neurol 1985;17:158–162.

229. Johnston I, Hawke S, Halmagyi M, et al. The pseudotumor syndrome. Disorders of cerebrospinal fluid circulation causing intracranial hypertension without ventriculomegaly. Arch Neurol 1991;48:740–747.

230. Malm J, Kristensen B, Markgren P, et al. CSF hydrodynamics in idiopathic intracranial hypertension. A long-term study. Neurology 1992;42:851–858.

231. Radhakrishnan K, Ahlskog JE, Garrity JA, et al. Idiopathic intracranial hypertension. Mayo Clinic Proc 1994;69:169–180.

232. Sugerman HJ, DeMaria EJ, Felton WL, et al. Increased intra-abdominal pressure and cardiac filling pressures in obesity-associated pseudotumor cerebri. Neurology 1997;49:507–511.

233. King JO, Mitchell PJ, Thomson KR, et al. Cerebral venography and manometry in idiopathic intracranial hypertension. Neurology 1995;45:2224–2228.

234. Farb RI, Vanek I, Scott JN, et al. Idiopathic intracranial hypertension. The prevalence and morphology of sinovenous stenosis. Neurology 2003;60:1418–1424.

235. Karahalios DG, Rekate HL, Khayata MH, et al. Elevated intracranial venous pressure as a universal mechanism in pseudotumor cerebri of varying etiologies. Neurology 1996;46:198–202.

236. King JO, Mitchell PJ, Thomson KR, et al. Manometry combined with cervical puncture in idiopathic intracranial hypertension. Neurology 2002;58:26–30.

237. McGonigal A, Bone I, Teasdale E. Resolution of transverse sinus stenosis in idiopathic intracranial hypertension after L-P shunt. Neurology 2004;62:514–515.

238. Baryshnik DB, Farb RI. Changes in the appearance of venous sinuses after treatment of disordered intracranial pressure. Neurology 2004;62:1445–1446.

239. Higgins JN, Pickard JD. Lateral sinus stenoses in idiopathic intracranial hypertension resolving after CSF diversion. Neurology 2004;62:1907–1908.

240. Bono F, Giliberto C, Mastrandrea C, et al. Transverse sinus stenoses persist after normalization of the CSF pressure in IIH. Neurology 2005;65:1090–1093.

241. Corbett JJ, Digre K. Idiopathic intracranial hypertension. An answer to, "the chicken or the egg?" [editorial]. Neurology 2002;58:5–6.

242. Friedman DI. Cerebral venous pressure, intra-abdominal pressure, and dural venous sinus stenting in idiopathic intracranial hypertension. J Neuroophthalmol 2006;26:61–64.

243. Corbett JJ. Increased intracranial pressure. Idiopathic and otherwise. J Neuroophthalmol 2004;24:103–105.

244. Dandy WE. Intracranial pressure without brain tumor. Diagnosis and treatment. Ann Surg 1937;106:492–513.

245. Sahs AL, Joynt RJ. Brain swelling of unknown cause. Neurology 1956;6:791–803.

246. Mathew NT, Meyer JS, Ott EO. Increased cerebral blood volume in benign intracranial hypertension. Neurology 1975;25:646–649.

247. Raichle ME, Grubb RL, Phelps ME, et al. Cerebral hemodynamics and metabolism in pseudotumor cerebri. Ann Neurol 1978;4:104–111.

248. Greer M. Benign intracranial hypertension. VI. Obesity. Neurology 1965;15:382–388.

249. Soelberg Sørensen P, Thomsen C, Gjerris F, et al. Brain water accumulation in pseudotumor cerebri demonstrated by MR-imaging of brain water self-diffusion. Acta Neurochir (Suppl) 1990;51:363–365.

250. Gideon P, Sørensen PS, Thomsen C, et al. Increased brain water self-diffusion in patients with idiopathic intracranial hypertension. AJNR Am J Neuroradiol 1995;16:381–387.

251. Wall M, Dollar JD, Sadun AA, et al. Idiopathic intracranial hypertension. Lack of histologic evidence for cerebral edema. Arch Neurol 1995;52:141–145.

252. Fishman RA. Diseases of intracranial pressure. Hydrocephalus, brain edema, pseudotumor, intracranial hypotension, and related disorders. In: Cerebrospinal Fluid in Diseases of the Nervous System, 2nd edn, pp 103–155. Philadelphia, W.B. Saunders, 1992.

253. Gideon P, Sørensen PS, Thomsen C, et al. Assessment of CSF dynamics and venous flow in the superior sagittal sinus by MRI in idiopathic intracranial hypertension. A preliminary study. Neuroradiology 1994;36:350–354.

254. Martin NA, Linfoot J, Wilson CB. Development of pseudotumor cerebri after the removal of an adrenocorticotropic hormone-secreting pituitary adenoma: case report. Neurosurgery 1981;8:699–702.

255. Weissman MN, Page LK, Bejar RL. Cushing's disease in childhood. Benign intracranial hypertension after trans-sphenoidal adenomectomy. Neurosurgery 1983;13:195–197.

256. Friedman DI, Streeten DH. Idiopathic intracranial hypertension and orthostatic edema may share a common pathogenesis. Neurology 1998;50:1099–1104.

257. Soelberg Sørensen P, Gjerris F, Svenstrup B. Endocrine studies in patients with pseudotumor cerebri. Estrogen levels in blood and cerebrospinal fluid. Arch Neurol 1986;43:902–906.

258. Sussman J, Leach M, Greaves M, et al. Potentially prothrombotic abnormalities of coagulation in benign intracranial hypertension. J Neurol Neurosurg Psychiatr 1997;62:229–233.

259. Dogulu CF, Kansu T, Leung MY, et al. Evidence for genetic susceptibility to thrombosis in idiopathic intracranial hypertension. Thromb Res 2003;111:389–395.

260. Dunkley S, Johnston I. Thrombophilia as a common predisposing factor in pseudotumor cerebri. Blood 2004;103:1972–1973.

261. Weksler B. Linking thrombophilia and idiopathic intracranial hypertension. J Lab Clin Med 2005;145:63–64.

262. Leker RR, Steiner I. Anticardiolipin antibodies are frequently present in patients with idiopathic intracranial hypertension. Arch Neurol 1998;55:817–820.

263. Selhorst JB, Kulkantrakorn K, Corbett JJ, et al. Retinol-binding protein in idiopathic intracranial hypertension (IIH). J Neuroophthalmol 2000;20:250–252.

264. Tabassi A, Salmasi AH, Jalali M. Serum and CSF vitamin A concentrations in idiopathic intracranial hypertension. Neurology 2005;64:1893–1896.

265. Warner JE, Larson AJ, Bhosale P, et al. Retinol-binding protein and retinol analysis in cerebrospinal fluid and serum of patients with and without idiopathic intracranial hypertension. J Neuroophthalmol 2007;27:258–262.

266. Warner JE, Bernstein PS, Yemelyanov A, et al. Vitamin A in the cerebrospinal fluid of patients with and without idiopathic intracranial hypertension. Ann Neurol 2002;52:647–650.

267. Fishman RA. Polar bear liver, vitamin A, aquaporins, and pseudotumor cerebri [editorial]. Ann Neurol 2002;52:531–533.

268. Libien J, Blaner WS. Retinol and retinol-binding protein in cerebrospinal fluid. Can vitamin A take the "idiopathic" out of idiopathic intracranial hypertension? [editorial]. J Neuroophthalmol 2007;27:253–257.

269. Rush JA. Pseudotumor cerebri. Clinical profile and visual outcome in 63 patients. Mayo Clinic Proc 1980;55:541–546.

270. Biousse V, Newman NJ, Lessell S. Audible pulsatile tinnitus in idiopathic intracranial hypertension. Neurology 1998;50:1185–1186.

271. Lee AG. Pulsatile tinnitus as a presenting symptom of pseudotumour cerebri. J Otolaryngol 1996;25:203–204.

272. O'Duffy D, James B, Elston J. Idiopathic intracranial hypertension presenting with gaze-evoked amaurosis. Acta Ophthalmol Scand 1998;76:119–120.

273. McCammon A, Kaufman HH, Sears ES. Transient oculomotor paralysis in pseudotumor cerebri. Neurology 1981;31:182–184.

274. Thapa R, Mukherjee S. Transient bilateral oculomotor palsy in pseudotumor cerebri. J Child Neurol 2008;23:580–581.

275. Speer C, Pearlman J, Phillips PH, et al. Fourth cranial nerve palsy in pediatric patients with pseudotumor cerebri. Am J Ophthalmol 1999;127:236–237.

276. Friedman DI, Forman S, Levi L, et al. Unusual ocular motility disturbances with increased intracranial pressure. Neurology 1998;50:1893–1896.

277. Davie C, Kennedy P, Katifi HA. Seventh nerve palsy as a false localising sign [letter]. J Neurol Neurosurg Psychiatr 1992;55:510–511.

278. Selky AK, Dobyns WB, Yee RD. Idiopathic intracranial hypertension and facial diplegia. Neurology 1994;44:357.

279. Selky AK, Purvin VA. Hemifacial spasm. An unusual manifestation of idiopathic intracranial hypertension. J Neuroophthalmol 1994;14:196–198.

280. Benegas NM, Volpe NJ, Liu GT, et al. Hemifacial spasm and idiopathic intracranial hypertension [letter]. J Neuroophthalmol 1996;16:70.

281. Davenport RJ, Will RG, Galloway PJ. Isolated intracranial hypertension presenting with trigeminal neuropathy [letter]. J Neurol Neurosurg Psychiatr 1994;57:381.

282. Arsava EM, Uluc K, Nurlu G, et al. Electrophysiological evidence of trigeminal neuropathy in pseudotumor cerebri. J Neurol 2002;249:1601–1602.

283. Dorman PJ, Campbell MJ, Maw AR. Hearing loss as a false localising sign in raised intracranial pressure [letter]. J Neurol Neurosurg Psychiatr 1995;58:516.

284. Round R, Keane JR. The minor symptoms of increased intracranial pressure. 101 patients with benign intracranial hypertension. Neurology 1988;38:1461–1464.

285. Miller NR. Walsh and Hoyt's Clinical Neuro-ophthalmology, 4th edn, pp 175–211. Baltimore, Williams and Wilkins, 1982.

286. Thambisetty M, Lavin PJ, Newman NJ, et al. Fulminant idiopathic intracranial hypertension. Neurology 2007;68:229–232.

287. Ney JJ, Volpe NJ, Liu GT, et al. Functional visual loss in idiopathic intracranial hypertension. Ophthalmology 2009;116:1808–1813.

288. Verplanck M, Kaufman DI, Parsons T, et al. Electrophysiology versus psychophysics in the detection of visual loss in pseudotumor cerebri. Neurology 1988;38:1789–1792.

289. Wall M, White WN. Asymmetric papilledema in idiopathic intracranial hypertension. Prospective interocular comparison of sensory visual function. Invest Ophthalmol Vis Sci 1998;39:134–142.

290. Yuh WT, Zhu M, Taoka T, et al. MR imaging of pituitary morphology in idiopathic intracranial hypertension. J Magn Reson Imaging 2000;12:808–813.

291. Mashima Y, Oshitari K, Imamura Y, et al. High-resolution magnetic resonance imaging of the intraorbital optic nerve and subarachnoid space in patients with papilledema and optic atrophy. Arch Ophthalmol 1996;114:1197–1203.

292. Gibby WA, Cohen M, Goldberg HI, et al. Pseudotumor cerebri. CT findings and correlation with vision loss. Am J Radiol 1993;160:143–146.

293. Brodsky MC, Glasier CM. Magnetic resonance visualization of the swollen optic disc in papilledema. J Neuroophthalmol 1995;15:122–124.

294. Brodsky MC, Vaphiades M. Magnetic resonance imaging in pseudotumor cerebri. Ophthalmology 1998;105:1686–1693.

295. Weisberg LA, Housepian EM, Saur DA. Empty sella syndrome and complication of benign intracranial hypertension. J Neurosurg 1975;43:177–180.

296. Foley KM, Posner JB. Does pseudotumor cerebri cause the empty sella syndrome? Neurology 1975;25:565–569.

297. Weisberg LA. Computerized tomography in benign intracranial hypertension. Neurology 1985;35:1075–1078.

298. Jacobson DM, Karanjia PN, Olson KA, et al. Computerized tomography ventricular size has no predictive value in diagnosing pseudotumor cerebri. Neurology 1990;40:1454–1455.

299. Rothwell PM, Gibson RJ, Sellar RJ. Computed tomographic evidence of cerebral swelling in benign intracranial hypertension. J Neurol Neurosurg Psychiatr 1994;57:1407–1409.

300. Sullivan HC. Fatal tonsillar herniation in pseudotumor cerebri. Neurology 1991;41:1142–1144.

301. Whiteley W, Al-Shahi R, Warlow CP, et al. CSF opening pressure: reference interval and the effect of body mass index. Neurology 2006;67:1960–1961.

302. Chandra V, Bellur SN, Anderson RJ. Low CSF protein concentration in idiopathic pseudotumor cerebri. Ann Neurol 1986;19:80–82.

303. Johnston PK, Corbett JJ, Maxner CE. Cerebrospinal fluid protein and opening pressure in idiopathic intracranial hypertension (pseudotumor cerebri). Neurology 1991;41:1040–1042.

304. Practice parameters. Lumbar puncture (summary statement). Neurology 1993;43:625–627.

305. Shuper A, Snir M, Barash D, et al. Ultrasonography of the optic nerves. Clinical application in children with pseudotumor cerebri. J Pediatr 1997;131:734–740.

306. Mulholland DA, Craig JJ, Rankin SJ. Use of scanning laser ophthalmoscopy to monitor papilloedema in idiopathic intracranial hypertension. Br J Ophthalmol 1998;82:1301–1305.

307. Tamburrelli C, Salgarello T, Caputo CG, et al. Ultrasonographic evaluation of optic disc swelling. Comparison with CSLO in idiopathic intracranial hypertension. Invest Ophthalmol Vis Sci 2000;41:2960–2966.

308. Newborg B. Pseudotumor cerebri treated by rice/reduction diet. Arch Intern Med 1974;133:802–807.

309. Sugerman HJ, Felton WL, Salvant JB, et al. Effects of surgically induced weight loss on idiopathic intracranial hypertension in morbid obesity. Neurology 1995;45:1655–1659.

310. Johnson LN, Krohel GB, Madsen RW, et al. The role of weight loss and acetazolamide in the treatment of idiopathic intracranial hypertension (pseudotumor cerebri). Ophthalmology 1998;105:2313–2317.

311. Kupersmith MJ, Gamell L, Turbin R, et al. Effects of weight loss on the course of idiopathic intracranial hypertension in women. Neurology 1998;50:1094–1098.

312. Smith JL. Pseudotumor cerebri. Trans Am Acad Ophth Otol 1958;62:432–440.

313. Kessler LA, Novelli PM, Reigel DH. Surgical treatment of benign intracranial hypertension—subtemporal decompression revisited. Surg Neurol 1998;50:73–76.

314. Gücer G, Viernstein L. Long-term intracranial pressure recording in the management of pseudotumor cerebri. J Neurosurg 1978;49:256–263.

315. Schoeman JF. Childhood pseudotumor cerebri. Clinical and intracranial pressure response to acetazolamide and furosemide treatment in a case series. J Child Neurol 1994;9:130–134.

316. Liu GT, Volpe NJ, Galetta SL. Pseudotumor cerebri and its medical treatment. Drugs of Today 1998;34:563–574.

317. Tomsak RL, Niffenegger AS, Remler BF. Treatment of psudotumor cerebri with Diamox (acetazolamide). J Clin Neuroophthalmol 1988;8:93–98.

318. Wandstrat TL, Phillips J. Pseudotumor cerebri responsive to acetazolamide [letter]. Ann Pharmacother 1995;29:318.

319. Strom BL, Schinnar R, Apter AJ, et al. Absence of cross-reactivity between sulfonamide antibiotics and sulfonamide nonantibiotics. N Engl J Med 2003;349:1628–1635.

320. Alward WLM. Medical management of glaucoma. N Engl J Med 1998;339:1298–1307.

321. Fraunfelder FT, Bagby GC. Monitoring patients taking oral carbonic anhydrase inhibitors. Am J Ophthalmol 2000;130:221–223.

322. Lichter PR. Reducing side effects of carbonic anhydrase inhibitors. Ophthalmology 1981;88:266–269.

323. Finsterer J, Földy D, Fertl E, et al. Topiramate resolves headache from pseudotumor cerebri [letter]. J Pain Symptom Manage 2006;32:401–402.

324. Shah VA, Fung S, Shahbaz R, et al. Idiopathic intracranial hypertension [letter]. Ophthalmology 2007;114:617.

325. Thompson PJ, Baxendale SA, Duncan JS, et al. Effects of topiramate on cognitive function. J Neurol Neurosurg Psychiatry 2000;69:636–641.

326. Gadde KM, Franciscy DM, Wagner HR, 2nd, et al. Zonisamide for weight loss in obese adults. A randomized controlled trial. JAMA 2003;289:1820–1825.

327. Banta JT, Farris BK. Pseudotumor cerebri and optic nerve sheath decompression. Ophthalmology 2000;107:1907–1912.

328. Smith JL, Hoyt WF, Newton TH. Optic nerve sheath decompression for relief of chronic monocular choked discs. Am J Ophthalmol 1969;68:633–639.

329. Brourman ND, Spoor TC, Ramocki JM. Optic nerve sheath decompression for pseudotumor cerebri. Arch Ophthalmol 1988;106:1378–1383.

330. Sergott RC, Savino PJ, Bosley TM. Modified optic nerve sheath decompression provides long-term visual improvement for pseudotumor cerebri. Arch Ophthalmol 1988;106:1384–1390.

331. Corbett JJ, Nerad JA, Tse DT, et al. Results of optic nerve sheath fenestration for pseudotumor cerebri. The lateral orbitotomy approach. Arch Ophthalmol 1988;106:1391–1397.

332. Pearson PA, Baker RS, Khorram R, et al. Evaluation of optic nerve sheath fenestration in pseudotumor cerebri using automated perimetry. Ophthalmology 1991;98:99–105.

333. Kelman SE, Heaps R, Wolf A, et al. Optic nerve decompression surgery improves visual function in patients with pseudotumor cerebri. Neurosurgery 1992;30:391–395.

334. Tse DT, Nerad JA, Anderson RL, et al. Optic nerve sheath fenestration in pseudotumor cerebri. A lateral orbitotomy approach. Arch Ophthalmol 1988;106:1458–1462.

335. Rizzuto PR, Spoor TC, Ramocki JM, et al. Subtenon's local anesthesia for optic nerve sheath fenestration. Am J Ophthalmol 1996;121:326–327.

336. Spoor TC, McHenry JG. Complications of optic nerve sheath decompression [letter]. Ophthalmology 1993;100:1432.

337. Plotnik JL, Kosmorsky GS. Operative complications of optic nerve sheath decompression. Ophthalmology 1993;100:683–690.

338. Rizzo JF, Lessell S. Choroidal infarction after optic nerve sheath fenestration. Ophthalmology 1994;101:1622–1626.

339. Flynn WJ, Westfall CT, Weisman JS. Transient blindness after optic nerve sheath fenestration [letter]. Am J Ophthalmol 1994;117:678–679.

340. Brodsky MC, Rettele GA. Protracted postsurgical blindness with visual recovery following optic nerve sheath fenestration. Arch Ophthalmol 1997;115:1473–1474.

341. Keltner JL. Optic nerve sheath decompression. How does it work? Has its time come [editorial]? Arch Ophthalmol 1988;106:1365–1369.

342. Seiff SR, Shah L. A model for the mechanism of optic nerve sheath fenestration. Arch Ophthalmol 1990;108:1326–1329.

343. Sallomi D, Taylor H, Hibbert J, et al. The MRI appearance of the optic nerve sheath following fenestration for benign intracranial hypertension. Eur Radiol 1998;8:1193–1196.

344. Tsai JC, Petrovich MS, Sadun AA. Histopathological and ultrastructural examination of optic nerve sheath decompression. Br J Ophthalmol 1995;79:182–185.

345. Hamed LM, Tse DT, Glaser JS, et al. Neuroimaging of the optic nerve after fenestration for management of pseudotumor cerebri. Arch Ophthalmol 1992;110:636–639.

346. Yazici Z, Yazici B, Tuncel E. Findings of magnetic resonance imaging after optic nerve sheath decompression in patients with idiopathic intracranial hypertension. Am J Ophthalmol 2007;144:429–435.

347. Burde RM, Karp JS, Miller RN. Reversal of visual deficit with optic nerve decompression in long-standing pseudotumor cerebri. Am J Ophthalmol 1974;77:770–772.

348. Kaye AH, Galbraith JFK, King J. Intracranial pressure following optic nerve decompression for benign intracranial hypertension. J Neurosurg 1981;55:453–456.

349. Spoor TC, Ramocki JM, Madion MP, et al. Treatment of pseudotumor cerebri by primary and secondary optic nerve sheath decompression. Am J Ophthalmol 1991;112:177–185.

350. Spoor TC, McHenry JG. Long-term effectiveness of optic nerve sheath decompression for pseudotumor cerebri. Arch Ophthalmol 1993;111:632–635.

351. Liu GT, Glaser JS, Schatz NJ. High-dose methylprednisolone and acetazolamide for visual loss in pseudotumor cerebri. Am J Ophthalmol 1994;118:88–96.

352. Mauriello JA, Shaderowfsky P, Gizzi M, et al. Management of visual loss after optic nerve sheath decompression in patients with pseudotumor cerebri. Ophthalmology 1995;102:441–445.

353. Eggenberger ER, Miller NR, Vitale S. Lumboperitoneal shunt for the treatment of pseudotumor cerebri. Neurology 1996;46:1524–1530.

354. Burgett RA, Purvin VA, Kawasaki A. Lumboperitoneal shunting for pseudotumor cerebri. Neurology 1997;49:734–739.

355. Brazis PW. Clinical review: the surgical treatment of idiopathic pseudotumour cerebri (idiopathic intracranial hypertension). Cephalalgia 2008;28:1361–1373.

356. Rosenberg ML, Corbett JJ, Smith C, et al. Cerebrospinal fluid diversion procedures in pseudotumor cerebri. Neurology 1993;43:1071–1072.

357. Tulipan N, Lavin PJ, Copeland M. Stereotactic ventriculoperitoneal shunt for idiopathic intracranial hypertension. Technical note. Neurosurgery 1998;43:175–176.

358. Bynke G, Zemack G, Bynke H, et al. Ventriculoperitoneal shunting for idiopathic intracranial hypertension. Neurology 2004;63:1314–1316.

359. Garton HJ. Cerebrospinal fluid diversion procedures. J Neuroophthalmol 2004;24:146–155.

360. Buchwald H, Avidor Y, Braunwald E, et al. Bariatric surgery. A systematic review and meta-analysis. JAMA 2004;292:1724–1737.

361. Curry WT, Jr., Butler WE, Barker FG, 2nd. Rapidly rising incidence of cerebrospinal fluid shunting procedures for idiopathic intracranial hypertension in the United States, 1988–2002. Neurosurgery 2005;57:97–108; discussion 197–108.

362. Donnet A, Metellus P, Levrier O, et al. Endovascular treatment of idiopathic intracranial hypertension. Clinical and radiologic outcome of 10 consecutive patients. Neurology 2008;70:641–647.

363. Digre KB, Varner MW, Corbett JJ. Pseudotumor cerebri and pregnancy. Neurology 1984;34:721–729.

364. Lee AG, Pless M, Falardeau J, et al. The use of acetazolamide in idiopathic intracranial hypertension during pregnancy. Am J Ophthalmol 2005;139:855–859.

365. Friedman DI, Jacobson DM. Idiopathic intracranial hypertension. J Neuroophthalmol 2004;24:138–145.

366. Rowe FJ, Sarkies NJ. Visual outcome in a prospective study of idiopathic intracranial hypertension [letter]. Arch Ophthalmol 1999;117:1571.

367. Bruce BB, Preechawat P, Newman NJ, et al. Racial differences in idiopathic intracranial hypertension. Neurology 2008;70:861–867.

368. Guy J, Johnston PK, Corbett JJ, et al. Treatment of visual loss in pseudotumor cerebri associated with uremia. Neurology 1990;40:28–32.

369. Kesler A, Hadayer A, Goldhammer Y, et al. Idiopathic intracranial hypertension. Risk of recurrences. Neurology 2004;63:1737–1739.

370. Taktakishvili O, Shah VA, Shahbaz R, et al. Recurrent idiopathic intracranial hypertension [letter]. Ophthalmology 2008;115:221.

371. Shah VA, Kardon RH, Lee AG, et al. Long-term follow-up of idiopathic intracranial hypertension. The Iowa experience. Neurology 2008;70:634–640.

372. Marcelis J, Silberstein SD. Idiopathic intracranial hypertension without papilledema. Arch Neurol 1991;48:392–399.

373. Mathew NT, Ravishankar K, Sanin LC. Coexistence of migraine and idiopathic intracranial hypertension without papilledema. Neurology 1996;46:1226–1230.

374. Krishna R, Kosmorsky GS, Wright KW. Pseudotumor cerebri sine papilledema with unilateral sixth nerve palsy. J Neuroophthalmol 1998;18:53–55.

375. Wang SJ, Silberstein SD, Patterson S, et al. Idiopathic intracranial hypertension without papilledema: a case-control study in a headache center. Neurology 1998;51:245–249.

376. Bono F, Messina D, Giliberto C, et al. Bilateral transverse sinus stenosis predicts IIH without papilledema in patients with migraine. Neurology 2006;67:419–423.

377. Vieira DS, Masruha MR, Goncalves AL, et al. Idiopathic intracranial hypertension with and without papilloedema in a consecutive series of patients with chronic migraine. Cephalalgia 2008;28:609–613.

378. Digre KB, Nakamoto BK, Warner JE, et al. A comparison of idiopathic intracranial hypertension with and without papilledema. Headache 2009;49:185–193.

379. Lessell S. Pediatric pseudotumor cerebri (idiopathic intracranial hypertension). Surv Ophthalmol 1992;37:155–166.

380. Dietz WH, Robinson TN. Clinical practice. Overweight children and adolescents. N Engl J Med 2005;352:2100–2109.

381. Hoppin AG, Katz ES, Kaplan LM, et al. Case records of the Massachusetts General Hospital. Case 31–2006. A 15-year-old girl with severe obesity. N Engl J Med 2006;355:1593–1602.

382. Couch R, Camfield PR, Tibbles JAR. The changing picture of pseudotumor cerebri in children. Can J Neurol Sci 1985;12:48–50.

383. Baker RS, Carter D, Hendrick EB, et al. Visual loss in pseudotumor cerebri of childhood. A follow-up study. Arch Ophthalmol 1985;103:1681–1686.

384. Babikian P, Corbett JJ, Bell W. Idiopathic intracranial hypertension in children. The Iowa experience. J Child Neurol 1994;9:144–149.

385. Gordon K. Pediatric pseudotumor cerebri. Descriptive epidemiology. Can J Neurol Sci 1997;24:219–221.

386. Scott IU, Siatkowski RM, Eneyni M, et al. Idiopathic intracranial hypertension in children and adolescents. Am J Ophthalmol 1997;124:253–255.

387. Cinciripini GS, Donahue S, Borchert MS. Idiopathic intracranial hypertension in prepubertal pediatric patients: characteristics, treatment, and outcome. Am J Ophthalmol 1999;127:178–182.

388. Balcer LJ, Liu GT, Forman S, et al. Pediatric pseudotumor cerebri. Relationship of age and obesity. Neurology 1999;52:870–872.

389. Salman MS, Kirkham FJ, MacGregor DL. Idiopathic "benign" intracranial hypertension. Case series and review. J Child Neurol 2001;16:465–470.

390. Distelmaier F, Sengler U, Messing-Juenger M, et al. Pseudotumor cerebri as an important differential diagnosis of papilledema in children. Brain Dev 2006;28:190–195.

391. Genizi J, Lahat E, Zelnik N, et al. Childhood-onset idiopathic intracranial hypertension. Relation of sex and obesity. Pediatr Neurol 2007;36:247–249.

392. Esmaili N, Bradfield YS. Pseudotumor cerebri in children with Down syndrome. Ophthalmology 2007;114:1773–1778.

393. Winner P, Bello L. Idiopathic intracranial hypertension in a young child without visual symptoms or signs. Headache 1996;36:574–576.

394. Johnston IH, Duff J, Jacobson EE, et al. Asymptomatic intracranial hypertension in disorders of CSF circulation in childhood—treated and untreated. Pediatr Neurosurg 2001;34:63–72.

395. Kesler A, Fattal-Valevski A. Idiopathic intracranial hypertension in the pediatric population. J Child Neurol 2002;17:745–748.

396. Weig SG. Asymptomatic idiopathic intracranial hypertension in young children. J Child Neurol 2002;17:239–241.

397. Youroukos S, Psychou F, Fryssiras S, et al. Idiopathic intracranial hypertension in children. J Child Neurol 2000;15:453–457.

398. Bassan H, Berkner L, Stolovitch C, et al. Asymptomatic idiopathic intracranial hypertension in children Acta Neurol Scand 2008;118:251–255.

399. Stiebel-Kalish H, Kalish Y, Lusky M, et al. Puberty as a risk factor for less favorable visual outcome in idiopathic intracranial hypertension. Am J Ophthalmol 2006;142:279–283.

400. Lee AG, Patrinely JR, Edmond JC. Optic nerve sheath decompression in pediatric pseudotumor cerebri. Ophthalmic Surg Lasers 1998;29:514–517.

401. Thuente DD, Buckley EG. Pediatric optic nerve sheath decompression. Ophthalmology 2005;112:724–727.

402. Rekate HL, Wallace D. Lumboperitoneal shunts in children. Pediatr Neurosurg 2003;38:41–46.

403. Gordon DL. The diagnosis and management of cerebral venous thrombosis. In: Adams HP (ed). Handbook of Cerebrovascular Diseases, pp 591–612. New York, Marcel Dekker, 1993.

404. Wechsler B, Vidailhet M, Piette JC, et al. Cerebral venous thrombosis in Behçet's disease. Clinical study and long-term follow-up of 25 cases. Neurology 1992;42:614–618.

405. Daif A, Awada A, Al-Rajeh S, et al. Cerebral venous thrombosis in adults. A study of 40 cases from Saudi Arabia. Stroke 1995;26:1193–1195.

406. Mokri B, Jack CR, Petty GW. Pseudotumor syndrome associated with cerebral venous sinus occlusion and antiphospholipid antibodies. Stroke 1993;24:469–472.

407. Confavreux C, Brunet P, Petiot P, et al. Congenital protein C deficiency and superior sagittal sinus thrombosis causing isolated intracranial hypertension. J Neurol Neurosurg Psychiatr 1994;57:655–657.

408. Cakmak S, Derex L, Berruyer M, et al. Cerebral venous thrombosis. Clinical outcome and systematic screening of prothrombotic factors. Neurology 2003;60:1175–1178.

409. Sébire G, Tabarki B, Saunders DE, et al. Cerebral venous sinus thrombosis in children. Risk factors, presentation, diagnosis and outcome. Brain 2005;128:477–489.

410. Purvin VA, Trobe JD, Kosmorsky G. Neuro-ophthalmic features of cerebral venous obstruction. Arch Neurol 1995;52:880–885.

411. Silberberg DS, Laties AM. Increased intracranial pressure in disseminated lupus erythematosus. Arch Neurol 1973;29:88–90.

412. Carlow TJ, Glaser JS. Pseudotumor cerebri syndrome in systemic lupus erythematosus. JAMA 1974;228:197–200.

413. Li EK, Ho PCP. Pseudotumor cerebri in systemic lupus erythematosus. J Rheumatol 1989;16:113–116.

414. Li EK, Chan MSY. Is pseudotumor cerebri in SLE a thrombotic event [letter]? J Rheumatol 1990;17:983–984.

415. Vidailhet M, Piette J-C, Wechsler B, et al. Cerebral venous thrombosis in systemic lupus erythematosus. Stroke 1990;21:1226–1231.

416. Al-Hakim M, Katirji MB, Osorio I, et al. Cerebral venous thrombosis in paroxysmal nocturnal hemogloblinuria. Report of two cases. Neurology 1993;43:742–746.

417. Hauser D, Barzilai N, Zalish M, et al. Bilateral papilledema with retinal hemorrhages in association with cerebral venous sinus thrombosis and paroxysmal nocturnal hemogloblinuria. Am J Ophthalmol 1996;122:592–593.

418. Case Records of the MGH. Case 20–1988. N Engl J Med 1988;318:1322–1328.

419. Cohen SM, Keltner JL. Thrombosis of the lateral transverse sinus with papilledema. Arch Ophthalmol 1993;111:274–275.

420. Cremer PD, Thompson EO, Johnston IH, et al. Pseudotumor cerebri and cerebral venous hypertension. Neurology 1996;47:1602–1603.

421. Kim AW, Trobe JD. Syndrome simulating pseudotumor cerebri caused by partial transverse venous sinus obstruction in metastatic prostate cancer. Am J Ophthalmol 2000;129:254–256.

422. Lam BL, Schatz NJ, Glaser JS, et al. Pseudotumor cerebri from cranial venous obstruction. Ophthalmology 1992;99:706–712.

423. Horton JC, Seiff SR, Pitts LH, et al. Decompression of the optic nerve sheath for vision-threatening papilledema caused by dural sinus occlusion. Neurosurgery 1992;31:203–212.

424. Angeli SI, Sato Y, Gantz BJ. Glomus jugulare tumors masquerading as benign intracranial hypertension. Arch Otolaryngol Head Neck Surg 1994;120:1277–1280.

425. Kikuchi M, Kudo S, Wada M, et al. Retropharyngeal rhabdomyosarcoma mimicking pseudotumor cerebri. Pediatr Neurol 1999;21:496–499.

426. Biousse V, Ameri A, Bousser M-G. Isolated intracranial hypertension as the only sign of cerebral venous thrombosis. Neurology 1999;53:1537–1542.

427. Ansari I, Crichlow B, Gunton KB, et al. A child with venous sinus thrombosis with initial examination findings of pseudotumor syndrome. Arch Ophthalmol 2002;120:867–869.

428. Lin A, Foroozan R, Danesh-Meyer HV, et al. Occurrence of cerebral venous sinus thrombosis in patients with presumed idiopathic intracranial hypertension. Ophthalmology 2006;113:2281–2284.

429. deVeber G, Andrew M, Adams C, et al. Cerebral sinovenous thrombosis in children. N Engl J Med 2001;345:417–423.

430. van den Bergh WM, van der Schaaf I, van Gijn J. The spectrum of presentations of venous infarction caused by deep cerebral vein thrombosis. Neurology 2005;65:192–196.

431. Kuehnen J, Schwartz A, Neff W, et al. Cranial nerve syndrome in thrombosis of the transverse/sigmoid sinuses. Brain 1998;121:381–388.

432. Crawford SC, Digre KB, Palmer CA, et al. Thrombosis of the deep venous drainage of the brain in adults. Arch Neurol 1995;52:1101–1108.

433. de Bruijn SF, Stam J. Randomized, placebo-controlled trial of anticoagulant treatment with low-molecular-weight heparin for cerebral sinus thrombosis. Stroke 1999;30: 484–488.

434. Crassard I, Bousser MG. Cerebral venous thrombosis. J Neuroophthalmol 2004;24: 156–163.

435. Stam J. Sinus thrombosis should be treated with anticoagulation. Arch Neurol 2008;65:984–985.

436. Horowitz M, Purdy P, Unwin H, et al. Treatment of dural sinus thrombosis using selective catheterization and urokinase. Ann Neurol 1995;38:58–67.

437. Stam J. Thrombosis of the cerebral veins and sinuses. N Engl J Med 2005;352:1791–1798.

438. Acheson JF, Green WT, Sanders MD. Optic nerve sheath decompression for the treatment of visual failure in chronic raised intracranial pressure. J Neurol Neurosurg Psychiatr 1994;57:1426–1429.

439. Cockerell OC, Lai HM, Ross-Russell RW. Pseudotumour cerebri associated with arteriovenous malformations. Postgrad Med J 1993;69:637–640.

440. Martin TJ, Bell DA, Wilson JA. Papilledema in a man with an "occult" dural arteriovenous malformation. J Neuroophthalmol 1998;18:49–52.

441. Chimowitz MI, Little JR, Awad IA, et al. Intracranial hypertension associated with unruptured cerebral arteriovenous malformations. Ann Neurol 1990;27:474–479.

442. Kühner A, Drastel A, Stoll W. Arteriovenous malformations of the transverse dural sinus. J Neurosurg 1976;45:12–19.

443. Cognard C, Gobin YP, Pierot L, et al. Cerebral dural arteriovenous fistulas. Clinical and angiographic correlation with a revised classification of venous drainage. Radiology 1995;194:671–680.

444. David CA, Peerless SJ. Pseudotumor syndrome resulting from a cerebral arteriovenous malformation: case report. Neurosurgery 1995;36:588–590.

445. Jozefowicz RF. Neurologic manifestations of pulmonary disease. Neurol Clin 1989;7: 605–616.

446. Kirkpatrick PJ, Meyer T, Sarkies N, et al. Papilloedema and visual failure in a patient with nocturnal hypoventilation [letter]. J Neurol Neurosurg Psychiatr 1994;57:1546–1547.

447. Waller EA, Bendel RE, Kaplan J. Sleep disorders and the eye. Mayo Clin Proc 2008;83: 1251–1261.

448. Wolin MJ, Brannon WL. Disk edema in an overweight woman. Surv Ophthalmol 1995;39:307–314.

449. Purvin VA, Kawasaki A, Yee RD. Papilledema and obstructive sleep apnea syndrome. Arch Ophthalmol 2000;118:1626–1630.

450. Fantin A, Feist RM, Reddy CV. Intracranial hypertension and papilloedema in chronic inflammatory demyelinating polyneuropathy. Br J Ophthalmol 1993;77:193.

451. Midroni G, Dyck PJ. Chronic inflammatory demyelinating polyradiculoneuropathy: unusual clinical features and therapeutic responses. Neurology 1996;46:1206–1212.

452. Ropper AH, Wijdicks EFM, Truax BT. Papilledema and pseudotumor cerebri. Clinical features of Guillain-Barré syndrome. In: Guillain-Barré Syndrome, pp 94–95. Philadelphia, F.A. Davis, 1991.

453. Michaud LJ, Ried SR, Liu GT, et al. Pseudotumor cerebri with loss of vision in Guillain-Barré syndrome [abstract]. Arch Phys Med Rehabil 1994;75:1050–1051.

454. Ersahin Y, Mutluer S, Yurtseven T. Hydrocephalus in Guillain-Barré syndrome. Clin Neurol Neurosurg 1995;97:253–255.

455. Weiss GB, Bajwa ZH, Mehler MF. Co-occurrence of pseudotumor cerebri and Guillain-Barré syndrome in an adult. Neurology 1991;41:603–604.

456. Gross FJ, Mindel JS. Pseudotumor cerebri and Guillain-Barré syndrome associated with human immunodeficiency virus infection. Neurology 1991;41:1845–1846.

457. Matzkin DC, Slamovits TL, Genis I, et al. Disc swelling. A tall tail? Surv Ophthalmol 1992;37:130–136.

458. Oikawa S, Kyoshima K, Takemae T, et al. Multiple spinal neurinomas presenting visual disturbance as the initial symptom: case report. Surg Neurol 1992;38:309–314.

459. Breen LA. Disk edema and peripheral neuropathy. Surv Ophthalmol 1994;38:467–474.

460. Phan TG, Krauss WE, Fealey RD. Recurrent lumbar ependymoma presenting as headache and communicating hydrocephalus. Mayo Clin Proc 2000;75:850–852.

461. Costello F, Kardon RH, Wall M, et al. Papilledema as the presenting manifestation of spinal schwannoma. J Neuroophthalmol 2002;22:199–203.

462. Ghazi NG, Jane JA, Lopes MB, et al. Capillary hemangioma of the cauda equina presenting with radiculopathy and papilledema. J Neuroophthalmol 2006;26:98–102.

463. Rekate HL. Why would a spinal tumor cause increased intracranial pressure? J Neuroophthalmol 2002;22:197–198.

464. Ko MW, Osborne B, Jung S, et al. Papilledema as a manifestation of a spinal subdural abscess. J Neurol Sci 2007;260:288–292.

465. Vaphiades MS, Eggenberger ER, Miller NR, et al. Resolution of papilledema after neurosurgical decompression for primary Chiari I malformation. Am J Ophthalmol 2002;133:673–678.

466. Avery RA, Shah SS, Licht DJ, et al. Reference range of cerebrospinal fluid opening pressure in children undergoing diagnostic lumbar puncture. NEJM (in press).

Vision loss: disorders of the chiasm

Chiasmal disorders are important in the differential diagnosis of anterior visual pathway dysfunction, particularly when the visual loss is gradually progressive. Involvement of the chiasm is suggested by (1) a monocular or bitemporal hemianopia or (2) visual loss of any type associated with endocrine dysfunction. The most common etiologies are compressive sellar masses, and therefore the diagnosis and management depends heavily on neuroimaging. These lesions produce visual acuity and field deficits by interfering with the optic nerves, chiasm, or optic tracts or, less often, by obstructing the third ventricle and causing chronic atrophic papilledema. Endocrinopathy is the result of pituitary, stalk, or hypothalamic dysfunction, while ocular motility abnormalities can result from lateral extension and involvement of the cavernous sinuses. Because sellar masses are so frequently associated with visual disturbances, neuro-ophthalmic evaluation often leads to their detection and is important for pretreatment assessment and subsequent follow-up.

Anatomic aspects of the chiasm and sellar and parasellar structures will be reviewed first, followed by a discussion of the neuro-ophthalmic signs and symptoms of chiasmal disease. Because of its clinical importance, pituitary and hypothalamic physiology also will be covered. The differential diagnosis of the various entities affecting the chiasm will then be discussed, in the context of the patient's age, clinical history, general physical findings, neuroimaging, and endocrine testing. Finally, the clinical features and treatment of these disorders will be detailed, with the greatest emphasis placed on the most common disorders: pituitary adenomas, craniopharyngiomas, meningiomas, aneurysms, and chiasmal/hypothalamic gliomas.

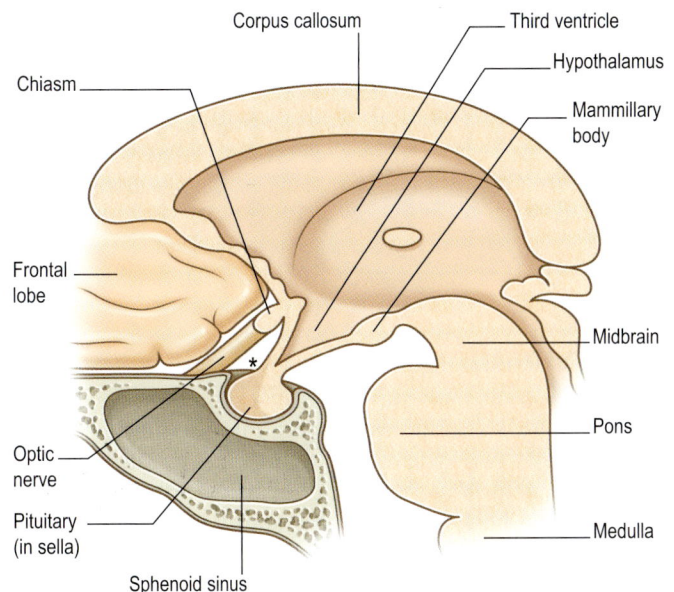

Figure 7–1. Sagittal view of the brain detailing the chiasm and surrounding structures. Note the optic nerves and chiasm rise at approximately 45 degrees. The chiasm lies in a cerebrospinal fluid-filled space called the suprasellar cistern (∗) bordered superiorly by the frontal lobe and inferiorly by the diaphragma sellae (which forms the roof of the sella above the pituitary gland). The chiasm is also located at the anterior and inferior part of the third ventricle, immediately inferior to the hypothalamus.

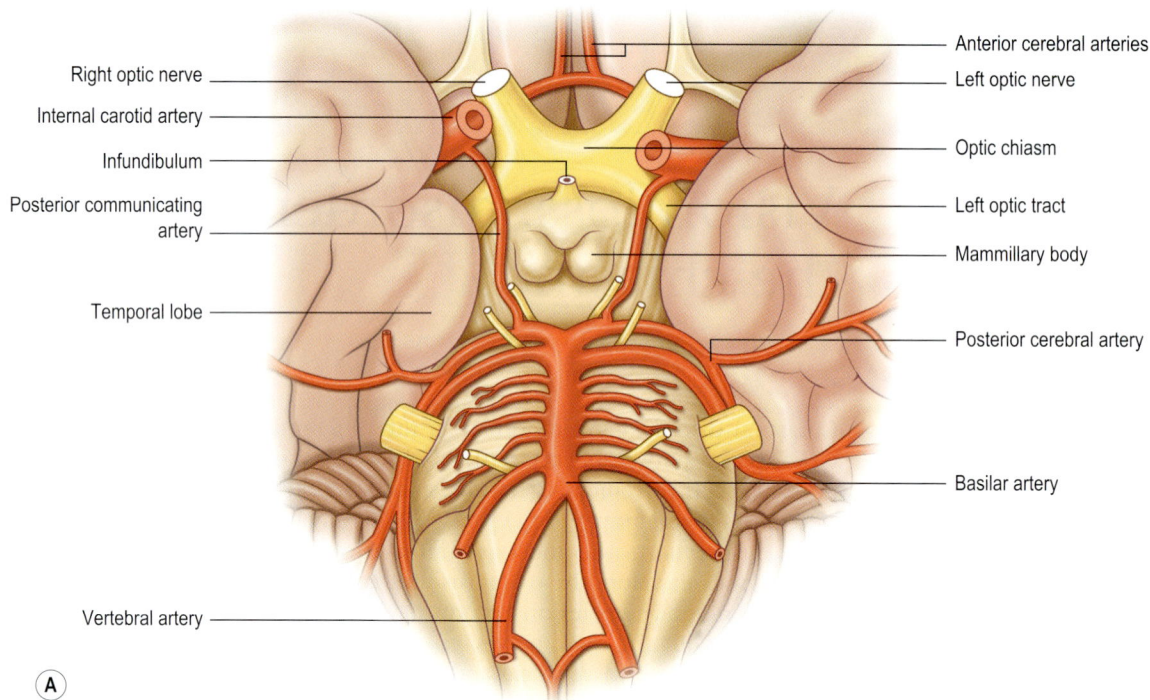

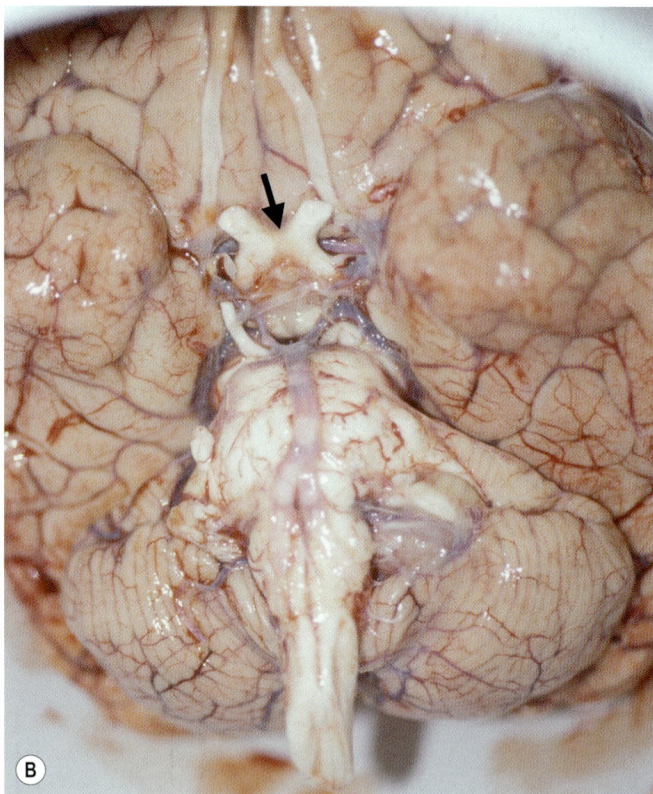

Figure 7–2. **A**. Ventral view of the brain detailing the chiasm and its relationship with the circle of Willis. Note the anterior cerebral and anterior communicating arteries lie superior (dorsal) to the optic nerves and chiasm, while the posterior communicating arteries lie inferior (ventral) to the chiasm and optic tracts. The infundibulum is immediately posterior to the body of the chiasm. **B**. Ventral side of autopsy specimen (view corresponds roughly to the drawing in part A). The arrow points to the chiasm.

Neuroanatomy

Intracranially, the optic nerves ascend and converge medially to join at the optic chiasm, which has the shape of the letter X when viewed from above or below. The chiasm tilts upward at an angle of 45 degrees and lies in the subarachnoid (cerebrospinal fluid (CSF) filled) space of the suprasellar cistern (**Fig. 7–1**). It is approximately 12 mm wide, 8 mm in anteroposterior diameter, and 4 mm thick.[1] Its posterior portion forms the anterior and inferior wall of the third ventricle. The chiasm lies inferior to the hypothalamus and third ventricle and anterior to the pituitary stalk (or infundibulum, which connects the hypothalamus and the pituitary) (**Fig. 7–2**). The pituitary gland sits 10 mm below the chiasm in a recess in the sphenoid bone called the sella turcica. The bony boundaries of the sella include the tuberculum sellae anteriorly, the dorsum sellae posteriorly, and

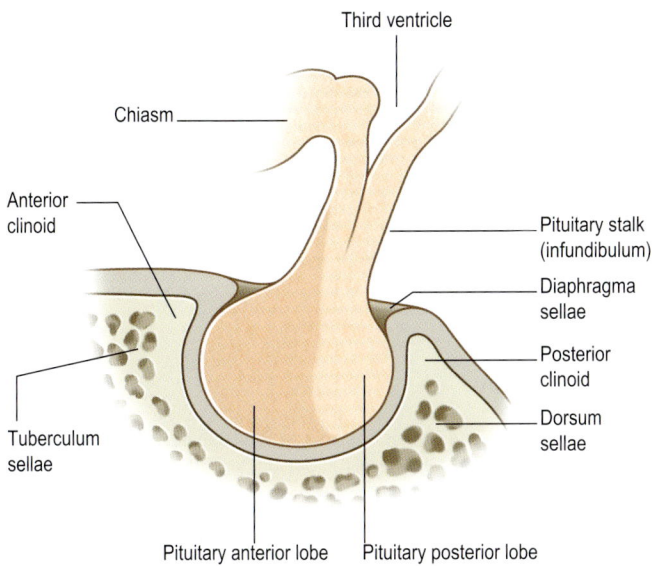

Figure 7–3. Sagittal view of the chiasm, pituitary gland, and sella.

the anterior and posterior clinoid processes superiorly (Fig. 7–3).[2] The cavernous sinuses, containing cranial nerves III, IV, V1, V2, and VI, the internal carotid arteries, and sympathetic fibers, form the lateral walls of the sella. The diaphragma sellae, penetrated only by the pituitary stalk, is a horizontal fold of dura mater which separates the pituitary gland from the suprasellar cistern (Fig. 7–3).[3] In 80% of individuals, the chiasm is located directly above the pituitary gland, while in 15% it lies over the tuberculum sellae (prefixed chiasm), and in 5% it is over the dorsum sellae (postfixed chiasm) (Fig. 7–4).[4–6]

Magnetic resonance imaging (MRI) provides exquisite detail of the sellar area (Fig. 7–5). Normally on T1-weighted MR coronal images the body of the chiasm has a dumbbell shape[7] and is located in the middle of the suprasellar cistern. More anteriorly the two optic nerves are visible; more posteriorly the chiasm lies sandwiched between the vertically oriented third ventricle above it and the pituitary stalk below it. On coronal images within the sella the pituitary gland appears flat, and the cavernous sinuses are lateral to it. The pituitary stalk and cavernous sinuses normally enhance with gadolinium. On sagittal sections, the tilted chiasm is easily identified above the pituitary. On T1-weighted images, the anterior pituitary is isointense with the pons, but the posterior portion of pituitary is bright.[8] Details of the chiasm and sellar region are less evident with CT scanning.[9]

At the chiasm, axons from the nasal retinal ganglion cells (temporal visual field) from both eyes cross, and the most ventral axons originating in the inferonasal retina bend temporarily up to 3 mm into axons of the contralateral optic nerve (Wilbrand's knee[10]) (Fig. 7–6). The knee's existence has been questioned[11,12] and one author attributed it to a histopathologic artifact of long-term monocular enucleation.[11] Fibers from the temporal retina (containing information from the nasal field) remain ipsilateral. The ratio of crossed to uncrossed fibers is 53:47. The fibers transmitting visual information from the superior retina remain superior in the chiasm; those from the inferior retina remain inferiorly situated. Approximately 90% of chiasmal fibers originate from the macula,[5] and, of these, those that cross lie superiorly and posteriorly within the chiasm.

Most of the ganglion cell axons travelling through the optic chiasm exit posteriorly and diverge to form the left and right optic tracts. Each tract is made up of ipsilateral temporal fibers and contralateral nasal fibers. In addition, retinal ganglion cell axons within the retinohypothalamic tract mediate the visual input responsible for diurnal variations of various neuroendocrine systems (circadian rhythms). These cells, which express melanopsin and respond to short-wavelength (blue) light, travel through the posterior chiasm then project to the hypothalamus, specifically the suprachiasmic nucleus or the supraoptic nucleus.[13]

The supraclinoid portions of the carotid arteries ascend lateral to the optic chiasm. The pre-communicating segments of the anterior cerebral arteries and the anterior communicating arteries are located anterior and superior (dorsal) to the chiasm. Because of the chiasm's upward tilt, the posterior portion of the circle of Willis lies behind and below it (ventral) (Fig. 7–2).[14] The chiasm derives its blood supply from an inferior and superior anastomotic group of vessels. The inferior group is made up of the superior hypophyseal arteries, which derive their blood supply from the internal carotid, posterior communicating, and posterior cerebral arteries. The superior group of vessels consists of pre-communicating branches of the anterior cerebral arteries.[14] There is evidence to suggest that the body of the chiasm receives its blood supply only from the inferior group, while the lateral parts of the chiasm are fed by branches from both inferior and superior groups.[15]

Neuro-ophthalmic symptoms and signs in chiasmal disorders

Visual symptoms

Because most chiasmal disturbances are caused by compressive lesions, the visual loss is usually insidious. Acute visual loss would imply a rapidly expanding mass, hemorrhage within a mass, or infectious, vascular, or inflammatory etiology, and these situations may mimic retrobulbar optic neuritis. Visual complaints are usually vague, often reflecting blurry or hazy vision or difficulty reading or focusing. Patients with slowly progressive chiasmal field loss may be without visual complaints unless acuity is abnormal, and a temporal field defect may not be apparent until the patient reads only the nasal half of the acuity chart. Others might describe double vision because of ocular motility dysfunction or difficulty aligning noncorresponding nasal fields (see Sensory double vision, below). Photophobia is a rare but reported visual symptom due to compressive lesions of the chiasm.[16]

Visual acuity, color vision, and afferent pupillary defects

When acuity is diminished, asymmetry is the rule.[5] Color vision may be altered only in defective fields, and asymmetric lesions may produce an afferent pupillary defect.

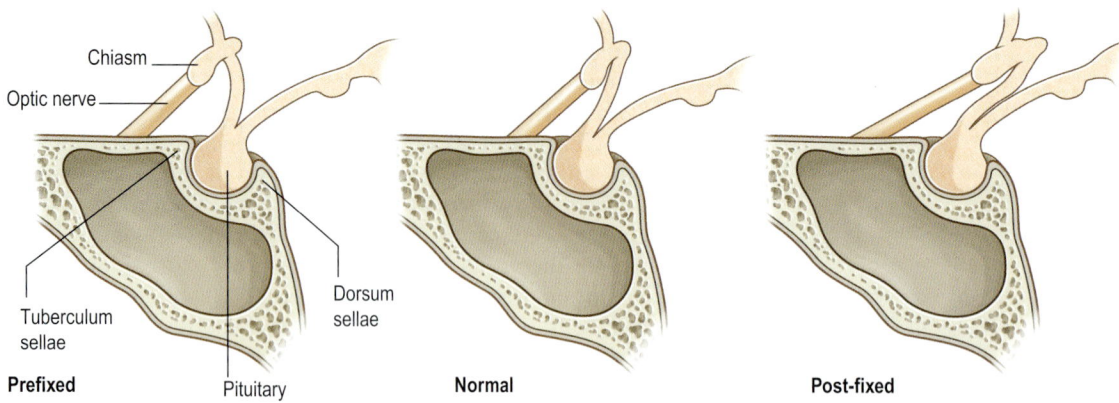

Figure 7–4. Relationship of the chiasm to the sella (sagittal views). Normally, in approximately 80% of individuals, the chiasm is directly above the pituitary gland. In 15% the chiasm is prefixed and over the tuberculum sella, and in the remaining 5% it is post-fixed and over the dorsum sella. (Redrawn from AL Rhoton, FS Harris, Renn WH. Neuro-ophthalmology Symposium of the University of Miami and the Bascom Palmer Eye Institute, JS Glaser (ed.), pp. 75–105. St. Louis, C.V. Mosby, 1973, with permission.)

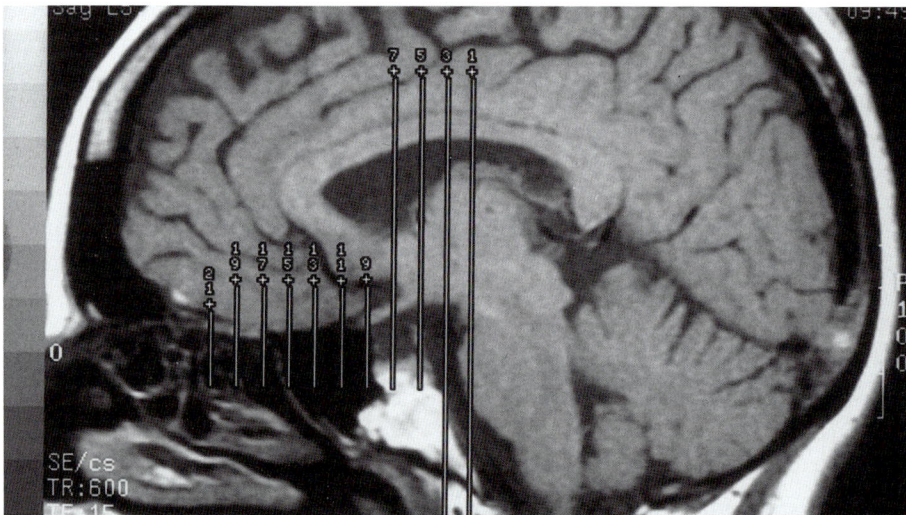

Figure 7–5. A. *Top:* Sagittal MRI (T1-weighted) through the chiasm (see Fig. 7–1 for corresponding illustration and labeling of structures. *Bottom:* Corresponding coronal sections (T1-weighted with gadolinium) through the optic nerves/anterior chiasm, body of chiasm, and posterior chiasm/optic tracts. The slice numbers are indicated in the sagittal image.

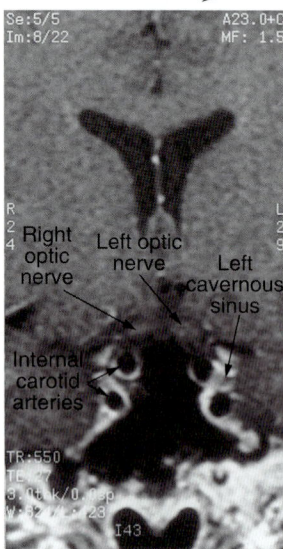

Slice 8. Optic nerves/ anterior chiasm

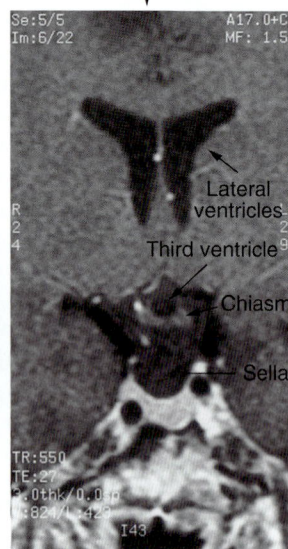

Slice 6. Body of chiasm

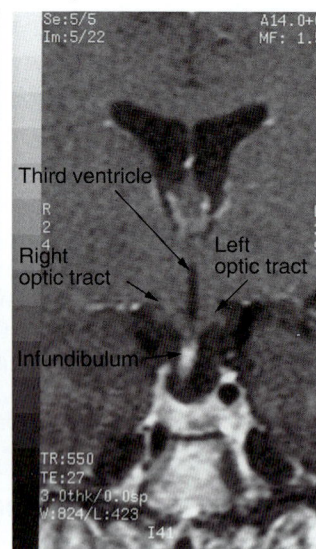

Slice 5. Posterior chiasm/ optic tracts

Ⓐ

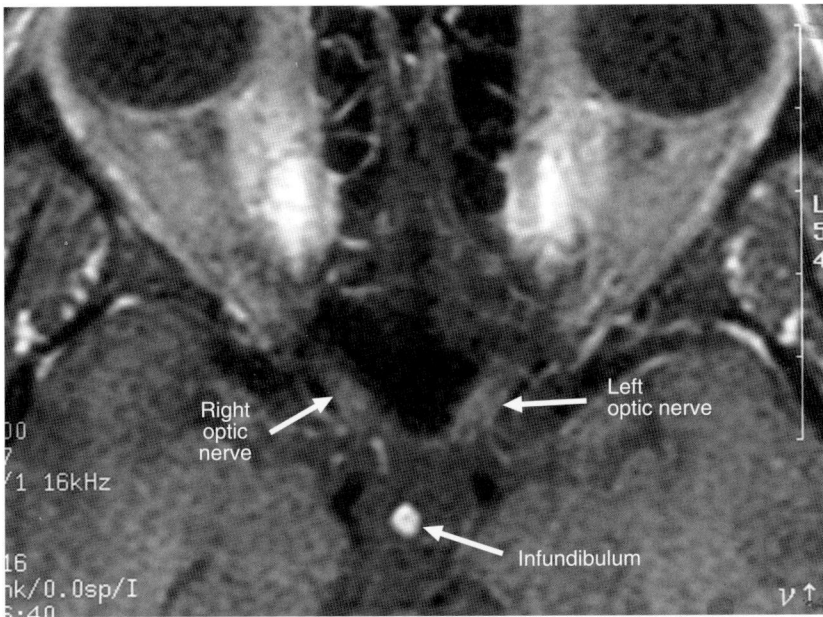

Anterior–inferior chiasm

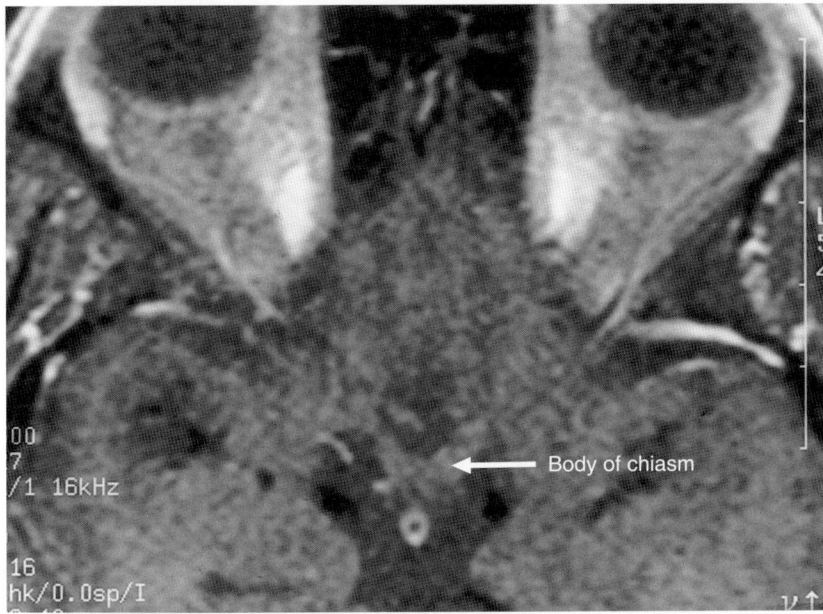

Mid-chiasm

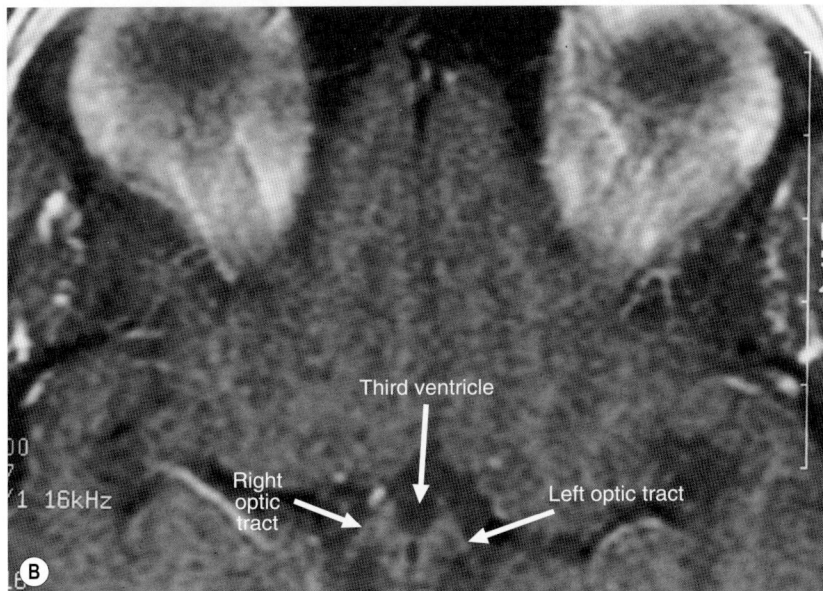

Posterior–superior chiasm

Figure 7–5. *Continued* **B**. Axial MRI scans (gadolinium enhanced) through the anterior–inferior, mid-, and posterior–superior chiasm.

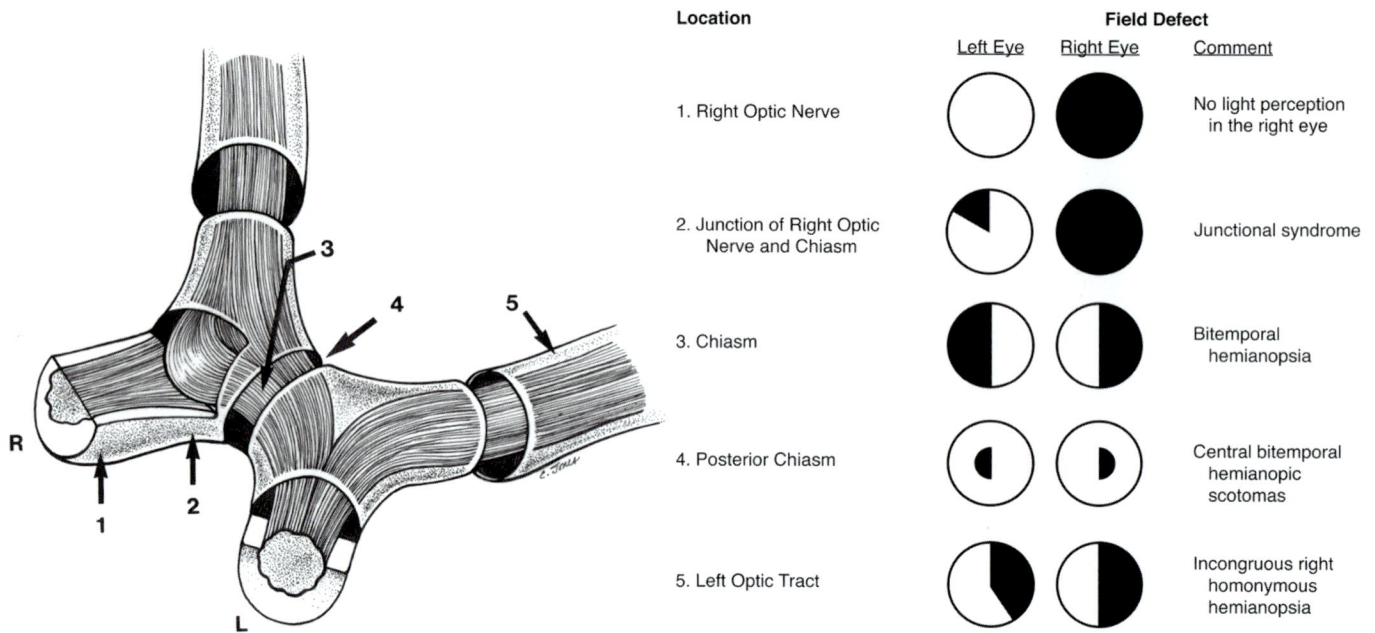

Figure 7–6. Optic chiasm: correlation of lesion site and field defect. Note the most ventral nasal fibers (mostly from inferior nasal retina) temporarily travel within the fellow optic nerve in Wilbrand's knee. (From Liu GT. Disorders of the eyes and eyelids. In: Samuels MA, Feske S (eds): The Office Practice of Neurology, p 46. New York, Churchill Livingstone, 1996, with permission. Adapted from Hoyt WF, Luis O, Arch Ophthalmol 1963;70:69–85, with permission (copyright 1963, American Medical Association).)

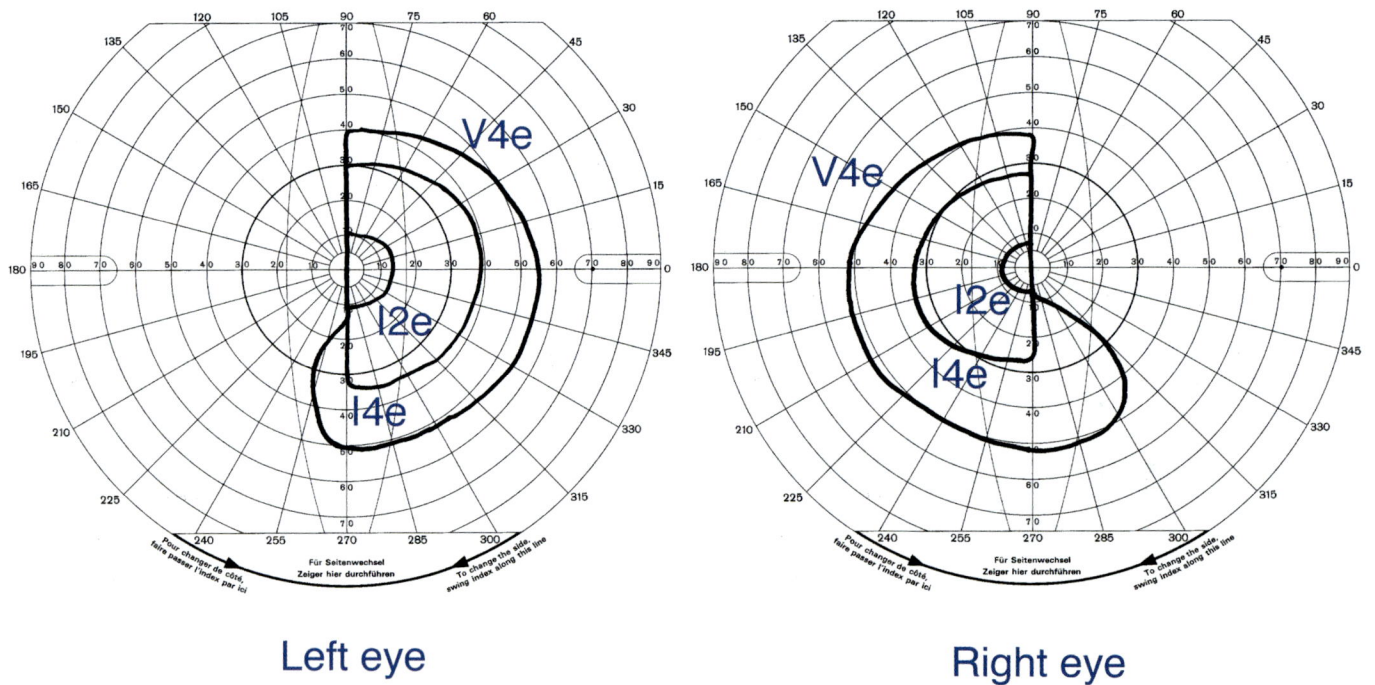

Figure 7–7. Bitemporal hemianopia documented on Goldmann perimetry in a patient with a craniopharyngioma compressing the chiasm from below. Note the preservation of a small amount of temporal field in each eye inferiorly, reflecting the sparing of some fibers in the superior portion of the chiasm.

Patterns of visual field loss

Temporal field defects respecting the vertical meridian, in one eye or both eyes, are the hallmarks of chiasmal dysfunction. The actual pattern of field loss depends on the chiasm's position and the exact location of the culprit lesion (**Fig. 7–6**). For instance, if the process affects the crossing nasal fibers in the body of the chiasm, in the case of sellar mass growing upward and impinging upon a normally situated chiasm, a classic bitemporal hemianopia is the result (**Fig. 7–7**). Incomplete and asymmetric bitemporal defects occur in the majority of cases (**Fig. 7–8**). Compression of the superior portion of the chiasm will result in visual field defects denser inferiorly (**Fig. 7–9**). More diffuse processes in this location can, of course, eventually cause nasal defects and acuity loss. However, it is a common observation that large

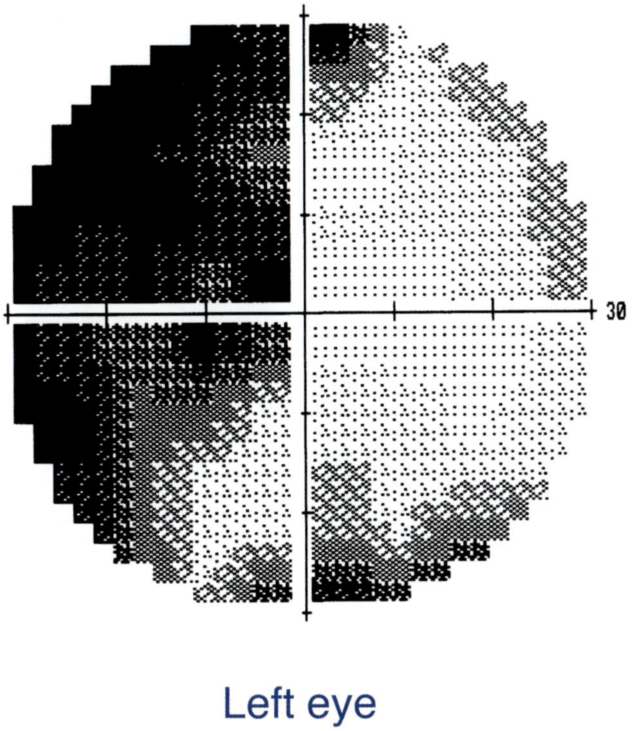

Left eye

Right eye

Figure 7–8. Incomplete, asymmetric bitemporal hemianopia, denser superiorly in each eye, documented on computerized threshold perimetry in a patient with inferior chiasmal compression by a pituitary adenoma.

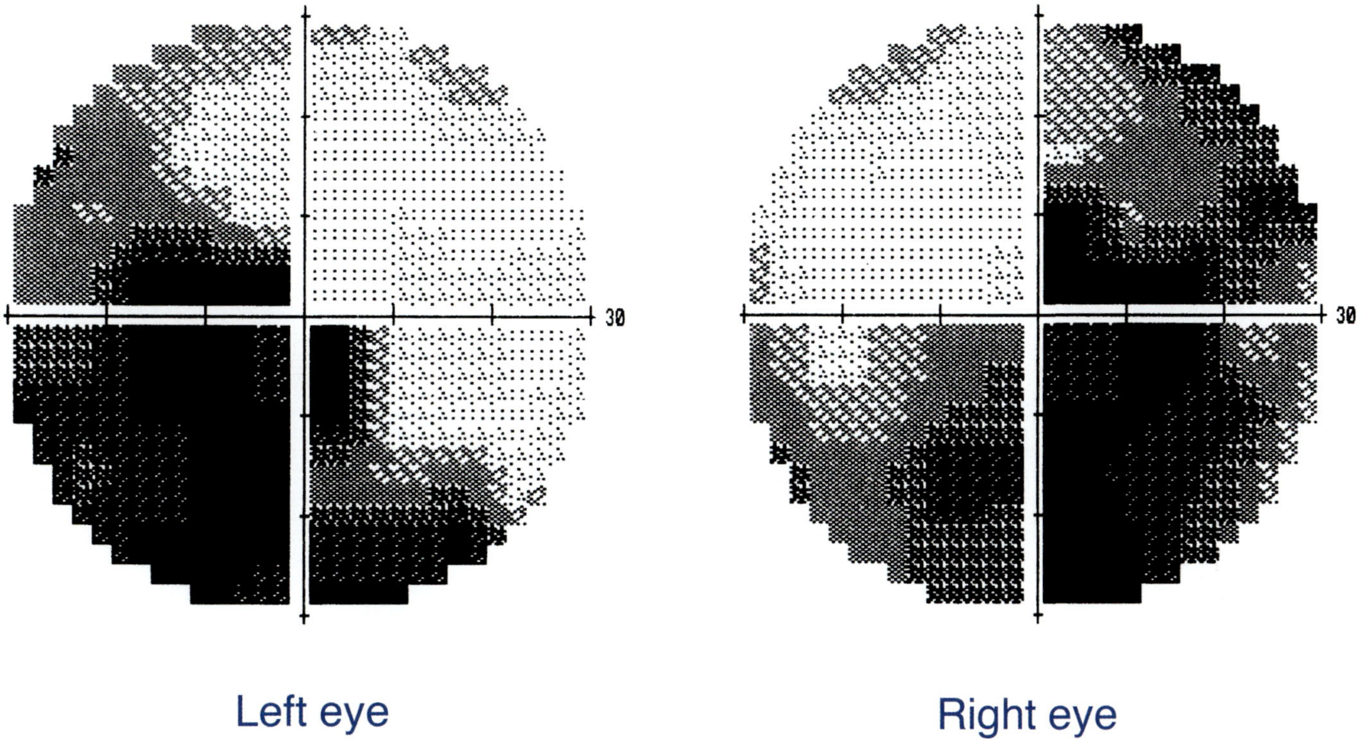

Left eye

Right eye

Figure 7–9. Computerized visual fields in a patient with an inferior bitemporal hemianopia, denser inferiorly in each eye, due to superior chiasmal compression by a craniopharyngioma.

sellar masses, despite compression, elevation, and flattening of the chiasm, as well as optic nerves and tracts in many instances, sometimes produce only a bitemporal hemianopia. It is unclear why the crossing fibers are so vulnerable. Mechanical distortion of nerve fiber bundles and impair-

ment of the extrinsic vascular supply are two possible explanations, but a combination of both is likely.[10,17] The crossing fibers may be more prone to deformation from a mass compressing the chiasm inferiorly.[18,19] Alternatively, an enlarging suprasellar mass might preferentially interrupt the inferior blood supply of the chiasm, affecting the body of the chiasm and crossing fibers,[15] and leave the more lateral and superior vascular supply of the lateral parts of the chiasm relatively spared. The relatively immediate improvement in visual fields following surgical decompression in some patients with chronic mass lesions is also enigmatic. In these instances, vascular compromise seems less likely than reversible axonal compression.

Patients with complete bitemporal hemianopias and *post-fixation blindness*[20] may have trouble performing near tasks and complain of abnormal depth perception. When the eyes converge on a near target, the blind temporal fields overlap behind it (**Fig. 7–10**). Objects behind the fixation point are therefore not seen. Affected patients will have difficulty threading a needle, for instance. One can investigate this by having the patient fixate on a near target, then test whether they see any objects directly behind it.

If the chiasm is post-fixed (**Fig. 7–4**) in relationship to a sellar mass, or the lesion affects the anterior portion of the chiasm, several patterns of field loss can be seen. Patients may present with a monocular arcuate or central scotoma if the process primarily affects one optic nerve, and these instances may be difficult to separate from glaucoma or optic neuritis. More characteristic of a chiasmal lesion is involvement of the ipsilateral optic nerve and Wilbrand's knee, resulting in a junctional scotoma.[21–23] This field deficit is characterized by a central scotoma or other optic nerve-related defect in the ipsilateral eye and a supratemporal defect in the other eye (**Fig. 7–11**). This pattern of visual field loss localizes to the proximal optic nerve whether Wilbrand's knee truly exists or not (see discussion above).[24] A monocu-

lar temporal field defect also localizes to the ipsilateral anterior chiasm and proximal optic nerve. Here a unilateral lesion is posterior enough to disrupt the ipsilateral crossing nasal fibers after they have segregated but is too anterior to involve the contralateral ones.[25] Since this pattern of field

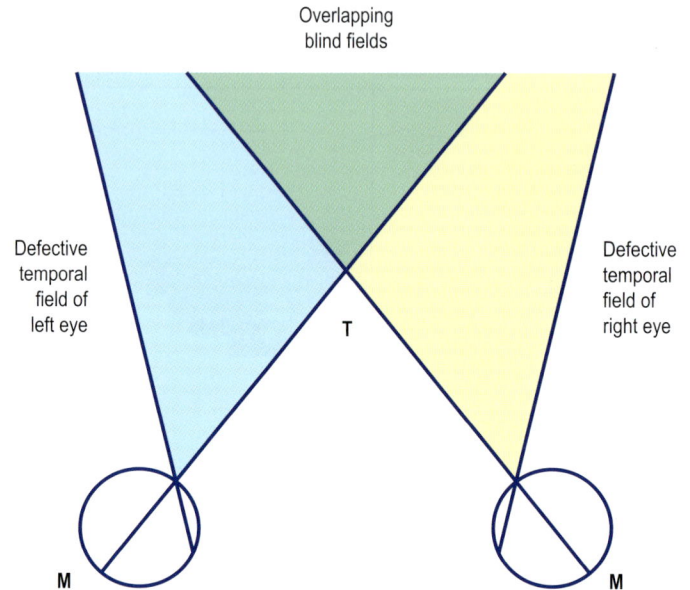

Figure 7–10. Post-fixation blindness associated with a complete bitemporal hemianopia. When the eyes converge and fix on a near target (T), the blind temporal fields overlap behind it. Objects directly behind the target are invisible. M, macula.

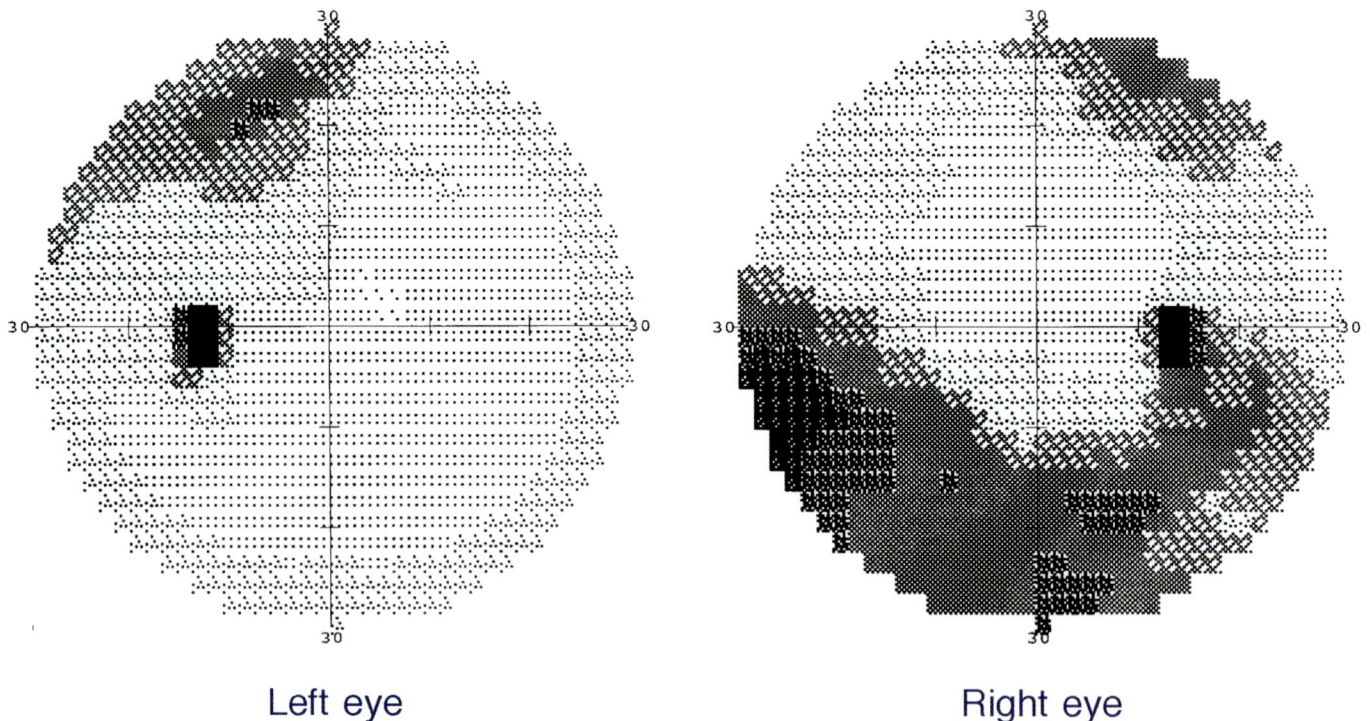

Left eye

Right eye

Figure 7–11. Junctional syndrome due to a pituitary adenoma affecting the anterior chiasm. The patient has an inferior arcuate defect in the right eye reflecting optic nerve dysfunction. The left eye has a superior temporal defect superiorly, owing to involvement of the Wilbrand's knee on the right.

loss is also often functional, patients with organic monocular temporal field defects should be distinguished by an associated ipsilateral afferent pupillary defect, sometimes with optic atrophy. Less commonly, a disturbance of the crossing nerve fiber bundle anteriorly may result in an arcuate scotoma emanating from the blind spot and ending abruptly at the vertical meridian (**Fig. 7–12**).[26] Central bitemporal hemianopic scotomas (**Fig. 7–13**) or optic tract syndromes may be the product of pre-fixed chiasms or more posteriorly situated lesions.

The examiner should be aware of processes which produce bitemporal defects which do not respect the vertical

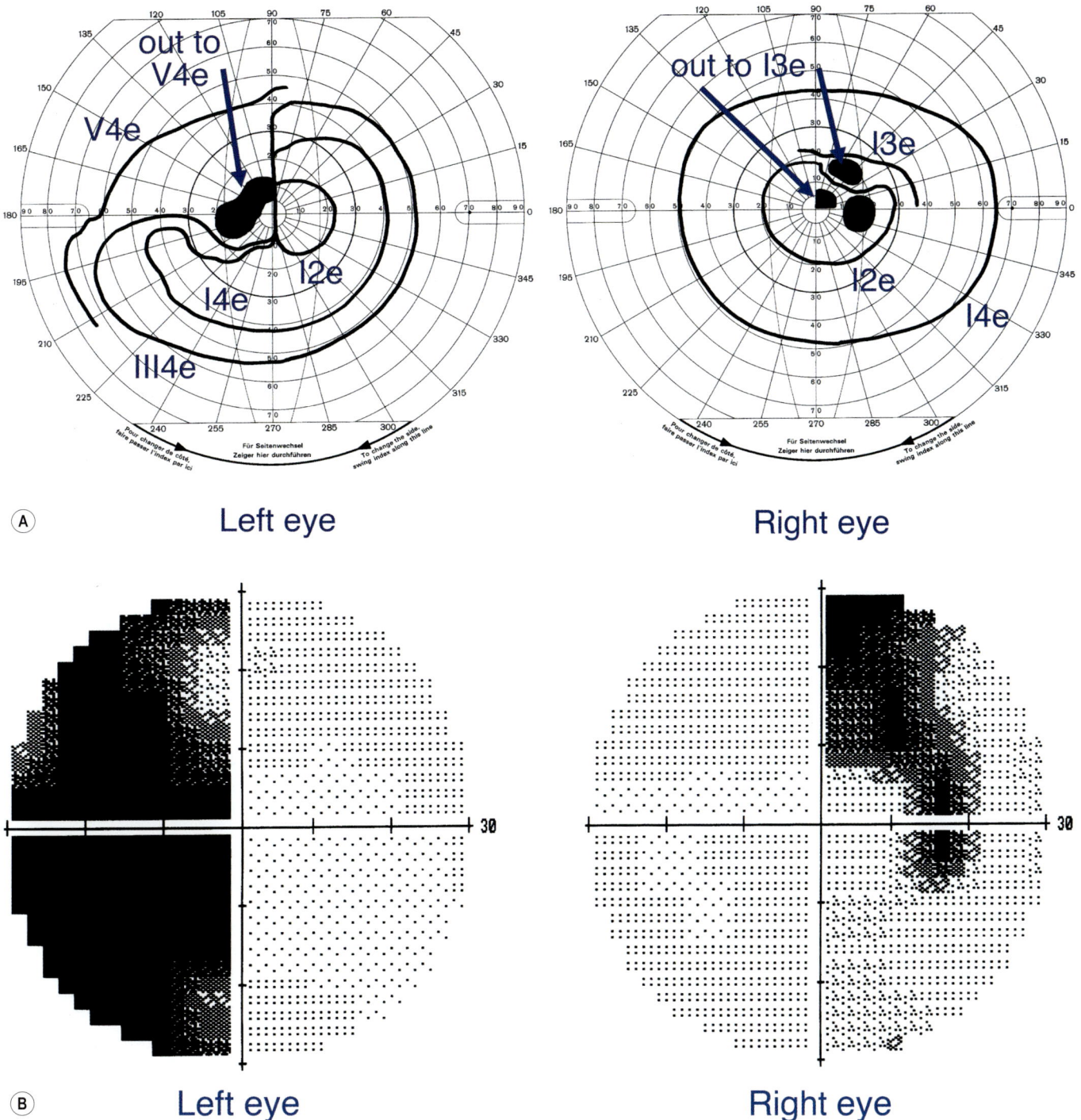

Figure 7–12. Arcuate scotomas in two patients ending abruptly at the vertical meridian due to chiasmal compression, a pattern that may result from a disturbance of the crossing optic nerve fibers anteriorly in the optic chiasm. **A**. Goldmann visual field demonstrating a superior bitemporal hemianopia due to tumor compression. A superior arcuate scotoma in the left eye respects the vertical meridian. **B**. Computerized visual field showing an asymmetric bitemporal hemianopia due to a prolactinoma compressing the chiasm from below. In the right eye a superior arcuate scotoma ends abruptly at the vertical meridian.

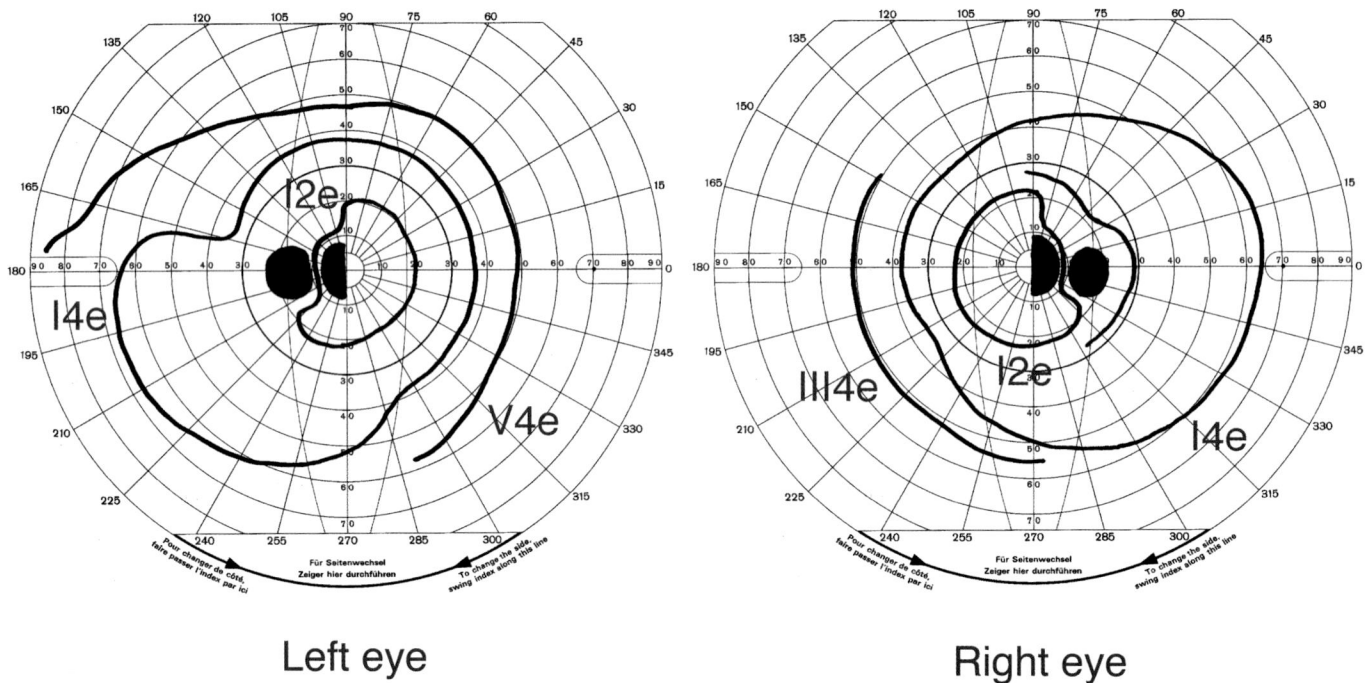

Left eye

Right eye

Figure 7–13. Goldmann visual field demonstrating central bitemporal hemianopic scotomas due to a posterior chiasmal lesion.

meridian. These include tilted or hypoplastic optic discs (see Chapter 5), sectoral (nasal) retinitis pigmentosa, and enlarged blind spots (see Chapter 6). In these cases, neuroimaging of the chiasm will be unremarkable.

Binasal defects respecting the vertical meridian due to chiasmal dysfunction are extremely unusual.[27] Theoretically this pattern can result from bilateral ectatic carotid artery compression of the lateral portions of the chiasm, compression from a variety of chiasmal region tumors, or from third ventricular enlargement (see below). Usually binasal defects have ocular causes such as glaucoma, retinitis pigmentosa, and ischemic optic neuropathy.[28] Uncommonly, altitudinal defects can occur when crossed and uncrossed fibers are affected equally by a process involving the inferior or superior portions of the chiasm.

Optic disc findings

Long-standing processes can lead to optic disc pallor, but this finding is variable and does not correlate with the degree of visual loss. Nevertheless, disc pallor and retinal nerve fiber layer loss[29,30] generally are associated with a poorer prognosis for visual improvement following treatment. Optic disc swelling in the setting of chiasmal dysfunction indicates either papilledema due to third ventricular compression by a sellar mass or an infiltrative or inflammatory process involving the anterior visual pathway. Cupping of the optic disc may occur due to chronic optic nerve compression.[31]

In patients with bitemporal hemianopias, a characteristic transverse "band" optic atrophy can result from chiasmal compression of crossing nasal fibers.[32] In each eye, ganglion cells and their axons degenerate in the blind nasal hemiretina, leading to a nasal wedge of optic atrophy. Fibers from the blind nasal half of the macula are similarly affected, resulting in a temporal wedge of optic atrophy. The nerve

fibers coming from "seeing" temporal macula and retina, entering the disc superiorly and inferiorly, are preserved.

Hemifield slide phenomena

Rarely, patients with complete bitemporal hemianopias may have odd complaints caused by an inability to align the noncorresponding nasal visual fields of each eye (hemifield slide phenomena[20]) (**Fig. 7–14**). With a hypertropia, a patient may describe vertical misalignment or slippage of nasal fields. In contrast, esodeviated eyes can result in horizontal separation of nasal fields. Exodeviated eyes may cause overlap of nasal fields and so-called nonparetic double vision.[33] One can test for these phenomena in patients with horizontal deviations by drawing a line of small dots or circles, then asking the patient to look quickly at the center of them and tell the examiner how many he or she sees (**Fig. 7–15**).

Eye movement abnormalities

Ocular motor palsies and nystagmoid eye movements can be associated with chiasmal disorders but are uncommon. Chiasmal field loss accompanied by an ocular motor palsy implies cavernous sinus involvement, sometimes also suggested by facial pain or numbness resulting from trigeminal nerve dysfunction. The sellar process which most commonly affects both the chiasm and cavernous sinuses, with overt clinical manifestations, is pituitary apoplexy (see below).

See-saw nystagmus can be a sign of a chiasmal process, and sellar masses and trauma are the usual culprits. In this unique motility disturbance one eye elevates and intorts while the other depresses and extorts, then vice versa in a pendular fashion (see **Fig. 17–13**).[34] The exact mechanism

Video 17.

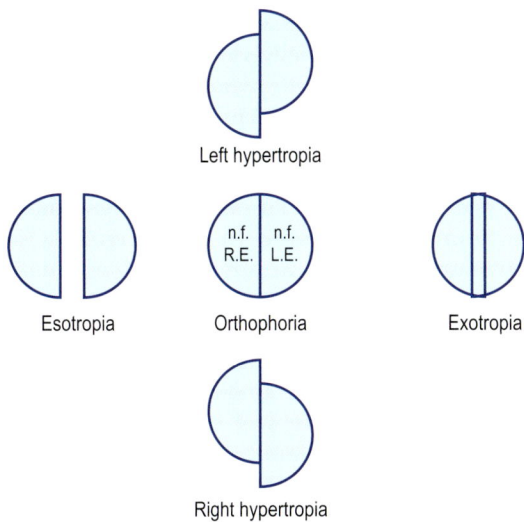

Figure 7–14. Hemifield slide phenomena associated with complete bitemporal hemianopias. The diagrams depict the visual fields from the patient's perspective with both eyes open (cyclopean view). If the eyes are orthophoric (no misalignment), then the nasal fields will align properly. n.f.R.E., nasal field of the right eye; n.f.L.E., nasal field of the left eye. However, because the nasal fields are noncorresponding, affected individuals will be unable to compensate for any tendency for ocular misalignment, and the nasal fields will drift if there is a hypertropia, esotropia, or exotropia.

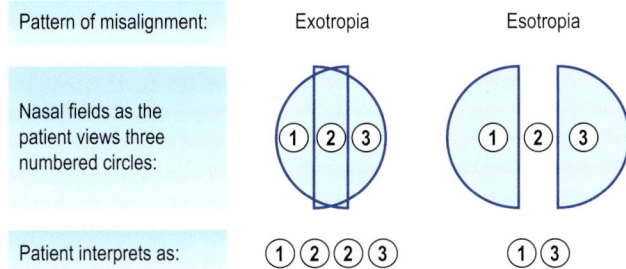

Figure 7–15. Sensory double vision and hemifield slide phenomena associated with complete bitemporal hemianopias. The diagrams depict the visual fields from the patient's perspective with both eyes open. As described in **Fig. 7–14**, if a patient with a bitemporal hemianopia and an exotropia views three numbered circles, he might think he is seeing four circles. The no. 2 circle is contained in each nasal field and is therefore duplicated ("double vision"). A patient with an esotropia might actually see only two of the circles, because neither nasal field contains the no. 2 circle.

is unclear, but almost all patients with acquired see-saw nystagmus have either a bitemporal hemianopia or bilateral involvement of the interstitial nuclei of Cajal (inC) in the mesencephalon.[35] Most sellar masses which exhibit see-saw nystagmus are large, causing both the field defect and midbrain compression. However, each factor by itself is sufficient for the development of this motility disorder. Patients with see-saw nystagmus and chiasmal trauma, for instance, usually have a bitemporal hemianopia, while those with midbrain infarction or hemorrhage involving the inC have no visual loss. Proposed explanations relating the bitemporal hemianopia and see-saw nystagmus include: (1) a tor-

sional adaptive process which attempts to increase the overlap of noncorresponding nasal fields[36] and (2) disruption of the visuovestibular connections between retina and inferior olive.[35] Rare achiasmatic and hemichiasmatic individuals, who may have normal fields, can also have see-saw nystagmus (see Anomalies of the chiasm, below).[37,38] See-saw nystagmus is also discussed in Chapter 17.

Asymmetric or monocular nystagmus

Young children with sellar masses such as gliomas or craniopharyngiomas in unusual instances may present with monocular or asymmetric nystagmus when the chiasm is involved. Sometimes the full triad of nystagmus, head nodding, and head tilt is present, mimicking the benign symptom complex of spasmus nutans.[39] Usually those with intracranial lesions will have reduced vision, optic atrophy, strabismus, or diencephalic syndrome,[40] and these findings will convince the examiner that neuroimaging should be performed. The mechanism by which sellar masses produce the motility disorder is not clear. For a more detailed discussion of spasmus nutans and its imitators, the reader is referred to the chapter on nystagmus and nystagmoid eye movements (Chapter 17).

Video 17.5

Visual field testing

Patients with suspected chiasmal disorders should undergo careful documentation of visual fields in addition to the neuro-ophthalmic examination. Subtle superior temporal defects respecting the vertical meridian may be the first sign of a compressive sellar mass, so examiners should look carefully in these areas.[41] Goldmann kinetic perimetry may be necessary in poorly cooperative patients and those with severe visual loss. However, we prefer computerized threshold perimetry in most patients with chiasmal disturbances, as they likely will require serial field examinations to monitor disease activity. We do not advocate the use of visual-evoked potentials (VEPs)[42] in the evaluation or follow-up of patients with chiasmal disorders.

Endocrine disturbances associated with chiasmal disorders

Pituitary gland, hormone physiology, and endocrinopathy

Traditionally, the pituitary gland is separated into the anterior (adenohypophysis) and posterior (neurohypophysis) lobes (see **Fig. 7–3**).[8] Laterally, the adenohypophysis contains cells which secrete prolactin and growth hormone (GH), while cells which produce thyroid-stimulating hormone (TSH), follicle-stimulating hormone (FSH), luteinizing hormone (LH), and adrenocorticotropic hormone (ACTH) are located medially. The hormones vasopressin (or antidiuretic hormone (ADH)) and oxytocin are synthesized in the supraoptic and periventricular nuclei in the hypothalamus, then transported to the posterior lobe via long axons within the pituitary stalk.

Prolactin stimulates production of breast milk in women. GH stimulates liver production of insulin-like growth factor I (IGF-I, also called somatomedin C). Corticotropin (ACTH) causes adrenal secretion of both cortisol and androgens. TSH stimulates thyroid production of triiodothyronine (T_3) and thyroxine (T_4). In women, FSH and LH lead to estradiol and progesterone secretion, folliculogenesis, and ovulation, while, in men, these two hormones stimulate testosterone secretion and spermatogenesis.[43] Hormone secretion in the adenohypophysis is regulated in part by proteins produced in the hypothalamus and brought to the pituitary via the hypophyseal portal venous system (**Fig. 7–16**). Dopamine tonically inhibits prolactin secretion, for example. End-organ hormone levels confer additional regulation by modulating the production of pituitary and hypothalamic releasing hormones. ADH, released in the neurohypophysis, stimulates free-water reabsorption in the collecting ducts of the kidney. Oxytocin stimulates uterine contraction and milk ejection.[43]

Because of the chiasm's proximity to the pituitary, stalk, and hypothalamus, chiasmal disorders, especially those due to mass lesions, often present concomitantly with endocrine dysfunction. In this setting, the endocrinopathies usually fall into two major categories: pituitary hormone deficiency (hypopituitarism) and hypersecretion. Hypopituitarism can be the result of compression of normal pituitary tissue, impaired blood flow of normal tissue, or interference with hypothalamic production or delivery of releasing hormones.[43] Symptoms consistent with hypopituitarism, which can vary according to sex, are outlined in **Table 7–1**. Of these, the most common are those associated with GH deficiency, but the most salient clinical features of hypopituitarism actually vary with age. In children, failure of normal linear growth is the dominant symptom; in adolescence, it is delayed sexual maturation; and in adults, it is secondary hypogonadism.[44]

On the other hand, pituitary hormone excess generally is caused either by hypersecreting pituitary adenomas or by target organ failure with secondary hypersecretion. In the one exception, mild degrees of hyperprolactinemia can be associated with hypothalamic dysfunction or stalk compression, both of which result in decreased delivery of dopamine, which normally inhibits prolactin secretion, to the pituitary gland. Clinical features of pituitary hormone hypersecretion due to adenomas are highlighted in **Table 7–2**. When chiasmal dysfunction due to a sellar mass is present, hypopituitarism is more common than hypersecretion, but patients can have elements of one or both (for instance, when a hypersecreting adenoma compresses and compromises adjacent normal pituitary tissue).

Hypopituitarism can also be an unavoidable side-effect of surgery or irradiation of sellar lesions. Thus, before and

Table 7–1 Typical features of hypopituitarism due to hypothalamic/pituitary dysfunction.[43,580] See text for explanation of abbreviations

	Hormones affected	**In women**	**In men**	**In women and men**
Hypogonadism	↓ or nl LH ↓ or nl FSH ↓ estradiol in women ↓ testosterone in men	Oligomenorrhea or amenorrhea Dyspareunia Vaginal dryness	↓ facial and body hair Testicular atrophy Erectile dysfunction Gynecomastia	↓ libido
Hypoprolactinemia	↓ prolactin	Failure to start and maintain lactation		
Hypothyroidism	↓ or nl TSH ↓ T_3, T_4			Fatigue, weakness, inability to lose weight, puffiness, constipation, cold intolerance, memory impairment, altered mentation, bradycardia, delayed relaxation of deep tendon reflexes
Growth hormone deficiency	↓ GH, IGF-I			Short stature in children ↓ vigor, ↓ exercise tolerance ↓ body muscle:fat ratio
Hypoadrenalism	↓ or nl ACTH ↓ cortisol	Loss of axillary and pubic hair		Fatigue and malaise, postural hypotension, pallor, anorexia, and nausea
Diabetes insipidus	↓ ADH			Polyuria Polydipsia Hypernatremia
Oxytocin deficiency		↓ milk ejection during lactation		

nl, normal.

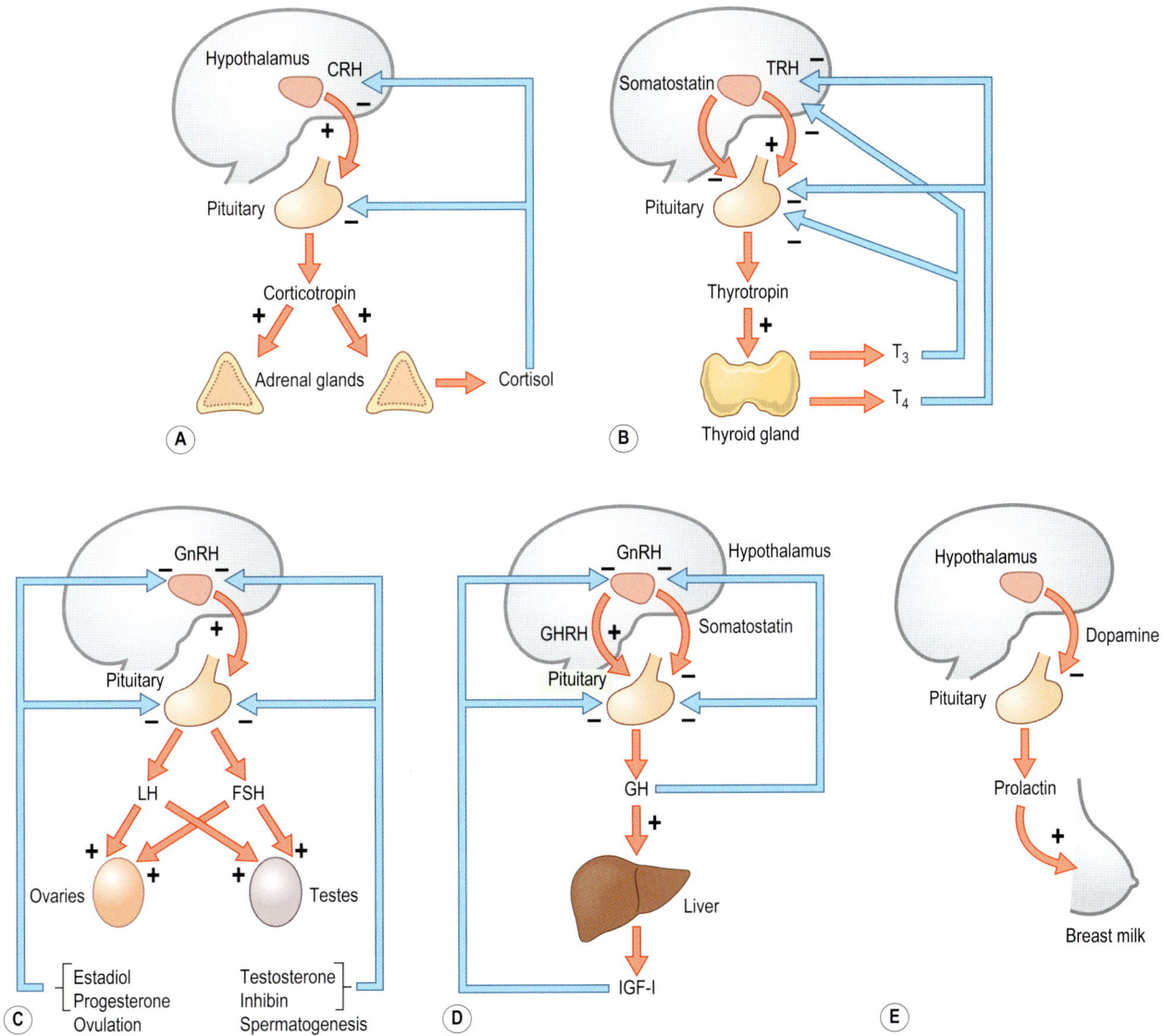

Figure 7–16. Interactions among the hypothalamus, pituitary, and target glands. **A**. The hypothalamic–pituitary–adrenal axis. **B**. The hypothalamic–pituitary–thyroid axis. **C**. The hypothalamic–pituitary–gonadal axis. **D**. The regulation of growth hormone (GH) secretion. **E**. The regulation of prolactin secretion. CRH, corticotropin-releasing hormone; TRH, thryrotropin-releasing hormone; T_3, triiodothyronine; T_4, thryroxine; GnRH, gonadotropin-releasing hormone; LH, luteinizing hormone; FSH, follicle-stimulating hormone; GHRH, growth hormone-releasing hormone; and IGF-I, insulin-like growth factor I. Plus signs denote stimulation, and minus signs inhibition.[43] Redrawn with permission from N Engl J Med 1994; 330: 1652.

Table 7–2 Typical features of hypersecreting syndromes associated with pituitary adenomas. See text for details and explanation of abbreviations

	Hormones affected	In women	In men	In women and men
Hyperprolactinemia	↑ prolactin	Amenorrhea Oligomenorrhea Infertility	Impotence Gynecomastia	↓ libido Galactorrhea (rare in men)
Growth hormone excess	↑ GH, IGF-I			Acromegaly Gigantism (children)
ACTH excess (Cushing disease)	↑ or nl ACTH ↑ cortisol	Oligomenorrhea Amenorrhea	↓ libido	Sudden weight gain Moon facies Buffalo hump Hypertension Hirsuitism Acne Glucose intolerance Muscle wasting and weakness[54]
Hyperthyroidism	↑ or nl TSH ↑ T_3, T_4			Thyrotoxicosis Goiter

Excess LH/FSH	↑ or nl LH
	↑ or nl FSH
	↑ or nl estradiol in women
	↑ testosterone in men
	  (variable)
		Amenorrhea
		Oligomenorrhea
				Precocious puberty in
				  childhood
				↓ libido in adults

nl, normal.

following treatment in many instances, hormone replacement will be required because cortisol and thyroxine are necessary for life, uncontrolled diabetes insipidus can be life-threatening, and gonadotropin deficiency is associated with osteoporosis and impaired reproductive and sexual functions. It is not uncommon for patients with sellar processes to require replacement regimens consisting of various combinations of corticosteroid, thyroxine, GH (in children), estrogen (for women), testosterone (for men), and DDAVP (desmopressin; 1-deamino-8-arginine vasopressin).

Hypothalamic syndromes

Two childhood endocrinopathies, Russell's diencephalic syndrome[45] and precocious puberty, are the most important clinical syndromes associated with hypothalamic lesions in the pediatric age group. The diencephalic syndrome has a typical age of onset between the newborn period to 4 years of age[46] and is characterized by emaciation, hyperkinesis, and euphoria (**Fig. 7–17**). The weight loss is the most salient trait, and it occurs after initially normal weight gain. Children are often evaluated for failure to thrive.[47] Linear growth and head circumference are unaltered.[48] An alert appearance (due to lid retraction), vomiting, pallor, and nystagmus are other common features.[49] Optic atrophy occurs in approximately one-quarter.[49] Hypothalamic chiasmal gliomas are the usual cause, and anterior hypothalamic dysfunction is one proposed mechanism for the syndrome.[49]

Precocious puberty is seen in boys more commonly than in girls, and affected children are tall for age and exhibit early gonadal maturation. Responsible lesions typically lie in the floor of the third ventricle, posterior hypothalamus, tuber cinereum, or median eminence. Common etiologies in these areas include hamartomas of the tuber cinereum, hypothalamic gliomas, and suprasellar germ cell tumors.[50] There may be several mechanisms, each resulting in a premature onset of puberty. Germ cell tumors, for instance (see below), produce β-human chorionic gonadotropin, which stimulates Leydig cells. Alternatively, hypothalamic infiltration might cause increased secretion of gonadotropin-releasing hormone.[46]

In children and adults following surgery in the hypothalamic region, for example for treatment of craniopharyngioma, weight gain and obesity are common. This likely results from injury to satiety centers in the hypothalamus.

Diagnosis/approach

It is often difficult on the basis of the neuro-ophthalmic signs and symptoms alone to arrive at the specific pathologic diagnosis. The visual complaints and field patterns facilitate chiasmal localization, but are usually nondiagnostic with regards to etiology. Only in rare instances, such as progressive superior bitemporal field deficits due to an expanding pituitary adenoma, does the pattern of visual loss suggest a specific entity. Rather, once a chiasmal disorder is suspected on neuro-ophthalmic grounds, the diagnosis is best established by considering the patient's age, clinical history, general physical findings, neuroimaging results, and endocrine testing.

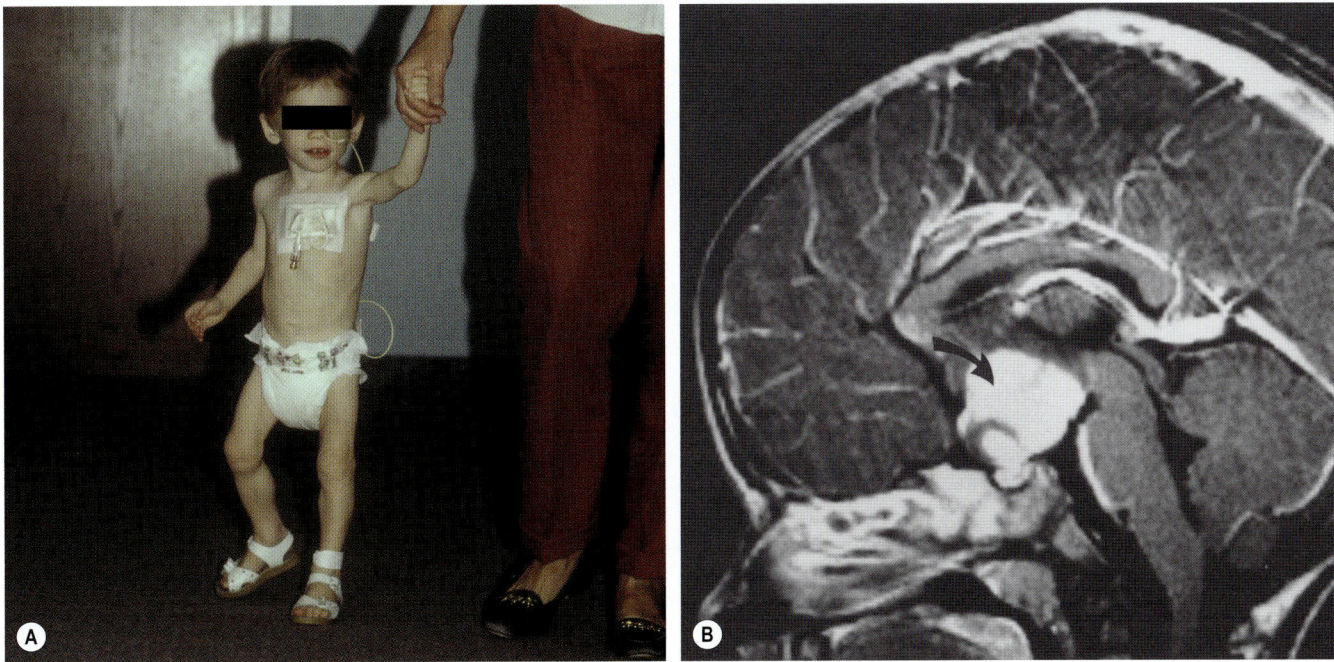

Figure 7–17. A. A young girl with emaciation as part of Russell's diencephalic syndrome due to a hypothalamic glioma, demonstrated in a contrast-enhanced MRI (**B**); arrow points to the lesion.

Age

Most chiasmal disorders are due to compressive lesions, many of which have a tendency to occur more frequently either in (1) children and young adults or in (2) middle age and elderly individuals. **Table 7–3** outlines the differential diagnosis of most sellar and suprasellar processes, based upon age predilection and frequency. In general, tumors and masses of congenital derivation are more common in childhood, and rarer vascular processes and metastases in late adulthood. The inflammatory, infectious, and infiltrative disorders occur at all ages.

Clinical history

Both the rate of onset of symptoms and presence and quality of endocrine features will be important. Because the most common etiology is a compressive sellar mass, most visual and endocrine symptoms will be insidious. Acute chiasmal syndromes can occur when tumors enlarge suddenly, due to cyst expansion or intratumor hemorrhage, as in pituitary apoplexy. However, sudden chiasmal field loss might also suggest chiasmal neuritis, ischemia, or an intrinsic vascular malformation. Patients should also be questioned about double vision or difficulty with depth perception.

Historical features suggestive of endocrine dysfunction should be investigated. In particular, the patient should be asked about symptoms consistent either with hypopituitarism or with pituitary hormone hypersecretion. While the former could be due to any sellar mass, the latter suggests a pituitary adenoma. Other types of endocrine dysfunction, such as diabetes insipidus, are characteristic of sellar sarcoidosis and germinoma, for instance. However, diabetes insipidus may be seen in many other suprasellar processes.

General physical findings

The examiner should look for evidence of endocrine dysfunction, and in some cases the diagnosis can be made on physical findings alone. Patients with gynecomastia, Cushingoid features, or acromegaly, for example, might harbor hypersecreting pituitary adenomas. Precocious puberty suggests hypothalamic dysfunction, while growth retardation might be due to GH deficiency. Features of neurofibromatosis, such as café au lait spots and neurofibromas, should also be excluded because of its association with optic pathway gliomas.

Diagnostic studies/neuroimaging

All patients suspected of having a chiasmal disorder should undergo enhanced and unenhanced MRI with special attention to the sellar area, including axial and 3 mm coronal and sagittal sections. If the clinical history and findings on examination suggest chronicity (long duration of symptoms and optic disc pallor, for example), neuroimaging can be performed over the next day or two. However, either sudden visual loss, indicating an acute process, or optic disc swelling, a sign of possible hydrocephalus, are indications for emergent scanning. MRI is far superior to computed tomography (CT) in the evaluation of this region because it provides excellent anatomic detail, sagittal views, and better soft-tissue imaging. The only disadvantage of MRI in this regard is its inability to demonstrate small amounts of calcification and changes in the sellar walls, which are made of cortical bone and separate the pituitary gland and cavernous sinuses. When MRI is contraindicated or intolerable, CT scanning can still be useful, especially if contrast images and coronal views (thin 1.5 mm sections) can be obtained.

Table 7–3 Sellar and suprasellar processes which can affect the chiasm, according to age group, etiology, and frequency. Adapted from Liu GT. In: Samuels MA, Feske S (eds): The Office Practice of Neurology, pp 40–74. New York, Churchill Livingston, 1995, with permission

Age group	More common	Less common
Pediatric–young adult	Chiasmal–hypothalamic glioma Craniopharyngioma	Arteriovenous malformation Dermoid Germ cell tumors 　Germinoma 　Teratoma 　Nongerminoma Lymphocytic hypophysitis Pituitary adenoma Suprasellar arachnoid cyst
Middle age–elderly	Pituitary adenoma Meningioma Craniopharyngioma Aneurysm (internal carotid)	Choristomas Empty sella syndrome Epidermoids Infarction Malignant optic glioma Metastases to chiasm, sella, 　or suprasellar region Pituitary apoplexy Rathke's cleft cyst Sphenoid sinus mucocele
No particular age predilection		Histiocytosis Meningitis 　Bacterial 　Tuberculous Sarcoidosis

In some instances CT scanning is adjunctive to MRI by outlining bony landmarks and possibly their erosion by a sellar mass. CT scanning can also identify calcification within suspected sellar lesions. When aneurysms are suspected because of MRI or CT findings, an MRI angiogram or a conventional angiogram is necessary.

Intrinsic disorders of the chiasm will be suggested by radiographically demonstrated chiasmal enlargement, signal abnormality, or gadolinium enhancement. Extrinsic compression will be evident if there is a mass lesion and distortion or displacement of the chiasm.

Diagnostic studies/endocrine testing

The outpatient endocrinologic panel should include serum prolactin, serum early morning cortisol, TSH, T4, LH, FSH, estradiol (in women), and testosterone (in men) levels. Other tests which should be ordered include GH (after a 75 g oral glucose load), insulin-like growth factor I (IGF-I), ACTH, and 24 hour urine free cortisol. Low values, and even normal ones in some instances, are consistent with hypopituitarism (**Table 7–1**). High values imply hypersecretion (**Table 7–2**). Some relevant details should be mentioned here:

1. As a rule, prolactin-secreting macroadenomas are associated with a serum prolactin level of greater than 150–200 ng/ml (normal 2–15 ng/ml), and elevated levels correlate with tumor size.[51] Microadenomas, hypothalamic dysfunction, pituitary stalk compression, or drugs such as neuroleptics and antidepressants lead to more modest elevations.[52] Physiologic hyperprolactinemia, also modest, occurs during pregnancy and postpartum lactation.

2. After a 75 g oral glucose load, the normal GH level is <2 ng/ml. Lack of suppression to this extent is the rule in acromegaly, and secretory spikes are frequent in this disorder. IGF-I levels are also elevated, but are more stable and correlate better with the severity of the acromegaly.[53]

3. If neuroimaging suggests a pituitary adenoma, and clinical features are consistent with ACTH hypersecretion despite normal or equivocal ACTH and cortisol levels, adjunctive testing may be required. In the overnight dexamethasone suppression test, 1 mg dexamethasone is given orally at midnight, then at 8 a.m. the following day the plasma cortisol level is measured, and should be less than 5 μg/dl. Elevated levels suggest pituitary ACTH hypersecretion. In a more definitive suppression test, 0.5 mg dexamethasone is administered every 6 hours for 2 days and urinary cortisol is measured for 24 hours. An unchanged urine cortisol level would be consistent with inappropriate cortisol secretion. Finally, petrosal venous[54] or cavernous sinus[55] ACTH sampling may be performed, but this is rarely necessary if an adenoma has already been demonstrated radiographically.

Table 7-4 Evaluation of patients with suspected chiasmal disorders

I. Consideration of patient's age
Childhood and young adulthood
Middle age and elderly

II. Clinical history
Visual symptoms
Endocrine symptoms

III. Neuro-ophthalmic examination
Including careful visual field testing

IV. General physical examination
Evidence of endocrine dysfunction
Evidence of underlying systemic disease

V. Neuroimaging
MRI, preferably, including sagittal and coronal thin cuts through
  the sellar region
CT, with coronal views

VI. Endocrine testing and evaluation
Serum prolactin, AM cortisol, TSH, T_4, LH, FSH, estradiol (in
  women), and testosterone (in men)
GH (after a 75 g oral glucose load) and IGF-I if acromegaly
  suspected; ACTH and dexamethasone suppression tests if
  inappropriate ACTH secretion suspected

VII. Other adjunctive tests
Lumbar puncture if neuroimaging suggests an infectious,
  inflammatory, or infiltrative disorder

A summary of evaluation of patients with suspected chiasmal disorders is outlined in **Table 7-4**. The discovery of a mass lesion requires neurosurgical consultation, while the presence of endocrine dysfunction, on either clinical or laboratory grounds, should prompt a formal endocrinologic evaluation as well. The remainder of this chapter discusses the various entities leading to chiasmal dysfunction. The clinical features and the management of each are emphasized.

Pituitary adenomas

These tumors are the most common cause of chiasmal dysfunction in adults, and they are very common, representing about 10–15% of all intracranial tumors.[44] Pituitary adenomas may be found in 3.1–22.5% of routine autopsies, but frequently these incidental lesions are smaller than 2 mm in size.[56,57] About 70% of pituitary adenomas occur in individuals aged 30–50, and only 3–7% occur in patients less than 20.[58–60] Pituitary adenomas are uncommon but can occur in children.[61,62]

There is disagreement whether adenomas arise from somatic mutation of a single cell or from hyperstimulation due to hypothalamic or hormonal dysregulation, or both.[60,63] In general, they are benign epithelial neoplasms which rarely metastasize; primary pituitary carcinomas are rare. Microadenomas are adenomas less than 10 mm in size, and these are rarely large enough to cause chiasmal compression, while macroadenomas are those larger than 10 mm. Pitui-

tary adenomas are usually isolated, but they can be associated with tumors of the parathyroid gland and pancreas, and less commonly with those of the thymus, in multiple endocrine neoplasia (MEN) type I syndrome.[64,65]

Pituitary adenomas can be classified functionally by their endocrine abnormality into two major groups: those with *nonfunctional enlargement* and those exhibiting *hormone hypersecretion*.[56] Approximately one-quarter to one-third of patients with clinically apparent pituitary adenomas are nonfunctioning or nonsecreting.[66,67] On the other hand, the two most common hypersecreting adenomas are prolactinomas and GH-secreting tumors,[68] but ACTH-, TSH-, and LH/FSH-secreting tumors are also clinically important. Modern morphologic techniques have rendered the classification of pituitary adenomas based upon staining characteristics, such as acidophilic, basophilic, and chromophobic, less helpful.[69]

The presentation of pituitary adenomas varies according to tumor subtype. Nonfunctioning adenomas are often asymptomatic until after they have extended beyond the sella, causing signs related to tumor enlargement and compression of surrounding structures: visual loss, headache, and hypopituitarism. Most (70%) of the large adenomas causing visual loss will be nonfunctioning.[70] In contrast, hypersecreting tumors present more commonly with characteristic endocrine symptoms, described in detail below. In all pituitary adenomas, diabetes insipidus at presentation is unusual.

Neuro-ophthalmic symptoms and signs

Chiasmal visual field loss is the most important neuro-ophthalmic manifestation of pituitary adenomas. Usually it is insidious and slowly progressive,[44] and often there is a delay of months or years between the onset of visual loss and diagnosis of the pituitary tumor.[71] Since the chiasm is located directly above the pituitary in most instances, the crossing inferonasal fibers are usually the first to be disturbed by upward growing adenomas, causing superotemporal defects respecting the vertical meridian. Further tumor enlargement results in more complete interruption of crossing fibers in the body of the chiasm, leading to a complete bitemporal hemianopia. Because of the distance between the diaphragm and the chiasm, only macroadenomas with significant suprasellar extension are associated with field loss. These principles are reflected in the excellent data from a review of 1000 cases by Hollenhorst and Younge.[72] Thirty percent of patients had no visual field abnormalities. Superotemporal field defects occurred in 10%, and bitemporal hemianopias in 30%. Junctional scotomas, central scotomas, and homonymous hemianopias were less frequent, consistent with the lower incidence of post-fixed and pre-fixed chiasms. Today, the percentage of patients presenting with field loss is probably lower, perhaps reflecting earlier tumor detection by more modern endocrinologic testing and neuroimaging.[73]

Acuity is affected less commonly (16%)[74] than visual fields. Disc pallor occurs in about 30% of patients[72] and correlates with the presence of decreased visual acuity better than with field loss or the severity of visual loss.[5] Papilledema is unusual unless the adenoma is large enough to cause

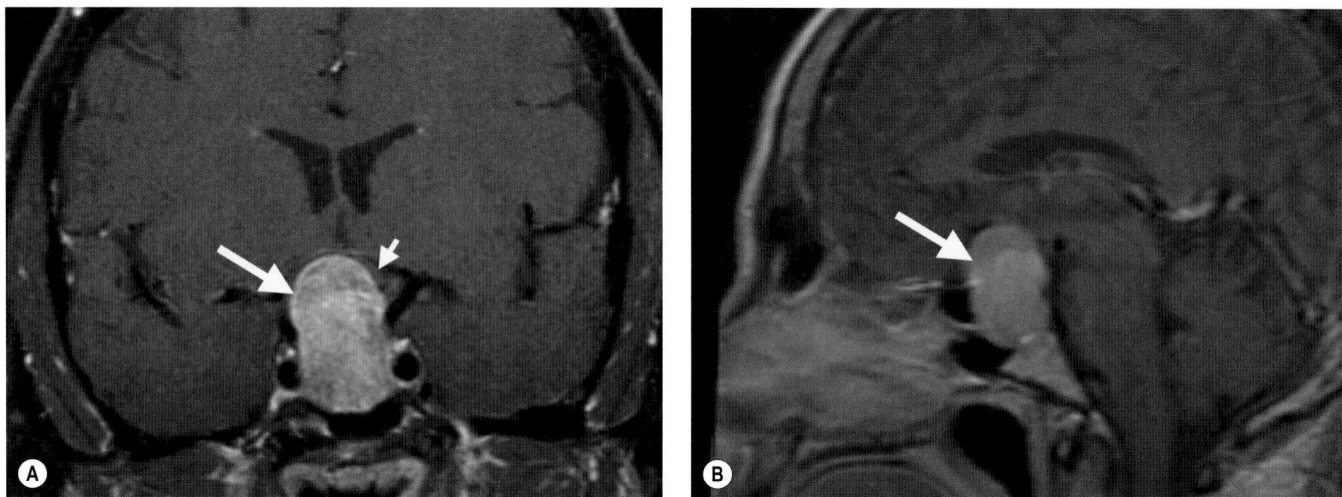

Figure 7–18. Enhancing, nonsecreting pituitary macroadenoma (long arrow) seen on gadolinium enhanced MR images. **A**. Coronal view. The short arrow points to the compressed, elevated chiasm. **B**. Sagittal view.

hydrocephalus[75] and instead suggests other sellar processes which have a greater tendency for causing third ventricular obstruction. Formed visual hallucinations, presumably release phenomena (see Chapter 12), have been reported in association with field loss due to pituitary adenomas.[76]

Cavernous sinus invasion,[77] following lateral erosion of the thin sellar wall, may lead to ocular motor palsies (in 1–5% of patients[17]) or trigeminal dysfunction. However, motility disturbances are much more common with pituitary apoplexy (see below). When ocular motor palsies occur, the IIIrd nerve is the most commonly affected.[17,72] Rarely, a IIIrd, IVth, or VIth nerve palsy is the sole presenting feature of the pituitary adenoma.[78,79] Orbital invasion[80] and extrasellar pituitary adenomas[81] have been reported but are uncommon growth patterns.

Traditionally headaches have been thought not to be caused by pituitary tumors. However, Levy et al.[82,83] analyzed a large number of patients with pituitary adenomas and headaches, many of which improved following medical or surgical treatment of the tumor. Headache types included migraine, trigeminal autonomic cephalalgias such as cluster headache, short-lasting unilateral neuralgiform headache attacks with conjuctival injection and tearing (SUNCT), and trigeminal neuralgia. SUNCT syndrome occurred usually in association with prolactinomas and GH-secreting adenomas. Large tumor size and cavernous sinus invasion may be[84] but are not always[82] associated with headache, suggesting dural stretching and trigeminal involvement, respectively, were not necessarily the cause.

Diagnostic studies/neuroimaging

In 80–95% of microadenomas, a hypointense lesion is evident within the normal pituitary on T1-weighted MR images.[85] A hyperintense region on T1-weighted images usually indicates a hemorrhagic component. Most of the time (75%) the hemorrhage is not associated with clinical apoplexy (see below).[86] In about one-third to one-half of cases, the adenoma is hyperintense on T2 images. Contrast may be helpful if the unenhanced images are equivocal. The

various types of adenomas usually cannot be distinguished by MRI, although prolactinomas and GH-secreting adenomas tend to be more lateral, while ACTH-, TSH-, and LH/FSH-secreting adenomas are usually more midline. This pattern reflects the normal location of the secreting cells.

Macroadenomas share similar MRI signal characteristics, but differ morphologically (**Fig. 7–18**). They are characterized frequently by suprasellar extension, enlargement of the sella turcica, and a dumbbell or figure-eight shape on sagittal and coronal images (caused by the limitations of the bony sella). In some instances there is demonstrable lateral extension into the cavernous sinus.[87] Approximately 20% of macroadenomas may exhibit radiographic evidence of cystic changes, necrosis, or hemorrhage, but only 1% are associated with a history of sudden clinical deterioration[85] (see Pituitary apoplexy, below). MRI should be sufficient to outline vascular structures and rule out coexisting aneurysms,[88–90] so routine angiography is unnecessary in most preoperative assessments. On CT scanning the pituitary adenomas are hypodense compared with the normal gland on both enhanced and unenhanced images.[8] Sellar erosion can be evident on CT with larger adenomas.

Although not part of the routine evaluation of patients with pituitary adenomas, those with thinning of the retinal nerve fiber layer demonstrated on optical coherence tomography (OCT) may have a relatively poorer visual prognosis.[29,30]

Diagnostic studies/laboratory tests

In addition to the MRI, endocrinologic studies are necessary to classify the tumor type and direct treatment (see **Table 7–4**). Abnormal results and their interpretation are outlined in **Tables 7–1** and **7–2**.

Treatment. Some generalizations regarding treatment, outcome, and management of pituitary adenomas can be made.

1. Except for prolactinomas, the first-line treatment of symptomatic adenomas is transsphenoidal neurosurgery. Advantages of this method versus a craniotomy include direct visualization of the pituitary gland and tumor, no external scars, and better tolerance of the surgery even by elderly and medically complicated individuals. Access to the sphenoid is usually via a sublabial or transnasal approach or combinations of both,[91] and tumors are removed with the aid of the operating microscope. When necessary, the sella floor is reconstructed with a plate of nasal bone or cartilage, and the sphenoid sinus is packed with muscle, fat, or Gelfoam.[92] Postoperative diabetes insipidus (usually transient), CSF leak, visual loss, ocular motor nerve palsy, hemorrhage, traumatic aneurysm, and cerebral ischemia are potential complications, but the morbidity and mortality rates are usually very low.[92–94] At some institutions, the sella is exposed transnasally or transseptally using an endoscope, and the tumor removal is accomplished also endoscopically[95] or with an operating microscope.[96,97] A pterional or transfrontal approach via craniotomy should be considered when there is extensive extrasellar tumor.[98]

2. The prognosis for visual improvement is excellent following surgical or medical decompression. Recovery to some degree may occur within days or weeks of treatment (**Fig. 7–19**). In Trautmann and Laws'[74] large series of patients who underwent transsphenoidal surgery, approximately half of those with reduced acuity experienced improvement in this parameter, while about three-quarters of those with field loss had restoration or improvement in visual fields. Slightly better results were reported in smaller studies.[99,100] Prognostic signs which are associated with lack of improvement included optic disc pallor, lengthy delay prior to diagnosis, and poor visual acuity.[5,101] Interestingly the degree of visual field loss has no predictive value, as patients with profound field defects still have a reasonable chance for improvement.

3. External beam radiotherapy is useful in instances of residual or recurrent tumor, but, in general, the effects are not seen for months or years.[102–104] Patients should be informed of the possible late side-effects of radiation, such as chiasmal or optic neuropathy in up to 3%,[105] hypopituitarism, brain parenchymal necrosis, and secondary neoplasms (meningiomas and sarcomatous transformation of the pituitary adenoma).[102,103,106,107] Fortunately, radiation optic neuropathy is becoming less common in this setting.[108] Stereotactic radiosurgery[109–114] allows more precise delivery of radiation to this area with less risk to surrounding tissues.

4. We recommend a neuro-ophthalmic examination, including visual field testing, within the first few weeks postoperatively, and Klibanski[66] recommends a follow-up MRI at this time to check for residual tumor. Serial neuroimaging and neuro-ophthalmic examinations then can be performed at 6 and 12 months postoperatively and, if stable, yearly intervals after that. Postradiation follow-up can be similar. Follow-up of prolactinomas is slightly different because the primary treatment is medical (see below). However, if surgery or radiation becomes part of the management of a prolactinoma, the above schedule may be applied. Endocrine follow-up is also necessary.

Rarely, a delayed visual loss months or years following transsphenoidal resection without radiation can occur. The visual deficits are slowly progressive, and possible mechanisms include chiasmal prolapse into an empty sella[115] or tethering scar tissue. Some authors have advocated surgical removal of adhesions and repair of the sellar floor.[116] Postoperative pneumatoceles causing visual loss have also been reported.[117]

The clinical features and treatment of nonfunctioning and hypersecreting pituitary adenomas

Nonfunctioning (nonsecreting) pituitary tumors. These are usually macroadenomas without clinical evidence of pituitary hormone hypersecretion.[67] In one report, visual loss occurred in 72%, hypopituitarism in 61%, headache in 36%, and cranial neuropathies in 10%.[92] Tumor compression of the normal residual pituitary gland or the stalk often leads to loss of normal LH/FSH, ACTH, and TSH secretion along with mild degrees of hyperprolactinemia.[66,92]

Although classically "nonfunctioning," immunocytochemical techniques have demonstrated that cells in the majority of these tumors are capable of producing a small amount of hormone, but not enough to elevate serum levels.[66,67] In one surgical series,[92] 82% were null-cell adenomas, while the rest were silent prolactinomas, gonadotropic adenomas, and corticotropic adenomas.

Transsphenoidal tumor removal is the treatment modality of choice. All patients with headache in the series of Ebersold et al.[92] were relieved of this symptom. However, the prognosis for recovery of pituitary function following transsphenoidal surgery of nonfunctioning tumors is fair to good.[118] Because these tumors are nonfunctioning, hormone levels are unhelpful in detecting residual tumor or recurrences. In younger patients with moderate residual tumor postoperatively, local irradiation should be considered.[67,119] Surgery is the preferred modality when tumors recur following radiotherapy.

Medical options are available to patients with nonfunctioning adenomas in whom surgery is contraindicated, or in whom postoperative recurrence is documented. Bromocriptine (see Prolactinomas, below), when taken long term, has been shown to decrease tumor size in a small number (16%) of patients with nonsecreting adenomas.[70,120] Octreotide (see GH-secreting tumors, below) may reduce the size of some nonsecreting tumors and improve visual symptoms, occasionally within days or even hours.[67,121,122] The effects are often transient, and only 30% of patients have long-lasting, stable visual improvement. Thus, Sassolas et al.[67] suggested using octreotide as a temporary alternative to surgery in patients with severe visual impairment. The mechanism of action of these medications in this setting is unclear. Our group has little personal experience with bromocriptine and octreotide in the treatment of nonsecreting tumors, so we would still recommend surgery when possible.

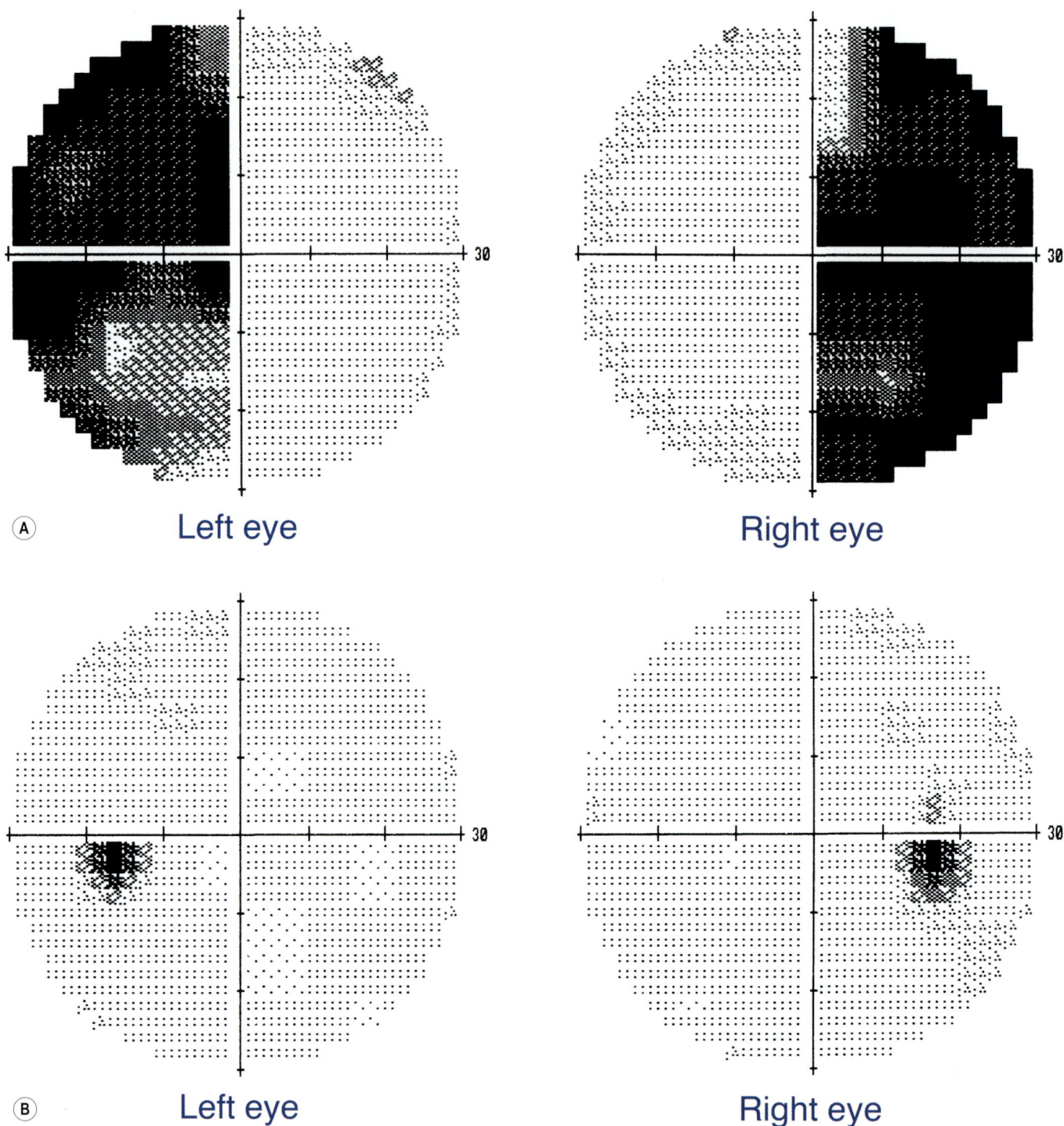

Figure 7–19. Marked improvement in visual fields following transsphenoidal resection of the pituitary adenoma shown in **Fig. 7–18. A.** Preoperative computerized visual fields demonstrating an almost complete bitemporal hemianopia. **B.** At 2.5 months postoperatively, the visual fields are near normal.

Prolactinomas. Prolactin-secreting tumors are the most common hormone-secreting pituitary adenomas. In women, endocrine symptoms caused by prolactinomas include galactorrhea and evidence of gonadal dysfunction such as decreased libido, amenorrhea, oligomenorrhea, or infertility (**Table 7–2**). In men, diminished libido, gynecomastia, or impotence are the most common manifestations, and galactorrhea is less frequent.[123] Prolactinomas have been reported in childhood and adolescence.[124]

Medical therapy with dopamine agonists, such as bromocriptine and cabergoline, which inhibit the synthesis and secretion of prolactin, are the first-line treatment of prolactinomas.[70] These medications can afford tumor shrinkage and reduction in serum prolactin level in the majority of patients with prolactinomas.[125] Common side-effects include nausea, vomiting, dizziness, and orthostatic hypotension, but sometimes these can be avoided by starting with lower dosages.[52] Cabergoline, now first-line treatment,[126] needs to be taken only twice a week and is better tolerated than bromocriptine.[127] Moster et al.[128] followed 10 patients with prolactinomas treated with bromocriptine. Improvement in visual acuity and fields and reduction in tumor size occurred in nine out of 10 patients, and in general the salutary effect was sustained. Other dopamine agonists such as pergolide and quinagolide (CV 205-502) have also been tried in patients with prolactinomas and visual loss.[129,130] Patients often noticed the visual improvement within days of starting the drug, and subsequent studies[131,132] have confirmed the potential for rapid visual recovery.

In patients who experience normalization of prolactin levels and whose MRIs show no evidence of residual tumor, cabergoline may be tapered with careful monitoring.[133,134] However, in many others the medication must be taken indefinitely. Chiasmal prolapse has been reported as a cause of visual loss following pergolide treatment.[135]

Transsphenoidal surgery of prolactinomas is less effective,[136] as hyperprolactinemia often recurs postoperatively.[125] Radiotherapy alone may reduce tumor mass effect and prevent further growth,[102] but it is generally an ineffective treatment of hyperprolactinemia.[123] Surgery and radiotherapy should be reserved for patients who do not tolerate or who fail medical therapy.

Besser[52] recommends biweekly neuro-ophthalmic follow-up and prolactin levels initially at the start of medical therapy in individuals with compromised vision. Neuroimaging can be repeated in 6 weeks if vision and prolactin levels have improved. Alternatively, repeat neuroimaging should be performed in 2–3 weeks in patients who do not improve, and surgery should be recommended in such cases.

A prolactinoma in the setting of pregnancy is a special situation. During pregnancy, the normal pituitary gland increases in size by 50–70% due to lactotroph hyperplasia,[70] but chiasmal compression is rarely an issue. On the other hand, pregnant women with microprolactinomas have a 1% chance of developing symptomatic pituitary enlargement, but those with macroprolactinomas have a 10–25% chance.[123] Although bromocriptine is probably safe during pregnancy, Vance and Thorner[123] suggest stopping the medication in women with prolactinomas who become pregnant, and then monitoring visual function carefully. If visual acuity or field abnormalities develop, either continued observation or restarting bromocriptine would be reasonable approaches. Finally, transsphenoidal surgery can also be carried out successfully during pregnancy if absolutely necessary.

Growth hormone (GH, somatotropin)-secreting pituitary tumors. According to Molitch's meta-analysis,[137] the mean age of affected patients at diagnosis is 42 years, and approximately half are women. Endocrine manifestations are the most common symptom, while visual field defects occur in approximately 20% of patients with this type of tumor.[138] Headaches occur in 55%, but their etiology is unclear because they correlate poorly with tumor size.

Gigantism and acromegaly are the two major medical conditions which result from GH hypersecretion. Characteristic bony and soft-tissue changes occur, primarily owing to GH-induced increases in IGF-I. GH oversecretion in childhood is associated with pituitary gigantism, and in this disorder longitudinal bone growth is still possible. In acromegaly, typified by overgrowth of acral segments (hands, feet, nose, chin, and forehead),[53] epiphyseal closure has already occurred, prohibiting bone elongation.[53] The disfiguring frontal bossing and enlargement of the mandible and hands are characteristic (**Fig. 7–20**). Because the changes are insidious, patients may notice only a gradual increase in glove or hat size. Furthermore, because acromegaly primarily occurs in middle-aged individuals, the changes are often attributed to "normal aging." In fact, the delay between onset of symptoms and diagnosis averages 8.7 years.[137]

In addition, bony and soft-tissue overgrowth commonly results in carpal tunnel syndrome and other entrapment neuropathies.[137] Myopathy, arthropathy, and depression are also seen in association with acromegaly. Patients with acromegaly have a higher mortality rate than the normal population, due in part to greater frequencies of hypertension, diabetes, cardiovascular disease, hypertrophic cardiomyopathy, upper and lower airway restrictive pulmonary disease, and gastrointestinal malignancies (colon, especially) occurring in individuals with this endocrinopathy.[137] GH hypersecretion can also cause ocular hypertension and exophthalmos.[44] Hypogonadism occurs in 30–40%, likely as the result of stalk compression and hyperprolactinemia (by inhibiting gonadotropin-releasing hormone secretion).[53] Some GH-secreting adenomas cosecrete prolactin.

Definitive treatment of GH-secreting adenomas is imperative because of their associated disfigurement and increased mortality. Transsphenoidal surgery is the primary treatment,[139] and successful surgery results in a rapid fall in the GH level, although usually not to normal levels.[53,140] Unfortunately, advanced acromegalic features are rarely reversible, but mild soft-tissue enlargement can be reduced.

Surgical, medical, and radiotherapeutic treatment options can be combined in an overall approach to patients with acromegaly. Octreotide, a somatostatin analogue can normalize growth hormone levels and decreased tumor size.[141,142] Octreotide alone can lead to marked improvement in chiasmal visual field defects.[121,122] The major side-effects are transient diarrhea and nausea, and less frequent ones are gallbladder sludge and asymptomatic gallstones. Melmed's treatment algorithm[141] is a reasonable one and suggests octreotide prior to surgery to facilitate removal[143] in patients with tumors >5 mm. A cure is considered a reduction in GH levels to <2 μg/l after an oral glucose challenge. Bromocriptine and cabergoline may be used but are not as effective as octreotide.[53,144] Cabergoline may be more efficacious than bromocriptine. Pegvisomant, a GH-receptor antagonist, can also be used.[145] Patients with persistently high GH levels in spite of these measures can be retreated with octreotide or receive radiotherapy.[102] Despite doses of 4000–5000 cGy, radiation can take years to lower GH levels.

Adrenocorticotropin (ACTH)-secreting pituitary tumors (Cushing disease). These adenomas occur primarily in women of childbearing age, and approximately three-quarters of cases of Cushing syndrome (excess circulating cortisol) are caused by ACTH-secreting pituitary tumors (Cushing disease).[54] Elevated ACTH levels result in adrenocortical hyperplasia and increased secretion of cortisol.

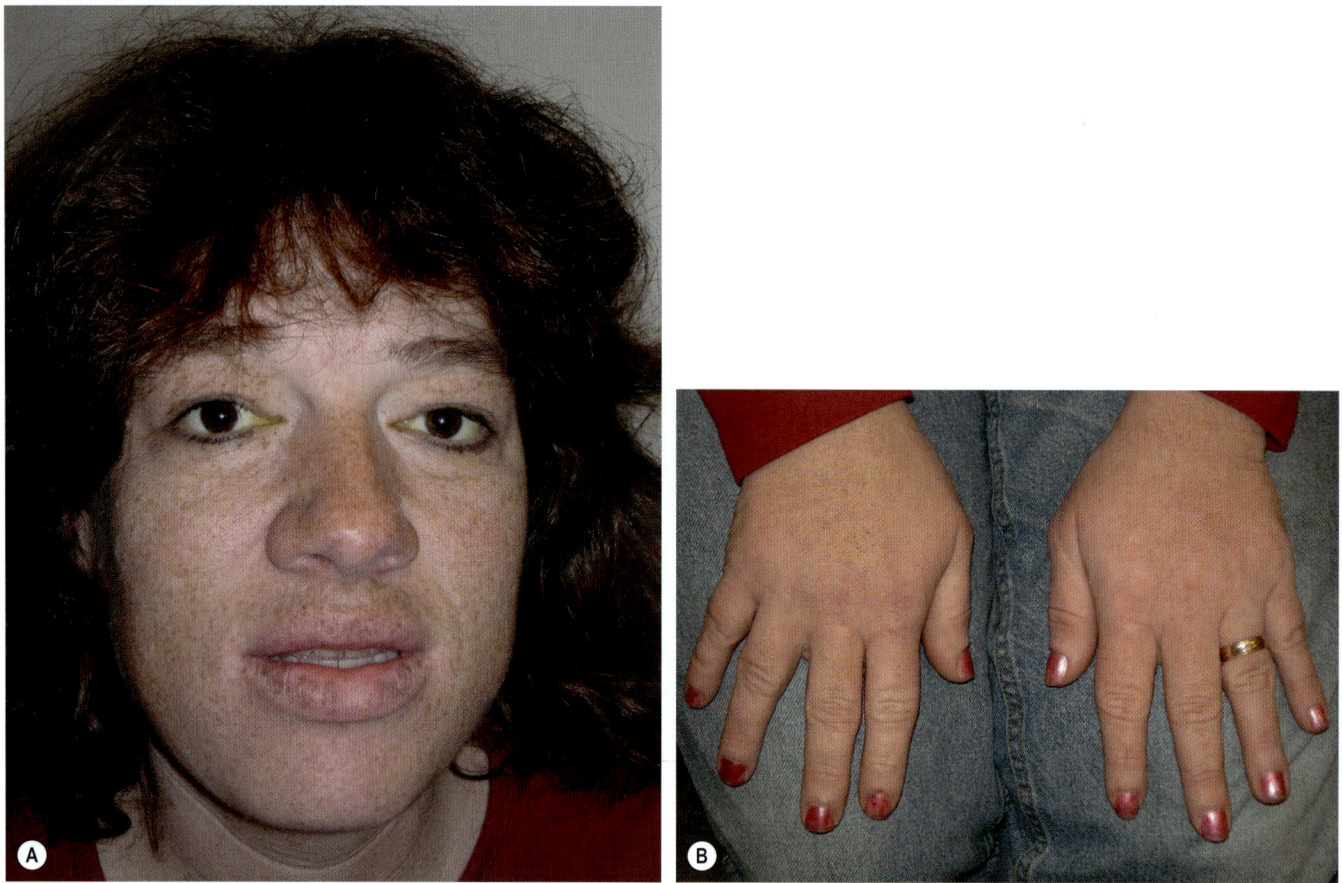

Figure 7–20. Acromegaly due to growth hormone-secreting adenoma. **A**. Coarse facial features and nasal and mandibular overgrowth. **B**. Enlargement of the hands. Note the enlargement of the left ring finger relative to the ring.

Common clinical features include obesity with moon facies and a buffalo hump, hypertension, hirsutism, striae, psychiatric symptoms, gonadal dysfunction, osteopenia, and glucose intolerance.[146] Usually these tumors are microadenomas without extrasellar involvement.

Transsphenoidal removal is the procedure of choice.[147–149] Radiotherapy can be used in patients with persistent or recurrent disease,[102,150] but cortisol levels may not be controlled until 1–2 years later. In the interim, drugs such as metyrapone, ketoconazole, and aminoglutethimide, which inhibit adrenal cortisol synthesis, or cyproheptadine, sodium valproate, bromocriptine, and octreotide, which can inhibit ACTH secretion, can be used short term to control symptoms.[63] As a last resort, those individuals failing both surgery and radiation are candidates for bilateral adrenalectomy to suppress the hypercortisolism, but this procedure has no effect on pituitary size.[54] Nelson syndrome, characterized by hyperpigmentation, elevated ACTH levels, and an enlarging pituitary gland, is the clinical progression of an ACTH-secreting pituitary adenoma following bilateral adrenalectomy for Cushing disease.[147]

Thyrotropin (TSH)-secreting pituitary tumors. These are uncommon, but occur in two varieties. In the first type, which is really not a tumor per se, primary hypothyroidism leads to compensatory hyperplasia of pituitary thyrotroph cells.[151] In one review,[152] one-third of affected patients developed visual defects (types unspecified) due to pituitary enlargement and chiasmal compression. Reduction in pituitary size and improvement in visual field deficits are often successful after thyroid replacement.[153]

In contrast, the second type, a thyrotropin-secreting adenoma (thyrotropinoma), is usually associated with thyrotoxicosis due to inappropriate TSH secretion. The diagnosis is established by demonstrating high circulating levels of T_3 and T_4, normal or elevated TSH, and a pituitary lesion. Fifty-four percent of affected individuals in Smallridge's[152] literature review had abnormal visual fields (again, types unspecified). In general, patients do not develop thyroid-associated ophthalmopathy. Transsphenoidal surgery, followed by radiation if necessary, is the treatment of choice. Thyroidectomy or radioactive iodine controls the hyperthyroidism but not the pituitary enlargement. Octreotide, which can improve chiasmal field defects in this setting, may also be considered.[121,154,155]

Gonadotropin (LH, FSH)-secreting pituitary tumors. Patients with these adenomas are typically male and older than 40, have normal gonadal function, and typically present with visual impairment due to chiasmal compression.[156] In Snyder's[156] series, 17% of 139 men with pituitary macroadenomas had this type of tumor. In a series of 100 patients from the Mayo Clinic,[157] 43% presented with visual loss, 22% with symptoms of hypopituitarism, and 8% with headache. Hypersecretion of FSH is the most common endocrinologic abnormality. Precocious puberty results when this tumor occurs in childhood. Transsphenoidal surgery usually results in some visual improvement,[157] and octreotide may have a beneficial effect with this type of adenoma as well.[121]

Three other situations related to pituitary adenomas—pituitary apoplexy, metastases to the pituitary, and incidental pituitary adenomas—deserve special mention.

Pituitary apoplexy. This clinical syndrome is characterized by sudden visual loss, headache, and ophthalmoplegia due to rapid expansion of a pituitary adenoma into the suprasellar space and cavernous sinuses (**Fig. 7–21**).[158,159] Defined in this way, pituitary apoplexy presents with headache in 95%, vomiting in 69%, ocular paresis in 78%, visual field deficits in 64%, and reduction in acuity in 52%.[160] Third nerve palsies are more common than IV and VI nerve deficits. When visual loss and headache are the primary symptoms, the condition can be confused with retrobulbar optic neuritis. Alteration in consciousness occurs in 30% of patients[161] due to diencephalic compression, and hypopituitarism, facial pain or numbness, and signs of meningeal irritation (blood or necrotic tumor tissue-induced) are common associated features. Other rare but reported clinical manifestations include retraction nystagmus,[162] presumably due to dorsal midbrain compression, and Horner syndrome caused by interference of the oculosympathetic fibers surrounding the cavernous internal carotid artery.[163] Diabetes insipidus is surprisingly uncommon in this setting. Most affected patients were previously unaware that they harbored a pituitary adenoma. The syndrome is uncommon, and only about 2% of pituitary adenomas will present apoplectically.[160]

Often pituitary apoplexy is the result of extensive tumor infarction or hemorrhage. Although most cases are associated solely with a pituitary adenoma, predisposing factors may include sudden trauma, anticoagulation, alteration of pressure gradients (angiography, for example), cardiac surgery,[164,165] diabetic ketoacidosis, and estrogen, bromocriptine, radiotherapy, and postpartum hemorrhage (Sheehan syndrome).[166]

The clinical suspicion of pituitary apoplexy mandates MRI as routine CT scanning may miss the lesion. MRI usually demonstrates a macroadenoma with heterogeneous signal characteristics due to the presence of blood, while CT scanning can reveals an unenhancing, hyperdense sellar mass. Hemorrhage, when present, can extend in the subarachnoid space and ventricles. Lumbar puncture may demonstrate an aseptic meningitis, sometimes accompanied by red blood cells. Since the sudden headache and ocular motor palsies associated with pituitary apoplexy may mimic aneurysmal subarachnoid hemorrhage, a CSF hemorrhagic component may warrant angiographic exclusion of an aneurysm if CT or MRI are inconclusive. Transsphenoidal surgery and emergent steroid and other hormonal replacement have facilitated the management of pituitary apoplexy. Some cases improve spontaneously.[167] The prognosis for visual improvement depends more upon early surgical decompression than upon the severity of the visual deficit.[168] One study found that patients with tumor infarction had a slightly better visual prognosis than those with hemorrhage.[169] Almost all patients undergoing surgery within 1 week will experience some improvement in acuity, fields, and ocular motility.[159,160] A conservative approach may be appropriate for stable or improving patients without visual loss or mental status changes who have a medical contraindication for surgery.

Metastatic tumors to the pituitary. These can have clinical and radiographic presentations similar to nonsecreting pituitary adenomas, except that patients with metastases to the pituitary are more likely to have diabetes insipidus and ocular motor palsies, and a more rapidly evolving clinical course is seen.[170–172] The most common primary sources are breast and lung.[173] The pituitary lesion may be the first indication of malignancy, and in these instances patients may undergo transsphenoidal surgery with an incorrect preoperative diagnosis of pituitary adenoma.

Incidental pituitary adenomas. Incidental identification of a pituitary lesion may occur in as many as 10% of patients undergoing neuroimaging for other reasons. All such individuals require endocrinologic screening, but those with macroadenomas also need neuro-ophthalmic evaluation. If endocrine and visual function are normal, neuroradiologic and neuro-ophthalmic assessments can be repeated on a semi-annual or annual basis. Surgery would be indicated if there is evidence of tumor compression or growth. Incidentally detected macroadenomas have approximately a one-third chance of enlarging, while only 15% of microadenomas will increase in size.[174–176]

Craniopharyngiomas

Craniopharyngiomas are cystic, calcified sellar-region tumors which constitute 1.2–3% of all intracranial neoplasms.[177] They may present at any age, but, in various series,[177–179] the peak age incidence occurred in either the first or second decade of life. Approximately half of all cases are seen in adults, and some present in patients in their sixth decade.[177] They are epithelial in origin and are thought to derive from remnants of Rathke's pouch, which ordinarily migrates upward from the primitive buccal cavity. Craniopharyngiomas can be found anywhere along the migratory path.[180,181] Others have suggested that craniopharyngiomas might originate from squamous metaplasia in cells of the adenohypophysis.[181] Although benign in histology, craniopharyngiomas may act aggressively by invading local structures and by recurring despite apparent complete resection.[182]

Pathology

There are two major histologic subtypes, adamantinomatous and squamous papillary, each with different age predilections. Although seen in all age groups, adamantinomatous craniopharyngiomas most often occur in childhood.[177] The microscopic appearance is characterized by angulated columnar cells, and keratin nodules and calcification are common.[181] Cysts are present in 90% and are mixed frequently with solid components. The cyst fluid has the

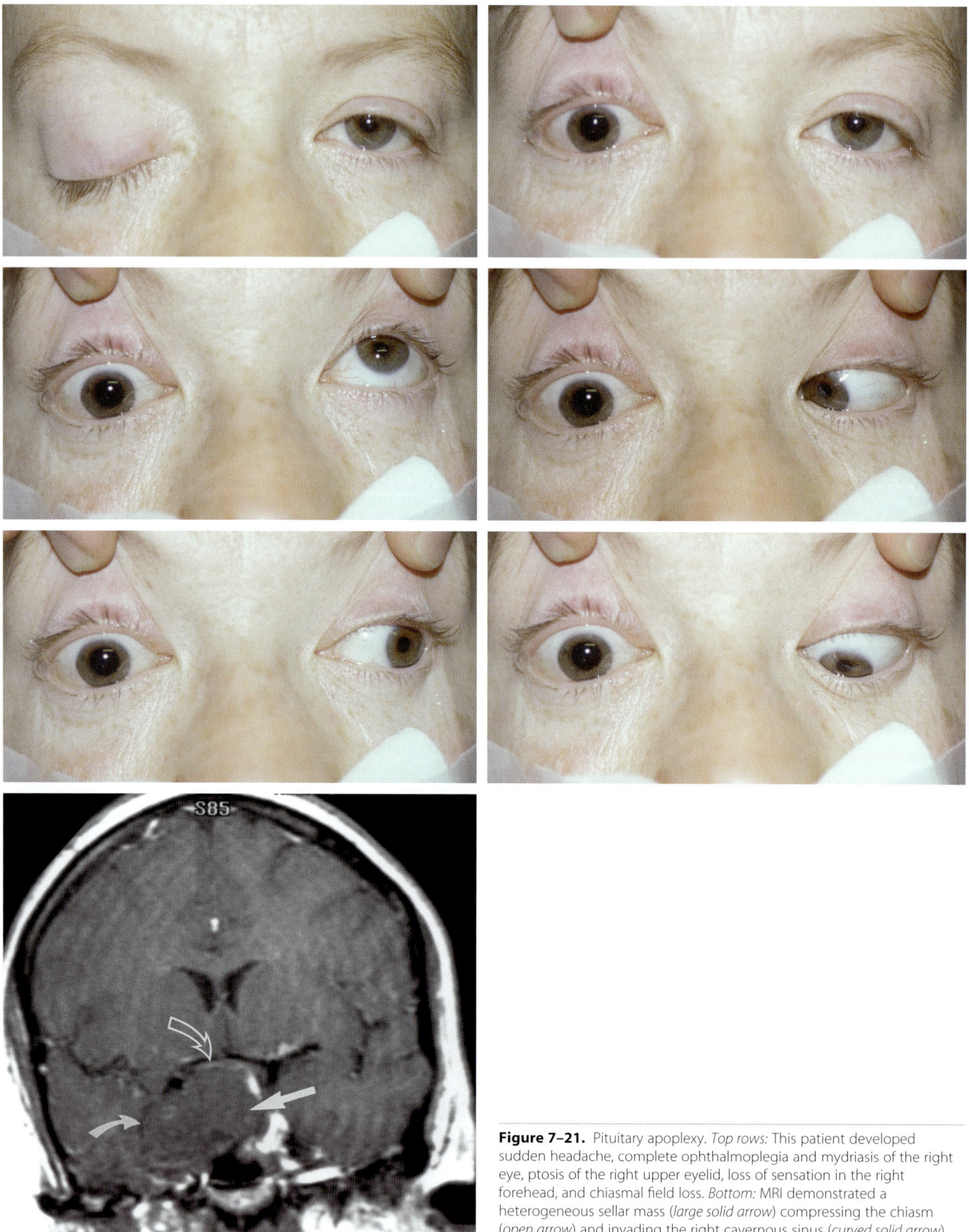

Figure 7–21. Pituitary apoplexy. *Top rows:* This patient developed sudden headache, complete ophthalmoplegia and mydriasis of the right eye, ptosis of the right upper eyelid, loss of sensation in the right forehead, and chiasmal field loss. *Bottom:* MRI demonstrated a heterogeneous sellar mass (*large solid arrow*) compressing the chiasm (*open arrow*) and invading the right cavernous sinus (*curved solid arrow*).

consistency of light machinery ("crank-case") oil and contains suspended cholesterol crystals. Although usually well defined, adamantinomatous craniopharyngiomas may adhere to surrounding brain and vascular structures.[181] Reactive gliosis and tumor islets[177] may be seen in adjacent brain tissue. These features may, in part, account for recurrences of adamantinomatous craniopharyngiomas despite "total" resection.[177]

Craniopharyngiomas in adulthood tend to be squamous papillary. Calcification, keratin nodule formation, and adamantinous epithelium are conspicuously absent in these tumors. Cysts occur in approximately 50% of cases.[177] Squamous papillary craniopharyngiomas tend to be well demarcated, and after complete resection they tend not to recur.[177,183]

Location and growth characteristics

Craniopharyngiomas may occur in the sella, suprasellar area, and third ventricle. Typically they traverse more than one of these spaces, and entirely intrasellar or intraventricular craniopharyngiomas are unusual.[184] Prechiasmatic tumors, when large, can protrude between the optic nerves and lift the A1 segments of the anterior cerebral arteries. Retrochiasmal tumors can extend posteriorly into the third ventricle and abut the basilar artery and midbrain.[185] Their size may vary from a few millimeters to several centimeters,[85] but the majority of tumors are 2–4 cm in greatest diameter.[183] Tumors may be densely adherent to the hypothalamus with small papillary projections.[181] Hydrocephalus, due to third ventricular compression, occurs in approximately 38% of patients.[183]

Craniopharyngiomas typically disrupt the anterior visual pathways by external compression. However, unusual instances of intrachiasmatic craniopharyngiomas, causing chiasmal thickening, have been described.[186-188] Tumor extension through the optic foramen and canal into the orbit is also rare, but has been reported.[189,190] Other unusual growth patterns include spread beyond the sellar area into the anterior, middle, and posterior fossas.[191] Midbrain,[192] hemispheric,[193] and cerebellopontine angle[194] involvement have also been reported.

Fluid leakage, from surgical or spontaneous cyst rupture, can result in a severe chemical arachnoiditis or meningitis.[181] Spontaneous hemorrhage with subarachnoid hemorrhage is a reported but unusual complication.[195]

Symptoms

Initial manifestations can be grouped into four major categories: visual, endocrinologic, and cognitive abnormalities, and headaches.[177,179,183] Visual symptoms are usually the most common manifestation, occurring in 61–77% of patients.[177,179,183,196,197] These and endocrinologic abnormalities are discussed in more detail below. Cognitive deficits include personality changes, memory loss, depression, and confusion. Headaches are nonspecific, but are sometimes accompanied by nausea and vomiting. Some authors have touted a varied presentation according to age group, with visual loss and endocrine symptoms seen at all ages, but with headaches and papilledema occurring more frequently in childhood and mental status changes more often in adult cases.[178,179]

Neuro-ophthalmic signs

In Repka et al.'s series,[198] visual acuity was less than 20/40 in 41% of eyes at presentation, and approximately 15% were worse than 20/400. Bitemporal hemianopias are commonly observed field abnormalities,[178,196] and asymmetry and incomplete defects appear to be the rule.[179,199] Homonymous hemianopias, due to optic tract compression,[200] are less frequent.[178,196] Usually visual impairment occurs gradually, but sudden unilateral or bilateral visual loss, mimicking retrobulbar optic neuritis, has been reported.[179,201] The majority of patients with visual loss will have optic atrophy.[178] Sixth nerve palsies are common, and are usually due to third ventricular compression and elevated intracranial pressure, but they can also result from infiltration of the cavernous sinuses. Children may present with comitant or incomitant esotropia.[178] See-saw nystagmus may also be an associated finding.[36]

Some authors[181] have written that children with craniopharyngiomas may be less apt to report visual loss, so visual deficits at presentation may be more severe than in adults. However, not all comparative data support this notion. In one analysis,[178] the difference was not statistically significant. In another series,[198] more children had subnormal acuities, but more adults had visual field deficits.

Endocrinologic manifestations

Kennedy and Smith's study,[178] in which 64% of patients had endocrine abnormalities, contains excellent data regarding the frequency of these symptoms. Twenty-seven percent had complaints consistent with diabetes insipidus, 22% experienced weight gain, 20% had short stature, 36% developed various manifestations of hypogonadism, 16% had myxedema, while 24% were somnolent. Other investigators have had similar results.[190] Thomsett et al.[202] found that 83% of children with craniopharyngioma had at least one hypothalamic–pituitary hormone deficiency after careful laboratory evaluation. Growth retardation is, of course, a symptom primarily of children and young adults. It is uncertain whether endocrinopathy is more frequent in adults or children, because different series give conflicting results.[177,178,183] The syndrome of inappropriate secretion of antidiuretic hormone (SIADH) at presentation can occur but is uncommon.[203]

Diagnostic studies/neuroimaging

The MRI appearance of craniopharyngiomas is characteristic.[204] They are discrete intra- or suprasellar masses which can be hyperintense on T1-weighted images. Increased amounts of cholesterol, protein, and keratin cause these tumors to be markedly hyperintense on T2-weighted images. Cysts appear as round masses which are hypointense on T1-weighted images (**Fig. 7–22**) and hyperintense on T2-weighted images. Areas of signal void within the tumor represent calcification, and on rare occasions the solid component is completely calcified. After administration of gadolinium, the solid portion may exhibit modest enhancement (**Fig. 7–22**).[85]

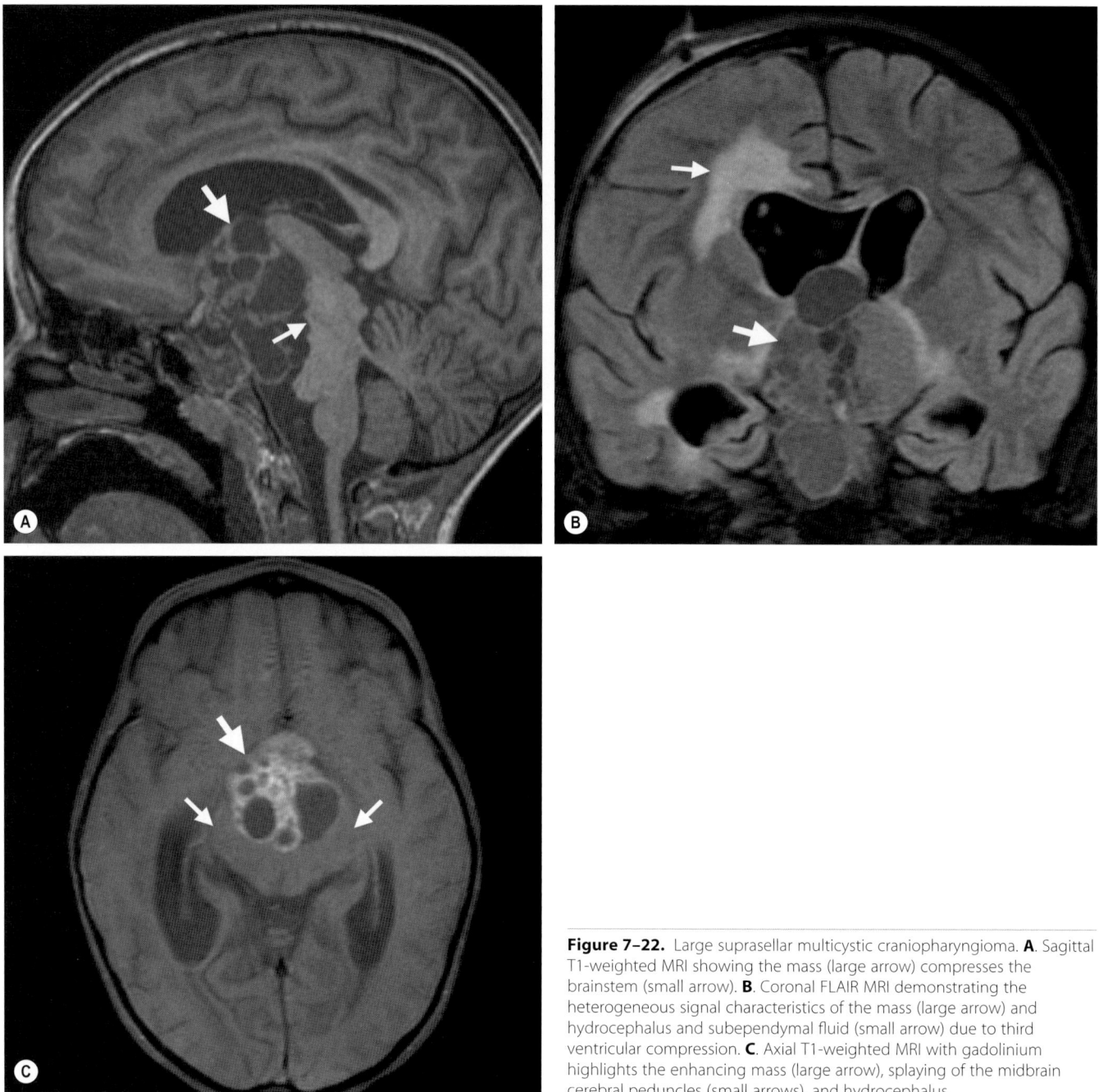

Figure 7–22. Large suprasellar multicystic craniopharyngioma. **A**. Sagittal T1-weighted MRI showing the mass (large arrow) compresses the brainstem (small arrow). **B**. Coronal FLAIR MRI demonstrating the heterogeneous signal characteristics of the mass (large arrow) and hydrocephalus and subependymal fluid (small arrow) due to third ventricular compression. **C**. Axial T1-weighted MRI with gadolinium highlights the enhancing mass (large arrow), splaying of the midbrain cerebral peduncles (small arrows), and hydrocephalus.

High signal within the optic tracts and posterior limbs of the internal capsules has been observed with MRI, producing a "moustache" appearance,[205] but resolution of this finding following tumor resection suggests perifocal edema rather than tumor invasion.[206,207] In some instances MRI angiography may be helpful in excluding an aneurysm[88] and defining the tumor's relationship to vascular structures within the circle of Willis, which can be either displaced or surrounded by the tumor.[193] Conventional invasive angiography, which may demonstrate absence of neovascularity or tumor staining,[208] is rarely necessary.

CT scanning, especially with coronal views, is complementary and often diagnostic when calcification is evident (**Fig. 7–23**). Cysts and solid components are easily distin-

guishable, and the solid portions variably enhance after administration of intravenous contrast. Cysts may ring enhance. Calcification within an intra- or suprasellar mass on CT is highly characteristic of craniopharyngiomas and occurs in approximately 80% of cases.[193] Thus, preoperatively many authorities would recommend MRI, with its sagittal views and emphasis on anatomic detail, as well as CT scanning.[181]

Treatment

The primary treatment of craniopharyngiomas is neurosurgical,[209,210] utilizing microsurgical techniques. Tumors which are primarily intrasellar or subdiaphragmatic may be

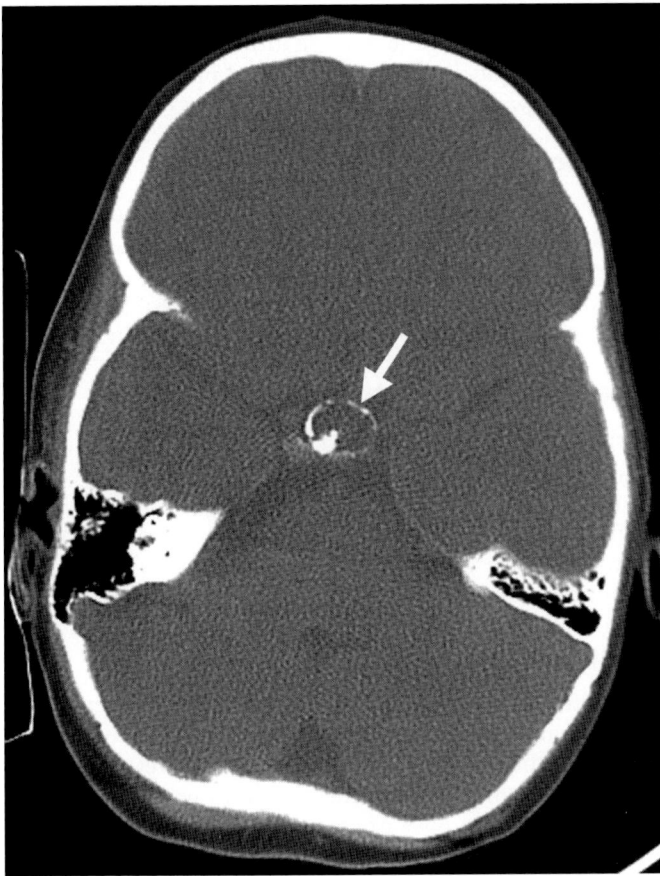

Figure 7–23. Craniopharyngioma exhibiting calcification (arrow) on axial, non-contrast CT scan.

amenable to transsphenoidal surgery,[74,211–213] which offers a lower surgical morbidity. However, the two most common approaches are unilateral pterional and subfrontal[180] craniotomies, which can be combined with a transcallosal approach if the tumor involves the third ventricle,[214] or transsphenoidal procedure when there is subdiaphragmatic extension.[190] Multiple procedures may be required for complete decompression of large and recurrent tumors.[196,215] Shunt placement may be necessary when hydrocephalus is present.[190]

Experts disagree whether the best treatment is complete excision or subtotal resection plus radiation.[190,196,197] The controversy exists in part because many authors espouse just one treatment approach.[196,216] Advocates of complete resection[185,190,217,218] argue that modern neuroimaging, microsurgical techniques, and hormonal replacement therapy allow aggressive surgery, and patients are spared the side-effects of radiation. However, extensive surgery can result in debilitating visual, endocrinologic, emotional, and cognitive deficits,[219,220] and has an operative mortality of up to 11%.[181] Accidental tears in the carotid artery, leading to cerebral infarction, have been reported when complete excision was attempted.[185] Furthermore, this approach does not guarantee a cure, as recurrence rates still range from 6% to 50% despite apparent complete removal.[185,190,197,217,218]

Proponents of subtotal resection plus external beam radiation readily emphasize a lower rate of operative morbidity

and mortality associated with this method of treatment.[180,196,221] Postoperative radiotherapy decreases the rate of recurrence and improves patient survival compared with partial removal alone.[222] Radiation doses usually range from 5000 to 5500 cGy, given in 180 cGy fractions.[197,223] Unfortunately, dose-related radiation toxicity, manifesting as endocrinopathy, optic neuropathy, vascular events, and secondary malignancies,[224] can occur in approximately 50% of patients treated in this fashion.[216]

In order to arrive at a sensible treatment approach, several investigators[181–183,197,202,223,225–228] compared the various treatment regimens, using retrospective analysis of patients treated at their institutions. In the one study[202] that specifically addressed endocrinologic issues, hypothalamic–pituitary dysfunction occurred least commonly in patients treated with limited excision plus radiotherapy. Tumor recurrence rate was similar in children and adults.[183] In all studies, subtotal resection alone had the highest rate of recurrence. Cyst aspiration plus radiation had reasonable outcomes, but was not included in most reviews. Except in one study,[183] subtotal resection combined with radiation was associated with a lower recurrence rate than total resection. Meta-analyses,[181,197,223] however, show that the recurrence rates for these two approaches are similar. Therefore, based upon these results, the most reasonable approach seems to be to attempt complete resection if possible, especially in young children, in whom radiation is less desirable. Most tumors can be handled in this way. When involvement of visual and endocrine structures precludes complete excision, and when neuroimaging indicates residual tumor following surgery, external beam irradiation should be performed postoperatively.[182,197,225,228,229] This is the treatment algorithm currently practiced by the neurosurgery service at The Children's Hospital of Philadelphia.[230]

Another recognized complication of surgery is fusiform enlargement of the supraclinoid internal carotid artery ipsilateral to the surgical approach.[231,232] The mechanism is thought to be related to surgical manipulation, but the abnormality has no clinical consequences.

Intracavitary brachytherapy, utilizing β-emitting radioactive colloids, is an alternative to surgical excision when craniopharyngiomas are primarily cystic or when they recur.[233] Radiation destroys the epithelial lining, leading to cyst collapse.[234] Because the cystic components are frequently the largest part of the tumor, reduction in cyst size may result in improvement in symptoms. The most common isotopes injected stereotactically include phosphorus-32, yttrium-90, rhenium-186, and gold-198.[199] Intratumoral bleomycin, an antineoplastic antibiotic, has also been used to reduce cyst size.[235]

Some craniopharyngiomas can be treated with either single dose (e.g., gamma-knife) or fractionated stereotactic radiosurgery, which deliver more concentrated radiation doses within narrower fields.[236,237] However, these modalities may not be suited for residual perichiasmal tumor. Ideal craniopharyngiomas for stereotactic radiosurgery are smaller than 2.5 cm and are sufficiently distant from the optic chiasm (>5 mm) to limit the chance of chiasmal radiation necrosis.[238]

Although survival in craniopharyngioma is excellent, the visual and endocrinologic complications can be devastating.[229,239] These are discussed separately.

Visual outcome. Dramatic visual recovery can occur,[240] but, in general, the prognosis for visual improvement following therapy for craniopharyngiomas is modest at best[74,230,241] and less sanguine than that associated with pituitary adenomas. Repka et al.[198] retrospectively compared pre- and postoperative visual examinations in 30 patients, most of whom underwent transcranial surgery for their craniopharyngiomas. The proportion of eyes with visual acuity worse than 20/40 fell from 41% preoperatively to 24% postoperatively, and those with visual field abnormalities decreased from 80% to 44%. Optic atrophy was associated with poorer postoperative visual acuities, whereas normal preoperative optic nerve appearance almost always predicted a postoperative visual acuity of 20/30 or better. Adults had a greater chance for improvement in acuity and fields compared with children, and the authors attributed this difference to longer periods of undetected visual loss in younger patients. A poorer visual prognosis in children was confirmed in other series.[230,242] Based on our personal experience, we agree with Repka and Miller[243] that "one should not be optimistic regarding postoperative visual outcome after removal of craniopharyngioma, particularly in children … cautious optimism may be appropriate for some adults, particularly those without ophthalmoscopic evidence of optic atrophy."

The visual outcome following intracavitary brachytherapy is similar. van den Berge et al.[199] concluded that intracavitary brachytherapy with yttrium-90 offered good radiologic results, but was not as efficacious in preserving vision. Anderson et al.[234] reported more encouraging results with phosphorus-32 although in some instances multiple injections were required.

Endocrine outcome. Post-treatment pituitary dysfunction is the rule, usually the result of surgery but occasionally due to radiation.[202,244] In one series,[245] 74% of patients post-treatment had diabetes insipidus, 100% were growth hormone deficient, 72% had ACTH deficiency, 65% TSH deficiency, and 93% gonadotrophin deficiency. Thus, after treatment most patients require some combination of GH, corticosteroid, thyroid, and gonadal steroid replacement and DDAVP. Diabetes insipidus, if not present preoperatively, usually manifests after surgery sometimes following a transient phase of SIADH. There may be slight improvement and a minority recover, but most affected patients develop permanent ADH deficiency.[46,246] Interestingly, even without GH replacement some patients experience normal or accelerated growth post-treatment, sometimes accompanied by obesity and hyperphagia.[245,247]

Rathke's cleft cysts

These lesions are similar to craniopharyngiomas in derivation, location, and symptoms, but there are some important differences. Although small incidental cysts are found commonly on neuroimaging and in the pars distalis or pars intermedia in 2–26% of routine autopsy cases, symptomatic Rathke's cleft cysts are unusual.[248,249] Patients are typically older; the average age at presentation is 38 years.[248] Other dissimilarities, including a better visual prognosis, are highlighted below.

Pathology

Rathke's cleft cysts also originate from Rathke's pouch, but histopathologically are less complex than craniopharyngiomas. The cysts are lined by a single layer of cuboidal or ciliated columnar epithelium and contain a gold-colored or white serous or mucinous fluid.[250,251] Calcification is rare.

Location and growth characteristics

Most cysts are intrasellar, and when symptomatic lead to headache and hypopituitarism. A prominent suprasellar component can result in chiasmal compression and hypothalamic dysfunction, and, in unusual situations, obstructive hydrocephalus.[252] Rarely, symptomatic Rathke's cleft cysts are entirely suprasellar.[252,253]

Symptoms

Voelker et al.[248] reviewed the findings in 155 patients with symptomatic Rathke's cleft cyst: eight from their institution and 147 other cases reported in the literature up to 1991. The most common presenting symptom was pituitary dysfunction, found in 69% of cases. Hypopituitarism, amenorrhea–galactorrhea, and diabetes insipidus occurred in decreasing order of frequency. Visual disturbances were present in 56% (see below), and headache in 49%. In another series,[254] the cysts were found incidentally in 14% of the patients.

Neuro-ophthalmic signs

Approximately one-half of patients have visual field deficits, and about one-quarter will have visual acuity loss.[248,255] Most visual field deficits indicate a chiasmal disturbance (i.e., bitemporal or monocular temporal field abnormalities).[251]

Diagnostic studies/neuroimaging

There are two characteristic patterns. Serous lesions are hypodense on CT, and on MRI they are hypointense in T1-weighted images and hyperintense on T2-weighted images, like CSF (**Fig. 7–24**).[256] On the other hand, mucoid cysts on CT are either isodense or hyperdense, compared with brain. On MRI they are hyperintense on T1-weighted images and iso- or hypointense on T2-weighted images.[257] The cyst wall (rim) may enhance, and blood or hemosiderin can also be evident.[258,259]

Treatment

Neurosurgical decompression is curative and often affords symptomatic improvement.[260] Because Rathke's cleft cysts are primarily intrasellar, transsphenoidal drainage and biopsy of the cyst wall is the favored surgical approach.[211,254,255,261] Associated morbidity and mortality is limited to diabetes insipidus. In one series,[261] headache was cured in all cases in which it was present preoperatively, but

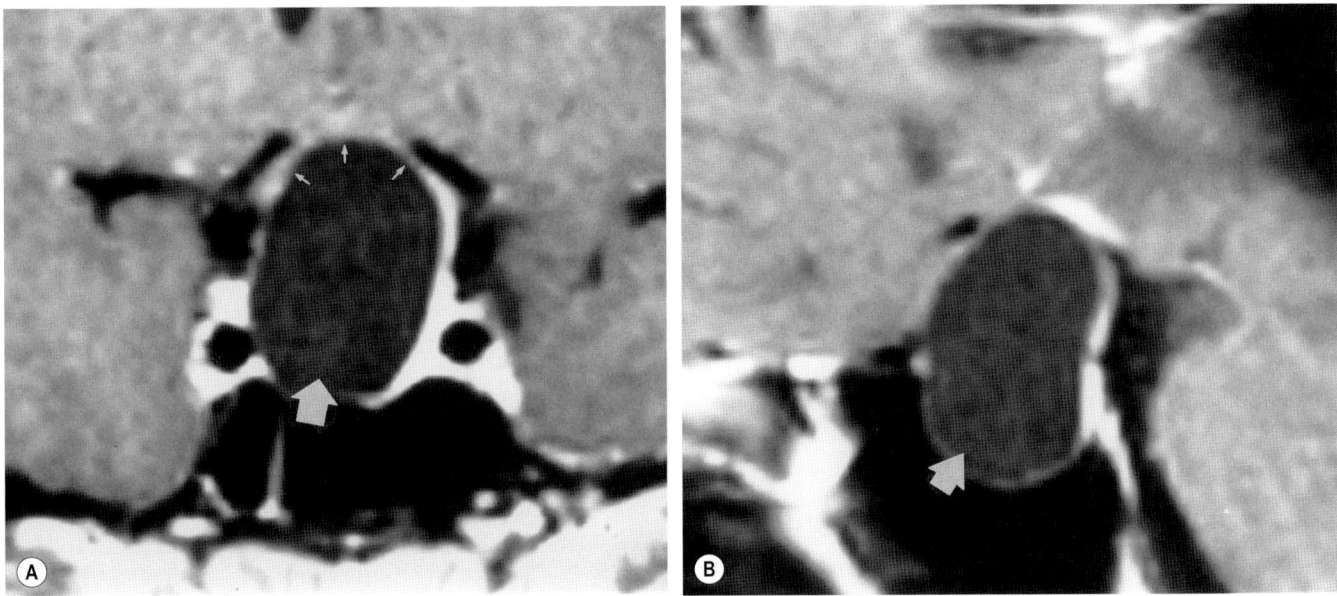

Figure 7–24. Symptomatic Rathke's cleft cyst (*thick arrow*), serous type, compressing the chiasm (*small arrows*). **A.** Coronal view. **B.** Sagittal view. The cyst contains fluid that is hypointense on these postcontrast T1-weighted MR images, and the cyst wall enhances. Like cerebrospinal fluid, the cyst fluid was bright on T2-weighted images (not shown). The patient had a bitemporal hemianopia. (Courtesy of Lawrence Gray, OD.)

endocrine outcomes were variable. Hypopituitarism and diabetes insipidus frequently persist.[248] Large suprasellar components may require removal via craniotomy.[254] Recurrences requiring repeat drainage can occur[262,263] but are uncommon, and adjunctive radiation or chemotherapy is unnecessary.

Visual outcome

In contrast to visual loss associated with craniopharyngiomas, the visual prognosis associated with Rathke's pouch cysts is excellent following decompression, with over two-thirds experiencing improvement in visual acuity or fields.[248,251,255]

Suprasellar arachnoid cysts

These are uncommon lesions, and they are thought to derive from an anomaly in Liliequist's membrane, either as a diverticulum or as a cleavage within the membrane and CSF secretion into the cavity.[264] On CT and MRI, suprasellar arachnoid cysts contain fluid with neuroimaging characteristics of CSF, and the cyst wall does not enhance. The cysts are usually noncommunicating, but in some instances may connect with the basal cisterns. Rare instances of intraluminal hemorrhage may give a cyst a "blue-domed" appearance.[265] Half of cases present before 6 years of age.[264] Common clinical features include signs and symptoms of slowly progressive obstructive hydrocephalus, visual impairment, endocrine dysfunction, spasticity, and gait disturbances.[266] Approximately 10% of patients will have a peculiar to-and-fro head bobbing.[266,267]

Asymptomatic suprasellar arachnoid cysts can be observed, but in symptomatic cases the treatment is neurosurgical.[268] Endoscopic ventriculocystosomy seems to be the safest and most effective technique.[266] Removal or fenestration via subfrontal craniotomy or fenestration of the cyst into the lateral ventricle and shunt insertion are other options.[264,266]

Meningiomas of the skull base

Meningiomas can affect the chiasm when they arise from the tuberculum sellae, anterior clinoid processes, or diaphragma sellae (see **Fig. 7–3**). Dorsum sellae meningiomas are rare.[269] When they become large enough, juxta- and parasellar meningiomas can also cause chiasmal compression, but these are discussed in the chapters dealing with their primary neuro-ophthalmic disturbance: planum sphenoidale, olfactory groove, and optic sheath meningiomas in Chapter 5, and middle and lateral sphenoid wing and cavernous sinus meningiomas in Chapter 15. This section will concentrate on the meningiomas that occur primarily in the suprasellar region, which account for approximately 8% of all intracranial meningiomas.[270]

Pathology

Meningiomas arise from the arachnoid mater,[270] and in particular suprasellar meningiomas derive from the meninges covering the medial portion of the sphenoid bone, tuberculum, and anterior clinoid processes. They tend to be vascular and firm in consistency.[271] Histologically they are usually of the "classic" variety, characterized by whorls and psammoma bodies.[272] "Classic" subtypes include meningotheliomatous, fibroblastic, transitional, psammomatous, and angiomatous.[273] Other classes of meningiomas, such as angioblastic,[273] are much less common in the sellar region. For the most part meningiomas grow slowly, are benign, and cause dysfunction by compressing adjacent structures. They generally do not invade brain. They can grow exclusively along a dural surface (en plaque meningioma) or a similar flat dural component can be attached to a more clearly defined soft-tissue mass (dural tail).

Associations

Progesterone and sometimes estrogen receptors can be found in meningiomas. The functional significance of these receptors is not clear, except meningiomas are more common in women than in men, can enlarge during pregnancy and during hormonal replacement, and are associated with breast carcinoma. They are found frequently in patients with neurofibromatosis type 2 and prior intracranial irradiation. They generally present in middle and older age. Metastases from distant systemic cancers are recognized to spread to meningiomas.[274]

Neuro-ophthalmic symptoms and signs

Painless, progressive visual loss is a feature of almost all symptomatic suprasellar meningiomas, and often it is the only manifestation.[271] The pattern of the visual deficit depends on the exact location of the meningioma in relationship to the optic nerve, chiasm, and tract (see below). Because meningiomas take years to enlarge, visual loss is usually accompanied by optic atrophy. Third ventricular obstruction and papilledema can occur in association with large meningiomas, but big asymmetric tumors involving the optic foramen may instead present with ipsilateral optic disc pallor and contralateral disc swelling (Foster–Kennedy syndrome; see Chapter 6). Optociliary shunt vessels would be more characteristic of intraorbital optic nerve sheath meningiomas, but in some rare instances they can occur with suprasellar meningiomas,[270] especially those associated with elevated intracranial pressure. Ocular motility deficits, proptosis, and eye pain can result when there is more lateral involvement of the superior orbital fissure or cavernous sinus.

Other symptoms and signs

Headache, usually frontal, occurs in about half of patients.[271] Much less frequent symptoms include changes in personality or mentation (due to frontal lobe dysfunction), anosmia, and seizures. Endocrine dysfunction is also uncommon, but when it occurs the symptoms are consistent with hypopituitarism.[271]

Diagnostic studies/neuroimaging

On CT meningiomas are round and isodense compared with brain on unenhanced scans, may be partially calcified, and enhance uniformly with contrast (**Fig. 7–25**).[272] Surrounding cerebral edema may be evident.[275] Hyperostosis, bony erosion, and calcification are best demonstrated by CT. On T1-weighted MR images, meningiomas are usually isointense to gray matter (see **Fig. 5–61**), and less commonly are hypointense. Half the time on T2-weighted images, they remain isointense, while in remaining instances they are hyperintense. Thickening of the dura, a wide dural base, a dural tail, and homogeneous gadolinium enhancement are also characteristic features (**Fig. 7–26**).[85] MR or conventional

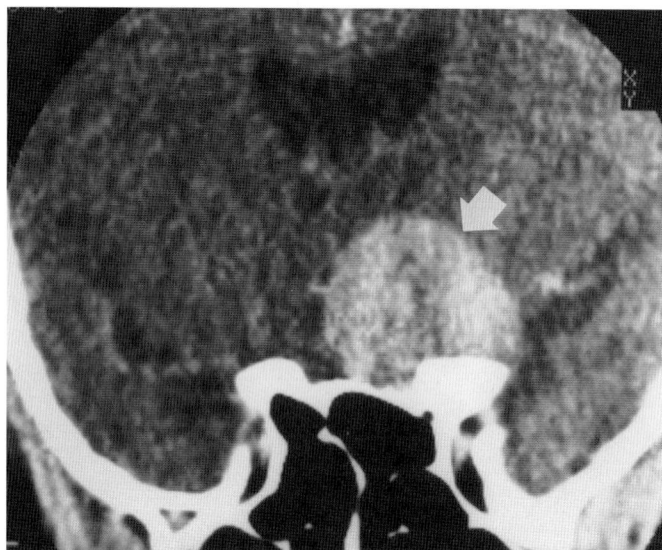

Figure 7–25. Meningioma (*arrow*) arising from the anterior clinoid evident on CT, coronal view with contrast. (Courtesy of Lawrence Gray, OD.)

angiography may be necessary to outline the tumor's relationship to vascular structures.[276] Angiography may be necessary in the preoperative evaluation of these meningiomas because large tumors commonly elevate and encase the proximal anterior cerebral arteries. Conventional angiography also may add more information regarding arterial supply and venous drainage, especially if embolization is considered.[277]

Treatment

Visual loss is the best indication for intervention, which is primarily neurosurgical. In some instances preoperative embolization facilitates removal, given the hypervascularity of these lesions.[278] Pterional or subfrontal craniotomies are the most popular surgical approaches.[279] When the tumor is densely adherent to the internal carotid or anterior cerebral arteries or the anterior visual pathway, a subtotal resection is recommended.[277,280] Smaller less complicated sellar meningiomas may be removed transsphenoidally using endoscopic techniques.[281] External beam radiation (5000 to 5500 cGy)[282] or gamma-knife stereotactic radiosurgery[283,284] should be considered when there is residual or recurrent tumor, or when surgery is contraindicated.

Alternatively, observation may be the best approach in some cases. Elderly patients or poor operative candidates with mild to minimal visual loss, for instance, may be better off with conservative management.[285] Hormonal therapy may be another option when tumors recur despite surgery or radiation, when they become unresectable because of location, or when these traditional approaches are contraindicated.[286] Experience with suprasellar meningiomas, however, is limited,[287] and some hormonal treatments such as RU-486 are poorly tolerated because of a flu-like side-effect.

Outcome

The chance for visual improvement following neurosurgical decompression is good and only slightly less than that of

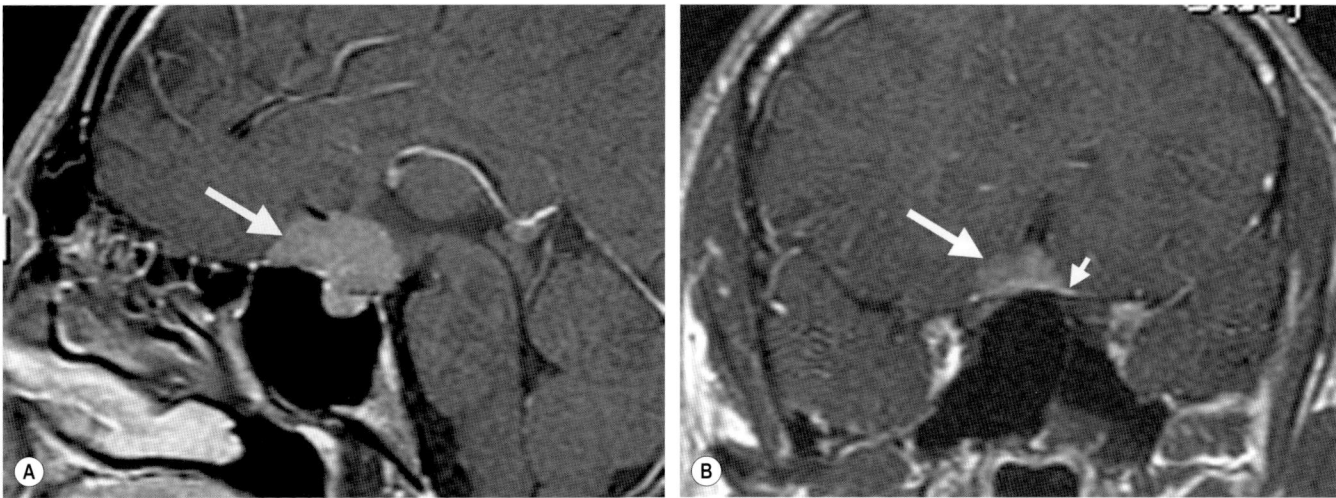

Figure 7–26. Tuberculum sella meningioma **A**. Enhanced T1-weighted sagittal MRI demonstrating an enhancing suprasellar mass (arrow). The mass extends anteriorly along the planum sphenoidale and posteroinferiorly into the sella turcica. **B**. Coronal enhanced view shows the meningioma (large arrow) and a characteristic dural tail (small arrow).

treated pituitary adenomas. However, this is tempered by the fact that suprasellar meningiomas have higher risk of recurrence, and their surgical removal is associated with much higher rates of visual loss, morbidity, and mortality. In a large series by Symon and Rosenstein,[271,288] 64% experienced some improvement in visual acuity or fields, while visual function remained unchanged in 12% and worsened in 24%. Other authors[279,289–292] have described similar results. Patients with large tumor size and long-standing or severe visual deficits tend to have the poorest visual prognosis,[288] but those factors do not preclude the chance for some visual recovery following surgery.[279,290] Radiation alone in some instances can afford visual improvement as well.[282] Symon and Rosenstein[271] found that one-third of partially resected tumors recurred, compared with only 1.4% of completely resected ones. Recurrences typically occurred years (average 3.7 years) after initial therapy, and were treated with either radiation or repeat craniotomy.

The three major types of suprasellar meningiomas, tuberculum sellae, anterior clinoidal, and diaphragma sellae, are considered separately below, as they differ slightly in presentation and treatment. They are named after the bony or meningeal structure from which they arise. There is considerable overlap, and when the tumors are large sometimes the distinction is artificial. The classification, however, is most useful regarding outcome. In general, meningiomas restricted to the tuberculum sellae have a more favorable visual prognosis following surgical decompression. On the other hand, those involving the anterior clinoid and diaphragma sellae are more difficult to remove completely and are associated with higher rates of operative visual loss, postoperative visual deterioration,[279] and surgical morbidity.

Tuberculum sellae meningiomas. The tuberculum sellae lies midline in the sphenoid bone, and is anterior and inferior to the chiasm (**Fig. 7–26**). Classically tuberculum sella meningiomas present in middle age, and interfere with the anterior portion of the chiasm, causing asymmetric bitemporal or junctional field defects and optic atrophy. Loss of vision is usually insidious and progressive. Grant and

Hedges[293] observed a characteristic pattern: the visual loss was "invariably asymmetric in its progression and accompanied initially by central hemianopic temporal visual field defects. Slowly developing blindness in one eye with diminution of acuity is then accompanied by a temporal field defect in the opposite eye." This temporal sequence of progressive monocular visual loss followed months later by fellow eye involvement was confirmed by Gregorius et al.[290] In some instances the visual loss may mimic retrobulbar optic neuritis or fluctuate.[289,294] Ocular motor palsies and proptosis are very unusual, reflecting the midline origin of the tumor.[293]

Because of their location, sometimes radical resection of tumor, dura, and bone is possible.[295] Smaller lesions may be amenable to transsphenoidal endoscopic removal.[281] Surgical morbidity consists of further visual impairment and hypopituitarism, including diabetes insipidus. Operative visual loss is usually the result of interruption of the blood supply of the chiasm or optic nerve. The small surgical mortality is in part due to the risk of pulmonary embolism.[294]

Anterior clinoidal meningiomas. The two anterior clinoid processes lie on the medial ridge of the lesser wings of the sphenoid bone. They look like two triangles pointing towards the back of the head. On each side of the midline, the intracranial and canalicular portions of the optic nerve, and the internal carotid artery, exiting from the cavernous sinus just below the nerve, lie just inferomedial to the anterior clinoid process. Meningiomas of the anterior clinoid can cause either an optic neuropathy or chiasmal disturbance. Foster–Kennedy syndrome and superior orbital fissure or cavernous sinus involvement are more common with this type, given its more lateral location.[296] Complete neurosurgical removal may be impossible when the tumor encases either the optic nerve or the internal carotid artery, and adjuvant radiotherapy is required in these instances. Surgical mortality, related to injury of the internal carotid or middle cerebral arteries, can be as high as 42%.[296] Visual recovery in general is poor.

Diaghragma sella meningiomas. A less common type of meningioma in this area arises from the diaphragma sellae.

Kinjo et al.[297] presented their personal experience with 12 such patients and reviewed 27 other reported cases. Visual field disturbances are still frequent with this variation. When these meningiomas originate from the diaphragm's upper leaf, they grow upward into the suprasellar cistern, so their presentation and management is similar to that of other suprasellar meningiomas. Those originating from the lower leaf, when they grow large enough, expand the sella, and can mimic a nonsecreting pituitary adenoma clinically and radiographically.[298] Some of the latter type may be amenable to a combined transsphenoidal–transcranial resection. In either type, however, complete resection may be limited when the tumor encases the chiasm or pituitary stalk.

Aneurysms

Because of the intimate relationship of the circle of Willis to the chiasm and sella (**Fig. 7–2**), large saccular aneurysms in this area can cause chiasmal visual loss and endo-crinopathy.[299,300] In some instances, their presentation may be clinically indistinguishable from a pituitary adenoma or craniopharyngioma.[301]

Pathology/demographics

Aneurysms most likely develop from congenital defects in arterial walls, and pathologically they are characterized by disruption of the media and fibrinoid changes.[302] Arterial bifurcations which are either sharp or give rise to a hypo-plastic branch may predispose to development of an aneu-rysm.[303] In addition, hypertension, hemodynamic stress, smoking, heavy alcohol use, cocaine abuse, and atherosclerosis are modifiable risk factors for their development.[304,305] Affected patients tend to be female and middle-aged.

Location and growth characteristics

Any aneurysm arising from the anterior circle of Willis may compress the chiasm, but chiasmal syndromes are most characteristic of those of the supraclinoid internal carotid artery. These tend to be large (several centimeters in diameter) with upward and medial growth, resulting in compression of the anterolateral portion of the chiasm.

Carotid–ophthalmic artery aneurysms are also frequently associated with chiasmal disturbances. This type of aneurysm arises in the first 2 mm of the internal carotid artery above the cavernous sinus. The overwhelming majority of individuals presenting with visual loss are women. There is up to a 20% incidence of bilateral carotid–ophthalmic aneurysms and many affected individuals have multiple aneurysms elsewhere.[302] When they enlarge superiorly, they can erode the ipsilateral anterior clinoid process, then grow upwards towards the chiasm. Anterior chiasmal compression is the likely cause of visual loss in these instances, and these aneurysms are similar to anterior clinoidal meningiomas in location and associated field defects.

When cavernous or anterior communicating artery aneurysms cause visual loss, the mechanism is usually optic nerve compression.[306] However, less commonly these two types can cause chiasmal disturbances, depending on their growth

pattern.[306] For instance, cavernous aneurysms can extend medially to invade the pituitary fossa, then superiorly to compress the chiasm. Anterior communicating aneurysms with downward extension (because the anterior communicating artery is above the chiasm) rarely can encroach upon the chiasm.[307]

Pregnancy may be associated with a higher risk of aneurysmal rupture, with subsequent high rates of morbidity and mortality for both the mother and the fetus. Thus, in their review of the management of a pregnant patient with aneurysmal visual loss, Shutter et al.[308] emphasized that pregnancy should not alter the neurosurgical management of symptomatic ruptured or unruptured aneurysms.

Symptoms

Some individuals have headache, although most patients with visually symptomatic aneurysms in this area will not.[309] Retro-orbital pain is also an occasional accompanying feature. Visual loss and endocrinopathy have already been alluded to, and will be discussed in more detail below. Although many patients will present with neuro-ophthalmic symptoms, others may present following aneurysmal rupture, and the visual loss is detected at that time. The ocular features of aneurysmal rupture and subarachnoid hemorrhage are discussed in the chapter on disc swelling (Chapter 6).

Neuro-ophthalmic signs

Their visual presentation is usually similar to that of other sellar masses, with chronic visual acuity and field loss and optic atrophy. However, the examiner should be alerted to the possibility of an aneurysm if the visual loss fluctuates. Sudden worsening or improvement can result from aneurysmal thrombosis or dilation, and acute visual loss might be the result of hemorrhage into the chiasm.[302] In addition, aneurysmal chiasmal disturbances tend to produce very asymmetric field loss. A symmetric bitemporal hemianopia caused by an aneurysm would be unusual and more suggestive of a pituitary adenoma.

Because of their varying location and growth patterns described above, the different aneurysmal subtypes are purported to have characteristic patterns of chiasmal visual loss.

1. *Supraclinoid carotid artery aneurysms.* These arise from the supraclinoid portion of the internal carotid artery. Visual loss is typically highly asymmetric and sequential, beginning in the ipsilateral eye.[310] Because the aneurysm is lateral to the chiasm, the visual loss in the ipsilateral eye is first nasal, then central and temporal. Vision is usually severely reduced in this eye, then, as the aneurysm enlarges, the crossing nasal fibers of the other eye are affected. The end result is a blind ipsilateral eye and a temporal defect in the fellow eye.[306] Uncommonly the aneurysms compress the chiasm from above rather than from the side. In these cases the patients can develop an asymmetric bitemporal hemianopia.

2. *Carotid–ophthalmic aneurysms.* In Ferguson and Drake's series[309] of 100 patients with carotid–ophthalmic

aneurysms, which arise from the origin of the ophthalmic artery, 32 (25 of 61 with intact aneurysms, seven of 39 with ruptured aneurysms) had visual abnormalities. Twenty-eight of the 32 patients harbored giant aneurysms (greater than 2.5 cm in diameter). Sixteen of the 32 patients had evidence of chiasmal compression, based upon the pattern of field loss (three of the 16 had bilateral aneurysms). The chiasmal field defects fell roughly into two groups: asymmetric bitemporal hemianopias and junctional field loss characterized by severe visual loss in the ipsilateral eye and a temporal field defect in the fellow eye. Carotid–ophthalmic aneurysms are discussed further in the chapter on optic neuropathies (Chapter 5).

3. *Cavernous carotid aneurysms.* The diagnosis is suggested by signs of cavernous sinus involvement: IIIrd, IVth, or VIth nerve palsies, ipsilateral facial pain or dysesthesias, or Horner syndrome. In the late stages of aneurysmal expansion, optic nerve and pituitary dysfunction may occur. These aneurysms receive more attention in Chapter 15.

4. *Anterior communicating aneurysms.* An aneurysm of the anterior communicating artery or of its junction with an anterior cerebral artery more commonly ruptures before becoming large enough to compress the optic apparatus.[306] When visual loss occurs, monocular or binocular inferior altitudinal defects can be observed because of the aneurysm's location above the anterior visual pathway. Chiasmal compression and bitemporal hemianopias are rare but can result from an aneurysm of this type growing downward between the optic nerves, then enlarging and forcing the chiasm upwards and backwards.[306,307,311]

5. *Posterior communicating aneurysms.* The most common neuro-ophthalmic presentation associated with an aneurysm at the junction of the internal carotid and posterior communicating artery is a pupil-involving IIIrd nerve palsy. Visual loss is unusual because the aneurysm usually points away from the optic pathways. However, when a giant posterior communicating aneurysm projects into the suprasellar region, the optic tract can be involved. Rarely, medial chiasmal compression and a bitemporal hemianopia can be observed.[312] These aneurysms also receive more attention in Chapters 13 and 15.

Endocrinologic manifestations

The frequency of endocrinopathy has not been well studied, but it is clear that hypopituitarism of varying degrees can occur due to pituitary or stalk compression by an adjacent suprasellar aneurysm.[313] Following treatment, it is interesting that few patients require endocrine replacement, in contrast to those with other types of sellar lesions.[302]

Diagnostic studies/neuroimaging

On MRI suprasellar aneurysms will appear as round lesions in this area (**Fig. 7–27**). The signal characteristics depend on the presence of clot. Nonthrombosed aneurysms have a telltale internal signal void (hypointense on T1) produced by rapid blood flow and disappearance of protons before they have a chance to emit a signal.[314] Aneurysmal blood flow can also cause a characteristic phase-encoded artifact which runs through the aneurysm and across the image.[85] Partially thrombosed aneurysms contain clot which can appear laminated and bright on T1- and T2-weighted images, mixed

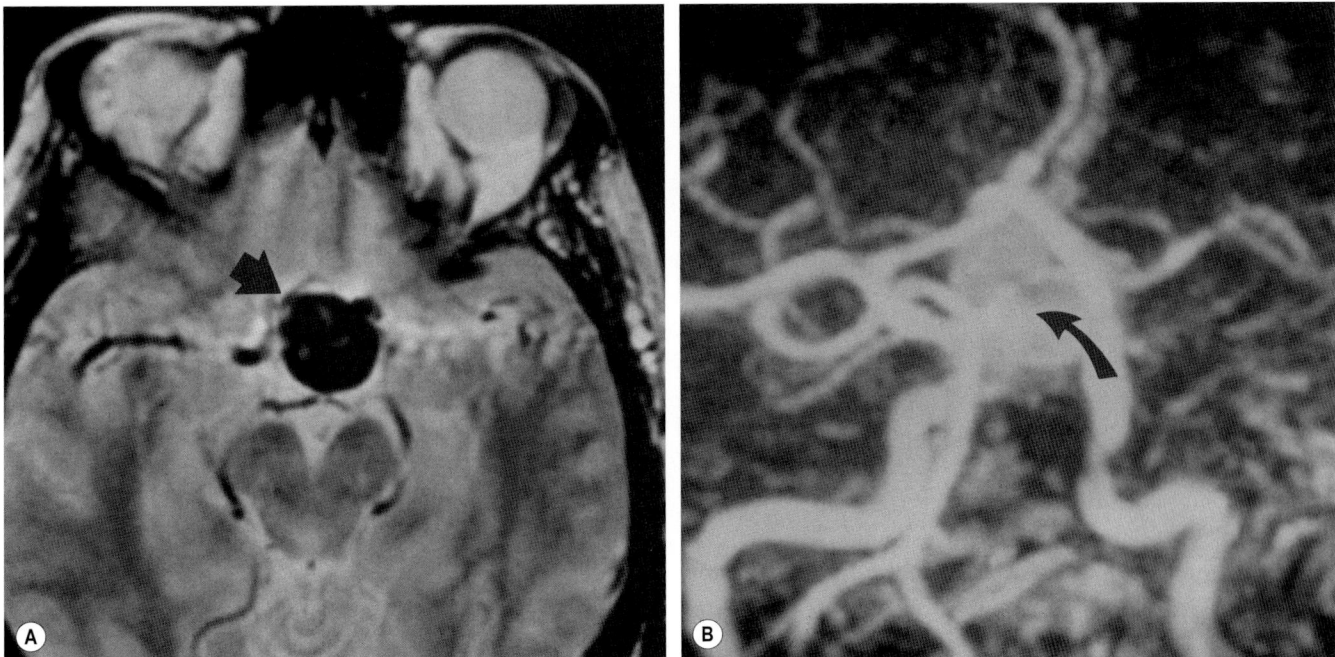

Figure 7–27. Internal carotid artery aneurysm that presented with an incomplete bitemporal hemianopia. **A**. T2-weighted MRI revealed a round flow-void (*arrow*). **B**. MR angiography confirmed a large internal carotid aneurysm (*arrow*).

with areas of signal void. Hemosiderin, evident as dark areas on T2-weighted images, may be visible outside of the aneurysm in adjacent tissues. Gradient-echo images may be helpful in demonstrating intraluminal flow in equivocal cases.[315]

On CT scanning aneurysmal calcification may be evident, and aneurysms contrast enhance. CT is better than MRI in detecting the presence of subarachnoid hemorrhage (when that is an issue) and in delineating the relationship of the aneurysm to bony structures.

When aneurysms are suspected, MRI or CT angiography should be performed. Since most of the suprasellar aneurysms which cause visual loss are giant ones, MRI angiography should provide a reasonable screening tool (**Fig. 7–27**). Treatment decisions will almost always require conventional angiography to locate the neck of the aneurysm and to delineate the aneurysm's exact blood supply and its relationship to surrounding vessels. Angiography also screens for the presence of other intracranial aneurysms. An aneurysm detected on MRI may appear smaller on angiography if it is partially thrombosed with a small lumen.[302]

Treatment

In general, aneurysms which cause compressive chiasmal syndromes should be treated.[316] A nonruptured aneurysm needs to be occluded to prevent symptom progression or subarachnoid hemorrhage, which is associated with an 8–60% mortality rate even before an affected individual reaches the hospital.[304] Even after admission to the hospital, the mortality rate following subarachnoid hemorrhage is 37%.[304] Patients whose aneurysms have ruptured, and who are salvageable, require definitive treatment to prevent rebleeding. On the other hand, two large studies[317,318] suggested that the morbidity and mortality associated with surgery greatly exceeded the risk of bleeding in unruptured aneurysms smaller than 0.7 cm in patients without any previous history of subarachnoid hemorrhage.[319]

Neurosurgical clipping of the aneurysm remains the most popular approach.[320–322] When feasible, a metal clip with a spring closure is placed around the aneurysmal neck to isolate it from the parent vessel. When small perforating arteries arise from the aneurysm, clipping may be undesirable. Percutaneous intra-arterial (endovascular) embolization of the aneurysm with balloons or metallic coils, or balloon occlusion of the parent artery, are two alternatives in patients with inoperable aneurysms.[323,324] A large study[325] concluded that coiling was superior to clipping in ruptured aneurysms. However, the choice between surgery and an endovascular procedure can be made on a case-by-case basis considering the age and medical condition of the patient, the location and size of the aneurysm, and the center's level of expertise with the two options.

Visual outcome

In Ferguson and Drake's series,[309] of those with visual deficits who survived and were treated, approximately half had some improvement in visual acuity or field, one-third remained unchanged, and about 15% worsened.

Vascular malformations intrinsic to the chiasm

Maitland et al.[326] used the term "chiasmal apoplexy" to describe sudden visual loss due to an intrachiasmal hematoma. Vascular malformations are the usual cause although in one case the hemorrhage was associated with an optic glioma[326] and in another a pituitary adenoma bled into the chiasm.[327] Characteristically, acute visual loss is accompanied by headache.[328] Because the hematomas distend but are usually confined to the chiasm, endocrine symptoms, meningismus, and focal neurologic signs are conspicuously absent. The various subtypes of vascular malformations intrinsic to the chiasm are discussed below.

Cavernous angiomas (cavernous hemangiomas, cavernomas)

Kupersmith[329] describes these histologically as "irregular sinusoids of vascular channels" without interposed neuronal tissue and without a major arterial supply or venous drainage. Usually they are sporadic, but in rare instances familial cavernous hemangiomas can present in the chiasm.[330] Symptoms are due to hemorrhage in the chiasm and are frequently sudden.[331] On MRI the chiasm is enlarged, and the cavernous angioma is usually heterogeneous on T1-weighted MR images (**Fig. 7–28**) and contains dark areas on gradient-echo images indicative of hemosiderin.[332,333] On CT scanning a calcified or enhancing suprasellar mass can be detected. Not infrequently, angiography fails to demonstrate these lesions because of their slow flow characteristics.

The best management of symptomatic cavernous angiomas in the chiasm is unclear.[334] Several authors[328,335] have advocated microsurgical removal of these lesions to prevent further hemorrhages. On the other hand, we have managed several patients with recurrent hemorrhages and visual loss which have resolved spontaneously over weeks following

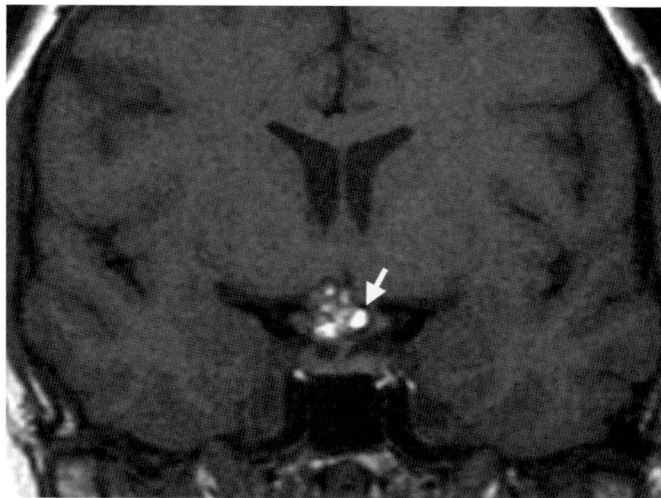

Figure 7–28. Cavernous hemangioma of the chiasm demonstrated on T1-weighted enhanced coronal MR image. Note heterogeneous signal characteristics with surrounding low signal (arrow), consistent with hemosiderin. The patient presented with a sudden headache and visual loss.

the ictus. It would seem unwise to subject all individuals with a chiasmal cavernous angioma to a craniotomy and unnecessary surgery involving the optic apparatus when some display a benign course.

Arteriovenous malformations (AVMs)

Rarely, AVMs, consisting of direct arterial communication with veins, occur in the chiasm and cause a bitemporal hemianopia when they bleed. Lavin et al.[336] reported two patients in whom formal angiography failed to demonstrate any vessel abnormalities, but chiasmal cryptic AVMs were confirmed histopathologically. The first presented with repeated episodes of visual loss which resolved either spontaneously or following surgical decompression of the hematomas. The second patient had just one acute episode of visual loss prior to surgery. CT in both patients revealed high-density suprasellar masses. Surgical removal of these AVMs should be considered. External compression of the chiasm by AVMs is discussed below. AVMs of the cerebral hemispheres, which are much more common, are discussed in Chapter 8.

Venous angiomas

These represent developmental anomalies of the venous system and are usually asymptomatic.[329] One rare case of a chiasmal venous angioma presenting apoplectically has been described.[337]

Others

Balcer et al.[338] reported the rare occurrence of a hemangioblastoma of the chiasm in a patient with von Hippel–Lindau disease. The chiasmal lesion was accompanied by retinal capillary hemangiomas and cervicomedullary hemangioblastomas.

Other vascular processes affecting the chiasm

Ischemic chiasmal syndrome

Patients with vasculopathic risk factors may develop small-vessel infarction of the chiasm.[339] However, for unclear reasons this is unusual. This diagnosis might be entertained in an elderly patient with diabetes or hypertension, with or without a previous history of small-vessel strokes, who develops a sudden bitemporal hemianopia or bilateral visual loss. Neuroimaging fails to reveal a sellar mass, but typical small-vessel-related white matter and basal ganglia lesions may be evident.

Like posterior ischemic optic neuropathy, atherosclerotic ischemic chiasmal syndrome must be a diagnosis of exclusion. Vasculitides such as giant cell arteritis can all cause infarction of the chiasm.[339] MRI may reveal chiasmal T2 high signal or enhancement. When vasculitis is suspected, appropriate studies should be obtained (see Atypical optic neuritis and Giant cell arteritis in Chapter 5, and Vasculitides in Chapter 8) and high-dose intravenous steroids should be considered.

Compression by atherosclerotic anterior cerebral and internal carotid arteries

In our opinion, this is even more uncommon. Dolichoectatic sclerotic anterior cerebral arteries may cause bitemporal field loss either by direct chiasmal compression[339–341] or by impairing the blood supply of the chiasm.[342] MRI and MRI angiography can confirm the diagnosis. It is unclear whether surgical decompression is the best treatment approach. In one case report,[343] atherosclerotic internal carotid artery compression of the optic nerves mimicked a sellar mass. The patient presented with a bitemporal hemianopia, and unroofing of the optic canals resulted in improvement in visual fields. The close anatomic relationship of the internal carotid artery and the optic nerves and chiasm predisposes to compressive neuropathy, even when the carotid artery is normal.[344]

Optic neuropathy due to these causes is discussed in Chapter 5.

Compression by an arteriovenous malformation

In contrast to the smaller cryptic chiasmal AVMs which present acutely, extrinsic compression by a larger AVM is more likely to cause insidious symptoms. Sibony et al.[345] described two patients with large, angiographically evident AVMs affecting the chiasm. One was suprasellar and fed by the right ophthalmic artery, while the other was a large frontal AVM. Both patients had long-standing evidence of decreasing vision. We have seen a similar case in which the AVM's draining vein compressed the chiasm.[346] Endocrine disturbances, mimicking those associated with a pituitary macroadenoma, may occur when the AVM is intrasellar.[347]

Chiasmal/hypothalamic gliomas

Chiasmal/hypothalamic gliomas, along with craniopharyngiomas, constitute the two most common sellar masses in children. In general, optic gliomas or optic pathway tumors are intrinsic, sometimes hamartoma-like tumors of the anterior visual pathways (optic nerve, chiasm, and tracts) and hypothalamus. These tumors are rare, but they constitute 5% of all childhood brain tumors and 30% of all brain tumors in children less than 5 years old at The Children's Hospital of Philadelphia.[348] Between 59% and 70% present before age 10, and another 20–22% by age 20.[349,350]

Optic nerve gliomas, which involve only the optic nerve, are reviewed in the chapter on optic neuropathies (Chapter 5). In general the greatest morbidity of optic nerve gliomas is visual loss, and the mortality rate is extremely low.[349] On the other hand, optic pathway tumors involving the chiasm and/or hypothalamus, given their location, often present with endocrine dysfunction and are associated with higher morbidity and mortality rates. Therefore, they must be managed differently. Chiasmal/hypothalamic gliomas constitute approximately 75% of all optic pathway gliomas.[350]

271

Association with neurofibromatosis type 1 (NF-1)

The incidence of neurofibromatosis 1 (NF-1, von Reckling-hausen's disease) among patients with optic gliomas is 10–70% (average 29%).[350] Because of the strong association, all patients with newly discovered optic gliomas should be screened for NF-1. Diagnostic criteria for NF-1 include two or more of the following (**Fig. 7–29**): (1) café au lait spots on the skin, (2) cutaneous neurofibromas, (3) axillary or inguinal freckling, (4) optic gliomas, (5) iris hamartomas (Lisch nodules), (6) bony lesion such as sphenoid wing dysplasia, and (7) family history of NF-1.[351] Thus, in a patient with an optic glioma, the presence of any other feature of NF-1 establishes the diagnosis. Although there have been a few reported individuals with neurofibromato-sis type 2 (bilateral acoustic neuromas) and optic pathway tumors,[352] an association has not been confirmed.

In one study by Lewis et al.,[353] 15% of patients with NF-1 were found to have optic pathway gliomas when screened with brain CT. Listernick et al.[354] found 19% of their NF-1 patients had optic gliomas. The slightly higher proportion in this study may have resulted from the fact that patients were screened with both CT and MRI, the latter of which may be more sensitive in detecting optic pathway involvement. Optic gliomas in NF-1 are more likely to involve the optic nerves, while those in patients without NF-1 more commonly involve the chiasm.[355] Bilateral optic nerve gliomas without chiasmal involvement is highly suggestive of NF-1 and unusual in its absence.

Only a portion of patients with NF-1 develop visual loss, usually at a young age. Lewis et al.[353] found that only one-

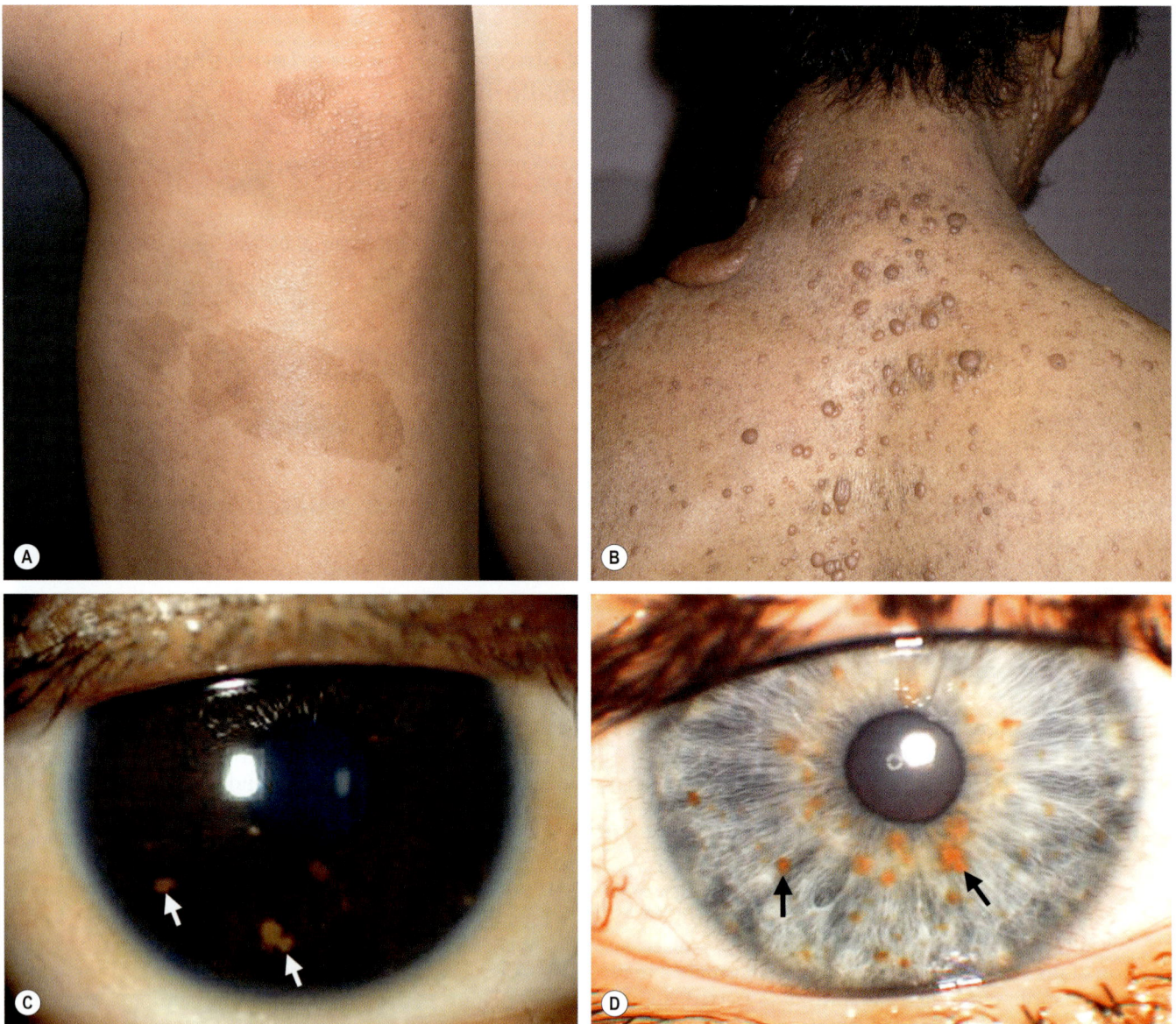

Figure 7–29. Systemic manifestations of neurofibromatosis type 1. **A**. Typical café au lait spots on the skin. **B**. Multiple cutaneous neurofibromas. **C**. Iris Lisch nodules (arrows), in an individual with a dark iris, evident on slit-lamp examination. The nodules are light-colored and appear like splattered putty or white paint. **D**. In contrast, individuals with light irises tend to have orange or brown round Lisch nodules (arrows).

third of their patients with radiographically demonstrated gliomas were symptomatic with either subnormal vision or optic atrophy. In Balcer et al.'s study,[356] approximately one-half of patients with NF-1 and optic gliomas developed vision loss, most often before age 10. All symptomatic optic pathway tumors in Listernick et al.'s[354] study were diagnosed before 6 years of age. New vision loss or visual progression can occur in adolescence but is less common.[356-358] A newly symptomatic optic pathway glioma would be very unusual in adulthood.[359]

There is considerable debate whether all children with NF-1 should undergo routine neuroimaging[360-363] or VEPs[364,365] to screen for optic pathway tumors.[366] Currently at The Children's Hospital of Philadelphia, the decision to perform an MRI is made on an individual basis. MRIs are obtained in NF-1 patients with an abnormal neurologic examination or learning disability, attentional deficit, endocrinopathy, or developmental delay or in those not cooperative for a visual assessment. Every patient with NF-1 receives at least an annual neuro-ophthalmologic examination, and unexplained acuity, color, or field loss, afferent pupillary defect, proptosis, or optic atrophy would also mandate neuroimaging.[367] Because there is no evidence that treating an asymptomatic optic glioma in patients with NF-1 prevents subsequent visual loss, in general there is no advantage in detecting these lesions at an early stage with screening neuroimaging. Even after a normal MRI, the neuro-ophthalmologic status of a young patient with NF-1 is still closely monitored, because optic gliomas may still develop despite the unremarkable initial neuroimaging.[368,369] Some authors[370-374] have suggested screening for and following gliomas in NF-1 with VEPs. However, our NF-1 patients do not undergo VEPs because the testing is associated with unacceptable false-positive[365] and false-negative rates[375] regarding tumor detection.[376] The neuro-ophthalmic examination in our opinion is a more reliable screen, even in young children.[366,377]

Pathology

Optic gliomas, like cystic cerebellar astrocytomas, are juvenile pilocytic astrocytomas.[378] In general, these are benign, low-grade glial tumors, which are grade 1 in the World Health Organization classification of gliomas.[379] Other pathologic features include eosinophilic Rosenthal fibers and the absence of mitotic figures. Extracellular accumulation of acid mucopolysaccharide may account for some instances of tumor enlargement,[380,381] and resorption of this mucosubstance may explain spontaneous shrinkage of some optic nerve and chiasmal gliomas. Other possible mechanisms for tumor growth include proliferation of neoplastic cells and reactive arachnoidal proliferation.[350] Optic gliomas should be distinguished from cerebral gliomas and malignant optic gliomas of adulthood, which are discussed in the subsequent section.

Location and growth characteristics

Gliomas involving the chiasm and the optic nerves are termed *anterior chiasmal gliomas,* while those with extension into the optic tracts or hypothalamus are classified as *posterior chiasmal gliomas.*

For decades, the growth potential of these optic gliomas has been a controversial issue.[382] Hoyt and Baghdassarian[383] advocated the notion that they are benign hamartomas: "optic gliomata are clinically indolent tumours that tend to enlarge, cause symptoms early in life, and remain static thereafter. Unlike the rare glioblastomata that arise in the adult optic nerve, childhood gliomata do not undergo malignant degeneration. They have features of congenital hamartomata." On the other hand, more recent histopathologic studies have suggested that optic gliomas are true neoplasms.[384,385]

It has been our personal experience that chiasmal/hypothalamic gliomas behave unpredictably, and their growth rates span a wide spectrum. Some do behave like hamartomas,[386] but some grow over years, then stop, while others continue to enlarge and cause progressive symptoms despite all interventions. In rare instances, spontaneous improvement in vision and radiographic appearance can also occur.[387-395] Central nervous system (CNS) and abdominal (via ventriculoperitoneal shunting) metastases also have been documented.[396-400] In general, the morbidity and mortality of anterior chiasmal gliomas is much less than those with posterior extension.[349,401,402]

Extension of an optic nerve glioma into a previously uninvolved chiasm is extremely rare.[403] Therefore we are not routinely recommending removal of a posteriorly situated optic nerve glioma to prevent "spread" into the chiasm.

In neurofibromatosis, there is a relatively high rate of second intracranial tumors such as cerebral gliomas.[404]

Symptoms

Because they are slow growing, chiasmal/hypothalamic gliomas tend to present insidiously with visual loss with optic atrophy and/or endocrine dysfunction. Headache can be a common complaint, especially when the third ventricle is obstructed by a large hypothalamic component.

Neuro-ophthalmic signs

Visual acuity varies at presentation, but profound acuity loss (worse than 20/200) is not uncommon.[350] Monocular or bitemporal field defects occur in about 40% of cases, and other patterns of field loss include unilateral or bilateral optic nerve-related deficits, homonymous defects due to optic tract involvement, or diffuse visual loss.[386] In general, it is difficult to correlate an optic glioma's location with the field defect, as dysfunction of anatomically involved structures does not always occur. Despite diffuse infiltration of the anterior visual pathway, an optic glioma may present solely with a bitemporal hemianopia or a unilateral central scotoma. In the extreme case of some patients with neurofibromatosis with large radiographically demonstrated lesions, there may be no visual field defect. In addition, optic gliomas may progress radiographically without change in visual function, and vision can worsen without any change in size of the lesion.[405]

Visual loss rarely can occur apoplectically,[406] and in some instances this behavior may reflect sudden cyst enlargement rather than tumor growth per se. Young children, who might not complain of visual loss, may present with strabismus owing to poor vision in one eye. Other presentations include monocular[407] or asymmetric nystagmus or the full triad of head nodding, head tilt, and nystagmus, mimicking spasmus nutans.[40,408] Optic atrophy is the rule, but optic nerve infiltration or third ventricular obstruction with hydrocephalus may be associated with optic disc swelling (**Fig. 7–30**). A large optic nerve component might also lead to proptosis. Cranial neuropathies in general are not associated with chiasmal/hypothalamic gliomas.

Endocrinologic manifestations

Endocrine signs and symptoms can be a prominent feature when the glioma either originates or extends into the hypothalamus.[409,410] Russell's diencephalic syndrome and precocious puberty are the two most common endocrinopathies at presentation (see **Fig. 7–17**),[47,400] while diabetes insipidus and hypopituitarism are uncommon initial symptoms.

Diagnostic studies/neuroimaging

MRI is preferable to CT in the evaluation of these tumors because of the availability of coronal images and its superior ability in imaging the optic tract/hypothalamic extent of the lesion.[411,412] Chiasmal gliomas are seen best on coronal images, and they appear as intrinsic enlargement of the chiasm (**Fig. 7–31**),[413] occasionally with a cystic component.[414] When the optic nerves are also involved and enlarged, the anterior chiasm looks like an upside-down pair of pants on axial images. Chiasmal/hypothalamic gliomas are usually

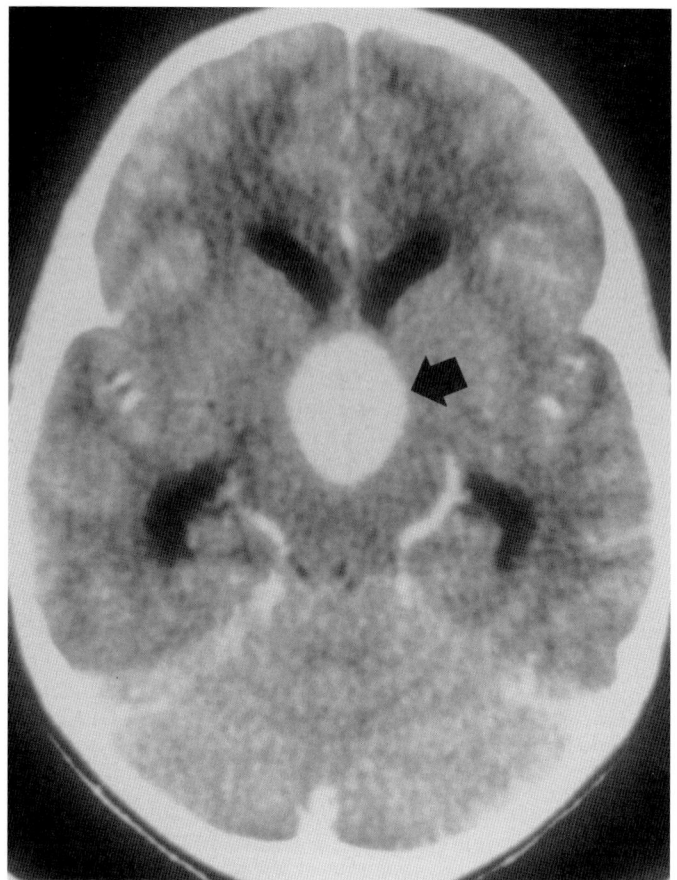

Figure 7–30. Axial CT scan showing contrast-enhancing globular chiasmal/hypothalamic glioma (*arrow*) obstructing the third ventricle and causing hydrocephalus and papilledema.

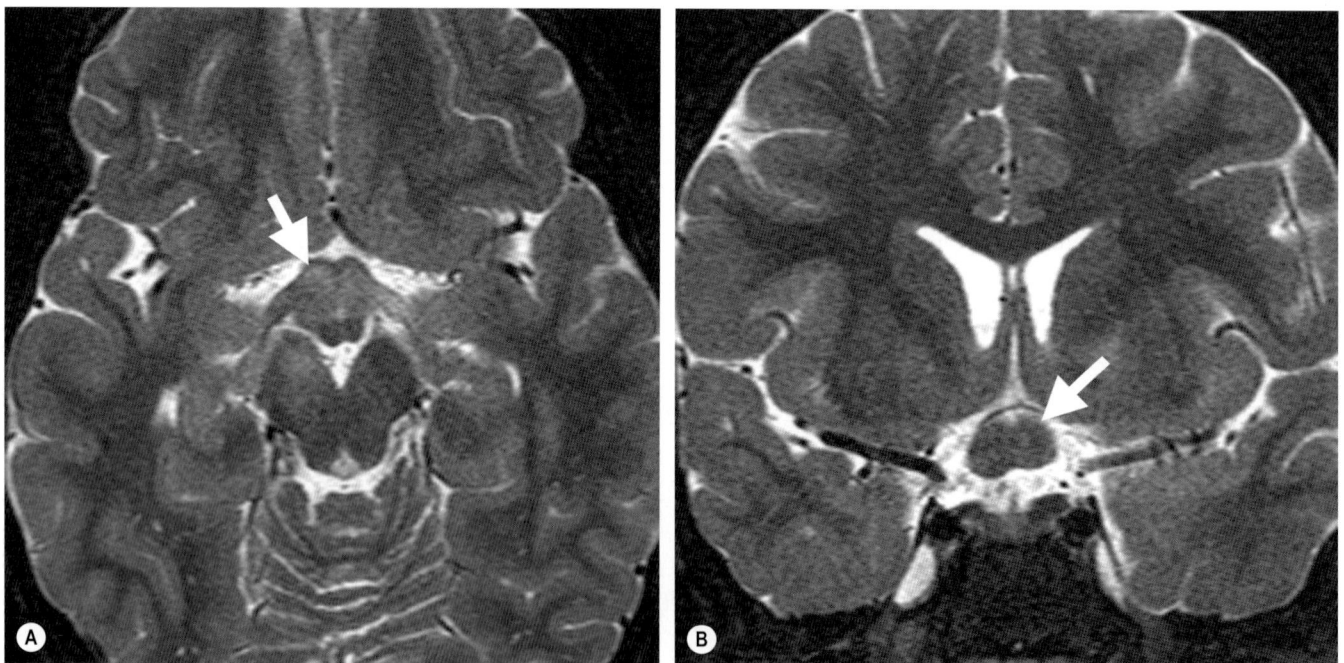

Figure 7–31. Chiasmal glioma. Intrinsic enlargement of the chiasm (arrow) demonstrated on T2-weighted MR images. **A**. Axial view. **B**. Coronal view.

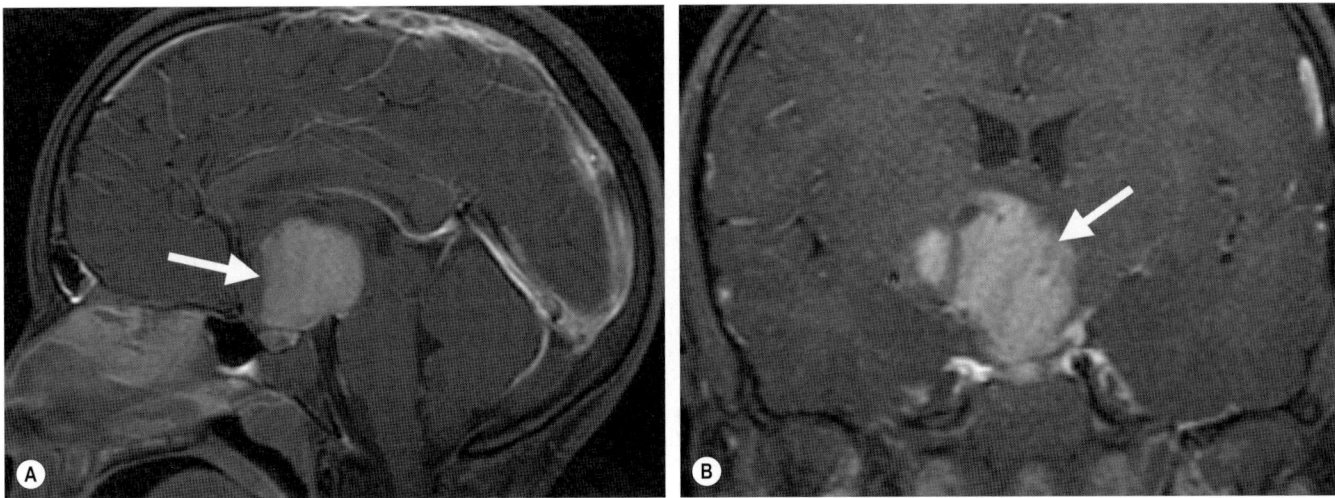

Figure 7–32. Chiasmal/hypothalamic glioma, depicted in enhanced T1-weighted MR images. The large enhancing mass (arrow) obliterates the chiasm, hypothalamus, and third ventricle. **A**. Sagittal view. **B**. Coronal view.

round suprasellar masses, and often it is difficult to tell whether the growth arises from the chiasm or hypothalamus (**Fig. 7–32**). The lesions are isointense or hypointense on T1-weighted images, hyperintense on T2-weighted images, and may enhance with gadolinium.[85] Optic tract involvement can be evident when the tracts are bright on T2 and enhanced images (**Fig. 7–33**).[415] Involvement of the optic radiations is rare but has been reported.[416]

When there is intrinsic enlargement of visual pathways in any child or an individual of any age with NF-1, the MRI appearance is almost pathognomonic. Masqueraders include gangliogliomas, germ cell tumors, sarcoidosis, and intrachiasmal craniopharyngiomas. Although chiasmal neuritis may have a similar neuroradiologic appearance, its sudden visual loss should easily distinguish that entity from a chiasmal glioma. Malignant optic gliomas can be distinguished clinically by rapidly progressive visual loss and onset in adulthood.

Fletcher et al.[405] outlined three characteristics of chiasmal gliomas evident on CT scanning: tubular thickening of the optic nerve and chiasm, a suprasellar tumor with contiguous optic nerve expansion, and a suprasellar tumor with optic tract involvement. The diagnosis cannot be made with certainty in the case of a globular suprasellar mass without optic nerve or tract extension.

Treatment

Despite the myriad of retrospective series and reviews by authorities on the subject,[349,350,366,383,386,401,402,417–438] the best treatment of chiasmal/hypothalamic gliomas is unfortunately still unclear. The controversy exists in part because the tumors are heterogeneous in terms of clinical presentation, location, and natural history, and each institution has its own bias with regards to treatment approach. Many studies failed to include complete neuro-ophthalmic data, and older studies were performed prior to the availability of MRIs, which have greatly improved tumor localization. Several studies analyzed the efficacy of radiation, previously a popular treatment, but today rarely used because of side-

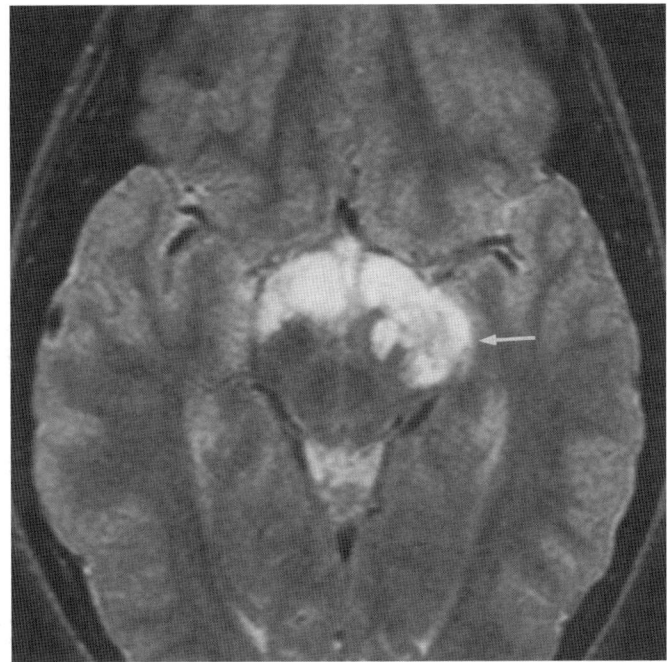

Figure 7–33. Optic tract involvement (arrow) by a chiasmal/hypothalamic glioma. T2-weighted axial MRI.

effects. A prospective, controlled trial is necessary to resolve these treatment issues, but such a study would have to account for tumor heterogeneity and include long follow-up. The tumors grow slowly, and in some instances many years may pass following treatment before they progress again.

Combined, the neuro-oncology and neuro-ophthalmology services at The Children's Hospital of Philadelphia[433,434,437] currently maintain an individualized approach to chiasmal/hypothalamic gliomas based upon (1) location of the tumor on MRI, (2) tumor size, (3) neuro-ophthalmic status, (4) endocrine status, and (5) the presence of NF-1. *Anterior chiasmal gliomas*, especially in patients with NF-1, do not require a biopsy, and without evidence of radiographic or clinical (visual or endocrine) progression, can be observed.[401] The MRI and neuro-ophthalmic examination, including visual fields, should be repeated in 6–18 weeks, then semiannually if stable. If the lesion is confined to the optic nerves and chiasm, biopsy or surgery carries the chance of causing further visual loss, and therefore should be avoided in such instances.

Evidence of progression on two successive neuro-ophthalmologic or radiologic examinations would be an indication for chemotherapy.[348,439,440] Currently vincristine and carboplatin (preferred now over actinomycin D) are first-line agents;[441] topotecan and oral etoposide (VP-16), procarbazine, vinblastine, N-(2-chloroethyl)-N-cyclohexyl-N-nitrosurea (CCNU), and thioguanine are other alternatives, especially when the tumors recur.[438,442] Furthermore, in the case of a very young child with a chiasmal/hypothalamic glioma and profound visual loss, it is reasonable to initiate chemotherapy without evidence of progression, as the child's age may preclude detection of small changes in vision.

External beam radiation (approximately 4500–5000 cGy in divided doses[443]) can halt tumor growth and the progression of visual loss.[426,427,444–447] Less commonly, vision improves.[448] However, major side-effects of cranial irradiation for optic gliomas include mental retardation, endocrinopathies, and cerebrovascular disease including moya-moya syndrome,[449–451] particularly in smaller children who are most vulnerable to these complications. Radionecrosis of the chiasm[452] and secondary tumors[453] have also been reported. Therefore, radiation is only uncommonly used now.

In young children with grossly asymmetric visual loss, part-time monocular patching of the better eye should also be considered when superimposed amblyopia may be present (see Chapter 5, Optic nerve gliomas).

Posterior chiasmal gliomas in patients with NF-1 may be observed, particularly when their neuro-ophthalmic examination is normal. In those without NF-1 and with hypothalamic involvement, a biopsy of that part should be performed because the differential diagnosis, which includes craniopharyngiomas or germinomas for instance, can be broad. Since these posterior gliomas have a poorer prognosis, it may be prudent in some cases then to institute chemotherapy right away, without requiring documentation of radiographic or clinical progression. It has been debated whether partial or radical resection of a globular hypothalamic component, in cases without extensive optic nerve or tract involvement, enhances the prognosis.[429,431,432,434] Large tumors, obstruction of the foramina of Monro, and cysts associated with visual progression are other reasonable indications for neurosurgical intervention.[454] However, it is unclear whether aggressive surgery, which can be associated with vascular occlusion, endocrinopathy, and further visual loss, is necessary in every instance.

Outcome

In patients with NF-1, those with gliomas involving the tract or hypothalamus have a worse visual prognosis than those with solely optic nerve or chiasmal involvement.[356] Chemotherapy may halt or reverse visual and radiographic progression in the majority of cases, but many patients continue to lose vision despite chemotherapy.[438,455] Outcome analyses of patients treated with radiation are no longer relevant.[350,402,444]

It has been our impression that children who present at a very young age in general have a poor prognosis, but that those with NF-1 have a better prognosis. While some authors have agreed with our observations,[423,431] analyses of larger numbers of patients have not arrived at the same conclusions regarding the protective effect of NF-1.[349,350,436]

Malignant optic chiasmal gliomas of adulthood

These uncommon tumors also primarily involve the anterior visual pathway, and occur primarily in middle-aged and elderly individuals. In contrast to the aforementioned pediatric optic gliomas, however, malignant optic chiasmal gliomas of adulthood cause rapidly progressive bilateral visual loss, and are uniformly lethal. Some cases have been associated with prior intracranial irradiation.[456] Only a handful of unusual cases in children have been reported.[457]

Pathology, location and growth characteristics

These tumors should be considered glioblastomas of the anterior visual pathway, although some would also include anaplastic astrocytomas in this location. Hoyt et al.[458] called these lesions a "common type of brain tumour in an uncommon location." Initially malignant optic gliomas affect just one optic nerve, then within several weeks spread to the chiasm and other optic nerve before reaching the optic tracts, hypothalamus, internal capsules, and basal ganglia.

Symptoms and signs

Initially, patients appear to have optic neuritis in one eye, with monocular visual loss occurring over a few weeks, and the optic disc is either normal or exhibits only mild disc swelling.[458] They may also complain of ocular pain exacerbated by eye movements. Within the ensuing weeks or months, visual loss progresses, often accompanied by ophthalmoscopic evidence of a central retinal artery or venous occlusion due to tumor infiltration of the proximal optic nerve. Later, vision in the other eye becomes involved, and eventually each eye suffers from severe visual loss. Cerebral extension is manifested by hypothalamic disturbances, hemiparesis, and altered mental status.

Diagnostic studies/neuroimaging

Typically on MRI, the chiasm is enlarged and enhances with gadolinium. As the lesion progresses, radiographic involvement of the optic tracts, hypothalamus, and other cerebral structures becomes evident (**Fig. 7–34**).[459,460] On CT scanning, adult chiasmal gliomas may appear cystic with ring

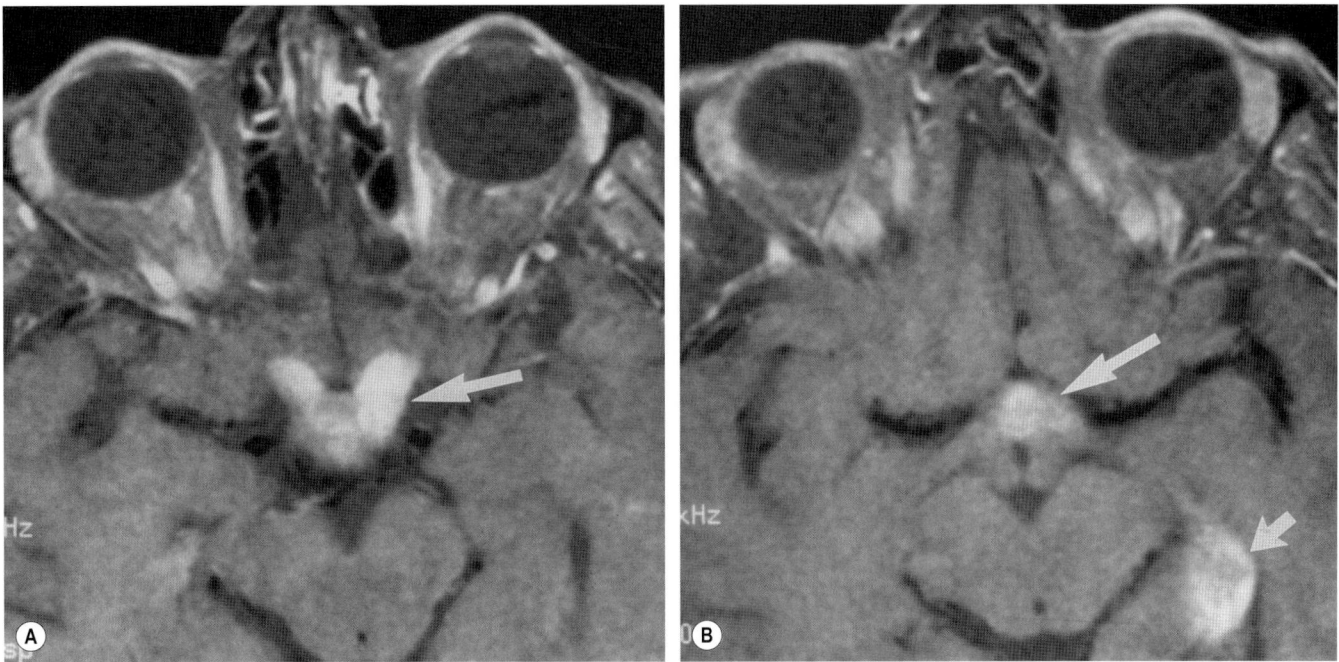

Figure 7–34. Malignant chiasmal glioma, which presented with rapidly progressive visual loss and was biopsy proven. **A**. Axial MRI scan with gadolinium demonstrates chiasmal enlargement and enhancement (*arrow*). **B**. Axial MRI scan with gadolinium, dorsal to the view in part A, revealing tumor involvement of the left optic tract (*larger arrow*) and lateral geniculate nucleus (*smaller arrow*).

enhancement and mimic other suprasellar masses.[461] Since the neuroimaging features are nonspecific, the diagnosis relies more on the patient's age and rapidly progressive symptoms.

Treatment

The results of most treatment modalities in this disorder are disappointing. Steroids usually have only some transient benefit. In exceptional instances, combined radiation and chemotherapy may prolong survival.[462]

Hypothalamic (tuber cinereum) hamartomas

These lesions present primarily with precocious puberty because they release luteinizing hormone-releasing hormone (LHRH), and other common clinical features can include gelastic seizures, mental retardation, and behavioral disturbances. However, when they grow large enough, they can compress the chiasm. Hypothalamic hamartomas are noninvasive, rarely grow in size, and microscopically are composed of neurons and glia. Radiographically, they appear as round sessile or pedunculated masses ("collar-buttons") attached to the posterior hypothalamus between the infundibulum and mamillary bodies.[463] They are isointense relative to gray matter on T1-weighted MR images and are homogeneous and hyperintense on T2-weighted images.

When the clinical, radiographic, and endocrinologic (e.g., LHRH levels) features are consistent with a hypothalamic hamartoma, observation with serial biannual or annual neuroimaging and examinations may be sufficient. Treatment of the precocious puberty consists of hormonal suppression therapy. Surgical management should be reserved for chias-

mal compression, atypical lesions, progressive enlargement, and instances where medical management fails to control endocrine dysfunction.[463,464]

Gangliogliomas

Gangliogliomas are CNS neoplasms which contain neuronal and glial elements. These tumors may arise anywhere in the neuroaxis but are more common in the cerebral hemispheres and spinal cord.[465] Patients usually present with intellectual and behavioral abnormalities, seizures, or focal neurologic deficits.[466]

Gangliogliomas involving the anterior visual pathways are uncommon but have been reported.[467–470] Mechanisms include medial extension of a temporal lobe ganglioglioma into the suprasellar area and tumor intrinsic to the hypothalamus and chiasm. Since the optic nerve and chiasm do not contain neuronal cell bodies, these gangliogliomas may have arisen from ectopic neural tissue or more primitive neurons, or spread from the floor of the third ventricle. Because of their indolent visual loss associated with optic nerve or chiasmal enlargement, gangliogliomas intrinsic to the anterior visual pathway may mimic optic gliomas clinically and radiologically.[471]

Gangliogliomas are usually slowly growing neoplasms, and occasionally behave like hamartomas. When surgically accessible, complete resection is usually curative, with radiation and chemotherapy reserved for cases with progression or recurrence.[472,473] However, when the chiasm and hypothalamus are involved, complete surgical resection is impossible. In these instances, patients should undergo subtotal removal followed by radiotherapy, but the visual prognosis is varied.

Germ cell tumors

Intracranially, these tumors arise in midline structures, particularly the suprasellar and pineal regions. The reason for the predilection for those areas is not clear, but these may be sites of primordial germ cell migration during ontogeny.[474] Most are diagnosed between 10 and 21 years of age,[464] and there is no sex preponderance for suprasellar lesions.[475] Actually, extracranial sites are more common and include the gonads (e.g., testicular seminomas and ovarian dysgerminomas), retroperitoneum, and mediastinum.[464]

There are three major groups of intracranial germ cell neoplasms: germinomas, teratomas, and nongerminoma germ cell tumors.[474] Suprasellar germinomas include tumors previously termed ectopic pinealomas,[476] atypical teratomas,[477] or dysgerminomas. They are composed of primordial, polygonal germ cells with lymphocytic infiltration, and these tend to have the best prognosis because of their radiosensitivity. Teratomas, on the other hand, consist of differentiated tissue of all three germ layers. Pure teratomas are benign and also have a good prognosis.[478] The nongerminoma germ cell tumors include embryonal carcinomas, yolk sac or endodermal sinus tumors, choriocarcinomas, and immature teratomas.[464] As these are radio-insensitive, they have the worst prognosis.

Location and growth characteristics

Suprasellar germ cell tumors tend to be located inferior and posterior to the chiasm. Frequently they infiltrate the hypothalamus, infundibulum, and optic nerves. Subarachnoid, intra-axial, and subependymal (ventricular) seeding unfortunately is not uncommon.[477] Germinomas can secrete human chorionic gonadotropin (HCG), α-fetoprotein, and carcinoembryonic antigen (CEA). In a minority of cases there is concomitant involvement of both the suprasellar region and the pineal gland, a presentation known as "multiple midline germinomas"[443] (**Fig. 7–35**).

Symptoms and signs

The symptom triad of diabetes insipidus, visual loss, and hypopituitarism is present in the majority of patients with suprasellar germ cell tumors.[475,476] Of these, diabetes insipidus is the most common, occurring in almost all patients.[477,479] It is usually the initial symptom and can be present for years prior to diagnosis. Visual deficits result either from tumor compression or from infiltration of the chiasm.[479] Thus bitemporal hemianopias as well as nondescript field loss can be observed,[477,480] and optic atrophy is very common. Papilledema due to elevated intracranial pressure and ocular motor palsies occur in only a very small minority.[481] Hypothalamic and pituitary dysfunction manifests as, in decreasing order of frequency, hypogonadism, panhypopituitarism, hypothyroidism, dwarfism, hypocortisolism, central hyperthermia, cachexia, and precocious puberty.[476] Tumor β-HCG production stimulates Leydig cells to secrete testosterone, leading to precocious puberty in males.

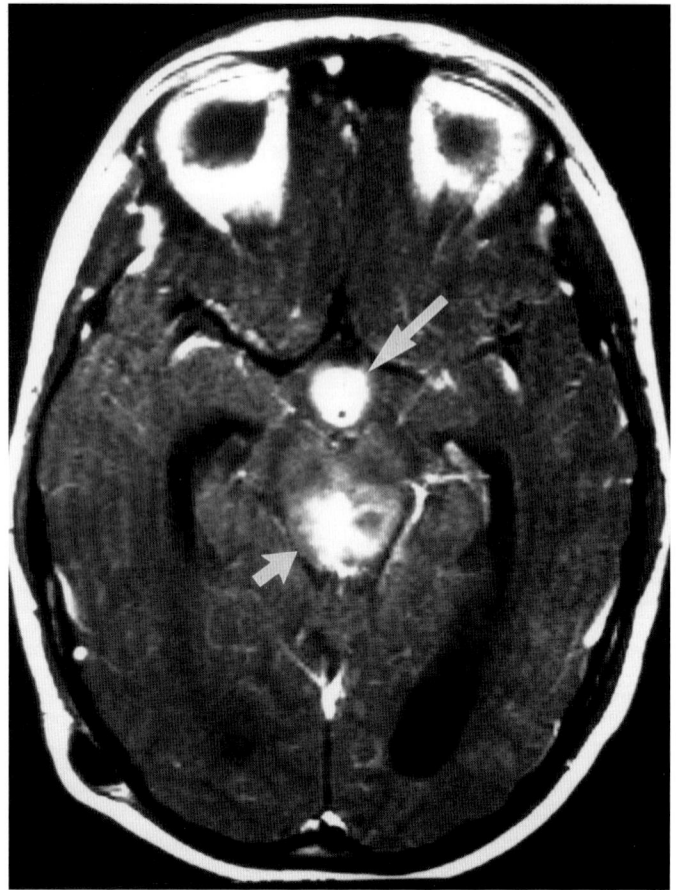

Figure 7–35. Enhanced axial MRI scan demonstrating multicentric germinoma involving the sella (*large arrow*) and pineal region (*small arrow*).

Diagnostic studies/neuroimaging

By the time they present, suprasellar germinomas are usually already large. They are homogeneous and only rarely have cystic components. On MRI they are mildly hypointense on T1-weighted images, hyperintense on T2-weighted images, and enhance with contrast. Teratomas tend to be more heterogeneous with evidence of fat or calcification.[85] On CT the lesions are iso- or high density, and they also contrast enhance.[480]

Diagnostic studies/laboratory tests

Along with the standard endocrinologic screening, serum and CSF β-HCG and α-fetoprotein levels should be evaluated. These tumor markers are helpful in monitoring treatment. High β-HCG levels suggest choriocarcinoma. Cerebrospinal fluid also should be sent for cytologic examination, which can reveal abnormal cells when there is a germ cell tumor.

Treatment

Previously, germinomas were empirically irradiated, sometimes supported by an abnormal CSF cytology.[480] However, modern neurosurgical techniques, a preference for histologic confirmation,[474] and the observation that decompression of the anterior visual pathways can result in visual improvement have made subtotal resection the preferable approach.[481] Benign teratomas require no further therapy, and pure germinomas respond well to postoperative radiation. Younger children may undergo chemotherapy to delay radiation. Recurrent disease may necessitate chemotherapy.[482] The more aggressive nongerminoma germ cell tumors require both craniospinal irradiation and adjuvant chemotherapy.[443]

Outcome

Recurrence and survival rates depend heavily on tumor histology. In one series,[481] intracranial germinomas had an 85% long-term survival rate, while those with intracranial nongerminoma germ cell tumors had only a 45% survival rate.

Miscellaneous growths

Epidermoids and dermoids

Epidermoids and dermoids are congenital inclusions of germ layers that occur at the time of neural tube closure.[483] Epidermoids consist of ectodermal germ cells, while dermoids contain both ectodermal and mesodermal germ layers. Visual disturbances, and less commonly hypopituitarism, diabetes insipidus, and cranial neuropathies, can occur when these lesions are in the suprasellar region.[85] On MRI suprasellar epidermoids and dermoids appear as round homogeneous masses which are hyperintense on T1- and T2 weighted images. Their signal characteristics are similar to subcutaneous fat, reflecting the presence of glandular tissue from hair follicles and sebaceous and apocrine glands.

Chiasmal metastases

Cohen and Lessell[484] described three such cases, each presenting with acuity loss and bitemporal hemianopia. Breast and lung cancer were the primary malignancies in two of the patients, while in the third no primary was found. Dexamethasone and radiation, with chemotherapy in one case, offered some visual recovery.

Sellar and chiasmal lymphoma

Primary B-cell CNS lymphoma should be considered when there is a sellar mass in any immunocompromised individual, especially one with acquired immunodeficiency syndrome (AIDS).[485] In addition, cases in immunocompetent individuals have been described.[486-488] In one, lymphoma intrinsic to the chiasm was discovered, and the lesion was steroid responsive.[486] Another reported patient presented with visual loss, impotence, decreased libido, diabetes insipidus, and hearing loss.[487] MRI revealed an enhancing suprasellar mass involving the infundibulum, mamillary bodies, chiasm, and fornix. Biopsy revealed lymphoma, and the patient was treated with high-dose methotrexate followed by radiation.

Granular cell and related tumors

When occurring in the suprasellar region, these masses clinically and radiographically act like pituitary adenomas, presenting with hypopituitarism and visual loss. However, typically they arise from the posterior pituitary or stalk. Other terms used for lesions highly related to sellar granular cell tumors include choristomas, gangliocytomas, myoblastomas, infundibulomas, pituicytomas, and posterior pituitary astrocytoma.[489-493] Technically, choristomas are composed of histologically normal tissue in an abnormal location (heterotopias). In one report of a patient with slowly progressive visual loss owing to a chiasmal choristoma, fibrous tissue and smooth muscle were found in the optic nerve and chiasm.[494] Pituicytomas arise from pituicytes, the parenchymal cells of the posterior lobe of the pituitary. Surgical removal seems to be the most reasonable approach for all these tumors.

Chordomas and chondrosarcomas

These skull base tumors more commonly present with ocular motor palsies so are discussed in more detail in Chapter 15. However, rarely chordomas and chondrosarcomas involving the central skull base can present with chiasmal interference and bitemporal hemianopias.[495,496]

Chiasmal neuritis

Autopsy studies of patients with multiple sclerosis commonly reveal demyelinating lesions in the chiasm. In addition, occasionally patients with optic neuritis with complaints in just one eye are found to have bitemporal field defects on formal perimetry.[497,498] However, clinically evident chiasmal neuritis occurs much less frequently than ordinary optic neuritis. Newman et al.[499] described five such patients and reviewed the reported cases with clinical correlation up to 1991. Most affected individuals were young adult or middle-aged females. The rate of onset of the visual loss was variable, and chiasmal field defects were often accompanied by evidence of optic nerve involvement. MRI typically showed chiasmal enlargement and enhancement, along with intrinsic bright T2 signal. Although most individuals improved with or without corticosteroids, for unclear reasons patients took longer (months) to recover than those with ordinary optic neuritis.

In an individual with a history of multiple sclerosis, no further workup is required. In other cases, systemic lupus erythematosus,[500] sarcoidosis, and other systemic disorders should be excluded by appropriate testing (antinuclear antibodies (ANA), angiotensin converting enzyme (ACE), erythrocyte sedimentation rate (ESR), and chest radiograph and/or gallium scan). Optic gliomas appear similar radiographically, but they can be distinguished clinically by their more insidious visual loss.

In the Optic Neuritis Treatment Trial,[501] patients with optic neuritis who were given corticosteroids recovered more quickly, but their visual outcomes at 1 year were similar to those given placebo. However, we consider chiasmal neuritis as a different situation because of the bilateral nature of the visual loss. If the field defects are subtle, then it might be reasonable to observe. On the other hand we treat those patients with dense bitemporal defects or severe acuity loss with 3–5 days of high-dose (1 g) intravenous methylprednisolone, followed by a short taper of oral prednisone over 5–10 days.

Inflammatory masses

Inflammatory suprasellar masses include sarcoidosis, histiocytosis X, lymphocytic adenohypophysitis, idiopathic granulomatous hypophysitis, and optochiasmatic arachnoiditis. Sarcoidosis is more common than the others. In unusual cases, these disorders can present with isolated sellar lesions without systemic involvement, thereby mimicking pituitary tumors or craniopharyngiomas. In such instances, a transsphenoidal or stereotactic biopsy is required to establish the diagnosis.

Sarcoidosis

Because of its tendency to involve the basal meninges, it is not uncommon for sarcoidosis to affect the chiasm, hypothalamus, or pituitary gland.[502,503] The typical scenario is a bitemporal hemianopia or some other pattern of bilateral visual loss, diabetes insipidus, obesity, and hypopituitarism—with or without systemic involvement.[504–506] Chronic cases usually present with optic atrophy, but concomitant optic nerve involvement may be associated with disc swelling. Concurrent uveitis or facial nerve or ocular motor palsies are highly suggestive of sarcoid. On MRI, suprasellar sarcoid appears as an irregular, infiltrative mass which is isointense to brain on T1-weighted images, hyperintense on T2-weighted images, and enhances with contrast (**Fig. 7–36** and see **Fig. 17–14**).[507] On CT scanning the suprasellar lesions contrast enhance.[508] Sarcoid can also be intrinsic to the chiasm and optic nerves, causing radiographic enlargement and gadolinium enhancement of the anterior visual pathway.[509] In one

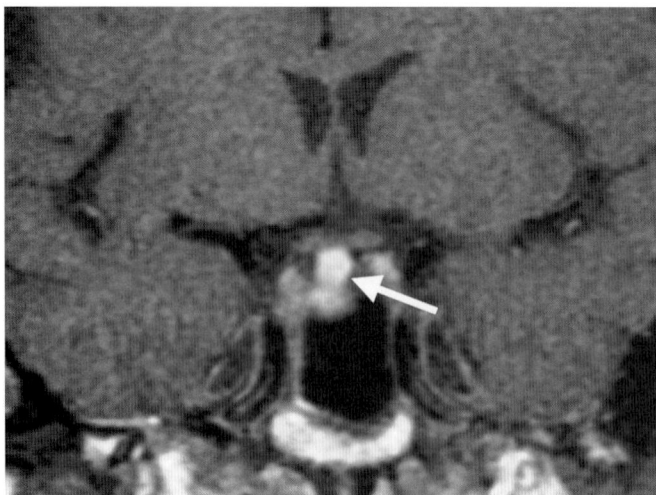

Figure 7–36. Coronal T1-weighted, gadolinism-enhanced MRI demonstrating sarcoidosis involving the sella and infundibulum (arrow), contiguous to the inferior chiasm.

series of chiasmal sarcoid,[510] four out of four patients had elevated CSF protein. Gelwan et al.[511] treated four patients with chiasmal sarcoid and visual loss with high-dose intravenous corticosteroids. Visual improvement was usually temporary, and subsequent deteriorations necessitated radiation, then immunosuppressive medications such as azathioprine or chlorambucil. Other steroid-sparing agents such as cyclophosphamide, methotrexate,[512] cyclosporine,[503] and cladribine[513] have been used in sarcoidosis in this region.

Further details regarding the histopathology, diagnosis, and treatment of sarcoidosis involving the anterior visual pathway are discussed in Chapter 5.

Langerhans cell histiocytosis (histiocytosis X)

Pathologically, this disorder is typified by distinctive granulomas resulting from idiopathic proliferation of histiocytes, plasma cells, and eosinophilic inflammatory cells.[514] Other terms for Langerhans cell histiocytosis have been used, depending upon its focality and severity. Eosinophilic granuloma is the preferred designation when the process is unifocal. Hand–Schüller–Christian disease, the multifocal type, has a classic triad of exophthalmos, diabetes insipidus, and skull lesions. The cells are well differentiated in these two types. In contrast, Letterer–Siwe disease is a more aggressive form characterized by poorly differentiated histiocytes and multiorgan involvement.

Intracranial Langerhans cell histiocytosis has a predilection for the hypothalamic–pituitary axis.[514–516] Endocrine disturbances are the most common manifestation, and the most frequent of these are diabetes insipidus, GH deficiency, and delayed puberty.[464] Histiocytosis should always be considered in an individual with diabetes insipidus and an enhancing mass involving the pituitary stalk.[517] Visual loss due to compression of the anterior visual pathway can occur.[518,519] Previous or concurrent skin, bone, or reticuloendothelial involvement should suggest the diagnosis, but cases can be isolated to the CNS. Surgical removal, chemotherapy, immunosuppression, and radiation therapy are all reasonable treatment options, depending upon the extent of CNS and systemic involvement.[520]

Lymphocytic adenohypophysitis

This entity occurs predominantly in younger women and is most common during pregnancy or in the postpartum period.[521,522] It is a presumed autoimmune disease,[44] as other associated conditions include Sjögren's disease, thyroiditis, pernicious anemia, rheumatoid arthritis, and insulin-dependent diabetes.[523] The disorder is characterized histopathologically by plasma cell and lymphocyte infiltration of the pituitary, and clinically by headaches and hyperprolactinemia or hypopituitarism out of proportion to the degree of radiographic pituitary enlargement.[524] Bitemporal field defects may occur when extrasellar extension involves the chiasm.[524–526] On MRI, lymphocytic adenohypophysitis appears as a symmetric, solid sellar mass which is isotense with gray matter on T1- and T2-weighted images and which gadolinium enhances.[524,527] The lesions are homogeneous and contrast enhancing on CT. Because the clinical and radiographic features can be confused with those of a pituitary adenoma,[528] a definitive diagnosis requires a biopsy. Chiasmal compression is an indication for partial resection, but complete removal, often resulting in unwarranted panhypopituitarism, should be avoided.[526] Adjunctive corticosteroid treatment is usually extremely effective.

Idiopathic granulomatous hypophysitis (giant cell granuloma)

This related disorder can involve the pituitary, infundibulum, and potentially the chiasm.[529-531] Granulomatous hypophysitis typically presents in middle-aged or older women with hypopituitarism and diabetes insipidus. The older age predilection, diabetes insipidus, MRI evidence of infundibular thickening, and granulomatous inflammation distinguish this disorder from lymphocytic adenohypophysitis. Lack of systemic involvement separates it from the aforementioned granulomatous processes. Transsphenoidal biopsy is usually necessary to establish the diagnosis, and corticosteroids are the treatment of choice. Rarely, granulomatous hypophysitis caused by a ruptured intrasellar Rathke's cleft cyst can be identified.[532]

Optochiasmatic arachnoiditis

An inflammatory response in the suprasellar space may occur idiopathically or in association with head trauma or infections such as tuberculosis and cysticercosis (see below). In addition, optochiasmatic arachnoiditis may be induced by muslin wrapping of intracranial aneurysms in this region.[533,534]

Infections

Because the chiasm is surrounded by cerebrospinal fluid, it is particularly vulnerable to any of the infectious meningitides. In addition to tuberculous meningitis, which is discussed in more detail below, purulent meningitis due to *Streptococcus pneumoniae, Staphylococcus, Pseudomonas aeruginosa,* cryptococcus, and syphilis infrequently can involve the chiasm. Other types of infections in this area are discussed below as well.

Tuberculosis

Pathologically, tuberculous meningitis is characterized by a thick grayish, gelatinous exudate at the base of the brain and cisterns,[535] consisting of polymorphonuclear cell infiltration, fibrin, endarteritis, and caseous necrosis.[536] With modern multidrug therapy, anterior visual pathway involvement in tuberculous meningitis has become exceedingly rare in developed nations.[537] However, we treated a previously healthy, immunocompetent 11-year-old boy who developed blindness, optic atrophy, and bilateral partial IIIrd nerve palsies as early sequelae of tuberculous meningitis. MRI revealed perichiasmal and basal cistern enhancement (**Fig. 7-37**).[538] Some authors have termed this process tuberculous optochiasmatic arachnoiditis.[539] When this occurs, visual field defects may be scotomatous or hemianopic, but more typically concentric contraction is present.[539] The diagnosis

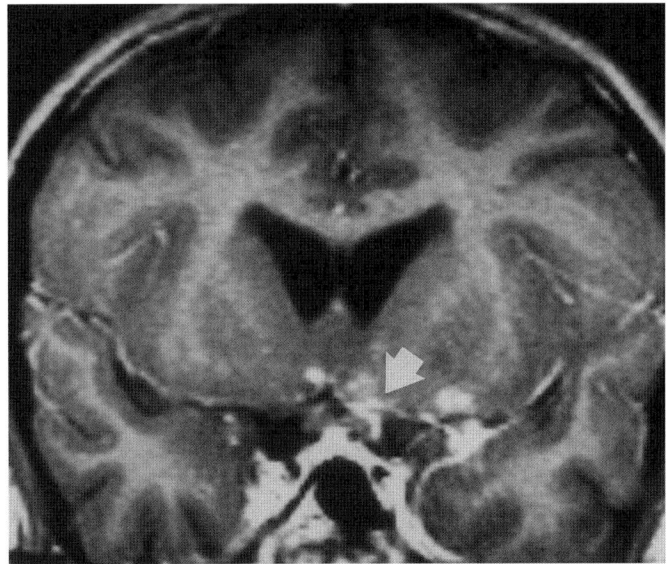

Figure 7-37. This patient with tuberculous meningitis presented with blindness, IIIrd nerve palsies, and altered mental status. The coronal MRI scan with gadolinium demonstrated perichiasmal enhancement (*arrow*), presumably due to arachnoiditis. (From Silverman IE, Liu GT, Bilaniuk LT, et al. Tuberculous meningitis with blindness and peri-chiasmal involvement on MRI. Pediatr Neurol 1995;12:65–67, with permission.)

is supported by MRI evidence of perichiasmal enhancement. CSF analysis should be consistent with tuberculous meningitis (low glucose, lymphocytic or polymorphonuclear pleocytosis, and elevated protein).[540] Unfortunately, CSF acid-fast bacilli smears are often negative, and tubercle bacilli cultures takes days or weeks. For those reasons, polymerase chain reaction (PCR) for rapid detection of *Mycobacterium tuberculosis* in the CSF can be used as a diagnostic tool.[541,542] Chest radiographs will reveal evidence of pulmonary tuberculosis in a majority of cases.[535] Antituberculous medication is the primary therapy in this disorder, at times in combination with neurosurgical lysis of adhesions.[539] Tuberculomas of the chiasm have also been described,[543] but are even more uncommon.

Pituitary abscesses

These are rare. Typically patients present with visual field loss and meningitis, or they appear as if they have a pituitary tumor: headache, bitemporal hemianopia, and hypopituitarism.[544,545] Etiologies of primary pituitary abscesses include contiguous sphenoid sinus or cavernous sinus infection, meningitis, bacteremia, and CSF leaks. They may also occur secondarily when existing lesions such as pituitary adenomas, craniopharyngiomas, or Rathke's cleft become infected.[489] Pituitary abscess are typically iso- or hypointense on T1-weighted MRI and rim enhance.[546] Antibiotics should be administered, and, if there is no response, the abscess can be drained transsphenoidally.[545]

Cysticercosis

In unusual instances cysticerci may infect the suprasellar cistern or sella and imitate a pituitary tumor.[547,548] On MRI or CT, calcified cysts may be evident, and if large enough the cysts can cause hydrocephalus due to third ventricular compression. Proximity to the meninges or ventricular system can result in lymphocytic or eosinophilic meningitis. The diagnosis should be suspected when the neuroradiologic findings are suggestive in an individual from an endemic area (e.g., Central America) or in a person who might have had direct contact with someone else who is infected with the parasite. Serum serologic testing for antibodies directed against the responsible tapeworm, *Taenia solium*, is the most sensitive and specific test for cysticercosis. Corticosteroids and anticysticercal drugs such as praziquantel or albendazole should be administered, and the presence of hydrocephalus may require a shunting procedure. Surgical removal is sometimes necessary for large lesions. Cisternal cysticercosis may have a poor prognosis despite treatment. Chronic inflammation of cysts and meninges can cause fibrosis and adhesions, leading to impairment of CSF flow and vasculitis with subsequent brain infarction.[547]

Side-effects of radiation

In the previous sections on pituitary adenomas and craniopharyngiomas, we alluded to the hazards of radiotherapy near the sellar area. This section will discuss in greater detail those which can cause chiasmal visual loss: radionecrosis of the chiasm and secondary neoplasms. Fortunately more modern techniques utilize more focused radiation, resulting in less damage to surrounding structures and thus fewer complications.

Chiasmal radionecrosis

This complication has been most frequently reported following radiation treatment of pituitary adenomas, craniopharyngiomas, meningiomas, and other tumors near the skull base. Risk factors include radiation dose exceeding 4800 cGy, fractional dosage greater than 200 cGy, overlapping treatment fields, and concurrent chemotherapy.[549] In one study, the time between completion of radiation therapy and onset of visual symptoms ranged from 4 to 35 months.[550] Visual loss is painless and can be either acute or gradual. Both eyes may be involved simultaneously or sequentially, with fellow eye involvement separated by weeks or months. Acutely the fundus appearance is normal, but eventually optic atrophy ensues.

Neuroimaging is required to confirm the diagnosis and exclude recurrent or secondary tumor. Typically, radionecrosis of the chiasm causes intrinsic enlargement and gadolinium enhancement on MRI.[551,552] Involvement of surrounding structures, such as the hypothalamus, frontal lobes, or pons, is often evident due to contrast enhancement or T2 signal abnormalities.[553] With a history of previous radiation, the MRI findings are virtually diagnostic and obviate the need for further testing or biopsy.[554] CT scanning, with or without enhancement, can be insensitive to subtle changes. In equivocal cases, positron emission tomography (PET) with ^{18}F-deoxyglucose may be helpful in distinguishing radiation necrosis from tumor. The former is hypometabolic on PET, while recurrent or secondary tumors are hypermetabolic.

The pathophysiology and relative merits of treatment with corticosteroids, hyperbaric oxygen, and anticoagulation are discussed under radiation optic neuropathy in the chapter on optic neuropathies (Chapter 5).

Secondary tumors

Radiation-induced tumors of the chiasm are unusual but have been reported. Hufnagel et al.[555] reported a 41-year-old man who developed rapidly progressive visual loss due to a malignant optic chiasmal glioma 8 years following radiotherapy for a prolactinoma.

Third ventricular enlargement

The neuro-ophthalmologic complications of third ventricular enlargement are described in an excellent review by Osher et al.[556] Rarely, third ventricle dilation causes downward chiasmal compression and a bitemporal hemianopia, owing to the intimate relationship of those two structures.[557] Optic tract and optic nerve disturbances can also occur if the chiasm is pre- or post-fixed, respectively. Proptosis, ocular motor palsies due to cavernous sinus compression, and Parinaud syndrome can be other complications. Posterior fossa tumors are the most common cause of the hydrocephalus in these instances, while aqueductal stenosis and postmeningitic adhesions are less frequent etiologies. Shunting procedures can improve visual field deficits and other symptoms.

Theoretically, binasal hemianopias may result from third ventricular enlargement if the chiasm and optic nerves are pushed downwards and laterally against the carotid arteries. We agree with Osher et al.[556] that binasal defects in the setting of hydrocephalus are much more commonly caused by papilledema.

Chiasmal trauma

In the setting of blunt head trauma, vision loss much less commonly localizes to the chiasm than to the optic nerve. Nonetheless, a traumatic chiasmal syndrome is well recognized. Blunt frontal head trauma is the usual cause, and patients wake up with a nonprogressive bitemporal hemianopia, often complete.[558] Common associated findings include ocular motility deficits, anosmia, deafness, CSF rhinorrhea and otorrhea, and diabetes insipidus due to trauma to the pituitary stalk.[559] In a few instances see-saw nystagmus is related to chiasmal trauma.[35] Neuroimaging may reveal longitudinal disruption of the chiasm (**Fig. 7–38**).[560,561] The mechanism of the bitemporal hemianopia is unclear, and proposed theories include stretching of the body of the chiasm,[559] a vascular insult, or contusion hemorrhage, necrosis, or tears.[562] Two patients with traumatic chiasmal syndrome were found to have midline basilar skull fractures through the midclivus, sella turcica floor, dorsum sellae, and sphenoid sinus, suggesting the chiasm was torn.[558] One case following autoenucleation and removal of the optic nerve and half of the chiasm has also been reported.[563]

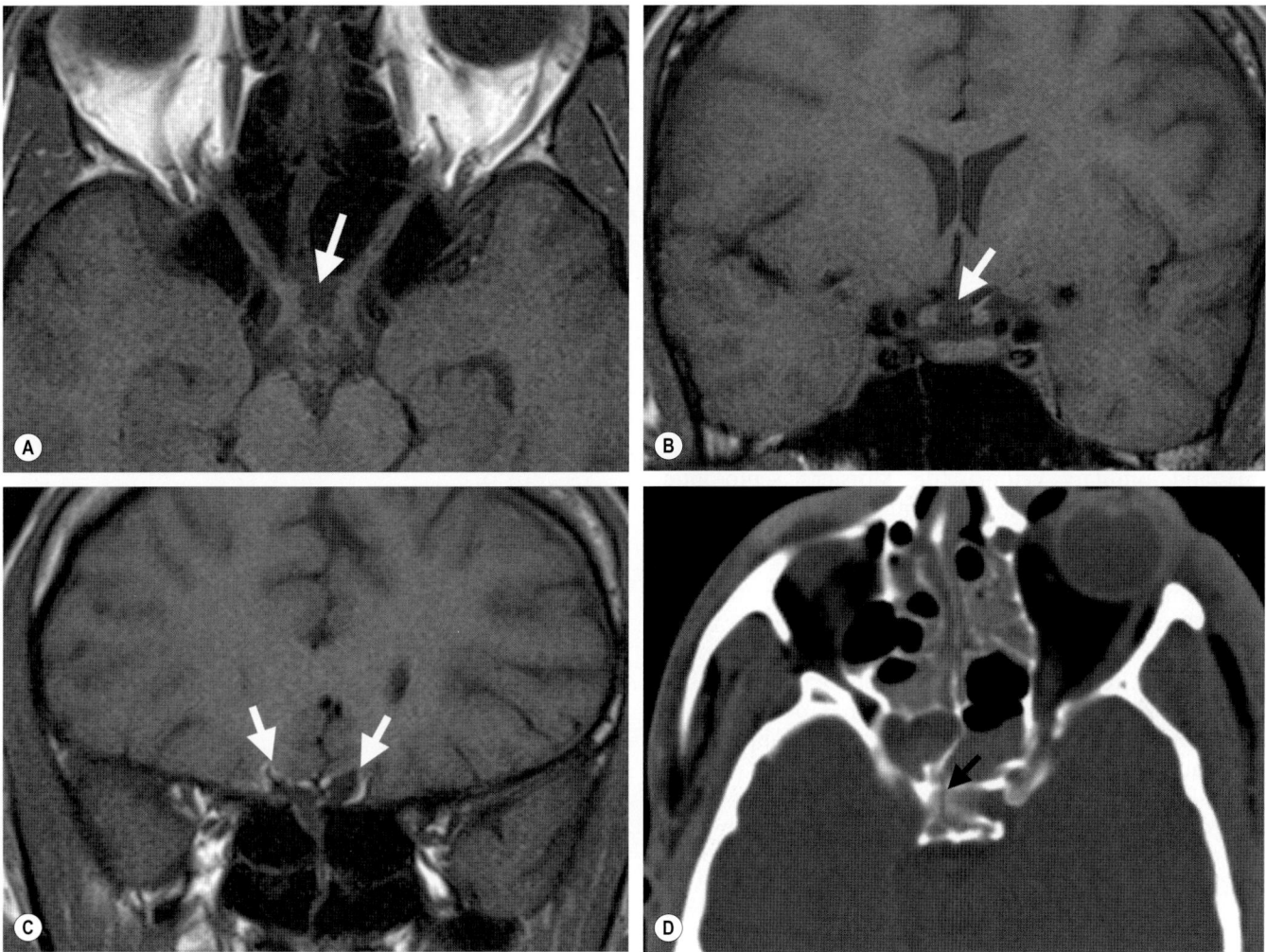

Figure 7–38. Chiasmal trauma following a fall and associated head trauma. The patient had a complete bitemporal hemianopia and was symptomatic with hemifield slide phenomena. The chiasm was almost completely transected (arrow) as demonstrated on (**A**) axial and (**B**) coronal T1-weighed MR images. **C**. Inferior frontal lobe contusions were also found (arrows). The patient had multiple base of skull fractures, including one through the sellar floor (arrow) shown on axial CT scan (**D**).

Empty sella syndrome

In this condition, the sella is enlarged and the pituitary flattened against the sellar floor because of arachnoid herniation through a defect in the diaphragm (see **Fig. 6–16**).[43] In primary empty sella, the defect is presumably congenital, while in secondary cases it results from surgery, radiation, infarction of a pituitary adenoma, or elevated intracranial pressure. In most instances when the sella is empty, it is CSF filled. However, occasionally the suprasellar portions of the optic nerves, chiasm, and tracts and anteroinferior third ventricle herniate into the space.[564] Bitemporal field deficits can occur in primary empty sellae,[565] but they are uncommon and seem unrelated to the amount of herniation.[564] Visual loss is usually nonprogressive, so surgical intervention is for the most part unnecessary. Endocrine function is usually preserved, but uncommonly hormone abnormalities are found. Visual acuity and field loss in secondary empty sella is multifactorial and more likely the result of the original process. An empty sella is commonly observed in patients with pseudotumor cerebri,[566] but generally does not contrib-

ute to visual loss or endocrine dysfunction because herniation of suprasellar structures does not occur.

Sphenoid sinus mucoceles

These can be considered retention cysts of the sinus, in many instances owing to inflammatory blockage of the draining ostium.[567] They consist of a sterile creamy fluid which is sometimes purulent.[489] Enlargement usually causes headache and orbital apex interference; however, chiasmal syndromes have been reported.[568] Surgical drainage of these mucoceles is best achieved via transnasal or transoral routes by an otolaryngologist.

Developmental anomalies of the chiasm

These are rare and include chiasms which either malformed or miswired.[569] Transsphenoidal encephaloceles, for instance, are characterized by congenital downward herniation of the optic nerves, chiasm, tract, and hypothalamus through the sphenoid bone.[570] Hypopituitarism, agenesis of the corpus callosum, and other cranial midline defects, such as hypertelorism, cleft lip, and cleft palate, are frequent accompanying features. Bitemporal hemianopias are the most common visual field defect. Disc atrophy is the usual fundus finding, but many patients instead have optic nerve colobomas or Morning glory disc anomalies (see **Fig. 5–23**). Indications for surgical intervention include progressive visual loss (uncommon), epipharyngeal respiratory obstruction, and CSF rhinorrhea. The surgeon is always careful to reduce rather than amputate the sac containing neural and endocrine structures.

Chiasmal aplasia or asymmetry can be associated with anophthalmia, which results from faulty development of one or both optic vesicles.[571] Chiasmal dysplasia can accompany optic nerve hypoplasia, absence of the septum pellucidum, and pituitary ectopia (de Morsier's septo-optic dysplasia).[10] A hereditary chiasmal optic neuropathy, without any major abnormalities on neuroimaging, has also been described.[572]

Miswiring of retinal fibers in the chiasm occurs almost exclusively in albinos, in whom some temporal ganglion cell axons can cross and project to the contralateral lateral geniculate nucleus. Greater activation of the contralateral occipital lobe following monocular stimulation has been demonstrated using VEPs[573] and functional MRI.[574] The appearance of the chiasm on MRI seems to be unaffected.[575]

Nonalbino patients without chiasms have been reported.[576-579] These individuals had optic nerves which projected solely ipsilaterally to the optic tracts. In typical examples, Apkarian and colleagues[576,577] described two individuals whose visual fields were normal, but they had reduced acuity, esotropia, torticollis, and head tremor. Eye movement recordings demonstrated congenital nystagmus waveforms in the horizontal plane and see-saw nystagmus in the vertical and torsional planes. Their MRIs demonstrated complete absence of the chiasm.

References

1. Hupp SL, Kline LB. Magnetic resonance imaging of the optic chiasm. Surv Ophthalmol 1991;36:207–216.
2. Lechan RM. Neuroendocrinology of pituitary hormone regulation. Endocrinol Metab Clin North Am 1987;16:475–501.
3. Ciric I. Pituitary tumors. Neurol Clin 1985;3:751–768.
4. Bergland RM, Ray BS, Torack RM. Anatomical variations in the pituitary gland and adjacent structures in 225 human autopsy cases. J Neurosurg 1968;28:93–99.
5. Melen O. Neuro-ophthalmologic features of pituitary tumors. Endocrinol Metab Clin North Am 1987;16:585–608.
6. Doyle AJ. Optic chiasm position on MR images. AJNR Am J Neuroradiol 1990;11:553–555.
7. Wagner AL, Murtagh FR, Hazlett KS, et al. Measurement of the normal optic chiasm on coronal MR images. AJNR Am J Neuroradiol 1997;18:723–726.
8. Elster AD. Modern imaging of the pituitary. Radiology 1993;187:1–14.
9. Kline LB, Vitek JJ, Acker JD. Computed tomography in the evaluation of the optic chiasm. Surv Ophthalmol 1983;27:387–396.
10. Hoyt WF. Correlative functional anatomy of the optic chiasm, 1969. Clin Neurosurg 1970;17:189–208.
11. Horton JC. Wilbrand's knee of the primate optic chiasm is an artefact of monocular enucleation. Trans Am Ophthalmol Soc 1997;95:579–609.
12. Lee JH, Tobias S, Kwon JT, et al. Wilbrand's knee: does it exist? Surg Neurol 2006;66:11–17; discussion 17.
13. Benarroch EE. Suprachiasmatic nucleus and melatonin: reciprocal interactions and clinical correlations. Neurology 2008;71:594–598.
14. Kupersmith MJ. Circulation of the eye, orbit, cranial nerves, and brain. In: Neurovascular Neuro-ophthalmology, pp 1–67. Berlin, Springer-Verlag, 1993.
15. Bergland R, Ray BS. The arterial supply of the human optic chiasm. J Neurosurg 1969;31:327–334.
16. Kawasaki A, Purvin VA. Photophobia as the presenting visual symptom of chiasmal compression. J Neuroophthalmol 2002;22:3–8.
17. Wray SH. Neuro-ophthalmic manifestations of pituitary and parasellar lesions. Clin Neurosurg 1977;24:86–117.
18. McIlwaine GG, Carrim ZI, Lueck CJ, et al. A mechanical theory to account for bitemporal hemianopia from chiasmal compression. J Neuroophthalmol 2005;25:40–43.
19. Kosmorsky GS, Dupps WJ, Jr., Drake RL. Nonuniform pressure generation in the optic chiasm may explain bitemporal hemianopsia. Ophthalmology 2008;115:560–565.
20. Kirkham TH. The ocular symptomatology of pituitary tumours. Proc R Soc Med 1972;65:1–2 (517–518).
21. Bird AC. Field loss due to lesions at the anterior angle of the chiasm. Proc R Soc Med 1972;65:3–4 (519–520).
22. Mojon DS, Odel JG, Rios RJ, et al. Pituitary adenoma revealed by paracentral junctional scotoma of Traquair. Ophthalmologica 1997;211:104–108.
23. Karanjia N, Jacobson DM. Compression of the prechiasmatic optic nerve produces a junctional scotoma. Am J Ophthalmol 1999;128:256–258.
24. Hickman SJ, Kupersmith MJ, Straga J, et al. Upper temporal visual field depressions in the fellow eye in posterior acute optic neuritis: 'knee' or no 'knee', Wilbrand's concept remains clinically significant. Neuroophthalmology 2002;28:69–75.
25. Hershenfeld SA, Sharpe JA. Monocular temporal hemianopia. Br J Ophthalmol 1993;77:424–427.
26. Trobe JD. Chromophobe adenoma presenting with a hemianopic temporal arcuate scotoma. Am J Ophthalmol 1974;77:388–392.
27. Nagai Y, Takamura T, Ando H, et al. A patient with GH-producing pituitary adenoma presenting with a binasal superior quadrantanopsia [letter]. Endocrine J 1999;46:345–346.
28. Salinas-Garcia RF, Smith JL. Binasal hemianopia. Surg Neurol 1978;10:187–194.
29. Danesh-Meyer HV, Papchenko T, Savino PJ, et al. In vivo retinal nerve fiber layer thickness measured by optical coherence tomography predicts visual recovery after surgery for parachiasmal tumors. Invest Ophthalmol Vis Sci 2008;49:1879–1885.
30. Jacob M, Raverot G, Jouanneau E, et al. Predicting visual outcome after treatment of pituitary adenomas with optical coherence tomography. Am J Ophthalmol 2009;147:64–70, e62.
31. Blumenthal EZ, Girkin CA, Dotan S. Glaucomatous-like cupping associated with slow-growing supra-sellar intracranial lesions. Neuroophthalmology 2006;30:111–115.
32. Unsold R, Hoyt WF. Band atrophy of the optic nerve. Arch Ophthalmol 1980;98:1637–1638.
33. Lyle TK, Clover P. Ocular symptoms and signs in pituitary tumours. Proc R Soc Med 1961;54:611–619.
34. Daroff RB. See-saw nystagmus. Neurology 1965;15:874–877.
35. Nakada T, Kwee IL. Seesaw nystagmus. Role of visuovestibular interaction in its pathogenesis. J Clin Neuroophthalmol 1988;8:171–177.
36. Arnott EJ, Miller SJH. See saw nystagmus. Trans Ophthalmol Soc UK 1970;90:491–496.
37. Dell'Osso LF. See-saw nystagmus in dogs and humans. Neurology 1996;47:1372–1374.
38. Dell'Osso LF, Daroff RB. Two additional scenarios for see-saw nystagmus: achiasma and hemichiasma. J Neuroophthalmol 1998;18:112–113.
39. Gottlob I, Zubcov A, Catalano RA, et al. Signs distinguishing spasmus nutans (with and without central nervous system lesions) from infantile nystagmus. Ophthalmology 1990;97:1166–1175.
40. Lavery MA, O'Neill JF, Chu FC, et al. Acquired nystagmus in early childhood: a presenting sign of intracranial tumor. Ophthalmology 1984;91:425–435.
41. Trobe JD, Acosta PC, Krischer JP. A screening method for chiasmal visual-field defects. Arch Ophthalmol 1981;99:264–271.
42. Kooi KA, Yamada T, Marshall RE. Field studies of monocularly evoked cerebral potentials in bitemporal hemianopsia. Neurology 1973;23:1217–1225.
43. Vance ML. Hypopituitarism. N Engl J Med 1994;330:1651–1661.
44. Abboud CF, Laws EJ. Diagnosis of pituitary tumors. Endocrinol Metab Clin North Am 1988;17:241–280.
45. Russell A. A diencephalic syndrome of emaciation in infancy and childhood. Arch Dis Child 1951;26:274.
46. Costin G. Endocrine disorders associated with tumors of the pituitary and hypothalamus. Pediatr Clin North Am 1979;26:15–31.
47. Poussaint TY, Barnes PD, Nichols K, et al. Diencephalic syndrome: clinical features and imaging findings. AJNR Am J Neuroradiol 1997;18:1499–1505.
48. Zafeiriou DI, Koliouskas D, Vargiami E, et al. Russell's diencephalic syndrome. Neurology 2001;57:93.
49. Burr IM, Slonim AE, Danish RK, et al. Diencephalic syndrome revisited. J Pediatr 1976;88:439–444.
50. Carel JC, Léger J. Clinical practice. Precocious puberty. N Engl J Med 2008;358:2366–2377.
51. Aron DC, Tyrrell JB, Wilson CB. Pituitary tumors. Current concepts in diagnosis and management. West J Med 1995;162:340–352.
52. Besser M. Criteria for medical as opposed to surgical treatment of prolactinomas. Acta Endocrinol (Copenh) 1993;129 (Suppl 1):27–30.
53. Baumann G. Acromegaly. Endocrinol Metab Clin North Am 1987;16:685–703.
54. Orth DN. Cushing's syndrome. N Engl J Med 1995;332:791–803.
55. Teramoto A, Yoshida Y, Sanno N, et al. Cavernous sinus sampling in patients with adrenocorticotrophic hormone-dependent Cushing's syndrome with emphasis on inter- and intracavernous adrenocorticotrophic hormone gradients. J Neurosurg 1998;89:762–768.
56. Post KD, Muraszko K. Management of pituitary tumors. Neurol Clin 1986;4:801–831.

57. Teramoto A, Hirakawa K, Sanno N, et al. Incidental pituitary lesions in 1,000 unselected autopsy specimens. Radiology 1994;193:161–164.

58. Di Rocco C, Maira G, Borelli P. Pituitary microadenomas in children. Child's Brain 1982;9:165–178.

59. Shalet SM. Pituitary adenomas in childhood. Acta Endocrinol Suppl (Copenh) 1986;279:434–439.

60. Faglia G. Epidemiology and pathogenesis of pituitary adenomas. Acta Endocrinol (Copenh) 1993;1:1–5.

61. Lee AG, Sforza PD, Fard AK, et al. Pituitary adenoma in children. J Neuroophthalmol 1998;18:102–105.

62. Abe T, Lüdecke DK, Saeger W. Clinically nonsecreting pituitary adenomas in childhood and adolescence. Neurosurgery 1998;42:744–750.

63. Alford FP, Arnott R. Medical management of pituitary tumours. Med J Aust 1992;157:57–60.

64. Keltner JL, Gittinger JW, Burde RM, et al. Endocrinological associations of pituitary tumors. Surv Ophthalmol 1980;25:31–36.

65. Simcic KJ, Moreno AJ. Tumors of the pituitary, pancreas, and parathyroid glands in a patient with multiple endocrine neoplasia type 1. N Engl J Med 1998;339:1602.

66. Klibanski A. Nonsecreting pituitary tumors. Endocrinol Metab Clin North Am 1987;16:793–804.

67. Sassolas G, Trouillas J, Treluyer C, et al. Management of nonfunctioning pituitary adenomas. Acta Endocrinol (Copenh) 1993;129 (Suppl 1):21–26.

68. Gsponer J, De Tribolet N, Déruaz JP, et al. Diagnosis, treatment, and outcome of pituitary tumors and other abnormal intrasellar masses. Retrospective analysis of 353 patients. Medicine 1999;78:236–269.

69. Kovacs K, Horvath E. Pathology of pituitary tumors. Endocrinol Metab Clin North Am 1987;16:529–551.

70. Bevan JS, Webster J, Burke CW, et al. Dopamine agonists and pituitary tumor shrinkage. Endocrine Rev 1992;13:220–240.

71. Elkington SG. Pituitary adenoma: preoperative symptomatology in a series of 260 patients. Br J Ophthalmol 1968;52:322–328.

72. Hollenhorst RW, Younge BR. Ocular manifestations produced by adenomas of the pituitary gland: analysis of 1,000 cases. In: Kohler PO, Ross GT (eds): Diagnosis and Treatment of Pituitary Tumors, pp 53–64. Amsterdam, Excerpta Medica-American Elsevier, 1973.

73. Anderson D, Faber P, Marcovitz S, et al. Pituitary tumors and the ophthalmologist. Ophthalmology 1983;90:1265–1270.

74. Trautmann JC, Laws ER. Visual status after transsphenoidal surgery at the Mayo Clinic, 1971–1982. Am J Ophthalmol 1983;96:200–208.

75. Zikel OM, Atkinson JL, Hurley DL. Prolactinoma manifesting with symptomatic hydrocephalus. Mayo Clinic Proc 1999;74:475–477.

76. Dawson DJ, Enoch BA, Shepherd DI. Formed visual hallucinations with pituitary adenomas. BMJ 1984;289:414.

77. Knosp E, Steiner E, Kitz K, et al. Pituitary adenomas with invasion of the cavernous sinus space: a magnetic resonance imaging classification compared with surgical findings. Neurosurgery 1993;33:610–617.

78. Saul RF, Hilliker JK. Third nerve palsy: the presenting sign of a pituitary adenoma in five patients and the only neurological sign in four patients. J Clin Neuroophthalmol 1985;5:185–193.

79. Petermann SH, Newman NJ. Pituitary macroadenoma manifesting as an isolated fourth nerve palsy. Am J Ophthalmol 1999;127:235–236.

80. Spiegel PH, Karcioglu ZA. Orbital invasion by pituitary adenoma. Am J Ophthalmol 1994:270–271.

81. Matsumura A, Meguro K, Doi M, et al. Suprasellar ectopic pituitary adenoma: case report and review of the literature. Neurosurgery 1990;26:681–685.

82. Levy MJ, Jager HR, Powell M, et al. Pituitary volume and headache: size is not everything. Arch Neurol 2004;61:721–725.

83. Levy MJ, Matharu MS, Meeran K, et al. The clinical characteristics of headache in patients with pituitary tumours. Brain 2005;128:1921–1930.

84. Gondim JA, de Almeida JP, de Albuquerque LA, et al. Headache associated with pituitary tumors. J Headache Pain 2009;10:15–20.

85. Kucharczyk W, Montanera WJ. The sella and parasellar region. In: Atlas SW (ed.): Magnetic Resonance Imaging of the Brain and Spine, pp 625–667. New York, Raven Press, 1991.

86. Ostrov SG, Quencer RM, Hoffman JC, et al. Hemorrhage within pituitary adenomas: how often associated with pituitary apoplexy syndrome? AJNR Am J Neuroradiol 1989;10:503–510.

87. Cottier JP, Destrieux C, Brunereau L, et al. Cavernous sinus invasion by pituitary adenoma: MR imaging. Radiology 2000;215:463–469.

88. Jakubowski J, Kendall B. Coincidental aneurysms with tumours of pituitary origin. J Neurol Neurosurg Psychiatr 1978;41:972–979.

89. Weir B. Pituitary tumors and aneurysms: case report and review of the literature. Neurosurgery 1992;30:585–591.

90. Pant B, Arita K, Kurisu K, et al. Incidence of intracranial aneurysm associated with pituitary adenoma. Neurosurg Rev 1997;20:13–17.

91. Laws ER. Pituitary surgery. Endocrinol Metab Clin North Am 1987;16:647–665.

92. Ebersold MJ, Quast LM, Laws ER, et al. Long-term results in transsphenoidal removal of nonfunctioning pituitary adenomas. J Neurosurg 1986;64:713–719.

93. Ciric I, Ragin A, Baumgartner C, et al. Complications of transsphenoidal surgery: results of a national survey, review of the literature, and personal experience. Neurosurgery 1997;40:225–236.

94. Dolenc VV, Lipovsek M, Slokan S. Traumatic aneurysm and carotid-cavernous fistula following transsphenoidal approach to a pituitary adenoma: treatment by transcranial operation. Br J Neurosurg 1999;13:185–188.

95. Jho HD, Carrau RL, Ko Y, et al. Endoscopic pituitary surgery: an early experience. Surg Neurol 1997;47:213–222.

96. Yaniv E, Rappaport ZH. Endoscopic transseptal transsphenoidal surgery for pituitary tumors. Neurosurgery 1997;40:944–946.

97. Sheehan MT, Atkinson JLD, Kasperbauer JL. Preliminary comparison of the endoscopic transnasal vs. the sublabial approach for clinically nonfunctioning pituitary macroadenomas. Mayo Clinic Proc 1999;74:661–670.

98. Adams CB, Burke CW. Current modes of treatment of pituitary tumours [editorial]. Br J Neurosurg 1993;7:123–127.

99. Lennestand G. Visual recovery after treatment for pituitary adenoma. Acta Ophthalmol 1983;61:1104–1117.

100. Cohen AR, Cooper PR, Kupersmith MJ, et al. Visual recovery after transsphenoidal removal of pituitary adenomas. Neurosurgery 1985;17:446–452.

101. Klauber A, Rasmussen P, Lindholm J. Pituitary adenoma and visual function. The prognostic value of clinical, ophthalmological and neuroradiological findings in 51 patients subjected to operation. Acta Ophthalmol 1978;56:252–263.

102. Halberg FE, Sheline GE. Radiotherapy of pituitary tumors. Endocrinol Metab Clin North Am 1987;16:667–684.

103. Capo H, Kupersmith MJ. Efficacy and complications of radiotherapy of anterior visual pathway tumors. Neurol Clin 1991;9:179–203.

104. Sasaki R, Murakami M, Okamoto Y, et al. The efficacy of conventional radiation therapy in the management of pituitary adenoma. Int J Radiat Oncol Biol Phys 2000;47:1337–1345.

105. Wen PY, Loeffler JS. Advances in the diagnosis and management of pituitary tumors. Curr Opin Oncol 1995;7:56–62.

106. Al-Mefty O, Kersh JE, Routh A, et al. The long-term side effects of radiation therapy for benign brain tumors in adults. J Neurosurg 1990;73:502–512.

107. Alexander MJ, DeSalles AA, Tomiyasu U. Multiple radiation-induced intracranial lesions after treatment for pituitary adenoma. Case report. J Neurosurg 1998;88:111–115.

108. van den Bergh AC, Schoorl MA, Dullaart RP, et al. Lack of radiation optic neuropathy in 72 patients treated for pituitary adenoma. J Neuroophthalmol 2004;24:200–205.

109. Kondziolka D, Lunsford LD, Flickinger JC. Gamma knife radiosurgery for pituitary tumors: imaging, visual, and endocrine results [abstract]. Acta Neurochir (Wien) 1993;122:148.

110. Pollock BE, Gorman DA, Schomberg PJ, et al. The Mayo Clinic gamma knife experience: indications and initial results. Mayo Clinic Proc 1999;74:5–13.

111. Mitsumori M, Shrieve DC, Alexander E, et al. Initial clinical results of LINAC-based stereotactic radiosurgery and stereotactic radiotherapy for pituitary adenomas. Int J Radiat Oncol Biol Phys 1998;42:573–580.

112. Jackson IM, Noren G. Role of gamma knife therapy in the management of pituitary tumors. Endocrinol Metab Clin North Am 1999;28:133–142.

113. Jalali R, Brada M, Perks JR, et al. Stereotactic conformal radiotherapy for pituitary adenomas: technique and preliminary experience. Clin Endocrinol 2000;52:695–702.

114. Kong DS, Lee JI, Lim do H, et al. The efficacy of fractionated radiotherapy and stereotactic radiosurgery for pituitary adenomas: long-term results of 125 consecutive patients treated in a single institution. Cancer 2007;110:854–860.

115. Dorotheo EU, Tang RA, Bahrani HM, et al. Her vision was tied down. Surv Ophthalmol 2005;50:588–597.

116. Czech T, Wolfsberger S, Reitner A, et al. Delayed visual deterioration after surgery for pituitary adenoma. Acta Neurochir 1999;141:45–51.

117. Lee AG, Van Gilder JC, White ML. Progressive visual loss because of a suprasellar pneumatocele after trans-sphenoidal resection of a pituitary adenoma. J Neuroophthalmol 2003;23:142–144.

118. Arafah BM, Brodkey JS, Manni A, et al. Recovery of pituitary function following surgical removal of large nonfunctioning pituitary adenomas. Clin Endocrinol 1982;17:213–222.

119. Breen P, Flickinger JC, Kondziolka D, et al. Radiotherapy for nonfunctional pituitary adenoma: analysis of long-term tumor control. J Neurosurg 1998;89:933–938.

120. Van Schaardenburg D, Roelfsema F, Van Seters AP, et al. Bromocriptine therapy for non-functioning pituitary adenomas. Clin Endocrinol 1989;30:475–484.

121. Warnet A, Timsit J, Chanson P, et al. The effect of somatostatin analogue on chiasmal dysfunction from pituitary macroadenomas. J Neurosurg 1989;71:687–691.

122. Warnet A, Harris AG, Renard E, et al. A prospective multicenter trial of octreotide in 24 patients with visual field defects caused by nonfunctioning and gonadotropin-secreting pituitary adenomas. Neurosurgery 1997;41:786–797.

123. Vance ML, Thorner MO. Prolactinomas. Endocrinol Metab Clin North Am 1987;16:731–753.

124. Colao A, Loche S, Cappa M, et al. Prolactinomas in children and adolescents. Clinical presentation and long-term follow-up. J Clin Endocrinol Metab 1998;83:2777–2780.

125. Serri O. Progress in the management of hyperprolactinemia [editorial]. N Engl J Med 1994;331:942–944.

126. Cannavò S, Curtò L, Squadrito S, et al. Cabergoline: a first-choice treatment in patients with previously untreated prolactin-secreting pituitary adenoma. J Endocrinol Invest 1999;22:354–359.

127. Webster J, Piscitelli G, Polli A, et al. A comparison of cabergoline and bromocriptine in the treatment of hyperprolactinemic amenorrhea. N Engl J Med 1994;331:904–909.

128. Moster ML, Savino PJ, Schatz NJ, et al. Visual function in prolactinoma patients treated with bromocriptine. Ophthalmology 1985;92:1332–1341.

129. Grochowicki M, Khafallah Y, Vighetto A, et al. Ophthalmic results in patients with macroprolactinomas treated with a new prolactin inhibitor CV 205–502. Br J Ophthalmol 1993;77:785–788.

130. Di Sarno A, Landi ML, Marzullo P, et al. The effect of quinagolide and cabergoline, two selective dopamine receptor type 2 agonists, in the treatment of prolactinomas. Clin Endocrinol 2000;53:53–60.

131. Lesser RL, Zheutlin JD, Boghen D, et al. Visual function improvement in patients with macroprolactinomas treated with bromocriptine. Am J Ophthalmol 1990;109:535–543.

132. Mbanya J-CN, Mendelow AD, Crawford PJ, et al. Rapid resolution of visual abnormalities with medical therapy alone in patients with large prolactinomas. Br J Neurosurg 1993;7:519–527.

133. Colao A, Di Sarno A, Cappabianca P, et al. Withdrawal of long-term cabergoline therapy for tumoral and nontumoral hyperprolactinemia. N Engl J Med 2003;349:2023–2033.

134. Schlechte JA. Clinical practice. Prolactinoma. N Engl J Med 2003;349:2035–2041.

135. Chuman H, Cornblath WT, Trobe JD, et al. Delayed visual loss following pergolide treatment of a prolactinoma. J Neuroophthalmol 2002;22:102–106.

136. van't Verlaat JW. The use of surgery for the treatment of prolactinomas. Acta Endocrinol (Copenh) 1993;129 (Suppl 1):34–37.

137. Molitch ME. Clinical manifestations of acromegaly. Endocrinol Metab Clin North Am 1992;21:597–614.

138. Rivoal O, Brezin AP, Feldman-Billard S, et al. Goldmann perimetry in acromegaly: a survey of 307 cases from 1951 through 1996. Ophthalmology 2000;107:991–997.

139. Melmed S. Medical progress: acromegaly. N Engl J Med 2006;355:2558–2573.

140. Davis DH, Laws ER, Ilstrup DM, et al. Results of surgical treatment for growth hormone-secreting pituitary adenomas. J Neurosurg 1993;79:70–75.

141. Melmed S. Medical management of acromegaly: what and when? Acta Endocrinol (Copenh) 1993;129 (Suppl 1):13–17.

142. Lamberts SWJ, van der Lely A-J, de Herder WW, et al. Octreotide. N Engl J Med 1996;334:246–254.

143. Stevenaert A. Presurgical octreotide treatment in acromegaly. Acta Endocrinol (Copenh) 1993;129 (Suppl 1):18–20.

144. Abs R, Verhelst J, Maiter D, et al. Cabergoline in the treatment of acromegaly: a study in 64 patients. J Clin Endocrinol Metab 1998;83:374–378.

145. Trainer PJ, Drake WM, Katznelson L, et al. Treatment of acromegaly with the growth hormone-receptor antagonist pegvisomant. N Engl J Med 2000;342:1171–1177.

146. Aron DC, Findling JW, Tyrell JB. Cushing's disease. Endocrinol Metab Clin North Am 1987;16:705–730.

147. Tyrell JB, Wilson CB. Cushing's disease. Therapy of pituitary adenomas. Endocrinol Metab Clin North Am 1994;23:925–938.

148. Utiger RD. Treatment, and retreatment of Cushing's disease [editorial]. N Engl J Med 1997;336:215–217.

149. Atkinson JL, Young WF, Jr., Meyer FB, et al. Sublabial transseptal vs transnasal combined endoscopic microsurgery in patients with Cushing disease and MRI-depicted microadenomas. Mayo Clin Proc 2008;83:550–553.

150. Estrada J, Boronat M, Mielgo M, et al. The long-term outcome of pituitary irradiation after unsuccessful transsphenoidal surgery in Cushing's disease. N Engl J Med 1997;336:172–177.

151. Young M, Kattner K, Gupta K. Pituitary hyperplasia resulting from primary hypothyroidism mimicking macroadenomas. Br J Neurosurg 1999;13:138–142.

152. Smallridge RC. Thyrotropin-secreting pituitary tumors. Endocrinol Metab Clin North Am 1987;16:765–792.

153. Yamamoto K, Saito K, Takai T, et al. Visual field defects and pituitary enlargement in primary hypothyroidism. J Clin Endocrinol Metab 1983;57:283–287.

154. Fukuda T, Yokoyama N, Tamai M, et al. Thyrotropin secreting pituitary adenoma effectively treated with octreotide. Intern Med 1998;37:1027–1030.

155. Iglesias P, Diez JJ. Long-term preoperative management of thyrotropin-secreting pituitary adenoma with octreotide. J Endocrinol Invest 1998;21:775–778.

156. Snyder PJ. Gonadotroph cell pituitary adenomas. Endocrinol Metab Clin North Am 1987;16:755–764.

157. Young WF, Scheithauer BW, Kovacs KT, et al. Gonadotroph adenoma of the pituitary gland: a clinicopathologic analysis of 100 cases. Mayo Clinic Proc 1996;71:649–656.

158. Cardoso ER, Peterson EW. Pituitary apoplexy: a review. Neurosurgery 1984;14:363–373.

159. Randeva HS, Schoebel J, Byrne J, et al. Classical pituitary apoplexy: clinical features, management and outcome. Clin Endocrinol 1999;51:181–188.

160. Bills DC, Meyer FB, Laws ER, et al. A retrospective analysis of pituitary apoplexy. Neurosurgery 1993;33:602–608.

161. Biousse V, Newman NJ, Oyesiku NM. Precipitating factors in pituitary apoplexy. J Neurol Neurosurg Psychiatr 2001;71:542–545.

162. Poisson M, Van Effentere R, Mashaly R. Pituitary apoplexy with retraction nystagmus. Ann Neurol 1980;7:286.

163. Shin RK, Cucchiara BL, Liebeskind DS, et al. Pituitary apoplexy causing optic neuropathy and Horner syndrome without ophthalmoplegia. J Neuroophthalmol 2003;23:208–210.

164. Tang-Wai DF, Wijdicks EF. Pituitary apoplexy presenting as postoperative stupor. Neurology 2002;58:500–501.

165. Thurtell MJ, Besser M, Halmagyi GM. Pituitary apoplexy causing isolated blindness after cardiac bypass surgery. Arch Ophthalmol 2008;126:576–578.

166. Vaphiades MS, Simmons D, Archer RL, et al. Sheehan syndrome: a splinter of the mind. Surv Ophthalmol 2003;48:230–233.

167. David NJ, Gargano FP, Glaser JS. Pituitary apoplexy in clinical perspective. In: Glaser JS, Smith JL (eds): Neuroophthalmology. Symposium of the University of Miami and the Bascom Palmer Eye Institute, Vol. VIII, pp 140–165. St. Louis, C.V. Mosby, 1975.

168. Muthukumar N, Rossette D, Soundaram M, et al. Blindness following pituitary apoplexy: timing of surgery and neuro-ophthalmic outcome. J Clin Neurosci 2008;15:873–879.

169. Semple PL, Jane JA, Lopes MB, et al. Pituitary apoplexy: correlation between magnetic resonance imaging and histopathological results. J Neurosurg 2008;108:909–915.

170. Juneau P, Schoene WC, Black P. Malignant tumors in the pituitary gland. Arch Neurol 1992;49:555–558.

171. Aaberg TM, Kay M, Sternau L. Metastatic tumors to the pituitary. Am J Ophthalmol 1995;119:779–785.

172. Weil RJ. Pituitary metastasis. Arch Neurol 2002;59:1962–1963.

173. Case Records of the MGH. N Engl J Med 2001;345:1483–1488.

174. Molitch ME. Incidental pituitary adenomas. Am J Med Sci 1993;306:262–264.

175. Molitch ME. Evaluation and treatment of the patient with a pituitary incidentaloma. J Clin Endocrinol Metab 1995;80:3–6.

176. Molitch ME. Approach to the incidentally discovered pituitary mass. In: Arnold A (ed.): Endocrine Neoplasms (Cancer Treatment & Research), Vol. 89, pp 73–90. Norwell, MA, Kluwer Academic, 1997.

177. Adamson TE, Wiestler OD, Kleihues P, et al. Correlation of clinical and pathological features in surgically treated craniopharyngiomas. J Neurosurg 1990;73:12–17.

178. Kennedy HB, Smith RJ. Eye signs in craniopharyngioma. Br J Ophthalmol 1975;59:689–695.

179. Crane TB, Yee RD, Hepler RS, et al. Clinical manifestations and radiologic findings in craniopharyngiomas in adults. Am J Ophthalmol 1982;94:220–228.

180. Shillito JJ. Craniopharyngiomas: the subfrontal approach, or none at all? Clin Neurosurg 1980;27:188–205.

181. Sanford RA, Muhlbauer MS. Craniopharyngioma in children. Neurol Clin 1991;9:453–465.

182. Cabezudo JM, Vaquero J, Areitio E, et al. Craniopharyngiomas: a critical approach to treatment. J Neurosurg 1981;55:371–375.

183. Weiner HL, Wisoff JH, Rosenberg ME, et al. Craniopharyngiomas: a clinicopathological analysis of factors predictive of recurrence and functional outcome. Neurosurgery 1994;35:1001–1010.

184. McLone DG, Raimondi AJ, Naidich TP. Craniopharyngiomas. Childs Brain 1982;9:188–200.

185. Hoffman HJ, De Silva M, Humphreys RP, et al. Aggressive surgical management of craniopharyngiomas in children. J Neurosurg 1992;76:47–52.

186. Duff TA, Levine R. Intrachiasmatic craniopharyngioma. Case report. J Neurosurg 1983;59:176–178.

187. Brodsky MC, Hoyt WF, Barnwell SL, et al. Intrachiasmatic craniopharyngioma: a rare cause of chiasmal thickening. Case report. J Neurosurg 1988;68:300–302.

188. Brummitt ML, Kline LB, Wilson ER. Craniopharyngioma: pitfalls in diagnosis. J Clin Neuroophthalmol 1992;12:77–81.

189. Block MA, Goree JA, Jimenez JP. Craniopharyngioma with optic canal enlargement simulating glioma of the optic chiasm. Case report. J Neurosurg 1973;39:523–527.

190. Yasargil MG, Curcic M, Kis M, et al. Total removal of craniopharyngiomas. Approaches and long-term results in 144 patients. J Neurosurg 1990;73:3–11.

191. Petito CK, DeGirolami U, Earle KM. Craniopharyngiomas: a clinical and pathological review. Cancer 1976;37:1944–1952.

192. Waga S, Morikawa A, Sakakura M. Craniopharyngioma with midbrain involvement. Arch Neurol 1979;36:319–320.

193. Young SC, Zimmerman RA, Nowell MA, et al. Giant cystic craniopharyngiomas. Neuroradiology 1987;29:468–473.

194. Altinors N, Senveli E, Erdogan A, et al. Craniopharyngioma of the cerebellopontine angle. Case report. J Neurosurg 1984;60:842–844.

195. Yamamoto T, Yoneda S, Funatsu N. Spontaneous haemorrhage in craniopharyngioma [letter]. J Neurol Neurosurg Psychiatr 1989;52:803–804.

196. Baskin DS, Wilson CB. Surgical management of craniopharyngiomas. A review of 74 cases. J Neurosurg 1986;65:22–27.

197. Weiss M, Sutton L, Marcial V, et al. The role of radiation therapy in the management of childhood craniopharyngioma. Int J Radiat Oncol Biol Phys 1989;17:1313–1321.

198. Repka MX, Miller NR, Miller M. Visual outcome after surgical removal of craniopharyngiomas. Ophthalmology 1989;96:195–199.

199. van den Berge JH, Blaauw G, Breeman WAP, et al. Intracavitary brachytherapy of cystic craniopharyngiomas. J Neurosurg 1992;77:545–550.

200. Savino PJ, Paris M, Schatz NJ, et al. Optic tract syndrome. A review of 21 patients. Arch Ophthalmol 1978;96:656–663.

201. Cappaert WE, Kiprov RV. Craniopharyngioma presenting as unilateral central visual loss. Ann Ophthalmol 1981;13:703–704.

202. Thomsett MJ, Conte FA, Kaplan SL, et al. Endocrine and neurologic outcome in childhood craniopharyngioma. J Pediatr 1980;97:728–735.

203. Gonzales-Portillo G, Tomita T. The syndrome of inappropriate secretion of antidiuretic hormone: an unusual presentation for childhood craniopharyngioma: report of three cases. Neurosurgery 1998;42:917–921.

204. Johnson LN, Hepler RS, Yee RD, et al. Magnetic resonance imaging of craniopharyngioma. Am J Ophthalmol 1986;102:242–244.

205. Nagahata M, Hosoya T, Kayama T, et al. Edema along the optic tract: a useful MR finding for the diagnosis of craniopharyngiomas. AJNR Am J Neuroradiol 1998;19:1753–1757.

206. Higashi S, Yamashita J, Fujisawa H, et al. "Moustache" appearance in craniopharyngiomas: unique magnetic resonance imaging and computed tomographic findings of perifocal edema. Neurosurgery 1990;27:993–996.

207. Youl BD, Plant GT, Stevens JM, et al. Three cases of craniopharyngioma showing optic tract hypersignal on MRI. Neurology 1990;40:1416–1419.

208. Numaguchi Y, Kishikawa T, Ikeda J, et al. Neuroradiological manifestations of suprasellar pituitary adenomas, meningiomas and craniopharyngiomas. Neuroradiology 1981;21:67–74.

209. Pierre-Kahn A, Sainte-Rose C, Renier D. Surgical approach to children with craniopharyngiomas and severely impaired vision: special considerations. Pediatr Neurosurg 1994;21 (Suppl 1):50–56.

210. Allen MB, Yaghmai F. Diagnosis and treatment of pituitary tumors and craniopharyngiomas. In: Allen MB, Miller RH (eds): Essentials of Neurosurgery. A Guide to Clinical Practice, pp 211–228. New York, McGraw-Hill, 1995.

211. Landolt AM, Zachmann M. Results of transsphenoidal extirpation of craniopharyngiomas and Rathke's cysts. Neurosurgery 1991;28:410–415.

212. Honegger J, Buchfelder M, Fahlbusch R, et al. Transsphenoidal microsurgery for craniopharyngioma. Surg Neurol 1992;37:189–196.

213. Norris JS, Pavaresh M, Afshar F. Primary transsphenoidal microsurgery in the treatment of craniopharyngiomas. Br J Neurosurg 1998;12:305–312.

214. Long DM, Leibrock L. The transcallosal approach to the anterior ventricular system and its application in the therapy of craniopharyngioma. Clin Neurosurg 1980;27:160–168.

215. Caldarelli M, di Rocco C, Papacci F, et al. Management of recurrent craniopharyngioma. Acta Neurochir 1998;140:447–454.

216. Regine WF, Mohiuddin M, Kramer S. Long-term results of pediatric and adult craniopharyngiomas treated with combined surgery and radiation. Radiother Oncol 1993;27:13–21.

217. Symon L, Sprich W. Radical excision of craniopharyngioma. Results in 20 patients. J Neurosurg 1985;62:174–181.

218. Symon L, Pell MF, Habib AH. Radical excision of craniopharyngioma by the temporal route: a review of 50 patients. Br J Neurosurg 1991;5:539–549.

219. Cavazzuti V, Fischer EG, Welch K, et al. Neurological and psychophysiological sequelae following different treatments of craniopharyngioma in children. J Neurosurg 1983;59:409–417.

220. De Vile CJ, Grant DB, Kendall BE, et al. Management of childhood craniopharyngioma: can the morbidity of radical surgery be predicted? J Neurosurg 1996;85:73–81.

221. Fischer EG, Welch K, Shillito J, et al. Craniopharyngiomas in children. Long-term effects of conservative surgical procedures combined with radiation therapy. J Neurosurg 1990;73:534–540.

222. Manaka S, Teramoto A, Takakura K. The efficacy of radiotherapy for craniopharyngioma. J Neurosurg 1985;62:648–656.

223. Wen BC, Hussey DH, Staples J, et al. A comparison of the roles of surgery and radiation therapy in the management of craniopharyngiomas. Int J Radiat Oncol Biol Phys 1989;16:17–24.

224. Sogg RL, Donaldson SS, Yorke CN. Malignant astrocytoma following radiotherapy of a craniopharyngioma. J Neurosurg 1978;48:622–627.

225. Shapiro K, Till K, Grant DN. Craniopharyngiomas in childhood. A rational approach to treatment. J Neurosurg 1979;50:617–623.

226. Fahlbusch R, Honegger J, Paulus W, et al. Surgical treatment of craniopharyngiomas: experience with 168 patients. J Neurosurg 1999;90:237–250.

227. Karavitaki N, Brufani C, Warner JT, et al. Craniopharyngiomas in children and adults: systematic analysis of 121 cases with long-term follow-up. Clin Endocrinol (Oxf) 2005;62:397–409.

228. Kawamata T, Amano K, Aihara Y, et al. Optimal treatment strategy for craniopharyngiomas based on long-term functional outcomes of recent and past treatment modalities. Neurosurg Rev 2010;33:71–81.

229. Puget S, Garnett M, Wray A, et al. Pediatric craniopharyngiomas: classification and treatment according to the degree of hypothalamic involvement. J Neurosurg 2007;106:3–12.

230. Stripp DC, Maity A, Janss AJ, et al. Surgery with or without radiation therapy in the management of craniopharyngiomas in children and young adults. Int J Radiat Oncol Biol Phys 2004;58:714–720.

231. Sutton LN, Gusnard D, Bruce DA, et al. Fusiform dilatations of the carotid artery following radical surgery of childhood craniopharyngiomas [see comments]. J Neurosurg 1991;74:695–700.

232. Linfante I, Tucci C, Andreone V. Fusiform dilatation of the internal carotid artery after craniopharyngioma resection. Pediatr Neurol 2008;39:139–140.

233. Voges J, Sturm V, Lehrke R, et al. Cystic craniopharyngioma: long-term results after intracavitary irradiation with stereotactically applied colloidal beta-emitting radioactive sources. J Neurosurg 1997;40:263–269.

234. Anderson DR, Trobe JD, Taren JA, et al. Visual outcome in cystic craniopharyngiomas treated with intracavitary phosphorus-32. Ophthalmology 1989;96:1786–1792.

235. Cavalheiro S, Sparapani FV, Franco JO, et al. Use of bleomycin in intratumoral chemotherapy for cystic craniopharyngioma. Case report. J Neurosurg 1996;84:124–126.

236. Kobayashi T, Tanaka T, Kida Y. Stereotactic gamma radiosurgery of craniopharyngiomas. Pediatr Neurosurg 1994;21 (Suppl 1):69–74.

237. Stieber VW. Radiation therapy for visual pathway tumors. J Neuroophthalmol 2008;28:222–230.

238. Stephanian E, Lunsford LD, Coffey RJ, et al. Stereotactic radiosurgery. Neurosurg Clin North Am 1992;3:207–218.

239. Fisher PG, Jenab J, Goldthwaite PT, et al. Outcomes and failure patterns in childhood craniopharyngiomas. Childs Nerv Syst 1998;14:558–563.

240. Mutlukan E, Cullen JF. Visual outcome after craniopharyngioma [letter]. Ophthalmology 1990;97:539–540.

241. Sorva R, Heiskanen O, Perheentupa J. Craniopharyngioma surgery in children: endocrine and visual outcome. Childs Nerv Syst 1988;4:97–99.

242. Abrams LS, Repka MX. Visual outcome of craniopharyngioma in children. J Pediatr Ophthalmol Strab 1997;34:223–228.

243. Repka MX, Miller NR. Visual outcome after craniopharyngioma [comment]. Ophthalmology 1990;97:539–540.

244. Newman CB, Levine LS, New MI. Endocrine function in children with intrasellar and suprasellar neoplasms: before and after therapy. Am J Dis Child 1981;135:259–266.

245. Lyen KR, Grant DB. Endocrine function, morbidity, and mortality after surgery for craniopharyngioma. Arch Dis Child 1982;57:837–841.

246. Honegger J, Buchfelder M, Fahlbusch R. Surgical treatment of craniopharyngiomas: endocrinological results. J Neurosurg 1999;90:251–257.

247. Tiulpakov AN, Mazerkina NA, Brook CG, et al. Growth in children with craniopharyngioma following surgery. Clin Endocrinol 1998;49:733–738.

248. Voelker JL, Campbell RL, Muller J. Clinical, radiographic, and pathological features of symptomatic Rathke's cleft cysts. J Neurosurg 1991;74:535–544.

249. Oka H, Kawano N, Suwa T, et al. Radiological study of symptomatic Rathke's cleft cysts. Neurosurgery 1994;35:632–636.

250. Kucharczyk W, Peck WW, Kelly WM, et al. Rathke cleft cysts: CT, MR imaging, and pathologic features. Radiology 1987;165:491–495.

251. Rao GP, Blyth CP, Jeffreys RV. Ophthalmic manifestations of Rathke's cleft cysts. Am J Ophthalmol 1995;119:86–91.

252. Barrow DL, Spector RH, Takei Y, et al. Symptomatic Rathke's cleft cysts located entirely in the suprasellar region: review of diagnosis, management, and pathogenesis. Neurosurgery 1985;16:766–772.

253. Itoh J, Usui K. An entirely suprasellar symptomatic Rathke's cleft cyst: case report. Neurosurgery 1992;30:581–584.

254. Ross DA, Norman D, Wilson CB. Radiologic characteristics and results of surgical management of Rathke's cysts in 43 patients. Neurosurgery 1992;30:173–178.

255. el-Mahdy W, Powell M. Transsphenoidal management of 28 symptomatic Rathke's cleft cysts, with special reference to visual and hormonal recovery. Neurosurgery 1998;42:7–16.

256. Maggio WW, Cail WS, Brookeman JR, et al. Rathke's cleft cyst: computed tomographic and magnetic resonance imaging appearances. Neurosurgery 1987;21:60–62.

257. Hayashi Y, Tachibana O, Muramatsu N, et al. Rathke cleft cyst: MR and biomedical analysis of cyst content. J Comput Assist Tomogr 1999;23:34–38.

258. Crenshaw WB, Chew FS. Rathke's cleft cyst. AJR Am J Roentgenol 1992;158:1312.

259. Kurisaka M, Fukui N, Sakamoto T, et al. A case of Rathke's cleft cyst with apoplexy. Childs Nerv Syst 1998;14:343–347.

260. Zada G, Ditty B, McNatt SA, et al. Surgical treatment of Rathke cleft cysts in children. Neurosurgery 2009;64:1132–1137.

261. Midha R, Jay V, Smyth HS. Transsphenoidal management of Rathke's cleft cysts. A clinicopathological review of 10 cases. Surg Neurol 1991;35:446–454.

262. Iraci G, Giordano R, Gerosa M, et al. Ocular involvement in recurrent cyst of Rathke's cleft: case report. Ann Ophthalmol 1979;11:94–98.

263. Mukherjee JJ, Islam N, Kaltsas G, et al. Clinical, radiological and pathological features of patients with Rathke's cleft cysts: tumors that may recur. J Clin Endocrinol Metab 1997;82:2357–2362.

264. Rappaport ZH. Suprasellar arachnoid cysts: options in operative management. Acta Neurochir (Wien) 1993;122:71–75.

265. Burnbaum MD, Harbison JW, Selhorst JB, et al. Blue-domed cyst with optic nerve compression. J Neurol Neurosurg Psychiatr 1978;41:987–991.

266. Pierre KA, Capelle L, Brauner R, et al. Presentation and management of suprasellar arachnoid cysts. Review of 20 cases. J Neurosurg 1990;73:355–359.

267. Benton JW, Nellhaus G, Huttenlocher PR, et al. The bobble-head doll syndrome. Report of unique truncal tremor associated with third ventricular cyst and hydrocephalus in children. Neurology 1966;16:725–729.

268. Chun BB, Lee AG, Coughlin WF, et al. Unusual presentations of sellar arachnoid cyst. J Neuroophthalmol 1998;18:246–249.

269. Abe T, Matsumoto K, Homma H, et al. Dorsum sellae meningioma mimicking pituitary macroadenoma: case report. Surg Neurol 1999;51:543–546.

270. Wilson WB. Meningiomas of the anterior visual system. Surv Ophthalmol 1981;26:109–127.

271. Symon L, Rosenstein J. Surgical management of suprasellar meningioma. Part 1. The influence of tumor size, duration of symptoms, and microsurgery on surgical outcome in 101 consecutive cases. J Neurosurg 1984;61:633–641.

272. Black PM. Meningiomas. Neurosurgery 1993;32:643–657.

273. Chou SM, Miles JM. The pathology of meningiomas. In: Al-Mefty O (ed.): Meningiomas, pp 37–57. New York, Raven Press, 1991.

274. Lee A, Wallace C, Rewcastle B, et al. Metastases to meningioma. AJNR Am J Neuroradiol 1998;19:1120–1122.

275. Brihaye J, Brihaye-van Geertruyden M. Management and surgical outcome of suprasellar meningiomas. Acta Neurochir (Suppl) (Wein) 1988;42:124–129.

276. Yeakley JW, Kulkarni MV, McArdle CB, et al. High-resolution MR imaging of juxtasellar meningiomas with CT and angiographic correlation. AJNR Am J Neuroradiol 1988;9:279–285.

277. Ojemann RG. Management of cranial and spinal meningiomas (honored guest presentation). Clin Neurosurg 1993;40:321–383.

278. Rodesch G, Lasjaunias P. Embolization and meningiomas. In: Al-Mefty O (ed.): Meningiomas, pp 285–297. New York, Raven Press, 1991.

279. Andrews BT, Wilson CB. Suprasellar meningiomas: the effect of tumor location on postoperative visual outcome. J Neurosurg 1988;69:523–528.

280. Probst C. Possibilities and limitations of microsurgery in patients with meningiomas of the sellar region. Acta Neurochir (Wien) 1987;84:99–102.

281. Kitano M, Taneda M, Nakao Y. Postoperative improvement in visual function in patients with tuberculum sellae meningiomas: results of the extended transsphenoidal and transcranial approaches. J Neurosurg 2007;107:337–346.

282. Kupersmith MJ, Warren FA, Newall J, et al. Irradiation of meningiomas of the intracranial anterior visual pathway. Ann Neurol 1987;21:131–137.

283. Kondziolka D, Lunsford LD, Coffey RJ, et al. Stereotactic radiosurgery of meningiomas. J Neurosurg 1991;74:552–559.

284. Hakim R, Alexander E, Loeffler JS, et al. Results of linear accelerator-based radiosurgery for intracranial meningiomas. Neurosurgery 1998;42:446–453.

285. Herscovici Z, Rappaport Z, Sulkes J, et al. Natural history of conservatively treated meningiomas. Neurology 2004;63:1133–1134.

286. Schrell UMH, Fahlbusch R. Hormonal manipulation of cerebral meningiomas. In: Al-Mefty O (ed.): Meningiomas, pp 273–283. New York, Raven Press, 1991.

287. Grunberg SM, Weiss MH, Spitz IM, et al. Treatment of unresectable meningiomas with the antiprogesterone agent mifepristone. J Neurosurg 1991;74:861–866.

288. Rosenstein J, Symon L. Surgical management of suprasellar meningioma. Part 2. Prognosis for visual function following craniotomy. J Neurosurg 1984;61:642–648.

289. Finn JE, Mount LA. Meningiomas of tuberculum sellae and planum sphenoidale: a review of 83 cases. Arch Ophthalmol 1974;92:23–27.

290. Gregorius FK, Hepler RS, Stern WE. Loss and recovery of vision with suprasellar meningioma. J Neurosurg 1975;42:69–75.

291. Rosenberg L, Miller NR. Visual results after microsurgical removal of meningioma involving the anterior visual system. Arch Ophthalmol 1984;102:1019–1023.

292. Chicani CF, Miller NR. Visual outcome in surgically treated suprasellar meningiomas. J Neuroophthalmol 2003;23:3–10.

293. Grant FC, Hedges TR. Ocular findings in meningiomas of the tuberculum sellae. Arch Ophthalmol 1956;56:163–170.

294. Al-Mefty O, Smith RR. Tuberculum sellae meningiomas. In: Al-Mefty O (ed.): Meningiomas, pp 395–411. New York, Raven Press, 1991.

295. Schick U, Hassler W. Surgical management of tuberculum sellae meningiomas: involvement of the optic canal and visual outcome. J Neurol Neurosurg Psychiatr 2005;76:977–983.

296. Al-Mefty O. Clinoidal meningiomas. In: Al-Mefty O (ed.): Meningiomas, pp 427–443. New York, Raven Press, 1991.

297. Kinjo T, Al-Mefty O, Ciric I. Diaphragma sellae meningiomas. Neurosurgery 1995;36:1082–1092.

298. Cappabianca P, Cirillo S, Alfieri A, et al. Pituitary macroadenoma and diaphragma sellae meningioma: differential diagnosis on MRI. Neuroradiology 1999;41:22–26.

299. Kasner SE, Liu GT, Galetta SL. Neuro-ophthalmologic aspects of aneurysms. Neuroimag Clin North Am 1997;7:679–692.

300. Date I, Asari S, Ohmoto T. Cerebral aneurysms causing visual symptoms: their features and surgical outcome. Clin Neurol Neurosurg 1998;100:259–267.

301. Walsh FB. Visual field defect due to aneurysms at the circle of Willis. Arch Ophthalmol 1964;71:15–27.

302. Kupersmith MJ. Aneurysms involving the motor and sensory visual pathways. In: Neurovascular Neuro-ophthalmology, pp 239–300. Berlin, Springer-Verlag, 1993.

303. Bor AS, Velthuis BK, Majoie CB, et al. Configuration of intracranial arteries and development of aneurysms: a follow-up study. Neurology 2008;70:700–705.

304. Meyer FB, Morita A, Puumala MR, et al. Medical and surgical management of intracranial aneurysms. Mayo Clin Proc 1995;70:153–172.

305. Suarez JI, Tarr RW, Selman WR. Aneurysmal subarachnoid hemorrhage. N Engl J Med 2006;354:387–396.

306. Peiris JB, Ross Russell RW. Giant aneurysms of the carotid system presenting as visual field defect. J Neurol Neurosurg Psychiatr 1980;43:1053–1064.

307. Højer-Pedersen E, Haase J. Giant anterior communicating artery aneurysm with bitemporal hemianopsia: case report. Neurosurgery 1981;8:703–706.

308. Shutter LA, Kline LB, Fisher WS. Visual loss and a suprasellar mass complicated by pregnancy. Surv Ophthalmol 1993;38:63–69.

309. Ferguson G, Drake CG. Carotid-ophthalmic aneurysms: visual abnormalities in 32 patients and the results of treatment. Surg Neurol 1981;16:1–8.

310. Bird AC, Nolan B, Gargano FP, et al. Unruptured aneurysm of the supraclinoid carotid artery. Neurology 1970;20:445–454.

311. Date I, Akioka T, Ohmoto T. Penetration of the optic chiasm by a ruptured anterior communicating artery aneurysm. Case report. J Neurosurg 1997;87:324–326.

312. Raymond LA, Tew J. Large suprasellar aneurysms imitating pituitary tumor. J Neurol Neurosurg Psychiatr 1978;41:83–87.

313. Heshmati HM, Fatourechi V, Dagam SA, et al. Hypopituitarism caused by intrasellar aneurysms. Mayo Clin Proc 2001;76:789–793.

314. Biondi A, Scialfa G, Scotti G. Intracranial aneurysms: MR imaging. Neuroradiology 1988;30:214–218.

315. Atlas SW, Mark AS, Fram EK, et al. Vascular intracranial lesions: applications of gradient-echo MR imaging. Radiology 1988;169:455–461.

316. Friedman JA, Piepgras DG, Pichelmann MA, et al. Small cerebral aneurysms presenting with symptoms other than rupture. Neurology 2001;57:1212–1216.

317. International Study of Unruptured Intracranial Aneurysms Investigators. Unruptured intracranial aneurysms: risk of rupture and risks of surgical intervention. N Engl J Med 1998;339:1725–1733.

318. Wiebers DO, Whisnant JP, Huston J, 3rd, et al. Unruptured intracranial aneurysms: natural history, clinical outcome, and risks of surgical and endovascular treatment. Lancet 2003;362:103–110.

319. Wiebers DO, Piepgras DG, Meyer FB, et al. Pathogenesis, natural history, and treatment of unruptured intracranial aneurysms. Mayo Clin Proc 2004;79:1572–1583.

320. Schievink WI. Intracranial aneurysms. N Engl J Med 1997;336:28–40.

321. De Jesús O, Sekhar LN, Riedel CJ. Clinoid and paraclinoid aneurysms: surgical anatomy, operative techniques, and outcome. Surg Neurol 1999;51:477–487.

322. Cawley CM, Zipfel GJ, Day AL. Surgical treatment of paraclinoid and ophthalmic aneurysms. Neurosurg Clin North Am 1998;9:765–783.

323. Guterman LR, Hopkins LN. Endovascular treatment of cerebral aneurysms. Diagnosis and treatment. Clin Neurosurg 1993;40:56–83.

324. Nichols DA, Meyer FB, Piepgras DG, et al. Endovascular treatment of intracranial aneurysms. Mayo Clin Proc 1994;69:272–285.

325. Molyneux A, Kerr R, Stratton I, et al. International Subarachnoid Aneurysm Trial (ISAT) of neurosurgical clipping versus endovascular coiling in 2143 patients with ruptured intracranial aneurysms: a randomised trial. Lancet 2002;360:1267–1274.

326. Maitland CG, Abiko S, Hoyt WF, et al. Chiasm apoplexy: report of four cases. J Neurosurg 1982;56:118–122.

327. Pakzaban P, Westmark K, Westmark R. Chiasmal apoplexy due to hemorrhage from a pituitary adenoma into the optic chiasm: case report. Neurosurgery 2000;46:1511–1513.

328. Hwang J-F, Yau C-W, Huang J-K, et al. Apoplectic optochiasmal syndrome due to intrinsic cavernous hemangioma. Case report. J Clin Neuroophthalmol 1993;13:232–236.

329. Kupersmith MJ. Vascular malformations of the brain. In: Neurovascular Neuro-ophthalmology, pp 301–351. Berlin, Springer-Verlag, 1993.

330. Corboy JR, Galetta SL. Familial cavernous angiomas manifesting with an acute chiasmal syndrome. Am J Ophthalmol 1989;108:245–250.

331. Mohr G, Hardy J, Gauvin P. Chiasmal apoplexy due to ruptured cavernous hemangioma of the optic chiasm. Surg Neurol 1985;24:636–640.

332. Tien R, Dillon WP. MR imaging of cavernous hemangioma of the optic chiasm. J Comput Assist Tomogr 1989;13:1087–1088.

333. Glastonbury CM, Warner JE, MacDonald JD. Optochiasmal apoplexy from a cavernoma. Neurology 2003;61:266.

334. Warner JEA, Rizzo JF, Brown EW, et al. Recurrent chiasmal apoplexy due to cavernous malformation. J Neuroophthalmol 1996;16:99–106.

335. Hassler W, Zentner J, Wilhelm H. Cavernous angiomas of the anterior visual pathways. J Clin Neuroophthalmol 1989;9:160–164.

336. Lavin PJM, McCrary JA, Roessmann U, et al. Chiasmal apoplexy: hemorrhage from a cryptic vascular malformation in the optic chiasm. Neurology 1984;34:1007–1011.

337. Fermaglich J, Kattah J, Manz H. Venous angioma of the optic chiasm. Ann Neurol 1978;4:470–471.

338. Balcer LJ, Galetta SL, Curtis M, et al. von Hippel-Lindau disease manifesting as a chiasmal syndrome. Surv Ophthalmol 1995;39:302–306.

339. Lee KF, Schatz NJ, Savino PJ. Ischemic chiasmal syndrome. In: Glaser JS, Smith JL (eds): Neuroophthalmology. Symposium of the University of Miami and the Bascom Palmer Eye Institute, Vol. VIII, pp 115–130. St. Louis, C.V. Mosby, 1975.

340. Jacobson DM. Symptomatic compression of the optic nerve by the carotid artery. Clinical profile of 18 patients with 24 affected eyes identified by magnetic resonance imaging. Ophthalmology 1999;106:1994–2004.

341. Chen CS, Gailloud P, Miller NR. Bitemporal hemianopia caused by an intracranial vascular loop. Arch Ophthalmol 2008;126:274–276.

342. Hilton GF, Hoyt WF. An arteriosclerotic chiasmal syndrome. Bitemporal hemianopia associated with fusiform dilatation of the anterior cerebral arteries. JAMA 1966;196:1018–1020.

343. Matsuo K, Kobayashi S, Sugita K. Bitemporal hemianopsia associated with sclerosis of the intracranial internal carotid arteries. J Neurosurg 1980;53:566–569.

344. Golnik KC, Hund PW, Stroman GA, et al. Magnetic resonance imaging in patients with unexplained optic neuropathy. Ophthalmology 1996;103:515–530.

345. Sibony PA, Lessell S, Wray S. Chiasmal syndrome caused by arteriovenous malformations. Arch Ophthalmol 1982;100:438–442.

346. Volpe NJ, Sharma MC, Galetta SL, et al. Orbital drainage from cerebral arteriovenous malformations. Neurosurgery 2000;46:820–824.

347. Gould TJ, Johnson LN, Colapinto EV, et al. Intrasellar vascular malformation mimicking a pituitary macroadenoma. J Neuroophthalmol 1996;16:199–203.

348. Packer RJ. Treatment of chiasmatic/hypothalamic gliomas of childhood with chemotherapy. In: Smith JL, Katz RS (eds): Neuroophthalmology Enters the Nineties, pp 145–151. Hialeah, Dutton, 1988.

349. Alvord EC, Lofton S. Gliomas of the optic nerve or chiasm: outcome by patients' age, tumor site, and treatment. J Neurosurg 1988;68:85–98.

350. Dutton JJ. Gliomas of the anterior visual pathways. Surv Ophthalmol 1994;38:427–452.

351. Ragge NK. Clinical and genetic patterns of neurofibromatosis 1 and 2. Br J Ophthalmol 1993;77:662–672.

352. Bouzas EA, Parry DM, Eldridge R, et al. Visual impairment in patients with neurofibromatosis 2. Neurology 1993;43:622–623.

353. Lewis RA, Gerson LP, Axelson KA, et al. von Recklinghausen neurofibromatosis. II. Incidence of optic gliomata. Ophthalmology 1984;91:929–935.

354. Listernick R, Charrow J, Greenwald M, et al. Natural history of optic pathway tumors in children with neurofibromatosis type 1: a longitudinal study. J Pediatr 1994;125:63–66.

355. Kornreich L, Blaser S, Schwarz M, et al. Optic pathway glioma: correlation of imaging findings with the presence of neurofibromatosis. AJNR Am J Neuroradiol 2001;22:1963–1969.

356. Balcer LJ, Liu GT, Heller G, et al. Visual loss in children with neurofibromatosis type 1 and optic pathway gliomas: relation to tumor location by magnetic resonance imaging. Am J Ophthalmol 2001;131:442–445.

357. Listernick R, Ferner RE, Piersall L, et al. Late-onset optic pathway tumors in children with neurofibromatosis 1. Neurology 2004;63:1944–1946.

358. Thiagalingam S, Flaherty M, Billson F, et al. Neurofibromatosis type 1 and optic pathway gliomas: follow-up of 54 patients. Ophthalmology 2004;111:568–577.

359. Créange A, Zeller J, Rostaing-Rigattieri S, et al. Neurological complications of neurofibromatosis type 1 in adulthood. Brain 1999;122:473–481.

360. Champion MP, Robinson RO. Screening for optic gliomas in neurofibromatosis type 1: the role of neuroimaging [letter]. J Pediatr 1995;127:507–508.

361. Listernick R, Louis DN, Packer RJ, et al. Optic pathway gliomas in children with neurofibromatosis 1: consensus statement from the NF1 optic pathway glioma task force. Ann Neurol 1997;41:143–149.

362. Blazo MA, Lewis RA, Chintagumpala MM, et al. Outcomes of systematic screening for optic pathway tumors in children with neurofibromatosis type 1. Am J Med Genet A 2004;127A:224–229.

363. Listernick R, Charrow J. Knowledge without truth: screening for complications of neurofibromatosis type 1 in childhood. Am J Med Genet A 2004;127A:221–223.

364. Jabbari B, Maitland CG, Morris LM, et al. The value of visual evoked potential as a screening test in neurofibromatosis. Arch Neurol 1985;42:1072–1074.

365. North K, Cochineas C, Tang E, et al. Optic gliomas in neurofibromatosis type 1: role of visual evoked potentials. Pediatr Neurol 1994;10:117–123.

366. Listernick R, Ferner RE, Liu GT, et al. Optic pathway gliomas in neurofibromatosis-1: controversies and recommendations. Ann Neurol 2007;61:189–198.

367. Listernick R, Charrow J. Screening for optic gliomas in neurofibromatosis type 1: the role of neuroimaging [reply]. J Pediatr 1995;127:507–508.

368. Listernick R, Charrow J, Greenwald M. Emergence of optic pathway gliomas in children with neurofibromatosis type 1 after normal neuroimaging results. J Pediatr 1992;121:584–587.

369. Massry GG, Morgan CF, Chung SM. Evidence of optic pathway gliomas after previously negative neuroimaging. Ophthalmology 1997;104:930–935.

370. Ng Y, North KN. Visual-evoked potentials in the assessment of optic gliomas. Pediatr Neurol 2001;24:44–48.

371. Wolsey DH, Larson SA, Creel D, et al. Can screening for optic nerve gliomas in patients with neurofibromatosis type I be performed with visual-evoked potential testing? J AAPOS 2006;10:307–311.

372. Kelly JP, Weiss AH. Comparison of pattern visual-evoked potentials to perimetry in the detection of visual loss in children with optic pathway gliomas. J AAPOS 2006;10:298–306.

373. Chang BC, Mirabella G, Yagev R, et al. Screening and diagnosis of optic pathway gliomas in children with neurofibromatosis type 1 by using sweep visual evoked potentials. Invest Ophthalmol Vis Sci 2007;48:2895–2902.

374. Falsini B, Ziccardi L, Lazzareschi I, et al. Longitudinal assessment of childhood optic gliomas: relationship between flicker visual evoked potentials and magnetic resonance imaging findings. J Neurooncol 2008;88:87–96.

375. Rossi LN, Pastorino G, Scotti G, et al. Early diagnosis of optic glioma in children with neurofibromatosis type 1. Childs Nerv Syst 1994;10:426–429.

376. Siatkowski RM. VEP testing and visual pathway gliomas: not quite ready for prime time. J AAPOS 2006;10:293–295.

377. Liu GT, Molloy PT, Needle M, et al. Optic gliomas in neurofibromatosis type 1: role of visual evoked potentials [letter]. Pediatr Neurol 1995;12:89–90.

378. Borit A, Richardson EP. The biological and clinical behaviour of pilocytic astrocytomas of the optic pathways. Brain 1982;105:161–187.

379. Coakley KJ, Huston J, Scheithauer BW, et al. Pilocytic astrocytomas: well-demarcated magnetic resonance appearance despite frequent infiltration histologically. Mayo Clinic Proc 1995;70:747–751.

380. Anderson DR, Spencer WH. Ultrastructural and histochemical observations of optic nerve gliomas. Arch Ophthalmol 1970;83:324–335.

381. Bilgiç S, Erbengi A, Tinaztepe B, et al. Optic glioma of childhood: clinical, histopathological, and histochemical observations. Br J Ophthalmol 1989;73:832–837.

382. Parsa CF, Givrad S. Juvenile pilocytic astrocytomas do not undergo spontaneous malignant transformation: grounds for designation as hamartomas. Br J Ophthalmol 2008;92:40–46.

383. Hoyt WF, Baghdassarian SA. Optic glioma of childhood: natural history and rationale for conservative management. Br J Ophthalmol 1969;53:793–798.

384. Burnstine MA, Levin LA, Louis DN, et al. Nucleolar organizer regions in optic gliomas. Brain 1993;116:1465–1476.

385. Miller NR. Optic pathway gliomas are tumors! Ophthal Plast Reconstr Surg 2008;24:433.

386. Glaser JS, Hoyt WF, Corbett J. Visual morbidity with chiasmal glioma. Arch Ophthalmol 1971;85:3–12.

387. Tym R. Piloid gliomas of the anterior optic pathways. Br J Surg 1961;49:322–331.

388. Venes JL, Latack J, Kandt RS. Postoperative regression of opticochiasmatic astrocytoma: a case for expectant therapy. Neurosurgery 1984;15:421–423.

389. Kanamori M, Shibuya M, Yoshida J, et al. Long-term follow-up of patients with optic glioma. Childs Nerv Syst 1985;1:272–278.

390. Brzowski A, Bazan C, Mumma J, et al. Spontaneous regression of optic glioma in a patient with neurofibromatosis. Neurology 1992;42:679–681.

391. Liu GT, Lessell S. Spontaneous visual improvement in chiasmal gliomas. Am J Ophthalmol 1992;114:193–201.

392. Takeuchi H, Kabuto M, Sato K, et al. Chiasmal gliomas with spontaneous regression: proliferation and apoptosis. Childs Nerv Syst 1997;13:229–233.

393. Gottschalk S, Tavakolian R, Buske A, et al. Spontaneous remission of chiasmatic/hypothalamic masses in neurofibromatosis type 1: report of two cases. Neuroradiology 1999;41:199–201.

394. Parsa CF, Hoyt CS, Lesser RL, et al. Spontaneous regression of optic gliomas: thirteen cases documented by serial neuroimaging. Arch Ophthalmol 2001;119:516–529.

395. Piccirilli M, Lenzi J, Delfinis C, et al. Spontaneous regression of optic pathways gliomas in three patients with neurofibromatosis type I and critical review of the literature. Childs Nerv Syst 2006;22:1332–1337.

396. Trigg ME, Swanson JD, Letellier MA. Metastasis of an optic glioma through a ventriculoperitoneal shunt. Cancer 1983;52:599–601.

397. Civitello LA, Packer RJ, Rorke LB, et al. Leptomeningeal dissemination of low-grade gliomas in childhood. Neurology 1988;38:562–566.

398. de Keizer RJW, de Wolff-Rouendaal D, Bots GTAM, et al. Optic glioma with intraocular tumor and seeding in a child with neurofibromatosis. Am J Ophthalmol 1989;108:717–725.

399. Bruggers CS, Friedman HS, Phillips PC, et al. Leptomeningeal dissemination of optic pathway gliomas in three children. Am J Ophthalmol 1991;111:719–723.

400. Perilongo G, Carollo C, Salviati L, et al. Diencephalic syndrome and disseminated juvenile pilocytic astrocytomas of the hypothalamic-optic chiasm region. Cancer 1997;80:142–146.

401. Miller NR, Iliff WJ, Green WR. Evaluation and management of gliomas of the anterior visual pathways. Brain 1974;97:743–754.

402. Jenkin D, Angyalfi S, Becker L, et al. Optic glioma in children: surveillance, resection, or irradiation? Int J Radiat Oncol Biol Phys 1993;25:215–225.

403. Walrath JD, Engelbert M, Kazim M. Magnetic resonance imaging evidence of optic nerve glioma progression into and beyond the optic chiasm. Ophthal Plast Reconstr Surg 2008;24:473–475.

404. Friedman JM, Birch P. An association between optic glioma and other tumours of the central nervous system in neurofibromatosis type 1. Neuropediatrics 1997;28:131–132.

405. Fletcher WA, Imes RK, Hoyt WF. Chiasmal gliomas: appearance and long-term changes demonstrated by computerized tomography. J Neurosurg 1986;65:154–159.

406. Pfaffenbach DD, Kearns TP, Hollenhorst RW. An unusual case of optic nerve-chiasmal glioma. Am J Ophthalmol 1972;74:523–525.

407. Schulman JA, Shults WT, Jones JM. Monocular vertical nystagmus as an initial sign of chiasmal glioma. Am J Ophthalmol 1979;87:87–90.

408. Kelly TW. Optic glioma presenting as spasmus nutans. Pediatrics 1970;45:295–296.

409. Brauner R, Malandry F, Rappaport R, et al. Growth and endocrine disorders in optic glioma. Eur J Pediatr 1990;149:825–828.

410. Cnossen MH, Stam EN, Cooiman LC, et al. Endocrinologic disorders and optic pathway gliomas in children with neurofibromatosis type 1. Pediatrics 1997;100:667–670.

411. Holman RE, Grimson BS, Drayer BP, et al. Magnetic resonance imaging of optic gliomas. Am J Ophthalmol 1985;100:596–601.

412. Haik BG, Saint Louis L, Bierly J, et al. Magnetic resonance imaging in the evaluation of optic nerve gliomas. Ophthalmology 1987;94:709–717.

413. Hollander MD, FitzPatrick M, O'Connor SG, et al. Optic gliomas. Radiol Clin North Am 1999;37:59–71.

414. Wilson WB, Finkel RS, McCleary L, et al. Large cystic optic glioma. Neurology 1990;40:1898–1900.

415. Brown EW, Riccardi VM, Mawad M, et al. MR imaging of optic pathways in patients with neurofibromatosis. AJNR Am J Neuroradiol 1987;8:1031–1036.

416. Liu GT, Brodsky MC, Phillips PC, et al. Optic radiation involvement in optic pathway gliomas in neurofibromatosis. Am J Ophthalmol 2004;137:407–414.

417. Wong IG, Lubow M. Management of optic glioma of childhood: a review of 42 cases. In: Smith JL (ed.): Neuroophthalmology. Symposium of the University of Miami and the Bascom Palmer Eye Institute, Vol. VI, pp 51–60. St. Louis, C.V. Mosby, 1972.

418. Glaser JS. Gliomas of the anterior visual pathway in childhood: rationale for conservative management. In: Brockhurst RJ, Boruchoff SA, Hutchinson BT, et al. (eds): Controversy in Ophthalmology, pp 897–906. Philadelphia, W.B. Saunders, 1977.

419. Oxenhandler DC, Sayers MP. The dilemma of childhood optic gliomas. J Neurosurg 1978;48:34–41.

420. Heiskanen O, Raitta C, Torsti R. The management and prognosis of gliomas of the optic pathways in children. Acta Neurochir 1978;43:193–199.

421. DeSousa AL, Kalsbeck JE, Mealey J, et al. Optic chiasmatic glioma in children. Am J Ophthalmol 1979;87:376–381.

422. Sung DI. Suprasellar tumors in children: a review of clinical manifestations and managements. Cancer 1982;50:1420–1425.

423. Rush JA, Younge BR, Campbell RJ, et al. Optic glioma: long-term follow-up of 85 histopathologically verified cases. Ophthalmology 1982;89:1213–1219.

424. Packer RJ, Savino PJ, Bilaniuk LT, et al. Chiasmatic gliomas of childhood. A reappraisal of natural history and effectiveness of cranial irradiation. Childs Brain 1983;10:393–403.

425. Imes RK, Hoyt WF. Childhood chiasmal gliomas: update on the fate of patients in the 1969 San Francisco study. Br J Ophthalmol 1986;70:179–182.

426. Wong JYC, Uhl V, Wara WM, et al. Optic gliomas: a reanalysis of the University of California, San Francisco experience. Cancer 1987;60:1847–1855.

427. Flickinger JC, Torres C, Deutsch M. Management of low-grade gliomas of the optic nerve and chiasm. Cancer 1988;61:635–642.

428. Gittinger JW. To image or not to image. Surv Ophthalmol 1988;32:350–356.

429. Rodriguez LA, Edwards MSB, Levin VA. Management of hypothalamic gliomas in children: an analysis of 33 cases. Neurosurgery 1990;26:242–247.

430. Cohen ME, Duffner PK. Optic pathway tumors. Neurol Clin 1991;9:467–477.

431. Hoffman HJ, Humphreys RP, Drake JM, et al. Optic pathway/hypothalamic gliomas: a dilemma in management. Pediatr Neurosurg 1993;19:186–195.

432. Nishio S, Takeshita I, Fujiwara S, et al. Optico-hypothalamic glioma: an analysis of 16 cases. Childs Nerv Syst 1993;9:334–338.

433. Janss AJ, Grundy R, Cnaan A, et al. Optic pathway and hypothalamic chiasmatic gliomas in children younger than age 5 years with a 6-year follow-up. Cancer 1995;75:1051–1059.

434. Sutton LN, Molloy PT, Sernyak H, et al. Long-term outcome of hypothalamic/chiasmatic astrocytomas in children treated with conservative surgery. J Neurosurg 1995;83:583–589.

435. Medlock MD, Madsen JR, Barnes PD, et al. Optic chiasm astrocytomas of childhood. 1. Long-term follow-up. Pediatr Neurosurg 1997;27:121–128.

436. Chan MY, Foong AP, Heisey DM, et al. Potential prognostic factors of relapse-free survival in childhood optic pathway glioma: a multivariate analysis. Pediatr Neurosurg 1998;29:23–28.

437. Liu GT. Optic gliomas of the anterior visual pathway. Curr Opin Ophthalmol 2006;17:427–431.

438. Nicolin G, Parkin P, Mabbott D, et al. Natural history and outcome of optic pathway gliomas in children. Pediatr Blood Cancer 2009;53:1231–1237.

439. Packer RJ, Sutton LN, Bilaniuk LT, et al. Treatment of chiasmatic/hypothalamic gliomas of childhood with chemotherapy: an update. Ann Neurol 1988;23:79–85.

440. Moghrabi A, Friedman HS, Burger PC, et al. Carboplatin treatment of progressive optic pathway gliomas to delay radiation. J Neurosurg 1993;79:223–227.

441. Packer RJ, Ater J, Allen J, et al. Carboplatin and vincristine chemotherapy for children with newly diagnosed progressive low-grade gliomas. J Neurosurg 1997;86:747–754.

442. Chamberlain MC. Recurrent chiasmatic-hypothalmic glioma treated with oral etoposide. Arch Neurol 1995;52:509–513.

443. Halperin EC, Constine LS, Tarbell NJ, et al. Supratentorial brain tumors except ependymoma; brain tumors in babies and very young children. In: Pediatric Radiation Oncology, 2nd edn, pp 40–89. New York, Raven Press, 1994.

444. Horwich A, Bloom HJG. Optic gliomas: radiation therapy and prognosis. Int J Radiat Oncol Biol Phys 1985;11:1067–1079.

445. Kovalic JJ, Grigsby PW, Shepard MJ, et al. Radiation therapy for gliomas of the optic nerve and chiasm. Int J Radiat Oncol Biol Phys 1990;18:927–932.

446. Tao ML, Barnes PD, Billett AL, et al. Childhood optic chiasm gliomas: radiographic response following radiotherapy and long-term clinical outcome. Int J Radiat Oncol Biol Phys 1997;39:579–587.

447. Cappelli C, Grill J, Raquin M, et al. Long-term follow up of 69 patients treated for optic pathway tumours before the chemotherapy era. Arch Dis Child 1998;79:334–338.

448. Adams C, Fletcher WA, Myles ST. Chiasmal glioma in neurofibromatosis type 1 with severe visual loss regained with radiation. Pediatr Neurol 1997;17:80–82.

449. Hirata Y, Matsukado Y, Mihara Y, et al. Occlusion of the internal carotid artery after radiation therapy for the chiasmal lesion. Acta Neurochir 1985;74:141–147.

450. Grill J, Couanet D, Cappelli C, et al. Radiation-induced cerebral vasculopathy in children with neurofibromatosis and optic pathway glioma. Ann Neurol 1999;45:393–396.

451. Ullrich NJ, Robertson R, Kinnamon DD, et al. Moyamoya following cranial irradiation for primary brain tumors in children. Neurology 2007;68:932–938.

452. Warman R, Glaser JS, Quencer RM. Radionecrosis of optico-hypothalamic glioma. Neuroophthalmology 1989;9:219–226.

453. Sharif S, Ferner R, Birch JM, et al. Second primary tumors in neurofibromatosis 1 patients treated for optic glioma: substantial risks after radiotherapy. J Clin Oncol 2006;24:2570–2575.

454. Medlock MD, Scott RM. Optic chiasm astrocytomas of childhood. 2. Surgical management. Pediatr Neurosurg 1997;27:129–136.

455. Dalla Via P, Opocher E, Pinello ML, et al. Visual outcome of a cohort of children with neurofibromatosis type 1 and optic pathway glioma followed by a pediatric neuro-oncology program. Neurol Oncol 2007;9:430–437.

456. Wilson WB, Feinsod M, Hoyt WF, et al. Malignant evolution of childhood chiasmal pilocytic astrocytoma. Neurology 1976;26:322–325.

457. Safneck JR, Napier LB, Halliday WC. Malignant astrocytoma of the optic nerve in a child. Can J Neurol Sci 1992;19:498–503.

458. Hoyt WF, Meshel LG, Lessell S, et al. Malignant optic glioma of adulthood. Brain 1973;96:121–132.

459. Millar WS, Tartaglino LM, Sergott RC, et al. MR of malignant optic glioma of adulthood. AJNR Am J Neuroradiol 1995;16:1673–1676.

460. Woiciechowsky C, Vogel S, Meyer R, et al. Magnetic resonance imaging of a glioblastoma of the optic chiasm. Case report. J Neurosurg 1995;83:923–925.

461. Barbaro NM, Rosenblum ML, Maitland CG, et al. Malignant optic glioma presenting radiologically as a "cystic" suprasellar mass: case report and review of the literature. Neurosurgery 1982;11:787–789.

462. Albers GW, Hoyt WF, Forno LS, et al. Treatment response in malignant optic glioma of adulthood. Neurology 1988;38:1071–1074.

463. Burton EM, Ball WS, Crane K, et al. Hamartomas of tuber cinereum: comparison of MR and CT findings in 4 cases. AJNR Am J Neuroradiol 1989;10:497–502.

464. Styne DM. The therapy for hypothalamic-pituitary tumors. Endocrinol Metab Clin North Am 1993;22:631–648.

465. Miller DC, Lang FF, Epstein FJ. Central nervous system gangliogliomas. Part 1. Pathology. J Neurosurg 1993;79:859–866.

466. Sutton LN, Packer RJ, Rorke LB, et al. Cerebral gangliogliomas during childhood. Neurosurgery 1983;13:124–128.

467. Chilton J, Caughron MR, Kepes JJ. Ganglioglioma of the optic chiasm: case report and review of the literature. Neurosurgery 1990;26:1042–1045.

468. Liu GT, Galetta SL, Rorke LB, et al. Gangliogliomas involving the optic chiasm. Neurology 1996;46:1669–1673.

469. Shuangshoti S, Kirsch E, Bannan P, et al. Ganglioglioma of the optic chiasm: case report and review of the literature. AJNR Am J Neuroradiol 2000;21:1486–1489.

470. Pant I, Suri V, Chaturvedi S, et al. Ganglioglioma of optic chiasma: case report and review of literature. Childs Nerv Syst 2006;22:717–720.

471. Sugiyama K, Goishi J, Sogabe T, et al. Ganglioglioma of the optic pathway. Surg Neurol 1992;37:22–25.

472. Johannsson JH, Rekate HL, Roessmann U. Gangliogliomas: pathological and clinical correlation. J Neurosurg 1981;54:58–63.

473. Lang FF, Epstein FJ, Ransohoff J, et al. Central nervous system gangliogliomas. Part 2. Clinical outcome. J Neurosurg 1993;79:867–873.

474. Allen JC. Controversies in management of intracranial germ cell tumors. Neurol Clin 1991;9:441–452.

475. Bowman CB, Farris BK. Primary chiasmal germinoma. J Clin Neuroophthalmol 1990;10:9–17.

476. Izquierdo JM, Rougerie J, Lapras C, et al. The so-called ectopic pinealomas. A cooperative study of 15 cases. Childs Brain 1979;5:505–512.

477. Camins MB, Mount LA. Primary suprasellar atypical teratoma. Brain 1974;97:447–456.

478. Muzumdar D, Goel A, Desai K, et al. Mature teratoma arising from the sella: case report. Neurol Med Chir (Tokyo) 2001;41:356–359.

479. Kageyama N, Belsky R. Ectopic pinealoma in the chiasmal region. Neurology 1961;11:318–327.

480. Takeuchi J, Handa H, Nagata I. Suprasellar germinoma. J Neurosurg 1978;49:41–48.

481. Hoffman HJ, Otsubo H, Hendrick EB, et al. Intracranial germ-cell tumors in children. J Neurosurg 1991;74:545–551.

482. Neuwelt EA, Frenkel EP, Smith RG. Suprasellar germinomas (ectopic pinealomas): aspects of immunological characterization and successful chemotherapeutic responses in recurrent disease. Neurosurgery 1980;7:352–358.

483. Houston LW, Hinke ML. Neuroradiology case of the day: suprasellar epidermoid. AJR Am J Radiol 1986;146:1094–1095.

484. Cohen MM, Lessell S. Chiasmal syndrome due to metastases. Arch Neurol 1979;36:565–567.

485. Lee AG, Tang RA, Roberts D, et al. Primary central nervous system lymphoma involving the optic chiasm in AIDS. J Neuroophthalmol 2001;21:95–98.

486. Gray RS, Abrahams JJ, Hufnagel TJ, et al. Ghost-cell tumor of the optic chiasm. Primary CNS lymphoma. J Clin Neuroophthalmol 1989;9:98–104.

487. Case Records of the MGH. N Engl J Med 1994;331:861–868.

488. Kuhn D, Buchfelder M, Brabletz T, et al. Intrasellar malignant lymphoma developing within pituitary adenoma. Acta Neuropathol 1999;97:311–316.

489. Post KD, McCormick PC, Bello JA. Differential diagnosis of pituitary tumors. Endocrinol Metab Clin North Am 1987;16:609–645.

490. Cone L, Srinivasan M, Romanul FC. Granular cell tumor (choristoma) of the neurohypophysis: two cases and a review of the literature. AJNR AM J Neuroradiol 1990;11:403–406.

491. Cohen-Gadol AA, Pichelmann MA, Link MJ, et al. Granular cell tumor of the sellar and suprasellar region: clinicopathologic study of 11 cases and literature review. Mayo Clin Proc 2003;78:567–573.

492. Shah B, Lipper MH, Laws ER, et al. Posterior pituitary astrocytoma: a rare tumor of the neurohypophysis: a case report. AJNR Am J Neuroradiol 2005;26:1858–1861.

493. Newnham HH, Rivera-Woll LM. Images in clinical medicine. Hypogonadism due to pituicytoma in an identical twin. N Engl J Med 2008;359:2824.

494. Kazim M, Kennerdell JS, Maroon J, et al. Choristoma of the optic nerve and chiasm. Arch Ophthalmol 1992;110:236–238.

495. Volpe NJ, Liebsch NJ, Munzenrider JE, et al. Neuro-ophthalmologic findings in chordoma and chondrosarcoma of the skull base. Am J Ophthalmol 1993;115:97–104.

496. Thodou E, Kontogeorgos G, Scheithauer BW, et al. Intrasellar chordomas mimicking pituitary adenoma. J Neurosurg 2000;92:976–982.

497. Keltner JL, Johnson CA, Spurr JO, et al. Baseline visual field profile of optic neuritis. The experience of the optic neuritis treatment trial. Optic Neuritis Study Group. Arch Ophthalmol 1993;111:231–234.

498. Beck RW, Kupersmith MJ, Cleary PA, et al. Fellow eye abnormalities in acute unilateral optic neuritis. Experience of the optic neuritis treatment trial. Ophthalmology 1993;100:691–697.

499. Newman NJ, Lessell S, Winterkorn JMS. Optic chiasmal neuritis. Neurology 1991;41:1203–1210.

500. Siatkowski RM, Scott IU, Verm AM, et al. Optic neuropathy and chiasmopathy in the diagnosis of systemic lupus erythematosus. J Neuroophthalmol 2001;21:193–198.

501. Beck RW, Cleary PA, Optic Neuritis Study Group. Optic neuritis treatment trial. One year follow-up results. Arch Ophthalmol 1993;111:773–775.

502. Case Records of the MGH. N Engl J Med 1996;335:1668–1674.

503. Zajicek JP, Scolding NJ, Foster O, et al. Central nervous system sarcoidosis-diagnosis and management. Q J Med 1999;92:103–117.

504. Shealy CN, Kahana L, Engel FL, et al. Hypothalamic pituitary sarcoidosis. Am J Med 1961;30:46–55.

505. Walsh TJ, Smith JL. Sarcoidosis and suprasellar mass. In: Smith JL (ed.): Neuroophthalmology. Symposium of the University of Miami and the Bascom Palmer Eye Institute, Vol. IV, pp 167–177. St. Louis, C.V. Mosby, 1968.

506. Guoth MS, Kim J, de Lotbiniere AC, et al. Neurosarcoidosis presenting as hypopituitarism and a cystic pituitary mass. Am J Med Sci 1998;315:220–224.

507. Hayes WS, Sherman JL, Stern BJ, et al. MR and CT evaluation of intracranial sarcoidosis. AJR Am J Radiol 1987;149:1043–1049.

508. Case Records of the MGH. N Engl J Med 1991;324:677–687.

509. Beck AD, Newman NJ, Grossniklaus HE, et al. Optic nerve enlargement and chronic visual loss. Surv Ophthalmol 1994;38:555–566.

510. Tang RA, Grotta JC, Lee KF, et al. Chiasmal syndrome in sarcoidosis. Arch Ophthalmol 1983;101:1069–1073.

511. Gelwan MJ, Kellen RI, Burde RM, et al. Sarcoidosis of the anterior visual pathway: successes and failures. J Neurol Neurosurg Psychiatr 1988;51:1473–1480.

512. Lower EE, Broderick JP, Brott TG, et al. Diagnosis and management of neurological sarcoidosis. Arch Intern Med 1997;157:1864–1868.

513. Tikoo RK, Kupersmith MJ, Finlay JL. Treatment of refractory neurosarcoidosis with cladribine [letter]. N Engl J Med 2004;350:1798–1799.

514. Tibbs PA, Challa V, Mortara RH. Isolated histiocytosis X of the hypothalamus. J Neurosurg 1978;49:929–934.

515. Czech T, Mazal PR, Schima W. Resection of a Langerhans cell histiocytosis granuloma of the hypothalamus: case report. Br J Neurosurg 1999;13:196–200.

516. Margo CE, Goldman DR. Langerhans cell histiocytosis. Surv Ophthalmol 2008;53:332–358.

517. Maghnie M, Cosi G, Genovese E, et al. Central diabetes insipidus in children and young adults. N Engl J Med 2000;343:998–1007.

518. Goodman RH, Post KD, Molitsch ME, et al. Eosinophilic granuloma mimicking a pituitary tumor. Neurosurgery 1979;5:723–725.

519. Job OM, Schatz NJ, Glaser JS. Visual loss with Langerhans cell histiocytosis: multifocal central nervous system involvement. J Neuroophthalmol 1999;19:49–53.

520. Halperin EC, Constine LS, Tarbell NJ, et al. Langerhans' cell histiocytosis. In: Pediatric Radiation Oncology, 2nd edn, pp 446–472. New York, Raven Press, 1994.

521. Kerrison JB, Lee AG. Acute loss of vision during pregnancy due to a suprasellar mass. Surv Ophthalmol 1997;41:402–408.

522. Tubridy N, Molloy J, Saunders D, et al. Postpartum pituitary hypophysitis. J Neuroophthalmol 2001;21:106–108.

523. Li J-Y, Lai P-H, Lam H-C, et al. Hypertrophic cranial pachymeningitis and lymphocytic hypophysitis in Sjögren's syndrome. Neurology 1999;52:420–423.

524. Case Records of the MGH. N Engl J Med 1995;333:441–447.

525. Baskin DS, Townsend JJ, Wilson CB. Lymphocytic adenohypophysitis of pregnancy simulating a pituitary adenoma: a distinct pathological entity. J Neurosurg 1982;56:148–153.

526. Levine SN, Benzel EC, Fowler MR, et al. Lymphocytic hypophysitis: clinical, radiological, and magnetic resonance imaging characterization. Neurosurgery 1988;22:937–941.

527. Saiwai S, Inoue Y, Ishihara T, et al. Lymphocytic adenohypophysitis: skull radiographs and MRI. Neuroradiology 1998;40:114–120.

528. Hungerford GD, Biggs PJ, Levine JH, et al. Lymphoid adenohypophysitis with radiologic and clinical findings resembling a pituitary tumor. AJNR Am J Neuroradiol 1982;3:444–446.

529. Case Records of the MGH. N Engl J Med 1985;312:297–305.

530. Case Records of the MGH. N Engl J Med 2000;343:1399–1406.

531. Arsava EM, Uluc K, Kansu T, et al. Granulomatous hypophysitis and bilateral optic neuropathy. J Neuroophthalmol 2001;21:34–36.

532. Roncaroli F, Bacci A, Frank G, et al. Granulomatous hypophysitis caused by a ruptured intrasellar Rathke's cleft cyst: report of a case and review of the literature. Neurosurgery 1998;43:146–149.

533. Lee AG, Cech DA, Rose JE, et al. Recurrent visual loss due to muslin-induced optochiasmatic arachnoiditis. Neuroophthalmology 1997;18:199–204.

534. Taravati P, Lee AG, Bhatti MT, et al. That's a wrap. Surv Ophthalmol 2006;51:434–444.

535. Donald PR, Schoeman JF. Tuberculous meningitis. N Engl J Med 2004;351:1719–1720.

536. Okazaki H. Infectious disease. In: Fundamentals of Neuropathology, 2nd edn, pp 115–147. New York, Igaku-Shoin, 1989.

537. Hepler RS. Miscellaneous optic neuropathies. In: Albert DM, Jakobiec FA (eds): Principles and Practice of Ophthalmology, pp 2604–2615. Philadelphia, W.B. Saunders, 1993.

538. Silverman IE, Liu GT, Bilaniuk LT, et al. Tuberculous meningitis with blindness and peri-chiasmal involvement on MRI. Pediatr Neurol 1995;12:65–67.

539. Navarro IM, Peralta VHR, Leon JAM, et al. Tuberculous optochiasmatic arachnoiditis. Neurosurgery 1981;9:654–660.

540. Fishman RA. CSF findings in diseases of the nervous system. In: Cerebrospinal Fluid in Diseases of the Nervous System, 2nd edn, pp 253–343. Philadelphia, W.B. Saunders, 1992.

541. Kox LFF, Kuijper S, Kolk AHJ. Early diagnosis of tuberculous meningitis by polymerase chain reaction. Neurology 1995;45:2228–2232.

542. Nguyen LN, Kox LFF, Pham LD, et al. The potential contribution of the polymerase chain reaction to the diagnosis of tuberculous meningitis. Arch Neurol 1996;53:771–776.

543. Sharma MC, Arora R, Mahapatra AK, et al. Intrasellar tuberculoma: an enigmatic pituitary infection: a series of 18 cases. Clin Neurol Neurosurg 2000;102:72–77.

544. Lindholm J, Rasmussen P, Korsgaard O. Intrasellar or pituitary abscess. J Neurosurg 1973;38:616–619.

545. Domingue JN, Wilson CB. Pituitary abscess. Report of seven cases and review of the literature. J Neurosurg 1977;46:601–608.

546. Wolansky LJ, Gallagher JD, Heary RF, et al. MRI of pituitary abscess: two cases and review of the literature. Neuroradiology 1997;39:499–503.

547. Case Records of the MGH. N Engl J Med 1993;328:566–573.

548. Chang GY, Keane JR. Visual loss in cysticercosis: analysis of 23 patients. Neurology 2001;57:545–548.

549. Ebner R, Slamovits TL, Friedland S, et al. Visual loss following treatment of sphenoid sinus carcinoma. Surv Ophthalmol 1995;40:62–68.

550. Roden D, Bosley TM, Fowble B, et al. Delayed radiation injury to the retrobulbar optic nerves and chiasm. Ophthalmology 1990;97:346–351.

551. Zimmerman CF, Schatz NJ, Glaser JS. Magnetic resonance imaging of radiation optic neuropathy. Am J Ophthalmol 1990;110:389–394.

552. Piquemal R, Cottier JP, Arsène S, et al. Radiation-induced optic neuropathy 4 years after radiation: report of a case followed up with MRI. Neuroradiology 1998;40:439–441.

553. Tachibana O, Yamaguchi N, Yamashima T, et al. Radiation necrosis of the optic chiasm, optic tract, hypothalamus, and upper pons after radiotherapy for pituitary adenomas, detected by gadolinium-enhanced T1-weighted magnetic resonance imaging: case report. Neurosurgery 1990;27:640–643.

554. Hudgins PA, Newman NJ, Dillon WP, et al. Radiation-induced optic neuropathy: characteristic appearances on gadolinium-enhanced MR. AJNR AM J Neuroradiol 1992;13:235–238.

555. Hufnagel TJ, Kim JH, Lesser R, et al. Malignant glioma of the optic chiasm eight years after radiotherapy for prolactinoma. Am J Ophthalmol 1988;106:1701–1705.

556. Osher RH, Corbett JJ, Schatz NJ, et al. Neuro-ophthalmological complications of enlargement of the third ventricle. Br J Ophthalmol 1978;62:536–542.

557. Bogdanovic MD, Plant GT. Chiasmal compression due to obstructive hydrocephalus. J Neuroophthalmol 2000;20:266–267.

558. Heinz GW, Nunery WR, Grossman CB. Traumatic chiasmal syndrome associated with midline basilar skull fractures. Am J Ophthalmol 1994;117:90–96.

559. Savino PJ, Glaser JS, Schatz NJ. Traumatic chiasmal syndrome. Neurology 1980;30:963–970.

560. Sharma R, Goyal M, Sharma A, et al. Traumatic transection of the optic chiasm: magnetic resonance evaluation. Aust Radiol 1998;42:80–82.

561. El-Hindy N, Lalchan S-A, Scullion D, et al. Traumatic chiasmal syndrome: a multidisciplinary challenge. Neuroophthalmology 2007;31:7–9.

562. Lindenberg R, Walsh FB, Sacks JG. The chiasm. In: Neuropathology of Vision: An Atlas, pp 197–313. Philadelphia, Lea & Febiger, 1973.

563. Dilly JS, Imes RK. Autoenucleation of a blind eye. J Neuroophthalmol 2001;21:30–31.

564. Kaufman B, Tomsak RL, Kaufman BA, et al. Herniation of suprasellar visual system and third ventricle into empty sellae: morphologic and clinical considerations. AJNR AM J Neuroradiol 1989;10:65–76.

565. Buckman MT, Husain M, Carlow TJ, et al. Primary empty sella syndrome with visual field defects. Am J Med 1976;61:124–128.

566. Weisberg LA, Housepian EM, Saur DA. Empty sella syndrome and complication of benign intracranial hypertension. J Neurosurg 1975;43:177–180.

567. Nugent GR, Sprinkle P, Bloor BM. Sphenoid sinus mucoceles. J Neurosurg 1970;32:443–451.

568. Goodwin JA, Glaser JS. Chiasmal syndrome in sphenoid sinus mucocele. Ann Neurol 1978;4:440–444.

569. Thompson DA, Kriss A, Chong K, et al. Visual-evoked potential evidence of chiasmal hypoplasia. Ophthalmology 1999;106:2354–2361.

570. Smith DE, Murphy MJ, Hitchon PW, et al. Transphenoidal encephaloceles. Surg Neurol 1983;20:471–480.

571. Brodsky MC, Frindik JP. Hypothalamic-hypophyseal dysgenesis as a neuroimaging correlate of pituitary hormone deficiency in anophthalmia. Am J Ophthalmol 1996;122:747–748.

572. Pomeranz HD, Lessell S. A hereditary chiasmal optic neuropathy. Arch Ophthalmol 1999;117:128–131.

573. Bouzas EA, Caruso RC, Drews-Bankiewicz MA, et al. Evoked potential analysis of visual pathways in human albinism. Ophthalmology 1994;101:309–314.

574. Hedera P, Lai S, Haacke EM, et al. Abnormal connectivity of the visual pathway in human albinos demonstrated by susceptibility-sensitized MRI. Neurology 1994;44:1921–1926.

575. Brodsky MC, Glasier CM, Creel DJ. Magnetic resonance imaging of the visual pathways in human albinos. J Pediatr Ophthalmol Strab 1993;30:382–385.

576. Apkarian P, Bour LJ, Barth PG, et al. Non-decussating retinal-fugal fibre syndrome. An inborn achiasmatic malformation associated with visuotopic misrouting, visual evoked potential ipsilateral asymmetry and nystagmus. Brain 1995;118:1195–1216.

577. Victor JD, Apkarian P, Hirsch J, et al. Visual function and brain organization in non-decussating retinal-fugal fibre syndrome. Cereb Cortex 2000;10:2–22.

578. Jansonius NM, van der Vliet TM, Cornelissen FW, et al. A girl without a chiasm: electrophysiologic and MRI evidence for the absence of crossing optic nerve fibers in a girl with a congenital nystagmus. J Neuroophthalmol 2001;21:26–29.

579. Hertle RW, Dell'Osso LF, FitzGibbon EJ, et al. Clinical, radiographic, and electrophysiologic findings in patients with achiasma or hypochiasma. Neuroophthalmology 2002;26:43–57.

580. Levy A, Lightman SL. Diagnosis and management of pituitary tumours. BMJ 1994;308:1087–1091.

CHAPTER **8**

Retrochiasmal disorders

The retrochiasmal afferent visual pathways include the optic tract, lateral geniculate nucleus, optic radiations, and striate cortex. The most common neuro-ophthalmic presentation of a unilateral retrochiasmal disturbance is a homonymous hemianopic field defect with normal acuity.

Important concepts in retrochiasmal disorders will be discussed first. The second part of this chapter will be subdivided by localization and progress from anterior to posterior structures, with neuroanatomy, clinical presentation, and common etiologies described in each section. The last portion of this chapter details the diagnosis and management of lesions in the optic radiations and occipital lobe. Emphasis will be placed on cerebrovascular disease, since it is seen most frequently.

Important concepts in retrochiasmal disorders

Etiology and localization in adults versus children

In adults, the most common cause of unilateral retrochiasmal visual loss is a stroke (**Table 8–1**).[1-3] In Zhang et al.'s[4] study of isolated and non-isolated hemianopias in adults, all of whom had undergone CT or MR imaging, 63% were caused by ischemic stroke, 12% by trauma, and 11% by hemorrhages.[5] The responsible lesion in adults is most commonly in the occipital lobe (47%).[5]

In contrast, Kedar et al.[5] found in children the most common causes of a hemianopia were trauma (34%) and tumor (27%). In our own experience from the Children's Hospital of Philadelphia,[6] brain neoplasms involving the visual pathways or their associated biopsy or removal were the most common etiology in pediatric patients (**Table 8–2**). The difference between the two studies likely reflects referral bias. Injury to the optic radiations is the most common localization in children (37%).[5] Cerebrovascular disease and cerebral hemorrhages are also responsible causes in children, but are seen less commonly.

Hemianopia congruity and localization

As discussed in Chapter 3, *congruity* refers to the symmetry of the homonymous visual field defects. Congruity can be assessed only in incomplete homonymous hemianopias not involving the whole half of the visual field. Isolated complete homonymous hemianopias are non-localizing.

In general, incongruous hemianopias localize to more anterior retrochiasmal lesions, for instance in the optic tract. More congruous hemianopias suggest more posterior disturbances, i.e., the occipital lobe. The explanation offered for the incongruity observed in more anterior lesions is anatomical. Uncrossed and crossed axons combine first in the optic tract, where fibers carrying information from corresponding areas within the contralateral homonymous hemifield may still be widely separated.[7,8] More posteriorly, the corresponding areas are subserved by fibers which are closer together or in the case of striate cortex in the occipital lobe, by single binocular neurons.

Table 8–1 Frequency of etiologies (by category and primary location) of hemifield loss in inpatient and outpatient adults seen by one of the authors (G.T.L.) from July 1993 to October 1996. All patients had CT or MRI confirmation of the lesion and localization

		Optic tract	Optic radiations	Occipital lobe	Total	
Vascular (68%)	Stroke (infarction)		6	17	23	(52%)
	Hemorrhage		1	5	6	(14%)
	Aneurysm	1			1	(2%)
Neoplasm (18%)	Pre-operative or following neurosurgical removal of neoplasm involving the visual pathways		7	1	8	(18%)
Trauma (4%)			1	1	2	(4%)
Other (9%)			3	1	4	(9%)
Total					44	

Table 8–2 Frequency of etiologies (by category and primary location) of hemifield loss in pediatric patients seen at the Children's Hospital of Philadelphia from July 1993 to February 1997 (reprinted with permission from Liu GT and Galetta SL. Neurology 1997;49:1748–1749).

		Optic tract	Optic radiations	Occipital lobe	Total	
Neoplasm (39%)	Pre-operative	5		1	6	(17%)
	Following neurosurgical removal of neoplasm involving the visual pathways	2	4	2	8	(22%)
Vascular (25%)	Stroke (infarction)		2	2	4	(11%)
	Hemorrhage	1	1	2	4	(11%)
	Following neurosurgical removal of hematoma involving anterior visual pathway			1	1	(3%)
Trauma (19%)	Nonsurgical		4	1	5	(14%)
	Neurosurgical-during operations that did not involve tumors in the visual pathways			2	2	(6%)
Other (17%)	Congenital		2		2	(6%)
	Other		3	1	4	(11%)
Total					36	

Thus a partial anterior lesion may affect the visual field in each eye asymmetrically, while posterior lesions are more likely to cause the same deficit in both eyes. However, these are guidelines rather than rules. Incongruous homonymous hemianopias may also be caused by optic radiation and occipital lobe lesions, and optic tract lesions may result in congruous visual field defects.[9]

LESIONS OF THE RETROCHIASMAL PATHWAYS

Optic tract

In adults, optic tract lesions are relatively uncommon and accounted for only 10% of hemianopias in the Zhang et al.

series.[4] The higher frequency of tract involvement in children (8/36 (22%), **Table 8–2**)[6] may in part owe to the higher incidence of sellar masses and the lower incidence of strokes in the pediatric patients.

Neuroanatomy

The afferent visual fibers (ganglion cell axons) exit the chiasm posteriorly and diverge to form the left and right optic tracts, each of which is made up of fibers from the ipsilateral temporal retinal and the contralateral nasal retina (see **Figs 3–1**, **3–2**, and **7–6**). The optic tracts sweep around and above the infundibulum, below the third ventricle, and superomedially to the uncal gyri (see **Figs 7–2** and **7–5**). They then turn posterolaterally to the interpenduncular cistern, just ventral to the rostral midbrain and cerebral peduncles.

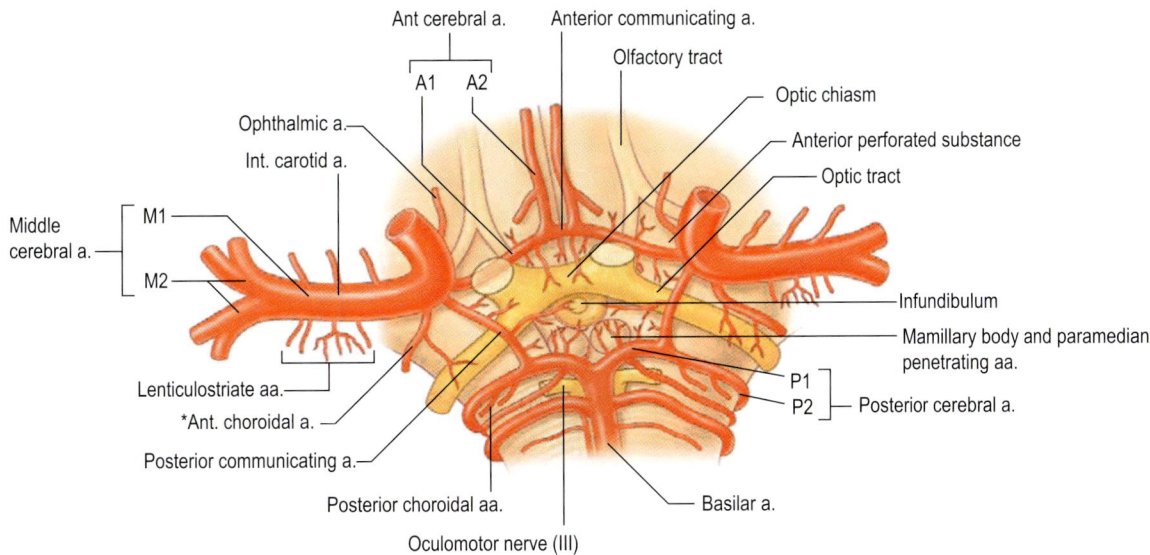

Figure 8–1. Relationship of the anterior choroidal artery (*) and the posterior choroidal arteries with the circle of Willis. The anterior choroidal artery is a branch of the internal carotid/middle cerebral artery complex, while the posterior choroidal artery is a branch of the posterior cerebral artery. a., artery; aa., arteries.

Most of the tract fibers synapse within the ipsilateral lateral geniculate nucleus; however, some axons depart from the optic tract to complete the afferent limb of the pupillary light reflex. These pupillary fibers pass ventral to the medial geniculate nucleus, and then continue through the brachium of the superior colliculi before reaching the pretectal nuclei, where they synapse. In turn, these nuclei connect bilaterally to the Edinger–Westphal nuclei in the oculomotor complex (see **Fig. 13–2**).

The blood supply of the optic tract is variable but typically comes from an anastamotic network of branches from the posterior communicating and anterior choroidal arteries (from the internal carotid artery (ICA)) (**Fig. 8–1**).[10]

Symptoms and signs

Visual field defects. Incongruous homonymous hemianopias are seen more frequently in association with optic tract lesions than with any other retrochiasmal localization.[9] Classically, incomplete optic tract lesions characteristically result in highly incongruous homonymous hemianopias of variable density and with sloping margins (**Fig. 8–2**).[7] If the lesion progresses to involve the entire optic tract, the result is a complete macular-splitting contralateral hemianopia.

Other neuro-ophthalmic signs. Acuity is preserved in an isolated tract lesion, but a relative afferent pupillary defect in the contralateral eye may be observed. In fact, a homonymous hemianopia accompanied by normal visual acuities but a relative afferent pupillary defect (RAPD) ipsilateral to the field defect is highly suggestive of an optic tract disturbance. If the chiasm or optic nerves are also involved, by a large sellar mass for instance, acuity may be reduced, and a RAPD may be evident in the eye with the greater visual field loss. In most cases, the RAPD is observed in the eye contralateral to the optic tract lesion as the temporal field loss is usually larger than the nasal field loss (also see Chapter 13, Pupillary disorders). One study[11] suggested the presence and

magnitude of an optic tract RAPD was related to this asymmetry of visual field loss rather than the classic explanation of a disturbance of more crossed then uncrossed fibers. Other described pupillary abnormalities include contralateral mydriasis (Behr's pupil), and hemianopic pupillary reactivity (Wernicke's pupil). However, both of these pupillary abnormalities are of uncertain clinical significance, and their existence is debated.[12]

Because presynaptic ganglion cell axons are interrupted, patients with isolated tract lesions may have bilateral optic atrophy with ipsilateral temporal pallor and contralateral "bow-tie" or "band" atrophy (**Fig. 8–3**). Larger lesions also affecting the chiasm or optic nerves may produce diffuse bilateral optic atrophy. A homonymous hemianopia accompanied by optic atrophy would be consistent with a disturbance of either the optic tract or lateral geniculate nucleus.

Other symptoms and signs. Because of its proximity to the optic tract, the cerebral peduncle can be simultaneously affected by compressive mass lesions, leading to a hemiparesis on the same side as the hemianopia. Endocrine disturbances, owing to involvement of the pituitary, stalk, or hypothalamus, may also be seen. In Bender and Bodis-Wollner's[13] series of patients with optic tract lesions, five of their 12 patients had memory problems, and three of these had visual hallucinations, and the authors attributed these symptoms to temporal lobe involvement.

Etiology

Because of the anatomic relationship between the two, any process which can involve the optic chiasm (**Table 7–3**) may also affect the optic tract, and therefore the differential diagnosis is similar. If the chiasm is prefixed (short intracranial optic nerves, see **Fig. 7–4**), an enlarging sellar mass is likely to cause a posterior chiasmal or optic tract interference. Sellar disturbances are discussed in detail in Chapter 7.

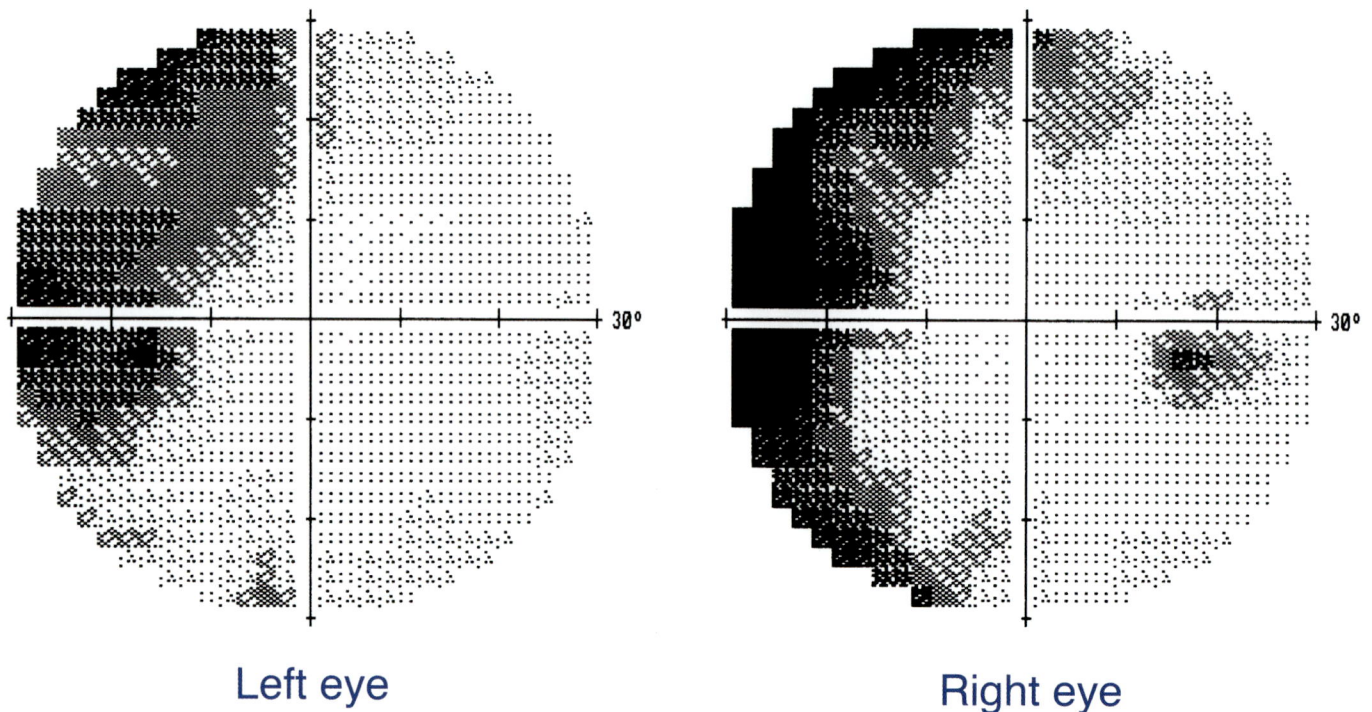

Left eye

Right eye

Figure 8–2. Incongruous homonymous hemianopia due to a hypothalamic glioma involving the optic tract. Computerized perimetry grayscale output.

In addition, temporal lobe masses may cause optic tract disturbances, but in these instances it may be difficult to distinguish pressure on the optic tract from involvement of the optic radiations.

Among 21 patients with optic tract syndromes in one series,[12] the most common etiologies were craniopharyngi-oma (8/21 (38%)), aneurysms (3/21 (14%)) (**Fig. 8–4a**), and pituitary adenomas (3/21 (14%)). Other less frequent causes seen were trauma, temporal lobe tumor, demyelination, meningioma, pinealoma, and malignant astrocytoma. In another series,[13] suprasellar masses were also the most common etiology. Because of the rich anastamotic blood supply from the anterior choroidal and posterior cerebral arteries, ischemic tract lesions were not seen in either study and are therefore considered unusual.[14] With the use of modern neuroimaging, more patients with demyelination of the optic tract have been recognized (**Fig. 8–4b**), often in the setting of multiple sclerosis.[15] In addition, individuals with homonymous hemianopias due to arteriovenous mal-formations,[16] basilar artery dolichoectasia,[17] and metastases[18] (**Fig. 8–4c**) involving the optic tract and congenital absence of the optic tract[19] have been described. Overall, these studies together serve to emphasize that an optic tract lesion is most often caused by a mass lesion.

Lateral geniculate nucleus

Ganglion cell axons traveling in the optic tract end in the lateral geniculate nucleus (LGN), where they synapse with neurons that form the optic radiations. Isolated disturbances of the lateral geniculate are even less common than those of the optic tract. However, when they occur, they are some-times recognized by the characteristic patterns of sectoral hemianopic field loss.

Neuroanatomy

The LGN, situated within the lateral recess of the choroidal fissure, above the ambient cistern,[20-22] is considered part of the thalamus (**Fig. 8–5**). Coronally, the LGN has six neuronal layers, and the input into each is monocular and retinotopi-cally organized (**Fig. 8–6**). Visual information from the ipsi-lateral eye synapses within laminae 2, 3, and 5, while that from the contralateral eye synapses within laminae 1, 4, and 6. Furthermore, macular vision is subserved by the middle wedge (hilum), while the medial and lateral horns carry information from the inferior and superior quadrants, respectively (**Fig. 8–7**).

Layers 1 and 2 contain large neurons (magnocellular LGN layers), while layers 3–6 contain smaller neurons (parvocel-lular LGN layers). There are at least two types of retinal ganglion cells (M and P, respectively) that project preferen-tially to each group, and that each layer may have distinct projections within the striate cortex as well. The M-group of retinal ganglion cells are important in motion detection while P-cells serve form and color vision (see Chapters 4, 5, and 9 for further discussion).

The LGN also has a rich anastomotic blood supply made up of the anterior and posterior choroidal arteries. While the anterior choroidal artery derives from the ICA, the posterior choroidal arteries, consisting of one medial and two lateral arteries, are branches of the posterior cerebral artery and arise distal to the thalamogeniculate arteries.[23] The medial and lateral horns of the LGN are supplied by the anterior choroidal artery, and the hilum by the posterior choroidal

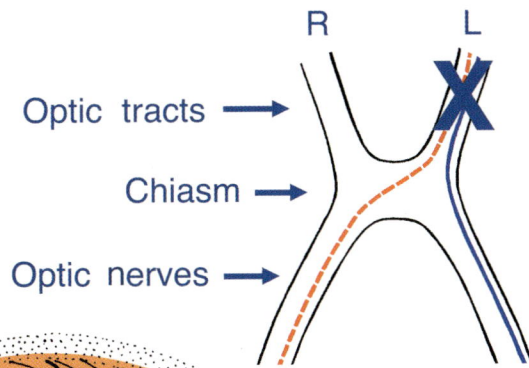

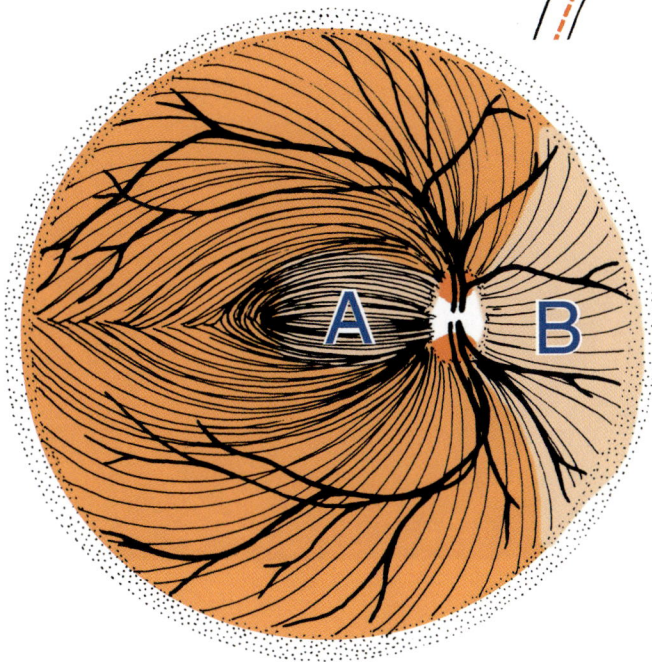

Right eye
"Bow-tie" optic nerve atrophy

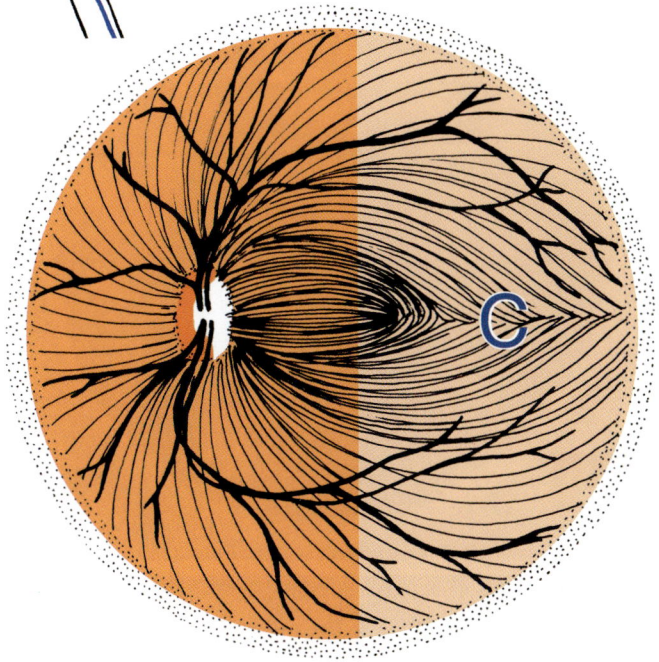

Left eye
Temporal optic nerve atrophy

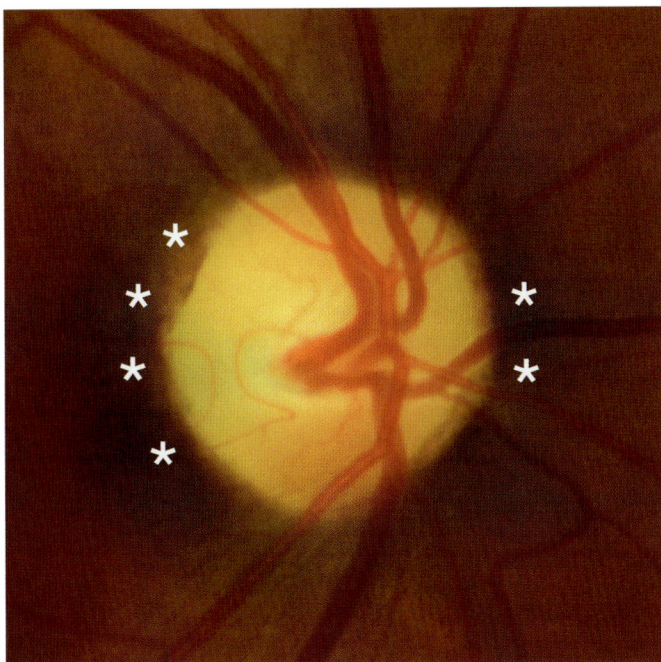

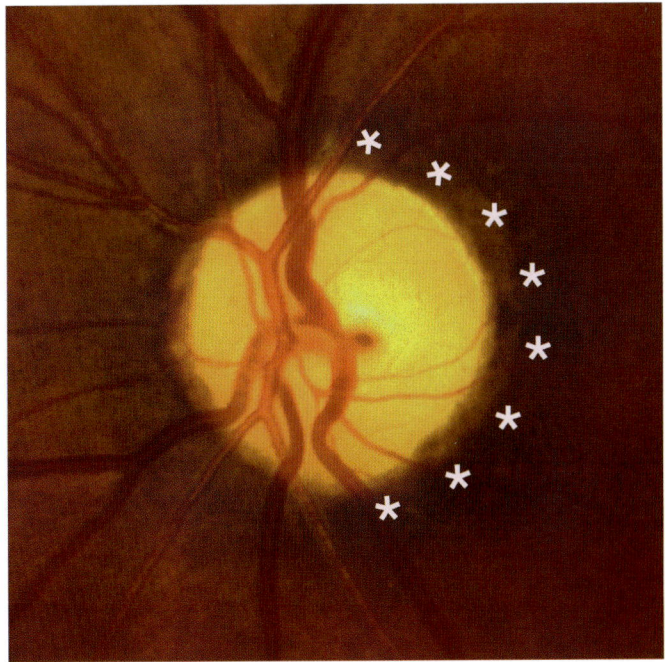

Figure 8–3. "Bow-tie atrophy" due to an optic tract lesion. **Top**. Following a chronic lesion ("X") in the left optic tract, three groups of retinal ganglion cell fibers atrophy: **Middle**. A, those from the nasal half of the macula in the right eye; B, those from the nasal retina in the right eye; and C, those from the temporal retina of the left eye. A and B result in a bow-tie or band pattern of optic atrophy (white areas) in the right disc, and C results in temporal atrophy of the left disc (white area). This pattern of optic atrophy is similar to that seen in homonymous hemioptic atrophy due to a congenital lesion of the geniculocalcarine pathway. Bottom: Right disc (**left**) and left disc (**right**) exhibiting "bow-tie" atrophy due to a left optic tract lesion. Atrophic areas are highlighted by the asterisks.

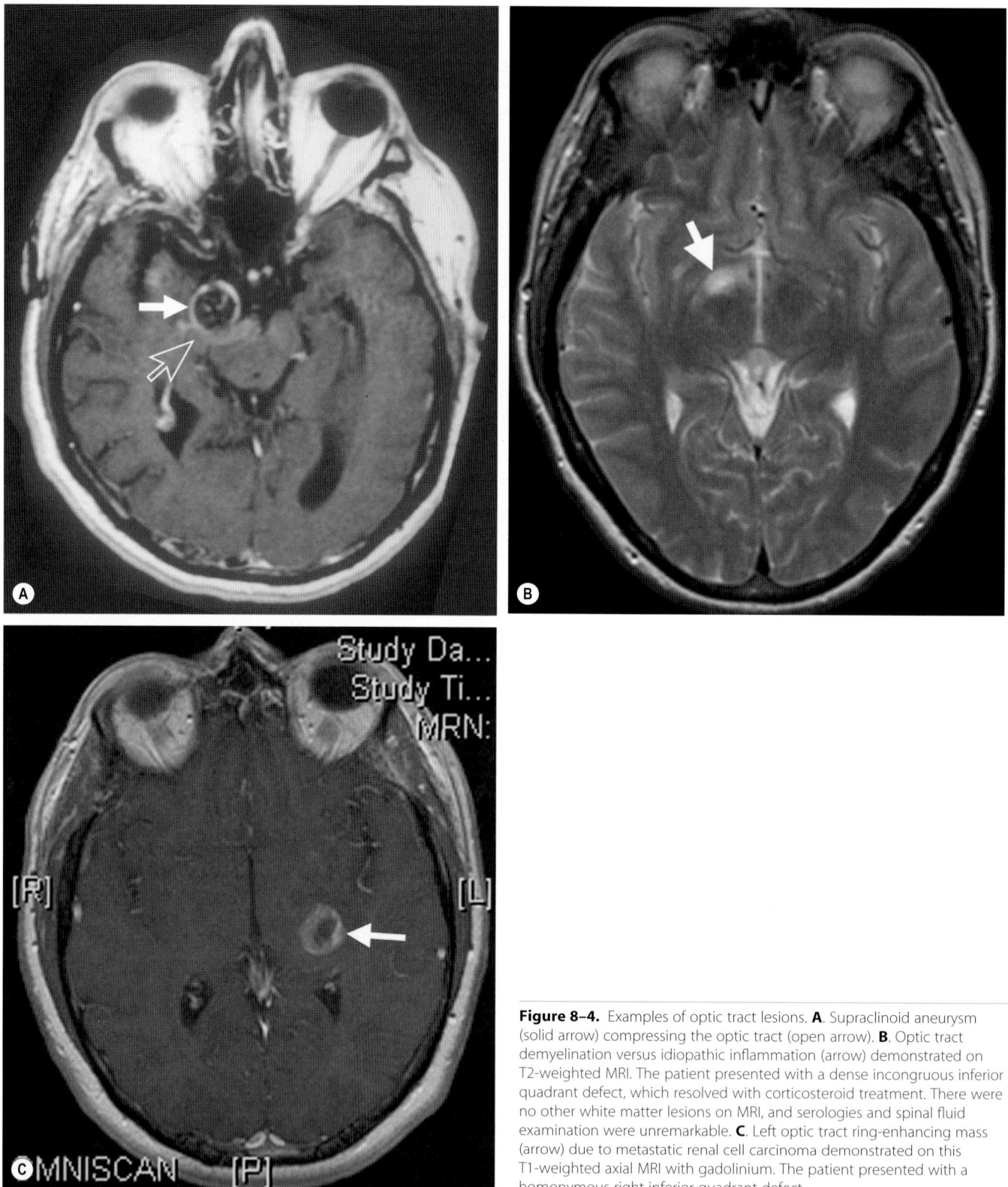

Figure 8–4. Examples of optic tract lesions. **A.** Supraclinoid aneurysm (solid arrow) compressing the optic tract (open arrow). **B.** Optic tract demyelination versus idiopathic inflammation (arrow) demonstrated on T2-weighted MRI. The patient presented with a dense incongruous inferior quadrant defect, which resolved with corticosteroid treatment. There were no other white matter lesions on MRI, and serologies and spinal fluid examination were unremarkable. **C.** Left optic tract ring-enhancing mass (arrow) due to metastatic renal cell carcinoma demonstrated on this T1-weighted axial MRI with gadolinium. The patient presented with a homonymous right inferior quadrant defect.

artery and its branches (**Fig. 8–1** and **Fig. 8–7**).[24] In about 50% of cases, small portions of the LGN receive blood from other small posterior cerebral artery branches. Ischemic lesions to the posterior portion of the optic tract and the LGN are considered rare due to their rich anastomotic blood supply.[10,25]

Symptoms and signs

Visual field defects. Compressive or infiltrative lesions of the LGN typically cause an incongruous contralateral homonymous hemianopia. When the disturbance involves the LGN completely, the result is a complete hemianopia.

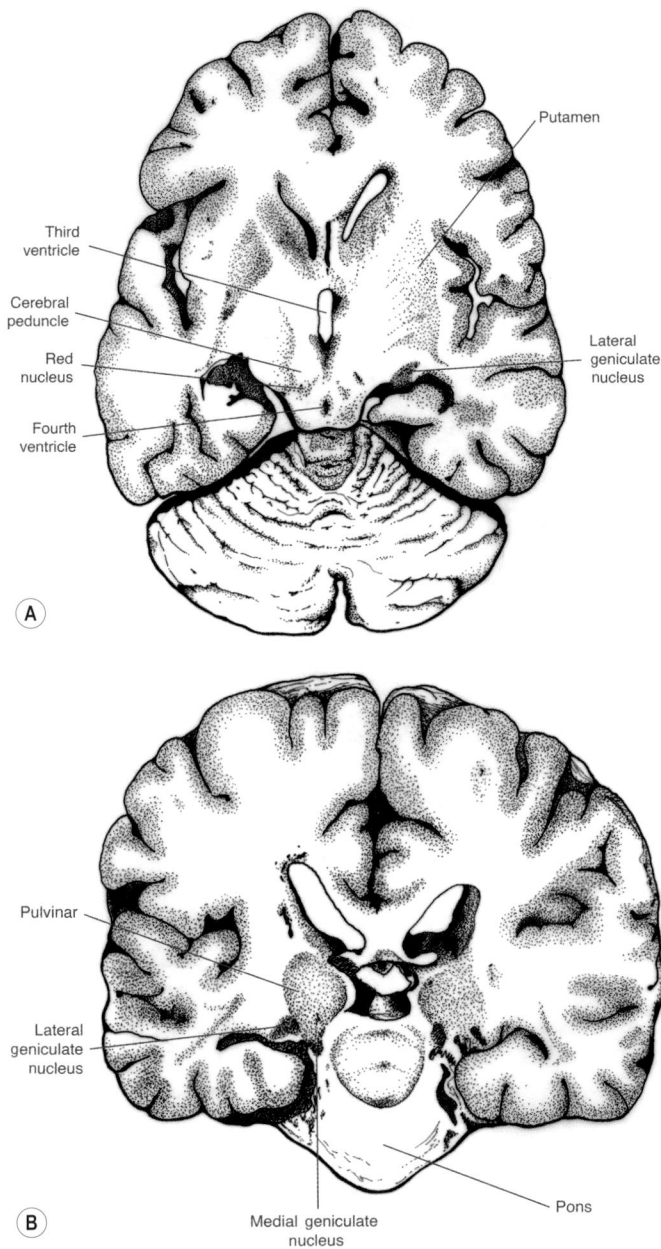

(A)

(B)

Figure 8–5. Location of lateral geniculate nucleus. **A.** Axial view at the level of the midbrain; **B.** coronal view through the pulvinar and basilar pons.

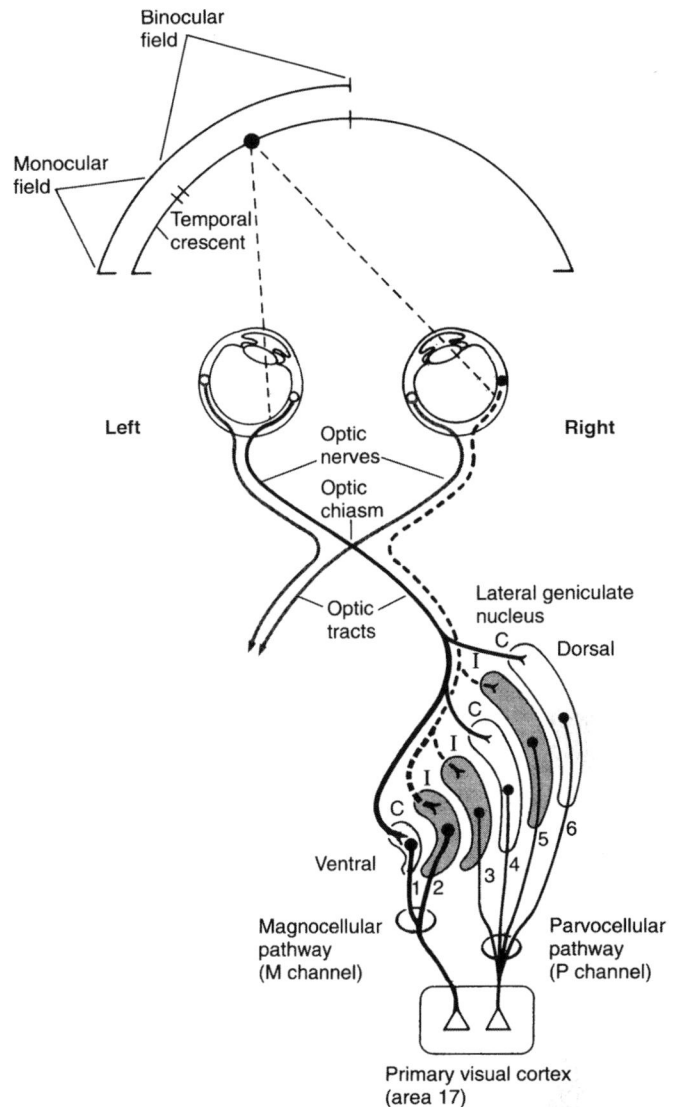

Figure 8–6. Inputs into and outputs from layers of lateral geniculate nucleus. Inputs from the right hemiretina of each eye project to different layers of the right lateral geniculate nucleus to create a complete representation of the left visual hemifield. Similarly, fibers from the left hemiretina of each eye project to the left lateral geniculate nucleus (not shown). Fibers subserving the temporal crescent of the left eye visual field project to the right (contralateral) lateral geniculate nucleus. There are no corresponding fibers coming from the right eye. Layers 1 and 2 comprise the magnocellular layers; layers 4–6 comprise the parvocellular layers. All of these project to area 17, the primary visual cortex (borrowed with permission from Mason C, Kandel ER. Central visual pathways, p. 425, Appleton & Lange, Norwalk, 1991).

Two patterns of field loss, although rare, are highly suggestive of LGN involvement and relate to its blood supply pattern and retinotopic organization:[26]

1. A *horizontal homonymous sectoranopia* is the hallmark of posterior choroidal artery territory infarction (**Fig. 8–8**).[24] The field defect, which characteristically points inward towards and involves fixation, results from involvement of the central hilum of the LGN.[27] Several authors, however, have cautioned that horizontal homonymous sectoranopias are nonspecific, and similar visual field abnormalities may result from lesions in the optic radiations[28,29] or occipital cortex.[30]

2. Also uncommon, but highly localizable is the "mirror image" field defect: an *upper and lower* homonymous

sectoranopia (**Fig. 8–9**). Sometimes, this field defect is referred to as a "quadruple sectoranopia."[31] This pattern of field loss results from anterior choroidal artery infarction, affecting the medial and lateral horns of the LGN.[32]

Other neuro-ophthalmic signs. Like optic tract lesions, acuity should be normal in processes involving only the LGN, and hemianopic patterns of optic atrophy may be evident.[32,33] However, because ganglion cell axons subserving the pupillary light reflex leave the anterior visual pathway prior to the LGN (see **Fig. 13–2**), lesions of the LGN only should have no influence on pupillary reactivity or size and should not cause a relative afferent pupillary defect.

Other signs and symptoms. Thalamic involvement due to posterior choroidal artery territory infarction may lead to contralateral sensory loss and language and memory disturbances.[24] Anterior choroidal artery infarction is typically also associated with hemiparesis and hemisensory loss ipsilateral to the hemianopia, and these symptoms are likely due to

involvement of the motor and sensory pathways in the posterior limb of the internal capsule.[34,35]

Etiology

Small-vessel occlusion in the territories of the anterior and posterior choroidal arteries may cause LGN-related field disturbances (**Fig. 8–10**).[36] Recognizing these visual field defects not only suggests the etiology of the lesion, but also predicts the circulation involved. Vascular accidents in these distributions have also been reported following intentional and inadvertent neurosurgical ligation.[32,34] In addition, LGN damage due to trauma[37,38] and bilateral quadruple sectoranopias from bilateral LGN involvement in central myelinolysis[39,40] have been described.

Optic radiations

Postsynaptic fibers from the LGN form the optic radiations, which are destined for the calcarine cortex.

Neuroanatomy

The optic radiations (geniculocalcarine fibers) exit dorsally from the LGN, then spread into two major bundles (see **Fig. 3–1**). The group of fibers containing contralateral superior quadrant visual information (inferior fascicle) curves in an anteroinferior direction into the anterior pole of the temporal lobe, forming Meyer's loop.[41] Since the fibers dedicated to the macula do not extend anteriorly, they may be spared in anterior temporal lobe lesions that involve the optic radiations. The anterior fibers of Meyer's loop subserve the superior visual field just lateral to the vertical meridian,

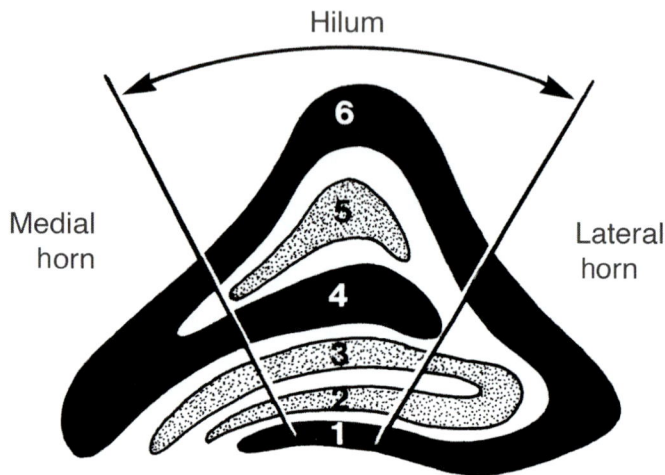

Figure 8–7. Coronal view of the lateral geniculate nucleus: layers, retinotopic organization, and vascular supply. Visual information from the ipsilateral eye synapses within laminae 2, 3, and 5, while that from the contralateral eye synapses within laminae 1, 4, and 6. Macular vision is subserved by the middle wedge (hilum), which is supplied by the posterior choroidal artery. The medial and lateral horns carry information from the inferior and superior quadrants, respectively, and are fed by anterior choroidal artery.

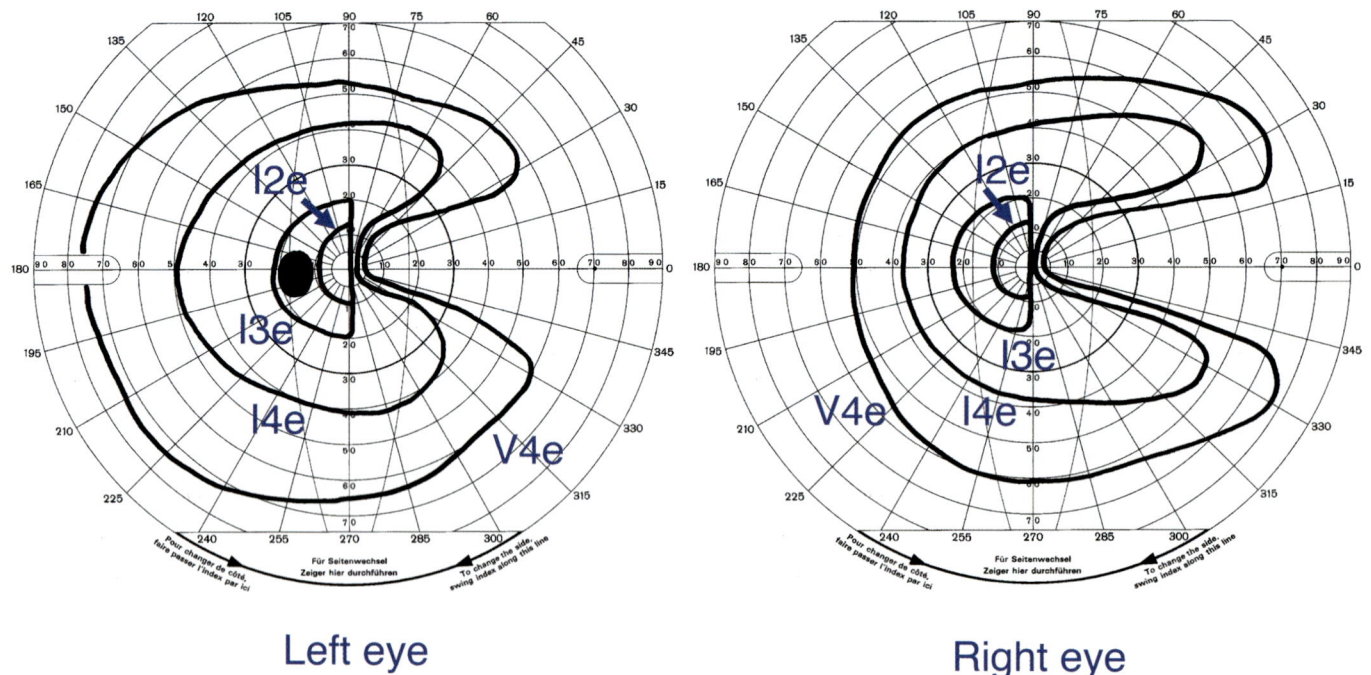

Left eye

Right eye

Figure 8–8. Wedge-shaped sectoranopia typical of left posterior choroidal infarction and involvement of the hilum of the left lateral geniculate nucleus. Goldmann visual field.

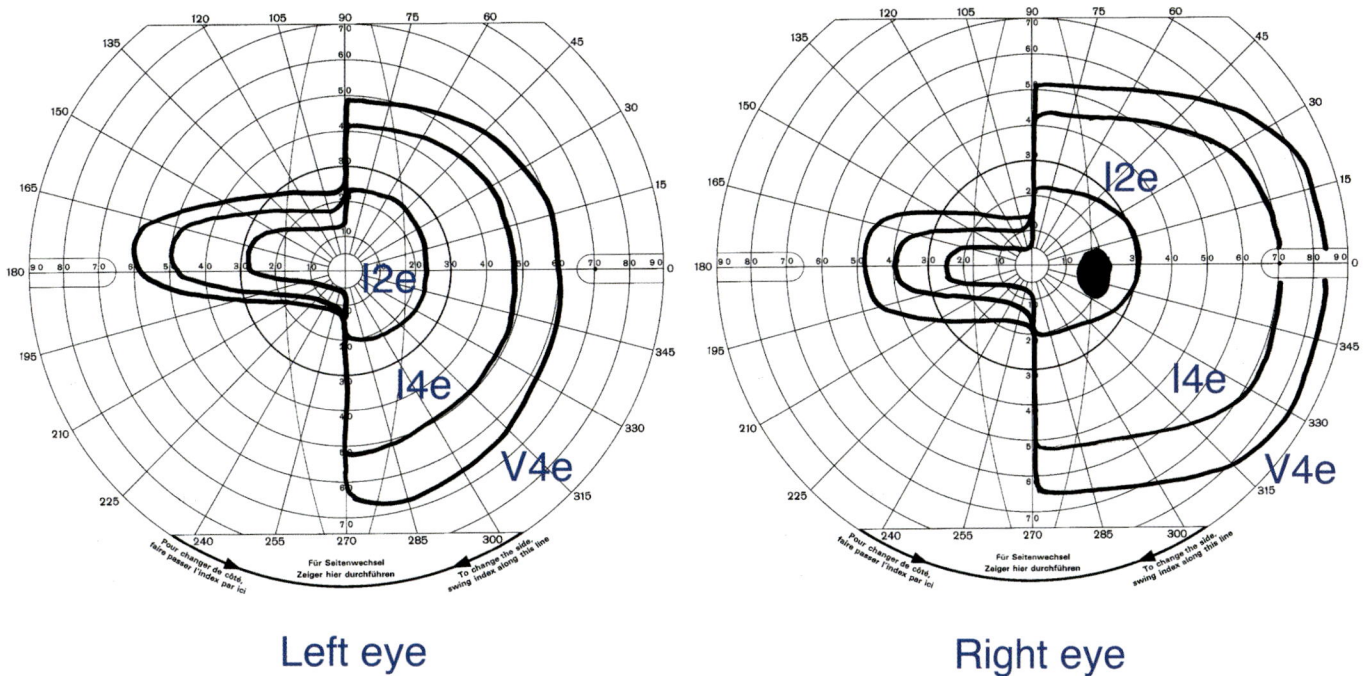

Left eye   Right eye

Figure 8–9. Upper and lower (quadruple) sectoranopia, characteristic of anterior choroidal infarction and involvement of the medial and lateral portions of the right lateral geniculate nucleus. Goldmann visual field.

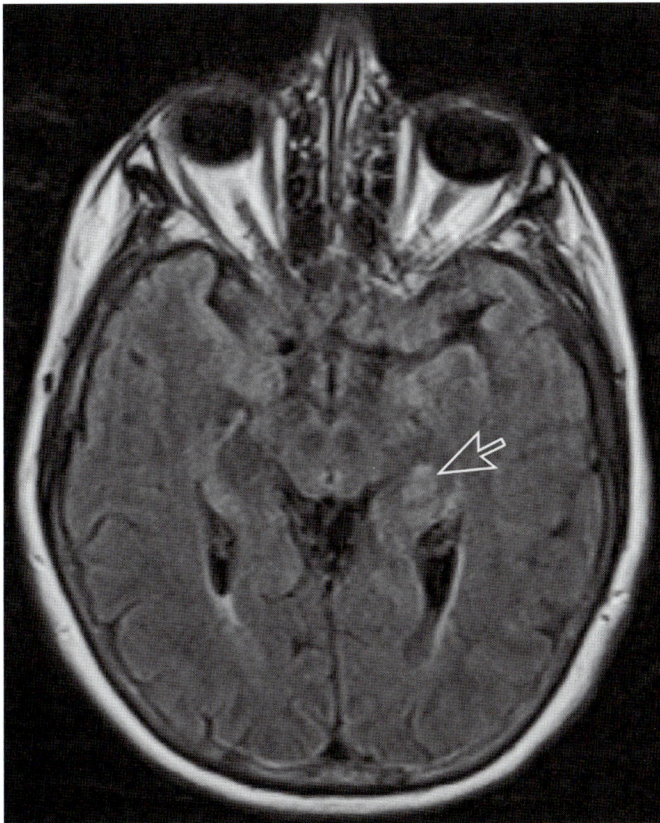

Figure 8–10. Axial fluid level attenuated inversion recovery (FLAIR) magnetic resonance imaging in a patient with an incongruous right homonymous hemianopia due to a left lateral geniculate infarction (arrow) in the left anterior choroidal artery distribution.

while the more posteriorly situated fibers carry visual field information just superior to the horizontal meridian.[42,43] The superior fascicle lies deep within the parietal lobe and subserves visual information from the contralateral inferior quadrant. The temporal and parietal fascicles project in a retinotopic fashion to the lower and upper banks of calcarine cortex, respectively.

The temporal portion of the optic radiations receives its blood supply from the anterior choroidal artery and other middle cerebral artery (MCA) branches within the sylvian fissure (**Fig. 8–11**), including the lenticulostriate and inferior temporo-occipital artery. The distal branches of the MCA, including the angular and posterior temporal arteries, supply the more superiorly situated parietal fascicles.[44] The most posterior portions of the optic radiations, just before their entry into the occipital lobe, are supplied by the superior temporo-occipital sylvian artery branch of the MCA, and the anterior temporal and calcarine arteries of the posterior cerebral artery (PCA).[10,25]

Symptoms and signs

Visual field defects. An isolated lesion of Meyer's loop will typically lead to an incongruous contralateral homonymous hemianopia denser superiorly ("pie in the sky defect") (**Fig. 8–12**).[42,43,45] In contrast, lesions of the parietal lobe characteristically will lead to incongruous defects more prominent inferiorly (**Fig. 8–13**), and rarely quadrantanopias respecting the horizontal meridian can be seen.[46,47] In clinical practice, there is significant variation in these findings, especially with regards to congruity. Complete interruption of the optic radiations will cause a dense homonymous

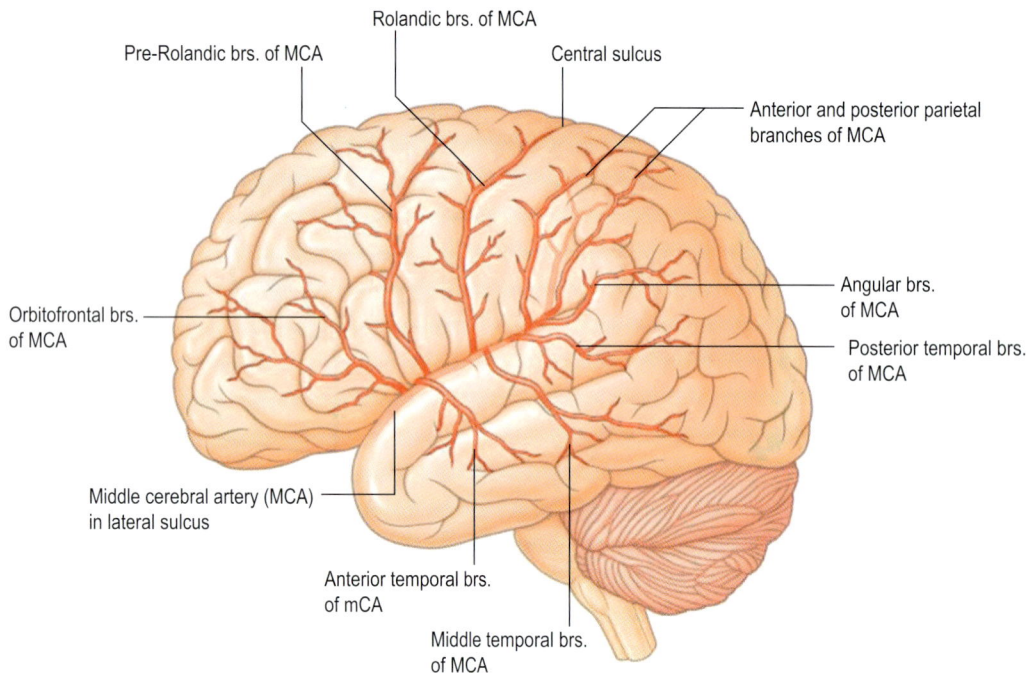

Figure 8–11. Branches of the middle cerebral artery (MCA). Lateral view of the left cerebral hemisphere showing the location and general branching pattern of the middle cerebral artery. The middle cerebral artery branches in the depths of the lateral sulcus.

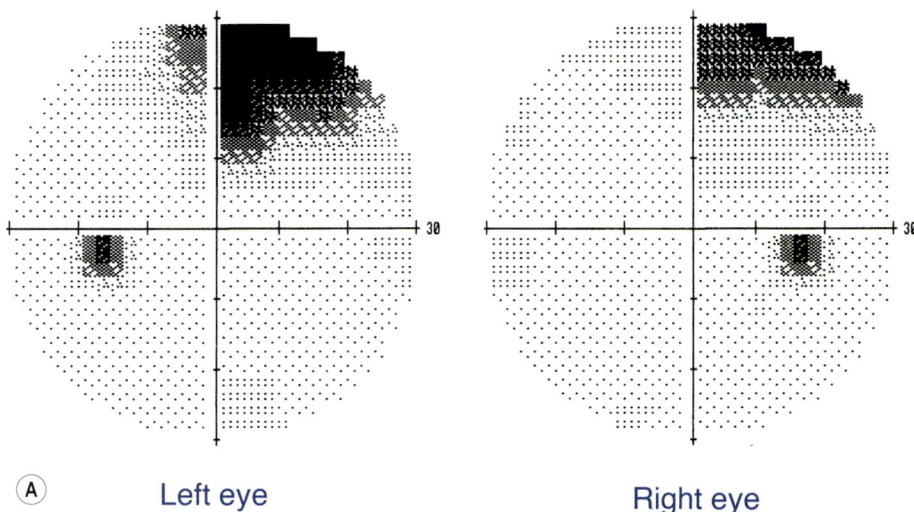

(A) Left eye   Right eye

Figure 8–12. A. Upper right visual field ("pie in the sky") defect (computerized perimetry grayscale output) following

hemianopia (**Fig. 8–14**). Bilateral lesions of the optic radiations will cause *cerebral blindness.*

Other neuro-ophthalmic signs. Visual acuity is spared in unilateral lesions, but can be impaired if bilateral lesions are present. Pupillary responses are normal in disturbances limited to the optic radiations. The optic discs are also normal unless the lesion is large enough to cause mass effect or obstruction of the ventricular system and lead to papilledema. In addition, optic radiation lesions which developed in utero or were acquired within the first week of life may be associated with optic atrophy as a result of transsynaptic degeneration.

A homonymous hemianopia or quadrantanopia due to deep parietal lobe lesions may be associated with a defective optokinetic response when the targets are drawn towards the side of the lesion (see Chapter 17, Nystagmus). Similarly, slow pursuit will be defective in the direction ipsilateral to the lesion (see Chapter 16, Gaze disorders). The combination of the hemianopia, defective optokinetic response, and poor tracking result from co-involvement of the optic radiations and adjacent descending corticobulbar fibers from the parieto-occipitotemporal pursuit area. In contrast, normal optokinetic responses would be expected in a hemianopia due to a lesion solely within the occipital lobe. Patients with a hemianopia or neglect may also have a gaze preference away from the visual deficit.

During attempted eye closure, normally each eye has an upward and outward trajectory (Bell's phenomenon). However, in the majority of hemispheric lesions, both eyes will deviate up and away from the side of the lesion. This

Video 9.1

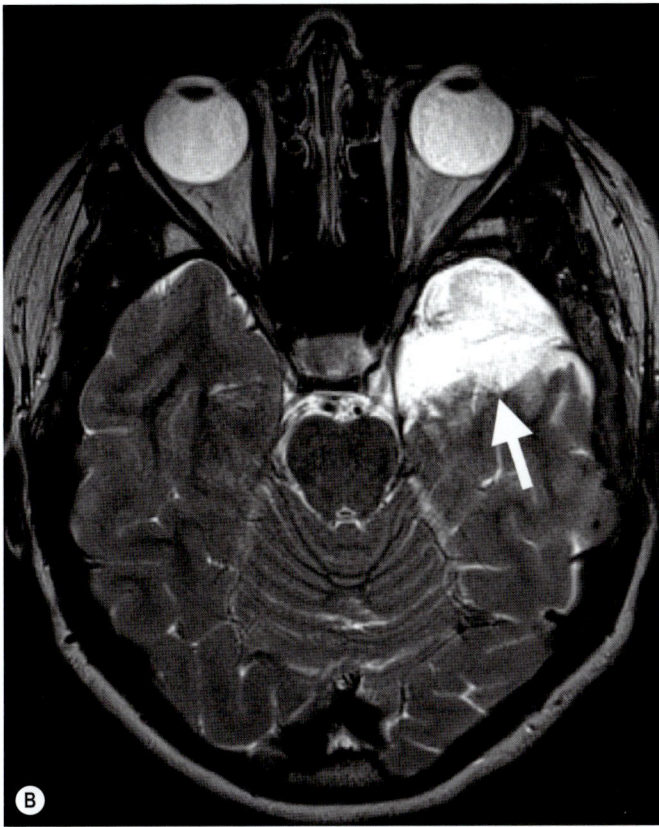

Figure 8–12. cont'd (**B**) resection (arrow) of a left temporal lobe ganglioglioma; T2-weighted axial MRI.

phenomena, known as *Cogan's spasticity of conjugate gaze*,[48,49] has been attributed to an increased tone in contralateral gaze deviation or a decreased ability to suppress attention to the contralateral hemispace.[50] Overall, we find this sign to be relatively unreliable since such lateral gaze deviations with eye closure may be seen with normal patients. Furthermore, patients with established parietal optic radiation lesions may have a normal Bell's phenomenon.

Other cortical signs and symptoms. Hemianopias that result from lesions of the optic radiations are often associated with other "cortically based" neurologic findings. Temporal lobe lesions may be accompanied by personality changes, complex partial seizures, memory deficits, fluent aphasia (if the dominant side is involved), or Klüver–Bucy syndrome (hypersexuality, placidity, hyperorality, visual and auditory agnosia, and apathy) with involvement of the anterior temporal lobes bilaterally. A conduction aphasia, Gerstmann syndrome (finger agnosia, agraphia, acalculia, and right–left disorientation), and tactile agnosia, all suggest a dominant parietal lobe process. Left-sided neglect, topographic memory loss, constructional and dressing apraxias, in association with a left hemianopia suggest a nondominant, parietal lesion.

Other signs and symptoms. Hemispheric lesions may produce a homonymous field defect and ipsilateral hemiparesis and hyperreflexia when the optic radiations and motor strip or descending motor fibers are disrupted. A homonymous field defect in combination with ipsilateral sensory loss, astereognosis, decreased two-point discrimination, or graphesthesia suggests a parietal lesion. A process

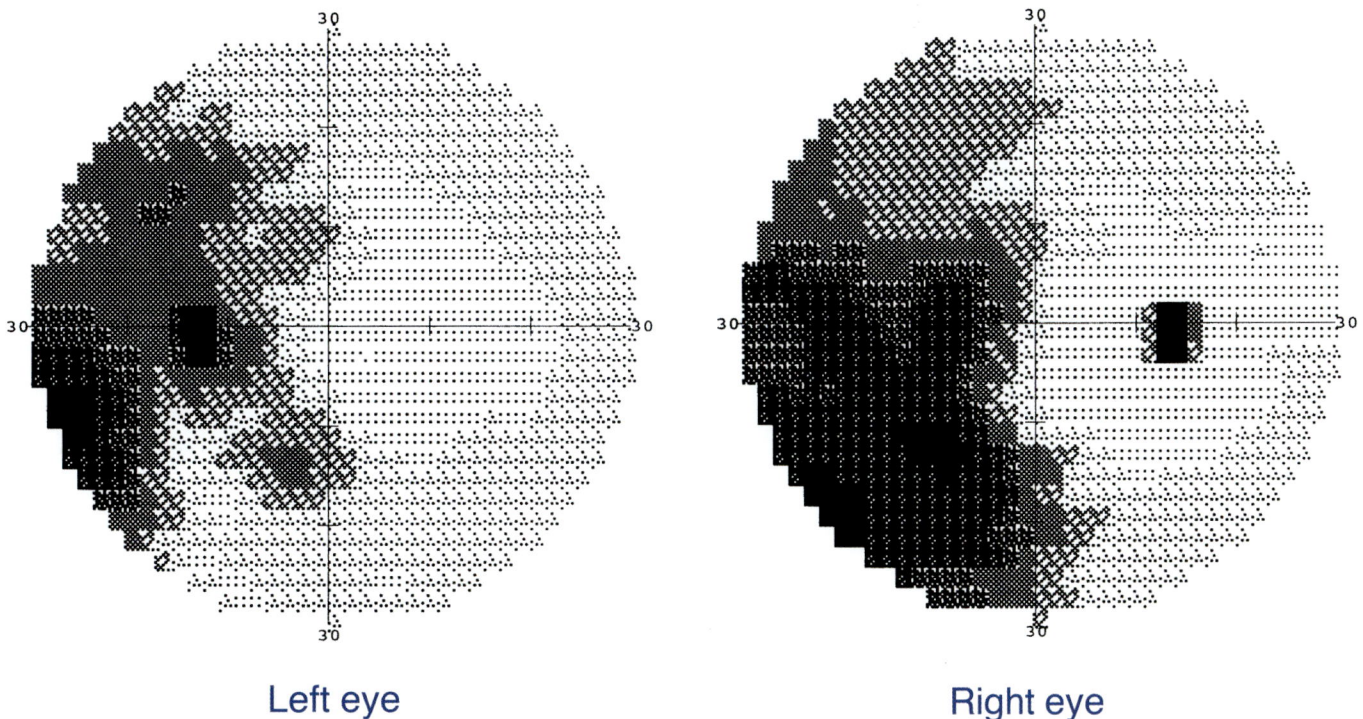

Left eye   Right eye

Figure 8–13. Incomplete left homonymous hemianopia, densest inferiorly, due to traumatic brain injury affecting primarily the right parietal lobe. Computerized perimetry grayscale output. The patient also had a left hemiparesis and defective optokinetic response when the targets were drawn to his right.

Left eye   Right eye

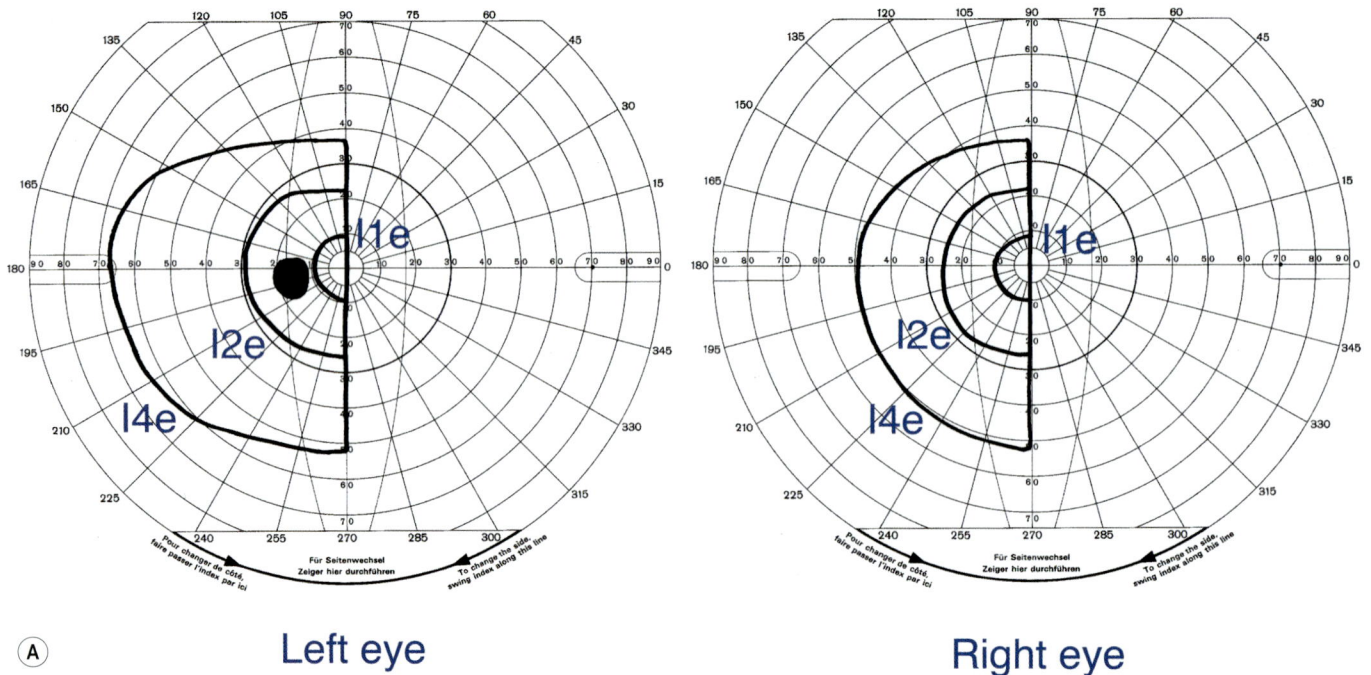

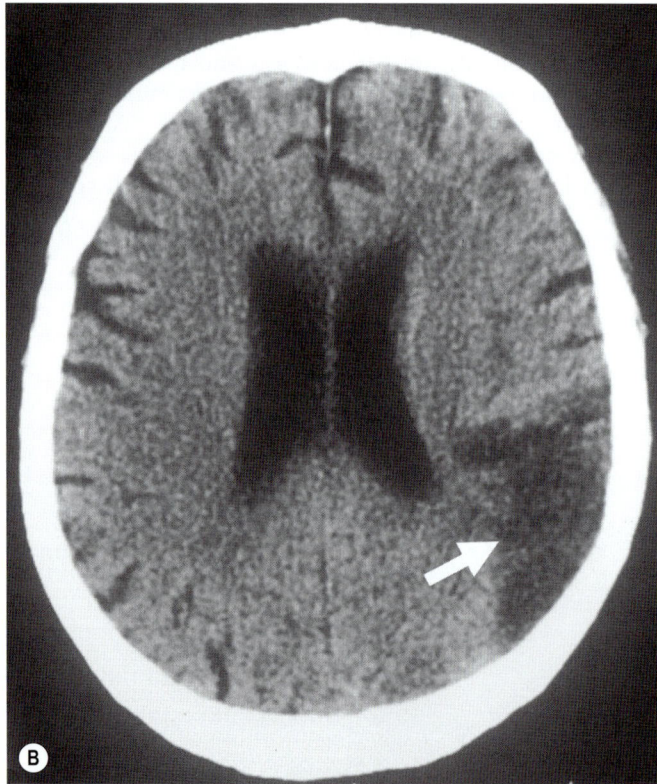

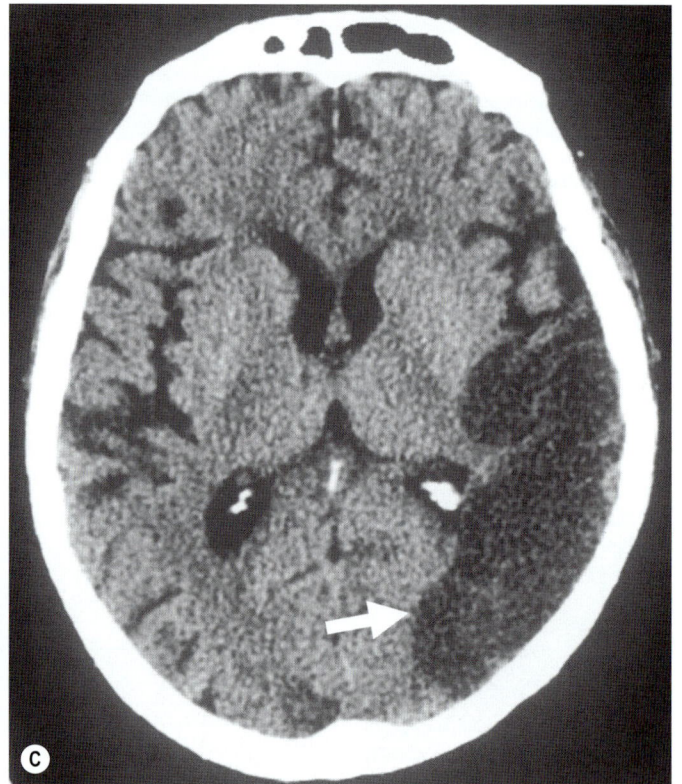

Figure 8–14. A. Complete, macular splitting right homonymous hemianopia (computerized perimetry grayscale output) due to large left middle cerebral artery infarction depicted in the axial CT scans in (**B**) and (**C**). **B** demonstrates the hypodense area (arrow) in the left parietal region, while (**C**), a more ventral slice, depicts the hypodense infarction (arrow) in the left temporal lobe. The patient was also aphasic.

within the nondominant (usually right) parietal lobe can also produce a contralateral neglect syndrome or hemianopia, accompanied by contralateral sensory inattention. Pain, hemianesthesia, or choreoathetoid movements and an ipsilateral homonymous field deficit imply co-involvement of the thalamus and optic radiations.

Etiology

Strokes in the MCA distribution (**Fig. 8–14**) and neoplasms are the most common causes of optic radiation hemianopias in adults (**Table 8–1**). Hemorrhages, trauma, infections, and degenerative diseases are also seen but are less common.

An occlusion of the proximal MCA would cause a contralateral hemianopia, a contralateral hemiparesis due to disturbance of the motor cortex or descending corticospinal tracts, and sensory loss resulting from involvement of the postcentral gyrus or ascending fibers from the thalamus. Aphasia or neglect may be observed in MCA occlusion, depending on whether the stroke affects the dominant or nondominant hemisphere, respectively. Anterior division MCA strokes can be recognized by the predominantly motor findings and nonfluent (Broca's) aphasia, while posterior division MCA strokes have more salient sensory and fluent (Wernicke's) language deficits. MCA strokes associated with hemianopias are either frontoparietal, parietal, or parietotemporal.

Isolated temporal lobe-related field loss is less common. Causes include neoplasms, particularly glial cell tumors, herpes encephalitis, and anterior temporal lobe resection for recalcitrant seizures due to mesial temporal sclerosis.[42,43,51,52]

The diagnosis and management of cerebrovascular disease, tumors, and other processes which affect the parietal and temporal lobes are discussed in more detail in the section following occipital lobe-related field loss, since there is considerable overlap.

Occipital lobe/striate cortex

Brodmann area 17 (or V1, primary, calcarine, or striate cortex) is the end organ of the afferent visual system and is situated in the occipital lobe on both sides of the brain.

Neuroanatomy

The upper bank of striate cortex lies superior to the calcarine fissure, and the lower bank below the fissure (see **Fig. 3–1** and **Fig. 8–15**). Other boundaries of striate cortex include the splenium of the corpus callosum anteriorly, the interhemispheric fissure medially, and the occipital pole posteriorly. Laterally, some striate cortex may be visible on the posterolateral outer surface of the occipital lobes.

Neuronal input arrives in a retinotopic fashion from fibers of the LGN and synapses within striate cortex, which is divided into six layers. Entry is primarily into the thick, light-colored layer 4, which is visible to the naked eye and has been termed the stria of Gennari.[53] Fibers from the medial aspect of the LGN, carrying information from superior retina, project to the upper bank of the calcarine cortex, while those from the lateral aspect, carrying information from the inferior retina, project to the lower bank. The inferior visual fields are thus represented within the upper bank, and the superior visual fields within the lower bank. Left and right visual fields are represented within right and left occipital lobes, respectively.

Macular projections from the central 10 degrees of vision synapse in the occipital pole and occupy 55–60% of the entire surface area of striate cortex.[54–57] The occipital tip is devoted to foveal vision. The anterior striate cortex, comprising approximately 8–10% of striate cortex,[58] is monocularly innervated[59] and subserves the temporal 30 degrees of the visual field of the contralateral eye (**Fig. 8–16**). The representation of the horizontal meridian of the visual field lies deep within the calcarine fissure at the calcarine bank while that of the vertical meridian lies along the calcarine lips (**Fig. 8–17**).[60]

The majority of the blood supply to striate cortex derives from branches of the PCA (**Fig. 8–18**): the calcarine artery, mostly, with lesser contributions from the posterior temporal and parieto-occipital arteries.[61] In most cases, small penetrating branches from the calcarine artery supply both the upper and lower banks of calcarine cortex. In up to one-third of cases, one major branch to each bank may be seen. At the occipital pole, there is an anastomosis between PCA vessels and the superior temporo-occipital sylvian artery from the MCA. This dual blood supply to the area responsible for central vision is one vascular explanation for macular sparing in the setting of PCA occlusion.

The PCAs are normally considered part of the posterior circulation of the brain, as usually both PCAs arise from the distal bifurcation of the basilar artery (**Fig. 8–1**). In some anomalous cases, however, a PCA may derive its blood supply from the anterior portion of the circle of Willis. These variations include (1) a persistent trigeminal artery,[62] and (2) persistence of the fetal origin of the PCA from the internal carotid artery.[63,64]

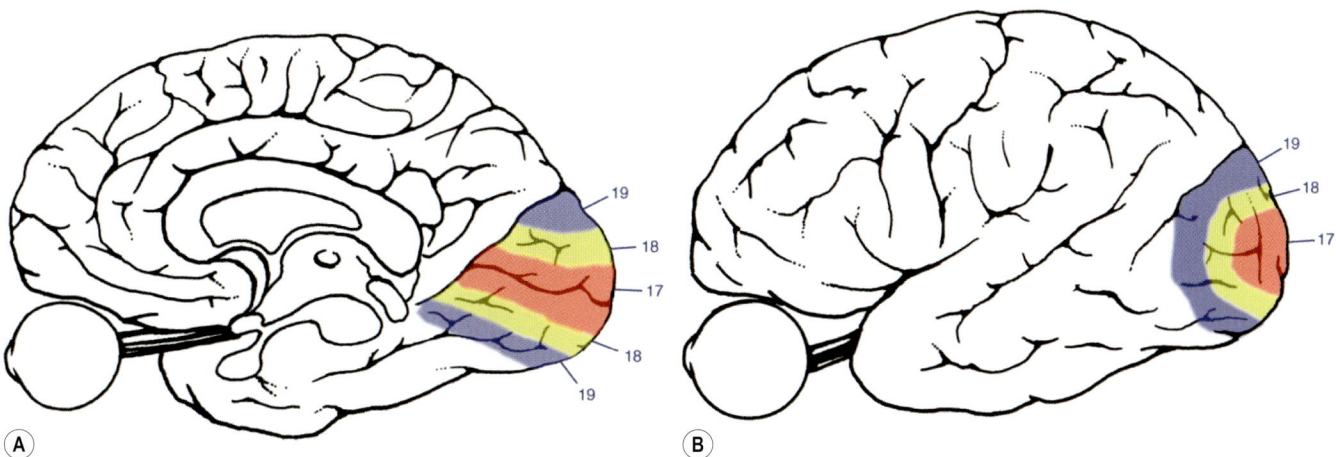

Figure 8–15. A. Medial and **B** lateral views of the occipital lobe in relationship to the rest of the brain. Areas 17, 18, and 19 are highlighted.

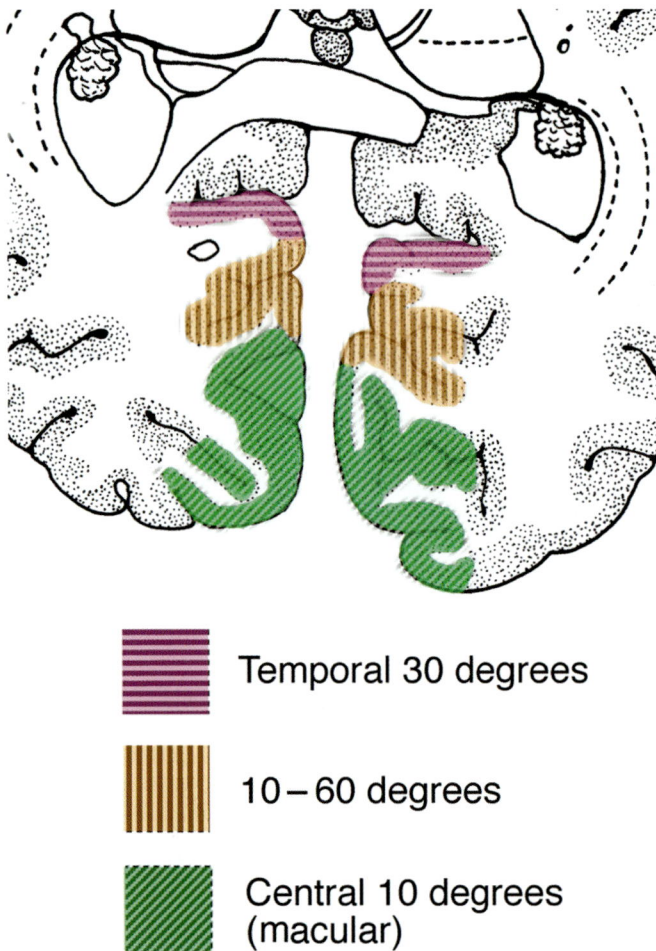

Temporal 30 degrees

10 – 60 degrees

Central 10 degrees (macular)

Figure 8–16. Retinotopic organization of the striate cortex (axial section at the level of the calcarine fissures, viewed inferiorly; the lower bank of the occipital lobe is cut away). Approximately 55–60% of the surface area of striate cortex, located posteriorly, is responsible for the central 10 degrees of vision. The anterior striate cortex subserves the temporal 30 degrees of the visual field of the contralateral eye.

Symptoms and signs

Visual field defects. Unilateral occipital lobe lesions may cause a contralateral congruous homonymous hemianopia respecting the vertical meridian. The following visual field features, when present, are specific to occipital lobe disturbances. These features are often more easily identified with Goldmann or tangent screen perimetry than with automated perimetry.[65]

1. *Macular sparing.* Posterior cerebral artery infarction may produce a hemianopia with macular sparing (**Fig. 8–19**) (as opposed to macular splitting), and this feature is characteristic of but not specific to occipital lobe-related hemianopias.[4] Proposed mechanisms include the dual vascular supply of the occipital poles, bilateral representation of the maculae, and test artifact due to poor central fixation by the patient.[66,67] However, a clinicoradiologic study[68] provided evidence for unilateral macular representation. In addition, a study using a scanning laser ophthalmoscope to stimulate the retina directly confirmed macular sparing in occipital lobe-related hemianopias.[69]

2. *Homonymous hemianopic central scotomas* are also a telltale sign of a unilateral occipital lobe tip disturbance (**Fig. 8–20**). In rare occasions these scotomas are paracentral.[70]

3. *Sparing or involvement of the temporal crescent.* If an occipital lobe lesion does not involve the anterior striate cortex, the temporal 30 degrees of the visual field of the contralateral eye may be spared (**Fig. 8–21**).[71,72] On the other hand, lesions restricted to the anterior striate cortex may selectively affect the temporal 30 degrees of vision of the contralateral eye.[73,74]

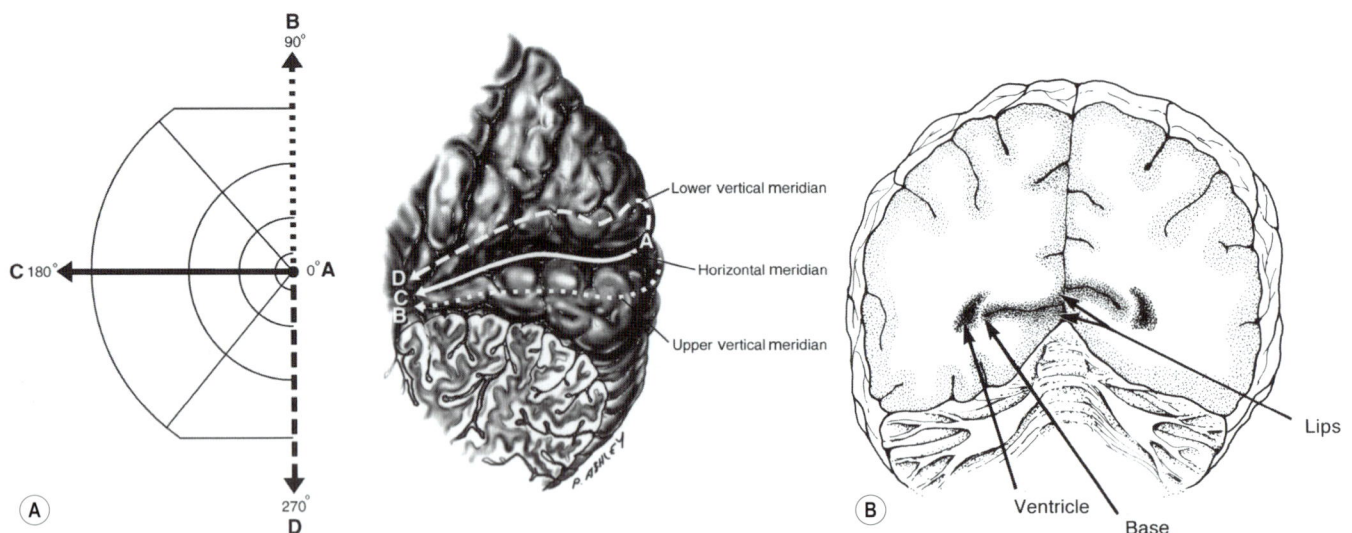

Figure 8–17. Occipital lobe representation of the vertical horizontal meridians. **A**. The left visual hemifield is demonstrated with the corresponding right calcarine fissure opened to reveal the fissure base and calcarine banks. The vertical hemianopic meridian is represented along the borders of the calcarine lips. The lower vertical meridian of the visual field, line AD, is represented along the perimeter of upper striate cortex, i.e., the margin of the upper calcarine lip. The upper vertical meridian of the visual field, line AB, is similarly represented along the border of the lower calcarine lip. The horizontal meridian of the visual field, line AC, follows the contour of the base of the calcarine fissure. **B**. This coronal section through the occipital region shows the relationship of the calcarine lips to the base of the calcarine sulcus that flanks the medial wall of the posterior ventricular horn. (Reprinted with permission from Gray LG, Galetta SL, Schatz NJ. Neurology 1998;50:1170–1173).

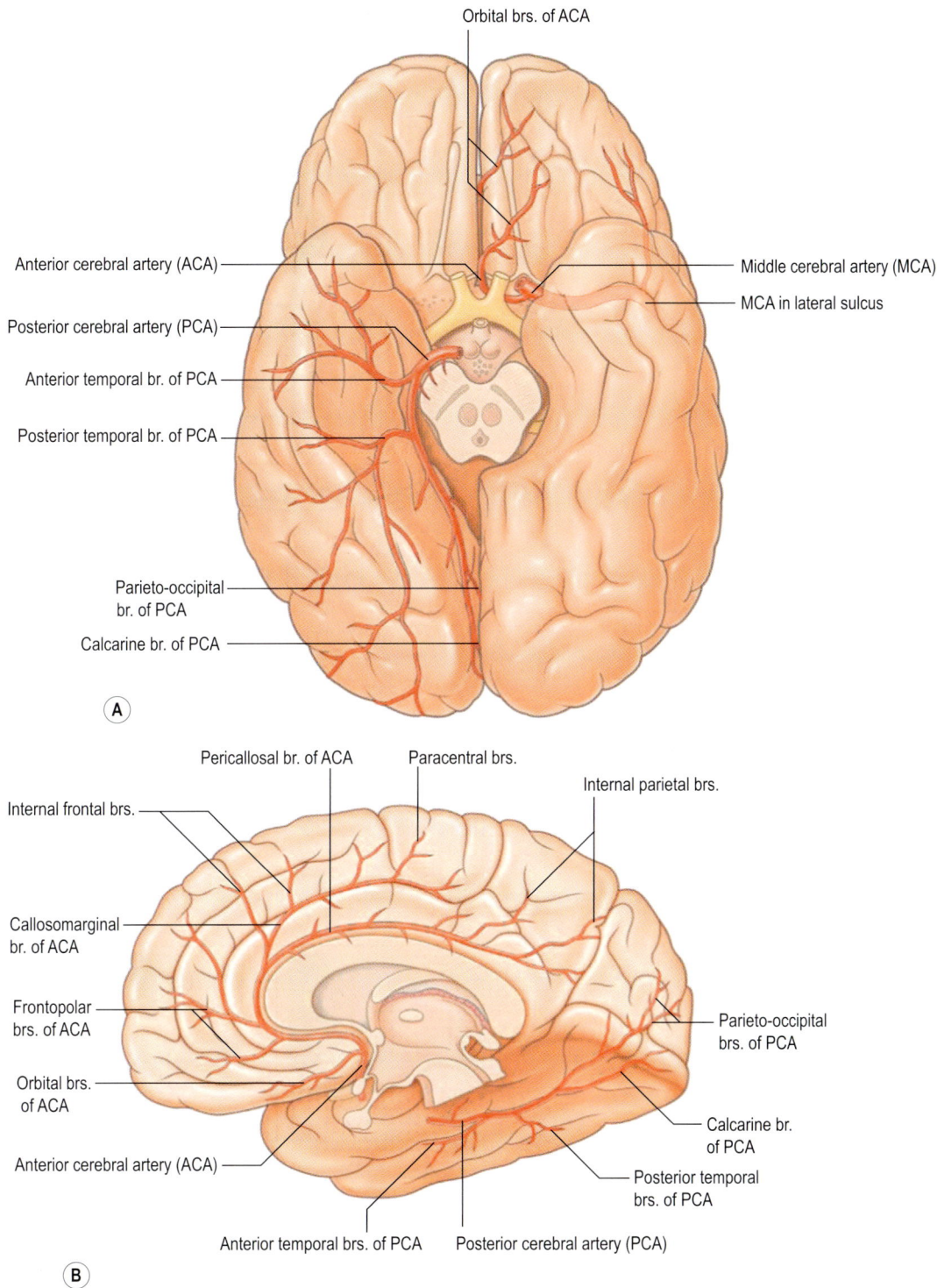

Figure 8–18. Posterior cerebral artery. **A**. Ventral view of the cerebral hemispheres with brain stem removed showing the branching pattern of the posterior cerebral artery (PCA) and some branches of the anterior (ACA) and middle cerebral arteries (MCA). **B**. Mid-sagittal view of the cerebral hemisphere showing the locations and branching patterns of the ACA and PCA.

Bilateral PCA infarction may lead to bilateral macular sparing hemianopias, with a "keyhole" residual visual field (**Fig. 8–22**). Patients are left with vision in the central 5–10 degrees. The preserved tunnel is often asymmetric with a vertical step off that helps to distinguish this field defect from ocular causes of field constriction.

Restricted lesions of the upper or lower banks of the calcarine cortex may cause quadrantic field defects (**Fig. 8–23**).[47]

It has been suggested that occipital lobe quadrantanopias with strict horizontal meridian sparing are more likely the result of an extrastriate lesion involving V2 (area 18) and V3 (area 19) (see **Fig. 8–15** and Chapter 9).[75] However, either a striate or extrastriate lesion can be responsible.[76] Crossed quadrantanopias may result from a lesion of one lower bank and the contralateral upper bank. This has been called the checkerboard visual field.[77]

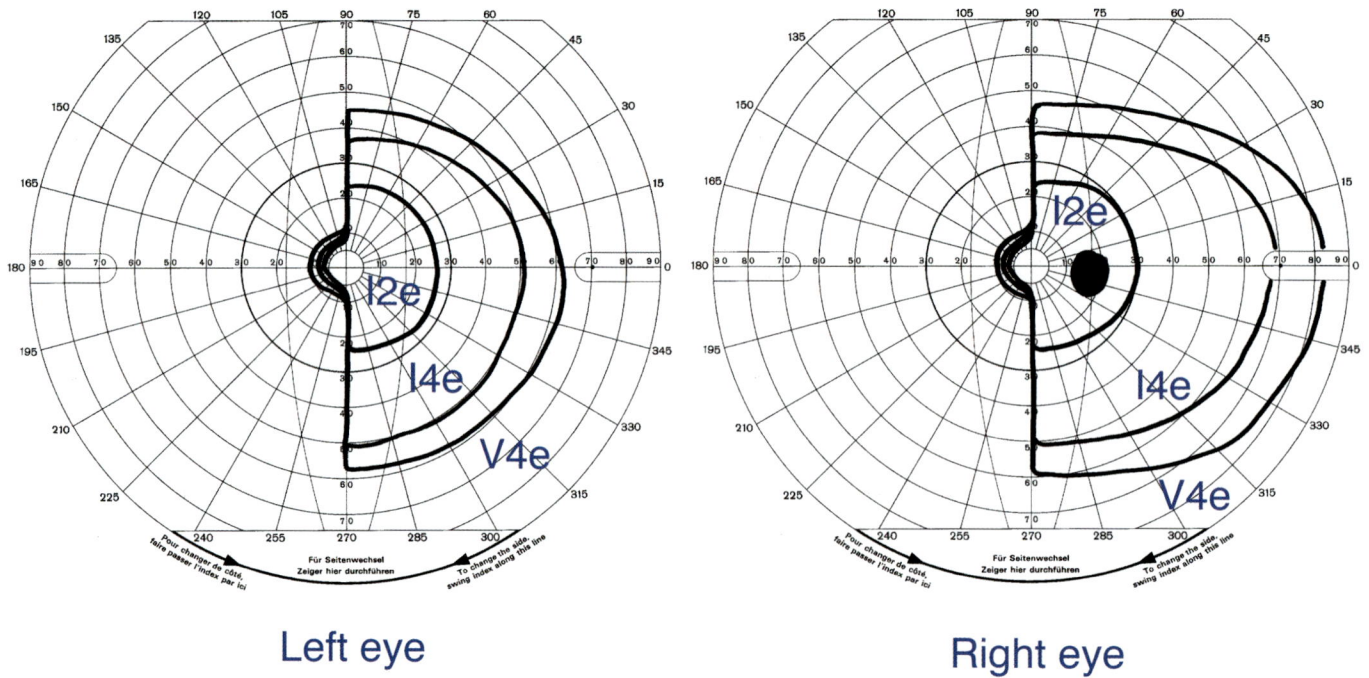

Left eye

Right eye

Figure 8–19. Macular sparing left homonymous hemianopia due to a right posterior cerebral artery stroke. Goldmann visual field.

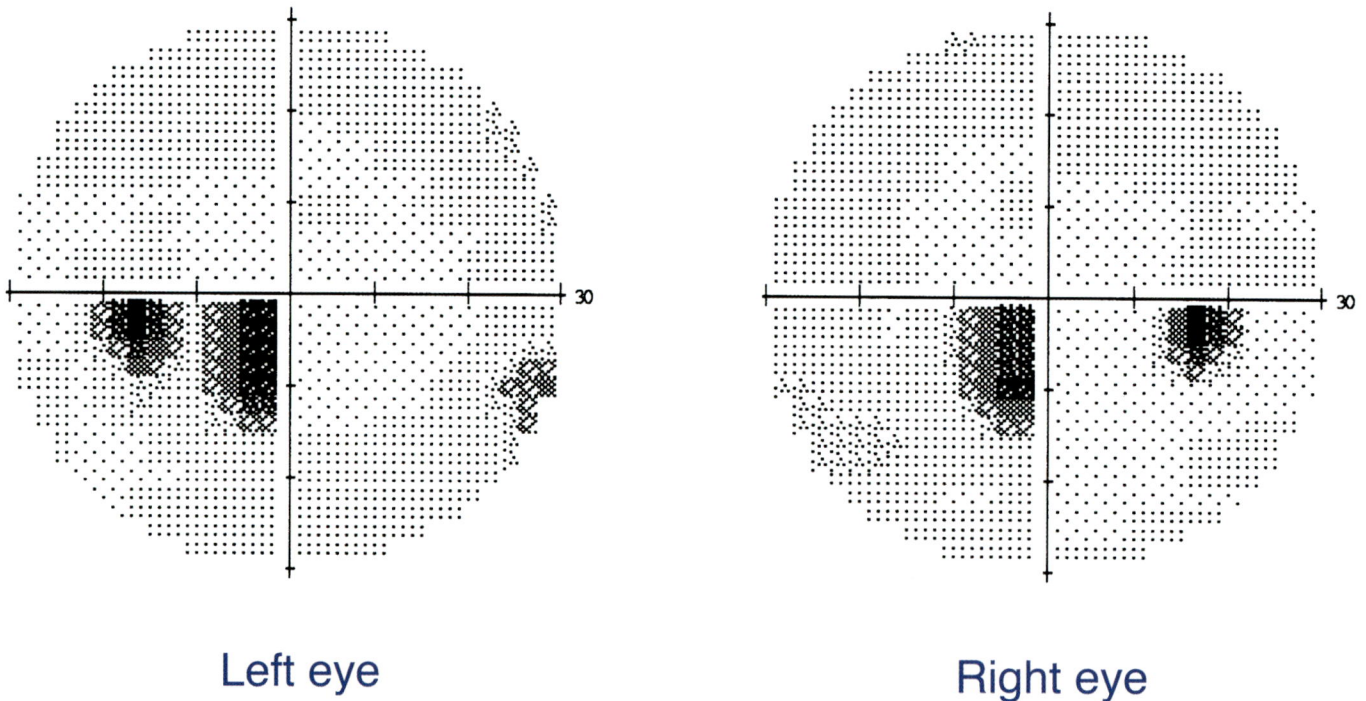

Left eye

Right eye

Figure 8–20. Left homonymous inferior quadrantic central scotomas due to a neoplasm of the right occipital tip. Goldmann visual field.

Bilateral upper or lower bank disturbances produce altitudinal hemianopias respecting the horizontal meridian (**Fig. 8–24**).[78] This pattern may be mistaken for similar visual field deficits caused by bilateral optic neuropathies. The vertical meridian can be spared if the calcarine lips are not involved, while horizontal meridian sparing may be seen if the base of the calcarine banks deep within the calcarine fissure is uninvolved.[60]

Cerebral blindness. This condition, characterized by blindness, absent blink to threat[79] and optokinetic responses, normal pupillary reactivity, and normal fundi, results from bilateral retrogeniculate dysfunction. When lesions to both occipital lobes are responsible, as opposed to bilateral involvement of the optic radiations, the term cortical blindness may be applied (**Fig. 8–25**). Clinically, patients with cerebral blindness can be distinguished from those with

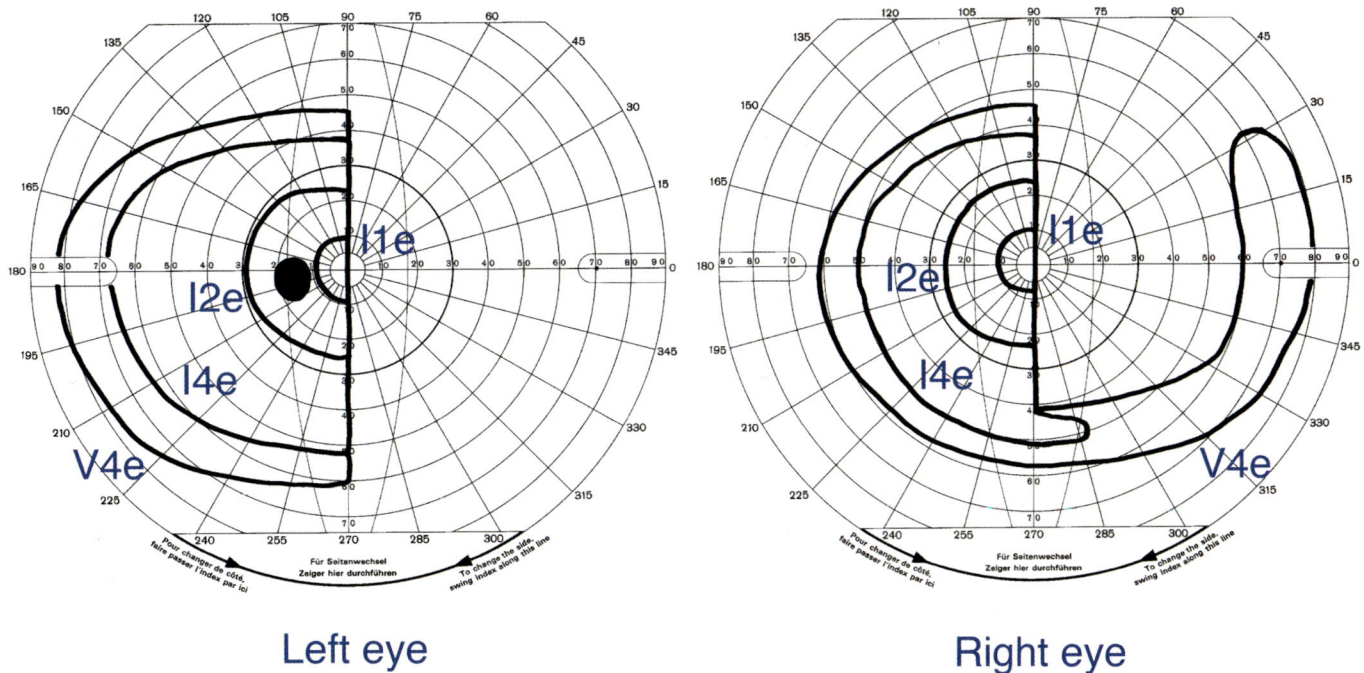

Left eye　　　　　　　　　Right eye

Figure 8–21. Right homonymous hemianopia with sparing of the temporal crescent in the right eye. This resulted from a left posterior cerebral artery infarction which spared the anterior striate cortex on that side. Goldmann visual field.

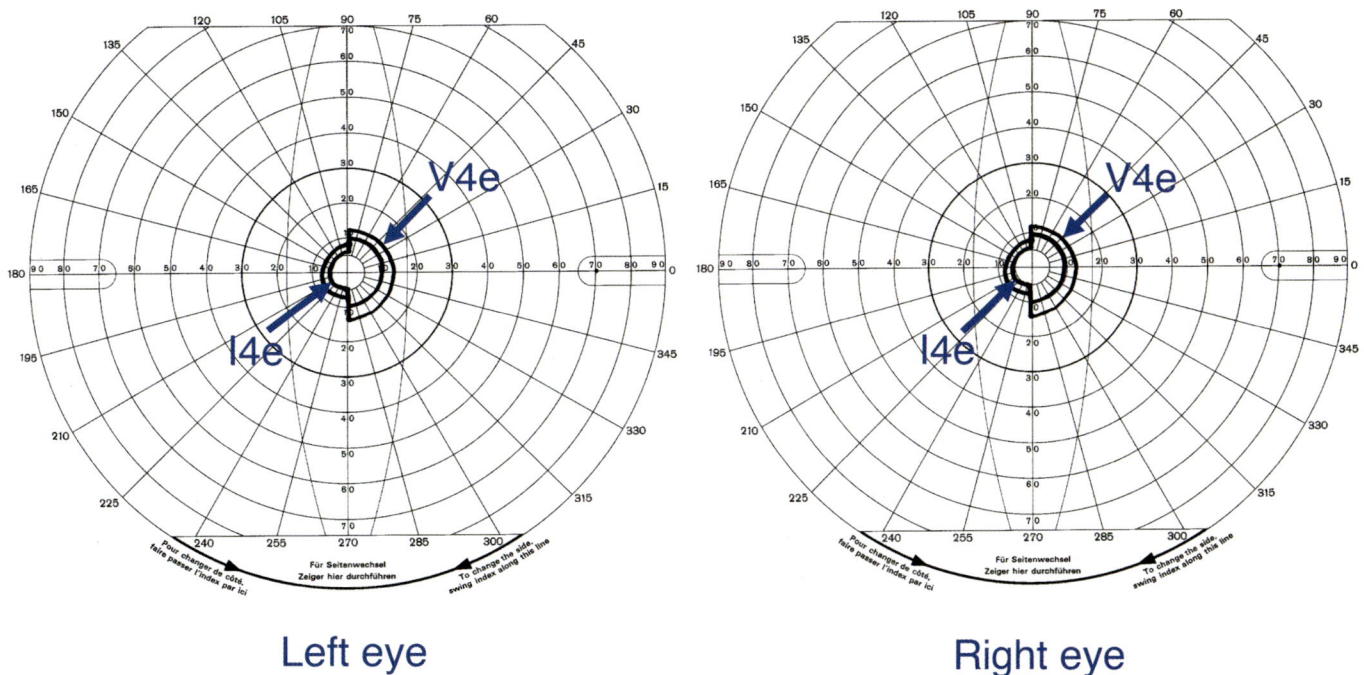

Left eye　　　　　　　　　Right eye

Figure 8–22. "Keyhole"-shaped spared central vision due to bilateral posterior cerebral artery infarctions. Sparing of central vision is greater in the right visual field than the left, and the demarcation (step off) between the two respects the vertical meridian. Goldmann visual field.

pregeniculate lesions by the presence of intact pupillary light responses. Cerebral blind patients may confabulate visual perceptions or deny their blindness (*Anton's syndrome*). Some of these patients have additional, contributory frontal or temporal lobe lesions that alter recognition, memory, and behavior.

The Riddoch phenomenon and blindsight. Riddoch[80] and Holmes[81] observed that individuals recovering from occipital lobe injuries first perceive moving objects but not stationary ones. The Riddoch phenomenon can be observed during confrontation field testing by comparing the patient's responses to moving and still targets. More recently it has been shown that rare patients with uni- or bilateral occipital lesions lose object recognition but in some instances may have "blindsight," an unconscious ability to locate light sources and detect moving targets in affected fields.[82–90] Some

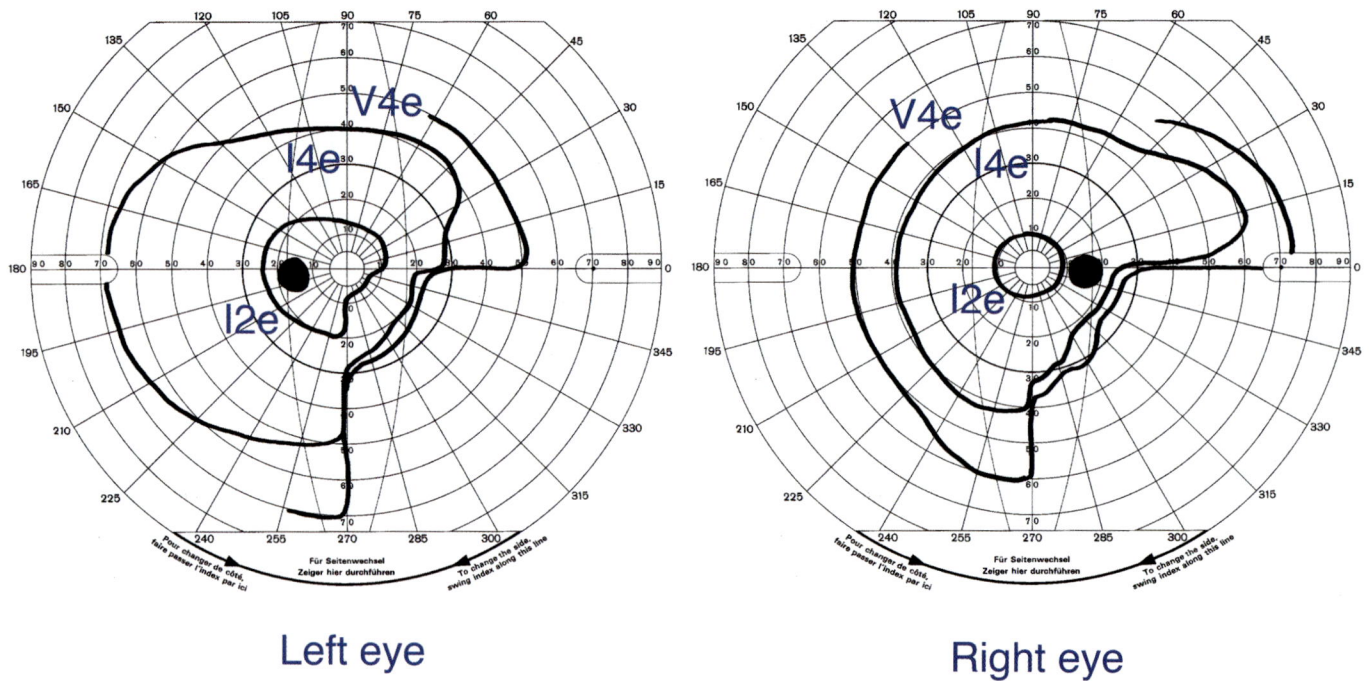

Left eye   Right eye

Figure 8–23. Right homonymous inferior quadrantanopia from left upper bank infarction of the occipital lobe. Note there is a suggestion of macular sparing. Goldmann visual field.

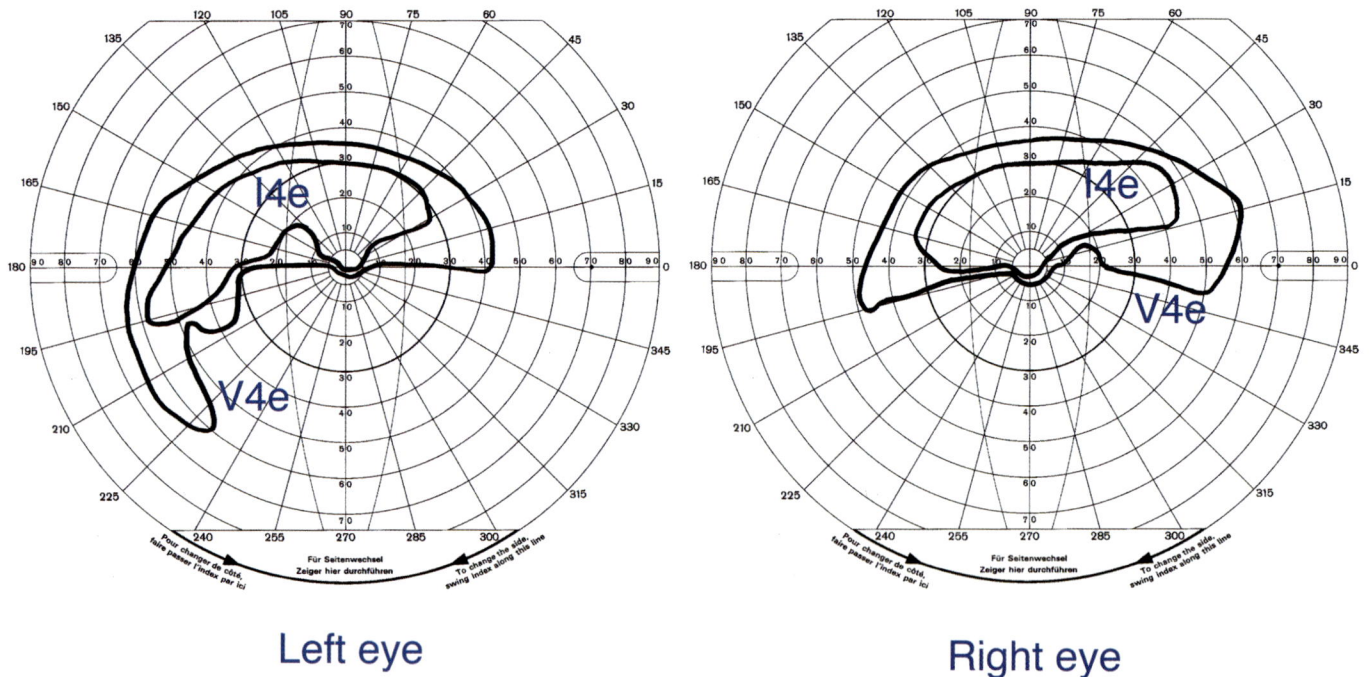

Left eye   Right eye

Figure 8–24. Bilateral inferior altitudinal hemianopia from bilateral parietal-occipital hemorrhages. The patient also had Balint's syndrome (see Chapter 9). Goldmann visual field.

have argued that patients with blindsight have some residual visual function in this apparent blind field, and it is merely conscious vision that is impaired. Extrageniculostriate vision resulting from a "second" more primitive, secondary visual pathway consisting of retino–tectal–pulvinar connections with parietal lobe[91] and with V5, the putative motion detection area (see Chapter 9 for further discussion of the role of V5), have been invoked to explain the Riddoch phenomenon and blindsight.[83–87,92–97] Tractography has confirmed the existence of such alternative visual pathways in patients with blindsight.[98,99] Other evidence, however, has suggested that residual subcortical connections with V5 are not necessary for[100,101] and may not entirely explain[102] these phenomena. Alternative mechanisms[103] include residual functioning areas

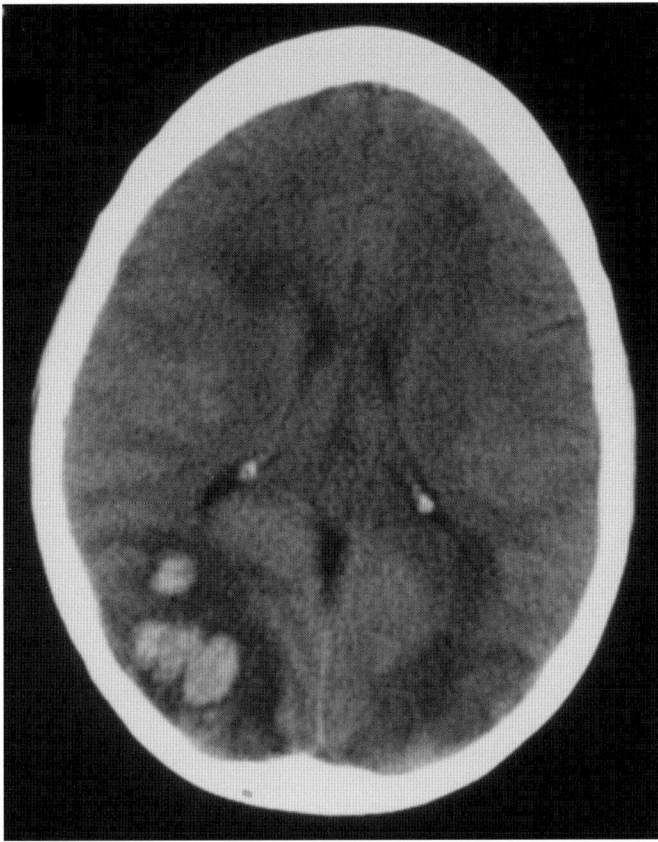

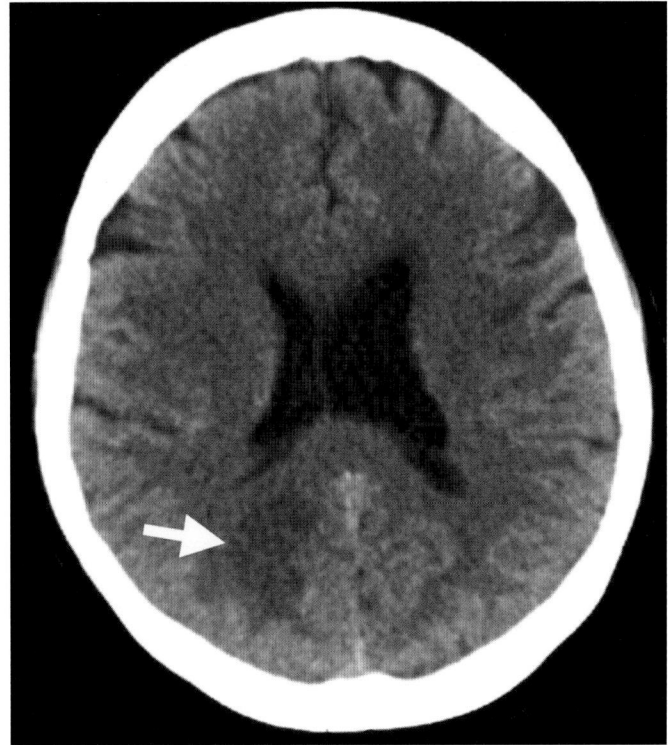

Figure 8–26. Axial CT scan showing a hypodense area (arrow) in the right occipital lobe consistent with a posterior cerebral artery infarction in a patient with left homonymous visual field loss.

Figure 8–25. CT-demonstrated bilateral occipital lobe hemorrhagic lesions and edema, presumably due to aspergillus, in a patient with leukemia and cortical blindness. Hypodense lesions in the subcortical white matter of the frontal lobes indicate widespread, multifocal involvement.

of visual cortex,[104,105] direct connections from the lateral geniculate nucleus to extrastriate areas V2 and V4[106] (see Chapter 9) or, less likely, light scatter in the retina.[107] It should be noted that the Riddoch phenomenon is not specific for lesions of the striate cortex and may be observed with lesions of the anterior visual pathway as well.[108]

Other neuro-ophthalmic signs. Visual acuity is affected only if bilateral lesions are present. Any level of visual acuity is possible with bilateral retrochiasmal lesions, but the acuities should be symmetric unless there is superimposed anterior visual pathway disease.

Occipital lobe hemianopias that are stroke related are often isolated, unless a proximal PCA occlusion leads to a third-nerve palsy. We have also seen several individuals with acute PCA strokes who complained of pain in the distribution of the ophthalmic division of the trigeminal nerve, ipsilateral to the vascular occlusion. One proposed mechanism is referred pain due to trigeminal innervation of the circle of Willis or the tentorium.[109]

A patient with a unilateral hemianopia due to occipital lobe infarction will have a normal optokinetic response. In contrast, one with a hemianopia due to an occipital lobe mass with edema extending into the parietal lobe might have an abnormal optokinetic response when the targets are drawn ipsilaterally to the lesion (Cogan's rule).

Upper bank occipital lobe lesions may be associated with Balint's syndrome. Lower bank lesions may be accompanied

by hemiachromatopsia, prosopagnosia, and object agnosias. Alexia without agraphia may follow a left occipital lesion with involvement of the splenium of the corpus callosum. These higher cortical disorders are discussed in Chapter 9.

Other unusual visual phenomena observed following occipital lobe injury include palinopsia (persistence of visual images) and optic allesthesia (abnormal object orientation in space). These symptoms are discussed in more detail in Chapter 12.

Other signs and symptoms. As alluded to above, a proximal PCA occlusion may cause a midbrain and occipital lobe infarction.[110,111] Resulting signs might include an ipsilateral third-nerve palsy, contralateral ataxia or hemiparesis, and contralateral hemianopia.[112] PCA occlusion may also lead to memory or personality changes from mesial–temporal or thalamic involvement.[113] Thalamic lesions may also lead to sensory loss.[114] The "top of the basilar syndrome"[115] (discussed in more detail in Chapters 15 and 16) often includes signs and symptoms of unilateral or bilateral PCA occlusion. Hemianopias related to occipital lobe infarction also may be associated with brain stem signs and other types of ocular motor dysfunction such as nystagmus, skew deviation, or gaze palsies, if the etiology is vertebrobasilar occlusion. Insidious field loss accompanied by language or cognitive decline suggests a mass lesion or dementing illness.

Etiology

In adults, the most common cause of an occipital lobe hemianopia is a PCA stroke (**Table 8–1**) (**Fig. 8–26**). A homonymous hemianopia, with or without macular

Table 8–3 Important causes of cortical blindness

Acquired
Vascular
  Bilateral posterior cerebral artery infarction
  Cardiac surgery
  Cerebral angiography
Hypoxia
Reversible leukoencephalopathies
  Hypertensive encephalopathy
  Peripartum state
  FK-501
  Cyclosporine
Carbon monoxide poisoning
Creutzfeldt–Jacob disease
Progressive multifocal leukoencephalopathy
Alzheimer's disease
Congenital
Hypoxemic-ischemic encephalopathy
Periventricular leukomalacia

sparing, unaccompanied by any other neurologic signs or symptoms, would be the most common presentation of a PCA stroke.[116]

In elderly patients, the differential diagnosis of occipital lobe dysfunction also includes lobar hemorrhage due to amyloid angiopathy. Infectious causes include abscesses, progressive multifocal leukoencephalopathy, and Creutzfeldt–Jakob disease (CJD). In children, adrenoleukodystrophy and MELAS (mitochondrial myopathy, encephalopathy, lactic acidosis, and stroke-like episodes) may be responsible for hemianopias. Ictal or postictal hemianopias, and complicated migraine leading to occipital lobe infarction are uncommon.

Important acquired and congenital causes of cortical blindness[117] are listed in **Table 8–3**.

DIAGNOSIS AND MANAGEMENT OF DISTURBANCES OF THE OPTIC RADIATIONS AND OCCIPITAL LOBE

Because processes which affect these locations are very similar, they are discussed together in the following section.

Cerebrovascular disease (ischemic stroke)

Occlusion of the MCA or PCA is suggested by the sudden onset of neurologic symptoms in an elderly individual with cerebrovascular risk factors such as atrial fibrillation, hypertension, diabetes, smoking, hypercholesterolemia, or sleep apnea. Classically defined, a transient ischemic attack (TIA) is a cerebrovascular event that lasts for a few minutes or hours, and a stroke is one that produces a fixed deficit that lasts for more than a day. However, more modern definitions of TIAs recognize that some transient neurological events as brief as 30–60 minutes may lead to cerebral infarc-

tion visible on magnetic resonance imaging (MRI) and therefore should be labeled a stroke.[118,119] TIAs are discussed in more detail in Chapter 10, Transient visual loss.

MCA strokes are associated with cardiogenic emboli, internal carotid occlusion, and internal carotid artery dissection. Common causes of PCA infarction include embolism from the heart and a more proximal vascular lesion in the vertebral or basilar arteries. Posterior division MCA strokes, leading to Wernicke's aphasia and hemianopia, and isolated PCA infarcts are frequently cardioembolic.[120] Less commonly, MCA and PCA infarction can result from local atherostenosis, migraine, or hypercoagulable state, and vertebral artery dissection can be associated with PCA strokes.[121,122]

Neuroimaging. Computed tomography (CT) scanning, which is fast and readily available, can be performed in the emergency setting to differentiate between an ischemic or hemorrhagic stroke. Small strokes may be more visible with MRI, especially on T2-weighted and fluid level attenuated inversion recovery (FLAIR) images. Neither CT nor conventional MR may show any abnormality within the first 6 hours after the stroke ictus. MRI techniques such as diffusion-weighted imaging (**Fig. 8–27**), which detects changes in the random motion of water molecules, and perfusion-weighted imaging, which may identify ischemic areas with low blood volume, may delineate brain ischemia before CT or routine MRI are able. Magnetic resonance angiography (MRA) of the carotid system and circle of Willis is frequently helpful when establishing the stroke mechanism.

Treatment. The best treatment for stroke is primary prevention according to the underlying medical or vascular condition.[123,124] Control of hypertension, lowering serum cholesterol, cessation of smoking, and exercise may reduce the risk of stroke.[125,126] The use of statin drugs (hydroxymethylglutaryl-coenzyme A reductase inhibitors), by mechanisms beyond reduction of cholesterol such as an anti-inflammatory effect, may also be protective.[127] Reducing glucose, dietary modification, and avoidance of obesity are also recommended, but these measures have not been proven to reduce the risk of cerebrovascular events.[125] Considerations regarding asymptomatic carotid stenosis are reviewed in Chapter 10. Treatment of underlying cardiac and hypercoagulable states and secondary prevention are discussed separately in more detail below.

While the details of the management of acute stroke patients are beyond the scope of this book, it is helpful to mention some basic points. Acute stroke therapy is aimed at limiting neuronal damage and re-establishing cerebral blood flow. Maintenance of cerebral perfusion pressure, lying the patient flat, delivering oxygen, and normalization of serum glucose, body temperature, and intravascular volume are recommended.[128,129]

At many centers, thrombolytic therapy in selected patients with acute ischemic stroke is given to allow reperfusion by rapid recanalization of occluded vessels.[130–132] Two large randomized studies[133,134] evaluated *intravenous* recombinant tissue plasminogen activator (t-PA) in patients with acute ischemic stroke and a clinically significant neurologic defect. Patients with small-vessel occlusive, large-vessel occlusive, and cardioembolic strokes were enrolled.[135] They had to

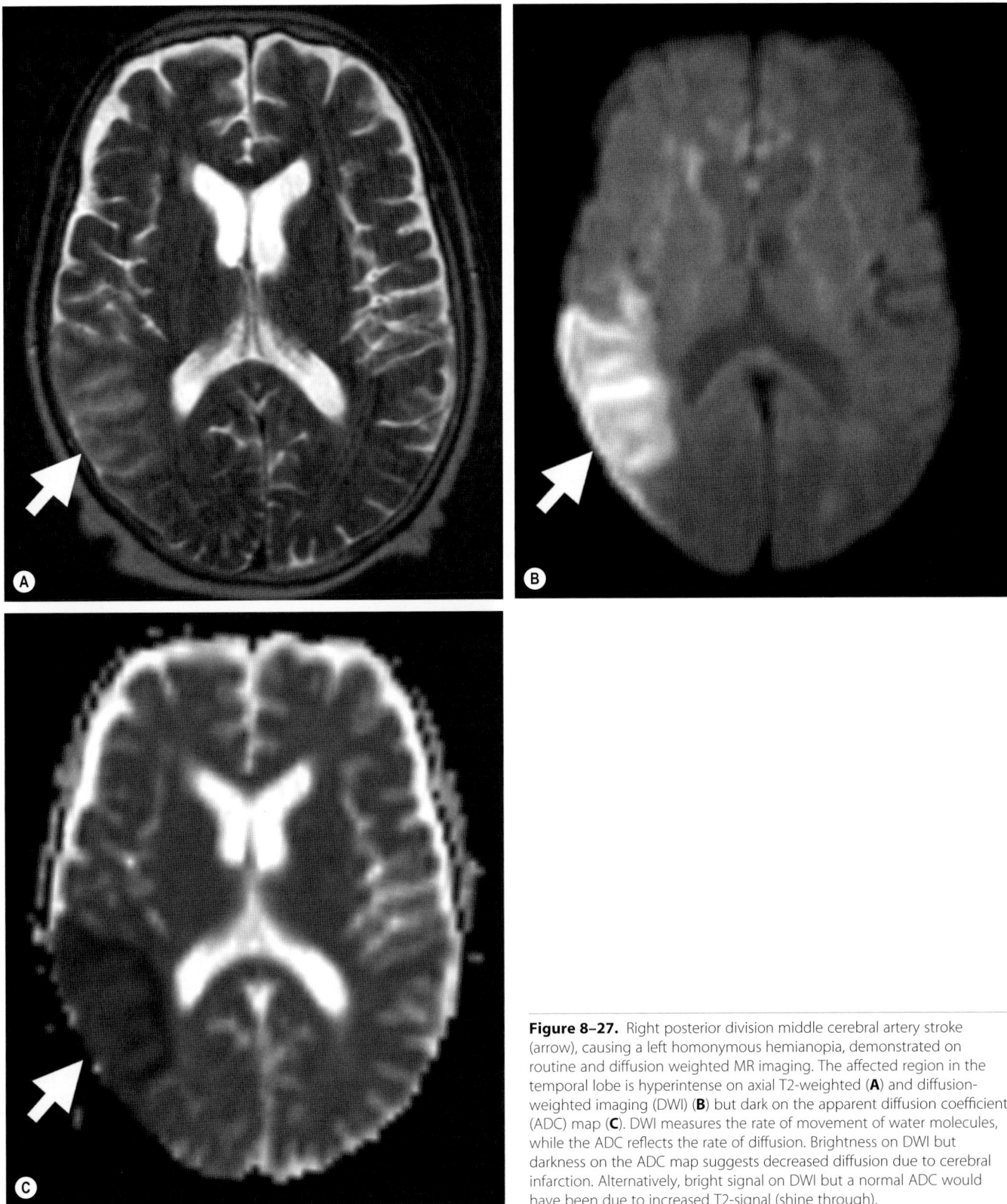

Figure 8–27. Right posterior division middle cerebral artery stroke (arrow), causing a left homonymous hemianopia, demonstrated on routine and diffusion weighted MR imaging. The affected region in the temporal lobe is hyperintense on axial T2-weighted (**A**) and diffusion-weighted imaging (DWI) (**B**) but dark on the apparent diffusion coefficient (ADC) map (**C**). DWI measures the rate of movement of water molecules, while the ADC reflects the rate of diffusion. Brightness on DWI but darkness on the ADC map suggests decreased diffusion due to cerebral infarction. Alternatively, bright signal on DWI but a normal ADC would have been due to increased T2-signal (shine through).

have been evaluated within 3 hours of onset of symptoms, and CT scanning had to demonstrate the absence of early infarction or hemorrhage.[135,136] Functional neurologic outcomes were improved and disability reduced in treated patients.[137] More recently, t-PA administered between 3 and 4.5 hours after stroke onset was also shown to improve clinical outcome.[138] Nevertheless, more frequent use of t-PA is limited by this narrow window of opportunity. In addition, enthusiasm for thrombolytic agents is always weighed against the high risk of associated cerebral hemorrhage. In patients for whom t-PA is contraindicated, aspirin can be used.[139]

Alternatively, selective *intra-arterial* catheter-based thrombolysis with prourokinase has been shown to improve reperfusion and patient outcomes in those with MCA occlusion.[140] Intra-arterial t-PA also can be used, and mechanically removing the clot in so-called thrombectomy or embolectomy has been employed.[141] The use of heparin and antiplatelet agents such as aspirin are discussed in more detail below in the sections on cardioembolic stroke and ischemic stroke, respectively. Neuroprotective agents have also been studied in stroke therapy, but none has proven to be both beneficial and safe.

In elderly patients, field deficits from cerebral infarction that persist for more than 48 hours have a relatively poor prognosis for recovery.[142] However, in children and young adults the prognosis is much better, as visual field improvement sometimes can be observed days or weeks following the ictus.

In addition to the treatments individualized according the various causes of stroke listed below, statins are generally advised for all patients with ischemic stroke to reduce the risk of recurrence.[143-146] Blood pressure management is another secondary preventative measure, and a diuretic or combination of a diuretic and angiotensin-converting enzyme (ACE) inhibitor is also recommended.[147]

Cardioembolism

Frequent cardioembolic causes of cerebral infarction include atrial fibrillation, regional or global wall hypokinesis, valvular disease, and patent foramen ovale. Less common causes include atrial myxoma and endocarditis.

Atrial fibrillation. Stroke occurs in 4.5% of untreated patients with atrial fibrillation per year.[148] In nonrheumatic atrial fibrillation, the risk of stroke is approximately five times that of the normal population, and in atrial fibrillation associated with rheumatic valvular disease, there is a 17-fold increase in risk.[149]

Although treatment should be individualized under the direction of a cardiologist, in general patients with atrial fibrillation should receive prophylaxis for thromboembolism. Warfarin, adjusted to maintain an international normalized ratio (INR) of 2.0–3.0,[150] has been proven to reduce the risk of stroke and secondary cerebrovascular events.[151-156] Cerebral hemorrhage is the most feared complication, but the risk is low at the aforementioned INRs. In patients with contraindications such as poorly controlled hypertension, inability to comply, gait instability, and history of bleeding, aspirin[157] or aspirin plus clopidogrel[158] may be used. Cardiac rate can be controlled by digoxin, beta-blockers, or calcium channel blockers.[148]

In acute stroke due to atrial fibrillation, when the infarct is non-hemorrhagic and mild to moderate in size, emergent anticoagulation with heparin,[159] followed by warfarin, should be considered to reduce the risk of re-embolus. Larger embolic infarctions have a greater tendency for spontaneous hemorrhagic transformation.[160] Nevertheless, some authors suggest heparin even in large[161] and hemorrhagic[162] embolic infarcts if the patient is relatively intact neurologically and at continued high risk for recurrent cardiac source emboli. Because of the greater ease of administration, treatment with subcutaneous unfractionated heparin instead of intravenous (IV) heparin before initiating long term warfarin is gaining in popularity.

Hypokinetic wall motion abnormalities. Especially within the first 2 weeks following a myocardial infarction, focal areas of left ventricular akinesia or dyskinesia may predispose to the development of mural thrombi with resultant cerebral and systemic emboli. The risk may extend for several years following myocardial infarction, and a decreased ejection fraction and older age were found to be independent predictors of an increased risk of stroke in one study.[163] Long-term anticoagulation, usually warfarin, is generally given to at-risk patients without contraindications. Treatment is similar in patients with low ejection fraction from dilated cardiomyopathy from myocarditis and amyloid, for example. In patients with acute ischemic events (see atrial fibrillation above) who are not already anticoagulated, emergent heparin followed by warfarin is recommended.

Patent foramen ovale and atrial septal aneurysm. In younger patients without other stroke risk factors and in those whose neurologic deficit followed Valsalva or cough, these mechanisms should be considered.[164] Asymptomatic deep venous thromboses may result in paradoxic emboli if clot material passes through a patent foramen ovale. The diagnosis may be established with a transesophageal echocardiogram bubble study, during which a small amount of air mixed in saline is injected into an antecubital vein. Excessive microbubbles detected in the left atrium in resting states or after Valsalva may indicate a right to left interatrial shunt. However, because patent foramen ovales are overrepresented in patients with cerebral infarcts of uncertain cause,[165] it is often difficult to correlate them with cerebrovascular events. Therefore, treatment, consisting of anticoagulation with warfarin or antiplatelet agents, or transcatheter or surgical closure of the defect,[166] should be determined on a case by case basis.[167-169]

Valvular disease. Mitral valve prolapse and mitral annulus calcification are also associated with higher risk of TIA and stroke.[170] However, like patent foramen ovale, they are such a common echocardiographic finding that it is sometimes hard to assign any clinical significance to them in a patient with a cerebrovascular event.[171] Nevertheless, antiplatelet therapy is frequently recommended. Prosthetic heart valves, because of their inherent thrombogenicity, require long-term warfarin anticoagulation.[172]

Atrial myxoma. Although histologically benign, these primary tumors of the heart may produce devastating effects when pieces detach and embolize to the brain or systemically. They are usually located within the left atrium, and are generally polypoid, pedunculated, round or oval, with a smooth or lobulated surface.[173] Myxomas typically present either with embolism or intracardiac obstruction. Transesophageal echocardiography, CT, or MRI of the chest may demonstrate these lesions, and surgical removal is the treatment of choice.

Endocarditis. Stroke due to septic emboli may complicate infective endocarditis in approximately 21% of cases (**Fig. 8–28**).[174] Typical organisms include *Staphylococcus aureus* and *Streptococcus*. Intracranial hemorrhages may also develop, some related to mycotic aneurysms.[175] The diagnosis of

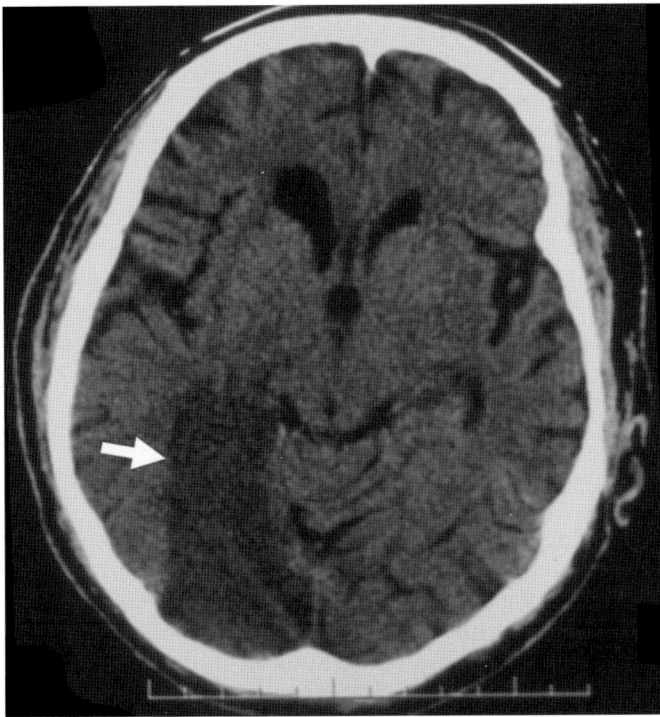

Figure 8–28. Axial CT scan showing a hypodensity (arrow) due to a right posterior cerebral artery embolic infarction in a patient with endocarditis and sudden left homonymous visual field loss.

infective endocarditis is established on the basis of a valvular vegetation seen on transthoracic or transesophageal echocardiography and positive blood cultures. Other systemic emboli, such as ocular Roth spots, often aid in the diagnosis. Other neurologic complications of infective endocarditis include encephalopathy, meningitis, brain abscess, seizures, and headache.[176,177] Most cerebral embolic phenomena occur early in the patient's course before the control of infection, so treatment is primarily antibiotics without anticoagulation.[174] Valve replacement may take place once the infection is controlled.

Other causes of ischemic stroke

Carotid artery disease. In the absence of cardioembolic phenomena, signs and symptoms of retinal or hemispheric ischemia demand exclusion of carotid artery stenosis. Infarction may result from carotid artery occlusion or emboli from an ulcerated atheromatous plaque. The evaluation and management of carotid stenosis is discussed in more detail in Chapter 10, Transient visual loss. Carotid artery dissection, which can produce ipsilateral Horner's syndrome, carotidynia (pain), dysgeusia (abnormal taste), and cortical ischemia or stroke, is discussed in more detail in Chapter 13, Pupillary disorders.

Vertebrobasilar disease. Ischemia in the PCA distribution may result from vertebral or basilar artery stenosis. Usually field defects due vertebrobasilar insufficiency are accompanied by other indications of brain stem or cerebellar ischemia such as diplopia, dysarthria, or ataxia.[178] Vertebral artery dissection,[179] due to trauma or chiropractic manipulation, for instance, may also result in upstream PCA ischemia. Alternatively, vertebral artery origin occlusive disease, similar to

carotid atheromatous plaques, may produce basilar or PCA strokes by intracranial intra-arterial embolism.[180] Not readily surgical amenable, in situ vertebrobasilar disease generally is best treated with antiplatelet agents, but vertebral artery dissection, stroke in evolution, and crescendo TIAs may require more aggressive anticoagulation with heparin and warfarin. Some authors have also used thrombolysis successfully in basilar artery stroke.[181,182]

Thrombosis in the circle of Willis (in situ thrombosis). Atherosclerosis of the MCA and PCA may be detected noninvasively using MRA, and symptomatic stenosis is usually treated medically with antiplatelet agents. Options to reduce the risk of recurrent stroke include aspirin (81–325 mg per day), the combination of extended-release dipyridamole and aspirin, and clopidogrel alone. Extended-release dipyridamole and aspirin was shown to be more protective than aspirin alone.[183] Another study showed no difference in efficacy between the combination of extended-release dipyridamole and aspirin versus clopidogrel alone.[184] Clopidrogrel, in one study, was slightly more effective than aspirin in reducing vascular events.[185,186] In patients failing antiplatelet agents, warfarin can be an alternative.[187] Intracranial angioplasty or arterial stenting can be also be considered in those failing medical therapy,[141] but perforator stroke, in lenticulostriate artery distributions associated with MCA angioplasty for instance, can be a complication.[147]

Hypercoagulable states. These conditions account for approximately 1% of ischemic strokes but up to 4% of strokes in young adults.[188] These include hematologic disorders such as protein C or S, factor V, or antithrombin III deficiency,[189] which are treated with chronic warfarin anticoagulation, and abnormalities of formed blood elements such as polycythemia vera, sickle cell anemia, sickle-C disease and essential thrombocythemia.[190] Prothombotic states such as oral contraceptive use,[191,192] pregnancy,[193] and cancer (Trousseau's syndrome) should also be considered.[194]

Autoantibody syndromes, due to antiphospholipid (e.g., anticardiolipin) antibodies and lupus anticoagulants, are also associated with hypercoagulability.[190] Several reports[195,196] have described the presence of these antibodies in patients with cerebral ischemia, even in those without systemic lupus erythematosus. However, their exact relationship with stroke is uncertain,[197,198] and the mechanism for the predisposition to thrombosis is unclear.[199] Furthermore, the best treatment, either aspirin or warfarin, is controversial,[200,201] but warfarin is preferred in patients with recurrent ischemic events.

Cardiac surgery. Open heart surgery remains the most common iatrogenic cause of stroke.[202] Perioperative mechanisms include (1) macroemboli from trauma to diseased brittle, atherosclerotic blood vessels or from intracardiac entrapment of air or particles; (2) microemboli produced by the cardiopulmonary bypass machinery; (3) alterations in blood pressure and oxygenation, and (4) pre-existing cerebrovascular or carotid disease.[203-205]

Aortic arch emboli. This is likely an underrecognized source of cerebral embolism.[206,207] In patients studied with transesophageal echocardiography, atherosclerotic plaques greater than 4 mm thick in the aortic arch were found to be associated with ischemic stroke[208] and to be predictors of recurrent brain infarction and other vascular events.[209] Aspirin may be recommended when these lesions are detected; however, the best treatment of aortic arch atherosclerosis is currently uncertain.[167]

Transtentorial herniation. Large neoplastic or hemorrhagic lesions causing downward transtentorial herniation may cause compression of the posterior cerebral arteries at the edge of the tentorium. Both unilateral hemianopias and cortical blindness may be produced.[210]

Migraine. Homonymous hemianopic field defects in migraine are usually transient and are therefore discussed in more detail in Chapter 10. However, if the deficit lasts for more than 7 days, or if a parietal or occipital lobe infarction is demonstrated on neuroimaging, the International Headache Society diagnosis of "migrainous cerebral infarction" is suggested.[211] The rest of the diagnostic criteria are (1) the patient has previously fulfilled the criteria for migraine with aura except that one or more aura symptoms persist for more than an hour, (2) the attack is typical of previous attacks, (3) other causes of infarction have been excluded.[211,212]

Epidemiologic studies have now confirmed migraine as an independent risk factor for stroke.[213,214] We strongly discourage our migraine patients from smoking or using oral contraception, in order to reduce the chance of stroke. Any combination of risk factors may be synergistic.

In patients with migraine-related occipital infarction, basilar artery or PCA stenosis or spasm may be evident on MRA. However, in some instances the stroke does not respect the usual MCA or PCA territories (see Fig. 19–2), suggesting that a strictly vascular mechanism is insufficient to explain all migraine-related stroke phenomena. The exact pathogenesis of migraine-related stroke is unclear, but a combination of coagulation, hemodynamic, and neuronal factors is likely to be responsible.[215]

The best treatment of patients with migraine-related stroke is unknown. Aspirin, exclusion of other causes of stroke, and migraine prophylaxis is one recommended approach. Migraine treatment is discussed in more detail in Chapter 19.

Stroke in young adults and children

Strokes in patients less than 40 years old are relatively uncommon. In young adults, cardiogenic emboli and atherosclerotic occlusive disease are the two most common identifiable causes of stroke.[216] Other etiologies which should be considered in this age group include hypercoagulable states, nonatherosclerotic vascular disease (dissection or moya-moya vessels, for instance), illicit drug use, and migraine. One study found that a cause may not be found in approximately one-third of patients despite an exhaustive search.[217] In children, cyanotic heart disease and sickle cell are seen more often as causes of stroke, and atherosclerosis is rarely considered.[218]

Hemorrhage

Table 8–4 highlights some of the more important causes of intracerebral hemorrhages.

Table 8–4 Important causes of intracerebral hemorrhage[488]

Hypertension
Amyloid angiopathy
Vascular malformations
Arteriovenous malformations
Cavernous angiomas
Saccular or mycotic aneurysms
Trauma
Hemorrhagic infarction
Anticoagulant treatment and bleeding diathesis
Hemorrhage into intracranial tumors
Drug related

Evaluation of patients with suspected intracerebral hemorrhage begins with an unenhanced CT scan. A CT scan is easily obtained and makes it possible to determine the size of the hemorrhage, the extent of mass effect, and whether the ventricular system is compromised. A follow-up MRI scan is often helpful to ensure that the hemorrhage is not from an underlying arteriovenous malformation or brain tumor. In addition, MRA provides a useful non-invasive way to screen for aneurysms. Because MRA may miss some aneurysms, conventional angiography is indicated when the etiology of the intracerebral hemorrhage remains uncertain. In most instances patients with intracerebral hemorrhages will be managed in a neuro-intensive care unit setting, with attention directed towards managing blood pressure and intracranial pressure. Although many studies have failed to demonstrate a difference in outcome between patients with supratentorial hemorrhage treated medically versus surgically,[219,220] neurosurgical evacuation is still often considered if the patient's condition deteriorates or if shunting is required.[221]

Hypertensive hemorrhage

In order of decreasing frequency, hemorrhages associated with long-standing hypertension arise in the putamen, thalamus, pons, cerebellum, and cerebral white matter. In contrast to hemorrhages associated with amyloid angiopathy, hypertensive hemorrhages are more likely to be subcortical.[222] When large enough, thalamic hemorrhages may cause hemianopias by involving the lateral geniculate nucleus (**Fig. 8–29**), while putaminal and lobar hemorrhages may disrupt the optic radiations. When the hemorrhages are limited to brain parenchyma, treatment is usually supportive. Intraventricular blood may lead to hydrocephalus and thus may require shunting.

Amyloid angiopathy

This entity should be strongly considered in any elderly individual with posteriorly situated lobar hemorrhages. In contrast to hypertensive hemorrhages, cerebral amyloid angiopathy tends to produce one or more episodes of lobar hemorrhage (**Fig. 8–30a**), with a propensity to affect the parieto-occipital regions.[223] The lobar distribution of hemorrhage in cerebral amyloid angiopathy reflects the preferential deposition of amyloid in the superficial and leptomeningeal

Arteriovenous malformations

Arteriovenous malformations (AVMs) are dysplastic vascular lesions in which the normal capillary bed is replaced by a convolution of abnormally connected arterial and venous channels.[234] Intracranial AVMs are thought to form secondarily to developmental arrest during cerebrovascular development. Usually intraparenchymal cerebral AVMs are supplied by large branches of the circle of Willis. Dural AVMs, which tend to be more superficially located, result from communications between the arteries that supply the dura mater and the intracranial venous sinuses. The afferent and efferent vessels of AVMs may vary considerably in their course, size, and number. In some instances, the entire lesion may be only a few millimeters in size, while in others, a whole cerebral lobe may be involved. The intervening cerebral tissue is often gliotic, and the surrounding neural tissue characteristically shows some degree of atrophy. Neurologic abnormalities and visual field defects are caused most commonly either by compression of local structures, ischemia, or hemorrhage.

The majority of AVMs are sporadic although familial cases have been documented.[235] Men are affected slightly more often than women (1.4 : 1),[236] and the majority of individuals do not present until their second or third decade. Malformations often become symptomatic during times of hormonal fluctuation, accelerating growth, or accentuated intravascular volume such as puberty or pregnancy.[237] Neurocutaneous syndromes linked with intracranial AVMs include Wyburn–Mason, Osler–Weber–Rendu, Sturge–Weber (see congenital conditions, below), and Klippel–Theraunay–Weber.[237]

The most common presentation of an intracranial AVM is an intraparenchymal or subarachnoid hemorrhage (**Fig. 8.31A**), often with a focal neurologic deficit. Seizures and headaches are the next most frequent presentations. Subjective bruits are more common with extracranial AVMs, and only sometimes is the bruit audible. Dural AVMs can cause cortical disturbances but also present with venous sinus congestion from obstruction or arterialization. Many individuals with unruptured occipital lobe AVMs present with transient visual field defects or positive visual phenomena (e.g., scintillating scotomas, fortification spectra, or spots) followed by headache, mimicking migraine.[238] Usually in these cases the distinguishing feature is an overwhelming headache or a residual field deficit, but sometimes differentiating between migraine and AVM is difficult on clinical grounds alone.

Radiographically, cerebral AVMs are usually identified by their serpiginous flow voids on T1- and T2-weighted images.[239] When patients present with large hemorrhages, AVMs may be masked and may not be evident on routine neuroimaging. MRA is often helpful in demonstrating the feeding arteries and abnormal tangle of vessels. Formal angiography is required for proper definition of the vascular anatomy (**Fig. 8–31B**).

Definitive treatment is neurosurgical removal of the AVM, especially when superficially located.[240] In some instances endovascular embolization of feeding vessels may reduce the size of the lesion, making it more surgically amenable.

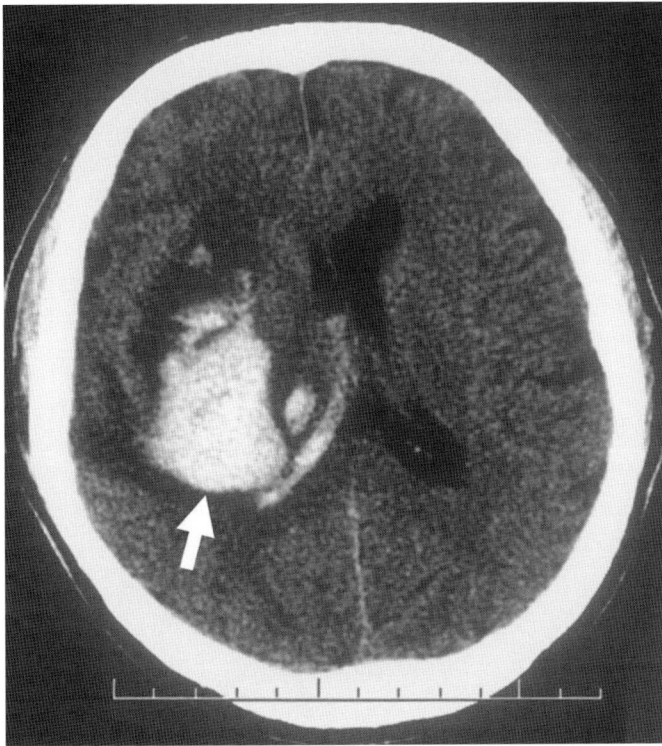

Figure 8–29. Hypertensive thalamic hemorrhage (arrow) on axial CT. The patient had a left homonymous hemianopia and left hemiplegia.

arteries.[223] Pathologically, vessel walls contain congophilic material which exhibits apple-green birefringence when viewed with polarized light, and fibrinoid necrosis is often seen (**Fig. 8–30B–D**).[224] It has been suggested that the amyloid in this vascular disorder is the same as the amyloid found in senile plaques in Alzheimer's disease.[225]

Autopsy studies have found a greater frequency of cerebral amyloid angiopathy with increasing age. Approximately 5% of individuals from 60 to 69 years of age have cerebral amyloid angiopathy, compared with more than 50% of patients in their 90s.[226] Despite this high frequency of vessel involvement, the reason hemorrhage is still relatively infrequent in the affected population remains unclear. Predisposition to hemorrhage may be related to the severity of amyloid deposition, the presence of fibrinoid necrosis,[227] and possession of the apolipoprotein E $\in$2 and $\in$4 alleles.[228–230]

Although a definitive diagnosis requires a pathological analysis of brain tissue, biopsy of the brain is rarely performed given the availability of neuroimaging to exclude other etiologies, the absence of effective therapy, and the advanced age of most patients with cerebral amyloid angiopathy. Most diagnoses are made postmortem. The clinical diagnosis of "probable cerebral amyloid angiopathy" can be made in a patient older than 55 years of age with multiple lobar hemorrhages with no other cause of bleeding.[231,232] Because of increased fragility of vessels affected by amyloid deposition, conservative management is preferred over surgical evacuation of the hematoma.[233] Antiplatelet agents or anticoagulants should be withdrawn.[231]

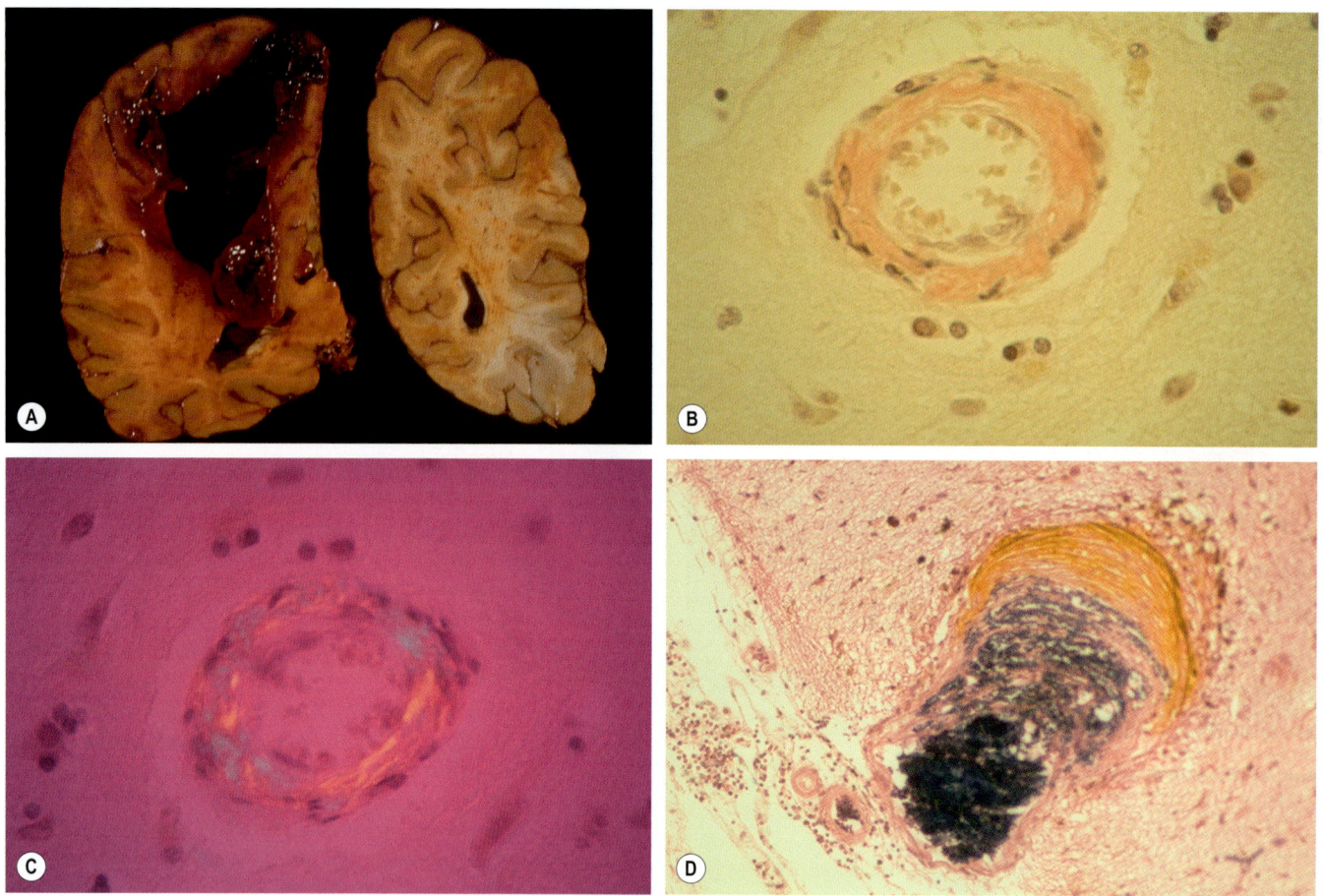

Figure 8–30. Cerebral hemorrhage due to amyloid angiopathy. **A**. Coronal pathologic section of the brain, showing a recent large right lobar hematoma. This 78-year-old man presented with an occipital headache, left homonymous hemianopia, right gaze preference, and left hemiplegia. Microscopic views of an involved cerebral blood vessel, which was thickened and stained positive with Congo red (**B**) and displayed "apple-green" birefringence (**C**). **D**. Vessel with fibrinoid necrosis (dark area), a feature likely predisposing to hemorrhage.

When they involve the optic radiations or occipital lobe with partial hemifield loss, unfortunately following embolization or surgical extirpation the field defects can worsen or become complete.[238,241] Stereotactic radiosurgery can be used to treat AVMs less than 3 cm in size, particularly those in eloquent areas.[242,243]

Cavernous angiomas (cavernomas)

Although these small vascular malformations often occur in the cortex and cerebral white matter, associated retrochiasmal field defects are relatively uncommon. They may present with signs and symptoms of acute hemorrhage.[244] Alternatively, asymptomatic cavernous angiomas may be detected on neuroimaging done for other reasons. They consist of dilated spaces filled with blood without intervening neural tissue, separated by fibrous collagenous bands.[245] Their histopathologic and radiographic features are discussed in more detail in the section on cavernous angiomas of the chiasm (Chapter 7). Cavernous angiomas may occur sporadically or as a familial autosomal dominant condition.[246]

Treatment of cavernous angiomas depends on their location and symptomatology. For symptomatic superficial

lesions, surgery is effective and safe, and should be considered to prevent rebleeding.[247,248] Deeper symptomatic lesions may also be removed, but in such cases observation is often a better option because of the morbidity associated with such surgery. Unfortunately recurrent bleeding often mandates surgical removal. Asymptomatic cavernous angiomas should be treated conservatively.

Vasculitis

Vasculitis is the broad term used to characterize those disorders associated with inflammation of blood vessels. Some of these conditions like giant cell arteritis purely affect vessels while others, like systemic lupus erthematosus, produce inflammation of connective tissue including blood vessels. It is helpful to divide central nervous system (CNS) vasculitis into two categories based on whether there is evidence of systemic disease. *Primary CNS vasculitis* is the term used to describe those entities in which the vasculitis process is limited to the CNS and eyes. Typically those patients with *systemic vasculitis*, such as temporal arteritis or systemic lupus

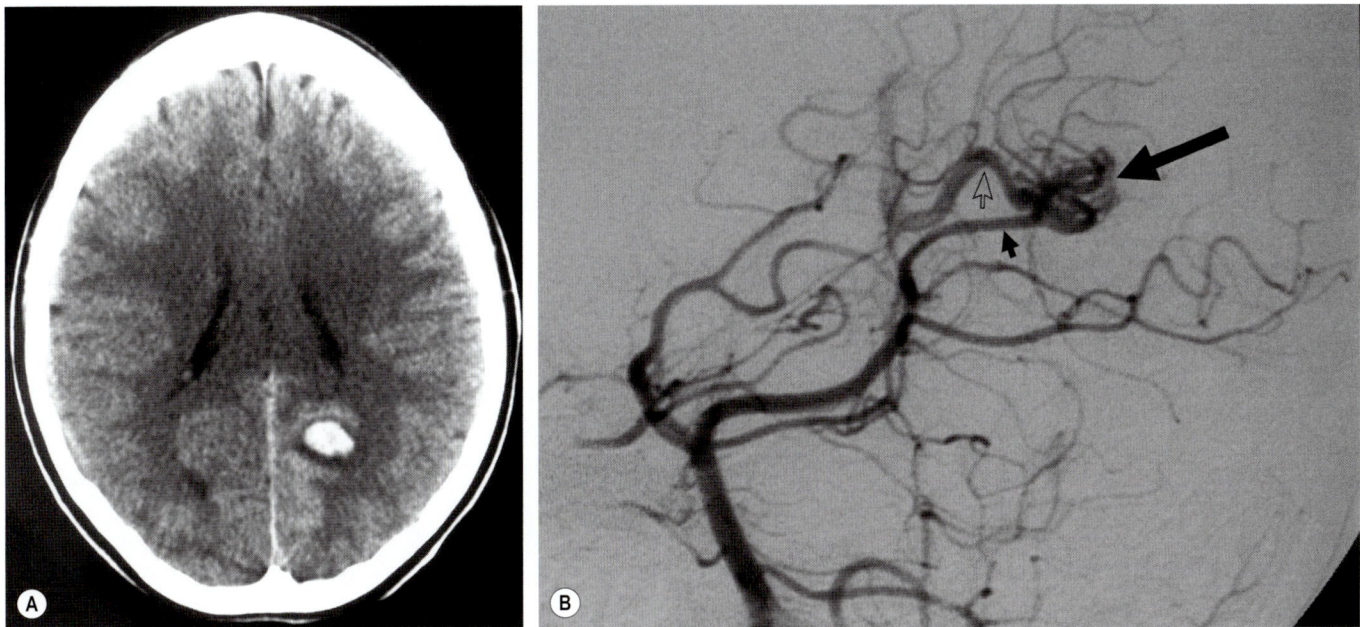

Figure 8–31. Arteriovenous malformation (AVM) of the left occipital lobe. **A**. CT scan demonstrates a hyperdense lesion in the left occipital lobe, consistent with hemorrhage. **B**. Selective right vertebral arteriogram shows an AVM (large solid arrow) supplied by the calcarine branch of the left posterior cerebral artery (small solid arrow) with a large vein (open arrow) which drains into the straight sinus.

erythematosus, will usually demonstrate signs and symptoms suggesting a more widespread angiitic process before the CNS is involved.

Primary CNS vasculitis (angiitis)

This idiopathic disorder is characterized by vasculitis restricted to the blood vessels of the brain and spinal cord.[249–258] Typically, there are multiple bilateral infarcts involving the cortex and subcortical white matter,[259,260] often in a young individual. Scattered punctate-enhancing lesions have also been observed.[261] CSF examination often reveals an elevated protein or white count, or both.

The diagnosis is suggested by demonstration of vascular abnormalities on angiography but is confirmed by biopsy.[262] Like conventional angiography,[259,263] MRA may show cut-off of vessels, aneurysms, and beading but may be particularly limited in cases where a small-vessel vasculitis like granulomatous angiitis (GANS) is suspected. Biopsy of the leptomeninges or parenchyma is the only definitive method to establish the diagnosis of primary angiitis of the CNS.[251,264] Pathologically, this disorder affects small and medium-size vessels. The cellular infiltrate is composed of lymphocytes, macrophages, and giant cells in all layers of the vessel wall.

Without treatment, patients usually suffer recurrent strokes and die within several years. The administration of prednisone and cyclophosphamide may produced remission and even cure.[251,252,254,256,265] Many patients require treatment for years. When repeat angiography shows normal findings, the immunosuppressive agent may be tapered.[263]

Other primary CNS vasculopathies, such as Susac and Cogan syndrome, and Eales disease, which are typified more by their retinal manifestations, are discussed in Chapter 4.

Systemic vasculitis

Giant cell (temporal) arteritis. The pathology, systemic associations, diagnosis, and treatment of giant cell arteritis, especially with regard to arteritic ischemic optic neuropathy, are reviewed in greater detail in Chapter 5.

Transient ischemic attacks and cerebral infarcts in giant cell arteritis may occur in any vascular distribution but there is a tendency for involvement of the posterior circulation.[266–271] Thus, from a neuro-ophthalmic perspective, hemifield defects and cortical blindness may ensue as the result of an occipital lobe infarction.[266,272,273] The preponderance of posterior circulation ischemia in giant cell arteritis reflects the predilection for arteritic involvement of the extracranial vertebral arteries.[274] The pathologic changes of ischemic brain injury related to giant cell arteritis include (1) inflammatory obstruction of vessels with a striking propensity for the arteritic involvement to cease as the vessel penetrates the dura intracranially; (2) embolism distal from an inflamed artery; and (3) a propagating thrombosis.[275,276] Intracranial vasculitis due to giant cell arteritis is rare but has been reported.[277]

Treatment of giant cell arteritis associated with brain ischemia has no established regimen. We advocate a high dose intravenous methylprednisolone pulse, but this regimen may also fail.[278] Since the mechanism of the brain ischemia may be inflammatory occlusive disease, consideration should be given to administration of anti-platelet agents, heparin, and overhydration to help evolving low flow or thromboembolic states.

Systemic lupus erythematosus (SLE). Permanent homonymous visual field defects may occur, evolving either acutely or over several days.[279–282] Occasionally, a homonymous field defect may herald the diagnosis of SLE.[283]

Potential causes of cortical ischemia in SLE include emboli from Libman–Sachs endocarditis, thrombotic infarction associated with antiphospholipid antibodies, vasospasm, and true vasculitis. Most pathologic studies of patients with ischemic visual or neurologic deficits have not demonstrated inflammation of the intracranial arteries. In the classic clinicopathologic study of 24 patients with SLE (18 with CNS manifestations), Johnson and Richardson[284] found true vasculitis in only 12.5%. Vascular necrosis was noted in 23%, fibrin thrombi in 12.5%, and microinfarction in 70%.[284] Similar findings were confirmed in other subsequent neuropathologic studies.[285,286]

Pulse IV methylprednisolone for 3 days followed by oral prednisone 1–2 mg/kg/day for at least 1 month, along with IV heparin with plans to convert to coumadin, are recommended in patients with SLE and cortical ischemia. It is also particularly important to look for a source of emboli and the presence of antiphospholipid antibodies. Finding antiphospholipid antibodies in this setting usually requires the patient to take long-term anticoagulation.

The optic neuropathy associated with SLE is discussed in Chapter 5.

Reversible posterior leukoencephalopathies

Reversible posterior leukoencephalopathy syndrome (RPLS), characterized by transient headache, seizures, hemianopia or cortical blindness, visual neglect, and mental status changes, is well recognized.[287,288] The condition occurs in adults as well as children.[289,290] Causes of RPLS usually fall into two groups. In the first group, consisting of malignant hypertension and eclampsia, the common feature is elevation in blood pressure. The second group comprises the immunosuppressive agents cyclosporine and FK-506 (tacrolimus),[291] and blood pressure is abnormal in only some of these cases. The final common pathway in both groups is felt to be capillary leak due to endothelial dysfunction.[292] Neuroimaging in this syndrome typically demonstrates extensive bilateral white matter edema and lesions which are hypodense on CT and high-signal on T2-weighted and FLAIR MR images (**Fig. 8–32**).[293] On diffusion-weighted MR images the lesions are usually isointense because the edema is vasogenic and not cytoxic, i.e., ischemia is not present. The lesions can be diffuse, but they predominate in the posterior portions of the hemispheres, which are thought to be more vulnerable because of decreased vascular sympathetic innervation in those areas.[294] Both the clinical symptoms and radiographic abnormalities in RPLS usually resolve within days to weeks following treatment of the hypertension or lowering of the dosage or cessation of the offending drug. In some instances gray matter is involved, and the term posterior reversible encephalopathy syndrome (PRES) has been used in such cases.[295–297]

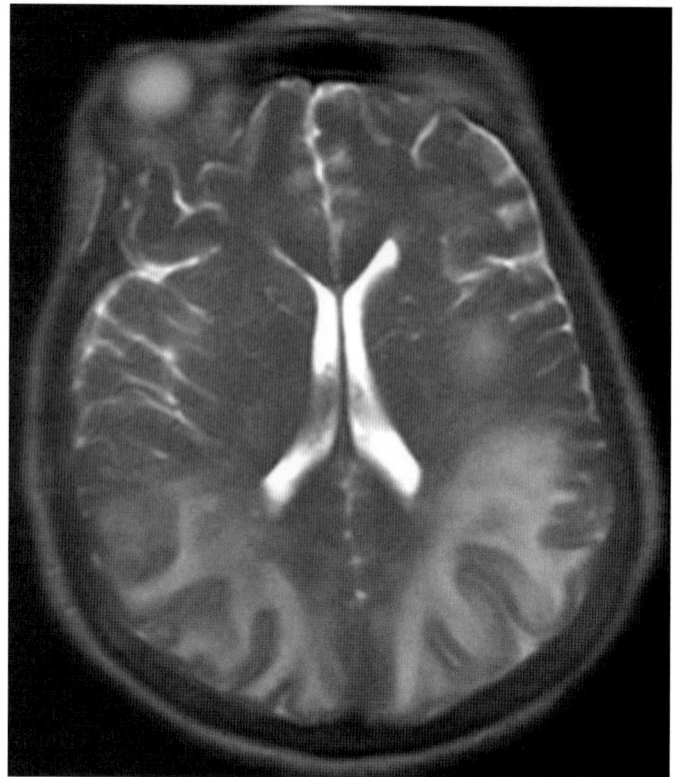

Figure 8–32. T2-weighted magnetic resonance imaging demonstrating diffuse white matter high signal abnormalities, with sparing of gray matter, in reversible posterior leukoencephalopathy syndrome (RPLS) due to cyclosporine toxicity.

Malignant hypertension and eclampsia

The mechanism in these cases is likely defective autoregulation of the brain vasculature caused by sudden elevations in blood pressure.[287] Resulting vasodilation and vasoconstriction cause breakdown of the blood–brain barrier with fluid transudation and petechial hemorrhages. Malignant hypertension with reversible leukoencephalopathy typically occurs in patients with a history of renal insufficiency.[298]

Reversible leukoencephalopathy in preeclampsia has been reported as a cause of temporary cortical blindness.[299,300] RPLS in association with pregnancy typically develops before delivery but has been reported up to 9 days postpartum.[301]

Drugs

Cyclosporine produces the reversible posterior leukoencephalopathy typically at toxic levels.[302,303] Aggravating factors appear to be cranial irradiation, hypomagnesemia, hypercholesterolemia, high-dose steroids, hypertension, and uremia.[303] The mechanism of this complication is unclear, but may reflect either direct neurotoxicity or a vasculopathy.[287] FK-501 (tacrolimus) is similar to cyclosporine in its action and toxic side-effects. Similar cortical blindness and white matter lesions have been observed.[304,305]

Neoplasms of the cerebral hemispheres

In adults, the cerebral hemispheres are the most common location of brain tumors. Patients with neoplastic mass

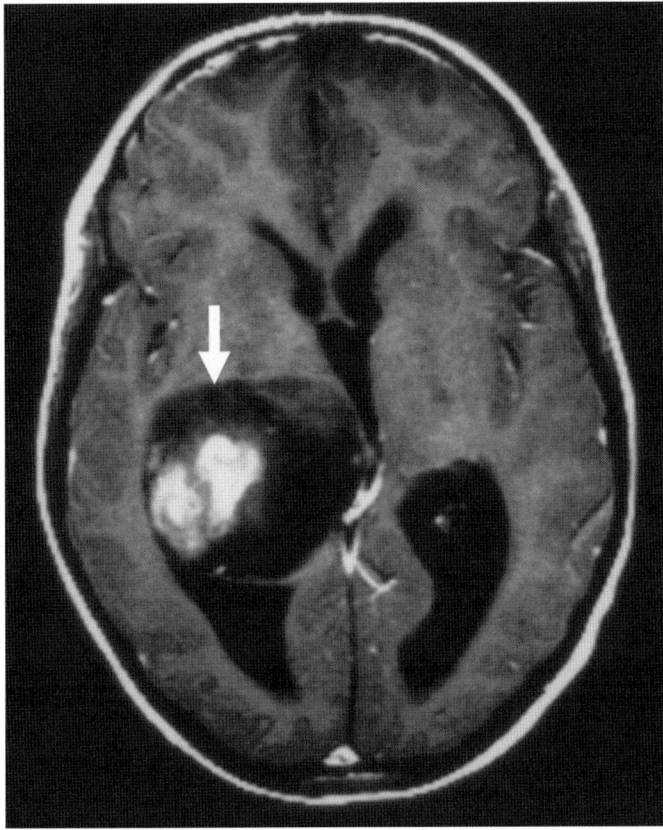

Figure 8–33. Magnetic resonance imaging demonstrating gadolinium-enhancing anaplastic astrocytoma of the right thalamus (arrow) and hydrocephalus in child who presented with headaches and a left homonymous hemianopia.

lesions of the parietal, temporal or occipital lobes can present subacutely (days) or chronically (weeks) with altered mentation, focal neurologic findings, seizures, or symptoms of elevated intracranial pressure such as headache, nausea, or vomiting.[306] Visual field defects caused by such tumors are insidious, and worsen slowly as the tumor enlarges. Acute neurologic symptoms are suggestive of hemorrhage within the tumor. Visual field loss may also result as complications of tumor treatment, as in neurosurgical removal or cranial irradiation.[307]

Tumor types can be subdivided by whether they arose from primary brain tissue or metastasized from a systemic neoplasm. In children, most brain tumors are primary (Fig. 8–33) and brain metastases are much less common.

Tumors in adults

Primary tumors. Common supratentorial primary tumors of the brain include those which are intrinsic and those which are extrinsic to the brain. Primary intraparenchymal tumors of the brain on MR or CT typically are heterogeneously enhancing masses with surrounding edema.

Gliomas are the most common primary intraparenchymal brain tumors.[308] They are subdivided into astrocytomas, oligodendrogliomas, gangliogliomas, and ependymomas. The astrocytomas are further categorized, in order of increasing malignancy, into low-grade astrocytomas such as pilo-

cytic ones (World Health Organization (WHO) grade I), fibrillary astrocytomas (WHO grade II), anaplastic astrocytomas (WHO grade III), and glioblastoma multiformes (WHO grade IV).[309,310] Generally, low-grade astrocytomas in the cerebral hemispheres are treated with complete resection, then observed without further treatment, but that is controversial. Anaplastic astrocytomas and glioblastomas are treated with surgery, followed by radiation and chemotherapy. The prognosis in glioblastomas is dismal, but age dependent: patients younger than 40 have an approximately 64% chance of survival at 18 months, while those over 60 have an 8% survival rate.[311] Methylation of the promoter of the MGMT gene in the tumor specimen predicts a better response to temozolomide chemotherapy.[312]

Intraventricular tumors, such as choroid plexus papillomas and meningiomas, can cause hemifield defects if they involve the posterior horn of the lateral ventricle. Extraparenchymal meningiomas may lead to hemianopias if they grow large enough and are located along the hemispheric convexities.

Primary CNS B-cell lymphoma should be considered when a cerebral mass develops in a patient immunocompromised due to human immunodeficiency virus (HIV) infection or iatrogenic causes. Most such patients have a depressed CD4 count and evidence of Epstein–Barr virus (EBV) exposure. However, CNS lymphomas have become well recognized in immunocompetent individuals as well.[313] CSF cytology is only sometimes helpful, and often stereotactic biopsy is necessary for a definitive diagnosis. A minority of individuals may develop intraocular spread and uveitis,[314] and in these patients intravitreal sampling may be helpful. Because the tumor is sensitive to corticosteroids, such treatment should be withheld prior to histopathological diagnosis. Except for biopsy, surgery is usually not recommended because CNS lymphomas tend to be infiltrating and deep seated. Methotrexate chemotherapy is the most effective treatment. Since radiation combined with methotrexate is associated with an unacceptably high risk of leukoencephalopathy, particularly in patients older than 60, the use of radiation in this disorder is diminishing.[315]

Metastatic tumors. The most common metastatic tumors to the brain originate from the lung and breast, but melanomas and genitourinary, gastrointestinal, and gynecological tumors should also be considered.[316,317] Only rarely do sarcomas, thyroid cancers, and head and neck tumors spread to the brain. MRI or CT typically demonstrates solitary or multiple ring-enhancing lesions at the gray–white matter junction with surrounding edema.

When metastases are suspected, but a systemic cancer is unknown, workup to detect a source would include at least a chest X-ray, chest, abdominal, and pelvis CT scan, carcinoembryonic antigen, stool guaiac, bone scan, and mammogram.[317] Brain biopsy is required when no source can be identified. When a systemic cancer is known, treatment may be presumptive. Treatment with corticosteroids is almost always beneficial, and seizure prophylaxis in many instances is also recommended. Whole-brain radiation is usually given, but there is evidence to suggest that patients with a solitary metastasis benefit from surgical resection plus radiation rather than surgery or radiation alone.[318] When the cerebral metastases are unresectable or multiple, stereotactic radiosurgery can be used instead of surgery prior to whole brain radiation.[319] The overall prognosis for patients with brain metastasis is still poor, but they tend to die of their systemic disease rather than from neurologic complications.[317]

Childhood tumors

In contrast to adults, only 25–40% of childhood brain tumors arise in the cerebral hemispheres. The tumor types are similar, except meningiomas are less common, and supratentorial primitive neuroectodermal tumors, gangliogliomas, and ependymomas are more frequently seen.

Effects of radiation

Altitudinal visual field loss has been reported in association with radionecrosis of the occipital lobes.[320] In addition, stroke-like migraine attacks after radiation therapy (SMART syndrome) can occur several years following posterior fossa radiation and present with periods of days of encephalopathy, focal sensory and motor deficits, and a hemianopia.[321]

Infections

Progressive multifocal leukoencephalopathy

This demyelinating viral infection is caused by reactivation of a human papovavirus, JC virus (the initials stand for the first patient in whom the virus was isolated).[322] The virus, normally latent in 80–90% of the normal population,[323] causes demyelination by lysing oligodendrocytes.[324] Progressive multifocal leukoencephalopathy (PML) is characterized pathologically by a triad of multifocal demyelination, hyperchromatic, enlarged oligodendroglial nuclei, and enlarged bizarre astrocytes with lobulated hyperchromatic nuclei.[325,326]

PML occurs primarily in immunocompromised individuals. Although originally described in patients with leukemia and lymphoma,[325] today most cases are seen in those infected with human immunodeficiency virus (HIV),[327] in whom 5% are likely to develop PML.[326] Other predisposing conditions include sarcoidosis, systemic lupus erythematosus,[328] macroglobulinemia, and immunosuppressive treatment following organ transplantation.[329] Recently, PML has been associated with a number of monoclonal antibody therapies including natalizumab, rituximab, and efalizumab and immunosuppressive drugs such as mycophenolate mofetil. The risk of PML associated with natalizumab use has been estimated as 1:1000 patients treated over an 18-month timeframe.[330]

PML presents insidiously with homonymous hemianopia, cortical blindness,[331,332] language disturbances, motor weakness, sensory loss, incoordination and dementia.[333] Posterior fossa involvement, which is less common, can lead to ataxia, dysarthria, and cranial nerve palsies.[331] While most patients suffer from an inexorably progressive decline followed by death within months of their diagnosis, occasionally some experience a spontaneously relapsing–remitting or static course.[333,334]

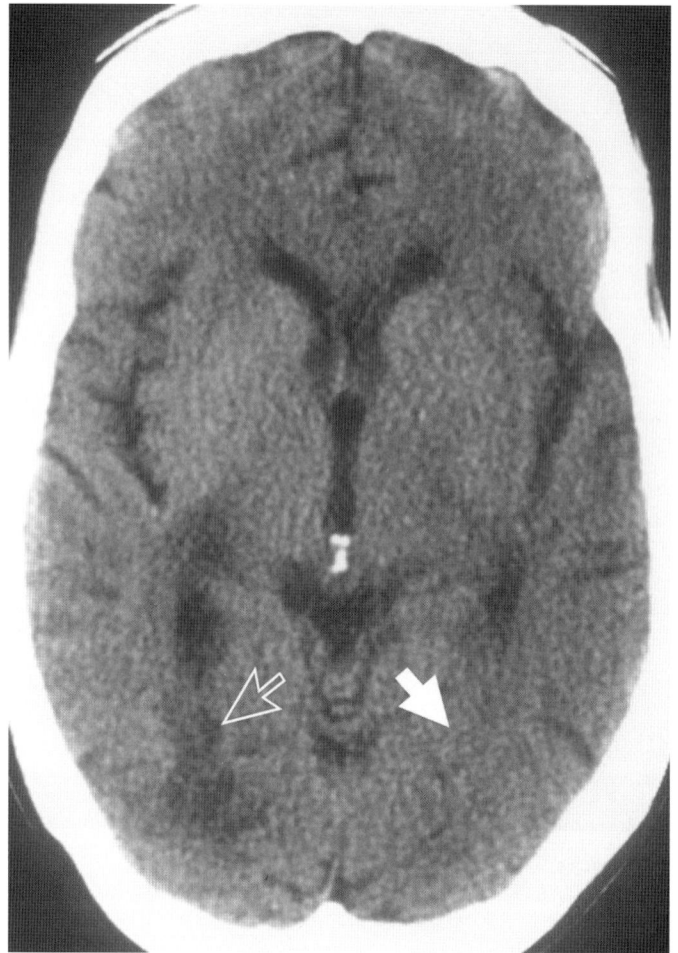

Figure 8–34. Progressive multifocal leukoencephalopathy in a patient with AIDS and a left homonymous hemianopia. The noncontrast CT scan demonstrates hypodensity of the optic radiations, affecting the right hemisphere (open arrow) more than the left (closed arrow).

CT scanning usually reveals diffuse white matter hypodensities in the posterior optic radiations (**Fig. 8–34**). MRI is best at demonstrating the extent and confluence of white matter involvement (see **Fig. 9–8**). The lesions are hypointense on T1-weighted MR images and hyperintense on T2-weighted images, and mass effect is typically absent. The lack of gadolinium enhancement usually distinguishes PML radiographically from CNS lymphoma.[335] However, a small number of cases of PML exhibit gadolinium enhancement, particularly around the lesion border. Magnetization transfer imaging, which is sensitive to demyelination, may aid in the radiologic diagnosis.[336] Routine cerebrospinal fluid examination is generally unhelpful although polymerase chain reaction testing for the JC virus in the CSF is highly sensitive and specific for PML.[337,338] If necessary, the diagnosis may be confirmed by stereotactic biopsy.

No direct treatment has been proven to be effective. Despite supportive anecdotal reports,[339] larger studies have demonstrated that neither intravenous nor intrathecal cytarabine improve survival in patients with PML.[340] Alpha-interferon,[323] cidofovir,[328] and mirtazapine[341] have also been used. However, the use of highly active antiretroviral therapy (HAART) aimed at reducing HIV load seems also to improve the prognosis of PML.[342] This regimen is sometimes combined with cidofovir, another antiviral agent.[343] Reversal of immunosuppression with HAART, on the other hand, within weeks may lead to immune reconstitution inflammatory syndrome (IRIS), a severe inflammatory reaction to the JC virus.[344,345] IRIS, characterized by clinical deterioration and contrast-enhancing lesions on MRI, is treated effectively with corticosteroids.[346] In patients who develop PML while on natalizumab, plasma exchange may accelerate drug clearance and restore lymphocyte function.[347]

Creutzfeldt–Jakob disease

Uncommonly, hemianopias or quadrantanopias may be the initial presentation of CJD in the Heidenhain (occipito-parietal) variant,[348–350] and the neuroimaging, neurological examination, and electroencephalography may be inconclusive in the early stages of the disease. However, usually by the time visual field loss is evident in patients with CJD, they are too demented for acuity and formal visual field testing. In the more advanced stages, patients with CJD often exhibit cortical blindness.[351] Like Alzheimer's disease, CJD is more commonly associated with higher cortical visual disorders, therefore it is discussed in more detail in Chapter 9.

Abscesses

The presence of infectious cerebral abscesses is suggested by fever, seizures, headache, acute or subacute focal neurologic signs and symptoms, and multiple rim-enhancing masses on MRI or CT. The differential diagnosis includes bacterial, fungal, and parasitic infections.[352] Although contiguous infection and penetrating trauma are two recognized mechanisms, hematogenous spread is the most common cause.

Causative bacterial agents include aerobes (e.g., *Streptococcus viridans* and *Staphylococcus aureus,*), anaerobes (e.g., *Peptostreptococcus*), treponemes (syphilitic gummas), and mycobacteria (tuberculomas). The usual settings for bacterial abscesses are endocarditis, dental procedures, sinus disease, trauma, and sepsis.[353] Fungal infections include aspergillus, cryptococcomas, histoplasmosis, coccidioidomycosis, and blastomycosis (**Fig. 8–25**). These infections, especially aspergillus, are well recognized in immunocompromised patients following bone marrow or liver transplantation.[354] Common parasitic abscesses include toxoplasmosis, which should be considered in any patients infected with HIV,[355,356] and cysticercosis, which should be suspected in individuals from endemic areas or with a travel history to central America or southeast Asia.

The diagnosis of a cerebral abscess usually can be established based upon blood cultures or serum serologies, but occasionally needle or open biopsy is required. The appropriate antibacterial, antifungal, or antiparasitic drug can then be administered.

Trauma

Hemianopias and other types of retrochiasmal field loss can result from intra-axial and extra-axial disturbances related to head trauma. The most common setting is a motor vehicle accident,[357] and one mechanism is diffuse and focal axonal injury affecting the optic radiations. Diffuse axonal injury, characterized by axonal stretching or tearing in the corpus callosum, subcortical white matter, cerebellar peduncles, and brain stem, results from shearing forces due to rotational acceleration and deceleration.[358,359] Radiographically, punctate hemorrhages and edema are frequently evident acutely, but later atrophy and encephalomalacia often supervene.

Occasionally, conventional neuroimaging studies may be normal despite the presence of traumatically induced homonymous hemianopia. In such situations functional neuroimaging such as positron emission tomography (PET) or single photon emission computerized tomography (SPECT) may confirm the localization of the suspected injury.[360]

If large enough, subdural and epidural hematomas overlying the cerebral convexities may compress the optic radiations. Intra-axial hematomas may also occur. Downward herniation in these settings may lead to impingement of the PCA and occipital lobe stroke. Other causes of injury include falls and penetration by sharp objects and gun shots.[357] In children, transient cortical visual loss may occur following minor or apparently trivial trauma. Blindness usually resolves within 24 hours, and neuroimaging is typically normal. Purported mechanisms include migrainous visual loss or vasospasm.[361]

Alzheimer's disease

Rarely, patients with Alzheimer's disease may present with a hemianopia (**Fig. 8–35**).[362–365] However, more commonly the visual deficits in Alzheimer's disease are visuospatial due to involvement of the visual association cortices, and the geniculocalcarine pathways are spared.[366,367] Thus this disorder is discussed in more detail in Chapter 9 (Disorders of higher cortical visual function).

Demyelination

Small lesions in the optic radiations, which are very common radiographically in multiple sclerosis, are usually clinically silent.[368] However, uncommonly a large demyelinating lesion in the optic radiations may cause a homonymous hemianopia.[15,46,369] This may occur in the setting of idiopathic demyelination, multiple sclerosis, or acute disseminated encephalomyelitis. Similar to optic neuritis, the prognosis for spontaneous visual recovery is good, with or without corticosteroids.[15]

Large demyelinating lesions, particularly when contrast enhancing with surrounding edema on MRI, may mimic a neoplasm in so-called *tumefactive multiple sclerosis* (**Fig. 8–36**).[370–373] Unfortunately some affected patients may undergo biopsy or surgical resection of the mass, resulting in permanent visual field deficits, before the correct diagnosis of a more benign demyelinating disorder is made histopathologically. More destructive demyelinating lesions

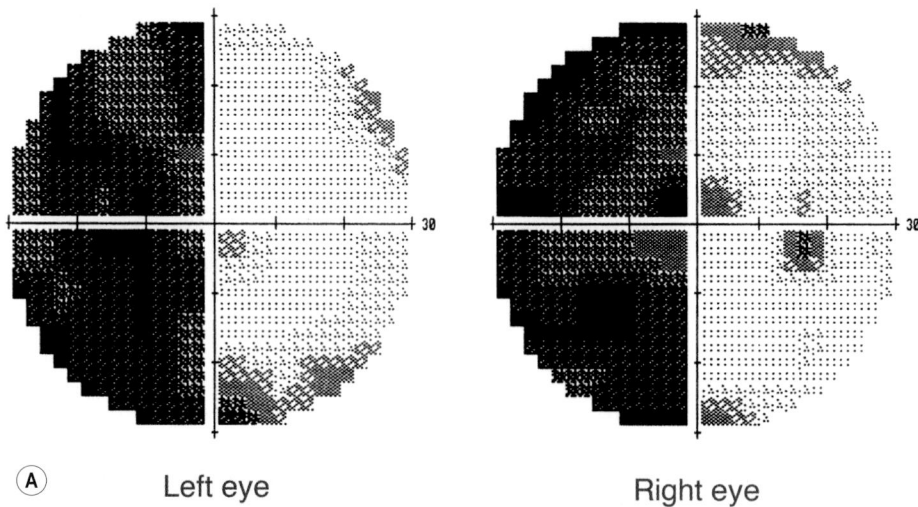

(A)   Left eye   Right eye

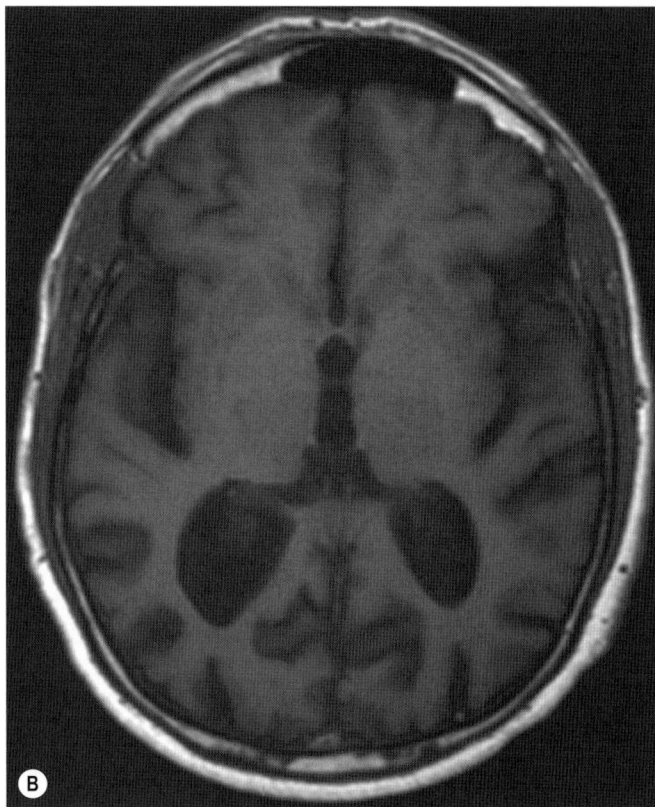

Figure 8–35. Left homonymous hemianopia (**A**) associated with posterior cortical atrophy due to the visual variant of Alzheimer's disease. Computerized perimetry grayscale output. **B**. This patient's T1-weighted MRI exhibited cortical atrophy posteriorly (bottom of figure) more than anteriorly (top of figure).

in the optic radiations may be seen in acute hemorrhagic leukoencephalitis (see **Fig.** 9–10).

Congenital/infantile disturbances

Most of the etiologies discussed here included those which occur in utero or due to birth injury. Children with unilateral hemianopias since birth are often without visual complaints and may escape detection.[374,375] On the other hand, if the visual loss is bilateral, children can present with poor fixation, nystagmus, or strabismus.[376] Visual acuity may be severely affected in bilateral cases, sometimes as poor as no light perception in both eyes.[377] The terms cortical blindness and cortical or cerebral visual impairment have been used to describe patients with visual loss due to retrogeniculate

lesions without major ocular disease.[378] We prefer the term *central visual impairment* because often both cortical and subcortical structures are affected and it allows for the term's use with various degrees of visual loss.

Because of the congenital nature of the retrochiasmal visual dysfunction, many affected patients develop an abnormal optic disc appearance resulting from transsynaptic degeneration. Commonly recognized subtypes of associated disc abnormalities in this setting include homonymous hemianopic hypoplasia associated with unilateral hemispheric injury (see Chapter 5),[379] optic nerve hypoplasia, dysplasia, or atrophy, and enlarged cupping.[380]

Associated esotropia or exotropia is common in children with central visual impairment.[381] Nystagmus may also be observed, but it is usually not a feature of isolated, congenital retrochiasmal lesions unless secondary optic disc abnor-

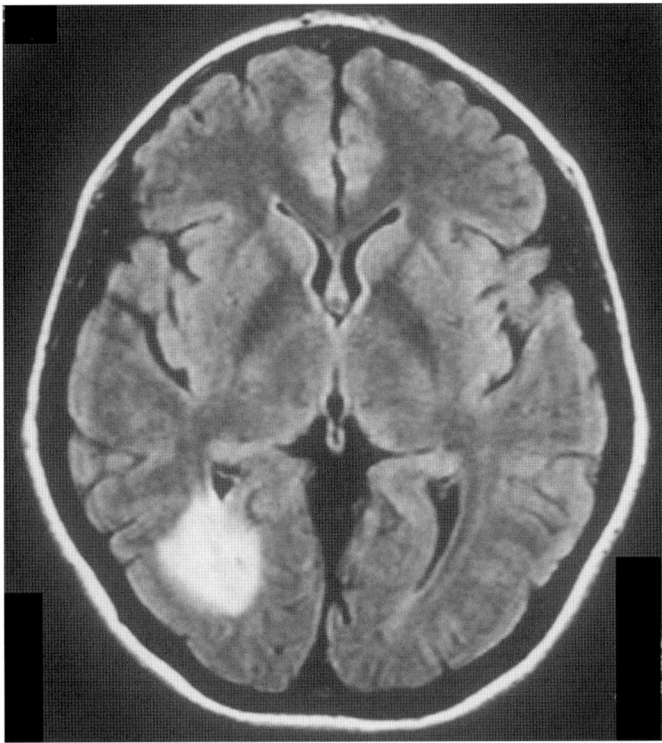

Figure 8–36. Tumefactive demyelination. Axial FLAIR MRI in a woman with an incomplete left homonymous hemianopia and a high signal lesion in the occipital lobe. Because the lesion was thought to be a tumor, a biopsy was performed and revealed macrophages and demyelination.

malities are also present.[382] Extrastriate lesions may result in optic ataxia and simultagnosia and other higher cortical visual perceptual disorders (see Chapter 9).[383–385]

Periventricular leukomalacia is the most common cause of central visual impairment in preterm infants, while hypoxic ischemic encephalopathy is the most common cause in term infants.[386,387] Because these two disorders are usually bilateral, they are less common etiologies in children with unilateral hemianopias, in whom neoplasms are more frequent.[6]

Periventricular leukomalacia

In premature and low birthweight infants, there is a predilection for ischemic injury of the posterior periventricular white matter. Immature vascular development, watershed ischemia, and disturbances of myelinogenesis have been suggested mechanisms to account for the prenatal vulnerability of the white matter in these locales.[388–390] CT and MRI frequently demonstrate reduced amounts of periventricular white matter and ventricular dilation, particularly where the optic radiations course around the occipital horn of the lateral ventricle. Affected areas are often hyperintense on T2-weighted MR images (**Fig. 8–37**),[391] but these changes may not be evident until the child is several months or a year old, once myelination has occurred. Usually the process is bilateral, but for unclear reasons occasionally one hemisphere can be involved much more than the other.[392] More severe cases, frequently resulting in central visual impairment,[393] may be associated with cystic leukomalacia or a history of intraventricular hemorrhage and hydrocephalus. Congenital nystagmus with mixed pendular and jerk

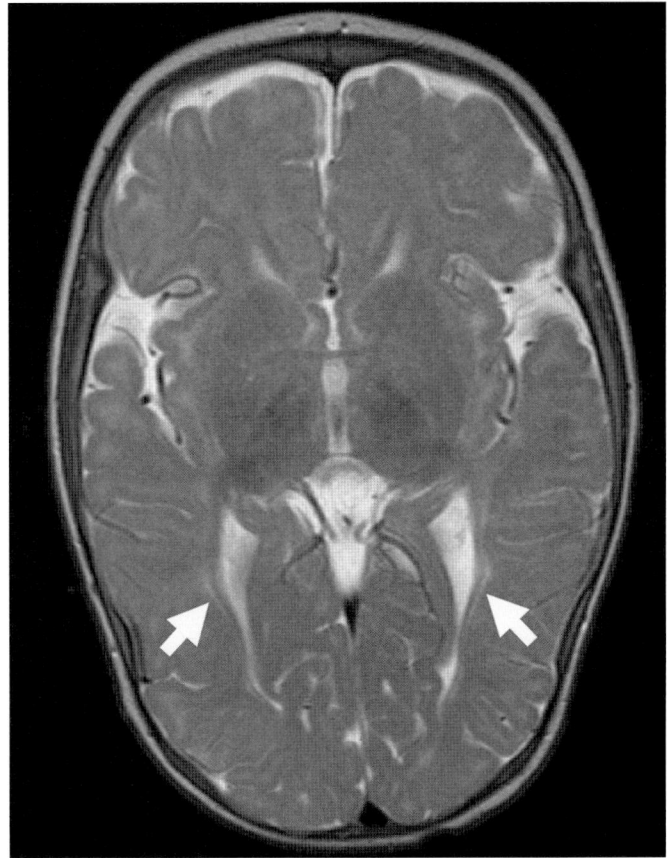

Figure 8–37. T2-weighted MRI showing periventricular leukomalacia in an infant born at prematurely at 32 weeks. High signal and thinning of the posterior periventricular white matter (arrows), with associated mild dilation of the adjacent posterior horns of the lateral ventricles, are seen.

waveforms can occur. In addition, for uncertain reasons latent nystagmus (see Chapter 17), which is usually not seen in association with specific neurologic lesions, may also be observed in patients with periventricular leukomalacia.[382,387,394]

Stroke in utero

Occasionally a child with a hemianopia is found to have a porencephalic (filled with CSF) lesion, which respects the MCA or PCA vascular territories.[395] An in utero vascular insult is presumed to have caused the cortical abnormality. In addition to the visual field defect, children with in utero MCA strokes usually have a hemiparesis and hemibody atrophy.[396] Often the etiology of the stroke is not found, and a placental embolus is a frequent presumed cause. Both the child and the mother should be evaluated for hypercoagulable disorders.[397]

Hypoxic ischemic encephalopathy

In contrast to the aforementioned prenatal disorders, hypoxic ischemic encephalopathy is more typically associated with perinatal birth asphyxia.[398,399] Neuroimaging typically demonstrates diffuse tissue loss involving white and gray matter structures with compensatory ventricular dilation (**Fig. 8–38**) The changes may be severe, resulting in cystic encephalomalacia. The children may exhibit microcephaly,

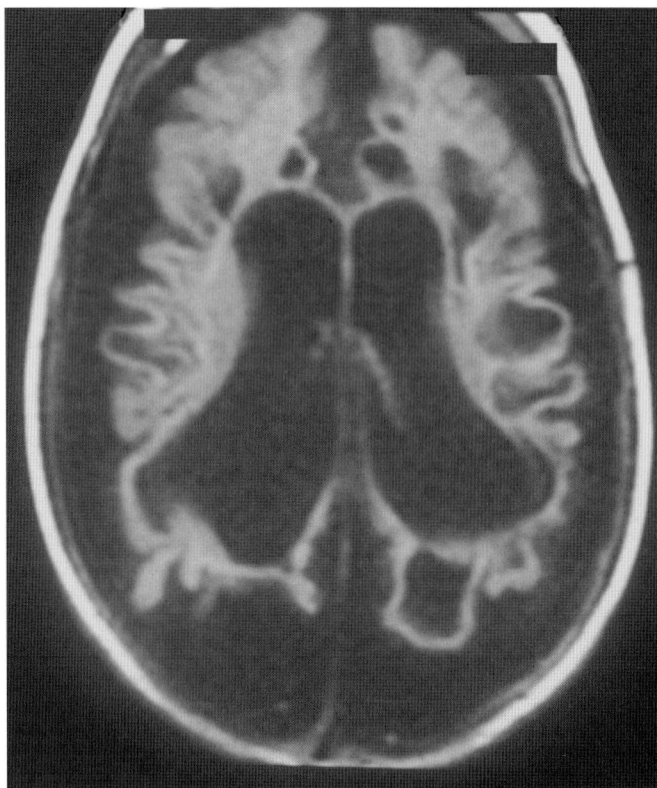

Figure 8–38. Hypoxemic–ischemic encephalopathy in a child with microcephaly, spasticity, developmental delay, and cortical blindness following perinatal asphyxia. The T1-weighted MRI shows severe encephalomalacia.

developmental delay, cortical visual loss, quadriparesis, spasticity, and seizures. Visual function may be as poor as "tunnel" vision, light perception only, and even no light perception.[400] The severity of visual dysfunction typically correlates with the amount of radiographically evident damage to the optic radiations and striate and parastriate cortices.[378,401,402]

Cortical dysplasia

Congenital retrochiasmal field loss may also be caused by cerebral cortex which is malformed and dysfunctional.[395,403] Dysplastic cortex, usually a disorder of cortical migration, is characterized radiographically by the absence of the normal gyral and sulcal pattern, seen best on MRI. Generalized developmental disorders of cerebral cortex include lissencephaly (agyria), pachygyria, band heterotopia, subependymal heterotopias, and hemimegalencephaly.[404] In addition to focal cortical dysplasias, other focal processes include polymicrogyria, focal subcortical heterotopias, schizencephaly, which is characterized by cerebral clefts,[405] and tuberous sclerosis (see Chapter 4, Retinal disorders).[404] The most common presentation of a cortical dysplasia is epilepsy.[406]

Delayed visual maturation

This well-recognized condition is characterized by abnormal visual function in the first year of life despite apparently normal and intact visual pathways.[407] Despite the absence of fixing or following, the child's pupillary reactivity, fundus appearance, visual evoked potentials, electroretinograms, and neuroimaging are all normal. Uniformly, vision improves spontaneously over weeks or months. Nystagmus rarely may also be seen at presentation, but this also resolves.[408] Delayed myelination of the posterior visual pathways, delayed dendrite and synapse formation in the striate cortex, and temporary visual inattention have been implicated.[409] Most of the children are neurologically normal, but some have developmental delays that improve along with the vision or persist.[409] Masqueraders, such as Leber's congenital amaurosis and saccadic disorders such as congenital ocular motor apraxia (see Chapter 16),[410] must be excluded.

Other childhood disorders

Mitochondrial myopathy, encephalopathy, lactic acidosis and stroke-like episodes

Mitochondrial myopathy, encephalopathy, lactic acidosis and stroke-like episodes (MELAS), first characterized by Pavlakis et al.,[411] is a mitochondrial disorder typified clinically by recurrent migraine or stroke-like episodes in children and young adults. Attacks usually consist of headache, nausea, vomiting, and focal and generalized seizures, followed by transient hemianopia, cortical blindness, or hemiparesis.[412,413] Other less commonly associated ophthalmologic features include bilateral ptosis, chronic external ophthalmoplegia, diffuse choroidal atrophy, atypical pigmentary retinopathy with macular involvement, optic atrophy, and patchy atrophy of the iris stroma.[414–416] However, the ocular findings are usually absent.

Onset is usually in childhood, and cases after age 40 are exceptional.[417–420] There is usually a history of normal early development, short stature, and exercise intolerance due to muscle weakness, and some patients may also have sensorineural hearing loss, diabetes mellitus, or cardiomyopathy.[421,422] However, progressive neurologic decline, dementia, and eventually death is the typical course. An earlier onset of symptoms (<2 years) is associated with more rapid progression.[423]

MELAS is a relatively uncommon disorder, and was not included in a childhood series of hemifield loss which spanned 3.5 years.[6] In a study of 38 patients between 18 and 45 years of age with an occipital lobe stroke, MELAS was diagnosed in one.[424]

Diagnostic studies. Eighty to ninety percent of patients with MELAS have an associated point mutation in the mitochondrial DNA at nucleotide 3243 of tRNA$^{Leu(UUR)}$.[417] Less common mutations are seen at nucleotide 3271 of tRNA$^{Leu(UUR)}$, in the subunits 4 and 5 of complex I (ND4 and ND5),[417,425] and at nucleotide 1642 of tRNA^{Val}.[426] The defective translation of leucine codons due to the tRNA mutation results in decreased normal synthesis of a number of mitochondrial proteins. These patients therefore demonstrate a number of mitochondrial biochemical defects, which result in impaired energy metabolism, excessive free radical generation, and dysregulated apoptosis.

Serum and cerebrospinal fluid lactate are typically elevated. MELAS, along with Kearn–Sayre syndrome, chronic external ophthalmoplegia (see Chapter 15), and MERRF (myoclonic epilepsy with ragged red fibers) are the mitochondrial myopathies associated with ragged red fibers on muscle biopsy. During stroke-like episodes, T2-weighted MRI can reveal hyperintensities in the temporal, parietal, and occipital cortices, not respecting the usual MCA or PCA vascular territories.[427] Acutely the lesions may be hyperintense on diffusion-weighted MRI with no or only a minor reduction in apparent diffusion coefficient.[420,428] MR spectroscopy may reveal increased lactate in the occipital and temporal lobes,[427,429] and on CT scanning basal ganglia calcification may be seen.[429]

Pathology. Affected cortical areas are characterized pathologically by spongy degeneration most prominent at the crests of gyri, and on electron microscopy the blood vessels contain abnormal mitochondria within the vascular smooth muscle and in endothelial cells.[427] Muscle biopsies may reveal ragged red fibers and other evidence of defective mitochondria.[420,430] The stroke-like episodes have been attributed to mitochondrial angiopathy or energy failure.[431]

Treatment. Vitamins, coenzymes (Q10 for example), riboflavin, nicotinamide,[432] dichloroacetate,[426] and L-arginine[433] have been associated with either anectodal improvement in clinical symptoms and signs or decrease in serum lactate.[421] However, most current treatments are unable to alter the ultimate progression of the disease.

Adrenoleukodystrophy

In this rare X-linked childhood disorder of young boys, CNS demyelination is caused by defective peroxisomal very long-chain fatty acid (VLCFA) metabolism.[434,435] The responsible mutations on Xp28 cause aberrations in the adrenoleukodystrophy (ALD) protein, which normally facilitates VLCFA-CoA synthetase enzyme function.[436] As a result, VLCFAs accumulate in the brain white matter and adrenal glands, leading to abnormal behavior and cognition, visual loss, gait disturbances, skin hyperpigmentation, and hypoadrenalism.[437] The neurologic and systemic abnormalities usually precede the visual manifestations by several years. Visual disturbances, which are either retrochiasmal or due to optic nerve demyelination with associated optic atrophy, are typically relentlessly progressive in untreated cases.[438,439] The diagnosis is suggested when elevated levels of serum VLCFAs are detected. MRI may reveal characteristic parieto-occipital white matter signal abnormalities (**Fig. 8–39**), and biochemical changes may be demonstrated on MR spectoscopy.[440] Treatments include Lorenzo oil or bone marrow transplantation.[441] An adult form[442,443] and an adrenomyeloneuropathic variant[444,445] have also been described.

Sturge–Weber (encephalotrigeminal angiomatosis)

This phakomatosis is characterized by a facial capillary hemangioma accompanied by an ipsilateral leptomeningeal vascular malformation (**Fig. 8–40**).[446] The inheritance pattern is sporadic.[447] The facial lesion has a port wine color and is usually unilateral on the upper part of the face. Port wine

stains which are bilateral or involve the eyelid or all three trigeminal distributions on one side are associated with a greater risk of eye or brain complications.[448] Commonly associated ocular findings include ipsilateral glaucoma and a "tomato ketchup" fundus due to choroidal involvement by the hemangioma. Infantile-onset glaucoma is likely due to chamber angle anomalies, while glaucoma which occurs later in life is attributed to hemangioma-associated elevated episcleral venous pressures.[449]

The intracranial vascular disturbance, leptomeningeal angiomatosis, is usually located in the posterior half of the brain. It can often cause a homonymous hemianopia, seizures, developmental delay, or hemiparesis.[450–452] On neuroimaging, cortical atrophy, leptomeningeal enhancement, and gyriform cortical calcification are pathognomonic.[449,453] Transient field defects may be the result of seizures or ischemia. Seizures refractory to medications may require focal cortical resection[454] or hemispherectomy.[455]

Meningitis

Cortical damage associated with bacterial meningitis may be caused by arterial occlusion or venous thrombosis. More severely affected children can develop encephalomalacia with loculated cysts.

Ictal

Both ictal homonymous hemianopias and ictal cortical blindness are well recognized but infrequent.[456] In this setting decreased visual attention due to sedation caused by anticonvulsants such as phenobarbital or benzodiazepines should also be considered. Also, occipital lobe seizures due to nonketotic hyperglycemia should be considered in a patient with a homonymous hemianopia but normal neuroimaging.[457–459] Postictal hemifield loss and cortical blindness are even less common and suggest an underlying, irritative structural lesion. Visual loss associated with seizures is discussed in more detail in Chapter 10, Transient visual loss.

Functional

Functional homonymous hemifield loss is unusual and is discussed in Chapter 11, Functional visual loss.

Diagnostic evaluation in patients with suspected retrochiasmal lesions

Neuroimaging

All patients with homonymous hemianopias require neuroimaging, preferably MRI. Attention to the sella and optic tract is required when the field defect is associated with optic atrophy or an afferent pupillary defect. When a stroke is suspected, because of the sudden onset of visual loss in a middle-aged or an elderly patient with vasculopathic risk factors, diffusion-weighted, FLAIR, and perfusion images can be obtained in addition to routine T1- and T2-weighted and gadolinium-enhanced scans. When MRI is contraindicated, due to claustrophobia, cardiac pacemaker, or aneurysm

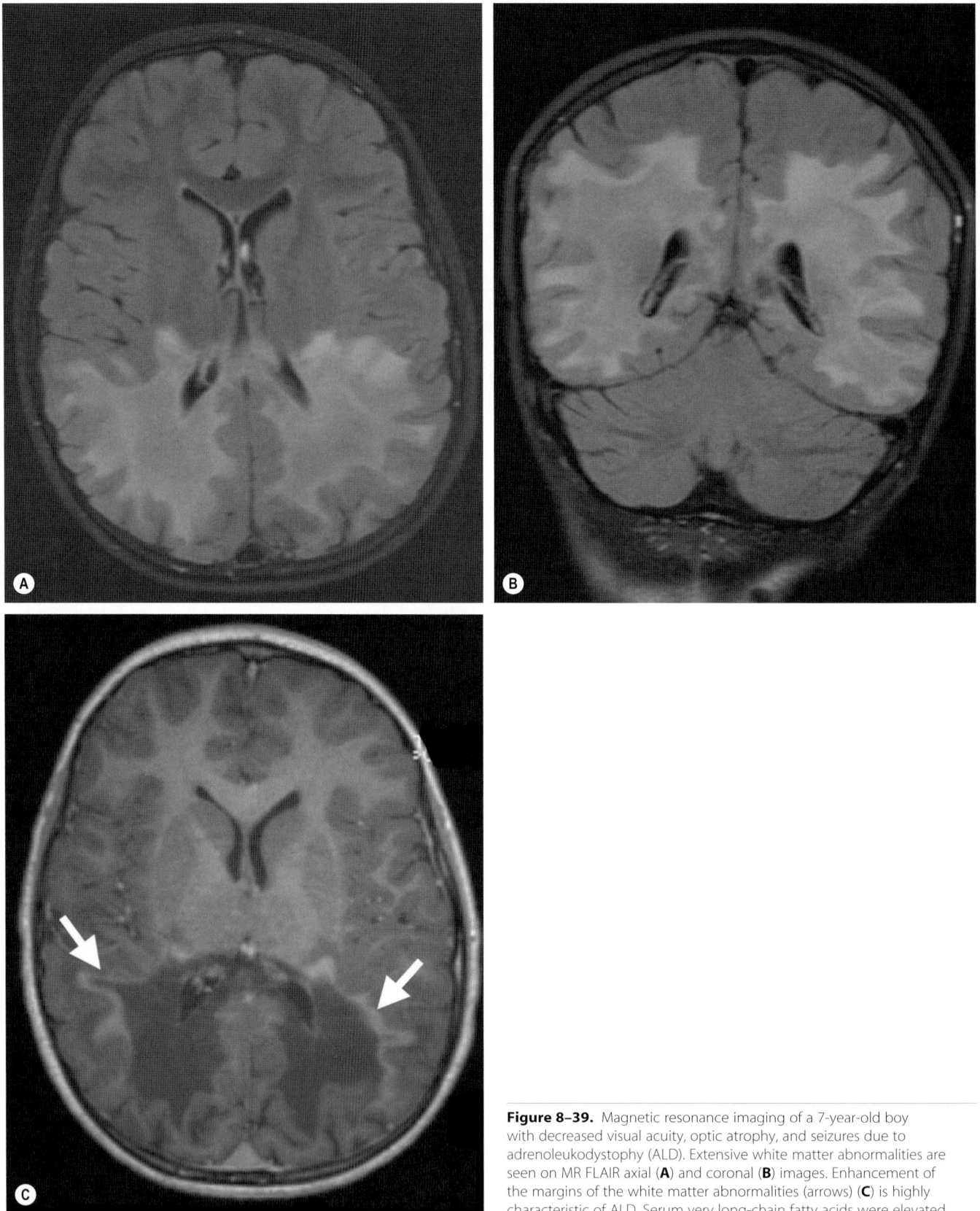

Figure 8–39. Magnetic resonance imaging of a 7-year-old boy with decreased visual acuity, optic atrophy, and seizures due to adrenoleukodystophy (ALD). Extensive white matter abnormalities are seen on MR FLAIR axial (**A**) and coronal (**B**) images. Enhancement of the margins of the white matter abnormalities (arrows) (**C**) is highly characteristic of ALD. Serum very long-chain fatty acids were elevated.

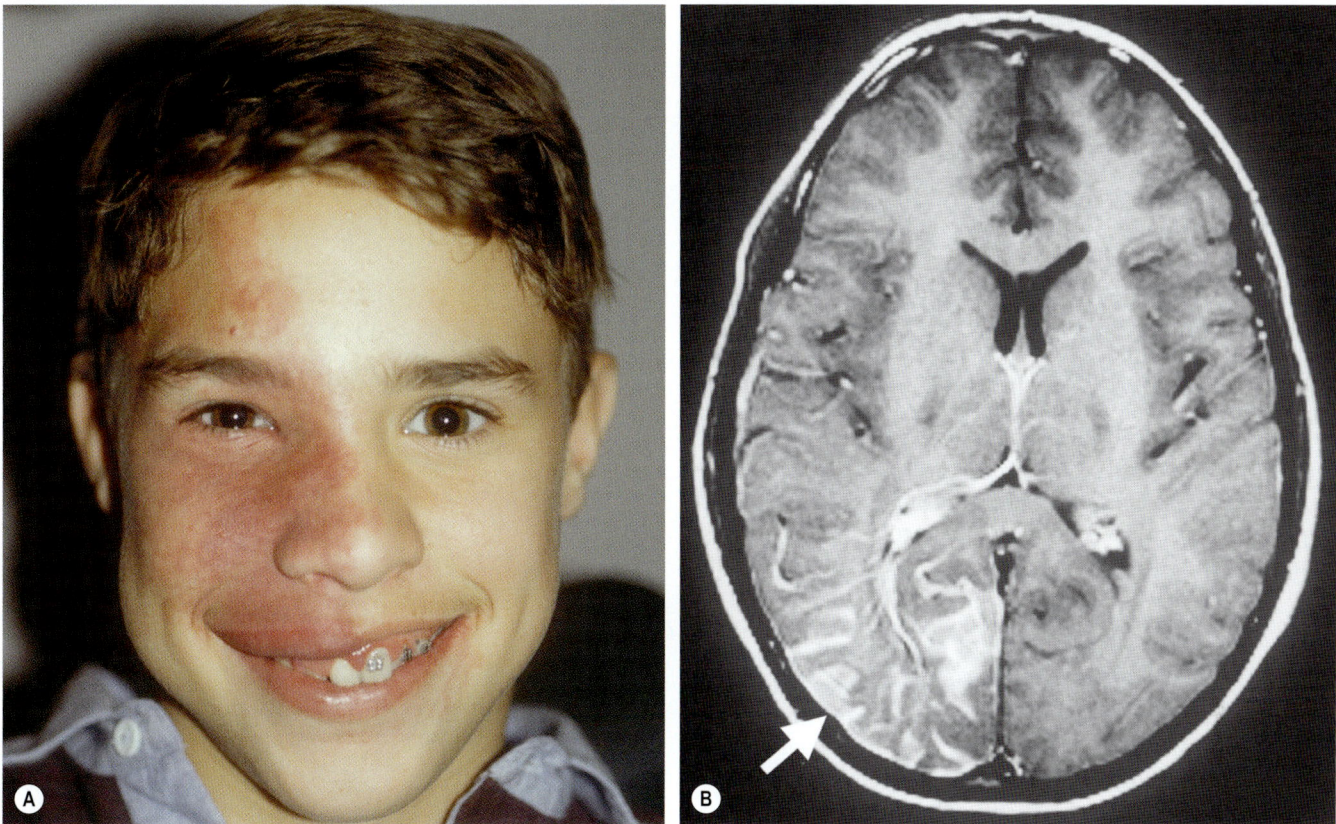

Figure 8–40. Sturge–Weber. This teenage boy with a (**A**) right facial angioma had a transient left homonymous hemianopia. **B**. Gyral enhancement (arrow) of the right occipital lobe was demonstrated on magnetic resonance imaging.

clips, for example, then CT with and without contrast can be performed.

Vascular anatomy may be assessed with MR or CT angiography of the circle of Willis, carotid arteries, and vertebral arteries. Cerebral angiography may be necessary for more definitive evaluation, such as prior to endarterectomy.

Some experimental functional neuroimaging techniques may be helpful in cases where MRI or CT is inconclusive. Using PET or SPECT techniques, hypoperfusion in visual cortex areas may be demonstrated in patients with unexplained visual field loss.[360,460,461] Functional MRI can highlight areas of cortical activation by detecting small changes in local blood flow.[462–465] This technique may be more helpful for localization of normally functioning areas of brain.

Other diagnostic studies

Blood studies are indicated when specific pathologic processes are suspected. Vascular events may require evaluation of the ESR, rapid plasmin reagin (RPR), anti-nuclear antibody (ANA), and coagulation indices such as prothrombin time, partial thromboplastin time (PT and PTT), and platelet count. The ESR and C-reactive protein are particularly important in the evaluation of transient or permanent visual loss in elderly people to rule out giant cell arteritis. In young individuals without an obvious risk factor for stroke, protein C, protein S, antithrombin III, factor V, antiphospholipid

antibody, and anticardiolipin antibody levels should be obtained. Cardiac source emboli can be excluded by an electrocardiogram, cardiac monitoring (telemetry or Holter), and transthoracic echocardiogram (TTE). If the TTE is unrevealing, and a patent foramen ovale or valvular abnormality is still highly suspected, then a transesophageal echocardiogram (TEE) can be ordered.

Other noninvasive vascular techniques may complement MRA in the patient with a suspected stroke. These include carotid Doppler studies, which are most helpful in the evaluation of extracranial carotid artery disease, and transcranial Doppler studies, which may aid in the detection of intracranial stenosis, collateral flow, and vasospasm.

A toxicology screen is necessary if drug use is suspected. Most intracranial mass lesions require either at least brain biopsy if a primary neoplasm is suspected, or a metastatic evaluation if multiple metastases are more likely. In many cases of demyelinating disease, other autoimmune, inflammatory, and infectious disorders should be excluded by evaluating the ANA, ACE, Lyme titer, and ESR for instance.

Visual evoked potentials (VEPs) may have a useful role in children with cortical visual impairment, as a normal study may be associated with a favorable visual outcome.[407] However, an abnormal VEP does not preclude visual improvement,[466] so they have not become part of our usual evaluation in such patients. Standard and even multifocal VEPs probable have no clinical utility in adults with retrochiasmal field loss.[467]

Practical advice, hemianopic prisms, and visual rehabilitation

Initially, patients with acquired homonymous hemianopias may not notice their field defect, especially if a right hemispheric lesion is responsible. Eventually, however, most adult patients become aware of their defective peripheral vision.

Those with dense field deficits may bump into objects in their blind hemifield. We caution affected patients that they must turn their head to see into the defective field, but most learn to do that anyway. We also instruct family members to approach the patient from within the intact hemifield, and keep food, utensils, and beverages within the patient's intact hemifield when eating. At least initially, patients with dense hemianopias should not be allowed to cross the street independently. Furthermore, their defective vision makes driving problematic, and in many states and countries illegal.

Many have difficult reading, because a left hemianopia may hamper their ability to find the beginning of the next line, and a right hemianopia may not allow them to appreciate the entire line of words (*hemianopic alexia*). Macular splitting and paracentral defects may make seeing individual words difficult. A colored piece of paper placed vertically along the left or right side of the page is often helpful when loss of the margins is source of difficulty. It can also be used horizontally and moved down the lines of the page. Other strategies include teaching patients with left hemianopias to shift their gaze to the left side of every line and to the first letter of every word, and instructing those with right hemianopias to reach the end of a word before going to the next.[142]

In a rare compensatory phenomenon, children with a congenital or early-onset hemianopia may develop an exotropic eye and head turn, both toward the field defect. An adaptive mechanism to increase the useful visual field has been postulated.[468]

Hemianopic prisms

Patients with chronic, dense homonymous hemianopias can be offered optical assistance from prisms,[469,470] but only a minority of them will find it beneficial. Base-out prism therapy should be attempted only in individuals who have normal mentation and in whom the hemianopia is isolated. A 15–45 (usually 30) diopter base out Fresnel press-on prism can be placed on the temporal half of an eyeglass ipsilateral to the hemianopia (**Fig. 8–41**). This optically displaces images in the blind half of vision toward the good hemifield. A central area can be trimmed from the Fresnel prism to reduce double vision. The patients who like the prism therapy are those who use the prism to notice novel objects in their blind field; they then turn their head in that direction to use their good field to see the objects more clearly. Unfortunately, most individuals find this too confusing and suboptimal and only 20–30% continue to use it. It certainly does not improve their vision to the point they can drive or read normally. Other prism combinations have been tried with some purported success.[471] Wide-angle lenses

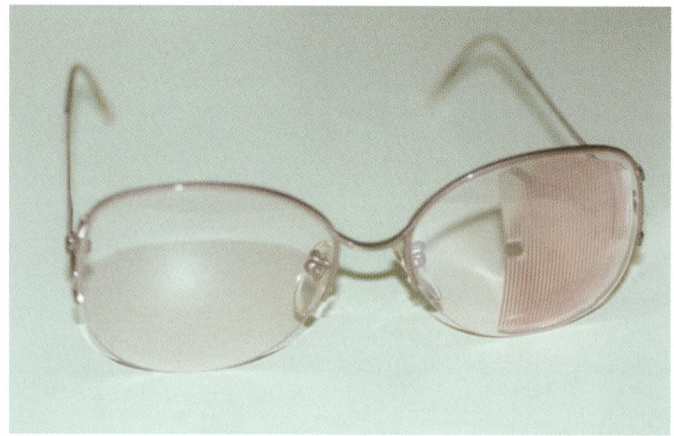

Figure 8–41. Hemianopic prism for an individual with a left homonymous visual field defect. A 30 diopter base out Fresnel prism is placed over the temporal half of the left lens. A notch was cut out over the optical center to reduce double vision.

or mirror devices attached to the spectacle frame have also been used with limited improvement.

Visual rehabilitation

We have found that visual occupational therapy and rehabilitation can be marginally helpful. Compensatory oculomotor strategies, designed to enhance visual saccades into and exploration within the defective hemifield, may be tried.[142,472] In one study of patients with homonymous hemianopia, explorative saccade training was associated with improved saccadic behavior, natural search and scene exploration.[473] In another, optokinetic therapy improved text reading in patients with hemianopic alexia.[474]

Training of blindsight and recovering some lost visual field have also been attempted.[142,475,476] One type, vision restoration therapy, is a costly home-based computerized treatment with repetitive stimulation on both sides of a border of a visual field defect. Many patients seem to benefit from these types of therapies in terms of reading and watching TV, for instance.[477] However, it is highly controversial whether this improvement is the result of learning to saccade or attend into blind fields, changes in cortical connections, or harnessing of extrastriate areas dedicated to vision such as those for color and motion.[478–484] Some authors have proposed that the recovery is mediated by different visual circuits outside of V1 such as those involving area V5. Nonetheless, the debate continues whether such improvements are the result of testing parameters that do not adequately control for fixation shifts or from small residual islands of residual V1 vision.[485] Actual expansion of the intact visual field does not seem to occur,[477,486] and some experts have argued that neuroplasticity is unlikely.[487] Therefore, we believe, further studies are needed to answer the questions about how visual rehabilitation works and the extent of its effectiveness. For many patients there is going to be a balance of the cost of the training versus the actual benefit.[482]

References

1. Smith JL. Homonymous hemianopia. A review of 100 cases. Am J Ophthalmol 1962;54:616–622.

2. Trobe JD, Lorber ML, Schlezinger NS. Isolated homonymous hemianopia. A review of 104 cases. Arch Ophthalmol 1973;89:377–381.

3. Fujino T, Kigazawa K, Yamada R. Homonymous hemianopia. A retrospective study of 140 cases. Neuro-ophthalmology 1986;6:17–21.

4. Zhang X, Kedar S, Lynn MJ, et al. Homonymous hemianopias. Clinical-anatomic correlations in 904 cases. Neurology 2006;66:906–910.

5. Kedar S, Zhang X, Lynn MJ, et al. Pediatric homonymous hemianopia. J AAPOS 2006;10:249–252.

6. Liu GT, Galetta SL. Homonymous hemifield loss in children. Neurology 1997;49: 1748–1749.

7. Harrington DO, Drake MV. Postchiasmal visual pathway. In: The Visual Fields. Text and Atlas of Clinical Perimetry, 7th edn, pp 311–361. St. Louis, Mosby, 1990.

8. Arnold A. Congruency in homonymous hemianopia. Am J Ophthalmol 2007;143: 856–858.

9. Kedar S, Zhang X, Lynn MJ, et al. Congruency in homonymous hemianopia. Am J Ophthalmol 2007;143:772–780.

10. Kupersmith MJ. Circulation of the eye, orbit, cranial nerves, and brain. In: Neurovascular Neuro-ophthalmology, pp 1–67. Berlin, Springer-Verlag, 1993.

11. Kardon R, Kawasaki A, Miller NR. Origin of the relative afferent pupillary defect in optic tract lesions. Ophthalmology 2006;113:1345–1353.

12. Savino PJ, Paris M, Schatz NJ, et al. Optic tract syndrome. A review of 21 patients. Arch Ophthalmol 1978;96:656–663.

13. Bender MB, Bodis-Wollner I. Visual dysfunctions in optic tract lesions. Ann Neurol 1978;3:187–193.

14. Archer JS, Gracies J-M, Tohver E, et al. Bilateral optic disk pallor after unilateral internal carotid artery occlusion. Neurology 1998;50:809–811.

15. Plant GT, Kermode AG, Turano G, et al. Symptomatic retrochiasmal lesions in multiple sclerosis. Clinical features, visual evoked potentials, and magnetic resonance imaging. Neurology 1992;42:68–76.

16. Kupersmith MJ, Vargas M, Hoyt WF, et al. Optic tract atrophy with cerebral arteriovenous malformations. Direct and transsynaptic degeneration. Neurology 1994;44:80–83.

17. Guirgis MF, Lam BL, Falcone SF. Optic tract compression from dolichoectatic basilar artery. Am J Ophthalmol 2001;132:283–286.

18. Groom M, Kay MD, Vicinanza-Adami C, et al. Optic tract syndrome secondary to metastatic breast cancer. Am J Ophthalmol 1998;125:115–118.

19. Margo CE, Hamed LM, McCarty J. Congenital optic tract syndrome. Arch Ophthalmol 1991;109:1120–1122.

20. Horton JC, Landau K, Maeder P, et al. Magnetic resonance imaging of the human lateral geniculate body. Arch Neurol 1990;47:1201–1206.

21. Miki A, Raz J, Haselgrove JC, et al. Functional magnetic resonance imaging of lateral geniculate nucleus at 1.5 tesla. J Neuroophthalmol 2000;20:285–287.

22. Fujita N, Tanaka H, Takanashi M, et al. Lateral geniculate nucleus. Anatomic and functional identification by use of MR imaging. AJNR Am J Neuroradiol 2001;22: 1719–1726.

23. Carpenter MB. Blood supply of the central nervous system. In: Core Text of Neuroanatomy, 4th edn, pp 391–416. Baltimore, Williams & Wilkins, 1991.

24. Neau J-P, Bogousslavsky J. The syndrome of posterior choroidal artery territory infarction. Ann Neurol 1996;39:779–788.

25. Glaser JS, Sadun AA. Anatomy of the visual sensory system. In: Glaser JS (ed). Neuro-ophthalmology, 2nd edn, pp 61–82. Philadelphia, J.B. Lippincott, 1990.

26. Gunderson CH, Hoyt WF. Geniculate hemianopia. Incongruous homonymous field defects in two patients with partial lesions of the lateral geniculate nucleus. J Neurol Neurosurg Psychiatr 1971;34:1–6.

27. Schaklett DE, O'Connor PS, Dorwart RH, et al. Congruous and incongruous sectorial visual field defects with lesions of the lateral geniculate nucleus. Am J Ophthalmol 1984;98:283–290.

28. Carter JE, O'Connor P, Shacklett D, et al. Lesions of the optic radiations mimicking lateral geniculate nucleus visual field defects. J Neurol Neurosurg Psychiatr 1985;48: 982–988.

29. Grochowicki M, Vighetto A. Homonymous horizontal sectoranopia. Report of four cases. Br J Ophthalmol 1991;75:624–628.

30. Grossman M, Galetta SL, Nichols CW, et al. Horizontal homonymous sectoral field defect after ischemic infarction of the occipital cortex. Am J Ophthalmol 1990;109: 234–236.

31. Osborne BJ, Liu GT, Galetta SL. Geniculate quadruple sectoranopia. Neurology 2006;66:E41–42.

32. Frisén L. Quadruple sectoranopsia and sectorial optic atrophy. A syndrome of the distal anterior choroidal artery. J Neurol Neurosurg Psychiatr 1979;42:590–594.

33. Frisén L, Homegaard L, Rosencrantz M. Sectorial optic atrophy and homonymous, horizontal sectoranopsia. A lateral choroidal artery syndrome. J Neurol Neurosurg Psychiatr 1978;41:374–380.

34. Suzuki H, Fujita K, Ehara K, et al. Anterior choroidal artery syndrome after surgery for internal carotid artery aneurysms. Neurosurgery 1992;31:132–136.

35. Palomeras E, Fossas P, Cano AT, et al. Anterior choroidal artery infarction. A clinical, etiologic and prognostic study. Acta Neurol Scand 2008;118:42–47.

36. Luco C, Hoppe A, Schweitzer M, et al. Visual field defects in vascular lesions of the lateral geniculate body. J Neurol Neurosurg Psychiatr 1992;55:12–15.

37. Borruat F-X, Maeder P. Sectoranopia after head trauma. Evidence of lateral geniculate body lesion on MRI. Neurology 1995;45:590–592.

38. Kosmorsky G, Lancione RR. When fighting makes you see black holes instead of stars. J Neuroophthalmol 1998;18:255–257.

39. Donahue SP, Kardon RH, Thompson HS. Hourglass-shaped visual fields as a sign of bilateral lateral geniculate myelinolysis. Am J Ophthalmol 1995;119:378–380.

40. Barton JJ. Bilateral sectoranopia from probable osmotic demyelination. Neurology 2001;57:2318–2319.

41. Sherbondy AJ, Dougherty RF, Napel S, et al. Identifying the human optic radiation using diffusion imaging and fiber tractography. J Vis 2008;8:1–11.

42. Egan RA, Shults WT, So N, et al. Visual field deficits in conventional anterior temporal lobectomy versus amygdalohippocampectomy. Neurology 2000;55:1818–1822.

43. Barton JJ, Hefter R, Chang B, et al. The field defects of anterior temporal lobectomy. A quantitative reassessment of Meyer's loop. Brain 2005;128:2123–2133.

44. Tatu L, Moulin T, Bogousslavsky J, et al. Arterial territories of the human brain: cerebral hemispheres. Neurology 1998;50:1699–1708.

45. Hughes TS, Abou-Khalil B, Lavin PJM, et al. Visual field defects after temporal lobe resection. A prospective quantitative analysis. Neurology 1999;53:167–172.

46. Borruat F-X, Siatkowski RM, Schatz NJ, et al. Congruous quadrantanopia and optic radiation lesion. Neurology 1993;43:1430–1432.

47. Jacobson DM. The localizing value of a quadrantanopia. Arch Neurol 1997;54:401–404.

48. Cogan DG. Neurologic significance of lateral conjugate deviation of the eyes on forced closure of the lids. Arch Ophthalmol 1948;39:37–42.

49. Smith JL, Gay AJ, Cogan DG. The spasticity of conjugate gaze phenomenon. Arch Ophthalmol 1959;62:694–696.

50. Sullivan HC, Kaminski HJ, Maas EF, et al. Lateral deviation of the eyes on forced lid closure in patients with cerebral lesions. Arch Ophthalmol 1991;48:310–311.

51. Tecoma ES, Laxer KD, Barbaro NM, et al. Frequency and characteristics of visual field deficits after surgery for mesial temporal sclerosis. Neurology 1993;43:1235–1238.

52. Chen X, Weigel D, Ganslandt O, et al. Prediction of visual field deficits by diffusion tensor imaging in temporal lobe epilepsy surgery. Neuroimage 2009;45:286–297.

53. Zeki S. The P and M pathways and the 'what and where' doctrine. In: A Vision of the Brain, pp 186–196. Oxford, Blackwell Scientific, 1993.

54. Horton JC, Hoyt WF. The representation of the visual field in human striate cortex. A revision of the classic Holmes map. Arch Ophthalmol 1991;109:816–824.

55. McFadzean R, Brosnahan D, Hadley D, et al. Representation of the visual field in the occipital striate cortex. Br J Ophthalmol 1994;78:185–190.

56. Wong AMF, Sharpe JA. Representation of the visual field in human occipital cortex. Arch Ophthalmol 1999;117:208–217.

57. McFadzean RM, Hadley DM, Condon BC. The representation of the visual field in the occipital striate cortex. Neuroophthalmology 2002;27:55–78.

58. Horton JC. Arrangement of ocular dominance columns in human visual cortex. Arch Ophthalmol 1990;108:1025–1031.

59. Miki A, Liu GT, Raz J, et al. Contralateral monocular dominance in anterior visual cortex confirmed by functional magnetic resonance imaging. Am J Ophthalmol 2000;130:821–824.

60. Gray LG, Galetta SL, Schatz NJ. Vertical and horizontal meridian sparing in occipital lobe homonymous hemianopia. Neurology 1998;50:1170–1173.

61. Smith CG, Richardson WFG. The course and distribution of the arteries supplying the visual (striate) cortex. Am J Ophthalmol 1966;61:1391–1396.

62. Gasecki AP, Fox AJ, Daneault N. Bilateral occipital infarctions associated with carotid stenosis in a patient with persistent trigeminal artery. Stroke 1994;25:1520–1523.

63. Balcer LJ, Galetta SL, Hurst RW, et al. Occipital lobe infarction from a carotid artery embolic source. J Neuroophthalmol 1996;16:33–35.

64. Cucchiara BL, Kasner SE. Carotid dissection causing occipital lobe infarction. Neurology 2005;65:1408.

65. Wong AMF, Sharpe JA. A comparison of tangent screen, Goldmann, and Humphrey perimetry in the detection and localization of occipital lesions. Ophthalmology 2000;107:527–544.

66. Bischoff P, Lang J, Huber A. Macular sparing as a perimetric artifact. Am J Ophthalmol 1995;119:72–80.

67. Leff A. A historical review of the representation of the visual field in primary visual cortex with special reference to the neural mechanisms underlying macular sparing. Brain Lang 2004;88:268–278.

68. Gray LG, Galetta SL, Siegal T, et al. The central visual field in homonymous hemianopia. Arch Neurol 1997;54:312–317.

69. Trauzettel-Klosinski S, Reinhard J. The vertical field border in hemianopia and its significance for fixation and reading. Invest Ophthalmol Vis Sci 1998;39:2177–2186.

70. Kölmel HW. Homonymous paracentral scotomas. J Neurol 1987;235:22–25.

71. Benton S, Levy I, Swash M. Vision in the temporal crescent in occipital infarction. Brain 1980;103:83–97.

72. Lepore FE. The preserved temporal crescent. The clinical implications of an "endangered" finding. Neurology 2001;57:1918–1921.

73. Landau K, Wichmann W, Valavanis A. The missing temporal crescent. Am J Ophthalmol 1995;119:345–349.

74. Chavis PS, Al-Hazmi A, Clunie D, et al. Temporal crescent syndrome with magnetic resonance correlation. J Neuroophthalmol 1997;17:151–155.

75. Horton JC, Hoyt WF. Quadrantic visual field defects. A hallmark of lesions in extrastriate (V2/V3) cortex. Brain 1991;114:1703–1718.

76. McFadzean RM, Hadley DM. Homonymous quadrantanopia respecting the horizontal meridian. A feature of striate and extrastriate cortical disease. Neurology 1997;49: 1741–1746.

77. Cross SA, Smith JL. Crossed-quadrant homonymous hemianopsia. The "checkerboard" field defect. J Clin Neuroophthalmol 1982;2:149–158.

78. Newman RP, Kinkel WR, Jacobs L. Altitudinal hemianopia caused by occipital infarctions. Clinical and computerized tomographic correlations. Arch Neurol 1984;41:413–418.

79. Liu GT, Ronthal M. Reflex blink to visual threat. J Clin Neuroophthalmol 1992;12: 47–56.

80. Riddoch G. Dissociation of visual perceptions due to occipital injuries, with especial reference to appreciation of movement. Brain 1917;40:15–57.

81. Holmes G. Disturbances of vision by cerebral lesions. Br J Ophthalmol 1918;2:353–384.

82. Pöppel E, Held R, Frost D. Residual visual function after brain wounds involving the central visual pathways in man. Nature 1973;243:295–296.

83. Sanders MD, Warrington EK, Marshall J, et al. "Blindsight" vision in a field defect. Lancet 1974;1:707–708.

84. Damasio AR, Damasio H, Ferro JM, et al. Recovery from hemianopia in man. Evidence for collicular vision? Lancet 1974;2:110.

85. Weiskrantz L, Warrington EK, Sanders MD, et al. Visual capacity in the hemianopic field following a restricted occipital ablation. Brain 1974;97:709–728.

86. Barbur JL, Ruddock KH, Waterfield VA. Human visual responses in the absence of the geniculo-calcarine projection. Brain 1980;103:905–928.

87. Blythe IM, Kennard C, Ruddock KH. Residual vision in patients with retrogeniculate leisons of the visual pathways. Brain 1987;110:887–905.

88. Stoerig P, Cowey A. Blindsight in man and monkey. Brain 1997;120:535–559.

89. Weiskrantz L, Cowey A, Barbur JL. Differential pupillary constriction and awareness in the absence of striate cortex. Brain 1999;122:1533–1538.

90. Morland AB, Jones SR, Finlay AL, et al. Visual perception of motion, luminance and colour in a human hemianope. Brain 1999;122:1183–1198.

91. Zihl J, Von Cramon D. The contribution of the "second" visual system to directed visual attention in man. Brain 1979;102:835–856.

92. Schneider GE. Two visual systems. Brain mechanisms for localization and discrimination are dissociated by tectal and cortical lesions. Science 1969;163:895–902.

93. Rafal R, Smith J, Krantz J, et al. Extrageniculate vision in hemianopic humans. Saccade inhibition by signals in the blind field. Science 1990;250:118–120.

94. Zeki S, Ffytche DH. The Riddoch syndrome. Insights into the neurobiology of conscious vision. Brain 1998;121:25–45.

95. Stoerig P, Kleinschmidt A, Frahm J. No visual responses in denervated V1. High-resolution functional magnetic resonance imaging of a blindsight patient. Neuroreport 1998;9:21–25.

96. Goebel R, Muckli L, Zanella FE, et al. Sustained extrastriate cortical activation without visual awareness revealed by fMRI studies of hemianopic patients. Vision Res 2001;41: 1459–1474.

97. Schoenfeld MA, Noesselt T, Poggel D, et al. Analysis of pathways mediating preserved vision after striate cortex lesions. Ann Neurol 2002;52:814–824.

98. Leh SE, Johansen-Berg H, Ptito A. Unconscious vision. New insights into the neuronal correlate of blindsight using diffusion tractography. Brain 2006;129:1822–1832.

99. Bridge H, Thomas O, Jbabdi S, et al. Changes in connectivity after visual cortical brain damage underlie altered visual function. Brain 2008;131:1433–1444.

100. Barton JJ, Sharpe JA. Smooth pursuit and saccades to moving targets in blind hemifields. A comparison of medial occipital, lateral occipital and optic radiation lesions. Brain 1997;120:681–699.

101. Barton JJ, Sharpe JA. Motion direction discrimination in blind hemifields. Ann Neurol 1997;41:255–264.

102. Azzopardi P, Cowey A. Motion discrimination in cortically blind patients. Brain 2001;124:30–46.

103. Farah M, Feinberg TE. Perception and awareness. In: Feinberg TE, Farah MJ (eds). Behavioral Neurology and Neuropsychology, pp 357–368. New York, McGraw-Hill, 1997.

104. Fendrich R, Wessinger CM, Gazzaniga MS. Residual vision in a scotoma: implications for blindsight. Science 1992;258:1489–1491.

105. Radoeva PD, Prasad S, Brainard DH, et al. Neural activity within area V1 reflects unconscious visual performance in a case of blindsight. J Cogn Neurosci 2008;20: 1927–1939.

106. Cowey A, Stoerig P. The neurobiology of blindsight. Trends Neurosci 1991;14:140–145.

107. Campion J, Latto R, Smith YM. Is blindsight an effect of scattered light, spared cortex, and near-threshold vision? Behav Brain Sci 1983;6:423–486.

108. Safran AB, Glaser JS. Statokinetic dissociation in lesions of the anterior visual pathways. A reappraisal of the Riddoch phenomenon. Arch Ophthalmol 1980;98:291–295.

109. Liu GT. Anatomy and physiology of the trigeminal nerve. In: Miller NR, Newman NJ (eds). Walsh and Hoyt's Clinical Neuro-ophthalmology, 4th edn., pp 1595–1648. Baltimore, Williams and Wilkins, 1998.

110. Hommel M, Besson G, Pollak P, et al. Hemiplegia in posterior cerebral artery occlusion. Neurology 1990;40:1496–1499.

111. Hommel M, Moreaud O, Besson G, et al. Site of arterial occlusion in the hemiplegic posterior cerebral artery syndrome. Neurology 1991;41:604–605.

112. Yamamoto Y, Georgiadis AL, Chang H-M, et al. Posterior cerebral artery territory infarcts in the New England Medical Center posterior circulation registry. Arch Neurol 1999;56: 824–832.

113. Chambers BR, Brooder RJ, Donnan GA. Proximal posterior cerebral artery occlusion simulating middle cerebral artery occlusion. Neurology 1991;41:385–390.

114. Georgiadis AL, Yamamoto Y, Kwan ES, et al. Anatomy of sensory findings in patients with posterior cerebral artery territory infarction. Arch Neurol 1999;56:835–838.

115. Caplan LR. "Top of the basilar syndrome". Neurology 1980;30:72–79.

116. Zhang X, Kedar S, Lynn MJ, et al. Homonymous hemianopia in stroke. J Neuroophthalmol 2006;26:180–183.

117. Aldrich MS, Alessi AG, Beck RW, et al. Cortical blindness. Etiology, diagnosis, and prognosis. Ann Neurol 1987;21:149–158.

118. Albers GW, Caplan LR, Easton JD, et al. Transient ischemic attack: proposal for a new definition. N Engl J Med 2002;347:1713–1716.

119. Warach S, Kidwell CS. The redefinition of TIA. The uses and limitations of DWI in acute ischemic cerebrovascular syndromes [editorial]. Neurology 2004;62:359–360.

120. Caplan LR, Wityk RJ, Glass TA, et al. New England Medical Center Posterior Circulation registry. Ann Neurol 2004;56:389–398.

121. Devereaux MW. The neuro-ophthalmologic complications of cervical manipulation. J Neuroophthalmol 2000;20:236–239.

122. Caplan LR. Dissections of brain-supplying arteries. Nat Clin Pract Neurol 2008;4:34–42.

123. Sacco RL. Risk factors, outcomes, and stroke subtypes for ischemic stroke. Neurology 1997;49(Suppl 4):S39–S44.

124. Sacco RL. Identifying patient populations at high risk for stroke. Neurology 1998;51(Suppl 3):S27–S30.

125. Bronner LL, Kanter DS, Manson JE. Primary prevention of stroke. N Engl J Med 1995;333:1392–1400.

126. Hebert PR, Gaziano JM, Chan KS, et al. Cholesterol lowering with statin drugs, risk of stroke, and total mortality. An overview of randomized trials. JAMA 1997;278: 313–321.

127. O'Regan C, Wu P, Arora P, et al. Statin therapy in stroke prevention. A meta-analysis involving 121,000 patients. Am J Med 2008;121:24–33.

128. Fulgham JR, Ingall TJ, Stead LG, et al. Management of acute ischemic stroke. Mayo Clin Proc 2004;79:1459–1469.

129. van der Worp HB, van Gijn J. Clinical practice. Acute ischemic stroke. N Engl J Med 2007;357:572–579.

130. Adams HP, Brott TG, Furlan AJ, et al. Guidelines for thrombolytic therapy for acute stroke. A supplement to the guidelines for the management of patients with acute ischemic stroke. A statement for healthcare professionals from a special writing group of the Stroke Council, American Heart Association. Circulation 1996;94:1167–1174.

131. Lyden PD, Grotta JC, Levine SR, et al. Intravenous thrombolysis for acute stroke. Neurology 1997;49:14–29.

132. Tanne D, Bates VE, Verro P, et al. Initial clinical experience with tissue plasminogen activator for acute ischemic stroke. A multicenter survey. Neurology 1999;53:424–427.

133. Hacke W, Kaste M, Fieschi C, et al. Intravenous thrombolysis with recombinant tissue plasminogen activator for acute hemispheric stroke. The European Cooperative Acute Stroke Study (ECASS). JAMA 1995;274:1017–1025.

134. The National Institute of Neurological Disorders and Stroke rt-PA Stroke Study Group. Tissue plasminogen activator for acute ischemic stroke. N Engl J Med 1995;333: 1581–1587.

135. Morgenstern LB. rtPA in acute ischemic stroke. The North American perspective. Neurology 1997;49(Suppl 4):S63–S65.

136. Hacke W. rtPA in acute ischemic stroke. European perspective. Neurology 1997;49(Suppl 4):S60–S62.

137. Kwiatkowski TG, Libman RB, Frankel M, et al. Effects of tissue plasminogen activator for acute ischemic stroke at one year. N Engl J Med 1999;340:1781–1787.

138. Hacke W, Kaste M, Bluhmki E, et al. Thrombolysis with alteplase 3 to 4.5 hours after acute ischemic stroke. N Engl J Med 2008;359:1317–1329.

139. Coull BM, Williams LS, Goldstein LB, et al. Anticoagulants and antiplatelet agents in acute ischemic stroke. Report of the Joint Stroke Guideline Development Committee of the American Academy of Neurology and the American Stroke Association (a division of the American Heart Association). Stroke 2002;33:1934–1942.

140. Furlan A, Higashida R, Wechsler L, et al. Intra-arterial prourokinase for acute ischemic stroke. The PROACT II study: a randomized controlled trial. Prolyse in Acute Cerebral Thromboembolism. JAMA 1999;282:2003–2011.

141. Caplan LR. Treatment of patients with stroke. Arch Neurol 2002;59:703–707.

142. Pambakian AL, Kennard C. Can visual function be restored in patients with homonymous hemianopia? Br J Ophthalmol 1997;81:324–328.

143. Ovbiagele B, Kidwell CS, Saver JL. Expanding indications for statins in cerebral ischemia. A quantitative study. Arch Neurol 2005;62:67–72.

144. Elkind MS, Benesch CG. Lowering cholesterol in patients with stroke. Raising the standard [editorial]. Neurology 2006;66:1140–1141.

145. Amarenco P, Bogousslavsky J, Callahan A, 3rd, et al. High-dose atorvastatin after stroke or transient ischemic attack. N Engl J Med 2006;355:549–559.

146. Sanossian N, Ovbiagele B. Drug insight. Translating evidence on statin therapy into clinical benefits. Nat Clin Pract Neurol 2008;4:43–49.

147. Adams HP, Jr. Secondary prevention of atherothrombotic events after ischemic stroke. Mayo Clin Proc 2009;84:43–51.

148. Blackshear JL, Kopecky SL, Litin SC, et al. Management of atrial fibrillation in adults. Prevention of thromboembolism and symptomatic treatment. Mayo Clinic Proc 1996;71:150–160.

149. Wolf PA, Dawber TR, Thomas HE, et al. Epidemiologic assessment of chronic atrial fibrillation and risk of stroke. Neurology 1978;28:973–977.

150. Hylek EM, Skates SJ, Sheehan MA, et al. An analysis of the lowest effective intensity of prophylactic anticoagulation for patients with nonrheumatic atrial fibrillation. N Engl J Med 1996;335:540–546.

151. Peterson P, Boysen G, Godtfredson J, et al. Placebo-controlled, randomised trial of warfarin and aspirin for prevention of thromboembolic complications in chromic atrial fibrillation. The Copenhagen AFASAK study. Lancet 1989;1:175–179.

152. The Boston Area Anticoagulation Trial for Atrial Fibrillation investigators. The effect of low-dose warfarin on the risk of stroke in patients with nonrheumatic atrial fibrillation. N Engl J Med 1990;323:1505–1511.

153. Stroke Prevention in Atrial Fibrillation investigators. Stroke Prevention in Atrial Fibrillation Study. Final results. Circulation 1991;84:527–539.

154. Ezelkowitz MD, Bridgers SL, James KE, et al. Warfarin in the prevention of stroke associated with nonrheumatic atrial fibrillation. N Engl J Med 1992;327:1406–1412.

155. EAFT (European Atrial Fibrillation Trial) study group. Secondary prevention in non-rheumatic atrial fibrillation after transient ischaemic attack or minor stroke. Lancet 1993;342:1255–1262.

156. Stroke Prevention in Atrial Fibrillation investigators. Warfarin versus aspirin for prevention of thromboembolism in atrial fibrillation. Lancet 1994;343:687–691.

157. Hart RG, Sherman DG, Easton JD, et al. Prevention of stroke in patients with nonvalvular atrial fibrillation. Neurology 1998;51:674–681.

158. The ACTIVE investigators. Effect of clopidogrel added to aspirin in patients with atrial fibrillation. N Engl J Med 2009.

159. Chamorro A, Vila N, Ascaso C, et al. Heparin in acute stroke with atrial fibrillation. Clinical relevance of very early treatment. Arch Neurol 1999;56:1098–1102.

160. Hart RG, Easton JD. Hemorrhagic infarcts. Stroke 1986;17:586–589.

161. Chamorro A, Vila N, Saiz A, et al. Early anticoagulation after large cerebral embolic infarction. A safety study. Neurology 1995;45:861–865.

162. Pessin MS, Estol CJ, Lafranchise F, et al. Safety of anticoagulation after hemorrhagic infarction. Neurology 1993;43:1298–1303.

163. Loh E, St. John Sutton M, Wun C-CC, et al. Ventricular dysfunction and the risk of stroke after myocardial infarction. N Engl J Med 1997;336:251–257.

164. Lechat P, Mas JL, Lascault G, et al. Prevalence of patent foramen ovale in patients with stroke. N Engl J Med 1988;318:1148–1152.

165. Petty GW, Khandheria BK, Chu CP, et al. Patent foramen ovale in patients with cerebral infarction. A transesophageal echocardiographic study. Arch Neurol 1997;54:819–822.

166. Devuyst G, Bogousslavsky J, Ruchat P, et al. Prognosis after stroke followed by surgical closure of patent foramen ovale. A prospective follow-up study with brain MRI and simultaneous transesophageal and transcranial Doppler ultrasound. Neurology 1996;47:1162–1166.

167. Saver JL. Emerging risk factors for stroke. Patent foramen ovale, proximal aortic atherosclerosis, antiphospholipid antibodies, and activated protein C resistance. J Stroke Cerebrovasc Dis 1997;6:167–172.

168. Messé SR, Silverman IE, Kizer JR, et al. Practice parameter. Recurrent stroke with patent foramen ovale and atrial septal aneurysm. Report of the Quality Standards Subcommittee of the American Academy of Neurology. Neurology 2004;62:1042–1050.

169. Messé SR, Kasner SE. Is closure recommended for patent foramen ovale and cryptogenic stroke? Patent foramen ovale in cryptogenic stroke. Not to close. Circulation 2008;118:1999–2004.

170. Cerebral embolism task force. Cardiogenic brain embolism. The second report of the cerebral embolism task force. Arch Neurol 1989;46:727–743.

171. Gilon D, Buonanno FS, Joffe MM, et al. Lack of evidence of an association between mitral-valve prolapse and stroke in young patients. N Engl J Med 1999;341:8–13.

172. Freeman WD, Aguilar MI. Stroke prevention in atrial fibrillation and other major cardiac sources of embolism. Neurol Clin 2008;26:1129–1160, x–xi.

173. Reynen K. Cardiac myxomas. N Engl J Med 1995;333:1610–1617.

174. Hart RG, Foster JW, Luther MF, et al. Stroke in infective endocarditis. Stroke 1990;21:695–700.

175. Brust JCM, Dickinson PCT, Hughes JEO, et al. The diagnosis and treatment of cerebral mycotic aneurysms. Ann Neurol 1990;27:238–246.

176. Pruitt AA, Rubin RH, Karchmer AW, et al. Neurologic complications of bacterial endocarditis. Medicine 1978;57:329–343.

177. Kanter MC, Hart RG. Neurologic complications of infective endocarditis. Neurology 1991;41:1015–1020.

178. Bogousslavsky J, Regli F, Maeder P, et al. The etiology of posterior circulation infarcts. A prospective study using magnetic resonance imaging and magnetic resonance angiography. Neurology 1993;43:1528–1533.

179. Hicks PA, Leavitt JA, Mokri B. Ophthalmic manifestations of vertebral artery dissection. Patients seen at the Mayo Clinic from 1976 to 1992. Ophthalmology 1994;101:1786–1792.

180. Caplan LR, Amarenco P, Rosengart A, et al. Embolism from vertebral artery origin occlusive disease. Neurology 1992;42:1505–1512.

181. Wijdicks EFM, Nichols DA, Thielen KR, et al. Intra-arterial thrombolysis in acute basilar artery thromboembolism. The initial Mayo Clinic experience. Mayo Clinic Proc 1997;72:1005–1013.

182. Grond M, Rudolf J, Schmülling S, et al. Early intravenous thrombolysis with recombinant tissue-type plasminogen activator in vertebrobasilar ischemic stroke. Arch Neurol 1998;55:466–469.

183. Halkes PH, van Gijn J, Kappelle LJ, et al. Aspirin plus dipyridamole versus aspirin alone after cerebral ischaemia of arterial origin (ESPRIT): randomised controlled trial. Lancet 2006;367:1665–1673.

184. Sacco RL, Diener HC, Yusuf S, et al. Aspirin and extended-release dipyridamole versus clopidogrel for recurrent stroke. N Engl J Med 2008;359:1238–1251.

185. CAPRIE Steering Committee. A randomised, blinded trial of clopidogrel versus aspirin in patients at risk of ischaemic events (CAPRIE). Lancet 1996;348:1329–1339.

186. Wilterdink JL, Easton JD. Dipyridamole plus aspirin in cerebrovascular disease. Arch Neurol 1999;56:1087–1092.

187. Mohr JP, Thompson JL, Lazar RM, et al. A comparison of warfarin and aspirin for the prevention of recurrent ischemic stroke. N Engl J Med 2001;345:1444–1451.

188. Samuels MA, Thalinger K. Cerebrovascular manifestations of selected hematologic diseases. Semin Neurol 1991;11:411–418.

189. High KA. Antithrombin III, protein C, and protein S. Naturally occurring anticoagulant proteins. Arch Pathol Lab Med 1988;112:28–36.

190. Hart RG, Kanter MC. Hematologic disorders and ischemic stroke. Stroke 1990;21:1111–1121.

191. Irey NS, McAllister HA, Henry JM. Oral contraceptives and stroke in young women. A clinicopathologic correlation. Neurology 1978;28:1216–1219.

192. Longstreth WT, Swanson PD. Oral contraceptives and stroke. Stroke 1984;15:747–750.

193. Kittner SJ, Stern BJ, Feeser BR, et al. Pregnancy and the risk of stroke. N Engl J Med 1996;335:768–774.

194. Schafer AI. The hypercoagulable states. Ann Intern Med 1985;102:814–828.

195. Levine SR, Deegan MJ, Futrell N, et al. Cerebrovascular and neurologic disease associated with antiphospholipid antibodies. 48 cases. Neurology 1990;40:1181–1189.

196. Brey RL, Hart RG, Sherman DG, et al. Antiphospholipid antibodies and cerebral ischemia in young people. Neurology 1990;40:1190–1196.

197. The Antiphospholipid Antibodies and Stroke Study Group (APASS). Anticardiolipin antibodies and the risk of recurrent thrombo-occlusive events and death. Neurology 1997;48:91–94.

198. Tanne D, D'Olhaberriague L, Schultz LR, et al. Anticardiolipin antibodies and their associations with cerebrovascular risk factors. Neurology 1999;52:1368–1373.

199. Coull BM, Goodnight SH. Antiphospholipid antibodies, prethrombotic states, and stroke. Stroke 1990;21:1370–1374.

200. Khamashta MA, Cuadrado MJ, Mujic F, et al. The management of thrombosis in the antiphospholipid-antibody syndrome. N Engl J Med 1995;332:993–997.

201. Lockshin MD. Answers to the antiphospholipid-antibody syndrome [editorial]? N Engl J Med 1995;332:1025–1027.

202. Roach GW, Kanchuger M, Mangano CM, et al. Adverse cerebral outcomes after coronary bypass surgery. N Engl J Med 1996;335:1857–1863.

203. Furlan AJ, Breuer AC. Central nervous system complications of open heart surgery. Stroke 1984;15:912–915.

204. Gilman S. Neurological complications of open heart surgery. Ann Neurol 1990;28:475–476.

205. Swain JA. Cardiac surgery and the brain [editorial]. N Engl J Med 1993;329:1119–1120.

206. Horowitz DR, Tuhrim S, Budd J, et al. Aortic plaque in patients with brain ischemia. Diagnosis by transesophageal echocardiography. Neurology 1992;42:1602–1604.

207. Amarenco P, Duyckaerts C, Tzourio C, et al. The prevalence of ulcerated plaques in the aortic arch in patients with stroke. N Engl J Med 1992;326:221–225.

208. Amarenco P, Cohen A, Tzourio C, et al. Atherosclerotic disease of the aortic arch and the risk of ischemic stroke. N Engl J Med 1994;331:1474–1479.

209. The French Study of Aortic Plaques in Stroke Group. Atherosclerotic disease of the aortic arch as a risk factor for recurrent ischemic stroke. N Engl J Med 1996;334:1216–1221.

210. Keane JR. Blindness following tentorial herniation. Ann Neurol 1980;8:186–190.

211. Headache classification subcommittee of the International Headache Society. The International Classification of Headache Disorders, 2nd edn. Cephalalgia 2004;24 (Suppl 1):9–160.

212. Welch KMA. Relationship of stroke and migraine. Neurology 1994;44(Suppl 7):S33–S36.

213. Buring JE, Hebert P, Romero J, et al. Migraine and subsequent risk of stroke in the physicians' health study. Arch Neurol 1995;52:129–134.

214. Merikangas KR, Fenton BT, Cheng SH, et al. Association between migraine and stroke in a large-scale epidemiological study of the United States. Arch Neurol 1997;54:362–368.

215. Welch KMA, Levine SR. Migraine-related stroke in the context of the International Headache Society classification of head pain. Arch Neurol 1990;47:458–462.

216. Bevan H, Sharma K, Bradley W. Stroke in young adults. Stroke 1990;21:382–386.

217. Kittner SJ, Stern BJ, Wozniak M, et al. Cerebral infarction in young adults. The Baltimore-Washington cooperative young stroke study. Neurology 1998;50:890–894.

218. Williams LS, Garg BP, Cohen M, et al. Subtypes of ischemic stroke in children and young adults. Neurology 1997;49:1541–1545.

219. Manno EM, Atkinson JL, Fulgham JR, et al. Emerging medical and surgical management strategies in the evaluation and treatment of intracerebral hemorrhage. Mayo Clin Proc 2005;80:420–433.

220. Mendelow AD, Gregson BA, Fernandes HM, et al. Early surgery versus initial conservative treatment in patients with spontaneous supratentorial intracerebral haematomas in the International Surgical Trial in Intracerebral Haemorrhage (STICH). A randomised trial. Lancet 2005;365:387–397.

221. Rabinstein AA, Wijdicks EF. Surgery for intracerebral hematoma. The search for the elusive right candidate. Rev Neurol Dis 2006;3:163–172.

222. Sessa M. Intracerebral hemorrhage and hypertension. Neurol Sci 2008;29 (Suppl 2):S258–259.

223. Kase CS. Intracerebral hemorrhage. Nonhypertensive causes. Stroke 1986;17:590–595.

224. Case records of the Massachusetts General Hospital. Case 27-1991. N Engl J Med 1991;325:42–54.

225. Case records of the Massachusetts General Hospital. Case 22-1996. N Engl J Med 1996;335:189–196.

226. Vinters HV, Gilbert JJ. Cerebral amyloid angiopathy. Incidence and complications in the aging brain. II. The distribution of amyloid vascular changes. Stroke 1983;14:924–928.

227. Vonsattel JPG, Myers RH, Hedley-Whyte ET, et al. Cerebral amyloid angiopathy without and with cerebral hemorrhages. A comparative histological study. Ann Neurol 1991;30:637–649.

228. Nicoll JAR, Burnett C, Leth S, et al. High frequency of apolipoprotein E epsilon 2 allele in hemorrhage due to cerebral amyloid angiopathy. Ann Neurol 1997;41:716–721.

229. Greenberg SM, Hyman BT. Cerebral amyloid angiopathy and apolipoprotein E: bad news for the good allele [editorial]? Ann Neurol 1997;41:701–702.

230. O'Donnell HC, Rosano J, Knudsen KA, et al. Apolipoprotein E genotype and the risk of recurrent lobar intracerebral hemorrhage. N Engl J Med 2000;342:240–245.

231. Greenberg SM. Cerebral amyloid angiopathy. Prospects for clinical diagnosis and treatment. Neurology 1998;51:690–694.

232. Knudsen KA, Rosand J, Karluk D, et al. Clinical diagnosis of cerebral amyloid angiopathy. Validation of the Boston criteria. Neurology 2001;56:537–539.

233. Greene GM, Godersky JC, Biller J, et al. Surgical experience with cerebral amyloid angiopathy. Stroke 1990;21:1545–1549.

234. Bennett J, Volpe NJ, Liu GT, et al. Neurovascular neuro-ophthalmology. In: Jakobiec FA, Albert D (eds). Principles of Ophthalmology, 2nd edn, pp 3238–3273. Philadelphia, W.B. Saunders, 1998.

235. Yokoyama K, Asano Y, Murakawa T, et al. Familial occurrence of arteriovenous malformation of the brain. J Neurosurg 1991;74:585–589.

236. Mingrino S. Supratentorial arteriovenous malformations of the brain. Adv Tech Stand Neurosurg 1978;5:93–123.

237. Kupersmith MJ. Vascular malformations of the brain. In: Neurovascular Neuro-ophthalmology, pp 301–351. Berlin, Springer-Verlag, 1993.

238. Kupersmith MJ, Vargas ME, Yashar A, et al. Occipital arteriovenous malformations. Visual disturbances and presentation. Neurology 1996;46:953–957.

239. Lee K, Holman BL. Images in clinical medicine. Cerebral arteriovenous malformation. N Engl J Med 1995;332:923.

240. The Arteriovenous Malformation Study Group. Arteriovenous malformations of the brain in adults. N Engl J Med 1999;340:1812–1818.

241. Bartolomei J, Wecht DA, Chaloupka J, et al. Occipital lobe vascular malformations. Prevalence of visual field deficits and prognosis after therapeutic intervention. Neurosurgery 1998;43:415–421.

242. Ogilvy CS, Stieg PE, Awad I, et al. AHA Scientific Statement. Recommendations for the management of intracranial arteriovenous malformations. A statement for healthcare professionals from a special writing group of the Stroke Council, American Stroke Association. Stroke 2001;32:1458–1471.

243. Friedlander RM. Clinical practice. Arteriovenous malformations of the brain. N Engl J Med 2007;356:2704–2712.

244. Tagle P, Huete I, Méndez J, et al. Intracranial cavernous angioma. Presentation and management. J Neurosurg 1986;64:720–723.

245. Bartlett JE, Kishore PRS. Intracranial cavernous hemangioma. Am J Roentgenol 1977;128:653–656.

246. Labauge P, Denier C, Bergametti F, et al. Genetics of cavernous angiomas. Lancet Neurol 2007;6:237–244.

247. Acciarri N, Padovani R, Giulioni M, et al. Intracranial and orbital cavernous angiomas. A review of 74 surgical cases. Br J Neurosurg 1993;7:529–539.

248. Tomlinson FH, Houser OW, Scheithauer BW, et al. Angiographically occult vascular malformations. A correlative study of features on magnetic resonance imaging and histological examination. Neurosurgery 1994;34:792–799.

249. Moore PM, Cupps TR. Neurological complications of vasculitis. Ann Neurol 1983;14:155–167.

250. Kattah JC, Cupps TR, Di Chiro G, et al. An unusual case of central nervous system vasculitis. J Neurol 1987;234:344–347.

251. Sigal LH. The neurologic presenation of vasculitic and rheumatologic syndromes. A review. Medicine 1987;66:157–180.

252. Moore PM. Diagnosis and management of isolated angiitis of the central nervous system. Neurology 1989;39:167–173.

253. Levin JR, Awerbuch G, Nigro MA, et al. Isolated angiitis of the central nervous system in children. Ann Neurol 1989;26:478.

254. Zimmerman RS, Young HG, Hadfield MG. Granulomatous angiitis of the nervous system. Surg Neurol 1990;33:206–212.

255. Calabrese LH, Furlan AJ, Gragg LA, et al. Primary angiitis of the central nervous system. Diagnostic criteria and clinical approach. Cleve Clin J Med 1992;59:293–306.

256. Calabrese LH, Gragg LA, Furlan AJ. Benign angiopathy. A distinct subset of angiographically defined primary angiitis of the central nervous system. J Rheumatol 1993;20:2046–2050.

257. Rhodes RH, Madelaire NC, Petrelli M, et al. Primary angiitis and angiopathy of the central nervous system and their relationship to systemic giant cell arteritis. Arch Pathol Lab Med 1995;119:334–349.

258. Ozawa T, Sasaki O, Sorimachi T, et al. Primary angiitis of the central nervous system. Report of two cases and review of the literature. Neurosurgery 1995;36:173–179.

259. Vollmer TL, Guarnaccia J, Harrington W, et al. Idiopathic angiitis of the central nervous system. Diagnostic challenges. Arch Neurol 1993;50:925–930.

260. Ehsan T, Hasan S, Powers JM, et al. Serial magnetic resonance imaging in isolated angiitis of the central nervous system. Neurology 1995;45:1462–1465.

261. Shoemaker E, Lin ZS, Rae Grant AD, et al. Primary angiitis of the central nervous system. Unusual MR appearance. AJNR Am J Neuroradiol 1994;15:331–334.

262. Jacobs DA, Liu GT, Nelson PT, et al. Primary central nervous system angiitis, amyloid angiopathy, and Alzheimer's pathology presenting with Balint's syndrome. Surv Ophthalmol 2004;49:454–459.

263. Alhalabi M, Moore PM. Serial angiography in isolated angiitis of the CNS. Neurology 1994;44:1221–1226.

264. Younger DS, Hays AP, Brust JCM, et al. Granulomatous angiitis of the brain. An inflammatory reaction of diverse etiology. Arch Neurol 1988;45:514–518.

265. Salvarani C, Brown RD, Jr., Calamia KT, et al. Primary central nervous system vasculitis. Analysis of 101 patients. Ann Neurol 2007;62:442–451.

266. Caselli RJ, Hunder GG, Whisnant JP. Neurologic disease in biopsy proven giant cell (temporal) arteritis. Neurology 1988;38:352–359.

267. Caselli RJ, Daube JR, Hunder GG, et al. Peripheral neuropathic syndromes in giant cell (temporal) arteritis. Neurology 1988;38:685–689.

268. Hunder GG. Polymyalgia rheumatica and giant cell arteritis. In: Cecil Textbook of Medicine, pp 1498–1500. Philadelphia, W. B. Saunders, 1996.

269. Caselli RJ, Hunder GG. Neurologic aspects of giant cell (temporal) arteritis. Rheum Dis Clin N Am 1990;19:941–953.

270. Thielen KR, Wijdicks EFM, Nichols DA. Giant cell (temporal) arteritis. Involvement of the vertebral and internal carotid arteries. Mayo Clinic Proc 1998;73:444–446.

271. Staunton H, Stafford F, Leader M, et al. Deterioration of giant cell arteritis with corticosteroid therapy. Arch Neurol 2000;57:581–584.

272. Chisholm IH. Cortical blindness in cranial arteritis. Br J Ophthalmol 1975;59:332–333.

273. Nevyas JY, Nevyas HJ. Giant cell arteritis with normal erythrocyte sedimentation rate. A management dilemma. Metab Pediatr Syst Ophthalmol 1987;10:18–21.

274. Wilkinson IMS, Russell RWR. Arteries of the head and neck in giant cell arteritis. A pathological study to show the pattern of arterial involvement. Arch Neurol 1972;27:378–391.

275. Cullen JF, Coleiro JA. Ophthalmic complications of giant cell arteritis. Surv Ophthalmol 1976;20:247–260.

276. Ronthal M, Gonzalez RG, Smith RN, et al. Case records of the Massachusetts General Hospital. Weekly clinicopathological exercises. Case 21–2003. A 72-year-old man with repetitive strokes in the posterior circulation. N Engl J Med 2003;349:170–180.

277. Salvarani C, Giannini C, Miller DV, et al. Giant cell arteritis. Involvement of intracranial arteries. Arthritis Rheum 2006;55:985–989.

278. Galetta SL, Balcer LJ, Liu GT. Giant cell arteritis with unusual flow related neuro-ophthalmologic manifestations. Neurology 1997;49:1463–1465.

279. Trevor RP, Sondheimer FK, Fessel WJ, et al. Angiographic demonstration of major cerebral vessel occlusion in systemic lupus erythematosus. Neuroradiology 1972;4:202–207.

280. Brandt KD, Lessell S, Cohen AS. Cerebral disorders of vision in systemic lupus erythematosus. Annals of Internal Medicine 1975;83:163–169.

281. Lessell S. The neuro-ophthalmology of systemic lupus erythematosus. Doc Ophthalmol 1979;47:13–42.

282. Honda Y. Scintillating scotoma as the first symptom of systemic lupus erythematosus. Am J Ophthalmol 1985;99:607.

283. Rubin BR, De Horatius RJ. Acute visual loss in systemic lupus erythematosus. J Am Optom Assoc 1989;89:73–77.

284. Johnson RT, Richardson EP. The neurological manifestations of systemic lupus erythematosus. A clinical-pathological study of 24 cases and review of the literature. Medicine 1968;47:337–369.

285. Ellis SG, Verity MA. Central nervous system involvement in systemic lupus erythematosus. A review of neuropathologic findings in 57 cases, 1955–1977. Semin Arth Rheum 1979;8:212–221.

286. Devinsky O, Petito CK, Alonso DR. Clinical and neuropathological findings in systemic lupus erythematosus. The role of vasculitis, heart emboli, and thrombotic thrombocytopenic purpura. Ann Neurol 1988;23:380–384.

287. Hinchey J, Chaves C, Appignani B, et al. A reversible posterior leukoencephalopathy syndrome. N Engl J Med 1996;334:494–500.

288. Lee VH, Wijdicks EF, Manno EM, et al. Clinical spectrum of reversible posterior leukoencephalopathy syndrome. Arch Neurol 2008;65:205–210.

289. Pavlakis SG, Frank Y, Kalina P, et al. Occipital-parietal encephalopathy. A new name for an old syndrome. Pediatr Neurol 1997;16:145–148.

290. Shin RK, Stern JW, Janss AJ, et al. Reversible posterior leukoencephalopathy during the treatment of acute lymphoblastic leukemia. Neurology 2001;56:388–391.

291. Torocsik HV, Curless RG, Post J, et al. FK506-induced leukoencephalopathy in children with organ transplants. Neurology 1999;52:1497–1500.

292. Hinchey JA. Reversible posterior leukoencephalopathy syndrome. What have we learned in the last 10 years [editorial]? Arch Neurol 2008;65:175–176.

293. Ay H, Buonanno FS, Schaefer PW, et al. Posterior leukoencephalopathy without severe hypertension. Utility of diffusion-weighted MRI. Neurology 1998;51:1369–1376.

294. Schwartz RB. A reversible posterior leukoencephalopathy syndrome. N Engl J Med 1996;334:1743; author reply 1746.

295. Casey SO, Sampaio RC, Michel E, et al. Posterior reversible encephalopathy syndrome. Utility of fluid-attenuated inversion recovery MR imaging in the detection of cortical and subcortical lesions. AJNR Am J Neuroradiol 2000;21:1199–1206.

296. Narbone MC, Musolino R, Granata F, et al. PRES. Posterior or potentially reversible encephalopathy syndrome? Neurol Sci 2006;27:187–189.

297. Gocmen R, Ozgen B, Oguz KK. Widening the spectrum of PRES. Series from a tertiary care center. Eur J Radiol 2007;62:454–459.

298. Beutler JJ, Koomans HA. Malignant hypertension. Still a challenge. Nephrol Dial Transplant 1997;12:2019–2023.

299. Do DV, Rismondo V, Nguyen QD. Reversible cortical blindness in preeclampsia. Am J Ophthalmol 2002;134:916–918.

300. Gregory DG, Pelak VS, Bennett JL. Diffusion-weighted magnetic resonance imaging and the evaluation of cortical blindness in preeclampsia. Surv Ophthalmol 2003;48:647–650.

301. Raps EC, Galetta SL, Broderick M, et al. Delayed peripartum vasculopathy. Cerebral eclampsia revisited. Ann Neurol 1993;33:222–225.

302. Rubin AM, Kang H. Cerebral blindness and encephalopathy with cyclosporin A toxicity. Neurology 1987;37:1072–1076.

303. Patchell RA. Neurological complications of organ transplantation. Ann Neurol 1994;36:688–703.

304. Shutter LA, Green JP, Newman NJ, et al. Cortical blindness and white matter lesions in a patient receiving FK506 after liver transplantation. Neurology 1993;43:2417–2418.

305. Lavigne CM, Shrier DA, Ketkar M, et al. Tacrolimus leukoencephalopathy. A neuropathologic confirmation. Neurology 2004;63:1132–1133.

306. Snyder H, Robinson K, Shah D, et al. Signs and symptoms of patients with brain tumors presenting to the emergency department. J Emerg Med 1993;11:253–258.

307. Pomeranz HD, Henson JW, Lessell S. Radiation-associated cerebral blindness. Am J Ophthalmol 1998;126:609–611.

308. Radhakrishnan K, Mokri B, Parisi PE, et al. The trends in incidence of primary brain tumors in the population of Rochester, Minnesota. Ann Neurol 1995;37:67–73.

309. DeAngelis LM. Brain tumors. N Engl J Med 2001;344:114–123.

310. Buckner JC, Brown PD, O'Neill BP, et al. Central nervous system tumors. Mayo Clin Proc 2007;82:1271–1286.

311. Black PM. Brain tumors. N Engl J Med 1991;324:1471–1476 (Part one), 1555–1564 (part two).

312. Hegi ME, Diserens AC, Gorlia T, et al. MGMT gene silencing and benefit from temozolomide in glioblastoma. N Engl J Med 2005;352:997–1003.

313. Case records of the Massachusetts General Hospital. Case 33–1988. N Engl J Med 1988;319:426–436.

314. Grimm SA, McCannel CA, Omuro AM, et al. Primary CNS lymphoma with intraocular involvement. International PCNSL Collaborative Group Report. Neurology 2008;71: 1355–1360.

315. Deangelis LM, Hormigo A. Treatment of primary central nervous system lymphoma. Semin Oncol 2004;31:684–692.

316. Cairncross JG, Kim J-H, Posner JB. Radiation therapy for brain metastases. Ann Neurol 1980;7:529–541.

317. Posner JB. Intracranial metastases. In: Neurologic Complications of Cancer, pp 77–110. Philadelphia, F.A. Davis, 1995.

318. Patchell RA, Tibbs PA, Walsh JW, et al. A randomized trial of surgery in the treatment of single metastases to the brain. N Engl J Med 1990;322:494–500.

319. Andrews DW, Scott CB, Sperduto PW, et al. Whole brain radiation therapy with or without stereotactic radiosurgery boost for patients with one to three brain metastases. Phase III results of the RTOG 9508 randomised trial. Lancet 2004;363:1665–1672.

320. Monheit BE, Fiveash JB, Girkin CA. Radionecrosis of the inferior occipital lobes with altitudinal visual field loss after gamma knife radiosurgery. J Neuroophthalmol 2004;24:195–199.

321. Pruitt A, Dalmau J, Detre J, et al. Episodic neurologic dysfunction with migraine and reversible imaging findings after radiation. Neurology 2006;67:676–678.

322. Koralnik IJ. Progressive multifocal leukoencephalopathy revisited. Has the disease outgrown its name? Ann Neurol 2006;60:162–173.

323. Manji H, Miller RF. Progressive multifocal leucoencephalopathy. Progress in the AIDS era. J Neurol Neurosurg Psychiatr 2000;69:569–571.

324. Greenlee JE. Progressive multifocal leukoencephalopathy—progress made and lessons relearned (editorial). N Engl J Med 1998;338:1378–1380.

325. Richardson EP. Progressive multifocal leukoencephalopathy 30 years later [editorial]. N Engl J Med 1988;318:315–317.

326. Berger JR, Concha M. Progressive multifocal leukoencephalopathy. The evolution of a disease once considered rare. J Neurovirol 1995;1:5–18.

327. Gillespie SM, Chang Y, Lemp G, et al. Progressive multifocal leukoencephalopathy in persons infected with human immunodeficiency virus, San Francisco, 1981–1989. Ann Neurol 1991;30:597–604.

328. Razonable RR, Aksamit AJ, Wright AJ, et al. Cidofovir treatment of progressive multifocal leukoencephalopathy in a patient receiving highly active antiretroviral therapy. Mayo Clin Proc 2001;76:1171–1175.

329. Case records of the Massachusetts General Hospital. Case 20–1995. N Engl J Med 1995;332:1773–1780.

330. Yousry TA, Major EO, Ryschkewitsch C, et al. Evaluation of patients treated with natalizumab for progressive multifocal leukoencephalopathy. N Engl J Med 2006;354:924–933.

331. Ormerod LD, Rhodes RH, Gross SA, et al. Ophthalmologic manifestations of acquired immune deficiency syndrome-associated progressive multifocal leukoencephalopathy. Ophthalmology 1996;103:899–906.

332. Downes SM, Black GC, Hyman N, et al. Visual loss due to progressive multifocal leukoencephalopathy in a congenital immunodeficiency disorder. Arch Ophthalmol 2001;119:1376–1378.

333. Berger JR, Levy RM. The neurologic complications of human immunodeficiency virus infection. Med Clin North Am 1993;77:1–23.

334. Berger JR, Levy RM, Flomenhoft D, et al. Predictive factors for prolonged survival in acquired immunodeficiency syndrome-associated progressive multifocal leukoencephalopathy. Ann Neurol 1998;44:341–349.

335. Weiss PJ, DeMarco JK. Images in clinical medicine. Progressive multifocal leukoencephalopathy. N Engl J Med 1994;330:1197.

336. Kasner S, Galetta SL, McGowan JC, et al. Magnetization transfer imaging in progressive multifocal leukoencephalopathy. Neurology 1997;48:534–536.

337. Major EO, Ault GS. Progressive multifocal leukoencephalopathy. Clinical and laboratory observations on a viral induced demyelinating disease in the immunodeficient patient. Curr Opin Neurol 1995;8:184–190.

338. Koralnik IJ, Boden D, Mai VX, et al. JC virus DNA load in patients with and without progressive multifocal leukoencephalopathy. Neurology 1999;52:253–260.

339. Garrels K, Kucharczyk W, Wortzman G, et al. Progressive multifocal leukoencephalopathy. Clinical and MR response to treatment. AJNR Am J Neuroradiol 1996;17:597–600.

340. Hall CD, Dafni U, Simpson D, et al. Failure of cytarabine in progressive multifocal leukoencephalopathy associated with human immunodeficiency virus infection. N Engl J Med 1998;338:1345–1351.

341. Cettomai D, McArthur JC. Mirtazapine use in human immunodeficiency virus-infected patients with progressive multifocal leukoencephalopathy. Arch Neurol 2009;66:255–258.

342. Clifford DB, Yiannoutsos C, Glicksman M, et al. HAART improves prognosis in HIV-associated progressive multifocal leukoencephalopathy. Neurology 1999;52: 623–625.

343. De Luca A, Fantoni M, Tartaglione T, et al. Response to cidofovir after failure of antiretroviral therapy alone in AIDS-associated progressive multifocal leukoencephalopathy. Neurology 1999;52:891–892.

344. Venkataramana A, Pardo CA, McArthur JC, et al. Immune reconstitution inflammatory syndrome in the CNS of HIV-infected patients. Neurology 2006;67:383–388.

345. McCombe JA, Auer RN, Maingat FG, et al. Neurologic immune reconstitution inflammatory syndrome in HIV/AIDS. Outcome and epidemiology. Neurology 2009;72:835–841.

346. Martinez JV, Mazziotti JV, Efron ED, et al. Immune reconstitution inflammatory syndrome associated with PML in AIDS: a treatable disorder. Neurology 2006;67: 1692–1694.

347. Khatri BO, Man S, Giovannoni G, et al. Effect of plasma exchange in accelerating natalizumab clearance and restoring leukocyte function. Neurology 2009;72:402–409.

348. Vargas ME, Kupersmith MJ, Savino PJ, et al. Homonymous field defect as the first manifestation of Creutzfeldt-Jakob disease. Am J Ophthalmol 1995;119:497–504.

349. Jacobs DA, Lesser RL, Mourelatos Z, et al. The Heidenhain variant of Creutzfeldt-Jakob disease. Clinical, pathologic, and neuroimaging findings. J Neuroophthalmol 2001;21: 99–102.

350. Nozaki I, Hamaguchi T, Noguchi-Shinohara M, et al. The MM2-cortical form of sporadic Creutzfeldt-Jakob disease presenting with visual disturbance. Neurology 2006;67:531–533.

351. Proulx AA, Strong MJ, Nicolle DA. Creutzfeldt-Jakob disease presenting with visual manifestations. Can J Ophthalmol 2008;43:591–595.

352. Case records of the Massachusetts General Hospital. Case 39–1996. N Engl J Med 1996;335:1906–1914.

353. Case records of the Massachusetts General Hospital. Case 31–1991. N Engl J Med 1991;325:341–350.

354. Boes B, Bashir R, Boes C, et al. Central nervous system aspergillosis. J Neuroimaging 1994;4:123–129.

355. Evaluation and management of intracranial mass lesions in AIDS. Report of the quality standards subcommittee of the American Academy of Neurology. Neurology 1998;50:21–26.

356. Ammassari A, Cingolani A, Pezzotti P, et al. AIDS-related focal brain lesions in the era of highly active antiretroviral therapy. Neurology 2000;55:1194–1200.

357. Bruce BB, Zhang X, Kedar S, et al. Traumatic homonymous hemianopia. J Neurol Neurosurg Psychiatr 2006;77:986–988.

358. Adelson PD, Kochanek PM. Head injury in children. J Child Neurol 1998;13:2–15.

359. Gennarelli TA, Thibault LE, Graham DI. Diffuse axonal injury. An important form of traumatic brain damage. Neuroscientist 1998;4:202–215.

360. Silverman IE, Grossman M, Galetta SL, et al. Understanding human visual cortex. The role of functional imaging. Neuropsychiatr, Neuropsych, Behav Neurol 1995;8:241–254.

361. Brodsky MC, Baker RS, Hamed LM. The apparently blind infant. In: Pediatric neuro-ophthalmology, pp 1–41. New York, Springer-Verlag, 1996.

362. Mendez MF, Tomsak RL, Remler B. Disorders of the visual system in Alzheimer's disease. J Clin Neuroophthalmol 1990;10:62–69.

363. Lee AG, Martin CO. Neuro-ophthalmic findings in the visual variant of Alzheimer's disease. Ophthalmology 2004;111:376–380.

364. Atchison M, Harrison AR, Lee MS. The woman who needed a pet. Surv Ophthalmol 2006;51:592–595.

365. Oda H, Ohkawa S, Maeda K. Hemispatial visual defect in Alzheimer's disease. Neurocase 2008;14:141–146.

366. Katz B, Rimmer S. Ophthalmologic manifestations of Alzheimer's disease. Surv Ophthalmol 1989;34:31–43.

367. Rizzo JF, Cronin-Golomb A, Growdon JH, et al. Retinocalcarine function in Alzheimer's disease. A clinical and electrophysiologic study. Arch Neurol 1992;49:93–101.

368. Hornabrook RS, Miller DH, Newton MR, et al. Frequent involvement of the optic radiation in patients with acute isolated optic neuritis. Neurology 1992;42:77–79.

369. Cesareo M, Pozzilli C, Ristori G, et al. Crossed quadrant homonymous hemianopsia in a case of multiple sclerosis. Clin Neurol Neurosurg 1995;97:324–327.

370. Kepes JJ. Large focal tumor-like demyelinating lesions of the brain. Intermediate entity between multiple sclerosis and acute disseminated encephalomyelitis? A study of 31 patients. Ann Neurol 1993;33:18–27.

371. Friedman DI. Multiple sclerosis simulating a mass lesion. J Neuroophthalmol 2000;20:147–153.

372. McAdam LC, Blaser SI, Banwell BL. Pediatric tumefactive demyelination. Case series and review of the literature. Pediatr Neurol 2002;26:18–25.

373. Lucchinetti CF, Gavrilova RH, Metz I, et al. Clinical and radiographic spectrum of pathologically confirmed tumefactive multiple sclerosis. Brain 2008;131:1759–1775.

374. Bajandas FJ, McBeath JB, Smith JL. Congenital homonymous hemianopia. Am J Ophthalmol 1976;82:498–500.

375. Bosley TM, Kiyosawa M, Moster M, et al. Neuro-imaging and positron emission tomography of congenital homonymous hemianopsia. Am J Ophthalmol 1991;111:413–418.

376. Fazzi E, Signorini SG, Bova SM, et al. Spectrum of visual disorders in children with cerebral visual impairment. J Child Neurol 2007;22:294–301.

377. Eken P, de Vries LS, van Nieuwenhuizen O, et al. Early predictors of cerebral visual impairment in infants with cystic leukomalacia. Neuropediatrics 1996;27:16–25.

378. Cioni G, Fazzi B, Ipata AE, et al. Correlation between cerebral visual impairment and magnetic resonance imaging in children with neonatal encephalopathy. Dev Med Child Neurol 1996;38:120–132.

379. Hoyt WF, Rios-Montenegro EN, Behrens MM, et al. Homonymous hemioptic hypoplasia. Fundoscopic features in standard and red-free illustration in three patients with congenital hemiplegia. Br J Ophthalmol 1972;56:537–545.

380. Jacobson L, Hellström A, Flodmark O. Large cups in normal-sized optic discs. A variant of optic nerve hypoplasia in children with periventricular leukomalacia. Arch Ophthalmol 1997;115:1263–1269.

381. Khetpal V, Donahue SP. Cortical visual impairment. Etiology, associated findings, and prognosis in a tertiary care setting. J AAPOS 2007;11:235–239.

382. Jacobson L, Ygge J, Flodmark O. Nystagmus in periventricular leucomalacia. Br J Ophthalmol 1998;82:1026–1032.

383. Good WV, Jan JE, Burden SK, et al. Recent advances in cortical visual impairment. Dev Med Child Neurol 2001;43:56–60.

384. Saidkasimova S, Bennett DM, Butler S, et al. Cognitive visual impairment with good visual acuity in children with posterior periventricular white matter injury. A series of 7 cases. J AAPOS 2007;11:426–430.

385. Drummond SR, Dutton GN. Simultanagnosia following perinatal hypoxia. A possible pediatric variant of Balint syndrome. J AAPOS 2007;11:497–498.

386. Flodmark O, Jan JE, Wong PKH. Computed tomography of the brains of children with cortical visual impairment. Dev Med Child Neurol 1990;32:611–620.

387. Brodsky MC, Fray KJ, Glasier CM. Perinatal cortical and subcortical visual loss. Mechanisms of injury and associated ophthalmologic signs. Ophthalmology 2002;109:85–94.

388. Takashima S, Iida K, Deguchi K. Periventricular leukomalacia, glial development and myelination. Early Human Development 1995;43:177–184.

389. Leviton A, Gilles F. Ventriculomegaly, delayed myelination, white matter hypoplasia, and "periventricular" leukomalacia. How are they related? Pediatr Neurol 1996;15:127–136.

390. Volpe JJ. Neurologic outcome of prematurity. Arch Neurol 1998;55:297–300.

391. Uggetti C, Egitto MG, Fazzi E, et al. Cerebral visual impairment in periventricular leukomalacia. MR correlation. AJNR Am J Neuroradiol 1996;17:979–985.

392. Ragge NK, Barkovich AJ, Hoyt WF, et al. Isolated congenital hemianopia caused by prenatal injury to the optic radiation. Arch Neurol 1991;48:1088–1091.

393. Cioni G, Fazzi B, Coluccini M, et al. Cerebral visual impairment in preterm infants with periventricular leukomalacia. Pediatr Neurol 1997;17:331–338.

394. Jacobson LK, Dutton GN. Periventricular leukomalacia. An important cause of visual and ocular motility dysfunction in children. Surv Ophthalmol 2000;45:1–13.

395. Lambert SR, Kriss A, Taylor D. Detection of isolated occipital lobe anomalies during early childhood. Dev Med Child Neurol 1990;32:451–455.

396. Mercuri E, Spano M, Bruccini G, et al. Visual outcome in children with congenital hemiplegia. Correlation with MRI findings. Neuropediatrics 1996;27:184–188.

397. Thorarensen O, Ryan S, Hunter J, et al. Factor V Leiden mutation. An unrecognized cause of hemiplegic cerebral palsy, neonatal stroke, and placental thrombosis. Ann Neurol 1997;42:372–375.

398. Hill A, Volpe JJ. Perinatal asphyxia. Clinical aspects. Clin Perinatology 1989;16:435–457.

399. Volpe JJ. Hypoxic-ischemic encephalopathy. In: Neurology of the Newborn, 3rd edn, pp 211–369. Philadelphia, W.B. Saunders, 1995.

400. van Hof-van Duin J, Mohn G. Visual defects in children after cerebral hypoxia. Behav Brain Res 1984;14:147–155.

401. Lambert SR, Hoyt CS, Jan JE, et al. Visual recovery from hypoxic cortical blindness during childhood. Computed tomographic and magnetic resonance imaging predictors. Arch Ophthalmol 1987;105:1371–1377.

402. Casteels I, Demaerel P, Spileers W, et al. Cortical visual impairment following perinatal hypoxia. Clinicoradiologic correlation using magnetic resonance imaging. J Ped Ophthalmol Strab 1997;34:297–305.

403. Tychsen L, Hoyt WF. Occipital lobe dysplasia. Magnetic resonance findings in two cases of isolated congenital hemianopsia. Arch Ophthalmol 1985;103:680–682.

404. Kuzniecky RI. Magnetic resonance imaging in developmental disorders of the cerebral cortex. Epilepsia 1994;35:S44–56.

405. Barkovich AJ, Kjos BO. Schizencephaly. Correlation of clinical findings with MR characteristics. AJNR 1992;13:85–94.

406. Raymond AA, Fish DR, Sisodiya SM, et al. Abnormalities of gyration, heterotopias, tuberous sclerosis, focal cortical dysplasia, microdysgenesis, dysembryoplastic neuroepithelial tumour and dysgenesis of the archicortex in epilepsy. Clinical, EEG and neuroimaging features in 100 adult patients. Brain 1995;118:629–660.

407. Good WV, Jan JE, DeSa L, et al. Cortical visual impairment in children. Surv Ophthalmol 1994;38:351–364.

408. Bianchi PE, Salati R, Cavallini A, et al. Transient nystagmus in delayed visual maturation. Dev Med Child Neurol 1998;40:263–265.

409. Hoyt CS. Constenbader Lecture. Delayed visual maturation. The apparently blind infant. J AAPOS 2004;8:215–219.

410. Weiss AH, Kelly JP, Phillips JO. The infant who is visually unresponsive on a cortical basis. Ophthalmology 2001;108:2076–2087.

411. Pavlakis SG, Phillips PC, DiMauro S, et al. Mitochondrial myopathy, encephalopathy, lactic acidosis, and strokelike episodes. A distinctive clinical syndrome. Ann Neurol 1984;16:481–488.

412. Newman NJ. Neuro-ophthalmology of mitochondrial disorders in children. Pediatric Neuro-ophthalmology course. American Academy of Neurology 1998. Minneapolis, MN.

413. DiMauro S, Schon EA. Mitochondrial DNA and diseases of the nervous system. The spectrum. Neuroscientist 1998;4:53–63.

414. Rummelt V, Folberg R, Ionasescu V, et al. Ocular pathology of MELAS syndrome with mitochondrial DNA nucleotide 3243 point mutation. Ophthalmology 1993;100:1757–1766.

415. Sue CM, Mitchell P, Crimmins DS, et al. Pigmentary retinopathy associated with the mitochondrial DNA 3243 point mutation. Neurology 1997;49:1013–1017.

416. Latkany P, Ciulla TA, Cacchillo PF, et al. Mitochondrial maculopathy. Geographic atrophy of the macula in the MELAS associated A to G 3243 mitochondrial DNA point mutation. Am J Ophthalmol 1999;128:112–114.

417. Hirano M, Pavlakis SG. Mitochondrial myopathy, encephalopathy, lactic acidosis, and strokelike episodes (MELAS). Current concepts. J Child Neurol 1994;9:4–13.

418. Kimata KG, Gordan L, Ajax ET, et al. A case of late-onset MELAS. Arch Neurol 1998;55:722–725.

419. Sharfstein SR, Gordon MF, Libman RB, et al. Adult-onset MELAS presenting as herpes encephalitis. Arch Neurol 1999;56:241–243.

420. Case records of the Massachusetts General Hospital. Case 36–2005. N Engl J Med 2005;353:2271–2280.

421. Thambisetty M, Newman NJ. Diagnosis and management of MELAS. Expert Rev Mol Diagn 2004;4:631–644.

422. Sproule DM, Kaufmann P. Mitochondrial encephalopathy, lactic acidosis, and strokelike episodes. Basic concepts, clinical phenotype, and therapeutic management of MELAS syndrome. Ann N Y Acad Sci 2008;1142:133–158.

423. Koo B, Becker LE, Chuang S, et al. Mitochondrial encephalomyopathy, lactic acidosis, stroke-like episodes (MELAS). Clinical, radiological, pathological, and genetic observations. Ann Neurol 1993;34:25–32.

424. Majamaa K, Turkka J, Kärppä M, et al. The common MELAS mutation A3243G in mitochondrial DNA among young patients with an occipital brain infarct. Neurology 1997;49:1331–1334.

425. Naini AB, Lu J, Kaufmann P, et al. Novel mitochondrial DNA ND5 mutation in a patient with clinical features of MELAS and MERRF. Arch Neurol 2005;62:473–476.

426. Saitoh S, Momoi MY, Yamagata T, et al. Effects of dichloroacetate in three patients with MELAS. Neurology 1998;50:531–534.

427. Clark JM, Marks MP, Adalsteinsson E, et al. MELAS. Clinical and pathologic correlations with MRI, xenon/CT, and MR spectroscopy. Neurology 1996;46:223–227.

428. Yonemura K, Hasegawa Y, Kimura K, et al. Diffusion-weighted MR imaging in a case of mitochondrial myopathy, encephalopathy, lactic acidosis, and strokelike episodes. AJNR Am J Neuroradiol 2001;22:269–272.

429. Bi WL, Baehring JM, Lesser RL. Evolution of brain imaging abnormalities in mitochondrial encephalomyopathy with lactic acidosis and stroke-like episodes. J Neuroophthalmol 2006;26:251–256.

430. Case records of the Massachusetts General Hospital. Case 39–1998. N Engl J Med 1998;339:1914–1923.

431. Iizuka T, Sakai F, Suzuki N, et al. Neuronal hyperexcitability in stroke-like episodes of MELAS syndrome. Neurology 2002;59:816–824.

432. Penn AMW, Lee JWK, Thuillier P, et al. MELAS syndrome with mitochondrial tRNA$^{Leu(UUR)}$ mutation. Correlation of clinical state, nerve conduction, and muscle ^{31}P magnetic resonance spectroscopy during treatment with nicotinamide and riboflavin. Neurology 1992;42:2147–2152.

433. Koga Y, Ishibashi M, Ueki I, et al. Effects of L-arginine on the acute phase of strokes in three patients with MELAS. Neurology 2002;58:827–828.

434. Moser HW. Adrenoleukodystrophy. Survey of 303 cases. Biochemistry, diagnosis, and therapy. Ann Neurol 1984;16:628–641.

435. Moser HW. Adrenoleukodystrophy. Phenotype, genetics, pathogenesis and therapy. Brain 1997;120:1485–1508.

436. Kaye EM. Update on genetic disorders affecting white matter. Pediatr Neurol 2001;24:11–24.

437. Schaumberg HH, Powers JM, Raine CS, et al. Adrenoleukodystrophy. A clinical and pathological study of 17 cases. Arch Neurol 1975;32:577–591.

438. Wray SH, Cogan DG, Kuwabara T, et al. Adrenoleukodystrophy with disease of the eye and optic nerve. Am J Ophthalmol 1976;82:480–485.

439. Traboulsi EI, Maumenee IH. Ophthalmologic manifestations of X-linked childhood adrenoleukodystrophy. Ophthalmology 1987;94:47–52.

440. Öz G, Tkác I, Charnas LR, et al. Assessment of adrenoleukodystrophy lesions by high field MRS in non-sedated pediatric patients. Neurology 2005;64:434–441.

441. Gess A, Christiansen SP, Pond D, et al. Predictive factors for vision loss after hematopoietic cell transplant for X-linked adrenoleukodystrophy. J AAPOS 2008;12:273–276.

442. Farrell DF, Hamilton SR, Knauss TA, et al. X-linked adrenoleukodystrophy. Adult cerebral variant. Neurology 1993;43:1518–1522.

443. Costello DJ, Eichler FS, Grant PE, et al. Case records of the Massachusetts General Hospital. Case 1–2009. A 57-year-old man with progressive cognitive decline. N Engl J Med 2009;360:171–181.

444. Griffin JW, Goren E, Schaumburg H, et al. Adrenomyeloneuropathy. A probable variant of adrenoleukodystrophy. Neurology 1977;27:1107–1113.

445. Kaplan PW, Kruse B, Tusa RJ, et al. Visual system abnormalities in adrenomyeloneuropathy. Ann Neurol 1995;37:550–552.

446. Brodsky MC, Baker RS, Hamed LM. Neuro-ophthalmologic manifestations of systemic and intracranial disease. In: Pediatric Neuro-ophthalmology, pp 399–465. New York, Springer-Verlag, 1996.

447. Richard JM. The phacomatoses. neurocutaneous disorders. In: Wright KW (ed). Pediatric Ophthalmology and Strabismus, pp 673–687. St. Louis, Mosby, 1995.

448. Tallman B, Tan OT, Morelli JG, et al. Location of port-wine stains and the likelihood of ophthalmic and/or central nervous system complications. Pediatrics 1991;87:323–327.

449. Thomas-Sohl KA, Vaslow DF, Maria BL. Sturge-Weber syndrome. A review. Pediatr Neurol 2004;30:303–310.

450. Pascual-Castroviejo I, Diaz-Gonzalez C, Garcia-Melian RM, et al. Sturge-Weber syndrome. Study of 40 patients. Pediatr Neurol 1993;9:283–288.

451. Maria BL, Neufeld JA, Rosainz LC, et al. High prevalence of bihemispheric structural and functional defects in Sturge-Weber syndrome. J Child Neurol 1998;13:595–605.

452. Maria BL, Neufeld JA, Rosainz LC, et al. Central nervous system structure and function in Sturge-Weber syndrome. Evidence of neurologic and radiologic progression. J Child Neurol 1998;13:606–618.

453. Udani V, Pujar S, Munot P, et al. Natural history and magnetic resonance imaging follow-up in 9 Sturge-Weber syndrome patients and clinical correlation. J Child Neurol 2007;22:479–483.

454. Arzimanoglou AA, Andermann F, Aicardi J, et al. Sturge-Weber syndrome. Indications and results of surgery in 20 patients. Neurology 2000;55:1472–1479.

455. Kossoff EH, Buck C, Freeman JM. Outcomes of 32 hemispherectomies for Sturge-Weber syndrome worldwide. Neurology 2002;59:1735–1738.

456. Brooks BP, Simpson JL, Leber SM, et al. Infantile spasms as a cause of acquired perinatal visual loss. J AAPOS 2002;6:385–388.

457. Harden CL, Rosenbaum DH, Daras M. Hyperglycemia presenting with occipital seizures. Epilepsia 1991;32:215–220.

458. Freedman KA, Polepalle S. Transient homonymous hemianopia and positive visual phenomena in nonketotic hyperglycemic patients. Am J Ophthalmol 2004;137:1122–1124.

459. Taban M, Naugle RI, Lee MS. Transient homonymous hemianopia and positive visual phenomena in patients with nonketotic hyperglycemia. Arch Ophthalmol 2007;125:845–847.

460. Moster MM, Galetta SL, Schatz NJ. Physiologic functional imaging in "functional" visual loss. Surv Ophthalmol 1996;40:395–399.

461. Wang A-G, Liu R-S, Liu J-H, et al. Positron emission tomography scan in cortical visual loss in patients with organophosphate intoxication. Ophthalmology 1999;106:1287–1291.

462. Miki A, Nakajima T, Abe A, et al. Occipital lobe dysfunction revealed by functional brain imaging in a patient with traumatic visual field loss. Neuroophthalmology 1999;22:127–132.

463. Lee YJ, Chung TS, Yoon YS, et al. The role of functional MR imaging in patients with ischemia in the visual cortex. AJNR Am J Neuroradiol 2001;22:1043–1049.

464. Miki A, Liu GT, Modestino EJ, et al. Functional magnetic resonance imaging of the visual system. Curr Opin Ophthalmol 2001;12:423–431.

465. Miki A, Haselgrove JC, Liu GT. Functional magnetic resonance imaging and its clinical utility in patients with visual disturbances. Surv Ophthalmol 2002;47:562–579.

466. Granet DB, Hertle RW, Quinn GE, et al. The visual-evoked response in infants with cerebral visual impairment. Am J Ophthalmol 1993;116:437–443.

467. Watanabe K, Shinoda K, Kimura I, et al. Discordance between subjective perimetric visual fields and objective multifocal visual evoked potential-determined visual fields in patients with hemianopsia. Am J Ophthalmol 2007;143:295–304.

468. Donahue SP, Haun AK. Exotropia and face turn in children with homonymous hemianopia. J Neuroophthalmol 2007;27:304–307.

469. Smith JL, Weiner IG, Lucero AJ. Hemianopic Fresnel prisms. J Clin Neuroophthalmol 1982;2:19–22.

470. Perlin RR, Dziadul J. Fresnel prisms for field enhancement of patients with constricted or hemianopic visual fields. J Am Optom Assoc 1991;62:58–64.

471. Bowers AR, Keeney K, Peli E. Community-based trial of a peripheral prism visual field expansion device for hemianopia. Arch Ophthalmol 2008;126:657–664.

472. Pambakian A, Currie J, Kennard C. Rehabilitation strategies for patients with homonymous visual field defects. J Neuroophthalmol 2005;25:136–142.

473. Roth T, Sokolov AN, Messias A, et al. Comparing explorative saccade and flicker training in hemianopia. A randomized controlled study. Neurology 2009;72:324–331.

474. Spitzyna GA, Wise RJ, McDonald SA, et al. Optokinetic therapy improves text reading in patients with hemianopic alexia. A controlled trial. Neurology 2007;68:1922–1930.

475. Zihl J, Von Cramen D. Restitution of visual function in patients with cerebral blindness. J Neurol Neurosurg Psychiatr 1979;42:312–322.

476. Zihl J, Von Cramen D. Visual field recovery from scotoma in patients with postgeniculate damage. A review of 55 cases. Brain 1985;108:335–365.

477. Reinhard J, Schreiber A, Schiefer U, et al. Does visual restitution training change absolute homonymous visual field defects? A fundus controlled study. Br J Ophthalmol 2005;89:30–35.

478. Hyvärinen L, Raninen AN, Näsänen RE. Visual rehabilitation in homonymous hemianopia. Neuroophthalmology 2002;27:97–102.

479. Poggel DA, Kasten E, Sabel BA. Attentional cueing improves vision restoration therapy in patients with visual field defects. Neurology 2004;63:2069–2076.

480. Sabel BA, Trauzettel-Klosinksi S. Improving vision in a patient with homonymous hemianopia. J Neuroophthalmol 2005;25:143–149.

481. Glisson CC. Capturing the benefit of vision restoration therapy. Curr Opin Ophthalmol 2006;17:504–508.

482. Glisson CC, Galetta SL. Visual rehabilitation. Now you see it; now you don't [editorial]. Neurology 2007;68:1881–1882.

483. Galetta SL, Glisson CC. Visual rehabilitation. Now you see it; now you don't [correspondence]. Neurology 2008;70:159.

484. Marshall RS, Ferrera JJ, Barnes A, et al. Brain activity associated with stimulation therapy of the visual borderzone in hemianopic stroke patients. Neurorehabil Neural Repair 2008;22:136–144.

485. Huxlin KR, Martin T, Kelly K, et al. Perceptual relearning of complex visual motion after V1 damage in humans. J Neurosci 2009;29:3981–3991.

486. Schreiber A, Vonthein R, Reinhard J, et al. Effect of visual restitution training on absolute homonymous scotomas. Neurology 2006;67:143–145.

487. Horton JC. Disappointing results from Nova Vision's visual restoration therapy. Br J Ophthalmol 2005;89:1–2.

488. Javeed N, Khan Z, Jayaram S, et al. Cerebral amyloid angiopathy. Res Staff Phys 1995;41:21–28.

CHAPTER **9**

Disorders of higher cortical visual function

While the anterior visual and geniculocalcarine pathways deliver the elemental visual data from the eyes to striate cortex, the higher cortical visual (or association) areas perform the more complex interpretation of this visual information.[1] Deficits caused by damage to these areas are characterized by abnormalities in visual processing or attention often despite otherwise relatively normal visual acuity and fields.[2,3] This chapter will detail the important higher cortical visual disorders (**Table 9–1**), then highlight some of the neurologic diseases which commonly cause them.

Neuroanatomical organization of higher cortical areas

Area V1 designates striate cortex (Brodmann area 17), while V2–V5 refer to higher cortical (or association) visual areas. The higher cortical visual areas are divided anatomically and functionally into ventral and dorsal pathways (**Fig. 9–1**, middle).[4] In general, the ventral stream (occipitotemporal) is more concerned with object recognition ("what") and represents the continuation of the parvocellular pathway (**Fig. 9–1**, bottom).[5] The area V4 complex, situated in the fusiform and lingual gyri, is responsible for color perception within the contralateral hemifield.[6] Bilateral mesial occipitotemporal regions are necessary for object and facial recognition.[7–9] On the other hand, the dorsal stream carries out functions related to spatial orientation[10] (the "where" pathway) and is the extension of the magnocellular pathway (**Fig. 9–1**, top). The parietal lobe is devoted to directed attention. Area V5, within the lateral occipitotemporal region, is important for motion perception. Areas V2 and V3 correspond roughly to Brodmann areas 18 and 19, respectively.

Important concepts in higher cortical visual disorders

The various higher cortical visual disorders will be discussed below by cerebral localization. However, two concepts, disconnection and simultaneous occurrence, should be considered in any review of these conditions.

Disconnection (versus direct damage)

While some of the higher cortical disorders result from direct damage to vital cortical areas, such as the color center in the inferior occipitotemporal lobe, others, for example, result from disconnecting the occipital lobe from visual association areas. This disconnection concept was popularized by Geschwind.[11–13] Examples would include a lesion involving white matter pathways connecting striate cortex and facial recognition centers or another

Table 9–1 Important higher cortical visual disturbances, their main and associated clinical features, and their most common localization. Whether or not the condition is a disconnection syndrome is also indicated

Syndrome	Main clinical features	Commonly associated clinical features	Most common localization	Disconnection?
Alexia without agraphia	Able to write but not read	Right homonymous hemianopia	Left occipital lobe and splenium of corpus callosum	Yes, usually
Hemi-achrom-atopsia	Loss of color vision in one hemifield	Ipsilateral homonymous upper quadrantanopia	Contralateral occipito-temporal lobe in the fusiform (and lingual) gyri (V4 complex)	No
Visual object agnosia	Inability to recognize visualized objects	Alexia without agraphia Prosopagnosia	Bilateral occipito-temporal lobes involving the inferior longitudinal fasciculi	Yes
Prosopagnosia	Inability to recognize faces	Alexia without agraphia Visual object agnosia	Bilateral occipito-temporal lobes involving the midfusiform gyri, rarely associated with unilateral lesions	Sometimes
Akinetopsia	Defective motion perception	None	Bilateral lateral occipito-temporal lobes (V5)	No
Visual hemi-inattention	Neglect of visual stimuli in left hemi-space	Inattention Left-sided sensory loss and weakness	Right inferior parietal lobule	No
Balint syndrome	Simultanagnosia Ocular apraxia Optic ataxia	Bilateral inferior altitudinal visual field defects	Bilateral parieto-occipital lobes	Yes for some features

connecting to language areas. **Table 9–1** indicates which higher cortical visual disorders are thought to be disconnection syndromes versus those which are due to direct damage to cortical structures.

Simultaneous occurrence

The higher cortical visual disorders are not mutually exclusive. Rather, because of the proximity of many of the important cortical areas and white matter tracts in the parietal, occipital, and temporal lobes, many syndromes occur simultaneously. For instance, a combination of visual field defects, visual recognition, and reading disorders often result from concomitant involvement of the occipital and occipito-temporal lobes (**Table 9–1**).

Symptoms and signs

Neuro-ophthalmic symptoms

Most subjective complaints due to involvement of visual association areas are vague, such as "I have blurry vision" or "I'm having trouble seeing." Rarely, patients will complain of difficulty seeing colors or recognizing faces. Many such patients have seen numerous eye specialists with reportedly normal examinations. Some individuals with inattention or dementia are unaware of their visual deficits, and the family

members are the ones who bring them to medical attention. Another group of patients is seen after a stroke or neurosurgical intervention. Visual field loss may cause the dominant symptoms but careful examination reveals that complaints of "trouble reading and seeing" may be the result of higher cortical dysfunction.

Neurologic symptoms

Higher cortical visual disturbances should be suspected when patients complain of loss of memory, confusion, disorientation, or behavioral changes suggestive of a dementing illness or hemispheric lesion. Their families may report that patients seem no longer able to take care of themselves or get lost frequently.

Signs on examination

Visual acuity is usually normal. Visual fields in each quadrant and with double simultaneous stimulation should be tested to exclude visual inattention. Color vision, reading, and writing should also be examined. In addition, magazine pictures with familiar faces and pictures with complex scenery can be used to screen for higher cortical dysfunction. Sometimes figure and clock drawings are also helpful. **Table 9–2** highlights the various examination techniques helpful in patients with suspected higher cortical visual disorders, and these methods are reviewed in detail in Chapter 2.

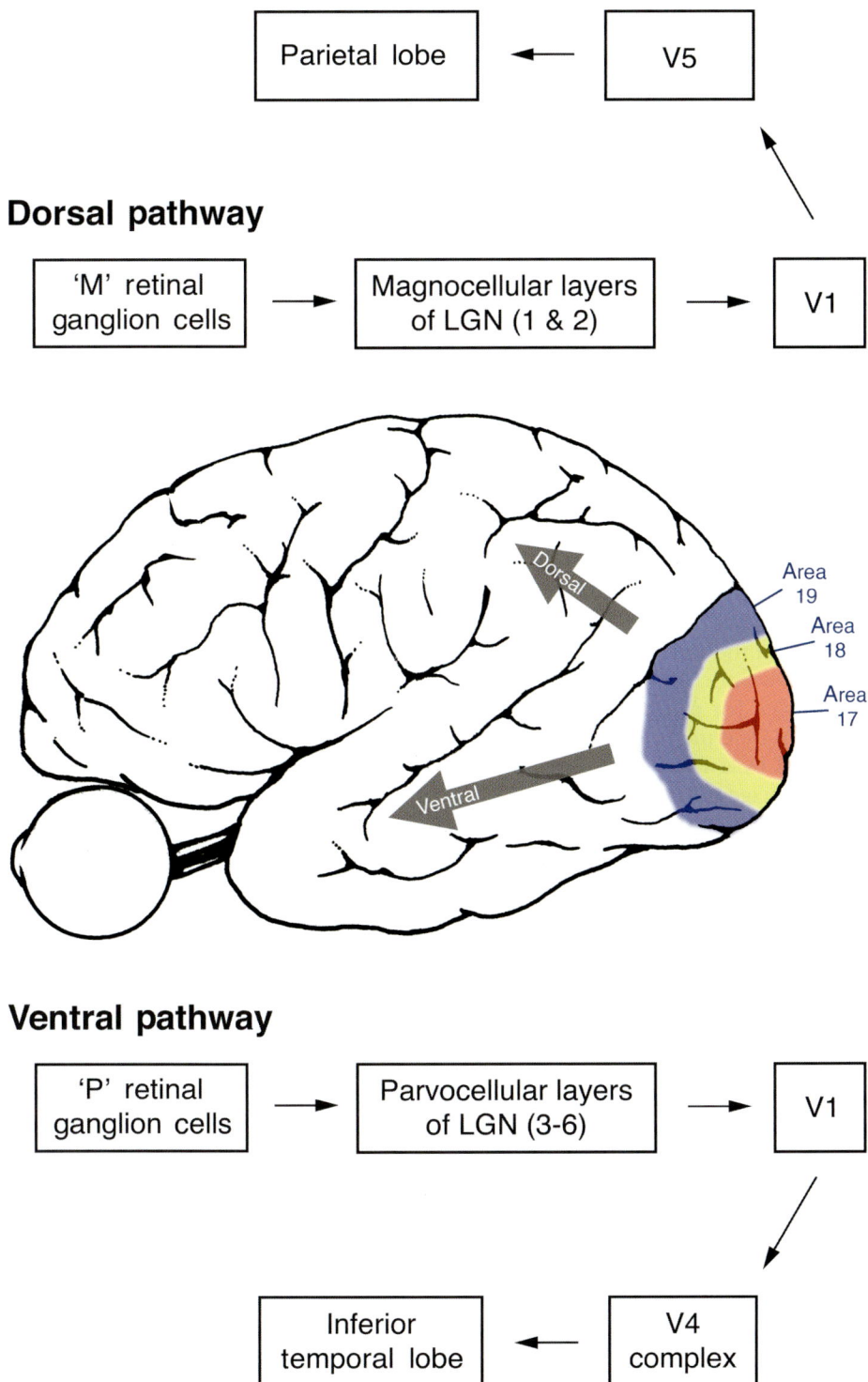

Figure 9–1. Diagram of dorsal and ventral higher cortical visual streams. **Middle**. Lateral view of the brain. In an oversimplification, after reaching area 17, visual information passes through areas 18 and 19, then dorsally for spatial analysis and ventrally for object analysis. Schematic diagrams of dorsal stream (magnocellular pathway) for spatial relations and "where" analysis (**Top**); and ventral stream (parvocellular pathway) for color and "what" analysis (**bottom**), from retina to higher cortical visual areas. LGN = lateral geniculate nucleus.

Occipital lobe disturbances

Disorders of V1 are described in Chapter 8. Areas V2 and V3 surround V1 above and below the calcarine sulcus (see Chapter 8). Isolated and clinically apparent lesions of V2 and V3 are unusual, but a combined lesion of V2 and V3 restricted to upper or lower bank typically causes a homonymous quadrantic visual field defect.[14]

Another condition, alexia without agraphia, is a more commonly recognized occipital lobe syndrome and is detailed below:

Table 9–2 Examination techniques helpful in patients with suspected higher cortical visual disorders. See Chapter 2 for detailed description of each test

Test	Result	Higher cortical disorder to suspect
Reading and writing	Able to write but not read	Alexia without agraphia
Ishihara color plates	Can see colors but not the numbers	Simultanagnosia
Ishihara color plates	Misses all the digits on one side	Hemi-achromatopsia
Magazine pictures	Identifies only part and not the whole scene	Simultanagnosia
Famous faces in pictures and familiar ones in identification cards	Cannot identify familiar faces	Prosopagnosia
Name objects presented visually	Unable to identify objects by sight but can with verbal description	Visual object agnosia

Alexia without agraphia

Often aphasic patients who have difficulty reading also have difficulty writing. However, patients with a left occipital lesion and ipsilateral simultaneous involvement of the splenium of the corpus callosum or adjacent periventricular white matter may develop *alexia without agraphia* (or *pure alexia* or *"word-blindness"*). First characterized by Dejerine,[15] this is a disconnection syndrome characterized by a right homonymous field deficit, sparing of key language areas, but an inability to access lexical visual information processed in the right occipital lobe (**Fig. 9–2**). Geschwind[11,12] emphasized that reading is impossible if the left angular gyrus, which is responsible for converting written to spoken language, is deprived of visual information. Affected patients are therefore unable to read words, but they are able to write, speak, comprehend, and repeat normally. Ironically, then, they are unable to read what they write. Patients have a common compensatory strategy, called letter-by-letter reading, during which they sequentially name each letter of a word.[16–18]

Many variations on the classic description of alexia without agraphia have been described.

1. *Other lesions.* Alexia without agraphia due to infarction of the left lateral geniculate body and splenium of the corpus callosum has been reported.[19]

2. *No hemianopia.* Less commonly patients have been described with alexia without agraphia but with normal visual fields.[20–24] It is possible that periventricular white matter lesions in the left occipital lobe alone may spare striate cortex but interfere with the transfer of visual information from both ipsilateral and contralateral striate cortex to the language areas by undercutting the angular gyrus.[25]

    In addition, recent evidence suggests the existence of a "visual word form area" (VWFA) in the posterior part of the left midfusiform gyrus in the occipitotemporal region.[26–28] Although this area is contested,[29,30] focal disturbances in this region theoretically could lead to an isolated inability to read the word as a whole: thus alexia alone without a hemianopia.[31]

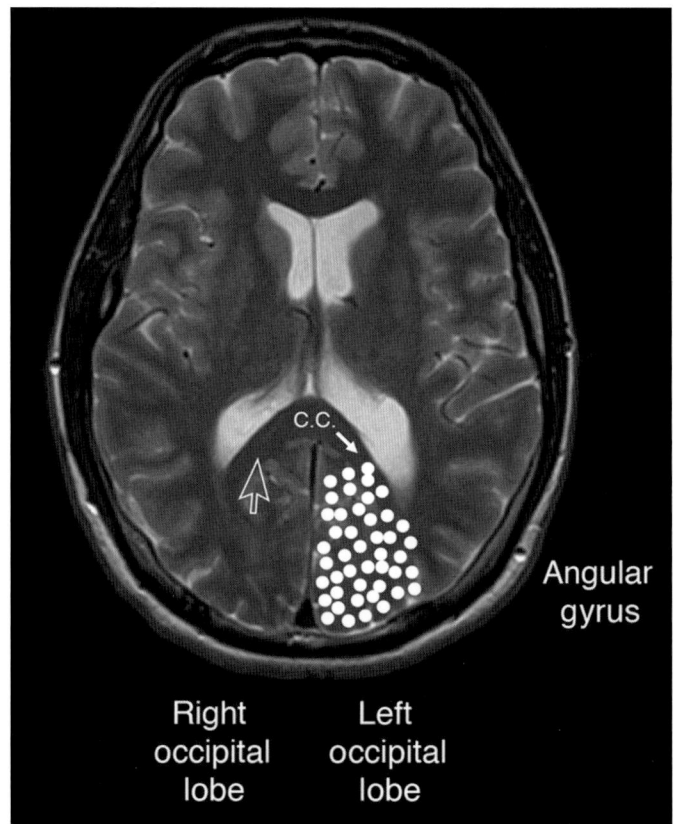

Figure 9–2. Classic localization of the left occipital lesion (dotted area) in patients with alexia without agraphia and right homonymous hemianopia. Because of the left lateral and mesial occipital lobe involvement, visual information (open arrow) can come only from the right occipital lobe. However, owing to disruption of the paraventricular white matter and the outflow of the corpus callosum (C.C.), this visual information (small arrow) cannot access the angular gyrus in the language areas.

3. *Left hemiparalexia.* Isolated lesions of the splenium of the corpus callosum may have intact visual fields, but inability to transfer visual information from the right occipital lobe to the left angular gyrus.[32] This may cause an inability to read the left side of words despite the absence of a hemianopia.

4. *Other associated higher cortical visual disturbances.* Several cases have been reported where alexia without agraphia

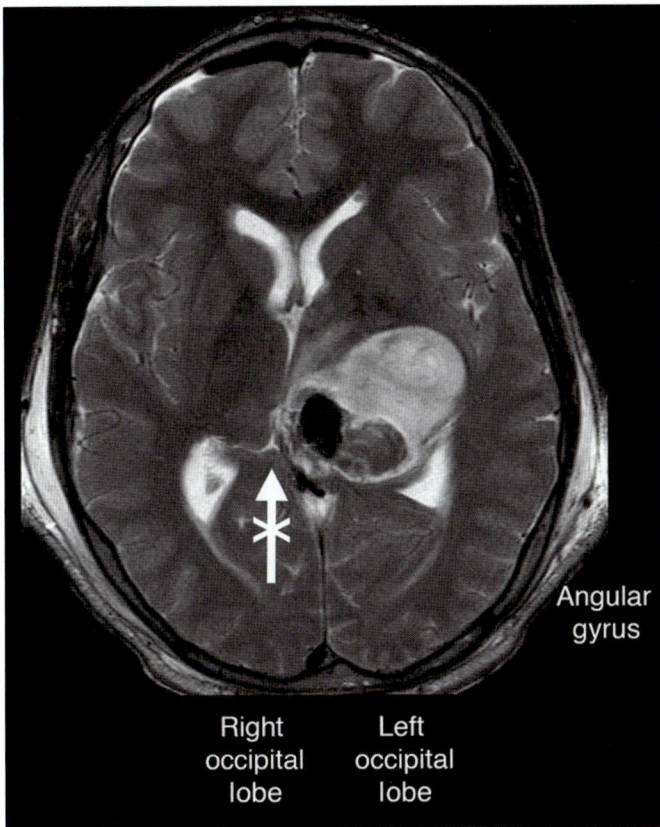

Figure 9–3. Alexia without agraphia and right homonymous hemianopia following biopsy of a left thalamic tumor. Postoperative T2-weighted MRI scan of the brain, showing an exophytic mass and hemorrhage in the surgical bed. The white arrow and cross refer to the inability of visual information from the right occipital lobe to reach the angular gyrus and language areas in the left hemisphere, owing to the disruption of the forceps major and splenium of the corpus callosum. (Reprinted from Tamhankar M et al. Pediatr Neurol 2004;30:140–142, with permission from Elsevier).

occurs together with various combinations of apperceptive visual agnosia, prosopagnosia,[33,34] visuospatial disorientation, optic ataxia, optic aphasia,[35] hemiachromatopsia, and color naming deficits (these are all discussed below).[25,36]

While the most common cause of alexia without agraphia is a posterior cerebral artery distribution stroke,[37] it has also been reported in association with intracerebral hemorrhages,[38] arteriovenous malformations,[39] tumors (Fig. 9–3),[40] abscesses, migraine, herpes encephalitis,[41] and demyelination.[42,43]

Other related reading disorders. In contrast, *alexia with agraphia* is a syndrome characterized by the inability to read or write without other obvious language deficits. Caused by an isolated lesion of the angular gyrus or the posterior left inferior temporal lobe, there is often an accompanying right homonymous hemianopia because of involvement of the adjacent optic radiations.

Alexia without agraphia should not be confused with *hemianopic alexia*, in which patients have difficulty reading because their right homonymous hemianopia, particularly if macular splitting, interferes with their ability to see the right side of a word.[44,45]

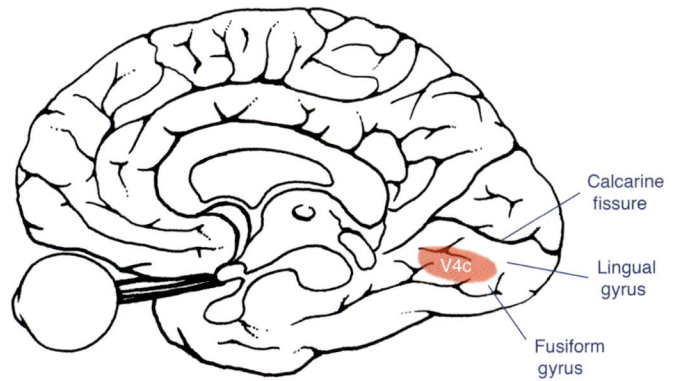

Figure 9–4. Medial view of the brain demonstrating location of area V4 complex, the human color center, which lies primarily in the posterior fusiform gyrus, with a lesser contribution from the lingual gyrus.

Occipitotemporal disturbances

Cerebral hemiachromatopsia

More than a century ago, Verrey[46] described hemiachromatopsia, the loss of color vision in one hemifield, and claimed that a functionally separate cortex existed for color processing. However, only in the past three decades has the notion of a neuroanatomically distinct region for color vision been accepted.[47] Initially, lesion studies in primates and humans have designated a region of the visual association cortex known as V4 to be critical for color processing.[48,49] In humans the V4 homologue resides in the lingual and fusiform gyri, located in the ventromedial occipitotemporal cortex (Fig. 9–4).[50] There is a similar area on both sides of the brain, and each mediates color vision in the opposite hemifield.

Functional neuroimaging has helped to confirm the specialization of V4 and has elucidated other adjacent areas responsible for mediating color vision in humans. Positron emission tomography (PET) studies of individuals viewing a multicolored abstract display show increased blood flow to V1/V2 and the lingual and fusiform gyri.[51] Studies using functional magnetic resonance imaging (MRI), comparing brain activation during colored versus black and white stimulus conditions, found the most significant changes in brain oxygenation occurred in the fusiform gyrus.[52,53] Likewise, electrical cortical stimulation studies in epilepsy patients confirm the presence of a specialized color center in humans.[54,55] A region in the fusiform gyrus anterior to V4, termed area V8, was found to mediate conscious perception of color and color afterimages[56] and color synesthesia.[57] In addition, other adjacent color-sensitive cortical regions termed VO[58,59] and V4-α[60] have been identified.[61] Herein, for the purposes of this chapter, these neighboring regions (V4, V8, VO-1, and V4-α) will be collectively termed area V4 complex.

Symptoms. Many patients with hemiachromatopsia are unaware of their color deficit, perhaps because the other hemifield has intact color vision, or because they ignore their deficit (anosognosia). Hemiachromatopsia can occur in the left or right hemifield. When bilateral V4 complex lesions occur, patients may develop central achromatopsia,

343

or defective color vision in both hemifields. Compared to those with hemiachromatopsia, bilaterally affected patients may be more likely to describe their color deficit, which may differ from a loss of brightness to a complete inability to perceive colors.[62] The described effect is a "graying" or "washing-out" of vision.[63] Some liken the impact to a switch from a color television to a black-and-white one.[64]

Signs. Since acquired cerebral color deficits tend to occur in quadrants or hemifields, they are best detected during confrontation field testing using colored swatches, sticks, or threads. Color plate testing may also reveal a hemi-defect in color vision if the patient consistently misses the left sided digits, for instance. However, color plate identification may be normal as may be more formal color testing, such as D-15 or Farnsworth–Munsell 100-Hue tests (see Chapter 2), for example, if color vision is normal within central fixation.

Associated signs. Cerebral hemiachromatopsia is rarely an isolated finding. More commonly a combination of a contralateral homonymous upper quadrantanopsia and defective color vision in the inferior quadrant is observed clinically (**Fig. 9–5**).[50] This pattern of deficits is likely the result of the proximity between the lingual and fusiform gyri and the inferior optic radiations, inferior striate cortex, and inferior extrastriate cortex (V2/V3).[14] Visual acuity is normal when the lesions are unilateral. Hemiachromatopsia may also be associated with alexia without agraphia (see above) when the lesion is left sided,[65] or prosopagnosia (see below) because the areas responsible for color and face processing are in close proximity in the occipitotemporal cortices.[6,66–68]

When isolated cerebral full-field hemiachromatopsia occurs, it is often in the setting of a developing or receding hemianopia.[67] Albert et al.[69] described a monocular man who suffered cortical blindness only to recover with a partial right superior quadrantanopia yet complete left-sided color vision loss. In Kölmel's two cases,[70] a homonymous hemianopia resolved eventually to an upper quadrant hemiachromatopsia, in one instance following a transient full-field hemiachromatopsia.

Etiology. Infarction in the distribution of the posterior temporal or common temporal arteries, branches of the posterior cerebral artery, is the most common cause of hemiachromatopsia. Other less common etiologies include removal of an arteriovenous malformation,[71] trauma,[72] neoplasm,[67] hemorrhage, multiple sclerosis,[73] abscess, subarachnoid hemorrhage, and carbon monoxide poisoning.[74] Transient full-field achromatopsia has been attributed to migraine,[75] occipital epilepsy (after the recovery of form vision), and vertebrobasilar insufficiency.[76]

Other cortical color processing deficits. Patients with *color anomia*, or *color name aphasia*, have an inability to name colors despite normal color perception, as evidenced by their intact ability to match colors and identify pseudo-isochromatic color plates.[3] They also have difficulty pointing to named colors. This disorder can be associated with alexia without agraphia (see above),[36] and patients commonly have a right homonymous hemianopia.[64] The usual etiology is a left posterior cerebral artery stroke involving the mesial occipitotemporal region.[77] Those with *color*

agnosia, or *color amnesia*, have trouble naming the specific color of common objects, such as blood or a stop sign, despite normal color perception and language function. In one published case,[78] color agnosia was acquired due to bilateral medial temporal and left inferotemporo-occipital infarctions, but in another the deficit was life-long without any obvious cortical lesions on MRI.[79,80] Both color anomia and color agnosia are rare.[81]

Visual agnosias

A *visual object agnosia* is an inability to recognize visualized objects despite relatively normal vision, memory, language, and intellectual function.[82,83] In this condition, naming function is intact, as patients are able to identify objects by touching and feeling them or by listening to a verbal description.[84] Functional neuroimaging studies suggest lateral occipital (LO) regions are used to recognize objects (**Fig. 9–6**).[85] Classically, a distinction between associative and apperceptive agnosias is made.[86–88]

Associative visual object agnosia. Patients with this type of agnosia have relatively normal vision within intact visual fields. They are able to draw or copy what they see, indicating their perception is relatively normal.[33] Upon request, they can also produce accurate drawings of objects they are unable to recognize visually, indicating intact visual memory and imagery.[33]

Associative visual object agnosia suggests bilateral medial inferior occipitotemporal lesions disrupting the inferior longitudinal fasciculus,[89,90] a white matter pathway connecting striate cortex with visual association areas in the temporal lobe. This is usually due to bilateral posterior cerebral artery occlusion and produces a "visual–verbal disconnection syndrome."[91] Many cases of associative visual object agnosia also exhibit alexia without agraphia,[33,92] likely reflecting concomitant involvement of the corpus callosum in such instances.[89] Many are also associated with prosopagnosia (see below).[33] Less commonly, isolated unilateral left or right hemispheric lesions can produce associative visual object agnosia.[92]

Apperceptive visual object agnosia. In this type, also termed *visual form agnosia*, patients have confounding deficits in shape and form perception although elemental acuity and fields are still relatively normal.[82,93] For instance, patients with apperceptive visual agnosia have difficulty copying geometric figures. In one study,[94] patients also had difficulty recognizing and naming line drawings, recognizing complex shapes, and mentally manipulating objects by rotation, for instance. The exact anatomic substrate is unclear, but some neuroimaging and PET studies have demonstrated lesions or hypoperfusion in bilateral temporo-occipital cortices.[95–98] A number of cases of apperceptive visual agnosia have been reported following carbon monoxide toxicity,[34,99,100] which has a predilection for causing occipital lobe damage.

Prosopagnosia

This section will review facial recognition and the related disorder, prosopagnosia, which is a dramatic visual agnosia for faces.[101] The observation that there are individuals with prosopagnosia but without visual agnosia for other objects

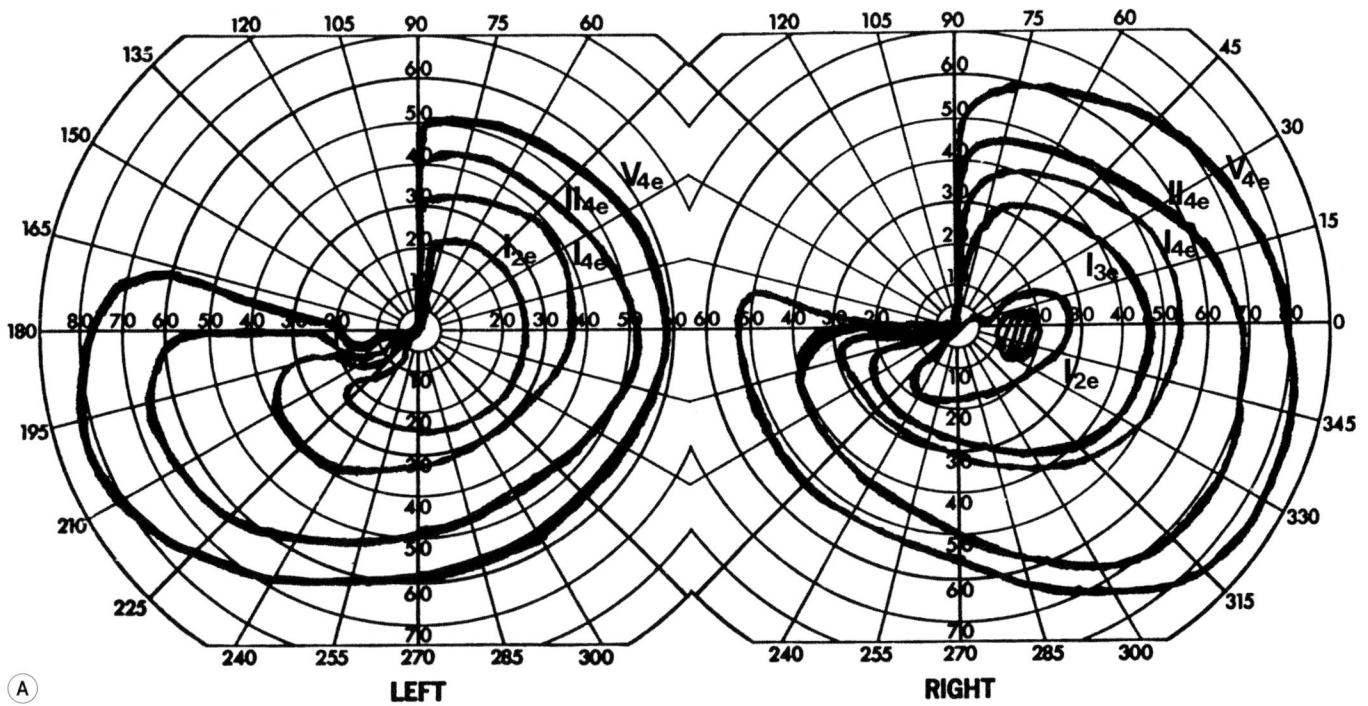

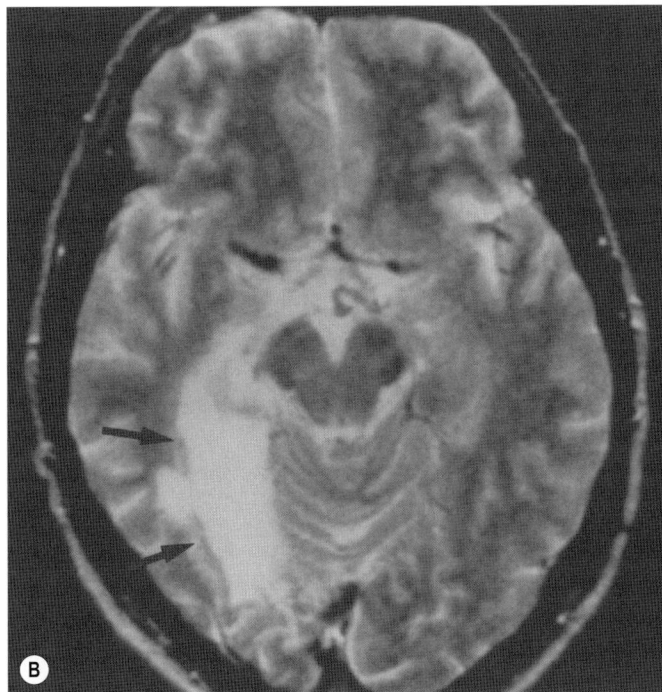

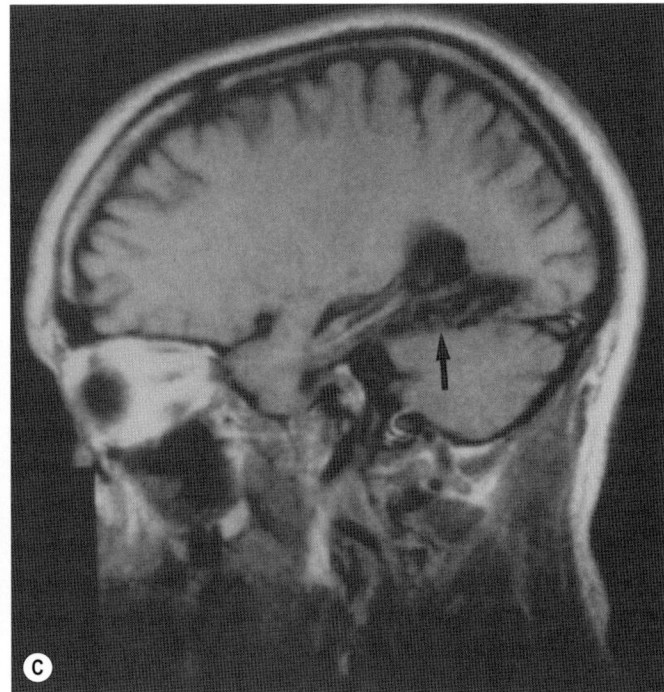

Figure 9–5. Visual field and neuroimaging in a patient with cerebral hemiachromatopsia of the left hemifield. **A.** Goldmann perimetry demonstrates a left homonymous superior quadrantanopia with an intact inferior quadrant. Axial (**B**) and sagittal (**C**) MRI reveals an infarction involving the right occipitotemporal gyri (arrows) (Reprinted from Paulson HL, Galetta SL, Grossman M, et al. Hemiachromatopsia of unilateral occipitotemporal infarcts. Am J Ophthalmol 1994;118:518–523, with permission from Elsevier Science).

suggests facial recognition is a modular specific task of the human brain.[102]

Facial recognition. The ability to recognize a familiar face is an extremely important behavior, used in almost every live interpersonal interaction. Even young infants have this ability, emphasizing its social and evolutionary importance. Facial recognition requires first perceiving the face, then ana-lyzing its features, matching it to stored faces, and in many instances, retrieving its name.[101]

Functional studies have established that occipitotemporal structures bilaterally are specialized, arguably specifi-cally, for human facial perception and recognition (**Fig. 9–6**). These areas include the fusiform and lingual gyri, in a region labeled as the fusiform face area (FFA),[103–105] one

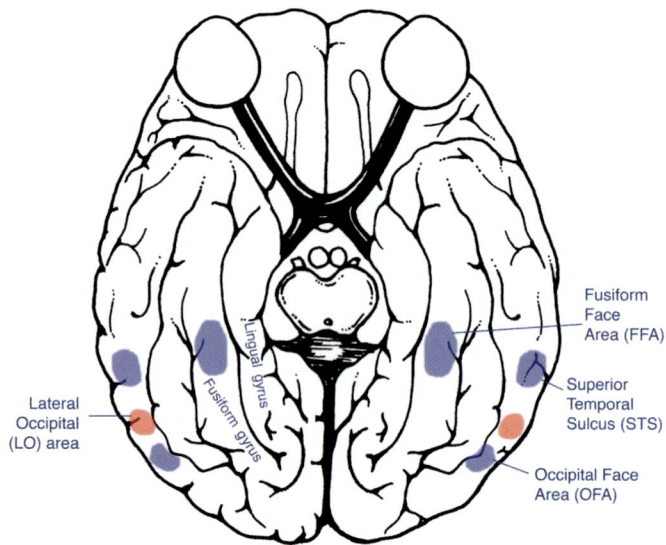

Figure 9–6. Underside view of the brain, highlighting the cortical areas active specifically during tasks of facial (FFA, STS, and OFA) and object recognition (LO).[105,116,168] Note V4 complex (not shown) lies more posteriorly in the fusiform gyrus (see Fig. 9–4). For simplicity, the highlighted areas, which are all bilateral, are labeled on only one side of the brain.

more posteriorly in the inferior occipital cortex in an area called the occipital face area (OFA),[27,106] and another in the superior temporal sulcus (STS).[107] These areas activate more strongly during viewing of faces when compared with seeing scrambled faces, common objects, houses, and human hands.[108] The FFA and OFA are likely more important for identification of faces, while the STS likely subserves processing of facial expression and gaze.[107] Less specifically, limbic structures such as the amygdala and hippocampus, in addition to anterior temporal cortex and right parahippocampal gyrus,[109–111] and the frontal lobe[112] also participate in facial recognition because of involvement of distributed emotional and memory networks necessary for this task.[113–116]

Signs and symptoms in prosopagnosia. Often very aware of their condition, patients with prosopagnosia commonly report the inability to recognize the faces of friends and family.[117] Functioning in society is difficult without the ability to recognize faces. A typical complaint is that the patient finds his or her own face in the mirror unfamiliar, but knows that the image must be theirs.[118] Likewise, prosopagnosics usually report knowing that they are looking at faces, and often they can identify the gender, race, and approximate age of the person.[117] Often patients use contextual clues such as posture, body movement,[118] and especially voices to identify familiar faces.[119] Most patients exhibit both a retrograde and anterograde defect, as they often cannot recognize old faces or learn new ones.[64] Sometimes the disorder is so striking and odd that affected patients may be mistakenly diagnosed with a psychiatric disease.[117]

Associated signs. Prosopagnosia may be isolated but more commonly is associated with elemental visual or other higher cortical deficits.[120] Unilateral homonymous hemianopias are typically present, but because the responsible lesions are typically occipitotemporal (see below), superior altitudinal or upper quadrantanopias are also seen.[7] Occasionally

bilateral visual field deficits and related visual acuity loss are observed. Associated higher cortical abnormalities include achromatopsia,[68,121] alexia without agraphia,[122,123] left hemispatial neglect,[124] visual memory deficits,[9] visual object agnosia,[125–127] visuospatial disorientation, impaired visual imagery,[34] color agnosia,[89] and anosognosia.[128]

Neuropsychological aspects. Because prosopagnosia is a type of visual agnosia, the condition is probably characterized by varying degrees of associative and apperceptive components (see visual agnosias, above).[129] Evidence for an associative component can be seen in patients with prosopagnosia but who can still correctly draw generic faces,[130] scan faces,[131,132] estimate a person's age[133] and gender,[130] and interpret and imitate facial expressions.[134,135] Patients with a more apperceptive type would be expected to have more difficulty with a face matching task, using for example a series of faces in the Benton–Van Allen facial recognition test,[133] than those with an associative type.[102,136,137] Further evidence of an apperceptive component can be seen in patients with prosopagnosia who have difficulty discerning curved stimuli[138] and face-related features such as eye gaze,[139] gender,[134] spatial relation of facial features,[140] and facial configuration.[141]

Similar to patients with blindsight (see Chapter 8), some patients with prosopagnosia report an inability to remember or distinguish faces, but careful testing may reveal some unconscious or covert ability to do so.[106,142,143]

Prosopagnosia may not be specific for human faces, as affected individuals may also have difficulty recognizing familiar animals. One former bird watcher lost the ability to identify birds with the onset of her prosopagnosia.[144] Likewise, a farmer reported the inability to recognize his cattle, although he was able to do so before the onset of prosopagnosia.[144] However, another patient began acquiring sheep after developing prosopagnosia. He was more successful on identification tasks involving his sheep than on identical tasks with human faces.[145]

Etiology and associations. The most common cause of prosopagnosia is a posterior cerebral artery stroke, although any process which can damage the occipitotemporal lobes may be responsible. Thus other etiologies include carbon monoxide poisoning,[34] temporal lobectomy, encephalitis,[131,146,147] neoplasms,[125] right temporal lobe atrophy,[148] trauma,[9] and Alzheimer's disease.[149] More diffuse processes include alcohol intoxication,[150] autism,[151] and psychosis due to schizophrenia and mescaline.[152] One epidemiological study found that prosopagnosia occurred significantly more frequently in men than in women,[153] which might be either a reflection of a higher incidence of stroke or a different lateralization of facial recognition in men.

Congenital prosopagnosia due to central nervous system insults due to meningitis or stroke in infancy has also been described.[119,143] In addition, there is a rare developmental variety of prosopagnosia in which individuals never acquire a normal ability to recognize faces.[154,155] In pure developmental cases there are no obvious visual abnormalities or lesions on neuroimaging,[156] and familial cases of developmental prosopagnosia have been reported.[157,158]

Localization and uni- versus bilaterality of the lesions. Most cases of prosopagnosia have bilateral lesions in the occipitotemporal region demonstrated at autopsy,[7,8,89,159] CT,[9,122,136,160] or MR imaging.[124] However, multiple cases have been reported of prosopagnosics with only right-sided lesions as uncovered by autopsy,[161] CT,[162,163] or MRI.[102,148,164–166] Prosopagnosia was also observed in a patient who had undergone a right hemispherectomy.[167] Thus it appears that bilateral lesions are often seen in patients with prosopagnosia, but in several instances a unilateral right-sided lesion was sufficient to cause the deficit.[101,168]

There is in fact evidence for a right-sided cerebral dominance for facial recognition in humans. One study compared the performance of right-lesioned to left-lesioned patients (both groups classified using CT data) on a facial identification task. Patients with right-sided lesions performed significantly worse than left-lesioned patients and controls.[169] Cases of prosopagnosia due to isolated left-sided lesions are extraordinary, and in one instance occurred in a left-handed individual, suggesting anomalous lateralization.[170]

Critical lesion. Most of the reported disturbances are localized within the right occipitotemporal region.[171] However, the critical structure involved in this area can vary between the inferior occipitotemporal cortex, the fusiform gyrus, and the hippocampal region.[172] A larger study correlated two separate extrastriate lesion positions to two cognitive deficits. Damage to the fusiform gyri, when accompanied with right-sided infarcts in the occipitotemporal or ventromedial regions, leads to problems in perceiving facial detail. Patients with damage to the right parahippocampal gyrus, and the accompanying occipitotemporal ventromedial damage in the right hemisphere, exhibited a deficit in connecting faces to memory stores.[110] Using more recent terminology, a meta-analysis[68] of published cases of prosopagnosia and detailed studies of a single patient[168,173,174] suggested damage to the occipital face area (OFA) was more critical than damage to the fusiform face area (FFA) in causing this syndrome.

Outcome. Although it may be an enduring condition, patients may eventually recover from prosopagnosia, especially if damage is confined to the right hemisphere.[136,175] A prosopagnosic with a right-sided lesion, as observed with MRI, regained the ability to recognize famous faces as well as friends and family 2 months after the onset of his symptoms. However, he remained unable to identify the faces of people whom he met after the onset of symptoms.[165] Bilateral damage may be necessary in order for the prosopagnosic symptoms to endure past the acute period.[64] Some affected patients may improve their facial recognition abilities with training to increase attention to specific facial features such as the eyes.[156]

Capgras and Frégoli syndromes. Prosopagnosia is similar in its presentation to Capgras syndrome, which is one of the delusional misidentification disorders.[120] A patient with Capgras syndrome feels that a friend or relative has been replaced by an impostor.[176,177] There are some authors who feel that some patients with Capgras syndrome have prosopagnosia.[176] Etiologies include neurodegenerative and psychiatric illnesses[178] and bilateral occipitotemporal lesions.[179] In the Frégoli syndrome, another delusional misidentification disorder, the affected individual feels that a stranger is a familiar person.

Other types of visual agnosias

Landmark agnosia and topographagnosia. In this unusual syndrome, affected individuals are unable to recognize previously familiar landmarks to orient themselves.[180] In fact, specialized occipitotemporal regions have been identified which are specific for building recognition.[85] In a related disorder, topographagnosia, patients can not recognize familiar scenes.[180] One reported patient had a right medial occipitotemporal stroke.[181]

Color agnosia is described above in the section on cerebral hemi-achromatopsia, while simultanagnosia is detailed in the section below on Balint syndrome.

Optic aphasia

In contrast, patients with optic aphasia, which is condition closely related to visual object agnosia, are unable to name visually presented material or point to named objects although they recognize it.[182] They are able to name and recognize what they may hear or feel. The responsible lesion is usually unilateral and involves the left posterior cerebral hemisphere. This disorder likely is another visual–verbal disconnection syndrome.[11] However, patients with optic aphasia may have better recognizing capabilities than those with object agnosia because of relatively preserved access to right hemispheric perceptual/semantic systems.[183]

Visual memory disturbances

The ability to remember visual information requires storing then retrieving it.[184] Functional MRI studies suggest that extrastriate cortical regions used for visual perception are also initially utilized in visual memory tasks.[185] Subsequently, a network involving temporal lobe, hippocampal, and ventrolateral prefrontal cortex mediates human visual working memory, which is the process of retaining visual information for a brief period so that is available for immediate use.[186–189] Then visual information is stored using long-term memory systems.

Clinical observations in brain damaged individuals support these notions. Ross[190] reported two patients with bilateral posterior temporal lobe infarctions and loss of visual recent memory. Tactile, verbal, and nonverbal auditory memory functions were normal, but they could not recognize faces. Attributing the visual memory deficit to a disconnection syndrome, he hypothesized the bilateral lesions disrupted tracts between primary visual cortex and structures important for memory, such as the medial temporal lobe. Other patients with similar bilateral temporal lobe lesions and prosopagnosia have been described,[8,9] suggesting recognition of faces and visual memory share similar mechanisms.

Evidence for lateralization and the role of the right temporal lobe in visual memory is provided by studies in right temporal lobectomy patients, who exhibit defective recognition of visual material;[191] a patient with damage to the right frontotemporal region following middle cerebral artery aneurysm rupture who had defective memory of new visual objects and faces;[192] and posterior cerebral artery amobarbital tests, which suggest the right temporal lobe is important for remembering visual aspects of an object, while the left temporal lobe is more critical for recalling the object's verbal representation.[193]

Other similar patients with impaired visual memory have been described following infarction of the right dorsomedial thalamic nucleus[194] and damage to the anterior commissure and right fornix,[195] structures also important in the formation and retrieval of visual information.

Akinetopsia

Lateral occipital-temporal lesions affecting area V5 (**Fig. 9–7**), which lies in the posterior bank of the superior temporal sulcus, may result in defective motion perception, or akinetopsia.[196] Animal experiments first suggested that the comparable location in monkeys, area MT, contains cells which receive direct connections from striate cortex and are highly motion selective.[197] Lesions to area MT impair motion perception in the contralateral hemifield.[198] Zihl et al.[199] then described a seminal patient with defective motion perception due to bilateral cortical venous infarctions involving the temporoparietal and occipital periventricular and subcortical white matter, posterior portion of the middle temporal gyrus, and lateral occipital gyri. Striate cortex was spared. When the patient poured tea or coffee into a cup, the fluid "appeared to be frozen, like a glacier." She was unable to judge the speed of a moving car, but could identify the car without difficulty. Follow-up studies[200,201] reported the patient's MRI, which confirmed the bilateral lesions involving the upper part of the occipital gyri and the

adjacent portion of the middle temporal gyri, with the main focus of damage in the upper banks of the anterior occipital sulcus. Subsequently, other patients with deficits in motion perception have been described in association with cortical disturbances, usually bilateral, in these regions due to strokes,[202–204] traumatic brain injury, and Alzheimer's disease.[205] Patients with unilateral V5 lesions have been shown to have defective motion perception in the contralateral but not the ipsilateral hemifield.[206] Thus both the animal and clinical literature suggested the existence of a cortical area, separate from striate cortex, which mediates visual motion perception.

Other experimental evidence in normal humans has continued to support this notion. PET studies of individuals viewing moving black and white random-square patterns show increased blood flow to the occipito-temporal-parietal junction.[51] Functional MRI studies demonstrate increased activation of lateral occipitotemporal cortex in association with viewing moving stimuli (**Fig. 9–7**).[207–209] Likewise, electrical cortical stimulation in epilepsy patients[54,55] and magnetoencephalography (MEG)[210] and transmagnetic stimulation (TMS)[211] in normal subjects have confirmed the presence of a specialized motion area in humans concentrated at the occipito-temporal-parietal junction.

Some drugs have been reported to cause akinetopsia. Two cases of akinetopsia related to use of nefazodone, an antidepressant that blocks serotonin (5-HT2) receptors and the reuptake of 5-HT, have been described.[212] Other conditions which may be associated with decreased motion perception include Williams syndrome, lesions of the cerebellar vermis, amblyopia,[209,213] and schizophrenia.[214] V5 activity may be

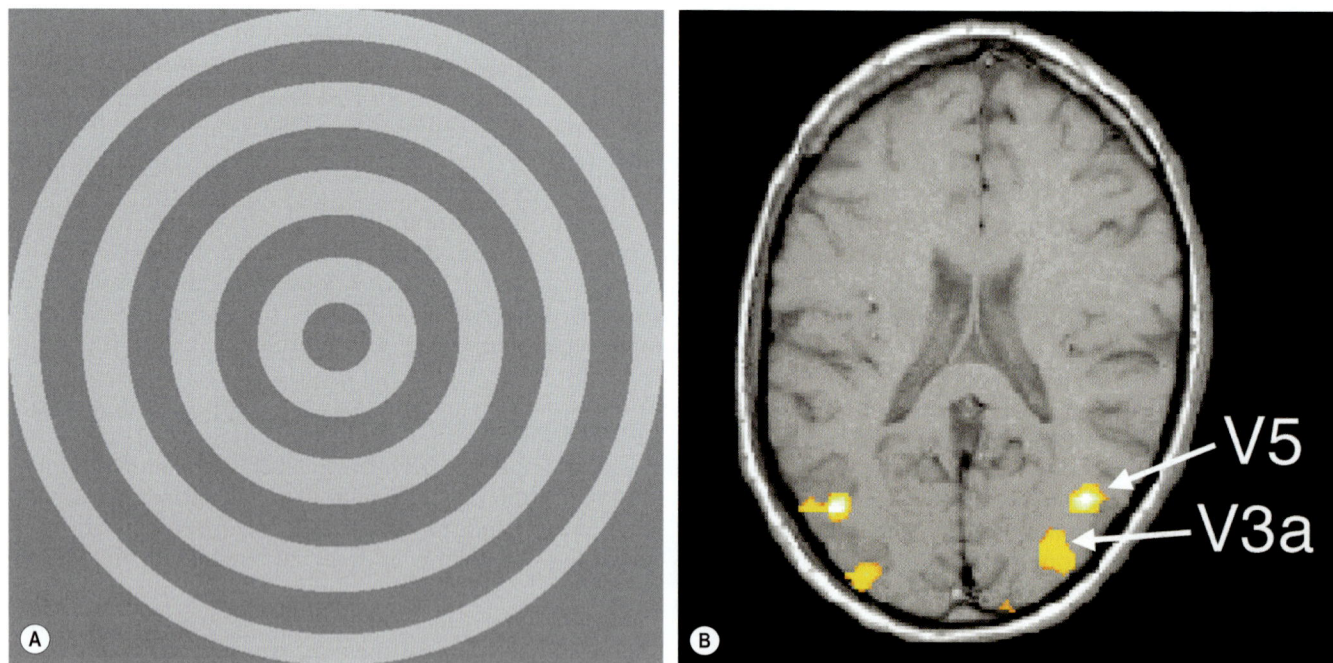

Figure 9–7. Functional magnetic resonance imaging (fMRI) demonstration of motion sensitive areas of the brain. **A.** Stimulus consisting of concentric rings, one cycle per degree of visual angle, which expanded and contracted at a speed of 1 degree of visual angle/second. The gray and light-gray ring contrast is 22%. The stimulus paradigm alternated eight cycles of 30 seconds of moving rings then 30 seconds of stationary rings. **B.** Areas (V5 and V3a) activated by the moving rings but not the stationary ones are superimposed on the subject's corresponding T1-weighted image. The height threshold of the activation map was set at p < 0.001 "(uncorrected)" (courtesy of G. R. Bonhomme, A. Miki, and G.T. Liu).

suppressed as an adaptive measure in patients with oscillopsia due to unilateral vestibular failure.[215]

Riddoch phenomenon, blindsight, and V5. The preservation of parallel retinotectalpulvinar connections with V5 is one possible explanation for the Riddoch phenomenon (ability to perceive motion) and for blindsight (unconscious vision) in individuals with field loss due to striate cortex damage (for further discussion of these phenomena see Chapter 8). In one study,[216] a patient with a left occipital lesion who was able to perceive fast but not slow moving stimuli within an otherwise blind hemifield underwent visual evoked potential testing. This demonstrated that V5 was activated despite the destruction of V1 (striate cortex), suggesting that in addition to the main pathway from V1 to V5, there existed another pathway to V5 which bypassed V1. Another study[217] suggested that in patients with visual field loss due to cerebral hemispheric lesions, those with preserved motion detection tended to have sparing of lateral temporo-occipital cortex, while those without motion detection usually had involvement of this area. In PET and functional MRI studies of patients with unilateral occipital lobe infarction, ipsilateral lateral temporo-occipital cortex is still activated during optokinetic stimulation[218] and when moving stimuli are presented in the blind hemifield.[219-221]

Parietal disturbances

Right parietal lesions (**Fig. 9–8**) may result in *sensory neglect* of visual, tactile, and auditory stimuli in left hemispace.[175] *Motor neglect*, a defect in exploration of and responding to stimuli in contralateral hemispace, may also occur.[222,223] When the left neglect is dense, affected patients may ignore everything to the left and have a right head turn and gaze preference. They sometimes also display visual or spatial disorientation, a difficulty in localizing objects visually, to their left.[224-226] However, visual disorientation occurs more commonly in bilateral lesions (see Balint syndrome, below). Other symptoms of right parietal injury include dressing and constructional apraxia, failure to recognize one side of the body (asomatognosia), and a denial of neurologic impairment (anosognosia). These deficits are unaccounted for by visual field loss, other primary sensory deficits, or motor weakness.[227,228] Unilateral spatial and motor neglect may occur even in young children.[229,230]

Parietal areas involved likely include the superior parietal lobule (human area 7) or inferior parietal lobule (human area 39 and 40, angular gyrus), or both.[231-233] According to one hypothesis, left neglect syndromes resulting from right-sided lesions are more common because the right hemisphere is dominant for the distribution of attention.[234] In other words, the left hemisphere attends to the right side of space, while the right hemisphere attends to both sides. Thus a left-sided lesion tends not to cause neglect because the intact right hemisphere is still able to attend to the right side. Nevertheless, neglect of the right side due to a left hemispheric lesion can occur,[235,236] but it tends to be less severe and recover more quickly than left neglect.[237]

The majority of this section will review sensory neglect of visual stimuli.

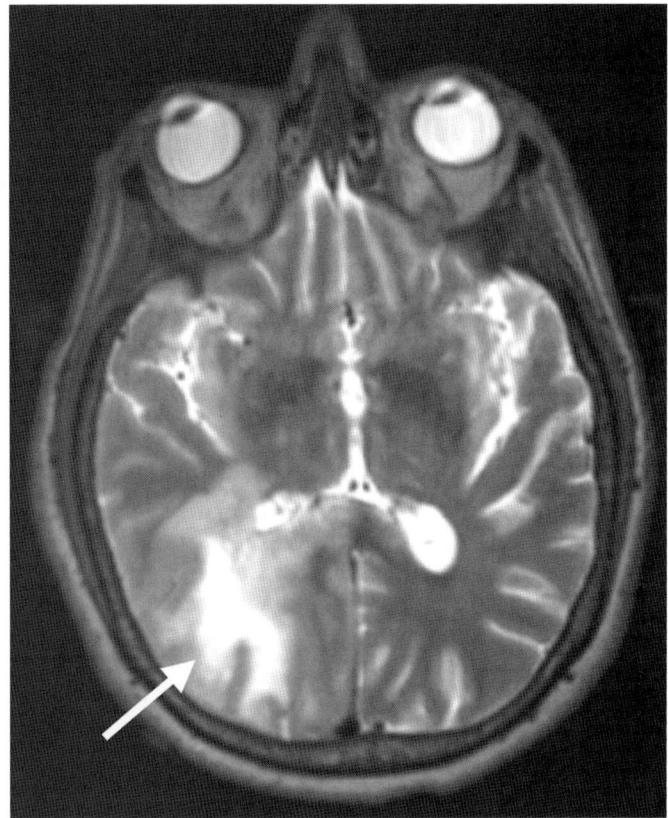

Figure 9–8. Axial T2-weighted MRI in an HIV-positive man with progressive multifocal leukoencephalopathy (PML) and dense left hemineglect due to a right parietal lesion (arrow). Note the MRI shows his eyes are deviated to the right, consistent with his gaze preference. When asked where his left hand was, he pointed to his right hand.

Visual neglect (hemi-inattention)

The term unilateral visual hemi-inattention describes the neglect of visual stimuli in a homonymous half-field despite an intact geniculostriate system. Clinically, patients with this phenomenon may be difficult to distinguish from those with a homonymous hemianopia, but unlike the latter, those with hemi-inattention will be more likely to detect the stimulus if their attention is directed to the neglected side (assuming central fixation is maintained).[238] In more subtle cases the visual fields will be normal to confrontation, but if comparable visual stimuli are presented simultaneously in right and left hemifields (double simultaneous stimulation), the one contralateral to the lesion will be ignored (visual extinction).[239] When the neglect is dense, however, the absence of a hemianopia is frequently difficult to prove. If the parietal lesion is large enough, often both the neglect and a hemianopia are present.

Bedside tests for hemi-inattention, such as line or letter cancellation, line bisection, or figure and clock drawing, are reviewed in Chapter 2. In line or letter cancellation, patients with left neglect tend to identify targets only in their right hemispace. During line bisection, when patients are asked to identify the middle of a horizontal line, those with left neglect often pick a point which is on the right side of the line. Copying of figures or the numbers of a clock may be drawn only on the right side (see **Figs. 2–16** and **2–17**).

Video 9.1

Patients with both left hemi-inattention and hemianopia tend to do more poorly on these tests than those with hemi-attention alone.[240]

Several theories have attempted to explain neglect.[241-244] Bisiach et al.[245] attributed unilateral neglect to a defect in the internal mental representation of the external world, as some patients with left hemineglect have defective mental imagery of the left side of space (*representational neglect*—see Visual imagery, below). Others[238,246-248] have proposed that an interruption in the corticolimbic-reticular loop causes a defect in the orienting response towards stimuli in the contralateral hemispace. Mesulam[249-252] hypothesized that a cortical network involving posterior parietal lobe, frontal lobe, and cingulate gyrus mediates directed attention. Damage to any one or more components could lead to a neglect syndrome (see frontal lobe lesions, below).[253] In Mesulam's scheme, the posterior parietal component provides an internal sensory map of extrapersonal space, the frontal component a mechanism for scanning and exploring, and the cingulate a spatial map for motivation. More recent studies have distinguished between personal neglect resulting from lesions of the right parietal lobe and extrapersonal neglect due to a disruption in a network involving right frontal regions and superior temporal gyrus.[254,255] Because these proposed mechanisms are not mutually exclusive, a combination of them may also apply.[244,256-258]

Interhemispheric rivalry, a concept in which the intact hemisphere suppresses the injured hemisphere, has been used to explain visual extinction as a phenomenon separate from neglect.[259] However, our clinical experience suggests visual extinction is simply a milder, more subtle form of visual hemi-attention or neglect.

Other cortical and subcortical lesions. Neglect may also occur in association with lesions affecting the frontal lobe (see below), right superior temporal gyrus,[254,260] and para-hippocampus.[233] Unilateral neglect behavior less commonly may result from subcortical lesions.[261] Examples include damage to the thalamus,[262,263] striatum (putamen and head of caudate) and adjacent deep white matter,[264-266] and corpus callosum.[267,268] These lesions may cause neglect by indirect effects on the parietal lobe by, for example, disrupting subcortical–cortical connections. Diaschisis, a poorly understood transient depression of function elsewhere in the brain due to a focal cerebral lesion, may be another explanation.[269]

Treatment. Patients with severe left-sided neglect can be some of the most difficult to rehabilitate, and their functional disability and prognosis for recovery is often poorer than individuals with global aphasia or hemiplegia.[270,271] Many patients with neglect are difficult to help because they are unaware of or deny their deficit. One study found that those with larger right sided lesions and with pre-existing cortical atrophy had a poorer prognosis for recovery.[272]

The treatment of visual hemi-inattention is largely adaptive. Like in patients with hemianopias, those with hemi-inattention should have their bed within their room arranged to face their non-neglected side. Similarly, family and friends should be instructed to approach the patient from the intact side. Visual hemi-inattention precludes driving, cooking, crossing the street unaided, or working with heavy machin-ery. A vertical colored strip of paper can be placed along the left margin of text to facilitate reading, with instructions given to the patient to find the paper when moving down to the next line.

Other treatment options, although touted because of their positive results during neuropsychological testing, are either unsatisfactory or unproven when improvement in activities of daily living is the goal,[242,270,273] or the effects are temporary. We have found hemianopic prisms[274] (see Chapter 8) relatively unhelpful in patients with left-sided neglect, particularly because of the confusion they cause in patients who likely also have visual disorientation. Prism adaptation, in which subjects are trained to point straight ahead while wearing base out OS and base in OD prisms, thus shifting vision to the right, has been studied extensively and been shown to improve neglect in some individuals,[275-279] albeit transiently.[280] The positive effects of training with virtual reality are also only temporary.[281] The use of hemispatial sunglasses, which shade the non-neglected side of each eye and force viewing into the neglected side, has been reported anecdotally as effective.[282] Another technique involves the use of visual imagery and trains the patient to pretend their eyes are like the light of a lighthouse, sweeping far to the left and right.[283] An alternative strategy, which trains the patient to turn their heads to the left, utilizes the intact right visual field for scanning. Phasic alerting, which uses a warning sound, can correct visual awareness[284] but is impractical outside of the experimental setting.

In addition, vestibular stimulation by cold water, for instance, may have some efficacy in patients with visual neglect.[285] This maneuver may train patients how to orient towards the affected hemispatial field. Lastly, noradrenergic agents[286] and dopamine agonists[287] have been shown anecdotally to improve neglect. However, these therapies have not been evaluated in a controlled fashion, and in one study bromocriptine actually worsened some aspects of hemispatial neglect.[288]

Parieto-occipital disturbances

Balint syndrome

Balint[289-292] first analyzed this symptom complex, and Holmes[291-293] later elaborated his description. It results most frequently from bilateral symmetric parieto-occipital cortical or white matter injury (**Figs. 9–9, 9–10**). In the minority of cases there is additional frontal lobe involvement.[294] In its most severe form, patients with Balint syndrome appear disabled and almost completely blind except for macular sparing: they bump into objects and often require assistance while walking in the room, they do not refixate on novel stimuli in their visual periphery, they do not blink to threat, but they become tremendously visually fixated on single objects.[295,296] The full syndrome consists of *simultanagnosia* (or simultaneous agnosia), *ocular apraxia* (a deficit in shifting gaze), and *optic ataxia* (a defect in reaching under visual guidance).[294,297] Each of these elements, which may be seen alone or in combination, will be briefly considered.

Simultanagnosia. A striking deficit in Balint syndrome, simultanagnosia is the element seen most often in isolation.

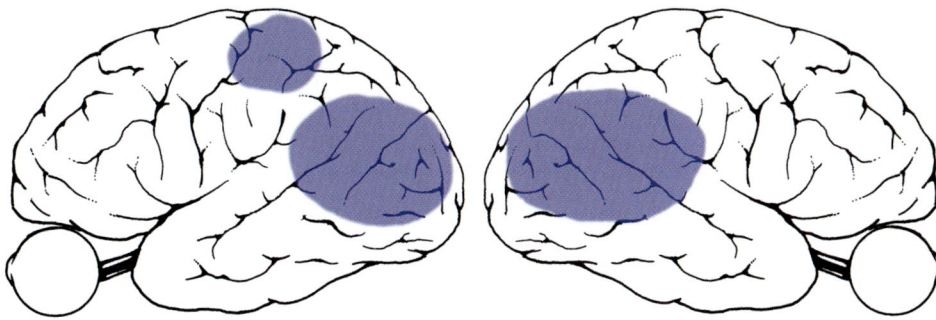

Figure 9–9. Location of lesions in Balint's original patient.[289] The two largest areas of damage were in the parietal lobes bilaterally, but there was also a lesion near the left central sulcus.

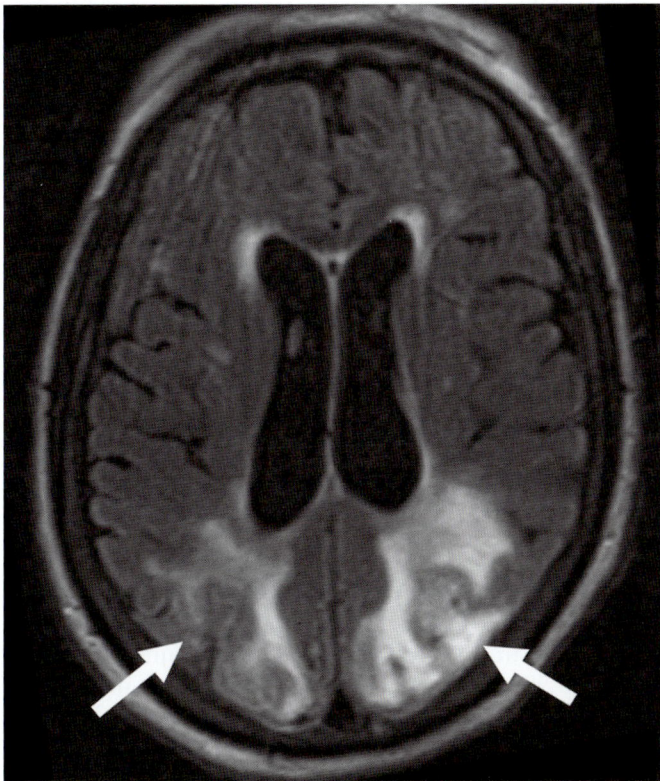

Figure 9–10. Balint syndrome due to acute hemorrhagic leukoencephalitis. Magnetic resonance MR fluid attenuated inversion recovery axial image demonstrates bilateral parieto-occipital lesions (arrows). In addition to simultanagnosia, optic ataxia, and ocular apraxia, the patient had a right homonymous hemianopia.

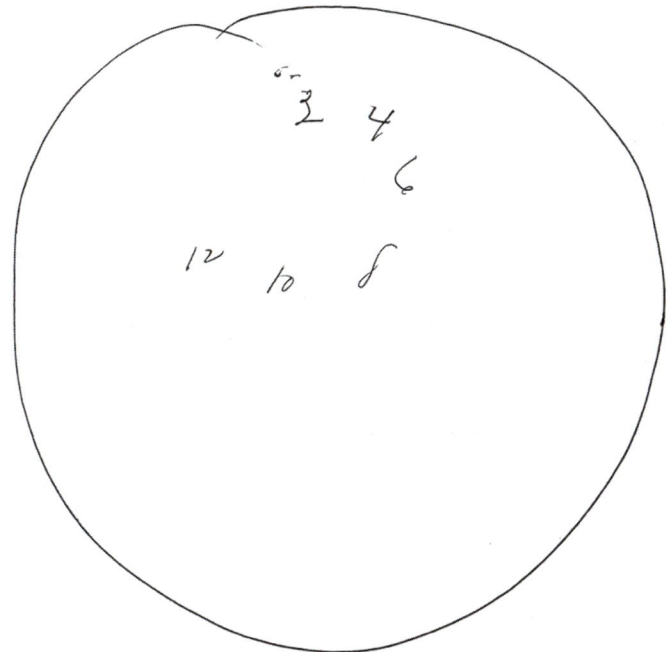

Figure 9–11. Disorganized clock drawn by a patient with Alzheimer's dementia, simultanagnosia, and spatial disorientation. The examiner drew the circle, and then the patient was asked to draw in the numbers of a clock face within the circle.

It is defined as an inability to grasp the entire meaning of a picture despite an intact capacity to recognize the picture's individual constituent elements.[64] Thus, affected patients may be unable to identify a picture of a landscape but are able to recognize a small tree within it. Such patients may be able to read single 20/20 letters but can read words only by spelling them out loud. Despite normal color vision, patients with simultanagnosia may also have difficulty with Ishihara color plates (see Chapter 2),[298] which requires them to identify colored numbers created by small dots. The Navon figure test (**Fig. 2–14**) is also an excellent method for assessing simultanagnosia, and attempts at drawing clocks (**Fig. 9–11**) and other figures[299] will often reveal the individual's inability to appreciate an entire scene.

Simultanagnosia may reflect bilaterally defective visual attention,[300–302] as the lesions in Balint syndrome typically involve Brodmann areas 7 (superior parietal lobule), 19 (dorsorostral occipital lobe) and sometimes 39 (inferior parietal lobule).[303] These are areas important for visual attention. Several authors have offered the absent blink to visual threat response as evidence for decreased visual attention in this disorder.[304,305] One authority[10] attributed the visual behavior to an "extreme narrowing of attention," referring to an inability to notice any object outside foveal vision. Impaired shifting of attention, defective visual exploration of extrapersonal space, leading to deficits in visual scanning,[306–308] and an impairment in linking structural descriptions and object location—a deficit of binding ventral and dorsal stream information, respectively,[309–311] have also been implicated.

Ocular apraxia. Patients with ocular apraxia are unable to generate voluntary saccades, but their involuntary reflexive saccades are normal. The terms *psychic gaze paralysis* and *spasm of fixation* have also been used. Possible mechanisms

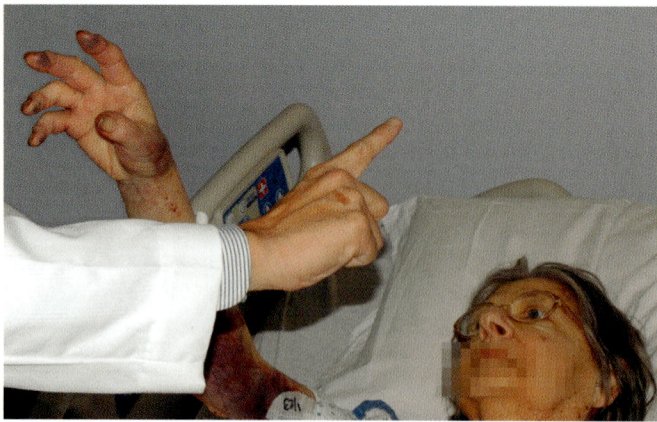

Figure 9–12. Optic ataxia in a patient with Balint syndrome due to Alzheimer's disease. Visual fields were normal, but the patient reached inaccurately when asked to touch the examiner's finger.

include a disconnection of the occipital lobe from the frontal eye fields or uncertainty about the target's location.[295] In its purest form, ocular apraxia is associated with normal pursuit eye movements, but in fact many patients have defective pursuit as well. Other clinical features and mechanisms of ocular apraxia, which is also seen in other disorders, are reviewed in Chapter 16.

Optic ataxia. Although patients with optic ataxia may be able to see an object of regard, they may reach for it inaccurately (**Fig. 9–12**). Optic ataxia, also known as *visuomotor ataxia*, is unassociated with any cerebellar dysfunction or motor weakness. Instead, optic ataxia may result from a disconnection of the occipital lobe from motor centers more anteriorly in the frontal lobe, where the reaching is programmed.[10,303,312,313] A defect in the internal representation of extrapersonal space, or damage to areas responsible for integrating panoramic visual information with proprioceptive information relating to the upper extremity,[303,314] or a specific impairment in visuomotor control without deficits in perception,[315–317] are alternative explanations.

Other neuro-ophthalmic signs. As alluded to earlier, the blink to threat response may be absent even within intact visual fields.[318] Spatial or visual disorientation, a difficulty in localizing and finding objects in extrapersonal space by sight alone, is another prominent feature in a number of cases.[293,294,319] Although the visual fields may be normal,[64] often bilateral inferior altitudinal defects are present[319,320] owing to the frequent involvement of the superior banks of the occipital lobes.

Etiology. The usual etiology is watershed infarction in the setting of hypoperfusion following cardiac or respiratory arrest, but patients with cardiogenic emboli, Alzheimer's disease,[321] Creutzfeldt–Jakob disease,[322] and progressive multifocal leukoencephalopathy[323] (see Retrochiasmal disorders, Chapter 8) may also present with complex visual disturbances manifesting with any or all of the elements of Balint syndrome. Less common but other reported causes include angiography,[324] central nervous system vasculitis,[325] adrenoleukodystrophy,[326] and perinatal hypoxic ischemic encephalopathy.[327] In addition, we have seen a case of Balint syndrome caused by acute hemorrhagic leukoencephalitis (**Fig. 9–10**).

Treatment. Aside from treating the underlying condition, the management of patients with Balint syndrome is largely adaptive. Like patients with parietal hemispatial neglect, visual cues such as colored strips of paper can be used to help them read and scan pages.[328] Some patients, however, are so severely affected that they are rendered visually disabled.

Posterior cortical atrophy

The label *"posterior cortical atrophy"* has been applied to a progressive dementing syndrome characterized primarily by higher cortical visual disorders.[329] Typically patients exhibit some combination of visual field defects, alexia with or without agraphia, visual agnosia, components of Balint syndrome, prosopagnosia, Gerstmann syndrome (left–right confusion, finger agnosia, acalculia, and agraphia), and transcortical sensory aphasia (fluent aphasia with intact ability to repeat).[330–335] Visual hallucinations can also occur.[336] Memory and frontal lobe functions such as judgment and insight are affected later in the course of the disease. Neuroimaging reveals cerebral atrophy, more severe posteriorly.

Etiologic considerations include Alzheimer's, Pick's, or Creutzfeldt–Jakob disease, corticobasal degeneration,[337] or Lewy body dementia.[332,333,338] Posterior cortical atrophy is felt to be a unique presentation of these conditions.[339] The notion that a degenerative disease can produce focal cortical findings is not without precedent. Primary progressive aphasia with left perisylvian atrophy can occur in the absence of memory difficulty, yet many affected patients will eventually develop a dementing illness such as Alzheimer's disease.

Visual imagery

Although visual imagery is not solely a parietal lobe function, lesions in this area may affect this cognitive function. Numerous neuropsychological and functional neuroimaging studies have suggested that many of the same areas of the brain that are responsible for viewing and interpreting an object are also important for imagining it.[340–346] For instance, patients with occipital lobe lesions and a contralateral hemianopia or quadrantanopia can have defective visual imagery on the side of the field defect.[347] In addition, PET studies have demonstrated that patients with acquired blindness due to anterior visual pathway lesions activate visual cortex during mental imagery.[348] Patients with prosopagnosia and achromatopsia may have an imagery disorder involving faces and colors of objects.[349] Individuals with visual agnosias for particular objects, living versus nonliving, for example, may have selective loss of visual imagery for the same types of items.[350]

Furthermore, imagining an object or scene requires the ability to generate an internal representation of objects and scenes in extrapersonal space. This is one of the tasks of the inferior parietal lobule. Thus patients with right parietal lobe lesions may neglect the left side during visual imagery (*so-called representational neglect*).[351] For instance, Bisiach and Luzzatti[352] asked patients with left hemineglect to imagine they were looking at the Piazza del Duomo in Milan. When they were asked to describe the view from the side of the square opposite the cathedral, they described fewer land-marks on the left side of their imagined scene. Then they were asked to recall the view of the square from the other side on the cathedral steps. Again they neglected more details on their left, but they described correctly objects on the right they had previously ignored from the other side. Other patients with visual disorientation and defective visual–spatial imagery have been reported.[349]

However, there are notable exceptions to this concept that perception, higher cortical function, and imagery are highly correlated. This implies the mechanism for imagery may be much more complicated. In fact, several cases have shown that perception and imagery can be dissociated. For instance, patients with hemianopias and cortical blindness have been reported with intact visual imagery.[345,346,353,354] Some patients with cerebral achromatopsia have preserved color imagery.[355,356] In addition, a patient with a right parietal lesion and left-sided representational neglect without visual perceptual neglect,[357] and others with visual agnosia but intact visual imagery,[95,358] have been reported.

Frontal lobe disturbances

Frontal lobe neglect is well recognized in humans.[359,360] It can be denser than parietal neglect and mimic a homony-mous hemianopia.[231] Cogan[361] in fact used the term "pseu-dohemianopsia" to refer to patients with this disorder. In contrast to those with a hemianopia from parietal or occipi-tal injury, however, the frontal defect is usually transient. Furthermore, frontal neglect may preferentially affect exploratory-motor rather than perceptual-sensory tasks.[222] Many patients will have a hemiparesis and mild difficulty with contraversive lateral gaze, consistent with adjacent involvement of the motor strip as well as the more anterior frontal eye fields. In one study[362] of patients with frontal neglect of the left hemispace, all lesions involved the inferior frontal gyrus (Brodmann's area 44) and the underlying white matter. Part of the premotor cortex, this area is the homologue of Broca's area in the right hemisphere.

Diseases commonly associated with higher cortical visual disturbances

The most common cause of a higher cortical visual distur-bance is a vaso-occlusive stroke. Typically the posterior cerebral artery or one of its branches is involved unilaterally or bilaterally, affecting the occipital, occipitotemporal and occipitoparietal areas. Middle cerebral artery strokes may cause parietal or frontal lobe syndromes. Other etiolo-gies include neoplasms, hemorrhages, multiple sclerosis, abscesses, trauma, progressive multifocal leukoencephalopa-thy, and carbon monoxide poisoning. The differential diag-nosis is similar to that of retrochiasmal disturbances (see Chapter 8).

However, two dementing illnesses, Alzheimer's disease and Creutzfeldt–Jakob disease, have a predilection for visual association cortices (see Posterior cortical atrophy, above).[363] Thus each condition will be reviewed here. In each section,

the neurologic, neuro-ophthalmic, laboratory, and patho-logic features, followed by treatment issues, will be discussed.

Alzheimer's disease

This chronic degenerative condition is highlighted by gradu-ally progressive dementia, which in turn is characterized by (i) a loss of intellect sufficient enough to interfere with social or occupational functions, (ii) memory loss, and (iii) a clear sensorium. The disease is considered probable if these fea-tures are present, the age of onset is between 40 and 90 years, and other neurologic diseases which could account for the deficits are absent.[364,365] The terms presenile and senile dementia refer to dementia which occurs either before or after age 65, respectively.

Alzheimer's disease is the most common cause of demen-tia in North America and Europe,[366] accounting for at least half of cases.[367] Its prevalence increases with age. In one population study,[368] of individuals 65–74 years of age, 3.0% had probable Alzheimer's disease, while 18.7% of persons 75–84 years old and 47.2% of those over 85 had the disor-der. Thus, as the general population ages, this disease is likely to become more prevalent.

Besides advanced age, other primary risk factors for the disease include family history, presence of the apolipopro-tein E $\in$4 allele, and trisomy 21.[369] Much less common autosomal dominant forms of early-onset Alzheimer's disease are associated with mutations in the amyloid precur-sor protein gene on chromosome 21 and presenilin 1 and 2 genes on chromosomes 14 and 1, respectively.[369–372] Possible risk factors include a history of head trauma and low intel-ligence.[373] Commonly, patients with a diagnosis of mild cognitive impairment later develop Alzheimer's disease.[365]

Neurologic symptoms and signs. Aside from the insidious memory loss which defines this condition,[374] patients with Alzheimer's disease may develop language deficits, particu-larly word-finding difficulties. Personality changes, prob-lems with concentration, and change in affect may also occur, and some patients become psychotic and agitated. In later stages deterioration in social skills and motor impair-ment may also become evident. In general though, the cranial nerve, motor strength, sensation, gait, and reflexes are all normal. Extrapyramidal signs such as bradykinesia and tremor may be observed, as some patients have coexist-ing Parkinson's disease. Job loss, home care, nursing home placement, then eventual demise is an inevitable progres-sion in most instances. Patient survival is usually between 5 and 12 years following disease onset.[366]

Differential diagnosis. Depression, multi-infarct demen-tia, extrapyramidal disorders, hypothyroidism, and toxic-metabolic disorders, for instance drug toxicity and B_{12} deficiency, are the most common conditions mistaken for Alzheimer's disease. Neurosyphilis should also be excluded. The reader is referred to published reviews[366,369,375,376] for lists and discussions of the less common disorders to be considered in the differential diagnosis of dementia.

Neuro-ophthalmic symptoms and signs. Occasionally visual deficits are the initial complaints and findings in the synony-mous "visual," "posterior," or "posterior cortical atrophy" variants of Alzheimer's disease. The visual disturbances tend to be higher cortical in nature.[363,377] In one study[378] of community based patients with Alzheimer's disease, approximately one-half had a visual object agnosia, while one-fifth had Balint syndrome. Prosopagnosia, visual hallucinations (see Chapter 12), defective visual motion perception,[379-381] abnormal form perception,[382] decreased visual attention,[383] poor performance on visuospatial tasks,[384,385] right-sided neglect, alexia without agraphia, poor visual memory,[386] and diminished curiosity of novel or unusual visual stimuli[387] may also occur. Because patients with Alzheimer's disease and higher cortical visual disturbances usually have normal visual acuity, relatively clear ocular media, and normal fundus appearance, many such patients have persistent visual complaints despite visits to several ophthalmologists and numerous changes in eyeglass prescriptions.

In addition, patients with Alzheimer's disease may also have more elementary visual deficits involving the primary visual pathways. Deficits in visual acuity,[388] visual fields including hemianopic field loss,[377,389-391] contrast sensitivity,[392] stereoacuity,[393,394] and color vision[395] have all been observed. However, some of these results are only inconsistently observed, and some studies are hampered by limitations in patient testing. For instance some authors[396,397] were unable to demonstrate any abnormalities in primary visual function that were not also observed in age-matched controls. In addition, in one study[398] of patients with Alzheimer's disease who underwent computerized perimetry, many had nonspecific visual field constriction. However, the numbers of fixation losses and false-negative and -positive responses for each patient were very high, making any conclusions difficult.

Diagnostic studies. The results of neuroradiologic studies, both anatomic and functional, tend to be nonspecific in patients with Alzheimer's disease. CT and MRI, although helpful in excluding a mass lesion, multiple infarcts, or normal pressure hydrocephalus, is usually either normal or reveals diffuse cortical atrophy. PET, single photon emission computed tomography (SPECT) and perfusion studies may demonstrate decreased rates of glucose metabolism and blood flow and in the posterior cingulate, parietal, parieto-occipital, temporal, and prefrontal regions.[399,400] When the symptoms are primarily visual, the abnormalities on anatomical and functional imaging tend to be more posterior.[389,390,401]

Lumbar puncture, which is often performed to exclude tertiary syphilis, for instance, is generally unremarkable. However, spinal fluid levels of tau may be elevated and those of beta-amyloid protein (see pathology, below) may be decreased in patients with Alzheimer's disease.[365,402,403] Sometimes an electroencephalogram, which is either normal or shows diffuse slowing in Alzheimer's disease, is performed when Creutzfeldt–Jakob disease is also considered.

Although their significance is unclear, abnormal visual evoked potentials[404] and electroretinograms[405,406] and reduction in nerve fiber layer[407] and optic nerve fibers[408] demonstrated by optic imaging have also been reported in patients with Alzheimer's disease.

Pathology. The diagnosis of Alzheimer's disease can be confirmed only histologically, either by biopsy or postmortem examination. The diagnostic pathologic features include neurofibrillary tangles, which are characterized by paired helical fibers composed of altered forms of the microtubule-associated protein tau; senile plaques, consisting of insoluble beta-amyloid protein; neuron degeneration; and loss of synapses.[369,409-412] Also seen are granulovacuolar degeneration, amyloid (congophilic) deposition in vessel walls, and Hirano bodies, which are eosinophilic filaments. Cell loss in the basal forebrain cholinergic complex and decreased choline acetyltranferase activity suggest defective cholinergic transmission may be associated with the disease.[413]

The visual deficits in Alzheimer's disease are usually attributed to neurofibrillary tangles in visual association areas[414-416] or striate cortex.[417] Levine et al.[418] described a patient with Alzheimer's, visual object agnosia, visual field constriction, and impaired contrast sensitivity. The postmortem examination revealed the density of tangles was highest in the occipitoparietal areas and lowest in the frontal lobes. A similar distribution of lesions was found in a group of Alzheimer's patients presenting with Balint syndrome.[419] Alzheimer's patients who are visually symptomatic are more likely to demonstrate tangles in the occipitoparietal regions than those who have normal visual function.[420]

Pathologic findings in the primary visual pathways have also been found,[404] but like analogous clinical observations, the results are inconsistent. For instance, the density of retinal ganglion cells subserving the central 11 degrees of vision was reduced in patients with Alzheimer's disease as well as in age-matched control patients.[421]

Treatment. A detailed overview of the various pharmacologic agents used in Alzheimer's disease is beyond the scope of this section, so the reader is referred to reviews on this topic.[369,422-427] However, some principles will be discussed here. In general, there is no cure and no method for halting disease progression, and these medications are only mildly effective, at best. Based upon notion that enhancing central cholinergic neurotransmission might improve the cognitive and behavioral aspects of Alzheimer's disease, cholinesterase inhibitors such as donepezil, rivastigmine, and galantamine can be used.[428] However, gastrointestinal side-effects such as nausea and diarrhea are common. Despite its proven efficacy, the use of another cholinesterase inhibitor, tacrine (tetrahydroaminoacridine) is limited because of the risk of hepatotoxicity.[429] Memantine, an N-methyl-D-aspartate (NMDA) antagonist, may be effective in Alzheimer's disease by interfering with glutamatergic excitotoxicity or its effect on hippocampal neurons.[426]

Medications or vitamins, such as selegiline or vitamin E (alpha-tocopherol), that increase the levels of brain catecholamines and protect against oxidative damage to neurons, have also been used.[430] Herbal supplements such as ginkgo biloba may have a small effect on cognition.[431] However, purported treatments such as anti-inflammatory agents, hormone-replacement therapy, and statins have shown no benefit after careful study.[426,432] Patients may also require medical treatment of agitation, depression, and psychosis, which may include visual hallucinations (see Chapter 12).

Creutzfeldt–Jakob disease

Creutzfeldt–Jakob disease, a relatively uncommon neurodegenerative disorder in adults, is characterized by rapidly progressive dementia and myoclonus. In contrast to patients with Alzheimer's disease, who deteriorate slowly over years, individuals with Creutzfeldt–Jakob tend to worsen quickly over weeks to months. In one large study,[433] the range of age of onset was wide, 16–82 years of age, but the most frequent age group affected was the 60–64 age bracket.

Creutzfeldt–Jakob disease, along with kuru, Gerstmann–Sträussler–Scheinker syndrome, and fatal familial insomnia, constitute a group of dementing illnesses known as human transmissible spongiform encephalopathies.[434] Clinically, kuru and Gerstmann–Sträussler–Scheinker syndrome present primarily with cerebellar syndromes, and dementia occurs at later stages. Scrapie and bovine spongiform encephalopathy (mad cow disease) are related neurodegenerative diseases seen more commonly in animals. The likely responsible agents in these conditions are proteinaceous particles called prions (PrP = prion protein), which are devoid of nucleic acids.[435] Disease results when the normal (cellular) prion protein PrP^C misfolds into the pathologic (scrapie) form, PrP^{Sc}.[436,437]

Eighty-five percent of cases of Creutzfeldt–Jakob are sporadic, and different classification schemes have been proposed based upon the molecular genetics of the PrP.[438] Ten to 15% of cases are familial, caused by a mutation in the prion protein gene (PRNP). Mutations in this gene are also responsible for Gerstmann–Sträussler–Scheinker syndrome and fatal familial insomnia. Much less commonly, Creutzfeldt–Jakob is iatrogenic due to growth hormone derived from human cadaveric pituitary glands,[439] reuse of stereotactic electroencephalography electrodes, and corneal[440] or cadaveric dural transplantation.[441–443] New-variant Creutzfeldt–Jakob results from consumption of beef from bovines with spongiform encephalopathy.[444]

Neurologic symptoms and signs. The disorder usually starts with gradual memory loss and behavioral abnormalities. Some patients present with additional sleep disturbances, depression, weight loss, anorexia, or anxiety. Cerebellar dysfunction, typified by ataxia and dysarthria, or pyramidal or extrapyramidal dysfunction may also be evident. Usually within a few weeks or months of onset, mental and motor function deteriorate rapidly. Global dementia, cerebellar incoordination, rigidity, akinetic mutism, and startle-induced or spontaneous myoclonic jerks typify the later stages of the illness.[433,444]

Neuro-ophthalmic symptoms and signs. Patients with the Heidenhain (occipitoparietal) variant may have visual field defects such as homonymous hemianopia or quadrantanopia.[445–447] Cortical blindness,[448] visual hallucinations, visual agnosia, palinopsia,[449] and Balint syndrome may also occur.[322,450] Usually the fundus is normal, but rare patients with optic atrophy have been reported.[451] Ocular motor disturbances, including supranuclear (e.g., Parinaud syndrome) and infranuclear gaze palsies,[452] nystagmus, and slow saccades,[453] and eyelid abnormalities such as ptosis and apraxia of eyelid opening, may also be observed.

Visual abnormalities may predate dementia or behavioral changes. However, frequently by the time visual signs and symptoms develop, patients with Creutzfeldt–Jakob disease are too confused and uncooperative for careful documentation and accurate testing of their visual function.

Pathology. Creutzfeldt–Jakob disease is characterized neuropathologically by neuronal loss, prominent gliosis, and spongiosis in cortex, thalamus, basal ganglia, and cerebellum.[433] Occasionally fine, radiating eosinophilic kuru amyloid plaques may be observed.[454] Immunohistochemistry with antibodies against the prion protein can provide additional confirmation of the disease.[455,456] In the Heidenhain variant, the neuropathologic abnormalities are most pronounced in the parietal and occipital lobes.[457] Although tissue damage is usually confined to the central nervous system, some reports have documented involvement of the optic nerve head[458] and retina.[459]

Diagnostic studies. The definitive diagnosis of Creutzfeldt–Jakob disease can be made only with a biopsy or autopsy. However, spinal fluid analysis for the 14-3-3 brain protein is a sensitive (53–97%) and specific (87–96%) laboratory test for the sporadic form of this disorder.[460–464] Caution in its use should be applied, because autopsy-proven false negatives can occur,[465] and false-positive 14-3-3 assay results have been reported in patients with herpes simplex encephalitis, hypoxic brain injury, intracerebral metastases, frontotemporal dementia, and Alzheimer's disease.[461,462,465] The 14-3-3 spinal fluid analysis is therefore recommended for use only in patients for whom the clinical suspicion of Creutzfeldt–Jakob disease is high.

Conventional T1-weighted MR images are frequently normal in patients with Creutzfeldt–Jakob disease. However, diffusion-weighted MR sequences may demonstrate otherwise undetectable high signal abnormalities in the cortex or basal ganglia (**Fig. 9–13**).[466–472] This modality may be useful in the detection of brain abnormalities in patients with early signs and symptoms.[473] Similarly, but with less sensitivity,

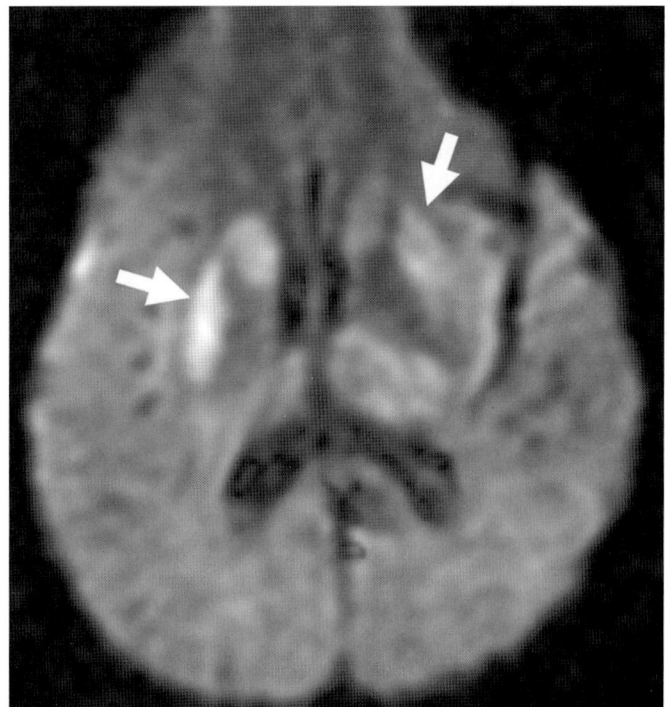

Figure 9–13. Diffusion-weighted MR imaging demonstrating signal abnormalities in the basal ganglia (arrows) in a patient with Creutzfeldt–Jakob disease who presented with supranuclear gaze and gait abnormalities.[452]

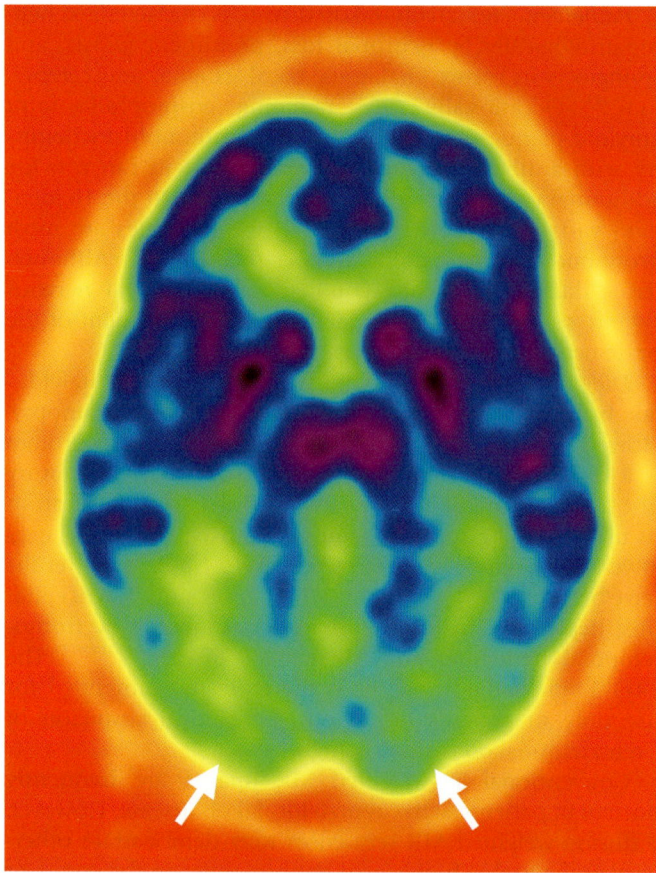

Figure 9–14. Fluorodeoxyglucose positron emission tomography (FDG-PET) scan demonstrating occipital lobe hypometabolism in a patient with the Heidenhain variant of Creutzfeldt–Jakob disease. Arrows point to green and yellow hypometabolic cortical regions in comparison to the anterior, blue relatively hypermetabolic regions. The patient had bilateral inferior visual defects, but the corresponding anatomical MRI scan of the brain was relatively normal.

T2-weighted[474] and fluid attenuated inversion recovery (FLAIR)[475] images may reveal similar changes. PET may demonstrate hypometabolism (**Fig. 9–14**) and SPECT may show hypoperfusion in the occipital lobes in patients with the Heidenhain variant of Creutzfeldt–Jakob disease.[476] Occasionally, the abnormalities on PET and SPECT will precede those found on MR imaging.

In moderately to severely affected patients, the electroencephalogram (EEG) may contain 1–2 Hz rhythmic periodic sharp wave complexes or a slow-wave burst-suppression pattern.[477] Some patients may have an abnormal electroretinogram (ERG) with a B1-wave decrease and relative preservation of the A wave.[459,478]

In practice, the combination of a clinical history of rapidly progressive dementia with myoclonus, pyramidal or extrapyramidal dysfunction, or visual deficits, and tests revealing the presence of 14-3-3 CSF protein, diffusion-weighted MR abnormalities, and periodic complexes on EEG would be highly suggestive of the diagnosis of Creutzfeldt–Jakob disease.[479–481] In contrast, a normal CSF, diffusion-weighted MRI, and EEG would make Creutzfeldt–Jakob disease extremely unlikely.[482]

Treatment. Unfortunately, Creutzfeldt–Jakob disease is uniformly fatal, usually within one year of onset.[483] Pres-

ently, there is no effective treatment although pharmacologic strategies are emerging based upon the current understanding of the molecular biology of disease.[484,485]

References

1. Zeki S. The visual association cortex. Current Opin Neurobiol 1993;3:155–159.
2. Girkin CA, Miller NR. Central disorders of vision in humans. Surv Ophthalmol 2001;45:379–405.
3. Stasheff SF, Barton JJ. Deficits in cortical visual function. Ophthalmol Clin North Am 2001;14:217–242.
4. Hodgson TL, Kennard C. Disorders of higher visual function and hemi-spatial neglect. Curr Opin Neurol 2000;13:7–12.
5. Zeki S. The P and M pathways and the "what and where" doctrine. In: A Vision of the Brain, pp 186–196. Oxford, Blackwell Scientific, 1993.
6. Damasio A, Yamada T, Damasio H, et al. Central achromatopsia. Behavioral, anatomic, and physiologic aspects. Neurology 1980;30:1064–1071.
7. Meadows JC. The anatomical basis of prosopagnosia. J Neurol Neurosurg Psychiatr 1974;37:489–501.
8. Damasio AR, Damasio H, Van Hoesen GW. Prosopagnosia: anatomic basis and behavioral mechanisms. Neurology 1982;32:331–341.
9. Bauer RM, Trobe JD. Visual memory and perceptual impairments in prosopagnosia. J Clin Neuroophthalmol 1984;4:39–46.
10. De Renzi E. Disorders of spatial orientation. In: Vinken PJ, Bruyn GW, Klawans HL (eds). Handbook of Clinical Neurology. Neuropsychology, pp 405–422. Amsterdam, Elsevier, 1985.
11. Geschwind N. Disconnection syndromes in animal and man. Brain 1965;88:237–294, 585–644.
12. Absher JR, Benson DF. Disconnection syndromes. An overview of Geschwind's contributions. Neurology 1993;43:862–867.
13. Catani M, ffytche DH. The rises and falls of disconnection syndromes. Brain 2005;128: 2224–2239.
14. Horton JC, Hoyt WF. Quadrantic visual field defects. A hallmark of lesions in extrastriate (V2/V3) cortex. Brain 1991;114:1703–1718.
15. Dejerine J. Contribution à l'étude anatomopathologique et clinique des differentes variétés de cécité verbale. Mem Soc Biol 1892;4:61–90.
16. Coslett HB, Saffran EM, Greenbaum S, et al. Reading in pure alexia. The effect of strategy. Brain 1993;116:21–37.
17. Arguin M, Bub DN. Pure alexia. Attempted rehabilitation and its implications for interpretation of the deficit. Brain & Language 1994;47:233–268.
18. Coslett HB. Acquired dyslexia. In: Feinberg TE, Farah MJ (eds). Behavioral Neurology and Neuropsychology, pp 197–208. New York, McGraw-Hill, 1997.
19. Stommel EW, Friedman RJ, Reeves AG. Alexia without agraphia associated with spleniogeniculate infarction. Neurology 1991;41:587–588.
20. Greenblatt SH. Alexia without agraphia or hemianopsia. Anatomical analysis of an autopsied case. Brain 1973;96:307.
21. Greenblatt SH. Subangular alexia without agraphia or hemianopsia. Brain Lang 1976;3: 229–245.
22. Vincent FM, Sadowsky CH, Saunders RL, et al. Alexia without agraphia, hemianopia or color-naming defect. A disconnection syndrome. Neurology 1977;27:689–691.
23. Henderson VW, Friedman RB, Teng EL, et al. Left hemisphere pathways in reading. Inferences from pure alexia without hemianopia. Neurology 1985;35:962–968.
24. Iragui VJ, Kritchevsky M. Alexia without agraphia or hemianopia in parietal infarction [letter]. J Neurol Neurosurg Psychiatr 1991;54:841–842.
25. Damasio AR, Damasio H. The anatomic basis of pure alexia. Neurology 1983;33: 1573–1583.
26. Hillis AE, Newhart M, Heidler J, et al. The roles of the "visual word form area" in reading. Neuroimage 2005;24:548–559.
27. Kleinschmidt A, Cohen L. The neural bases of prosopagnosia and pure alexia. Recent insights from functional neuroimaging. Curr Opin Neurol 2006;19:386–391.
28. Mani J, Diehl B, Piao Z, et al. Evidence for a basal temporal visual language center. Cortical stimulation producing pure alexia. Neurology 2008;71:1621–1627.
29. Price CJ, Devlin JT. The myth of the visual word form area. Neuroimage 2003;19: 473–481.
30. Cohen L, Dehaene S. Specialization within the ventral stream. The case for the visual word form area. Neuroimage 2004;22:466–476.
31. Sakurai Y. Varieties of alexia from fusiform, posterior inferior temporal and posterior occipital gyrus lesions. Behav Neurol 2004;15:35–50.
32. Binder JR, Lazar RM, Tatemichi TK, et al. Left hemiparalexia. Neurology 1992;42:562–569.
33. Rubens AB, Benson DF. Associative visual agnosia. Arch Neurol 1971;24:305–316.
34. Sparr SA, Jay M, Drislane FW, et al. A historic case of visual agnosia revisited after 40 years. Brain 1991;114:789–800.
35. Lhermitte F, Beauvois MF. A visual-speech disconnexion syndrome. Report of a case with optic aphasia, agnosic alexia and colour agnosia. Brain 1973;96:695–714.
36. Geschwind N, Fusillo M. Color naming defects in association with alexia. Arch Neurol 1966;15:137–146.
37. Quint DJ, Gilmore JL. Alexia without agraphia. Neuroradiology 1992;34:210–214.
38. Weisberg LA, Wall M. Alexia without agraphia. Clinical-computed tomographic correlations. Neuroradiology 1987;29:283–286.

39. Paquier PF, De Smet HJ, Marien P, et al. Acquired alexia with agraphia syndrome in childhood. J Child Neurol 2006;21:324–330.

40. Tamhankar MA, Coslett HB, Fisher MJ, et al. Alexia without agraphia following biopsy of a left thalamic tumor. Pediatr Neurol 2004;30:140–142.

41. Erdem S, Kansu T. Alexia without either agraphia or hemianopia in temporal lobe lesion due to herpes simplex encephalitis. J Neuroophthalmol 1995;15:102–104.

42. Dogulu CF, Kansu T, Karabudak R. Alexia without agraphia in multiple sclerosis [letter]. J Neurol Neurosurg Psychiatr 1996;61:528.

43. Little RD, Goldstein JL. Alexia without agraphia in a child with acute disseminated encephalomyelitis. Neurology 2006;67:725.

44. Leff AP, Crewes H, Plant GT, et al. The functional anatomy of single-word reading in patients with hemianopic and pure alexia. Brain 2001;124:510–521.

45. Leff AP, Spitsyna G, Plant GT, et al. Structural anatomy of pure and hemianopic alexia. J Neurol Neurosurg Psychiatr 2006;77:1004–1007.

46. Verrey D. Hémiachromatopsie droite absolue. Arch d'Ophthalmol (Paris) 1888;8:289–301.

47. Zeki S. A century of cerebral achromatopsia. Brain 1990;113:1721–1777.

48. Rizzo M, Nawrot M, Blake R, et al. A human visual disorder resembling area V4 dysfunction in the monkey. Neurology 1992;42:1175–1180.

49. Heywood CA, Kentridge RW. Achromatopsia, color vision, and cortex. Neurol Clin 2003;21:483–500.

50. Paulson HL, Galetta SL, Grossman M, et al. Hemiachromatopsia of unilateral occipitotemporal infarcts. Am J Ophthalmol 1994;118:518–523.

51. Zeki S, Watson JDG, Lueck CJ, et al. A direct demonstration of functional specialization in human visual cortex. J Neurosci 1991;11:641–649.

52. Sakai K, Watanabe E, Onodera Y, et al. Functional mapping of the human colour centre with echo-planar magnetic resonance imaging. Proceedings of the Royal Society of London—Series B. Biological Sciences 1995;261:89–98.

53. McKeefry DJ, Zeki S. The position and topography of the human colour centre as revealed by functional magnetic resonance imaging. Brain 1997;120:2229–2242.

54. Galetta SL. A stimulating view of human visual cortex [editorial]. Neurology 2000;54:785–786.

55. Lee HW, Hong SB, Seo DW, et al. Mapping of functional organization in human visual cortex. Electrical cortical stimulation. Neurology 2000;54:849–854.

56. Hadjikhani N, Liu AK, Dale AM, et al. Retinotopy and color sensitivity in human visual cortical area V8. Nat Neurosci 1998;1:235–241.

57. Nunn JA, Gregory LJ, Brammer M, et al. Functional magnetic resonance imaging of synesthesia. Activation of V4/V8 by spoken words. Nat Neurosci 2002;5:371–375.

58. Wade AR, Brewer AA, Rieger JW, et al. Functional measurements of human ventral occipital cortex: retinotopy and colour. Philos Trans R Soc Lond B Biol Sci 2002;357:963–973.

59. Brewer AA, Liu J, Wade AR, et al. Visual field maps and stimulus selectivity in human ventral occipital cortex. Nat Neurosci 2005;8:1102–1109.

60. Zeki S, Bartels A. The clinical and functional measurement of cortical (in)activity in the visual brain, with special reference to the two subdivisions (V4 and V4 alpha) of the human colour centre. Philos Trans R Soc Lond B Biol Sci 1999;354:1371–1382.

61. Murphey DK, Yoshor D, Beauchamp MS. Perception matches selectivity in the human anterior color center. Curr Biol 2008;18:216–220.

62. Rizzo M, Smith V, Pokorny J, et al. Color perception profiles in central achromatopsia. Neurology 1993;43:995–1001.

63. Meadows JC. Disturbed perception of colours associated with localized cerebral lesions. Brain 1974;97:615–632.

64. Damasio AR. Disorders of complex visual processing. agnosias, achromatopsia, Balint's syndrome, and related difficulties of orientation and construction. In: Mesulam M-M (ed). Principles of Behavioral Neurology, pp 259–288. Philadelphia, F. A. Davis, 1985.

65. Freedman L, Costa L. Pure alexia and right hemiachromatopsia in posterior dementia. J Neurol Neurosurg Psychiatr 1992;55:500–502.

66. Brazis PW, Biller J, Fine M. Central achromatopsia [letter]. Neurology 1981;31:920–921.

67. Green GJ, Lessell S. Acquired cerebral dyschromatopsia. Arch Ophthalmol 1977;95:121–128.

68. Bouvier SE, Engel SA. Behavioral deficits and cortical damage loci in cerebral achromatopsia. Cereb Cortex 2006;16:183–191.

69. Albert ML, Reches A, Silverberg R. Hemianopic colour blindness. J Neurol Neurosurg Psychiatr 1975;38:546–549.

70. Kölmel HW. Pure homonymous hemiachromatopsia. Findings with neuro-ophthalmologic examination and imaging procedures. Eur Arch Psychiatr Neurol Sci 1988;237:237–243.

71. Silverman IE, Galetta SL. Partial color loss in hemiachromatopsia. Neuroophthalmology 1995;15:127–134.

72. Heywood CA, Wilson B, Cowey A. A case study of cortical colour "blindness" with relatively intact achromatic discrimination. J Neurol Neurosurg Psychiatr 1987;50:22–29.

73. Müller T, Büttner T, Kuhn W, et al. Achromatopsia as a symptom of multiple sclerosis. Neuroophthalmology 1994;14:277–278.

74. Fine RD, Parker GD. Disturbance of central vision after carbon monoxide poisoning. Aust NZ J Ophthalmol 1996;24:137–141.

75. Lawden MC, Cleland PG. Achromatopsia in the aura of migraine. J Neurol Neurosurg Psychiatr 1993;56:708–709.

76. Lapresle J, Metreau R, Annabi A. Transient achromatopsia in vertebrobasilar insufficiency. J Neurol 1977;215:155–158.

77. Mohr JP, Leicester J, Stoddard LT, et al. Right hemianopia with memory and color deficits in circumscribed left posterior cerebral artery territory infarction. Neurology 1971;21:1104–1113.

78. Schnider A, Landis T, Regard M, et al. Dissociation of color from object in amnesia. Arch Neurol 1992;49:982–985.

79. Nijboer TC, Van Der Smagt MJ, Van Zandvoort MJ, et al. Colour agnosia impairs the recognition of natural but not of non-natural scenes. Cogn Neuropsychol 2007;24:152–161.

80. van Zandvoort MJ, Nijboer TC, de Haan E. Developmental colour agnosia. Cortex 2007;43:750–757.

81. Tranel D. Disorders of color processing (perception, imagery, recognition, and naming). In: Feinberg TE, Farah MJ (eds). Behavioral Neurology and Neuropsychology, pp 257–265. New York, McGraw-Hill, 1997.

82. Farah MJ, Feinberg TE. Visual object agnosia. In: Feinberg TE, Farah MJ (eds). Behavioral Neurology and Neuropsychology, pp 239–255. New York, McGraw-Hill, 1997.

83. Biran I, Coslett HB. Visual agnosia. Curr Neurol Neurosci Rep 2003;3:508–512.

84. Bender MB, Feldman M. The so-called "visual agnosias." Brain 1972;95:173–186.

85. Hasson U, Harel M, Levy I, et al. Large-scale mirror-symmetry organization of human occipito-temporal object areas. Neuron 2003;37:1027–1041.

86. De Renzi E. Disorders of visual recognition. Semin Neurol 2000;20:479–485.

87. Riddoch MJ, Humphreys GW. Visual agnosia. Neurol Clin 2003;21:501–520.

88. Riddoch MJ, Humphreys GW, Akhtar N, et al. A tale of two agnosias. Distinctions between form and integrative agnosia. Cogn Neuropsychol 2008;25:56–92.

89. Benson DF, Segarra J, Albert ML. Visual agnosia-prosopagnosia. A clinicopathologic correlation. Arch Neurol 1974;30:307–310.

90. Albert ML, Soffer D, Silverberg R, et al. The anatomic basis of visual agnosia. Neurology 1979;29:876–879.

91. Albert ML, Reches A, Silverberg R. Associative visual agnosia without alexia. Neurology 1975;25:322–326.

92. Feinberg TE, Schindler RJ, Ochoa E, et al. Associative visual agnosia and alexia without prosopagnosia. Cortex 1994;30:395–411.

93. Devinsky O, Farah MJ, Barr WB. Chapter 21. Visual agnosia. Handb Clin Neurol 2008;88:417–427.

94. Grossman M, Galetta S, D'Esposito M. Object recognition difficulty in visual apperceptive agnosia. Brain Cogn 1997;33:306–342.

95. Shelton PA, Bowers D, Duara R, et al. Apperceptive visual agnosia. A case study. Brain Cogn 1994;25:1–23.

96. Grossman M, Galetta S, Ding X-S, et al. Clinical and positron emission tomography studies of visual apperceptive agnosia. Neuropsychiatr Neuropsychol Behav Neurol 1996;9:70–77.

97. Ferreira CT, Ceccaldi M, Giusiano B, et al. Separate visual pathways for perception of actions and objects. Evidence from a case of apperceptive agnosia. J Neurol Neurosurg Psychiatr 1998;65:382–385.

98. de-Wit LH, Kentridge RW, Milner AD. Object-based attention and visual area LO. Neuropsychologia 2009;47:1483–1490.

99. Benson DF, Greenberg JP. Visual form agnosia. A specific defect in visual discrimination. Arch Neurol 1969;20:82–89.

100. Campion J, Latto R. Apperceptive agnosia due to carbon monoxide poisoning. An interpretation based on critical band masking from disseminated lesions. Behav Brain Res 1985;15:227–240.

101. Goldsmith ZG, Liu GT. Facial recognition and prosopagnosia. Past and present concepts. Neuroophthalmology 2001;25:177–192.

102. Riddoch MJ, Johnston RA, Bracewell RM, et al. Are faces special? A case of pure prosopagnosia. Cogn Neuropsychol 2008;25:3–26.

103. Allison T, McCarthy G, Nobre A, et al. Human extrastriate visual cortex and the perception of faces, words, numbers, and colors. Cereb Cortex 1994;4:544–554.

104. Puce A, Allison T, Gore JC, et al. Face-sensitive regions in human extrastriate cortex studied by functional MRI. J Neurophysiol 1995;74:1192–1199.

105. Kanwisher N, Yovel G. The fusiform face area. A cortical region specialized for the perception of faces. Philos Trans R Soc Lond B Biol Sci 2006;361:2109–2128.

106. Barton JJ, Cherkasova M. Face imagery and its relation to perception and covert recognition in prosopagnosia. Neurology 2003;61:220–225.

107. Engell AD, Haxby JV. Facial expression and gaze-direction in human superior temporal sulcus. Neuropsychologia 2007;45:3234–3241.

108. Kanwisher N, McDermott J, Chun MM. The fusiform face area. A module in human extrastriate cortex specialized for the perception of faces. J Neurosci 1997;17:4302–4311.

109. Sergent J, Ohta S, MacDonald B. Functional neuroanatomy of face and object processing. Brain 1992;115:15–36.

110. Sergent J, Signoret JL. Functional and anatomical decomposition of face processing. Evidence from prosopagnosia and PET study of normal subjects. Phil Trans Royal Soc London—Series B. Biol Sci 1992;335:55–61.

111. Andreasen NC, O'Leary DS, Arndt S, et al. Neural substrates of facial recognition. J Neuropsychiatry Clin Neurosci 1996;8:139–146.

112. Rapcsak SZ, Nielsen L, Littrell LD, et al. Face memory impairments in patients with frontal lobe damage. Neurology 2001;57:1168–1175.

113. Seeck M, Mainwaring N, Ives J, et al. Differential neural activity in the human temporal lobe evoked by faces of family members and friends. Ann Neurol 1993;34:369–372.

114. Seeck M, Schomer D, Mainwaring N, et al. Selectively distributed processing of visual object recognition in the temporal and frontal lobes of the human brain. Ann Neurol 1995;37:538–545.

115. Chatterjee A, Farah MJ. Face module, face network. The cognitive architecture of the brain revealed through studies of face processing. Neurology 2001;57:1151–1152.

116. Fox CJ, Iaria G, Barton JJ. Disconnection in prosopagnosia and face processing. Cortex 2008;44:996–1009.

117. De Renzi E. Prosopagnosia. In: Feinberg TE, Farah MJ (eds). Behavioral Neurology and Neuropsychology, pp 245–255. New York, McGraw-Hill, 1997.

118. Damasio AR, Tranel D, Damasio H. Face agnosia and the neural substrates of memory. Annu Rev Neurosci 1990;13:89–109.

119. Farah MJ, Rabinowitz C, Quinn GE, et al. Early commitment of neural substrates for face recognition. Cogn Neuropsychol 2000;17:117–124.

120. Barton JJ. Disorders of face perception and recognition. Neurol Clin 2003;21:521–548.

121. Adachi-Usami E, Tsukamoto M, Shimada Y. Color vision and color pattern visual evoked cortical potentials in a patient with acquired cerebral dyschromatopsia. Doc Ophthalmol 1995;90:259–269.

122. Aptman M, Levin H, Senelick RC. Alexia without agraphia in a left-handed patient with prosopagnosia. Neurology 1977;27:533–536.

123. De Renzi E, di Pellegrino G. Prosopagnosia and alexia without object agnosia. Cortex 1998;34:403–415.

124. Takahashi N, Kawamura M, Hirayama K, et al. Prosopagnosia. A clinical and anatomical study of four patients. Cortex 1995;31:317–329.

125. Levine DN. Prosopagnosia and visual object agnosia. A behavioral study. Brain & Language 1978;5:341–365.

126. Habib M. Visual hypoemotionality and prosopagnosia associated with right temporal lobe isolation. Neuropsychologia 1986;24:577–582.

127. Farah MJ, Levinson KL, Klein KL. Face perception and within-category discrimination in prosopagnosia. Neuropsychologia 1995;33:661–674.

128. Jacome DE. Subcortical prosopagnosia and anosognosia. Am J Med Sci 1986;292:386–388.

129. De Renzi E, Faglioni P, Grossi D, et al. Apperceptive and associative forms of prosopagnosia. Cortex 1991;27:213–221.

130. Bruyer R, Laterre C, Seron X, et al. A case of prosopagnosia with some preserved covert remembrance of familiar faces. Brain Cogn 1983;2:257–284.

131. Rizzo M, Corbett JJ, Thompson HS, et al. Spatial contrast sensitivity in facial recognition. Neurology 1986;36:1254–1256.

132. Rizzo M, Hurtig R, Damasio AR. The role of scanpaths in facial recognition and learning. Ann Neurol 1987;22:41–45.

133. Benton AL, Van Allen MW. Prosopagnosia and facial discrimination. J Neurol Sci 1972;15:167–172.

134. Young AW, Ellis HD. Childhood prosopagnosia. Brain Cogn 1989;9:16–47.

135. Roudier M, Marcie P, Grancher AS, et al. Discrimination of facial identity and of emotions in Alzheimer's disease. J Neurol Sci 1998;154:151–158.

136. Malone DR, Morris HH, Kay MC, et al. Prosopagnosia. A double dissociation between the recognition of familiar and unfamiliar faces. J Neurol Neurosurg Psychiatr 1982;45:820–822.

137. Davidoff J, Landis T. Recognition of unfamiliar faces in prosopagnosia. Neuropsychologia 1990;28:1143–1161.

138. Kosslyn SM, Hamilton SE, Bernstein JH. The perception of curvature can be selectively disrupted in prosopagnosia. Brain Cogn 1995;27:36–58.

139. Campbell R, Heywood CA, Cowey A, et al. Sensitivity to eye gaze in prosopagnosic patients and monkeys with superior temporal sulcus ablation. Neuropsychologia 1990;28:1123–1142.

140. Barton JJ, Cherkasova MV. Impaired spatial coding within objects but not between objects in prosopagnosia. Neurology 2005;65:270–274.

141. Barton JJ, Press DZ, Keenan JP, et al. Lesions of the fusiform face area impair perception of facial configuration in prosopagnosia. Neurology 2002;58:71–78.

142. De Haan EHF, Young AW, Newcombe F. Covert and overt recognition in prosopagnosia. Brain 1991;11:2575–2591.

143. Barton JJ, Cherkasova M, O'Connor M. Covert recognition in acquired and developmental prosopagnosia. Neurology 2001;57:1161–1168.

144. Bornstein B, Sroka H, Munitz H. Prosopagnosia with animal face agnosia. Cortex 1969;5:164–169.

145. McNeil JE, Warrington EK. Prosopagnosia. a face-specific disorder. Q J Exp Psychol. A, Human Exp Psychol 1993;46:1–10.

146. McCarthy RA, Evans JJ, Hodges JR. Topographic amnesia. Spatial memory disorder, perceptual dysfunction, or category specific semantic memory impairment? J Neurol Neurosurg Psychiatr 1996;60:318–325.

147. Carlesimo GA, Sabbadini M, Loasses A, et al. Analysis of the memory impairment in a post-encephalitic patient with focal retrograde amnesia. Cortex 1998;34:449–460.

148. Evans JJ, Heggs AJ, Antoun N, et al. Progressive prosopagnosia associated with selective right temporal lobe atrophy. A new syndrome? Brain 1995;118:1–13.

149. Mendez MF, Martin RJ, Smyth KA, et al. Disturbances of person identification in Alzheimer's disease. A retrospective study. J Nerv Ment Dis 1992;180:94–96.

150. Werth R, Steinbach T. Symptoms of prosopagnosia in intoxicated subjects. Perceptual & Motor Skills 1991;73:399–412.

151. Kracke I. Developmental prosopagnosia in Asperger syndrome. Presentation and discussion of an individual case. Dev Med Child Neurol 1994;36:873–886.

152. Harrington A, Oepen G, Spitzer M. Disordered recognition and perception of human faces in acute schizophrenia and experimental psychosis. Comprehensive Psychiatry 1989;30:376–384.

153. Mazzucchi A, Biber C. Is prosopagnosia more frequent in males than in females? Cortex 1983;19:509–516.

154. De Haan EH, Campbell R. A fifteen year follow-up of a case of developmental prosopagnosia. Cortex 1991;27:489–509.

155. Galaburda AM, Duchaine BC. Developmental disorders of vision. Neurol Clin 2003;21:687–707.

156. Schmalzl L, Palermo R, Green M, et al. Training of familiar face recognition and visual scan paths for faces in a child with congenital prosopagnosia. Cogn Neuropsychol 2008;25:704–729.

157. De Haan EH. A familial factor in the development of face recognition deficits. J Clin Exp Neuropsychol 1999;21:312–315.

158. Behrmann M, Avidan G. Congenital prosopagnosia. Face-blind from birth. Trends Cogn Sci 2005;9:180–187.

159. Cohn R, Neumann MA, Wood DH. Prosopagnosia. a clinicopathological study. Ann Neurol 1977;1:177–182.

160. Kay MC, Levin HS. Prosopagnosia. Am J Ophthalmol 1982;94:75–80.

161. Landis T, Regard M, Bliestle A, et al. Prosopagnosia and agnosia for noncanonical views. An autopsied case. Brain 1988;111:1287–1297.

162. Landis T, Cummings JL, Christen L, et al. Are unilateral right posterior cerebral lesions sufficient to cause prosopagnosia? Clinical and radiological findings in six additional patients. Cortex 1986;22:243–252.

163. De Renzi E. Prosopagnosia in two patients with CT scan evidence of damage confined to the right hemisphere. Neuropsychologia 1986;24:385–389.

164. De Renzi E, Perani D, Carlesimo GA, et al. Prosopagnosia can be associated with damage confined to the right hemisphere—an MRI and PET study and a review of the literature. Neuropsychologia 1994;32:893–902.

165. Tohgi H, Watanabe K, Takahashi H, et al. Prosopagnosia without topographagnosia and object agnosia associated with a lesion confined to the right occipitotemporal region. J Neurol 1994;241:470–474.

166. Mendez MF, Ghajarnia M. Agnosia for familiar faces and odors in a patient with right temporal lobe dysfunction. Neurology 2001;57:519–521.

167. Sergent J, Villemure JG. Prosopagnosia in a right hemispherectomized patient. Brain 1989;112:975–995.

168. Sorger B, Goebel R, Schiltz C, et al. Understanding the functional neuroanatomy of acquired prosopagnosia. Neuroimage 2007;35:836–852.

169. Rösler A, Lanquillon S, Dippel O, et al. Impairment of facial recognition in patients with right cerebral infarcts quantified by computer aided "morphing." J Neurol Neurosurg Psychiatr 1997;62:261–264.

170. Barton JJ. Prosopagnosia associated with a left occipitotemporal lesion. Neuropsychologia 2008;46:2214–2224.

171. Whiteley AM, Warrington EK. Prosopagnosia. a clinical, psychological, and anatomical study of three patients. J Neurol Neurosurg Psychiatr 1977;40:395–403.

172. Clarke S, Lindemann A, Maeder P, et al. Face recognition and postero-inferior hemispheric lesions. Neuropsychologia 1997;35:1555–1563.

173. Rossion B, Caldara R, Seghier M, et al. A network of occipito-temporal face-sensitive areas besides the right middle fusiform gyrus is necessary for normal face processing. Brain 2003;126:2381–2395.

174. Dricot L, Sorger B, Schiltz C, et al. The roles of "face" and "non-face" areas during individual face perception. Evidence by fMRI adaptation in a brain-damaged prosopagnosic patient. Neuroimage 2008;40:318–332.

175. Hier DB, Mondlock J, Caplan LR. Recovery of behavioral abnormalities after right hemisphere stroke. Neurology 1983;33:337–344.

176. Shraberg D, Weitzel WD. Prosopagnosia and the Capgras syndrome. J Clin Psychiatry 1979;40:313–316.

177. Gibbs A, Andrewes D. Capgras' syndrome or prosopagnosia? [letter]. Br J Psychiatry 1988;153:853.

178. Josephs KA. Capgras syndrome and its relationship to neurodegenerative disease. Arch Neurol 2007;64:1762–1766.

179. Lewis SW. Brain imaging in a case of Capgras' syndrome. Br J Psychiatry 1987;150:117–121.

180. Aguirre GK, D'Esposito M. Topographical disorientation. A synthesis and taxonomy. Brain 1999;122:1613–1628.

181. Mendez MF, Cherrier MM. Agnosia for scenes in topographagnosia. Neuropsychologia 2003;41:1387–1395.

182. Hillis AE. Aphasia. progress in the last quarter of a century. Neurology 2007;69:200–213.

183. Schnider A, Benson DF, Scharre DW. Visual agnosia and optic aphasia: are they anatomically distinct? Cortex 1994;30:445–457.

184. Rubin DC, Greenberg DL. Visual memory-deficit amnesia. A distinct amnesic presentation and etiology. Proceedings of the National Academy of Sciences USA 1998;95:5413–5416.

185. Slotnick SD. Visual memory and visual perception recruit common neural substrates. Behav Cogn Neurosci Rev 2004;3:207–221.

186. Ungerleider LG, Courtney SM, Haxby JV. A neural system for human visual working memory. Proceedings of the National Academy of Sciences USA 1998;95:883–890.

187. Ranganath C, D'Esposito M. Directing the mind's eye. Prefrontal, inferior and medial temporal mechanisms for visual working memory. Curr Opin Neurobiol 2005;15:175–182.

188. Ranganath C. Working memory for visual objects. Complementary roles of inferior temporal, medial temporal, and prefrontal cortex. Neuroscience 2006;139:277–289.

189. Zimmer HD. Visual and spatial working memory: from boxes to networks. Neurosci Biobehav Rev 2008;32:1373–1395.

190. Ross ED. Sensory-specific and fractional disorders of recent memory in man. I. Isolated loss of visual recent memory. Arch Neurol 1980;37:193–200.

191. Kimura D. Right temporal-lobe damage. Arch Neurol 1963;8:48–55.

192. Hanley JR, Pearson NA, Young AW. Impaired memory for new visual forms. Brain 1990;113:1131–1148.

193. Kaplan RF, Meadows M-E, Verfaellie M, et al. Lateralization of memory for the visual attributes of objects. Evidence from the posterior cerebral artery amobarbital test. Neurology 1994;44:1069–1073.

194. Speedie LJ, Heilman KM. Anterograde memory deficits for visuospatial material after infarction of the right thalamus. Arch Neurol 1983;40:183–186.

195. Botez-Marquard T, Botez MI. Visual memory deficits after damage to the anterior commissure and right fornix. Arch Neurol 1992;49:321–324.

196. Zeki S. Cerebral akinetopsia (visual motion blindness). A review. Brain 1991;114:811–824.

197. Zeki SM. Functional organization of a visual area in the posterior bank of the superior temporal sulcus of the rhesus monkey. J Physiol 1974;236:549–573.

198. Newsome WT, Paré EB. A selective impairment of motion perception following lesions of the middle temporal visual area (MT). J Neurosci 1988;8:2201–2211.

199. Zihl J, Von Cramon D, Mai N, et al. Selective disturbance of movement vision after bilateral brain damage. Brain 1983;106:313–340.

200. Zihl J, Von Cramon D, Mai N, et al. Disturbance of movement vision after bilateral posterior brain damage. Further evidence and follow up observations. Brain 1991;114:2235–2252.

201. Shipp S, de Jong BM, Frackowiak RSJ, et al. The brain activity related to residual motion vision in a patient with bilateral lesions of V5. Brain 1994;117:1023–1038.

202. Vaina LM, Lemay M, Bienfang DC, et al. Intact "biological motion" and "structure from motion" perception in a patient with impaired motion mechanisms. A case study. Vis Neurosci 1990;5:353–369.

203. Vaina LM, Cowey A, Eskew RT, Jr., et al. Regional cerebral correlates of global motion perception. Evidence from unilateral cerebral brain damage. Brain 2001;124:310–321.

204. Vaina LM, Cowey A, Jakab M, et al. Deficits of motion integration and segregation in patients with unilateral extrastriate lesions. Brain 2005;128:2134–2145.

205. Pelak VS, Hoyt WF. Symptoms of akinetopsia associated with traumatic brain injury and Alzheimer's disease. Neuroophthalmology 2005;29:137–142.

206. Moo LR, Emerton BC, Slotnick SD. Functional MT + lesion impairs contralateral motion processing. Cogn Neuropsychol 2008;25:677–689.

207. Tootell RB, Reppas JB, Kwong KK, et al. Functional analysis of human MT and related visual cortical areas using magnetic resonance imaging. J Neurosci 1995;15:3215–3230.

208. Barton JJS, Simpson T, Diriakopoulos E, et al. Functional MRI of lateral occipitotemporal cortex during pursuit and motion perception. Ann Neurol 1996;40:387–398.

209. Bonhomme GR, Liu GT, Miki A, et al. Decreased cortical activation in response to a motion stimulus in anisometropic amblyopic eyes using functional magnetic resonance imaging. JAAPOS 2006;10:540–546.

210. Sofue A, Kaneoke Y, Kakigi R. Physiological evidence of interaction of first- and second-order motion processes in the human visual system. A magnetoencephalographic study. Hum Brain Mapp 2003;20:158–167.

211. Cattaneo Z, Silvanto J. Investigating visual motion perception using the transcranial magnetic stimulation-adaptation paradigm. Neuroreport 2008;19:1423–1427.

212. Horton JC, Trobe JD. Akinetopsia from nefazodone toxicity. Am J Ophthalmol 1999;128:530–531.

213. Donahue SP, Wall M, Stanek KE. Motion perimetry in anisometropic amblyopia. Elevated size thresholds extend into the midperiphery. JAAPOS 1998;2:94–101.

214. Nawrot M. Disorders of motion and depth. Neurol Clin 2003;21:609–629.

215. Deutschländer A, Hüfner K, Kalla R, et al. Unilateral vestibular failure suppresses cortical visual motion processing. Brain 2008;131:1025–1034.

216. ffytch DH, Guy CN, Zeki S. Motion specific responses from a blind hemifield. Brain 1996;119:1971–1982.

217. Barton JJS, Sharpe JA, Raymond JE. Retinotopic and directional defects in motion discrimination in humans with cerebral lesions. Ann Neurol 1995;37:665–675.

218. Brandt T, Bucher SF, Seelos KC, et al. Bilateral functional MRI activation of the basal ganglia and middle temporal/medial superior temporal motion-sensitive areas. Arch Neurol 1998;55:1126–1131.

219. Barbur J, Watson JDG, Frackowiak RSJ, et al. Conscious visual perception without V1. Brain 1993;116:1293–1302.

220. Zeki S, ffytche DH. The Riddoch syndrome. Insights into the neurobiology of conscious vision. Brain 1998;121:25–45.

221. Stoerig P, Kleinschmidt A, Frahm J. No visual responses in denervated V1. High resolution functional magnetic resonance imaging of a blindsight patient. Neuroreport 1998;9:21–25.

222. Liu GT, Bolton AK, Price BH, et al. Dissociated perceptual-sensory and exploratory-motor neglect. J Neurol Neurosurg Psychiatr 1992;55:701–714.

223. Buxbaum LJ, Ferraro MK, Veramonti T, et al. Hemispatial neglect. Subtypes, neuroanatomy, and disability. Neurology 2004;62:749–756.

224. Riddoch G. Visual disorientation in homonymous half-fields. Brain 1935;5:376–382.

225. Brain WR. Visual disorientation with special reference to lesions of the right cerebral hemisphere. Brain 1941;64:244–272.

226. Cole M, Schutta HS, Warrington EK. Visual disorientation in homonymous half-fields. Neurology 1962;12:257–263.

227. Baynes K, Holtzman JD, Volpe BT. Components of visual attention. Alterations in response pattern to visual stimuli following parietal lobe infarction. Brain 1986;109:99–114.

228. Vallar G, Sandroni P, Rusconi ML, et al. Hemianopia, hemianesthesia, and spatial neglect. A study with visual evoked potentials. Neuropsychologia 1991;24:609–622.

229. Laurent-Vannier A, Pradat-Diehl P, Chevignard M, et al. Spatial and motor neglect in children. Neurology 2003;60:202–207.

230. Smith SE, Chatterjee A. Visuospatial attention in children. Arch Neurol 2008;65:1284–1288.

231. Mesulam M-M. Attention, confusional states, and neglect. In: Mesulam M-M (ed). Principles of Behavioral Neurology, pp 125–168. Philadelphia, F.A. Davis, 1985.

232. Vallar G, Perani D. The anatomy of unilateral neglect after right-hemisphere stroke lesions. A clinical/CT-scan correlation study in man. Neuropsychologia 1986;24:609–622.

233. Mort DJ, Malhotra P, Mannan SK, et al. The anatomy of visual neglect. Brain 2003;126:1986–1997.

234. Weintraub S, Mesulam M-M. Right cerebral dominance in spatial attention. Further evidence based on ipsilateral neglect. Arch Neurol 1987;44:621–625.

235. Beis JM, Keller C, Morin N, et al. Right spatial neglect after left hemisphere stroke. Qualitative and quantitative study. Neurology 2004;63:1600–1605.

236. Kleinman JT, Newhart M, Davis C, et al. Right hemispatial neglect. Frequency and characterization following acute left hemisphere stroke. Brain Cogn 2007;64:50–59.

237. Ringman JM, Saver JL, Woolson RF, et al. Frequency, risk factors, anatomy, and course of unilateral neglect in an acute stroke cohort. Neurology 2004;63:468–474.

238. Heilman KM, Valenstein E, Watson RT. The neglect syndrome. In: Vinken PJ, Bruyn GW, Klawans HL (eds). Handbook of Clinical Neurology, vol. 1 (45) Clinical Neuropsychology, pp 153–183. Amsterdam, Elsevier, 1985.

239. Becker E, Karnath HO. Incidence of visual extinction after left versus right hemisphere stroke. Stroke 2007;38:3172–3174.

240. Doricchi F, Angelelli P. Misrepresentation of horizontal space in left unilateral neglect. Role of hemianopia. Neurology 1999;52:1845–1852.

241. Milner AD, McIntosh RD. The neurological basis of visual neglect. Curr Opin Neurol 2005;18:748–753.

242. Adair JC, Barrett AM. Spatial neglect. Clinical and neuroscience review. A wealth of information on the poverty of spatial attention. Ann N Y Acad Sci 2008;1142:21–43.

243. Hillis AE. Neurobiology of unilateral spatial neglect. Neuroscientist 2006;12:153–163.

244. Bartolomeo P. Visual neglect. Curr Opin Neurol 2007;20:381–386.

245. Bisiach E, Luzzatti C, Perani D. Unilateral neglect, representational schema and consciousness. Brain 1979;102:609–618.

246. Heilman KM, Valenstein E. Mechanisms underlying hemispatial neglect. Ann Neurol 1979;5:166–170.

247. Heilman KM, Bowers D, Coslett HB, et al. Directional hypokinesia. Prolonged reaction times for leftward movements in patients with right hemisphere lesions and neglect. Neurology 1985;35:855–859.

248. Meador KJ, WAtxon RT, Bowers D, et al. Hypometria with hemispatial and limb motor neglect. Brain 1986;109:293–305.

249. Mesulam M-M. A cortical network for directed attention and unilateral neglect. Ann Neurol 1981;10:309–325.

250. Daffner KR, Ahern GL, Weintraub S, et al. Dissociated neglect behavior following sequential strokes in the right hemisphere. Ann Neurol 1990;28:97–101.

251. Mesulam M-M. Large-scale neurocognitive networks and distributed processing for attention, language, and memory. Ann Neurol 1990;28:597–613.

252. Mesulam MM. Spatial attention and neglect. Parietal, frontal and cingulate contributions to the mental representation and attentional targeting of salient extrapersonal events. Philos Trans R Soc Lond B Biol Sci 1999;354:1325–1346.

253. Watson RT, Heilman KM, Cauthen JC, et al. Neglect after cingulectomy. Neurology 1973;23:1003–1007.

254. Karnath HO, Ferber S, Himmelbach M. Spatial awareness is a function of the temporal not the posterior parietal lobe. Nature 2001;411:950–953.

255. Committeri G, Pitzalis S, Galati G, et al. Neural bases of personal and extrapersonal neglect in humans. Brain 2007;130:431–441.

256. Coslett HB, Bowers D, Fitzpatrick E, et al. Directional hypokinesia and hemispatial inattention in neglect. Brain 1990;113:475–486.

257. D'Esposito M, McGlinchey-Berroth M, Alexander MP, et al. Dissociable cognitive and neural mechanisms of unilateral visual neglect. Neurology 1993;43:2638–2644.

258. Bartolomeo P, D'Erme P, Perri R, et al. Perception and action in hemispatial neglect. Neuropsychologia 1998;36:227–237.

259. Fink GR, Driver J, Rorden C, et al. Neural consequences of competing stimuli in both visual hemifields. A physiological basis for visual extinction. Ann Neurol 2000;47:440–446.

260. Hillis AE, Newhart M, Heidler J, et al. Anatomy of spatial attention. Insights from perfusion imaging and hemispatial neglect in acute stroke. J Neurosci 2005;25:3161–3167.

261. Karnath HO, Himmelbach M, Rorden C. The subcortical anatomy of human spatial neglect. Putamen, caudate nucleus and pulvinar. Brain 2002;125:350–360.

262. Watson RT, Heilman KM. Thalamic neglect. Neurology 1979;29:690–694.

263. Watson RT, Valenstein E, Heilman KM. Thalamic neglect. Possible role of the medial thalamus and nucleus reticularis in behavior. Arch Neurol 1981;38:501–506.

264. Healton EB, Navarro C, Bressman S, et al. Subcortical neglect. Neurology 1982;32:776–778.

265. Chamorro A, Sacco RL, Ciecierski K, et al. Visual hemineglect and hemihallucinations in a patient with a subcortical infarction. Neurology 1990;40:1463–1464.

266. Sakashita Y. Visual attentional disturbance with unilateral lesions in the basal ganglia and deep white matter. Ann Neurol 1991;30:673–677.

267. Kashiwagi A, Kashiwagi T, Nishikawa T, et al. Hemispatial neglect in a patient with callosal infarction. Brain 1990;113:1005–1023.

268. Heilman KM, Adams DJ. Callosal neglect. Arch Neurol 2003;60:276–279.

269. Perani D, Vallar G, Cappa S, et al. Aphasia and neglect after subcortical stroke. A clinical/cerebral perfusion correlation study. Brain 1987;110:1211–1229.

270. D'Esposito M. Specific stroke syndromes. In: Mills VM, Cassidy JW, Katz DI (eds). Neurologic Rehabilitation. A Guide to Diagnosis, Prognosis, and Treatment Planning, pp 59–103. Malden, Blackwell Science, 1997.

271. Kalra L, Perez I, Gupta S, et al. The influence of visual neglect on stroke rehabilitation. Stroke 1997;28:1386–1391.

272. Levine D, Warach JD, Benowitz L, et al. Left spatial neglect. Effects of lesion size and premorbid brain atrophy on severity and recovery following right cerebral infarction. Neurology 1986;36:362–366.

273. Bowen A, Lincoln NB. Cognitive rehabilitation for spatial neglect following stroke. Cochrane Database Syst Rev 2007:CD003586.

274. Rossi PW, Kheyfets S, Reding MJ. Fresnel prisms improve visual perception in stroke patients with homonymous hemianopia or unilateral visual neglect. Neurology 1990;40:1597–1599.

275. Frassinetti F, Angeli V, Meneghello F, et al. Long-lasting amelioration of visuospatial neglect by prism adaptation. Brain 2002;125:608–623.

276. Maravita A, McNeil J, Malhotra P, et al. Prism adaptation can improve contralesional tactile perception in neglect. Neurology 2003;60:1829–1831.

277. Ferber S, Danckert J, Joanisse M, et al. Eye movements tell only half the story. Neurology 2003;60:1826–1829.

278. Luauté J, Michel C, Rode G, et al. Functional anatomy of the therapeutic effects of prism adaptation on left neglect. Neurology 2006;66:1859–1867.

279. Pisella L, Rode G, Farne A, et al. Prism adaptation in the rehabilitation of patients with visuo-spatial cognitive disorders. Curr Opin Neurol 2006;19:534–542.

280. Rossetti Y, Rode G, Pisella L, et al. Prism adaptation to a rightward optical deviation rehabilitates left hemispatial neglect. Nature 1998;395:166–169.

281. Castiello U, Lusher D, Burton C. Improving left hemispatial neglect using virtual reality. Neurology 2004;62:1958–1962.

282. Arai T, Ohi H, Sasaki H, et al. Hemispatial sunglasses. Effect on unilateral spatial neglect. Arch Phys Med Rehab 1997;78:230–232.

283. Niemeier JP. The Lighthouse Strategy. Use of a visual imagery technique to treat visual inattention in stroke patients. Brain Injury 1998;12:399–406.

284. Robertson IH, Mattingley JB, Rorden C, et al. Phasic alerting of neglect patients overcomes their spatial deficit in visual awareness. Nature 1998;395:169–172.

285. Rubens AB. Caloric stimulation and unilateral visual neglect. Neurology 1985;35:1019–1024.

286. Malhotra PA, Parton AD, Greenwood R, et al. Noradrenergic modulation of space exploration in visual neglect. Ann Neurol 2006;59:186–190.

287. Fleet WS, Valenstein E, Watson RT, et al. Dopamine agonist therapy for neglect in humans. Neurology 1987;37:1765–1771.

288. Grujic Z, Mapstone M, Gitelman DR, et al. Dopamine agonists reorient visual exploration away from the neglected hemispace. Neurology 1998;51:1395–1398.

289. Bálint R. Seelenlähmung des "Schauens," optische Ataxie, räumliche Störung der Aufmerksamkeit. Monatsschr Psychiatr Neurol 1909;25:51–81.

290. Husain M, Stein J. Rezsö Balint and his most celebrated case. Arch Neurol 1988;45:89–93.

291. Rizzo M, Vecera SP. Psychoanatomical substrates of Balint's syndrome. J Neurol Neurosurg Psychiatr 2002;72:162–178.

292. Moreaud O. Balint syndrome. Arch Neurol 2003;60:1329–1331.

293. Holmes G. Disturbances of visual orientation. Br J Ophth 1918;2:449–486, 506–518.

294. Hausser CO, Robert F, Giard N. Balint's syndrome. Can J Neurol Sci 1980;7:157–161.

295. Rafal RD. Balint syndrome. In: Feinberg TE, Farah MJ (eds). Behavioral Neurology and Neuropsychology, pp 337–356. New York, McGraw-Hill, 1997.

296. Vallar G. Spatial neglect, Balint-Holmes' and Gerstmann's syndrome, and other spatial disorders. CNS Spectr 2007;12:527–536.

297. Rizzo M. "Balint's syndrome" and associated visuospatial disorders. Baillière's Clinical Neurology 1993;2:415–437.

298. Brazis PW, Graff-Radford NR, Newman NJ, et al. Ishihara color plates as a test for simultanagnosia. Am J Ophthalmol 1998;126:850–851.

299. McMonagle P, Kertesz A. Exploded drawing in posterior cortical atrophy. Neurology 2006;67:1866.

300. Rizzo M, Hurtig R. Looking but not seeing. Attention, perception, and eye movements in simultanagnosia. Neurology 1987;37:1642–1648.

301. Rizzo M, Robin DA. Simultanagnosia: a defect of sustained attention yields insights on visual information processing. Neurology 1990;40:447–455.

302. Demeyere N, Rzeskiewicz A, Humphreys KA, et al. Automatic statistical processing of visual properties in simultanagnosia. Neuropsychologia 2008;46:2861–2864.

303. Damasio AR, Benton AL. Impairment of hand movements under visual guidance. Neurology 1979;29:170–178.

304. Pierrot-Deseilligny C, Gray F, Brunet P. Infarcts of both inferior parietal lobules with impairment of visually guided eye movements, peripheral visual inattention and optic ataxia. Brain 1986;109:81–97.

305. Watson RT, Rapcsak SZ. Loss of spontaneous blinking in a patient with Balint's syndrome. Arch Neurol 1989;46:567–570.

306. Tyler HR. Abnormalities of perception with defective eye movements (Bálint's syndrome). Cortex 1968;4:154–171.

307. De Renzi E. Disorders of Space Exploration and Cognition, pp 57–137. Chichester, John Wiley & Sons, 1982.

308. Verfaellie M, Rapcsak SZ, Heilman KM. Impaired shifting of attention in Balint's syndrome. Brain Cog 1990;12:195–204.

309. Coslett HB, Saffran E. Simultanagnosia: to see but not two see. Brain 1991;113:1523–1545.

310. Coslett HB, Lie G. Simultanagnosia: when a rose is not red. J Cogn Neurosci 2008;20:36–48.

311. Coslett HB, Lie E. Simultanagnosia: effects of semantic category and repetition blindness. Neuropsychologia 2008;46:1853–1863.

312. Rondot P, De Recondo J, Ribadeau Dumas JL. Visuomotor ataxia. Brain 1977;100:355–376.

313. Nagaratnam N, Grice D, Kalouche H. Optic ataxia following unilateral stroke. J Neurol Sci 1998;155:204–207.

314. Levine DN, Kaufman KJ, Mohr JP. Inaccurate reaching associated with a superior parietal lobe tumor. Neurology 1978;28:556–561.

315. Rossetti Y, Pisella L, Vighetto A. Optic ataxia revisited. Visually guided action versus immediate visuomotor control. Exp Brain Res 2003;153:171–179.

316. Pisella L, Binkofski F, Lasek K, et al. No double-dissociation between optic ataxia and visual agnosia. Multiple sub-streams for multiple visuo-manual integrations. Neuropsychologia 2006;44:2734–2748.

317. Gaveau V, Pelisson D, Blangero A, et al. Saccade control and eye-hand coordination in optic ataxia. Neuropsychologia 2008;46:475–486.

318. Liu GT, Ronthal M. Reflex blink to visual threat. J Clin Neuroophthalmol 1992;12:47–56.

319. Holmes G, Horrax G. Disturbances of spatial orientation and visual attention with loss of stereoscopic vision. Arch Neurol Psychiatr 1919;1:385–407.

320. Godwin-Austen RB. A case of visual disorientation. J Neurol Neurosurg Psychiatr 1965;28:453–458.

321. Graff-Radford NR, Bolling JP, Earnest F, et al. Simultanagnosia as the initial sign of degenerative dementia. Mayo Clinic Proc 1993;68:955–964.

322. Ances BM, Ellenbogen JM, Herman ST, et al. Balint syndrome due to Creutzfeldt–Jakob disease. Neurology 2004;63:395.

323. Moulingnier A, de Saint Martin L, Mahieux F, et al. Balint's syndrome [letter]. Neurology 1995;45:1030–1031.

324. Merchut MP, Richie B. Transient visuospatial disorder from angiographic contrast. Arch Neurol 2002;59:851–854.

325. Jacobs DA, Liu GT, Nelson PT, et al. Primary central nervous system angiitis, amyloid angiopathy, and Alzheimer's pathology presenting with Balint's syndrome. Surv Ophthalmol 2004;49:454–459.

326. Uyama E, Iwagoe H, Maeda J, et al. Presenile-onset cerebral adrenoleukodystrophy presenting as Balint's syndrome and dementia. Neurology 1993;43:1249–1251.

327. Drummond SR, Dutton GN. Simultanagnosia following perinatal hypoxia. a possible pediatric variant of Balint syndrome. JAAPOS 2007;11:497–498.

328. Perez FM, Tunkel RS, Lachmann EA, et al. Balint's syndrome arising from bilateral posterior cortical atrophy or infarction. Rehabilitation strategies and their limitation. Disabil Rehabil 1996;18:300–304.

329. Benson DF, Davis RJ, Snyder BD. Posterior cortical atrophy. Arch Neurol 1988;45:789–793.

330. Ardila A, Rosselli M, Arvizu L, et al. Alexia and agraphia in posterior cortical atrophy. Neuropsychiatry Neuropsychol Behav Neurol 1997;10:52–59.

331. Mendez MF, Cherrier MM. The evolution of alexia and simultanagnosia in posterior cortical atrophy. Neuropsychiatry Neuropsychol Behav Neurol 1998;11:76–82.

332. Tang-Wai DF, Graff-Radford NR, Boeve BF, et al. Clinical, genetic, and neuropathologic characteristics of posterior cortical atrophy. Neurology 2004;63:1168–1174.

333. Renner JA, Burns JM, Hou CE, et al. Progressive posterior cortical dysfunction. a clinicopathologic series. Neurology 2004;63:1175–1180.

334. McMonagle P, Deering F, Berliner Y, et al. The cognitive profile of posterior cortical atrophy. Neurology 2006;66:331–338.

335. Kirshner HS, Lavin PJ. Posterior cortical atrophy. A brief review. Curr Neurol Neurosci Rep 2006;6:477–480.

336. Josephs KA, Whitwell JL, Boeve BF, et al. Visual hallucinations in posterior cortical atrophy. Arch Neurol 2006;63:1427–1432.

337. Tang-Wai DF, Josephs KA, Boeve BF, et al. Pathologically confirmed corticobasal degeneration presenting with visuospatial dysfunction. Neurology 2003;61:1134–1135.

338. Tang-Wai D, Mapstone M. What are we seeing? Is posterior cortical atrophy just Alzheimer disease? Neurology 2006;66:300–301.

339. Freedman L, Selchen DH, Black SE, et al. Posterior cortical dementia with alexia. Neurobehavioural, MRI, and PET findings. J Neurol Neurosurg Psychiatr 1991;54:443–448.

340. Farah MJ. The neurologic basis of mental imagery. A componential analysis. Cognition 1984;18:245–272.

341. Farah MJ, Peronnet F, Gonon MA, et al. Electrophysiological evidence for a shared representational medium for visual images and visual percepts. J Exp Psychol Gen 1988;117:248–257.

342. Farah MJ. Is visual imagery really visual? Overlooked evidence from neuropsychology. Psychol Rev 1988;95:307–317.

343. Kosslyn SM, Alpert NM, Thompson WL, et al. Visual mental imagery activates topographically organized visual cortex. PET investigations. J Cogn Neurosci 1993;5:263–287.

344. Kosslyn SM, Thompson WL, Alpert NM. Neural systems shared by visual imagery and visual perception. A positron emission tomography study. Neuroimage 1997;6:320–334.

345. Bartolomeo P. The relationship between visual perception and visual mental imagery. A reappraisal of the neuropsychological evidence. Cortex 2002;38:357–378.

346. Bartolomeo P. The neural correlates of visual mental imagery. An ongoing debate. Cortex 2008;44:107–108.

347. Butter CM, Kosslyn S, Mijovic-Prelec D, et al. Field-specific deficits in visual imagery following hemianopia due to unilateral occipital infarcts. Brain 1997;120:217–228.

348. Büchel C, Price C, Frackowiak RSJ, et al. Different activation patterns in the visual cortex of late and congenitally blind subjects. Brain 1998;121:409–419.

349. Levine DN, Warach J, Farah M. Two visual systems in mental imagery. Dissociation of "what" and "where" in imagery disorders due to bilateral posterior cerebral lesions. Neurology 1985;35:1010–1018.

350. Mehta Z, Newcombe F, De Haan E. Selective loss of imagery in a case of visual agnosia. Neuropsychologia 1992;30:645–655.

351. Rode G, Revol P, Rossetti Y, et al. Looking while imagining. The influence of visual input on representational neglect. Neurology 2007;68:432–437.

352. Bisiach E, Luzzatti C. Unilateral neglect of representational space. Cortex 1978;14:129–133.

353. Chatterjee A, Southwood MH. Cortical blindness and visual imagery. Neurology 1995;45:2189–2195.

354. Goldenberg G, Müllbacher W, Nowak A. Imagery without perception—a case study of anosognosia for cortical blindness. Neuropsychologia 1995;33:1373–1382.

355. Shuren JE, Brott TG, Schefft BK, et al. Preserved color imagery in an achromatopsic. Neuropsychologia 1996;34:485–489.

356. Bartolomeo P, Bachoud-Lévi A-C, Denes G. Preserved imagery for colours in a patient with cerebral achromatopsia. Cortex 1997;33:369–378.

357. Beschin N, Cocchini G, Della Sala S, et al. What the eyes perceive, the brain ignores. A case of pure unilateral representational neglect. Cortex 1997;33:3–26.

358. Behrmann M, Moscovitch M, Winocur G. Intact visual imagery and impaired visual perception in a patient with visual agnosia. J Exp Psychol. Hum Percept Perform 1994;20:1068–1087.

359. Heilman KM, Valenstein E. Frontal lobe neglect in man. Neurology 1972;22:660–664.

360. Stein S, Volpe BT. Classical "parietal" neglect syndrome after subcortical right frontal lobe infarction. Neurology 1983;33:797–799.

361. Cogan DG. Neurology of the ocular muscles, pp 104–105. Springfield, Thomas, 1956.

362. Husain M, Kennard C. Visual neglect associated with frontal lobe infarction. J Neurol 1996;243:652–657.

363. Caselli RJ. Visual syndromes as the presenting feature of degenerative brain disease. Semin Neurol 2000;20:139–144.

364. McKhann G, Drachman D, Folstein M, et al. Clinical diagnosis of Alzheimer's disease. Report of the NINCDS-ADRDA Work Group under the auspices of the Department of Health and Human Services Task Force on Alzheimer's disease. Neurology 1984;34:939–944.

365. Dubois B, Feldman HH, Jacova C, et al. Research criteria for the diagnosis of Alzheimer's disease. Revising the NINCDS-ADRDA criteria. Lancet Neurol 2007;6:734–746.

366. Friedland RP. Alzheimer's disease. Clinical features and differential diagnosis. Neurology 1993;43 (Suppl 4):S45–S51.

367. Skoog I, Nilsson L, Palmertz B, et al. A population-based study of dementia in 85-year olds. N Engl J Med 1993;328:153–158.

368. Evans DE, Funkenstein HH, Albert MS, et al. Prevalence of Alzheimer's disease in a community population of older persons. Higher than previously reported. JAMA 1989;262:2551–2556.

369. Desai AK, Grossberg GT. Diagnosis and treatment of Alzheimer's disease. Neurology 2005;64:S34–39.

370. Roses AD. Genetic testing for Alzheimer disease. Arch Neurol 1997;54:1226–1229.

371. Blacker D, Tanzi RE. The genetics of Alzheimer disease. Current status and future prospects. Arch Neurol 1998;55:294–296.

372. Martin JB. Molecular basis of the neurodegenerative disorders. N Engl J Med 1999;340:1970–1980.

373. Cummings JL, Vinters HV, Cole GM, et al. Alzheimer's disease. Etiologies, pathophysiology, cognitive reserve, and treatment opportunities. Neurology 1998;51(Suppl 1):S2–S17.

374. Hodges JR. Alzheimer's centennial legacy: origins, landmarks and the current status of knowledge concerning cognitive aspects. Brain 2006;129:2811–2822.

375. Fleming KC, Adams AC, Petersen RC. Dementia: diagnosis and evaluation. Mayo Clinic Proc 1995;70:1093–1107.

376. Geldmacher DS, Whitehouse PJ. Evaluation of dementia. N Engl J Med 1996;335:330–336.

377. Mendez MF, Tomsak RL, Remler B. Disorders of the visual system in Alzheimer's disease. J Clin Neuroophthalmol 1990;10:62–69.

378. Mendez MF, Mendez MA, Martin R, et al. Complex visual disturbances in Alzheimer's disease. Neurology 1990;40:439–443.

379. Trick GL, Silverman SE. Visual sensitivity to motion. Age-related changes and deficits in senile dementia of the Alzheimer type. Neurology 1991;41:1437–1440.

380. Silverman SE, Tran DB, Zimmerman KM, et al. Dissociation between the detection and perception of motion in Alzheimer's disease. Neurology 1994;44:1814–1818.

381. Fernandez R, Kavcic V, Duffy CJ. Neurophysiologic analyses of low- and high-level visual processing in Alzheimer disease. Neurology 2007;68:2066–2076.

382. Rizzo M, Nawrot M. Perception of movement and shape in Alzheimer's disease. Brain 1998;121:2259–2270.

383. Rizzo M, Anderson SW, Dawson J, et al. Visual attention impairments in Alzheimer's disease. Neurology 2000;54:1954–1959.

384. Trobe JD, Butter CM. A screening test for integrative visual dysfunction in Alzheimer's disease. Arch Ophthalmol 1993;111:815–818.

385. Butter CM, Trobe JD, Foster NL, et al. Visual-spatial deficits explain visual symptoms in Alzheimer's disease. Am J Ophthalmol 1996;122:97–105.

386. Kawas CH, Corrada MM, Brookmeyer R, et al. Visual memory predicts Alzheimer's disease more than a decade before diagnosis. Neurology 2003;60:1089–1093.

387. Daffner KR, Scinto LFM, Weintraub S, et al. Diminished curiosity in patients with probable Alzheimer's disease as measured by exploratory eye movements. Neurology 1992;42:320–328.

388. Sadun AA, Borchert M, De Vita E, et al. Assessment of visual impairment in patients with Alzheimer's disease. Am J Ophthalmol 1987;104:113–120.

389. Lee AG, Martin CO. Neuro-ophthalmic findings in the visual variant of Alzheimer's disease. Ophthalmology 2004;111:376–380.

390. Atchison M, Harrison AR, Lee MS. The woman who needed a pet. Surv Ophthalmol 2006;51:592–595.

391. Oda H, Ohkawa S, Maeda K. Hemispatial visual defect in Alzheimer's disease. Neurocase 2008;14:141–146.

392. Hutton JT, Morris JL, Elias JW, et al. Contrast sensitivity dysfunction in Alzheimer's disease. Neurology 1993;43:2328–2330.

393. Mendola JD, Cronin-Golomb A, Corkin S, et al. Prevalence of visual deficits in Alzheimer's disease. Optom Vis Sci 1995;72:155–167.

394. Cronin-Golomb A. Vision in Alzheimer's disease. Gerontologist 1995;3:370–376.

395. Cronin-Golomb A, Sugiura R, Corkin S, et al. Incomplete achromatopsia in Alzheimer's disease. Neurobiol Aging 1993;14:471–477.

396. Cronin-Golomb A, Corkin S, Rizzo JF, et al. Visual dysfunction in Alzheimer's disease. Relation to normal aging. Ann Neurol 1991;29:41–52.

397. Rizzo JF, Cronin-Golomb A, Growdon JH, et al. Retinocalcarine function in Alzheimer's disease. A clinical and electrophysiologic study. Arch Neurol 1992;49:93–101.

398. Trick GL, Trick LR, Morris P, et al. Visual field loss in senile dementia of the Alzheimer's type. Neurology 1995;45:68–74.

399. Reiman EM, Caselli RJ, Yun LS, et al. Preclinical evidence of Alzheimer's disease in persons homozygous for the Œ4 allele for apolipoprotein E. N Engl J Med 1996;334:752–758.

400. Sandson TA, O'Connor M, Sperling RA, et al. Noninvasive perfusion MRI in Alzheimer's disease. Neurology 1996;47:1339–1342.

401. Bokde AL, Pietrini P, Ibanez V, et al. The effect of brain atrophy on cerebral hypometabolism in the visual variant of Alzheimer disease. Arch Neurol 2001;58:480–486.

402. Galasko D, Chang L, Motter R, et al. High cerebrospinal fluid tau and low amyloid ß42 levels in the clinical diagnosis of Alzheimer disease and relation to apolipoprotein E genotype. Arch Neurol 1998;55:937–945.

403. Andreasen N, Hesse C, Davidsson P, et al. Cerebrospinal fluid beta-amyloid (1–42) in Alzheimer disease. Differences between early-and late-onset Alzheimer disease and stability during the course of the disease. Arch Neurol 1999;56:673–680.

404. Katz B, Rimmer S. Ophthalmologic manifestations of Alzheimer's disease. Surv Ophthalmol 1989;34:31–43.

405. Katz B, Rimmer S, Iragui V, et al. Abnormal pattern electroretinogram in Alzheimer's disease. Evidence for retinal ganglion cell degeneration? Ann Neurol 1989;26:221–225.

406. Trick GL, Barris MC, Bickler-Bluth M. Abnormal pattern electroretinograms in patients with senile dementia of the Alzheimer type. Ann Neurol 1989;26:226–231.

407. Berisha F, Feke GT, Trempe CL, et al. Retinal abnormalities in early Alzheimer's disease. Invest Ophthalmol Vis Sci 2007;48:2285–2289.

408. Danesh-Meyer HV, Birch H, Ku JY, et al. Reduction of optic nerve fibers in patients with Alzheimer disease identified by laser imaging. Neurology 2006;67:1852–1854.

409. Rumble B, Retallack R, Hilbich C, et al. Amyloid A4 protein and its precursor in Down's syndrome and Alzheimer's disease. N Engl J Med 1989;320:1446–1452.

410. Selkoe DJ. Aging, amyloid, and Alzheimer's disease [editorial]. N Engl J Med 1989;320:1484–1487.

411. Yankner BA, Mesulam M-M. ß-amyloid and the pathogenesis of Alzheimer's disease. N Engl J Med 1991;325:1849–1857.

412. Masters CL, Beyreuther K. Alzheimer's disease. BMJ 1998;316:446–448.

413. Mayeux R. Therapeutic strategies in Alzheimer's disease. Neurology 1990;40:175–180.

414. Lewis DA, Campbell MJ, Terry RD, et al. Laminar and regional distributions of neurofibrillary tangles and neuritic plaques in Alzheimer's disease. A quantitative study of visual and auditory cortices. J Neurosci 1987;7:1799–1808.

415. Arnold SE, Hyman BT, Flory J, et al. The topographical and neuroanatomical distribution of neurofibrillary tangles and neuritic plaques in the cerebral cortex of patients with Alzheimer's disease. Cereb Cortex 1991;1:103–116.

416. Giannakopoulos P, Gold G, Duc M, et al. Neuroanatomical correlates of visual agnosia in Alzheimer's disease. A clinicopathological study. Neurology 1999;52:71–77.

417. Galton CJ, Patterson K, Xuereb JH, et al. Atypical and typical presentations of Alzheimer's disease. A clinical, neuropsychological, neuroimaging and pathological study of 13 cases. Brain 2000;123:484–498.

418. Levine DN, Lee JM, Fisher CM. The visual variant of Alzheimer's disease. Neurology 1993;43:305–313.

419. Hof PR, Bouras C, Constantinidis J, et al. Balint's syndrome in Alzheimer's disease. Specific disruption of the occipito-parietal visual pathway. Brain Res 1989;493:368–375.

420. Hof PR, Bouras C, Constantinidis J, et al. Selective disconnection of specific visual association pathways in cases of Alzheimer's disease presenting with Balint's syndrome. J Neuropathol Exp Neurol 1990;49:168–184.

421. Curcio CA, Drucker DN. Retinal ganglion cells in Alzheimer's and aging. Ann Neurol 1993;33:248–257.

422. Borson S, Raskind MA. Clinical features and pharmacologic treatment of behavioral symptoms of Alzheimer's disease. Neurology 1997;48(Suppl 6):S17–S24.

423. Aisen PS, Davis KL. The search for disease-modifying treatment for Alzheimer's disease. Neurology 1997;48(Suppl 6):S35–S41.

424. Farlow MR, Evans RM. Pharmacologic treatment of cognition in Alzheimer's dementia. Neurology 1998;51(Suppl 1):S36–S44.

425. Mayeux R, Sano M. Treatment of Alzheimer's disease. N Engl J Med 1999;341:1670–1679.

426. Cummings JL. Alzheimer's disease. N Engl J Med 2004;351:56–67.

427. Klafki HW, Staufenbiel M, Kornhuber J, et al. Therapeutic approaches to Alzheimer's disease. Brain 2006;129:2840–2855.

428. Birks J. Cholinesterase inhibitors for Alzheimer's disease. Cochrane Database Syst Rev 2006:CD005593.

429. Gautheir S, Bouchard R, Lamontagne A, et al. Tetrahydroaminoacridine-lecithin combination treatment in patients with intermediate-stage Alzheimer's disease. N Engl J Med 1990;322:1272–1276.

430. Sano M, Ernesto C, Thomas RG, et al. A controlled trial of selegiline, alpha-tocopherol, or both as treatment for Alzheimer's disease. N Engl J Med 1997;336:1216–1222.

431. Kelley BJ, Knopman DS. Alternative medicine and Alzheimer disease. Neurologist 2008;14:299–306.

432. Hüll M, Berger M, Heneka M. Disease-modifying therapies in Alzheimer's disease. How far have we come? Drugs 2006;66:2075–2093.

433. Brown P, Gibbs CJ, Rodgers-Johnson P, et al. Human spongiform encephalopathy. The National Institutes of Health series of 300 cases of experimentally transmitted disease. Ann Neurol 1994;35:513–529.

434. Haywood AM. Transmissible spongiform encephalopathies. N Engl J Med 1997;337:1821–1828.

435. Prusiner SB, Hsiao KK. Human prion diseases. Ann Neurol 1994;35:385–395.

436. Prusiner SB. Shattuck lecture–neurodegenerative diseases and prions. N Engl J Med 2001;344:1516–1526.

437. Brown P. Transmissible spongiform encephalopathy in the 21st century: neuroscience for the clinical neurologist. Neurology 2008;70:713–722.

438. Cali I, Castellani R, Yuan J, et al. Classification of sporadic Creutzfeldt–Jakob disease revisited. Brain 2006;129:2266–2277.

439. Brandel J-P, Peoc'h K, Beaudry P, et al. 14-3-3 protein cerebrospinal fluid detection in human grown hormone-treated Creutzfeldt–Jakob disease patients. Ann Neurol 2001;49:257–260.

440. Heckmann JG, Lang CJG, Petruch F, et al. Transmission of Creutzfeldt–Jakob disease via a corneal transplant. J Neurol Neurosurg Psychiatr 1997;63:388–390.

441. Hoshi K, Yoshino H, Urata J, et al. Creutzfeldt–Jakob disease associated with cadaveric dura mater grafts in Japan. Neurology 2000;55:718–721.

442. Brown P, Preece M, Brandel J-P, et al. Iatrogenic Creutzfeldt–Jakob disease at the millennium. Neurology 2000;55:1075–1081.

443. Hannah EL, Belay ED, Gambetti P, et al. Creutzfeldt–Jakob disease after receipt of a previously unimplicated brand of dura mater graft. Neurology 2001;56:1080–1083.

444. Tyler KL. Creutzfeldt–Jakob disease. N Engl J Med 2003;348:681–682.

445. Vargas ME, Kupersmith MJ, Savino PJ, et al. Homonymous field defect as the first manifestation of Creutzfeldt–Jakob disease. Am J Ophthalmol 1995;119:497–504.

446. Jacobs DA, Lesser RL, Mourelatos Z, et al. The Heidenhain variant of Creutzfeldt–Jakob disease. Clinical, pathologic, and neuroimaging findings. J Neuroophthalmol 2001;21:99–102.

447. Nozaki I, Hamaguchi T, Noguchi-Shinohara M, et al. The MM2-cortical form of sporadic Creutzfeldt–Jakob disease presenting with visual disturbance. Neurology 2006;67:531–533.

448. Proulx AA, Strong MJ, Nicolle DA. Creutzfeldt–Jakob disease presenting with visual manifestations. Can J Ophthalmol 2008;43:591–595.

449. Purvin V, Bonnin J, Goodman J. Palinopsia as a presenting manifestation of Creutzfeldt–Jakob disease. J Clin Neuroophthalmol 1989;9:242–246.

450. Neetens A, Martin JJ. Neuro-ophthalmologic aspects of prion diseases. Neuroophthalmology 1998;19:137–144.

451. Lesser RL, Albert DM, Bobowick AR, et al. Creutzfeldt–Jakob disease and optic atrophy. Am J Ophthalmol 1979;87:317–321.

452. Prasad S, Ko MW, Lee EB, et al. Supranuclear vertical gaze abnormalities in sporadic Creutzfeldt–Jakob disease. J Neurol Sci 2007;253:69–72.

453. Grant MP, Cohen M, Peterson RB, et al. Abnormal eye movements in Creutzfeldt–Jakob disease. Ann Neurol 1993;34:192–197.

454. Case Records of the MGH. Case 17-1993. N Engl J Med 1993;328:1259–1266.

455. Kretzschmar HA, Ironside JW, DeArmond SJ, et al. Diagnostic criteria for sporadic Creutzfeldt–Jakob disease. Arch Neurol 1996;53:913–920.

456. Case Records of the MGH. Case 27-2005. N Engl J Med 2005;353:1042–1050.

457. Furlan AJ, Henry CE, Sweeney PJ, et al. Focal EEG abnormalities in Heidenhain's variant of Jakob-Creutzfeldt disease. Arch Neurol 1981;38:312–314.

458. Roth AM, Keltner JL, Ellis WG, et al. Virus-simulating structures in the optic nerve head in Creutzfeldt–Jakob disease. Am J Ophthalmol 1979;87:827–833.

459. de Seze J, Hache JC, Vermersch P, et al. Creutzfeldt–Jakob disease. Neurophysiologic visual impairments. Neurology 1998;51:962–967.

460. Hsich G, Kenney K, Gibbs CJ, et al. The 14-3-3 brain protein in cerebrospinal fluid as a marker for transmissible spongiform encephalopathies. N Engl J Med 1996;335:924–930.

461. Zerr I, Bodemer M, Gefeller O, et al. Detection of 14-3-3 protein in the cerebrospinal fluid supports the diagnosis of Creutzfeldt–Jakob disease. Ann Neurol 1998;43:32–40.

462. Lemstra AW, van Meegen MT, Vreyling JP, et al. 14-3-3 testing in diagnosing Creutzfeldt–Jakob disease. A prospective study in 112 patients. Neurology 2000;55:514–516.

463. Green AJ. Cerebrospinal fluid brain-derived proteins in the diagnosis of Alzheimer's disease and Creutzfeldt–Jakob disease. Neuropathol Appl Neurobiol 2002;28:427–440.

464. Geschwind MD, Martindale J, Miller D, et al. Challenging the clinical utility of the 14-3-3 protein for the diagnosis of sporadic Creutzfeldt–Jakob disease. Arch Neurol 2003;60:813–816.

465. Chapman T, McKeel DW, Jr., Morris JC. Misleading results with the 14-3-3 assay for the diagnosis of Creutzfeldt–Jakob disease. Neurology 2000;55:1396–1397.

466. Bahn MM, Kido DK, Lin W, et al. Brain magnetic resonance diffusion abnormalities in Creutzfeldt–Jakob disease. Arch Neurol 1997;54:1411–1415.

467. Demaerel P, Heiner L, Robberecht W, et al. Diffusion-weighted MRI in sporadic Creutzfeldt–Jakob disease. Neurology 1999;52:205–208.

468. Na DL, Suh CK, Choi SH, et al. Diffusion-weighted magnetic resonance imaging in probable Creutzfeldt–Jakob disease. Arch Neurol 1999;56:951–957.

469. Case Records of the MGH. Case 28-1999. N Engl J Med 1999;341:901–908.

470. Bahn MM, Parchi P. Abnormal diffusion-weighted magnetic resonance images in Creutzfeldt–Jakob disease. Arch Neurol 1999;56:577–583.

471. Mittal S, Farmer P, Kalina P, et al. Correlation of diffusion-weighted magnetic resonance imaging with neuropathology in Creutzfeldt–Jakob disease. Arch Neurol 2002;59:128–134.

472. Rabinstein AA, Whiteman ML, Shebert RT. Abnormal diffusion-weighted magnetic resonance imaging in Creutzfeldt–Jakob disease following corneal transplantations. Arch Neurol 2002;59:637–639.

473. Shiga Y, Miyazawa K, Sato S, et al. Diffusion-weighted MRI abnormalities as an early diagnostic marker for Creutzfeldt–Jakob disease. Neurology 2004;63:443–449.

474. Meissner B, Köhler K, Körtner K, et al. Sporadic Creutzfeldt–Jakob disease. Magnetic resonance imaging and clinical findings. Neurology 2004;63:450–456.

475. Vrancken AFJE, Frijns CJM, Ramos LMP. FLAIR MRI in sporadic Creutzfeldt–Jakob disease. Neurology 2000;55:147–148.

476. Jibiki I, Fukushima T, Kobayashi K, et al. Utility of 123-I-IMP SPECT brain scans for the early detection of site-specific abnormalities in Creutzfeldt–Jakob disease (Heidenhain type). A case study. Neuropsychobiology 1994;1994:29.

477. Steinhoff BJ, Räcker S, Herrendorf G, et al. Accuracy and reliability of periodic sharp wave complexes in Creutzfeldt–Jakob disease. Arch Neurol 1996;53:162–166.

478. Katz BJ, Warner JE, Digre KB, et al. Selective loss of the electroretinogram B-wave in a patient with Creutzfeldt–Jakob disease. J Neuroophthalmol 2000;20:116–118.

479. Zerr I, Pocchiari M, Collins S, et al. Analysis of EEG and CSF 14-3-3 proteins as aids to the diagnosis of Creutzfeldt–Jakob disease. Neurology 2000;55:811–815.

480. Collins SJ, Sanchez-Juan P, Masters CL, et al. Determinants of diagnostic investigation sensitivities across the clinical spectrum of sporadic Creutzfeldt–Jakob disease. Brain 2006;129:2278–2287.

481. Geschwind MD, Josephs KA, Parisi JE, et al. A 54-year-old man with slowness of movement and confusion. Neurology 2007;69:1881–1887.

482. Zeidler M, Green A. Advances in diagnosing Creutzfeldt–Jakob disease with MRI and CSF 14-3-3 protein analysis. Neurology 2004;63:410–411.

483. Brown P, Cathala F, Castaigne P, et al. Creutzfeldt–Jakob disease. Clinical analysis of a consecutive series of 230 neuropathologically verified cases. Ann Neurol 1986;20:597–602.

484. Korth C, Peters PJ. Emerging pharmacotherapies for Creutzfeldt–Jakob disease. Arch Neurol 2006;63:497–501.

485. Stewart LA, Rydzewska LH, Keogh GF, et al. Systematic review of therapeutic interventions in human prion disease. Neurology 2008;70:1272–1281.

CHAPTER **10**

Transient visual loss

Transient loss or blurring of vision lasting for seconds or minutes are common visual complaints. This chapter suggests one approach to patients with these symptoms: to distinguish (1) the more innocent nonischemic ocular conditions from (2) those premonitory events that may be harbingers of potentially catastrophic retinal or cerebral ischemia, (3) migraine, and (4) other unique causes. The diagnosis and treatment of the neuro-ophthalmic causes of transient visual loss will be detailed, with particular emphasis on the presentation and management of carotid disease.

Approach: nonischemic, ischemic, and other causes

The distinction between nonischemic, ischemic, migraine, and other causes of transient visual loss can often be made on historical grounds.[1]

Nonischemic causes

Patients with nonischemic causes of transient visual loss may be recognized by their longstanding, vague, and often innocuous visual complaints. The term *transient visual blurring* is more accurate as these patients generally have only mild visual changes. Most often they are concerned by a reduced quality to their vision with a superimposed, momentary, worsening or change that causes their vision to vary during the course of the day. They often have difficulty determining which eye is having the problem. Patients will typically report problems under one specific set of circumstances such as with reading small print or seeing words on the television or computer screen. They rarely describe a visual field defect. Other neurologic complaints or new headaches are absent.

Ischemic causes

Sudden, transient loss of central or peripheral vision with full or partial recovery would be more consistent with an ischemic cause. Patients tend to be more definitive in their description of the visual loss with regard to the onset of symptoms, the number of episodes, and their duration. When field deficits occur, they may respect the vertical or horizontal meridian ("shade coming down"), and when bilateral may be homonymous, consistent with a vascular cause. Bruno et al.[2] found that patients with altitudinal or lateralized transient monocular visual loss were likely to have identifiable ischemic causes. Pain, headache, scalp tenderness, jaw claudication, accompanying neurologic signs or symptoms, or the presence of cerebrovascular risk factors suggest an ischemic (embolic, thrombotic, or vasculitic) cause of the transient visual loss.

Migraine

Migrainous transient visual loss, suggested by accompanying symptoms of headache, nausea, or vomiting, should also be considered. Previous migraines, a history of affected family members, or accompanying positive phenomena such as scintillations, prisms, or colored lights also support the diagnosis of migrainous visual loss. When numerous, recurrent, unexplained episodes of visual loss occur, particularly in young people, a migrainous cause should also be considered.

Other causes

A history of seizures, loss of consciousness, or abnormal motor activity would suggest ictal or postictal visual loss. The patient with a history of optic neuritis might complain of transient visual loss with a rise in body temperature (Uhthoff's phenomenon). Vision loss with eye movements is consistent with gaze-evoked amaurosis and suggests an underlying orbital mass. Patients with papilledema may have transient visual obscurations that are often elicited by changes in posture, such as standing up, or head position.

Examination of the patient with transient visual loss

In addition to documenting afferent visual function, particular attention should be paid to the slit-lamp examination to search for any tear film or corneal surface abnormalities and to the fundus examination for evidence of retinal emboli, cotton-wool spots, or disc swelling. Focal signs on the neurologic examination should also be excluded. On the general examination, palpation of the temporal arteries and auscultation of the carotid arteries and heart should be performed.

Nonischemic transient vision loss

Many patients who describe variable blurring of their vision have an ocular (nonischemic) cause (**Table 10–1**). While the symptoms may be quite disruptive and difficult to treat, there are almost no critical diagnoses to make except transient elevation of intraocular pressure or corneal edema.

Ocular surface abnormalities

Tear film or corneal abnormalities are probably the most common nonischemic causes of transient visual loss. Patients with tear film abnormalities typically describe a pattern in which visual blurring occurs for hours many times per week, often at the end of the day, and often under one environmental circumstance. For instance, symptoms occur in the afternoon at work, in the evening when sitting down to read, or after a walk on a windy day. Repeat blinking or lubrication of the eyes in this setting will often improve the vision. On slit-lamp biomicroscopy there may be abnormal tear film break up, blepharitis, or corneal and conjunctival fluorescein staining. Patients with blepharitis may have the greatest problem in the morning with increased accumulation of abnormal meibomian gland secretions overnight. Bathing the eyes usually leads to prompt improvement. If dryness or tear film abnormality leads to epithelial breakdown, there may be associated foreign body sensation, pain,

Table 10–1 Nonischemic causes of transient visual loss

Tear film abnormalities
Dry eye
Blepharitis
Corneal epithelial disease
Dry eye
Epithelial irregularity
Corneal endothelial dysfunction
Recurrent corneal erosions
Transient elevation of intraocular pressure
Intermittent angle closure
Uveitis
Fluctuating blood sugar
Anterior chamber abnormalities
Uveitis
Hyphema
Vitreous floaters
Afterimages
Optic disc anomalies (transient visual obscurations)
Optic nerve head drusen (transient visual obscurations)

or redness. Those with dry eyes will frequently have an abnormal Schirmer's test (see Chapter 2).

In addition, patients with corneal endothelial dysfunction can develop blurred vision from corneal epithelial and stromal edema. These episodes often last for hours and occur most commonly in the morning. The diagnosis can be made by examining patients during symptomatic periods.

Other ocular causes

Subacute transient attacks of narrow-angle glaucoma may cause episodes of transient visual blurring accompanied by halos.[3] During asymptomatic periods intraocular pressure may be normal, but slit-lamp examination and gonioscopy will reveal shallow or occluded anterior chamber angles. Recurrent spontaneous anterior chamber hemorrhages (hyphema) may also cause episodic visual blurring.[4] Such recurrent hemorrhages can occur in patients with juvenile xanthogranuloma, those with a malpositioned intraocular lens with iris contact, and patients with iris neovascularization.

Osmotic changes in the lens can occur with widely fluctuating blood glucose levels, such as in patients with diabetes or those taking corticosteroids. This blurring is associated with a change in refractive error, for instance an increase in myopia with hyperglycemia, without visible lens alterations. Pinholes usually improve the visual acuities in these cases. Vitreous abnormalities, particularly acute posterior vitreous detachments and opacities associated with uveitis, can also cause transient visual blurring. Posterior opacities can move or float over the macula and alter visual acuity, but some patients report a more fixed opacity that blurs vision.

Table 10–2 Ischemic causes of transient vision loss

Carotid embolic disease
Cardiac embolic disease
Valvular disease
Mural thrombus (atrial fibrillation)
Atrial myxoma
Aortic arch embolic disease
Vasospasm
Migraine (?)
Temporal arteritis
Vertebrobasilar insufficiency
Hematologic abnormalities
Hypercoaguable state
Polycythemia

Ischemic transient visual loss

In these instances vision is lost due to temporary interruption of the blood supply of the retina, optic nerve, or retrochiasmal visual pathways (**Table 10-2**). In patients with transient monocular blindness (amaurosis fugax or "fleeting blindness"), carotid disease, cardiac emboli, and giant cell arteritis should be considered and distinguished from migraine or vasospasm. Bilateral visual loss may be due to involvement of both eyes, but hemianopic visual loss due to middle cerebral artery or vertebrobasilar ischemia should also be excluded. Since many of these patients are at risk for permanent visual loss or stroke, they must be identified and treated expeditiously.

Vascular anatomy. The aortic arch gives rise to the great vessels supplying the head and neck. The first branch of the aorta is the innominate (brachiocephalic) artery, which divides to form the right subclavian and right common carotid arteries. The next branch off the aorta is the left common carotid artery. Each carotid artery enters the neck, eventually traveling through the temporal bone to enter the cavernous sinus (**Fig. 10–1**). The sympathetic pathway finds its way to the eye by following the carotid and its branches (see Chapter 13). Upon exiting the cavernous sinus, the carotid gives off its first major branch, the ophthalmic artery. In 10% of patients, the ophthalmic artery originates from the cavernous carotid. The ophthalmic artery provides the blood supply to the optic nerve, retina, and other structures of the eye. The muscular branches supply the extraocular muscles. The central retinal artery enters the substance of the optic nerve to supply the most anterior portion of the optic nerve head and retina (see **Fig. 4–1**). Most of the optic nerve head derives its supply from two or more long posterior ciliary arteries. The optic nerve head represents a potential watershed area between these posterior ciliary arteries (see Chapter 5 for more details).

The blood supplies of the optic radiations and occipital cortex are reviewed in detail in Chapter 8.

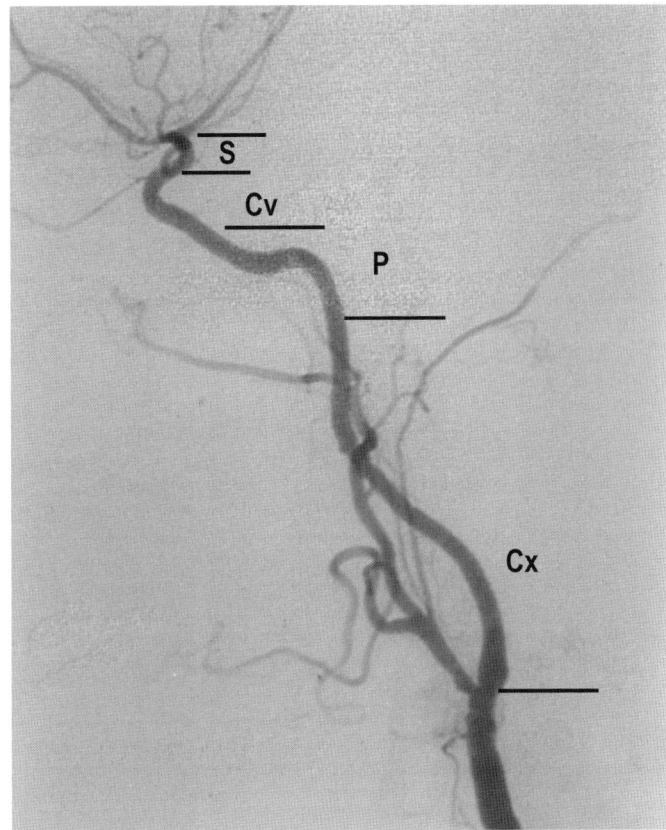

Figure 10–1. Angiogram of a normal carotid artery. S, supraclinoid; Cv, cavernous; P, petrous; and Cx, cervical portions. (From Bennett J, Volpe NJ, Liu GT, Galetta SL. Neurovascular neuro-ophthalmology. In Albert D, Jakobiec FA (eds): Principles of Ophthalmology, pp 4238–4274. Philadelphia, WB Saunders, 2000, with permission.)

Carotid disease

Extracranial internal carotid artery stenosis or occlusion is the most common cause of the ischemic form of transient visual loss.[5,6] In this setting, transient visual loss is more often labeled as transient monocular blindness, amaurosis fugax, or a retinal transient ischemic attack (TIA).[7] The origin of the internal carotid artery at the bifurcation may be narrowed by atherosclerotic plaque formation (**Fig. 10–2**) and related mural thrombi, plaque ulceration, and intraplaque hemorrhage.[8,9] Nonatherosclerotic causes of carotid disease include carotid dissection (see Chapter 13), fibromuscular dysplasia, Takayasu's arteritis, carotid trauma, and radiation arteritis.[10]

Carotid-related amaurosis fugax most frequently results from emboli from the diseased proximal internal carotid artery segment to the retinal artery circulation.[11] Another mechanism for monocular visual loss due to occlusive carotid disease is low flow,[12] particularly when collateral circulation to the eye from the circle of Willis and external carotid artery circulation are also compromised. In these cases symptoms may be induced when carotid blood flow is decreased because of changes in posture or eating,[13] or when distal blood flow is insufficient, as in chronic ocular ischemia or bright-light amaurosis (see below).

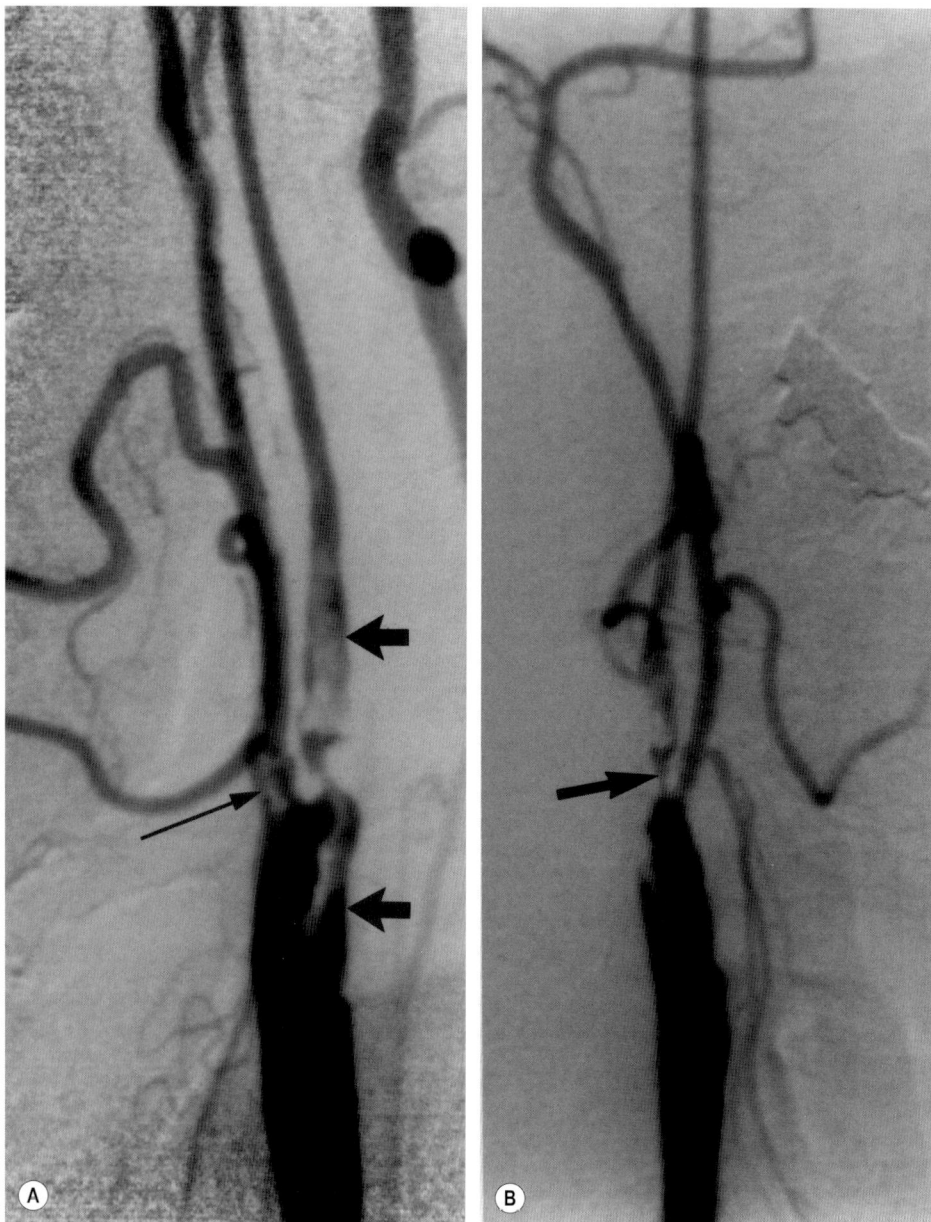

Figure 10–2. Right common carotid artery angiogram in a patient with amaurosis fugax and carotid artery stenosis. **A**. Magnified view of the right common carotid artery injection demonstrating filling defects within the common carotid (lower arrow), internal carotid (upper arrow), and external carotid arteries (thin arrow). These filling defects represent extensive clots within the carotid circulation. **B**. Oblique view showing the high-grade stenosis of the internal carotid artery (arrow) with the filling defect from the clot above. The small caliber of the cervical portion of the right internal carotid artery extending superiorly should be noted. (From Balcer LJ, Galetta SL, Yousem DM, et al. Pupil-involving third nerve palsy and carotid stenosis: rapid recovery following endarterectomy. Ann Neurol 1997;41:273–276, with permission.)

The risk of stroke from carotid-related amaurosis fugax is lower than that associated with hemispheric TIAs. The risk of stroke from amaurosis fugax per annum had been previously estimated to be 2%, with a 1% risk of permanent visual loss.[14] This compares with the 5–8% yearly risk of stroke associated with cerebral TIAs.[15] More recent prospective data confirmed that the risk in retinal TIAs was approximately half.[16] It is unclear why transient monocular visual loss has less of a stroke risk than those with hemispheric TIAs.[17] Possible explanations include that (1) local ophthalmic disease (nonischemic disease) rather than carotid disease might have been the cause of some cases of transient vision loss[18] and (2) mechanisms of transient visual loss other than

arteriosclerotic disease such as vasospasm, (3) smaller emboli, and (4) the retina may be more vulnerable to reduced flow (highly energy dependent), making more patients likely to be symptomatic and presenting before a hemispheric event occurs.[19]

Symptoms. The characteristics of this type of vision loss are summarized in **Table 10–3**. Its onset is usually sudden and is often described as a shade or curtain that obscures vision in one eye. Visual loss may be altitudinal, peripheral, central, or even vertical.[15] A nasal visual field defect may suggest an embolic mechanism because of the tendency of these particles to lodge in the temporal retinal circulation.[20] Most episodes last 5 minutes or less. Rarely, scintillating

Table 10–3 Typical features of embolic transient monocular blindness

Abrupt onset
Painless
Typically lasts 1–5 minutes
Darkening or fogging (not blurring) of visual field
Altitudinal pattern (shade closing) of vision loss
Vision returns gradually over minutes

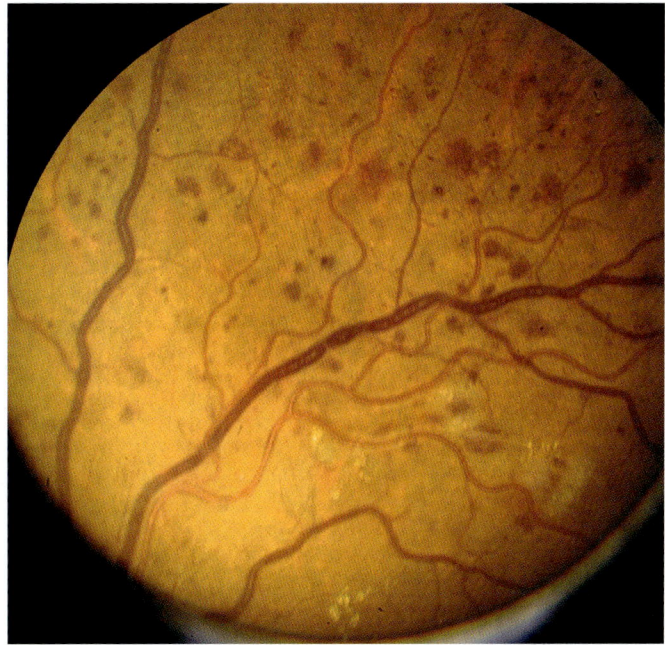

Figure 10–3. Midperipheral venous stasis retinopathy in a patient with ocular ischemic syndrome due to ipsilateral 95% carotid artery stenosis (courtesy of Dr. Albert Maguire).

scotomas or tiny bright lights may be experienced.[21] Pain is uncommon and its presence should raise the possibility of temporal arteritis (see below).

Rarely, patients may complain of transient monocular blindness after exposure to sunlight or even after viewing a white wall.[22] This phenomenon of bright-light-induced amaurosis fugax in patients with carotid occlusive disease is well documented.[23,24] Presumably, impaired blood flow to the outer retinal segment compromises the regeneration of retinal pigments required for visual perception. In one study,[25] the visual evoked response was attenuated when the patients were exposed to a light source for 30 seconds or more.

In patients with carotid stenosis, ipsilateral eye symptoms may be accompanied by those of ipsilateral cerebral ischemia. These include contralateral hemiparesis, sensory loss, or even hemianopia. Ischemia of the dominant hemisphere may cause language deficits.

Other history. A screening history for other evidence of arteriosclerotic vascular disease, hypertension, smoking, diabetes, and cardiac arrhythmias should be obtained. In addition, symptoms suggestive of temporal (giant cell) arteritis (see below) should be excluded.

Neuro-ophthalmic signs. Retinal emboli are the most common associated finding, and there are two main types seen in carotid disease: (1) cholesterol (Hollenhorst plaques), which have a refractile, metallic gold appearance and are typically a sign of carotid disease;[26] and (2) platelet–fibrin emboli, which are creamy white/gray longitudinal intravascular opacifications that fill the entire lumen.[20,26] Platelet–fibrin emboli are likely a result of either carotid thrombosis or thrombosis associated with recent myocardial infarction. Retinal emboli and their clinical characteristics and implications are discussed in more detail in Chapter 4.

Severe carotid disease may produce hypoperfusion of the globe and *chronic ocular ischemia*. This is associated with a variety of signs involving the anterior and posterior segments of the eye. Anterior ischemia may lead to episcleral and conjunctival injection. Corneal edema may obscure vision, and while cells and flare in the anterior chamber may be mistaken for an inflammatory process. If new iris vessels form, neovascular glaucoma may ensue. In the retina, a venous stasis retinopathy characterized by microaneurysms and midperipheral dot and blot hemorrhages may be evident (**Fig. 10–3**). The retinal abnormalities are similar to those seen in diabetic retinopathy and retinal vein occlusion, except they are located in the midperiphery instead of the posterior pole and they tend to be unilateral, corresponding to the side of the more obstructed carotid.[27] Optic nerve head swelling is typically not seen until the very late stages of posterior segment ischemia. When vision is severely affected, the visual prognosis is poor.[28]

Rarely, signs of *orbital ischemia* may follow severe carotid disease, with proptosis, chemosis, conjunctival injection, ophthalmoparesis, and retinal ischemia heralding its onset.[29,30] Orbital ischemia and infarction are uncommon because of the rich anastomoses between the ophthalmic and external carotid arteries.

Other neuro-ophthalmic findings associated with carotid disease include retinal artery occlusions (see Chapter 4) and Horner syndrome (see Chapter 13). Ocular motor palsies have been reported following carotid occlusion and dissection.[29,31,32] Presumably, ischemia of the extraocular muscles or nerves is responsible for the ophthalmoparesis, which may be transient, usually resolving within days to weeks. These motility disturbances do not occur in isolation as patients typically have severe unilateral visual loss and hemispheric signs of variable degree. Although anterior ischemic optic neuropathy (AION) has also been described in association with carotid disease,[33,34] a causative relationship is unlikely because AION is more likely the result of small vessel posterior ciliary artery occlusion rather than artery-to-artery emboli or a low-flow state resulting from large vessel occlusive disease.

General examination. The presence or absence of a carotid bruit is generally not helpful for diagnosing significant carotid stenosis or predicting a carotid source of emboli. The incidence of carotid bruits increases with age. They may be predictive of future cardiac and cerebrovascular events,[35,36] especially when further evaluation reveals an underlying carotid stenosis.[37] However, the accuracy of this physical finding is low, and therefore the presence of a bruit cannot be used to diagnose carotid stenosis. Furthermore, in one study[38] over one-third of patients with high-grade carotid stenosis did not have a bruit. Thus the absence of a bruit cannot be used to exclude operable carotid artery disease.[39,40]

Diagnostic tests. The laboratory evaluation of the patient with suspected ischemic monocular visual loss begins with noninvasive assessment of the carotid using either ultrasound or magnetic resonance imaging–angiography (MRA). Carotid ultrasound and Doppler (**Fig. 10–4**) are effective screening tools for identification and estimation of the degree of internal carotid artery stenosis.[41] When athero-sclerotic plaques are present, B-mode ultrasound can often provide morphologic details.[42] Doppler waveforms allow analysis of blood flow velocity.[43] Because of technical limitations, one major drawback is the technique's relative

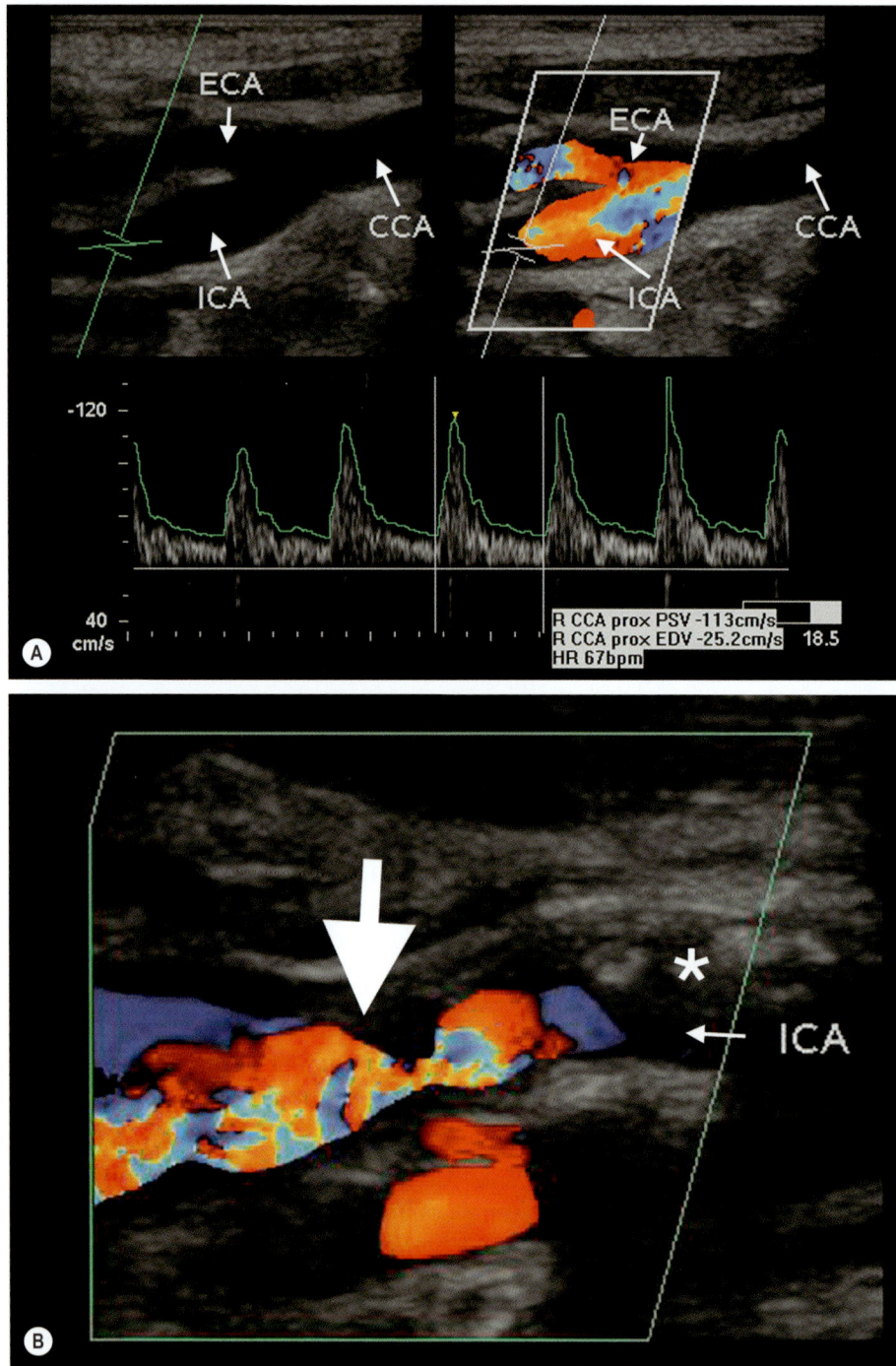

Figure 10–4. Carotid ultrasound and Doppler in the evaluation of carotid disease. **A**. Normal carotid ultrasound (upper left), and corresponding color Doppler (upper right) and Doppler velocity waveforms (bottom). **B**. Ultrasound and color Doppler demonstrating internal carotid narrowing due to plaque (asterisk) and turbulent flow (large arrow) distal to the stenosis. CCA, common carotid artery; ECA, external carotid artery; and ICA, internal carotid artery (courtesy of Maria Stierheim, RVT).

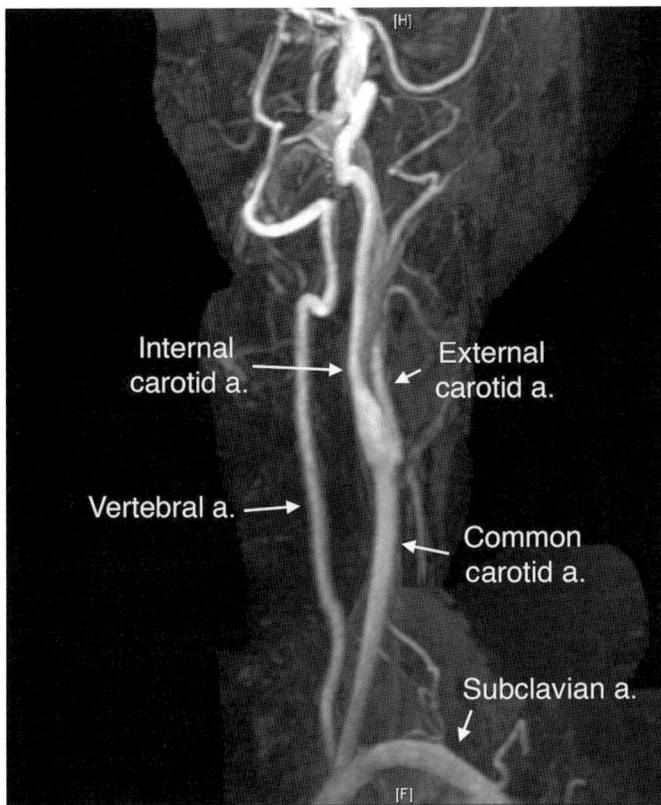

Figure 10–5. Normal contrast-enhanced magnetic resonance imaging–angiogram of the neck, demonstrating the right carotid artery, in a patient with monocular transient visual loss.

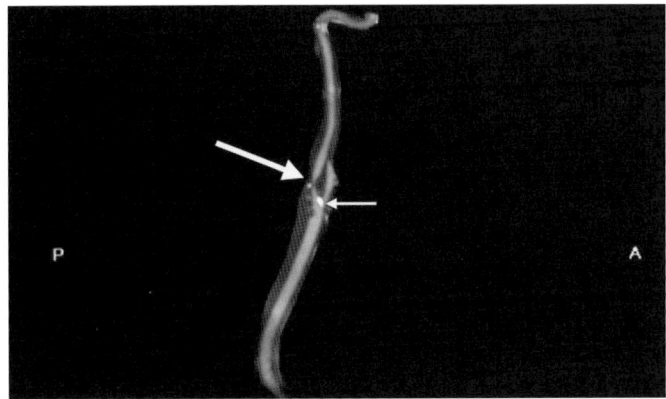

Figure 10–6. Computed tomography–angiogram of the neck, contrast enhanced, demonstrating an approximately 60% narrowing of the right internal carotid artery (large arrow). Hyperdense calcium is seen (small arrow).

inability to differentiate between 99% stenosis and total occlusion.[44]

Magnetic resonance imaging-angiography, either time of flight or contrast-enhanced methods,[45] is another effective noninvasive test available to detect carotid disease. Results are generally reported within a range: mild (0–30% occluded), moderate (30–70% occluded), and severe (70–99% occluded). Sometimes the occlusion is complete, and the source is presumed to be a stump embolus. MRA in particular is best at identifying ulcerative areas with stenotic plaques. Unlike carotid ultrasound, MRA also provides a view of the intracranial circulation. Its major limitation is that it tends to overestimate stenoses.[46] However, a normal MRA (**Fig. 10–5**) is very helpful because it makes any clinically important carotid disease very unlikely. Computed tomographic angiography (CTA) (**Fig. 10–6**) is a suitable alternative screening test and it may be used to confirm the MRA or carotid ultrasound findings.[47,48]

Conventional angiography still remains the most accurate method for the evaluation and quantification of carotid stenoses (**Fig. 10–2**).[45,49–51] The specificity and sensitivity of angiography exceed those of any noninvasive test. Disadvantages of angiography include potential allergy to intravenous contrast and risk of stroke and renal failure. In one study,[52] the angiographic stroke rate was 1.2%. Many surgeons prefer formal angiography prior to endarterectomy, although some may operate on stenotic arteries when the ultrasound, CTA, or MRA examinations are in agreement.

Other useful studies in the evaluation of retinal ischemia include a complete blood count and cholesterol, triglyceride, and serum glucose levels. A careful historical review and erythrocyte sedimentation rate should always be obtained in an elderly patient with amaurosis, which may be the initial manifestation of giant cell arteritis (see below). A cardiac source embolus should be excluded (see below). In select patients, neuroimaging of the brain and transcranial Doppler studies may be obtained.

In many elderly patients the workup outlined above will be unrevealing. In this setting atheroma may be arising from the more proximal vessels such as the aorta, or acephalgic migraine should be considered. In younger patients vasospasm and hypercoagulable states, due to abnormal antiphospholipid antibodies, protein C, protein S, and antithrombin III levels, need to be excluded.

Treatment (medical). If not contraindicated, antiplatelet therapy with aspirin (81 or 325 mg) should be begun in all patients with amaurosis fugax to reduce the risk of stroke. If episodes continue to occur, then larger doses of aspirin (doses may vary between 40 and 1300 mg), clopidogrel (75 mg p.o. q.d.), aspirin and extended release dipyridamole, and warfarin can be considered as alternatives in patients without surgical carotid disease (see below).[53] If crescendo TIAs are present or suspected, then heparinization and an inpatient workup and treatment should be considered.[53] Medical treatment or stenting (see below) are alternatives in patients with moderate to high-grade stenosis in which medical problems prohibit endarterectomy.

Treatment (surgical). Together the North American Symptomatic Carotid Endarterectomy Trial (NASCET),[54,55] the European Carotid Surgery Trial,[56] and the Veterans Administration Cooperative Symptomatic Carotid Stenosis Trial[57] established a benefit for carotid surgery, during which occlusive lesions are removed, for stenoses greater than 70% in individuals suffering a retinal or hemisphere TIA. The procedure should also be considered in selected symptomatic men with 50–70% stenosis, particularly those without underlying medical complications and with a life expectancy greater than 5 years.[55] Patients with both symptomatic extracranial and mild to moderate intracranial internal carotid artery stenoses may still benefit from endarterectomy.[58,59] Technical details of the procedure are discussed elsewhere.[60] Aspirin (81 or 325 mg) should be given before and after carotid endarterectomy to reduce the risk of stroke, myocardial infarction, and death.[61]

Compared with carotid endarterectomy in patients with hemispheric TIAs, the procedure may be more beneficial in those with amaurosis fugax who are 75 years or older and male, and have a history of hemispheric TIA or stroke, a history of intermittent claudication, carotid stenosis of 80–94%, and no collateral circulation.[16] In patients in other categories, for instance a 60-year-old woman with transient monocular blindness and 65% ipsilateral internal carotid stenosis, medical therapy is probably best.[19,62]

The perioperative complication rate for major stroke and death was 2.1% in the NASCET study, emphasizing the importance of the skills of the angiographer, anesthetist, and vascular or neurosurgeon in patients requiring carotid endarterectomy.[63] The low complication rate in the NASCET study likely reflects the exclusion of patients greater than 80 years of age and those with significant intracranial disease, cardiac emboli, and life-threatening disease.[64] In addition to stroke[65] and TIA, other recognized complications of carotid endarterectomy include seizures,[66] intracerebral hemorrhage,[67] and cerebral edema[68] from hyperperfusion,[69] hypertension,[70] and lower cranial nerve palsies.[71]

In contrast, the surgical management of *asymptomatic* carotid stenosis is extremely controversial.[72–76] Previous studies[77,78] had produced conflicting results, but in two more definitive studies[52,79] endarterectomy was shown to benefit patients with asymptomatic carotid stenosis of greater than 60% and 70%, respectively. A meta-analysis suggested that endarterectomy in patients with asymptomatic stenosis reduced the incidence of ipsilateral stroke, but the absolute benefit was small.[80] Individuals with asymptomatic retinal emboli or carotid bruits detected on a routine examination, or vascular disease elsewhere (cardiac or peripheral vascular disease), should probably undergo noninvasive examination of the carotids. Endarterectomy may be considered in those with greater than 60% stenosis, taking into account the age and general health of the patient (at least a 5-year life expectancy) as well as the operative statistics of the surgeon (the complication rate should be less than 3%).[61]

Also controversial, percutaneous transluminal angioplasty and stenting of the internal carotid artery are currently being considered as possible alternatives to carotid endarterectomy to prevent stroke.[81–83] Neither requires general anesthesia or a surgical incision; therefore, these procedures may be ideal for patients with coexisting coronary disease, who may be poor surgical candidates. On the other hand, angioplasty is associated with the theoretical possibilities of dislodging a thrombus, which can embolize to the cerebral circulation, or causing a carotid dissection. Restenosis may also occur. The results of large studies of patients treated for symptomatic carotid disease with stenting and use of an emboli-protection device compared with endarterectomy have been inconsistent,[84] with some[85,86] demonstrating similar efficacy and others[87] showing surgery to be superior.

In eyes with ocular ischemia, the intraocular pressure should be lowered if high. Carotid endarterectomy can be performed in surgical candidates with high-grade stenosis.[88] Extracranial–intracranial arterial bypass, external carotid endarterectomy, angioplasty, and stenting have been occasionally performed with anecdotal success.[89] Panretinal photocoagulation to prevent iris neovascularization is controversial,[28] but most authors favor it. Occasionally the signs of ocular ischemia will spontaneously regress without specific therapy.

Cardiac emboli

Less commonly, cardiac emboli, due to atrial fibrillation,[90,91] valvular disease, atrial myxomas,[92] and mitral valve prolapse,[93] for instance, can reach the retinal circulation. Retinal *calcific emboli* are usually seen in patients with cardiac valvular disease. These emboli are gray-white and ovoid in appearance and usually lodge near the optic nerve head (see Chapter 4). They usually result in retinal infarction. Less commonly they arise from a carotid source.

A careful cardiac examination should be directed at detection of an irregular pulse suggestive of atrial fibrillation or a murmur consistent with significant cardiac valvular disease. Cardiac evaluation, including electrocardiography, 24-hour cardiac monitoring, and transthoracic echocardiography (TTE), is also suggested. If the TTE is unrevealing but a cardiac source embolus is still highly suspected, transesophageal echocardiography (TEE) may be useful in certain patients with unexplained ocular ischemia.[94] TEE has particular advantages over conventional echocardiography in viewing the left atrial appendage, the aorta, and the interatrial septum and in detecting a patent foramen ovale.

Nonmigrainous retinal vasospasm

Vasospastic vision loss may also occur outside of the context of migraine. These patients will have no associated pain or headache, and they may complain of several episodes of monocular visual loss per day. Rarely during an event, temporary narrowing of the retinal vessels may be witnessed.[95,96] The diagnosis is one of exclusion with negative cardiac and carotid evaluations. However, retinal vasospasm may occur with increased frequency in patients with connective tissue disorders such as systemic lupus erythematosus. If a vasospastic cause of the vision loss is suspected, symptoms may be improved with calcium channel blockers.[97,98] We prefer using verapamil 120–360 mg per day, but amlodipine or propranolol are alternative medications that may be effective in this situation. If necessary, aspirin may also be added to the regimen.

Retinal vasospasm and transient monocular visual loss have also been reported in association with exercise[99] and cocaine abuse.[100]

Amaurosis fugax in adolescents and young adults

In patients under age 45, the ischemic ocular causes of transient blurring are relatively uncommon. Most of these patients have migraine, and almost none of them will go on to develop significant visual or neurologic deficits.[101] That being said, important diagnoses to exclude in young patients with transient monocular blindness include atrial septal defect, cardiac valvular disease, carotid dissection, hypercoagulable states,[102] and connective tissue disorders such as fibromuscular dysplasia.[103]

Giant cell arteritis

In patients over the age of 55 with transient monocular or binocular vision loss, the diagnosis of giant cell (temporal) arteritis must be considered. Many patients with temporal arteritis who develop infarction of the optic nerve and blindness report multiple episodes of blurring or darkening of their vision prior to the permanent event.[104,105] In fact, repeated episodes of amaurosis make embolic causes less likely and temporal arteritis more likely. Transient visual loss may be positional in the setting of tenuous blood flow[106] or as a result of viewing bright light (bright-light amaurosis, see above).[107] A careful historical review with attention to headaches, scalp tenderness, jaw claudication, fever, weight loss, and polymyalgia symptoms must be performed. In patients with giant cell arteritis and amaurosis fugax, the fundus is usually normal but on occasion a cotton-wool spot (nerve fiber infarct) may be seen.[108] Fluorescein angiography may demonstrate abnormal choroidal perfusion in some cases.

Further details regarding the pathology, diagnosis, and management of giant cell arteritis are discussed in Chapter 5.

Cortical transient ischemic attacks

In the traditional time-based definition, TIAs last anywhere from minutes to hours, but less than a day—any neurologic deficit of a vascular nature that persists for more than 24 hours is considered a stroke. However, several experts have proposed that TIAs should be redefined using tissue-based guidelines.[109] They suggest that symptoms related to focal brain or retinal ischemia are "brief," typically less than 1 hour, without evidence of acute infarction on neuroimaging. Thus, even if a symptom lasts 2 hours, if an infarct is seen on MRI, then a stroke should diagnosed.

TIAs characterized by isolated homonymous hemianopias are uncommon and most cases of transient hemianopic vision loss are migrainous. Most are accompanied by evidence of ischemia to neighboring structures in the same vascular distribution.

In addition to cardiogenic emboli and hypercoagulable states, other causes are discussed below by location.

Anterior circulation. Other responsible causes in this distribution include extracranial or intracranial (cavernous) internal carotid artery stenosis and middle cerebral artery atheromatous disease. Ischemia in this distribution typically also leads to motor, sensory, or language disturbances.

Posterior circulation. Vertebrobasilar insufficiency, due to vertebral or basilar artery stenosis, for example, can be associated with transient visual loss that is fleeting and bilateral. In this setting there is reduced perfusion to the occipital lobes resulting in momentary altered vision. These TIAs are often associated with other symptoms of posterior circulation blood flow insufficiency such as ataxia, vertigo, slurred

speech, and double vision. However, in some instances the visual loss may be isolated.

In one large meta-analysis,[110] the pooled short-term risk of stroke was 3.5%, 8.0%, and 9.2% at 2, 30, and 90 days, respectively, after a TIA. Thus, following exclusion of carotid or vertebrobasilar disease or cardiac source emboli, as well as a hypercoagulable state, patients with cortical TIAs usually receive anticoagulation using aspirin or another antiplatelet agent to reduce the risk of a subsequent stroke.[53,111]

Migraine

Transient visual loss in migraine is exceedingly common and takes many different forms. The three most frequently encountered are scintillating scotomas, hemianopias, and monocular visual loss. Purely negative phenomena, while they can occur in the aura of migraine, are usually accompanied by positive phenomena (**Table 10–4**). The exact cause of transient visual loss associated with migraine is not known exactly, but likely mechanisms include spreading depression (nonischemic; see Chapter 18) and vasospasm (ischemic). The reader is referred to Chapter 19 for a detailed discussion of the pathophysiology, diagnosis, and treatment of migraine.

In migraine with aura (classic migraine), a typical migraine headache with hemicranial throbbing, nausea, and photophobia follows the visual disturbance. Older patients, many with a history of migraine as a younger adult, can develop migrainous visual auras without headache (acephalgic migraine). Often these events are difficult to distinguish from the ischemic embolic events described above. When positive visual phenomena and gradual build up of aura symptoms over 15–30 minutes occurs, migraine is more readily differentiated from an occipital lobe TIA.

Scotomas. The best example of combined negative and positive visual phenomena in migraine is an enlarging scintillating scotoma (see **Fig. 12–1**). An area of blurry, wavy, or absent vision surrounded by teichopsia is characteristic. Scintillating scotomas and positive visual phenomena associated with migraine are described in detail in Chapter 12.

Hemianopias. Other migraine patients may develop a true hemianopia in the aura phase without positive visual phenomena. Fortunately, transient isolated hemianopias,

Table 10–4 Typical features of migraine-related transient vision loss

Gradual onset and duration of up to 1 hour
Positive visual phenomena
Photopsias
Scintillating scotoma
Often followed by headache but may be acephalgic
Associated photophobia and nausea
Previous history of migraine
May have recognized "trigger" such as stress or hunger

Table 10–5 Other causes of transient visual loss

Type of vision loss	Symptom	Most common setting	Alternative settings
Transient visual obscuration	Fleeting graying of vision associated with postural change	Papilledema	Other elevated optic disc anomalies
Uhthoff's symptom	Loss of vision associated with increased body temperature	Optic neuritis (active or recovered)	Other optic neuropathies
Gaze-evoked amaurosis	Loss of vision associated with eye movement in one direction	Orbital intraconal mass	Other orbital lesions

particularly in young patients, are more commonly the result of migraine and less frequently the result of a hemispheric embolic TIA. In the migraine setting they often build up over several minutes then resolve over 15–30 minutes. Many patients with migrainous transient hemianopia will recognize the disturbance in only one eye, typically the one with the temporal visual field defect, making their condition sometimes difficult to discern from transient monocular visual loss.

Retinal migraine. The last important migraine variant of transient visual loss, retinal migraine, is the least common but the most difficult to distinguish from amaurosis fugax. The typical symptom is a scotoma or complete loss of vision in one eye for seconds or minutes.[112,113] Patients generally do not describe a shade coming down over their vision as occurs with emboli. Since the symptoms of retinal migraine may be difficult to distinguish from embolic amaurosis fugax, it remains a diagnosis of exclusion. One feature of retinal migraine is its propensity to occur repetitively in a stereotyped fashion over years without residual vision loss. Such a pattern without visual or neurologic sequelae would be very atypical for embolic transient monocular blindness. The diagnosis of retinal migraine is best made in an individual with repeated episodes of monocular visual loss associated with headache, an otherwise typical history of migraine (headaches with nausea, vomiting, photophobia, and phonophobia), and a normal examination.[114]

Experts disagree whether retinal migraine is a rare or common cause of transient monocular visual loss, and whether the mechanism is spreading depression or vasospasm. In their literature review, Hill et al.[115] concluded the condition was "exceedingly rare," an opinion shared by others,[116–118] and questioned whether spreading depression could occur in the retina. On the other hand, Grosberg et al.[119,120] suggested that retinal migraine may be underdiagnosed and that many such patients may have permanent visual loss from retinovascular or optic nerve injury.

Our clinical experience suggests that (1) retinal migraine is a relatively common phenomenon, as we frequently see patients in whom that diagnosis is the most logical, and (2) permanent visual loss is an extraordinarily uncommon sequela of retinal migraine. While spreading depression might not occur in the retina, migraine-related retinal vasospasm may account for some of the episodes of visual loss. Ophthalmoscopy may reveal the constricted retinal vessels, although usually it is very difficult to make such an observation. One such example is given in Chapter 19, where retinal migraine is also discussed.

Treatment. Migraine therapies are discussed in detail in Chapter 19.

Other causes of transient visual loss

Table 10–5 summarizes other causes of transient vision loss that may be confused with vascular amaurosis fugax. This last section will discuss these and other causes of transient visual loss.

Transient visual obscurations

Papilledema may be associated with episodes of gray, black, or white vision lasting for seconds (Fig. 10–7). The hallmark of this type of transient visual loss is its fleeting nature and its association with changes in posture, such as sitting up, or head position, by turning side to side, for instance. These transient visual obscurations also occur in patients with pseudopapilledema due to optic nerve head drusen or colobomas, for instance.[121] The mechanism in papilledema and pseudopapilledema is likely transient ischemia or axonal compression at the elevated, crowded optic nerve head. Transient visual obscurations are also discussed in Chapter 6.

Uhthoff's phenomenon

Patients with optic neuropathy, resolved or otherwise, may complain of transient visual loss in the affected eye when body temperature is elevated. Symptoms improve when the body temperature normalizes, and there are no permanent visual sequelae. This phenomenon is most common following optic neuritis, and is discussed in more detail in Chapter 5.

Gaze-evoked amaurosis

Eye movements may cause temporary visual loss due to intraorbital optic nerve or ophthalmic artery compression. Responsible lesions include optic nerve sheath meningiomas, optic gliomas, papilledema,[122] orbital fractures,[123] and intraconal masses such as cavernous hemangiomas[124] and foreign bodies.[123,125] Either horizontal or vertical eye movements may induce visual loss,[126] depending on the location of the culprit lesion. Vision typically decreases seconds after eccentric gaze and returns to normal seconds after returning to straight-ahead gaze.[127] One report[128] described reading-induced visual dimming. Either transient axonal or vascular compression have been suggested as possible mechanisms,[127]

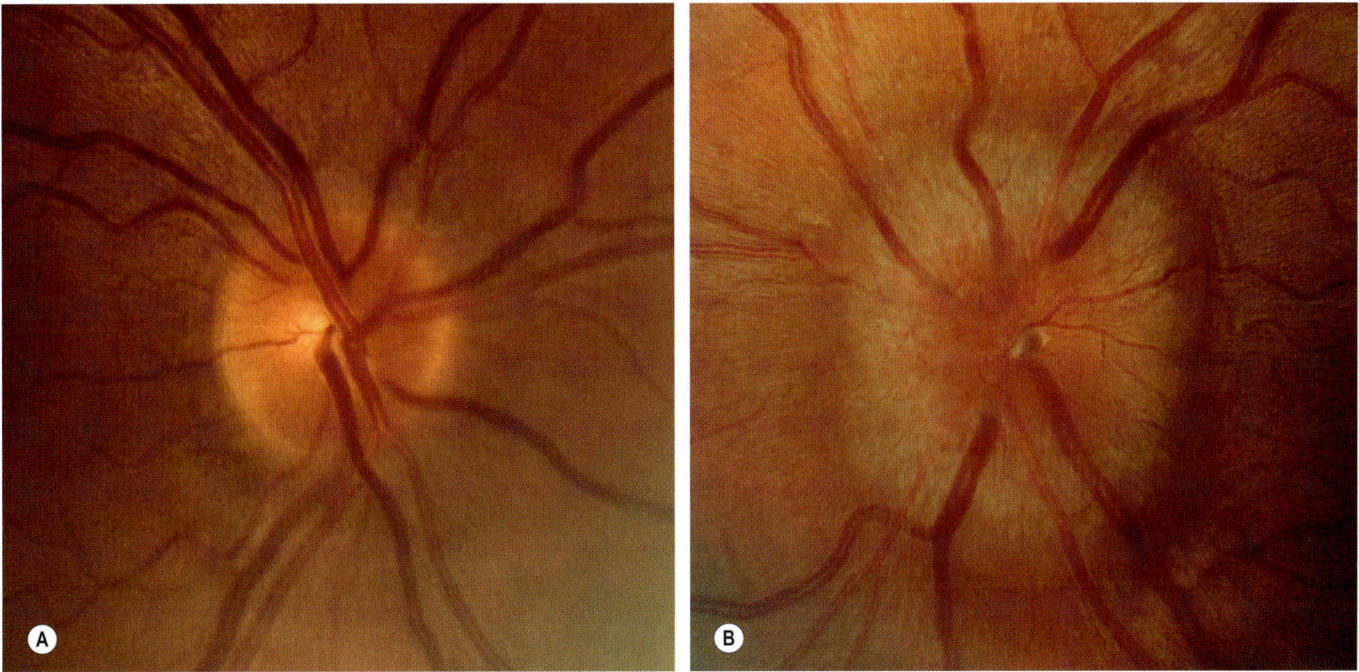

Figure 10–7. Monocular transient visual obscurations due to highly asymmetric papilledema. Fundus photographs of the (**A**) hyperemic right disc and (**B**) edematous left disc in a woman with unilateral papilledema due to pseudotumor cerebri. She complained of multiple episodes of dark-gray vision in her left eye lasting seconds, precipitated by getting up to go to the bathroom or changes in head position. The visual disturbance would resolve first in the center then improve in the periphery.

and one study demonstrated reduced central retinal artery blood flow on orbital color Doppler imaging in a patient with gaze-evoked amaurosis.[129]

Epileptic visual loss

Although ictal and postictal visual loss is unusual, the phenomenon is well recognized. The visual deficits are almost always binocular, and patients may complain of homonymous hemianopias or complete blindness. In the absence of other seizure activity or a history of epilepsy, clinically these patients can be difficult to differentiate from those with migrainous visual loss.

Ictal visual loss. Ictal amaurosis is highly characteristic of benign occipital lobe epilepsy, a childhood seizure condition.[130–132] The average age of onset is 6 years, and other clinical features include postictal headache, nausea, and vomiting; psychomotor or hemiclonic seizures; occipital spike- and slow-wave activity with eyes closed; good response to anticonvulsant medication; and spontaneous remission by age 19.[133] Neuroimaging is typically normal.

Other varieties of ictal visual loss can also occur. Gilliam et al.[134] reported ictal visual loss in children or young adults with seizures related to stroke, trauma, or neoplasm. Interictal vision was normal, but interictal electroencephalography demonstrated posterior spike- and slow-wave complexes limited to the occipital, parieto-occipital, or temporo-occipital regions.[134] Middle aged and elderly patients have been described with hemianopias or complete cortical blindness lasting for minutes, hours, or days.[135,136] Barry et al.[135] used the term *status epilepticus amauroticus* to describe the patients with the longer lasting symptoms. Most had other clinical evidence of seizures such as mental status change or

forced eye deviation, and ictal occipital or temporo-occipital discharges were recorded. Finally, occipital lobe seizures and transient cortical visual loss may be a manifestation of nonketotic hyperglycemia.[137,138]

Postictal visual loss. Similar to a Todd's paralysis, visual loss may occur for hours or days following a seizure. In hemianopic cases, the visual deficit is usually contralateral to the cortical seizure focus. Postictal visual loss is much less common than the ictal variety.

References

1. Volpe NJ, Liu GT, Galetta SL. Transient visual loss. Curr Conc Ophthalmol 1998;6:55–59.
2. Bruno A, Corbett JJ, Biller J, et al. Transient monocular visual loss patterns and associated vascular abnormalities. Stroke 1990;21:34–39.
3. Ravits J, Seybold M. Transient monocular visual loss from narrow-angle glaucoma. Arch Neurol 1984;41:991–993.
4. Kosmorsky GS, Rosenfeld SL, Burde RM. Transient monocular obscuration? Amaurosis fugax: a case report. Br J Ophthalmol 1985;69:688–690.
5. Adams HP, Putnam SF, Corbett JJ, et al. Amaurosis fugax: the results of arteriography in 59 patients. Stroke 1983;14:742–744.
6. Donders RCJM. Clinical features of transient monocular blindness and the likelihood of atherosclerotic lesions of the internal carotid artery. J Neurol Neurosurg Psychiatry 2001;71:247–249.
7. Biousse V, Trobe JD. Transient monocular visual loss. Am J Ophthalmol 2005;140: 717–721.
8. Hayward JK, Davies AH, Lamont PM. Carotid plaque morphology: a review. Eur J Vasc Endovasc Surg 1995;9:368–374.
9. Garcia JH, Khang-Loon H. Carotid atherosclerosis. Definition, pathogenesis, and clinical significance. Neuroimaging Clin N Am 1996;6:801–810.
10. Russo CP, Smoker WRK. Nonatheromatous carotid artery disease. Neuroimaging Clin N Am 1996;6:811–830.
11. Fisher CM. Observation of the fundus oculi in transient monocular blindness. Neurology 1959;9:333–336.
12. Lepore FE. Visual obscurations: evanescent and elementary. Semin Neurol 1986;6:167–175.
13. Levin LA, Mootha VV. Postprandial transient visual loss. A symptom of critical carotid stenosis. Ophthalmology 1997;104:397–401.

14. Poole CJM, Russell RWR. Mortality and stroke after amaurosis fugax. J Neurol Neurosurg Psychiatr 1985;48:902–905.

15. Wray SH. Visual aspects of extracranial internal carotid artery disease. In: Bernstein EF (ed): Amaurosis Fugax, pp 72–80. New York, Springer-Verlag, 1988.

16. Benavente O, Eliasziw M, Streifler JY, et al. Prognosis after transient monocular blindness associated with carotid-artery stenosis. N Engl J Med 2001;345:1084–1090.

17. Streifler JY, Eliasziw M, Benavente OR, et al. The risk of stroke in patients with first-ever retinal vs. hemispheric transient ischemic attacks and high-grade carotid stenosis. Arch Neurol 1995;52:246–249.

18. Nakajima N, Kimura K, Minematsu K, et al. A case of frequently recurring amaurosis fugax with atherothrombotic ophthalmic artery occlusion. Neurology 2004;62:117–118.

19. Wolintz RJ. Carotid endarterectomy for ophthalmic manifestations: is it ever indicated? J Neuroophthalmol 2005;25:299–302.

20. Arruga J, Saunders MD. Ophthalmologic findings in 70 patients with evidence of retinal embolism. Ophthalmology 1982;89:1336–1347.

21. Burde RM. Amaurosis fugax. An overview. J Clin Neuroophthalmol 1989;9:185–189.

22. Sempere AP, Duarte J, Coria F, et al. Loss of vision induced by the color white: a sign of carotid occlusive disease (letter). Stroke 1992;23:1179.

23. Furlan AJ, Whisnant JP, Kearns TP. Unilateral visual loss in bright light: an unusual symptom of carotid artery occlusive disease. Arch Neurol 1979;36:675–676.

24. Kaiboriboon K, Piriyawat P, Selhorst JB. Light-induced amaurosis fugax. Am J Ophthalmol 2001;131:674–676.

25. Donnan GA, Sharbrough FW, Whisnant JP. Carotid occlusive disease: effect of bright light on visual evoked response. Arch Neurol 1982;1982:687–689.

26. Howard RS, Russell RW. Prognosis of patients with retinal embolism. J Neurol Neurosurg Psychiatr 1987;50:1142–1147.

27. McCrary JA. Venous stasis retinopathy of stenotic or occlusive carotid origin. J Clin Neuroophthalmol 1989;9:195–199.

28. Mizener JB, Podhajsky P, Hayreh SS. Ocular ischemic syndrome. Ophthalmology 1997;104:859–864.

29. Galetta SL, Leahey A, Nichols CW, et al. Orbital ischemia, ophthalmoparesis, and carotid dissection. J Clin Neuroophthalmol 1991;11:284–287.

30. Borruat F-X, Bogousslavsky J, Uffer S, et al. Orbital infarction syndrome. Ophthalmology 1993;100:562–568.

31. Wilson WB, Leavengood JM, Ringel SP, et al. Transient ocular motor paresis associated with acute internal carotid artery occlusion. Ann Neurol 1989;25:286–290.

32. Balcer LJ, Galetta SL, Yousem DM, et al. Pupil-involving third nerve palsy and carotid stenosis: rapid recovery following endarterectomy. Ann Neurol 1997;41:273–276.

33. Waybright EA, Selhorst JB, Combs J. Anterior ischemic optic neuropathy with internal carotid artery occlusion. Am J Ophthalmol 1982;93:42–47.

34. Kim SK, Volpe NJ, Stoltz RA. Contemporaneous retinal and optic nerve infarcts, choroidal non-perfusion, and Hollenhorst plaque: are these all embolic events? J Neuroophthalmol 2006;26:113–116.

35. Roederer GO, Langlois YE, Jager KA, et al. The natural history of carotid arterial disease in asymptomatic patients with cervical bruits. Stroke 1984;15:605–613.

36. Chambers BR, Norris JW. Outcome in patients with asymptomatic neck bruits. N Engl J Med 1986;315:860–865.

37. Mackey AE, Abrahamowicz M, Langlois Y, et al. Outcome of asymptomatic patients with carotid disease. Neurology 1997;48:896–903.

38. Sauvé JS, Thorpe KE, Sackett DL, et al. Can bruits distinguish high-grade from moderate symptomatic carotid stenosis? The North American Symptomatic Carotid Endarterectomy Trial. Ann Intern Med 1994;120:633–637.

39. David TE, Humphries AW, Young JR, et al. A correlation of neck bruits and arteriosclerotic carotid arteries. Arch Surg 1973;107:729–734.

40. Sauvé J-S, Laupacis A, Østbye T, et al. Does this patient have a clinically important carotid bruit? JAMA 1993;270:2843–2845.

41. Carroll BA. Carotid ultrasound. Neuroimag Clin North Am 1996;6:875–897.

42. Sidhu PS, Allan PL. The extended role of carotid artery ultrasound. Clin Radiol 1997;52:643–653.

43. Prestigiacomo CJ, Connolly ES, Jr., Quest DO. Use of carotid ultrasound as a preoperative assessment of extracranial carotid artery blood flow and vascular anatomy. Neurosurg Clin N Am 1996;7:577–587.

44. Sidhu PS, Allan PL. Ultrasound assessment of internal carotid artery stenosis. Clin Radiol 1997;52:654–658.

45. U-King-Im JM, Trivedi RA, Graves MJ, et al. Contrast-enhanced MR angiography for carotid disease: diagnostic and potential clinical impact. Neurology 2004;62:1282–1290.

46. Rosovsky MA, Litt AW, Krinsky G. Magnetic resonance carotid angiography of the neck. Clin Implications 1996;6:863–874.

47. Gandhi D. Computed tomography and magnetic resonance angiography in cervicocranial vascular disease. J Neuroophthalmol 2004;24:306–314.

48. Josephson SA, Bryant SO, Mak HK, et al. Evaluation of carotid stenosis using CT angiography in the initial evaluation of stroke and TIA. Neurology 2004;63:457–460.

49. Norris JW, Rothwell PM. Noninvasive carotid imaging to select patients for endarterectomy: is it really safer than conventional angiography? Neurology 2001;56:990–991.

50. Johnston DC, Goldstein LB. Clinical carotid endarterectomy decision making: noninvasive vascular imaging versus angiography. Neurology 2001;56:1009–1015.

51. Powers WJ. Carotid arteriography: still golden after all these years? Neurology 2004;62:1246–1247.

52. Executive Committee for the Asymptomatic Carotid Atherosclerosis Study. Endarterectomy for asymptomatic carotid artery stenosis. JAMA 1995;273:1421–1428.

53. Johnston SC, Nguyen-Huynh MN, Schwarz ME, et al. National Stroke Association guidelines for the management of transient ischemic attacks. Ann Neurol 2006;60:301–313.

54. North American Symptomatic Carotid Endarterectomy Trial Collaborators. Beneficial effect of endarterectomy in symptomatic patients with high-grade carotid stenosis. N Engl J Med 1991;325:445–453.

55. Barnett HJM, Taylor DW, Eliasziw M, et al. Benefit of carotid endarterectomy in patients with symptomatic moderate or severe stenosis. N Engl J Med 1998;339:1415–1425.

56. European Carotid Surgery Trialists' Collaborative Group. MRC European Carotid surgery trial: interim results for symptomatic patients with severe (70–99%) or with mild (0–29%) carotid stenosis. Lancet 1991;337:1235–1243.

57. Mayberg MR, Wilson SE, Yatsu F, et al. Carotid endarterectomy and prevention of cerebral ischemia in symptomatic carotid stenosis. JAMA 1991;266:3289–3294.

58. Kappelle LJ, Eliasziw M, Fox AJ, et al. Importance of intracranial atherosclerotic disease in patients with symptomatic stenosis of the internal carotid artery. The North American Symptomatic Carotid Endarterectomy Trial. Stroke 1999;30:282–286.

59. Barnett HJ, Meldrum HE, Eliasziw M. The appropriate use of carotid endarterectomy. CMAJ 2002;166:1169–1179.

60. Curtis JA, Johansen K. Techniques in carotid artery surgery. Neurosurg Focus 2008;24:E18.

61. Chaturvedi S, Bruno A, Feasby T, et al. Carotid endarterectomy—an evidence-based review: report of the Therapeutics and Technology Assessment Subcommittee of the American Academy of Neurology. Neurology 2005;65:794–801.

62. Rothwell PM, Mehta Z, Howard SC, et al. Treating individuals. 3. From subgroups to individuals: general principles and the example of carotid endarterectomy. Lancet 2005;365:256–265.

63. Feasby TE, Quan H, Ghali WA. Hospital and surgeon determinants of carotid endarterectomy outcomes. Arch Neurol 2002;59:1877–1881.

64. North American Symptomatic Carotid Endarterectomy Trial (NASCET) Steering Committee. North American Symptomatic Carotid Endarterectomy Trial. Methods, patient characteristics, and progress. Stroke 1991;22:711–720.

65. Ruckley CV. Stroke after carotid endarterectomy. Br J Surg 1999;86:3–4.

66. Kieburtz K, Ricotta JJ, Moxley RT. Seizures following carotid endarterectomy. Arch Neurol 1990;47:568–570.

67. Mansoor GA, White WB, Grunnet M, et al. Intracerebral hemorrhage after carotid endarterectomy associated with ipsilateral fibrinoid necrosis: a consequence of the hyperperfusion syndrome? J Vasc Surg 1996;23:147–151.

68. Breen JC, Caplan LR, DeWitt LD, et al. Brain edema after carotid surgery. Neurology 1996;46:175–181.

69. Sundt TM, Sharbrough FW, Piepgras DG, et al. Correlation of cerebral blood flow and electroencephalographic changes during carotid endarterectomy. With results of surgery and hemodynamics of cerebral ischemia. Mayo Clinic Proc 1981;56:533–543.

70. Biller J, Feinberg WM, Castaldo JE, et al. Guidelines for carotid endarterectomy: a statement for healthcare professionals from a Special Writing Group of the Stroke Council, American Heart Association. Circulation 1998;97:501–509.

71. Ballotta E, Da Giau G, Renon L, et al. Cranial and cervical nerve injuries after carotid endarterectomy: a prospective study. Surgery 1999;125:85–91.

72. Barnett HJM, Eliasziw M, Meldrum HE, et al. Do the facts and figures warrant a 10-fold increase in the performance of carotid endarterectomy on asymptomatic patients? Neurology 1996;46:603–608.

73. Perry JR, Szalai JP, Norris JW, et al. Consensus against both endarterectomy and routine screening for asymptomatic carotid artery stenosis. Arch Neurol 1997;54:25–28.

74. Inzitari D, Eliasziw M, Gates P, et al. The causes and risk of stroke in patients with asymptomatic internal-carotid-artery stenosis. North American Symptomatic Carotid Endarterectomy Trial Collaborators. N Engl J Med 2000;342:1693–1700.

75. Thijs V. Does surgery have a role in the management of asymptomatic carotid artery stenosis? Yes, but. Nat Clin Pract Neurol 2008;4:2–3.

76. Abbott A. Asymptomatic carotid artery stenosis: it's time to stop operating. Nat Clin Pract Neurol 2008;4:4–5.

77. The Casanova Study Group. Carotid surgery versus medical therapy in asymptomatic carotid stenosis. Stroke 1991;22:1229–1235.

78. Hobson RW, Weiss DG, Fields WS, et al. Efficacy of carotid endarterectomy for asymptomatic carotid stenosis. N Engl J Med 1993;328:221–227.

79. Halliday A, Mansfield A, Marro J, et al. Prevention of disabling and fatal strokes by successful carotid endarterectomy in patients without recent neurological symptoms: randomised controlled trial. Lancet 2004;363:1491–1502.

80. Benavente O, Moher D, Pham B. Carotid endarterectomy for asymptomatic carotid stenosis: a meta-analysis. BMJ 1998;317:1477–1480.

81. Chaturvedi S, Fessler R. Angioplasty and stenting for stroke prevention: good questions that need answers. Neurology 2002;59:664–668.

82. Brott TG, Brown RD, Jr., Meyer FB, et al. Carotid revascularization for prevention of stroke: carotid endarterectomy and carotid artery stenting. Mayo Clin Proc 2004;79:1197–1208.

83. Meschia JF, Brott TG, Hobson RW, II. Diagnosis and invasive management of carotid atherosclerotic stenosis. Mayo Clin Proc 2007;82:851–858.

84. Coward LJ, Featherstone RL, Brown MM. Safety and efficacy of endovascular treatment of carotid artery stenosis compared with carotid endarterectomy: a Cochrane systematic review of the randomized evidence. Stroke 2005;36:905–911.

85. Yadav JS, Wholey MH, Kuntz RE, et al. Protected carotid-artery stenting versus endarterectomy in high-risk patients. N Engl J Med 2004;351:1493–1501.

86. Gurm HS, Yadav JS, Fayad P, et al. Long-term results of carotid stenting versus endarterectomy in high-risk patients. N Engl J Med 2008;358:1572–1579.

87. Mas JL, Chatellier G, Beyssen B, et al. Endarterectomy versus stenting in patients with symptomatic severe carotid stenosis. N Engl J Med 2006;355:1660–1671.

88. Kawaguchi S, Okuno S, Sakaki T, et al. Effect of carotid endarterectomy on chronic ocular ischemic syndrome due to internal carotid artery stenosis. Neurosurgery 2001;48:328–332.

89. Marx JL, Hreib K, Choi IS, et al. Percutaneous carotid artery angioplasty and stenting for ocular ischemic syndrome. Ophthalmology 2004;111:2284–2291.

90. Anderson DC, Kappelle LJ, Eliasziw M, et al. Occurrence of hemispheric and retinal ischemia in atrial fibrillation compared with carotid stenosis. Stroke 2002;33:1963–1967.

91. Mead GE, Lewis SC, Wardlaw JM, et al. Comparison of risk factors in patients with transient and prolonged eye and brain ischemic syndromes. Stroke 2002;33:2383–2390.

92. Furlong BR, Verdile VP. Myxomatous embolization resulting in unilateral amaurosis. Am J Emerg Med 1995;13:46–49.

93. Lesser RL, Heineman M-H, Borkowski H, et al. Mitral valve prolapse and amaurosis fugax. J Clin Neuroophthalmol 1981;1:153–160.

94. Wisotsky BJ, Engel HM. Transesophageal echocardiography in the diagnosis of branch retinal artery obstruction. Am J Ophthalmol 1993;115:653–656.

95. Burger SK, Saul RF, Selhorst JB, et al. Transient monocular blindness caused by vasospasm. N Engl J Med 1991;12:870–873.

96. Petzold A, Islam N, Plant GT. Video reconstruction of vasospastic transient monocular blindness. N Engl J Med 2003;348:1609–1610.

97. Winterkorn JMS, Teman AJ. Recurrent attacks of amaurosis fugax treated with calcium channel blocker. Ann Neurol 1991;30:423–425.

98. Winterkorn JMS, Kupersmith MJ, Wirtschafter JD, et al. Treatment of vasospastic amaurosis fugax with calcium channel blockers. N Engl J Med 1993;329:396–398.

99. Jehn A, Frank Dettwiler B, Fleischhauer J, et al. Exercise-induced vasospastic amaurosis fugax. Arch Ophthalmol 2002;120:220–222.

100. Libman RB, Masters SR, de Paola A, et al. Transient monocular blindness associated with cocaine abuse. Neurology 1993;43:228–229.

101. Tippin J, Corbett JJ, Kerber RE, et al. Amaurosis fugax and ocular infarction in adolescents and young adults. Ann Neurol 1989;26:69–77.

102. Winterkorn JM, Mack P, Eggenberger E. Transient visual loss in a 60-year-old man. Surv Ophthalmol 2008;53:301–305.

103. Slavin ML, Wall M, Weinstein J. Amaurosis fugax in the young. Surv Ophthalmol 1997;41:481–487.

104. Liu GT, Glaser JS, Schatz NJ, et al. Visual morbidity in giant cell arteritis: clinical characteristics and prognosis for vision. Ophthalmology 1994;101:1779–1785.

105. Finelli P. Alternating amaurosis fugax and temporal arteritis. Am J Ophthalmol 1997;123:850–851.

106. Diego M, Margo CE. Postural visual loss in giant cell arteritis. J Neuroophthalmol 1998;18:124–126.

107. Galetta SL, Balcer LJ, Liu GT. Giant cell arteritis with unusual flow related neuro-ophthalmologic manifestations. Neurology 1997;49:1463–1465.

108. Melberg MS, Grand MG, Dieckert JP, et al. Cotton wool spots and the early diagnosis of giant cell arteritis. Ophthalmology 1995;102:1611–1614.

109. Albers GW, Caplan LR, Easton JD, et al. Transient ischemic attack: proposal for a new definition. N Engl J Med 2002;347:1713–1716.

110. Wu CM, McLaughlin K, Lorenzetti DL, et al. Early risk of stroke after transient ischemic attack: a systematic review and meta-analysis. Arch Intern Med 2007;167:2417–2422.

111. Johnston SC. Clinical practice. Transient ischemic attack. N Engl J Med 2002;347:1687–1692.

112. Robertson DM. I am a retinal migraineur [letter]. J Neuroophthalmol 2008;28:81–82.

113. Evans RW, Grosberg BM. Retinal migraine: migraine associated with monocular visual symptoms. Headache 2008;48:142–145.

114. Headache Classification Subcommittee of the International Headache Society. The International Classification of Headache Disorders, 2nd edition. Cephalalgia 2004;24(Suppl 1):9–160.

115. Hill DL, Daroff RB, Ducros A, et al. Most cases labeled as "retinal migraine" are not migraine. J Neuroophthalmol 2007;27:3–8.

116. Winterkorn JM. "Retinal migraine" is an oxymoron [editorial]. J Neuroophthalmol 2007;27:1–2.

117. Daroff RB. Retinal migraine [letter]. J Neuroophthalmol 2007;27:83.

118. Lepore FE. Retinal migraine [letter]. J Neuroophthalmol 2007;27:242–243.

119. Grosberg BM, Solomon S, Friedman DI, et al. Retinal migraine reappraised. Cephalalgia 2006;26:1275–1286.

120. Solomon S, Grosberg BM, Friedman DI, et al. Retinal migraine [letter]. J Neuroophthalmol 2007;27:243–244.

121. Sadun AA, Currie JN, Lessell S. Transient visual obscurations with elevated optic discs. Ann Neurol 1984;16:489–494.

122. O'Duffy D, James B, Elston J. Idiopathic intracranial hypertension presenting with gaze-evoked amaurosis. Acta Ophthalmol Scand 1998;76:119–120.

123. Otto CS, Coppit GL, Mazzoli RA, et al. Gaze-evoked amaurosis: a report of five cases. Ophthalmology 2003;110:322–326.

124. McDonald WI. The symptomatology of tumours of the anterior visual pathway. Can J Neurol Sci 1982;8:381–390.

125. Danesh-Meyer HV, Savino PJ, Bilyk JR, et al. Gaze-evoked amaurosis produced by intraorbital buckshot pellet. Ophthalmology 2001;108:201–206.

126. Manor RS, Ben Sira I. Amaurosis at downward gaze. Surv Ophthalmol 1987;31:411–416.

127. Orcutt JC, Tucker WM, Mills RP, et al. Gaze-evoked amaurosis. Ophthalmology 1987;94:213–218.

128. Manor RS, Yassur Y, Hoyt WF. Reading-evoked visual dimming. Am J Ophthalmol 1996;121:212–214.

129. Knapp ME, Flaharty PM, Sergott RC, et al. Gaze-induced amaurosis from central retinal artery compression. Ophthalmology 1992;99:238–240.

130. Jaffe SJ, Roach ES. Transient cortical blindness with occipital lobe epilepsy. J Clin Neuroophthalmol 1988;8:221–224.

131. Andermann F, Zifkin B. The benign occipital epilepsies of childhood: an overview of the idiopathic syndromes and of the relationship to migraine. Epilepsia 1998;39:S9–S23.

132. Shahar E, Barak S. Favorable outcome of epileptic blindness in children. J Child Neurol 2003;18:12–16.

133. Gastaut H. A new type of epilepsy: benign partial epilepsy of childhood with occipital spike-waves. Clin Electroencephalogr 1982;13:13–22.

134. Gilliam F, Wyllie E. Ictal amaurosis: MRI, EEG, and clinical features. Neurology 1995;45:1619–1621.

135. Barry E, Sussman NM, Bosley TM, et al. Ictal blindness and status epilepticus amauroticus. Epilepsia 1985;26:577–584.

136. Kattah JC, Gujrati M, Hui ET, et al. Bilateral occipital lobe hyperperfusion demonstrated by single photon emission computed tomography during seizure-related cortical blindness. J Neuroophthalmol 2004;24:24–26.

137. Harden CL, Rosenbaum DH, Daras M. Hyperglycemia presenting with occipital seizures. Epilepsia 1991;32:215–220.

138. Taban M, Naugle RI, Lee MS. Transient homonymous hemianopia and positive visual phenomena in patients with nonketotic hyperglycemia. Arch Ophthalmol 2007;125:845–847.

CHAPTER **11**

Functional visual loss

Functional (nonorganic) visual loss is frequently encountered in ophthalmic and neurologic practice, occurring in 0.5–5%[1] of patients presenting with vision loss according to some estimates.[2,3] Patients with functional visual loss may be misdiagnosed because of the paucity of objective findings on examination. Identifying such patients is extremely important in order to avoid unnecessary laboratory testing and secondary gain. Likewise, it is also imperative to be able to identify those patients with organic vision loss with superimposed functional vision loss. Although the characterization of the psychological profile of patients with functional vision loss is helpful, for the ophthalmologist or neurologist a familiarity with diagnostic strategies used to identify functional vision loss is more important. In this chapter, terminology will be clarified, then patient types and their potential interactions with the examiner will be described. The methods used to diagnose functional vision loss will be reviewed in detail, followed by a brief description of other neuro-ophthalmologic manifestations of nonorganic disease.

Terminology

Historically, numerous terms have been used to describe functional visual loss, including hysteria, hysterical visual loss, malingering, nonphysiologic visual loss, factitious visual loss, nonorganic visual loss, psychogenic visual loss, Münchausen syndrome, and conversion disorder of vision. Ambiguity results for two different reasons. First, there has been no universal agreement about a term to describe nonorganic visual loss. The term functional visual loss denotes the symptomatic and measured loss of vision that is unassociated with an identifiable lesion of the visual pathways. Furthermore, in patients with functional visual loss there is no explanation for their complaints on the basis of contemporary knowledge of the visual pathways. Thus the term functional visual loss is equivalent to factitious, nonorganic, and nonphysiologic visual loss.

The second level of confusion exists when the terminology attempts to identify the underlying cause or circumstance of the nonorganicity. For instance, *malingering* implies that there is a willful alteration of subjective symptoms and responses on examination. Usually this is an attempt to secure secondary gain such as time away from work or monetary gain from an insurance settlement. Such patients with volitional alteration of the examination can be labeled as malingerers if the examiner chooses to begin a long and arduous confrontation between him- or herself, the patient, lawyers, and insurance companies. The examiner may simply report the vision loss as functional and incompatible with a specific organic lesion. This approach is particularly wise when the initial factors driving the feigned loss are unclear.

Other diagnoses, such as hysteria, conversion disorder, Münchausen syndrome, hypochondriasis, or somatization disorder, may be considered in patients who are not clearly seeking secondary gain. The use of each of these terms is dependent on an understanding of the patient's potential

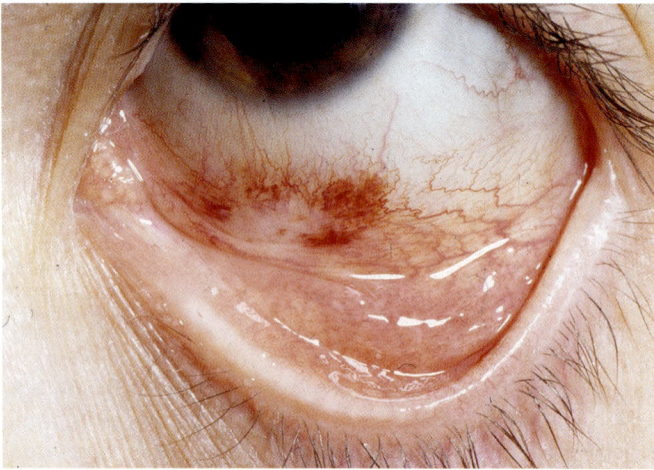

Figure 11–1. Conjunctival injection and abrasion secondary to digital trauma in a patient with Münchausen syndrome and associated functional visual loss.

psychiatric problems. For instance, Münchausen syndrome is a factitious disorder in which the patient intentionally produces physical signs and symptoms.[4] When Münchausen syndrome is associated with visual loss, patients can have associated eyelid swelling, conjunctival injection, or hemorrhages (**Fig. 11–1**). This may be the result of self-inflicted trauma or self-instilled eye irritant. These patients generally have some psychogenic factor driving them to assume the role of a sick person.

The physical symptoms of a patient with a conversion disorder and vision loss may reflect an inner conflict. The label *conversion disorder* incorporates many of the patients who, in the past, were diagnosed as having hysteria or hysterical vision loss. *Hysteria* derives from the root "hyst," referring to the uterus. This terminology had its beginnings in ancient Greece, where many conditions were thought to occur only in women, and the uterus was thought to have a will of its own. Until the 19th century this was a popular notion. Charcot was the first to ascribe "hysterical symptoms" to a mental disorder, and he felt it was likely that a specific brain lesion was present in these patients.[5] Babinski expanded on the notion that these symptoms were likely "caused by suggestion and cured by persuasion." Freud popularized the concept that like all else, "hysterical" vision loss had its basis in the inner unconscious battle between the ego, id, and superego. He then popularized the term *conversion disorder*, implying that an emotional symptom led to a physical finding.[5] These patients, although less deliberate than the malingerer, may realize both primary (reduction of stress from inner conflict) and secondary (more attention) gain.[6,7]

Finally, *hypochondriacs* are patients who excessively report signs and symptoms and believe they are seriously ill. They also attempt to convince the examiner that their symptoms and problems are serious. In somatization disorders, patients who are depressed or suffering from an anxiety disorder report numerous vague complaints. These may include symptoms of vision loss that ultimately prove to be nonorganic.

Since the terminology is inexact and overlapping, we prefer the umbrella term of *functional visual loss* and during

the interview and examination attempt to determine if there is any secondary gain. It is important to understand the terminology used to identify each of the types of psychogenic illness associated with functional visual loss, but we prefer that ultimately others more expert in psychiatric illness apply the specific label. Although the techniques used to identify patients that are malingering versus those that are truly suffering from some psychogenic process are the same, the interventions or treatment required may differ immensely.

Clinical presentation

Setting

Some insight into and understanding of types of patients with functional visual loss, as well as the attitudes of both the examiner and the patient toward their interaction, are essential. This understanding will help to make a potentially difficult interaction tolerable and non-confrontational.

The distortion of the patient–physician relationship in this setting may be very difficult for the physician to accept and manage. Instead of using knowledge and skill to diagnose and treat a real problem, the examiner instead often becomes frustrated and confrontational as he or she becomes increasingly suspicious regarding the nature of the patient's disorder. To paraphrase Thompson,[5] what usually is an allied relationship between doctor and patient against the common enemy of vision loss becomes an adversarial relationship in which the patient complains of vision loss, and the physician is out to prove otherwise. Many times the physician fails to make the correct diagnosis because of this distortion in the doctor–patient relationship. More concerning is the fact that as many as half of the patients with functional visual loss have this superimposed upon true or organic pathology. Any underlying problems may be unrecognized because the examiner is so put off by the patient's behavior.[8]

Patient characteristics

Patients with functional visual loss can come from any socioeconomic group. There is no clear sex or race predilection. A large proportion of one series consisted of blue-collar workers.[8] Another series found a high prevalence of functional visual loss in Cambodians living in California, and the authors postulated a relationship to previous stress during incarceration in prison camps.[9] In adults there is a high prevalence of pre-existing psychiatric disorders.[10] Although it is to some extent linked to the above discussion of terminology, the types of patients encountered, along with the type of interaction they are likely to have with the examiner, have been characterized by Thompson[5] under a slightly different scheme. He offered descriptive subgroups: the *deliberate malingerer, worried impostor, impressionable exaggerator,* and *suggestible innocent.* Characteristics of each of these patients are summarized in **Table 11–1**. This schema is useful in distinguishing patients as it avoids the term *hysteria.* It can assist with the interaction with the patient and can guide the examiner when giving advice to the patient, the family, and the referring doctor.

Table 11–1 Types of patients encountered with functional visual loss

	Patient's feelings	Patient's behavior	Characteristics of interaction
Deliberate malingerer	Malicious intent	Deliberate nonorganic responses	Confrontational; contest between patient and doctor
Worried impostor	Concerned that something is being missed	Aware of symptom exaggeration; self-doubt leads patient to believe symptoms	Tries to convince examiner of severity; often will accept diagnosis of "healthy eyes"
Impressionable exaggerator	Certain something is wrong with eyes	Does not want to hide serious problem; awareness of nonorganic symptoms is result of wanting to be sure nothing is missed	Wants to help by making diagnosis easy; yields poor effort, might improve with suggestion
Suggestible innocent	Convinced that something is wrong after minor injury	Indifferent about inconsistencies of exam or behavior ("la belle indifference")	Complacent; open to suggestions about improvement

From Thompson HS: Functional visual loss. Am J Ophthalmol 1985;100:209–213.

Classically, "la belle indifference" has been described as an important feature in all patients with hysterical vision loss (and used to distinguish it from malingering). However, we agree with other series[11,12] that suggest this finding is present only in a minority of patients and is most likely to occur in those characterized by the "suggestible innocent" profile. These patients with more subtle manifestations of functional visual loss might improve simply by reducing the amount of stress in their lives. Keltner[8] found that 51 of 59 adults with functional vision loss were clearly seeking financial gain. They presumably fit best in the "deliberate malingerer" subgroup, but some patients may have been "worried impostors," afraid they might miss some deserved benefit. Many adults with functional visual loss are consciously aware of their alteration of their examination. In children, triggering factors are often related to social issues while adults have often suffered some traumatic event.[10]

Types of complaints

The diagnosis of functional visual loss will be made only if the examiner has a high degree of suspicion. Therefore, unless the patient comes with functional visual loss as the referring diagnosis or the patient is being seen for an insurance company or lawyer, the examiner must depend on the history then the examination. With increasing experience, recognition of typical settings for organic and inorganic disease often suggests to the clinician that functional visual loss should be highly considered. For instance, head trauma is an important cause of traumatic optic neuropathy (see Chapter 5) and also is a common setting for functional visual loss. However, the characteristic severe blow to the brow or cheek that causes traumatic optic neuropathy is usually not described by the patient with functional visual loss. Similarly, a blow to the back of the head or a whiplash-type injury is unlikely to produce a traumatic optic neuropathy. In this setting, the examiner knows to be on guard.

Patients with functional visual loss often offer rather alarming chief complaints that frequently identify the potential for secondary gain; for instance, "I am blind in my eye since the accident" or "I cannot see since I got that chemical in my eye." However, as the examiner investigates further, the complaints become very vague, and patients are often unable to characterize the vision loss as anything more than absent or "blurry." They will often answer, "I do not know" or "I cannot be sure" to questions directed at better characterizing the nature of the vision loss. They less commonly describe the symptoms characteristic of true optic neuropathy, such a loss of brightness, darkening, pieces of vision missing, central blind spots, and altitudinal visual field loss. They are very unlikely to report metamorphopsia as patients with maculopathies might.

Impact

The major societal impact of functional visual loss is financial, in the form of undeserved benefits paid for fraudulent claims, missed work, and unnecessary testing. Most of the patients in Keltner's series[8] were unemployed. Convincing the examiner of a visual defect could result in a lifetime disability check as opposed to either dependency on public assistance or ultimate need to secure employment. The exact monetary amount is difficult to estimate. Keltner[8] noted that as many as one-third of claims from the Workers Compensation program may have been fraudulent. The problem is likely one that costs society millions of dollars per year. Ophthalmologists and optometrists can declare a patient legally blind, and because of the financial impact are obligated to be absolutely certain that functional visual loss is not present.

Functional visual loss in children

The presentation of functional visual loss in children is often different from that in adults. First, the clinical suspicion for true or organic vision loss in children must be higher since the pediatric eye examination may be marked by poor cooperation or a lack of understanding of test procedures. Even when functional visual loss is "confidently" diagnosed the patients must be followed closely for development of organic findings over time. Second, malingering, confrontational behavior, and pending insurance claims are infrequent in children. Lastly, children are less sophisticated and highly suggestible.

Clinical setting

Functional visual loss has been estimated to occur in approximately one child per 1000 per year, and the most commonly encountered demographic group is pubescent girls (ages 9–11).[1,8,13–16] There are often other accompanying symptoms, such as headache, eye pain and face pain.[10,13,17] As with adults, functional visual loss may accompany organic visual loss. Rada et al.[18] reported that one-fourth of children with functional visual loss have some true underlying organic disease.

Causes

Mantyjarvi[16] found that only a few children had an underlying psychological illness causing the functional visual loss. In some children functional visual loss resulted from a lack of parental attention or conflict with parents. Divorce or relocation to a different school or city are common external stresses. Although not malingering, many children realize the secondary gain of increased parental attention as a result of their complaints of defective vision. In others, deterioration in school performance may trigger complaints of functional visual loss.[13] In this setting there is often a mismatch between visual difficulty encountered at school and that noted at home. For instance, when the child is observed unknowingly, there may be no visual difficulty watching television or at play. Similar behavior may be seen in children who want to have glasses because their friends have them.

A true conversion disorder may be present when the child is conscious neither of the loss of function nor of the potential secondary gain. Thus the functional visual loss allows the child to avoid a situation in which conflict occurs. Physicians should be alerted to the possibility of childhood physical or sexual abuse in this setting.[10,13] In unusual circumstances, a parent drives the complaint of functional visual loss, thereby indirectly assuming the sick role (*Münchausen's by proxy*).

Approach to the patient with functional visual loss

Subjectivity

Every measure of visual function that requires the patient to respond or describe something is, by definition, subjective. In other words, patient cooperation and effort are required to obtain optimal results, especially with regard to testing of visual acuity, stereopsis, color vision, and visual fields.

Diagnosis

The diagnosis of functional visual loss is suggested when the examiner can demonstrate that a patient's behavior and responses to testing are inconsistent with an organic lesion. The diagnosis is confirmed when the examiner is able to

prove, by some of the methods described below, that the patient has better vision than he or she claims. Although often tempting, the diagnosis of functional visual loss should not be made unless normal acuity and visual fields can be established, and the pupillary and ophthalmoscopic examinations are also normal.

Alteration of the patient–physician relationship

Often the examiner can immediately recognize that a patient's behavior is inappropriate. This type of behavior frequently suggests the vision loss is functional and often sets the tone of the patient–physician interaction. The patient may be overly stoic or dramatic. Hostile, suspicious, flirtatious, or excessively cooperative behavior should make the examiner suspicious of functional visual loss. However, prejudices should not interfere with or alter the examiner's empathetic attitude. The caring and genuinely concerned examiner will be the most successful at applying the tests that ultimately prove functional visual loss. Disbelieving or confrontational behavior is likely to make the patient uncooperative with testing.[8,19]

Patterns of functional visual loss

In most patients with nonorganic loss of vision, acuity and visual fields are both affected to some extent.[1,7,20,21] However, several studies have suggested that the most common pattern is visual acuity loss with normal visual fields.[8,17,19] Although it is somewhat artificial, the various techniques used to identify functional visual loss will be described according to the level of visual dysfunction and whether the visual loss is monocular or binocular. It is essential that the examiner becomes familiar and comfortable with a few of the techniques that are used to identify functional visual loss. The testing should be performed in a routine and skillful manner without making the patient suspicious that the agenda is to prove functional visual loss.

It is important for the reader to note that while these techniques aim to prove that the vision is better than the patient claims, some of them are able to establish the actual level of vision in the supposed bad eye or eyes.

Total blindness

Observation. Throughout the course of the doctor–patient encounter the examiner must carefully observe the patient for behavior incompatible with the degree of alleged vision loss. Truly blind persons will always proceed cautiously around office furniture and equipment. They feel their way, and they will often bump into objects. Patient with functional visual loss, particularly deliberate malingerers, will move quickly and purposely bump objects but never fall or harm themselves. The examiner might intentionally line up the room with obstacles in the patient's direct path to see how they navigate the room. Most truly blind patients will look at the examiner in the direction of the examiner's voice. The deliberate malingerer might not look at or even avoid eye contact with the examiner, assuming that without vision, auditory clues would be inadequate to locate the other individuals in the room. Patients with functional vision loss may wear sunglasses for no apparent reason, and such individuals have a high rate of seeking secondary gain and often a diffusely positive review of systems.[22,23] We have seen patients who took on the physical appearance, behavior, and head movements of famous blind people commonly seen in the media.

Pupillary reactions. Patients who are bilaterally blind (no light perception) because of retinal, optic nerve, chiasmal, or optic tract disturbances will have pupils that are unreactive to light. Only cortical blindness is associated with normal pupillary reactivity. Therefore a patient who complains of total blindness, with intact pupillary responses, but no cortical lesion, is likely to be functional. A complaint of photophobia with orbicularis contraction when the bright indirect ophthalmoscope light is shone in the eye is incompatible with an ocular cause of blindness.

Optokinetic nystagmus (OKN). An optokinetic stimulus such as a drum or tape (see Chapter 2) produces a horizontal jerk nystagmus in patients with intact vision and an ocular motor system. The patient must look at and be able to see the figures or stripes on the drum or tape. The response is involuntary and implies a level of acuity equal to that necessary to resolve the stripes or other targets. Patients can voluntarily block this response if they look away from or beyond the stimulus. Excessive convergence on the part of the patient may also dampen the response. The use of a +3.00-diopter lens in front of the eye may force attention to the near stimulus and elicit a response. In the majority of cases, an intact OKN response confirms visual acuity to be at least 20/400. Although it is potentially possible to estimate a level of acuity by reducing the size of the object or stripe or using neutral density filters,[24] we do not recommend this approach.[23]

Tests of proprioception. Truly blind patients have no difficulty performing tests that appear to require vision but are actually proprioceptive tasks. For instance, a patient can be asked to simply look at his or her hand. A blind person can do this easily, but a patient with functional visual loss will often look away from his or her hand. The patient also can be asked to bring the tips of the first finger from each hand together from a distance.[7] This can be done without any vision and is easily performed by most blind patients. Patients with functional visual loss will often miss by inches. Finally, a blind person asked to sign his or her name will have no difficulty signing, while a functional patient will often produce a signature that is unlike his or her true signature and clearly is not along a horizontal line.

Mirror test. When a large mirror is placed in front of the face of a sighted person and rocked back and forth, an involuntary nystagmoid movement that results from forced fixation on the image in the mirror is produced.[25] A patient with functional visual loss will be unable to avoid this movement provided he or she is looking at the image in the mirror. Acuity better than hand motions is present if this response occurs.

Surprise. Although generally too confrontational to recommend in most settings, actions that are designed to surprise and elicit a response from a patient can be quite effective. Various techniques have been described, and all generally involve some behavior atypical in a normal physician–patient interaction. The examiner can make faces or write shocking words and watch the patient for a response. A smile, gasp, or surprised look by the patient confirms that he or she can see and often ends with a "you got me, doc."

Visual evoked potentials and electroretinograms. Electrophysiologic testing has an important role in the evaluation of patients with functional visual loss. In a patient with purported complete blindness, the flash evoked visual potential can be used to document intact visual pathways.[21,26–28] In cooperative but functional patients, a pattern-reversal visual evoked potential can provide an estimate of the individual's true visual acuity.[29–31] McBain et al.[29] found that in 88/100 patients with functional vision loss, normal Snellen acuity could be demonstrated with a short duration, pattern onset visual evoked potential. Massicotte et al.[32] used multifocal visual evoked responses to demonstrate normal responses in patients with functional vision loss and abnormal computerized perimetry. However, in patients with suspected functional visual loss, an abnormal visual evoked potential is difficult to interpret.[27] The patient can voluntarily alter the amplitude and latency of the P100 peak by defocusing, not wearing corrective lenses, or looking away from the stimulus.[33–35] Unfortunately, the opposite is also true, as normal responses have been documented in patients with organic visual loss.[36]

Severe unilateral vision loss

Techniques used on patients with severe bilateral vision loss can be applied to patients with severe unilateral vision loss by patching or covering the "good" eye. In fact, gross differences in behavioral observations and tests of proprioception when the examiner tests each eye separately are often the most compelling findings in this situation. The methods outlined below tend to emphasize the advantage the examiner has because of his or her understanding of binocularity and afferent visual pathway anatomy. It is most important to observe the patient carefully while performing these tests since a "smart" patient may close the "good" eye periodically to try to figure out what the examiner is trying to do.

Afferent pupillary defect. Most patients with severe unilateral vision loss, with no history of amblyopia and with clear media, have a relative afferent pupillary defect (RAPD). Regardless of the localization of unilateral vision loss (optic nerve or chiasm), if the level of acuity is 20/200 or worse, an RAPD is usually present. Certainly nearly all patients with counting fingers or worse vision in one eye, with normal vision in the other, will have an RAPD. The examiner should exercise caution because the RAPD in many ways is a subjective observation and may be absent in asymmetric but bilateral cases of optic neuropathy with very disparate levels of acuity. The absence of an RAPD should not be used to rule out an optic neuropathy, especially if there is a chance of pre- or coexisting optic neuropathy in the other eye.

Stereopsis. In cooperative but unsuspecting patients, measurement of stereopsis can be invaluable in testing for

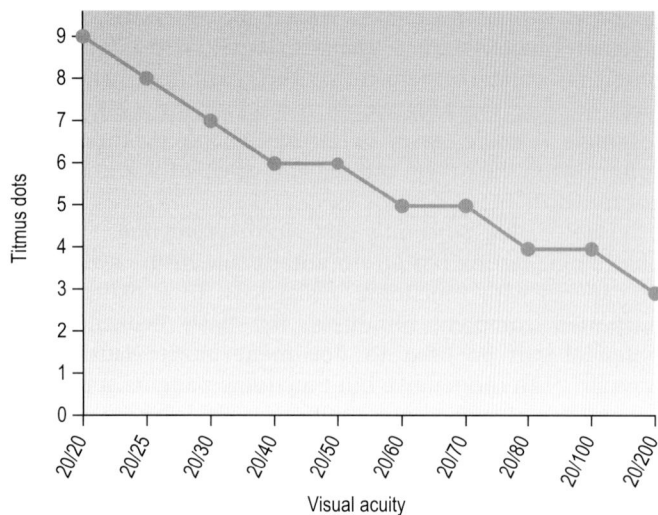

Figure 11–2. Correlation of level of stereoacuity with visual acuity. Individuals who can perceive the eighth of nine Titmus stereo dots must have at least 20/25 acuity in each eye. Similarly, the ability to perceive the first six of nine stereo dots correctly requires at least 20/50 in each eye. (Adapted from Levy NS, Glick EB: Stereoscopic perception and Snellen visual acuity, Am J Ophthalmol 1974;78:722–724, with permission from Elsevier.)

functional visual loss because the results may prove the patient has better vision than he or she claims.[25] Levy and Glick[37] have determined the minimum level of acuity in each eye required to achieve each of the levels of stereoacuity on the Titmus test (**Fig. 11–2**). Therefore, a patient with a claim of reduced acuity to the 20/400 level in one eye but who sees eight or nine circles in stereo on the Titmus test certainly has functional visual loss. Unfortunately, some patients quickly close an eye and realize the test requires binocular vision and subjectively further alter their responses. As with the visual acuity testing strategy described below, it is often effective to begin the stereoacuity testing with the most difficult circles (the ninth) and act somewhat surprised if the patient denies appreciation of elevation of the circle. The great advantages of the stereoacuity testing are its widespread availability and the fact that a specific level of acuity can be proven.

Duochrome test. Several variations of the duochrome test have been described. Two pieces of equipment commonly available in eye lanes are required. The first is the red/green overlay on the projector eye chart (**Fig. 11–3**). This overlay is commonly used to refine refraction but in this setting is used to separate the right and left portions of the chart (left is green and right is red). Next the red/green glasses used for the Worth 4 dot response are utilized. The test takes advantage of the fact that the eye looking through the red lens will see only the red (right) side of the chart. The eye looking through the green lens will see only the letters on the green (left) side of the chart. The red lens is typically placed over the right eye and the green over the left, but the orientation can be switched. If the patient reads the entire line better than their alleged level of visual acuity, then the examiner knows that the affected eye is seeing at least as well as the good eye at that level. The test depends on compatible colors on the eye charts and the red/green glasses for complete

filtering of the other color. Therefore, the examiner should check what the normal patient should see on their setup before administering the test to the patient.

A "poor man's" version of the duochrome test can be performed by simply writing letters in red or with a pink highlighter. These letters cannot be seen with the eye that has the red lens and therefore the green lens is placed over the bad eye. If the patient reads the letters, then they were seen with the "affected" eye. This technique, using a somewhat objectionable series or words, is a powerful combination.

Color plates and the red/green lenses. Another test that takes advantage of the readily available red/green lenses and can be used to prove at least 20/400 vision involves use of the Ishihara color plates.[38] These plates cannot be seen through a green lens, therefore if the red lens is put on over the "bad" eye and the patient reads the plates, then at least 20/400 vision is present in the eye that the patient claims has poor vision.

Polarized eye chart. Some commercially available projector charts come with a slide containing polarized letters. These charts along with the readily available polarized glasses used for stereoacuity testing can be used to dissociate the eyes and demonstrate that each eye is reading the letters.[39] The projected letters can be seen by the right eye, left eye, or both eyes and if the examiner moves quickly before the patient tries closing the good eye (not easily seen by the examiner because of the glasses) better acuity with the bad eye can usually be demonstrated.

Prism shift test. A normal prism shift test depends on the presence of binocular vision. To perform this test the examiner chooses a Snellen letter that is smaller than the acuity at which the patient alleges to see in the affected eye. For example, if the patient sees 20/200 with the affected eye, the test can be performed with a 20/50 letter or smaller. The patient then views the target binocularly, and a 4-diopter base-in loose prism is placed in front of the alleged bad eye. If the patient truly sees the target with both eyes then a compensatory movement of both eyes toward the apex of the prism is followed by a convergence movement of the fellow eye back toward center as the patient refuses the image. If the alleged bad eye is truly defective, a prism over it will not result in any compensatory eye movements because the patient is fixing only with the other eye.

Prism dissociation. Several variations of the prism dissociation test have been described.[40,41] This test uses a vertical prism to separate the images from the two eyes, and the goal is to have the patient unknowingly read the letters that correspond to the line seen by the bad eye. To perform this test the examiner needs to fool the patient into believing that both images are being seen by the good eye. This can be accomplished by momentarily holding the vertical prism only partially over the visual axis over the good eye, while covering the bad eye, intermittently causing monocular diplopia. The prism is then completely moved over the good eye while the bad eye is uncovered. This results in true binocular diplopia with each eye seeing the same but separate lines of Snellen acuity. For example, if an 8-diopter base-up prism is held over the good eye, the patient is then asked to read the higher line. If the patient reads the upper line, the examiner has established the acuity of the bad eye at that

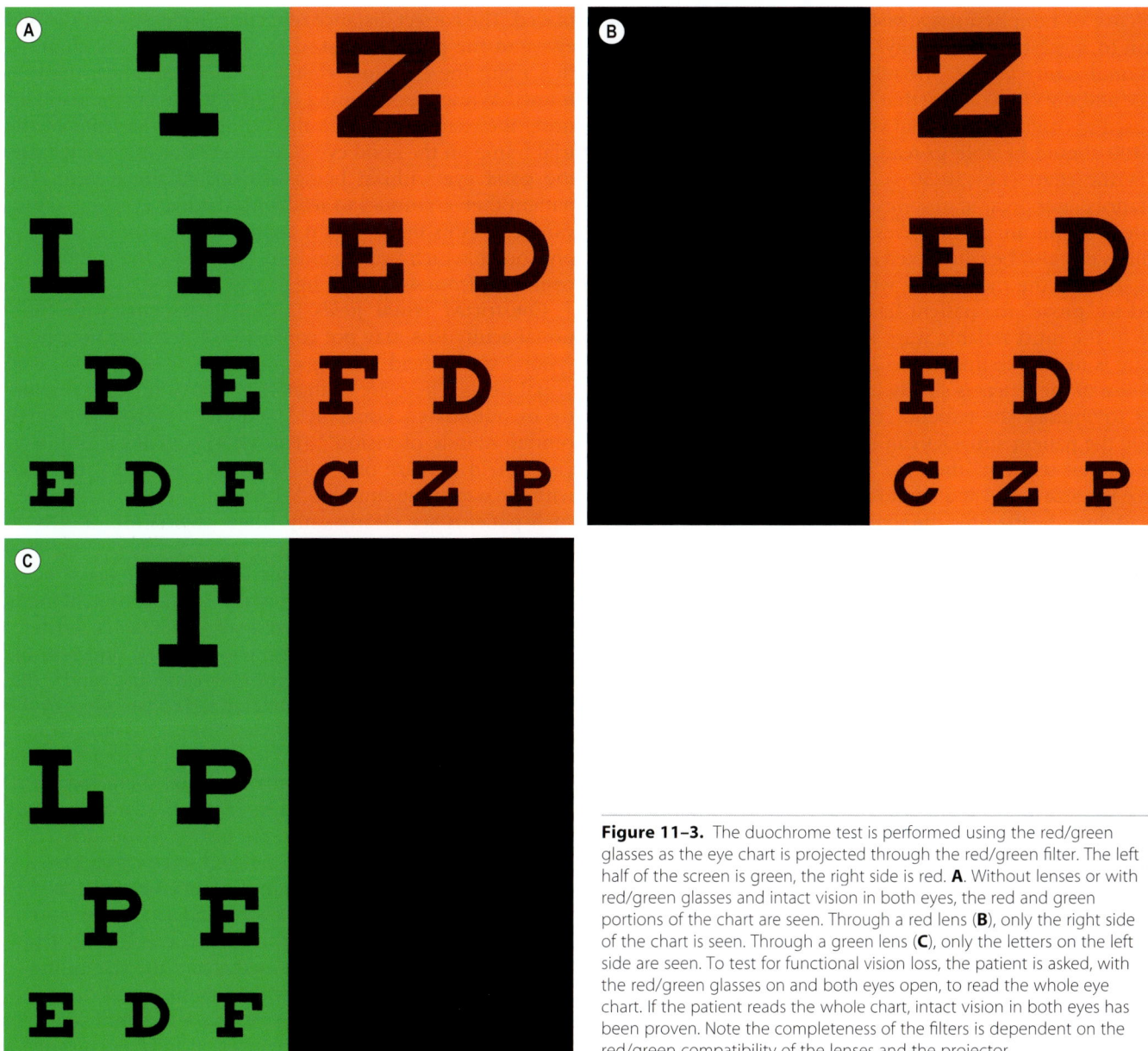

Figure 11–3. The duochrome test is performed using the red/green glasses as the eye chart is projected through the red/green filter. The left half of the screen is green, the right side is red. **A**. Without lenses or with red/green glasses and intact vision in both eyes, the red and green portions of the chart are seen. Through a red lens (**B**), only the right side of the chart is seen. Through a green lens (**C**), only the letters on the left side are seen. To test for functional vision loss, the patient is asked, with the red/green glasses on and both eyes open, to read the whole eye chart. If the patient reads the whole chart, intact vision in both eyes has been proven. Note the completeness of the filters is dependent on the red/green compatibility of the lenses and the projector.

level. Golnik et al.[40] have demonstrated that a simplified version of this test, in which a 4-diopter vertical prism is placed in front of the better eye and the patient is asked if they see one image or two vertically separated images, can be used as a simplified screening tool. In their study, patients with normal vision always saw two images; patients with poor vision only saw one image and 31/35 with suspected nonorganic vision loss reported seeing two images. The other four were found to have occult organic pathology.

Magic drop test. "Suggestible innocent" patients[5] (Table 11–1) may believe that a magic drop placed in their eye is going to temporarily improve their vision. It is important to emphasize that the improvement is only temporary since many patients are not going to be ready to "give up" their "poor" vision immediately. A topical anesthetic, with the bottle's label hidden, can be used. As it is instilled, it may be helpful for the examiner to say that if the vision improves with this drop, it will "help to understand better what part of the eye is having the problem." Putting the patient's distance refraction and a pinhole in a trial frame while the patient reads with the "magic drop" often helps the patient to see even better. This test is very effective in children because of their suggestibility, as moments later vision amazingly improves and then reverts to the predrop level. This is another test that establishes a better level of vision that what the patient claims.

Moderate monocular vision loss

Each of the methods outlined above for more severe unilateral vision loss is helpful in patients with complaints of more moderate visual acuity loss in the range of 20/40 to 20/100. However, in this situation the examiner often encounters a more sophisticated patient and finds the job of "proving" that the patient has better vision more difficult. Many times better acuity cannot be demonstrated, and the presence of nonphysiologic visual field loss must be relied upon to suggest nonorganicity.

Visual acuity testing. The relationship of the testing distance and the visual acuity that the patient is able to see can be used to confirm functional visual loss. A person who sees 20/100 should be able to read the 20/50 line from 10 feet from the chart (i.e., 10/50 = 20/100). By varying testing distances, nonorganic responses can usually be demonstrated. Significant mismatches between distance and near acuities can also be considered evidence of functional visual loss. Finally, the method by which acuity is tested may be used to "prove" the patient has better vision. For instance, one of the most reliable ways to demonstrate better visual acuity is to start testing at the 20/10 line of the chart. Then the size of the letters is slowly increased while the examiner tries to "outlast the patient." Prolonged periods of silence while the patient struggles can be followed by "are you sure you cannot see that" then by "OK, the letters will become twice the size now." If a chart is used that has three or four 20/20 lines, by the time the sixth line (20/25) is reached the patient often tires, acquiesces, and reads the line. "Counting" acuity may also be helpful in proving patients with moderate acuity loss see better. For this test the patient is asked to count the number of letters on a given line even if they are unable to read them. Levy et al.[42] determined that being able to count the 20/10 line requires acuity at least equal to 20/30 or better, counting 20/25 requires 20/80 acuity and counting between 20/30 and 20/60 meant an acuity of at least 20/200.

Another relatively simple test of visual acuity can be performed while testing near vision. A reading card with a paragraph of prose is used, and the patient is asked to read 20/20 size print with both eyes and near correction. The patient reads smoothly because the good eye is open. The patient is then asked to do the same thing with a pen held vertically between the eyes and the reading material. If the patient continues to read smoothly without having to move his or her head to look around the pen, then both eyes must have been able to see.

Fogging. The fogging technique involves blurring the good eye with lenses while the patient views the acuity chart binocularly. The acuity level achieved thereby represents the function of the supposed bad eye. One technique uses the phoropter, and the examiner makes numerous lens changes for several seconds involving the dials for both eyes. Eventually a small amount of sphere or cylinder over the bad eye and a +6.00-diopter lens over the good eye are in place. This maneuver blurs the vision of the good eye. The patient is then asked quietly but quickly to read the Snellen line in question. This technique is outstanding with suggestible patients, but in our experience many patients are sophisticated enough to be aware of the blurring of the good eye and close it.

An alternative method of using paired cylinders is subtler and may be more effective.[5,15] The blurring of the good eye is less obvious to the patient with this technique than with high-plus lenses. To perform this test a trial frame is used, and a plus and minus cylinders of 3.00 diopters each are placed on the same axis over the good eye with one lens in the posterior, nonrotating slot where spheres are usually placed. The correct distance refraction is placed over the bad eye, and the patient is asked to start reading the chart. At that point the examiner claims to need to "adjust the trial frame." While repositioning the trial frame on the patient's nose, the examiner rotates the cylinder in the front of the trial frame on the good eye 20 degrees. This effectively blurs the good eye without being obvious to the patient. The patient then continues to read with the bad eye. One disadvantage of this test is that it cannot be performed with the phoropter, which usually aids in distracting the patient and confusing from which eye he or she is seeing.

Constricted visual fields. Although patients with functional acuity loss may not complain of defective peripheral vision, visual field testing commonly reveals constricted visual fields. These are characterized on Goldmann perimetry or automated visual field analysis by preserved small central islands of vision[43] (**Fig. 11-4**). On the Goldmann visual field the size of the field often does not vary much with the size of the stimulus. With confrontation techniques, such patients see clearly only when objects are directly in front of their face.

Nonspecific generalized constriction of the visual fields with central visual field sparing is also characteristic of many organic conditions including end-stage glaucoma, bilateral occipital lobe damage, atrophic papilledema, and retinitis pigmentosa. Patients with functional visual loss can be distinguished from true cases of generalized constriction by the following maneuvers:

1. *Tubular visual fields.* The test is based on the principle that the normal visual field increases in size as the eye is moved farther away from the testing plane. It is generally performed with a tangent screen (**Fig. 11-5**), although simple confrontation methods can also be used. A monocular field is tested first at 1 meter, and the screen is marked with the patient's responses. The patient is then moved to 2 meters and the size of the stimulus is doubled. The field is retested, and many patients with functional visual loss will demonstrate tunneling without physiologic visual field expansion. A novel version of this test, using a computerized Goldmann perimeter and a reverse telescope to simulate an increase in test distance, effectively distinguishes true central islands of vision in organic disease from functional fields.[44] In nonorganic patients with only a central island of vision, the field, like with the tangent screen test, did not expand or even constricted when the reverse telescope was used. In contrast, patients with real field loss demonstrated expansion of the visual field when looking through the reverse telescope.

2. *Pantomime.* Patients who claim to have a small central visual field can often be fooled with the "Simon says trick." In this test the examiner claims to be doing a neurologic examination, and the patient's vigilance decreases because it appears as if vision is not being tested. The examiner holds both of his or her hands up beyond the central 30 degrees of the patient's visual field as they face each other. The examiner then begins with verbal commands such as "open and close your

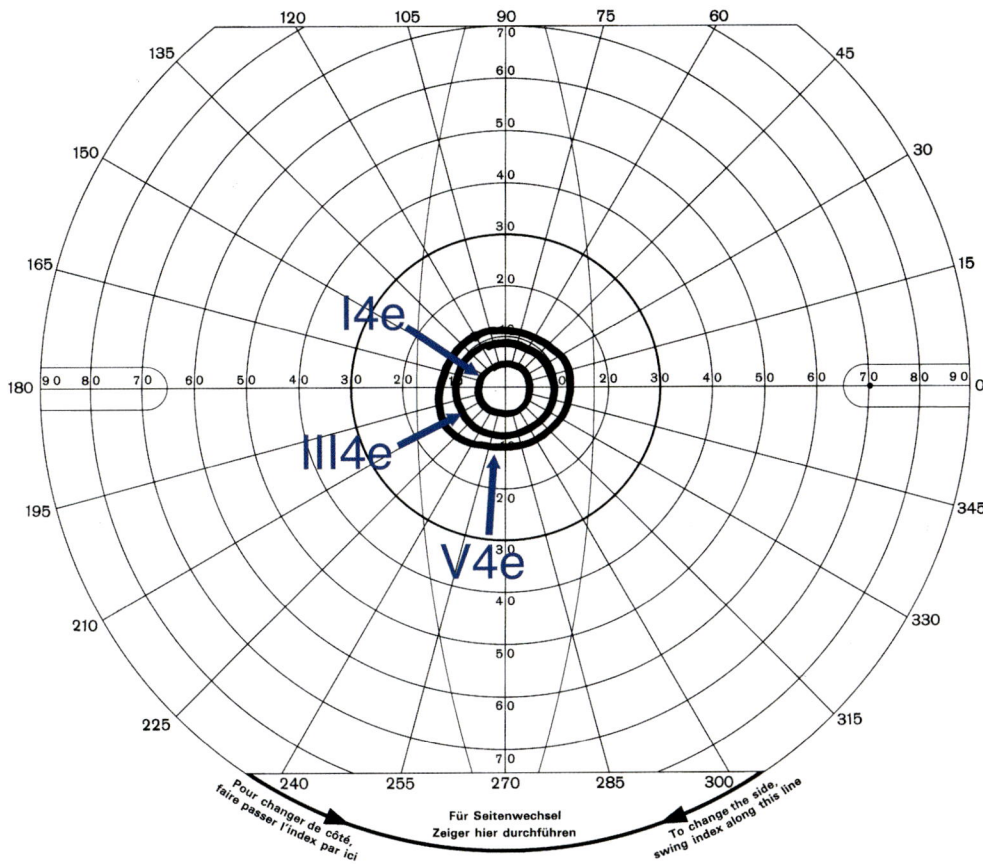

Figure 11–4. Goldmann visual field demonstrating generalized constriction. Note that each stimulus is associated with approximately the same size visual field.

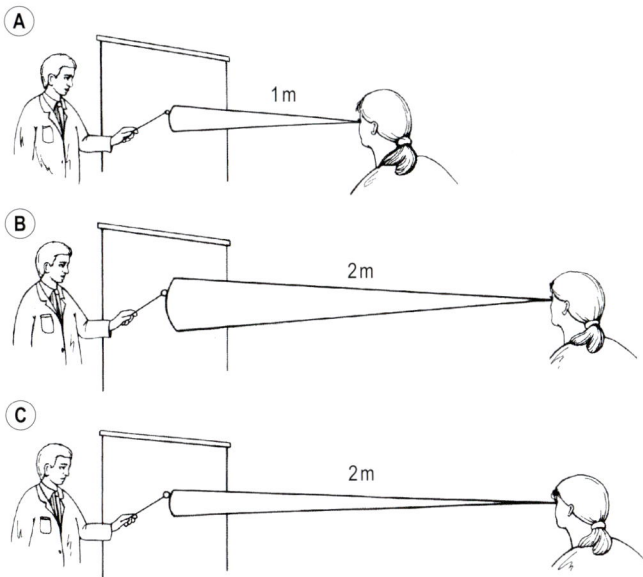

Figure 11–5. Testing for tubular visual fields with the tangent screen. **A**. The field is tested at one meter with a 9-mm white object and the results marked on the screen with chalk. **B**. When the patient with organic visual field loss is moved to 2 meters from the screen and the stimulus size doubled (18-mm white), the field expands to twice the size. **C**. The patient with functional visual loss demonstrates tubular fields as the field does not expand even though the testing distance is increased from 1–2 meters and the target size is doubled.

hands" or "hold up two fingers on each hand." At the same time the examiner is doing what he or she has asked the patient to perform. Suddenly the examiner makes a different type of hand or finger movement without a verbal command to the patient. If the patient mimics the movement accurately, intact visual fields beyond the central 30 degrees are confirmed.

3. *Nonphysiologic constriction.* Some patients may demonstrate nonphysiologic constriction of isopters with a field associated with larger stimuli actually smaller than the field with smaller stimuli (**Fig. 11–6**). It is occasionally helpful to begin perimetry with the smallest isopter so the examiner can demonstrate a normal-sized visual field before the patient begins voluntarily to constrict the field. For instance, a patient with an intact 10-degree Ile (the smallest, dimmest stimulus) field in the Goldmann perimeter is unlikely to be suffering from organic visual loss. The test can also be repeated with encouragement, such as telling the patient that he or she does not have to wait until the entire stimulus is seen with certainty before pushing the buzzer. A different result on retest is suggestive of functional visual loss. Nonphysiologic constriction of the visual field on computerized perimetry can take on a characteristic pattern called a "clover leaf" visual field defect (**Fig. 11–7**). Generally, rounded areas of visual field sparing with peripheral defects in all four quadrants resulting in a clover leaf

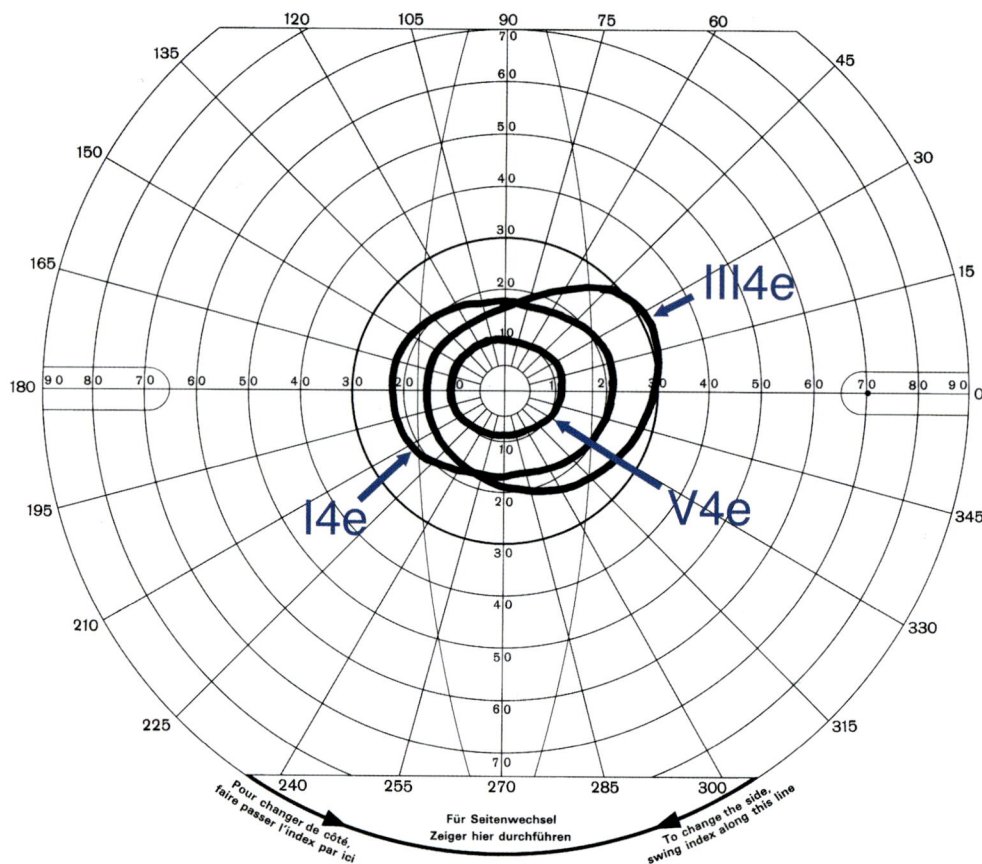

Figure 11–6. Goldmann visual field demonstrating "criss-crossing" of isopters. Note that there are parts of the visual field that are larger when testing with the smaller III4e stimulus compared to the larger V4e stimulus, and the 14e field is larger than the V4e field. This is nonphysiologic.

appearance on the gray scale are seen along with a high false positive rate. Visual field constriction which resolves with suggestion or varies over time is also suggestive of functional visual loss (**Fig. 11–7**).

4. *Spiraling*. A classic alteration of the visual field on Goldmann perimetry in patients with functional visual loss is called *spiraling* (**Fig. 11–8**). In this case the patient, often the "worried impostor" type[5] (Table 11–1), becomes more and more hesitant to respond to the same stimulus as it is sequentially presented along radial angles. The resultant field nonphysiologically spirals to the center as responses are delayed.

Moderate binocular vision loss

Patients with mild to moderate functional visual acuity loss of 20/40 to 20/60 in both eyes can be some of the most difficult patients to deal with. This slight level of acuity reduction is often sufficient to qualify for disability benefits, yet the patient is able to continue with daily activities, including driving and recreation. They claim binocular vision loss, and the patients are simply unwilling ever to report being able to see the smaller lines on the eye chart. Tests described above that depend on the tricking the patient with purported monocular visual loss into using the supposed bad eye cannot be used effectively. Except for the potential acuity meter technique, for the most part the examiner must depend largely on nonphysiologic responses

during visual acuity and field testing as described above to make the diagnosis.

Potential acuity meter. The potential acuity meter can be used in this setting to demonstrate better vision.[45] This apparatus projects the Snellen acuity letters directly onto the retina and is more commonly used to establish the potential visual acuity in patients with cataracts. The functional patient is informed that a problem has been found and that the diagnosis will be confirmed with this next test. It can be explained that the problem is likely in the retina, and it will be "bypassed with the potential acuity meter and the eye chart will be shone directly on the optic nerve." The patient will often read at a normal level in this circumstance.

Functional visual field loss

Tunneling of the visual fields and spiraling are often associated with functional visual loss, and as described above suggest the nonorganic nature of vision loss in many patients. However, in some patients, visual field deficits are the sole or primary manifestation of functional visual loss.

Perimetry. Visual field defects can be presented or "created" on any type of perimeter. That is, functional visual fields can be found in patients tested with sophisticated automated threshold perimetry as well as standard kinetic perimetry.[46–53] Visual field defects such as hemianopias (**Fig. 11–7**) and quadrantanopias can be fabricated on the automated

Central 30-2 Threshold Test

Fixation Monitor: Gaze/Blindspot
Fixation Target: Central
Fixation Losses: 2/22
False POS Errors: 5 %
False NEG Errors: 46 %
Test Duration: 10:24

Fovea: 35 dB

Stimulus: III, White
Background: 31.5 ASB
Strategy: SITA-Standard

Pupil Diameter: 4.5 mm
Visual Acuity:
RX: +1.50 DS   DC X

GHT
Outside normal limits

MD   -11.28 dB P < 0.5%
PSD   13.54 dB P < 0.5%

Total Deviation

Pattern Deviation

(A)

(B)

+0.12 lens

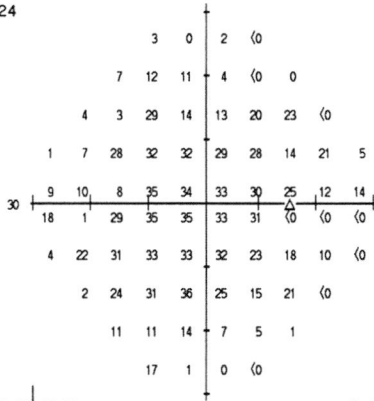

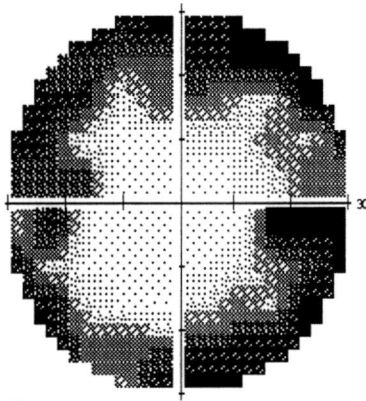

Figure 11-7. Examples of functional responses on computerized testing in three different patients with visual field constriction. **A**. Computerized visual fields demonstrating typical "cloverleaf" pattern of generalized constriction often seen in nonorganic vision loss. A high false positive rate is seen as well. **B**. Left eye inferior field loss and superior constriction which resolved with a +0.12 (negligible) lens which the patient was told would improve her visual field deficit.

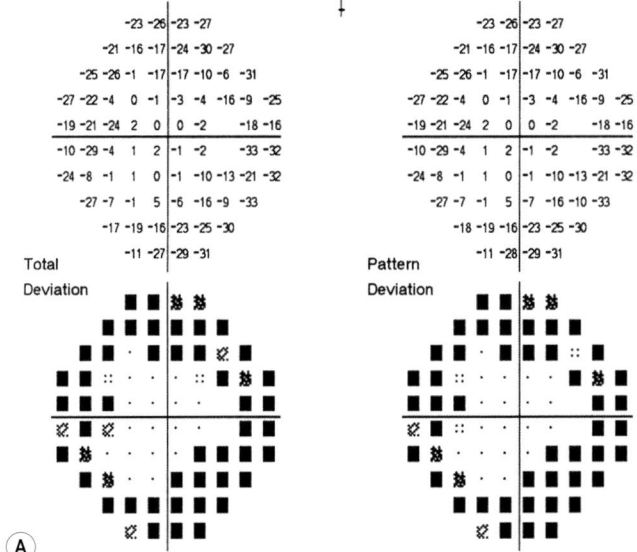

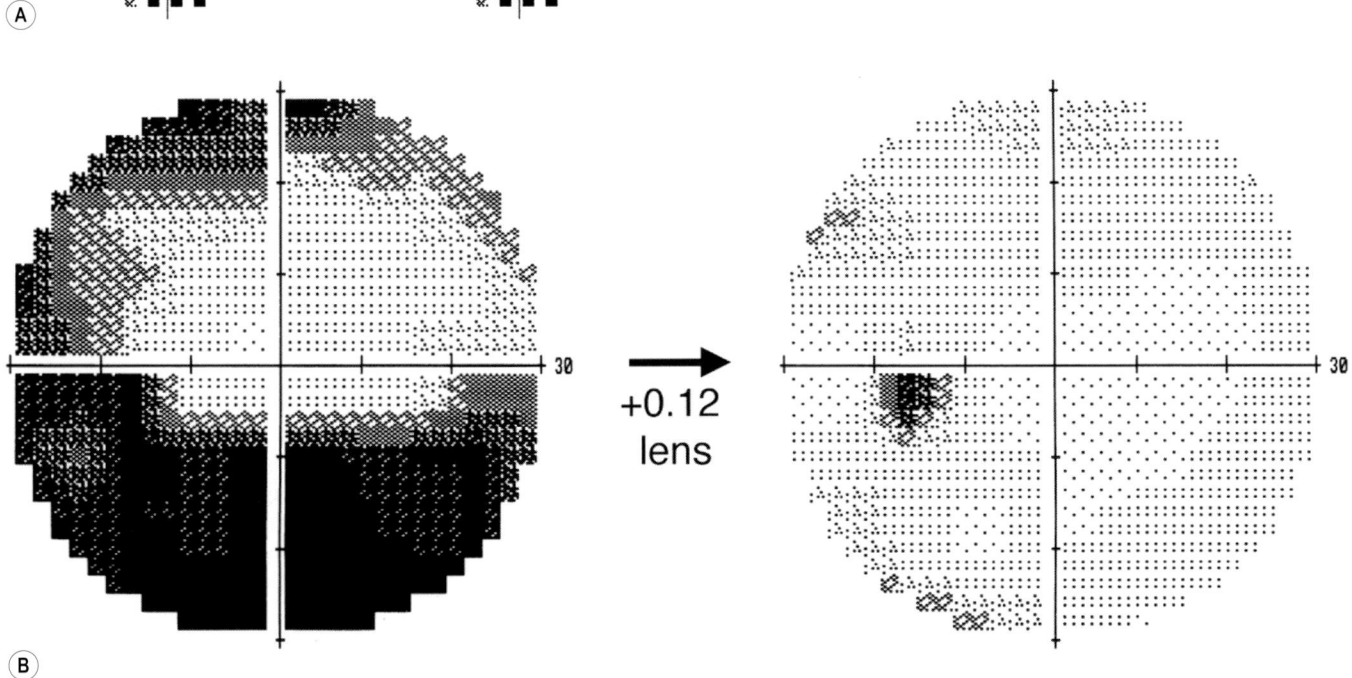

387

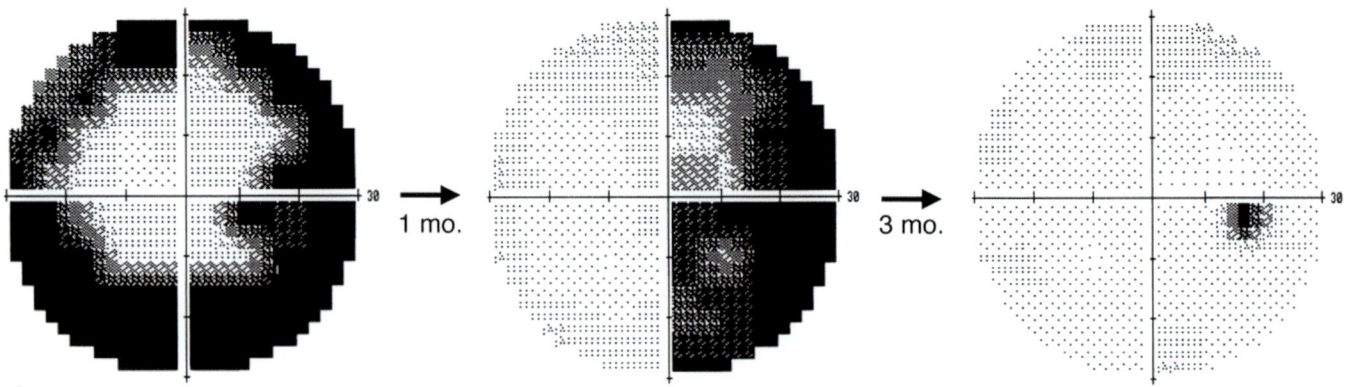

Figure 11–7. cont'd C. Right eye visual field constriction. One month later there was a temporal field defect, and three months after that the field defect spontaneously resolved.

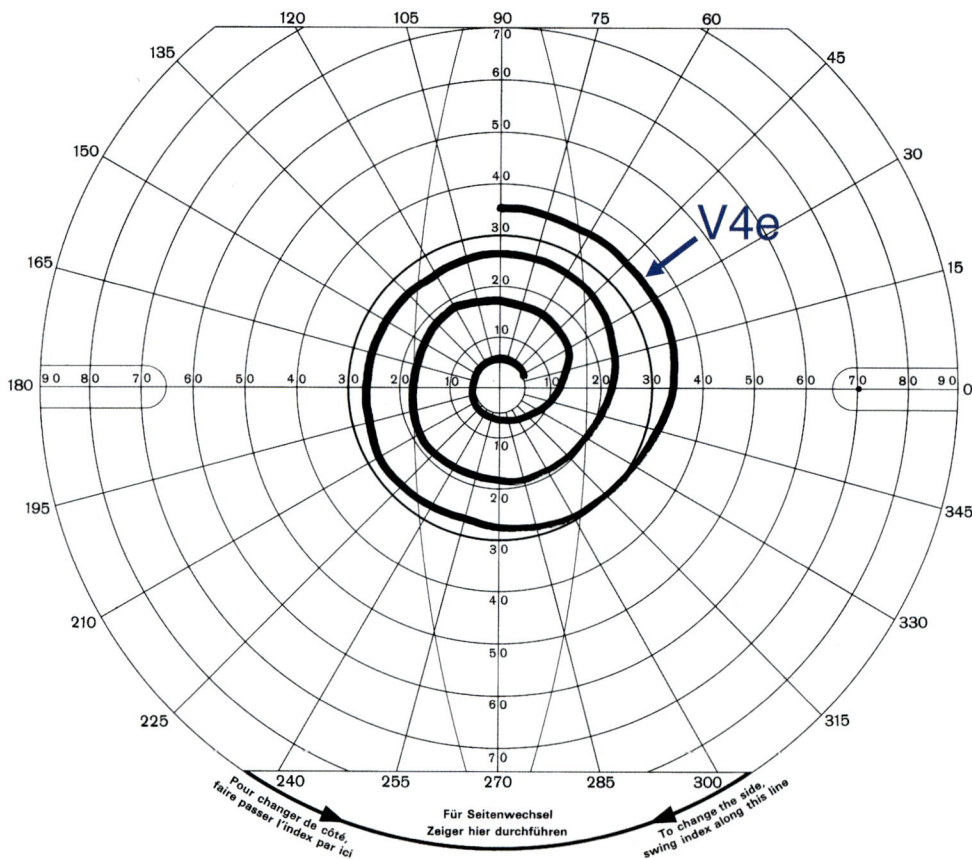

Figure 11–8. Goldmann visual field demonstrating nonphysiologic spiraling. As the test proceeds along adjacent radii, the patient responds later and later. The field "spirals" to the center.

perimeter, and in such cases the reliability parameters such as false positives and negatives are not helpful in identifying a voluntary alteration of the field.[51] However, the presence of an inter-eye difference in the mean threshold light sensitivity of 8.7 dB in patients with organic visual loss has been shown nearly always to produce an RAPD.[54] Therefore if such a difference exists, and there is no RAPD, functional visual field loss is likely present.

Bitemporal hemianopia. Functional visual loss can present as a bitemporal hemianopia[47,55] Patients, presumably unaware of the anatomic basis of the visual fields and the

localization of bitemporal hemianopia to the chiasm, may complain of loss of side vision, loss of peripheral vision, or tunnel vision. The key to the diagnosis here is the discrepancy between visual field tests when performed monocularly versus binocularly.[48,50,55] Standard perimetry is performed on each eye and results in a bitemporal hemianopia. The test is then repeated with both eyes open. Patients do not typically realize the extent of the nasal field of the contralateral eye. This area of intact vision disappears when the eyes are tested together because they assume the temporal visual field is only seen by the ipsilateral eye.

Monocular temporal hemianopia. Similar strategies can be applied in patients complaining of only monocular temporal visual field defects, the so-called missing half defect.[48,50,55,56] Despite the full nasal field of the normal other eye, binocular visual field testing fails to show an intact temporal field on the side of the "affected" eye (**Fig. 11–9**).[57] A similar strategy may be employed using computerized perimetry as well.[58] Such nonphysiologic results confirm there is some nonorganicity to the complaints. However, they do not prove necessarily that the monocular field defect is not real.

Saccades. The presence of accurate saccadic movement by an eye into an allegedly blind hemifield suggests nonorganic

visual field loss. The examiner tells the patient that eye movements are next to be tested. The patient is first asked to follow the examiner's finger with pursuit movements. Then the patient is asked to look quickly at the examiner's finger presented in the blind hemifield; if the saccade is accurate, an intact field is implied. The patient will often hesitate and say "I cannot see it that well in my peripheral vision." The examiner responds by saying "I know, therefore I want you to look at it with your central vision" and precise saccadic eye movements sometimes follow.

Central scotomas. Central scotomas are exceedingly rare manifestations of functional visual loss,[17] but they have been

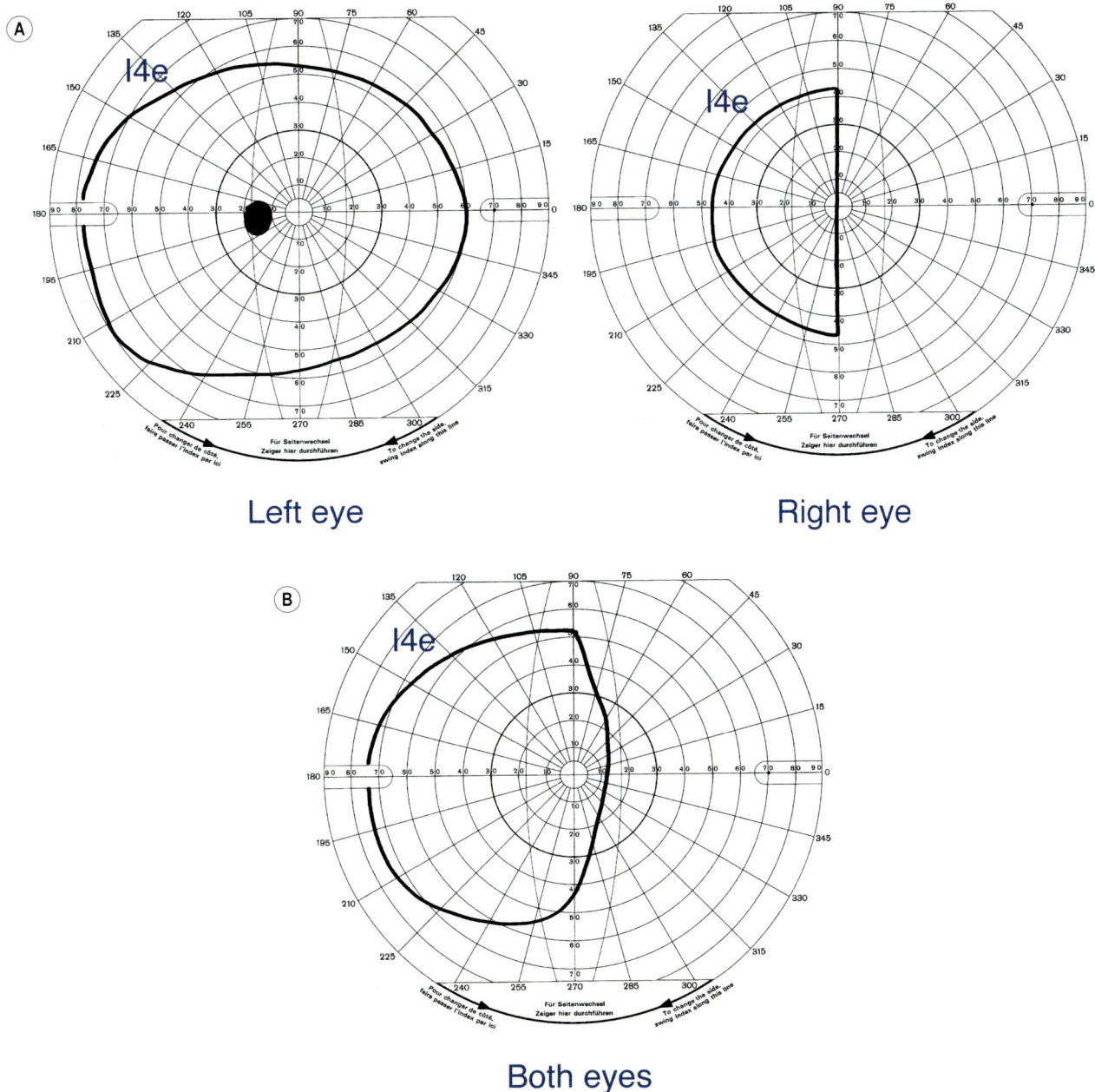

Figure 11–9. Testing for nonorganic temporal visual field defect using binocular Goldmann visual fields. The patient complains of temporal field loss in the right eye, which is documented in **A**. Note the visual field of the left eye is normal. **B**. The patient is then tested binocularly and believes that the right side of the visual field is seen only by the right eye. Therefore, a persistent temporal defect is present despite the presence of intact right-sided (nasal) visual field in the left eye.

reported. Patients with functional visual loss for the most part lack the sophistication required to know that a profound reduction of central acuity may occur despite intact peripheral fields. When a central scotoma is found, an extensive search for a maculopathy or optic neuropathy must be undertaken. Finally, patients complaining only of paracentral visual field defects can be tested using the red Amsler's grid and the red/green glasses.[59] If the scotoma disappears when the red lens is over the affected eye, and the green lens is over the good eye, then the patient is functional. The grid can only be seen through the red lens, and the patient's assumption that he or she can see it because the good eye is being used is incorrect.

Findings and diagnosis of functional visual loss in children

Children with functional visual loss most commonly present with moderate binocular deficits, with visual acuities in the range of 20/40 to 20/100. The child often seems to exert tremendous effort as he or she attempts to read the eye chart. Guesses are often completely wrong.

Diagnosis. In contrast to adults, who often have to be "tricked" into seeing better, children are much more easily coaxed into exhibiting normal visual acuity or visual fields with relatively simple maneuvers such as plano lenses or verbal encouragement. Many of the tests outlined above are also effective in children with functional visual loss. The technique described above in which the examiner starts with the smallest letters and acts surprised as he or she moves slowly up the chart to letters of increasing size (frequently combined with a low-power lens) often demonstrates better vision. "Magic drops" such as topical anesthetics, with the appropriate convincing, will often be quite effective. Stereo-acuity testing is another very effective way to demonstrate better vision since most young patients fail to realize the test requires binocular vision.

Overview of efferent nonorganic neuro-ophthalmic disorders

Efferent nonorganic neuro-ophthalmic disorders are much less common than afferent problems and can affect ocular motility or alignment, the eyelids, or the pupil. Commonly encountered problems are voluntary nystagmus and convergence spasm.[60] These topics will be mentioned briefly, as they are described in more detail in other chapters.

Factitious pupillary abnormalities. Nonorganic pupillary abnormalities can only result from the patient instilling something in the eye to make the pupil either larger or smaller. The distinction of pharmacologic dilation of the pupil from other causes of a fixed dilated pupil such as a third nerve palsy or Adie's pupil is described in Chapter 13. The key features of the pharmacologically dilated pupil are the wide dilation to 7–8 mm and the absence of constriction when 1% pilocarpine is instilled. The majority of pharmacologically dilated pupils are due to a chemical (often never identified) getting into an eye inadvertently. This is in contradistinction to a patient who knowingly places something in the eye in an attempt to create concern. These

patients often have knowledge of various available drops that can dilate pupils and also know that this examination finding will likely be interpreted as a neurologic emergency. For these reasons, many of these patients are health care workers.

Factitious ptosis. Factitious ptosis is relatively easily distinguished from true ptosis by the position of the eyebrow. Patients with true ptosis will be struggling to hold their eye open and will use the frontalis muscle to try and elevate the lid, thereby elevating the brow. The patient with factitious ptosis creates it with orbicularis contraction, thereby lowering the brow toward the eye.[61] Ptosis is discussed in greater detail in Chapter 14.

Factitious ophthalmoplegia: convergence spasm. Spasm of the near reflex, or convergence spasm, is characterized by esotropia (intermittent convergence), abduction limitation, accommodation (blurred distance vision), and miosis.[62–64] The condition is often associated with ocular discomfort and is always intermittent. Its differentiation from sixth nerve palsies and its differential diagnosis and management are reviewed in Chapter 15.

Video 15.3

Factitious nystagmus. Voluntary "nystagmus" occurs when a patient willingly initiates rapid back-to-back saccadic eye movements.[65] The movement, unlike true nystagmus, can be produced on command and can usually be sustained for only a few moments. The condition is recognized by its voluntary nature and by the frequently associated orbicularis contraction, blinking, eyelid flutter, and convergence. This eye movement disorder is also discussed in Chapter 17.

Video 17.1

Management of the patient with nonorganic symptoms

Differential diagnosis. It is paramount in this setting to be absolutely certain about the diagnosis of functional visual loss and to exclude any true disease that requires treatment.[17] When normal vision can be proven, and the examination is otherwise normal, the examiner may be more comfortable regarding the absence of organicity. However, in many instances a true underlying disorder cannot be excluded, particularly when normal vision cannot be proven.

The most common diseases that need to be considered in the differential diagnosis of functional visual loss include amblyopia, optic neuropathies, retinal degenerations and dystrophies, and cortical visual loss. Thus, when the diagnosis is uncertain, magnetic resonance imaging with contrast should be performed. Electroretinography should then be considered in all patients to exclude retinal dysfunction. When unrevealing, neuroimaging with nuclear medicine techniques to assess brain function (single proton emission computed tomography (SPECT) or positron emission tomography (PET)) can be performed. Moster et al.[66] reported two cases of cortical visual loss that were initially thought to be functional because of normal conventional neuroimaging. Ultimately the patients were determined to have cortical dysfunction based on occipital lobe hypoperfusion on SPECT. In addition, more occult forms of optic neuropathy, including hereditary conditions, inflammations associated with systemic illness, and nutritional causes, should be excluded. These can be screened for by examining family members, careful systemic evaluation by an internist, and appropriate blood tests.

Management of functional visual loss in adults. The successful management of patients with nonorganic neuro-ophthalmic symptoms begins with physician empathy and encouragement. For the most part, there is nothing to gain by confronting the patient. The best approach for the examiner is to acknowledge to the patient that a thorough examination of his or her eyes suggests that he or she is healthy. In particular, emphasis can be placed on statements that the patient is likely to agree with, such as the peripheral vision seems good, and the optic nerves appear healthy. The examiner can continue along these lines by saying that there is no evidence of serious neurologic illness such as a brain tumor, stroke, or multiple sclerosis. Finally, the examiner can state that he or she has seen similar patients who often improve with time as the "brain" once again realizes the visual potential of the eye.

Specific interventions have been reported to "improve" vision in patients with functional visual loss. These include the use of various drops, low-power spectacle prescription, contact lenses, and "retinal rest." Retinal rest[25] was a treatment used by physicians in the military after a diagnosis of a strained or tired retina was made. The patient's eyes were patched, the eyes covered, and the patient isolated from all auditory stimuli with minimal contact with others. Vision was checked every day and usually improved spontaneously. Outside of a military structure, it seems unlikely that this strategy could be applied. However, for some highly suggestible patients this treatment option seems ideal. Hypnosis and psychoanalysis have also been reported to be successful treatments of functional visual loss.[67,68] In Kathol et al.'s series,[69] 22 of the 42 patients had a diagnosable psychiatric condition or personality disorder. In contrast, in our experience (given the high prevalence of deliberate malingerers) and that of others,[5,15,18] the vast majority of patients neither require nor benefit from psychiatric intervention.

Fortunately, many patients with functional visual loss do not continue to revisit the physician demanding an explanation or pleading for help. Kathol et al.[15] found that most of the patients that were seen in follow-up were less bothered by their "vision loss" although they continued to demonstrate nonphysiologic responses on testing. Sletteberg et al.[1] found that half of their patients had spontaneous resolution, but 22% of their patients were still "disabled" because of their vision loss.

Patients who indeed have organic visual deficits but have superimposed nonphysiologic vision loss are often the most problematic. Scott and Egan[17] found that 71/133 (56%) of their patients with functional vision loss had organic findings on examination, indicating that functional findings were superimposed on true disease. Lim et al[10] found organic disease was present in 17% of their 138 pediatric and adult patients with functional vision loss. In such patients it can be very difficult to determine the exact amount of organic vision loss, making diagnostic and therapeutic decisions very difficult. There are no easy guidelines to help manage such patients. This may be the one time when discussion with the patient about concerns about his or her nonphysiologic responses is worthwhile (particularly for the "worried impos-

tor," see **Table 11–1**). Explaining to the patient that avoiding a risky treatment or intervention might result in improvement of the nonorganic component of the vision loss.

Management of functional visual loss in children. As with adults, the most productive interaction between the child with functional visual loss and the examiner occurs when the latter demonstrates empathetic, optimistic, and encouraging behavior. Once the diagnosis of functional visual loss without organicity in child has been made, we often speak to the parents without the child present. We explain that we cannot find anything wrong with the child's eyes or visual pathways. We tell them that we believe the child is not "making this up," but rather may have the visual problem as a result of some external trigger or stress. We emphasize to the parents that they should optimistically encourage their child, rather than accuse the child of dragging them to unnecessary doctor's visits and tests. Then we talk to the child in front of the parents, and explain to the child in an encouraging manner that we believe his or her vision will improve over the next few weeks. We schedule a follow-up visit in approximately 3 months, and suggest to the child the vision will likely improve by then. We have found this approach in children with suspected functional visual loss to be extremely successful both therapeutically and diagnostically. Lack of any visual improvement or worsening of vision at the 3-month follow-up is suggestive of an underlying organic disorder, and as such at a minimum neuroimaging, visual evoked potentials, and an electroretinogram should be considered.

In general, the prognosis for "visual recovery" in children with functional visual loss is excellent.[10,70] In Mantyjarvi's series of children,[16] one-third improved spontaneously. Catalano et al[13] found that one third of their patients were better within 1 day, and three-quarters were better by 2 months.

References

1. Sletteberg O, Bertelsen T, Hovding G. The prognosis of patients with hysterical visual impairment. Acta Ophthalmol (Copenh) 1989;67:159–163.
2. Rowland WD, Rowe AW. Marked concentric contraction of the visual fields: a study of 100 consecutive cases. Trans Am Acad Ophthalmol 1929;34;107–114.
3. Schaegel TF, Jr., Quilala FV. Hysterical amblyopia. Statistical analysis of forty-two cases found in a survey of eight hundred unselected eye patients at a university medical center. Arch Ophthalmol 1955;54;875–884.
4. Asher R. Munchausen's syndrome. Lancet 1951;1:339–341.
5. Thompson HS. Functional visual loss. Am J Ophthalmol 1985;100:209–213.
6. Rada RT, Meyer GG, Kellner R. Visual conversion reaction in children and adults. J Nerv Ment Dis 1978;166:580–587.
7. Weller M, Wiedemann P. Hysterical symptoms in ophthalmology. Doc Ophthalmol 1989;73:1–33.
8. Keltner JL. The California syndrome. A threat to all. Arch Ophthalmol 1988;106:1053–1054.
9. Drinnan MJ, Marmor MF. Functional visual loss in Cambodian refugees: a study of cultural factors in ophthalmology. Eur J Ophthalmol 1991;1:115–118.
10. Lim SA, Siatkowski RM, Farris BK. Functional visual loss in adults and children patient characteristics, management, and outcomes. Ophthalmology 2005;112:1821–1828.
11. Stephens JH, Kamp M. On some aspects of hysteria: a clinical study. J Nerv Ment Dis 1962;134:305–315.
12. Ziegler FJ, Imboden JB, Meyer E. Contemporary conversion reactions: a clinical study. Am J Psychiatry 1960;116:901–910.
13. Catalono RA, Simon JW, Krohel GB, et al. Functional visual loss in children. Ophthalmology 1986;93:385–390.
14. Clarke WN, Noel LP, Bariciak M. Functional visual loss in children: a common problem with an easy solution. Can J Ophthalmol 1996;31:311–313.
15. Kathol RG, Cox TA, Corbett JJ, et al. Functional visual loss. Follow-up of 42 cases. Arch Ophthalmol 1983;101:729–735.
16. Mantyjarvi MI. The amblyopic schoolgirl syndrome. J Pediatr Ophthalmol Strabismus 1981;18:30–33.

17. Scott JA, Egan RA. Prevalence of organic neuro-ophthalmologic disease in patients with functional visual loss. Am J Ophthalmol 2003;135:670–675.

18. Rada RT, Krill AE, Meyer GG, et al. Visual conversion reaction in children. II. Follow-up. Psychosomatics 1973;14:271–276.

19. Newman NJ. Neuro-ophthalmology and psychiatry. Gen Hosp Psychiatry 1993;15: 102–114.

20. Barris MC, Kaufman DI, Barberio D. Visual impairment in hysteria. Doc Ophthalmol 1992;82:369–382.

21. Kathol RG, Cox TA, Corbett JJ, et al. Functional visual loss: I. A true psychiatric disorder? Psychol Med 1983;13:307–314.

22. Bengtzen R, Woodward M, Lynn MJ, et al. The "sunglasses sign" predicts nonorganic visual loss in neuro-ophthalmologic practice. Neurology 2008;70:218–221.

23. Miller NR, Keane JR. Neuro-ophthalmologic manifestations of nonorganic disease. In: Miller NR, Newman NJ (eds). Walsh and Hoyt's Clinical Neuro-ophthalmology, 5th edn. Baltimore: Williams and Wilkins, 1998: 1765–1786.

24. Gruber H. Decrease of visual acuity in patients with clear media and normal fundi. Objective screening methods for differentiation and documentation. Doc Ophthalmol 1984;56:327–335.

25. Kramer KK, La Piana FG, Appleton B. Ocular malingering and hysteria: diagnosis and management. Surv Ophthalmol 1979;24:89–96.

26. Steele M, Seiple WH, Carr RE, et al. The clinical utility of visual-evoked potential acuity testing. Am J Ophthalmol 1989;108:572–577.

27. Towle VL, Sutcliffe E, Sokol S. Diagnosing functional visual deficits with the P300 component of the visual evoked potential. Arch Ophthalmol 1985;103:47–50.

28. Wildberger H, Huber C. [Visual evoked potentials in the evaluation of suspected simulation and aggravation]. Klin Monatsbl Augenheilkd 1980;176:704–707.

29. McBain VA, Robson AG, Hogg CR, et al. Assessment of patients with suspected non-organic visual loss using pattern appearance visual evoked potentials. Graefes Arch Clin Exp Ophthalmol 2007;245:502–510.

30. Xu S, Meyer D, Yoser S, et al. Pattern visual evoked potential in the diagnosis of functional visual loss. Ophthalmology 2001;108:76–80.

31. Gundogan FC, Sobaci G, Bayer A. Pattern visual evoked potentials in the assessment of visual acuity in malingering. Ophthalmology 2007;114:2332–2337.

32. Massicotte EC, Semela L, Hedges TR, 3rd. Multifocal visual evoked potential in nonorganic visual field loss. Arch Ophthalmol 2005;123:364–367.

33. Bumgartner J, Epstein CM. Voluntary alteration of visual evoked potentials. Ann Neurol 1982;12:475–478.

34. Morgan RK, Nugent B, Harrison JM, et al. Voluntary alteration of pattern visual evoked responses. Ophthalmology 1985;92:1356–1363.

35. Uren SM, Stewart P, Crosby PA. Subject cooperation and the visual evoked response. Invest Ophthalmol Vis Sci 1979;18:648–652.

36. Hess CW, Meienberg O, Ludin HP. Visual evoked potentials in acute occipital blindness. Diagnostic and prognostic value. J Neurol 1982;227:193–200.

37. Levy NS, Glick EB. Stereoscopic perception and Snellen visual acuity. Am J Ophthalmol 1974;78:722–724.

38. Savir H, Segal M. A simple test for detection of monocular functional visual impairment. Am J Ophthalmol 1988;106:500.

39. Fahle M, Mohn G. Assessment of visual function in suspected ocular malingering. Br J Ophthalmol 1989;73:651–654.

40. Golnik KC, Lee AG, Eggenberger ER. The monocular vertical prism dissociation test. Am J Ophthalmol 2004;137:135–137.

41. Slavin ML. The prism dissociation test in detecting unilateral functional visual loss. J Clin Neuroophthalmol 1990;10:127–130.

42. Levy AH, McCulley TJ, Lam BL, et al. Estimating visual acuity by character counting using the Snellen visual acuity chart. Eye 2005;19:622–624.

43. Linhart WO. Field findings in functional disease; report of 63 cases. Am J Ophthalmol 1956;42:75–84.

44. Pineles SL, Volpe NJ. Computerized kinetic perimetry detects tubular visual fields in patients with functional visual loss. Am J Ophthalmol 2004;137:933–935.

45. Levi L, Feldman RM. Use of the potential acuity meter in suspected functional visual loss. Am J Ophthalmol 1992;114:502–503.

46. Ellenberger C, Jr. Tunnel vision. Neurology 1984;34:129.

47. Fish RH, Kline LB, Hanumanthu VK, et al. Hysterical bitemporal hemianopia "cured" with contact lenses. J Clin Neuro-ophthalmol 1990;10:76–78.

48. Gittinger JW, Jr. Functional monocular temporal hemianopsia. Am J Ophthalmol 1986;101:226–231.

49. Glovinsky Y, Quigley HA, Bissett RA, et al. Artificially produced quadrantanopsia in computed visual field testing. Am J Ophthalmol 1990;110:90–91.

50. Keane JR. Hysterical hemianopia. The 'missing half' field defect. Arch Ophthalmol 1979;97:865–866.

51. Smith TJ, Baker RS. Perimetric findings in functional disorders using automated techniques. Ophthalmology 1987;94:1562–1566.

52. Stewart JF. Automated perimetry and malingerers. Can the Humphrey be outwitted? Ophthalmology 1995;102:27–32.

53. Thompson JC, Kosmorsky GS, Ellis BD. Field of dreamers and dreamed-up fields: functional and fake perimetry. Ophthalmology 1996;103:117–125.

54. Johnson LN, Hill RA, Bartholomew MJ. Correlation of afferent pupillary defect with visual field loss on automated perimetry. Ophthalmology 1988;95:1649–1655.

55. Mills RP, Glaser JS. Hysterical bitemporal hemianopia. Arch Ophthalmol 1981;99: 2053.

56. Gittinger JW, Jr. Functional hemianopsia: a historical perspective. Surv Ophthalmol 1988;32:427–432.

57. Keane JR. Patterns of hysterical hemianopia. Neurology 1998;51:1230–1231.

58. Martin TJ. Threshold perimetry of each eye with both eyes open in patients with monocular functional (nonorganic) and organic vision loss. Am J Ophthalmol 1998;125:857–864.

59. Slavin ML. The use of the red Amsler grid and red-green lenses in detecting spurious paracentral visual field defects. Am J Ophthalmol 1987;103:338–339.

60. Miller NR. Neuro-ophthalmologic manifestations of psychogenic disease. Semin Neurol 2006;26:310–320.

61. Keane JR. Neuro-ophthalmic signs and symptoms of hysteria. Neurology 1982;32:757–762.

62. Goldstein JH, Schneekloth BB. Spasm of the near reflex: a spectrum of anomalies. Surv Ophthalmol 1996;40:269–278.

63. Kung FT, Lai CW. Convergence spasm. Neurology 1983;33:1636–1637.

64. Sarkies NJ, Sanders MD. Convergence spasm. Trans Ophthalmol Soc U K 1985; 104(Pt 7):782–786.

65. Shults WT, Stark L, Hoyt WF, et al. Normal saccadic structure of voluntary nystagmus. Arch Ophthalmol 1977;95:1399–1404.

66. Moster ML, Galetta SL, Schatz NJ. Physiologic functional imaging in "functional" visual loss. Surv Ophthalmol 1996;40:395–399.

67. Greenleaf E. The Red House: hypnotherapy of hysterical blindness. Am J Clin Hypn 1971;13:155–161.

68. Wilkins LG, Field PB. Helpless under attack: hypnotic abreaction in hysterical loss of vision. Am J Clin Hypn 1968;10:271–275.

69. Kathol RG, Cox TA, Corbett JJ, et al. Functional visual loss: II. Psychiatric aspects in 42 patients followed for 4 years. Psychol Med 1983;13:315–324.

70. Bain KE, Beatty S, Lloyd C. Non-organic visual loss in children. Eye 2000;14(Pt 5): 770–772.

CHAPTER **12**

Visual hallucinations and illusions

Visual hallucinations and illusions comprise some of the most vivid and sometimes bizarre symptoms in neuro-ophthalmology. *Hallucinations* are defined as perceptions that occur in the absence of a corresponding external sensory stimulus.[1] Visual hallucinations can be classified as unformed/simple (e.g., dots, flashes, zig-zags) or formed/complex (actual objects or people). In contrast, *illusions* are misinterpretations of a true sensory stimulus.[2] Visual hallucinations and illusions are generally positive phenomena, in contrast to visual loss, which is a negative phenomenon.

The causes of visual hallucinations and illusions can be grouped into several major categories: migraine, release phenomena (in the setting of impaired vision), entoptic (ocular) phenomena, alcohol and drug-related, seizures, neurodegenerative disease, central nervous system lesions, psychiatric disease, and narcolepsy. These are summarized in **Table 12–1**, which also describes distinguishing features of each. This chapter will detail the various categories, but first theories on the pathogenesis of hallucinations and the history, examination, and diagnostic and therapeutic considerations in patients with hallucinations and illusions will be reviewed.

Hallucinations: theories on pathogenesis

Hughlings Jackson proposed that the central nervous system is organized into three levels: the higher cortical level; the middle structures (e.g., the basal ganglia), and the lowest level, of which the spinal cord is one part.[1] In this scheme, hallucinations were thought to occur when damage to the cortical level disinhibited activity of the middle level.

Subsequent authorities refined this notion that hallucinations can be release phenomena. West[3] theorized that in the normal waking state, the constant bombardment of external and internal stimuli inhibits the emergence of "previous perceptions." However, "impairment of information (sensory) input then permits the emergence or release of previously recorded percepts which can be woven into hallucinations." Cogan[4] presented patients with various ocular, optic nerve, chiasmal, tract, and occipital lesions who developed formed and complex visual sensations, and, like West, concluded that "a major factor in releasing the hallucinations is loss of the normally inhibiting visual control through blindness, hemianopia, or loss of cognitive functions." Similarly, in Fischer's "sensory/motor ratio" theory, an imbalance between internal and external sensory input is a necessary and sufficient condition for hallucinations.[5] ffytche and Howard[6] suggested that the quality of the release hallucinations is often reflective of dysfunction (and sometimes normal function) of striate and extrastriate cortex. For instance, color hallucinations may originate from area V4.

All hallucinations are not necessarily release phenomena, however. Clearly, some are due to abnormal biochemical states in the setting of alcohol, drugs, hallucinogens, or metabolic disturbances.[7] Dysfunction

Table 12–1 Major causes of visual hallucinations and illusions and their distinguishing features and clinical setting

Cause	Distinguishing feature(s) of visual hallucinations or illusions	Clinical setting
Migraine	Fortification spectra	Headache
	Scintillating scotomas	Personal or family history of migraine
	Develops and migrates over minutes	
	Persistent positive visual phenomena	
Release phenomena	Continuous	Visual loss
	Variable over time	
Entoptic phenomena	Phosphenes and photopsias	Observation of normal phenomena or ocular pathology
Alcohol and drugs	Colors	Accompanying auditory or tactile hallucinations
	Small insects or animals	History of substance abuse
	"Flashbacks"	
Seizures	Stereotyped	Other motor or sensory manifestations of seizures
	Brief	Abnormal EEG
Neurodegenerative		Clinical evidence of Parkinson's disease, dementia with Lewy bodies, or Alzheimer's disease
Focal neurologic lesions		
Peduncular hallucinations		Other evidence of a midbrain lesion
Palinopsia		Other evidence of an occipital lobe lesion
Cerebral diplopia and polyopia		Other evidence of an occipital lobe lesion
Upside down vision		Other evidence of a vestibular lesion
Psychiatric		Auditory hallucinations
		Delusions
		History of psychiatric disease
Narcolepsy		Sleep attacks
		Daytime somnolence

of the centrally acting neurotransmitters norepinephrine, dopamine, and serotonin has been implicated in the pathogenesis of visual hallucinations.[7] In Marrazzi's "neurophysiological dissociation" theory, it is proposed that hallucinogenic drugs have their effect by producing a functional dissociation between primary sensory cortex and cortical association areas.[5]

Other mechanisms for hallucinations include irritation of cortical neurons, as in epilepsy, and cognitive deficits, which can cause confusion between real stimuli and imagination.[2] Visual hallucinations related to migraine are thought to result from neuronal depression, without frank visual loss. Entoptic visual phenomena are images produced by normal physiologic events in the eye. For instance, some individuals become aware of the normal pulsation of their retinal vessels or are able to see white blood cells passing through retinal vasculature. Brainstem lesions causing visual hallucinations may affect ascending cholinergic and serotonergic pathways, resulting in associated sleep disturbances.[8] In the psychodynamic approach, hallucinations are thought to be similar to dreams, and Freud thought impairment of the ego allowed unconscious or preconscious material to enter consciousness and be misinterpreted as an external stimulus.[1,2]

More recent theories now account for the varied causes for visual hallucinations. ffytche[9] has proposed a classification scheme based upon three visual pathways in which the defect may occur: deafferentation (Charles Bonnet—see below), acetylcholine, or serotonin. Celesia[10] divided the etiologies into three other cateories: excitatory phenomena, release phenomena, and spreading depression.

History and examination in patients with visual hallucinations or illusions

The history is paramount in these patients because the diagnosis is frequently made based on the clinical setting and the detailed description of the visual symptoms. All too often the examination is unrevealing. The patient should be asked to detail the hallucinations or illusions, with particular attention to their content, complexity, and static or dynamic features. For illustrative purposes, it is often helpful to have him or her draw on paper or on the computer what is perceived.[11,12] One can ask whether the visual symptoms are monocular or binocular, but usually the patient has never checked or cannot make this distinction. In addition, their frequency, duration, and repetitiveness should be established. In some instances, patients with hallucinations or illusions are reluctant or ashamed to admit they have them because they fear a diagnosis of psychosis or dementia. With such individuals, encouragement from family members is often helpful.

Accompanying neurologic symptoms also can be very helpful in the diagnosis. For instance, a visual hallucination followed by a headache suggests migraine, while one followed by limb twitching and then loss of consciousness is suspicious of a seizure. The patient should be asked whether he or she knows if the perception is a hallucination or not. Insight is characteristic of release visual hallucinations (see below), for instance, while a schizophrenic with psychotic hallucinations might not be able to differentiate the hallucination from reality. Investigation into predisposing underlying conditions, such as metabolic disturbances, visual loss, psychiatric illnesses, alcohol intake, and drug use (illicit, recreational, or otherwise), is also extremely important.

The neuro-ophthalmic examination of a patient with visual hallucinations or illusions is directed toward excluding afferent pathway disease or another responsible lesion of the nervous system. Particular attention should be paid to visual acuity, color vision, pupillary reactivity, and the ophthalmoscopic examination. Even mild visual loss in the setting of macular degeneration or optic atrophy can be associated with release hallucinations, and these may be missed without a careful examination. We also prefer to perform formal visual field testing in almost every patient with a visual hallucination or illusion to exclude a field deficit. The neurologic examination, for example, should exclude an altered sensorium due to a mass lesion or toxic/metabolic disturbance; a hemiparesis or hemisensory loss suggestive of a hemispheric mass lesion; ataxia, third nerve palsy, or vertical gaze paresis consistent with a mesencephalic process (see peduncular hallucinations, below); nystagmus and imbalance associated with a brainstem or vestibular lesion; or evidence of Parkinson's or Alzheimer's disease.

Diagnostic and treatment considerations (overview)

Diagnosis

In one approach to the patient with visual hallucinations and illusions, the general categories (**Table 12–1**) should be considered first. Then, the patient's description of the visual phenomena is often very suggestive of a particular cause. Finally, the history and examination give the clinical setting and frequently supply clues to establish the proper diagnosis. For example, in a patient with a normal examination, a crescent of pulsating zig-zag lines seen in visual periphery, followed by a headache with nausea and vomiting, is most likely the result of a migraine. Brief episodes of flashing lights followed by loss of consciousness are more consistent with epilepsy. An individual with dense cataracts who complains of seeing people or objects that are not there may suffer from sensory deprivation associated with bilateral visual loss. This patient most likely has release hallucinations.

Treatment overview

In hallucinations due to migraine or epilepsy, the treatment is directed at the underlying disorder. In psychiatric and neurodegenerative disorders, treatment of the primary disorder is also important, but the addition of a neuroleptic is often required in these two conditions. In general, hallucinations associated with illicit or prescription drug use should be treated by removing the offending agent. In contrast, release visual hallucinations are very difficult to treat. Rarely affected patients require low-dose neuroleptics, but most often patient reassurance is the best management.

Migraine

A variety of visual hallucinations are characteristic of migraine.[13] These include enlarging scintillating scotomas and fortification spectra, or stars, sparks, flashes, or simple geometric forms. Visual illusions, experienced less commonly by migraineurs than hallucinations, include palinopsia (persistence of visual images), polyopia (multiple images), micropsia (shrunken images), macropsia (enlarged images), metamorphopsia (distortion of shape), and Alice in Wonderland syndrome (distortion of bodily image). These are summarized in **Table 12–2**.

The visual hallucinations and illusions associated with migraine are typically part of the aura. Previously termed *classic migraine*, the International Headache Society (IHS) now terms the condition *migraine with aura*.[14] The IHS defines a typical migraine aura as one that develops over more than 5 minutes, lasts less than 1 hour, and precedes (within 1 hour) or accompanies the headache (see Chapter 19, **Table 19–2**).[14] Usually the migraine headache occurs contralateral to the hemifield containing the visual aura.[15] A "prolonged aura" lasts more than 60 minutes but no longer than 7 days, and the IHS classifies such cases as *probable migraine with aura*.[14] When auras persist longer than 1 week, the term *persistent aura without infarction* is used.[14] If an aura occurs with a radiographically demonstrated infarction, a diagnosis of *migrainous infarction* is satisfied.[14]

Aura occurs in approximately one-third of adult patients with migraine.[16] It is our impression and that of some experienced pediatric neurologists[17] that auras are relatively less common in children with migraine.

Traditional theories proposed that vasoconstriction-induced cortical ischemia caused migraine aura, and experiments measuring regional cerebral blood flow and volume have confirmed decreased regional cerebral blood flow during the aura phase.[18,19] More recent theories,

Table 12–2 Hallucinations, illusions, and distortions associated with migraine

Hallucinations
Complex
Dots
Fortification spectra
Halos
Heat waves
Lights
Lines
Prisms
Scintillating scotomas
Shapes (geometric)
Sparkles
Squiggles
Illusions/distortions
Alice in Wonderland syndrome
Macropsia
Metamorphopsia
Micropsia
Palinopsia
Polyopia

however, attribute migraine aura to neuronal dysfunction resulting from cortical spreading depression.[20] The pathophysiology of migraine and aura is discussed in more detail in Chapter 19.

The remainder of this section will first detail the various visual hallucinations and illusions associated with migraine. For the most part, the hallucinations and illusions in migraine are positive visual phenomena. Negative visual phenomena associated with migraine, such as transient monocular blindness or hemifield loss, are detailed in Chapter 10. The treatment of migraine is discussed in Chapter 19.

Fortification spectra and scintillating scotomas

A visual aura consisting of fortification spectra or a scintillating scotoma, followed by a headache, is almost pathognomonic of migraine. The *fortification spectra* phenomenon, the most common visual aura, is characterized by an arc of jagged, serrated, or zig-zag lines (**Fig. 12–1**).[21] Patients often relate that the lines, also termed *teichopsia*, shimmer, scintillate, vibrate, flicker, or pulse at 3–30 Hz. The term *fortification* refers to the similarity of the visual phenomena with early European military fortifications.[13] The term *spectra* is used because many patients will describe colored jagged edges. The shimmering aspect gives the appearance of light reflecting off of small prisms and produces the various colors of a rainbow.

In addition to the typical appearance, the "buildup" or "march" of the fortification spectra is also highly characteristic (**Fig. 12–1**).[12] Patients usually notice the visual phenomenon paracentrally, and the open part of the arc of the fortification spectra faces centrally. Often vision within the arc is scotomatous or defective, and patients will describe this area as gray, cloudy, blurry, or water-like. The combination of the positive fortification spectra on the outside and the negative area in the middle is termed a *scintillating scotoma*. These are often circular, but may also be kidney-bean shaped. Over minutes, the diameter of the arc enlarges, and drifts toward the periphery, and the scotoma, when present, also enlarges. Often the entire visual field is affected, as the fortification spectra or scintillating scotoma frequently crosses the vertical and horizontal meridians. The entire sequence may take 15–20 minutes, after which the fortification spectra or scintillating scotoma breaks up and disappears. The phenomenon is usually homonymous but also can be monocular. However, often it is difficult for even the best observers to describe whether the phenomenon is perceived in one or both eyes.

Although highly suggestive of migraine, fortification spectra and scintillating scotomas may also be triggered by cerebral lesions such as arteriovascular malformations (AVMs), neoplasms, or abcesses,[22] with or without seizure activity. In some instances, after the hallucination resolves, the patient with an underlying mass lesion will have a residual visual field defect. Rarely, scintillations without "buildup" also can be associated with posterior cerebral artery ischemia.[13] There should be a low threshold for neuroimaging to rule out a structural cause in any patient with an accelerated frequency, intensity, or duration of homonymous positive visual phenomenon (particularly if they are always on the same side), and if these present late in life without a previous history of migraine.

Simple positive visual phenomena in migraine

Many patients with migraine report seeing less complex phenomena, some of which are listed in **Table 12–2**. Unlike fortification spectra and scintillating scotomas, these simple hallucinations tend not to "build up." For instance, patients may describe "dancing lights," "shapes," or a "flash bulb."[13] In some, the flashes of light last only fractions of a second; however, they may migrate across the visual field (**Fig. 12–2**). Patients with these complaints should not be confused with those with photopsias and phosphenes associated with disorders of the anterior visual pathway (see entoptic phenomena, below).

Complex visual hallucinations in migraine

Visual hallucinations containing complex objects such as people and animals (*zoopsia*) are unusual in migraine visual aura, but are well described. Hachinski et al.[23] described an 18-year-old girl with migraine who saw herself lying on a railroad track while a train passed over her. In her left visual field she experienced irregular multicolored scotomas. The visual hallucinations lasted 10 minutes and the accompanying migraine headache lasted 3 hours. Out-of-body

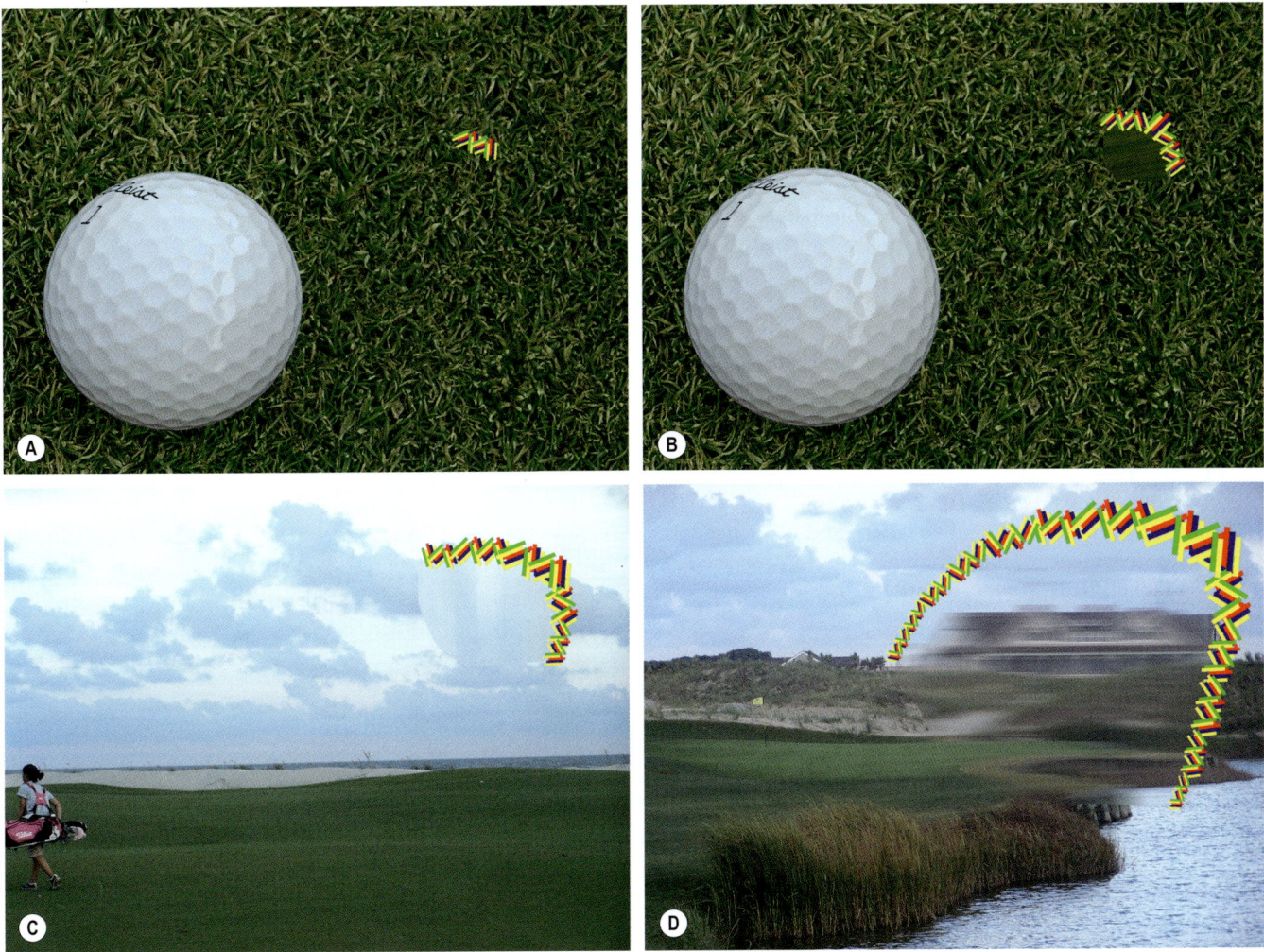

Figure 12–1. Characteristic buildup of a migrainous scintillating scotoma experienced by one of the authors while playing golf. **A**. Suddenly while he was "looking at the golf ball and about to putt," he noticed a small pulsating object in the upper right quadrant of both eyes. **B**. One minute later, it became more obvious to him that the object was gradually enlarging and the border of it consisted of small, jagged, and shimmering yellow, blue, green, and red prisms which flickered and pulsed at high frequency. Towards the center, there was an area of blurry, but not absent, vision (as if looking through water). **C**. Ten minutes later the visual disturbance continue to enlarge within the right upper homonymous quadrant. **D**. The blurry area and border of prisms gradually enlarged and crossed the vertical and horizontal meridians. Eventually it consumed the entire visual field then disintegrated at its borders and within the blurry center (not shown). Its resolution was followed one hour later by a holocephalic headache accompanied by nausea.

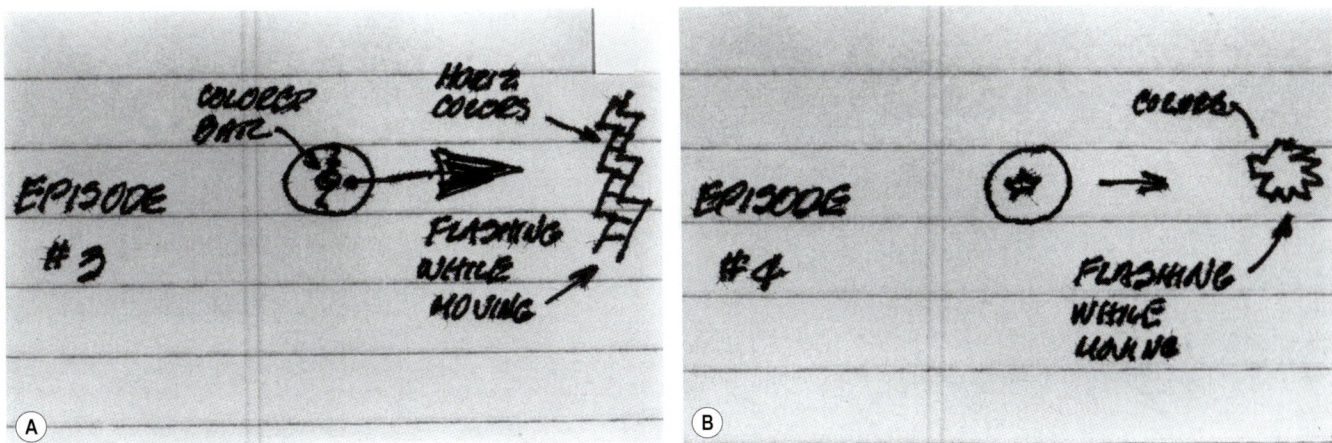

Figure 12–2. Migration of characteristic simple visual phenomena drawn and described by a migraineur. He wrote that in one episode (**A**), "a colored bar appeared at the center of the eye and began flashing and flickering, then moved from the center of the eye to the left. This lasted about 10 minutes. After the bar reached the side of the eye, it took the shape of an arc and continued to flicker for about 10 minutes." In another episode (**B**), "when looking down on the floor, eight-pointed colorful star-like figures appeared (one at a time), flickering and bright. One of the star-like figures (depicted in drawing), appeared at the center of the eye and worked itself toward the left outside of the eye, blinking and flickering as it moved."

experiences, including those in which the individual views his or her own body (*autoscopy*), although more common in seizures (see below), have also been reported in migraine.[24]

When complex visual hallucinations occur in migraine, they are usually unaccompanied by auditory and abnormal thought content;[15] however, Fuller et al.[25] reported an exceptional 69-year-old man with migraine and complex visual and auditory hallucinations as well as paranoid delusions. He felt his wife and brother-in-law had been killed, and the "ward staff were systematically butchering other patients on the ward." He saw "red and squirmy piranha fish on the floor of his room and would try to stamp on them, after which they would disappear." This history would be more suggestive of a psychiatric disorder or drug use, and migraine would have to be a diagnosis of exclusion.

A unique patient with migraine auras characterized by complete *achromatopsia* (no perception of color), *prosopagnosia* (inability to recognize faces), and *visual agnosia* (inability to recognize objects) has also been described.[26] These higher cortical visual disorders are discussed in Chapter 9.

Visual distortions and illusions in migraine

Metamorphopsia. Distortion of the shapes of objects may be experienced by patients with migraine (objects may appear too fat, too thin, too short, or too tall, for instance); however, metamorphopsia is a much more common complaint among patients with macular disease.

Micropsia/macropsia. In a variation of metamorphopsia, patients with migraine may complain that objects appear too small (*micropsia*) or too large (*macropsia*). We have seen a patient who described one episode in which a telephone, which was located across the room, appeared as if it were right next to her because is looked much larger than normal. In *teleopsia*, objects seem too far away. People may appear too small in *lilliputianism*. These symptoms can also be caused by seizures.

Alice in Wonderland syndrome. Lippman[27] described seven patients with classic migraine who experienced episodes of distorted body image. Each had fascinating hallucinations characterized by enlargement, diminution, or distortion of part of or the whole body, and each patient knew the sensations were not real. One 38-year-old woman reported attacks of feeling "about 1 foot high" accompanied by headache. Another elderly woman complained of migraine headaches preceded by the feeling of her left ear "ballooning out 6 inches or more." His Patient 7 reported headaches accompanied by sensations of body size distortion "as if someone had drawn a vertical line separating the two halves; the right half seems to be twice the size of the left half."

Lippman[27] recalled that Lewis Carroll (Charles Lutwidge Dodgson), also a migraineur, had described similar hallucinations in his book *Alice in Wonderland*. It has been speculated that Dodgson had experienced distortions in body image during his migraine events, and incorporated the hallucinations into the fictional story about the young girl who, during her adventures in Wonderland, shrinks and grows numerous times. Todd[28] then coined the condition *Alice in Wonderland syndrome*. Rolak[29] pointed out the similarity

between original illustrations in Dodgson's book (**Figs. 12–3 and 12–4**) and some of the descriptions catalogued by Lippman.[27]

For unclear reasons, metamorphopsia, micropsia/macropsia, and this syndrome occur much more commonly in

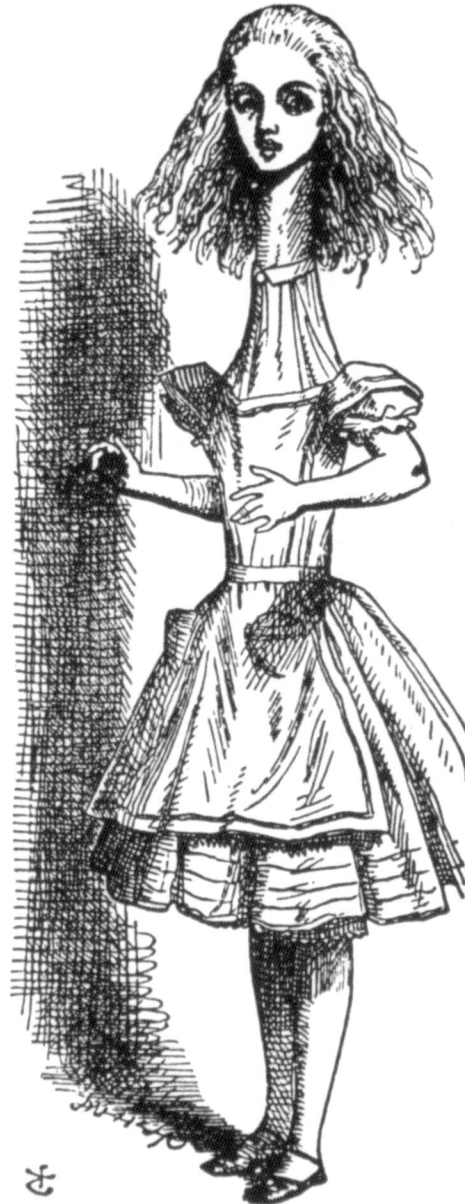

Figure 12–3. This original illustration from Lewis Carroll's "Alice in Wonderland" matches the descriptions of two of Lippman's[27] patients who experienced distortions in body image, in particular, excessive height. Patient 3, a 23-year-old woman, described the following: "I experienced the sensation that my head had grown to tremendous proportions and was so light that it floated up to the ceiling, although I was sure it was still attached to my neck. I used to try to hold it down with my hands. This sensation would pass with the migraine but would leave me with a feeling that I was very tall. When walking down the street I would think I would be able to look down on the tops of others' heads, and it was very frightening and annoying not to see as I was feeling. The sensation was so real that when I would see myself in a window or full-length mirror, it was quite a shock to realize that I was still my normal height of under five feet." Patient 6 said "I get tired out from pulling my head down from the ceiling. My head feels like a balloon; my neck stretches and my head goes to the ceiling. I've been pulling it down all night long." (Illustration borrowed with permission from Dover Publications, Mineola, NY.)

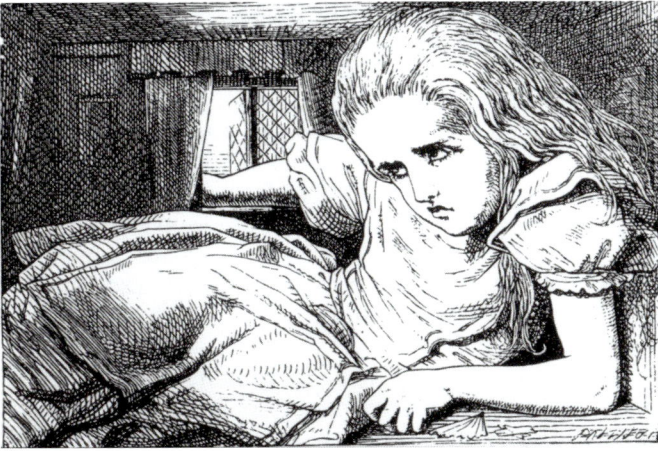

Figure 12–4. This original illustration from Lewis Carroll's "Alice in Wonderland" matches the descriptions of one of Lippmann's[27] patients who experienced distortions in body image, in particular, excessive height. (Illustration borrowed with permission from Dover Publications, Mineola, NY.)

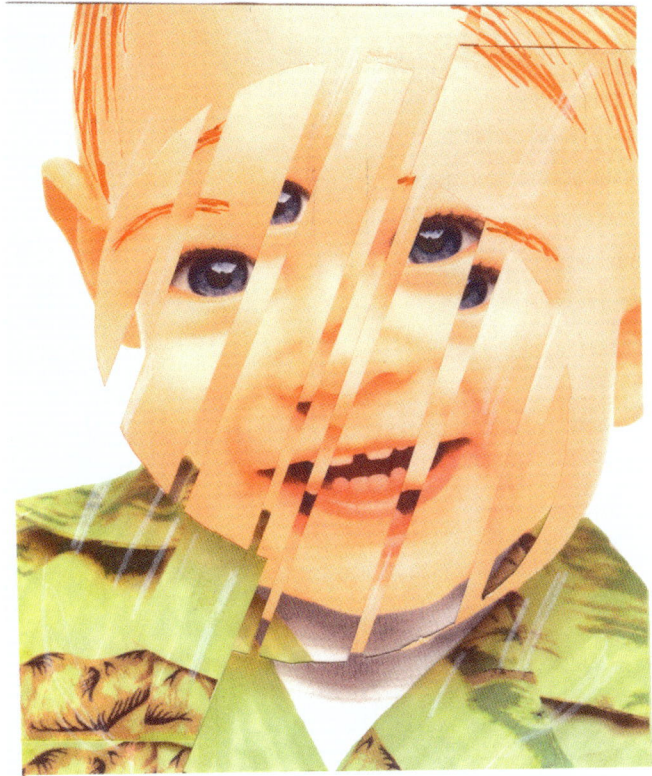

Figure 12–5. Illustration by a 42-year-old female graphic artist with migraine depicting her own visual aura. She described central vision loss in the left eye with breaking up of vision with skewed diagonal lines "like a prism." It was accompanied by a headache, which was fairly severe, but by the next day, the vision had improved.

children than adults with migraine.[15,23,30] Hachinski et al.[23] described a 6-year-old child who thought people around her were smaller than normal. Once, while playing in the snow, this same child felt that she was "unusually large" and that an ordinary snowball had become "huge and turned blue."

Metamorphopsia, micropsia/macropsia, and Alice in Wonderland syndrome have been attributed to migrainous cortical dysfunction in the nondominant posterior parietal lobule.[31] In contrast, SPECT (single photon emission computed tomography) imaging in one report[32] demonstrated occipital and temporal lobe abnormalities. Almost all cases of Alice in Wonderland syndrome have been associated with migraine, but frontal lobe epilepsy,[33] encephalopathy due to infectious mononucleosis,[34] topiramate use,[35] and varicella infection have also been reported causes.

Other distortions and illusions. Migraine may also produce the perception of multiple images, and should be included in the differential diagnosis of cerebral diplopia.[36] Kosmorsky,[37] in a report of his own acephalgic migraine, described the duplication of images within a scintillating scotoma. The double vision was present with either eye covered, and did not change with either monocular or binocular viewing. Migraineurs may also complain of *palinopsia* (see below), the persistence of visual images. However, palinopsia is more characteristically a symptom of parieto-occipital lobe damage. **Fig. 12–5** illustrates one patient's depiction of her visual illusion associated with migraine.

Persistent positive visual phenomena and migraine aura status

In these uncommon prolonged migraine aura conditions, the visual phenomena is either (1) continuous, full-field, unaccompanied by visual loss, and not visually disabling (*persistent positive visual phenomena*), or (2) similar to a more classic visual aura but is continuous or recurrent (*migraine aura status*).[38] The visual phenomena in each type are temporally unrelated to headaches and standard neuroimaging is negative without cerebral infarction.

Persistent positive visual phenomena. Ten patients with migraine who developed persistent positive visual phenom-

ena without visual loss lasting months to years were the subject of the original report.[39] None had major psychiatric disease. The visual complaints were similar in their simplicity and involvement of the entire visual field and usually consisted of diffuse small particles such as TV static, snow, lines of ants, dots, and rain (**Table 12–3** and **Fig. 12–6**). Some patients reported greater awareness of the visual phenomena when looking at the sky or at a light-colored wall. Complex phenomena such as palinopsia, micropsia, and formed hallucinations were exceptional. Some characterized these unformed visual hallucinations as bothersome, uncomfortable, or emotionally disabling, but not interfering with visual function. Other patients were unconcerned by them. Neurologic and ophthalmologic examinations were normal in all patients, and electroencephalograms were normal in eight of eight patients tested. Magnetic resonance imaging (MRI) was normal without evidence of infarction in all patients, except one who had nonspecific biparietal white matter lesions and another with a small venous angioma. In this series, medications such as tricyclic agents, calcium channel and beta blockers, and analgesics were unhelpful.

Persistent positive visual phenomena may result from spontaneous cortical discharges. Alternatively, selective dysfunction of inhibitory and modulating neurons in extrastriate areas, as evidenced by occipital hypoperfusion demonstrated by SPECT imaging,[40] may have allowed spontaneous discharges from the lateral geniculate or visual cortex. This could result in release visual hallucinations

Table 12-3 Persistent positive visual phenomena in migraine

Simple, unformed
A million dots
Black cracks and lines
Blobs of white and gray
Blue squares
Bubbles
Carpet background
Circles
Clouds
Comets
Dots
Black and white
Colored
Grainy vision
Heat waves
Lights
Flashing
Flickering
Lines of ants
Photopsias
Rainlike pattern
Snow
Squiggles
TV static
Complex
Micropsia
Palinopsia
People's heads

From Liu GT et al: Neurology 1995;45:664–668, with permission.

(see below), as suggested by West[3] and Cogan.[4] Normal diffusion- and perfusion-weighted MRIs suggest ischemia does not play a role.[38]

Migraine aura status. In this condition, a more classic aura persists, typically in just one part of the visual field, and sometimes with a combination of positive and negative visual phenomena. Haas[41] reported two individuals with "prolonged migraine aura status"; the first was a 70-year-old man with a long-standing history of migraine headaches who developed a constant "pinwheel of bright whirling color, mainly yellow and red" in the left homonymous hemifield accompanied by left hand paresthesias and clumsiness. The episode lasted 5 weeks, and resolved with aspirin and cyproheptadine. The second patient was an 18-year-old boy with a history of migraine with aura who experienced 7 months of "concentric gray circles like ripples in a pond" and "clustered sets of concentric circles in the right visual field," unaccompanied by headache. Both patients had normal neurologic and ophthalmologic examinations, but only the first had computed tomography of the brain and encephalography (EEG), both of which were normal. Luda et al.[42] reported a 65-year-old woman with "sustained visual aura" who had a 50-year history of migraine with aura who then developed 12 months of "scintillating geometric figures (in the shape of either rings or chains)" in the right visual hemifield. Carbamazepine, diazepam, flunarizine, nimodipine, and citicoline were unhelpful. Examination, EEG, and brain MRI were normal.

In our experience treatment of patients with either persistent positive visual phenomena of migraine or migraine aura status is usually ineffective with most migraine medications, anticonvulsants, and antidepressants. However, Rothrock[43] and Chen et al.[40] reported the successful management of patients with each type with divalproex sodium and lamotrigine, respectively. In addition, acetazolamide effectively treated three reported patients with migraine aura status,[44] while others were treated successfully with intravenous furosemide[45] and nimodipine.[46]

Acephalgic migraine

In patients with *acephalgic migraine*, the aura is unaccompanied by headache. In Alvarez's study,[47] 12% of men and 0.7% of women had "scotomas without a headache." The diagnosis of acephalgic migraine is suggested by a previous history of migraine, the occurrence of a positive or negative visual phenomenon typical of migraine, and the absence of cerebrovascular causes for the event. Both visual hallucinations and illusions as well as transient monocular and binocular visual loss can occur.[48] We have observed a common pattern in lifelong migraineurs of typical headaches without aura in adolescence and early adulthood then predominantly acephalgic migraines in middle age and afterwards. Fisher[49] detailed such a change in his own migraines.

When acephalgic migraine is experienced by older adults, distinguishing the event from a transient ischemic attack may be very difficult.[50] Fisher[51] described a group of patients over 40 years of age who experienced visual symptoms initially thought to be transient ischemic attacks. However, 50% had headache, the visual symptoms were more consistent with migraine, and angiography was unrevealing. He emphasized that in adults with positive and negative visual phenomena seemingly consistent with a vascular event, migraine can be considered but must be a diagnosis of exclusion. The gradual buildup of the visual disturbance typically favors the diagnosis of migraine. Acephalgic migraine in children is very unusual, occurring in only 31 of 1106 (3%) pediatric migraineurs in one series.[52]

The workup and treatment of acephalgic migraine are discussed in Chapter 19.

Visual loss (release hallucinations and the Charles Bonnet syndrome)

Cogan[4] re-emphasized the notion that visual hallucinations may be associated with loss of vision. In his report entitled

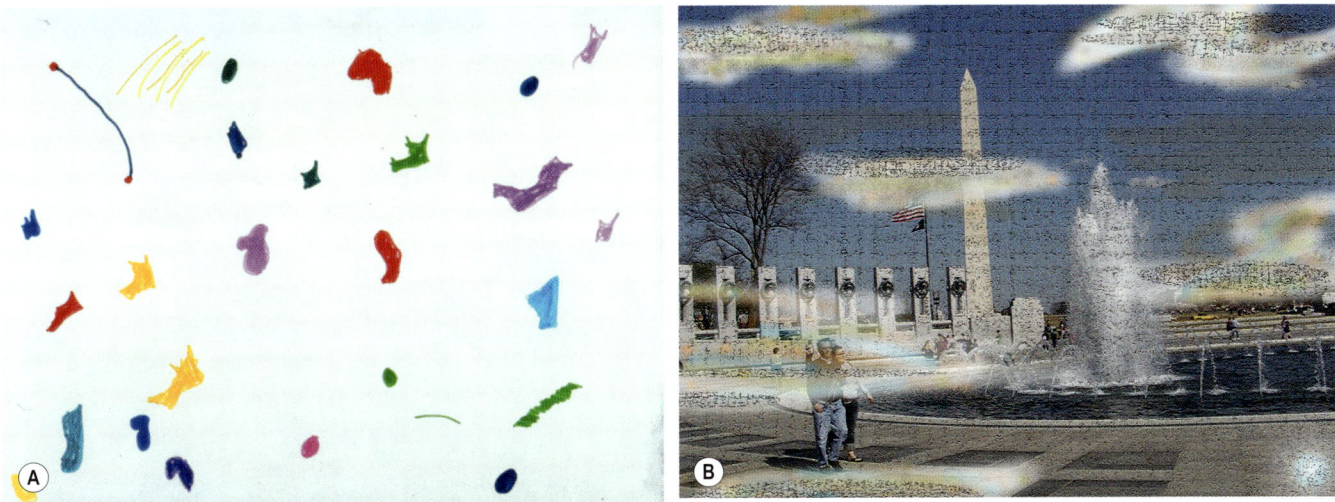

Figure 12–6. Persistent positive visual phenomena associated with migraine. **A**. A young girl's depiction of colored constant and full-field objects she perceived. This patient is one in the series by Liu et al.[39] **B**. An adult patient prepared this illustration which depicts her persistent positive visual phenomena. She described "flashes and blotches of light that had many different colors and "noise" in them, almost like TV static. These lights would come from the left and go to the right; there were always several in my field of vision at any given time."

"Visual hallucinations as release phenomena," he presented patients with blindness of varying degree and cause, including monocular blindness due to optic neuropathy, chiasmal visual loss affecting both eyes, and homonymous hemianopia due to retrochiasmal lesions. Each had formed or unformed visual hallucinations, typically within the defective area of vision. For instance, one woman with a right homonymous hemianopia complained of "zig-zag lines, colored triangles, and formed images suggesting that people and traffic were moving in on her from the right side." In general, the complexity of the hallucinations had no localizing value. When present, the hallucinations in his patients were usually continuous, variable, and more intense when the eyelids were closed (**Table 12–4**). He contrasted these from the episodic stereotyped visual hallucinations associated with seizure activity. Cogan suggested that interference of the normal visual input, from any lesion in the afferent visual pathway, might allow a "release of brain activity."

Lepore[53] studied 104 patients with retinal or neural afferent pathway disease, and found 57% reported spontaneous visual phenomena. Elementary disturbances such as photopsias and geometric forms, as well as complex ones such as people, animals, or vehicles were described. Like Cogan,[4] Lepore found their complexity did not correlate with lesion site. Furthermore, hallucinations occurred even in individuals with only minor amounts of visual loss. For example, spontaneous visual phenomena were described by three of Lepore's patients with pseudotumor cerebri, 20/20 vision, and only minimal enlargement of the physiologic blind spot. Many patients in his series were relieved when informed that the visual phenomena were common sequelae of visual loss and not reflective of any psychiatric disturbance.

The suggestions that vision loss of any degree due to lesions anywhere along the visual axis can lead to release hallucinations has been confirmed by several others. For instance, detailed descriptions of simple[54] and complex[55] visual hallucinations within homonymous hemianopias

Table 12–4 Visual symptoms and patient characteristics in release visual hallucinations

Visual symptoms

Both simple and complex

Complexity nonlocalizing

Typically, but not always within the defective area of vision

Usually continuous

Nonstereotyped

More intense when eyes closed

Can arise suddenly and unexpectedly

Patient characteristics

Vision loss to any degree from any cause

Insight into the unreal nature of the hallucinations

Intact sensorium

Absence of delusions

No hallucinations in any other sensory modality

have been reported. Patients with complex visual hallucinations and illusions associated with visual loss due to ocular diseases were described in another study.[6] Normal visual acuity but glaucomatous visual field loss may cause hallucinations.[56] Visual hallucinations of all types were found in 15% of patients seen in a retina clinic,[57] and have been described in association with retinal vascular occlusions,[58] macular photocoagulation,[59] and macular translocation surgery.[60] Visual hallucinations can also occur after enucleation.[61] Release visual hallucinations usually occur within the blind scotoma but occasionally can be full-field (**Fig. 12–7**).[62]

The concept that spontaneous visual phenomena may be released by a lack of inhibitory input may also explain visual

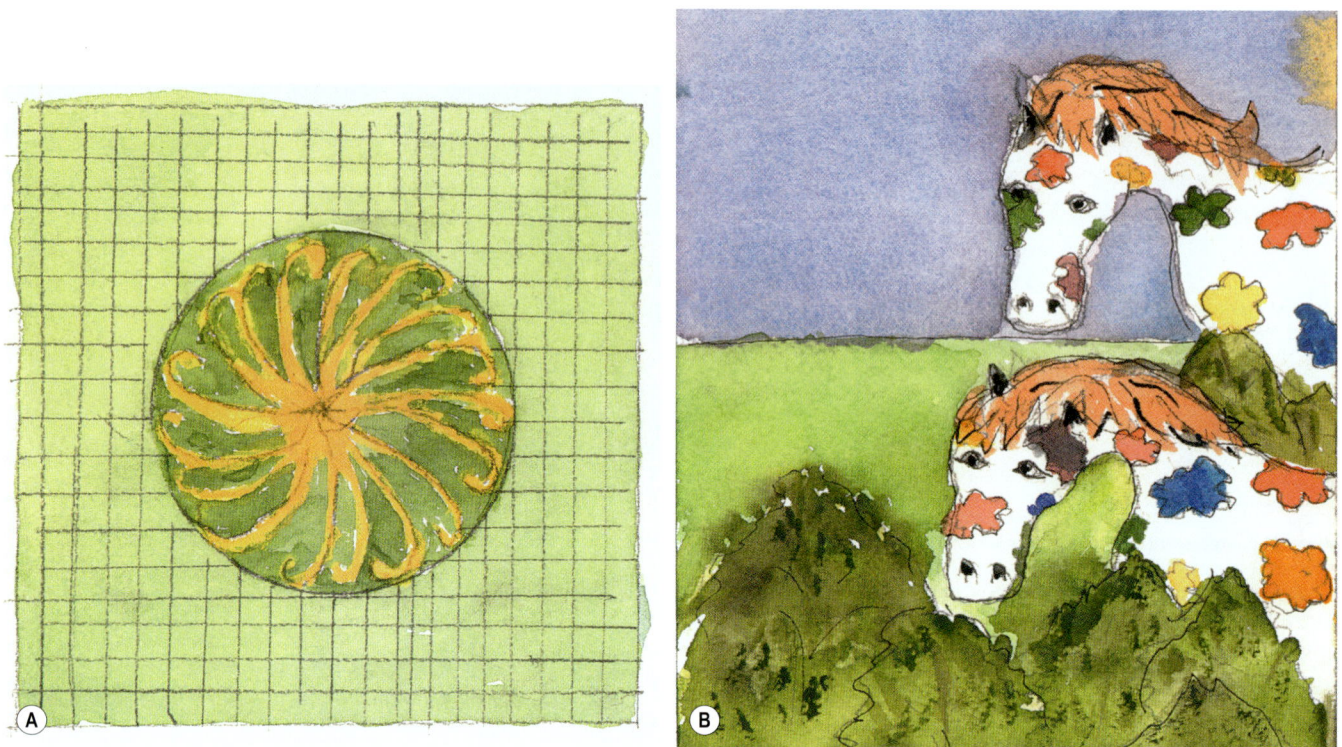

Figure 12–7. An 81-year-old woman's rendering of her release visual hallucinations associated with macular degeneration and central visual field deficits. **A**. "The hallucinations are similar in color and content: green background lined or gridded in black with a central figure.." As one example, she saw "yellow figures in the center spinning very fast." **B**. Sometimes the hallucinations were full field as in this "vision" with "cartoon horses."

hallucinations associated with severe sensory deprivation in prisoners of war or in normal volunteers blindfolded for extended periods of time,[61] for instance. In addition, patients with dense, bilateral cataracts, despite being alert and lucid, may experience vivid, pleasurable visual hallucinations.[63] Many of the cataract-associated hallucinations seem to occur when the patient is not receiving external stimuli, such as in a quiet room or just before the patient goes to sleep. In further support of the sensory deprivation concept, the hallucinations often resolve following cataract extraction.

Release visual hallucinations rarely can occur in children as well. A 3 and a half-year-old boy with an optic pathway glioma became completely blind following tumor debulking surgery, and 1 week later reported he saw his brother, Santa Claus, and animals for 3 days.[64]

In some cases the release hallucinations are the presenting symptom of new visual loss.[65,66] We examined a 51-year-old woman who complained of seeing "a picture within a picture—like the new kind of television sets" in her lower left visual field (**Fig. 12–8**) as a presentation of a new incomplete left inferior quadrantanopia due to a right parieto-occipital infarction.[67] She described a rectangular scene with a red background filled with several people milling about, and it differed completely from what she saw in her larger intact field. Multiple broad horizontal lines swept upward over the scene, and the patient said this effect mimicked a television set with malfunctioning "vertical hold."

The eponym *Charles Bonnet syndrome* has been applied to some patients with visual hallucinations associated with visual loss.[62] However, the use of the term is hampered by varying definitions. Charles Bonnet was a Swiss naturalist

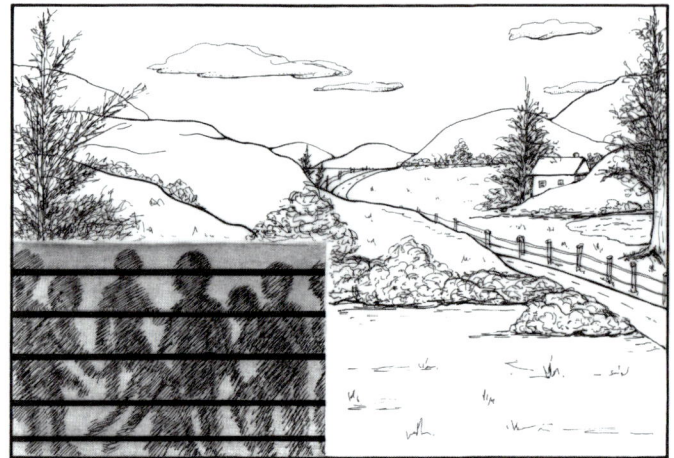

Figure 12–8. Artist's rendition of a patient's "picture within a picture" release hallucination due to a right parieto-occipital infarction. She complained of seeing "people milling about" and malfunctioning "vertical hold" in the lower left quadrant of vision. (From Benegas NM et al. Neurology 1996;47:1347–1348, with permission.)

and philosopher who, in 1769, described his 89-year-old grandfather's symptom complex of cataracts, blindness, and visions of men, women, birds, and buildings.[68] Initially used to designate elderly patients with eye-related visual loss and hallucinations, the label Charles Bonnet syndrome has been used as a "wastebasket" term to describe patients with visual hallucinations without psychiatric disease or drug use (so-called isolated visual hallucinations) but with insight into the artificial nature of their visions.[69,70] Most patients with

Charles Bonnet syndrome are elderly and have visual deficits of varying degree due to age-related macular degeneration, diabetic retinopathy, glaucoma, cataracts, and corneal disease.[71,72] However, visual loss has not been a consistent criterion for the diagnosis,[6,62] and patients with homonymous hemianopias[73] and children[74,75] have also been labeled with the name. Therefore, to describe visual hallucinations due to visual loss of any cause, we favor the use of the term *release visual hallucinations* rather than the Charles Bonnet syndrome.

The exact pathophysiology of release visual hallucinations is unclear, but one functional MRI study[76] of affected patients demonstrated cortical activity in ventral extrastriate areas. In addition, the hallucinations corresponded with activity in the region's functional specialization, e.g., visions of faces was associated with activity in the fusiform face area.

Evaluation

In a patient with visual hallucinations with known visual loss, release phenomena should be suspected but is a diagnosis of exclusion. Stereotyped images and accompanying motor activity or autonomic symptoms suggest seizures. Any history of psychiatric disease or drug use should be excluded. The patient's mentation should be normal, and ideally he or she should have complete insight into the unreal nature of the hallucinations.

There should be a low threshold for an electroencephalogram to rule out seizure activity. Neuroimaging is unnecessary if the cause of visual loss is ocular. However, if the cause of the visual loss is not ocular in origin, we would recommend neuroimaging to ensure there was no change in the original lesion, such as a hemorrhage, new stroke, or tumor growth. Neuroimaging would also be indicated if the electroencephalogram were abnormal. Finally, because release hallucinations can be the presenting symptoms of new visual loss, careful assessment of afferent visual function, such as acuity, color vision, and visual fields, should be performed, and the appropriate workup should be undertaken if a new visual deficit is detected.

Treatment

Many affected patients, particularly if they are elderly, find the hallucinations frightening or embarrassing, and are concerned about a diagnosis of insanity or dementia.[77] Therefore the best treatment of release visual hallucinations is physician recognition, patient education, and reassurance, which most patients find extremely comforting.[62,78] Vision loss should be corrected, if possible. Patients with depressive symptoms may benefit from appropriate pharmacologic therapy. Psychotherapy and medications in general are unhelpful in this disorder, but antipsychotic medications in some instances may diminished the hallucinations.[79,80]

Ironically, in some patients with hallucinations associated with progressive visual loss, the hallucinations resolve as their vision worsens. Some patients experience reduction of symptoms with increased lighting, which perhaps increases visual stimuli. Similarly, rapid eye movements, which may help release hallucinations by filling in scotomas in visual scenes, can be helpful.

Table 12–5 Entoptic phenomena

Normal physiologic entoptic phenomena
Real images
Scheerer's phenomena
Purkinje figures
Haidinger's brush
Hallucinations
Flick phosphenes
Pressure phosphenes
Accommodative phosphenes of Czermak
Entoptic phenomena due to ocular pathology
Real images
Floaters
Halos and light streaks
Hallucinations
Phosphenes and photopsias
Moore's lightning streak

Entoptic (ocular) phenomena

Entoptic phenomena, visual images produced by the structures of the eye,[81] can be divided into those which are normal physiologic events and those that are pathologic (**Table 12–5**). Then they can be further subdivided into those that are real visual images versus those that are truly hallucinogenic, where images are perceived in the absence of any true visual stimulus.

Normal physiologic entoptic phenomena

The diagnosis of these physiologic events is made in a well patient with a typical history and normal examination, including a dilated view of the fundus. These are common etiologies in normal adults complaining of floaters and in children reporting circles and dots throughout their vision.[82] They may become "suddenly" apparent to patients despite their physiologic nature.

Real images. Scheerer's phenomenon is the normal perception of moving stars or small lights, particularly when an individual looks at a bright field of snow or blue sky,[83] and is thought to be the result of leukocytes traveling in the retinal capillaries.[84] Purkinje figures are images of the vessels of the eye, best seen when a bright light is pressed and moved against a closed eyelid, casting shadows of the retinal circulation on the photoreceptors. These images are seen only when retinal and optic nerve function are normal, and therefore can be used as a gross screening test for visual potential in the setting of media opacities such as cataract and vitreous hemorrhage. *Haidinger's brush,* frequently described as a brownish-yellow hourglass with a blue bow-tie lying perpendicularly across its center, can be experienced by individuals looking at light through polarized lenses.

Hallucinations. Flick phosphenes are flashes of light occurring during eye movements. The phenomenon is best observed by dark-adapted eyes and while the eyelids are closed.[83] One possible mechanism is deformation of the posterior face of the vitreous and mechanical stimulation of the retina.[81] This explanation may also account for *pressure phosphenes*, which can occur when mechanical pressure is applied to the eye. *Accommodative phosphenes of Czermak* may be seen during prolonged accommodation, perhaps due to ciliary muscle traction on the peripheral retina[81]

Entoptic phenomena due to ocular pathology

Real images. Floaters, due to shadows on the retina cast by vitreous opacities, are typically reported as dust, cobwebs, or hair-like images which float and move as the eye looks in different directions. Common benign causes of floaters are posterior vitreous detachments and vitreous condensation and strands associated with normal aging, while more worrisome etiologies would include inflammatory cells (vitritis) and hemorrhages. *Halos* and *light streaks* can be experienced by patients with cataracts.

Hallucinations. Pathologic photopsias and phosphenes are unformed flashes of light witnessed in patients with a blow to the eye, traction on the retina, retinal inflammation, detachment, or degeneration, outer retinal disease (see Chapter 4), and optic neuropathy (particularly optic neuritis and papilledema).[63] These phenomena sometimes can be difficult to distinguish from the photopsias seen in migraine. *Moore's lightning streak* is a brief vertical lightning flash usually appearing in the temporal field. It is a special type of phosphene attributed to vitreoretinal traction related to advancing vitreous changes and shrinkage.[81] The streak is often seen as the individual walks into a dark room.

Alcohol and drugs

Alcohol, illicit drug use (cocaine, lysergic acid diethylamide (LSD), phencyclidine (PCP)) and medications (digoxin, levodopa) may also cause visual hallucinations and illusions. The discussion below is not intended to be exhaustive, but instead the goal is to highlight substances that are commonly responsible for these visual disturbances.

Alcohol withdrawal

Following prolonged or heavy ethanol consumption, periods of abstinence may be characterized by alcohol withdrawal. Symptoms include generalized tremor, hallucinosis, delirium tremens, and withdrawal seizures. Tremor and hallucinations tend to be the earliest withdrawal symptoms, typically occurring within hours of withdrawal and becoming most pronounced at 24–36 hours.[85] Hallucinations may be auditory or visual and usually occur with a clear sensorium, in contrast to the confusion associated with delirium tremens, which is a later withdrawal symptom. Zoopsia (see above), e.g., pink elephants, is commonly depicted in popular culture as a manifestation of alcohol related hallucinations, but is certainly not specific for them. Resumption of alcohol intake, and administration of benzodiazepines, beta-adrenergic receptor antagonists, or alpha-2-adrenergic receptor agonists are effective means of suppressing the tremor and hallucinations.[85]

Hallucinogens

Cocaine, LSD, psilocybin, psilocin, and PCP are drugs classified as a "hallucinogens," "illusionogens," or "psychedelics" because, in addition to mood alteration, their ingestion often produces hallucinations and distortion of sensory stimuli.[86] The effects occur at nontoxic doses and without alteration in consciousness. Synesthetic hallucinations are also associated with psychedelic use, and these are characterized by colorful visual phenomena induced by a loud noise, or an auditory hallucination in response to a bright light.[1]

Some visual phenomena associated with hallucinogen use can persist. So-called hallucinogen persisting perception disorder is associated with visual phenomena occurring well after discontinuation of the drug.[87] For instance, "flashbacks" are visual images that recur after the hallucinogen has worn off, and many are repetitions of previous hallucinations experienced during drug use. Levi and Miller[88] reported similar individuals with persistent visual hallucinations and illusions months to years after marijuana, LSD, or cocaine use. Visual complaints included shimmering of images, visual perseveration of stationary objects, streaking of moving objects, and strobe-light-like images. We have also seen such patients, and neuro-ophthalmic examinations, neuroimaging, EEG, and single photon emission tomography were all unrevealing. It is not uncommon for this syndrome to be provoked by a prescribed medication with central nervous system side effects. Hallucinogen persisting perception disorder has been treated successfully with clonazepam,[89] clonidine, anticonvulsants, and neuroleptics.[87]

Cocaine. The classic hallucination associated with chronic cocaine use is the sensation of animals, bugs, or insects moving under the skin ("cocaine bugs," or parasitosis).[90] However, other purely visual hallucinations and illusions can occur with cocaine, and these were experienced by 15% of cocaine users in Siegel's study.[91] "Snow lights" refers to the sensation of sunlight reflecting off of snow crystals. This phenomenon, and others such as vibrating or pulsating geometric shapes, and polyopia and dysmorphia, have an uncanny resemblance to migraine visual aura (see above). Cocaine use is also associated with olfactory, tactile, and gustatory hallucinations. One possible mechanism for the hallucinations and illusions in cocaine use implicates cocaine's excitatory affect on cortical structures.[91] Caution should applied when individuals using cocaine complain of photophobia, halos around lights, and difficulty focusing. These symptoms are more likely the result of pupillary mydriasis caused by a cocaine-related increase in sympathetic tone.

LSD. Common visual hallucinations associated with LSD use include moving patterns of bright color[92] and pulsating geometric shapes. Individuals may experience complex hallucinations consisting of people and scenes against a background of geometric forms. About one-fifth of LSD users report having seen Satan's face floating freely or over someone else's body, while about one-tenth report having seen rapid aging of their friend's or a stranger's face.[93] Flashbacks occurred in 64% of LSD users in one study,[93] and halos of light around objects, light following moving objects, geometric designs within familiar objects, and distortion in the sizes and shapes of faces and images were reported. In addition, Kawasaki and Purvin[94] described three patients with persistent palinopsia up to 3 years following LSD ingestion. LSD can inhibit serotonin in the central nervous system, and it also has an effect on postsynaptic dopamine receptors,[86] but the exact mechanism for producing hallucinations is unclear.

Psilocybin and psilocin. These are the active ingredients in hallucinogenic mushrooms. Hallucinations are usually visual, but can also be tactile or auditory.[95] Faces of friends or strangers can be reported to change shape or color or age dramatically.[96] Kaleidoscopic images or flashes of colors may be seen, but fully formed visual hallucinations consisting of people and Martians have also been described.[97]

PCP. A toxic psychosis, characterized by auditory or visual hallucinations, delusions, abnormal behavior, and sometimes disorientation, may occur with PCP use.[98] The visual hallucinations often consist of brightly colored objects. Although PCP-induced psychosis resembles acute schizophrenia, PCP use can often be recognized by the accompanying hypertension and nystagmus.[99]

Others. Mescaline,[100] amphetamines, cannabinoids, opiate agonists, and synthetic opioids may also be associated with visual hallucinations.[86] Cannabinoid, the active ingredient in marijuana and hashish, typically causes hallucinations only when there is excessive intoxication.

Digoxin

Toxic and sometimes even normal levels of the cardiac glycoside digoxin are characteristically associated with xanthopsia, the illusion of objects exhibiting abnormal colors. Yellow and green are typical colors in digoxin toxicity. Patients may also complain about blurry or snowy vision or photopsias,[101] and their visual symptoms are typically worse in brighter lighting conditions. On examination, patients with digoxin toxicity may actually have decreased acuity, central scotomas, generalized visual field depression, color vision defects, and pupillary mydriasis.[102] Electroretinography (ERG) often reveals evidence of cone dysfunction, suggesting the retina is the site of toxicity, perhaps at the level of Na^+K^+-ATPase pumps in retinal cells.[103] Symptoms and ERG abnormalities usually improve following lowering of the digoxin dose. Several elderly patients have been described with visual symptoms consistent with digoxin toxicity, despite serum concentrations of digoxin which were below or within the usual therapeutic range.[104,105]

Levodopa

Levodopa is the mainstay of treatment for Parkinson's disease; however, its use may be complicated by visual hallucinations in 5–30% of patients.[106] In some instances individuals taking levodopa can develop a pure psychosis.[107] Their underlying Parkinson's disease, elderly age, and use of other potentially psychotropic medications likely predispose

them to hallucinations. Patients often report seeing people in the room who are not really there, and animals may be described.[108] The mechanism is likely related to its effect on central dopamine receptors.

Levodopa-induced hallucinations can produce a vexing management dilemma, often necessitating a compromise between lowering the dose, adding another dopamine agonist, or treating with an atypical antipsychotic agent with few or no extrapyramidal side effects.[109] Sometimes the patient chooses to accept a lower dose of levodopa to resolve the hallucinations and accepts a minor amount of motor worsening.

Other prescription medications

Clomiphene citrate[110] and cyclosporine[111] have been reported to cause visual hallucinations. Sildenafil can cause subjective halos, blue tinge to vision, blurry vision, and increased brightness of lights.[112] Mild phosphodiesterase-6 inhibition by sildenafil in the retina at the level of the rod and cone photoreceptors may be responsible.[113] In addition, visual hallucinations and schizophrenia-like psychoses may occur in patients taking lamotrigine.[114]

Seizures

Visual hallucinations due to irritative cortical foci tend to be brief, intermittent, and stereotypically repetitive, and are often accompanied by other motor and sensory phenomena.[63] Secondary generalization, loss of consciousness, and ictal discharges on EEG also support a diagnosis of epilepsy. It is a useful guideline that occipital lobe seizures tend to be associated with simple visual hallucinations, while complex visual hallucinations are more likely the result of temporal lobe foci. Negative visual phenomena in epilepsy, in particular ictal and postictal visual loss, are discussed in Chapter 10.

Visual hallucinations are much more common in occipital lobe epilepsy than in seizures produced by temporal and parietal lobe foci. In general, they have no lateralizing value. Frontal lobe discharges are only rarely associated with visual hallucinations.[33,115] The following discussion will be subdivided by cerebral localization, with particular emphasis on hallucinations associated with occipital lobe epilepsy.

Occipital lobe epilepsy

Simple visual hallucinations were the most common presentation (60%) in patients with occipital lobe epilepsy in Williamson et al.'s study.[116] These individuals reported flashing colored lights, white phosphenes, and steady white or colored lights. In the series of patients with occipital lobe epilepsy by Salanova et al.,[117] simple visual hallucinations such as flashes, colored lights, stars, wheels, or triangles were frequently reported, and they were usually seen contralateral to the epileptogenic focus. Complex hallucinations, thought to represent seizure spread to the temporal lobe, were reported by less than 10% in this study, and these consisted of familiar faces, pictures, and people. Other reports have subsequently confirmed the predominance of simple versus complex visual hallucinations in occipital lobe epilepsy.[118,119] Although typically lasting just for seconds or minutes, occipital lobe seizures with hallucinations can also last for hours or days.[120,121]

In these large series,[116–118] the visual phenomena were often accompanied by other manifestations of seizures, such as rapid bilateral blinking or eye flutter or eye deviation with or without head deviation. When automatisms or motor manifestations appeared, seizure spread to the temporal lobe or motor cortex, respectively, was thought to have occurred. Visual field defects were detected in approximately 60%, but patients were often unaware of their visual field deficits. The majority of patients in these series had an identifiable lesion in the occipital lobe, usually a neoplasm, but scarring related to old trauma, cysts, old strokes, and cortical dysplasia were also found. Non-ketotic hyperglycemia may cause occipital-region partial seizures and prolonged hemianopias.[122] Children with occipital seizures may have cerebral dysgenesis, a genetic disorder, hypoxic ischemic encephalopathy,[123] or neonatal hypoglycemia[124] as underlying causes, often accompanied by some visual field loss.[125,126]

Since occipital lobe seizures may present solely with visual hallucinations, without other neurologic manifestations, the hallucination may be very difficult to distinguish clinically from those seen in acephalgic migraine or release phenomena.[121] Panayiotopoulos[127] compared the visual hallucinations of 50 migraine patients with those of 20 patients with occipital epilepsy. He concluded the following: (1) the hallucinations produced by seizures tended to be more multicolored with circular or spherical patterns; (2) in contrast, the hallucinations in the migraineurs were more often black and white, with occasional color on the borders, and linear or zig-zag; and (3) no seizure patients experienced scintillating scotomas or fortification spectra. The author believed these observations could be helpful in distinguishing hallucinations between the two groups. However, we would use these as only general guidelines, as we have seen several exceptions to these observations. In cases such as these, formal visual field testing may also be useful, as a hemianopic visual field defect would be suggestive of a structural lesion and a possible ictal focus.

Benign childhood epilepsy with occipital paroxysms is one of the benign, location-related seizure disorders in the pediatric age group.[128–130] This subtype made up 4.2% of all epilepsies with onset before age 13 in one study.[131] Nocturnal seizures with tonic deviation of the eyes and vomiting were the typical presenting features in younger children, while visual hallucinations and diurnal fits were more common in older children. The characteristic EEG finding is repetitive spike and slow-wave occipital discharges that diminish with open eyelids.[131] Overall, the prognosis for spontaneous remission is good. The visual hallucinations are typically unformed, but Gastaut and Zifkin[132] described three unusual children who experienced ictal visualization of numbers.

Temporal lobe epilepsy

Visual hallucinations in temporal lobe epilepsy are less common (**Fig. 12–9**). In two large reviews[133,134] of patients

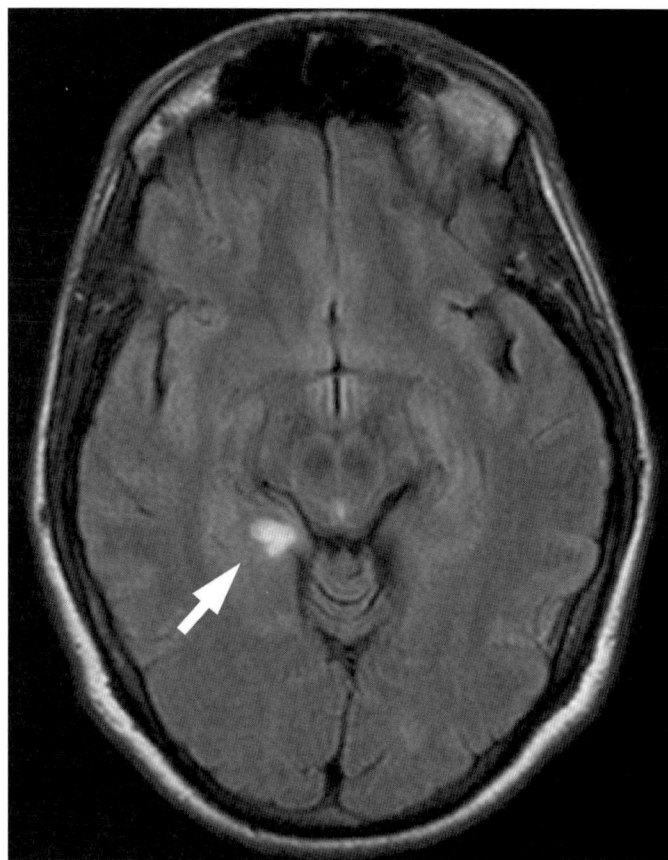

Figure 12–9. T2-weighted FLAIR magnetic resonance axial image from a man with presumed epileptic, simple positive visual phenomena in his left visual field as presentation of a right temporal lobe glioma (*arrow*). He described black and white jagged lines, television "fuzz," shadows of a ceiling fan, all to his left. He also reported that he sometimes saw other objects with "extra" depth and hyperperception associated with déjà vu. The surface encephalography was normal, but the visual phenomena resolved with anticonvulsant medication. He had no visual field defect.

with temporal lobe epilepsy, visual hallucinations occurred in 18% and 16%, respectively. Compared with patients with occipital lobe epilepsy, those with temporal lobe discharges are less likely to present solely with visual hallucinations, but both simple and complex visual phenomena can be described.[119,135] Visual hallucinations consisting of recently or distantly remembered scenes can occur.[136] Auras consisting of bad smells or tastes, visceral sensations, or feelings of déjà vu are frequent accompaniments. Temporal lobe seizures are also characterized by focal motor activity (e.g., eye deviation, head turning, limb movements) in 80%, automatisms (e.g., lip pursing, chewing, swallowing, finger movements, gesturing, verbalizations) in 95%, and autonomic changes (e.g., pupillary dilation, salivation, blushing, pallor, urinary incontinence) in 83%.[134]

Visual illusions reported in association with temporal lobe seizures include (1) distortions of bodily image, such as missing body parts and autoscopic phenomena (see below);[137] (2) ictal *hemimacropsia*, the illusory enlargement of half of the visual field, due to discharges from temporal[138] and occipito-temporal[139] regions; and (3) ictal illusory perception of motion (*epileptic kinetopsia*), presumably from activation of area V5, the cortical region subserving motion perception (see Chapter 9).[140]

Parietal lobe epilepsy

Visual hallucinations due to parietal lobe seizure foci are very uncommon,[141] but illusions of change or distortion in body shape, similar to Alice in Wonderland syndrome of migraine, can be associated with parietal lobe discharges. Elongation, shortening, swelling, or shrinking of a body part or the whole body may be experienced. The phenomenon is thought to arise from epileptic involvement of the nondominant inferior parietal lobule and superior part of the postcentral gyrus.[142]

Rousseaux et al.[143] described a teenager with left parietal epileptiform discharges who complained of visual hallucinations containing written words. He had a fluent aphasia due to head trauma 6 months earlier, and neuroimaging had demonstrated a porencephalic cavity area resulting from a hemorrhage in the left temporoparietal area.

Other unusual ictal visual hallucinations

Seizures rarely may also cause *macropsia, micropsia,* and *palinopsia,*[144] visual illusions described elsewhere in this chapter.

Autoscopic phenomena. Devinsky et al.[145] described 10 patients and reviewed 33 previously reported patients with seizures and *autoscopic phenomena,* in which the individual sees a copy of his or her body (mirror-image type), or in which the individual leaves his or her body to view it from another vantage point. In the first type, the body double is usually wearing the same clothing, has the same facial expression, and has the same gesticulations as the patient. The latter type is also known as an "out-of-body experience," and the person's body is typically viewed from above. Autoscopic phenomena are not associated with any particular seizure type, as patients with tonic–clonic, simple partial, and complex partial seizures were reported in this review. Post-ictal autoscopy has also been described.[146] Autoscopic phenomena are also associated with cocaine or alcohol addiction; schizophrenia; migraine; focal lesions of the parietal, temporal, and occipital lobes; near-death experiences; and release phenomena.[147]

Visual allesthesia. This phenomenon, in which visual information from one homonymous field is transferred to the other, may have several causes, but in one well-documented case by Jacobs,[148] epileptogenic activity was implicated. The patient had a right parieto-occipital AVM and an incomplete left homonymous hemianopia, and intermittently saw images in the defective left field transposed from the good right field. Sometimes the images were palinopic, persisting in the left field up to 15 minutes after the real objects were no longer visible. A right parieto-occipital focus was demonstrated, and anticonvulsants led to resolution of the visual allesthesia. Jacobs attributed the visual phenomena to interhemispheric transfer of visual information from the good to the irritated parieto-occipital lobe. We have seen a patient with a left occipital lobe meningioma who experienced visual allesthesia while reading. The right page of her book would often shift to the left.

Neurodegenerative disease

Parkinson's disease and dementia with Lewy bodies

As many as one-quarter to one-third of patients with Parkinson's disease may complain of visual hallucinations.[149–151] Typically they describe complex images of familiar or strange people,[152] and the hallucinations are usually non-threatening and recognized as not real. Although the use of levodopa is the most common cause of visual hallucinations in patients with Parkinson's disease, other contributory factors include the disease itself,[150] vision and visual perception impairments,[153] anticholinergic medications, advancing age, sleep disturbances,[154,155] psychoses, and dementia.[149,156,157] Hallucinations in this group of patients can be severely disabling,[158] and are often predictive of the need for nursing home placement.[159]

Recurrent, complex visual hallucinations, along with fluctuating cognitive impairment and parkinsonism, are clinical hallmarks of dementia with Lewy bodies. This uncommon condition is characterized pathologically by Lewy bodies, which are pathologic aggregations of alpha-synuclein, throughout the cortex and limbic system.[160]

Alzheimer's disease

Visual hallucinations occur in 3–33% of patients with Alzheimer's disease, and they are the most common type (up to 85%) of hallucination (others include auditory and tactile) associated with the disorder.[161,162] The visual hallucinations in Alzheimer's disease tend to be complex, as in one report[163] patients were reported to see "people in the backyard," "ducks sitting in the backyard," "animals at home and babies in bed." As in Parkinson's disease, visual hallucinations are associated with cognitive and functional decline, and predict a greater risk for institutionalization and mortality.[164] This association with poorer cognition may explain why the patients with Alzheimer's disease and visual hallucinations also frequently display delusional and paranoid ideation, auditory hallucinations, and verbal outbursts.[161] Alzheimer's disease is discussed in more detail in Chapter 9.

Low doses of neuroleptics, such as haloperidol, fluphenazine, risperidone, and aripiprazole can be used to treat hallucinations in patients with Alzheimer's disease. Anticholinergic and extrapyramidal side effects should be monitored.

Special visual hallucinations and illusions related to central nervous system lesions

Peduncular hallucinations

Peduncular hallucinations, consisting of vivid and lifelike visual images of concrete objects, are rare sequelae of ventral midbrain injury. Affected patients often report seeing animals, and the hallucinations are frequently accompanied by signs of third nerve dysfunction, ataxia, and sleep and cognitive disturbances. The usual cause is infarction in the distribution of the paramedian penetrating arteries arising from the proximal posterior cerebral arteries. However, peduncular hallucinations due to extrinsic masses compressing the midbrain have also been reported.[165,166] The term *peduncular* refers to the French "pédonculaire," meaning the midbrain,[167] rather than the cerebral peduncles, per se.

The original description is attributed to Lhermitte,[168] who reported a patient with visual hallucinations containing cats, chickens, and people, left ophthalmoplegia, and dysmetria suggestive of a destructive lesion of the midbrain and pons. However, there was no pathologic verification. Later van Bogaert described the clinical[169] and pathologic[170] findings in a similar patient who developed bilateral ptosis, a complete right third nerve palsy, a sluggish left pupil, left dysmetria, gait ataxia, and mildly increased reflexes and Babinski sign on the left. She complained of seeing a dog's head on her pillow, a horse's picture on the wall, a green serpent, and lines crossing the wall. The objects did not move, and they appeared and disappeared spontaneously. Occasionally she said white walls appeared pink and yellow, and sometimes her hands looked black. She was not frightened by the perceptions, but was convinced they were real. On pathologic examination, the patient was found to have a paramedian midbrain infarction involving the left red nucleus, left third nerve root, and left cerebral peduncle. Only the left side of the brain was studied. Attributing the abnormal visual perceptions to the midbrain damage, van Bogaert coined the term *peduncular hallucinations* (translation of van Bogaert's papers[169,170] courtesy of Dr. François-Xavier Borruat). Others[165,167,171–173] have subsequently reported similar patients.

The mechanism, other than the association with a ventral midbrain lesion, is unclear. van Bogaert's[169,170] and Geller and Bellur's[171] patients had relatively large lesions involving the red nuclei, third nerve fascicles, and cerebral peduncles. In contrast, in the clinicopathologic study by McKee et al.[172] the patient had only bilateral destruction of the medial substantia nigra pars reticulata, suggesting that involvement of this structure is crucial for the development of peduncular hallucinations. The substantia nigra pars reticulata, owing to connections with the pedunculopontine nucleus, may have a role in regulating REM sleep, and via connections with the striatum and limbic structures, may also participate in cognitive functions. McKee et al.[172] hypothesized disruption of these connections may be responsible for the sleep and cognitive disturbances sometimes seen in association with peduncular hallucinations. Other authors have considered peduncular hallucinations as release phenomena,[4,165] but afferent vision is usually unaffected.

The best treatment for peduncular hallucinations is uncertain, but in one report[173] agitation was treated with "a moderate dose of neuroleptic agent."

Palinopsia

Palinopsia (or *palinopia*) is an illusory visual phenomenon that Bender et al.[174] defined as "the persistence or recurrence of visual images after the exciting stimulus object has been

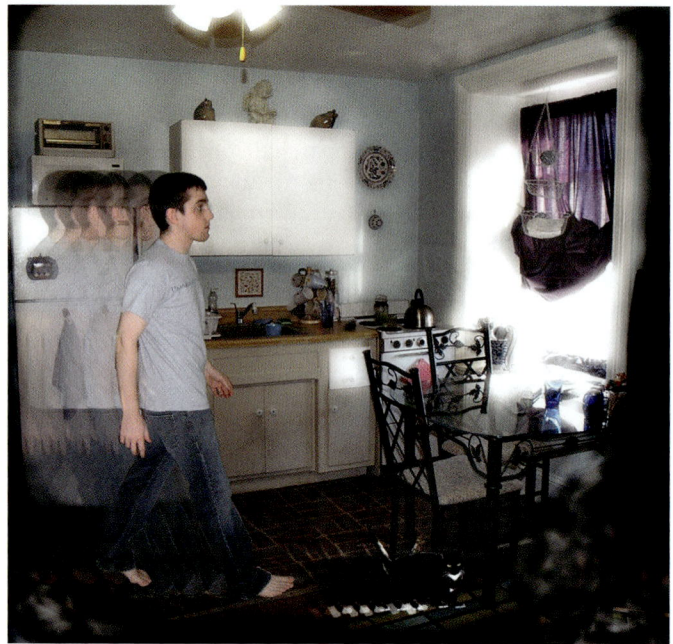

Figure 12–10. A patient's depiction of her palinopsia, which she describes as "a trailing effect behind moving objects" (the person and cat, for example).

removed." Alternatively, having looked at an object then turned away from it, they may report the image of the object follows their visual tracking (*visual perseveration*), like a "movie" or "strobe light" (**Fig. 12–10**). The persistent image may be incorporated appropriately into the scene being perceived, as in Meadows and Munro's[175] patient who saw a Santa Claus beard superimposed upon people's faces at a party. *Illusory visual spread* is an associated phenomenon in which objects or patterns enlarge to involve adjacent structures. Palinopic images should be distinguished from common afterimages produced by retinal over stimulation by a bright light, for example.

The most common cause of palinopsia is parieto-occipital damage with incomplete homonymous hemianopic field loss (**Fig. 12–11**). The abnormal visual phenomenon typically, but not always, appears within the field defect. Some authors have observed that palinopsia occurs early in the course of a progressive field defect, or as a severe visual field defect resolved.[174] The right hemisphere is most commonly affected, and the damage may be caused by vascular insults, trauma, and neoplasms.[176] Palinopsia rarely occurs during migraine aura, and it may also be associated with drugs such as trazodone,[177] clomiphene,[110] topiramate,[35] mescaline, or LSD (see above).[94] Palinopsia has also been reported in otherwise normal individuals and in patients with eye and optic nerve disease but without drug use or cerebral lesions.[178]

The mechanism of palinopsia is uncertain. Epileptic discharges have been implicated but seem unlikely in most cases because affected patients typically lack seizure activity on EEG and do not respond to anticonvulsants. It is possible they represent a type of hallucinatory release phenomenon in the defective visual field, although not all patients with palinopsia have identifiable field defects.[179] The predilection

Video 12.1

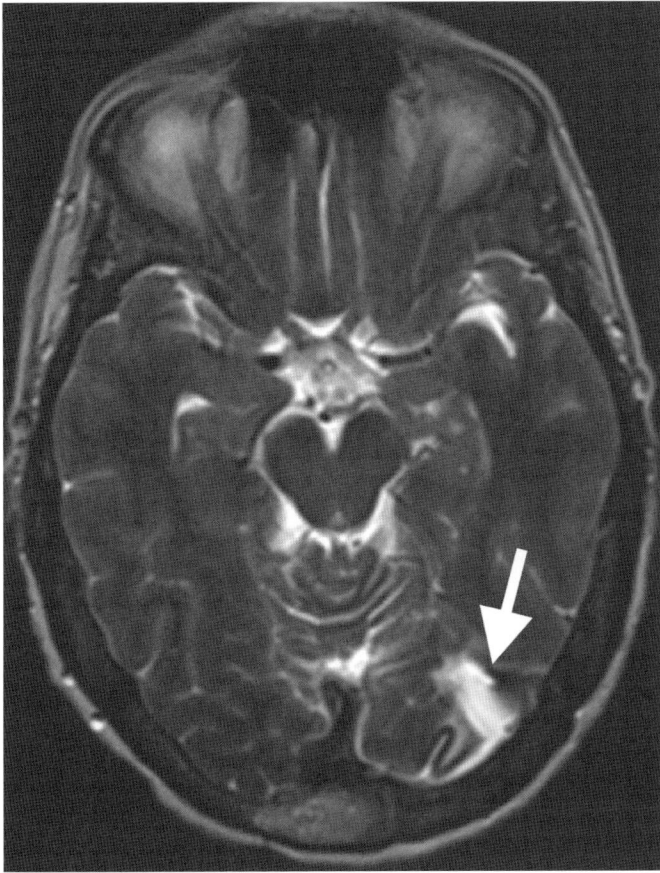

Figure 12–11. From a woman with palinopsia, a T2-weighted MR axial image demonstrates a left occipital–temporal post-surgical defect (arrow) following removal of an arteriovenous malformation (AVM). Two years following surgery, she complained of episodes of persistence of visual images lasting for minutes before fading. Her examination was remarkable for a central right homonymous upper quadrantanopia and right hemidyschromatopsia. Encephalography was normal.

for responsible parieto-occipital lesions to be right-sided may be artifactual because similar left-sided lesions may render patients too aphasic to communicate the abnormal visual phenomenon.

Cerebral diplopia and polyopia

Occipital lesions may rarely cause multiplicity of visual images, in either monocular or binocular viewing conditions. The visual disturbance is unrelated to ocular misalignment and does not resolve with use of a pinhole occluder. Specifically, the term *cerebral diplopia* refers to the duplication of images on a cortical basis, while *cerebral polyopia* describes the perception of multiple images.[180] In the outpatient setting, we have found organic polyopia to be a rare isolated phenomenon without other neurologic dysfunction. Homonymous field defects are frequently associated findings because the etiology is typically an occipital disturbance.[181,182] However, cerebral diplopia and polyopia may also be described by migraineurs and patients with epilepsy. The exact mechanism is uncertain. Although this phenomenon and palinopsia are similar and likely share common mechanisms,[183] technically cerebral diplopia and polyopia

refer to the multiplicity of a viewed image, while palinopsia describes the persistence of an image that is no longer being viewed.

Tilted and upside-down vision associated with vestibular disease

Because otolith receptors play an important role in the perception of verticality, an illusion that the environment is tilted or upside-down may follow damage to the peripheral or central vestibular system or its cortical connections. Visual images may be rotated or flipped 180 degrees.[184] Affected patients with posterior fossa lesions also usually have telltale ocular motor evidence of otolith dysfunction, such as skew deviation, ocular tilt, or ocular torsion (see Chapter 15). Their subjective visual vertical may be misaligned when compared with the true vertical defined by the earth's gravitational force.

Lesions causing the illusion that the room is tilted or upside-down are usually in the brain stem and are vascular in nature. Reported causes include transient vertebrobasilar ischemia,[185–188] compression of the lateral medulla by a dolichoectatic vertebral artery,[189] midbrain cavernoma,[190] basilar migraine,[184] and infarctions involving the lateral medulla (Wallenberg syndrome),[191] the territory of the medial branch of the posterior inferior cerebellar artery,[192] and the pons.[185,190]

Cortical and subcortical processes may also be responsible for tilted or upside-down vision. Migraine and epilepsy should always be considered when evidence of a posterior fossa lesion is lacking, although responsible supratentorial lesions have also been reported from bifrontal,[193] parieto-occipital,[194] and thalamic[195] disturbances. In addition, Brandt et al.[196] found that 23 of 52 patients with middle cerebral artery infarctions developed subjective visual vertical tilts. The authors attributed the altered perception of verticality to damage to the posterior insula, likely the homologue to parietoinsular vestibular cortex in monkeys.

Psychiatric disease

When hallucinations or illusions occur with delusions (false beliefs), primary psychiatric illnesses are the most likely diagnosis.[197] Of all psychiatric disorders with psychotic features, schizophrenia is the one most commonly associated with visual hallucinations. Psychosis in schizophrenia is suggested when complex visual hallucinations are accompanied by auditory hallucinations, particularly voices.[83] The visual hallucinations are characteristically formed, and are present with eyes opened or closed.[1] Affected individuals typically have a clear consciousness, but they display lack of insight into the unreal nature of their hallucinations. Hallucinations are less common in affective disorders such as depression and mania; however, psychosis can occur in a small minority of patients.[198] Antipsychotic medication is the mainstay of treatment for hallucinations in psychiatric diseases.

Sundowning, characterized by confusion, agitation, and visual hallucinations, can be seen in elderly patients, most typically in the late afternoon or evening. Most affected individuals have some degree of baseline dementia or cognitive decline.

Hypnagogic hallucinations in narcolepsy

Narcolepsy is characterized by the clinical tetrad of (1) *sleep attacks*, which are episodes of unwanted sleep; (2) *cataplexy*, an abrupt and reversible decrease or loss of muscle tone; (3) *sleep paralysis*, which occurs during sleep–wake transitions; and (4) *hypnagogic hallucinations*, which can be auditory or visual. Patients usually find hypnagogic hallucinations unpleasant or dreadful, and a common sensation is a threatening person at the door. Hypnagogic hallucinations occur at sleep onset, either at night or during daytime sleep episodes, and are frequently accompanied by sleep paralysis.[199]

Patients with narcolepsy also typically exhibit excessive daytime somnolence. The age range of affected patients is 5–55 years, but most individuals are in their second decade. The diagnosis is usually a straightforward one, but cases should be confirmed with polysomnography to document REM sleep at the onset of daytime or nighttime sleep episodes. Central nervous system stimulants, such as methylphenidate and modafinil, are the mainstay of treatment.[199,200]

Hypnagogic hallucinations are not necessarily pathologic. Normal individuals may experience both formed and unformed visual images upon wakening (*hypnopompic*) or upon going to sleep (*hypnagogic*).[201]

Metabolic

In unexplained cases, and in hospitalized patients with altered mental status, electrolyte imbalance, hypoxemia, and fevers should be considered as causes of visual hallucinations. Endocrine abnormalities and toxic levels of various chemicals, such as carbon dioxide, mercury, and bromide, can also produce hallucinations.[1]

Visual hallucinations in normal individuals

Aside from the aforementioned hypnagogic and hypnopompic phenomena associated with sleep/wake states, other visual hallucinations can occur in normal people. In a *grief reaction*, individuals may perceive the image of the spouse or close friend who recently died.[202] Life-threatening stress and fatigue may be other causes.[1]

References

1. Asaad G, Shapiro B. Hallucinations: theoretical and clinical overview. Am J Psychiatry 1986;143:1088–1097.
2. Carter JL. Visual, somatosensory, olfactory, and gustatory hallucinations. Psychiatr Clin North Am 1992;15:347–358.
3. West LJ. A general theory of hallucinations and dreams. In: West LJ (ed): Hallucinations, pp 275–291. New York, Grune & Stratton, 1962.
4. Cogan DG. Visual hallucinations as release phenomena. Albrecht von Graefes Arch klin exp Ophthalmol 1973;188:139–150.
5. Slade P. Hallucinations [editorial]. Psychol Med 1976;6:7–13.
6. ffytche DH, Howard RJ. The perceptual consequences of visual loss: 'positive' pathologies of vision. Brain 1999;122:1247–1260.
7. Weller M, Wiedemann P. Visual hallucinations. An outline of etiological and pathogenetic concepts. Int Ophthalmol 1989;13:193–199.
8. Manford M, Andermann F. Complex visual hallucinations. Clinical and neurobiological insights. Brain 1998;121:1819–1840.
9. ffytche DH. Visual hallucinatory syndromes: past, present, and future. Dialogues Clin Neurosci 2007;9:173–189.
10. Celesia GG. The mystery of photopsias, visual hallucinations, and distortions. Suppl Clin Neurophysiol 2006;59:97–103.
11. Kesari S. Digital rendition of visual migraines. Arch Neurol 2004;61:1464–1465.
12. Schott GD. Exploring the visual hallucinations of migraine aura: the tacit contribution of illustration. Brain 2007;130:1690–1703.
13. Hupp SL, Kline LB, Corbett JJ. Visual disturbances of migraine. Surv Ophthalmol 1989;33:221–236.
14. Headache classification subcommittee of the International Headache Society: The International Classification of Headache Disorders, 2nd edn. Cephalalgia 2004;24(Suppl 1):9–160.
15. Kaufman DM, Solomon S. Migraine visual auras. A medical update for the psychiatrist. Gen Hosp Psychiatry 1992;14:162–170.
16. Lipton RB, Stewart WF, Diamond S, et al. Prevalence and burden of migraine in the United States: data from the American Migraine Study II. Headache 2001;41:646–657.
17. Barlow CF. The expression of childhood migraine. In: Headache and Migraine in Childhood, pp 46–75. Philadelphia, JB Lippincott, 1984.
18. Olesen J, Friberg L, Olsen TS, et al. Timing and topography of cerebral blood flow, aura, and headache during migraine attacks. Ann Neurol 1990;28:791–798.
19. Cutrer FM, Sorensen AG, Weisskoff RM, et al. Perfusion-weighted imaging defects during spontaneous migrainous aura. Ann Neurol 1998;43:25–31.
20. Cutrer FM, Huerter K. Migraine aura. Neurologist 2007;13:118–125.
21. Plant GT. The fortification spectra of migraine. Br Med J 1986;293:1613–1617.
22. Sharma K, Wahi J, Phadke RV, et al. Migraine-like visual hallucinations in occipital lesions of cysticercosis. J Neuro-ophthalmol 2002;22:82–87.
23. Hachinski VC, Porchawka J, Steele JC. Visual symptoms in the migraine syndrome. Neurology 1973;23:570–579.
24. Podoll K, Robinson D. Out-of-body experiences and related phenomena in migraine art. Cephalalgia 1999;19:886–896.
25. Fuller GN, Marshall A, Flint J, et al. Migraine madness: recurrent psychosis after migraine. J Neurol Neurosurg Psychiatr 1993;56:416–418.
26. Lawden MC, Cleland PG. Achromatopsia in the aura of migraine. J Neurol Neurosurg Psychiatr 1993;56:708–709.
27. Lippman CW. Certain hallucinations peculiar to migraine. J Nerv Ment Dis 1952;116:346–351.
28. Todd J. The syndrome of Alice in Wonderland. Can Med Assoc J 1955;73:701–704.
29. Rolak LA. Literary neurologic syndromes. Alice in Wonderland. Arch Neurol 1991;48:649–651.
30. Golden GS. The Alice in Wonderland syndrome in juvenile migraine. Pediatrics 1979;63:517–519.
31. Evans RW, Rolak LA. The Alice in Wonderland Syndrome. Headache 2004;44:624–625.
32. Kuo YT, Chiu NC, Shen EY, et al. Cerebral perfusion in children with Alice in Wonderland syndrome. Pediatr Neurol 1998;19:105–108.
33. Zwijnenburg PJ, Wennink JM, Laman DM, et al. Alice in Wonderland syndrome: a clinical presentation of frontal lobe epilepsy. Neuropediatrics 2002;33:53–55.
34. Copperman SM. 'Alice in Wonderland' syndrome as a presenting symptom of infectious mononucleosis in children. Clin Pediatr 1977;16:143–146.
35. Evans RW. Reversible palinopsia and the Alice in Wonderland syndrome associated with topiramate use in migraineurs. Headache 2006;46:815–818.
36. Sinoff SE, Rosenberg M. Permanent cerebral diplopia in a migraineur. Neurology 1990;40:1138–1139.
37. Kosmorsky G. Unusual visual phenomenon during acephalgic migraine [letter]. Arch Ophthalmol 1987;105:613.
38. Jäger HR, Giffin NJ, Goadsby PJ. Diffusion- and perfusion-weighted MR imaging in persistent migrainous visual disturbances. Cephalalgia 2005;25:323–332.
39. Liu GT, Schatz NJ, Galetta SL, et al. Persistent positive visual phenomena in migraine. Neurology 1995;45:664–668.
40. Chen WT, Fuh JL, Lu SR, et al. Persistent migrainous visual phenomena might be responsive to lamotrigine. Headache 2001;41:823–825.
41. Haas DC. Prolonged migraine aura status. Ann Neurol 1982;11:197–199.
42. Luda E, Bo E, Sicuro L, et al. Sustained visual aura: a totally new variation of migraine. Headache 1991;31:582–583.
43. Rothrock JF. Successful treatment of persistent migraine aura with divalproex sodium. Neurology 1997;48:261–262.
44. Haan J, Sluis P, Sluis LH, et al. Acetazolamide treatment for migraine aura status. Neurology 2000;55:1588–1589.
45. Rozen TD. Treatment of a prolonged migrainous aura with intravenous furosemide. Neurology 2000;55:732–733.
46. San-Juan OD, Zermeno PF. Migraine with persistent aura in a Mexican patient: case report and review of the literature. Cephalalgia 2007;27:456–460.
47. Alvarez WC. The migrainous scotoma as studied in 618 persons. Am J Ophthalmol 1960;49:489–504.

48. O'Connor PS, Tredici TJ. Acephalgic migraine: fifteen years experience. Ophthalmology 1981;88:999–1003.

49. Fisher CM. Late-life (migrainous) scintillating zigzags without headache: one person's 27-year experience. Headache 1999;39:391–397.

50. Wijman CAC, Wolf PA, Kase CS, et al. Migrainous visual accompaniments are not rare in late life. The Framingham study. Stroke 1998;29:1539–1543.

51. Fisher CM. Late-life migraine accompaniments as a cause of unexplained transient ischemic attacks. Can J Neurol Sci 1980;7:9–17.

52. Al-Twaijri WA, Shevell MI. Pediatric migraine equivalents: occurrence and clinical features in practice. Pediatr Neurol 2002;26:365–368.

53. Lepore FE. Spontaneous visual phenomena with visual loss: 104 patients with lesions of the retinal and neural afferent pathways. Neurology 1990;40:444–447.

54. Kölmel HW. Coloured patterns in hemianopic fields. Brain 1984;107:155–167.

55. Kölmel HW. Complex visual hallucinations in the hemianopic field. J Neurol Neurosurg Psychiatr 1985;48:29–38.

56. Madill SA, Ffytche DH. Charles Bonnet syndrome in patients with glaucoma and good acuity. Br J Ophthalmol 2005;89:785–786.

57. Scott IU, Schein OD, Feuer WJ, et al. Visual hallucinations in patients with retinal disease. Am J Ophthalmol 2001;131:590–598.

58. Tan CS, Sabel BA, Goh KY. Visual hallucinations during visual recovery after central retinal artery occlusion. Arch Neurol 2006;63:598–600.

59. Cohen SY, Safran AB, Tadayoni R, et al. Visual hallucinations immediately after macular photocoagulation. Am J Ophthalmol 2000;129:815–816.

60. Au Eong KG, Fujii GY, Ng EW, et al. Transient formed visual hallucinations following macular translocation for subfoveal choroidal neovascularization secondary to age-related macular degeneration. Am J Ophthalmol 2001;131:664–666.

61. Merabet LB, Maguire D, Warde A, et al. Visual hallucinations during prolonged blindfolding in sighted subjects. J Neuro-ophthalmol 2004;24:109–113.

62. Menon GJ, Rahman I, Menon SJ, et al. Complex visual hallucinations in the visually impaired: the Charles Bonnet Syndrome. Surv Ophthalmol 2003;48:58–72.

63. Gittinger JW, Miller NR, Keltner JL, et al. Sugarplum fairies. Visual hallucinations. Surv Ophthalmol 1982;27:42–48.

64. White CP, Jan JE. Visual hallucinations after acute visual loss in a young child. Dev Med Child Neurol 1992;34:259–261.

65. Hoksbergen I, Pickut BA, Mariën P, et al. SPECT findings in an unusual case of visual hallucinosis. J Neurol 1996;243:594–598.

66. Flint AC, Loh JP, Brust JC. Vivid visual hallucinations from occipital lobe infarction. Neurology 2005;65:756.

67. Benegas NM, Liu GT, Volpe NJ, et al. "Picture within a picture" visual hallucinations. Neurology 1996;47:1347–1348.

68. Hedges TR, Jr. Charles Bonnet, his life, and his syndrome. Surv Ophthalmol 2007;52: 111–114.

69. Gold K, Rabins PV. Isolated visual hallucinations and the Charles Bonnet syndrome: a review of the literature and presentation of six cases. Comp Psychiatr 1989;30: 90–98.

70. Teunisse RJ, Zitman FG, Raes DCM. Clinical evaluation of 14 patients with the Charles Bonnet syndrome (isolated visual hallucinations). Comp Psychiatr 1994;35:70–75.

71. Teunisse RJ, Cruysberg JRM, Verbeek AL, et al. The Charles Bonnet syndrome: a large prospective study in the Netherlands. A study of the prevalence of the Charles Bonnet syndrome and associated factors in 500 patients attending the University Department of Ophthalmology at Nijmegen. Br J Psychiatr 1995;166:254–257.

72. Teunisse RJ, Cruysberg JR, Hoefnagels WH, et al. Visual hallucinations in psychologically normal people: Charles Bonnet's syndrome. Lancet 1996;347:794–797.

73. Ashwin PT, Tsaloumas MD. Complex visual hallucinations (Charles Bonnet syndrome) in the hemianopic visual field following occipital infarction. J Neurol Sci 2007;263: 184–186.

74. Schwartz TL, Vahgei L. Charles Bonnet syndrome in children. JAAPOS 1998;2:310–313.

75. Mewasingh LD, Kornreich C, Christiaens F, et al. Pediatric phantom vision (Charles Bonnet) syndrome. Pediatr Neurol 2002;26:143–145.

76. ffytche DH, Howard RJ, Brammer MJ, et al. The anatomy of conscious vision: an fMRI study of visual hallucinations. Nat Neurosci 1998;1:738–742.

77. Menon GJ. Complex visual hallucinations in the visually impaired: a structured history-taking approach. Arch Ophthalmol 2005;123:349–355.

78. Fernandez A, Lichtshein G, Vieweg WV. The Charles Bonnet syndrome: a review. J Nerv Ment Dis 1997;185:195–200.

79. Siatkowski RM, Zimmer B, Rosenberg PR. The Charles Bonnet syndrome. Visual perceptive dysfunction in sensory deprivation. J Clin Neuro-ophthalmol 1990;10:215–218.

80. Rovner BW. The Charles Bonnet syndrome: a review of recent research. Curr Opin Ophthalmol 2006;17:275–277.

81. Adamczyk DT. Visual phenomena, disturbances, and hallucinations. Optom Clin 1996;5:33–52.

82. Wright JD, Jr., Boger WP, 3rd. Visual complaints from healthy children. Surv Ophthalmol 1999;44:113–121.

83. Lessell S. Higher disorders of visual function: positive phenomena. In: Glaser JS, Smith JL (eds): Neuro-Ophthalmology, pp 27–44. St. Louis, C.V. Mosby, 1975.

84. Sinclair SH, Azar-Cavanagh M, Soper KA, et al. Investigation of the source of the blue field entoptic phenomenon. Invest Ophthalmol Vis Sci 1989;30:668–673.

85. Charness ME, Simon RP, Greenberg DA. Ethanol and the nervous system. N Engl J Med 1989;321:442–454.

86. Leikin JB, Krantz AJ, Zell-Kanter M, et al. Clinical features and management of intoxication due to hallucinogenic drugs. Med Toxicol Adverse Drug Exp 1989;4: 324–350.

87. Halpern JH, Pope HG, Jr. Hallucinogen persisting perception disorder: what do we know after 50 years? Drug Alcohol Depend 2003;69:109–119.

88. Levi L, Miller NR. Visual illusions associated with previous drug abuse. J Clin Neuro-ophthalmol 1990;10:103–110.

89. Lerner AG, Gelkopf M, Skladman I, et al. Clonazepam treatment of lysergic acid diethylamide-induced hallucinogen persisting perception disorder with anxiety features. Int Clin Psychopharmacol 2003;18:101–105.

90. Mitchell J, Vierkant AD. Delusions and hallucinations of cocaine abusers and paranoid schizophrenics: a comparative study. J Psychol 1991;125:301–310.

91. Siegel RK. Cocaine hallucinations. American Journal of Psychiatry 1978;135:309–314.

92. Kulig K. LSD. Emerg Med Clin North Am 1990;8:551–558.

93. Schwartz RH, Comerci GD, Meeks JE. Clinical and laboratory observations. LSD: patterns of use by chemically dependent adolescents. J Pediatr 1987;111:936–938.

94. Kawasaki A, Purvin V. Persistent palinopsia following ingestion of lysergic acid diethylamide (LSD). Arch Ophthalmol 1996;114:47–50.

95. Francis J, Murray VSG. Review of enquiries made to the NPIS concerning psilocybe mushroom ingestion. 1978–1981. Human Toxicology 1983;2:349–352.

96. Schwartz RH, Smith DE. Hallucinogenic mushrooms. Clin Pediatr 1988;27:70–73.

97. Peden NR, Macaulay KEC, Bissett AF, et al. Clinical toxicology of magic mushroom ingestion. Postgrad Med J 1981;57:543–545.

98. McCarron MM, Schulze BW, Thompson GA, et al. Acute phencyclidine intoxication: clinical patterns complications and treatment. Ann Emerg Med 1981;10:290–297.

99. McCarron MM, Schulze BW, Thompson GA, et al. Acute phencyclidine intoxication: incidence of clinical finding in 1000 cases. Ann Emerg Med 1981;10:237–242.

100. Schwartz RH. Mescaline: a survey. Am Fam Physician 1988;37:122–124.

101. Oishi A, Miyamoto K, Kashii S, et al. Photopsia as a manifestation of digitalis toxicity. Can J Ophthalmol 2006;41:603–604.

102. Piltz JR, Wertenbaker C, Lance SE, et al. Digoxin toxicity. J Clin Neuro-ophthalmol 1993;13:275–280.

103. Weleber RG, Shults WT. Digoxin retinal toxicity. Clinical and electrophysiologic evaluation of a cone dysfunction syndrome. Arch Ophthalmol 1981;99:1568–1572.

104. Butler VP, Odel JG, Rath E, et al. Digitalis-induced visual disturbances with therapeutic serum digitalis concentrations. Ann Intern Med 1995;123:676–680.

105. Wolin MJ. Digoxin visual toxicity with therapeutic blood levels of digoxin. Am J Ophthalmol 1998;125:406–407.

106. Banerjee AK, Falkai PG, Savidge M. Visual hallucinations in the elderly associated with the use of levodopa. Postgrad Med J 1989;65:358–361.

107. Friedman JH. The management of the levodopa psychoses. Clin Neuropharmacol 1991;14:283–295.

108. Cummings JL. Behavioral complications of drug treatment of Parkinson's disease. J Am Geriatr Soc 1991;39:708–716.

109. The Parkinson Study Group. Low-dose clozapine for the treatment of drug-induced psychosis in Parkinson's disease. N Engl J Med 1999;340:757–763.

110. Purvin VA. Visual disturbance secondary to clomiphene citrate. Arch Ophthalmol 1995;113:482–484.

111. Steg RE, Garcia EG. Complex visual hallucinations and cyclosporine neurotoxicity. Neurology 1991;41:1156.

112. Gabrieli CB, Regine F, Vingolo EM, et al. Subjective visual halos after sildenafil (Viagra) administration: electroretinographic evaluation. Ophthalmology 2001;108:877–881.

113. Laties A, Zrenner E. Viagra (sildenafil citrate) and ophthalmology. Prog Retin Eye Res 2002;21:485–506.

114. Brandt C, Fueratsch N, Boehme V, et al. Development of psychosis in patients with epilepsy treated with lamotrigine: report of six cases and review of the literature. Epilepsy Behav 2007;11:133–139.

115. La Vega-Talbot M, Duchowny M, Jayakar P. Orbitofrontal seizures presenting with ictal visual hallucinations and interictal psychosis. Pediatr Neurol 2006;35:78–81.

116. Williamson PD, Thadani VM, Darcey TM, et al. Occipital lobe epilepsy: clinical characteristics, seizure spread patterns, and results of surgery. Ann Neurol 1992;31: 3–13.

117. Salanova V, Andermann F, Olivier A, et al. Occipital lobe epilepsy: electroclinical manifestations, electrocorticography, cortical stimulation and outcome in 42 patients treated between 1930 and 1991. Brain 1992;115:1655–1680.

118. Aykut-Bingol C, Bronen RA, Kim JH, et al. Surgical outcome in occipital lobe epilepsy: implications for pathophysiology. Ann Neurol 1998;44:60–69.

119. Bien CG, Benninger FO, Urbach H, et al. Localizing value of epileptic visual auras. Brain 2000;123:244–253.

120. Thomas P, Barrè P, Chatel M. Complex partial status epilepticus of extratemporal origin: report of a case. Neurology 1991;41:1147–1149.

121. Walker MC, Smith SJM, Sisodiya SM, et al. Case of simple partial status epilepticus in occipital lobe misdiagnosed as migraine: clinical, electrophysiological, and magnetic resonance imagining characteristics. Epilepsia 1995;36:1233–1236.

122. Lavin PJ. Hyperglycemic hemianopia: a reversible complication of non-ketotic hyperglycemia. Neurology 2005;65:616–619.

123. Oguni H, Sugama M, Osawa M. Symptomatic parieto-occipital epilepsy as sequela of perinatal asphyxia. Pediatr Neurol 2008;338:345–352.

124. Caraballo RH, Sakr D, Mozzi M, et al. Symptomatic occipital lobe epilepsy following neonatal hypoglycemia. Pediatr Neurol 2004;31:24–29.

125. Libenson MH, Caravale B, Prasad AN. Clinical correlations of occipital epileptiform discharges in children. Neurology 1999;53:265–269.

126. Taylor I, Scheffer IE, Berkovic SF. Occipital epilepsies: identification of specific and newly recognized syndromes. Brain 2003;126:753–769.

127. Panayiotopoulos CP. Elementary visual hallucinations in migraine and epilepsy. J Neurol Neurosurg Psychiatr 1994;57:1371–1374.

128. Deonna T, Ziegler A-L, Despland PA. Paroxysmal visual disturbances of epileptic origin and occipital epilepsy in children. Neuropediatrics 1984;15:131–135.

129. Panayiotopoulos CP, Michael M, Sanders S, et al. Benign childhood focal epilepsies: assessment of established and newly recognized syndromes. Brain 2008;131:2264–2286.

130. Taylor I, Berkovic SF, Kivity S, et al. Benign occipital epilepsies of childhood: clinical features and genetics. Brain 2008;131:2287–2294.

131. Panayiotopoulos CP. Benign childhood epilepsy with occipital paroxysms. A 15-year prospective clinical and electroencephalographic study. Ann Neurol 1989;26:51–56.

132. Gastaut H, Zifkin BG. Ictal visual hallucinations of numerals. Neurology 1984;34:950–953.

133. Currie S, Heathfield KWG, Henson RA, et al. Clinical course and prognosis of temporal lobe epilepsy. Brain 1971;94:173–190.

134. King DW, Ajmone Marsan C. Clinical features and ictal patterns in epileptic patients with EEG temporal lobe foci. Ann Neurol 1977;2:138–147.

135. Sowa MV, Pituck S. Prolonged spontaneous complex visual hallucinations and illusions as ictal phenomena. Epilepsia 1989;30:524–526.

136. Vignal JP, Maillard L, McGonigal A, et al. The dreamy state: hallucinations of autobiographic memory evoked by temporal lobe stimulations and seizures. Brain 2007;130:88–99.

137. Ionasescu V. Paroxysmal disorders of the body image in temporal lobe epilepsy. Acta Psychiatr Scand 1960;35:171–181.

138. Mendez MF. Ictal hemimacropsia. Neurology 1992;42:1119–1120.

139. Kawai M, Cherches IM, Goldsmith IL. Visual illusory and hallucinatory phenomena in a patient with left occipital seizures. Neurology 2006;67:1457.

140. Laff R, Mesad S, Devinsky O. Epileptic kinetopsia: ictal illusory motion perception. Neurology 2003;61:1262–1264.

141. Williamson PD, Boon PA, Thadani VM, et al. Parietal lobe epilepsy: diagnostic considerations and results of surgery. Ann Neurol 1992;31:193–201.

142. Sveinbjornsdottir S, Duncan JS. Parietal and occipital lobe epilepsy: a review. Epilepsia 1993;34:493–521.

143. Rousseaux M, Debrock D, Cabaret M, et al. Visual hallucinations with written words in a case of left parietotemporal lesion. J Neurol Neurosurg Psychiatr 1994;57:1268–1271.

144. Müller T, Büttner T, Kuhn W, et al. Palinopsia as sensory epileptic phenomenon. Acta Neurol Scand 1995;91:433–436.

145. Devinsky O, Feldmann E, Burrowes K, et al. Autoscopic phenomena with seizures. Arch Neurol 1989;46:1080–1088.

146. Tadokoro Y, Oshima T, Kanemoto K. Postictal autoscopy in a patient with partial epilepsy. Epilepsy Behav 2006;9:535–540.

147. Blanke O, Mohr C. Out-of-body experience, heautoscopy, and autoscopic hallucination of neurological origin. Implications for neurocognitive mechanisms of corporeal awareness and self-consciousness. Brain Res Brain Res Rev 2005;50:184–199.

148. Jacobs L. Visual allesthesia. Neurology 1980;30:1059–1063.

149. Sanchez-Ramos JR, Ortoll R, Paulson GW. Visual hallucinations associated with Parkinson disease. Arch Neurol 1996;53:1265–1268.

150. Holroyd S, Currie L, Wooten GF. Prospective study of hallucinations and delusions in Parkinson's disease. J Neurol Neurosurg Psychiatry 2001;70:734–738.

151. Biousse V, Skibell BC, Watts RL, et al. Ophthalmologic features of Parkinson's disease. Neurology 2004;62:177–180.

152. Frucht SJ, Bernsohn L. Visual hallucinations in PD. Neurology 2002;59:1965.

153. Mosimann UP, Mather G, Wesnes KA, et al. Visual perception in Parkinson disease dementia and dementia with Lewy bodies. Neurology 2004;63:2091–2096.

154. Arnulf I, Bonnet AM, Damier P, et al. Hallucinations, REM sleep, and Parkinson's disease. a medical hypothesis. Neurology 2000;55:281–288.

155. Manni R, Pacchetti C, Terzaghi M, et al. Hallucinations and sleep-wake cycle in PD: a 24-hour continuous polysomnographic study. Neurology 2002;59:1979–1981.

156. Fénelon G, Mahieux F, Huon R, et al. Hallucinations in Parkinson's disease: prevalence, phenomenology and risk factors. Brain 2000;123:733–745.

157. Barnes J, David AS. Visual hallucinations in Parkinson's disease: a review and phenomenological survey. J Neurol Neurosurg Psychiatry 2001;70:727–733.

158. Goetz CG, Fan W, Leurgans S, et al. The malignant course of "benign hallucinations" in Parkinson disease. Arch Neurol 2006;63:713–716.

159. Goetz CG, Stebbins GT. Mortality and hallucinations in nursing home patients with advanced Parkinson's disease. Neurology 1995;45:669–671.

160. McKeith IG, Dickson DW, Lowe J, et al. Diagnosis and management of dementia with Lewy bodies: third report of the DLB Consortium. Neurology 2005;65:1863–1872.

161. Lerner AJ, Koss E, Patterson MB, et al. Concomitants of visual hallucinations in Alzheimer's disease. Neurology 1994;44:523–527.

162. Wilson RS, Gilley DW, Bennett DA, et al. Hallucinations, delusions, and cognitive decline in Alzheimer's disease. J Neurol Neurosurg Psychiatry 2000;69:172–177.

163. Lopez OL, Becker JT, Brenner RP, et al. Alzheimer's disease with delusions and hallucinations: neuropsychological and electroencephalographic correlates. Neurology 1991;41:906–912.

164. Scarmeas N, Brandt J, Albert M, et al. Delusions and hallucinations are associated with worse outcome in Alzheimer disease. Arch Neurol 2005;62:1601–1608.

165. Dunn DW, Weisberg LA, Nadell J. Peduncular hallucinations caused by brainstem compression. Neurology 1983;33:1360–1361.

166. Maiuri F, Iaconetta G, Sardo L, et al. Peduncular hallucinations associated with large posterior fossa meningiomas. Clin Neurol Neurosurg 2002;104:41–43.

167. Caplan LR. "Top of the basilar" syndrome. Neurology 1980;30:72–79.

168. Lhermitte J. Syndrome de la calotte du pédoncule cérébral. Les troubles psycho-sensoriels dans les lésions due mésocéphale. Rev Neurol (Paris) 1922;38:1359–1365.

169. van Bogaert L. Syndrome inférieur du noyau rouge, troubles psycho-sensoriels d'origine mésocéphalique. Rev Neurol (Paris) 1924;40:417–423.

170. van Bogaert L. L'hallucinose pédonculaire. Rev Neurol (Paris) 1927;47:608–617.

171. Geller TJ, Bellur SN. Peduncular hallucinosis: magnetic resonance imaging confirmation of mesencephalic infarction during life. Ann Neurol 1987;21:602–604.

172. McKee AC, Levine DN, Kowall NW, et al. Peduncular hallucinosis associated with isolated infarction of the substantia nigra pars reticulata. Ann Neurol 1990;27:500–504.

173. Kölmel HW. Peduncular hallucinations. J Neurol 1991;238:457–459.

174. Bender MB, Feldman M, Sobin AJ. Palinopsia. Brain 1968;91:321–328.

175. Meadows JC, Munro SSF. Palinopsia. J Neurol Neurosurg Psychiatr 1977;40:5–8.

176. Michel EM, Troost BT. Palinopsia: cerebral localization with computed tomography. Neurology 1980;30:887–889.

177. Hughes MS, Lessell S. Trazodone-induced palinopsia. Arch Ophthalmol 1990;108:399–400.

178. Pomeranz HD, Lessell S. Palinopsia and polyopia in the absence of drugs or cerebral disease. Neurology 2000;54:855–859.

179. Ritsema ME, Murphy MA. Palinopsia from posterior visual pathway lesions without visual field defects. J Neuro-ophthalmol 2007;27:115–117.

180. Lopez JR, Adornato BT, Hoyt WF. "Entomopia": a remarkable case of cerebral polyopia. Neurology 1993;43:2145–2146.

181. Cornblath WT, Butter CM, Barnes LL, et al. Spatial characteristics of cerebral polyopia: a case study. Vision Res 1998;38:3965–3978.

182. Jones MR, Waggoner R, Hoyt WF. Cerebral polyopia with extrastriate quadrantopia: report of a case with magnetic resonance documentation of V2/V3 cortical infarction. J Neuro-ophthalmol 1999;19:1–6.

183. Gottlieb D. The unidirectionality of cerebral polyopia. J Clin Neuro-ophthalmol 1992;12:257–262.

184. River Y, Ben Hur T, Steiner I. Reversal of vision metamorphopsia. Clinical and anatomical characteristics. Arch Neurol 1998;55:1362–1368.

185. Ropper AH. Illusion of tilting of the visual environment: report of five cases. J Clin Neuro-ophthalmol 1983;3:147–151.

186. Steiner I, Shahin R, Melamed E. Acute upside down reversal of vision in transient vertebrobasilar ischemia. Neurology 1987;37:1685–1686.

187. Mehler MF. Complete visual inversion in vertebrobasilar ischaemic disease. J Neurol Neurosurg Psychiatry 1988;51:1236–1237.

188. Stracciari A, Guarino M, Ciucci G, et al. Acute upside down reversal of vision in vertebrobasilar ischaemia [letter]. J Neurol Neurosurg Psychiatry 1993;56:423.

189. Slavin ML, LoPinto RJ. Isolated environmental tilt associated with lateral medullary compression by dolichoectasia of the vertebral artery. Is there a cause and effect relationship? J Clin Neuro-ophthalmol 1987;7:29–33.

190. Tiliket C, Ventre-Dominey J, Vighetto A, et al. Room tilt illusion. A central otolith dysfunction. Arch Neurol 1996;53:1259–1264.

191. Hörnsten G. Wallenberg's syndrome. Part I, General symptomatology with special references to visual disturbances and imbalance. Acta Neurol Scand 1974;50:434–446.

192. Charles N, Froment C, Rode G, et al. Vertigo and upside down vision due to an infarct in the territory of the medial branch of the posterior inferior cerebellar artery caused by dissection of a vertebral artery. J Neurol Neurosurg Psychiatry 1992;55:188–189.

193. Solms M, Kaplan-Solms K, Saling M, et al. Inverted vision after frontal lobe disease. Cortex 1988;24:499–509.

194. Girkin CA, Perry JD, Miller NR. Visual environmental rotation: a novel disorder of visiospatial integration. J Neuro-ophthalmol 1999;19:13–16.

195. Aldridge AJ, Kline LB, Girkin CA. Environmental tilt illusion as the only symptom of a thalamic astrocytoma. J Neuro-ophthalmol 2003;23:145–147.

196. Brandt T, Dieterich M, Danek A. Vestibular cortex lesions affect the perception of verticality. Ann Neurol 1994;35:403–412.

197. Norton JW, Corbett JJ. Visual perceptual abnormalities: hallucinations and illusions. Semin Neurol 2000;20:111–121.

198. Black DW, Nasrallah A. Hallucinations and delusions in 1715 patients with unipolar and bipolar affective disorders. Psychopathology 1989;22:28–34.

199. Billiard M. Narcolepsy. Clinical features and aetiology. Ann Clin Res 1985;17:220–226.

200. Nishino S. Clinical and neurobiological aspects of narcolepsy. Sleep Med 2007;8:373–399.

201. Manni R. Rapid eye movement sleep, non-rapid eye movement sleep, dreams, and hallucinations. Curr Psychiatry Rep 2005;7:196–200.

202. Schneck JM. S. Weir Mitchell's visual hallucinations as a grief reaction [letter]. Am J Psychiatry 1989;146:409.

Part **Three**

Efferent neuro-ophthalmic disorders

CHAPTER **13**

Pupillary disorders

Pupillary disorders usually fall into one of three major categories: (1) abnormally shaped pupils, (2) abnormal pupillary reaction to light, or (3) unequally sized pupils (anisocoria). Occasionally pupillary abnormalities are isolated findings, but in many cases they are manifestations of more serious intracranial pathology.

The pupillary examination is discussed in detail in Chapter 2. Pupillary neuroanatomy and physiology will be reviewed here, and then the various pupillary disorders, grouped roughly into one of the three categories listed above, will be discussed.

Neuroanatomy and physiology

The major functions of the pupil are to vary the quantity of light reaching the retina, to minimize the spherical aberrations of the peripheral cornea and lens, and to increase the depth of field (the depth within which objects will appear sharp).[1] In most individuals the two pupils are equal in size, and each is situated slightly nasal and inferior to the center of the cornea and iris (**Fig. 13–1**).

The iris contains the two muscles that control the size of the pupil. Contraction of the dilator muscle leads to pupillary enlargement (mydriasis), while sphincter muscle contraction causes pupillary constriction (miosis). The sphincter muscle wraps 360 degrees around the pupillary margin, and the dilator muscle similarly encircles the pupil but is more peripherally located.

Normally, light directed at either eye leads to bilateral pupillary constriction, and this pupillary light reflex is mediated by a parasympathetic pathway (see **Fig. 13–2** for details). Light entering the eye causes retinal photoreceptors to hyperpolarize, in turn causing activation of retinal interneurons and ultimately the retinal ganglion cells, the axons of which travel through the optic nerve, chiasm, and optic tract to reach the pretectal nuclei (afferent arc). Interneurons then connect the pretectal nuclei to the Edinger–Westphal nuclei. Although these connections are bilateral, the input into the Edinger–Westphal nuclei is predominantly from the contralateral pretectal nucleus. Since the afferent pupillary fibers leave the optic tract before the lateral geniculate nucleus, isolated lesions of the geniculate, optic radiations, and visual cortex generally do not affect pupillary size or reactivity. Efferent parasympathetic fibers, arising from the Edinger–Westphal nucleus, exit the midbrain within the third nerve (efferent arc). Within the subarachnoid portion of the third nerve, pupillary fibers tend to run on the external surface, making them more vulnerable to compression or infiltration and less susceptible to vascular insult. Within the anterior cavernous sinus, the third nerve divides into two portions. The pupillary fibers follow the inferior division into the orbit, where they then synapse at the ciliary ganglion, which lies in the posterior part of the orbit between the optic nerve and lateral rectus muscle (**Fig. 13–3**). The ciliary ganglion issues postganglionic

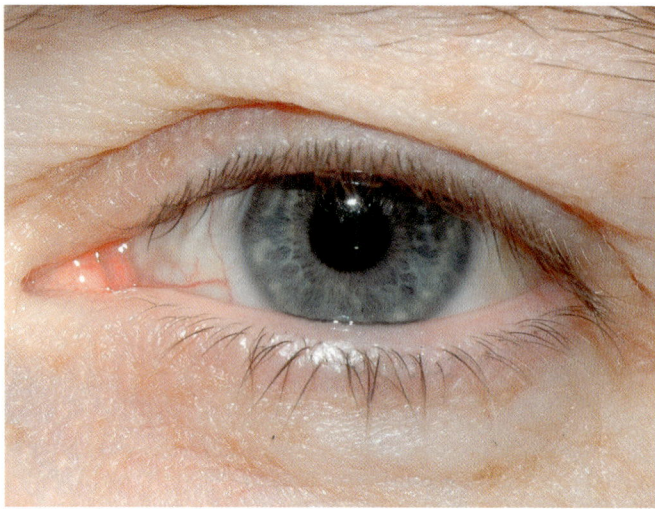

Figure 13–1. A normal left eye. Note the pupil is slightly nasal to the center of the cornea and iris.

cholinergic short ciliary nerves, which initially travel to the globe with the nerve to the inferior oblique muscle, then between the sclera and choroid, to innervate the ciliary body and iris sphincter muscle. Fibers to the ciliary body outnumber those to the iris sphincter muscle by 30:1.

The near response consists of pupillary constriction, accommodation (change in the shape of the lens), and convergence of the eyes (see Chapter 2). Although the pathways are uncertain, the supranuclear control for the near response likely arises from diffuse cortical locations. Stimulation of the peristriate cortex (areas 19 and 22) in primates can evoke a near reponse,[2] but more recent evidence suggests the lateral suprasylvian area is also related to the control of lens accommodation.[3] The signals converge in the rostral superior colliculus, near which a group of midbrain near-response neurons coordinates the pretectum for accommodation and miosis, the mesencephalic reticular formation for accommodation and vergence, and the raphe interpositus for visual fixation.[3,4] The final signal for pupillary miosis at near is still mediated by the Edinger–Westphal nuclei.

Pupillary dilation is the function of the oculosympathetic system (the ocular part of the sympathetic nervous system), which consists of three neurons beginning in the posterolateral hypothalamus and ending at the iris and eyelids (see **Fig. 13–4** for details). The first-order neuron projects from the hypothalamus through ill-defined brain stem pathways to synapse on the intermediolateral cell column in the spinal cord at C8–T2 (ciliospinal center of Budge). The second-order neuron (preganglionic) leaves the spinal cord and travels over the apex of the lung before ascending with the internal carotid artery to synapse at the superior cervical ganglion. In the region of the lung apex, the sympathetic pathway lies in close proximity to the lower brachial plexus. The third-order neuron (postganglionic) travels along the internal carotid into the cavernous sinus, after which the sympathetic pathways follow the sixth nerve, then the nasociliary nerve (a branch of the first division of the trigeminal nerve), then the long ciliary nerve into the orbit.[5] This

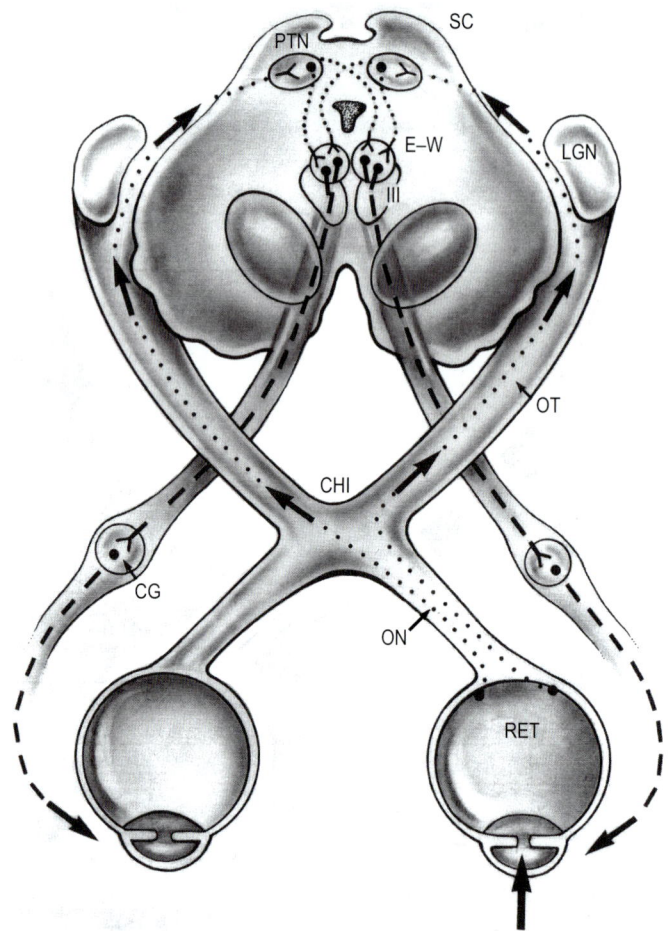

Figure 13–2. Pupillary light reflex–parasympathetic pathway. Light entering one eye (*straight black arrow*, bottom right) stimulates the retinal photoreceptors (RET), resulting in excitation of ganglion cells, whose axons travel within the optic nerve (ON), partially decussate in the chiasm (CHI), then leave the optic tract (OT) (before the lateral geniculate nucleus (LGN)) and pass through the brachium of the superior colliculus (SC) before synapsing at the mesencephalic pretectal nucleus (PTN). This structure connects bilaterally, but predominantly contralaterally, to the oculomotor nuclear complex at the Edinger–Westphal (E-W) nuclei, which issue parasympathetic fibers that travel within the third nerve (inferior division) and terminate at the ciliary ganglion (CG) in the orbit. Postsynaptic cells innervate the pupillary sphincter, resulting in miosis. Note light in one eye causes bilaterally pupillary constriction. (From Liu GT: Disorders of the eyes and eyelids: Disorders of the pupil. In Samuels MA, Feske S (eds): The Office Practice of Neurology, p 61. New York, Churchill Livingstone, 1996, with permission. Adapted from Slamovits TL, Glaser JS. The pupils and accommodation. In: Glaser JS (ed): Neuro-ophthalmology, 2nd edition, p 460. Philadelphia, JB Lippincott, 1990, with permission.)

neuron releases the neurotransmitter norepinephrine at the iris dilator muscle.

Pharmacologic testing of the pupils

As will be discussed, pharmacologic testing helps confirm the clinical diagnosis of many pupillary abnormalities. Some general guidelines need to be followed in this regard. By disrupting the corneal epithelium, corneal reflex evaluation and applanation tonometry may alter corneal permeability of the drug (especially cocaine) and therefore should not be

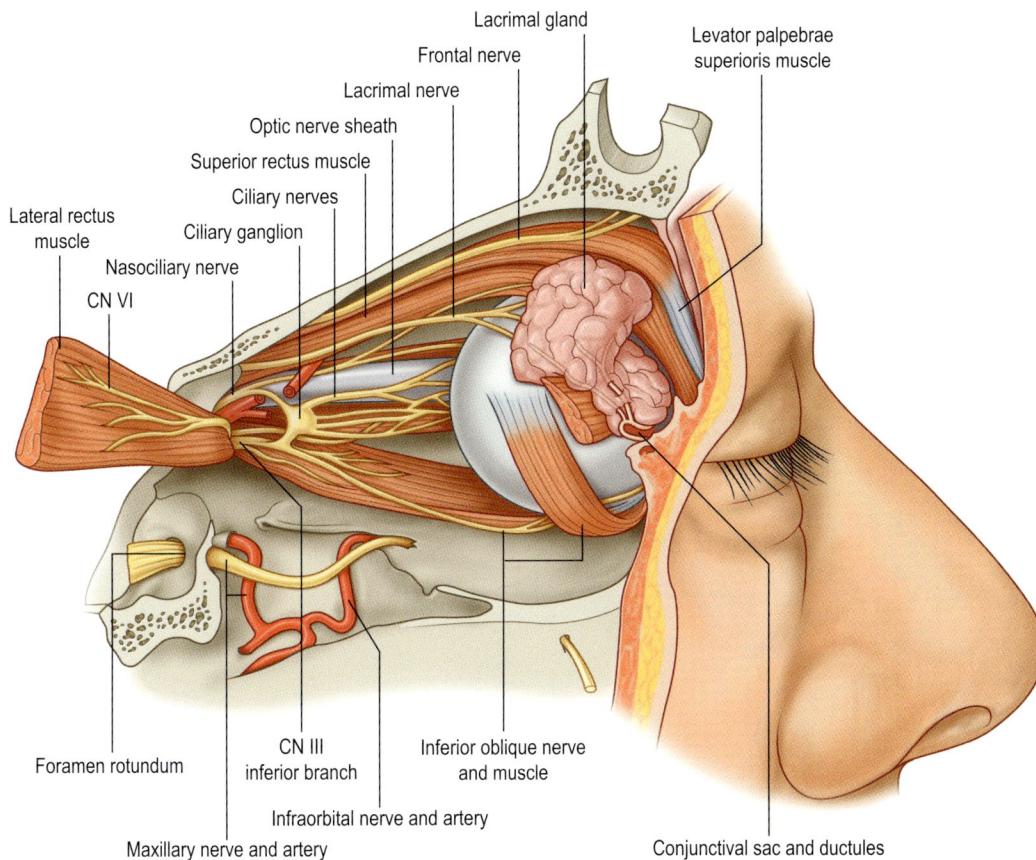

Figure 13–3. Ciliary ganglion depicted in a lateral view of a dissection of the orbit. Note the ciliary ganglion lies between the optic nerve and the lateral rectus muscle, receives fibers from the inferior branch of the third nerve, and issues short ciliary nerves to the orbit, orbital muscles, and lacrimal gland.

performed on the same day as pharmacologic testing. In general, the drops should be instilled in the inferior cul-de-sac, with care taken to use the same size drop in each eye. Drop administration should be repeated 1–5 minutes later. The pupil sizes then can be measured 30–45 minutes after instillation of the last set of drops. Baseline and test pupillary sizes are best measured in the same lighting conditions, and photographic documentation can be helpful.

Abnormally shaped pupils

Irregularly shaped pupils may be congenital or acquired (**Table 13–1**). Congenital conditions include:

1. *Aniridia*, in which the iris is hypoplastic, creating a large pupillary opening. Associated ocular findings often include cataracts, glaucoma, and impaired vision due to macular or optic nerve hypoplasia. Patients with aniridia, genitourinary anomalies, mental retardation, and a defect in the PAX6 gene on chromosome 11p13 are predisposed to Wilms' tumor.[6–8]
2. *Ectopia lentis et pupillae*, a rare heritable condition limited to the eyes in which lens dislocations may be associated with oval, ellipsoid, or slit-like displaced pupils.[6,9]
3. An *iris coloboma* is a notch inferiorly or infranasally in the iris (**Fig. 13–5**). This anomaly may be accompanied

Table 13–1 Causes of abnormally shaped pupils

Congenital causes
Aniridia
Ectopia lentis et pupillae
Iris coloboma
Anterior chamber cleavage anomalies
Ectopic pupils
Persistent pupillary membranes
Acquired causes
Iritis
Trauma (accidental or surgical)
Iris Atrophy (e.g., Diabetes, herpetic disease)
Neurologic (e.g., tonic pupils, midbrain damage (corectopia), tadpole-shaped pupils)

by chorioretinal or optic nerve colobomas, which like the iris abnormality are defects in closure of the embryonic fissure.[10] Colobomas may occur in isolation in healthy individuals or in patients with chromosomal duplication or deletions. They may also be seen in complex congenital disorders such as CHARGE syndrome (C, coloboma; H, heart disease; A, atresia or stenosis of the choanae; R, retarded growth and

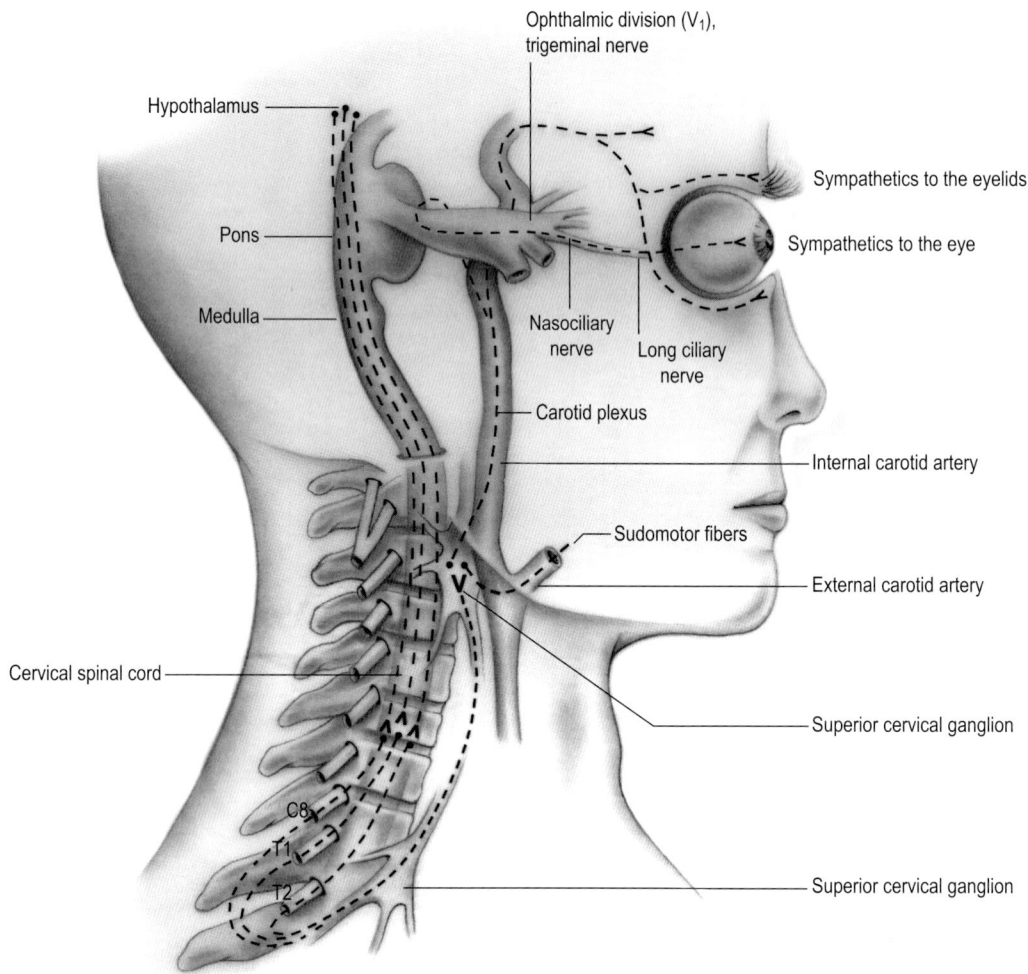

Figure 13–4. Sympathetic innervation of the pupil and eyelids. First-order hypothalamic (central) neurons descend through the brain stem (midbrain, pons, medulla) and cervical spinal cord. These fibers then synapse with preganglionic neurons, whose cell bodies lie in the intermediolateral gray column and whose axons exit the cord ipsilaterally at C8, T1, and T2 via the ventral roots. These second-order fibers then travel rostrally via the sympathetic chain, traverse the superior mediastinum, pass through the stellate ganglion (the fusion of the inferior cervical ganglion and the first thoracic ganglion), and terminate in the superior cervical ganglion, which lies posterior to the angle of the mandible. The postganglionic axons ascend within the carotid plexus, which surrounds the internal carotid artery, to reach the cavernous sinus. The sympathetic branches ultimately reach the iris by first joining the sixth nerve (not shown), then the nasociliary nerve, a branch of the first division of the trigeminal nerve, and then the long ciliary nerve. Sudomotor fibers (e.g., for sweating) to the lower face follow the external carotid and then the facial arteries. Sympathetic fibers to Müller's muscles (upper eyelid elevators and lower eyelid depressors) also travel within the carotid plexus into the cavernous sinus, then may join branches of the third nerve before reaching the upper and lower eyelids (Redrawn from Liu GT: Disorders of the eyes and eyelids: Disorders of the pupil. In Samuels MA, Feske S (eds): The Office Practice of Neurology, p 62. New York, Churchill Livingstone, 1996, with permission.)

development or central nervous system anomalies; G, genital hypoplasia; and E, ear anomalies or deafness).[11,12]

4. *Anterior chamber cleavage anomalies*, such as Peters (central corneal defects) or Rieger syndrome (peripheral corneal defects), also may be associated with misshapen pupils accompanied by abnormal adhesions between the cornea and iris.[13]

5. *Ectopic pupils* (misplaced—also called *corectopia*) may be inherited as an isolated ocular finding. Patients with these anomalies may require further genetic evaluation. An idiopathic tractional corectopia, in which a fibrous structure tethers the pupillary margin to the peripheral cornea and causes a misplaced pupil, has also been described.[14]

6. *Persistent pupillary membranes* may cause spoke-like opacities across the pupil. These derive from persistence of the tunica vasculosa lentis, which supplies blood to the developing crystalline lens and normally disappears by the 34th week of gestation.[15]

Acquired causes of abnormally shaped pupils include:

1. *Iritis.* Inflammation of the iris (iritis) may lead to adhesions between the iris and lens (posterior synechiae) and cause pupillary distortion (**Fig. 13–6A**).

2. *Trauma* may result in an iris tear or rupture of the iris sphincter. The ocular trauma may be accidental (**Fig. 13–6B**), or the iris may be damaged during anterior segment surgery.

3. *Neurologic causes* such as tonic pupils, neurosyphilis, severe damage to the midbrain, which can rarely cause pupillary corectopia (**Fig. 13–7**), tadpole-shaped pupils, and other conditions (e.g., herniation) associated with coma. These entities are all described in more detail below.

Defective pupillary light reaction associated with vision loss

In these cases the direct pupillary reaction to light is abnormal because of a disturbance within the afferent arc of the pupillary light reflex. In most such instances, there is associated visual loss.

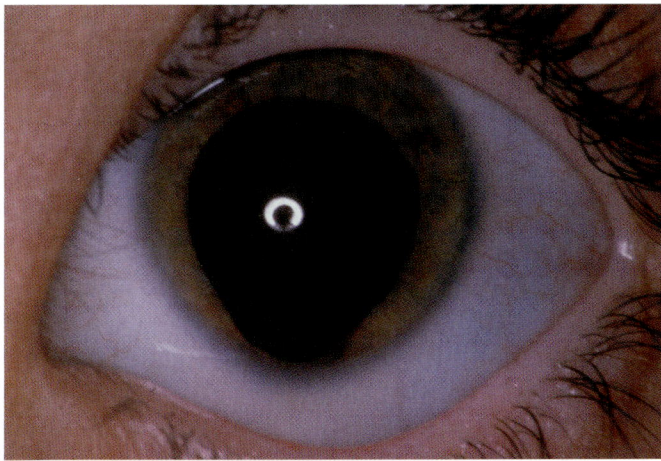

Figure 13–5. Iris coloboma, characterized by the inferior iris defect. (Photo courtesy of Dr. David Kozart. From Liu GT: Pupillary abnormalities in childhood. Contemp Pediatr 1995;12 (Nov):83–98, with permission.)

Relative afferent pupillary defect

The swinging flashlight test and the detection and grading of relative afferent pupillary defects (RAPDs) are discussed in Chapter 2. Abnormal visual acuity and color vision, a central scotoma, and an RAPD collectively are highly suggestive of an optic neuropathy, although a large macular lesion could produce similar findings. In bilateral optic nerve disease, an RAPD may not be present unless the visual loss is asymmetric. An individual with severe unilateral visual loss, no RAPD, and a normal ocular examination may have nonorganic visual loss.[16] An RAPD is not associated with visual loss due to corneal, lens, and vitreous opacities and refractive errors, but an amblyopic eye may have a mild RAPD.[17] Nevertheless, an amblyopic eye with an RAPD generally requires further investigation to exclude an acquired optic neuropathy. When anisocoria is present, care should be taken to avoid overcalling an RAPD.[18] In this setting, the false RAPD can be seen on the side of the smaller pupil as less light enters this eye than the fellow eye.

Asymmetric chiasmal syndromes may be associated with an RAPD, especially if an eye has subnormal visual acuity. Isolated optic tract lesions may have a contralateral RAPD, despite normal visual acuities, because the defective temporal field in the contralateral eye is 61–71% larger than the nasal field of the ipsilateral eye, the nasal retina has a greater photoreceptor density, and the ratio of crossed to uncrossed fibers in the chiasm is 53:47.[19] The magnitude of the RAPD in this setting may reflect the relative light sensitivity of the intact temporal versus nasal field.[20] Less commonly, when an optic tract lesion is associated with an incongruous homonymous hemianopia with greater involvement of the nasal field, the RAPD will be in the ipsilateral eye. *Behr's pupil* (a large contralateral pupil) and *Wernicke's hemianopic pupil*, one which reacts more briskly to light projected from within the intact hemifield than to

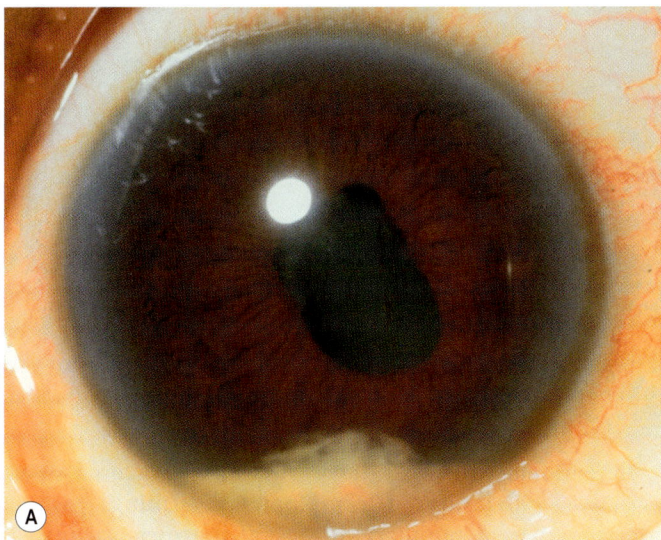

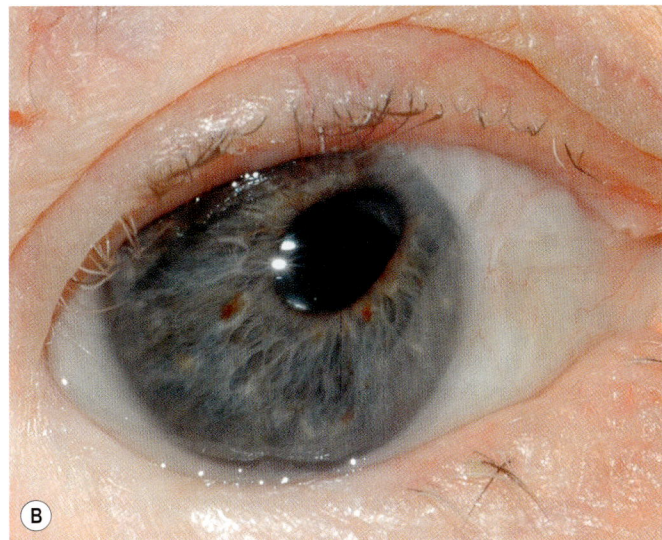

Figure 13–6. Misshapen pupils due to iritis (**A**) and trauma (**B**). **A**. Inflammation of the iris (iritis or anterior uveitis) can cause abnormal attachments between the iris and lens (iris synechiae). Note the pus layered out at the bottom of the anterior chamber (hypopyon). (Photo courtesy of Dr. Stephen Orlin. From Liu GT: Pupillary abnormalities in childhood. Contemp Pediatr 1995;12 (Nov):83–98, with permission.) **B**. Ocular trauma resulted in this oval, misshapen pupil in a patient's right eye.

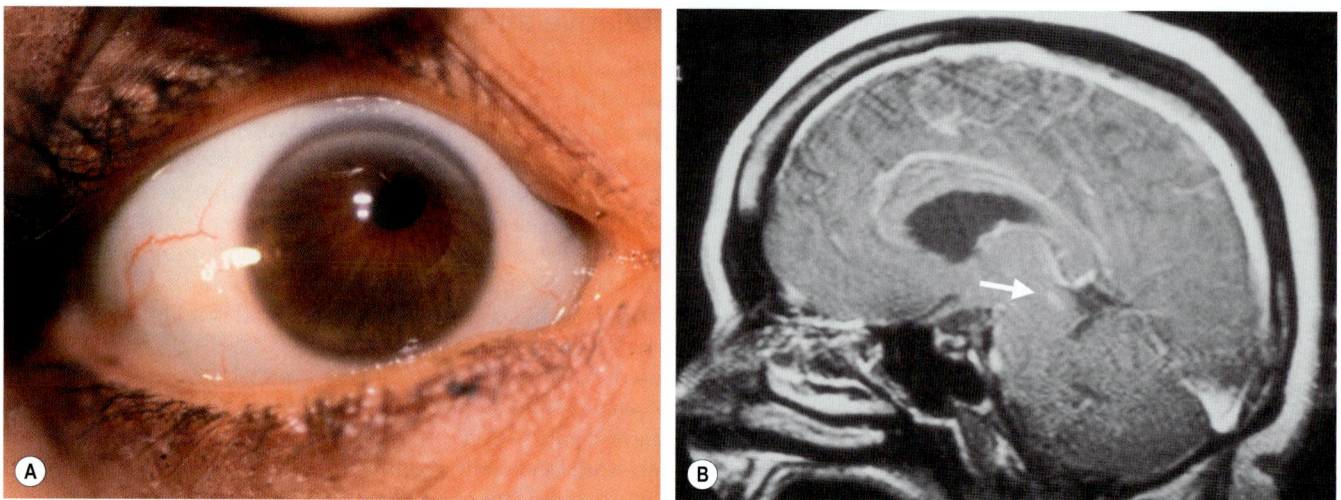

Figure 13–7. Pupil corectopia due to cysticercosis. **A**. The pupil of the right eye is displaced supranasally. **B**. T1-weighted gadolinium-enhanced sagittal magnetic resonance imaging scan from the same patient shows enhancement (*arrow*) in the Sylvian aqueduct.

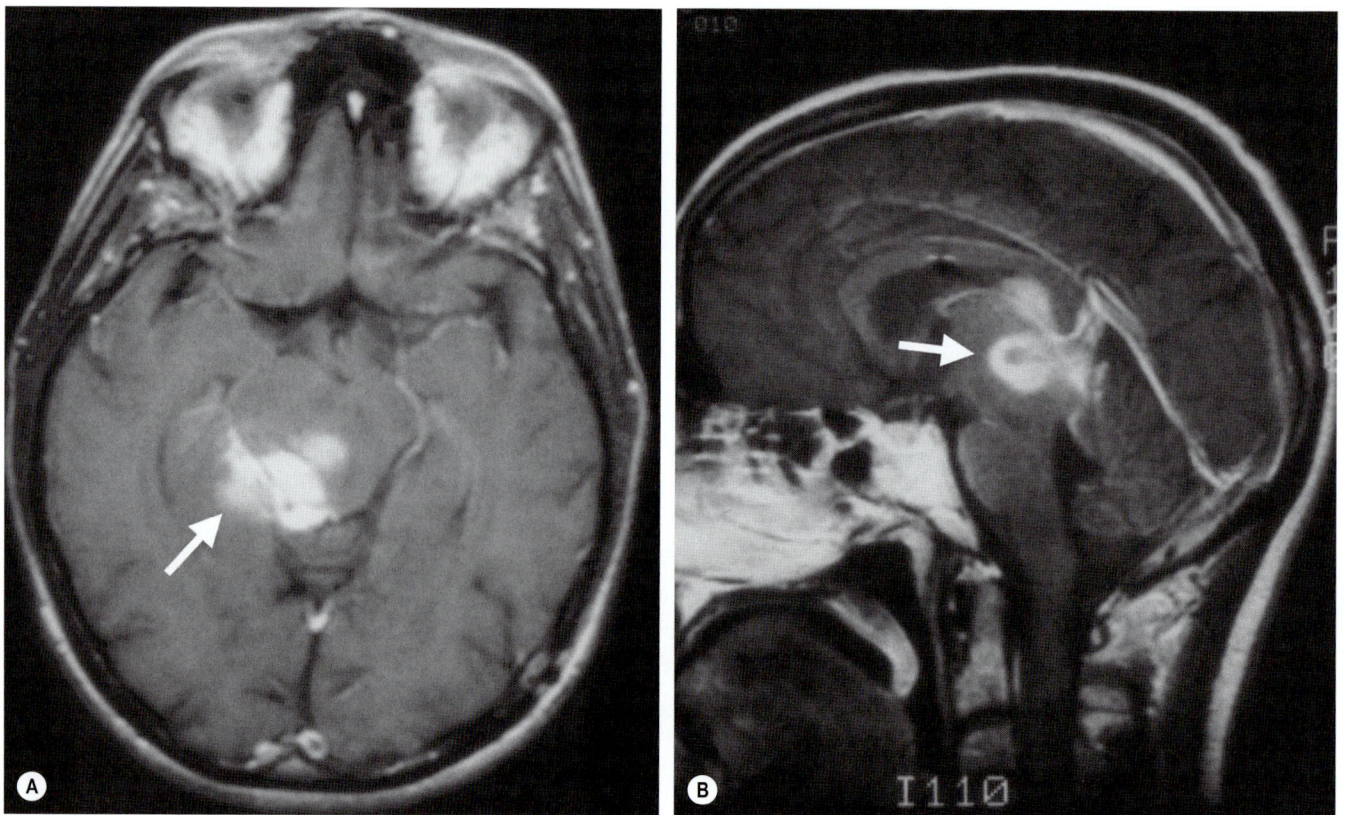

Figure 13–8. Thalamic and midbrain glioma responsible for a relative afferent pupillary defect with normal vision. T1-weighted gadolinium-enhanced axial magnetic resonance imaging (MRI) scan, and (**A**) sagittal T1-weighted gadolinium enhanced MRI scan (**B**) showing tumor (*arrows*) and edema involving the dorsal midbrain, thalamus, and anterior medullary velum. (From King JT, Galetta SL, Flamm ES: Relative afferent pupillary defect with normal vision in a glial brain stem tumor. Neurology 1991;41:945–946, with permission.)

light within the abnormal field, have been associated with optic tract syndromes. However, in clinical practice they are rarely identified, and the reliability of both signs has been questioned.[21] RAPDs in patients with hemianopias due to retrogeniculate lesions have been reported,[22] but in those cases concomitant optic tract involvement was not convincingly excluded.

Exceptional cases of RAPDs without visual loss can be associated with lesions in the midbrain pretectum,[23–26] which contains afferent pupillary fibers and the pretectal nuclei, but no visual fibers (**Fig. 13–8**). The RAPD is usually contralateral to the lesion.[27] Most of these patients have other signs of dorsal midbrain involvement, such as upgaze paresis, ataxia, or fourth nerve dysfunction.

Table 13–2 Important causes of pupillary light-near dissociation

Cause	Distinguishing feature(s)
Deafferention	Associated visual loss
Tonic pupil	Tonic redilation; denervation hypersensitivity (see Table 13–4)
Tectal lesions (Parinaud syndrome)	Associated upgaze paresis
Argyll Robertson pupils	Small; no pupillary response to direct or consensual light stimulation
Aberrant regeneration of the third nerve	Miosis during adduction; other signs of third nerve paresis
Diabetes	Irregularly shaped pupil; history of retinal photocoagulation; other evidence of autonomic neuropathy

Table 13–3 Causes of defective pupillary reactions to light generally unassociated with visual loss

Anatomic location	Cause
Dorsal midbrain	Tectal pupil (Parinaud syndrome)
	Argyll Robertson pupil
Third nerve	Third nerve palsy
Ciliary ganglion	Tonic pupil (Adie syndrome, for example)
	Miller Fisher syndrome
Synapse	Pharmacologic dilation
	Botulism
Iris sphincter	Trauma
	Angle-closure glaucoma
	Iritis

Anatomically, responsible lesions can be located in the dorsal midbrain or anywhere along the efferent parasympathetic pathway of the pupillary light reflex (see Fig. 13–2).

Pupillometry studies have demonstrated that some individuals with normal visual function can have subtle RAPDs[28] which may fluctuate (up to 0.3 log units) when tested over years.[29] Whether the RAPDs were due to test artifact or reflective of asymmetry in the visual pathways was unclear.[28]

Amaurotic (deafferented) pupil

In the absence of any optic nerve or retinal function, or both, the eye is completely blind (i.e., has no light perception (NLP)). The pupil is unreactive to even the brightest direct light stimuli because it is deafferented. If the fellow eye is normal and light is directed at it, the pupillary reaction in the affected eye (consensual) should be intact. An amaurotic pupil confirms blindness if the patient claims not to see anything out of that eye. However, if the pupil reacts to direct light in an eye with purported blindness, the visual loss is either nonorganic or has a cortical basis, or the patient is a poor observer. Bilateral deafferentiation will result in an increase in the resting size of both pupils as less total light is able to reach the midbrain pretectum.

Deafferented pupils can also react during attempted gaze at near targets, and thus exhibit light-near dissociation (**Table 13–2**). Even individuals who are bilaterally blind can attempt to look at their thumb placed a few inches in front of their face and stimulate the near reflex, as this task can be accomplished using proprioceptive clues.

Defective pupillary light reaction unassociated with vision loss

Defective pupillary light reactivity in most of these cases owes to dysfunction within the efferent arc of the pupillary light reflex, a so-called motor pupil. Lesions in the midbrain pretectum may also cause similar dysfunction. The major causes of this pupillary abnormality are highlighted in **Table 13–3**. A dilated pupil accompanied by eye movement or eyelid abnormalities suggests a lesion proximal to the ciliary ganglion (preganglionic), while an isolated dilated pupil would be more likely associated with a postganglionic process.

Pretectal pupils

Lesions affecting the dorsal midbrain, causing the pretectal, or Parinaud, syndrome (see Chapter 16), may interfere with pupillary reactivity by disrupting ganglion cell axons entering the pretectal region. The pretectal nuclei may also be involved. Bilaterally the pupils may be midposition to large and exhibit light-near dissociation due to intact supranuclear influences upon midbrain accommodative centers (**Fig. 13–9**). Usually both pupils are involved, although size and light reactivity may be asymmetric. Occasionally the near response may also be defective, as accommodative and convergence insufficiency can be observed. The diagnosis is suggested when other features of Parinaud syndrome, such as upgaze paresis, convergence retraction nystagmus, and eyelid retraction, are evident. Common causes include pineal region tumors and hydrocephalus, so abnormal pupils suggestive of a tectal lesion mandate neuroimaging.

Video 13.1

Argyll Robertson pupils

Argyll Robertson pupils[30,31] also exhibit light-near dissociation with a brisk near response, but typically are miotic, are slightly irregular, and dilate poorly in the dark (**Fig. 13–10**). The pupil does not react to light regardless of which eye is stimulated. Technically, to have an Argyll Robertson pupil, the involved eye must have some vision, to ensure the light-near dissociation is not due to a deafferented pupil. This pupillary abnormality is highly suggestive of syphilis and should therefore prompt serologic and fluorescent treponemal antibody absorption (FTA-ABS) testing. However, it is nonspecific and may also be caused by diabetes. The lesion responsible for Argyll Robertson pupils is uncertain but may result either from a disturbance in the midbrain light-reflex pathway between the pretectal and Edinger–Westphal nuclei or from damage to the ciliary ganglia.[32]

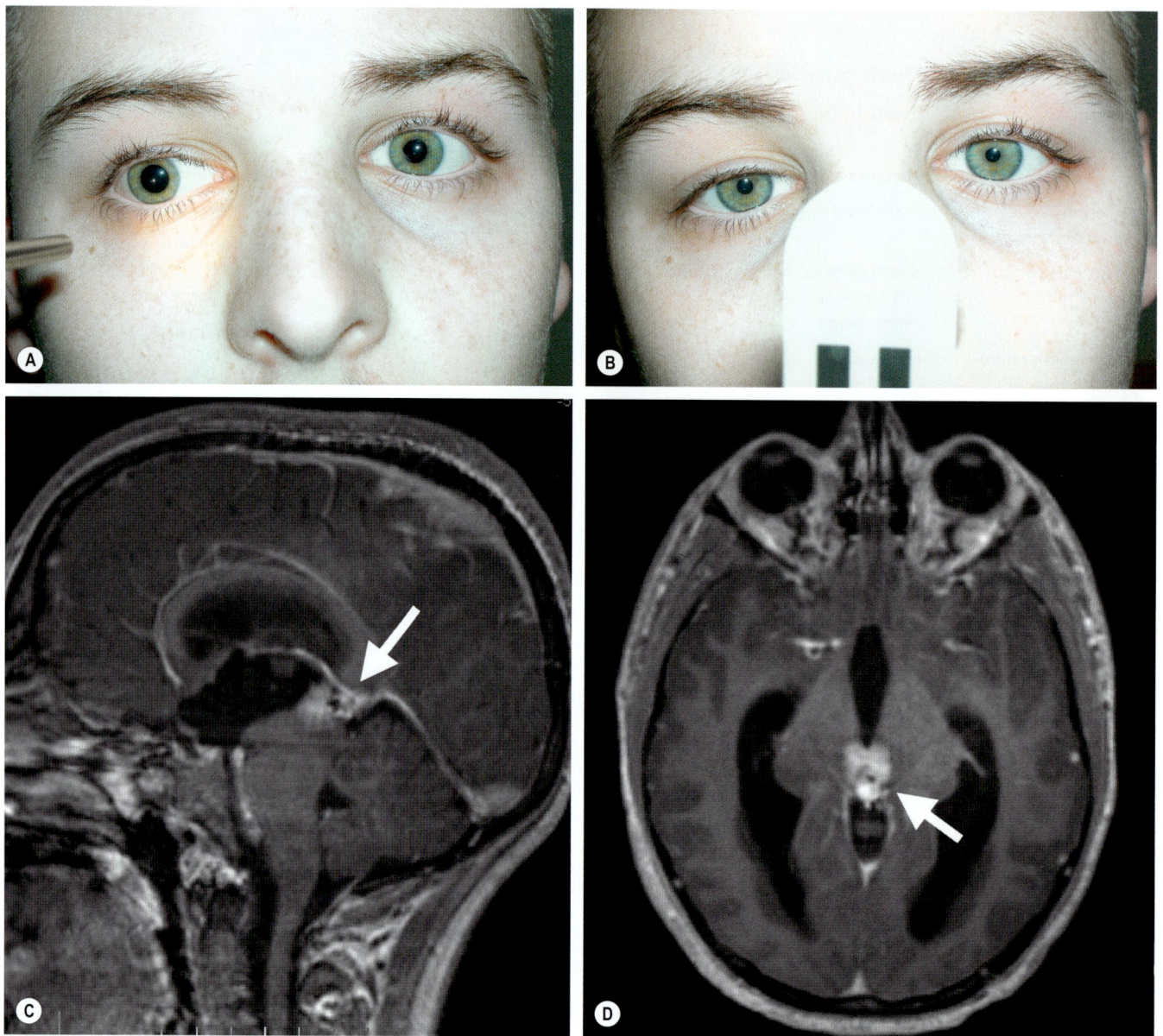

Figure 13–9. Tectal pupils associated with Parinaud syndrome due to a pineal region germinoma. **A**. On examination this 15-year-old boy was found to have upgaze paresis, ocular tilt reaction (right superior rectus skew deviation and head tilt), papilledema, and anisocoria. The pupils were moderate in size and poorly reactive to light, but (**B**) reactive to near stimuli (light-near dissociation). **C**. Sagittal and **D**. axial gadolinium-enhanced magnetic resonance images demonstrated hydrocephalus and a large enhancing pineal region mass (*arrows*) compressing the dorsal midbrain.

Third nerve palsy

Because the third nerve carries parasympathetic fibers originating from the Edinger–Westphal nuclei, injury to the third nerve often results in an ipsilateral poorly reactive or unreactive pupil.

Signs and symptoms. In a *pupil-involving third nerve palsy*, the pupil is large and does not constrict to light, either directly or consensually, or near stimuli (internal ophthalmoplegia) (**Fig. 13–11**). Usually either ptosis or a deficit in adduction, depression, or elevation of the eye, or a combination of these findings (external ophthalmoplegia), will assist in the diagnosis of a third nerve palsy, but in very rare instances a dilated pupil is the only manifestation. In inferior division third nerve palsies, the pupil and inferior rectus muscles are involved. In a *pupil-sparing third nerve palsy*, the eye movements or lid are affected, but the pupil retains normal size and reactivity.

Because a dilated pupil exposes spherical aberrations of the lens and cornea, some patients with pupil-involving third nerve palsies complain of blurry vision in that eye. Because this is a refractive problem, a pinhole occluder may resolve the visual symptom. This simple maneuver helps exclude other causes of visual loss associated with common scenarios causing third nerve palsies, such as vitreous hemorrhage (Terson syndrome) with a subarachnoid hemorrhage after aneurysm rupture or an or optic neuropathy from a lesion around the orbital apex or intracranial optic nerve.

Abnormal miosis during attempted ocular adduction or depression may be a sign of *aberrant regeneration* (*synkinesis*

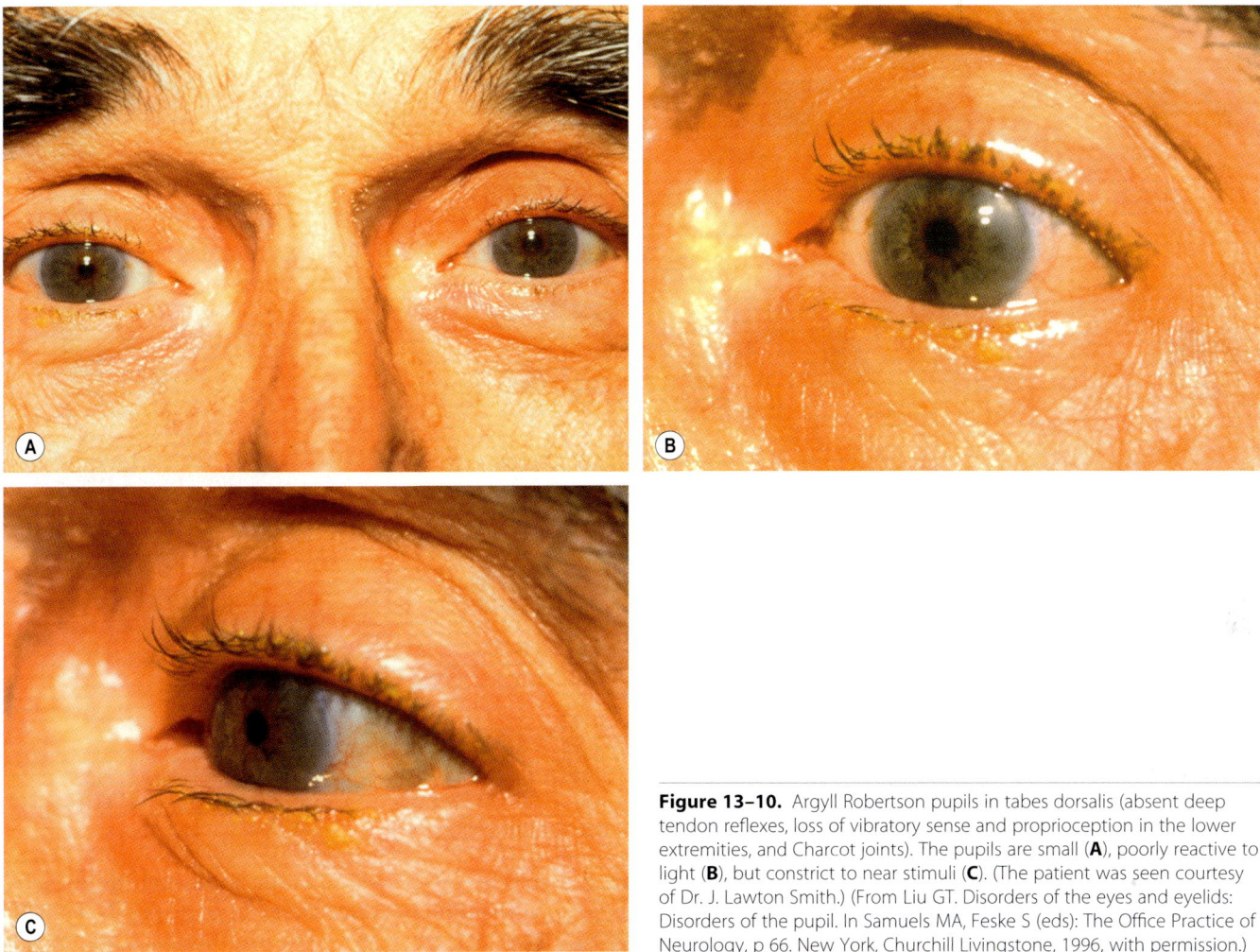

Figure 13–10. Argyll Robertson pupils in tabes dorsalis (absent deep tendon reflexes, loss of vibratory sense and proprioception in the lower extremities, and Charcot joints). The pupils are small (**A**), poorly reactive to light (**B**), but constrict to near stimuli (**C**). (The patient was seen courtesy of Dr. J. Lawton Smith.) (From Liu GT. Disorders of the eyes and eyelids: Disorders of the pupil. In Samuels MA, Feske S (eds): The Office Practice of Neurology, p 66. New York, Churchill Livingstone, 1996, with permission.)

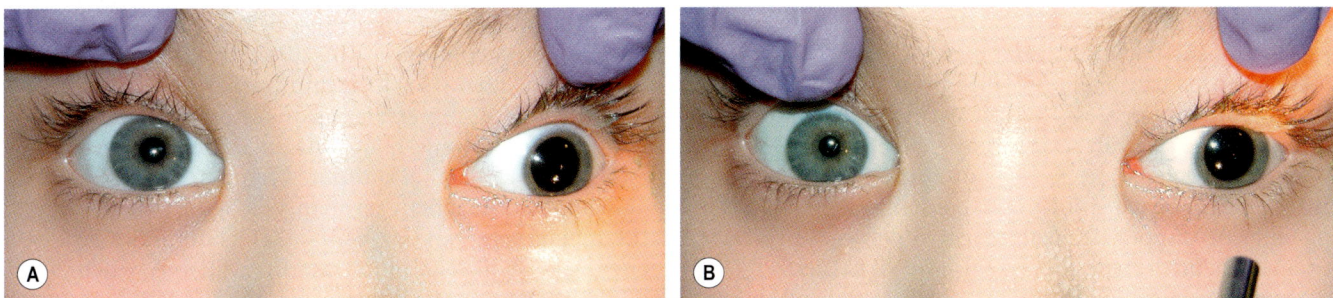

Figure 13–11. Pupil-involving left third nerve palsy due to head trauma. **A.** The ptotic left eyelid is being elevated, revealing the exotropic and hypotropic left eye and dilated left pupil. The right eyelid is also being elevated for photographic purposes. The left pupil is fixed, i.e., it does not react to direct light (**B**). Notice the intact right pupil constricts to light shone in the left eye (consensual response).

or *misdirection*) following a third nerve palsy (**Fig. 13–12**).[33] The phenomenon results when fibers that had previously supplied the medial rectus or inferior rectus regenerate and accidentally reach the ciliary ganglion, then connect with post-ganglionic neurons, which innervate the pupil. In these situations the pupil does not react to direct or consensual light stimulation but contracts during ocular adduction or depression. Segmental contraction of the iris sphincter during eye movements (Czarnecki's sign[34]) may also be observed in these instances. Furthermore, because postganglionic accommodative fibers far outnumber those dedi-

cated to the pupillary light reflex (see tonic pupil, below), pupillary miosis during accommodation is more likely to recover than constriction to direct light (light-near dissociation). These pupillary signs are sometimes accompanied by other manifestations of aberrant regeneration of the third nerve, such as elevation of the ptotic eyelid during adduction or depression of the eye.

Etiology. Pupil involvement is commonly seen in nuclear, fascicular, and especially subarachnoid third nerve palsies. As alluded to earlier, the external location of the pupillary fibers of the third nerve renders them particularly vulnerable

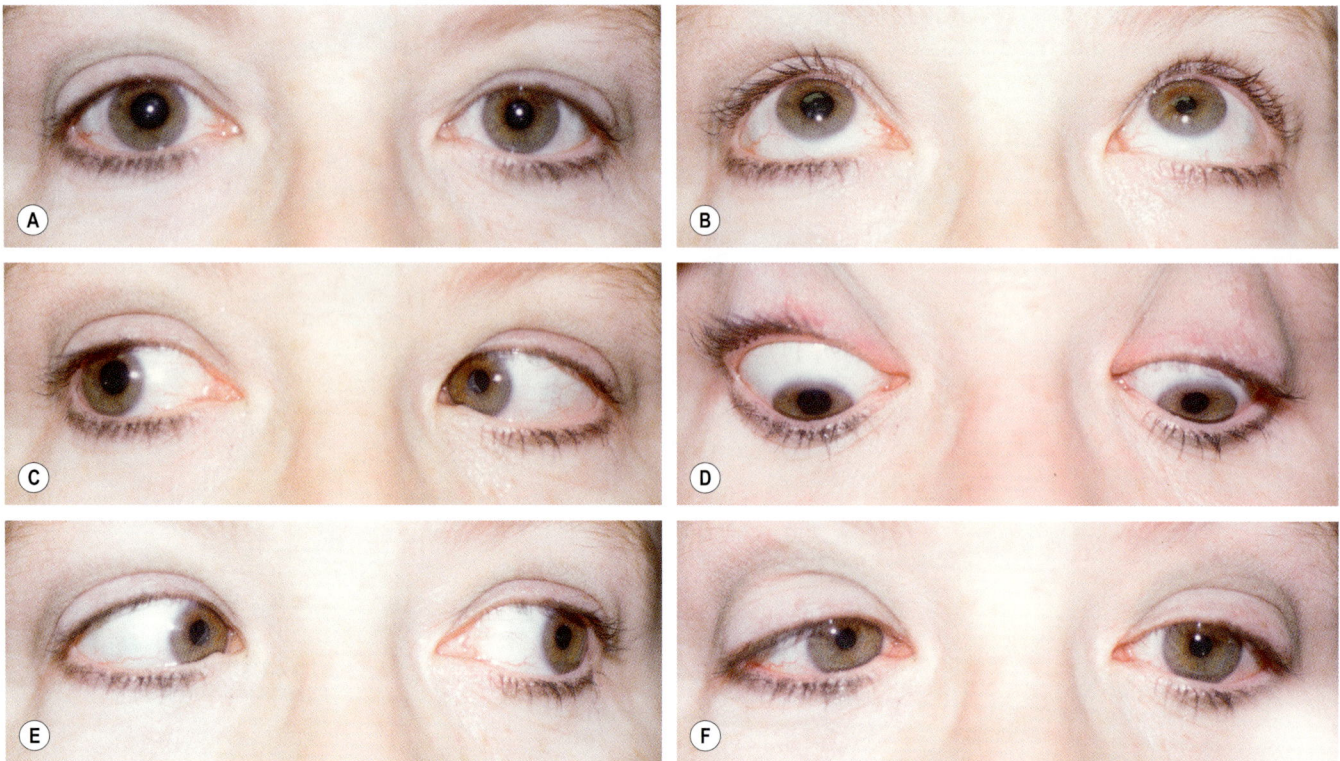

Figure 13–12. Pupillary constriction in adduction due to aberrant regeneration of the right third nerve. Pituitary apoplexy had caused ptosis and complete ophthalmoplegia of the right eye (see Chapter 7 for MRI of same patient), which recovered. The right pupil remained slightly enlarged, but was reactive to light. When the eyes are in (**A**) primary gaze, (**B**) upgaze, (**C**) rightward gaze, and (**D**) downgaze, the right pupil is larger than the left. However, (**E**) the right pupil constricts during adduction of the right eye and (**F**) constricts more than the left when viewing a near target.

to compression and infiltration in subarachnoid processes such as meningitis, aneurysmal compression (posterior communicating or internal carotid), and uncal herniation (Hutchinson's pupil). *Pupil-sparing third nerve palsies* in middle-aged to elderly patients are usually related to diabetes or hypertension, but occasionally can be seen even in fascicular or subarachnoid third nerve palsies from other causes. However, an aneurysm that presents initially with external ophthalmoparesis or ptosis alone typically will involve the pupil within several days.[35]

Aberrant regeneration most commonly occurs in traumatic or compressive third nerve palsies, sometimes with congenital or tumor-related third nerve palsies, but *almost never* in diabetic or hypertensive third nerve palsies.

Pharmacologic testing. A chronically dilated pupil due to a third nerve palsy may be difficult to distinguish from a tonic pupil (see below). Although the latter redilates slowly after constriction, both may exhibit light-near dissociation, segmental paresis of the iris sphincter, and denervation hypersensitivity.[36–38] The last characteristic, demonstrated by pupillary constriction following instillation of dilute (0.125%) pilocarpine eye drops, does not seem to depend on whether the lesion is anatomically before or after the ciliary ganglion (i.e., pre- or postganglionic), or whether there is aberrant regeneration. Jacobson[39–41] has offered the following explanations for denervation hypersensitivity in preganglionic third nerve lesions: (1) transsynaptic degeneration of post-ganglionic axons; (2) the greater sensitivity of larger pupils than smaller ones to dilute pilocarpine; and (3) upregulation of acetylcholine receptors because of

decreased cholinergic stimulation following third nerve injury. Denervation hypersensitivity in acute pupil-involving third nerve palsies, due to unclear mechanisms, is less common but has been observed.[42]

Management. If the patient has isolated pupillary dilation along with other signs of a third nerve palsy, an aneurysm of the posterior communicating artery should be considered until proven otherwise. To minimize risk and to screen for other possible compressive lesions, noninvasive angiography as well as routine brain imaging should be performed first. Either an emergent computed tomography (CT) and CT angiography or magnetic resonance imaging (MRI) scan and MRI angiography can be obtained. The choice of CT or MRI depends on which is more rapidly available, whether the patient is allergic to CT contrast, or whether MRI is contraindicated because of a pacemaker or metal in the body. If the scans are negative, conventional angiography is still necessary as small symptomatic aneurysms can still be missed by CT or MRI angiography.[43]

The reader is referred to a more detailed discussion regarding the differential diagnosis and management of third nerve palsies, in addition to issues regarding pupil-involving versus pupil-sparing third nerve palsies as well as aberrant regeneration in Chapter 15.

Tonic pupils

Clinical symptoms and signs. (See **Table 13–4**) Patients with a tonic pupil often discover that they have a unilateral, partially dilated pupil while looking in the mirror, or a friend notices the pupillary inequality. Affected individuals are usually otherwise healthy and more commonly female. They may be symptomatic with photophobia or difficulty reading with that eye. In general, the disorder is painless although

Table 13–4 Clinical features of tonic pupils

Presentation
Anisocoria noticed by the patient or others
Painless
Difficulty reading
Difficulty refocusing from near to far stimuli
Photophobia
More common in women
Examination
Initially large in size, but in chronic cases can become more miotic
Light-near dissociation (sometimes miosis at near response is also lost acutely)
Tonic redilation
Anisocoria worse in the dark (when unilateral)
Sectoral paralysis
Vermiform movements of the iris
Loss of pupillary ruff
Accommodative insufficiency
Depressed corneal sensation
Bilateral in 10% of cases
Pharmacologic testing
Denervation sensitivity, demonstrated by pupillary constriction following instillation of dilute (0.125%) pilocarpine

occasionally patients will complain of a cramping sensation in the affected eye resulting from ciliary body spasm.

Characteristically the pupil is initially large, exhibits light-near dissociation (**Fig. 13–13**), and redilates slowly after constriction (hence the term "tonic"). In some patients, especially in early cases, the near response may also be defective, or the individual may have difficulty refixing from near to far visual targets ("tonic" accommodation). Corneal sensation may be depressed. On a slit-lamp examination, the pupil may be irregular, with sectoral paralysis (immobility of parts of the pupil during light stimulation),[44] vermiform movements, and loss of pupillary ruff (the normal border of the pupil).[45] After 1 or 2 months, a tonic pupil may become miotic and smaller than the fellow pupil. In most patients the disorder is unilateral, but in about 10% of cases, the other pupil may become involved months or years later.[46]

Pathophysiology. The pupillary abnormality results from damage to the ciliary ganglion or the postganglionic short ciliary nerves (see **Fig. 13–3**), which innervate the pupillary sphincter and ciliary muscles (the latter is important for accommodation). Partial preservation of the pupil's parasympathetic innervation results in areas of segmental contraction adjacent to sector paralysis. When normal portions of the pupil contract, they pull and twist paralyzed segments toward them. Accommodation paresis accounts for the difficulty with near vision, and the photophobia results from the poor pupillary constriction to light. The light-near dissociation can be explained by the 30:1 ratio of accommodative fibers arising from the ciliary ganglion relative to those responsible for pupillary constriction.[46] Hence damage to the ciliary ganglion or short ciliary nerves would have a greater chance of disabling pupillary constriction to light than disrupting miosis associated with accommodation. Furthermore, as neuronal cell bodies in the ciliary

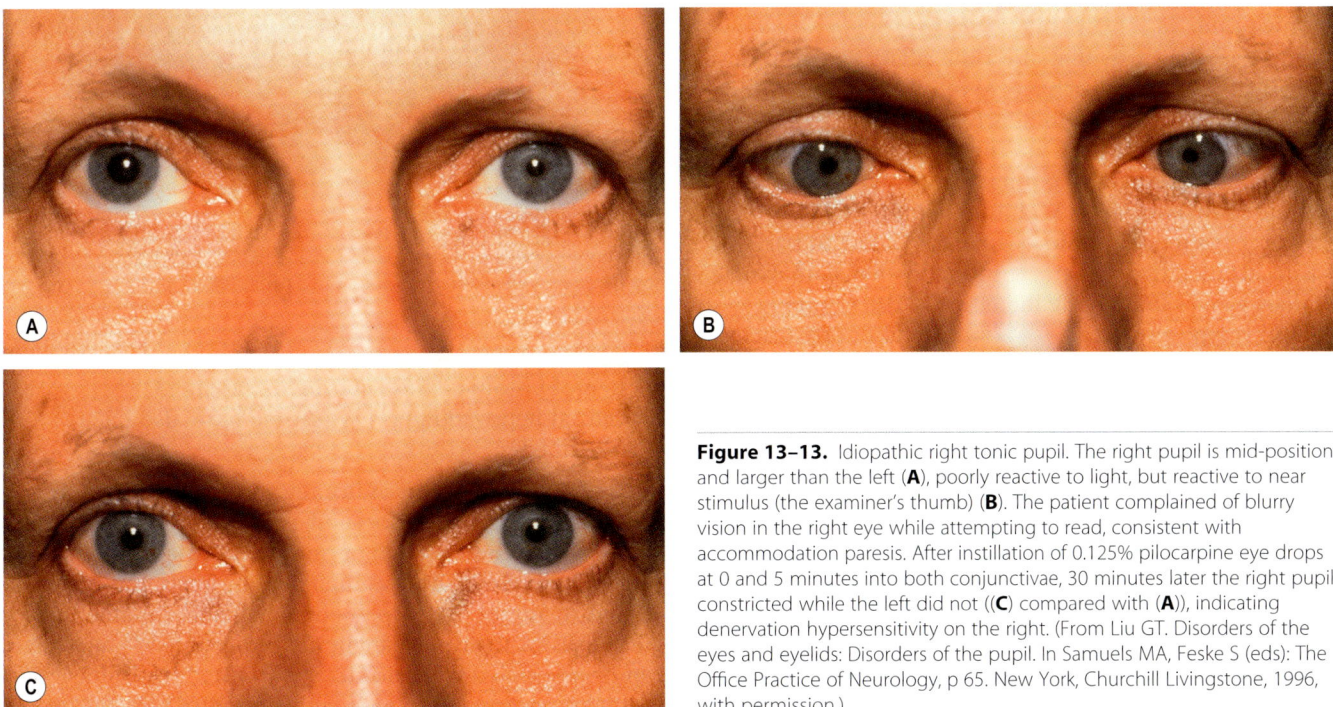

Figure 13–13. Idiopathic right tonic pupil. The right pupil is mid-position and larger than the left (**A**), poorly reactive to light, but reactive to near stimulus (the examiner's thumb) (**B**). The patient complained of blurry vision in the right eye while attempting to read, consistent with accommodation paresis. After instillation of 0.125% pilocarpine eye drops at 0 and 5 minutes into both conjunctivae, 30 minutes later the right pupil constricted while the left did not ((**C**) compared with (**A**)), indicating denervation hypersensitivity on the right. (From Liu GT. Disorders of the eyes and eyelids: Disorders of the pupil. In Samuels MA, Feske S (eds): The Office Practice of Neurology, p 65. New York, Churchill Livingstone, 1996, with permission.)

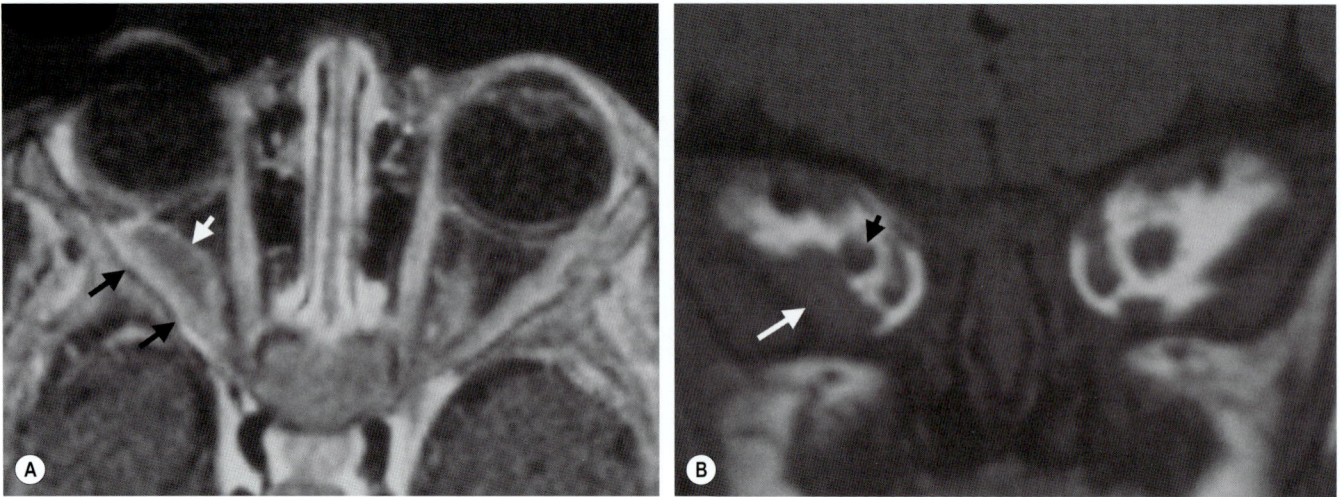

Figure 13–14. Posterolateral orbital mass that caused a tonic pupil in an infant. The lesion, which presumably compressed the ciliary ganglion or short ciliary nerves, was demonstrated to be a glial–neural hamartoma at biopsy. **A**. Axial contrast-enhanced magnetic resonance imaging (MRI) scan (TR = 600, TE with fat saturation) reveals enhancement on the periphery (*white arrow*) of the mass. There is normal contrast enhancement of the rectus muscles, and thus the right lateral rectus (*black arrows*) can be distinguished from the mass that lies along it. **B**. Coronal MRI scan (TR = 700, TE = 15) reveals the mass (*white arrow*) in the inferolateral aspect of the right orbit and obscuring the inferior and lateral rectus muscles, which are visible in the normal left orbit. The mass abuts the optic nerve sheath complex (*black arrow*), which is slightly displaced superiorly. (From Brooks-Kayal AR, Liu GT, Menacker SJ, et al. Tonic pupil and orbital glial-neural hamartoma in infancy. Am J Ophthalmol 1995;119:809–811, with permission from Elsevier Science.)

ganglion sprout new axons following injury, postganglionic accommodative fibers may mistakenly reinnervate the iris sphincter. This misdirection results in excess pupillary constriction during accommodation.

Etiology. The causes of tonic pupils fall into three major groups:

1. *Adie (or Holmes Adie) syndrome*, which is a symptom complex consisting of tonic pupil(s) and absent deep tendon reflexes.[47] The cause has yet to be elucidated, but the disorder may be explained by concurrent involvement of the ciliary and dorsal root ganglia or root entry zone. This is the most common cause of a tonic pupil.

2. *Local ocular processes* that affect the ciliary ganglion or short ciliary nerves, such as eye or orbital trauma, sarcoidosis,[48] or viral illnesses (e.g., varicella), or ischemia (e.g., giant cell arteritis,[49,50] other vasculitides[51] or strabismus surgery). Orbital tumors have also been reported in association with tonic pupils (**Fig. 13–14**).[52,53] Panretinal photocoagulation (laser) in patients with proliferative diabetic retinopathy may damage the ciliary nerves underlying the retina.[54] The resultant pupil is typically irregularly shaped and poorly reactive to light (**Fig. 13–15**). Other factors contributing to a poorly reactive pupil in diabetics can include iris ischemia, iris neovascularization, and associated autonomic neuropathy.

3. Reflecting *autonomic dysfunction*, tonic pupils uncommonly may occur in association with neurosyphilis, advanced diabetes mellitus, dysautonomias (e.g., Shy–Drager and Riley–Day syndromes), amyloidosis, Guillain–Barré syndrome, Miller Fisher variant (see below), Charcot–Marie–Tooth and Dejerine–Sottas neuropathies,[46,55] Lambert–Eaton myasthenic syndrome,[56,57] and paraneoplastic anti-Hu

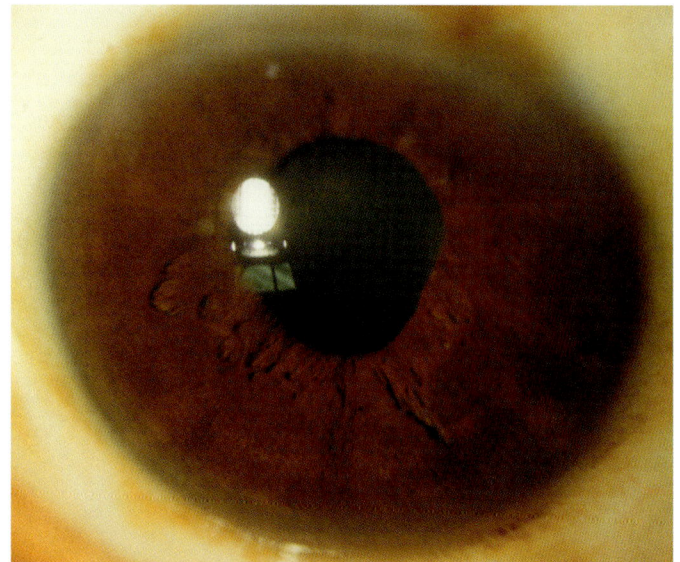

Figure 13–15. Irregularly shaped pupil in a diabetic patient who had undergone panretinal photocoagulation and whose diabetes was complicated by peripheral and autonomic neuropathy.

syndrome.[58,59] Two patients with congenital neuroblastoma, Hirschsprung disease, and central hypoventilation syndrome have also been described.[60]

Ross and harlequin syndromes are two rare focal dysautonomias frequently associated with pupillary abnormalities. Ross syndrome is characterized by the triad of tonic pupil, hyporeflexia, and segmental anhidrosis. It is probably related to injury to sympathetic and parasympathetic ganglion cells or their postganglionic projections[61,62] and rarely can be associated with Horner syndrome.[63] In contrast, harlequin syndrome, in which only half the face flushes or sweats,[64] is more frequently characterized by either normal pupils or oculosympathetic paresis. However, in some instances tonic pupils and areflexia can occur.[65]

Pharmacologic testing. Because of iris sphincter denervation cholinergic hypersensitivity, chronically tonic pupils will constrict following administration of dilute (0.125%) pilocarpine (see **Fig. 13–13**).[66] Pilocarpine is a cholinergic substance that can act directly on the iris sphincter muscle at higher concentrations. However, normal pupils typically have little or no response to dilute pilocarpine. The test should be considered positive when the pupil in question constricts more than the fellow pupil (assuming the fellow pupil is normal). The solution can be premixed or made readily by combining 0.1 ml of 1% pilocarpine with 0.7 ml of sterile saline in a 1-ml tuberculin syringe. With the needle removed, the syringe can be used as a dropper, with care taken to administer the same size drops into each eye. More dilute concentrations of pilocarpine such as 0.0625% can be used to reduce the chance of a false-positive result.[67]

Some caution is also necessary in interpreting the dilute pilocarpine test since some patients with preganglionic parasympathetic dysfunction (see above) will also respond to dilute pilocarpine.[41]

Management. The presence or absence of deep tendon reflexes should be noted. The ocular motility and orbital exam should be done carefully to exclude any evidence of a third nerve palsy or orbital tumor.

Since tonic pupils may be a manifestation of neurosyphilis, FTA-ABS or microhemagglutination assay–*Treponema pallidum* (MHA–TP) testing should be obtained in those patients without a defined cause for their dilated pupil.[68] In the elderly patient with a new onset tonic pupil we would suggest obtaining an erythrocyte sedimentation rate (ESR) and C-reactive protein (CRP) to screen for giant cell arteritis. No further laboratory workup is indicated, as tonic pupils otherwise usually have a benign cause.

Symptomatic treatment is sometimes helpful. Refractive correction may be prescribed for reading in those with accommodative insufficiency, for instance. Rarely, some patients find the anisocoria bothersome cosmetically, and these individuals might find pupil-forming contact lenses or dilute pilocarpine helpful. Dilute pilocarpine may also aid accommodation, and in addition may relieve photophobia. However, some patients find the induced pupillary miosis intolerably painful.

Pharmacologically dilated pupils

Pupils dilated surreptitiously or as part of an ophthalmic evaluation with anticholinergic agents such as atropine, tropicamide, or cyclopentolate or sympathomimetic agents such as phenylephrine or neosynephrine, are generally large (>7–8 mm) and unreactive to light or near stimulation.[69] Pharmacologically dilated pupils can also occur accidentally in an individual who has contact with atropine-like drugs, a scopolamine patch, ipratropium,[70] or plants such as jimson weed ("corn picker's pupil"), blue nightshade, or Angel's Trumpet,[71] who then touches his eye or if nasal vasoconstrictor sprays get into the eye. Other patients may consciously place mydriatic solutions in their eye as part of a functional

illness (Münchausen syndrome, for example). In many cases the actual cause of the pharmacological dilation cannot be identified despite careful review of the patient's history. Pupils that are overly generous and unreactive but appear normal on slit-lamp examination should suggest pharmacologic dilation, because third nerve-related and tonic pupils tend to be smaller. In addition, unlike tonic pupils, pharmacologically dilated pupils do not react to near targets. The lack of ptosis or ophthalmoplegia would exclude a third nerve palsy.

Pharmacologic testing. One percent pilocarpine drops will fail to constrict pharmacologically dilated pupils (examined after 30 minutes) because the postsynaptic receptors have been blocked.[72] However, 1% pilocarpine would be effective in normal pupils, as well as third nerve-related mydriasis, tonic pupils, and other pre- and postganglionic parasympathetic disorders because in these cases the receptors at the iris constrictor muscle are either normal or hypersensitive. This test should be applied with caution, as dilated pupils due to traumatic iridoplegia and acute narrow-angle glaucoma would also fail to constrict with 1% pilocarpine (see below).[69] The 1% pilocarpine test should also be interpreted carefully if it is performed near the termination of pharmacologic blockade, since the affected pupil may constrict.

Neuromuscular junction blockade

Patients with botulism, who have defective release of acetylcholine, can develop bilaterally dilated pupils and accommodative paresis with varying degrees of ptosis and ophthalmoparesis. The eye findings are often accompanied by bulbar or generalized weakness.[73,74] In general, the pupils are unaffected in myasthenia gravis, which affects nicotinic and not muscarinic cholinergic synapses. Both botulism and myasthenia gravis are discussed in more detail in Chapter 14.

Ocular causes of unreactive pupils

The clinical history or slit-lamp examination may suggest the following conditions. Depending on disease severity, the pupillary constriction with 1% pilocarpine may be defective.

1. *Ocular trauma.* Following trauma to the eye, the pupil may be fixed and unreactive (traumatic iridoplegia). Responsible mechanisms include tears or trauma to the iris sphincter muscle, tearing of short ciliary nerves, or compression of the ciliary nerves or ganglion by blunt trauma or a retrobulbar hemorrhage.

2. *Angle-closure glaucoma.* This disorder, an ophthalmic emergency, should be considered when the pupil is mid-dilated and fixed, and the patient acutely complains of visual loss, nausea, vomiting, eye pain, and a rainbow-colored halo seen around lights. Ocular pressures can be very high (>60 mm Hg), and visual acuity may be markedly impaired. Slit-lamp examination will identify the characteristic shallow anterior chamber, cornea edema, and ciliary or conjunctival injection. Pupillary nonreactivity is the

result of sphincter muscle ischemia. If left untreated, the pupil may remain fixed, and the iris can become atrophic.

3. *Iritis.* When affected by iritis, the pupil can be small, irregular, poorly reactive (see **Fig. 13–6A**) or demonstrate impaired dilation in the dark. Cells and flare in the anterior chamber, iris synechiae, and keratic precipitates seen on slit-lamp examination help establish the diagnosis. Photophobia is the major complaint, and there is less pain and the onset is more gradual than in angle-closure glaucoma. Because of the synechiae, the pupil dilates poorly and irregularly, even with mydriatics.

4. *Congenital mydriasis.* Albeit rare, in this condition children are born with fixed and dilated pupils that are unreactive to dilute or 1% pilocarpine. Accommodation is also affected. Two children with congenital mydriasis in association with patent ductus arteriosus have been reported,[75] and we have also seen such a case. The cause is unknown.

Anisocoria

The most common cause of asymmetric pupils (anisocoria) is nonpathologic *simple (essential, physiologic) anisocoria* (**Fig. 13–16**). The latter occurs in 15–30% of the normal population,[76,77] and is characterized by normal pupillary constriction and dilation as well as little change in the net amount of anisocoria under light and dark conditions.[1] The pupillary inequality in some cases may be larger in the dark (see below).[78] Also, the difference is rarely more than 1 mm.[79] Often the simple anisocoria will be evident on old photographs or a driver's license, which can be viewed critically with a slit-lamp or 20-diopter lens. No further testing is necessary in these instances. Rarely, the pupil asymmetry can reverse from day to day in this condition[80] (also see idiopathic alternating anisocoria, below). The cause of simple anisocoria is thought to be asymmetric supranuclear inhibition of the Edinger–Westphal nuclei.[78]

If the anisocoria is not physiologic, the next issue to resolve is which pupil is the abnormal one, assuming the problem is unilateral. The process combines examination of the pupillary light reactions and measurements of the anisocoria in light and dark.[79] If the pupillary inequality is

Video 13.2

greater in the light, and if one pupil is sluggish to light stimulation, then this pupil is the abnormal one. Likely the lesion lies in the efferent arc of the pupillary light reflex, or there may be pharmacologic blockade or iris damage. These pupillary abnormalities are discussed above in the sections on pupils with defective reactions to light, and the differential diagnosis includes those entities listed in Table 13–3.

A greater difference in darkness, with normal pupillary reactivity to light, implies either oculosympathetic paresis on the side with the smaller pupil or, less commonly, simple anisocoria, which may be less evident in light due to mechanical limitations of the iris.[81]

Figure 13–17 outlines an algorithm for evaluating anisocoria when only one pupil is abnormal.

Disorders of pupillary dilation: oculosympathetic disruption (Horner syndrome)

Horner syndrome, characterized primarily by unilateral miosis, facial anhidrosis, and mild upper and lower eyelid ptosis (**Fig. 13–18**),[82] is the most important neuro-ophthalmic cause of a small pupil that dilates poorly in the dark. **Table 13–5** lists the differential diagnosis of other entities which should be considered, and most of them have been discussed previously in other sections of this chapter.

Horner syndrome is a unique clinical sign, indicative of a remote process interrupting one of a series of three oculosympathetic neurons (see Fig. 13–4) that starts in the brain, descends to the upper chest, then ascends back to the eye. The benign nature of the ocular findings in Horner syn-

Table 13–5 Differential diagnosis of a small pupil that dilates poorly

Oculosympathetic paresis (Horner syndrome)
Iritis
Pharmacologic miosis
Tonic pupil (chronic)
Argyll Robertson pupil

Figure 13–16. Physiologic anisocoria. The amount of pupillary inequality is roughly the same in (**A**) bright light, (**B**) in ambient light, and (**C**) in the dark.

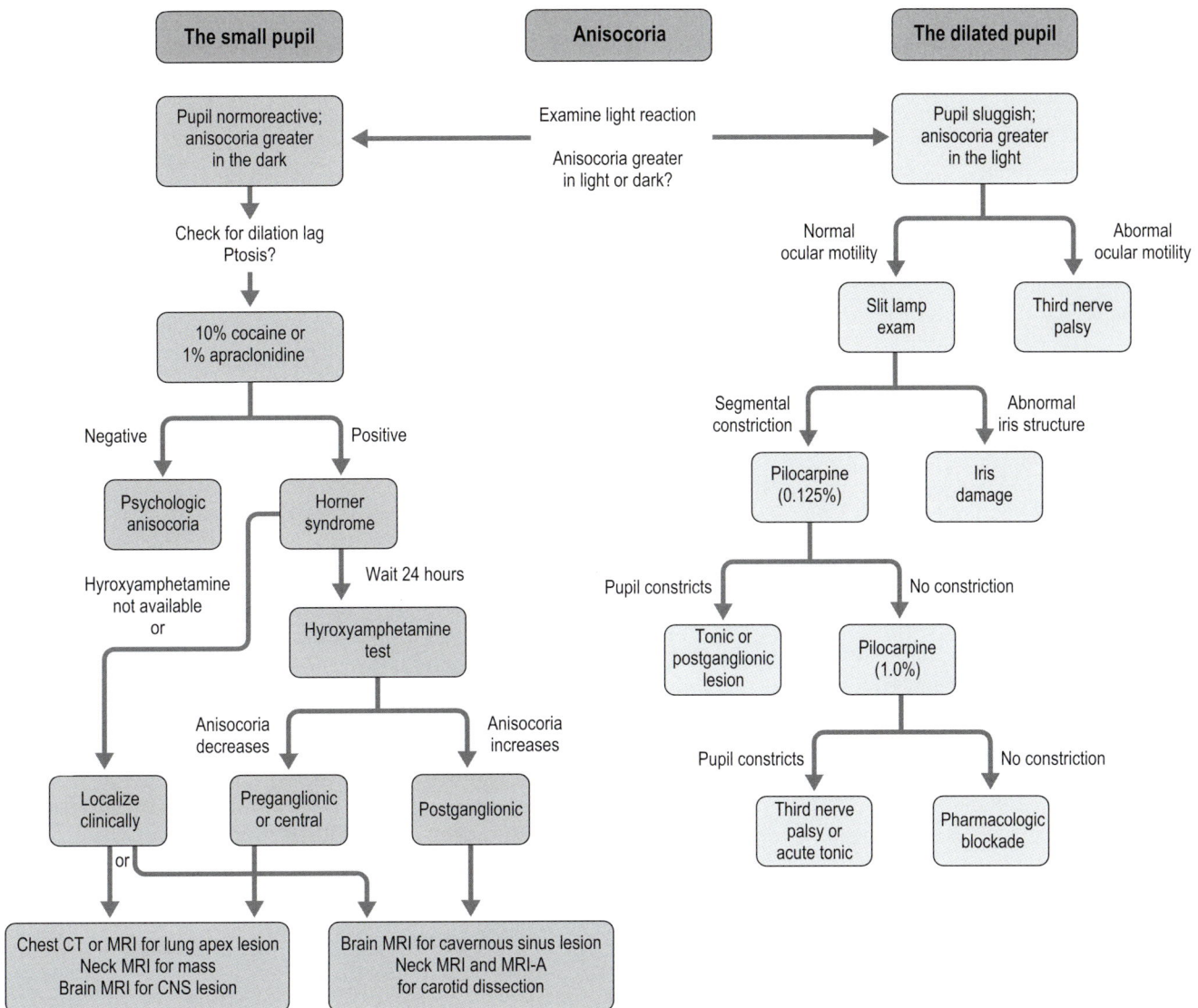

Figure 13–17. A diagnostic approach to anisocoria. The chart guides the workup of an abnormal pupil and assumes the other pupil is normal. See text for details, particularly "Management of Horner Syndrome" for issues regarding hydroxyamphetamine testing. (Adapted from Galetta SL, Liu GT, Volpe NJ. Neuro-ophthalmology. In: Evans R (ed): Diagnostic Testing in Neurology, Neurol Clinics, Vol. 14, 1996, p 212, with permission. Adapted from Thompson HS, Pilley SF: Unequal pupils: a flow chart for sorting out the anisocorias. Surv Ophthalmol 1976;21:45, with permission.)

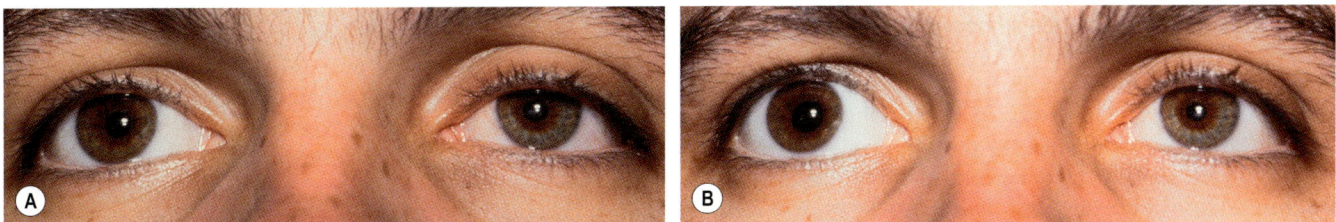

Figure 13–18. Left Horner syndrome due to cervical spinal cord trauma. **A**. In room light, the left pupil is miotic, and there is left upper lid ptosis. The left iris is lighter in color than the right (acquired heterochromia). **B**. After instillation of 10% cocaine into both conjunctivae at 0 and 1 minutes, then checked 45 minutes later, the normal right pupil dilated and the left did not, and the difference in sizes was greater than 1 mm, confirming oculosympathetic paresis on the left. (From Liu GT. Disorders of the eyes and eyelids: Disorders of the pupil. In Samuels MA, Feske S (eds): The Office Practice of Neurology, p 67. New York, Churchill Livingstone, 1996, with permission.)

drome, affecting appearance but not visual function, sometimes belies the seriousness of the underlying etiology. The causes and management will be discussed according to which neuron has been affected, and the management of Horner syndrome in childhood also will be reviewed.

Clinical signs and symptoms in Horner syndrome

Because of the lack of sympathetic input to the iris dilator muscle, Horner syndrome is strongly suggested when the

Table 13–6 Clinical features of oculosympathetic paresis (Horner syndrome)

Presentation
Anisocoria noticed by the patient or others
Unassociated with visual loss
Examination[64]
Pupillary miosis
Anisocoria worse in the dark
Pupillary dilation lag
Minimal ptosis of the upper lid
"Inverse" or "upside-down" ptosis of the lower lid
Pseudoenophthalmos
Anhidrosis
Conjunctival injection
Ocular hypotony, transient
Iris heterochromia (in congenital cases, typically)
Pharmacologic testing
Greater than 1 mm of relative anisocoria following instillation of 10% cocaine eye drops into both eyes
In postganglionic lesions, increase in the relative anisocoria by at least 1 mm following instillation of 1% hydroxyamphetamine drops into both eyes

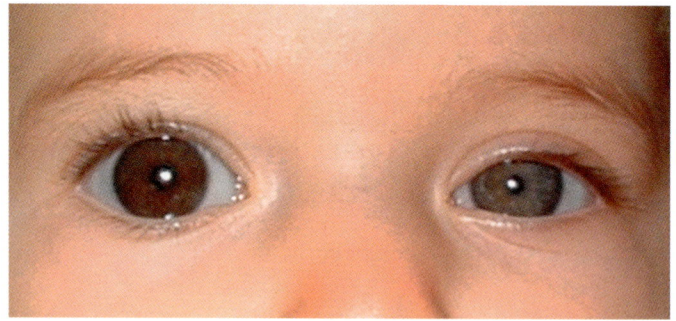

Figure 13–19. Iris heterochromia in idiopathic congenital Horner syndrome. The affected left eye has ptosis, miosis, and a lighter colored iris than the right eye. Imaging and urine catecholamine metabolite testing were unremarkable.

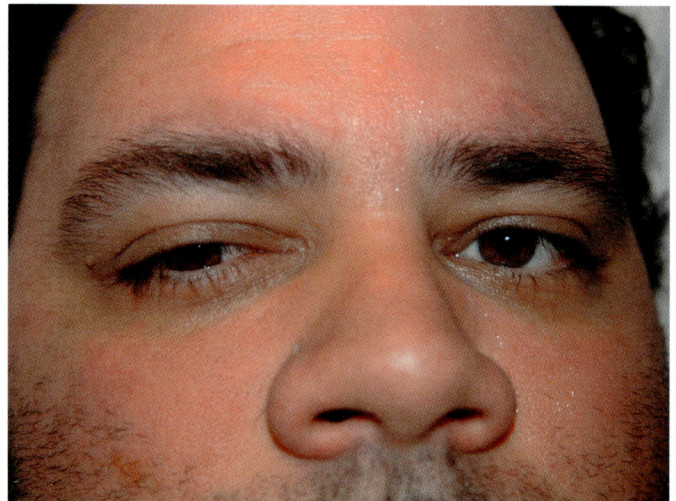

Figure 13–20. Right Horner syndrome with right ptosis, miosis and facial anhidrosis due to right lateral medullary infarction. The patient sweats on the left side of the face but not on the right.

Video 13.3

anisocoria increases in the dark or if dilation lag of the miotic pupil is observed (**Table 13–6**). Dilation lag may be demonstrated at the bedside by turning the lights off and observing the pupils with a dim light directed from below the nose. The normal pupil dilates briskly, but it takes time for the sympathetically denervated pupil to reach its final resting state in the dark.[83] Typically, measurements of pupil size are made at 5 and 15 seconds to document this dilation disparity in darkness, and there is usually more anisocoria at the earlier measurement. However, the absence of dilation lag does not exclude Horner syndrome.[84] The pupil in Horner syndrome reacts normally to light and near stimuli.

The upper lid ptosis is always mild and rarely ever covers the visual axis. The lower lid may be slightly elevated (lower eyelid, or upside-down, ptosis). The upper and lower eyelid ptosis (narrow palpebral fissure) may give the false impression that the eye is set back in the orbit (pseudoenophthalmos).

Horner syndrome by itself does not cause visual symptoms. However, disruption in sympathetic input to the eye may produce several other ocular signs. There may be conjunctival congestion or transient ocular hypotony. Because iris melanocytes require oculosympathetic input during development in early infancy, congenital Horner syndromes can be associated with an ipsilateral lighter colored iris (*iris heterochromia*) (**Fig. 13–19**).[85] In rare instances, heterochromia may also result from acquired instances of Horner syndrome (**Fig. 13–18**).[86] Also, neurotrophic corneal endothelial

failure has been reported in association with Horner syndrome.[87]

Theoretically, lesions of the third-order neuron distal to the carotid bifurcation result in loss of sweating or flushing on the medial aspect of the forehead and side of the nose, while more proximal lesions, including those of the first- and second-order neurons, decrease sweating or flushing in the whole half of the face (**Fig. 13–20**).[88,89] Hemibody sweating would also be anticipated from first-order neuron dysfunction. However, the expected patterns are present inconsistently, and the air conditioning in most hospitals and offices often masks any anhidrosis, making it a less important practical sign of Horner syndrome than the ptosis and miosis. If desired, the exact pattern of sweating may be outlined with alizarin powder, which turns dark purple when it comes in contact with perspiration.[62]

Etiology and localization of Horner syndrome

Table 13–7 outlines the differential diagnosis of Horner syndrome according to localization and frequency. The various causes have been analyzed in large series, and the most common localization varies, most likely due to selection bias. In a study of inpatients with acquired oculosympathetic palsy,[90] 63% had involvement of the first-order neuron, reflecting a large proportion of patients with strokes. The second-order neuron (preganglionic) was the most common lesion site in two other studies,[91,92] while the third-order neuron (post-ganglionic) was most frequent in another, reflecting the authors' interest in headaches.[93] The ganglion

Table 13–7 Causes of oculosympathetic paresis (Horner syndrome) according to affected neuron and frequency

	Common	Uncommon
First-order (central) neuron	Lateral medullary stroke	Hypothalmic, midbrain, or pontine injury
		Spinal cord lesion
Second-order (preganglionic) neuron	Pancoast tumor	Cervical disc disease
	Brachial plexus injury	
	Iatrogenic trauma	
	Neuroblastoma	
Third-order (postganglionic) neuron	Carotid dissection	Intraoral trauma
	Carotid thrombosis	
	Cluster headache	
	Cavernous sinus lesion	
	Small vessel ischemia	

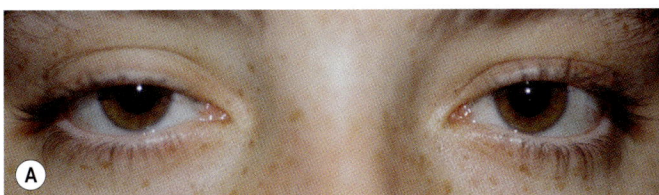

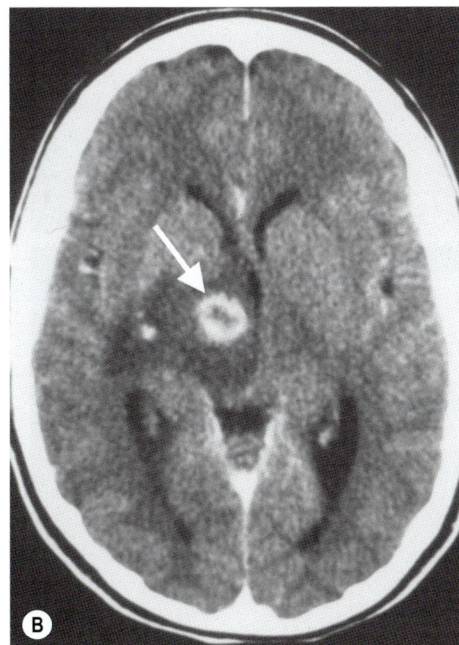

referred to is the superior cervical ganglion, thus "preganglionic" refers to the second-order neuron, "postganglionic" to the third-order neuron.

The presence of other clinical signs or symptoms may help localize the Horner syndrome. Sweat patterns have been mentioned already. Brain stem or spinal cord signs suggest involvement of the first-order neuron. Arm pain, or a history of neck or shoulder trauma, surgery, or catheterization point to injury of the second-order neuron. Horner syndrome accompanied by ipsilateral facial pain or headache is characteristic of disorders that affect the third-order neuron.

The ciliospinal reflex may also help with localization in Horner syndrome. The reflex consists of bilateral pupillary dilation in response to a noxious stimulus, such as a pinch, on the face, neck, or upper trunk. Reeves and Posner[94] showed that when there is a lesion of the first-order oculosympathetic neuron, the reflex is still intact. In contrast, in patients with injury to the second- or third-order neurons, which contain the efferent arm of the reflex, the pupil usually fails to dilate ipsilaterally.

Injury of the first-order neuron (central Horner syndrome)

Central Horner syndrome can be caused by lesions involving the descending oculosympathetic pathway in the hypothalamus, brain stem, or spinal cord.

Hypothalamic lesions. Injury to the neuronal cell bodies in the hypothalamus is a relatively infrequent etiology of Horner syndrome. The most common causes of dysfunction in this area are tumors or hemorrhages involving the thalamus or hypothalamus (**Fig. 13–21**). Less commonly, a Horner syndrome is the result of hypothalamic infarction,[95,96] occasionally combined with contralateral ataxic hemiparesis.[97]

Figure 13–21. A. Right Horner syndrome due to T-cell lymphoma involving the right thalamus and hypothalamus. **B**. Ring-enhancement (*arrow*) and edema are seen on the axial CT scan.

431

Isolated infarction of the hypothalamus is an unusual event because of a rich blood supply to the hypothalamus, consisting of branches from the anterior cerebral artery and thalamoperforating arteries arising from the proximal portions of the posterior cerebral arteries near the basilar bifurcation, as well as short hypothalamic arteries that derive from the posterior segment of the posterior communicating artery. However, in some individuals with persistence of the fetal circulation, the hypothalamus is supplied directly by branches of the internal carotid artery.[95,96] In such cases, large, deep cerebral infarcts may involve the hypothalamus when this artery is occluded, and these patients may have prominent sensory or motor signs or a hemianopia contralateral to the Horner syndrome.

Mesencephalic and pontine lesions. A lesion in the dorsal midbrain at the pontomesencephalic junction may cause a Horner syndrome and a contralateral fourth nerve palsy by interrupting the descending sympathetic tract and adjacent fourth nerve nucleus or fascicle (**Fig. 13–22**).[98] In a large series of isolated pontine infarcts,[99] for unclear reasons Horner syndrome was not a feature in any of the cases. However, large pontine hemorrhages may affect the descending sympathetic fibers, causing uni- or bilateral pinpoint pupils.

Wallenberg syndrome. The most common central cause of a Horner syndrome is a lateral medullary stroke (Wallenberg syndrome), due to either the infarction in lateral medullary (**Fig. 13–23**) or posterior inferior cerebellar artery (PICA) distributions. Horner syndrome, ipsilateral to the lesion, occurs in at least three-quarters of cases.[100,101] Ocular motor abnormalities are very frequent and are reviewed in detail in other chapters. These include skew deviation (Chapter 15), lateropulsion and defective smooth pursuit (Chapter 16), and torsional or horizontal nystagmus (Chapter 17). Other characteristic findings are (1) ipsilateral appendicular and gait ataxia, due to involvement of the inferior cerebellar peduncle, (2) ipsilateral corneal and facial anesthesia, owing to damage to the trigeminal spinal nucleus and tract, (3) contralateral body anesthesia, resulting from involvement of the ascending spinothalamic tract, (4) vertigo, caused by damage to the vestibular nuclei, and (5) nausea and vomiting, dysphagia, and ipsilateral palate, pharyngeal, and vocal cord paralysis due to involvement of the nucleus ambiguus.[102] Not infrequently the infarct extends rostrally into the lower pons, producing abducens and facial weakness, due to involvement of the sixth and seventh cranial nerves, respectively. Motor and tongue weakness and corticospinal tract signs are uncommon and would reflect medial medullary involvement.

Typically in patients with Wallenberg syndrome, MRI reveals a wedge-shaped defect in the lateral medulla (**Fig. 13–23**), and in a minority of cases (approximately

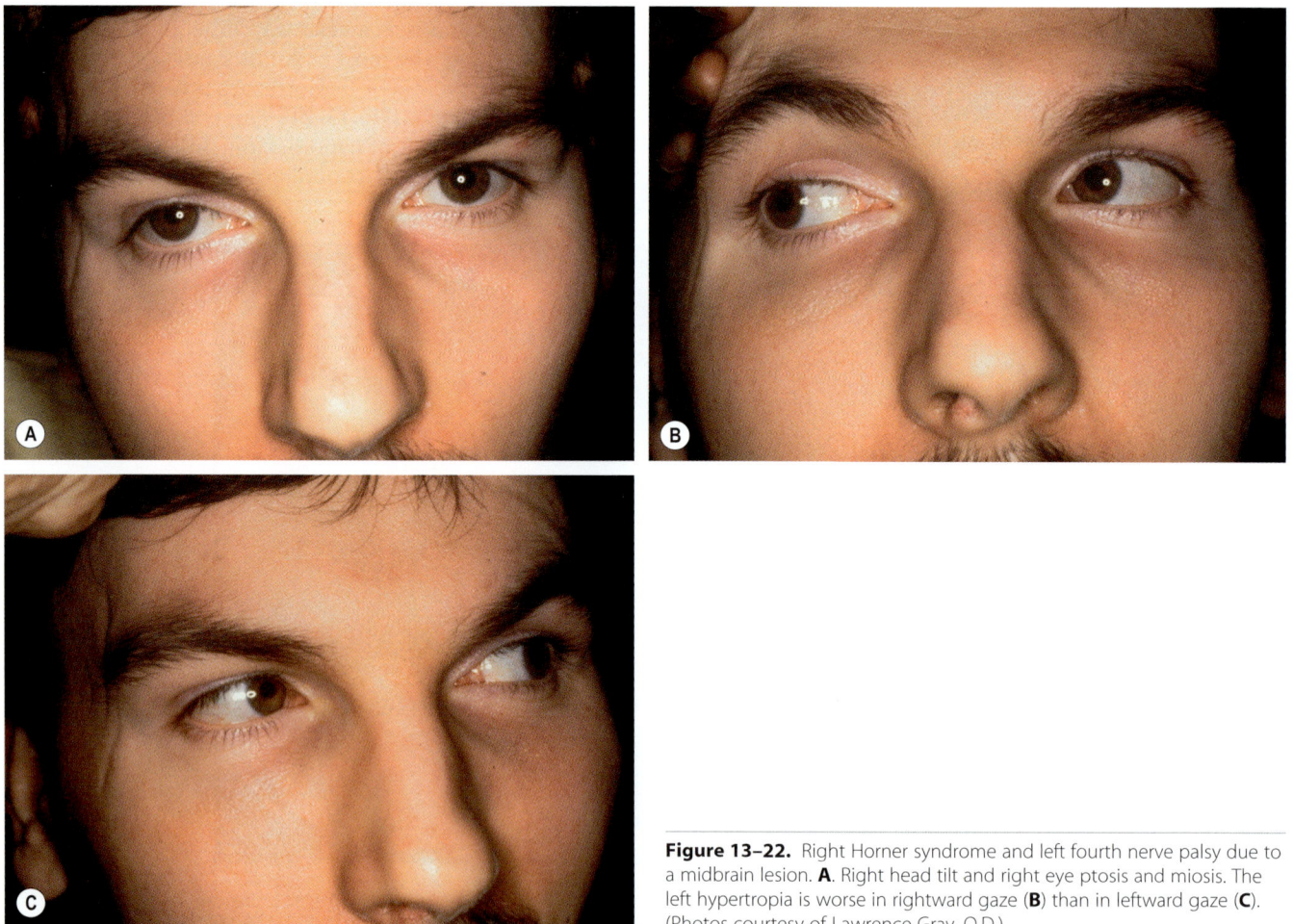

Figure 13–22. Right Horner syndrome and left fourth nerve palsy due to a midbrain lesion. **A**. Right head tilt and right eye ptosis and miosis. The left hypertropia is worse in rightward gaze (**B**) than in leftward gaze (**C**). (Photos courtesy of Lawrence Gray, O.D.)

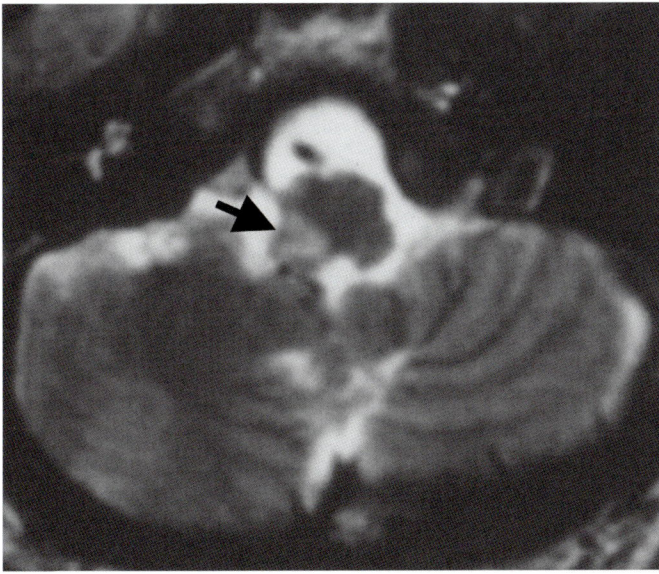

Figure 13–23. Wallenberg stroke. Axial T2-weighted MRI scan demonstrating a lateral medullary infarction (*arrow*) on the right. The patient had an ipsilateral Horner syndrome, skew deviation, lateropulsion to the right, left-beating nystagmus in left gaze, right face hypesthesia, and diminished pain and temperature sensation on the left side of the body. (From Galetta SL, et al. Cyclodeviation in skew deviation. Am J Ophthalmol 1994;118:509–514, with permission from Elsevier Science.)

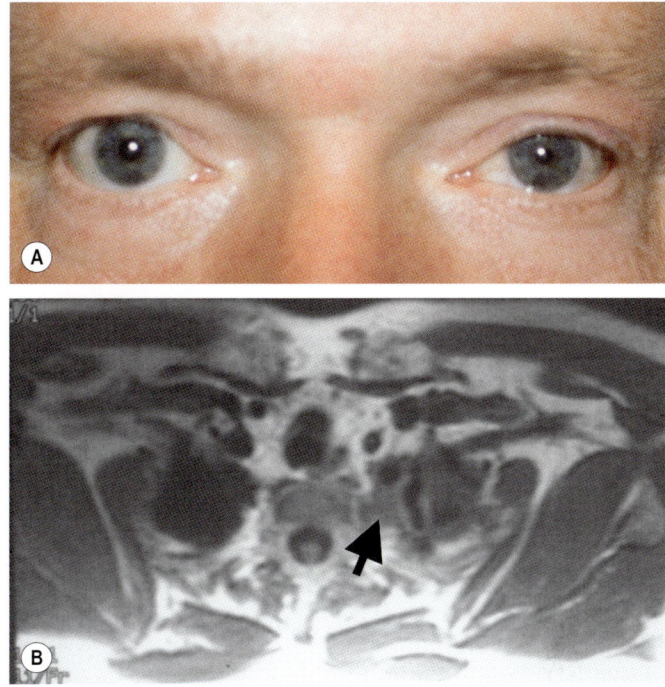

Figure 13–24. **A**. Left Horner syndrome due to apical lung (Pancoast) tumor. **B**. The lesion (*arrow*) in the upper thorax is demonstrated on the axial CT scan. (From Balcer LJ, Galetta SL. Pancoast syndrome. N Engl J Med 1997;337:1359, with permission from the Massachusetts Medical Society.)

20%) there is also a cerebellar infarction in the distal PICA territory.[100] Most cases result from occlusion of the intracranial vertebral artery or one of its branches due to local atheromatous disease.[103,104] However, emboli from the heart, proximal vertebral artery, or aortic arch should also be considered.

Spinal cord injury. Any injury to the spinal cord that affects the descending sympathetic pathway or the ciliospinal center of Budge at C8 through T2 can cause a Horner syndrome ipsilateral to the lesion (**Figs. 13–18**). The most common causes are syringomyelia[105,106] and trauma to the cord, but other recognized causes include myelitis, tumors, multiple sclerosis, and infarction.[107] Quadra- or paraparesis, a sensory level, bladder and bowel difficulty, hyperreflexia, and extensory plantar responses will aid in localization. In Brown–Séquard hemicord syndrome, Horner syndrome may be present ipsilateral to the weakness and loss of light touch sensation, and contralateral to the pain and temperature sense loss.[108] In cases with cervical injury associated with a cyst, very rarely the Horner syndrome may alternate when the patient turns from side to side[107] (see also oculosympathetic spasm, below).

Injury of the second-order neuron (preganglionic Horner syndrome)

Thoracic (lung and mediastinal) and neck tumors, brachial plexus or radicular injury, and iatrogenic trauma are the most common causes of impairment of this neuron. Maloney et al.[92] emphasized the association of Horner syndrome and ipsilateral arm pain as a presentation of a tumor in the superior pulmonary sulcus (Pancoast syndrome[109]) (**Fig. 13–24**). Owing to irritation of the sympathetic chain, some patients

with Pancoast syndrome may exhibit ipsilateral facial flushing and hyperhydrosis of the face before developing Horner syndrome.[110]

Iatrogenic causes of second-order Horner syndrome include radical neck dissection, lung or mediastinal surgery,[111] coronary artery bypass surgery,[112,113] chest tube placement,[111,114–116] internal jugular,[117] Swan–Ganz,[118] or central venous catheterization,[119,120] and lumbar epidural anesthesia.[121]

Injury of the third-order neuron (postganglionic Horner syndrome)

Many of the processes that affect the third-order neuron produce Horner syndrome and ipsilateral facial pain or headache, and this combination has been loosely termed *Raeder's paratrigeminal syndrome or neuralgia*.[122] Carotid artery dissection or thrombosis, vascular headache syndromes, and cavernous sinus lesions are the major disorders to consider in this subgroup.

Carotid dissection. This disorder should always be considered in the setting of Horner syndrome associated with ipsilateral headache or pain, carotidynia, and dysgeusia, as well as signs and symptoms consistent with ipsilateral ocular or cerebral ischemia.[123–126] Dissection of the carotid artery results when intraluminal blood enters the arterial wall and separates its component layers.[127] Accumulation of blood in the resulting dissecting aneurysm may compromise the true arterial lumen (**Fig. 13–25**). Ischemic symptoms result either from carotid stenosis or from embolism of thrombotic fragments; the latter is probably more common.[128] About 5–10% of cases are bilateral,[129] and dissection is the cause of at least

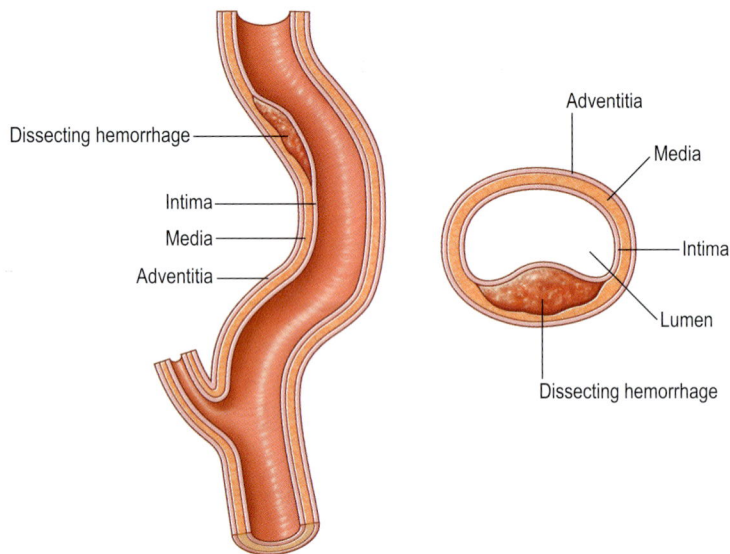

Figure 13–25. Dissection depicted in lateral (left) and cross-sectional (right) schematic views of the internal carotid artery. In this example, blood dissects within the media between the intima and adventitia. As the hemorrhage enlarges, the true lumen of the carotid artery can be compromised, leading to distal hypoperfusion or formation of thromboembolic material.

Table 13–8 Neuro-ophthalmic complications of carotid dissection, according to frequency[127]

Common	Uncommon
Horner syndrome	Anterior ischemic optic neuropathy
Amaurosis fugax	Posterior ischemic optic neuropathy
	Central retinal artery occlusion
	Ophthalmic artery occlusion
	Transient ophthalmoparesis
	Third, fourth, or sixth nerve palsy
	Ocular ischemic syndrome
	Homonymous field defects
	Monocular or binocular scintillations

5% of cerebral ischemic episodes in young adults.[130] Cases in children are uncommon but have been reported.[131]

Arterial dissections may be spontaneous or secondary to minor trauma such as chiropractic manipulation.[132–134] Prolonged periods of neck extension during cycling,[135] or painting a ceiling[136] have been reported to cause dissections. Some result from obvious blunt and penetrating trauma to the head and neck, and motor vehicle accidents are the most common cause in such cases.[137] They may also arise in the setting of fibromuscular dysplasia, cystic medial necrosis, syphilis, pharyngeal infection, extension of aortic dissection, atheromatous disease, or cerebral aneurysm.[129,138] Other predisposing conditions include collagen disorders such as Marfan syndrome or Ehlers–Danlos syndrome.[139]

Abrupt facial, ear, or neck pain usually signifies the onset of dissection of the extracranial carotid artery and may precede symptomatic ischemia to the eye or brain by hours to days. Patients may also complain of subjective bruits or pulsatile tinnitus.

The neuro-ophthalmic manifestations of carotid dissection are listed in **Table 13–8**.[127,140–149] Of these, Horner syndrome is most common, occurring in approximately 50% of patients.[125,129,138] In some instances Horner syndrome with ipsilateral headache is the only manifestation.[123,150] Cranial nerve palsies are not uncommon, and in one large series[146] occurred in 12% of patients. Lower cranial nerve (IX through XII) involvement can be explained by the geographic proximity of these structures to the carotid artery in the neck (see Fig 13–29). For example, tongue weakness and dysgeusia may result from ischemia, stretching, or compression of the hypoglossal nerve (XII) and chorda tympani, respectively.[151,152] On the other hand, ocular motor (III, IV, and VI)[145,153] and trigeminal (V)[154] nerve palsies are likely ischemic due to emboli into nutrient vessels.[146] Some authors have attributed cases of ischemic optic neuropathy[155] and other cranial neuropathies[156] associated with carotid dissection to a low-flow state. This mechanism, however, seems less likely in the absence of concomitant cerebral hemispheric signs.

Conventional (**Fig. 13–26B**) or MRI angiogram (**Fig. 13–27**) is essential for establishing the diagnosis and defining the extent of dissection. Lumen narrowing of the internal carotid usually begins 2 cm distal to the carotid bifurcation and extends rostrally for a variable distance. Dissection of the extracranial ICA almost always ends before the artery enters the petrous bone, where mechanical support limits further dissection.[129] The most common finding is a long narrow irregular lumen ("string sign"[157]), but other patterns are highlighted in **Figure 13–28**. Axial MR T1- and T2-weighted images through the neck may demonstrate a characteristic crescentic hyperintensity, representing a mural hematoma, constricting the true lumen of the internal carotid artery (**Fig. 13–26B**).[158] CT angiography and Doppler ultrasound can also detect the arterial dissection. However, both are inferior to MRI-a combined with MRI,[159] which can show both the dissection and the mural hematoma, often making conventional angiography unnecessary.[160] Spontaneous intracranial dissection of the supraclinoid ICA has been reported,[161] but Horner syndrome is not typically one of the associated features.

Management options for carotid dissection include anticoagulation with heparin, antiplatelet agents, superficial

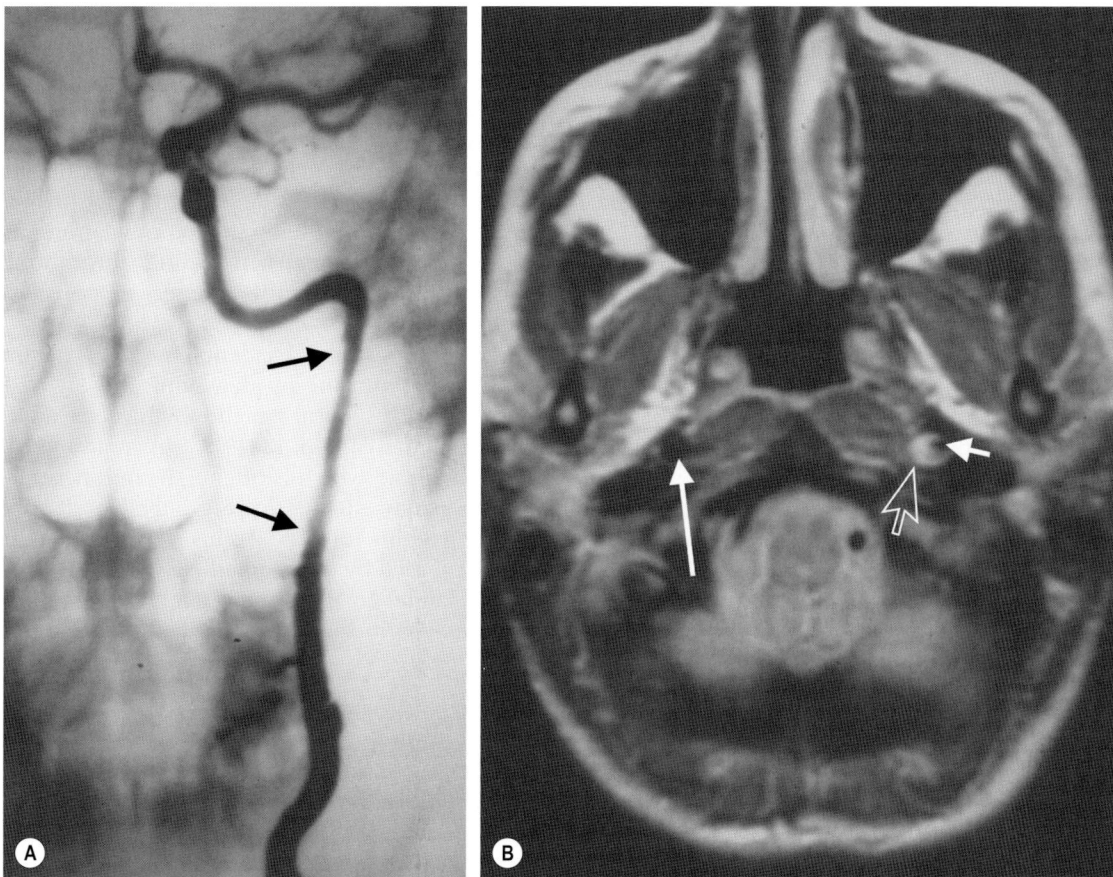

Figure 13–26. Painful Horner syndrome due to carotid dissection. **A**. Digital subtraction angiogram of the left carotid showing long narrowing (*arrows*) of the artery ("string-sign"). **B**. Axial MRI (TR = 2700, TE = 17) through the neck demonstrating crescent-shaped hyperintensity (*open arrow*), consistent with dissecting hemorrhage and narrowing of the lumen of the left internal carotid artery (*small arrow*) compared with the artery on the other side (*long arrow*).

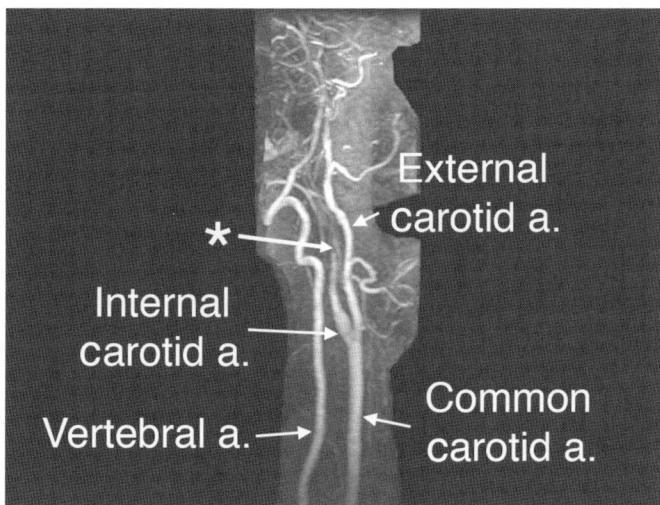

Figure 13–27. MRI angiogram of the neck in a patient with Horner syndrome due to carotid dissection. There is no flow in the internal carotid artery distal to the occlusion (asterisk). For comparison, see normal MRI angiogram of neck in Fig. 10–5.

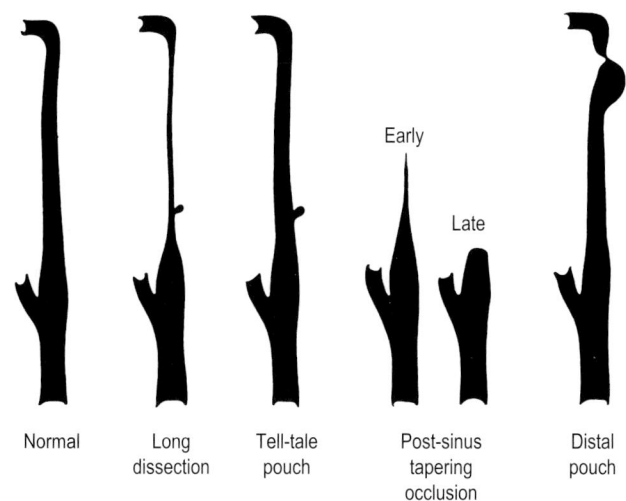

Figure 13–28. Diagrams of angiographic profiles in carotid dissection. (From Fisher CM, Ojemann RG, Robinson GH. Spontaneous dissection of cervico-cerebral arteries. Can J Neurol Sci 1978;5:9–19, with permission.)

temporal artery to middle cerebral artery anastomosis, direct exploration of the dissected internal carotid artery, carotid stenting, and observation.[125,138,162,163] In patients with acute carotid dissection, treatment with intravenous heparin for 5–7 days followed by 3–6 months of warfarin is one popular approach.[129,164] In individuals in whom long-term anticoagulation is contraindicated, heparin therapy can be followed by an antiplatelet agent such as aspirin. In otherwise asymptomatic patients whose dissection is several weeks old, aspirin alone can be given. However, the effectiveness of these medical therapies has not been established in any randomized clinical trials.[165] In fact, we have had several patients with acute symptomatic carotid dissections, treated successfully with aspirin alone. In general, surgical and endovascular options are risky and probably unnecessary.[125,166] Acute hemispheric strokes related to dissection can be treated with tissue plasminogen activator (t-PA).[164]

Mokri et al.[138] found excellent or complete clinical recovery in 85% of their patients, regardless of the treatment modality chosen, and overall mortality is less than 5%.[125] Angiographically demonstrated stenosis also completely resolved or markedly improved in 85%. Recurrence, which usually affects another artery, is uncommon. After the first month, the risk of recurrent dissection is only 1% per year,[167] and the risk of recurrent stroke is also extremely low.[166,168]

Carotid thrombosis. Carotid thrombosis, by interrupting the blood supply to the superior cervical ganglion or carotid plexus, can cause oculosympathetic paresis ipsilaterally, with or without pain.[169–171] The superior cervical ganglion derives its blood supply from small branches of the carotid artery

and from the ascending pharyngeal and superior thyroid arteries, both of which arise from the external carotid artery. The sympathetic carotid plexus is supplied by small direct branches from the internal carotid artery. Hemispheric signs, such as weakness, sensory loss, and hemianopia, may be present contralaterally, and in such situations it may difficult to tell whether the Horner syndrome is third order or due to deep cerebral infarction involving the hypothalamus (as described above). Further details regarding thrombotic carotid disease are discussed in the chapter on transient visual loss (Chapter 10).

Intraoral trauma. Iatrogenic or accidental intraoral trauma may cause a Horner syndrome by damaging the internal carotid artery or superior cervical ganglion, which are adjacent to the peritonsillar area (**Fig. 13–29**).[172] In an adult, the superior cervical ganglion, which is often 2–3 cm longitudinally, lies approximately 30–40 degrees lateral and only 1.5 cm behind the palatine tonsil.[173] At this level the internal carotid artery, surrounded by the sympathetic plexus, is situated immediately lateral to the superior cervical ganglion (**Fig. 13–29**). Other neighboring structures include the inter-

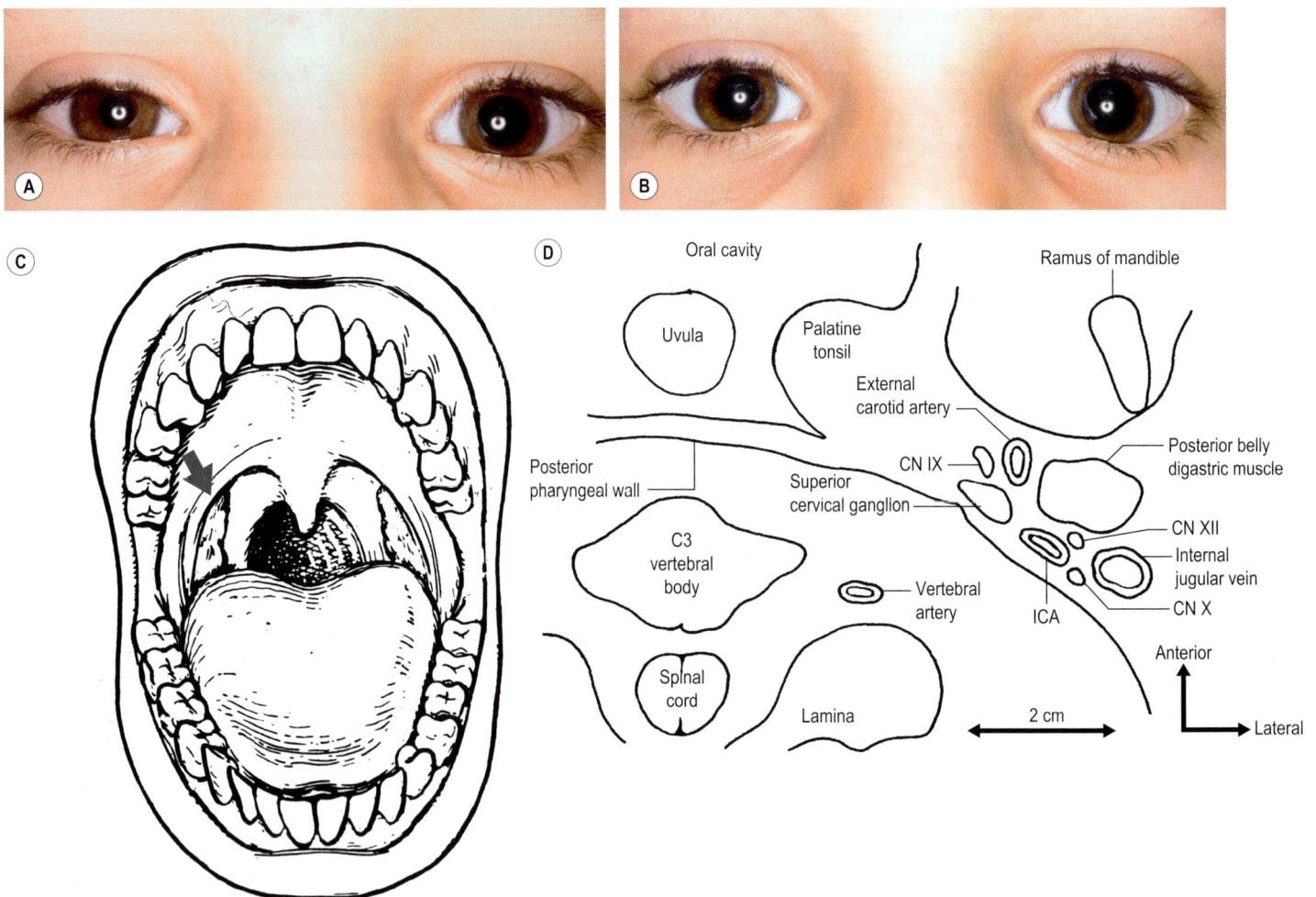

Figure 13–29. A. Horner syndrome, characterized by right upper eyelid ptosis, lower lid inverse ptosis (lower lid elevated), and miosis, due to intraoral trauma. **B**. After two drops of 1% hydroxyamphetamine in each eye, the right pupil dilates relatively more than the left, implying a preganglionic oculosympathetic lesion. **C**. View of the oral cavity. The arrow points to the area where a stick punctured this boy's right peritonsillar soft palate after he slipped on the ice. **D**. Vascular and nervous structures posterior and lateral to the palatine tonsil (axial view). a, Artery; CN, cranial nerve; ICA, internal carotid artery; v, vein. (From Liu GT, Deskin RW, Bienfang DC. Horner's syndrome due to intraoral trauma. J Clin Neuro-ophthalmol 1992;12:110–115, with permission.)

nal jugular vein, external carotid artery, and the glossopharyngeal (IX), vagus (X), and hypoglossal (XII) nerves. Alternatively, trauma to the internal carotid artery with intimal disruption could subsequently lead to thrombus formation or dissection, then sympathetic plexus ischemia. Accidental injury usually results from penetration by pencils,[174] sticks, or other sharp objects.[175] Iatrogenic causes include tonsillectomy[176] or other intraoral surgery, and peritonsillar anesthesia.[177,178] Horner syndrome following trauma to the peritonsillar region may be an ominous sign, alerting the clinician to the possibility of internal carotid injury, thrombus formation, or dissection.

Cluster headaches. These are characterized by "clusters" of ipsilateral headache or eye pain accompanied by ipsilateral Horner syndrome, rhinorrhea, conjunctival injection, and tearing. Although the oculosympathetic paresis is presumptively postganglionic, pharmacologic testing is often inconsistent.[179-181] The Horner syndrome may be intermittent or chronic.[182] Imaging should be performed to exclude mimickers such as carotid dissection.[183] More details regarding the clinical features, pathophysiology, and treatment of this disorder are discussed in Chapter 19.

Small-vessel ischemia. Not uncommonly, individuals with atherosclerosis associated with hypertension or diabetes, for instance, may develop a painless Horner syndrome. The mechanism is likely small-vessel ischemia involving the carotid plexus or vasa vasorium. Horner syndrome can also occur in the setting of giant cell arteritis.[184,185]

Cavernous sinus, superior orbital fissure, and orbital apex. A Horner syndrome and any combination of ipsilateral third, fourth, V_1, V_2, or sixth nerve involvement suggests a cavernous sinus process.[186,187] Alternating anisocoria in light and dark is unique to this localization.[188] If, for example, a right-sided cavernous sinus mass causes a right Horner syndrome and a right third nerve palsy, in the light, because of the third nerve palsy, the right pupil may be *larger* than the left. In the dark, however, because of the oculosympathetic paresis, the right pupil may become *smaller* than the left. Rarely Horner syndrome can be the only manifestation of a cavernous sinus process.[189]

Except for sparing of V_2, lesions of the superior orbital fissure are clinically difficult to distinguish from those of the cavernous sinus, and the causes are similar. The orbital apex syndrome consists of any combination of third, fourth, and sixth nerve paresis, V_1 distribution sensory loss, Horner syndrome, and visual loss due to optic nerve involvement.[190] The differential diagnosis and management of lesions of the cavernous sinus, superior orbital fissure, and orbital apex are discussed in more detail in Chapters 15 and 18.

Autonomic neuropathies. Unilateral and bilateral Horner syndrome due to sympathetic ganglion dysfunction may be a manifestation of autonomic neuropathy. Responsible underlying systemic disorders would include diabetes[191] and amyloidosis, for instance. Oculosympathetic autonomic neuropathy may be a feature of Ross[62] or harlequin[65,192] syndromes (see above), hereditary sensory and autonomic neuropathy (HSAN) type II, Anderson–Fabry disease, familial dysautonomia, multiple-system atrophy, pure autonomic failure, and dopamine-beta-hydroxylase deficiency.[193]

Others. Neck masses and trauma may also affect the postganglionic sympathetic fibers. Horner syndrome in association with middle ear infection has also been reported.[194]

Congenital and acquired causes of Horner syndrome in childhood

The most important identifiable cause in young children with congenital or acquired Horner syndrome is occult neuroblastoma. While birth trauma should always be considered, this is a relatively uncommon cause of Horner syndrome in an infant. Iris heterochromia, although an excellent sign of congenital oculosympathetic paresis,[85] is not always present. In many cases of Horner syndrome in infants, no cause can be found despite extensive history taking and investigation.[195,196] Weinstein et al.[197] speculated that these idiopathic cases might result from a congenital malformation or vascular insult of the superior cervical ganglion or some other structure in the oculosympathetic pathway. Spontaneous regression of a congenital neuroblastoma is another possibility in idiopathic cases.[196] Like others,[198-200] we have found idiopathic cases to be the most common group in childhood (**Table 13–9**).[196] Congenital malformations of the carotid artery may also be responsible.[201,202]

Neuroblastoma. Horner syndrome was found in 3.5% of neuroblastomas in one large series.[203] Neuroblastomas, believed to be of neural crest origin, are among the most common childhood solid tumors. When arising in the upper thorax or cervical sympathetic chain (**Fig. 13–30**), this tumor can present with Horner syndrome as well as stridor due to tracheal displacement, dysphagia owing to esophageal compression, or rarely lower cranial nerve involvement.[204,205] In some instances, they may grow large enough to present as a visible neck mass.[206] There have been rare cases with Horner syndrome associated with neuroblastomas arising from the adrenal glands and in the lower thoracic sympathetic chain.[207] How distant tumors affect the oculosympathetic pathway is uncertain, but a more generalized disorder of sympathetic neuronal maturation has been proposed.[207,208] Alternatively, a small cervical metastasis may have been missed without MRI. A more differentiated, benign form of the tumor, termed *ganglioneuroma*[208] or *ganglioneuroblastoma*,[209] may also be associated with Horner syndrome when it occurs in the neck and upper thorax.

The adrenal glands are the most common location, being the site of tumor in about one-half of cases.[210] Approximately one-quarter of neuroblastomas present in the cervical region or mediastinum, and these tumors may have a better prognosis.[211] Thus Musarella et al.[203] found patients with neuroblastoma associated with Horner syndrome to have an excellent survival rate of 78.6% at 3 years, due to the predominance of localized disease and favorable location among these patients. Histology in the setting of Horner syndrome is often "low risk," and treatment in such instances generally consists of surgical resection, then observation without chemo- or radiation therapy.[212] The treatment and prognosis of neuroblastoma is discussed in more detail in the discussion of opsoclonus/myoclonus in Chapter 17.

Table 13–9 Horner syndrome in childhood: differential diagnosis according to location, cause, and frequency as seen in various series

Localization	Cause	Cleveland (1976)[215]	Iowa (1980)[197]	Toronto (1988)[198]	USCF (1998)[200]	Toronto/ Hopkins (1998)[199]	Philadelphia CHOP (2006)[196]
Idiopathic			4 (36%)	4 (40%)	16 (70%)	31 (42%)	21 (36%)
First-order (central) neuron	Neoplasm involving: hypothalmus brain stem, or spinal cord	1 (14%)					5 (9%)
	Trauma						3 (5%)
	Syringomyelia						
	Arachnoid cyst			1 (10%)			
	Cerebral palsy			1 (10%)			
	Klippel–Feil						1 (2%)
	Infection						2 (4%)
Second-order (preganglionic) neuron	Neuroblastoma	1 (14%)		2 (20%)	2 (9%)	3 (5%)	5 (9%)
	Chest surgery		2 (18%)	2 (20%)			3 (5%)
	Birth-related injury of nerve roots or brachial plexus	1 (14%)	1 (9%)				
	Metastatic disease	1 (14%)					
	Intrathoracic aneurysm	1 (14%)					
	Infection						3 (5%)
	Cervical lymphadenopathy					2 (3%)	1 (2%)
	Neck surgery						4 (7%)
	Ganglioneuroma and other tumors				1 (4%)		3 (5%)
	Xanthogranuloma						1 (2%)
Third-order (postganglionic) neuron	Birth-related injury		4 (36%)		4 (17%)		1 (2%)
	Otitis media						
	Intraoral trauma						
	Nasopharyngeal tumor	1 (14%)				1 (1%)	
	Carotid artery occlusion	1 (14%)					
	Autonomic dysregulation						1 (2%)
	Carotid malformation						2 (4%)
Total		7	11	10	23	73	56

In the Cleveland series,[215] the presenting age was 10 years or younger. The Iowa[197] and University of California, San Francisco (UCSF), series[200] included only those patients with onset of Horner syndrome in the first year of life, while in the Toronto (1988) series,[198] all patients were 8 years of age or less. The Philadelphia series[196] consists of all cases in patients less than 18 years of age seen by one of us (GTL) at the Children's Hospital of Philadelphia (CHOP) from July 1993 through July 2005. The Toronto/Hopkins series,[199] which was also made up of patients less than 18 years of age, provided insufficient information to localize all cases. Thus, the list for that series is incomplete. All cases in the Iowa and Toronto (1988) series were confirmed with cocaine testing. In the Philadelphia series all idiopathic cases were confirmed pharmacologically and had unremarkable imaging and negative urine catecholamine screening.

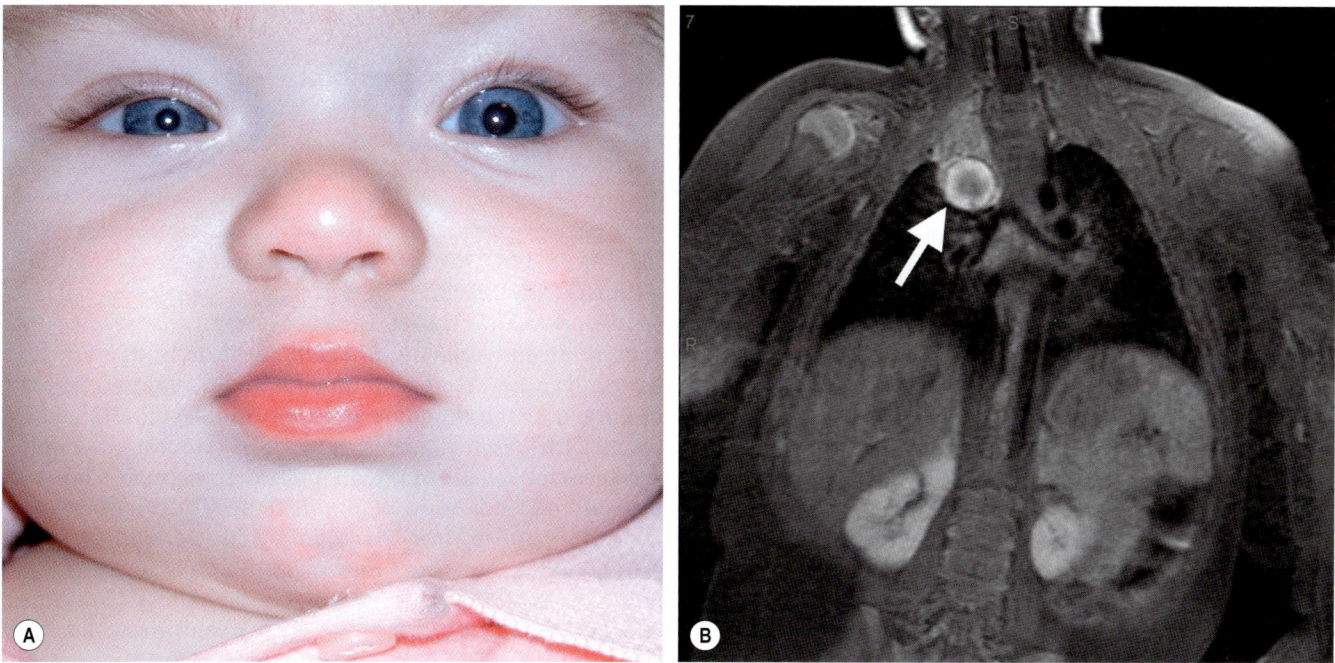

Figure 13–30. **A**. Right Horner syndrome in an infant due to a neuroblastoma (**B**) (*arrow*) of the lung apex demonstrated in a coronal gadolinium-enhanced chest magnetic resonance image.

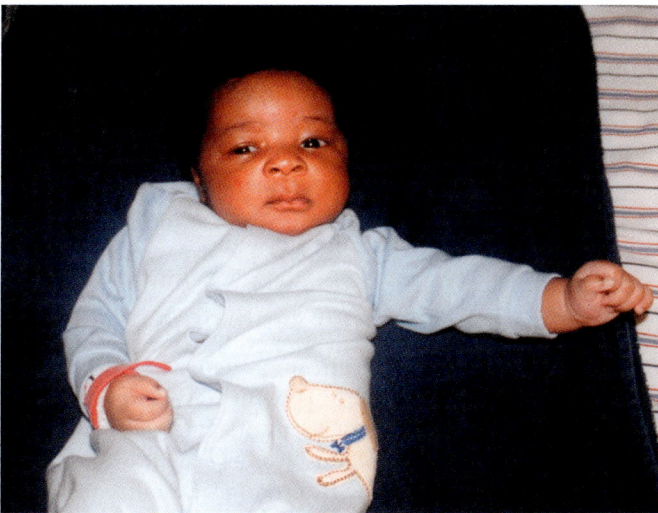

Figure 13–31. Infant with birth-related right brachial plexus injury resulting in right Horner syndrome and right arm weakness.

Birth trauma. A forceful pull of a child's arm during vaginal delivery may result in injury to the lower trunk of the brachial plexus (Klumpke's palsy).[213] In such instances Horner syndrome may result from dislocation of the C8 and T1 dorsal and ventral nerve roots. In addition, muscles and skin supplied by the C8 and T1 nerve roots are affected, leading to weakness of wrist flexion and intrinsic muscles of the hand as well as anesthesia in the ulnar aspect of the forearm and hand. Alternatively, one histopathologic report suggested C7 injury was the cause,[214] and in some instances Horner syndrome in the setting of more diffuse brachial plexus injury is seen (**Fig. 13–31**). Traction on the carotid plexus during difficult forceps delivery is another birth-related injury that may cause Horner syndrome.[197] Importantly, a history of birth trauma does not preclude the possibility of an underlying neoplasm such as neuroblastoma.[196]

Acquired Horner syndrome in childhood. The differential diagnosis of acquired causes of Horner syndrome in children is different than that in adults (**Table 13–9**).[196,215] Brain stem infarction, spontaneous carotid dissection, pulmonary tumors, and cluster headache are much less frequent in this age group. A child with Horner syndrome following implantation of a vagus nerve stimulator has been reported.[216]

Pharmacologic testing in Horner syndrome

Cocaine and apraclonidine confirmation. The diagnosis of a Horner syndrome associated with a lateral medullary stroke, brachial plexus injury, or spinal cord trauma, for instance, is often straightforward because of the accompanying signs and symptoms. However, the distinction between ipsilateral ptosis and miosis due to oculosympathetic paresis and other causes, such as physiologic anisocoria combined with levator dehiscence–disinsertion on the side of the miotic pupil (so-called pseudo-Horner syndrome[217]), may require pharmacologic testing.

Cocaine, which blocks reuptake of norepinephrine at the sympathetic nerve terminal in the iris dilator muscle, allows a relative increase of neurotransmitter available for the post-synaptic receptors. Iris dilator tone depends on the intactness of each neuron in the oculosympathetic pathway. Normally, cocaine will dilate the pupil and widen the palpebral fissure, and the pupillary dilation is more pronounced in individuals with light irises than in those with dark ones. However, interruption of any one of the three neurons results in decreased norepinephrine released by the third-order neuron, so cocaine will have little or no effect in such

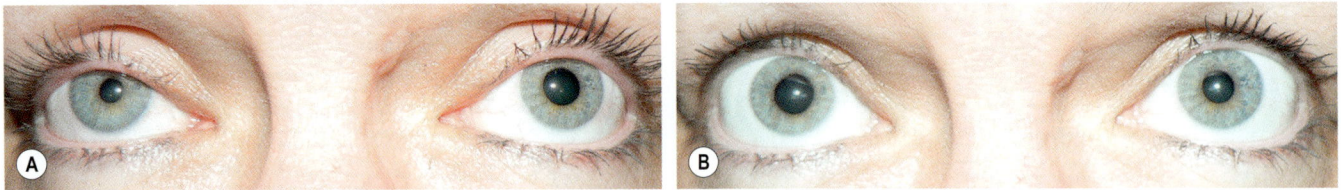

Figure 13–32. Apraclonidine test in Horner syndrome. **A**. The right eye exhibits ptosis and miosis. **B**. After topical administration of 1% apraclonidine to both eyes, the right pupil is larger and the ptosis has disappeared due to sympathetic stimulation of suprasensitive, upregulated receptors.

cases. Cocaine testing helps confirm the presence of a Horner syndrome, but does not aid in localization.

A 10% solution should be used since cocaine is a relatively weak pupillary dilator, and drop administration should be repeated 1–5 minutes later. Pupil sizes should be assessed at baseline and 40–60 minutes after the cocaine eye drops have been instilled. Sometimes neither pupil has responded, and this requires a readministration of drops and further observation for another 30 minutes. In a positive test, cocaine fails to dilate a sympathetically impaired pupil or does so very poorly, while the unaffected pupil dilates normally (see Fig. 13–18). Kardon and colleagues[218] and Van der Wiel and Van Gijn[219] suggest the most accurate way to interpret the cocaine test is to measure the postcocaine anisocoria. If the pupillary inequality following cocaine is greater than 1.0 mm, the test should be considered positive, and the greater the size difference, the more likely the positive result is correct. In simple anisocoria, both pupils will dilate with cocaine, but the pupillary inequality following cocaine should be small. Patients should be told urine samples may be positive for cocaine for a few days following eye drop testing.[220]

Apraclonidine, an alpha-adrenergic receptor agonist, also can be used to confirm Horner syndrome, based upon sympathetic denervation hypersensitivity of alpha-1 receptors on the pupillary dilator muscle.[221] Apraclonidine is commercially and widely available. After topical administration of 1% or 0.5% apraclonidine eye drops, the smaller Horner pupil will dilate, but a normal pupil will not (reversal of anisocoria) (**Fig. 13–32**).[222–224] The test's effectiveness requires the Horner syndrome to have been present long enough for receptor upregulation to have occurred.[225] False negatives can occur if the test is administered in acute Horner syndrome or even in long-standing cases if strict adherence to "reversal of anisocoria" as an endpoint is employed.[226] As cocaine is a controlled substance, has strict regulations regarding locked storage, and is becoming more difficult to acquire, apraclonidine's popularity will likely increase. However, at this time cocaine testing in Horner syndrome is still the gold standard, and more experience with apraclonidine is needed before cocaine is replaced (particularly in children, see below).[227]

Hydroxyamphetamine localization. Because many postganglionic Horner syndromes tend to be benign, while preganglionic (first and second order) Horner syndromes may reflect an underlying neoplasm, the distinction between pre- and postganglionic lesions may have important management implications. If the cocaine test indicates oculosympathetic paresis, 24–48 hours later 1% hydroxyam-

phetamine drops can be applied topically to both eyes to aid in localization. Drop administration is repeated after 1 minute, and the pupillary sizes 45 minutes later are compared with baseline measurements. Hydroxyamphetamine enhances the release of presynaptic norepinephrine, and this property depends only on the intactness of the third-order neuron.[228] In normal individuals, hydroxyamphetamine produces a symmetric 2-mm mean increase in the size of pupils,[229] and the drug dilates lighter irises faster and more effectively than dark ones.[230] Hydroxyamphetamine also normally widens the palpebral fissure.

As a rule, in first or second-order Horner syndrome, both pupils will also dilate with hydroxyamphetamine, and sometimes the involved pupil actually dilates more than the normal one (see **Fig. 13–29A,B**).[231] In contrast, in third-order sympathetic interruption, the involved pupil theoretically should not dilate. However, in order to establish a Horner syndrome as third order, in practice it is probably more helpful to determine if the relative anisocoria *increases* by more than 1 mm following administration of hydroxyamphetamine.[231,232] Unfortunately, the hydroxyamphetamine test is imperfect, as evidenced by the false-negative and positive results seen in several studies.[92,231,232]

Management of Horner syndrome

The diagnosis of Horner syndrome is usually a clinical one based upon examination findings, with cocaine used only to confirm equivocal cases. Hydroxyamphetamine is becoming more difficult to acquire because of decreasing commercial availability. This, coupled with the high false-negative and positive rate of the hydroxyamphetamine test, will encourage clinicians in most instances to localize the Horner syndrome and make management decisions clinically, based upon clues in the history or examination (**Fig. 13–17**). Imaging of some type typically will be pursued next, and the localization and clinical setting will dictate the modality and region to be evaluated.[233,234]

In adults with Horner syndrome, there are two situations that mandate radiologic investigation regardless of clinical or pharmacologic localization (because neither is perfect). First, in any middle-aged or elderly patient, especially one with a history of smoking, with an isolated, unexplained Horner syndrome, chest CT or MRI should be performed to rule out an apical lung tumor. Second, Horner syndrome accompanied by ipsilateral headache or eye pain, with or without ipsilateral cerebral or ocular ischemic symptoms, requires MRI and MRA of the neck to exclude a carotid dissection or thrombosis. Axial T1-weighted MR images through the neck are especially important in this setting.

Other situations can be governed by suspected localization:

1. *First-order neuron.* If the process is thought to be first order because of the presence of cerebral, posterior fossa, or spinal cord signs, then the neurologic findings should guide the investigation. For instance, accompanying hemianesthesia or ataxia mandate brain MRI to exclude a brain stem lesion. On the other hand, a sensory level or paraparesis accompanying a Horner syndrome should be evaluated with spine MRI.

2. *Second-order neuron.* If a presumed preganglionic Horner syndrome is isolated or associated with brachial plexopathy, screening chest roentgenography or chest CT or MRI with attention to the lung apex and neck is indicated.

3. *Third-order neuron.* If the lesion can be localized to the postganglionic neuron, in addition to an MRI and MRA of the neck to exclude a carotid dissection or thrombosis, we recommend an MRI of the brain to exclude a cavernous sinus lesion. The additional presence of a third, fourth, or sixth nerve palsy or trigeminal neuropathy ipsilateral to the Horner syndrome would be highly suggestive of such a localization. However, the evaluation of postganglionic Horner syndromes is often unrevealing as many have a benign cause (e.g., small vessel vasculopathy). Because of the proximity between sympathetic and vascular structures in the lateral and parapharyngeal space, Horner syndrome in the setting of intraoral trauma should also prompt evaluation of the neck and internal carotid artery.

Most individuals with Horner syndrome do not find the ptosis bothersome, as it is usually very mild and rarely affects vision. Cosmetic surgery may be considered in patients who find their appearance undesirable. The pupil abnormality should not cause subjective symptoms.

Horner syndrome in children. The neck and axillary regions should be palpated for masses or lymphadenopathy. To decide upon further management, cocaine testing should be used to confirm the Horner syndrome in unexplained cases in young children. When positive, diagnostic testing should be performed to exclude neuroblastoma and other responsible mass lesions.[196] Even children with a history of birth trauma or those with Horners at birth ("congenital") should be evaluated, as these patients may still harbor an underlying neoplasm.[235,236] MRI with and without gadolinium of the head, neck, and upper chest, as well as urinary catecholamine metabolite screening (vanillylmandelic acid (VMA) and homovanillic acid (HVA)) is one recommended protocol.[196] Only "spot" urine samples, rather than large collections, are needed. In one study of children with Horner syndrome of unknown etiology,[196] responsible mass lesions, such as neuroblastoma, Ewing sarcoma, and juvenile xanthogranuloma, were found in 33% of patients. Of interest, the MRI is more sensitive than urine testing in this setting, as all the newly diagnosed neuroblastomas in this study were detected on imaging but had normal VMA and HVA levels.[196]

Although excess production of catecholamines or their metabolites occurs in 90% of all neuroblastomas,[237] in low-risk neuroblastomas such as those causing Horner syndrome, as few as 40% may be associated with abnormal VMA and HVA levels.[238] Children with cocaine-confirmed oculosympathetic paresis with no obvious cause and normal imaging and urine testing are given the diagnosis of idiopathic Horner syndrome.

Testing with apraclonidine has been suggested in children with Horner syndrome,[239,240] but reports of drowsiness and unresponsiveness in infants tested with this agent,[241] and in those treated for glaucoma with the similar drug brimonidine,[242] have discouraged us from using it in this population. In our experience dry eye and mild irritability are the only side effects from the use of cocaine eye drops in children.

Caution also should be applied when hydroxyamphetamine is used in children with Horner syndrome. The normal development of the third-order oculosympathetic neuron and its synaptic connections depends on the integrity of the first and second neuron. In congenital preganglionic lesions, therefore, it is possible that hydroxyamphetamine will completely or partially fail to dilate the involved pupil because of transsynaptic degeneration of postganglionic fibers.[197]

Pupils in other neurologic conditions

Coma

Pupillary signs may be extremely important in the evaluation of comatose patients, especially with regard to diagnosis and localization (**Fig. 13–33**). As a rule, metabolic coma is more likely to be associated with normally reactive pupils than coma due to a structural lesion, although there are exceptions (see systemic medications, below).[243]

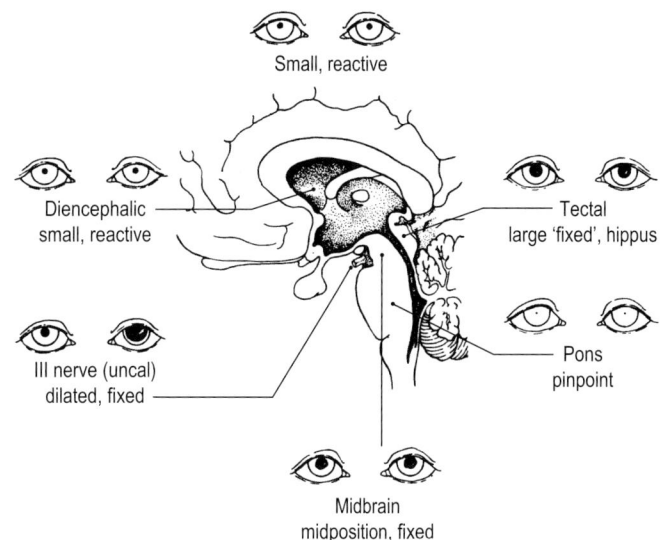

Figure 13–33. Pupils in comatose patients. (From Plum F, Posner JB. Pupils: In: The Diagnosis of Stupor and Coma, 3rd edition, p 46. New York, Oxford University Press, 1980, with permission.)

As stated above, hypothalamic lesions may cause small but reactive pupils due to oculosympathetic paresis, while thalamic and mesencephalic lesions may result in third nerve palsies, midposition or large pupils or, less likely, pupillary corectopia. Destructive lesions of the pons may disrupt the descending oculosympathetic pathways and result in bilateral pinpoint pupils. Diffuse anoxic brain damage can cause midbrain dysfunction and dilated pupils. Initially in brain death, the pupils can be midposition or dilated and unreactive to light. With more time after death, however, all pupils become midposition, reflecting the equal parasympathetic and sympathetic dysfunction.

Ipsilateral pupillary dilation may be the first sign of transtentorial uncal herniation before other signs of third nerve paresis develop. In this setting, mechanisms for third nerve dysfunction include direct compression by the herniating uncus beneath the tentorial edge, compression by the posterior cerebral artery or hippocampal gyrus, compression of the oculomotor complex in the midbrain, or displacement and kinking of the nerve over the clivus.[244] Further clinical progression may be monitored by examining the opposite pupil, which initially may be midposition with a depressed light reaction, then slightly miotic, and finally dilated.[245] Transiently the pupils may acquire an oval shape.[246] Uncommonly in transtentorial herniation, the opposite pupil is paradoxically the first to dilate.[247]

In metabolic encephalopathies, the pupils may be small but remain reactive to light until midbrain dysfunction ensues. In hepatic encephalopathy, for example, oculocephalic eye movements and pupillary reactivity are normal despite severe alteration in consciousness. However, in stage IV hepatic encephalopathy, cerebral edema and downward herniation can cause coma, fixed and dilated pupils, and ophthalmoplegia.[248,249]

Systemic medications

Opiate intoxication causes pinpoint pupils resembling those seen with large pontine lesions. Theoretically in these instances the pupils should be reactive to light, but they can be so miotic that any constriction is difficult to appreciate, even with a magnifying glass.

Poisoning with any substance, such as atropine or a tricyclic antidepressant with anticholinergic properties may cause dilated and fixed pupils. These pupils will not react to 1% pilocarpine. Glutethimide and barbiturate intoxication can also fix the pupils.[243]

Migraine

A dilated pupil and ipsilateral headache may be alarming for both the patient and physician, and certainly in these instances a third nerve palsy should be excluded. However, transient isolated mydriasis or so-called *benign episodic mydriasis*, with normal vision and pupillary reactivity to light, may occasionally accompany migraine headaches (**Fig. 13–34**).[250] Eyelid or motility disturbances, which might otherwise suggest ophthalmoplegic migraine, are absent. The dilated pupil is due either to parasympathetic insufficiency of the iris sphincter or sympathetic hyperactivity of

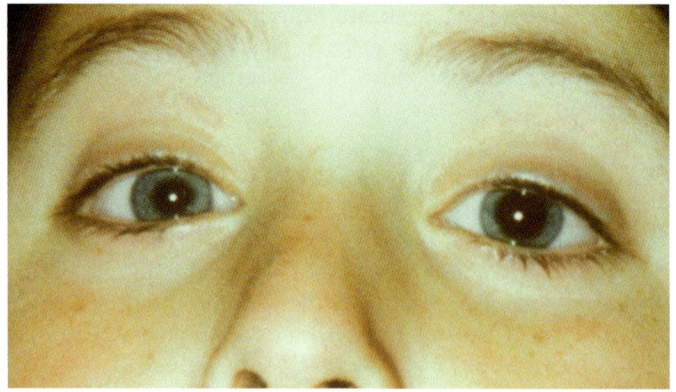

Figure 13–34. Benign episodic mydriasis in migraine. This boy developed transient episodes of left unilateral pupillary dilation accompanied by ipsilateral headache. Ocular motility, pupillary reactivity, and eyelids were normal. The photo was taken by his mother during one such episode.

the iris dilator.[251] In unusual cases, the mydriasis can have the clinical and pharmacologic characteristics of a tonic pupil,[252,253] or be tadpole shaped (see below).[254]

Several studies suggest that the pupils of migraineurs may be abnormal even in the days following an attack. For instance, pupil asymmetry was found to be greater in the migraine sufferers than in controls, but there was no correlation with the side of miotic pupil and of the headache.[255,256] Oculosympathetic defects were suggested by observations that migraineurs had smaller pupils than controls,[257] that their pupils exhibit dilation lag,[255] an inability to dilate after instillation of cocaine[255] or tyramine eye drops,[258] and denervation hypersensitivity.[258] Drummond[255] hypothesized that vasodilation or swelling of the arterial wall in the carotid canal could lead to minor oculosympathetic deficits in patients with frequent or severe migraine attacks. Slower velocities and lower amplitudes of constriction, implying parasympathetic dysfunction, have also been demonstrated.[256,257]

The neuro-ophthalmic complications of migraine are discussed in more detail in Chapters 11 and 19.

Seizures

Presumably because of diffuse stimulation of the sympathetic system, generalized tonic–clonic seizures may be associated with bilateral mydriasis. Ictal unilateral mydriasis may be observed ipsilateral or contralateral to a cortical epileptic focus.[259–261] Rarely, unilateral pupillary dilation (without other signs of third nerve palsy) may persist for a few hours postictally.[262] Ictal miosis has also been described, both bilaterally and unilaterally, contralateral to the seizure focus.[263,264] Proposed explanations implicate stimulation or inhibition of cortical centers with parasympathetic or sympathetic connections to the eye.[263,264]

Other neuromuscular diseases

Pupillary abnormalities in neuromuscular junction disorders have been described above in the section on unreactive pupils.

Guillain–Barré syndrome and the Miller Fisher variant. Pupillary dysfunction is purportedly uncommon in

Guillain–Barré syndrome, but this may reflect insufficient attention to the pupils in patients with this syndrome without ophthalmoplegia.[265] Reported patients have had either completely unreactive[266] or tonic[267] pupils, and postganglionic parasympathetic as well as sympathetic disturbances were felt to be responsible.

In contrast, pupillary abnormalities occur in approximately 40%[268] of patients with the Miller Fisher variant (ophthalmoplegia, ataxia, and areflexia). Two of Fisher's first three patients had pupils that were poorly reactive to light.[269] The abnormal pupils are most commonly either dilated and fixed or exhibit light-near dissociation.[270–274] Sympathetic and parasympathetic abnormalities have been described.[270,271,274] Some patients[272,273] were found to have circulating antibodies to GQ1b gangliosides, which may involve the ciliary ganglia. These disorders are detailed in Chapter 14.

Other pupillary phenomena

Westphal–Piltz reflex

Pupillary constriction in darkness is a normal occurrence when individuals close their eyes to go to sleep (Westphal–Piltz reflex). This phenomenon is thought to be secondary to decreased inhibition of the oculomotor complex.

Paradoxic pupillary constriction in the dark

Pupillary miosis followed by slow redilation when the lights are turned off may suggest a retinal dystrophy such as in congenital stationary night blindness or congenital achromatopsia.[275,276] The mechanism is uncertain, but a transient delay or "noise" in the rod bleaching signal, allowing the small but normal cone bleaching signal to constrict the pupils when the lights are turned off, has been proposed.[277] A child with paradoxic pupillary constriction, poor vision, nystagmus, or a family history of retinal disorders should undergo electroretinography.

Tournay's pupillary phenomenon

Anisocoria induced by lateral gaze, which occurs in no more than 10% of the normal population, is referred to as *Tournay's pupillary phenomenon*.[278,279] The pupil of the abducting eye is larger, and either that pupil has dilated or the pupil of the adducting eye has constricted. The mechanism is unclear, but an anomalous connection between the medial rectus subnucleus and the Edinger–Westphal nucleus may be responsible.[280]

Abduction miosis

In this rare phenomenon, the pupil constricts during ocular abduction. The finding may be congenital, perhaps due to an anastomosis between the sixth nerve and ciliary ganglion, or acquired following concurrent injury to the third and sixth nerves with aberrant regeneration of abducens fibers into the parasympathetic pupillary pathway.[281,282] Miosis is also an important feature of abduction limitation associated with convergence spasm (see below).

Oculosympathetic spasm

Irritation of the oculosympathetic pathway may result in unilateral pupillary mydriasis, occasionally accompanied by ipsilateral facial flushing, lid retraction, and hyperhydrosis. Oculosympathetic spasm is typically a delayed phenomenon associated with chronic cervical cord lesions such as syringomyelia or infarction, and the cause is unknown.[283] Cysts in this area may cause alternating anisocoria characterized by the presence of a Horner syndrome when the patient lies on the side of the lesion. The anisocoria reverses, presumably because of oculosympathetic spasm, when the patient lies on the other side.[107]

Cyclic oculomotor spasms

This disorder, which is also discussed in Chapter 15, is characterized by a complete or partial third nerve palsy that alternates with lid elevation, miosis, and a downward and inward movement of the eye.[284] Most cases are seen in congenital third nerve palsies, and a cause is found only infrequently.[285]

Idiopathic alternating anisocoria

In this rare condition, one pupil dilates, then several hours later the pupil returns to normal size, but the other pupil dilates.[80,286] The cycle can occur several times in one day. The eyelids and ocular motility remain normal, and there are no other neurologic abnormalities. The mechanism is unclear.

Tadpole-shaped pupils

Thompson et al.[254] described an unusual group of patients who exhibited episodic mydriasis with segmental pupillary distortion but intact constriction to light. This phenomenon occurred over minutes and was frequently accompanied by an ache or other abnormal sensations in the affected eye. The authors coined the descriptive term *tadpole-shaped pupils* and attributed them to abnormal segmental spasm of the iris dilator muscle. Clinical settings included ipsilateral Horner syndrome,[287,288] tonic pupils, and migraine.

Spasm of the near reflex

In this condition, miosis is associated with convergence, accommodation, and pseudo-(induced) myopia.[289] It is usually indicative of a functional disorder,[290] but can occur following head trauma.[291] The esotropia tends to be variable, and the myopia usually resolves after cycloplegia. The miosis upon attempted abduction is highly characteristic and may resolve upon occlusion of the fellow eye by disrupting the binocular input necessary for convergence.[292] Spasm of the near reflex is discussed in more detail in Chapter 15.

References

1. Slamovits TL, Glaser JS. The pupils and accommodation. In: Glaser JS (ed): Neuro-ophthalmology, 3rd edn., pp 527–552. Philadelphia, Lippincott Williams & Wilkins, 1999.
2. Jampel RS. Representation of the near-response in the cerebral cortex of the Macaque. Am J Ophthalmol 1959;48:573–582.
3. Ohtsuka K, Sato A. Descending projections from the cortical accommodation area in the cat. Invest Ophthalmol Vis Sci 1996;37:1429–1436.

4. Mays LE, Gamlin PD. Neuronal circuitry controlling the near response. Curr Opin Neurobiol 1995;5:763–768.

5. Parkinson D. Further observations on the sympathetic pathways to the pupil. Anat Rec 1988;220:108–109.

6. Martyn LJ, DiGeorge A. Selected eye defects of special importance in pediatrics. Pediatr Clin N Am 1987;34:1517–1542.

7. Guercio JR, Martyn LJ. Congenital malformations of the eye and orbit. Otolaryngol Clin North Am 2007;40:113–140, vii.

8. Brauner SC, Walton DS, Chen TC. Aniridia. Int Ophthalmol Clin 2008;48:79–85.

9. Byles DB, Nischal KK, Cheng H. Ectopia lentis et pupillae. A hypothesis revisited. Ophthalmology 1998;105:1331–1336.

10. Onwochei BC, Simon JW, Bateman JB, et al. Ocular colobomata. Surv Ophthalmol 2000;45:175–194.

11. Hayashi N, Valdes-Dapena M, Green WR. CHARGE association: histopathological report of two cases and a review. J Ped Ophthalmol Strab 1998;35:100–106.

12. Jongmans MC, Admiraal RJ, van der Donk KP, et al. CHARGE syndrome: the phenotypic spectrum of mutations in the CHD7 gene. J Med Genet 2006;43:306–314.

13. Alward WL. Axenfeld-Rieger syndrome in the age of molecular genetics. Am J Ophthalmol 2000;130:107–115.

14. Atkinson CS, Brodsky MC, Hiles DA, et al. Idiopathic tractional corectopia. J Ped Ophthalmol Strab 1994;31:387–390.

15. Burton BJ, Adams GG. Persistent pupillary membranes [letter]. Br J Ophthalmol 1998;82:711–712.

16. Bremner FD. Pupil assessment in optic nerve disorders. Eye 2004;18:1175–1181.

17. Portnoy JZ, Thompson HS, Lennarson L, et al. Pupillary defects in amblyopia. Am J Ophthalmol 1983;96:609–614.

18. Lam BL, Thompson HS. An anisocoria produces a small relative afferent pupillary defect in the eye with the smaller pupil. J Neuro-ophthalmol 1999;19:153–159.

19. Bell RA, Thompson HS. Relative afferent pupillary defect in optic tract hemianopsias. Am J Ophthalmol 1978;85:538–540.

20. Kardon R, Kawasaki A, Miller NR. Origin of the relative afferent pupillary defect in optic tract lesions. Ophthalmology 2006;113:1345–1353.

21. Savino PJ, Paris M, Schatz NJ, et al. Optic tract syndrome. A review of 21 patients. Arch Ophthalmol 1978;96:656–663.

22. Papageorgiou E, Ticini LF, Hardiess G, et al. The pupillary light reflex pathway: cytoarchitectonic probabilistic maps in hemianopic patients. Neurology 2008;70: 956–963.

23. Forman S, Behrens MM, Odel JG, et al. Relative afferent pupillary defect with normal visual function. Arch Ophthalmol 1990;108:1074–1075.

24. King JT, Galetta SL, Flamm ES. Relative afferent pupillary defect with normal vision in a glial brainstem tumor. Neurology 1991;41:945–946.

25. Eliott D, Cunningham ET, Miller NR. Fourth nerve paresis and ipsilateral relative afferent pupillary defect without visual sensory disturbance. A sign of contralateral dorsal midbrain disease. J Clin Neuro-ophthalmol 1991;11:169–172.

26. Girkin CA, Perry JD, Miller NR. A relative afferent pupillary defect without any visual sensory deficit. Arch Ophthalmol 1998;116:1544–1545.

27. Chen CJ, Scheufele M, Sheth M, et al. Isolated relative afferent pupillary defect secondary to contralateral midbrain compression. Arch Neurol 2004;61:1451–1453.

28. Wilhelm H, Peters T, Lüdtke H, et al. The prevalence of relative afferent pupillary defects in normal subjects. J Neuro-ophthalmol 2007;27:263–267.

29. Kawasaki A, Moore P, Kardon RH. Long-term fluctuation of relative afferent pupillary defect in subjects with normal visual function. Am J Ophthalmol 1996;122:875–882.

30. Ravin JG. Argyll Robertson. 'Twas better to be his pupil than to have his pupil. Ophthalmology 1998;105:867–870.

31. Pearce JM. The Argyll Robertson pupil. J Neurol Neurosurg Psychiatry 2004;75:1345.

32. Thompson HS, Kardon RH. The Argyll Robertson pupil. J Neuro-ophthalmol 2006;26: 134–138.

33. Sebag J, Sadun AA. Aberrant regeneration of the third nerve following orbital trauma. Synkinesis of the iris sphincter. Arch Neurol 1983;40:762–764.

34. Czarnecki JSC, Thompson HS. The iris sphincter in aberrant regeneration of the third nerve. Arch Ophthalmol 1978;96:1606–1610.

35. Kissel JT, Burde RM, Klingele TG, et al. Pupil-sparing oculomotor palsies with internal carotid-posterior communicating artery aneurysms. Ann Neurol 1983;13:149–154.

36. Coppeto JR, Monteiro MLR, Young D. Tonic pupils following oculomotor nerve palsies. Ann Ophthalmol 1985;17:585–588.

37. Cox TA. Tonic pupil and Czarnecki's sign following third nerve palsy [letter]. J Clin Neuro-ophthalmol 1991;11:217.

38. Ashker L, Weinstein JM, Dias M, et al. Arachnoid cyst causing third cranial nerve palsy manifesting as isolated internal ophthalmoplegia and iris cholinergic supersensitivity. J Neuro-ophthalmol 2008;28:192–197.

39. Jacobson DM. Pupillary responses to dilute pilocarpine in preganglionic 3rd nerve disorders. Neurology 1990;40:804–808.

40. Jacobson DM, Olson KA. Influence of pupil size, anisocoria, and ambient light on pilocarpine miosis. Implications for supersensitivity testing. Ophthalmology 1993;100: 275–280.

41. Jacobson DM. A prospective evaluation of cholinergic supersensitivity of the iris sphincter in patients with oculomotor nerve palsies. Am J Ophthalmol 1994;118:377–383.

42. Slamovits TL, Miller NR, Burde RM. Intracranial oculomotor nerve paresis with anisocoria and pupillary parasympathetic hypersensitivity. Am J Ophthalmol 1987;104:401–406.

43. Vaphiades MS, Cure J, Kline L. Management of intracranial aneurysm causing a third cranial nerve palsy: MRA, CTA or DSA? Semin Ophthalmol 2008;23:143–150.

44. Thompson HS. Segmental palsy of the iris sphincter in Adie's syndrome. Arch Ophthalmol 1978;96:1615–1620.

45. Gilmore PC, Carlow TJ. Diabetic oculomotor paresis with pupil fixed to light. Neurology 1980;30:1229–1230.

46. Loewenfeld IE. Lesions in the ciliary ganglion and short ciliary nerves: the tonic pupil ("Adie's" syndrome). In: The Pupil. Anatomy, Physiology, and Clinical Applications. Vol 1., pp 1080–1130. Detroit, Wayne State University Press, 1993.

47. Martinelli P. Holmes-Adie syndrome. Lancet 2000;356:1760–1761.

48. Bowie EM, Givre SJ. Tonic pupil and sarcoidosis. Am J Ophthalmol 2003;135:417–419.

49. Currie J, Lessell S. Tonic pupil with giant cell arteritis. Br J Ophthalmol 1984;68: 135–138.

50. Foroozan R, Buono LM, Savino PJ, et al. Tonic pupils from giant cell arteritis. Br J Ophthalmol 2003;87:510–512.

51. Bennett JL, Pelak VA, Mourelatos Z, et al. Acute sensorimotor polyneuropathy with tonic pupils and an abduction deficit: an unusual presentation of polyarteritis nodosa. Surv Ophthalmol 1999;43:341–344.

52. Brooks-Kayal AR, Liu GT, Menacker SJ, et al. Tonic pupil and orbital glial-neural hamartoma in infancy. Am J Ophthalmol 1995;119:809–811.

53. Goldstein SM, Liu GT, Edmond JC, et al. Orbital neural-glial hamartoma associated with a congenital tonic pupil. JAAPOS 2002;6:54–55.

54. Rogell GD. Internal ophthalmoplegia after argon laser panretinal photocoagulation. Arch Ophthalmol 1979;97:904–905.

55. Toth C, Fletcher WA. Autonomic disorders and the eye. J Neuro-ophthalmol 2005;25: 1–4.

56. O'Neill JH, Murray NMF, Newsom-Davis J. The Lambert-Eaton myasthenic syndrome. A review of 50 cases. Brain 1988;111:577–596.

57. Wirtz PW, de Keizer RJ, de Visser M, et al. Tonic pupils in Lambert-Eaton myasthenic syndrome. Muscle Nerve 2001;24:444–445.

58. Bruno MK, Winterkorn JM, Edgar MA, et al. Unilateral Adie pupil as sole ophthalmic sign of anti-Hu paraneoplastic syndrome. J Neuro-ophthalmol 2000;20:248–249.

59. Müller NG, Prass K, Zschenderlein R. Anti-Hu antibodies, sensory neuropathy, and Holmes-Adie syndrome in a patient with seminoma. Neurology 2005;64:164–165.

60. Lambert SR, Yang LL, Stone C. Tonic pupil associated with congenital neuroblastoma, Hirschsprung disease, and central hypoventilation syndrome. Am J Ophthalmol 2000;130:238–240.

61. Drummond PD, Edis RH. Loss of facial sweating and flushing in Holmes-Adie syndrome. Neurology 1990;40:847–849.

62. Wolfe GI, Galetta SL, Teener JW, et al. Site of autonomic dysfunction in a patient with Ross' syndrome and postganglionic Horner's syndrome. Neurology 1995;45:2094–2096.

63. Shin RK, Galetta SL, Ting TY, et al. Ross syndrome plus: beyond Horner, Holmes-Adie, and harlequin. Neurology 2000;55:1841–1846.

64. Drummond PD, Lance JW. Site of autonomic deficit in harlequin syndrome: local autonomic failure affecting the arm and face. Ann Neurol 1993;34:814–819.

65. Bremner F, Smith S. Pupillographic findings in 39 consecutive cases of harlequin syndrome. J Neuro-ophthalmol 2008;28:171–177.

66. Bourgon P, Pilley SFJ, Thompson HS. Cholinergic supersensitivity of the iris sphincter in Adie's tonic pupil. Am J Ophthalmol 1978;85:373–377.

67. Leavitt JA, Wayman LL, Hodge DO, et al. Pupillary response to four concentrations of pilocarpine in normal subjects: application to testing for Adie tonic pupil. Am J Ophthalmol 2002;133:333–336.

68. Fletcher WA, Sharpe JA. Tonic pupils in neurosyphilis. Neurology 1986;36:188–192.

69. McCrary JA, Webb NR. Anisocoria from scopolamine patches. JAMA 1982;248:353–354.

70. Openshaw H. Unilateral mydriasis from ipratropium in transplant patients. Neurology 2006;67:914.

71. Firestone D, Sloane C. Not your everyday anisocoria: angel's trumpet ocular toxicity. J Emerg Med 2007;33:21–24.

72. Thompson HS, Newsome DA, Loewenfield IE. The fixed dilated pupil: sudden iridoplegia or mydriatic drops? A simple diagnostic test. Arch Ophthalmol 1971;86: 21–27.

73. Miller NR, Moses H. Ocular involvement in wound botulism. Arch Ophthalmol 1977;95:1788–1789.

74. Terranova W, Palumbo JN, Breman JG. Ocular findings in botulism type B. JAMA 1979;241:475–477.

75. Gräf MH, Jungherr A. Congenital mydriasis, failure of accommodation, and patent ductus arteriosus. Arch Ophthalmol 2002;120:509–510.

76. Lam BL, Thompson HS, Corbett JJ. The prevalence of simple anisocoria. Am J Ophthalmol 1987;104:69–73.

77. Roarty JD, Keltner JL. Normal pupil size and anisocoria in newborn infants. Arch Ophthalmol 1990;108:94–95.

78. Kawasaki A, Kardon RH. Disorders of the pupil. Ophthalmol Clin North Am 2001;14: 149–168.

79. Thompson HS, Pilley SFJ. Unequal pupils. A flow chart for sorting out the anisocorias. Surv Ophthalmol 1976;21:45–48.

80. Bremner FD, Booth A, Smith SE. Benign alternating anisocoria. Neuro-ophthalmology 2004;28:129–135.

81. Lam BL, Thompson HS, Walls RC. Effect of light on the prevalence of simple anisocoria. Ophthalmology 1996;103:790–793.

82. Thompson HS. Johann Friedrich Horner (1831–1886). Am J Ophthalmol 1986;102: 792–795.

83. Pilley SF, Thompson HS. Pupillary "dilatation lag" in Horner's syndrome. Brit J Ophthalmol 1975;59:731–735.

84. Crippa SV, Borruat FX, Kawasaki A. Pupillary dilation lag is intermittently present in patients with a stable oculosympathetic defect (Horner syndrome). Am J Ophthalmol 2007;143:712–715.

85. Jaffe N, Cassady JR, Filler RM, et al. Heterochromia and Horner syndrome associated with cervical and mediastinal neuroblastoma. J Pediatr 1975;87:75–77.

86. Diesenhouse MC, Palay DA, Newman NJ, et al. Acquired heterochromia with Horner syndrome in two adults. Ophthalmology 1992;99:1815–1817.

87. Zamir E, Chowers I, Banin E, et al. Neurotrophic corneal endothelial failure complicating acute Horner syndrome. Ophthalmology 1999;106:1692–1696.

88. Morris JGL, Lee J, Lim CL. Facial sweating in Horner's syndrome. Brain 1984;107: 751–758.

89. Morrison DA, Bibby K, Woodruff G. The "harlequin" sign and congenital Horner's syndrome. J Neurol Neurosurg Psychiatry 1997;62:626–628.

90. Keane JR. Oculosympathetic paresis. Analysis of 100 hospitalized patients. Arch Neurol 1979;36:13–16.

91. Giles CL, Henderson JW. Horner's syndrome: an analysis of 216 cases. Am J Ophthalmol 1958;46:289–296.

92. Maloney WF, Younge BR, Moyer NJ. Evaluation of the causes and accuracy of pharmacologic localization in Horner's syndrome. Am J Ophthalmol 1980;90:394–402.

93. Grimson BS, Thompson HS. Drug testing in Horner's syndrome. In: Glaser JS, Smith JL (eds): Neuro-ophthalmology. Symposium of the University of Miami and the Bascom Palmer Eye Institute. Vol. VIII, pp 265–270. St. Louis, C.V. Mosby, 1975.

94. Reeves AG, Posner JB. The ciliospinal response in man. Neurology 1969;19:1145–1152.

95. Stone WM, de Toledo J, Romanul FCA. Horner's syndrome due to hypothalamic infarction. Clinical, radiologic, and pathologic correlations. Arch Neurol 1986;43: 199–200.

96. Austin CP, Lessell S. Horner's syndrome from hypothalamic infarction. Arch Neurol 1991;48:332–334.

97. Rossetti AO, Reichhart MD, Bogousslavsky J. Central Horner's syndrome with contralateral ataxic hemiparesis: a diencephalic alternate syndrome. Neurology 2003;61:334–338.

98. Guy J, Day AL, Mickle JP, et al. Contralateral trochlear nerve paresis and ipsilateral Horner's syndrome. Am J Ophthalmol 1989;107:73–76.

99. Bassetti C, Bogousslavsky J, Barth A, et al. Isolated infarcts of the pons. Neurology 1996;46:165–175.

100. Sacco RL, Freddo L, Bello JA, et al. Wallenberg's lateral medullary syndrome. Arch Neurol 1993;50:609–614.

101. Kim JS, Lee JH, Suh DC, et al. Spectrum of lateral medullary syndrome. Correlation between clinical findings and magnetic resonance imaging in 33 subjects. Stroke 1994;25:1405–1410.

102. Brazis PW. Ocular motor abnormalities in Wallenberg's lateral medullary syndrome. Mayo Clinic Proc 1992;67:365–368.

103. Norrving B, Cronqvist S. Lateral medullary infarction: prognosis in an unselected series. Neurology 1991;41:244–248.

104. Kim JS. Pure lateral medullary infarction: clinical-radiological correlation of 130 acute, consecutive patients. Brain 2003;126:1864–1872.

105. Kerrison JB, Biousse V, Newman NJ. Isolated Horner's syndrome and syringomyelia. J Neurol Neurosurg Psychiatry 2000;69:131–132.

106. Pomeranz H. Isolated Horner syndrome and syrinx of the cervical spinal cord. Am J Ophthalmol 2002;133:702–704.

107. Loewenfeld IE. Impairment of sympathetic pathways. In: The Pupil. Anatomy, Physiology, and Clinical Applications. Vol 1., pp 1131–1187. Detroit, Wayne State University Press, 1993.

108. Liu GT, Greene JM, Charness ME. Brown-Séquard syndrome in a patient with systemic lupus erythematosus. Neurology 1990;40:1474–1475.

109. Balcer LJ, Galetta SL. Pancoast syndrome. N Engl J Med 1997;337:1359.

110. Arcasoy SM, Jett JR. Superior pulmonary sulcus tumors and Pancoast's syndrome. N Engl J Med 1997;337:1370–1376.

111. Kaya SO, Liman ST, Bir LS, et al. Horner's syndrome as a complication in thoracic surgical practice. Eur J Cardiothorac Surg 2003;24:1025–1028.

112. Barbut D, Gold JP, Heinemann MH, et al. Horner's syndrome after coronary artery bypass surgery. Neurology 1996;46:181–184.

113. Imamaki M, Ishida A, Shimura H, et al. A case complicated with Horner's syndrome after off-pump coronary artery bypass. Ann Thorac Cardiovasc Surg 2006;12:113–115.

114. Bertino RE, Wesbey GE, Johnson RJ. Horner syndrome occurring as a complication of chest tube placement. Radiology 1987;164:745.

115. Shen SY, Liang BC. Horner's syndrome following chest drain migration in the treatment of pneumothorax. Eye 2003;17:785–788.

116. Levy M, Newman-Toker D. Reversible chest tube Horner syndrome. J Neuro-ophthalmol 2008;28:212–213.

117. Garcia EG, Wijdicks EFM, Younge BR. Neurologic complications associated with internal jugular vein cannulation in critically ill patients: a prospective study. Neurology 1994;44:951–952.

118. Teich SA, Halprin SL, Tay S. Horner's syndrome secondary to Swan-Ganz catheterization. Am J Med 1985;78:168–170.

119. Milam MG, Sahn SA. Horner's syndrome secondary to hydromediastinum. A complication of extravascular migration of a central venous catheter. Chest 1988;94:1093–1094.

120. Sulemanji DS, Candan S, Torgay A, et al. Horner syndrome after subclavian venous catheterization. Anesth Analg 2006;103:509–510.

121. Biousse V, Guevara RA, Newman NJ. Transient Horner's syndrome after lumbar epidural anesthesia. Neurology 1998;51:1473–1475.

122. Grimson BS, Thompson HS. Raeder's syndrome. A clinical review. Surv Ophthalmol 1980;24:199–210.

123. Kline LB, Vitek JJ, Raymon BC. Painful Horner's syndrome due to spontaneous carotid artery dissection. Ophthalmology 1987;94:226–230.

124. Kline LB. The neuro-ophthalmologic manifestations of spontaneous dissection of the internal carotid artery. Semin Ophthalmol 1992;7:30–37.

125. Schievink WI. Spontaneous dissection of the carotid and vertebral arteries. N Engl J Med 2001;344:898–906.

126. Caplan LR, Biousse V. Cervicocranial arterial dissections. J Neuro-ophthalmol 2004;24:299–305.

127. Galetta SL, Leahey A, Nichols CW, et al. Orbital ischemia, ophthalmoparesis, and carotid dissection. J Clin Neuro-ophthalmol 1991;11:284–287.

128. Lucas C, Moulin T, Deplanque D, et al. Stroke patterns of internal carotid artery dissection in 40 patients. Stroke 1998;29:2646–2648.

129. Hart RG, Easton JD. Dissections of cervical and cerebral arteries. Neurol Clin 1983;1: 155–182.

130. Hart RG, Easton JD. Dissections [editorial]. Stroke 1985;16:925–927.

131. Schievink WI, Mokri B, Piepgras DG. Spontaneous dissections of cervicocephalic arteries in childhood and adolescence. Neurology 1994;44:1607–1612.

132. Parwar BL, Fawzi AA, Arnold AC, et al. Horner's syndrome and dissection of the internal carotid artery after chiropractic manipulation of the neck. Am J Ophthalmol 2001;131:523–524.

133. Jeret JS, Bluth M. Stroke following chiropractic manipulation. Report of 3 cases and review of the literature. Cerebrovasc Dis 2002;13:210–213.

134. Khan AM, Ahmad N, Li X, et al. Chiropractic sympathectomy: carotid artery dissection with oculosympathetic palsy after chiropractic manipulation of the neck. Mt Sinai J Med 2005;72:207–210.

135. Lanczik O, Szabo K, Gass A, et al. Tinnitus after cycling. Lancet 2003;362:292.

136. Caso V, Paciaroni M, Bogousslavsky J. Environmental factors and cervical artery dissection. Front Neurol Neurosci 2005;20:44–53.

137. Mokri B, Piepgras DG, Houser OW. Traumatic dissections of the extracranial internal carotid artery. J Neurosurg 1988;68:189–197.

138. Mokri B, Sundt TM, Houser OW, et al. Spontaneous dissection of the cervical internal carotid artery. Ann Neurol 1986;19:126–138.

139. Brandt T, Orberk E, Weber R, et al. Pathogenesis of cervical artery dissections: association with connective tissue abnormalities. Neurology 2001;57:24–30.

140. Maitland CG, Black JL, Smith WA. Abducens nerve palsy due to spontaneous dissection of the internal carotid artery. Arch Neurol 1983;40:448–449.

141. Duker JS, Belmont JB. Ocular ischemic syndrome secondary to carotid artery dissection. Am J Ophthalmol 1988;106:750–752.

142. Newman NJ, Kline LB, Leifer D, et al. Ocular stroke and carotid artery dissection. Neurology 1989;39:1462–1464.

143. Rivkin MJ, Hedges TR, Logigian EL. Carotid dissection presenting as posterior ischemic optic neuropathy. Neurology 1990;40:1469.

144. Ramadan NM, Tietjen GE, Levine SR, et al. Scintillating scotomata associated with internal carotid artery dissection: report of three cases. Neurology 1991;41:1084–1087.

145. Schievink WI, Mokri B, Garrity JA, et al. Ocular motor nerve palsies in spontaneous dissections of the cervical internal carotid artery. Neurology 1993;43:1938–1941.

146. Mokri B, Silbert PL, Schievink WI, et al. Cranial nerve palsy in spontaneous dissection of the extracranial internal carotid artery. Neurology 1996;46:356–359.

147. Biousse V, Touboul P-J, D'Anglejan-Chatillon J, et al. Ophthalmologic manifestations of internal carotid artery dissection. Am J Ophthalmol 1998;126:565–577.

148. Lee SK, Kwon SU, Ahn H, et al. Acute isolated monocular blindness and painless carotid artery dissection. Neurology 1999;53:1155–1156.

149. Mokhtari F, Massin P, Paques M, et al. Central retinal artery occlusion associated with head or neck pain revealing spontaneous internal carotid artery dissection. Am J Ophthalmol 2000;129:108–109.

150. Leira EC, Bendixen BH, Kardon RH, et al. Brief, transient Horner's syndrome can be the hallmark of a carotid artery dissection. Neurology 1998;50:289–290.

151. Lieschke GJ, Davis S, Tress BM, et al. Spontaneous internal carotid artery dissection presenting as hypoglossal nerve palsy. Stroke 1988;19:1151–1155.

152. Guy N, Deffond D, Gabrillargues J, et al. Spontaneous internal carotid artery dissection with lower cranial nerve palsy. Can J Neurol Sci 2001;28:265–269.

153. Vargas ME, Desrouleaux JR, Kupersmith MJ. Ophthalmoplegia as a presenting manifestation of internal carotid artery dissection. J Clin Neuro-ophthalmol 1992;12: 268–271.

154. Francis KR, Williams DP, Troost BT. Facial numbness and dysesthesia. New features of carotid artery dissection. Arch Neurol 1987;44:345–346.

155. Biousse V, Schaison M, Touboul P-J, et al. Ischemic optic neuropathy associated with internal carotid artery dissection. Arch Neurol 1998;55:715–719.

156. Koennecke H-C, Seyfert S. Mydriatic pupil as the presenting sign of common carotid artery dissection. Stroke 1998;29:2653–2655.

157. Fisher CM, Ojemann RG, Robinson GH. Spontaneous dissection of cervico-cerebral arteries. Can J Neurol Sci 1978;5:9–19.

158. Goldberg HI, Grossman RI, Gomori JM, et al. Cervical internal carotid artery dissecting hemorrhage: diagnosis using MR. Radiology 1986;158:157–161.

159. Arnold M, Baumgartner RW, Stapf C, et al. Ultrasound diagnosis of spontaneous carotid dissection with isolated Horner syndrome. Stroke 2008;39:82–86.

160. Shah GV, Quint DJ, Trobe JD. Magnetic resonance imaging of suspected cervicocranial arterial dissections. J Neuro-ophthalmol 2004;24:315–318.

161. Chaves C, Estol C, Esnaola MM, et al. Spontaneous intracranial internal carotid artery dissection: report of 10 patients. Arch Neurol 2002;59:977–981.

162. Guillon B, Brunereau L, Biousse V, et al. Long-term follow-up of aneurysms developed during extracranial internal carotid artery dissection. Neurology 1999;53: 117–122.

163. Baumgartner RW. Stroke prevention and treatment in patients with spontaneous carotid dissection. Acta Neurochir Suppl 2008;103:47–50.

164. Shah Q, Messe SR. Cervicocranial arterial dissection. Curr Treat Options Neurol 2007;9:55–62.

165. Lyrer P, Engelter S. Antithrombotic drugs for carotid artery dissection. Cochrane Database Syst Rev 2003:CD000255.

166. Kremer C, Mosso M, Georgiadis D, et al. Carotid dissection with permanent and transient occlusion or severe stenosis: Long-term outcome. Neurology 2003;60: 271–275.

167. Schievink WI, Mokri B. Recurrent spontaneous cervical-artery dissection. N Engl J Med 1994;330:393–397.

168. Touzé E, Gauvrit JY, Moulin T, et al. Risk of stroke and recurrent dissection after a cervical artery dissection: a multicenter study. Neurology 2003;61:1347–1351.

169. Sears ML, Kier L, Chavis RM. Horner's syndrome caused by occlusion of the vascular supply to sympathetic ganglia. Am J Ophthalmol 1974;77:717–724.

170. Monteiro MLR, Coppeto JR. Horner's syndrome associated with carotid artery atherosclerosis. Am J Ophthalmol 1988;105:93–94.

171. Bollen AE, Krikke AP, de Jager AEJ. Painful Horner syndrome due to arteritis of the internal carotid artery. Neurology 1998;51:1471–1472.

172. Liu GT, Deskin RW, Bienfang DC. Horner's syndrome due to intra-oral trauma. J Clin Neuro-ophthalmol 1992;12:110–115.

173. Schnitzlein HN, Murtagh FR. Imaging anatomy of the head and spine. A photographic atlas of MRI, CT, gross, and microscopic anatomy in axial, coronal, and sagittal planes, pp 77. Baltimore, Urban & Schwarzenberg, 1985.

174. Woodhurst WB, Robertson WD, Thompson GB. Carotid injury due to intraoral trauma; case report and review of the literature. Neurosurgery 1980;6:559–563.

175. Bazak I, Miller A, Uri N. Oculosympathetic paresis caused by foreign body perforation of pharyngeal wall. Postgraduate Medical Journal 1987;63:681–683.

176. Shissas CG, Golnik KC. Horner's syndrome after tonsillectomy. Am J Ophthalmol 1994;117:812–813.

177. Campbell RL, Mercuri LG, Van Sickels J. Cervical sympathetic block following intraoral local anesthesia. Oral Surg Oral Med Oral Pathol 1979;47:223–226.

178. Hobson JC, Malla JV, Kay NJ. Horner's syndrome following tonsillectomy. J Laryngol Otol 2006;120:800–801.

179. Salvesen R, Bogucki A, Wysocka-Bakowska MM, et al. Cluster headache pathogenesis: a pupillometric study. Cephalalgia 1987;7:273–284.

180. Salvesen R, Sand T, Zhao J-M, et al. Cluster headache: pupillometric patterns as a function of the degree of anisocoria. Cephalalgia 1989;9:131–138.

181. Khurana RK. Bilateral Horner's syndrome in cluster type headaches. Headache 1993;33:449–451.

182. Havelius U. A Horner-like syndrome and cluster headache. What comes first? Acta Ophthalmol Scand 2001;79:374–375.

183. Rigamonti A, Iurlaro S, Reganati P, et al. Cluster headache and internal carotid artery dissection: two cases and review of the literature. Headache 2008;48:467–470.

184. Arunagiri G, Santhi S, Harrington T. Horner syndrome and ipsilateral abduction deficit attributed to giant cell arteritis. J Neuro-ophthalmol 2006;26:231–232.

185. Shah AV, Paul-Oddoye AB, Madill SA, et al. Horner's syndrome associated with giant cell arteritis. Eye 2007;21:130–131.

186. Kurihara T. Abducens nerve palsy and ipsilateral incomplete Horner syndrome: a significant sign of locating the lesion in the posterior cavernous sinus. Intern Med 2006;45:993–994.

187. Tsuda H, Ishikawa H, Kishiro M, et al. Abducens nerve palsy and postganglionic Horner syndrome with or without severe headache. Intern Med 2006;45:851–855.

188. Trobe JD, Glaser JS, Post JD. Meningiomas and aneurysms of the cavernous sinus. Arch Ophthalmol 1978;96:457–467.

189. Talkad AV, Kattah JC, Xu MY, et al. Prolactinoma presenting as painful postganglionic Horner syndrome. Neurology 2004;62:1440–1441.

190. Shin RK, Cucchiara BL, Liebeskind DS, et al. Pituitary apoplexy causing optic neuropathy and Horner syndrome without ophthalmoplegia. J Neuro-ophthalmol 2003;23:208–210.

191. Koc F, Kansu T, Kavuncu S, et al. Topical apraclonidine testing discloses pupillary sympathetic denervation in diabetic patients. J Neuro-ophthalmol 2006;26:25–29.

192. Galvez A, Ailouti N, Toll A, et al. Horner syndrome associated with ipsilateral facial and extremity anhydrosis. J Neuro-ophthalmol 2008;28:178–181.

193. Smith SA, Smith SE. Bilateral Horner's syndrome: detection and occurrence. J Neurol Neurosurg Psychiatry 1999;66:48–51.

194. Spector RH. Postganglionic Horner syndrome in three patients with coincident middle ear infection. J Neuro-ophthalmol 2008;28:182–185.

195. Leung A. Congenital Horner's syndrome. Ala J Med Sci 1986;23:204–205.

196. Mahoney NR, Liu GT, Menacker SJ, et al. Pediatric Horner syndrome: etiologies and roles of imaging and urine studies to detect neuroblastoma and other responsible mass lesions. Am J Ophthalmol 2006;142:651–659.

197. Weinstein JM, Zweifel TJ, Thompson HS. Congenital Horner's syndrome. Arch Ophthalmol 1980;98:1074–1078.

198. Woodruff G, Buncic JR, Morin JD. Horner's syndrome in children. J Ped Ophthalmol Strab 1988;25:40–44.

199. Jeffery AR, Ellis FJ, Repka MX, et al. Pediatric Horner syndrome. JAAPOS 1998;2: 159–167.

200. George NDL, Gonzalez G, Hoyt CS. Does Horner's syndrome in infancy require investigation? Br J Ophthalmol 1998;82:51–54.

201. Ryan FH, Kline LB, Gomez C. Congenital Horner's syndrome resulting from agenesis of the internal carotid artery. Ophthalmology 2000;107:185–188.

202. Tubbs RS, Oakes WJ. Horner's syndrome resulting from agenesis of the internal carotid artery: report of a third case. Childs Nerv Syst 2005;21:81–82.

203. Musarella M, Chan HSL, DeBoer G, et al. Ocular involvement in neuroblastoma: prognostic implications. Ophthalmology 1984;91:936–940.

204. Ogita S, Tokiwa K, Takahashi T, et al. Congenital cervical neuroblastoma associated with Horner syndrome. J Pediatr Surg 1988;23:991–992.

205. Abramson SJ, Berdon WE, Ruzal-Shapiro C, et al. Cervical neuroblastoma in eleven infants—a tumor with favorable prognosis. Clinical and radiologic (US, CT, MRI) findings. Pediatr Radiol 1993;23:253–257.

206. Casselman JW, Smet MH, Van Damme B, et al. Primary cervical neuroblastoma: CT and MR findings. JCAT 1988;12:684–686.

207. Gibbs J, Appleton RE, Martin J, et al. Congenital Horner syndrome associated with non-cervical neuroblastoma. Dev Med Child Neurol 1992;34:642–644.

208. McRae D, Shaw A. Ganglioneuroma, heterochromia iridis, and Horner's syndrome. J Pediatr Surg 1979;14:612–614.

209. Al-Jassim AHH. Cervical ganglioneuroblastoma. J Laryngol Otol 1987;101:296–301.

210. Coldman AJ, Fryer CJH, Elmwood JM, et al. Neuroblastoma: influence of age at diagnosis, stage, tumor site, and sex on prognosis. Cancer 1980;46:1896–1901.

211. Carlsen NLT, Schroeder H, Bro PV, et al. Neuroblastomas treated at the four major child oncologic clinics in Denmark 1943–1980: an evaluation of 180 cases. Med Pediatr Oncol 1985;13:180–186.

212. Park JR, Eggert A, Caron H. Neuroblastoma: biology, prognosis, and treatment. Pediatr Clin North Am 2008;55:97–120.

213. Zafeiriou DI, Psychogiou K. Obstetrical brachial plexus palsy. Pediatr Neurol 2008;38: 235–242.

214. Huang YG, Chen L, Gu YD, et al. Histopathological basis of Horner's syndrome in obstetric brachial plexus palsy differs from that in adult brachial plexus injury. Muscle Nerve 2008;37:632–637.

215. Sauer C, Levinsohn MW. Horner's syndrome in childhood. Neurology 1976;26:216–220.

216. Kim W, Clancy RR, Liu GT. Horner syndrome associated with implantation of a vagus nerve stimulator. Am J Ophthalmol 2001;131:383–384.

217. Thompson BM, Corbett JJ, Kline LB, et al. Pseudo-Horner's syndrome. Arch Neurol 1982;39:108–111.

218. Kardon RH, Denison CE, Brown CK, et al. Critical evaluation of the cocaine test in the diagnosis of Horner's syndrome. Arch Ophthalmol 1990;108:384–387.

219. Van der Wiel HL, Van Gijn J. The diagnosis of Horner's syndrome. Use and limitations of the cocaine test. J Neurol Sci 1986;73:311–316.

220. Jacobson DM, Berg R, Grinstead GF, et al. Duration of positive urine for cocaine metabolite after ophthalmic administration: implications for testing patients with suspected Horner syndrome using ophthalmic cocaine. Am J Ophthalmol 2001;131: 742–747.

221. Martin TJ. Horner's syndrome, Pseudo-Horner's syndrome, and simple anisocoria. Curr Neurol Neurosci Rep 2007;7:397–406.

222. Morales J, Brown SM, Abdul-Rahim AS, et al. Ocular effects of apraclonidine in Horner syndrome. Arch Ophthalmol 2000;118:951–954.

223. Brown SM, Aouchiche R, Freedman KA. The utility of 0.5% apraclonidine in the diagnosis of Horner syndrome. Arch Ophthalmol 2003;121:1201–1203.

224. Freedman KA, Brown SM. Topical apraclonidine in the diagnosis of suspected Horner syndrome. J Neuro-ophthalmol 2005;25:83–85.

225. Bohnsack BL, Parker JW. Positive apraclonidine test within two weeks of onset of Horner syndrome caused by carotid artery dissection. J Neuro-ophthalmol 2008;28: 235–236.

226. Kawasaki A, Borruat FX. False negative apraclonidine test in two patients with Horner syndrome. Klin Monatsbl Augenheilkd 2008;225:520–522.

227. Kardon R. Are we ready to replace cocaine with apraclonidine in the pharmacologic diagnosis of Horner syndrome? J Neuro-ophthalmol 2005;25:69–70.

228. Thompson HS, Mensher JH. Adrenergic mydriasis in Horner's syndrome. Am J Ophthalmol 1971;72:472–480.

229. Cremer SA, Thompson HS, Digre KB, et al. Hydroxyamphetamine mydriasis in normal subjects. Am J Ophthalmol 1990;110:66–70.

230. Heitman K, Bode DD. The paredrine test in normal eyes. J Clin Neuro-ophthalmol 1986;6:228–231.

231. Cremer SA, Thompson HS, Digre KB, et al. Hydroxyamphetamine mydriasis in Horner's syndrome. Am J Ophthalmol 1990;110:71–76.

232. Van der Wiel HL, Van Gijn J. Localization of Horner's syndrome. Use and limitations of the hydroxyamphetamine test. J Neurol Sci 1986;59:229–235.

233. Lee JH, Lee HK, Lee DH, et al. Neuroimaging strategies for three types of Horner syndrome with emphasis on anatomic location. AJR Am J Roentgenol 2007;188: W74–81.

234. Reede DL, Garcon E, Smoker WR, et al. Horner's syndrome: clinical and radiographic evaluation. Neuroimaging Clin N Am 2008;18:369–385.

235. Rabady DZ, Simon JW, Lopasic N. Pediatric Horner syndrome: etiologies and roles of imaging and urine studies to detect neuroblastoma and other responsible mass lesions [letter]. Am J Ophthalmol 2007;144:481–482.

236. Liu GT. Pediatric Horner syndrome: etiologies and roles of imaging and urine studies to detect neuroblastoma and other responsible mass lesions [letter]. Am J Ophthalmol 2007;144:482.

237. Halperin EC, Constine LS, Tarbell NJ, et al. Neuroblastoma. In: Pediatric radiation oncology, 2nd ed., pp 171–214. New York, Raven Press, 1994.

238. De Bernardi B, Conte M, Mancini A, et al. Localized resectable neuroblastoma: results of the second study of the Italian Cooperative Group for Neuroblastoma. J Clin Oncol 1995;13:884–893.

239. Bacal DA, Levy SR. The use of apraclonidine in the diagnosis of Horner syndrome in pediatric patients. Arch Ophthalmol 2004;122:276–279.

240. Chen PL, Hsiao CH, Chen JT, et al. Efficacy of apraclonidine 0.5% in the diagnosis of Horner syndrome in pediatric patients under low or high illumination. Am J Ophthalmol 2006;142:469–474.

241. Watts P, Satterfield D, Lim MK. Adverse effects of apraclonidine used in the diagnosis of Horner syndrome in infants. JAAPOS 2007;11:282–283.

242. Al-Shahwan S, Al-Torbak AA, Turkmani S, et al. Side-effect profile of brimonidine tartrate in children. Ophthalmology 2005;112:2143.

243. Plum F, Posner JB. Pupils. In: The diagnosis of stupor and coma, 3rd edn., pp 41–47. Philadelphia, F. A. Davis, 1980.

244. Ropper AH, Cole D, Louis DN. Clinicopathologic correlation in a case of pupillary dilation from cerebral hemorrhage. Arch Neurol 1991;48:1166–1169.

245. Ropper AH. The opposite pupil in herniation. Neurology 1990;40:1707–1709.

246. Fisher CM. Oval pupils. Arch Neurol 1980;37:502–503.

247. Chen R, Sahjpaul R, Del Maestro RF, et al. Initial enlargement of the opposite pupil as a false localising sign in intraparenchymal frontal haemorrhage. J Neurol Neurosurg Psychiatry 1994;57:1126–1128.

248. Rothstein JD, Herlong HF. Neurologic manifestations of hepatic disease. Neurol Clinics 1989;7:563–578.

249. Liu GT, Urion DK, Volpe JJ. Cerebral edema in acute fulminant hepatic failure: clinicopathologic correlation. Pediatr Neurol 1993;9:224–226.

250. Woods D, O'Connor PS, Fleming R. Episodic unilateral mydriasis and migraine. Am J Ophthalmol 1984;98:229–234.

251. Jacobson DM. Benign episodic unilateral mydriasis. Ophthalmology 1995;102:1623–1627.

252. Purvin VA. Adie's tonic pupil secondary to migraine. J Neuro-ophthalmol 1995;15:43–44.

253. Jacome DE. Status migrainosus and Adie's syndrome. Headache 2002;42:793–795.

254. Thompson HS, Zackon DH, Czarnecki JSC. Tadpole shaped pupils caused by segmental spasm of the iris dilator muscle. Am J Ophthalmol 1983;96:467–477.

255. Drummond PD. Cervical sympathetic deficit in unilateral migraine headache. Headache 1991;31:669–672.

256. Harle DE, Wolffsohn JS, Evans BJ. The pupillary light reflex in migraine. Ophthalmic Physiol Opt 2005;25:240–245.

257. Mylius V, Braune HJ, Schepelmann K. Dysfunction of the pupillary light reflex following migraine headache. Clin Auton Res 2003;13:16–21.

258. De Marinis M, Assenza S, Carletto F. Oculosympathetic alterations in migraine patients. Cephalalgia 1998;18:77–84.

259. Pant SS, Benton JN, Dodge PR. Unilateral pupillary dilatation during and immediately following seizures. Neurology 1966;16:837–840.

260. Zee DS, Griffen J, Price DL. Unilateral pupillary dilatation during adversive seizures. Arch Neurol 1974;30:403–405.

261. Lance JW. Pupillary dilatation and arm weakness as negative ictal phenomena. J Neurol Neurosurg Psychiatry 1995;58:261–262.

262. Gadoth N, Margalith D, Bechar M. Unilateral pupillary dilatation during focal seizures. J Neurol 1981;225:227–230.

263. Afifi AK, Corbett JJ, Thompson HS, et al. Seizure-induced miosis and ptosis: association with temporal lobe magnetic resonance imaging abnormalities. J Child Neurol 1990;5:142–146.

264. Rosenberg ML, Jabbari B. Miosis and internal ophthalmoplegia as a manifestation of partial seizures. Neurology 1991;41:737–739.

265. Ropper AH, Wijdicks EFM, Truax BT. Pupillary abnormalities. Clinical features of the typical syndrome. In: Guillain-Barré syndrome, pp 92. Philadelphia, F.A. Davis, 1991.

266. Williams D, Brust JC, Abrams G, et al. Landry-Guillain-Barre syndrome with abnormal pupils and normal eye movements: a case report. Neurology 1979;29:1033–1040.

267. Anzai T, Uematsu D, Takahashi K, et al. Guillain-Barré syndrome with bilateral tonic pupils. Intern Med 1994;33:248–251.

268. Mori M, Kuwabara S, Fukutake T, et al. Clinical features and prognosis of Miller Fisher syndrome. Neurology 2001;56:1104–1106.

269. Fisher M. An unusual variant of acute idiopathic polyneuritis (syndrome of ophthalmoplegia, ataxia and areflexia). N Engl J Med 1956;255:57–65.

270. Okajima T, Imamura S, Kawasaki S, et al. Fisher's syndrome: a pharmacological study of the pupils. Ann Neurol 1977;2:63–65.

271. Keane JR. Tonic pupils with acute ophthalmoplegic polyneuritis. Ann Neurol 1977;2:393–396.

272. Radziwill AJ, Steck AJ, Borruat F-X, et al. Isolated internal ophthalmoplegia associated with IgG anti-GQ1b antibody. Neurology 1998;50:307.

273. Caccavale A, Mignemi L. Acute onset of a bilateral areflexical mydriasis in Miller-Fisher syndrome: a rare neuro-ophthalmologic disease. J Neuro-ophthalmol 2000;20:61–62.

274. Nitta T, Kase M, Shinmei Y, et al. Mydriasis with light-near dissociation in Fisher's Syndrome. Jpn J Ophthalmol 2007;51:224–227.

275. Price MJ, Thompson HS, Judisch GF, et al. Pupillary constriction to darkness. Br J Ophthalmol 1985;69:205–211.

276. Myers GA, Barricks ME, Stark L. Paradoxic pupillary constriction in a patient with congenital stationary night blindness. Invest Ophthalmol Vis Sci 1985;26:736–740.

277. Barricks ME, Flynn JT, Kushner BJ. Paradoxical pupillary responses in congenital stationary night blindness. Arch Ophthalmol 1977;95:1800–1804.

278. Sharpe JA, Glaser JS. Tournay's phenomenon - a reappraisal of anisocoria in lateral gaze. Am J Ophthalmol 1974;77:250–255.

279. Loewenfeld IE, Friedlaender RP, McKinnon PFM. Pupillary inequality associated with lateral gaze (Tournay's phenomenon). Am J Ophthalmol 1974;78:449–469.

280. Cox TA, Law FCH. The clinical significance of Tournay's pupillary phenomenon. J Clin Neuro-ophthalmol 1991;11:186–189.

281. Pfeiffer N, Simonsz HJ, Kommerell G. Misdirected regeneration of abducens nerve neurons into the parasympathetic pupillary pathway. Graefes Arch Clin Exp Ophthalmol 1992;230:150–153.

282. Wilhelm H, Wilhelm B, Mildenberger I. Primary aberrant regeneration of abducens nerve fibers into the pupillary pathway. Neuro-ophthalmology 1994;14:85–89.

283. Kline LB, McCluer SM, Bonikowski FP. Oculosympathetic spasm with cervical spinal cord injury. Arch Neurol 1984;41:61–64.

284. Loewenfeld IE, Thompson HS. Oculomotor paresis with cyclic spasms. A critical review of the literature and a new case. Surv Ophthalmol 1975;20:81–124.

285. Bateman DE, Saunders M. Cyclic oculomotor palsy: description of a case and hypothesis of the mechanism. J Neurol Neurosurg Psychiatr 1983;46:451–453.

286. Brodsky MC, Sharp GB, Fritz KJ, et al. Idiopathic alternating anisocoria. Am J Ophthalmol 1992;114:509–510.

287. Balaggan KS, Hugkulstone CE, Bremner FD. Episodic segmental iris dilator muscle spasm: the tadpole-shaped pupil. Arch Ophthalmol 2003;121:744–745.

288. Koay KL, Plant G, Wearne MJ. Tadpole pupil. Eye 2004;18:93–94.

289. Goldstein JH, Schneekloth BB. Spasm of the near reflex: a spectrum of anomalies. Surv Ophthalmol 1996;40:269–278.

290. Griffin JF, Wray SH, Anderson DP. Misdiagnosis of spasm of the near reflex. Neurology 1976;26:1018–1020.

291. Chan RV, Trobe JD. Spasm of accommodation associated with closed head trauma. J Neuro-ophthalmol 2002;22:15–17.

292. Newman NJ, Lessell S. Pupillary dilatation with monocular occlusion as a sign of nonorganic oculomotor dysfunction. Am J Ophthalmol 1989;108:461–462.

CHAPTER 14

Eyelid and facial nerve disorders

The eyelids protect the eye and help maintain the corneal tear film. *Ptosis* (drooping), *retraction* (abnormal elevation), *facial weakness* (causing insufficient eyelid closure), *abnormal blinking* (absent or excessive), and other *abnormal eyelid and facial movements* are the most important eyelid and facial nerve disorders in neuro-ophthalmology. This chapter will review the relevant neuroanatomy, examination of the eyelids and facial nerve, and differential diagnosis of these and other eyelid abnormalities. At the end of the chapter, diseases which are commonly associated with ptosis or facial weakness will be discussed.

Neuroanatomy

Upper eyelid

Upper eyelid muscles and their innervations. The *levator palpebrae superioris muscle*, with minor contributions from *Müller's* and the *frontalis muscles*, maintains the normal position of the upper eyelid. The aponeurosis of the levator muscle attaches to the anterior surface and the superior edge of the superior tarsal plate (**Fig. 14–1**). Both levator muscles are controlled by the central caudal nucleus (CCN) of the oculomotor nuclear complex (cranial nerve III) (see Chapter 15), while the frontalis is innervated by the facial nerve (see below). Within the CCN, which is a single midline subnucleus, neurons to both levators are intermixed. Müller's muscle is innervated by oculosympathetic neurons (see Chapter 13), while the frontalis receives fibers from the facial nerve. Eyelid position depends mainly on the resting tone of the levator muscles, which varies according to the patient's state of arousal, with individuals having wider palpebral fissures when they are alert than when they are drowsy. Experimental lesions of the frontal lobes, angular gyrus, and temporal lobes may produce ptosis, and experimental stimulation of areas within frontal, temporal, and occipital lobes may produce eyelid opening, but the exact nature of the cortical control of the eyelids is unclear.[1] There is some evidence to suggest that the right hemisphere may be dominant for this function (see Cerebral ptosis, below).

Coordination with vertical eye movements. With only some minor differences in speed and conjugacy, the eyelids move with the eyes during both slow and rapid vertical eye movements.[2] The major nonpathological exception to this occurs while the eyelids blink, at which time the levator is temporarily inhibited and the orbicularis oculi contracts. Recent evidence suggests that vertical eye movements and lid position are coordinated through the M-group (supraoculomotor area or supra III) in the midbrain (**Fig. 14–2**).[3–5] In upgaze, M-group neurons excite the CCN, causing the levator muscles to contract and the eyelids to open. During downgaze, neurons from the interstitial nucleus of Cajal (inC) inhibit the M-group neurons and the CCN, resulting in levator relaxation and eyelid lowering.

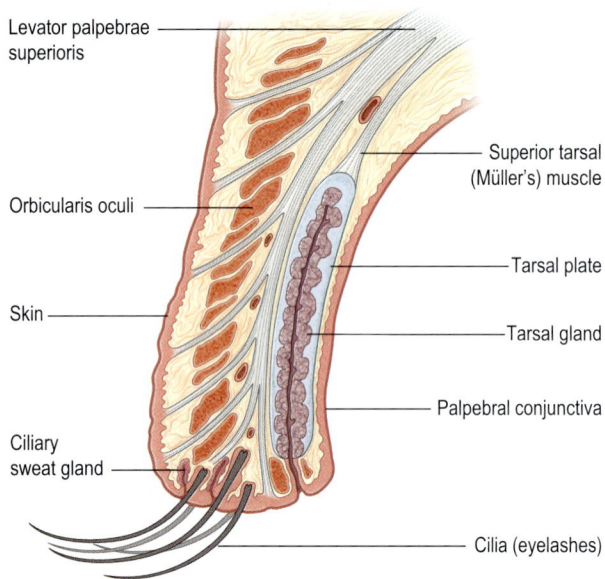

Figure 14–1. Drawing of sagittal section of the upper eyelid. The levator palpebrae superioris muscle attaches to the anterior surface and superior edge of the superior tarsal plate.[446]

The nuclei of the posterior commissure (nPC), which lie dorsolaterally to the IIIrd nerve nuclei, may also be important in control of lid–eye coordination. Interconnecting neurons between the nPC on each side travel through the posterior commissure in the dorsal midbrain. More details regarding the anatomy of the IIIrd nerve are discussed in Chapter 15.

Facial nerve

Supranuclear pathways. The supranuclear neurons destined to innervate the facial nerve nucleus lie in the precentral gyrus of the frontal lobe (**Fig. 14–3**). Discharges from this region initiate voluntary movements to command such as smiling or puckering of the lips. Somatotopically, these supranuclear neurons are located most laterally in the frontal cortex just below the representation for the hand. One functional imaging study demonstrated activation of the right primary motor cortex and supplementary motor area during voluntary blinking.[6]

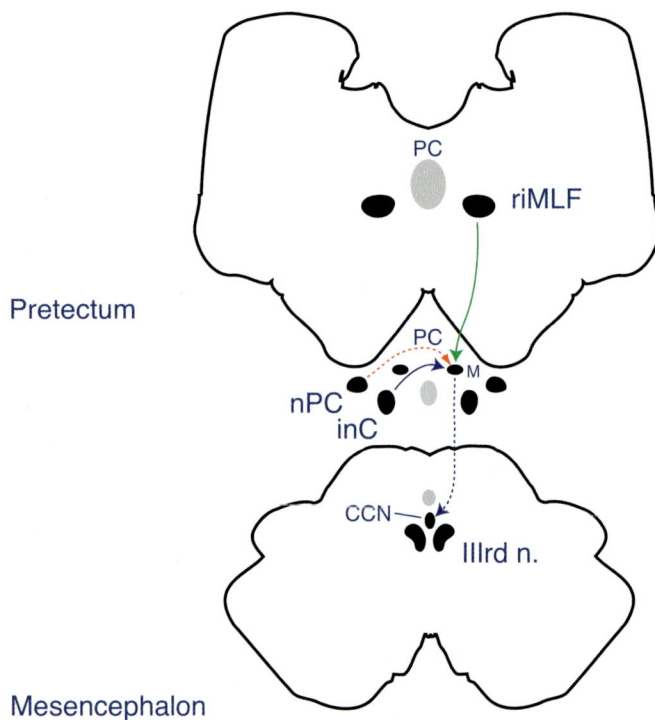

Figure 14–2. Theoretical scheme of lid–eye coordination.[5] An area called the M-group (M) (supraoculomotor area, or supra III), which is located medial to the rostral interstitial nucleus of the medial longitudinal fasciculus (riMLF), appears to be important in lid–eye coordination. This region receives input from the riMLF and the interstitial nucleus of Cajal (inC). The M-group exerts control over the central caudal nucleus (CCN) in the oculomotor nuclear complex (IIIrd n.). The riMLF may excite the M-group during upward saccades to drive the eyelids upward. On the other hand, the M-group may be inhibited by the inC during downgaze, resulting in relaxation of the eyelids. The nucleus of the posterior commissure (nPC) may also be important in control of lid–eye coordination. Note that fibers from the inC mediating vertical gaze (see also Fig. 16–18) also pass through the posterior commissure before innervating the IIIrd and IVth nerve nuclei. Thus lesions of the posterior commissure may cause both vertical gaze paresis and eyelid retraction.

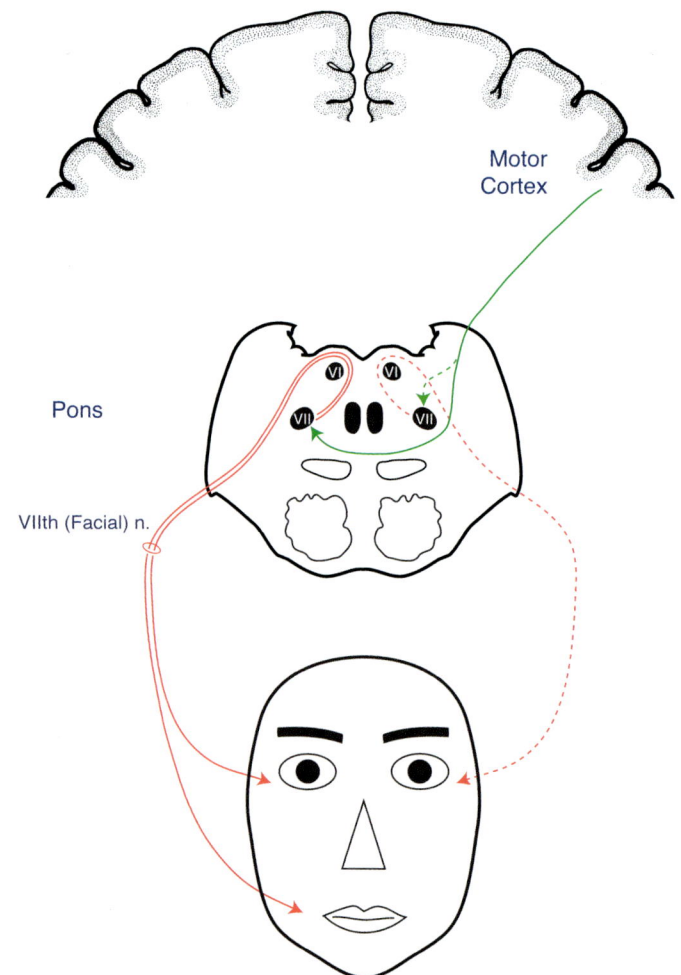

Figure 14–3. Cortical innervation of the facial nerve. Axons from the motor strip in the precentral gyrus descend within the corticobulbar tracts. Most supranuclear fibers cross to innervate the contralateral facial nerve nucleus. However, some fibers destined to innervate the upper face also synapse in the ipsilateral facial nucleus. Thus, the upper face is innervated by both hemispheres, which explains why supranuclear lesions result in weakness of the lower face only.

Leaving the precentral gyrus, the axons of the facial motor area coalesce and become part of the corticobulbar tracts that descend through the middle of the internal capsule on their way to the medial part of the cerebral peduncle. In the majority of individuals, at the level of the facial nerve nucleus in the pons, most of the supranuclear fibers cross over to the opposite side to innervate the facial nucleus.[7] However, in some individuals, the supranuclear fibers descend into the ventral medulla before looping rostrally, then crossing to innervate the contralateral facial nucleus.[7,8] In either case, other corticobulbar fibers medicating ipsilateral upper facial function synapse on the ipsilateral facial nerve nucleus, providing the upper face with innervation from both cerebral hemispheres. This unusual anatomic feature explains why supranuclear lesions involving the descending motor pathways result in weakness of the contralateral lower face only (**Fig. 14–3**).

Nuclear and infranuclear. The motor nucleus of the facial nerve resides in the lateral midpons.[9] Motor axons leaving the facial nucleus course dorsomedially toward the fourth ventricle to loop around the VIth nerve nucleus; thus forming the facial colliculus. After bending around the VIth nerve nucleus the motor fibers extend laterally to exit the pons (**Fig. 14–4**). The parasympathetic component of the facial nerve originates from the superior salvatory nucleus, which lies just superior to the facial motor nucleus. This nucleus supplies the sublingual, submandibular, and lacrimal glands and forms one part of the nervus intermedius (**Fig. 14–5**). The other component of the nervus intermedius is sensory, containing those fibers subserving taste to the anterior two-thirds of the tongue and somatic sensation to the external auditory meatus and postauricular region. Taste fibers synapse in the nucleus solitarius, while those of somatic sensation terminate in the spinal tract of the Vth nerve. Afferents to the facial nucleus are also derived from the trigeminal nucleus as part of the corneal reflex and the acoustic pathways as part of the stapedius reflex, in which the eyes blink reflexively to a loud noise (see below).

Cerebellopontine angle. At the ventrolateral angle of the pons, the facial motor root and the vestibuloacoustic nerve exit the brain stem together. Between these two nerves lies the nervus intermedius carrying sensory and parasympathetic information. In the cerebellopontine angle, the anterior inferior cerebellar artery (AICA) courses between the VIIth and VIIIth nerves in its course to supply the lateral pons and anterior cerebellum.[10] The close proximity of the Vth, VIIth, and VIIIth nerves in the cerebellopontine angle helps predict their involvement in tumors in this region. As the facial nerve motor branch enters the internal auditory meatus, it is joined to the nervus intermedius and lies superior and anterior to the vestibuloacoustic nerve. After exiting the internal auditory meatus, the facial nerves separate from the acoustic nerve to enter their own canal, the fallopian or facial canal[11] (**Fig. 14–6**). Here the facial nerve incorporates the geniculate ganglion and the first branch of the facial nerve known as the greater superficial petrosal nerve.[12] This nerve travels forward along the floor of the middle cranial

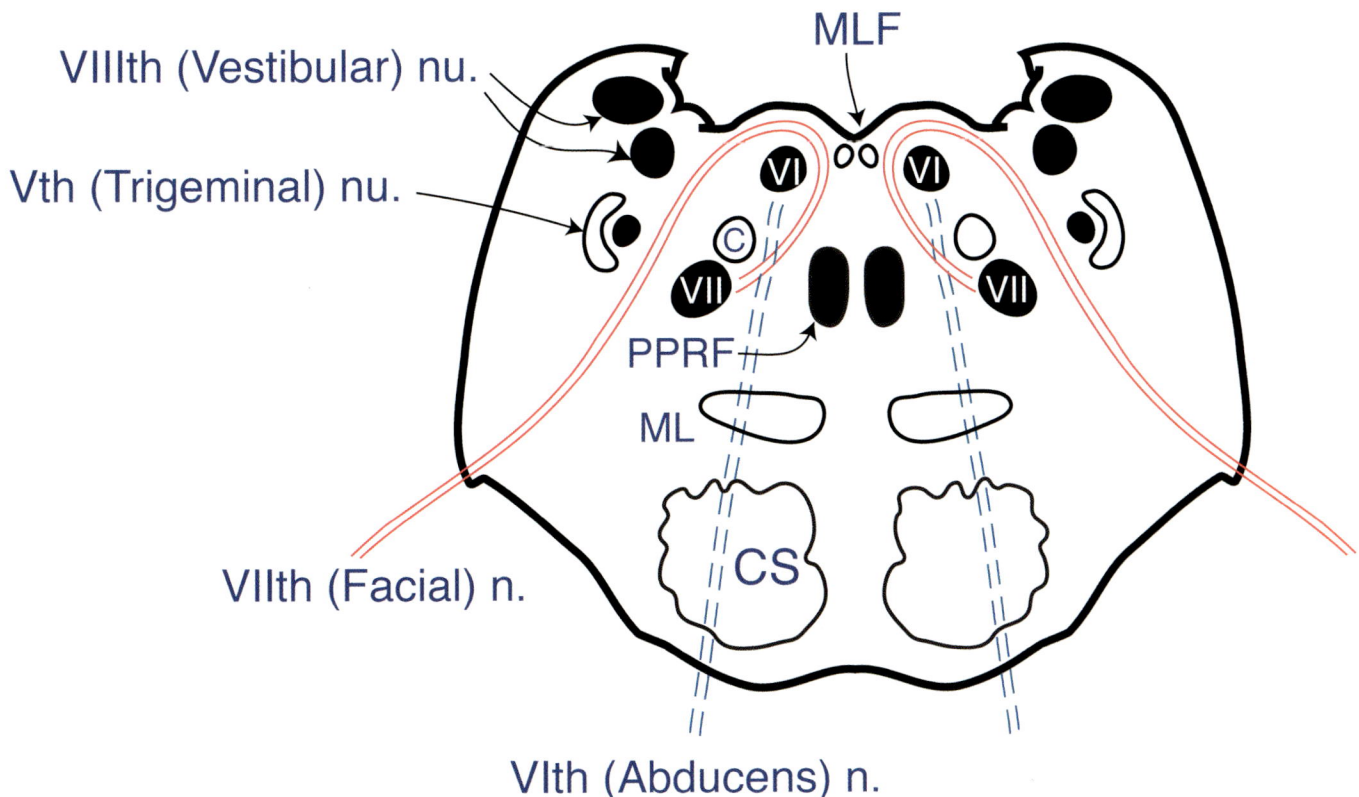

Figure 14–4. Cross-section of the lower pons, highlighting the proximity of the VIth, VIIth, and VIIIth cranial nerve nuclei; the pyramidal or corticospinal tracts should also be noted. C, central tegmental tract; CS, corticospinal tract; ML, medial lemniscus; MLF, medial longitudinal fasciculus; PPRF, paramedian pontine reticular formation.

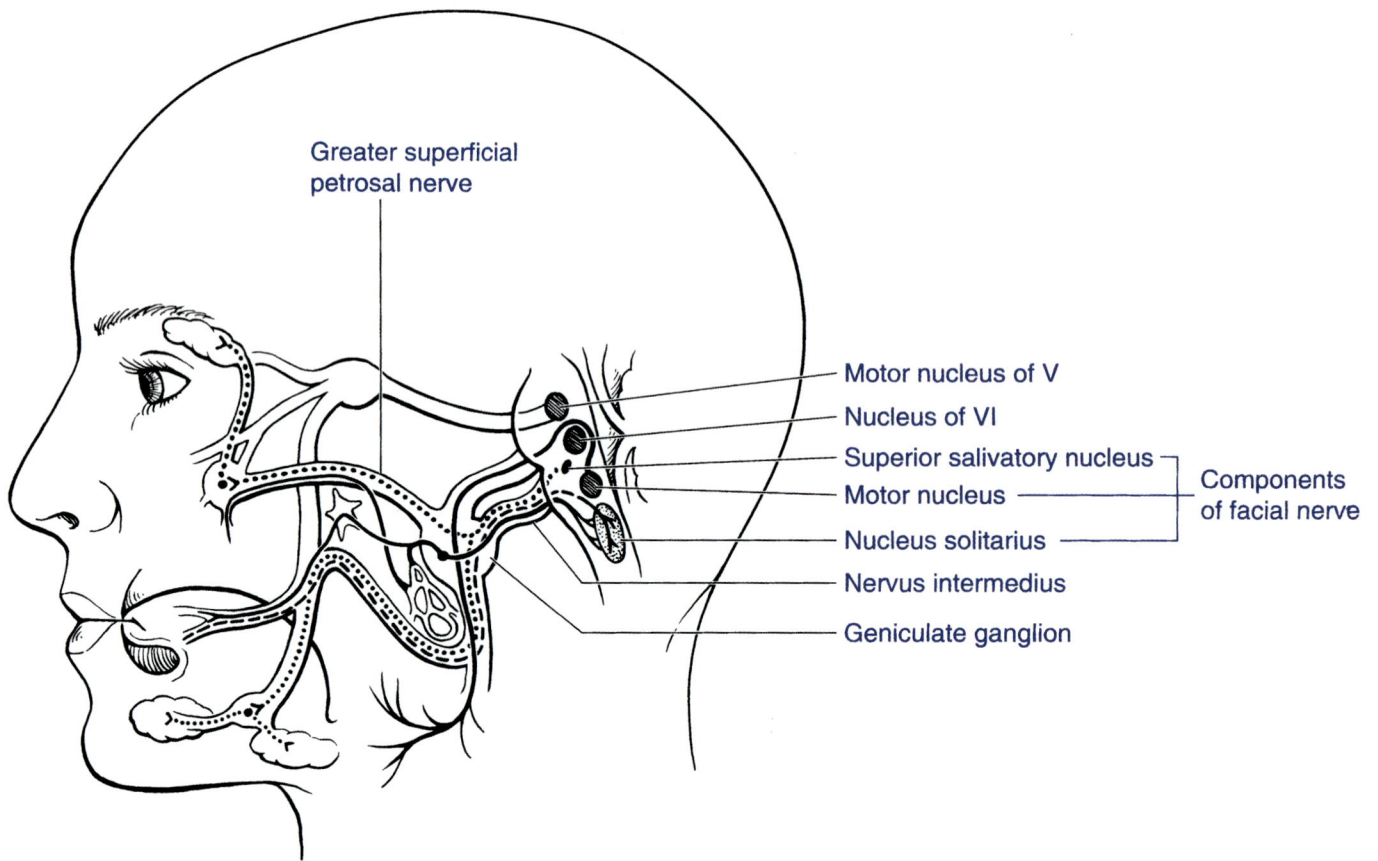

Figure 14–5. Facial nerve separated into motor fibers and nervus intermedius. The nervus intermedius contains both parasympathetic and sensory fibers. (From Handler LF, Galetta SL, Wulc AE, et al. Facial paralysis: diagnosis and management. In: Bosniak S (ed): Principles and Practice of Ophthalmic Plastic and Reconstructive Surgery, p 467. Philadelphia, WB Saunders, 1996, with permission.)

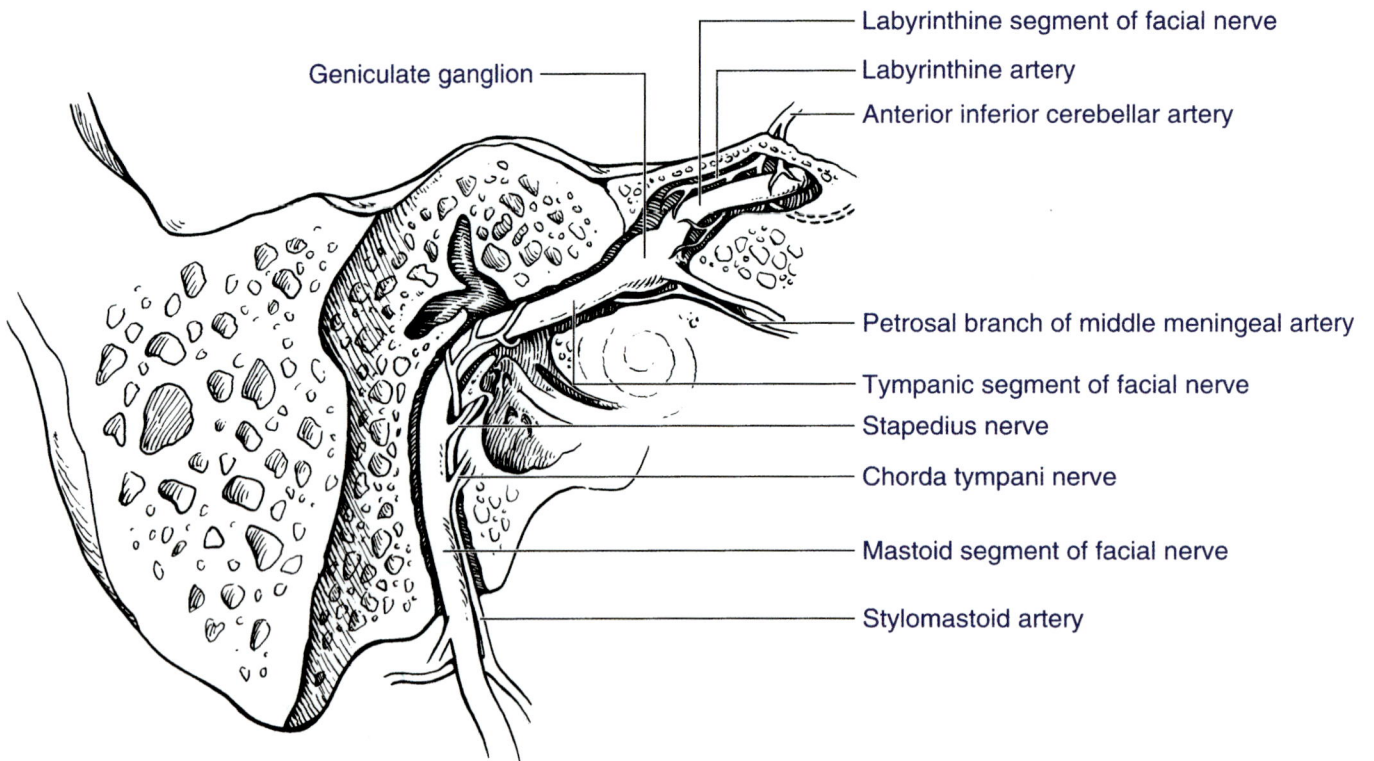

Figure 14–6. Intracanalicular facial nerve. Within the facial canal the nerve is divided into three segments: labyrinthine, tympanic, and mastoid. (From Handler LF, Galetta SL, Wulc AE, et al. Facial paralysis: diagnosis and management. In: Bosniak S (ed): Principles and Practice of Ophthalmic Plastic and Reconstructive Surgery, p 468. Philadelphia, WB Saunders, 1996, with permission.)

fossa to synapse in the sphenopalatine ganglion. Postganglionic parasympathetic fibers continue forward to innervate the lacrimal gland and nasopalatine glands.[13]

At the level of the lateral semicircular canal, the nerve to the stapedius takes its origin at the proximal portion of this segment while the chorda tympani nerve branches off more distally.[11] The chorda tympani nerve is a mixed nerve carrying taste fibers from the anterior two-thirds of the tongue, parasympathetic fibers to the submaxillary and sublingual glands, and pain and temperature sensation from the external auditory meatus.[13]

Extracranial course. The motor branches of the facial nerve exit the skull base via the stylomastoid foramen. Nerve twigs are immediately provided to the posterior auricular, posterior belly of the digastric and stylohyoid muscles. The facial nerve then bends again to proceed forward to penetrate the posterior aspect of the parotid gland. Within the substance of the parotid gland, the facial nerve divides into upper and lower divisions. These divisions may be further subdivided from top to bottom into temporal, zygomatic, buccal, mandibular, and cervical branches (**Fig. 14–7**).[14] The

vast interconnections amongst these branches provide the substrate for aberrant regeneration to ensue after facial palsy (see below).[12]

Vascular supply. From the brain stem to the internal auditory meatus, the facial nerve derives its blood supply from the AICA. The labyrinthine artery, a branch of the AICA, supplies the nerve in the internal auditory meatus. More distally, the petrosal branch of the middle meningeal artery enters the facial canal at the level of the geniculate ganglion and supplies blood to the tympanic portion of the nerve (**Fig. 14–6**). Anastomotic connections are made to the tympanic region by the stylomastoid artery, which extends up the vertically oriented mastoid segment. The weakest link in the arterial supply to the facial nerve is just proximal to the geniculate ganglion and this region represents the most likely site for ischemic injury to the nerve.

Muscles innervated by the facial nerve. All the muscles of facial expression are supplied by the facial nerve (**Fig. 14–8**).[15] The major muscles are the *frontalis*, which lifts the eyebrows, the *orbicularis oculi*, which closes the eyelids, the *orbicularis oris*, which closes the mouth and purses the lips, and the

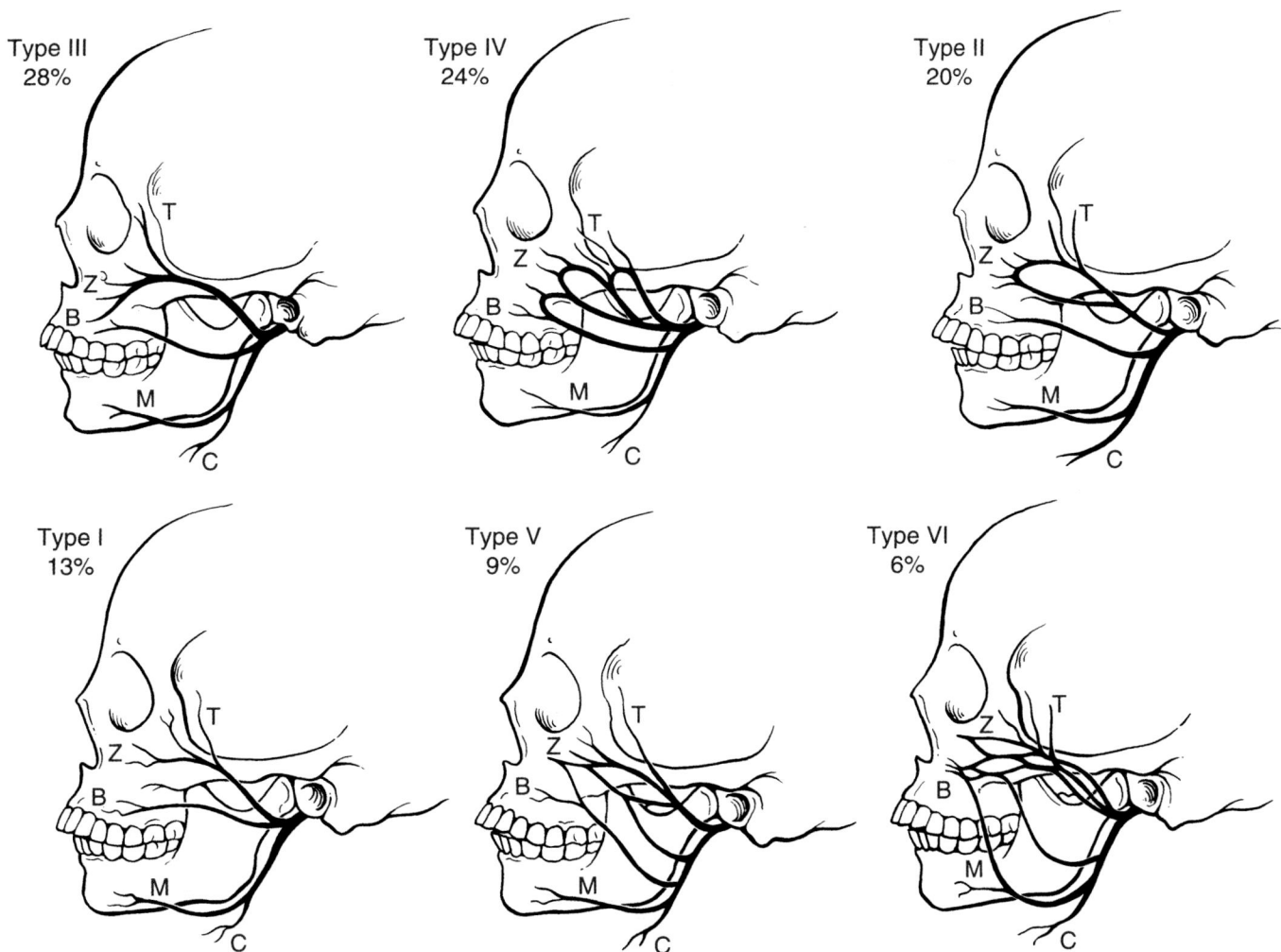

Figure 14–7. Branches of the facial nerve. Initially, the facial nerve divides into upper and lower segments within the parotid gland. The facial nerve then divides to form the temporal (T), zygomatic (Z), buccal (B), mandibular (M), and cervical (C) branches. The facial nerve divides into six common patterns. The frequency of each pattern is listed.[14] (From Handler LF, Galetta SL, Wulc AE, et al. Facial paralysis: diagnosis and management. In: Bosniak S (ed): Principles and Practice of Ophthalmic Plastic and Reconstructive Surgery, p. 468. Philadelphia, WB Saunders, 1996, with permission.)

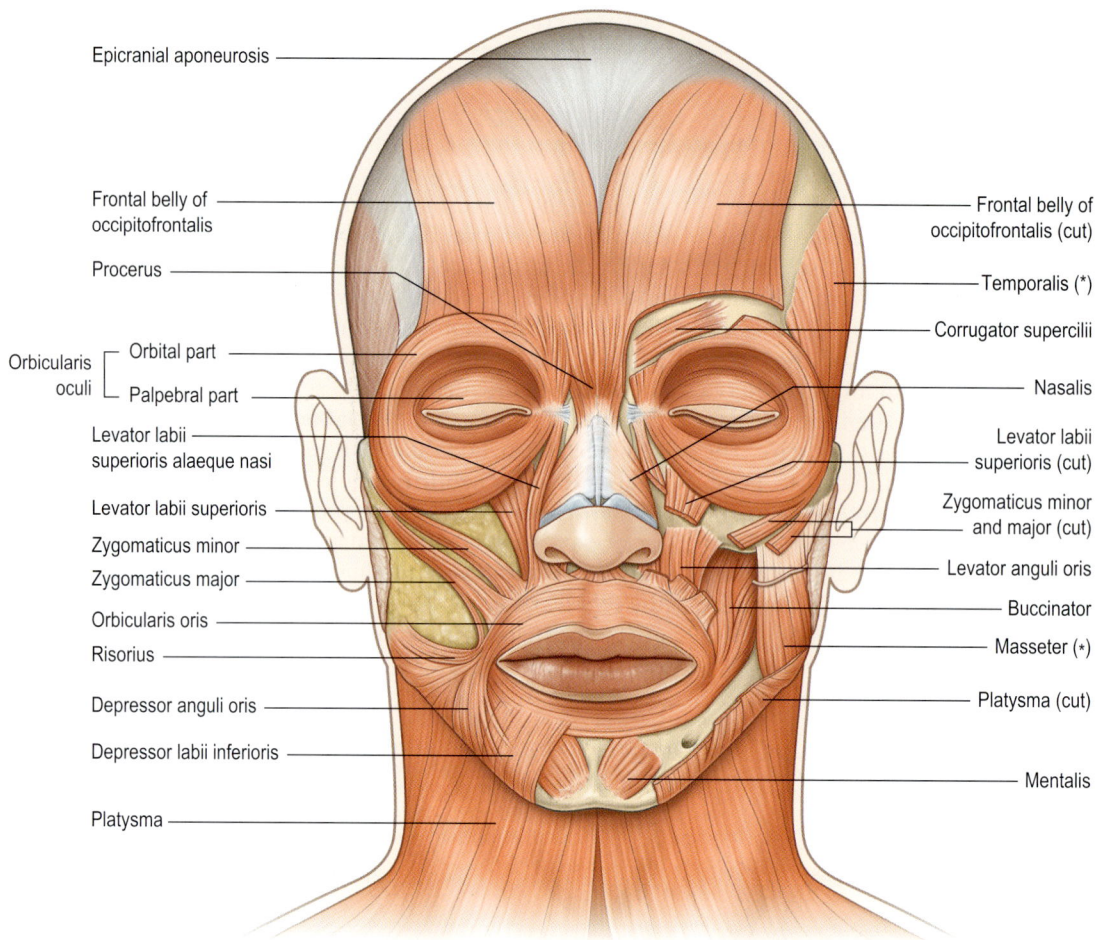

Figure 14–8. Muscles of the face, all of which are innervated by the facial nerve except*.

zygomaticus major, which lifts the angle of the mouth upward. The orbicularis oculi acts as a sphincter muscle around the eye, as it is organized in concentric circles around the orbital margin and the eyelids. There are three major parts of the orbicularis oculi: (1) the thick orbital part, for the most vigorous eyelid closure; (2) the thin palpebral part, for closing the eyelids lightly, and (3) the lacrimal part, which pulls the eyelids and lacrimal puncta medially to aid tear flow.[15]

History and examination

When a patient complains of ptosis, historical details such as duration, acuteness of symptoms, presence of eye pain, or diplopia are important considerations in making the diagnosis. Qualities such as fatiguability and associated dysarthria, and swallowing or breathing difficulty may suggest underlying myasthenia gravis. Patients with eyelid retraction should be asked about symptoms such as temperature intolerance, tachycardia, or proptosis which might indicate underlying thyroid-associated ophthalmopathy. Headache or difficulty with upgaze, consistent with a dorsal midbrain syndrome, should be excluded. Individuals with facial palsy should be asked about medical conditions, such as diabetes,

hypertension, sarcoidosis, Lyme disease, or pregnancy, which may predispose them to acquired VIIth nerve injury. In those with abnormal blinking or facial movements, historical evidence of basal ganglia diseases, old Bell's palsy, or multiple sclerosis, for example, should be investigated. A history consistent with allergies, photophobia, dry eye, or corneal damage may suggest an ocular cause of excessive eyelid closure.

The techniques of the eyelid and facial nerve examination are detailed in Chapter 2. However, some important guidelines will be discussed here. The eyelids and facial nerve should first be observed at rest. Eyelid position in relationship to the limbus and corneal light reflex should be noted, and the palpebral fissures measured. The position of the nasolabial fold and the nostrils should be evaluated because the nasolabial fold may disappear or be displaced in facial palsy, and the nostril may be ptotic or decreased circumferentially.

Eyelid fatigue, curtaining, and lid twitch should be tested for if the eyelid is ptotic. Although these signs are suggestive of myasthenia gravis, they are not specific for the disease.[16] Hering's Law of equal innervation, referring to the yoking of agonist muscles, applies to both levator muscles. Thus ptosis on one side may be accompanied by lid retraction on the other due to the excess tonus required to keep the ptotic lid

Video 14

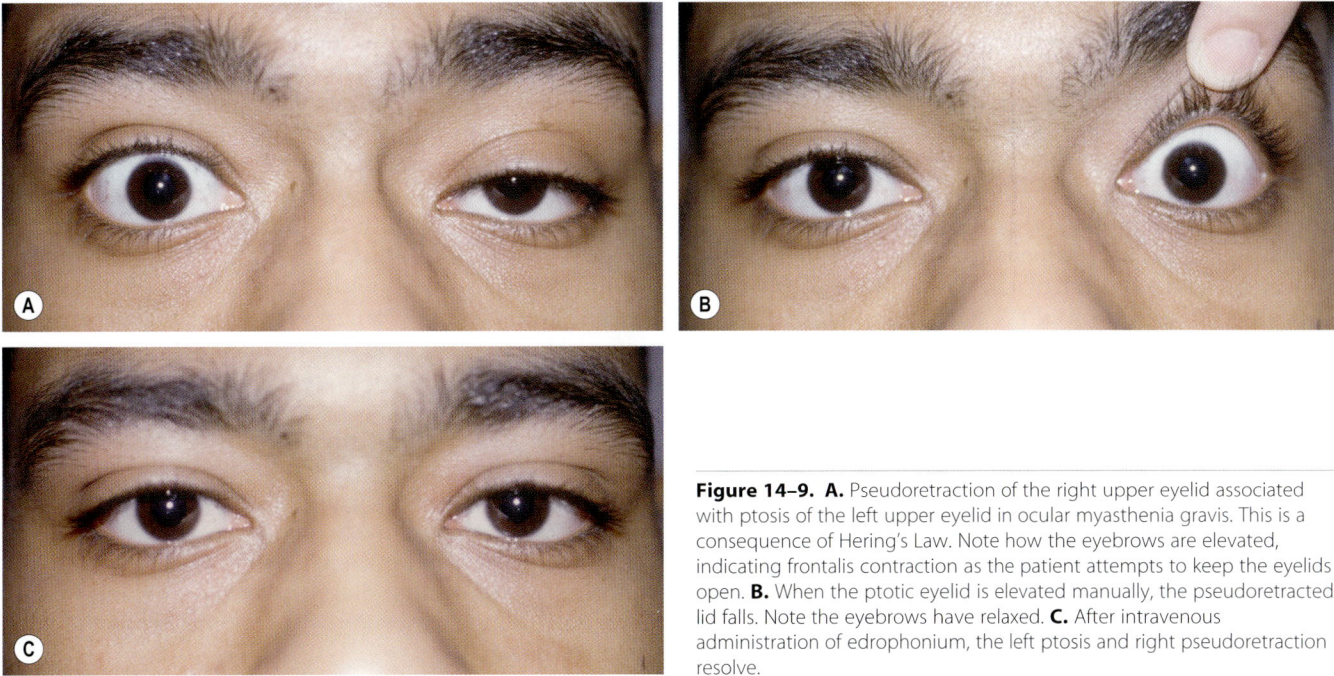

Figure 14–9. A. Pseudoretraction of the right upper eyelid associated with ptosis of the left upper eyelid in ocular myasthenia gravis. This is a consequence of Hering's Law. Note how the eyebrows are elevated, indicating frontalis contraction as the patient attempts to keep the eyelids open. **B.** When the ptotic eyelid is elevated manually, the pseudoretracted lid falls. Note the eyebrows have relaxed. **C.** After intravenous administration of edrophonium, the left ptosis and right pseudoretraction resolve.

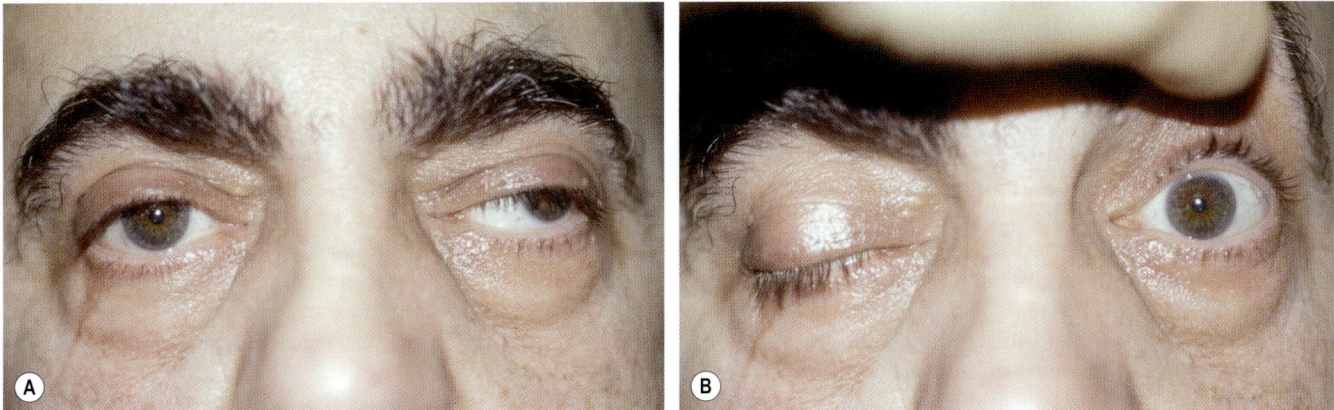

Figure 14–10. Enhanced ptosis in myasthenia gravis. **A.** Bilateral ptosis and exotropia. **B.** When a ptotic eyelid is manually elevated, the contralaterally retracted eyelid droops as a consequence of Hering's Law.

open (**Fig. 14–9A**). This is the case especially if the ptotic eye is the dominant and fixating one. In addition, if the ptotic eyelid is manually elevated, the retracted eyelid of the fellow eye drops (curtaining) (**Fig. 14–9B**). Similarly, when the ptosis is bilateral, if either eyelid is manually elevated, the ptosis on the other side worsens (enhanced ptosis) (**Fig. 14–10**). Hering's Law applies to ptosis caused by neuromuscular junction deficits as well as to ptosis resulting from oculomotor and other more proximal lesions.[17,18] Conversely, there may be pseudo-ptosis associated with contralateral pathologic eyelid retraction (**Fig. 14–11**).

The pupils and eye movements should also be observed. Levator and orbicularis oculi function should be assessed. Facial nerve function can be tested by having the patient lift the eyebrows, close the eyelids, and smile. In facial palsies, the ear should be examined for the presence of vesicles

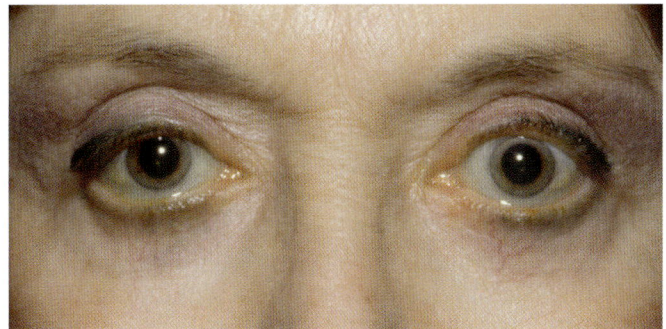

Figure 14–11. Pseudoptosis of the right upper eyelid associated with pathologic upper eyelid retraction of the left upper eyelid in thyroid-associated ophthalmopathy. This is a consequence of Hering's Law.

indicative of herpetic disease. When there are involuntary facial movements, the presence of subtle facial weakness or movements of other head and neck structures should be excluded. As suggested above, corneal abrasion or ulceration, iritis with photophobia, blepharitis, dry eye, or eyelid follicles should be ruled out in patients with excessive blinking. The tarsal conjunctiva should be examined for follicles in all patients with ptosis and ocular irritation.

When the width of a palpebral fissure is reduced, either upper eyelid ptosis or orbicularis spasm can be considered. The position of the involved eye's eyebrow compared with the other eye's may help differentiate between ptosis or spasm. For instance, because the frontalis muscle is usually contracted to elevate the eyelid to compensate for ptosis, the ipsilateral eyebrow in ptosis is typically elevated. In contrast, in blepharospasm, the ipsilateral eyebrow is typically lower, because the frontalis is relaxed and the orbicularis oculi is contracted.

Physiologic blink reflexes. In the *corneal blink reflex*, bilateral eyelid closure is elicited by touching one cornea with cotton, for instance. The ophthalmic division of the trigeminal nerve (V1) is the afferent limb of this reflex, with first-order neurons synapsing primarily in the chief sensory nucleus within the pontine tegmentum. Second-order neurons project from the chief sensory nucleus to both facial nerve nuclei. Tactile stimulation of the eyelids or eyelashes or tapping the forehead (*glabellar reflex*), which also elicit bilateral eyelid closure, are likely mediated by the same pathway.[19] These reflexes normally habituate with repetitive stimulation.[20] In the *corneomandibular reflex*, corneal stimulation elicits a bilateral eyelid blink and a brisk anterolateral jaw movement (palpebromandibular synkinesia).[21]

The *reflex blink to visual threat*, useful for evaluating visual fields in young children or uncooperative adults, can be elicited by a threatening gesture such as a menacing hand. Care should be taken not to push air onto the cornea, thereby provoking a corneal blink reflex. The reflex blink to visual threat requires an intact afferent visual pathway and occipital lobe as well as parietal and frontal lobe areas which mediate visual attention.[22] The reflex is likely a learned one,[23] as infants younger than 2–4 months of age may not exhibit it.[24] Patients in a vegetative state may have an intact blink to visual threat,[25] so it is not clear whether consciousness is necessary for an intact response.

Other normal blink reflexes include *blinking to sudden bright light or dazzle*, which is entirely brain stem mediated.[26–28] In the *stapedius reflex*, the eyes blink reflexively to a loud noise.

Ptosis

Approach

The etiologies of ptosis should be considered according to age (congenital vs acquired in adulthood), abruptness of onset, the appearance of the eyelid, the severity of the ptosis, pupillary size, and accompanying neurologic signs.[29] Acquired, painless ptosis of sudden onset strongly suggests a neurologic cause such as Horner syndrome or IIIrd nerve

palsy, especially in unilateral cases with pupillary involvement. Gradually progressive bilateral ptosis would be more consistent with a myopathic or neuromuscular junction disorder. Non-neurologic causes of ptosis, such as levator dehiscence, are more common than the etiologies listed above, and these disorders should be suspected in isolated cases. In addition, ptosis may be suspected incorrectly when in fact the upper eyelid of the other eye is pathologically retracted. When the ptosis is severe, a IIIrd nerve palsy or myasthenia gravis are the more likely etiologies as the lid droop of a Horner syndrome, for instance, is quite mild.

Measurement of levator palpebrae superioris function is also frequently helpful in narrowing the differential diagnosis (see **Fig. 2–22**). Ptosis produced by levator dehiscence and Horner syndrome is usually associated with normal levator function. In contrast, levator function is reduced in ptosis associated with myasthenia gravis, congenital ptosis, IIIrd nerve palsies, and myopathic conditions.

A detailed differential diagnosis of ptosis is outlined in **Table 14–1**,[30] but this section will concentrate on the most common causes.

Congenital

Isolated and with elevator palsy. Isolated, nonprogressive ptosis in the neonate or child is usually due to congenital maldevelopment of the levator palpebrae or its tendon. This also causes incomplete lowering of the eyelid in downgaze, resulting in lid lag (**Fig. 14–12**). The upper eyelid crease is typically shallow or absent. Commonly the involved eye has superior rectus or complete elevator palsy, and if both eyes are ptotic, neither eye may have normal upgaze. This frequent association between the eyelid and motility deficit has been attributed to a common embryological origin of and insult to the levator palpebrae and superior rectus muscles.[31] Some studies have demonstrated myopathic or dysgenetic features in the levator muscle.[32] Alternatively, a neurogenic cause has been proposed.[33] Familial cases have been reported.[34]

Marcus Gunn jaw-winking. Patients with *Marcus Gunn jaw-winking* have a ptotic eyelid which retracts during contraction of the external pterygoid muscle (e.g., nursing, chewing, mouth opening, or moving the jaw forward or side to side), presumably from anomalous innervation of the levator by the trigeminal nucleus (trigemino-oculomotor synkinesis). Cases are usually unilateral, but rarely patients are bilaterally affected. We have seen bilateral involvement where one eyelid was retracted and the other ptotic, and this pattern alternated when the child sucked a pacifier (**Fig. 14–13**). Associated ophthalmologic abnormalities include amblyopia, superior rectus weakness, double elevator palsy, and anisometropia.[35,36] Eyelid surgery can be considered when the jaw-winking or ptosis creates a functional or cosmetic problem.[37]

Other congenital causes. Neurofibromas (**Fig. 14–14**) and lid tumors such as hemangiomas should also be suspected in children with ptosis. Usually there is a palpable upper eyelid mass in these cases. Congenital oculomotor palsies (see Chapter 15), Horner syndrome (see Chapter 13), and

Video 14

Table 14–1 Differential diagnosis of ptosis[30]

Congenital

Isolated
With double-elevator palsy
Anomalous synkineses (including Marcus Gunn jaw-winking)
Lid or orbital tumors (hemangioma, dermoid)
Birth trauma (IIIrd nerve palsy, Horner's syndrome)
Neurofibromatosis (neurofibroma)
Neonatal myasthenia (transient)
Congenital fibrosis syndrome

Acquired

Myogenic
Chronic progressive external ophthalmoplegia (CPEO)
Kearns–Sayre syndrome (CPEO "plus")
Myotonic dystrophy
Oculopharyngeal dystrophy
Topical steroid eyedrops

Disorder of neuromuscular transmission
Myasthenia gravis
Lambert–Eaton syndrome
Botulism

Neurogenic
Horner's syndrome
Oculomotor nerve palsy
"Cortical" ptosis
Obtundation, drowsiness, coma
Apraxia of eyelid opening

Mechanical
Inflammatory (edema, allergy, chalazion, hordeolum, blepharitis, conjunctivitis)
Cicatricial
Tumor (lid, orbit)
Blepharochalasis

Levator dehiscence–disinsertion syndrome
Aging
Inflammation (ocular, lids, orbit)
Surgery (ocular, orbital, post-cataract)
Trauma
Contact lens use

Pseudo-ptosis
Dermatochalasis
Duane's retraction syndrome
Microphthalmos/phthisis bulbi
Enophthalmos
Pathologic lid retraction of the opposite eye
Chronic (old) Bell's palsy
Voluntary blepharospasm
Hypotropia
Hysteria

congenital fibrosis syndromes (see Chapter 15) should also be considered in this age group.

Acquired

Myopathic. Patients with myopathic ptosis often give a long history of droopy lids. Occasionally the ptosis will be the

only manifestation of a myopathic condition. However, many patients have other neurologic signs. These patients often have levator function between 5 and 11 mm. Important myogenic causes of ptosis include the mitochondrial disorders chronic progressive external ophthalmoplegia and Kearns–Sayre syndrome, myotonic dystrophy, and oculopharyngeal dystrophy. These entities are discussed in detail at the end of this chapter.

Neuromuscular junction. Fatiguable or variable unilateral or bilateral ptosis suggests a disorder of neuromuscular transmission, such as myasthenia gravis, Lambert–Eaton myasthenic syndrome, and botulism. These are also discussed in detail at the end of this chapter.

Neuropathic. IIIrd nerve palsy. Prominent unilateral ptosis with adduction, elevation, and depression deficits, with or without pupillary mydriasis, suggests an infranuclear IIIrd nerve palsy (see Chapter 15). A posterior communicating aneurysm manifesting as unilateral ptosis in isolation is rare.[38] A unilateral nuclear oculomotor lesion causes bilateral ptosis (nuclear ptosis), worse ipsilaterally, ipsilateral IIIrd nerve dysfunction, and contralateral superior rectus weakness (see Chapter 15).[39]

In the setting of a resolved IIIrd nerve palsy, a ptotic eyelid which elevates (retracts) when the eye infraducts or adducts implies aberrant regeneration of the eyelid. This levator synkinesis phenomenon is discussed in more detail in Chapter 15.

Horner syndrome. Mild unilateral ptosis accompanied by miosis and pupillary dilation lag in the dark implies Horner syndrome (see Chapter 13). The ptosis never completely covers the eye in Horner syndrome. The lower eyelid may be elevated in so-called lower eyelid ptosis. The small palpebral fissure due to the combination of the upper and lower eyelid ptosis gives the eye a pseudoenophthalmic appearance.

Cerebral (or cortical) ptosis. A unilateral cerebral hemispheric lesion may uncommonly cause unilateral or bilateral ptosis without IIIrd nerve or sympathetic involvement or apraxia (see below).[1,40] The side of the unilateral ptosis or the lower lid in bilateral cases can be either ipsilateral or contralateral to the lesion. The ptosis is usually transient, lasting only for a few days. In a series of 13 patients with bilateral cerebral ptosis, all patients had an acute right frontotemporoparietal lobe lesion and conjugate gaze deviation to the right.[41] Three other patients with right-sided lesions were reported who had bilateral ptosis and upgaze palsy.[42] These and other similar observations[43,44] suggest some supranuclear cortical control of the levator muscles, perhaps with right hemispheric dominance.

Apraxia of eyelid opening. Nonparalytic, deficient voluntary eyelid elevation (*apraxia of eyelid opening*) can mimic levator paralysis until the patient opens the eyes without ptosis after a sudden command or stimulation.[45] Patients contract their frontalis muscles while attempting to open their eyes. No ocular myopathy or sympathetic dysfunction is present.[46] This disorder should be distinguished from blepharospasm, which often accompanies it.[47,48] In blepharospasm (see Facial nerve section) there is obvious contraction of the orbicularis oculi, which does not visibly occur in apraxia of eyelid opening. However, in some patients with apraxia of

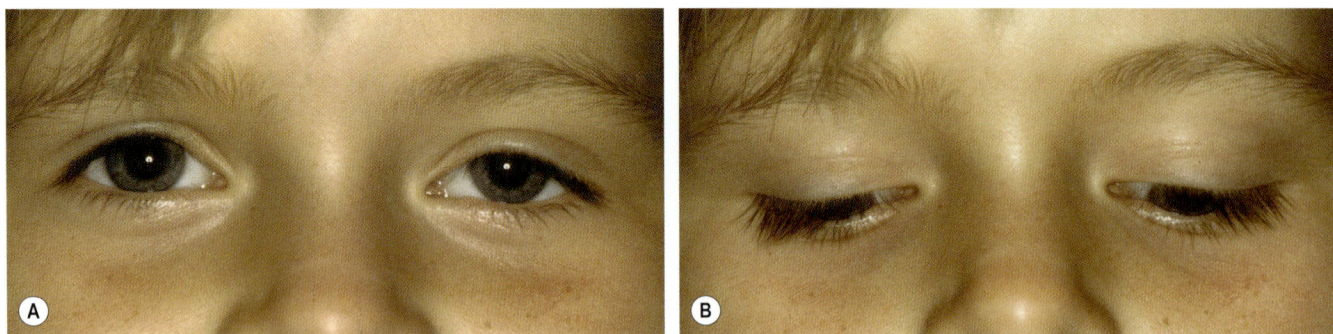

Figure 14–12. Congenital left ptosis characterized by a droopy eyelid (**A**), which incompletely lowers in downgaze (**B**).

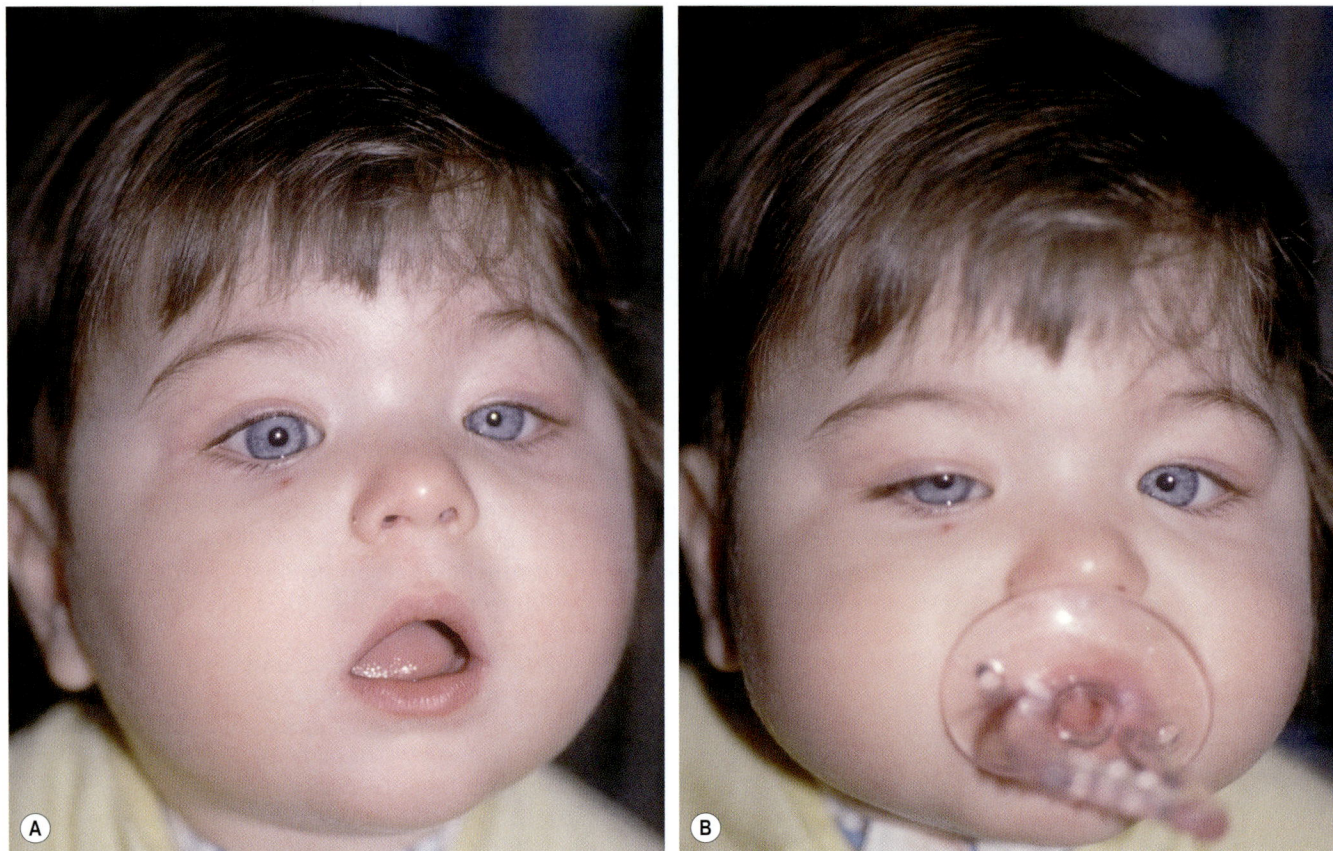

Figure 14–13. Bilateral Marcus Gunn jaw-winking phenomenon. **A.** This baby had left ptosis with the mouth open. **B.** When she sucked on a pacifier, the left ptosis alternated with right ptosis.

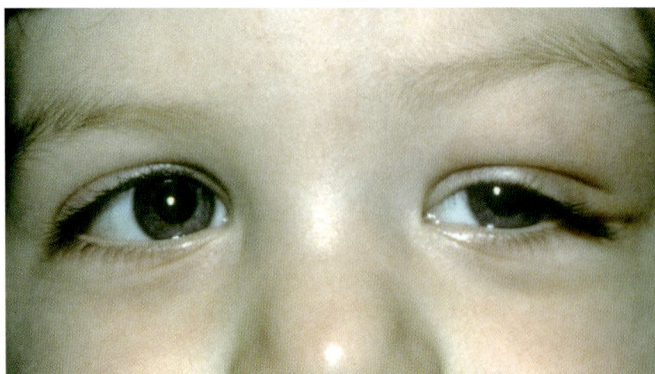

Figure 14–14. S-shaped left ptosis due to an eyelid neurofibroma in neurofibromatosis type 1.

eyelid opening, there may be electromyographically demonstrable (but not visible) orbicularis oculi contractions of the pretarsal portion during attempted eyelid opening.[49,50]

Apraxia of eyelid opening occurs insidiously in association with extrapyramidal disorders such as progressive supranuclear palsy (PSP),[51,52] Parkinson disease (PD), Shy–Drager syndrome,[46] Huntington disease,[45] and Wilson disease. Rarely this disorder can be seen in association with subthalamic nucleus deep brain stimulation for Parkinson disease[53] and paraneoplastic encephalitis,[54] acutely with dominant[55] and nondominant[56,57] hemispheric lesions, bifrontal lobe disease,[58] and chronically with amyotrophic lateral sclerosis.[59] The exact lesions responsible for apraxia of eyelid opening are uncertain.[47]

In patients with pyramidal and extrapyramidal diseases, some authors have questioned the use of the term apraxia, which should be used only in the context of intact motor systems. Therefore a more appropriate term such as "involuntary levator palpebrae inhibition of supranuclear origin" has been suggested.[46] Others have termed it an eyelid dystonia,[60] particularly if abnormal orbicularis oculi contraction is implicated.[61]

Botulinum injections of the pretarsal portion of the orbicularis oculi are sometimes recommended,[62,63] based upon the motor persistence of this muscle alluded to above.[49,50] Levodopa has been used in some isolated cases.[64,65] Upper eyelid myectomy has been performed in patients with blepharospasm with associated apraxia of eyelid opening refractory to botulinum toxin treatment.[66]

Levator dehiscence–disinsertion syndrome (aponeurotic ptosis). This is the most common cause of acquired ptosis in adults. In many elderly patients the aponeurosis of the levator muscle may spontaneously dehisce or disinsert from the tarsal plate of the upper eyelid (**Fig. 14–1**). The upper eyelid crease is often high or indistinct, and levator function is relatively preserved (**Fig. 14–15**). In younger and middle-aged patients, the most common etiology of levator dehiscence is contact lens wear.[67] Eyelid manipulation during lens removal is thought to cause or exacerbate the disinsertion, but pathologic studies have also shown fibrosis of Müller's muscle.[68] Other important causes of levator dehiscence include trauma, ocular surgery (such as cataract or orbital surgery), allergies, and eyelid edema.

Pseudo-ptosis. Disorders in this group are characterized by an eyelid which falsely appears to be drooping and therefore mimics ptosis. The various causes are listed in **Table 14–1**, but the most important ones include contralateral lid retraction and ipsilateral eyelid relaxation secondary to Hering's Law (see **Fig. 14–11**), enophthalmos, hypotropia, and dermatochalasis, the hanging of skin over the eyelid due to loss of skin elasticity and orbital fat herniation.

Treatment

Other than treating the primary cause, ptosis can be managed with taping the eyelids open or with eyelid "crutches" attached to eyeglasses. Most patients find the latter uncomfortable. Surgical management of ptosis is more effective in chronic cases, and popular procedures include shortening of the levator muscle or aponeurosis, or Müller's muscle resection.

Eyelid retraction

In primary gaze, the upper eyelid normally reaches just below the limbus. Eyelid retraction is diagnosed if there is sclera showing between the lower edge of the upper eyelid and the limbus. **Table 14–2** lists a differential diagnosis of eyelid retraction.[69,70] The three most important neuro-

Table 14–2 Differential diagnosis of eyelid retraction[70]

Neurogenic
  Dorsal midbrain syndrome
  Collier's eyelid retraction
  Eyelid lag in downgaze
 Contralateral ptosis
 Marcus Gunn jaw-winking
 Aberrant regeneration of the IIIrd nerve
 Ocular neuromyotonia
 IIIrd nerve palsy with cyclic spasms
 Facial nerve paresis
 Eyelid nystagmus
 Extrapyramidal disease
 Ipsilateral superior rectus weakness and enhanced innervation to
  the superior rectus/levator complex
 Hypo- and hyperkalemic periodic paralysis

Myogenic
  Thyroid associated ophthalmopathy (Grave's)
  Congenital

Mechanical
  Proptosis
  Axial myopia
  Ocular or orbital surgery
  Eyelid scarring

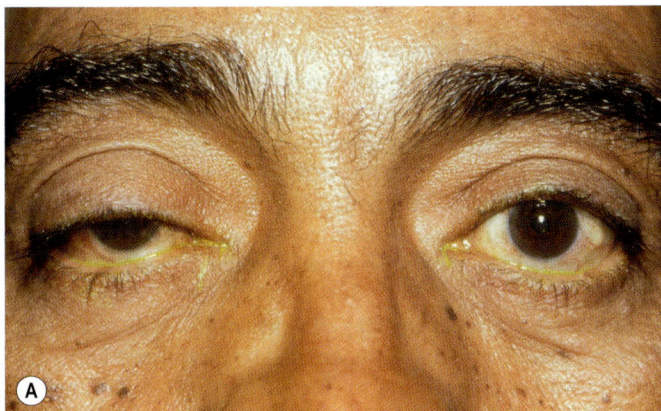

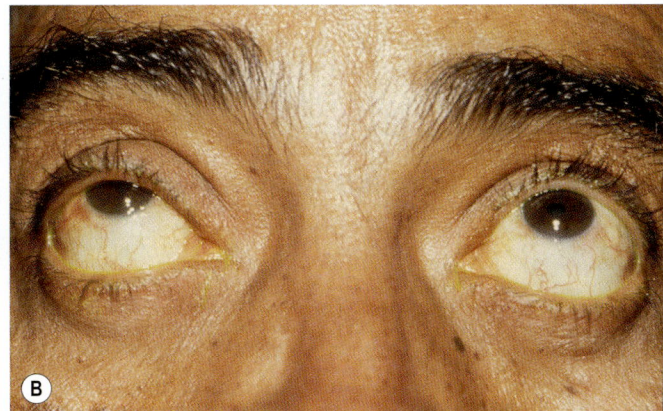

Figure 14–15. Levator dehiscence–disinsertion syndrome (aponeurotic ptosis). **A.** Ptosis of the right upper eyelid with a high upper eyelid crease. **B.** Relative preservation of right levator function.

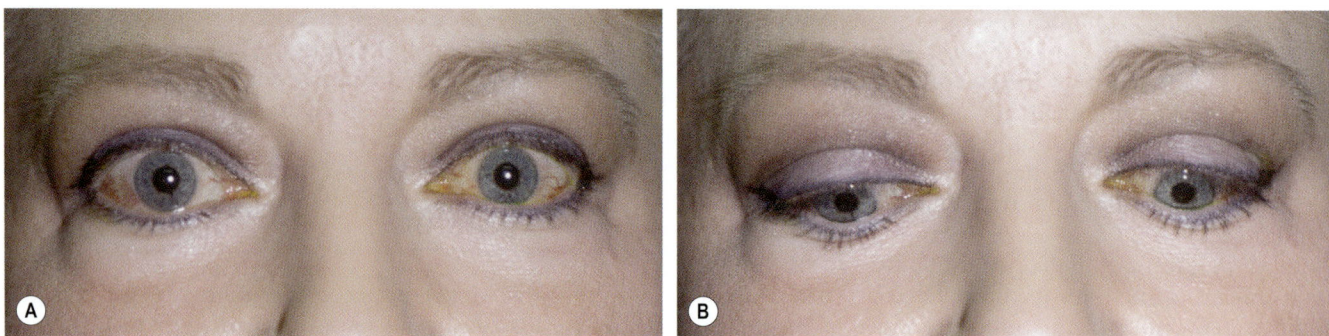

Figure 14–16. Eyelid retraction (**A**) and lid lag (**B**)—the lids fail to relax in downgaze—related to thyroid-associated ophthalmopathy. Note the characteristic upper and lower eyelid swelling and conjunctival injection.

ophthalmic causes of eyelid retraction are thyroid-associated ophthalmopathy, dorsal midbrain lesions, and contralateral ptosis. This section will discuss the first two. Eyelid retraction due to contralateral ptosis is a consequence of Hering's Law and has already been discussed above. Based on this relatively small differential diagnosis, we recommend that any patient with acquired eyelid retraction without contralateral ptosis or known thyroid disease to undergo thyroid function testing (TFT). If the thyroid workup is unrevealing, or if there is a history of headache, blurred vision, or ataxia, and there are other signs of dorsal midbrain disease, then neuroimaging of the brain is warranted.

Thyroid-associated ophthalmopathy

Upper eyelid retraction may be the only ocular abnormality in these patients. The retraction can either be uni- or bilateral (**Fig. 14–16A**). The eyelid tends to be more retracted temporally than medially. The exact mechanism of the eyelid retraction is unclear, but (1) fibrous contraction, thickening, shortening, or hyperactivity of the levator palpebrae muscle; (2) sympathetic overdrive and overaction of Müller's muscle; (3) proptosis; and (4) secondary upper eyelid retraction due to a restricted inferior rectus and limited upgaze have all been proposed as contributory factors.[71,72] Retraction is often accompanied by lid lag (von Graefe's sign), in which the upper eyelid fails or is slow to follow the eye in downgaze (**Fig. 14–16B**).[73] In thyroid-associated ophthalmopathy, the etiology of lid lag is likely related to the causes of the lid retraction. The lower lid is also frequently retracted.

Exposure keratopathy and dry eye can complicate thyroid-related lid retraction and lag, especially in individuals with infrequent blinking. Artificial tears are usually sufficient, but some thyroid patients with lid retraction require surgical levator recession or division, aponeurosis division, or excision of Müller's muscle.[71]

Further details regarding the features, diagnosis, and management of thyroid-associated ophthalmopathy are discussed in Chapter 18.

Pretectal eyelid retraction (Collier's sign)

Eyelid retraction may be a prominent sign in the pretectal (or Parinaud's or dorsal midbrain) syndrome. The patients have a characteristic stare (**Fig. 14–17**), often accompanied by upgaze paresis. The lid retraction is typically symmetric,

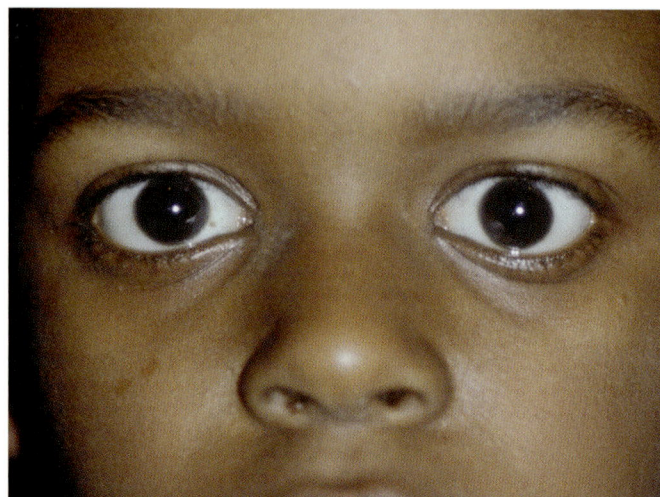

Figure 14–17. Eyelid retraction due to dorsal midbrain astrocytoma (Collier's sign).

except in the plus–minus lid syndrome (see below). Also, it usually is exacerbated on attempted upgaze, and normally the lids relax on downgaze. However, in some exceptional instances there is lid lag in downgaze (see below).

The other elements of the pretectal syndrome, which include supranuclear vertical gaze paresis (Chapter 16), pupillary light-near dissociation (Chapter 13), and convergence retraction nystagmus (Chapter 17) are discussed elsewhere.

Because the lid retraction typically occurs in patients with upgaze paresis, some authors have attributed the finding to combined excess superior rectus innervation and levator activity.[74] However, Schmidtke and Büttner-Ennever[3] postulated that neurogenic lid retraction can result either from a unilateral lesion of the nPC or from interruption of the posterior commissure, both of which would result in decreased inhibition of levator neurons in the CCN (see Fig. 14–2).

Eyelid lag in downgaze. As described earlier in this chapter, eyelid position is normally coordinated with vertical eye movements so that in upgaze the eyelids elevate, and in downgaze the eyelids typically relax and fall. In dorsal midbrain lesions, this relationship can be disrupted, causing the eyelids to remain elevated while the eyes infraduct.[75]

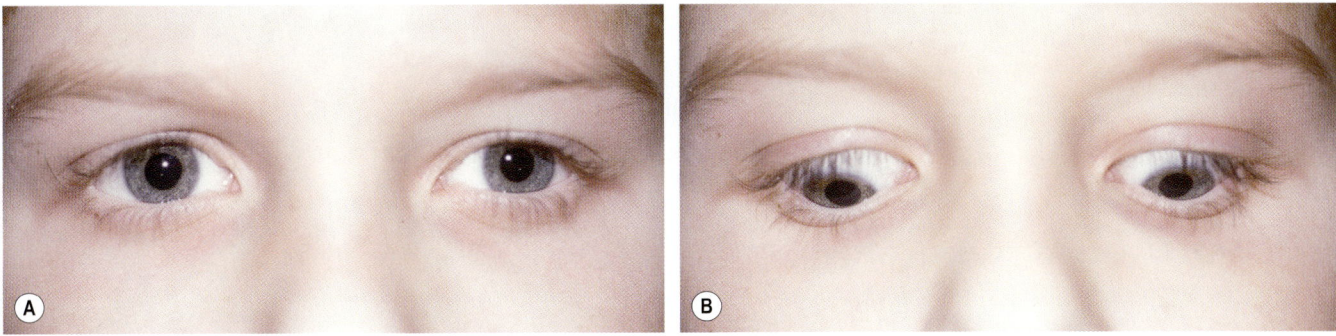

Figure 14–18. Child with pineal region germinoma and supranuclear upgaze paresis with normal lid position in primary gaze (**A**) but lid lag in downgaze (**B**).

Dramatic examples include the setting-sun sign (tonic downward eye deviation with lid retraction) in infants with hydrocephalus, thalamic hemorrhage (see Chapter 16), and rare comatose patients with phasic vertical eye movements and persistent eyelid elevation.[76] Lid lag in some instances may be difficult to detect because patients with pretectal dysfunction may have downgaze paralysis early in their course that precludes the ability to detect lid lag.

Although lid lag and lid retraction in such instances may share the same mechanism, patients have been observed who do not have lid retraction in primary gaze but have lid lag in downgaze (**Fig. 14–18**).[77] This suggests that there may be separate central mechanisms for these eyelid abnormalities. One possible lesion for lid lag without retraction involves the inhibitory connections from the supranuclear downgaze centers to the CCN (see **Fig. 14–2**).

Plus–minus eyelid syndrome. A unilateral lesion involving nPC and the oculomotor fascicle would produce an ipsilateral IIIrd nerve palsy with ptosis and contralateral lid retraction (*plus–minus lid syndrome*) (**Fig. 14–19**).[78] The ipsilateral lid retraction is masked by the infranuclear IIIrd nerve palsy. This eyelid pattern of ptosis and contralateral lid retraction can be mimicked in an individual with ptosis who fixates with the ptotic eye, thereby increasing the innervation to both levators (Hering's Law). In this case manual elevation of the ptotic eyelid would eliminate the contralateral lid retraction. It may also be seen in a patient with ptosis and contralateral superior rectus weakness who is fixating with the non-ptotic eye and increasing the innervation to the levator/superior rectus complex. This possibility can be investigated by covering the fixating non-ptotic eye.

Miscellaneous causes

Eyelid retraction in association with Marcus Gunn jaw-winking and aberrant regeneration of the IIIrd nerve with levator synkinesis have already been mentioned in the section on ptosis. Other neuro-ophthalmic causes include extrapyramidal diseases, neuromyotonia, and oculomotor paresis with cyclic spasm[79] (see Chapter 15). Mechanistic etiologies such as proptosis, axial myopia, eyelid scarring, and ocular or orbital surgery (such as overcorrection of ptosis) should be considered. A congenital, idiopathic variety has also been described.[80]

Facial weakness

Although idiopathic Bell's palsy is a common cause of facial weakness, it is important to explore the differential diagnosis of facial palsies. This was emphasized in a study by May,[81] in which only 53% of patients who were referred to one practice with a diagnosis of Bell's palsy had the disorder. Approximately 10% had a treatable, progressive, or life-threatening lesion. Bell's palsy is a diagnosis of exclusion, and other supranuclear, nuclear, infranuclear, and neuromuscular causes of facial weakness must be considered.

Approach

When weakness of the face is present, determining whether the palsy is central or peripheral is the first important diagnostic consideration. Asking the patient to look up or raise the eyebrows causes contraction of the frontalis muscle. If frontalis function is intact, a central palsy is likely, while impaired frontalis contraction suggests a peripheral cause (see **Figs 14–3** and **14–20**).

The clinical setting and accompanying signs then aid in refining the localization and determining the exact etiology. For example, nuclear facial nerve palsies are usually associated with other pontine disturbances. Also, peripheral facial nerve palsies are frequently accompanied by defective taste and tearing as well as hyperacusis. Furthermore, synkinesis or misdirection phenomenon (see next section) are late sequelae of peripheral rather than central facial palsies. In addition, idiopathic Bell's palsy rarely may affect both sides of the face, but acquired bilateral facial weakness should alert the examiner to the possibility of Lyme disease, sarcoidosis, carcinomatous meningitis, Guillain–Barré syndrome (GBS), and myasthenia gravis.[82] Congenital causes of bilateral facial weakness include Möbius syndrome and myotonic dystrophy.

The remainder of this section highlights some of the important causes of facial weakness, grouped by localization.

Central

Supranuclear. Supranuclear cortex and internal capsule lesions that produce lower facial weakness are usually associated with weakness of the ipsilateral arm. Since the

Video 14.3

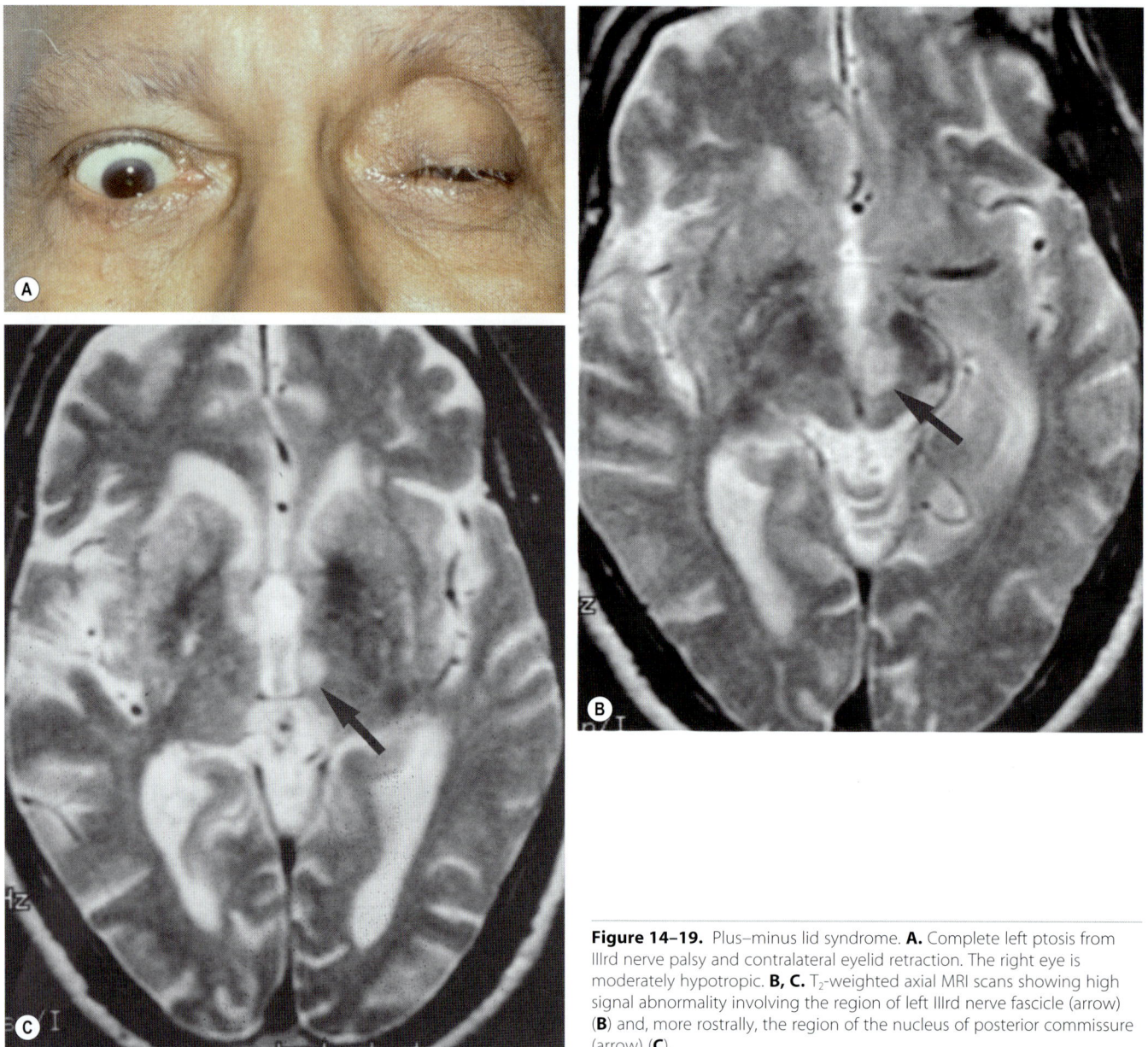

Figure 14–19. Plus–minus lid syndrome. **A.** Complete left ptosis from IIIrd nerve palsy and contralateral eyelid retraction. The right eye is moderately hypotropic. **B, C.** T_2-weighted axial MRI scans showing high signal abnormality involving the region of left IIIrd nerve fascicle (arrow) (**B**) and, more rostrally, the region of the nucleus of posterior commissure (arrow) (**C**).

facial nucleus also receives input from the basal ganglia region there may be a dissociation of voluntary and spontaneous facial movements. Thus, patients with lower facial weakness resulting from corticobulbar tract dysfunction typically show better facial movement when told a joke rather than simply asking them to smile.[83] On the other hand, pontine, thalamic, basal ganglia, dorsal midbrain, and supplementary motor area lesions may lead to normal voluntary smiling, but defective contralateral facial nerve function during reflex (emotional) smiling.[84–86]

A supranuclear paralysis of voluntary eyelid closure has been described. Lessell[87] reported a patient with presumed amyotrophic lateral sclerosis, with evidence of bilateral pyramidal tract involvement, who could not close his eyelids voluntarily but blinked to visual threat. Ross Russell[88] described three individuals with Creutzfeldt–Jakob disease with pyramidal tract degeneration documented on postmor-

tem who similarly could not blink on command but blinked to threat. In both reports, the patients also continued to blink spontaneously and in response to corneal stimulation and loud noise. In another reported case, a right anterior cerebral artery infarction led to defective voluntary closure of the left eyelid.[89] Lessell[87] and Ross Russell[88] argued that the deficiency in voluntary eyelid closure resulted from bilateral damage to cortical motor neurons and not from a facial dyspraxia (i.e., difficulty with motor planning or initiation).

Nuclear. *Möbius syndrome.* Congenital facial diplegia is the hallmark of this syndrome (**Fig. 14–21**). Abducens palsy is the most commonly associated feature, occurring in 82% of cases in the series reported by Henderson.[90] In addition, total external ophthalmoplegia was present in 25% of the cases in this series, oculomotor palsy in 21%, and bilateral ptosis in 10%. The abducens weakness is almost always bilateral,

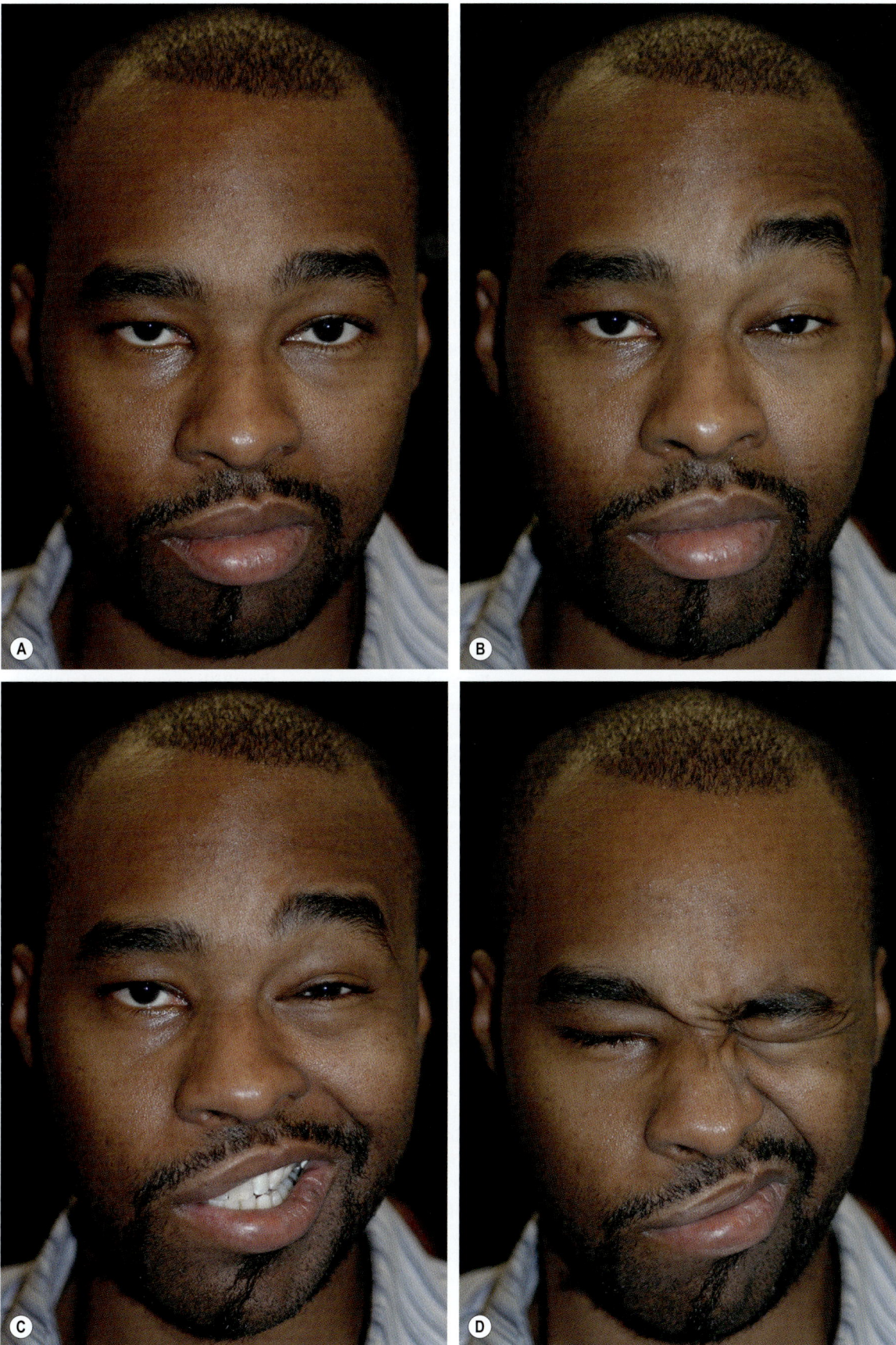

Figure 14–20. Idiopathic right peripheral facial palsy. **A.** At rest, the patient exhibits facial asymmetry, particularly of the right lower face. When asked to lift the eyebrows (**B**), smile (**C**), or close the eyelids (**D**), weakness on the right is seen.

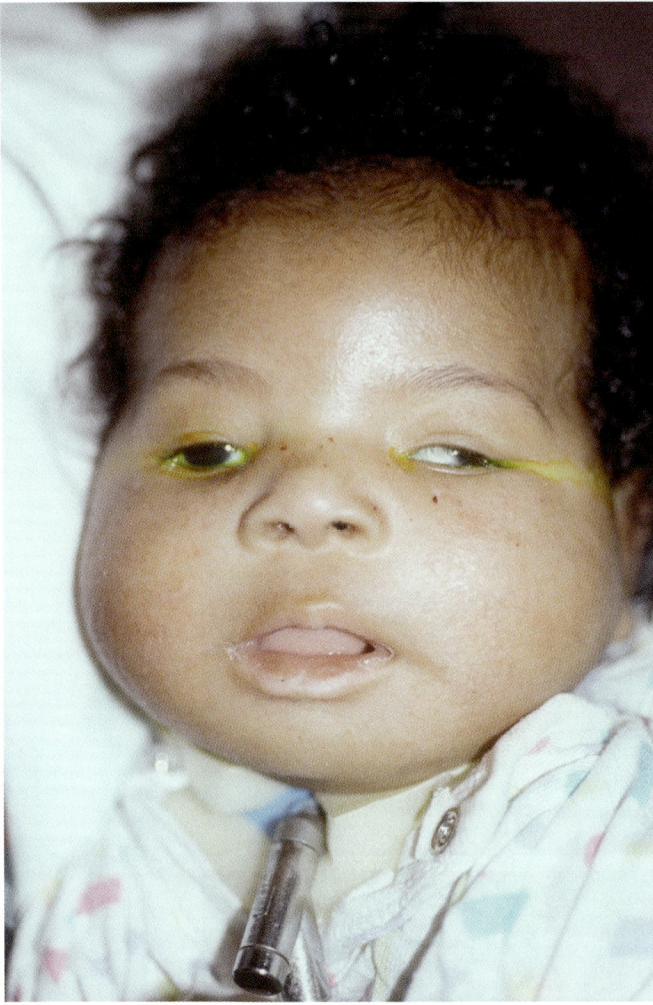

Figure 14–21. Child with Möbius syndrome characterized by bifacial weakness. In contrast to most patients with Möbius syndrome, this patient had bilateral oculomotor palsies but sparing of the abducens nerves. At autopsy, neurons were diminished within the VIIth nerve nuclei but not the VIth nerve nuclei.[93]

but of varying degree. When the lateral rectus palsy is severe, there is usually complete conjugate gaze paresis.

Parents may not notice the facial weakness if it is subtle, and often the child is brought to medical attention solely because of an esotropia. When the disorder involves only ocular motility and the upper face, the major issues—strabismus surgery, amblyopia, corneal surface protection, and cosmesis—can be handled primarily by ophthalmologists and plastic surgeons. However, lower facial weakness may complicate an infant's ability to suck a bottle or nipple. Less commonly lower cranial nerves, such as IX, X, and XII, are involved, causing dysphagia, arrhythmias, and aspiration for instance.[91] In such cases the disorder can be associated with much higher morbidity and mortality rates.[92,93] Pectoralis muscle defects and limb malformations (e.g., Poland anomaly) are also frequently associated with Möbius syndrome.[94]

No single theory can satisfactorily explain all cases of Möbius syndrome, as the disorder is usually sporadic and likely has many possible causes and localizations.[95–97] In

one subset of patients, electrophysiologic studies[98] have suggested, and pathologic studies[93,99,100] have demonstrated, aplasia or hypoplasia of cranial nerve nuclei. The cause in this group may be a genetically determined disruption in the formation of cranial nuclei or nerves. In a second group, abnormal peripheral portions of the cranial nerves are suspected.[97] In the third subset, more widespread destruction of the brain stem, perhaps due to a prenatal vascular insult, has been suggested radiologically and neuropathologically.[101,102] Neuroimaging in this group can demonstrate brain stem hypoplasia[103] and calcification,[104] and brain stem atrophy and mineralized necrotic foci have been found histopathologically.[105] These studies support the notion that Möbius syndrome in some cases could be the result of in utero brain stem vascular insufficiency. In one hypothesis, during the development of the posterior circulation, a potential transient watershed area within the brain stem exists while the blood flow in the basilar artery changes from a rostrocaudal to a caudal-to-rostral pattern. Brain stem ischemia may result if the blood flow during this transition is disrupted.[105] Alternatively, a more widespread syndrome of rhombencephalic maldevelopment has been theorized.[106–108]

Uncommonly the disorder is inherited, and one family harbored a defective gene in chromosome 3q.[109] Also, attempted abortion with misoprostol, a synthetic prostaglandin analogue also used to prevent and treat gastrointestinal ulcers, is associated with an increased risk of Möbius syndrome in infants.[110–113]

Fascicular. In the pons, the VIIth nerve fascicle may be disrupted dorsally in the facial colliculus syndrome (see **Fig. 16–5**), which is characterized by an ipsilateral "peripheral" facial palsy and conjugate gaze paresis.[114] Facial weakness in combination with ipsilateral deafness, facial numbness, and a Horner syndrome signifies a lesion in the lateral pons. More ventral pontine injury, where the VIIth nerve fascicle travels near the corticospinal tracts, may lead to ipsilateral facial paresis and contralateral hemiparesis (Millard–Gubler syndrome).[115] More lateral pontine lesions may result in "peripheral" facial nerve palsies without other brain stem signs (**Fig. 14–22**).

Peripheral

Cerebellopontine angle. Acoustic neuroma. These usually present with a VIIth cranial nerve palsy either late in their course as the facial nerve is displaced and compressed by an expanding cerebellopontine tumor or as a postoperative complication after neurosurgical resection. Common symptoms of acoustic neuromas include tinnitus, hearing loss, and cerebellar and vestibular signs. On magnetic resonance imaging (MRI), the mass is hypointense on T1-weighted images, hyperintense on T2-weighted images, and diffusely enhances. Treatment consists of neurosurgical excision.

Subarachnoid. Lyme disease. Lyme disease, caused by the tick-borne spirochete *Borrelia burgdorferi*, may cause unilateral or bilateral facial palsy at some point in its course in approximately 10% of patients.[116] This diagnosis should be considered as a cause of the facial palsy in endemic areas. Approximately 60% of patients will recall the diagnostic skin lesion of erythema chronicum migrans lesion, an erythema-

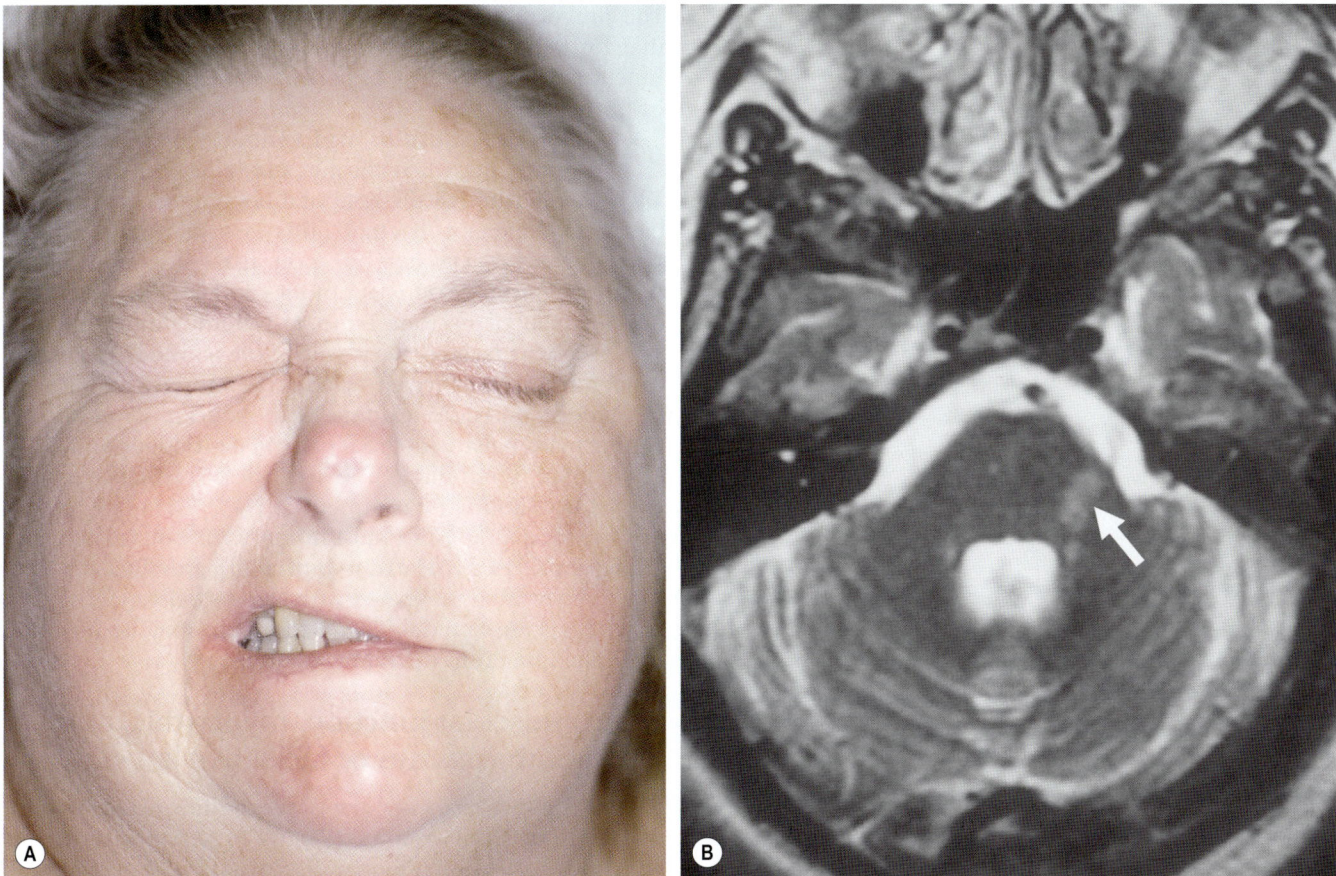

Figure 14–22. Left "peripheral" facial palsy (**A**), characterized by upper and lower facial weakness, caused by a lateral pontine infarction (arrow) seen on (**B**) T2 weighted axial MRI scan.

tous raised area that spreads centripetally, leaving a central clear zone and lasting several weeks if left untreated. Flu-like symptoms, including chills, fever, arthralgias, headaches, and myalgias, may occur concomitant with the lesion. The diagnosis may be made by finding a positive serum enzyme-linked immunosorbent assay titer and may be confirmed by the results of a western blot. A spinal tap can direct treatment in one suggested approach to patients with facial palsy and a positive Lyme titer: those with normal spinal fluid can be treated with oral doxycycline, while those with pleocytosis have meningitis and can be given either oral doxycycline or a course of intravenous ceftriaxone. The facial palsy has an excellent prognosis regardless of the antibiotic regimen chosen.

Sarcoidosis. Unilateral and bilateral facial nerve palsies may be a presenting symptom of neurosarcoidosis.[117] MRI may demonstrate meningeal enhancement, and cerebrospinal fluid examination may reveal elevated protein or lymphocytosis, or both. A serum angiotensin-converting enzyme (ACE) level and chest radiograph may be helpful in establishing sarcoidosis as the etiology of the facial palsy. The diagnosis and treatment of neurosarcoid is discussed in more detail in Chapters 5 and 7. Sarcoidosis may also cause a peripheral facial nerve palsy by involving the parotid gland (Heerfordt syndrome).

Metastatic lesions. A history of cancer and the presence of a rapidly progressive facial palsy are highly suggestive of a metastatic lesion. The nerve or the meninges may be infiltrated. MRI may show enhancement of the dura or of the facial nerve, or disruption of the blood–brain barrier, or both. Serial lumbar punctures may be necessary for the cytologic diagnosis of meningeal carcinomatosis.

Transtemporal bone. *Trauma.* The facial nerve is vulnerable in its bony course within the temporal bone at its exit point from the stylomastoid foramen and along its course to innervate the muscles of facial expression. The nerve itself can be either lacerated or traumatized bluntly. Fractures parallel to the long aspect of the petrous portion of the temporal bone (**Fig. 14–23**) are often accompanied by fractures of the ossicles or the labyrinth.

The facial nerve may be injured by mandibular fractures or during surgery of the mandible. The facial nerve branches are particularly vulnerable to undermining in the vicinity of the zygoma and lateral orbit during a face lift.

Bell's palsy. This is an idiopathic facial palsy that may have a viral cause. Presenting symptoms may include a combination of ipsilateral ear pain, numbness, or hyperacusis. Diabetes may be a risk factor, as is pregnancy.[118] Fortunately, the prognosis is excellent in most cases of Bell's palsy, with full recovery of function occurring in approximately 84% of patients.[119,120] Most patients begin to recover within 3 weeks of onset. Prognostically, the sooner the palsy begins to recover, the better the outcome. As the palsy becomes more complete, the likelihood of aberrant regeneration increases.[81]

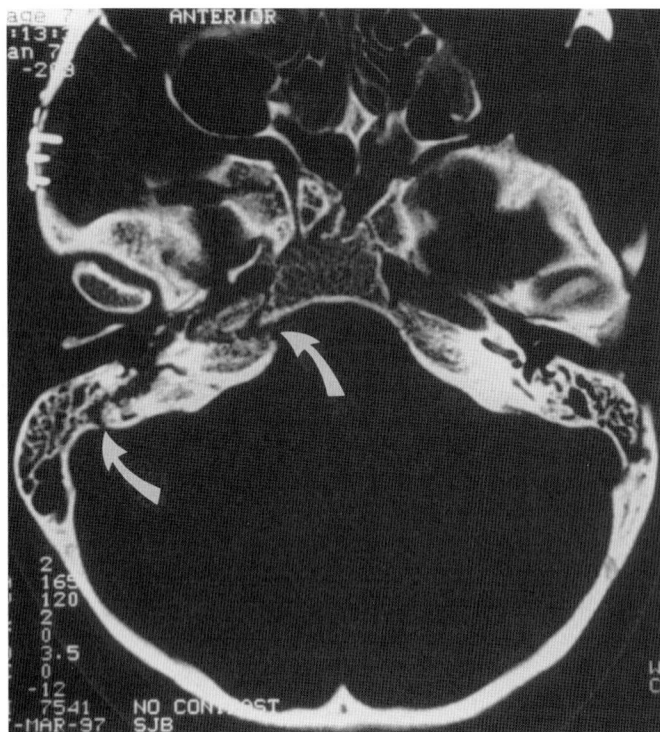

Figure 14–23. CT-demonstrated temporal bone traumatic fractures (arrows) causing the facial nerve palsy in the patient depicted in Fig. 2–25.

The prognosis for recovery in Bell's palsy is worse in patients with hyperacusis, decreased tearing, age greater than 60 years, diabetes, hypertension, and psychiatric disease.[121] Bell's palsy may recur in 10–20% of affected people.

The treatment of idiopathic Bell's palsy remains controversial. Most improve spontaneously, but experts disagree as to whether corticosteroids result in better facial outcomes[122] or whether corticosteroids have any proven effect on the natural course of the disorder.[119,123] Because of the purported viral etiology of Bell's palsy, in some patients acyclovir has also been used. However, one large study failed to show any benefit from acyclovir alone or acyclovir added to corticosteroids.[124] Facial nerve surgical decompression is not widely used and there is currently insufficient evidence to advocate its widespread use.[122,123] Until definitive data are available, in our practice we tend to use prednisone (60 mg p.o. per day for 5 days, then tapered over the next 5 days) when the patient is seen early in his or her course.[125] Treatment may be particularly effective if initiated within several days of symptom onset. If there is any concern regarding the possibility of Lyme disease, we would use acyclovir alone pending further studies (see below).

Neuroimaging is not necessary in typical cases, but when performed an MRI may show enhancement of peripheral portions of the facial nerve.[125]

Ramsay Hunt syndrome. Ramsay Hunt syndrome, or cephalic herpes zoster, is characteristically preceded by a prodrome of severe pain in the affected ear and is followed by a vesicular rash involving the pinna and external auditory canal.[126] The facial palsy may be accompanied by hearing loss, vestibular impairment, or encephalitis in severe cases.

The prognosis for herpes zoster cephalicus is poorer than that for Bell's palsy in terms of complete recovery of facial function, with only 60% of patients having complete return of function.[127]

Otitis media. Acute otitis media with or without mastoiditis may occur and, when chronic, may affect the facial nerve as it courses through the temporal bone. In elderly diabetic patients, malignant external otitis is usually caused by a necrotizing *Pseudomonas* infection that progresses fulminantly. Both intravenous antibiotics and surgery, with wide debridement of necrotic bone and granulation tissue, are necessary. The facial nerve is vulnerable within the fallopian canal and can be affected by adjacent suppuration, abscess formation, or cholesteatoma. The association of a VIth cranial nerve palsy with facial palsy in petrous apex infection (Gradenigo syndrome[128]) is well described and usually responds to antibiotic treatment.

Congenital facial palsy. Most instances of isolated congenital facial palsies are related to birth trauma to the peripheral VIIth nerve, often associated with forceps delivery. However, some cases are familial,[129] and the cause may be neuronal maldevelopment in the brain stem.[130]

Neuromuscular junction, myopathic, and neuropathic causes of facial weakness

Patients with myasthenia gravis and botulism may present with bilateral facial weakness (**Fig. 14–24**). Almost all patients with ptosis or ophthalmoparesis due to myasthenia gravis also have orbicularis oculi weakness. Myotonic dystrophy is also characterized by bilateral weakness of the facial muscles. Facial weakness is also commonly seen in GBS and Miller Fisher syndrome. These disorders are discussed in more detail at the end of this chapter.

Evaluation

One suggested approach is given in **Table 14–3**. A central facial palsy always requires neuroimaging in the workup. The evaluation of peripheral palsies, on the other hand, is usually directed towards excluding inflammatory and infectious causes. The history and examination are critical in determining the extent of the evaluation performed in patients with an isolated facial palsy.

Treatment

Aside from diagnosis and treatment of the underlying cause of the facial palsy, from an ocular standpoint, the major concern with facial paralysis is poor eyelid closure and exposure keratitis.[131] The cornea may become compromised, and corneal pathology may extend from mild drying to ulceration and the potential for visual loss. Many of the functional abnormalities seen with facial nerve palsy are age related. It is not unusual to have a young child with a mild congenital facial nerve palsy or a young individual with a mild acquired palsy completely adapt to their paralysis and require no medical or surgical intervention. On the other hand, reduction of the quality and quantity of the tear film with aging makes the older patient much more susceptible to exposure keratitis. Additionally, there are various degrees of facial

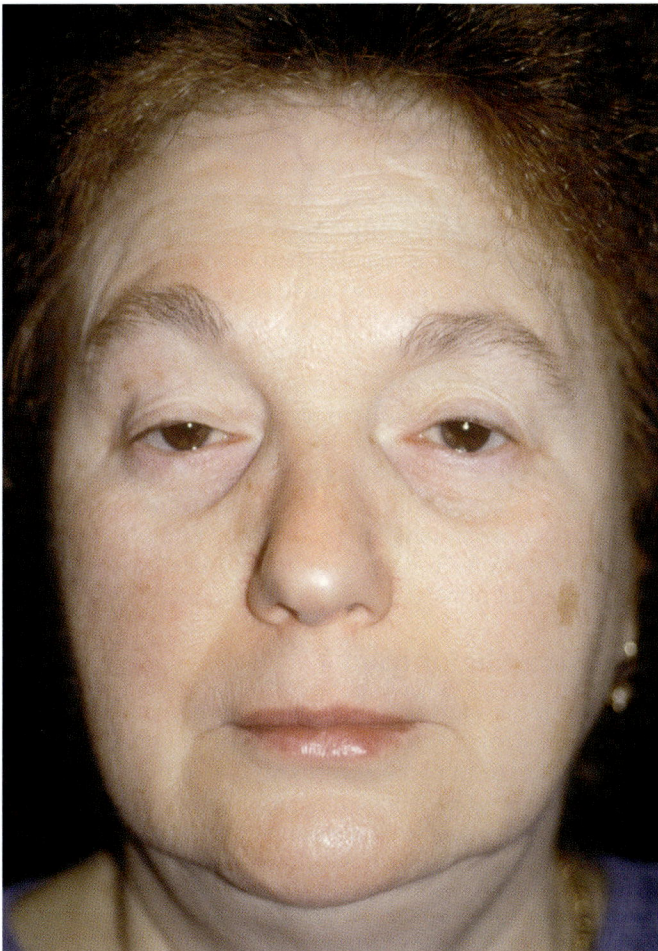

Figure 14–24. Bilateral facial weakness and ptosis in myasthenia gravis. Note the smooth lower face and lack of facial expression.

Table 14–3 Diagnostic considerations in facial nerve palsy (adapted with permission from Handler LF, Galetta SL, Wulc AE, et al. Facial paralysis: diagnosis and management. In: Bosniak S (ed): Principles and Practice of Ophthalmic Plastic and Reconstructive Surgery, pp 465–483, Philadelphia, W.B. Saunders, 1996, with permission)

Clinical problem	Test
Central facial palsy	Brain MRI
Peripheral facial palsy	
Bilateral palsy	Brain MRI, lumbar puncture, EMG (exclude Guillain–Barré syndrome, myotonia), edrophonium test or AchRAb level (exclude myasthenia)
Progressive palsy, dizziness, or associated hearing loss	MRI of cerebellopontine angle
Acute unilateral palsy	Blood glucose level, syphilis serology, and CBC; Lyme titer (endemic area or exposure history); angiotensin-converting enzyme (exclude sarcoid)
Chronic palsy	Chest radiograph (exclude sarcoid, tumor), brain MRI

AchRAb, acetylcholine receptor antibody; CBC, complete blood count; EMG, electromyography; MRI, magnetic resonance imaging.

palsy from partial to complete. Obviously a partial facial palsy may not present any functional or aesthetic problems for the patient other than occasional drying, whereas a complete loss of facial function would make the individual more susceptible to exposure and its related complications. Keratitis is more severe in patients who have neurotrophic keratitis (caused by trigeminal dysfunction, see Chapter 19), and such patients should be observed even more closely. In this section we review the medical and surgical management of facial nerve palsy.

Medical. The treatment of all patients with facial nerve palsy includes some type of topical eye lubricant. An over-the-counter artificial tear product should be the primary treatment in all cases. Some patients will need topical lubrication throughout the course of their disease regardless of any additional medical or surgical treatment. Some patients will want to try several different tear film products as their comfort level varies widely between each type of drop. Also, the dosage schedule will need to be tailored to the individual's needs. Patients can start with a four times a day regimen, but the unpreserved drops can be used as frequently as every 1/2 hour to 1 hour based on the patient's need for lubrication. Initial bedtime coverage would include a petroleum based ointment. Individuals who have severe keratitis may need day- and night-time applications of the ointment. Once

the keratitis has begun to heal the patient may be switched to drops daily and ointment at night. The advantage to this regimen is that the ointment is quite disruptive to visual acuity whereas the less viscous drops are not. Certain environmental aberrations such as windy weather and dry air may prompt the patient to switch ointments for short periods of time in order to maintain corneal comfort.

The next level of management involves additional coverage to the eye at bedtime. As mentioned above, these individuals should be using a protective ointment. Sometimes patients need to have a "moisture bubble" taped over the eye at night after applying the ointment. Options include standard swimming goggles or a small oval of cellophane wrap. Taping the eyelid closed is not always successful. The tape comes off, and if the patient is not skilled at taping the lids, they might tape the lids in an open position. This unfortunate situation might precipitate further irritation of the cornea. Moisture chambers, which are fitted to standard glass frames and molded to the face to create a tight seal, may eventually be required for day-time protection as well.

Surgical. When medical therapies are ineffective or not tolerated or when corneal damage makes more definitive measures imperative, surgical intervention may be indicated. Initial surgical therapy is usually with a temporary tarsorrhaphy, in which the eyelids are temporarily sewn together either partially or completely.[132] We have a low threshold for performing temporary tarsorrhaphies in patients with newly acquired VIIth nerve palsies with severe keratitis, especially those with defective trigeminal nerve function as well. If the VIIth nerve defect persists, then consideration can be given to permanent lateral tarsorrhaphy, medial tarsorrhaphy, lateral canthoplasty, or ectropion repair. These may produce scarring and reduced peripheral vision. Another group of procedures have been developed using various prosthetic devices to improve eyelid function and closure. These include silicone bands, eyelid springs, and eyelid gold weight implants.[133] Silicone bands have been abandoned because of difficulty in assessing the balance between eyelid closing and opening forces. Eyelid springs work well but are often complicated by infection, extrusion, local granuloma formation, and need for readjustment.

Implantation of a gold or platinum eyelid weight is a commonly performed procedure for or platinium eyelid animation, and it is our preferred procedure.[134] During this procedure a small weight (usually around 1 g) is sutured to the orbital septum or upper eyelid tarsus to aid passively in gravity-assisted eyelid closure. Preoperatively, test weights can be taped to the upper eyelid to determine the effects of various sized gold weights. The key is to have adequate weight to close the eye but not enough to cause severe ptosis. Implantation is accomplished through a small upper eyelid incision and the implant is sutured directly to the tarsus[135] or orbital septum through preplaced holes in the implant. Gold is the ideal material because it is heavy, and the color matches the color of fat, rendering it difficult to see through the skin. As well, gold weight implants are compatible with MRI since they are non-magnetic. This is particularly important in patients with VIIth nerve palsy secondary to an intracranial tumor that will require serial neuroimaging studies. Low-profile, thinner gold and platinum weights are also available. Success rates for this procedure are reported to be as high as 90%[133,135–137] with failures generally falling into two groups: unacceptable ptosis or inadequate closure. More rare complications include infections, eyelid contour changes and ectropion.[138] Gold weights rarely spontaneously extrude.[134] They can, however, be surgically removed relatively easily.

Abnormal blinking

A blink is a temporary closure of both eyelids and normally does not interfere with the continuity of vision. The mean ± standard deviation (SD) spontaneous blink rate is 16 ± 9 blinks per minute. Physiologic blinking helps keep the cornea moist and protects the eye from excess light and foreign objects. This section will be subdivided into two opposite parts: absent or decreased blinking and excessive blinking.

Absent or decreased blinking

Spontaneous blinking. Decreased spontaneous blink rates may be characteristic of thyroid-associated ophthalmopathy or parkinsonism (e.g., PD and PSP).[52,139] In patients with parkinsonism, however, reflex blink rates may be increased (see below).

Corneal and supraorbital blink reflexes. If the left ophthalmic division is defective, neither eye will blink to left corneal or forehead stimulation; if the right cornea or forehead is

stimulated in this setting, both eyes will blink. This scenario must be contrasted with the case of a left facial nerve palsy in which only the right eye will blink fully, regardless of which cornea or forehead is stimulated.

In a well-studied phenomenon,[140,141] patients with acute unilateral hemispheric lesions may have a diminished blink reflex when the contralateral cornea or forehead is stimulated. The responsible lesions tend to be large strokes. The defective blink reflex is usually temporary, lasting only 1 or 2 weeks following the ictus. These observations suggest the contralateral hemisphere exerts a supranuclear influence upon the blink reflex, and a cortical lesion may inhibit it.

Blink to visual threat. Patients with hemianopias from occipital and parietal lesions may not blink when approached with a menacing gesture in the defective field. A cardinal feature of cortical blindness is a completely absent blink to visual threat. Those with left-sided visual attention from a right parietal or frontal lesion or with diffusely decreased visual attention from Balint syndrome (see Chapter 9) may have decreased blink to threat in their inattentive fields.[22]

Excessive blinking

Increased blink rates are associated with schizophrenia and Tourette syndrome (see below). In addition, reflex blinking can be increased in parkinsonism. In this setting, the glabellar or Myerson's sign, elicited by tapping on the forehead, is characterized by persistent blinks with each tap.[142] Excessive blinking in childhood is typically benign when the history and examination are unremarkable.[143]

Blepharospasm and hemifacial spasm

Blepharospasm. Essential blepharospasm is an idiopathic dystonic disorder characterized by involuntary intermittent bilateral eyelid closure. It ranges from increased blink frequency to severe, sustained spasms of the orbicularis oculi. Initially only one eye may be affected, but eventually both orbicularis oculi are involved within weeks to months. Wind, sunlight, or stress may exacerbate the spasms,[144] but more chronic cases are characterized by spontaneous eyelid closure. Some more severely affected patients complain of functional blindness. Women are affected more than men, and blepharospasm usually begins in the fourth to sixth decades of life.[145] The cause is unclear, but enhanced blink reflex excitability, perhaps due to a loss of supranuclear inhibition, has been proposed.[146] In one functional imaging study, striatal activation was demonstrated;[147] however, activation of other cortical and basal ganglia regions has also been shown.[148–150] Usually the patient has no underlying cause for the disorder, but blepharospasm may occur in parkinsonism (e.g., PD and PSP),[52] months or years following an episode of Bell's palsy,[151] and in association with a lower pontine lesion.[152] Blepharospasm accompanied by dystonic movements of the lower face or neck (oromandibular dystonia) is termed *Meige syndrome.*

Hemifacial spasm. In hemifacial spasm, the whole face on one side contracts, with eyelid closure and elevation of the corner of the mouth. The movement disorder is thought to be due to either (1) hyperexcitability of the facial motor nucleus, either idiopathically or because of ischemia or a

Video 14.4

Video 14.5

mass lesion in the pons, or (2) compression of the facial nerve near its exit from the brain stem, causing myelin sheath injury and ephaptic transmission between individual nerve fibers.[153] A tortuous AICA or dolichoectatic artery of the posterior circulation is believed to be responsible for the majority of patients with hemifacial spasm.[154] MRI and magnetic resonance (MR) angiography are helpful in demonstrating vascular compression of the pons or facial nerve.[155,156]

Treatment. The treatment of choice in patients with debilitating blepharospasm or hemifacial spasm is localized subcutaneous injections of botulinum-A toxin around the eyelids to weaken the orbicularis oculi, other muscles involved in eyelid closure, and facial movements.[62,152,157–160] Botulinum-A is produced by *Clostridium botulinum* and causes temporary paralysis of injected muscles by interfering with acetylcholine release from nerve terminals. Injection of botulinum into the eyebrow and upper and lower eyelid in patients with blepharospasm, and into these same structures and into the lower facial musculature in patients with hemifacial spasm, has a high degree of initial success with relief of eyelid spasm and patient acceptance.

We usually begin with injections of 2.5 units of botulinum per injection site (**Fig. 14–25**) and agree that avoidance of the middle portion of the upper eyelid reduces the risk of ptosis. The exact sites of the injections can be varied from patient to patient depending on in which areas the patient has the most spasms. One study evaluated these standard injection sites and compared them with injection sites

further from the eyelid margin and in the brow.[161] This study found that, for blepharospasm patients, standard injections had the longest duration but were associated with increased transient ocular side-effects including irritation and epiphora. In the hemifacial spasm patients, brow treatment was as effective as standard treatment.

Clinical experience has traditionally been that initial treatments are the most successful and, with time, the effect of each injection may be less or tend to last for a shorter period. Reduced efficacy may be the result of antitoxin development, binding of the non-active large protein chain, or a resprouting of motor end plates.[162,163] In this setting a larger amount of botulinum can be given with each injection (5 units). Other studies, however, have failed to demonstrate a reduced effectiveness or shorter duration of treatment with time.[164,165] Greater than 90% of patients report a marked decrease in the squeezing action of the eyelids and twitching in lower part of the face.[157,166–171] The effect generally lasts between 1 and 4 months and tends to persist longer in hemifacial spasm than in blepharospasm. Because of its transient effect, the procedure must be repeated indefinitely.

Complications of botulinum injections include lagophthalmos and exposure keratitis which generally lasts several days and can be treated with lubricants and taping if necessary. Patients may develop tearing from keratitis or poor tear pump function. Sagging of the eyelid skin and brow may occur. More concerning complications result from deep penetration and include ptosis and double vision.[161] Ptosis develops in about 8% of patients.[172] Double vision occurs in 2% of patients and the inferior oblique muscle is the most commonly affected muscle.[173] Systemic complications do not occur, although systemic antibody production has been reported in patients receiving botulinum injections for hemifacial spasm or blepharospasm.[174]

If botulinum toxin fails, medications such as benzodiazepines, anticholinergic agents, dopamine agonists, anticonvulsants, and presynaptic dopamine-depleting agents may help some patients,[175] but their use is usually limited by side-effects. In patients with refractory hemifacial spasm, a Teflon sponge can be placed between the AICA and facial nerve. Other more drastic measures include myectomy, during which the orbicularis oculi and other muscles used in eyelid closure are excised (either surgically[171] or chemically[176]), or neurectomy, a procedure in which branches of the facial nerve are cut.[169]

The importance of support groups for these patients has recently been emphasized in a report by Anderson and associates,[171] who found support group intervention was the most effective therapy in blepharospasm. Ultimately, most patients (70%) continue to receive botulinum injections while a few (7%) spontaneously improve, and others benefit from pharmacotherapy, surgery, or psychotherapy.[170] Tinted lenses to ameliorate photophobia in patients with blepharospasm have also been recommended.[144,177]

Other causes of excessive blinking

Physiologic facial synkineses. Following injury of the peripheral facial nerve, abnormal reinnervation patterns may be observed as motor function recovers. Eyelid closure upon smiling or vice versa (**Fig. 14–26**) are caused by incorrect

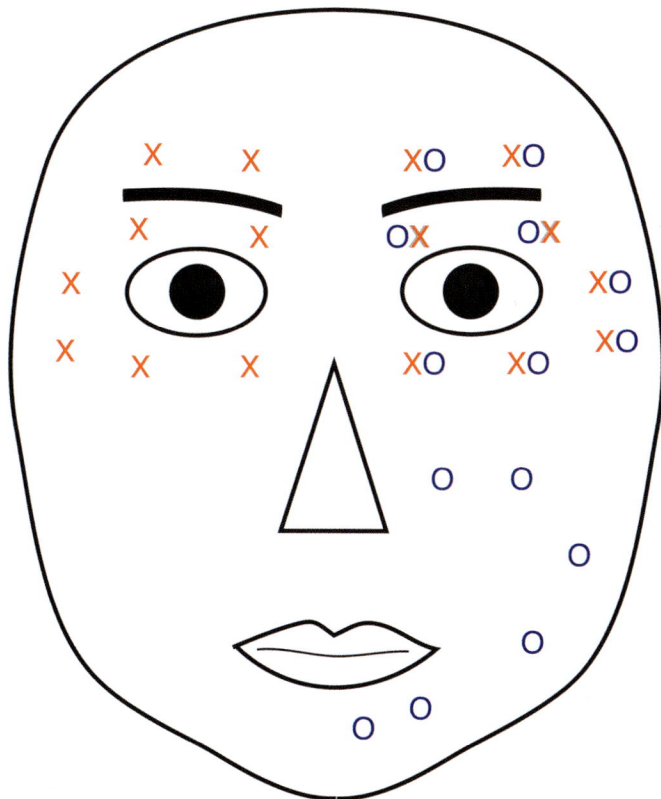

Figure 14–25. Injection sites for botulinum A toxin in patients with blepharospasm (Xs) and hemifacial spasm (Os). Injection volume is usually 0.1 ml and initial dose is 2.5 units of botulinum A toxin per injection site.

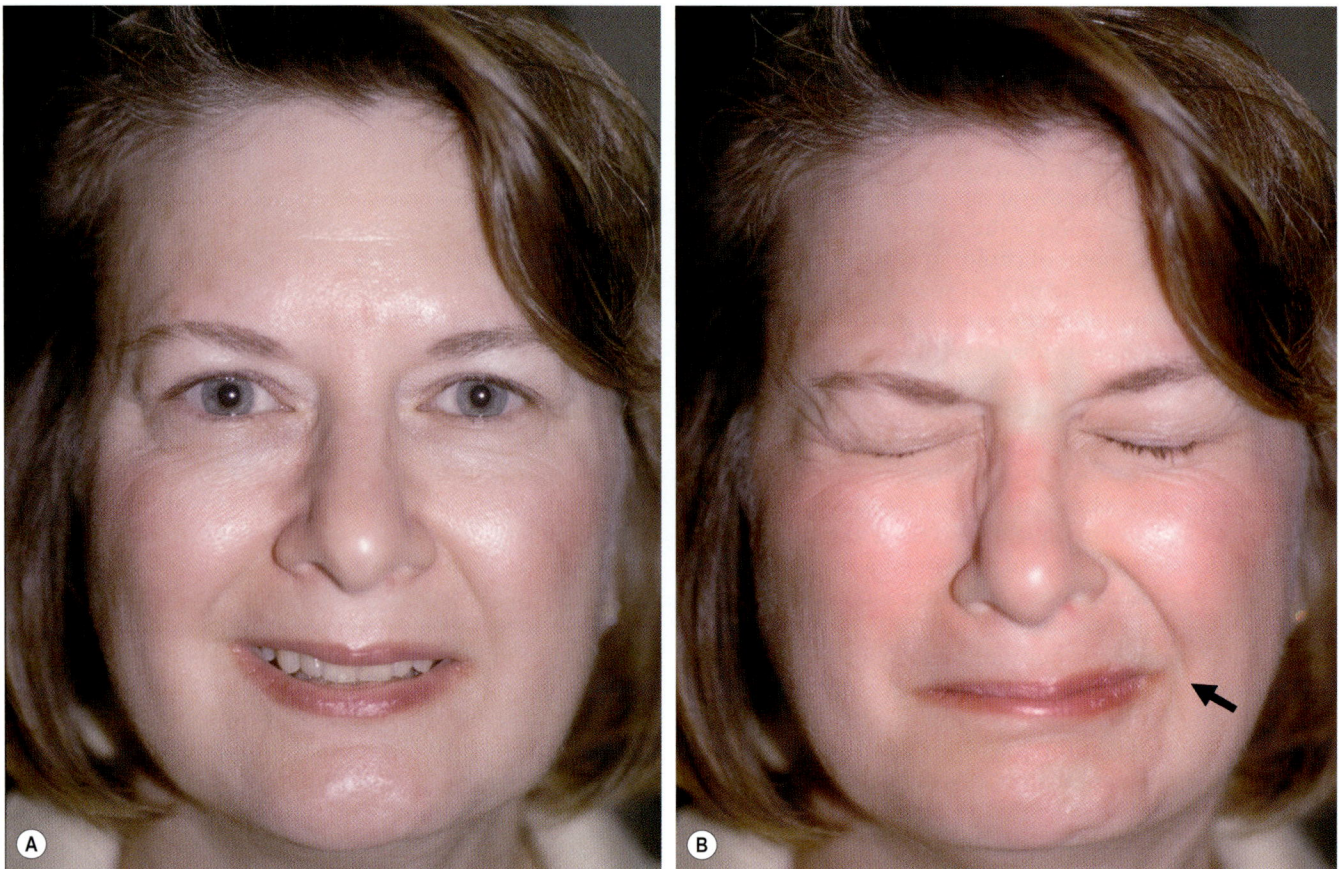

Figure 14–26. Facial synkinesis (aberrant regeneration). **A.** Patient with old left facial palsy following removal of left acoustic neuroma. **B.** Upon attempted eyelid closure, the orbicularis oris on the left (arrow) also contracts.

reinnervation by orbicularis oculi and zygomaticus motor neurons.[178] Tearing in anticipation of eating food (crocodile tears) occurs when nerve fibers destined to supply the salivary glands are misdirected to the lacrimal gland. Other proposed mechanisms, such as ephaptic transmission and central reorganization of synaptic inputs to facial motor neurons, are unlikely (see discussion of oculomotor synkinesis, Chapter 15).

Eyelid tics. These are brief, stereotyped, repetitive, and involuntary eyelid blinks, winks, or blepharospasm.[175] Affected patients may have a preceding urge before their tics, and they may be able to suppress them. Often idiopathic and considered benign motor tics, they can also be associated with encephalitis, drugs, toxins, stroke, head trauma, and static encephalopathies. Usually they do not require treatment. However, in some instances eyelid tics are a first manifestation of Tourette syndrome. This is a childhood disorder, affecting boys more than girls, in which eyelid and facial tics can be associated with tics in the limbs or body.[179] Characteristic behavioral manifestations of Tourette syndrome include obsessive–compulsive disorder, grunting, throat clearing, barking, copralalia, and echolalia.[180,181]

Myokymia and neuromyotonia. Small unilateral contractions of the facial muscles characterize *facial myokymia*, which, when associated with ipsilateral facial contracture and weakness (spastic–paretic facial contracture), indicates a pontine lesion rostral to the VIIth nerve nucleus. Multiple

sclerosis and brain stem tumors are the typical etiologies.[182,183] Other causes of facial myokymia include stroke, syringobulbia, hydrocephalus, acoustic neuroma, GBS, hypoxic injury, and meningitis. *Eyelid myokymia*, which are small, annoying twitches of the upper or lower eyelids, are very common. They are benign and usually due to stress, fatigue, nicotine, or caffeine. Most patients require only reassurance, as eyelid myokymia usually abates spontaneously. Occasionally it persists and in such instances can be treated with benzodiazepines or botulinum.[184] *Facial neuromyotonia*, which is similar to myokymia but is defined as a delay in muscle relaxation after a voluntary contraction, has been reported as a complication of radiation and responds to carbemazepine.[185]

Abnormal facial movements in other movement disorders. Blepharospasm and other involuntary movements of the face may be seen in Parkinson disease, progressive supranuclear palsy, Huntington disease, and Wilson disease.

Drug-induced facial dyskinesias. Use of antiemetics such as metoclopramide, neuroleptics including haloperidol, as well as antihistamines may lead to tardive dyskinesia, which may involve the face and eyes.[186] In such cases, patients develop a stereotyped, writhing unilateral or bilateral eyelid closure. The diagnosis is usually evident after eliciting the medication history. Treatment consists of withdrawing the offending agent, sometimes combined with the use of botulinum injections in refractory cases.

Focal motor seizures. Unilateral facial movements or eyelid closure which is repetitive, brief, and followed by weakness (Todd's paralysis) would suggest a focal motor seizure involving the face. Spread to the hands or limbs, or generalization to involve the other side of the face or body with loss of consciousness, would make this diagnosis obvious. Evaluation would consist of an electroencephalogram (EEG) and neuroimaging to detect a structural seizure focus, followed by treatment with anticonvulsants.

Palpebromandibular synkinesia. Spontaneous eyelid blinking associated with anterolateral jaw movements may be seen in bilateral cortical disease or upper brain stem lesions sparing the pons.[21]

Other abnormal eyelid and facial movements

Oculomasticatory myorhythmia. This movement disorder is characterized by slow (1 Hz) pendular convergent–divergent nystagmus associated with rhythmic movements of the muscles of mastication, face, and extremities. It is considered virtually pathognomonic of Whipple disease, which is caused by the bacillus *Tropheryma whippelii* (see Chapter 16).

Eyelid nystagmus. A slow downward drift of the eyelids followed by a quick corrective upward flick may be observed in myasthenia gravis and brain stem lesions, particularly mesencephalic ones.[187] Naturally, eyelid nystagmus may also be observed with vertical nystagmus of the eyes, particularly upbeat. Eyelid nystagmus may be observed in medullary lesions with lateral gaze shifts. Other terms for this phenomenon include lid hopping and upper lid jerks. The mechanism is unclear, but typically eyelid nystagmus is evoked by convergence[188] or horizontal gaze.[3]

Others. Paroxysmal eyelid movements such as fluttering can occur during seizures.[189] Seesaw-like eyelid movements have also been reported in a child with trisomy 2p.[190]

Diseases commonly associated with ptosis and/or facial weakness

Diseases to be discussed here include three neuromuscular junction disorders: myasthenia gravis, Lambert–Eaton myasthenic syndrome, and botulism; several myopathic disorders: chronic external ophthalmoplegia and Kearns–Sayre syndrome, myotonic dystrophy, and oculopharyngeal dystrophy; and polyneuropathies such as GBS, Miller Fisher syndrome, and chronic inflammatory demyelinating polyneuropathy. These are all neuromuscular conditions whose neuro-ophthalmic presentation can be predominantly ptosis and/or facial weakness.

Myasthenia gravis

This neurotransmission disorder is characterized by fatiguable muscular weakness. The eyelids and extraocular muscles are involved in over 90% of patients. Fifty percent present with ptosis or ocular motility abnormalities only,[191] and, of this group, approximately half will remain "ocular myasthenics," while the other half will develop generalized symptoms, usually within 2 years.[192] There is an approximately 22% spontaneous remission rate.[193]

Myasthenia has a prevalence of 50–125 cases per million population, with a sex- and age-related bimodal distribution consisting of women in their twenties and thirties and men in their sixties and seventies.[194] The incidence of later onset myasthenia may be increasing.[195] One study[196] suggested younger patients had a better prognosis than those who presented when older than 50. Rarely, another member of the family also has a history of myasthenia.

Pathophysiology. A reduction in the number of available acetylcholine receptors of skeletal muscles (**Fig. 14–27**) results in a defect in neuromuscular transmission and weakness. A humorally mediated autoimmune attack directed against acetylcholine receptors causes their

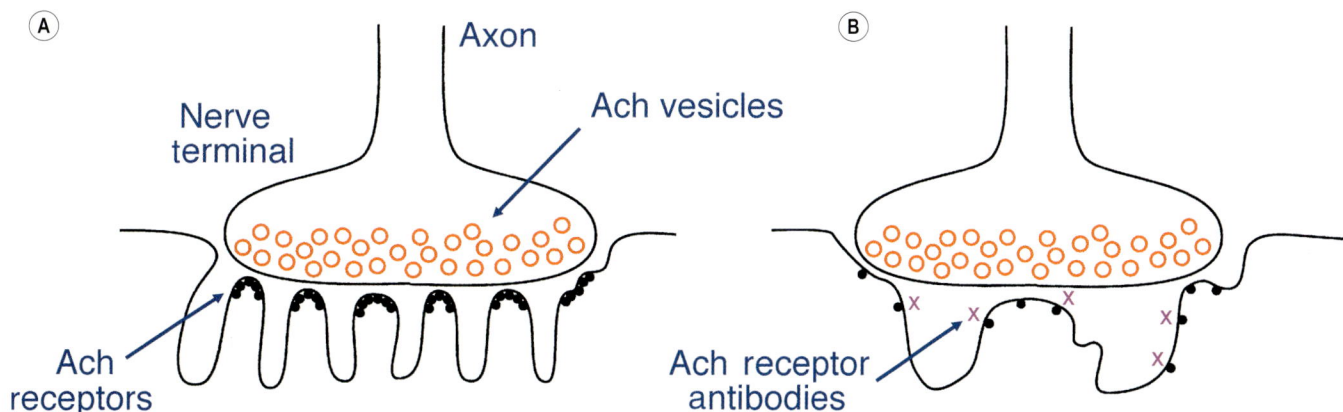

Figure 14–27. Drawing of the neuromuscular junction (Ach, acetylcholine). **A.** Normally, presynaptic nerve depolarization causes calcium influx then release of vesicles containing acetylcholine into the synaptic cleft. Acetylcholine binds to acetylcholine receptors at the junctional folds of the postsynaptic muscle membrane. This triggers ion channel opening and generation of an endplate potential, which in turn creates a muscle membrane action potential. Acetylcholinesterase (not shown) breaks down acetylcholine. **B.** In myasthenia gravis, a humorally mediated autoimmune attack by antibodies (Xs) directed against acetylcholine receptors causes their blockade, accelerated degradation, and complement-mediated damage. This results in a defect in neuromuscular transmission and muscle weakness.

blockade, accelerated degradation, and complement-mediated damage.[194,197,198] Both production of high-affinity IgG antibodies and sensitization of anti-acetylcholine receptor antibody CD4+ T-helper cells are observed.[199]

Usually the cause of this autoimmune disorder is unknown. However, in some cases it is drug-induced in association with the use of D-penicillamine, for instance. Anti-acetylcholine receptor antibodies may be produced, and, when the D-penicillamine is removed, often symptoms and receptor antibody levels normalize.[200] Drug-induced, antibody-positive myasthenia has also been reported in association with atorvastatin.[201] Several drugs, such as aminoglycosides, nitrofurantoin, beta-blockers, and quinidine, may exacerbate myasthenia gravis by their direct effects on the neuromuscular junction and neuromuscular blockade.[202–205]

Thymus hyperplasia and thymoma, the latter in approximately 15% of adult patients, are related findings. Myasthenia gravis also occurs frequently in association with other autoimmune disturbances such as hyperthyroidism (3–8% of patients with myasthenia[194]) and systemic lupus erythematosus.

Preferential involvement of extraocular muscles. Kaminski and colleagues[206,207] have reviewed the possible reasons why the eye muscles are frequently involved and sometimes solely affected in myasthenia gravis. These include (1) only mild extraocular muscle weakness is enough to cause ocular misalignment and symptomatic diplopia, (2) the high firing frequencies of extraocular muscles may predispose them to myasthenic fatigue, (3) extraocular muscle fibers may be more susceptible to neuromuscular blockade, and (4) extraocular muscles may contain antigens specific to them which make them more susceptible to immune attack. Although the fetal gamma subunit of the acetylcholine receptor in extraocular muscles was proposed as one such antigen,[208] in one study[209] the frequency of this subunit was found to be as common in eye as in other muscles. Alternatively, it is possible that there is another, yet unidentified, autoantibody in myasthenia gravis which preferentially affects the extraocular muscles.[210]

Symptoms and signs. Symptoms. Variable and fatiguable ptosis, diplopia, chewing difficulties, dysarthria, dysphagia, dyspnea, and systemic weakness are the hallmarks of myasthenia gravis. Most patients' symptoms exhibit diurnal variation, as their weakness is better in the morning or after sleep than at the end of the day, when they are weakest.

Neuro-ophthalmic signs. Eyelid abnormalities are frequently the most prominent ocular sign, and these include ptosis, fatiguability, Cogan's lid twitch, curtaining, and orbicularis oculi weakness (**Table 14–4**). None of these are pathognomonic of myasthenia,[211,212] but, when they are all present, this diagnosis should be strongly considered. Pupil-sparing ophthalmoplegia of any pattern may also be seen.

Video 14.1

1. *Ptosis.* Myasthenic eyelid drooping, due to weakness of the levator palpebrae muscles, can be symmetric or asymmetric. The patient may adopt a chin-up position to look underneath the ptotic eyelids and raise the eyebrows and furrow the brow to keep the eyelids open (**Fig. 14–28**). When asymmetric, the eyelid which is

Table 14–4 Common eyelid signs in ocular myasthenia gravis

Ptosis—asymmetric or symmetric
Cogan's lid twitch
Curtaining (enhanced ptosis)
Fatigue
Weakness of eyelid closure

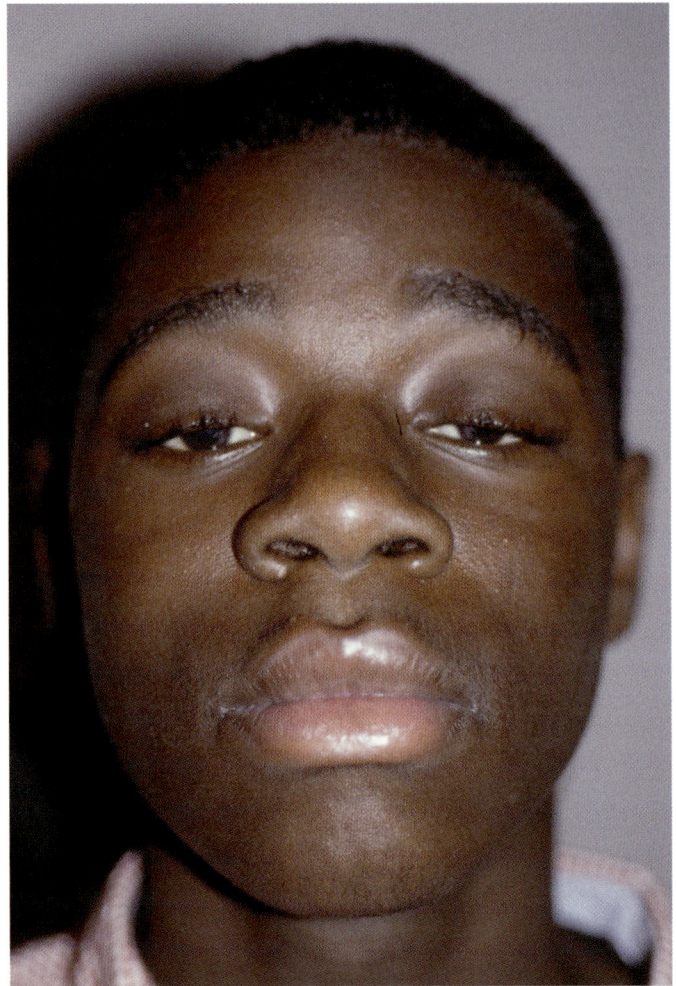

Figure 14–28. Severe bilateral ptosis in myasthenia gravis with chin-up position. In an attempt to lift the eyelids, the frontalis muscle is contracted and the brow is elevated.

affected more may alternate over time (so-called "alternating ptosis") (**Fig. 14–29**). The pattern of ptosis and contralateral pseudo-retraction reflects Hering's Law and the patient's increased effort to elevate both levator muscles.

Levator function in myasthenia is related to the amount of ptosis; those with prominent ptosis will have the most impaired levator function. Normal levator function in the setting of marked ptosis argues against the diagnosis of myasthenia.[213] Documentation of a change in levator function is one objective method to assess an improvement of ptosis.

2. *Fatiguability.* If the patient is asked to maintain upgaze, the eyelids may tire and droop because of levator

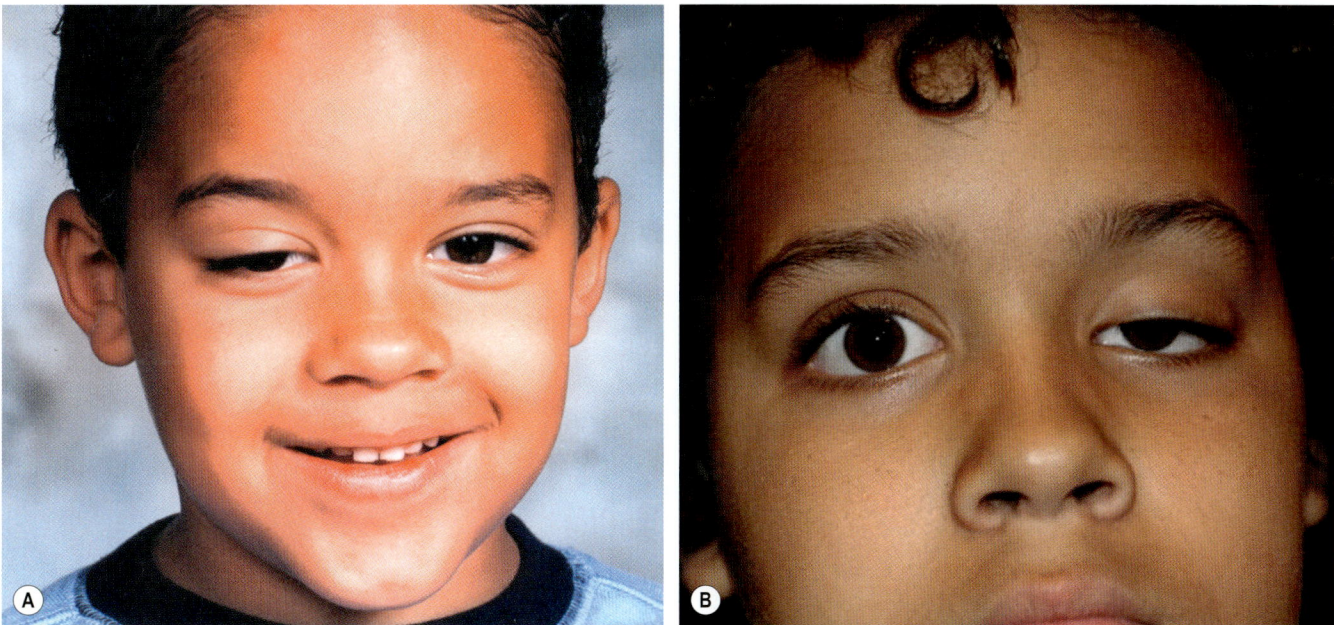

Figure 14–29. Alternating ptosis in ocular myasthenia gravis. This patient developed ptosis in the right eye (**A**), which resolved, then several years later developed ptosis in the left eye (**B**).

fatigue. Although characteristic of myasthenia, fatiguable ptosis may sometimes also be seen in other causes of ptosis.[214]

3. *Cogan's lid twitch*. If a patient with myasthenic ptosis looks downward for 3–5 seconds, then looks up quickly into primary gaze, the eyelid appears to overshoot upwards, then quickly falls.[212,215] One purported mechanism for the overshoot is a build-up of acetylcholine in the neuromuscular junctions of levator muscle fibers while the eyelid is resting in downgaze. Following upward refixation, the levator quickly fatigues, and the eyelid droops.

4. *Curtaining and enhanced ptosis*. In asymmetric ptosis, when the more ptotic eyelid is manually elevated, the fellow eyelid often droops (curtaining) (see **Fig. 14–9**). This sign is nonspecific, and can be seen in many other situations with asymmetric ptosis such as IIIrd nerve palsy. When the ptosis is symmetric, elevation of one eyelid will worsen the other eyelid (enhanced ptosis) (see **Fig. 14–10**). As discussed earlier, these eyelid signs are consequences of Hering's Law, as manual elevation of a ptotic eyelid reduces the patient's required effort to elevate the eyelids, and the other eyelid falls.

5. *Orbicularis oculi weakness*. In almost all patients with myasthenic ptosis or ophthalmoplegia, the orbicularis oculi are also weak, causing deficient eyelid closure (**Fig. 14–30**). In the related *lid peak sign*, if a patient with myasthenic weakness of the orbicularis oculi is asked to maintain vigorous closure of the eyelids, the orbicularis may tire, allowing the palpebral fissures to open.

6. *Lid hopping*. During attempted lateral gaze, the eyelids may appear to hop or jump.[216]

The pupils are normal, and this should distinguish myasthenic ptosis from that of Horner syndrome or a IIIrd nerve palsy.

Ophthalmoparesis. Myasthenic ocular motility abnormalities, which are very common, are reviewed in Chapter 15. These can mimic any pupil-sparing IIIrd nerve palsy, or IVth or VIth nerve palsy, or supranuclear or nuclear gaze paresis.

Other signs. The lower facial muscles may be sufficiently involved so the patient is unable to smile, whistle, pucker, or hold air in the cheeks.[217] Chewing difficulties may occur secondary to masseter weakness. When the oropharyngeal muscles are affected, speech may be nasal, and tongue protrusion may be weak. Neck flexor muscles are typically affected more than neck extensors in myasthenia. Any limb muscle may be weak. Deep tendon reflexes are decreased only in patients with severe weakness. Since myasthenia involves only the neuromuscular system, mental status and sensation are normal. Myasthenic crisis refers to life-threatening impairment of respiration.[194]

Although more useful for clinical studies than in everyday practice, the Osserman grading scheme can be used to classify severity of myasthenia: grade I, ocular involvement only; IIa, mild generalized; IIb, moderate generalized; III, acute fulminant; or IV, severe late.

Diagnostic testing. The diagnosis of myasthenia gravis should be confirmed by at least one of the following tests: antibody levels, repetitive stimulation, single fiber electromyography, or edrophonium testing.[218] Ice or rest testing can be performed and may be suggestive of the diagnosis, but they are not as definitive as the other tests.

Antibody testing. Anti-acetylcholine receptor antibodies are detected in 50–75% of ocular myasthenic patients and in 80–90% with generalized disease.[219–221] These antibodies are entirely specific for myasthenia gravis,[219] but their levels do

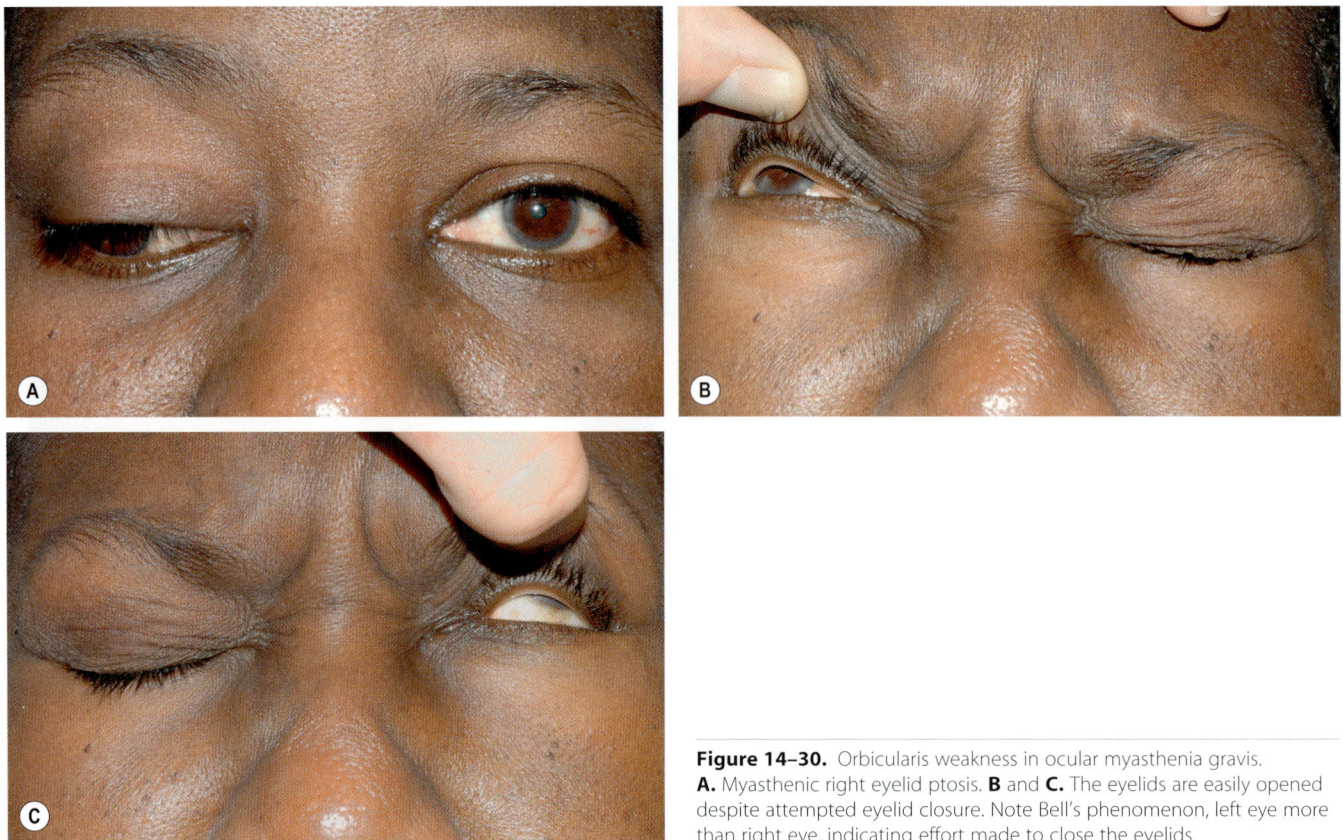

Figure 14–30. Orbicularis weakness in ocular myasthenia gravis. **A.** Myasthenic right eyelid ptosis. **B** and **C.** The eyelids are easily opened despite attempted eyelid closure. Note Bell's phenomenon, left eye more than right eye, indicating effort made to close the eyelids.

not necessarily correlate with the presence or severity of the disease. Antibody tests that measure the accelerated degradation or blockage of acetylcholine receptors may occasionally be positive in seronegative individuals.[194] Also, antibodies against components of striated muscle may be detected in myasthenia gravis. They have a low sensitivity but high specificity for myasthenia gravis,[198] and they also suggest the presence of thymoma. In addition, some presumably seronegative patients may in fact have low-affinity anti-acetylcholine receptor antibodies.[222]

Other patients without demonstrable anti-acetylcholine receptor antibodies may be found to have antibodies to muscle-specific kinase (MuSK). The exact mechanism by which MuSK antibodies cause myasthenic symptoms is unclear.[223,224] In contrast to those with anti-acetylcholine receptor antibodies, myasthenic patients positive for MuSK have more bulbar symptoms and facial and tongue muscle weakness and atrophy,[225,226] their disease may be more severe, more difficult to treat,[227,228] and may correlate with antibody levels.[229] Ocular manifestations are less common, and solely ocular myasthenia is very rare in those positive for MuSK antibodies.[230]

Electromyography. A decrement of the compound muscle action potential during repetitive nerve stimulation (2–5 Hz) of limb or facial muscles is diagnostic in many cases of myasthenia gravis.[231] Additional single fiber electromyographic (EMG) studies may be helpful in ocular myasthenia if the repetitive stimulation, edrophonium test, and antibody studies are nondiagnostic or cannot be performed. Normally, two muscle fibers innervated by the same motor axon will exhibit a variation, called jitter, in the time interval between their two action potentials during successive impulses. Jitter, detected by single fiber electromyography, can be increased in myasthenia gravis and other disorders of neuromuscular transmission.[232] Normally, a limb muscle is studied first, and, if negative, one of the facial muscles, for instance the orbicularis oris, oculi, or frontalis, is next evaluated. Patients who have only ocular symptoms but have an abnormal EMG when a limb muscle is tested are still considered to have only ocular myasthenia. By testing the orbicularis oculi muscles, one study found abnormal findings in 13 out of 14 (93%) myasthenic patients.[233] However, caution should be used when using single fiber electromyography to distinguish between ocular myasthenia gravis and chronic progressive external ophthalmoparesis (CPEO). One study[234] found that patients with CPEO may have abnormal jitter, while none of the patients with CPEO had an abnormal single fiber EMG in another study.[233] Although extraocular muscles and the levator muscle can be evaluated using single fiber electromyography,[235] they are not normally investigated by this technique in most neurophysiology laboratories. In patients with mild myasthenia, the combination of single fiber electromyography, anti-acetylcholine receptor antibody studies, and the edrophonium test should provide the laboratory confirmation of myasthenia gravis in at least 95% of patients.[236]

Edrophonium test. Edrophonium, an acetylcholinesterase inhibitor with rapid onset and short duration of effect, may be administered to slow the breakdown and increase the availability of acetylcholine in the neuromuscular junction.

In patients with myasthenia gravis, many of the eyelid, ocular motor, or systemic signs may objectively improve, thereby verifying the diagnosis (see **Fig. 14–9**).[237] The edrophonium test is positive in 80–90% of patients with myasthenia gravis.[233,236] The test should be performed only in those with obvious ptosis or ophthalmoparesis, in whom improvement can easily be observed.[238]

Edrophonium may be drawn up in a 1 ml tuberculin syringe and administered intravenously in 2 mg increments separated by 30–60 seconds up to a total of 10 mg. The advantage of the incremental method of edrophonium administration is that the full 10 mg dose may not be required to produce a positive response. Furthermore, over-medicating the patient and occasionally missing the point of ocular recovery can be avoided. The test can be terminated at any point or after the patient has received the full 10 mg dose if no response has occurred. If an intravenous line is used instead of a tuberculin syringe, flushing the line with normal saline is necessary to ensure that the edrophonium has been delivered to the bloodstream.

Optimally, an edrophonium test requires a team effort with one individual administering the drug, another documenting the clinical findings, and a third monitoring the blood pressure and pulse. Occasionally patients develop salivation and mild gastrointestinal discomfort. Atropine 0.4 mg should be ready in a separate syringe and administered intravenously if symptomatic bradycardia occurs. Cardiac monitoring or avoiding the test is suggested in patients with a history of heart disease or arrhythmia. Because of these potential side-effects, the increasing popularity of the more simple ice and rest tests (see below), and the increasing difficulty in obtaining edrophonium, many clinicians now only rarely perform the test.

In patients with myasthenic ptosis, the response to edrophonium is often dramatic and occurs within seconds or minutes of injection. Paradoxical worsening of ptosis should not be considered a positive test. The edrophonium test in patients with ocular dysmotility is discussed in more detail in Chapter 15. Eyelid twitching, tearing, and abdominal cramping are signs that the edrophonium has taken effect.[239] The edrophonium lasts for just a few minutes. Placebo injections are not necessary in patients with ptosis, which is almost never functional.

The edrophonium test unfortunately has many false negatives and positives. For unclear reasons, some individuals with myasthenia, confirmed by other test parameters (see below), may have an equivocal or no response to edrophonium. In contrast, clinical improvement with edrophonium may be observed in other disorders of neuromuscular transmission such as Lambert–Eaton myasthenic syndrome (see below), botulism, and organophosphate toxicity. In addition, patients whose ptosis and eye movements unequivocally improved with edrophonium, who later were found to have skull base tumors, have been described.[211] Therefore, a positive edrophonium test should not be the sole basis for making a diagnosis of myasthenia gravis.

Intramuscular neostigmine may be used instead of edrophonium in children who may be uncooperative for an intravenous infusion or too agitated to monitor over a short period of time or in adults whose signs are subtle and a longer period of observation is desired.[239,240] For adults, 1.5 mg of neostigmine and 0.6 mg of atropine sulfate are drawn up into a syringe and injected intramuscularly. The dose for children of neostigmine is 0.04 mg/kg, not to exceed a total of 1.5 mg.[241] The effect of intramuscular neostigmine usually begins by 15 minutes and is maximal by 30 minutes.[241]

Ice pack, rest, and sleep tests. If the patient has a cardiac history, one could try the noninvasive ice pack or sleep tests.[242,243] In the ice pack test, a bag of ice is placed over the affected lid for 1 minute and then whether there is improvement in ptosis or not is noted. The ice test has a relatively high (80%) sensitivity and specificity (100%) for myasthenia gravis, and even patients with a negative edrophonium test may have a positive ice pack test, demonstrating its added benefit as a diagnostic test.[242,244] The precise mechanism by which cooling improves myasthenic weakness is unclear. Enhanced transmitter release, reduced acetylcholinesterase activity, and increased receptor sensitization with lower temperature are possible mechanisms.[242] However, similar improvement of ptosis may occur with warm packs as well,[245] suggesting it is the resting, rather than the temperature, which is important. Nevertheless, one study showed that the ice test resulted in greater improvement in myasthenic ptosis than rest alone.[246] In the rest or sleep tests, the patient is allowed to rest, relax, or sleep for approximately 30 minutes to see if rest improves the ptosis (**Fig. 14–31**).[243]

Imaging. If there is any concern that the eyelid and ocular motility abnormalities are suggestive of more central rather

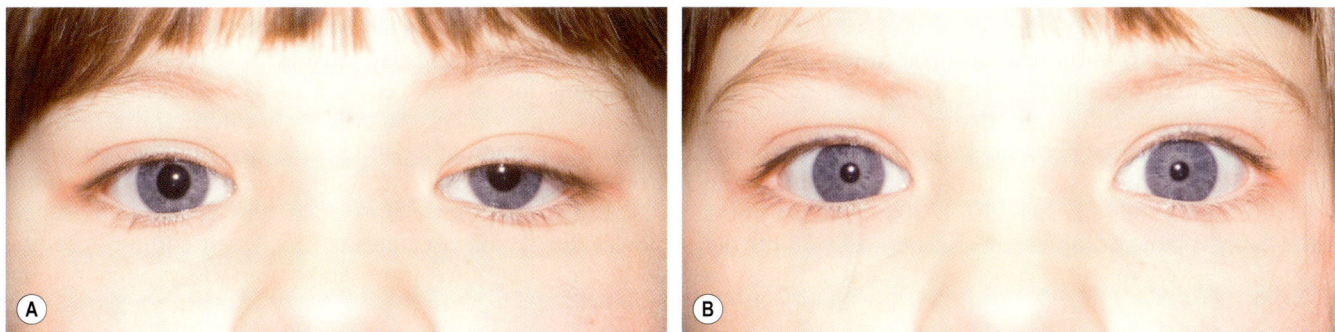

Figure 14–31. Positive rest test in myasthenia gravis. **A.** This girl with ocular myasthenia gravis exhibited ptosis in both eyes, left more than right. **B.** After resting in a dimly lit room with the eyelids gently closed for 20 minutes, both eyelids elevated and returned to normal.

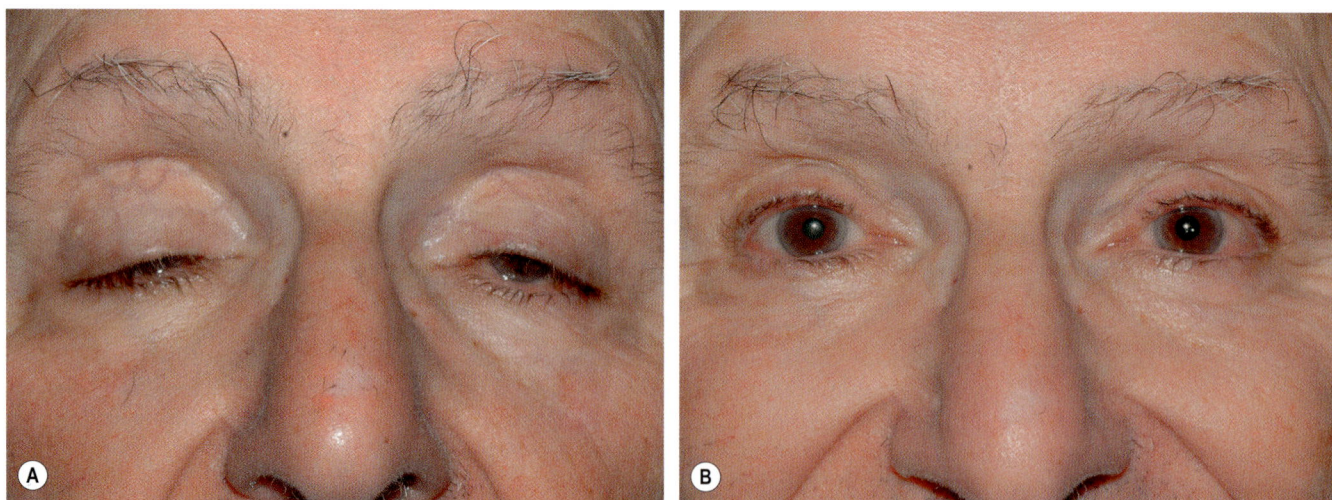

Figure 14–32. Ocular myasthenia treated with corticosteroids. **A.** Severe bilateral ptosis at presentation. **B.** The ptosis resolved completely after 1 month of corticosteroids. The patient also presented with ophthalmoplegia (not shown), which also improved with the corticosteroid treatment.

Table 14–5 Therapeutic options in ocular myasthenia gravis

1.	Symptomatic relief—pharmacologic Pyridostigmine
2.	Symptomatic relief—conservative Eyelid crutches Patching
3.	Disease suppression Corticosteroids Azathioprine Cyclosporine Mycophenolate mofetil
4.	Potential cure Thymectomy

than neuromuscular origin, then an MRI of the brain is mandatory. Computed tomography (CT)or MRI of the chest should be performed to exclude a thymoma in all cases.

Treatment. Patients with myasthenia gravis are treated with acetylcholinesterase inhibitors, plasmapheresis, intravenous gammaglobulin, immunodulators, or thymectomy, either alone or in combination (**Table 14–5**).[247] Treatment decisions are based upon the presence of bulbar or generalized symptoms, age, and disease severity. Unfortunately the treatment of ocular myasthenia has not been studied with rigorous randomized, controlled, clinical trials.[248,249]

Medical treatment. Although corticosteroids are more effective in ocular myasthenia than pyridostigmine,[250] the latter is typically used first in patients with ocular or mild generalized myasthenia because of its milder side-effect profile. Pyridostigmine, an acetylcholinesterase inhibitor, can be given orally at a starting dose of 30 mg every 4 hours while awake. The medication can be increased by 30 mg per dose, up to 120–150 mg every 4 hours, and a timespan preparation can be given at night-time to aid breathing, bulbar function, and weakness overnight and upon awakening. The response to pyridostigmine is variable, and it seems most effective at alleviating many of the bulbar and systemic symptoms, somewhat effective at improving ptosis, but relatively ineffective for diplopia. Tachyphylaxis and overmedication, inducing cholinergic crisis, rarely occur.[251] The most common side-effects are diarrhea and cramping, which resolves with lowering the dosage or can be alleviated with loperamide, glycopyrrolate, or diphenoxylate with atropine. The last two drugs decrease respiratory secretions.

In patients who fail or who cannot tolerate pyridostigmine, corticosteroids, the most effective immunosuppressive agent for myasthenia gravis,[252] can be tried next. Their use, however, must be weighed against the possible short- and long-term steroid-related side-effects. One suggested regimen starts patients at low alternate day doses (e.g., prednisone 10 mg q.o.d.), with slow weekly increases to achieve 60 mg q.o.d.[198] H_2-blockers for ulcer prophylaxis are often added. The prednisone dose can be tapered once therapeutic efficacy is reached, typically after a few months (**Fig. 14–32**). Starting with lower doses decreases the potential for steroid-induced worsening of symptoms in moderate to severe generalized myasthenia, but this complication rarely occurs in patients with predominantly ocular findings.[253] Therefore, in patients with purely ocular myasthenia, another alternative is to start patients at higher initial doses at 40–80 mg q.d.[254] Symptoms usually begin to improve more rapidly within the first 2–4 weeks. When the maximal effect, which may not be evident for 3–6 months, is reached, the dose can be tapered slowly. Every other dose is reduced by 5 mg per week, until a complete alternate day dosing is achieved. Then the remaining dose is reduced by 5 mg per week as well. Most patients on corticosteroids chronically require a small amount of alternate day dosing. A critical dose where worsening may occur is usually around 20 mg every other day. Failed attempts at dose reduction can be followed by slower dose reduction rates, an increased ending dose, the addition of another immunosuppressive, or thymectomy (see below).[255]

Some authorities have argued that lid crutches for ptosis or patching for diplopia are better conservative measures than corticosteroids in patients with ocular myasthenia,[256] or that the benefits (proven or otherwise) do not outweigh the risks of treatment.[257] However, we have found that many patients find these alternatives unacceptable, especially those who require stereoscopic vision for their occupation and for whom external appearance is an issue, and prefer using corticosteroids as long as side-effects are monitored and kept to a minimum.[258] Corticosteroids might also reduce the risk of conversion to generalized myasthenia (see below).[259] Surgical correction of ptosis in general is not recommended because of the variability of the eyelid drooping. However, select patients with ptosis stable for years may benefit from ptosis surgery.[260]

In patients with severe refractory symptoms or in those who seem dependent on large doses of corticosteroids, other immunosuppressants such as azathioprine, cyclosporine, or mycophenolate mofetil may be used as supplementary agents or for steroid-sparing effects. Azathioprine is given in 2–3 mg/kg/day doses, with a time to onset of effect of 3–12 months and time to maximal effect of 1–2 years.[194,261] Bone marrow and liver function should be monitored for possible side-effects. Cyclosporine can be given at 2.5 mg/kg b.i.d., with a time to onset of effect of 4–12 weeks[262] and a time to maximal effect of 3–6 months. For this drug, blood pressure, renal function, and drug levels should be monitored.[263] Some authors[264] have advocated their judicious use with corticosteroids in patients with difficult-to-manage ocular myasthenia. The use of mycophenolate mofetil at doses of 1–2 g per day has been recommended,[265–268] but the medication's effectiveness in myasthenia recently has been questioned.[269] One report suggested treatment of severely refractory myasthenia with high-dose cyclophosphamide followed by granulocyte colony-stimulating factor to "reboot" the bone marrow.[270]

Because of the cost, requirement of an inpatient stay, and frequent need for repeated treatments, we have not used plasmapheresis or intravenous gamma globulin[271,272] in patients with solely ocular myasthenia. These modalities are more appropriate for patients whose generalized symptoms of dyspnea, dysphagia, and systemic weakness are debilitating enough to require hospitalization.[273]

Preliminary studies suggest that myasthenia may also be successfully treated with oral antisense suppression of acetylcholinesterase activity by limiting the enzyme's synthesis.[274]

Surgical. Besides spontaneous remission, thymectomy represents the only potential cure for myasthenia gravis.[275] Possible mechanisms for improvement include: eliminating a source of continued antigenic stimulation,[276] removing a possible reservoir of B cells which secrete acetylcholine receptor antibodies, and correcting a disturbance of immune regulation.[194] The procedure traditionally is performed via a trans-sternal approach.[277,278] The transcervical approach, which requires only a incision at the base of the neck, has become popular because of less associated discomfort and quicker recovery.[279,280] Pathologically the thymus typically exhibits lymphoid hyperplasia.

Patients without thymoma less than 60 years of age who have generalized symptoms are ideal candidates for thymectomy. Those with bulbar or respiratory weakness may require preoperative plasmapheresis to reduce the postoperative

recovery period. Sixty percent of patients will experience complete remission without symptoms or need for medication over several years.[232,281] Another 30% are able to reduce their dose of pyridostigmine or immunosuppressive agent. Surgery earlier in the disease course and less severe disease appear to be associated with better outcomes.[282] As the morbidity associated with thymectomy, especially via the transcervical route, decreases with improvement in surgical techniques, we have lowered our threshold for recommending this procedure in patients with solely ocular myasthenia to aid medical therapy and possibly reduce the risk of generalization.[280,283–285] In addition, it has recently been suggested that patients older than 60 may safely undergo and benefit from the procedure.[286]

Thymoma associated with myasthenia is another indication for thymectomy, which is usually performed trans-sternally to insure complete removal of the tumor. Postoperatively the myasthenia in these patients tends to be more unstable, severe, and difficult to manage, and such patients often require a combination of different medical therapies. However, one study[287] suggested the long-term outcome in myasthenic patients with thymoma was no different than in those without thymoma.

Does treatment of ocular myasthenia reduce the risk of conversion to generalized myasthenia? Several retrospective studies have suggested that treatment of patients with ocular myasthenia gravis with corticosteroids,[288,289] azathioprine,[290] or thymectomy[280] may reduce the risk of conversion to generalized myasthenia. This topic is highly controversial.[249,257,259] In our experience, patients with ocular myasthenia who have undergone thymectomy do appear to have a lower incidence of generalization.[280] On the other hand, we have seen patients with ocular myasthenia gravis treated with corticosteroids or azathioprine who had no generalized symptoms at presentation or during treatment. However, when treatment was withdrawn, either accidentally or at the patient's request, the patients exhibited generalized symptoms. Therefore, it is unclear, at least in some instances, whether chronic immunosuppression simply masked the conversion to generalized myasthenia.

Myasthenia gravis in children. *Juvenile (or infantile) myasthenia gravis* has the same pathophysiology as the adult type, with idiopathic production of acetylcholine receptor antibodies.[291] In one study 14–30% of children experienced spontaneous remission,[292] and in another study[293] this always occurred within 40 months of disease onset in prepubertal patients. In one small exceptional series,[294] all of four children with solely ocular myasthenia had a spontaneous remission. As in adults, about one-third[295] to one-half[296] of children presenting with ocular myasthenia will eventually generalize (**Fig. 14–33**). Forty percent of children with ocular myasthenia have detectable acetylcholine receptor antibodies, whereas 70% of children with generalized symptoms are seropositive.[296] Younger prepubertal children have a higher incidence of seronegativity.[297] MuSK antibodies may be seen in children with myasthenia.[298,299] When an edrophonium test is performed, a total of 0.2 mg/kg can be infused intravenously in divided doses, not exceeding 10 mg.

Pyridostigmine is first-line therapy in ocular or generalized juvenile myasthenia, but, like with adults, the results are

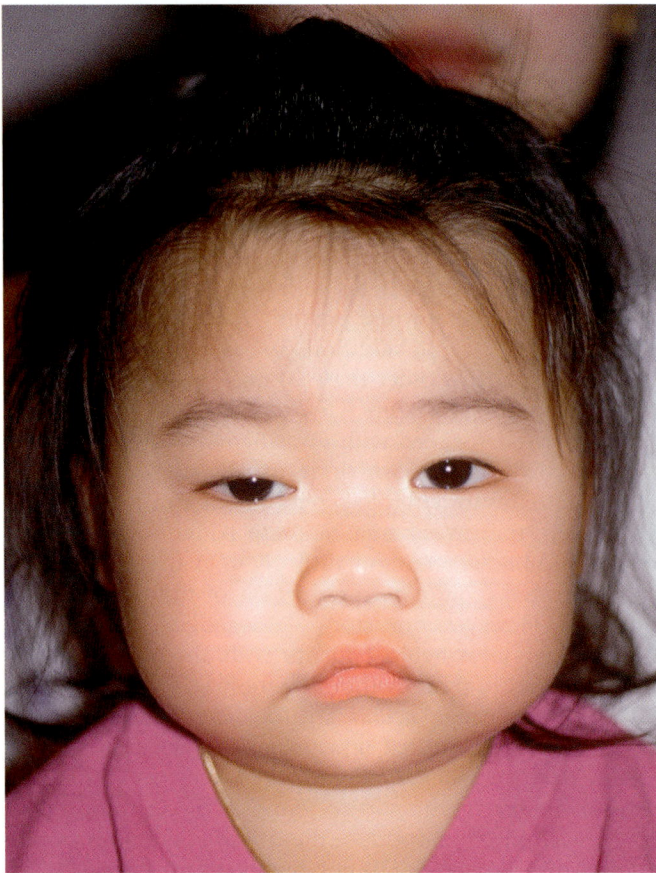

Figure 14–33. Two-year-old girl with generalized myasthenia gravis symptomatic with right eyelid ptosis, swallowing difficulty, and limb weakness.

often unsatisfactory. Long-term corticosteroids are often added when pyridostigmine is insufficient,[300] but the doses must be kept small because of steroid's possible effect on bone growth. Prevention of strabismic or deprivational (from ptosis) amblyopia is the reason for aggressive treatment of children with ocular myasthenia.[301] Chronic immunosuppression with azathioprine or cyclosporine are problematic in young patients because of side-effects, but may be necessary in patients with refractory systemic or bulbar symptoms.

Trans-sternal thymectomy has been performed in children with generalized myasthenia gravis with a remission rate of approximately 67%,[302–305] but controversy exists because some authors have opined that the thymus may be important for proper development of the immune system,[306] especially within the first year of life. However, Herrmann et al.[307] cite numerous studies in which no subsequent immunodeficiency was found in children undergoing thymectomy for myasthenia gravis, as part of early cardiac surgery, and for suspected thymoma. At many centers, including our own, thymectomy in young children can be performed trans-thorascopically, a procedure which leaves only small scars on the lateral chest wall.[308] Thus, we have a low threshold for thymectomy, even in children with solely ocular myasthenia gravis. Thymomas in children with myasthenia are extremely uncommon.

In transient *neonatal myasthenia gravis*, about 12% of infants of mothers with myasthenia may exhibit poor sucking, a weak cry, and hypotonia due to passive transfer of acetylcholine receptor antibodies. As the antibody titer declines over the first days or weeks of life, the child spontaneously improves.

Congenital myasthenic syndromes. These conditions share a different mechanism from antibody-mediated myasthenia gravis, although children present similarly with weakness evident shortly after birth.[309] These syndromes have been traced to genetic abnormalities of the presynaptic, synaptic, or postsynaptic portions of the neuromuscular junction.[310] Neither circulating autoantibodies nor abnormal thymus glands are found. Engel and colleagues[311–317] and others[318] have characterized several congenital myasthenic syndromes, and examples include: (1) a defect in acetylcholine resynthesis and packaging (presynaptic), (2) a congenital endplate acetylcholinesterase deficiency (synaptic), (3) a slow-channel syndrome (postsynaptic), (4) a congenital endplate acetylcholine receptor deficiency (postsynaptic), and (5) high conductance and fast closure of the acetylcholine receptor channel (postsynaptic). Except for the slow-channel syndrome, which is autosomal dominant, the congenital myasthenic syndromes have autosomal recessive inheritance.[319] Treatment options include low-dose pyridostigmine, fluoxetine,[320] and ephedrine.[321]

Lambert–Eaton myasthenic syndrome

Lambert–Eaton myasthenic syndrome (LEMS), which is much rarer than myasthenia gravis, is a presynaptic neurotransmission disorder. The syndrome has two major forms: paraneoplastic and primary autoimmune, but their presentations and pathophysiology are similar. Most patients are elderly, but individuals in all age groups can be affected. LEMS is commonly mistaken for myasthenia gravis because patients with both disorders may present with weakness and ptosis. However, LEMS is distinguished clinically by the presence of autonomic symptoms and lack of obvious ophthalmoplegia.

About half of all newly diagnosed patients with LEMS have the paraneoplastic form with an underlying malignancy.[322] Most of these patients harbor a small cell carcinoma of the lung, but LEMS is also associated with large cell neuroendocrine carcinomas and adenocarcinomas of the lung, lymphoproliferative disorders, renal cell carcinoma, and parotid tumors. As in many paraneoplastic disorders, the presentation of LEMS may precede or follow the cancer diagnosis. Rare individuals with LEMS and paraneoplastic cerebellar degeneration[323–325] and others with LEMS and antibody-positive myasthenia gravis[326] have been reported. LEMS can also be seen in association with other autoimmune diseases such as systemic lupus erythematosus, pernicious anemia, diabetes mellitus, and thyroid disease.[327] LEMS due to diltiazem, a calcium channel blocker, has also been described.[328]

Pathophysiology. In both the paraneoplastic or primary autoimmune types, LEMS is caused by antibodies directed against voltage-gated calcium channels on the presynaptic portion of the neuromuscular junction.[329,330] Various subtypes of these antibodies, designated P/Q, L, N, T, and MysB, have been described.[331] Acetylcholine release, which is dependent upon the influx of calcium into the nerve terminal, is therefore impaired. Exercise or high rates of stimulation increase the intracellular calcium concentration, thereby enhancing acetylcholine release.

Symptoms. Most patients present with progressive fatiguable proximal weakness, usually starting in their legs. Autonomic symptoms are also common and include dry mouth, impotence, blurred vision, dry eyes, and constipation. Neuro-ophthalmic symptoms are typically not prominent but may consist of droopy eyelids and transient diplopia. Respiratory difficulty and bulbar symptoms such as dysphagia and dysarthria are also uncommon.

Signs. The neurologic examination in LEMS is characterized by proximal muscle weakness and absent or depressed reflexes most apparent in the weakest limbs.[332] The increase in muscle strength after exercise is actually difficult to demonstrate clinically. An improvement in deep tendon reflexes after sustained contraction is more easily found. Sensation is typically normal.

Neuro-ophthalmic signs. Patients with LEMS may have mild bilateral ptosis, usually without noticeable ophthalmoparesis. In contrast to patients with myasthenia gravis, some patients may have improvement in their ptosis, mimicking lid retraction, with sustained upgaze.[333,334] In various series,[327,335] about one-half of patients had ptosis, and half had diplopia, although obvious eye movement abnormalities were usually not found. Two studies of patients with LEMS, with normal eye movements on neuro-ophthalmic examination, had improvement in saccadic velocity after exercise documented with oculography.[336,337] Autonomic dysfunction may be reflected in dry eye and sluggish pupillary reactivity. Isolated ocular involvement is rare but has been reported.[338]

Diagnosis. Although the characteristic combination of clinical signs and symptoms may suggest LEMS, the diagnosis must be confirmed by EMG. A decreased resting compound muscle action potential (CMAP) which increases with maximal voluntary contraction is the classic EMG finding. Repetitive stimulation at 3 Hz, which is typically performed to demonstrate decrement of the CMAP amplitude in myasthenia gravis, may also show a decremental response in LEMS. However, repetitive stimulation at 50 Hz may produce an incremental response. Single fiber electromyography may demonstrate jitter (see above) and neuromuscular blockade. Immunoassay for the antibodies directed against voltage-gated calcium channels may also be performed and is sensitive but not specific for LEMS.[330] Edrophonium testing, which is also nonspecific, may lead to some improvement in weakness. CT and MRI of the chest and abdomen, followed by bronchoscopy in smokers, is recommended to exclude cancer.[339]

Treatment. Management of patients with LEMS typically has three forms: identification and treatment of the underlying malignancy, enhancement of neurotransmission, and immunomodulation.[332,339,340] Treatment of the cancer, via chemotherapy, surgery, or radiation, is the most important step.[341] Although not widely available, 3,4-diaminopyridine, which prolongs the activation of voltage-gated calcium channels at the nerve terminal, thereby enhancing the release of acetylcholine, has been reported as an effective treatment

in LEMS.[322,342,343] Guanidine, which has a similar mechanism of action, and acetylcholinesterase inhibitors also may be used to enhance neurotransmission. Immunomodulation may be achieved with plasmapheresis, intravenous immunoglobulin,[344,345] or immunosuppression with prednisone or azathioprine.[346] Neurologic improvement can be observed in many cases, with survival over months to years after treatment.

Botulism

Botulism is caused by a clostridia toxin from *C. botulinum* that blocks the release of acetylcholine from the presynaptic nerve terminal. Breast-fed infants less than 1 year of age living in endemic areas are most commonly affected. Ingestion of honey or home-canned or -bottled products which have not been sterilized,[347] or wounds,[348] can result in clostridia infection.

The time from onset of symptoms to medical presentation is usually days to a week. Infants usually present with generalized hypotonia and poor suck for several days. In all ages, pharyngeal weakness, respiratory difficulty, and decreased limb strength may occur. Patients are treated with botulism immune globulin.[349–351]

Neuro-ophthalmic complications such as bifacial weakness, ophthalmoplegia, ptosis, blurry vision, and diplopia are very common.[348,352–355] Poorly reactive pupils are also frequently seen, and this finding and constipation often help differentiate patients with botulism in the emergency setting from myasthenia gravis or Guillain-Barré syndrome, the two major other disorders in the differential diagnosis of acute paralysis. High-frequency repetitive stimulation studies demonstrating post-tetanic potentiation and stool tests for botulinum toxin and culture can help confirm the diagnosis.

Chronic progressive external ophthalmoplegia, Kearns–Sayre syndrome, and related mitochondrial disorders

Chronic progressive external ophthalmoplegia and Kearns–Sayre syndrome

In CPEO, the ptosis is usually symmetric and accompanied by bilateral ophthalmoparesis and orbicularis oculi weakness. Patients with Kearns–Sayre syndrome (KSS) have the combination of (1) CPEO, (2) onset before age 20, (3) pigmentary retinopathy, and (4) at least one of the following: heart block, ataxia, or cerebrospinal fluid (CSF) protein above 100 mg/dl. CPEO and KSS are both mitochondrial myopathies.

Pathophysiology. These disorders are caused by mitochondrial DNA deletions.[356,357] Most cases are sporadic, and these are associated with single, large deletions which vary in size from 1.3 to 9.1 kilobases. The most common deletion is 4.9 kb from positions 8470–13460.[358]

Less common, familial varieties of CPEO have also been described that are inherited either autosomal dominantly or recessively. Mutations in nuclear genes, adenine nucleotide translocator 1 (ANT1), C10ORF (Twinkle), and polymerase gamma (POLG), have been associated with autosomal

Video 14.8

dominant progressive external ophthalmoplegia.[359] POLG mutations may also lead to autosomal recessive progressive external ophthalmoplegia.[360,361] Uncommonly, these mitochondrial DNA deletions may be responsible for sporadic cases as well.[362,363]

Symptoms. Except in KSS, symptoms can start at almost any age. Slowly progressive ptosis can be a patient's prominent complaint. Because the ophthalmoplegia is typically symmetric and chronically progressive, usually there is no diplopia. Family members or friends may be the first to notice the difficulty with eye movements. Visual loss due to retinal complications in KSS is uncommon but mild when it occurs. Historical evidence of longstanding muscle weakness, such as difficulty with running, jumping, or climbing, may be present.

Signs. In CPEO, symmetric ptosis with levator dysfunction and diffuse ophthalmoparesis are the most common features (**Fig. 14–34**). The pupils are spared. Patients often have asymptomatic orbicularis, neck, and limb weakness.[358] The pigmentary retinopathy in KSS (**Fig. 14–35**), which has been described as salt-and-pepper in appearance, is discussed in more detail in Chapter 4. Patients with KSS may have sensorineural hearing loss, dementia, or ataxia.

Systemic complications in Kearns–Sayre syndrome. The major systemic complication in KSS is heart block, but short stature and hypoparathyroidism have also been observed.[364,365]

Diagnosis. A definitive diagnosis of CPEO or KSS can be made by genetic testing for specific mitochondrial DNA deletions using muscle biopsies or blood. Muscle biopsy, usually of a deltoid or quadriceps muscle, may also demonstrate histological and ultrastructural abnormalities of skeletal muscle mitochondria.[366] Ragged-red fibers, which are red-staining granules in the subsarcolemmal zones and within the muscle fibers,[365] can be seen on modified Gomori trichrome staining (**Fig. 14–36**). Electron microscopy may reveal excessive proliferation of normal-looking mitochondria, giant mitochondria with disoriented cristae, intramitochondrial paracrystalline inclusions ("parking lots"), and electron-dense osmiophilic inclusions.[367]

Other ancillary testing may provide supportive evidence before the muscle biopsy is performed and test results are available. Conventional electromyography usually demonstrates myopathic patterns. However, as alluded to earlier in the section on myasthenia gravis, single fiber electromyography in CPEO may also show increased jitter.[234] This highlights the difficulty in using single fiber electromyography to differentiate CPEO from myasthenia gravis.

In KSS, nonspecific MR findings such as atrophy and white matter and basal ganglia hyperintensities on

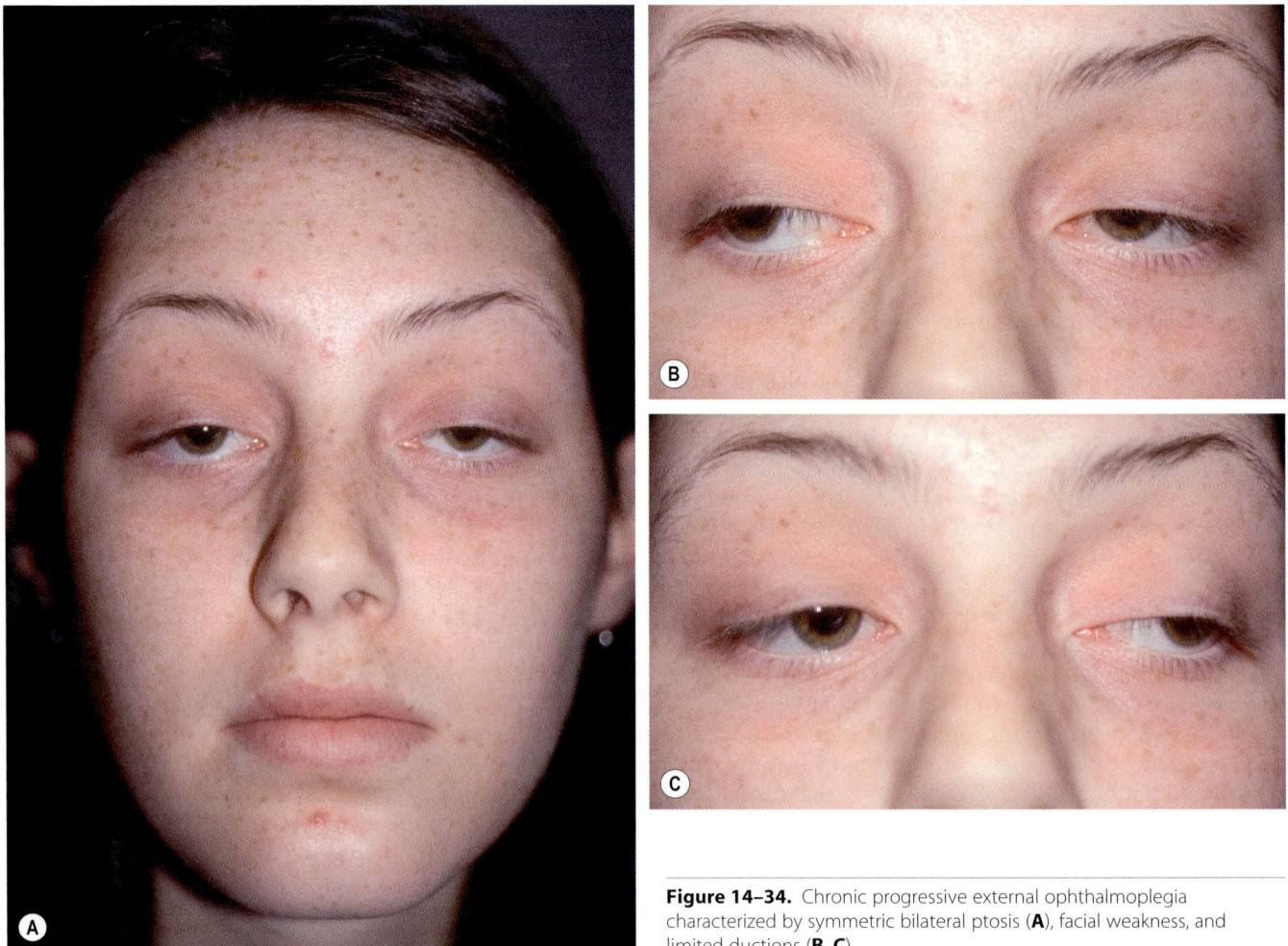

Figure 14–34. Chronic progressive external ophthalmoplegia characterized by symmetric bilateral ptosis (**A**), facial weakness, and limited ductions (**B**, **C**).

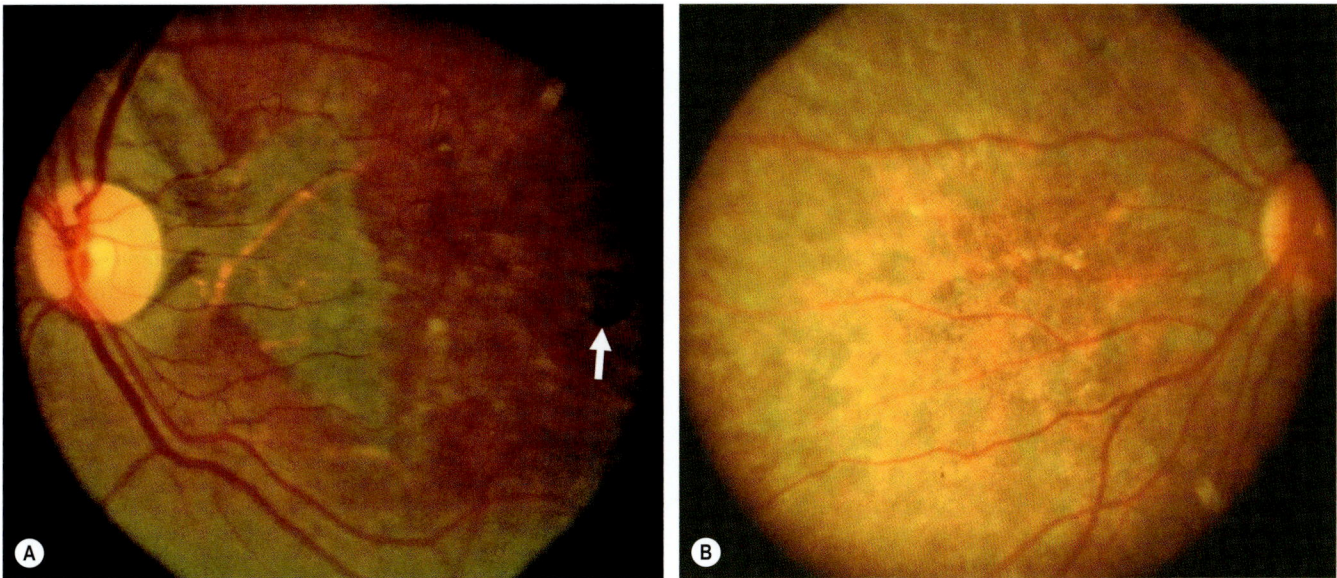

Figure 14–35. Fundus photographs in Kearns–Sayre syndrome. **A.** Posterior pole photograph demonstrating a healthy-appearing optic nerve but extensive pigmentary degeneration with atrophy and pigment clumping (arrow). **B.** Photograph of nasal periphery demonstrating diffuse pigmentary mottling with atrophy and hyperpigmentation ("salt and pepper" appearance).

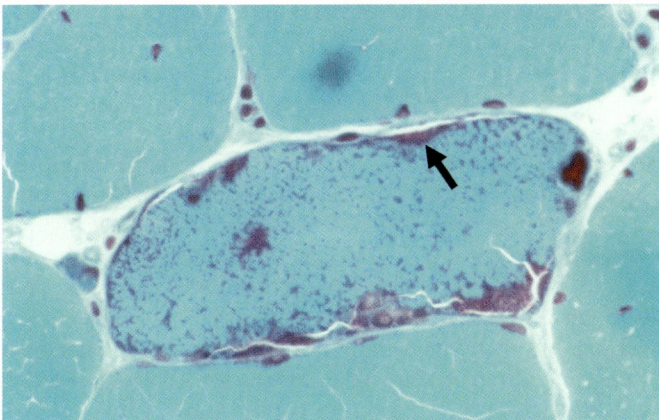

Figure 14–36. Muscle biopsy (modified Gomori trichrome) demonstrating ragged red fibers (arrow) in Kearns–Sayre syndrome.

T2-weighted images may be seen.[368,369] MR spectroscopy may reveal elevated brain lactate levels, which have been attributed to the impairment in oxidative metabolism.[370–372] CT may demonstrate basal ganglia hypointensities[365] or calcification.

Other abnormalities on diagnostic evaluation include elevation of serum lactate and abnormally increased CSF protein in KSS. At postmortem, spongy degeneration of the brain may be seen histopathologically.

Treatment. Treatment measures are symptomatic and biochemical. Ptosis surgery is often helpful.[373] However, overwidening of the palpebral fissures should be avoided in individuals who are unable to elevate their eye under the upper eyelid to protect the cornea, thereby risking exposure keratopathy.[374] Strabismus surgery can be performed in the rare individual with chronic strabismus and diplopia.[375] Vitamins and coenzyme Q can be given but often are of little benefit.

Mitochondrial neurogastrointestinal encephalopathy syndrome (MNGIE)

A familial *m*itochondrial *n*eurogastro*i*ntestinal *e*ncephalomyopathy (MNGIE) syndrome, caused by multiple mitochondrial DNA deletions, is now well recognized.[376–382] It is an autosomal recessive disorder caused by mutations in the nuclear gene for thymidine phosphorylase.[383] Other acronyms, such as POLIP (for polyneuropathy, ophthalmoplegia, leukoencephalopathy, and intestinal pseudo-obstruction), had also been used previously.[384] Affected patients are usually young to middle-aged adults. Characteristic clinical features are symmetric ptosis, ophthalmoparesis, intestinal pseudo-obstruction, and a mixed demyelinating and axonal neuropathy. Short stature, deafness, cachexia, white matter abnormalities on MRI, optic atrophy, and retinal pigmentary degeneration have also been observed.[381,382]

Myotonic dystrophy

Myotonic dystrophy is a hereditary bilateral myopathy that is associated with weakness and atrophy of the muscles of the face and extremities. This disorder, however, is distinguished from other neuromuscular disorders by muscle myotonia, a continued contraction despite attempted relaxation, and multiorgan involvement.

Pathophysiology. Myotonic dystrophy is inherited in an autosomally dominant fashion, typically from the mother. It is caused by an unstable cytosine–thymine–guanine trinucleotide (CTG triplet) repeat on chromosome 19q13.3. Anticipation among successive generations is observed, as the offspring are typically more severely affected than the parent. This phenomenon is explained by an increase in the number of triplet repeats among more affected offspring. The abnormal gene codes for a cyclic AMP-dependent protein kinase enzyme. A defect in phosphorylation of skeletal muscle ion channels may affect the excitability of the muscle membranes and result in myotonia.[385]

Symptoms. Patients often complain of progressive distal and proximal weakness. Neuro-ophthalmic symptoms include ptosis, lack of facial expression, and, rarely, diplopia. They may have a history of heart disease and cognitive deficits. Patients may present in the neonatal period with weakness and difficulty sucking and swallowing.

Signs. Bilateral ptosis is associated with bifacial weakness and "hatchet facies" due to temporalis muscle wasting. The upper lip may be "tented."[386] Ocular motor abnormalities have been described, including external ophthalmoplegia.[387] Subclinical saccadic slowing has been demonstrated oculographically, but it is controversial whether this phenomenon is a peripheral or central one.[388-392] A characteristic Christmas tree cataract, consisting of multicolored iridescent flecks, is found in almost all adult patients and can cause visual acuity loss. Less commonly, central macular lesions, pigmentary retinal degeneration, and hypotony may occur.[393]

Patients with myotonic dystrophy are diffusely weak. Action myotonia is elicited by having the patient grasp an object then have difficulty relaxing. Percussion myotonia can be observed following mechanical depression of the tongue or thenar eminence, for example. Many have cognitive delay, decreased IQ, or other mental status abnormalities. Typical systemic findings in males include temporal balding and testicular atrophy. Patients also may have cardiac abnormalities such as arrhythmias, conduction defects, and congestive heart failure.

Diagnosis. The diagnosis is suspected clinically in a patient with weakness, myotonia, the typical facies, and similarly affected family members. Electrical myotonia can be elicited during electromyography. Characteristic, there is a "dive bomber" sound, reflecting continuous discharges and difficulty with muscle relaxation.

The disorder should be distinguished from other myotonic neuromuscular disorders such as hyperkalemic period paralysis, paramyotonia congenita, and myotonia congenita.[385] Except for lid retraction and lag in hyperkalemic periodic paralysis, neuro-ophthalmic signs and symptoms in these conditions are less prominent than in myotonic dystrophy.

Other muscular dystrophies

Oculopharyngeal muscular dystrophy. Patients with this disorder usually present in middle age with progressive bilateral ptosis and dysphagia. Several subtypes have been described, including:

1. An autosomal dominant oculopharyngeal muscular dystrophy is recognized among French Canadian and Bukhara Jewish families. Ptosis and mild to moderate ophthalmoplegia may be presenting features,[394] and facial weakness and proximal limb weakness may also develop. The pathologic hallmark is a filamentous intranuclear inclusion in affected muscles. The genetic defect has been mapped to chromosome 14q11.2–13, and a guanine–cytosine–guanine (GCG) triplet repeat has been demonstrated.[395]

2. In another type, ophthalmoplegia is more prominent, and affected patients display clinical, electrophysiologic, and pathologic evidence of myopathy and neuropathy.[396]

Guillain-Barré syndrome and related polyneuropathies

Guillain-Barré syndrome

Today GBS is the most common cause of acute flaccid paralysis in the USA. Facial paresis occurs in approximately 50%.[397]

Pathophysiology. Most cases of GBS are caused by acute inflammatory demyelination of peripheral nerves (AIDP), the pathogenesis of which is likely to be autoimmune. Areas of demyelination are typically segmental and characterized by focal, perivascular infiltrates of lymphocytes and macrophages.[398,399] However, less common forms such as acute motor axonal neuropathy (AMAN), acute motor and sensory axonal neuropathy (AMSAN), and the Miller Fisher variant (discussed separately below) are well recognized.[400-402] Central nervous system involvement is uncommon.[403]

Up to three-quarters of patients with GBS have a preceding infection, which is usually gastrointestinal or respiratory.[402] Approximately one-quarter of patients have serologic or stool-culture evidence of recent *Campylobacter jejuni* infection, and a majority of these had diarrhea in the weeks before the onset of GBS. Patients with *C. jejuni* infection and GBS also have a greater likelihood of testing positive for GM_1 antibodies directed against gangliosides in peripheral nerve,[404] having AMAN or secondary axonal degeneration in association with AIDP,[405] as well as exhibiting slower recovery and greater residual neurologic disability.[406,407] Other common antecedent infections include human immunodeficiency virus (HIV), cytomegalovirus, Epstein–Barr virus, and *Mycoplasma pneumoniae*.[408] Associated diseases include Hodgkin's lymphoma[409] and systemic lupus erythematosus. A history of recent surgery is also a risk factor for GBS, although infrequent.

Symptoms. Patients usually present with motor weakness, often ascending, which progresses over days to weeks. Paresthesias in affected limbs occur frequently, but are usually a less prominent complaint. Pain in the thighs or back may occur.

Signs. GBS is highlighted by areflexia and symmetric motor weakness affecting the limbs and trunk. Bulbar and respiratory muscles are often involved. Sensory loss is mild.[410] Uni- or bilateral facial weakness occurs in about one-half of patients. The IIIrd, IVth, and VIth nerves may be affected, leading to ophthalmoplegia in about 15%.[397] Ptosis, when it occurs, is usually a result of IIIrd nerve palsy. However, in one series[411] 8% of patients with GBS had ptosis without ophthalmoparesis or pupillary abnormalities. When the spinal fluid protein level is very high, elevated intracranial pressure and papilledema may develop (see discussion in Chapter 6). Rare cases of optic neuritis have been reported.[412] Pupillary abnormalities, due most often to parasympathetic dysfunction, can be seen (see discussion in Chapter 13).

Respiratory failure may require mechanical ventilatory support in about one-third of cases.[397] Medical complications include pneumonia, urinary tract infections, sepsis, cardiac arrhythmias, blood pressure fluctuations, cardiac arrest from autonomic instability,[413] and deep vein thromboses and pulmonary emboli from immobility.

Diagnosis. Spinal fluid examination is helpful and classically demonstrates an elevated protein without pleocytosis (albumino-cytological dissociation). The typical nerve conduction study (NCS) findings of AIDP are conduction block or slowing of motor nerve conduction velocity.[414] However, both the spinal fluid examination and NCS may be normal within the first few days of the illness, and therefore in such cases they should be repeated approximately 1 week later if GBS is still strongly suspected. Detection of specific ganglioside autoantibodies, such as GM_1, GT_{1a}, GQ_{1b} (see below), and GD_{1b}, for instance, is often helpful.[415] Anti-GQ_{1b} can be detected in patients with GBS and ophthalmoparesis and usually not in those with normal eye movements.[416] The differential diagnosis for acute flaccid paralysis includes myasthenia gravis, poliomyelitis, botulism, tick bite paralysis, porphyria, hexacarbon abuse, diphtheria, or lead toxicity.[417]

Treatment. Large studies have demonstrated that patients with acute respiratory deficiency or inability to walk improve more rapidly with early plasmapheresis.[418] Alternatively, intravenous immunoglobulin therapy (IVIG), which is safer and easier to use, may also be administered. Several studies suggest that IVIG is as effective plasmapheresis.[419–422] Plasmapheresis is aimed at reducing, and IVIG, at neutralizing circulating neuromuscular blocking antibodies.[423] A number of other advances have improved the morbidity and mortality of patients with GBS. These include hospitalization of patients in intensive care settings, ventilatory management and pulmonary toilet, nutrition, pain control, deep vein thrombosis prophylaxis, blood pressure and cardiac monitoring, avoidance of decubiti with positioning, and improved bowel and bladder care.

Most patients recover over weeks to months,[424] although some require hospitalization for up to a year. Many patients have persistent minor weakness, areflexia, or paresthesias which do not interfere with ordinary activities.[397]

Miller Fisher syndrome

This variant of GBS, first characterized by Miller Fisher in 1956,[425] is highlighted by ataxia, ophthalmoplegia, and areflexia. In contrast to the usual AIDP form of GBS, eye movement abnormalities are prominent in the Miller Fisher syndrome, and diplopia is often the first complaint.[411] The ophthalmoplegia typically consists of various combinations of IIIrd, IVth, and VIth nerve involvement, and some patients develop complete loss of eye movements. In some patients, ophthalmoplegia is the only clinical finding. Pupillary dysfunction can also occur (see discussion in Chapter 13). Facial nerve palsy is frequently observed,[426] but usually systemic weakness is less salient than in AIDP. However, similar areflexia, electrophysiologic abnormalities, cytoalbuminal dissociation in the CSF, association with antecedent infections, and clinical course justify Miller Fisher as a subgroup of GBS.

Over 90% of patients with Miller Fisher syndrome have GQ_{1b} IgG autoantibodies in their serum, and titers decrease during clinical improvement.[416,427] In some cases this autoantibody is produced following *C. jejuni* infection,[428] and there is evidence for GQ_{1b}-like lipopolysaccharides on *C. jejuni* which could be the immunogens for their synthesis.[429,430]

There is considerable debate whether the lesions responsible for Miller Fisher syndrome are entirely peripheral or if the central nervous system is also affected.[431] Extra-axial enhancement of the ocular motor nerves on MRI suggests that in some cases the external ophthalmoplegia is caused by a peripheral process.[432,433] GQ_{1b} gangliosides are found in the paranodal regions of the extramedullary portions of the ocular motor nerves,[416] suggesting a basis for attack at this site. However, other MRI studies[434] have showed white matter lesions in the brain stem, implying that the process may be both central and peripheral in some cases. Furthermore, one report demonstrated that GQ_{1b} and GT_{1b} antibodies from sera of patients with Miller Fisher syndrome binds to cells in the molecular layer of human cerebellum.[435] This may be the mechanism for the ataxia seen in these patients. Cases with brain stem lesions but without peripheral nerve involvement (i.e., normal reflexes and electromyography) probably do not fall under the rubric of GBS. Instead these patients might be more appropriately diagnosed with Bickerstaff's brain stem encephalitis (see Chapter 15).[436]

Patients with Miller Fisher syndrome are treated with the same modalities such as IVIG and plasmapheresis, as those with AIDP.[437] The prognosis for full recovery after weeks to months is excellent.[426,438]

Chronic inflammatory demyelinating polyneuropathy (CIDP)

Patients with CIDP develop slowly progressive symmetric distal and proximal weakness, sensory loss, and areflexia in patterns similar to those with GBS. Facial weakness may be present in about 15%,[439,440] and rarely the ocular motor nerves are affected.[441] Progression occurs over several months, and approximately half have a monophasic course while the other half experience relapses and remissions.[440] Rarely there is clinical evidence of central nervous system demyelination and optic atrophy.[442] Papilledema may occur when the protein level is severely elevated in the CSF (see discussion in Chapter 6).

In about one-third of patients there may be a history of an antecedent viral illness or vaccination.[439] Concurrent illnesses such as Hodgkin disease, benign monoclonal gammopathy, inflammatory bowel disease, chronic hepatitis, diabetes, and HIV, for instance, may also occur. Either demyelinating or axonal features or both on NCS or sural nerve biopsy can confirm the diagnosis. As in GBS, the spinal fluid protein is elevated without pleocytosis. Treatment options include corticosteroids, azathioprine, cyclosporine, plasmapheresis, and intravenous immunoglobulin.[443–445]

References

1. Caplan LR. Ptosis. J Neurol Neurosurg Psychiatry 1974;37:1–7.
2. Wouters RJ, van den Bosch WA, Stijnen T, et al. Conjugacy of eyelid movements in vertical eye saccades. Invest Ophthalmol Vis Sci 1995;36:2686–2694.
3. Schmidtke K, Büttner-Ennever JA. Nervous control of eyelid function. A review of clinical, experimental and pathological data. Brain 1992;115:227–247.
4. Büttner-Ennever JA, Jenkins C, Armin-Parsa H, et al. A neuroanatomical analysis of lid-eye coordination in ptosis and downgaze paralysis. Clin Neuropathol 1996;15:313–318.
5. Horn AK, Buttner-Ennever JA. Brainstem circuits controlling lid-eye coordination in monkey. Prog Brain Res 2008;171:87–95.
6. van Eimeren T, Boecker H, Konkiewitz EC, et al. Right lateralized motor cortex activation during volitional blinking. Ann Neurol 2001;49:813–816.

7. Urban PP, Wicht S, Vucorevic G, et al. The course of corticofacial projections in the human brainstem. Brain 2001;124:1866–1876.

8. Terao S, Miura N, Takeda A, et al. Course and distribution of facial corticobulbar tract fibres in the lower brain stem. J Neurol Neurosurg Psychiatry 2000;69:262–265.

9. Carpenter M. Core Text of Neuro-anatomy, pp 151. Baltimore, Williams & Wilkins, 1985.

10. Martin RG, Grant JL, Peace D. Microsurgical relationship of the anterior inferior cerebellar artery and the facial-vestibulocochlear nerve complex. Neurosurgery 1980;6:483.

11. Malone B, Maisel RH. Anatomy of the facial nerve. Am J Otol 1988;9:494–504.

12. May M, Galetta SL. The facial nerve and related disorders of the face. In: Glaser JS (ed): Neuro-ophthalmology, 3rd edn, pp 293–326. Philadelphia, Lippincott, Williams, and Wilkins, 1999.

13. Miehike A. Surgery of the Facial Nerve, pp 7–21. Philadelphia, W.B. Saunders, 1973.

14. Davis RA, Anson BJ, Puddinger JM, et al. Surgical anatomy of the facial nerve and parotid gland based upon a study of 350 cervical facial halves. Surg Gynecol Obstet 1956;102:385–412.

15. Moore KL. Clinically Oriented Anatomy, 4th edn, p 853. Baltimore, Lippincott, Williams & Wilkins, 1999.

16. Ragge NK, Hoyt WF. Midbrain myasthenia: fatigable ptosis, "lid twitch" sign, and ophthalmoparesis from a dorsal midbrain glioma. Neurology 1992;42:917–919.

17. Averbuch-Heller L, Poonyathalang A, von Maydell RD, et al. Hering's law for eyelids: still valid. Neurology 1995;45:1781–1783.

18. Eggenberger E, Kayabasi N. Hering's law for eyelids [letter]. Neurology 1996;47:1352.

19. Fine EJ, Sentz L, Soria E. The history of the blink reflex. Neurology 1992;42:450–454.

20. Zametkin AJ, Stevens JR, Pittman R. Ontogeny of spontaneous blinking and of habituation of the blink reflex. Ann Neurol 1979;5:453–457.

21. Pullicino PM, Jacobs L, McCall WD, et al. Spontaneous palpebromandibular synkinesia: a localizing clinical sign. Ann Neurol 1994;35:222–228.

22. Liu GT, Ronthal M. Reflex blink to visual threat. J Clin Neuroophthalmol 1992;12:47–56.

23. Bracha V, Zhao L, Wunderlich DA, et al. Patients with cerebellar lesions cannot acquire but are able to retain conditioned eyeblink reflexes. Brain 1997;120:1401–1403.

24. Mac Keith RC. The eye and vision in the newborn infant. In: Gardiner P, MacKeith RC, Smith V (eds): Aspects of Developmental and Paediatric Ophthalmology. Clinics in Developmental Medicine, pp 9–14. London, Spastics International, 1969.

25. Vanhaudenhuyse A, Giacino J, Schnakers C, et al. Blink to visual threat does not herald consciousness in the vegetative state. Neurology 2008;71:1374–1375.

26. Hill K, Cogan DG, Dodge PR. Ocular signs associated with hydranencephaly. Am J Ophthalmol 1961;51:267–275.

27. Keane JR. Blinking to sudden illumination. A brain stem reflex present in neocortical death. Arch Neurol 1979;36:52–53.

28. Tavy DLJ, van Woerkom CAM, Bots GTAM, et al. Persistence of the blink reflex to sudden illumination in a comatose patient. Arch Neurol 1984;41:323–324.

29. Oosterhuis HJ. Acquired blepharoptosis. Clin Neurol Neurosurg 1996;98:1–7.

30. Thompson BM, Corbett JJ, Kline LB, et al. Pseudo-Horner's syndrome. Arch Neurol 1982;39:108–111.

31. Sevel D. Ptosis and underaction of the superior rectus muscle. Ophthalmology 1984;91:1080–1085.

32. Clark BJ, Kemp EG, Behan WMH, et al. Abnormal extracellular material in the levator palpebrae superioris complex in congenital ptosis. Arch Ophthalmol 1995;113:1414–1419.

33. Brodsky MC. The doctor's eye: seeing through the myopathy of congenital ptosis [editorial]. Ophthalmology 2000;107:1973–1974.

34. Pavone P, Barbagallo M, Parano E, et al. Clinical heterogeneity in familial congenital ptosis: analysis of fourteen cases in one family over five generations. Pediatr Neurol 2005;33:251–254.

35. Doucet TW, Crawford JS. The quantification, natural course, and surgical results in 57 eyes with Marcus-Gunn (jaw-winking) syndrome. Am J Ophthalmol 1981;92:702–707.

36. Pratt SG, Beyer CK, Johnson CC. The Marcus Gunn phenomenon. A review of 71 cases. Ophthalmology 1984;90:27–30.

37. Khwarg SI, Tarbet KJ, Dortzbach DK, et al. Management of moderate-to-severe Marcus-Gunn jaw-winking ptosis. Ophthalmology 1999;106:1191–1196.

38. Good EF. Ptosis as the sole manifestation of compression of the oculomotor nerve by an aneurysm of the posterior communicating artery. J Clin Neuroophthalmol 1990;10:59–61.

39. Barton JJ, Kardon RH, Slagel D, et al. Bilateral central ptosis in acquired immunodeficiency syndrome. Can J Neurol Sci 1995;22:52–55.

40. Krohel GB, Griffen JF. Cortical blepharoptosis. Am J Ophthalmol 1978;85:632–634.

41. Lepore F. Bilateral cerebral ptosis. Neurology 1987;37:1043–1046.

42. Averbuch-Heller L, Stahl JS, Remler BF, et al. Bilateral ptosis and upgaze palsy with right hemispheric lesions. Ann Neurol 1996;40:465–468.

43. Averbuch-Heller L, Leigh RJ, Mermelstein V, et al. Ptosis in patients with hemispheric strokes. Neurology 2002;58:620–624.

44. Blacker DJ, Wijdicks EF. Delayed complete bilateral ptosis associated with massive infarction of the right hemisphere. Mayo Clin Proc 2003;78:836–839.

45. Goldstein JE, Cogan DG. Apraxia of lid opening. Arch Ophthalmol 1965;73:155–159.

46. Lepore FE, Duvoisin RC. "Apraxia" of eyelid opening: an involuntary levator inhibition. Neurology 1985;35:423–427.

47. Boghen D. Apraxia of lid opening: a review. Neurology 1997;48:1491–1494.

48. Forget R, Tozlovanu V, Iancu A, et al. Botulinum toxin improves lid opening delays in blepharospasm-associated apraxia of lid opening. Neurology 2002;58:1843–1846.

49. Aramideh M, Ongerboer de Visser BW, Koelman JHTM, et al. Motor persistence of orbicularis oculi muscle in eyelid-opening disorders. Neurology 1995;45:897–902.

50. Micheli F, Scorticati C, Diaz S. Lid-opening apraxia [letter]. Neurology 1995;45:1788–1789.

51. Dehaene I. Apraxia of eyelid opening in progressive supranuclear palsy [letter]. Ann Neurol 1984;15:115–116.

52. Golbe LI, Davis PA, Lepore FE. Eyelid movement abnormalities in progressive supranuclear palsy. Mov Disord 1989;4:297–302.

53. Shields DC, Lam S, Gorgulho A, et al. Eyelid apraxia associated with subthalamic nucleus deep brain stimulation. Neurology 2006;66:1451–1452.

54. Wagner J, Schankin C, Birnbaum T, et al. Ocular motor and lid apraxia as initial symptom of anti-Ma1/Ma2-associated encephalitis. Neurology 2009;72:466–467.

55. Kaiboriboon K, Oliveira GR, Leira EC. Apraxia of eyelid opening secondary to a dominant hemispheric infarction [letter]. J Neurol 2002;249:341–342.

56. Johnston JC, Rosenbaum DM, Picone CM, et al. Apraxia of eyelid opening secondary to right hemispheric infarction. Ann Neurol 1989;25:622–624.

57. Verghese J, Milling C, Rosenbaum DM. Ptosis, blepharospasm, and apraxia of eyelid opening secondary to putaminal hemorrhage. Neurology 1999;53:652.

58. Adair JC, Williamson DJG, Heilman KM. Eyelid opening apraxia in focal cortical degeneration [letter]. J Neurol Neurosurg Psychiatry 1995;58:508–509.

59. Abe K, Fujimura H, Tatsumi C, et al. Eyelid "apraxia" in patients with motor neuron disease. J Neurol Neurosurg Psychiatry 1995;59:629–632.

60. Krack P, Marion MH. "Apraxia of lid opening," a focal eyelid dystonia: clinical study of 32 patients. Mov Disord 1994;9:610–615.

61. Tozlovanu V, Forget R, Iancu A, et al. Prolonged orbicularis oculi activity: a major factor in apraxia of lid opening. Neurology 2001;57:1013–1018.

62. Aramideh M, Ongerboer de Visser BW, Brans JWM, et al. Pretarsal application of botulinum toxin for treatment of blepharospasm. J Neurol Neurosurg Psychiatry 1995;59:309–311.

63. Jankovic J. Pretarsal injection of botulinum toxin for blepharospasm and apraxia of eyelid opening. J Neurol Neurosurg Psychiatry 1996;60:704.

64. Dewey RB, Maraganore DM. Isolated eyelid-opening apraxia: report of a new levodopa-responsive syndrome. Neurology 1994;44:1752–1754.

65. Yamada S, Matsuo K, Hirayama M, et al. The effects of levodopa on apraxia of lid opening. A case report. Neurology 2004;62:830–831.

66. Georgescu D, Vagefi MR, McMullan TF, et al. Upper eyelid myectomy in blepharospasm with associated apraxia of lid opening. Am J Ophthalmol 2008;145:541–547.

67. Kersten RC, de Conciliis C, Kulwin DR. Acquired ptosis in the young and middle-aged adult population. Ophthalmology 1995;102:924–928.

68. Watanabe A, Araki B, Noso K, et al. Histopathology of blepharoptosis induced by prolonged hard contact lens wear. Am J Ophthalmol 2006;141:1092–1096.

69. Stout AU, Borchert M. Etiology of eyelid retraction in children: a retrospective study. J Pediatr Ophthalmol Strabismus 1993;30:96–99.

70. Bartley GB. The differential diagnosis and classification of eyelid retraction. Ophthalmology 1996;103:168–176.

71. Olver JM, Fells P. "Henderson's" relief of eyelid retraction revisited. Eye 1995;9:467–471.

72. Guimarães FC, Cruz AAV. Palpebral fissure height and downgaze in patients with Graves upper eyelid retraction and congenital blepharoptosis. Ophthalmology 1995;102:1218–1222.

73. Gaddipati RV, Meyer DR. Eyelid retraction, lid lag, lagophthalmos, and von Graefe's sign quantifying the eyelid features of Graves' ophthalmopathy. Ophthalmology 2008;115:1083–1088.

74. Keane JR. The pretectal syndrome: 206 patients. Neurology 1990;40:684–690.

75. Galetta SL, Gray LG, Raps EC, et al. Pretectal eyelid retraction and lag. Ann Neurol 1993;33:554–557.

76. Keane JR. Spastic eyelids: failure of levator inhibition in unconscious states. Arch Neurol 1975;32:695–698.

77. Galetta SL, Raps EC, Liu GT, et al. Eyelid lag without eyelid retraction in pretectal disease. J Neuroophthalmol 1996;16:96–98.

78. Gaymard B, Lafitte C, Gelot A, et al. Plus-minus lid syndrome. J Neurol Neurosurg Psychiatry 1992;55:846–848.

79. Lam BL, Nerad JA, Thompson HS. Paroxysmal eyelid retractions. Am J Ophthalmol 1992;114:105–107.

80. Collin JR, Allen L, Castronuovo S. Congenital eyelid retraction. Br J Ophthalmol 1990;74:542–544.

81. May M. The Facial Nerve, pp 1–50. New York, Thieme Stratton, 1986.

82. Keane JR. Bilateral seventh nerve palsy: analysis of 43 cases and review of the literature. Neurology 1994;44:1198–1202.

83. Urban PP, Wicht S, Marx J, et al. Isolated voluntary facial paresis due to pontine ischemia. Neurology 1998;50:1859–1862.

84. Hopf HC, Müller-Forell W, Hopf NJ. Localization of emotional and volitional facial paresis. Neurology 1992;42:1918–1923.

85. Ross RT, Mathiesen R. Volitional and emotional supranuclear facial weakness. N Engl J Med 1998;338:1515.

86. Hopf HC, Fitzek C, Marx J, et al. Emotional facial paresis of pontine origin. Neurology 2000;54:1217.

87. Lessell S. Supranuclear paralysis of voluntary lid closure. Arch Ophthalmol 1972;88:241.

88. Ross Russell RW. Supranuclear palsy of eyelid closure. Brain 1980;103:71.

89. Korn T, Reith W, Becker G. Impaired volitional closure of the left eyelid after right anterior cerebral artery infarction: apraxia due to interhemispheric disconnection? Arch Neurol 2004;61:273–275.

90. Henderson JL. The congenital facial diplegia syndrome: clinical features, pathology, and etiology. Brain 1939;62:381–403.

91. Carr MM, Ross DA, Zuker RM. Cranial nerve defects in congenital facial palsy. J Otolaryngol 1997;26:80–87.
92. Igarashi M, Rose DF, Storgion SA. Moebius syndrome and central respiratory dysfunction. Pediatr Neurol 1997;16:237–240.
93. Tran DB, Wilson MC, Fox CA, et al. Möbius syndrome with oculomotor nerve paralysis but without abducens paralysis. J Neuroophthalmol 1998;18:281–283.
94. Abramson DL, Cohen MM, Mulliken JB. Möbius syndrome: classification and grading system. Plastic Reconstr Surg 1998;102:961–967.
95. Sudarshan A, Goldie WD. The spectrum of congenital facial diplegia (Moebius syndrome). Pediatr Neurol 1985;1:180–184.
96. Kumar D. Moebius syndrome. J Med Genet 1990;27:122–126.
97. Cattaneo L, Chierici E, Bianchi B, et al. The localization of facial motor impairment in sporadic Mobius syndrome. Neurology 2006;66:1907–1912.
98. Jaradeh S, D'Cruz O, Howard JF, Jr., et al. Mobius syndrome: electrophysiologic studies in seven cases. Muscle Nerve 1996;19:1148–1153.
99. Lammens M, Moerman P, Fryns JP, et al. Neuropathological findings in Moebius syndrome. Clin Genet 1998;54:136–141.
100. Peleg D, Nelson GM, Williamson RA, et al. Expanded Möbius syndrome. Pediatr Neurol 2001;24:306–309.
101. Saint-Martin C, Clapuyt P, Duprez T, et al. Möbius sequence and severe pons hypoplasia: a case report. Pediatr Radiol 1998;28:932.
102. Ghabrial R, Versace P, Kourt G, et al. Möbius' syndrome: features and etiology. J Pediatr Ophthalmol Strabismus 1998;35:304–311.
103. Pedraza S, Gamez J, Rovira A, et al. MRI findings in Möbius syndrome: correlation with clinical features. Neurology 2000;55:1058–1060.
104. Dooley JM, Stewart WA, Hayden JD, et al. Brainstem calcification in Mobius syndrome. Pediatr Neurol 2004;30:39–41.
105. D'Cruz OF, Swisher CN, Jaradeh S, et al. Möbius syndrome: evidence for a vascular etiology. J Child Neurol 1993;8:260–265.
106. Verzijl HT, van der Zwaag B, Cruysberg JR, et al. Möbius syndrome redefined: a syndrome of rhombencephalic maldevelopment. Neurology 2003;61:327–333.
107. Verzijl HT, Padberg GW, Zwarts MJ. The spectrum of Möbius syndrome: an electrophysiological study. Brain 2005;128:1728–1736.
108. Verzijl HT, Valk J, de Vries R, et al. Radiologic evidence for absence of the facial nerve in Möbius syndrome. Neurology 2005;64:849–855.
109. Kremer H, Kuyt LP, van den Helm B, et al. Localization of a gene for Möbius syndrome to chromosome 3q by linkage analysis in a Dutch family. Hum Mol Genet 1996;5:1367–1371.
110. Pastuszak AL, Schüler L, Speck-Martins CE, et al. Use of misoprostol during pregnancy and Möbius syndrome in infants. N Engl J Med 1998;338:1881–1885.
111. Gonzalez CH, Marques-Dias MJ, Kim CA, et al. Congenital abnormalities in Brazilian children associated with misoprostol misuse in first trimester of pregnancy. Lancet 1998;351:1624–1627.
112. Goldberg AB, Greenberg MB, Darney PD. Misoprostol and pregnancy. N Engl J Med 2001;344:38–47.
113. da Silva Dal Pizzol T, Knop FP, Mengue SS. Prenatal exposure to misoprostol and congenital anomalies: systematic review and meta-analysis. Reprod Toxicol 2006;22:666–671.
114. Lew SM, Khoshyomn S, Hamill RW, et al. Cavernous malformation of the facial colliculus. Neurology 2002;58:459.
115. Silverman IE, Liu GT, Volpe NJ, et al. The crossed paralyses: the original brainstem syndromes of Millard-Gubler, Foville, Weber, and Raymond-Cestan. Arch Neurol 1995;52:635–638.
116. Clark JR, Carlson RD, Sasak CT. Facial paralysis in Lyme disease. Laryngoscope 1985;95:1341–1345.
117. Zajicek JP, Scolding NJ, Foster O, et al. Central nervous system sarcoidosis: diagnosis and management. Q J Med 1999;92:103–117.
118. Paolino E, Granieri E, Tola MR. Predisposing factor in Bell's palsy: a case control study. J Neurol 1985;232:363–365.
119. Wolf SM, Wagner JH, Davidson S, et al. Treatment of Bell palsy with prednisone: a prospective, randomized study. Neurology 1978;28:158–161.
120. Peitersen E. The natural history of Bell's palsy. Am J Otol 1982;4:107–111.
121. Adour KK, Wingerd J. Idiopathic facial paralysis (Bell's palsy): factors affecting severity and outcome in 446 patients. Neurology 1974;24:1112–1116.
122. Grogan PM, Gronseth GS. Practice parameter. Steroids, acyclovir, and surgery for Bell's palsy (an evidence-based review): report of the Quality Standards Subcommittee of the American Academy of Neurology. Neurology 2001;56:830–836.
123. May M, Klein SR, Taylor FH. Idiopathic (Bell's) facial palsy: natural history defies steroid or surgical treatment. Laryngoscope 1985;95:406–409.
124. Sullivan FM, Swan IR, Donnan PT, et al. Early treatment with prednisolone or acyclovir in Bell's palsy. N Engl J Med 2007;357:1598–1607.
125. Gilden DH. Clinical practice. Bell's palsy. N Engl J Med 2004;351:1323–1331.
126. Hunt JR. On herpetic inflammations of the geniculate ganglion. A new syndrome and its complications. J Nerve Ment Dis 1907;34:73–96.
127. Portenoy RK, Duma C, Foley KM. Acute herpetic and postherpetic neuralgia. Clinical review and current management. Ann Neurol 1986;20:651–664.
128. Gradenigo G. A special syndrome of endocranial otitic complications. Ann Otol Rhinol Laryngol 1904;13:637.
129. Kondev L, Bhadelia RA, Douglass LM. Familial congenital facial palsy. Pediatr Neurol 2004;30:367–370.
130. Verzijl HT, van der Zwaag B, Lammens M, et al. The neuropathology of hereditary congenital facial palsy vs Möbius syndrome. Neurology 2005;64:649–653.
131. Rahman I, Sadiq SA. Ophthalmic management of facial nerve palsy: a review. Surv Ophthalmol 2007;52:121–144.
132. Seiff SR, Chang J. Management of ophthalmic complications of facial nerve palsy. Otolaryngol Clin North Am 1992;25:669–690.
133. May M. Gold weight and wire spring implants as alternatives to tarsorrhaphy. Arch Otolaryngol Head Neck Surg 1987;113:656–660.
134. Catalano PJ, Bergstein MJ, Biller HF. Comprehensive management of the eye in facial paralysis. Arch Otolaryngol Head Neck Surg 1995;121:81–86.
135. Seiff SR, Sullivan JH, Freeman LN, et al. Pretarsal fixation of gold weights in facial nerve palsy. Ophthal Plast Reconstr Surg 1989;5:104–109.
136. Kartush JM, Linstrom CJ, McCann PM, et al. Early gold weight eyelid implantation for facial paralysis. Otolaryngol Head Neck Surg 1990;103:1016–1023.
137. Townsend DJ. Eyelid reanimation for the treatment of paralytic lagophthalmos: historical perspectives and current applications of the gold weight implant. Ophthal Plast Reconstr Surg 1992;8:196–201.
138. Dinces EA, Mauriello JA, Jr., Kwartler JA, et al. Complications of gold weight eyelid implants for treatment of fifth and seventh nerve paralysis. Laryngoscope 1997;107:1617–1622.
139. Karson CN, LeWitt PA, Calne DB, et al. Blink rates in parkinsonism. Ann Neurol 1982;12:580–583.
140. Kimura J. Effect of hemispheral lesions on the contralateral blink reflex. A clinical study. Neurology 1974;24:168–174.
141. Berardelli A, Accornero N, Cruccu G, et al. The orbicularis oculi response after hemispheral damage. J Neurol Neurosurg Psychiatry 1983;46:837–843.
142. Brodsky H, Dat Vuong K, Thomas M, et al. Glabellar and palmomental reflexes in parkinsonian disorders. Neurology 2004;63:1096–1098.
143. Coats DK, Paysse EA, Kim DS. Excessive blinking in childhood: a prospective evaluation of 99 children. Ophthalmology 2001;108:1556–1561.
144. Adams WH, Digre KB, Patel BC, et al. The evaluation of light sensitivity in benign essential blepharospasm. Am J Ophthalmol 2006;142:82–87.
145. Castelbuono A, Miller NR. Spontaneous remission in patients with essential blepharospasm and Meige syndrome. Am J Ophthalmol 1998;126:432–435.
146. Hasan S, Baker RS, Sun WS, et al. The role of blink adaptation in the pathophysiology of benign essential blepharospasm. Arch Ophthalmol 1997;115:631–636.
147. Schmidt KE, Linden DE, Goebel R, et al. Striatal activation during blepharospasm revealed by fMRI. Neurology 2003;60:1738–1743.
148. Kerrison JB, Lancaster JL, Zamarripa FE, et al. Positron emission tomography scanning in essential blepharospasm. Am J Ophthalmol 2003;136:846–852.
149. Hallett M. Blepharospasm: recent advances. Neurology 2002;59:1306–1312.
150. Hallett M, Evinger C, Jankovic J, et al. Update on blepharospasm: report from the BEBRF International Workshop. Neurology 2008;71:1275–1282.
151. Baker RS, Sun WS, Hasan SA, et al. Maladaptive neural compensatory mechanisms in Bell's palsy-induced blepharospasm. Neurology 1997;49:223–229.
152. Aramideh M, Ongerboer de Visser BW, Holstege G, et al. Blepharospasm in association with a lower pontine lesion. Neurology 1996;46:476–478.
153. Ishikawa M, Ohira T, Namiki J, et al. Electrophysiological investigation of hemifacial spasm after microvascular decompression: F waves of the facial muscles, blink reflexes, and abnormal muscle response. J Neurosurg 1997;86:654–661.
154. Rahman EA, Trobe JD, Gebarski SS. Hemifacial spasm caused by vertebral artery dolichoectasia. Am J Ophthalmol 2002;133:854–856.
155. Adler CH, Zimmerman RA, Savino PJ, et al. Hemifacial spasm: evaluation by magnetic resonance imaging and magnetic resonance tomographic angiography. Ann Neurol 1992;32:502–506.
156. Ho SL, Cheng PW, Wong WC, et al. A case-controlled MRI/MRA study of neurovascular contact in hemifacial spasm. Neurology 1999;53:2132–2139.
157. Osako M, Keltner JL. Botulinum A toxin (Oculinum) in ophthalmology. Surv Ophthalmol 1991;36:28–46.
158. Price J, O'Day J. Efficacy and side effects of botulinum toxin treatment for blepharospasm and hemifacial spasm. Aust N Z J Ophthalmol 1994;22:255–260.
159. Defazio G, Abbruzzese G, Girlanda P, et al. Botulinum toxin A treatment for primary hemifacial spasm: a 10-year multicenter study. Arch Neurol 2002;59:418–420.
160. Dutton JJ, Fowler AM. Botulinum toxin in ophthalmology. Surv Ophthalmol 2007;52:13–31.
161. Price J, Farish S, Taylor H, et al. Blepharospasm and hemifacial spasm. Randomized trial to determine the most appropriate location for botulinum toxin injections. Ophthalmology 1997;104:865–868.
162. Holds JB, Alderson K, Fogg SG, et al. Motor nerve sprouting in human orbicularis muscle after botulinum A injection. Invest Ophthalmol Vis Sci 1990;31:964–967.
163. Alderson K, Holds JB, Anderson RL. Botulinum-induced alteration of nerve-muscle interactions in the human orbicularis oculi following treatment for blepharospasm. Neurology 1991;41:1800–1805.
164. Jankovic J, Schwartz KS. Longitudinal experience with botulinum toxin injections for treatment of blepharospasm and cervical dystonia. Neurology 1993;43:834–836.
165. Ainsworth JR, Kraft SP. Long-term changes in duration of relief with botulinum toxin treatment of essential blepharospasm and hemifacial spasm. Ophthalmology 1995;102:2036–2040.
166. Elston JS. Long-term results of treatment of idiopathic blepharospasm with botulinum toxin injections. Br J Ophthalmol 1987;71:664–668.
167. Engstrom PF, Arnoult JB, Mazow ML, et al. Effectiveness of botulinum toxin therapy for essential blepharospasm. Ophthalmology 1987;94:971–975.
168. Dutton JJ, Buckley EG. Long-term results and complications of botulinum A toxin in the treatment of blepharospasm. Ophthalmology 1988;95:1529–1534.
169. Kennedy RH, Bartley GB, Flanagan JC, et al. Treatment of blepharospasm with botulinum toxin. Mayo Clin Proc 1989;64:1085–1090.

170. Mauriello JA, Jr., Dhillon S, Leone T, et al. Treatment selections of 239 patients with blepharospasm and Meige syndrome over 11 years. Br J Ophthalmol 1996;80:1073–1076.

171. Anderson RL, Patel BC, Holds JB. Blepharospasm: past, present, and future. Ophthal Plast Reconstr Surg 1998;14:305–317.

172. Kalra HK, Magoon EH. Side effects of the use of botulinum toxin for treatment of benign essential blepharospasm and hemifacial spasm. Ophthalmic Surg 1990;21:335–338.

173. Wutthiphan S, Kowal L, O'Day J, et al. Diplopia following subcutaneous injections of botulinum A toxin for facial spasms. J Pediatr Ophthalmol Strabismus 1997;34:229–234.

174. Siatkowski RM, Tyutyunikov A, Biglan AW, et al. Serum antibody production to botulinum A toxin. Ophthalmology 1993;100:1861–1866.

175. Evidente VGH, Adler CH. Hemifacial spasm and other craniofacial movement disorders. Mayo Clin Proc 1998;73:67–71.

176. Wirtschafter JD, McLoon LK. Long-term efficacy of local doxorubicin chemomyectomy in patients with blepharospasm and hemifacial spasm. Ophthalmology 1998;105:342–346.

177. Herz NL, Yen MT. Modulation of sensory photophobia in essential blepharospasm with chromatic lenses. Ophthalmology 2005;112:2208–2211.

178. Baker RS, Stava MW, Nelson KR, et al. Aberrant reinnervation of facial musculature in a subhuman primate: a correlative analysis of eyelid kinematics, muscle synkinesis, and motoneuron localization. Neurology 1994;44:2165–2173.

179. Jankovic J. The neurology of tics. In: Marsden CD, Fahn S (eds): Movement Disorders 2, pp 383–405. London, Butterworths, 1987.

180. Jankovic J, Stone L. Dystonic tics in patients with Tourette's syndrome. Mov Disord 1991;6:248–252.

181. Jankovic J. Tourette's syndrome. N Engl J Med 2001;345:1184–1192.

182. Andermann F, Cosgrove JBR, Lloyd-Smith DL, et al. Facial myokymia in multiple sclerosis. Brain 1961;84:31–44.

183. Jacobs L, Kaba S, Pullicino P. The lesion causing continuous facial myokymia in multiple sclerosis. Arch Neurol 1994;51:1115–1119.

184. Banik R, Miller NR. Chronic myokymia limited to the eyelid is a benign condition. J Neuroophthalmol 2004;24:290–292.

185. Màrit-Fabregas J, Montero J, López-Villegas D, et al. Post-irradiation neuromyotonia in bilateral facial and trigeminal nerve distribution. Neurology 1997;48:1107–1109.

186. Mauriello JA, Carbonaro P, Dhillon S, et al. Drug-associated facial dyskinesias: a study of 238 patients. J Clin Neuroophthalmol 1998;18:153–157.

187. Brodsky MC, Boop FA. Lid nystagmus as a sign of intrinsic midbrain disease. J Neuroophthalmol 1995;5:236–240.

188. Sanders MD, Hoyt WF, Daroff RB. Lid nystagmus evoked by ocular convergence: an ocular electromyographic study. J Neurol Neurosurg Psychiatry 1968;31:368–371.

189. Camfield CS, Camfield PR, Sadler M, et al. Paroxysmal eyelid movements: a confusing feature of generalized photosensitive epilepsy. Neurology 2004;63:40–42.

190. Ishikawa T, Inukai K, Kanayama M. Paradoxical eyelid movement in trisomy 2p. Pediatr Neurol 2002;26:236–238.

191. Grob D, Arsura EL, Brunner G, et al. The course of myasthenia gravis and therapies affecting outcome. Ann N Y Acad Sci 1987;505:472–499.

192. Bever C, Aquino AV, Penn AS, et al. Prognosis of ocular myasthenia gravis. Ann Neurol 1983;14:516–519.

193. Oosterhuis HJGH. The natural course of myasthenia gravis: a long term follow up study. J Neurol Neurosurg Psychiatry 1989;52:1121–1127.

194. Drachman DB. Myasthenia gravis. N Engl J Med 1994;330:1797–1810.

195. Somnier FE. Increasing incidence of late-onset anti-AChR antibody-seropositive myasthenia gravis. Neurology 2005;65:928–930.

196. Donaldson DH, Ansher M, Horan S, et al. The relationship of age to outcome in myasthenia gravis. Neurology 1990;40:786–790.

197. Drachman DB, Adams RN, Josifek LF, et al. Functional activities of autoantibodies to acetylcholine receptors and the clinical severity of myasthenia gravis. N Engl J Med 1982;307:769–795.

198. Seybold ME. Myasthenia gravis: diagnostic and therapeutic perspectives in the 1990's. Neurologist 1995;1:345–360.

199. Wang Z-Y, Okita DK, Howard J, et al. Th1 epitope repertoire on the α subunit of human muscle acetylcholine receptor in myasthenia gravis. Neurology 1997;48:1643–1653.

200. Liu GT, Bienfang DC. Penicillamine-induced ocular myasthenia gravis in rheumatoid arthritis. J Clin Neuroophthalmol 1990;10:201–205.

201. Negevesky GJ, Kolsky MP, Laureno R, et al. Reversible atorvastatin-associated external ophthalmoplegia, anti-acetylcholine receptor antibodies, and ataxia. Arch Ophthalmol 2000;118:427–428.

202. Argov Z, Mastaglia FL. Disorders of neuromuscular transmission caused by drugs. N Engl J Med 1979;301:409–413.

203. Barrons RW. Drug-induced neuromuscular blockade and myasthenia gravis. Pharmacotherapy 1997;17:1220–1232.

204. Wittbrodt ET. Drugs and myasthenia gravis. An update. Arch Intern Med 1997;157:399–408.

205. Wasserman BN, Chronister TE, Stark BI, et al. Ocular myasthenia and nitrofurantoin. Am J Ophthalmol 2000;130:531–533.

206. Kaminski HJ, Maas E, Spiegel P, et al. Why are eye muscles frequently involved in myasthenia gravis? Neurology 1990;40:1663–1669.

207. Ubogu EE, Kaminski HJ. The preferential involvement of extraocular muscles by myasthenia gravis. Neuroophthalmology 2001;25:219–227.

208. Kaminski HJ, Ruff RL. Ocular muscle involvement by myasthenia gravis [editorial]. Ann Neurol 1997;41:419–420.

209. MacLennan C, Beeson D, Buijs A-M, et al. Acetylcholine receptor expression in human extraocular muscles and their susceptibility to myasthenia gravis. Ann Neurol 1997;41:423–431.

210. Newsom-Davis J. Myasthenia gravis and the Miller-Fisher variant of Guillain-Barré syndrome. Curr Opin Neurol 1997;10:18–21.

211. Moorthy G, Behrens MM, Drachman DB, et al. Ocular pseudomyasthenia or ocular myasthenia "plus": a warning to clinicians. Neurology 1989;39:1150–1154.

212. Schmidt D. Signs in ocular myasthenia and pseudomyasthenia. Differential diagnostic criteria. A clinical review. Neuroophthalmology 1995;15:21–58.

213. Nunery WR, Cepela M. Levator function in the evaluation and management of blepharoptosis. Ophthalmol Clin North Am 1991;4:1–16.

214. Kao Y-F, Lan M-Y, Chou M-S, et al. Intracranial fatigable ptosis. J Neuroophthalmol 1999;19:257–259.

215. Cogan DG. Myasthenia gravis: a review of the disease and a description of lid twitch as a characteristic sign. Arch Ophthalmol 1965;74:217–221.

216. Weinberg DA, Lesser RL, Vollmer TL. Ocular myasthenia: a protean disorder. Surv Ophthalmol 1994;39:169–210.

217. Massey JM. Acquired myasthenia gravis. Neurol Clin 1997;15:577–595.

218. Benatar M. A systematic review of diagnostic studies in myasthenia gravis. Neuromuscul Disord 2006;16:459–467.

219. Lindstrom JM, Seybold ME, Lennon VA, et al. Antibody to acetylcholine receptor in myasthenia gravis. Prevalence, clinical correlates, and diagnostic value. Neurology 1976;26:1054–1059.

220. Soliven BC, Lange DT, Penn AS. Seronegative myasthenia gravis. Neurology 1988;38:514.

221. Vincent A, Newsom DJ. Anti-acetylcholine receptor antibodies. J Neurol Neurosurg Psychiatry 1980;43:590–600.

222. Leite MI, Jacob S, Viegas S, et al. IgG1 antibodies to acetylcholine receptors in "seronegative" myasthenia gravis. Brain 2008;131:1940–1952.

223. Lindstrom J. Is "seronegative" MG explained by autoantibodies to MuSK? [editorial]. Neurology 2004;62:1920–1921.

224. Selcen D, Fukuda T, Shen XM, et al. Are MuSK antibodies the primary cause of myasthenic symptoms? Neurology 2004;62:1945–1950.

225. Evoli A, Tonali PA, Padua L, et al. Clinical correlates with anti-MuSK antibodies in generalized seronegative myasthenia gravis. Brain 2003;126:2304–2311.

226. Farrugia ME, Robson MD, Clover L, et al. MRI and clinical studies of facial and bulbar muscle involvement in MuSK antibody-associated myasthenia gravis. Brain 2006;129:1481–1492.

227. Hatanaka Y, Hemmi S, Morgan MB, et al. Nonresponsiveness to anticholinesterase agents in patients with MuSK-antibody-positive MG. Neurology 2005;65:1508–1509.

228. Deymeer F, Gungor-Tuncer O, Yilmaz V, et al. Clinical comparison of anti-MuSK- vs anti-AChR-positive and seronegative myasthenia gravis. Neurology 2007;68:609–611.

229. Bartoccioni E, Scuderi F, Minicuci GM, et al. Anti-MuSK antibodies: correlation with myasthenia gravis severity. Neurology 2006;67:505–507.

230. Sanders DB, El-Salem K, Massey JM, et al. Clinical aspects of MuSK antibody positive seronegative MG. Neurology 2003;60:1978–1980.

231. Lange DJ. Electrophysiologic testing of neuromuscular transmission. Neurology 1997;48 (Suppl 5):S18–S22.

232. Herrmann C, Lindstrom JM, Keesey JC, et al. Myasthenia gravis: current concepts. West J Med 1985;142:797–809.

233. Milone M, Monarco ML, Evoli A, et al. Ocular myasthenia: diagnostic value of single fiber EMG in the orbicularis oculi muscle. J Neurol Neurosurg Psychiatry 1993;56:720–721.

234. Krendel DA, Sanders DB, Massey JM. Single fiber electromyography in chronic progressive external ophthalmoplegia. Muscle Nerve 1987;10:299–302.

235. Uyama J, Mimura O, Ikeda N, et al. Single fiber electromyography of extraocular muscles in myasthenia gravis. Neuroophthalmology 1993;13:253–261.

236. Kelly JJ, Daube J, Lennon VA. The laboratory diagnosis of mild myasthenia gravis. Ann Neurol 1982;12:238–242.

237. Seybold ME. The office tensilon test for ocular myasthenia. Arch Neurol 1986;43:842–843.

238. Daroff RB. The office Tensilon test for myasthenia gravis. Arch Neurol 1986;43:843–844.

239. Glaser JS, Bachynski B. Infranuclear disorders of eye movement. In: Glaser JS (ed): Neuro-Ophthalmology, pp 396–397. Philadelphia, J.B. Lippincott, 1990.

240. Miller NR, Morris JE, Maguire M. Combined use of neostigmine and ocular motility measurements in the diagnosis of myasthenia. Arch Ophthalmol 1982;100:761–763.

241. Hyder DJ, Liu GT. Myasthenia gravis. In: Schwartz MW (ed): CHOP's 5 Minute Pediatric Consult, pp 508–509. Baltimore, Williams & Wilkins, 1997.

242. Sethi K, Rivner MH, Swift TR. Ice pack test for myasthenia gravis. Neurology 1987;37:1383–1385.

243. Odel JG, Winterkorn JMS, Behrens MM. The sleep test for myasthenia gravis: a safe alternative to tensilon. J Clin Neuroophthalmol 1991;11:228–292.

244. Golnik KC, Pena R, Lee AG, et al. An ice test for the diagnosis of myasthenia gravis. Ophthalmology 1999;106:1282–1286.

245. Movaghar M, Slavin ML. Effect of local heat versus ice on blepharoptosis resulting from ocular myasthenia. Ophthalmology 2000;107:2209–2214.

246. Kubis KC, Danesh-Meyer HV, Savino PJ, et al. The ice test versus the rest test in myasthenia gravis. Ophthalmology 2000;107:1995–1998.

247. Sanders DB, Scoppetta C. The treatment of patients with myasthenia gravis. Neurol Clin 1994;12:343–368.

248. Benatar M, Kaminski H. Medical and surgical treatment for ocular myasthenia. Cochrane Database Syst Rev 2006:CD005081.

249. Benatar M, Kaminski HJ. Evidence report: the medical treatment of ocular myasthenia (an evidence-based review): report of the Quality Standards Subcommittee of the American Academy of Neurology. Neurology 2007;68:2144–2149.

250. Bhanushali MJ, Wuu J, Benatar M. Treatment of ocular symptoms in myasthenia gravis. Neurology 2008;71:1335–1341.

251. Rowland LP. Controversies about the treatment of myasthenia gravis. J Neurol Neurosurg Psychiatry 1980;43:644–659.

252. Lewis RA, Selwa JF, Lisak RP. Myasthenia gravis: immunological mechanisms and immunotherapy. Ann Neurol 1995;37:S51–S62.

253. Kupersmith MJ, Moster M, Bhuiyan S, et al. Beneficial effects of corticosteroids on ocular myasthenia gravis. Arch Neurol 1996;53:802–804.

254. Richman DP, Agius MA. Treatment of autoimmune myasthenia gravis. Neurology 2003;61:1652–1661.

255. Miano MA, Bosley TM, Heiman-Patterson TD, et al. Factors influencing outcome of prednisone dose reduction in myasthenia gravis. Neurology 1991;41:919–921.

256. Kaminski HJ, Daroff RB. Treatment of ocular myasthenia: steroids only when compelled. Arch Neurol 2000;57:752–753.

257. Gilbert ME, De Sousa EA, Savino PJ. Ocular myasthenia gravis treatment: the case against prednisone therapy and thymectomy. Arch Neurol 2007;64:1790–1792.

258. Agius MA. Treatment of ocular myasthenia with corticosteroids: yes. Arch Neurol 2000;57:750–751.

259. Chavis PS, Stickler DE, Walker A. Immunosuppressive or surgical treatment for ocular myasthenia gravis. Arch Neurol 2007;64:1792–1794.

260. Bradley EA, Bartley GB, Chapman KL, et al. Surgical correction of blepharoptosis in patients with myasthenia gravis. Trans Am Ophthalmol Soc 2000;98:173–180; discussion 180–171.

261. Palace J, Newsom-Davis J, Lecky B, et al. A randomized double-blind trial of prednisolone alone or with azathioprine in myasthenia gravis. Neurology 1998;50:1778–1783.

262. Ciafaloni E, Nikhar NK, Massey JM, et al. Retrospective analysis of the use of cyclosporine in myasthenia gravis. Neurology 2000;55:448–450.

263. Tindall RSA, Rollins JA, Phillips JT, et al. Preliminary results of a double-blind, randomized, placebo-controlled trial of cyclosporine in myasthenia gravis. N Engl J Med 1987;316:719–724.

264. Sommer N, Sigg B, Melms A, et al. Ocular myasthenia gravis: response to long term immunosuppressive treatment. J Neurol Neurosurg Psychiatry 1997;62:156–162.

265. Chaudhry V, Cornblath DR, Griffin JW, et al. Mycophenolate mofetil: a safe and promising immunosuppressant in neuromuscular diseases. Neurology 2001;56:94–96.

266. Ciafaloni E, Massey JM, Tucker-Lipscomb B, et al. Mycophenolate mofetil for myasthenia gravis: an open-label pilot study. Neurology 2001;56:97–99.

267. Mowzoon N, Sussman A, Bradley WG. Mycophenolate (CellCept) treatment of myasthenia gravis, chronic inflammatory polyneuropathy and inclusion body myositis. J Neurol Sci 2001;185:119–122.

268. Schneider C, Gold R, Reiners K, et al. Mycophenolate mofetil in the therapy of severe myasthenia gravis. Eur Neurol 2001;46:79–82.

269. Muscle Study Group. A trial of mycophenolate mofetil with prednisone as initial immunotherapy in myasthenia gravis. Neurology 2008;71:394–399.

270. Drachman DB, Jones RJ, Brodsky RA. Treatment of refractory myasthenia: "rebooting" with high-dose cyclophosphamide. Ann Neurol 2003;53:29–34.

271. Gajdos P, Chevret S, Clair B, et al. Clinical trial of plasma exchange and high-dose intravenous immunoglobulin in myasthenia gravis. Ann Neurol 1997;41:789–796.

272. Howard JF. Intravenous immunoglobulin for the treatment of acquired myasthenia gravis. Neurology 1998;51 (Suppl 5):S30–S36.

273. Zinman L, Ng E, Bril V. IV immunoglobulin in patients with myasthenia gravis: a randomized controlled trial. Neurology 2007;68:837–841.

274. Argov Z, McKee D, Agus S, et al. Treatment of human myasthenia gravis with oral antisense suppression of acetylcholinesterase. Neurology 2007;69:699–700.

275. Gronseth GS, Barohn RJ. Practice parameter: thymectomy for autoimmune myasthenia gravis (an evidence-based review): report of the Quality Standards Subcommittee of the American Academy of Neurology. Neurology 2000;55:7–15.

276. Levinson AI, Wheatley LM. The thymus and the pathogenesis of myasthenia gravis. Clin Immunol Immunopathol 1996;78:1–5.

277. Mulder DG. Extended transsternal thymectomy. Chest Surg Clin N Am 1996;6:95–105.

278. Jaretzki A. Thymectomy for myasthenia gravis: analysis of the controversies regarding technique and results. Neurology 1997;48 (Suppl 5):S52–S63.

279. Ferguson MK. Transcervical thymectomy. Chest Surg Clin N Am 1996;6:105–115.

280. Shrager JB, Deeb ME, Mick R, et al. Transcervical thymectomy for myasthenia gravis achieves results comparable to thymectomy by sternotomy. Ann Thorac Surg 2002;74:320–326; discussion 326–327.

281. Mulder DG, Herrmann C, Keesey JC, et al. Thymectomy for myasthenia gravis. Am J Surg 1983;146:61–66.

282. Nieto IP. Prognostic factors for myasthenia gravis treated by thymectomy. Ann Thorac Surg 1999;67:1568–1571.

283. Schumm F, Wiethölter H, Fateh-Moghadam A, et al. Thymectomy in myasthenia with pure ocular symptoms. J Neurol Neurosurg Psychiatry 1985;48:332–337.

284. Lanska DJ. Indications for thymectomy in myasthenia gravis. Neurology 1990;40:1828–1829.

285. Roberts PF, Venuta F, Rendina E, et al. Thymectomy in the treatment of ocular myasthenia gravis. J Thorac Cardiovasc Surg 2001;122:562–568.

286. Tsuchida M. Efficacy and safety of extended thymectomy for elderly patients with myasthenia gravis. Ann Thorac Surg 1999;67:1563–1567.

287. Bril V, Kojic J, Dhanani A. The long-term clinical outcome of myasthenia gravis in patients with thymoma. Neurology 1998;51:1198–1200.

288. Kupersmith MJ, Latkany R, Homel P. Development of generalized disease at 2 years in patients with ocular myasthenia gravis. Arch Neurol 2003;60:243–248.

289. Monsul NT, Patwa HS, Knorr AM, et al. The effect of prednisone on the progression from ocular to generalized myasthenia gravis. J Neurol Sci 2004;217:131–133.

290. Mee J, Paine M, Byrne E, et al. Immunotherapy of ocular myasthenia gravis reduces conversion to generalized myasthenia gravis. J Neuroophthalmol 2003;23:251–255.

291. Fenichel GM. Myasthenia gravis. Pediatr Ann 1989;18:432–438.

292. Anlar B, Ozdirim E, Renda Y, et al. Myasthenia gravis in childhood. Acta Paediatr 1996;85:838–842.

293. Andrews PI, Massey JM, Howard JF, et al. Race, sex, and puberty influence onset, severity, and outcome in juvenile myasthenia gravis. Neurology 1994;44:1208–1214.

294. Schmidt D. Prognosis of ocular myasthenia in childhood. Neuroophthalmology 1983;3:117–124.

295. Mullaney P, Vajsar J, Smith R, et al. The natural history and ophthalmic involvement in childhood myasthenia gravis at the hospital for sick children. Ophthalmology 2000;107:504–510.

296. Afifi AK, Bell WE. Tests for juvenile myasthenia gravis: comparative diagnostic yield and prediction of outcome. J Child Neurol 1993;8:403–411.

297. Andrews PI, Massey JM, Sanders DB. Acetylcholine receptor antibodies in juvenile myasthenia gravis. Neurology 1993;43:977–982.

298. Murai H, Noda T, Himeno E, et al. Infantile onset myasthenia gravis with MuSK antibodies. Neurology 2006;67:174.

299. Saulat B, Maertens P, Hamilton WJ, et al. Anti-musk antibody after thymectomy in a previously seropositive myasthenic child. Neurology 2007;69:803–804.

300. Kim JH, Hwang JM, Hwang YS, et al. Childhood ocular myasthenia gravis. Ophthalmology 2003;110:1458–1462.

301. Ortiz S, Borchert M. Long-term outcomes of pediatric ocular myasthenia gravis. Ophthalmology 2008;115:1245–1248.

302. Seybold ME, Howard FM, Duane DD, et al. Thymectomy in juvenile myasthenia gravis. Arch Neurol 1971;25:385–392.

303. Ryniewicz B, Badurska B. Follow-up study of myasthenic children after thymectomy. J Neurol 1977;217:133–138.

304. Rodriguez M, Gomez MR, Howard FM, et al. Myasthenia gravis in children: long-term follow-up. Ann Neurol 1983;13:504–510.

305. Adams C, Theodorescu D, Murphy EG, et al. Thymectomy in juvenile myasthenia gravis. J Child Neurol 1990;5:215–218.

306. Sarnat HB, McGarry JD, Lewis JE. Effective treatment of infantile myasthenia gravis by combine prednisone and thymectomy. Neurology 1977;27:550–553.

307. Herrmann DN, Carney PR, Wald JJ. Juvenile myasthenia gravis: treatment with immune globulin and thymectomy. Pediatr Neurol 1998;18:63–66.

308. Kolski HK, Kim PC, Vajsar J. Video-assisted thoracoscopic thymectomy in juvenile myasthenia gravis. J Child Neurol 2001;16:569–573.

309. Gurnett CA, Bodnar JA, Neil J, et al. Congenital myasthenic syndrome: presentation, electrodiagnosis, and muscle biopsy. J Child Neurol 2004;19:175–182.

310. Vincent A, Newland C, Croxen R, et al. Genes at the junction: candidates for congenital myasthenic syndromes. Trends Neurosci 1997;20:15–22.

311. Engel AG. Congenital myasthenic syndromes. J Child Neurol 1988;3:233–246.

312. Engel AG, Uchitel OD, Walls TJ, et al. Newly recognized congenital myasthenic syndrome associated with high conductance and fast closure of the acetylcholine receptor channel. Ann Neurol 1993;34:38–47.

313. Engel AG, Ohno K, Milone M, et al. Congenital myasthenic syndromes caused by mutations in acetylcholine receptor genes. Neurology 1997;48 (Suppl 5):S28–S35.

314. Engel AG, Ohno K, Wang H-L, et al. Molecular basis of congenital myasthenic syndromes: mutations in the acetylcholine receptor. Neuroscientist 1998;4:185–194.

315. Engel AG, Ohno K, Sine SM. Congenital myasthenic syndromes. Recent advances. Arch Neurol 1999;56:163–167.

316. Engel AG, Ohno K, Shen XM. Congenital myasthenic syndromes: multiple molecular targets at the neuromuscular junction. Ann N Y Acad Sci 2003;998:138–160.

317. Milone M, Fukuda T, Shen XM, et al. Novel congenital myasthenic syndromes associated with defects in quantal release. Neurology 2006;66:1223–1229.

318. Sieb JP, Dörfler P, Tzartos S, et al. Congenital myasthenic syndromes in two kinships with end-plate acetylcholine receptor and utrophin deficiency. Neurology 1998;50:54–61.

319. Beeson D, Palace J, Vincent A. Congenital myasthenic syndromes. Curr Opin Neurol 1997;10:402–407.

320. Harper CM, Fukodome T, Engel AG. Treatment of slow-channel congenital myasthenic syndrome with fluoxetine. Neurology 2003;60:1710–1713.

321. Bestue-Cardiel M, Saenz de Cabezón-Alvarez A, Capablo-Liesa JL, et al. Congenital endplate acetylcholinesterase deficiency responsive to ephedrine. Neurology 2005;65:144–146.

322. Tim RW, Massey JM, Sanders DB. Lambert-Eaton myasthenic syndrome: electrodiagnostic findings and response to treatment. Neurology 2000;54:2176–2178.

323. Satoyoshi E, Kowa H, Fukunaga N. Subacute cerebellar degeneration and Eaton-Lambert syndrome with bronchogenic carcinoma. A case report. Neurology 1973;23:764–768.

324. Blumenfeld AM, Recht LD, Chad DA, et al. Coexistence of Lambert-Eaton myasthenic syndrome and subacute cerebellar degeneration: differential effects of treatment. Neurology 1991;41:1682–1685.

325. Mason WP, Graus F, Lang B, et al. Small-cell lung cancer, paraneoplastic cerebellar degeneration and the Lambert-Eaton myasthenic syndrome. Brain 1997;120:1279–1300.

326. Fettel MR, Shin HS, Penn AS, et al. Combined Eaton-Lambert syndrome and myasthenia gravis [abstract]. Neurology 1978;28:398.

327. O'Neill JH, Murray NMF, Newsom-Davis J. The Lambert-Eaton myasthenic syndrome. A review of 50 cases. Brain 1988;111:577–596.

328. Ueno S, Hara Y. Lambert-Eaton myasthenic syndrome without anti-calcium channel antibody: adverse effect of calcium antagonist diltiazem. J Neurol Neurosurg Psychiatry 1992;55:409–410.

329. Lennon VA, Kryzer TJ, Griesmann GE, et al. Calcium-channel antibodies in the Lambert-Eaton syndrome and other paraneoplastic syndromes. N Engl J Med 1995;332:1467–1474.

330. Motomura M, Johnston I, Lang B, et al. An improved diagnostic assay for Lambert-Eaton myasthenic syndrome. J Neurol Neurosurg Psychiatry 1995;58:85–87.

331. Dalmau JO, Posner JB. Paraneoplastic syndromes. Arch Neurol 1999;56:405–408.

332. McEvoy KM. Diagnosis and treatment of Lambert-Eaton myasthenic syndrome. Neurol Clin N Am 1994;12:387–399.

333. Breen LA, Gutmann L, Brick JF, et al. Paradoxical lid elevation with sustained upgaze: a sign of Lambert-Eaton syndrome. Muscle Nerve 1991;14:863–866.

334. Brazis PW. Enhanced ptosis in Lambert-Eaton myasthenic syndrome. J Neuroophthalmol 1997;17:202–203.

335. Burns TM, Russell JA, LaChance DH, et al. Oculobulbar involvement is typical with Lambert-Eaton myasthenic syndrome. Ann Neurol 2003;53:270–273.

336. Cruciger MP, Brown B, Denys EH, et al. Clinical and subclinical oculomotor findings in the Lambert-Eaton syndrome. J Clin Neuroophthalmol 1983;33:1157–1163.

337. Dell'Osso LF, Ayyar DR, Daroff RB, et al. Edrophonium test in Lambert-Eaton syndrome: quantitative oculography. Neurology 1983;33:1157–1163.

338. Rudnicki SA. Lambert-Eaton myasthenic syndrome with pure ocular weakness. Neurology 2007;68:1863–1864.

339. Sanders DB. Lambert-Eaton myasthenic syndrome: clinical diagnosis, immune-mediated mechanisms, and update on therapies. Ann Neurol 1995;37(S1):S63–S73.

340. Case records of the Massachusetts General Hospital. Case 32-1994. N Engl J Med 1994;331:528–535.

341. Chalk CH, Murray NMF, Newsom-Davis J, et al. Response of the Lambert-Eaton myasthenic syndrome to treatment of associated small-cell lung carcinoma. Neurology 1990;40:1552–1556.

342. McEvoy KM, Windebank AJ, Daube JR, et al. 3,4-Diaminopyridine in the treatment of Lambert-Eaton-myasthenic syndrome. N Engl J Med 1989;321:1567–1571.

343. Sanders DB, Massey JM, Sanders LL, et al. A randomized trial of 3,4-diaminopyridine in Lambert-Eaton myasthenic syndrome. Neurology 2000;54:603–607.

344. Bird SJ. Clinical and electrophysiologic improvement in Lambert-Eaton syndrome with intravenous immunoglobulin therapy. Neurology 1992;42:1422–1423.

345. Rich MM, Teener JW, Bird SJ. Treatment of Lambert-Eaton syndrome with intravenous immunoglobulin. Muscle Nerve 1997;20:614–615.

346. Grisold W, Drlicek M, Liszka-Setinek U, et al. Anti-tumour therapy in paraneoplastic neurological disease. Clin Neurol Neurosurg 1995;97:106–111.

347. Case records of the Massachusetts General Hospital. Case 22-1997. N Engl J Med 1997;337:184–190.

348. Miller NR, Moses H. Ocular involvement in wound botulism. Arch Ophthalmol 1977;95:1788–1789.

349. Thompson JA, Filloux FM, Van Orman CB, et al. Infant botulism in the age of botulism immune globulin. Neurology 2005;64:2029–2032.

350. Arnon SS, Schechter R, Maslanka SE, et al. Human botulism immune globulin for the treatment of infant botulism. N Engl J Med 2006;354:462–471.

351. Tseng-Ong L, Mitchell WG. Infant botulism. 20 years' experience at a single institution. J Child Neurol 2007;22:1333–1337.

352. Terranova W, Palumbo JN, Breman JG. Ocular findings in botulism type B. JAMA 1979;241:475–477.

353. Hedges TR, Jones A, Stark L, et al. Botulin ophthalmoplegia. Clinical and oculographic observations. Arch Ophthalmol 1983;101:211–213.

354. Caya JG. Clostridium botulinum and the ophthalmologist: a review of botulism, including biological warfare ramifications of botulinum toxin. Surv Ophthalmol 2001;46:25–34.

355. Penas SC, Faria OM, Serrao R, et al. Ophthalmic manifestations in 18 patients with botulism diagnosed in Porto, Portugal between 1998 and 2003. J Neuroophthalmol 2005;25:262–267.

356. Zeviani M, Moraes CT, DiMauro S, et al. Deletions of mitochondrial DNA in Kearns-Sayre syndrome. Neurology 1988;38:1339–1346.

357. Moraes CT, DiMauro S, Zeviani M, et al. Mitochondrial DNA deletions in progressive external ophthalmoplegia and Kearns-Sayre syndrome. N Engl J Med 1989;30:1293–1299.

358. Newman NJ. Mitochondrial disease and the eye. Ophthalmol Clin North Am 1992;5:405–424.

359. Hirano M, DiMauro S. ANT1, Twinkle, POLG, and TP: new genes open our eyes to ophthalmoplegia [editorial]. Neurology 2001;57:2163–2165.

360. Lamantea E, Tiranti V, Bordoni A, et al. Mutations of mitochondrial DNA polymerase gammaA are a frequent cause of autosomal dominant or recessive progressive external ophthalmoplegia. Ann Neurol 2002;52:211–219.

361. Mancuso M, Filosto M, Bellan M, et al. POLG mutations causing ophthalmoplegia, sensorimotor polyneuropathy, ataxia, and deafness. Neurology 2004;62:316–318.

362. Agostino A, Valletta L, Chinnery PF, et al. Mutations of ANT1, Twinkle, and POLG1 in sporadic progressive external ophthalmoplegia (PEO). Neurology 2003;60:1354–1356.

363. Hudson G, Deschauer M, Taylor RW, et al. POLG1, C10ORF2, and ANT1 mutations are uncommon in sporadic progressive external ophthalmoplegia with multiple mitochondrial DNA deletions. Neurology 2006;66:1439–1441.

364. Pellock JM, Behrens M, Lewis L, et al. Kearns-Sayre syndrome and hypoparathyroidism. Ann Neurol 1978;3:455–458.

365. Case records of the Massachusetts General Hospital. Case 34-1987. N Engl J Med 1987;317:493–501.

366. Mitsumoto H, Aprille JR, Wray SH, et al. Chronic progressive external ophthalmoplegia (CPEO): clinical, morphologic, and biochemical studies. Neurology 1983;33:452–461.

367. DiMauro S, Bonilla E, Lombes A, et al. Mitochondrial encephalomyopathies. Neurol Clin 1990;8:483–506.

368. Leutner C, Layer G, Zierz S, et al. Cerebral MR in ophthalmoplegia plus. AJNR Am J Neuroradiol 1994;15:681–687.

369. Kamata Y, Mashima Y, Yokoyama M, et al. Patient with Kearns-Sayre syndrome exhibiting abnormal magnetic resonance imaging of the brain. J Neuroophthalmol 1998;18:284–288.

370. Matthews PM, Andermann F, Silver K, et al. Proton MR spectroscopic differences in regional brain metabolic abnormalities in mitochondrial encephalomyopathies. Neurology 1993;43:2484–2490.

371. Kuwabara T, Watanabe H, Tanaka K, et al. Mitochondrial encephalomyopathy: elevated visual cortex lactate unresponsive to photic stimulation—a localized ^{1}H-MRS study. Neurology 1994;44:557–559.

372. Koenig MK. Presentation and diagnosis of mitochondrial disorders in children. Pediatr Neurol 2008;38:305–313.

373. Wong VA, Beckingsale PS, Oley CA, et al. Management of myogenic ptosis. Ophthalmology 2002;109:1023–1031.

374. Daut PM, Steinemann TL, Westfall CT. Chronic exposure keratopathy complicating surgical correction of ptosis in patients with chronic progressive external ophthalmoplegia. Am J Ophthalmol 2000;130:519–521.

375. Sorkin JA, Shoffner JM, Grossniklaus HE, et al. Strabismus and mitochondrial defects in chronic progressive external ophthalmoplegia. Am J Ophthalmol 1997;123:235–242.

376. Faber J, Fich A, Steinberg A, et al. Familial intestinal pseudoobstruction dominated by a progressive neurologic disease at a young age. Gastroenterology 1987;92:786–790.

377. Cervera R, Bruix J, Bayes A, et al. Chronic intestinal pseudoobstruction and ophthalmoplegia in a patient with mitochondrial myopathy. Gut 1988;29:544–547.

378. Case records of the Massachusetts General Hospital. Case 12-1990. N Engl J Med 1990;322:829–841.

379. Threlkeld AB, Miller NR, Golnik KC, et al. Ophthalmic involvement in myo-neuro-gastrointestinal encephalopathy syndrome. Am J Ophthalmol 1992;114:322–328.

380. Johns DR, Threlkeld AB, Miller NR, et al. Multiple mitochondrial DNA deletions in myo-neuro-gastrointestinal encephalopathy syndrome [letter]. Am J Ophthalmol 1993;115:108–109.

381. Hirano M, Silvestri G, Blacke DM, et al. Mitochondrial neurogastrointestinal encephalomyopathy (MNGIE): clinical, biochemical, and genetic features of an autosomal recessive mitochondrial disorder. Neurology 1994;44:721–727.

382. Papadimitriou A, Comi GP, Hadjigeorgiou GM, et al. Partial depletion and multiple deletions of muscle mtDNA in familial MNGIE syndrome. Neurology 1998;51:1086–1092.

383. Chinnery PF, Vissing J. Treating MNGIE: is reducing blood nucleosides the first cure for a mitochondrial disorder? [editorial]. Neurology 2006;67:1330–1332.

384. Simon LT, Horoupian DS, Dorman LJ, et al. Polyneuropathy, ophthalmoplegia, leukoencephalopathy, and intestinal pseudo-obstruction: POLIP syndrome. Ann Neurol 1990;28:349–360.

385. Ptacek LJ, Johnson KJ, Griggs RC. Genetics and physiology of the myotonic muscle disorders. N Engl J Med 1993;328:482–489.

386. Dyken PR, Harper PS. Congenital dystrophia myotonica. Neurology 1973;23:465–473.

387. Yamashita T, Matsubara E, Nagano I, et al. Bilateral extraocular muscle atrophy in myotonic dystrophy type 1. Neurology 2004;63:759–760.

388. Verhagen WIM, ter Bruggen JP, Huygen PL. Oculomotor, auditory, and vestibular responses in myotonic dystrophy. Arch Neurol 1992;49:954–960.

389. Anastasopoulos D, Kimmig H, Mergner T, et al. Abnormalities of ocular motility in myotonic dystrophy. Brain 1996;119:1923–1932.

390. Verhagen WI, Huygen PL. Abnormalities of ocular motility in myotonic dystrophy [letter]. Brain 1997;120:1907–1909.

391. Versino M, Romani A, Bergamaschi R, et al. Eye movement abnormalities in myotonic dystrophy. Electroencephalogr Clin Neurophysiol 1998;109:184–190.

392. Osanai R, Kinoshita M, Hirose K. Saccadic slowing in myotonic dystrophy and CTG repeat expansion. J Neurol 1998;245:674–680.

393. Winchester CL, Ferrier RK, Sermoni A, et al. Characterization of the expression of DMPK and SIX5 in the human eye and implications for pathogenesis in myotonic dystrophy. Hum Mol Genet 1999;8:481–492.

394. Hill ME, Creed GA, McMullan TF, et al. Oculopharyngeal muscular dystrophy: phenotypic and genotypic studies in a UK population. Brain 2001;124:522–526.

395. Blumen SC, Brais B, Korczyn AD, et al. Homozygotes for oculopharyngeal muscular dystrophy have a severe form of the disease. Ann Neurol 1999;46:115–118.

396. Hardiman O, Halperin JJ, Farrell MA, et al. Neuropathic findings in oculopharyngeal muscular dystrophy. A report of seven cases and a review of the literature. Arch Neurol 1993;50:481–488.

397. Ropper AH. The Guillain-Barré syndrome. N Engl J Med 1992;326:1130–1136.

398. Asbury AK, Arnason BG, Adams RD. The inflammatory lesion in idiopathic polyneuritis. Medicine 1969;48:173–215.

399. Prineas JW. Pathology of the Guillain-Barré syndrome. Ann Neurol 1981;9(Suppl):6–19.

400. Feasby TE, Gilbert JJ, Brown WF, et al. An acute axonal form of Guillain-Barré polyneuropathy. Brain 1986;109:1115–1126.

401. Griffin JW, Li CY, Ho TW, et al. Guillain-Barré syndrome in northern China: the spectrum of neuropathological changes in clinically defined cases. Brain 1995;118:577–595.

402. Asbury AK. Guillain-Barré syndrome. In: Stern MB, Brown MJ, Galetta SL, Asbury AK (eds): Penn Neurology 2000: Management of Common Neurological Problems, pp 99–114. Irvington, AlphaMedica Press, 2000.

403. Maier I, Schmidbauer M, Pfausler B, et al. Central nervous system pathology in patients with the Guillain-Barré syndrome. Brain 1997;120:451–464.

404. Sheikh KA, Nachamkin I, Ho TW, et al. *Campylobacter jejuni* lipopolysaccharides in Guillain-Barré syndrome. Molecular mimicry and host susceptibility. Neurology 1998;51:371–378.

405. Hadden RDM, Cornblath DR, Hughes RAC, et al. Electrophysiological classification of Guillain-Barré syndrome: clinical associations and outcome. Ann Neurol 1998;44: 780–788.

406. Rees JH, Soudain SE, Gregson NA, et al. *Campylobacter jejuni* infection in Guillain-Barré syndrome. N Engl J Med 1995;333:1374–1379.

407. Hadden RD, Karch H, Hartung HP, et al. Preceding infections, immune factors, and outcome in Guillain-Barre syndrome. Neurology 2001;56:758–765.

408. Jacobs BC, Rothbarth PH, van der Meché FGA, et al. The spectrum of antecedent infections in Guillain-Barré syndrome. A case-control study. Neurology 1998;51: 1110–1115.

409. Case records of the Massachusetts General Hospital. Case 39-1990. N Engl J Med 1990;323:895–908.

410. Asbury AK. Diagnostic considerations in Guillain-Barré syndrome. Ann Neurol 1981;9(Suppl):1–5.

411. Ropper AH, Wijdicks EFM, Truax BT. Clinical features of Guillain-Barré syndrome. In: Guillain-Barré Syndrome, pp 56–152. Philadelphia, F.A. Davis, 1991.

412. Nadkarni N, Lisak RP. Guillain-Barré syndrome (GBS) with bilateral optic neuritis and central white matter disease. Neurology 1993;43:842–843.

413. Ropper AH, Wijdicks EFM. Blood pressure fluctuations in the dysautonomia of Guillain-Barré syndrome. Arch Neurol 1990;47:706–708.

414. Ropper AH, Wijdicks EFM, Shahani BT. Electrodiagnostic abnormalities in 113 consecutive patients with Guillain-Barré syndrome. Arch Neurol 1990;47: 881–887.

415. Case records of the Massachusetts General Hospital. Case 39-1999. N Engl J Med 1999;341:1996–2003.

416. Chiba A, Kusunoki S, Obata H, et al. Serum anti-GQ_{1b} antibody is associated with ophthalmoplegia in Miller Fisher syndrome and Guillain-Barré syndrome. Clinical and immunohistochemical studies. Neurology 1993;43:1911–1917.

417. Asbury AK, Cornblath DR. Assessment of current diagnostic criteria for Guillain-Barré syndrome. Ann Neurol 1990;27(Suppl):S21–S24.

418. Guillain-Barré Syndrome Study Group. Plasmapheresis and acute Guillain-Barré syndrome. Neurology 1985;35:1096–1104.

419. van der Meché FGA, Schmitz PIM, Dutch Guillain-Barré Study Group. A randomized trial comparing intravenous immune globulin and plasma exchange in Guillain-Barré syndrome. N Engl J Med 1992;326:1123–1129.

420. Plasma Exchange/Sandoglobulin Guillain-Barré Syndrome Trial Group. Randomised trial of plasma exchange, intravenous immunoglobulin, and combined treatments in Guillain-Barré syndrome. Lancet 1997;349:225–230.

421. Hughes RA, Wijdicks EF, Barohn R, et al. Practice parameter: immunotherapy for Guillain-Barré syndrome. Report of the Quality Standards Subcommittee of the American Academy of Neurology. Neurology 2003;61:736–740.

422. Hughes RA, Swan AV, Raphael JC, et al. Immunotherapy for Guillain-Barré syndrome: a systematic review. Brain 2007;130:2245–2257.

423. Buchwald B, Ahangari R, Weishaupt A, et al. Intravenous immunoglobulins neutralize blocking antibodies in Guillain-Barré syndrome. Ann Neurol 2002;51:673–680.

424. Italian Guillain-Barré Study Group. The prognosis and main prognostic indicators of Guillain-Barré syndrome. A multicentre prospective study of 297 patients. Brain 1996;119:2053–2061.

425. Fisher M. An unusual variant of acute idiopathic polyneuritis (syndrome of ophthalmoplegia, ataxia and areflexia). N Engl J Med 1956;255:57–65.

426. Mori M, Kuwabara S, Fukutake T, et al. Clinical features and prognosis of Miller Fisher syndrome. Neurology 2001;56:1104–1106.

427. Yuki N, Sato S, Tsuji S, et al. Frequent presence of anti-G_{Q1b} antibody in Fisher's syndrome. Neurology 1993;43:414–417.

428. Ohtsuka K, Nakamura Y, Hashimoto M, et al. Fisher syndrome associated with IgG antiGQ_{1b} antibody following infection by a specific serotype of *Campylobacter jejuni*. Ophthalmology 1998;105:1281–1285.

429. Yuki N, Taki T, Takahashi M, et al. Molecular mimicry between GQ_{1b} ganglioside and lipopolysaccharides of *Campylobacter jejuni* isolated from patients with Fisher's syndrome. Ann Neurol 1994;36:791–793.

430. Jacobs BC, Endtz HPH, van der Meche FGA, et al. Serum anti-GQ_{1b} IgG antibodies recognize surface epitopes on *Campylobacter jejuni* isolated from patients with Miller Fisher syndrome. Ann Neurol 1995;37:260–264.

431. Vaphiades MS. The double vision decision. Surv Ophthalmol 2003;48:85–91.

432. Nagaoka U, Kato T, Kurita K, et al. Cranial nerve enhancement on three-dimensional MRI in Miller Fisher syndrome. Neurology 1996;47:1601–1602.

433. Tanaka H, Yuki N, Hirata K. Trochlear nerve enhancement on three-dimensional magnetic resonance imaging in Fisher syndrome. Am J Ophthalmol 1998;126:322–324.

434. Fargus A, Roig M, Vazquez E, et al. Brainstem involvement in a child with ophthalmoplegia, ataxia, areflexia syndrome. Pediatr Neurol 1998;18:73–75.

435. Kornberg AJ, Pestronk A, Blume GM, et al. Selective staining of the cerebellar molecular layer by serum IgG in Miller-Fisher and related syndromes. Neurology 1996;47:1317–1320.

436. Al-din AN, Anderson M, Bickerstaff ER, et al. Brainstem encephalitis and the syndrome of Miller Fisher. A clinical study. Brain 1982;105:481–495.

437. Mori M, Kuwabara S, Fukutake T, et al. Intravenous immunoglobulin therapy for Miller Fisher syndrome. Neurology 2007;68:1144–1146.

438. Berlit P, Rakicky J. The Miller Fisher syndrome. Review of the literature. J Clin Neuroophthalmol 1992;12:57–63.

439. McCombe PA, Pollard JD, McLeod JG. Chronic inflammatory demyelinating polyradiculoneuropathy. Brain 1987;110:1617–1630.

440. Barohn RJ, Kissel JT, Warmolts JR, et al. Chronic inflammatory demyelinating polyradiculopathy. Clinical characteristics, course, and recommendations for diagnostic criteria. Arch Neurol 1989;46:878–884.

441. Arroyo JG, Horton JC. Acute, painful, pupil-sparing third nerve palsy in chronic inflammatory demyelinating polyneuropathy. Neurology 1995;45:846–847.

442. Lee AG, Galetta SL, Lepore FE, et al. Optic atrophy and chronic acquired polyneuropathy. J Neuroophthalmol 1999;19:67–69.

443. Faed JM, Day B, Pollock M, et al. High-dose intravenous human immunoglobulin in chronic inflammatory demyelinating polyneuropathy. Neurology 1989;39:422–425.

444. van Doorn PA, Vermeulen M, Mulder PGH, et al. Intravenous immunoglobulin treatment in patients with chronic inflammatory demyelinating polyneuropathy. Clinical and laboratory characteristics associated with improvement. Arch Neurol 1991;48:217–220.

445. Gorson KC, Allam G, Ropper AH. Chronic inflammatory demyelinating polneuropathy: clinical features and response to treatment in 67 consecutive patients with and without a monoclonal gammopathy. Neurology 1997;48:321–328.

446. Moore KL. Clinically Oriented Anatomy, 4th edn, p 900. Baltimore, Williams & Wilkins, 1999.

CHAPTER 15

Eye movement disorders: third, fourth, and sixth nerve palsies and other causes of diplopia and ocular misalignment

This chapter will cover the diagnosis and management of the causes of double vision and ocular misalignment. Although the bulk of the discussion will concentrate on third, fourth, and sixth nerve palsies, other supranuclear, nuclear, neuromuscular junction, myopathic, and restrictive disorders will be detailed or alluded to. The relevant anatomy of the ocular motor system will be discussed first, followed by signs and symptoms in patients with diplopia, then the diagnosis and management. The differential diagnosis of the major entities that cause diplopia or ocular misalignment will then be reviewed.

Note: the following terms will be interchanged throughout this chapter: oculomotor = third = IIIrd nerve; trochlear = fourth = IVth nerve; abducens = sixth = VIth nerve. Also, the term "ocular motor nerves" refers to the IIIrd, IVth, and VIth nerves together.

Anatomy

Overview

The three ocular motor cranial nerves (IIIrd, IVth, and VIth) innervate the six extraocular muscles of each eye (**Fig. 15-1**), the major eyelid elevator, and the pupillary constrictor. The *oculomotor (IIIrd) nerve* activates the medial rectus (adduction), inferior rectus (depression), superior rectus, and inferior oblique (elevation) muscles as well as the pupillary sphincter muscle (constriction) and levator palpebrae of the upper lid. The *trochlear (IVth) nerve* supplies the superior oblique muscle, which intorts the eye and depresses it in adduction. The *abducens (VIth) nerve* innervates the lateral rectus muscle, which abducts the eye (**Fig. 15-2**).

From central nervous system to the orbit

Supranuclear control of III, IV, and VI. In a logical, hierarchical control of eye movements, the supranuclear centers in the cortex and brainstem direct the actions of the ocular motor nerves. For horizontal saccades (see **Fig. 16-2**), the frontal and cortical eye fields inhibit the contralateral omnipause neurons (OPNs), thereby disinhibiting the paramedian pontine reticular formation (PPRF). Neurons of the PPRF, in turn, excite the adjacent VIth nerve nucleus, which, via the ascending medial longitudinal fasciculus (MLF), innervates the contralateral medial rectus subnucleus in the mesencephalon. Supranuclear centers for pursuit lie in the ipsilateral frontal and

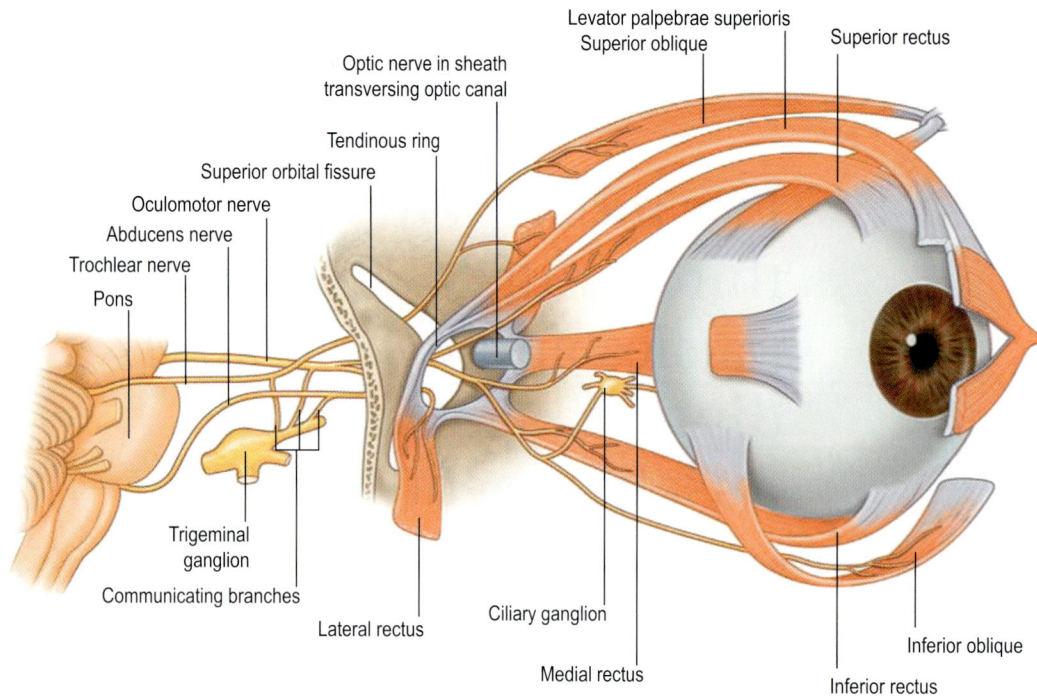

Figure 15–1. Innervation of the extraocular muscles. The oculomotor (III), trochlear (IV), and abducens (VI) nerves enter the orbit through the superior orbital fissure. The trochlear nerve supplies the superior oblique, the abducens nerve supplies the lateral rectus, and the oculomotor nerve supplies the remaining five muscles. Note the inferior oblique muscle attaches to the inferior bony orbit.

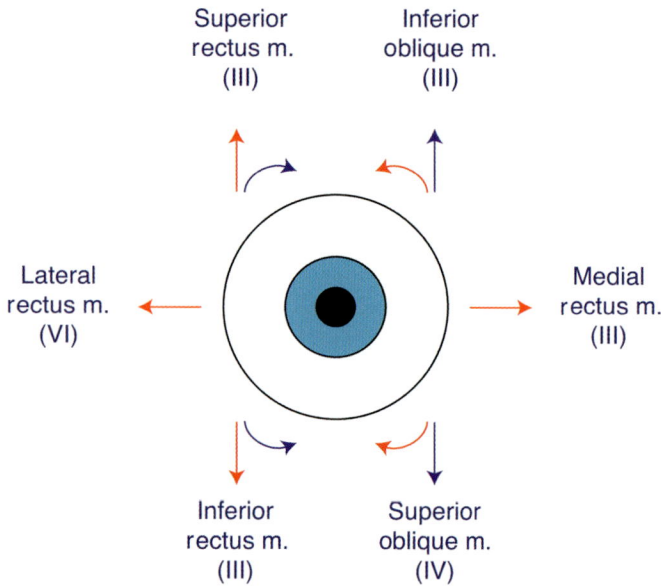

Figure 15–2. Diagram of right eye (examiner's view) showing direction of primary (red) and secondary (blue) actions of the six extraocular muscles (m.) and the ocular motor nerve (III, IV, or VI) that innervates each.

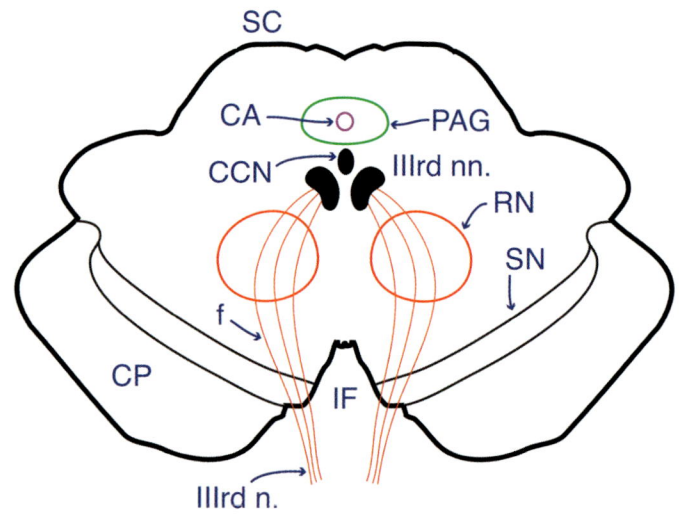

Figure 15–3. Diagram of axial section of the midbrain through the superior colliculus. CA, cerebral aqueduct; CCN, central caudal nucleus; CP, cerebral peduncle; SN, substantia nigra; f, oculomotor nerve fascicle; IIIrd nn., oculomotor nerve nucleus; IIIrd n., oculomotor nerve; IF, interpeduncular fossa; PAG, periaqueductal gray; SC, superior colliculus; and RN, red nucleus.

supplementary eye fields and V5 (see **Fig. 16–3**). Upgaze and downgaze saccades, also under voluntary control by the frontal and cortical eye fields, are initiated by neurons in the mesencephalic rostral interstitial nucleus of the medial longitudinal fasciculus (riMLF) and regulated by cells in the interstitial nucleus of Cajal (INC), areas which exert supra-nuclear control over the IIIrd and IVth nerve nuclei (see **Fig. 16–18**). The vestibular nuclei have direct connections with the IIIrd and IVth nerve nuclei, via the MLF. These and other supranuclear gaze centers are reviewed in detail in Chapter 16.

Nuclear and fascicular structures. The oculomotor (IIIrd) nuclear complex lies in the midbrain, anterior to the cerebral aqueduct (**Fig. 15–3**).[1] Each muscle innervated by the IIIrd

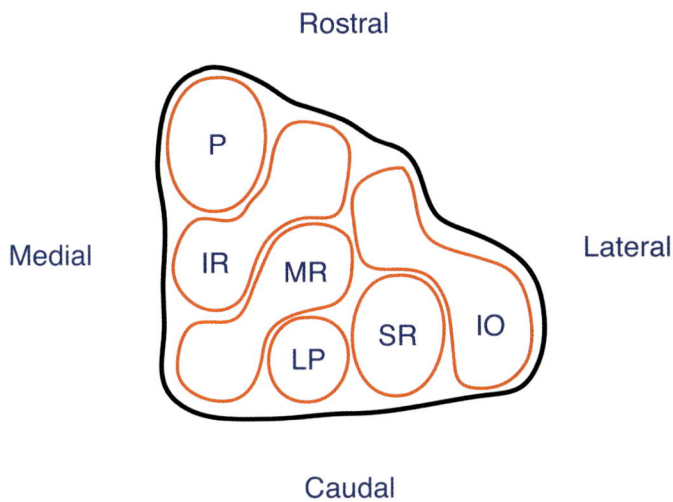

Figure 15–4. Cross-sectional diagram of topographic organization of the IIIrd nerve fascicle.[159,162] Labeled fiber distributions: P, pupillary; IR, inferior rectus; MR, medial rectus; LP, levator palpebrae; SR, superior rectus; IO, inferior oblique.

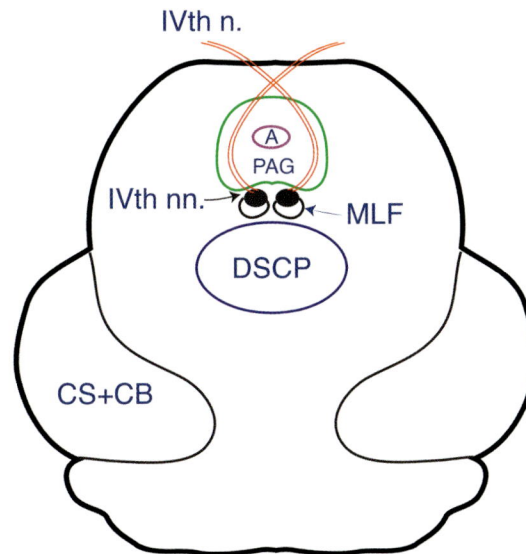

Figure 15–5. Axial section through the IVth nerve nuclei at the level of the pontomesencephalic junction. A, aqueduct; PAG, periaqueductal gray matter; IVth n., fourth nerve; IVth nn., fourth nerve nucleus; MLF, medial longitudinal fasciculus; CS + CB, corticospinal and corticobulbar tracts; DSCP, decussation of the superior cerebellar peduncle (brachium conjunctivum).

nerve is subserved by individual subnuclei.[2,3] Unique features, however, include the central caudal subnucleus, which subserves both levator muscles; the superior rectus subnuclei, which each innervate the contralateral superior rectus muscle; and the Edinger–Westphal nuclei, which supply the preganglionic cholinergic neurons of the pupil. Fibers from the superior rectus subnuclei are thought to pass through the contralateral superior rectus subnucleus before joining the contralateral IIIrd nerve fascicle.[4] Pupillary and eyelid function and related abnormalities are discussed in Chapters 13 and 14, respectively. The paired oculomotor fascicles travel ventrally through the midbrain, each passing through the red nuclei and then the medial portion of the cerebral peduncles before exiting into the interpeduncular fossa (**Fig. 15–3**). The neurons of each IIIrd nerve-innervated muscle are topographically organized within the fascicle (**Fig. 15–4**).

The trochlear nucleus lies ventral to the aqueduct in the pontomesencephalic junction (**Fig. 15–5**), caudal to the oculomotor complex. Fourth nerve axons decussate near the roof of the aqueduct and exit the brainstem dorsally just beneath the inferior colliculi, in an area called the anterior medullary vellum. Thus, each trochlear nucleus innervates the contralateral superior oblique muscle.

The abducens nucleus lies immediately ventral to the genu of the facial nerve (facial colliculus in dorsal pons) (**Fig. 15–6**). This nucleus contains cell bodies for the motor neurons which will innervate the ipsilateral VIth nerve and interneurons which will climb within the MLF to innervate the contralateral medial rectus subnucleus (see **Fig. 16–2**). The fascicles travel ventrally, passing through the cortical spinal tracts, before exiting anterolaterally at the pontomedullary junction.

It should be emphasized that, except for the superior rectus subnucleus and the trochlear nuclei, the ocular motor nuclei innervate ipsilateral eye muscles.

Extra-axial structures. The three ocular motor nerves traverse the subarachnoid space at the skull base before reaching the cavernous sinus (**Fig. 15–7**). The IIIrd nerve

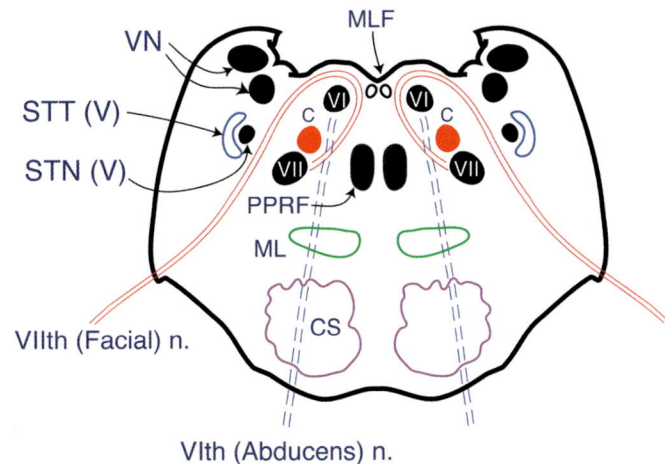

Figure 15–6. Axial section through the pons at the level of the VIth nerve nuclei. VI, sixth nerve nucleus; VII, seventh nerve nucleus; C, central tegmental tract; CS, corticospinal tract; VN, vestibular nuclei; ML, medial lemniscus; MLF, medial longitudinal fasciculus; PPRF, paramedian pontine reticular formation; STT (V), spinal trigeminal tract of the Vth nerve; STN (V), spinal trigeminal nucleus of the Vth nerve.

enters the cavernous sinus by piercing the dura in its most superior portion just lateral to the posterior clinoid process. The IVth nerve travels for about 3.5 cm from behind the brainstem, running under the free edge of the tentorium before piercing the dura to lie immediately inferior to the IIIrd nerve.[5] The VIth nerve ascends the clivus then travels underneath the petroclinoidal (Grüber's) ligament through Dorello's canal to enter the cavernous sinus. The transition from petrous to intracavernous segments of the internal carotid artery occurs as the vessel passes the petrolingual ligament, which is the posteroinferior attachment of the lateral wall of the cavernous sinus.

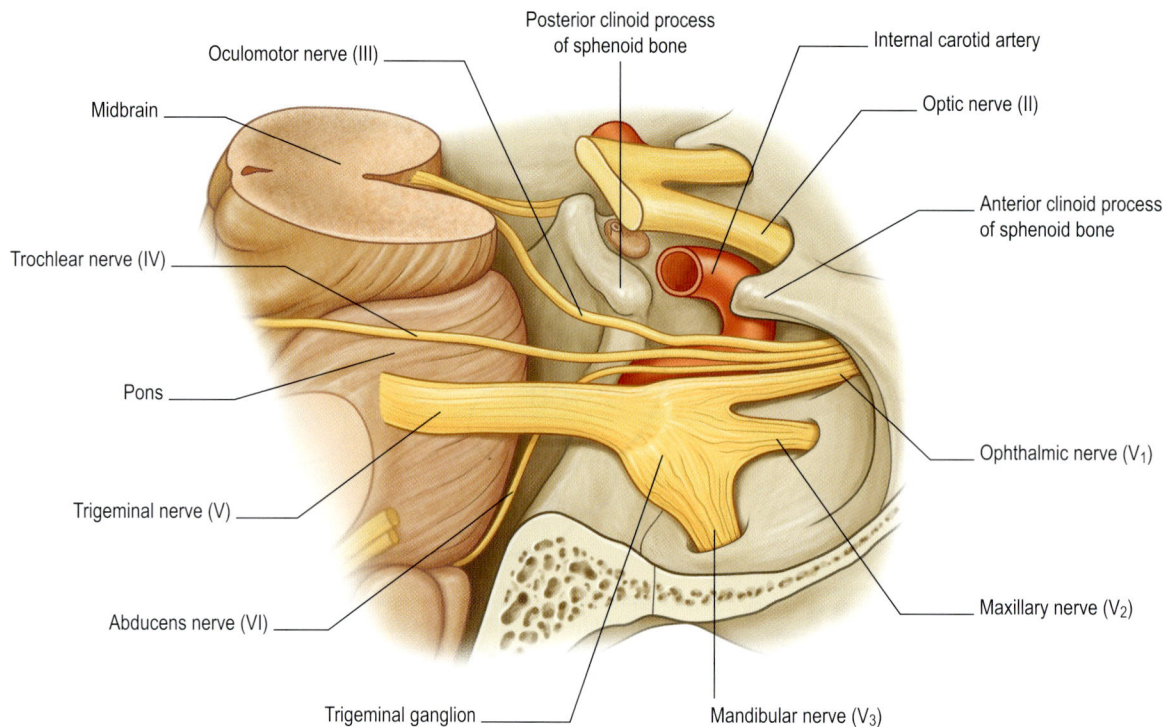

Figure 15–7. Lateral view of the right cavernous sinus with the temporal lobe and lateral wall dissected. The optic chiasm and third ventricle lie superomedially to this region and the divisions of the trigeminal nerve are entering their respective foramina. The IIIrd, IVth, and VIth nerves exit the brainstem (*left*), traverse the subarachnoid space, then enter the cavernous sinus along with V1 and V2.

The cavernous sinuses are triangular-shaped interconnecting structures that flank the lateral sides of the sella turcica. The walls of each sinus are created by dura mater extending from the superior orbital fissure to the posterior wall of the sella known as the dorsum sella. Inferiorly, the cavernous sinus region and pituitary fossa are in close proximity to the sphenoid and maxillary sinuses while the optic chiasm lies superomedially (see **Fig. 7–5**). Each cavernous sinus contains a plexus of veins that drains the inferior and superior ophthalmic veins of the orbit and funnel posteriorly to the inferior and superior petrosal sinuses.[6] Communications are established to the opposite cavernous sinus by channels that cross the midline. Inferiorly, connections are made to the pterygoid plexus that subsequently drain into the internal jugular vein while lateral anastomoses are made to the middle cerebral vein.[7,8]

The S-shaped intracavernous carotid artery gives rise to multiple important branches including: (1) the meningohypophyseal trunk that supplies blood to the tentorium and inferior pituitary gland; (2) the inferior lateral trunk that nourishes the ocular motor nerves;[9] and (3) the superior hypophyseal artery that provides blood to the rostral portion of the pituitary gland.[10]

The IIIrd and IVth nerves and the first and second divisions of the trigeminal nerve (V1 and V2) lie along the lateral wall of the cavernous sinus, while the internal carotid artery, the VIth nerve, and third-order oculosympathetic fibers from the superior cervical ganglion lie more medially (**Fig. 15–8**).[11] In the anterior portion of the cavernous sinus, the IIIrd nerve

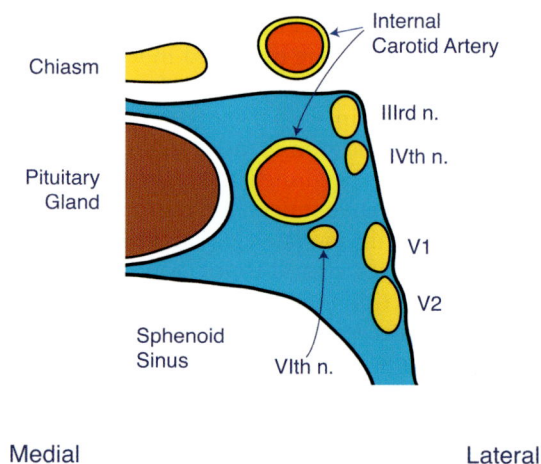

Figure 15–8. Diagram of the coronal view of the cavernous sinus (orange area). The IIIrd, IVth, and V1 and V2 cranial nerves line up vertically in the lateral wall of the cavernous sinus, whereas the VIth nerve lies freely closer to the carotid artery.

anatomically separates into superior and inferior divisions. The superior division innervates the superior rectus and levator muscles, while the inferior division supplies the inferior rectus, inferior oblique, medial rectus, and pupillary sphincter muscles. Within the anterior cavernous sinus, the IVth nerve crosses above the IIIrd nerve just before both nerves enter the superior orbital fissure. Within the cavernous sinus network, the VIth nerve lies freely just lateral to

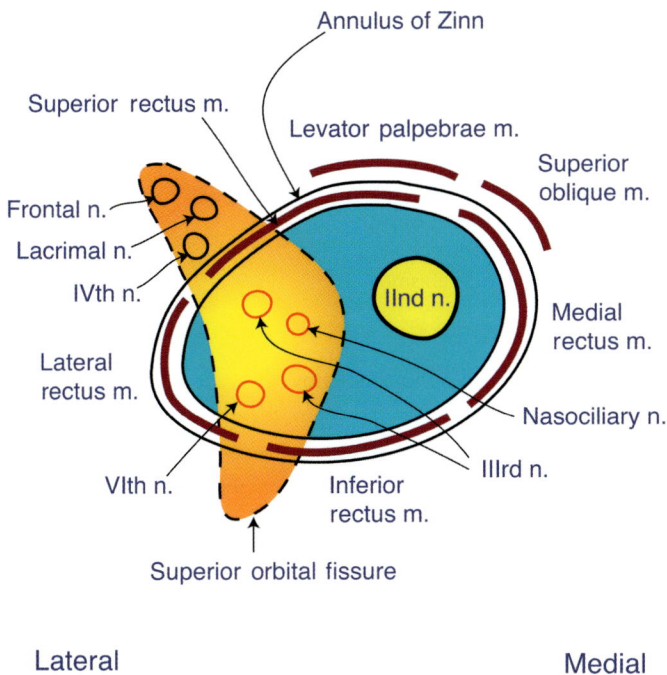

Figure 15–9. Diagram of the contents of the superior orbital fissure (orange area) and annulus of Zinn in a coronal view of the back of the orbit.

tion. Pupilloconstrictor fibers from the IIIrd nerve synapse in the ciliary ganglion, which lies within the lateral muscle cone (see **Fig. 13–3**) and issues postsynaptic fibers that innervate the pupil. Other details regarding orbital anatomy, including that of the extraocular muscles, are discussed in Chapter 18. Readers interested in detailed reviews of the anatomy and physiology of the extraocular muscles are referred to the reviews and articles by Porter, Baker, and their colleagues.[13-15]

Blood supply of the extra-axial ocular motor nerves. The nutrient circulation to the IIIrd nerve[16,17] arises from (1) small thalamomesencephalic perforators arising from the basilar and posterior cerebral arteries and the posterior circle of Willis, in the proximal subarachnoid space;[18] (2) as alluded to earlier, microscopic branches of the inferior lateral trunk of the intracavernous carotid within the cavernous sinus;[19] and (3) recurrent branches of the ophthalmic artery intraorbitally. A watershed region of the IIIrd nerve may exist between the proximal and intracavernous portions.[20] The cavernous and orbital blood supply of the IVth and VIth nerves is likely similar. The subarachnoid segment of the IVth nerve derives its blood supply from branches of the superior cerebellar artery.[21] The subarachnoid segment of the VIth nerve is likely supplied by branches from the posterior cerebral and superior cerebellar arteries.

the cavernous carotid artery and enters the superior orbital fissure as it courses anteriorly. The postganglionic sympathetic fibers travel up the carotid artery and briefly join the VIth nerve within the cavernous sinus. This anatomical relationship accounts for the occasional case of an abducens palsy and Horner syndrome associated with lesions of the cavernous sinus.[12]

Knowledge of the anatomy of the trigeminal nerve (see Chapter 19) is critical for localizing lesions within the parasellar region. Since the mandibular branch of the trigeminal nerve travels through the foramen ovale, involvement of this branch indicates a process posterior to cavernous sinus. More anteriorly, the maxillary division leaves the skull base at the level of the cavernous sinus via the foramen rotundum. The ophthalmic branch of the trigeminal, along with the IIIth, IVth, VIth nerves and the oculosympathetic fibers, leave the anterior cavernous sinus and enter the orbit through the superior orbital fissure (**Figs 15–1** and **15–9**).

Orbit. Once in the orbit (**Fig. 15–1**), the ocular motor nerves reach their respective extraocular muscles. The IIIrd and VIth nerves along with the optic nerve lie within the annulus of Zinn and muscle cone (**Fig. 15–9**). Like the frontal and lacrimal nerves (branches of V1), the trochlear nerve passes above the annulus of Zinn. However, the orbital apex syndrome is usually considered to consist of optic nerve, IIIrd, IVth, VIth, and V1 dysfunction. In contrast to the more direct orientation and attachments of the lateral, inferior, and superior rectus and inferior oblique muscles, the superior oblique muscle tendon courses through a pulley attached to the superonasal orbital wall then attaches to the globe on its posterior and temporal aspect (**Fig. 15–1**). This arrangement accounts for the down and in movement and intorsion of the eye produced by superior oblique contrac-

Symptoms

Patients with diplopia should be asked whether their double vision is (1) binocular, (2) horizontal or vertical, and (3) worse in left-, right-, up-, or downgaze, or distance or near.

1. *Binocular vs. monocular double vision.* This can be assessed by inquiring, "Does the double vision go away when you cover either eye?" Neurologic ocular misalignment causes binocular diplopia which disappears with either eye covered, whereas ocular causes such as refractive error, for instance, lead to monocular double vision which persists in one eye with the other eye covered.

2. *Horizontal or vertical.* Horizontal double vision suggests dysfunction of the medial or lateral rectus muscles. Vertical diplopia implies an abnormality of the vertically acting muscles such as the inferior rectus, superior rectus, inferior oblique, or superior oblique. Because the vertically acting muscles also tort the eye, their dysfunction can cause diplopia with tilted images.

3. *Directionality.* In a patient with diplopia caused by extraocular muscle paralysis, the double vision will worsen when the patient attempts to look in the direction of action of the paretic muscle. For example, attempted leftward gaze worsens the horizontal diplopia due to weakness of the right medial rectus muscle. Thus, in some instances, history alone is often helpful in localizing the problem.

Some patients with ocular misalignment complain of blurry vision instead of frank diplopia, especially if the two images are close together or the person has intermittent fusion. Asking if the blurry vision resolves with one eye covered is helpful in this regard.

Individuals with ocular misalignment who have no diplopia usually have either (1) defective vision in one or both eyes due to refractive error, cataract, optic neuropathy, or maculopathy, for instance, (2) long-standing childhood strabismus with strabismic amblyopia (defined as loss of two Snellen lines of visual acuity in the bad eye compared with the good one) or suppression (the ability to ignore one of the images), (3) ptosis of one eyelid, or (4) a large angle of strabismus, making the second image less confusing and easy to ignore.

The examiner should investigate other historical details such as duration of onset, whether the patient has had the motility deficit since childhood, presence of pain, fatigability, other neurologic symptoms such as dysphagia or weakness, underlying illnesses such as hypertension, diabetes, cerebrovascular disease, cardiac atherosclerotic disease, or multiple sclerosis, and habits such as smoking or alcohol use.

Signs

The ocular motility examination is detailed in Chapter 2. It should consist of testing for:

1. Obvious misalignment, ptosis, or pupillary abnormalities, first by inspection.
2. Ductions, which are movements of each eye separately.
3. Vergences, which are coordinated movements of both eyes in opposite directions.
4. Saccades and pursuit.
5. Oculocephalic maneuver.
6. Ocular misalignment, assessed qualitatively or quantitatively using cover/uncover, alternate cover, Maddox rod, or Krimsky or Hirschberg techniques. Often the motility disturbance will be obvious after inspection and testing of vergences. However, more subtle problems will require quantification of the misalignment using prism-alternative cover or Maddox rod techniques. Although there are many exceptions, acquired incomitant deviations (in which the ocular misalignment is different in different directions) are usually a neurologic problem, while comitant deviations (same in every direction) are typically long-standing, often dating to childhood.
7. Other clues such as head, face, and chin position (e.g., head tilt), or orbital signs such as proptosis or eyelid swelling.
8. Forced ductions when restrictive abnormalities are suspected.

Monocular diplopia that resolves with a pinhole is likely due to refractive error, media opacity, or retinal abnormality, but psychogenic disturbances should also be considered.

Approach

Using the clues from the history and examination, the examiner's goals are to decide:

Table 15–1 Horizontal vs. vertical diplopia: major causes

Horizontal diplopia
 VIth nerve palsy
 IIIrd nerve palsy
 Convergence insufficiency
 Divergence insufficiency
 Internuclear ophthalmoplegia
 Myasthenia gravis
 Decompensated Strabismus

Vertical diplopia
 IVth nerve palsy
 Thyroid-associated ophthalmopathy
 Myasthenia gravis
 Skew deviation
 Third nerve palsy

1. Whether the diplopia or misalignment is a neurologic, ocular, or a childhood strabismus problem. If it is neurologic, then a lesion affecting the structures outlined in the anatomic pathways above, from supranuclear ones to muscle, may be implicated.
2. Which extraocular muscles are involved.
3. The cause. We suggest considering the most common causes of acquired misalignment by whether they typically cause horizontal[22] or vertical diplopia[23,24] (**Table 15–1**).

Often the ophthalmoparesis and abnormal motility pattern is characteristic, and other historical features or accompanying neurologic findings aid in localization and diagnosis. A complete, isolated infranuclear IIIrd nerve palsy causes ipsilateral elevation, adduction, and depression weakness accompanied by abduction, hypodeviation, pupillary mydriasis, and ptosis. Patients with superior oblique paresis complain of vertical diplopia, often with a torsional component, and they have an ipsilateral hypertropia worse on contraversive (contralateral conjugate) horizontal gaze and ipsilateral head tilt. Patients with a lateral rectus palsy complain of binocular horizontal double vision worse on ipsiversive gaze and at distance. In many cases the limitation of abduction is evident, but, in more subtle instances, alternate cover or Maddox rod testing would confirm an esotropia largest on ipsiversive gaze. Small vertical deviations, consistent with normal hyperphorias, can be seen in VIth nerve palsies.[25] Restrictive diplopia, due to orbital processes such as thyroid-associated ophthalmopathy, are associated with limited movements with normal saccadic velocity but positive forced duction testing. Proptosis and periorbital swelling are also usually present in such cases.

Another important consideration when determining the etiology of the diplopia is the age of the patient. In adults, diabetes, hypertension, trauma, and aneurysms are common causes of ocular motor palsies (**Table 15–2**).[26–28] In contrast, in most pediatric series, the most common causes of acquired IIIrd, IVth, and VIth nerve palsies are trauma and neoplasms. Vascular and aneurysmal causes of ocular motor palsies are uncommon in children.[29]

Table 15–2 Causes of acquired IIIrd, IVth, and VIth nerve palsies in adults. "Vascular" refers to associated diabetes mellitus, hypertension, or atherosclerosis. * = most common group; # = most common group with an identifiable cause. Data from Richards et al.[28]

Etiology	IIIrd (%)	IVth (%)	VIth (%)	Multiple (any combination of IIIrd, IVth, or VIth) (%)
Undetermined	24*	32*	26*	12
Vascular	20#	18	13	4
Head trauma	15	29#	15	17
Aneurysm	16	1	3	9
Neoplasm	12	5	22#	35*#
Other	13	15	22	23

Treatment overview

The ophthalmoparesis in some of the disorders described, such as ischemic and traumatic ocular motor palsies, will often resolve spontaneously. Other cases, such as those due to myasthenia gravis or bacterial meningitis, will improve as the underlying cause is treated. In the meantime, patients with diplopia can wear an eyepatch over one eye to resolve the double vision, or one lens of a pair of eyeglasses can be taped over. Some authors have advocated botulinum toxin injections into the antagonist muscle of a paretic one, even in supranuclear ocular motility disorders.[30] For instance, in a left lateral rectus palsy, the left medial rectus palsy is injected with botulinum to decrease adduction tone. Prisms may be used to facilitate image alignment, and are best for patients with relatively comitant deviations. Temporary Fresnel paste-on prisms can be used initially, followed by ground-in prisms in chronic cases. Individuals with ophthalmoparesis who do not improve spontaneously, and whose examinations remain stable for at least 6 months, may be candidates for corrective eye muscle surgery.

Children with ocular motor palsies, especially those under age 8 years, have the potential for developing strabismic amblyopia. Third nerve palsies have the complicating feature of ptosis with the potential for deprivational amblyopia. These children, when able, should be referred to a pediatric ophthalmologist for patching or lid elevation. Children patched for symptomatic diplopia should have the patch alternated daily between eyes to prevent occlusion amblyopia.

Monocular double vision

Ophthalmic causes of monocular double vision

Most patients with monocular double vision have an optical problem, a macular abnormality, or a non-organic symptom. Generally, the description of double vision that persists with one eye closed is different in each of these circumstances. Patients with optical causes of monocular double vision generally describe blurring and a "ghost image" or extra line to things they are viewing. They do not see a discrete, second image but a lighter, partial second image that is attached to the main image and separates from it in one direction. The symptom almost always improves or disappears when the same object is viewed through a pinhole. Common causes of this type of double vision include cataracts, irregular astigmatism (particularly keratoconus), corneal scars, and tear film irregularities. If refraction with a rigid contact lens improves the double vision then the cause is likely to be an irregular corneal surface. Treatment of this type of double vision is etiology specific, i.e., refraction, rigid contact lens use, cataract extraction, or laser keratectomy.

Patients with macular causes of monocular double vision generally describe a break, bend, or distortion of the viewed edge leading to a double or distorted image. This type of monocular double vision generally does not improve with pinhole, and, in fact, vision is often worse through a pinhole in this setting. Common macular causes of monocular double vision include epiretinal membranes and retinal or choroidal folds. In addition, it should be noted that binocular diplopia can result from macular disease as well. In one mechanism, macular disease leads to significant image distortion or difference in image size compared with the other eye (aniseikonia). This image size or shape discrepancy prevents fusion of images despite normal alignment.[31,32] Alternatively, double vision may result from macular displacement by vitreoretinal traction or epiretinal membrane, for instance.[33,34]

Finally, patients with non-organic or functional vision loss often complain of monocular double vision. In our experience this is an ill-defined symptom which cannot be further characterized by the patient and may affect one or both eyes. Double vision may be reported only after the examiner asks specifically about it when trying to characterize a complaint of "blurred vision." In this setting, patients may also complain of triple or quadruple vision. The symptom does not improve with pinhole or any other maneuver on the part of the examiner. Non-organic vision loss is discussed further in Chapter 11.

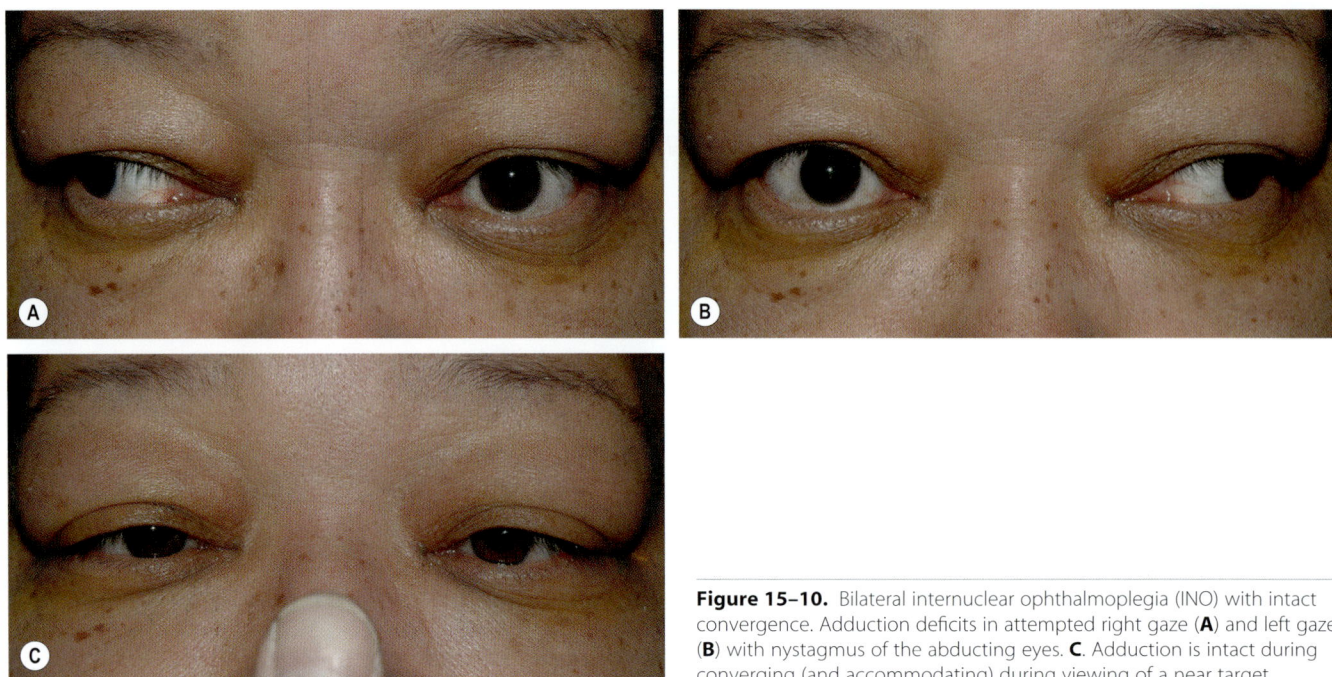

Figure 15-10. Bilateral internuclear ophthalmoplegia (INO) with intact convergence. Adduction deficits in attempted right gaze (**A**) and left gaze (**B**) with nystagmus of the abducting eyes. **C**. Adduction is intact during converging (and accommodating) during viewing of a near target.

Neurologic causes of monocular double vision

Rarely, acquired occipital lobe lesions or drugs may cause multiple images, akin to palinopsia. These types of visual hallucinations are discussed in Chapter 12.

Supranuclear causes of diplopia, including vergence disorders

This section will review diplopia caused by supranuclear lesions: internuclear ophthalmoplegia and the major vergence disorders (abnormalities of moving the eyes in opposite directions): convergence spasm, convergence and divergence insufficiency, and pseudoabducens palsy, which cause horizontal diplopia; and skew deviation and monocular elevator palsy, which lead to vertical diplopia.

Internuclear ophthalmoplegia

Disruption of the MLF in the pons or midbrain results in an *internuclear ophthalmoplegia (INO)* typified by an ipsilateral adduction deficit and contralateral abducting nystagmus (**Figs 15-10 and 15-11**). The side of the adduction deficit determines the side of the INO.

Symptoms. Patients with internuclear ophthalmoplegia (INO) may complain of horizontal diplopia, particularly when the adduction weakness is profound. Those patients with subtle paresis may have no symptoms or complain of blurred vision with eccentric gaze or quick shifts in horizontal gaze only. Since a skew deviation (see below)

Video 15.1

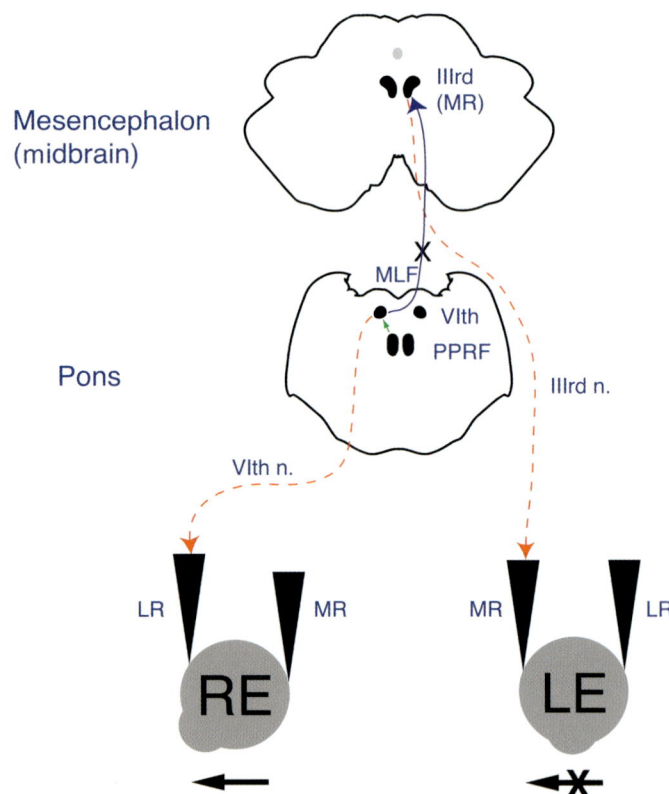

Figure 15-11. Diagram of the pathways and lesion for an internuclear ophthalmoplegia (INO). Interneurons from the VIth nerve nucleus cross in the pons and ascend within the medial longitudinal fasciculus (MLF) to innervate the contralateral medial rectus subnucleus. A lesion within the MLF (X) will cause an ipsilateral adduction deficit. LE, left eye; LR, medial rectus muscle; MR, medial rectus muscle; PPRF, paramedian pontine reticular formation; RE, right eye.

is frequently associated with lesions of the medial longitudinal fasciculus (MLF), vertical diplopia may be another complaint.[35] Oscillopsia may result from either the abduction nystagmus or an impaired vertical vestibular ocular reflex.[35]

Signs. The hallmark finding of INO is impaired adduction of the eye (**Fig. 15–10**). There is a wide range of medial rectus dysfunction in INO. Subtle cases may be evident only with fast eye movements from eccentric gaze to midline ("medial rectus float"). An optokinetic flag pulled along the horizontal plane may reveal slow adducting saccades in the affected eye during the fast phase of the nystagmus.[36] The demonstration of intact convergence in INO establishes the supranuclear localization of the medial rectus weakness and usually signifies a lesion of the MLF within the pons. In contrast, patients with MLF lesions close to the IIIrd nerve nucleus may have impaired convergence. However, some patients with INO have poor convergence because of the vertical misalignment produced by the associated skew deviation.[35] Therefore, the absence of convergence may not be a totally reliable sign to localize the lesion in a discrete part of the MLF pathway.

The eye that is contralateral to the MLF lesion typically exhibits an abducting nystagmus in end gaze. Evidence suggests that this abducting nystagmus is an adaptive phenomenon in an attempt to increase the innervation to the weak adducting eye.[35,37]

Since the otolith pathways project through the MLF, a skew deviation and ocular tilt reaction is commonly observed with an INO (see below).[38] Typically, the hypertropic eye is on the same side as the adduction weakness. A dissociated form of vertical torsional nystagmus may also be observed because of disrupted connections from the posterior semicircular canal. This results in a downbeating nystagmus in the eye ipsilateral to the MLF lesion and torsional nystagmus in the contralateral eye.[39,40] Bilateral lesions of the MLF often produce additional eye findings including impaired vertical pursuit and upbeat nystagmus in both eyes in upgaze.[41] Severe bilateral INOs may also result in a large angle exotropia in primary gaze in so-called "WEBINO" (*w*all-*e*yed *b*ilateral *INO*).[42]

Pathophysiology. Axons for the MLF arise from interneurons intermingled within the abducens nucleus (**Fig. 15–11**). These axons immediately cross the midline and ascend in the medial longitudinal fasciculus. Lesions of the medial longitudinal fasciculus produce impaired adduction of the ipsilateral eye. Since other important pathways travel in the MLF, a variety of other neuro-ophthalmologic signs may be found. The utricular pathway arising from the vestibular nucleus ascends in the MLF. Interruption of these vestibular connections results in an ipsilateral hypertropia. Vestibular information also travels to and from the interstitial nucleus of Cajal.[35,37,41] Interruption of these connections in the MLF, particularly when bilateral, will impair (1) vertical pursuit; (2) the vertical vestibular ocular reflex; and (3) vertical gaze-holding mechanisms.

Diagnosis. The diagnosis of internuclear ophthalmoplegia is usually straightforward, especially when there is impaired medial rectus dysfunction in lateral gaze with normal convergence. One should carefully search for other orbital signs since isolated medial rectus lesions may occur from local conditions such as extraocular muscle entrapment. Third nerve palsy should be considered, and ptosis, mydriasis, and vertical eye movement impairment should be carefully excluded. Exotropia resulting from strabismus can be distinguished by the presence of full extraocular movements in lateral gaze and normal saccades on gaze or optokinetic testing. Caution should be applied in this regard, however, because some patients with long-standing large angle exotropia may develop adduction weakness, perhaps on a restrictive basis, which may mimic an INO. Myasthenia gravis can rarely mimic an internuclear ophthalmoplegia (see Myasthenia gravis, below). In such patients there are often eyelid signs to suggest this diagnosis.

Differential diagnosis. A unilateral INO in an older patient usually results from a brainstem infarction, while bilateral internuclear ophthalmoplegia in a young patient typically signifies a demyelinating process such as multiple sclerosis (**Fig. 15–12**). INOs due to infarcts may result from small vessel (penetrator) occlusion or large vessel disease involving the posterior cerebral artery, superior cerebellar artery, or even the basilar artery.[43] In both ischemic[44,45] and demyelinating causes, the prognosis for spontaneous improvement over weeks is excellent.

However, a variety of lesions may be associated with INOs including vascular malformations, tumors, head trauma,[46,47] infections, vasculitis such as systemic lupus erythematosus,[48] Behçet disease,[49] and giant cell arteritis,[50] nutritional disorders including Wernicke disease, metabolic disorders such hepatic encephalopathy, structural abnormalities (Arnold–Chiari malformation),[51] drug intoxications such as toluene abuse,[52] and degenerative conditions, particularly progressive supranuclear palsy. We have seen transient internuclear ophthalmoplegia in a variety of other metabolic disorders causing coma.

In many patients with an INO, a lesion of the MLF in the midbrain or pons can be demonstrated on MRI,[53] but for unclear reasons often the brainstem appears normal.

Variations. The combination of an INO with an ipsiversive conjugate palsy is a *pontine "one-and-a-half" syndrome* due to simultaneous ipsilateral involvement of the PPRF (or VIth nerve nucleus) and the MLF (see Chapter 16, and **Figs 16–7 and 16–8**). Damage to the MLF in addition to the corticospinal tracts results in the *Raymond–Cestan syndrome,* characterized by an internuclear ophthalmoplegia and contralateral hemiparesis.[54] Rarely patients with impaired abduction will have adducting nystagmus. This has been sometimes referred to as a posterior INO of Lutz.[55] This combination of eye signs most likely results from an abducens palsy with the adducting nystagmus representing an adaptive response. A lesion of the medial longitudinal fasciculus seems unlikely with this combination of eye signs.[35]

Convergence spasm

This condition, characterized by convergence, accommodation, bilateral pupillary miosis, and pseudomyopia, may

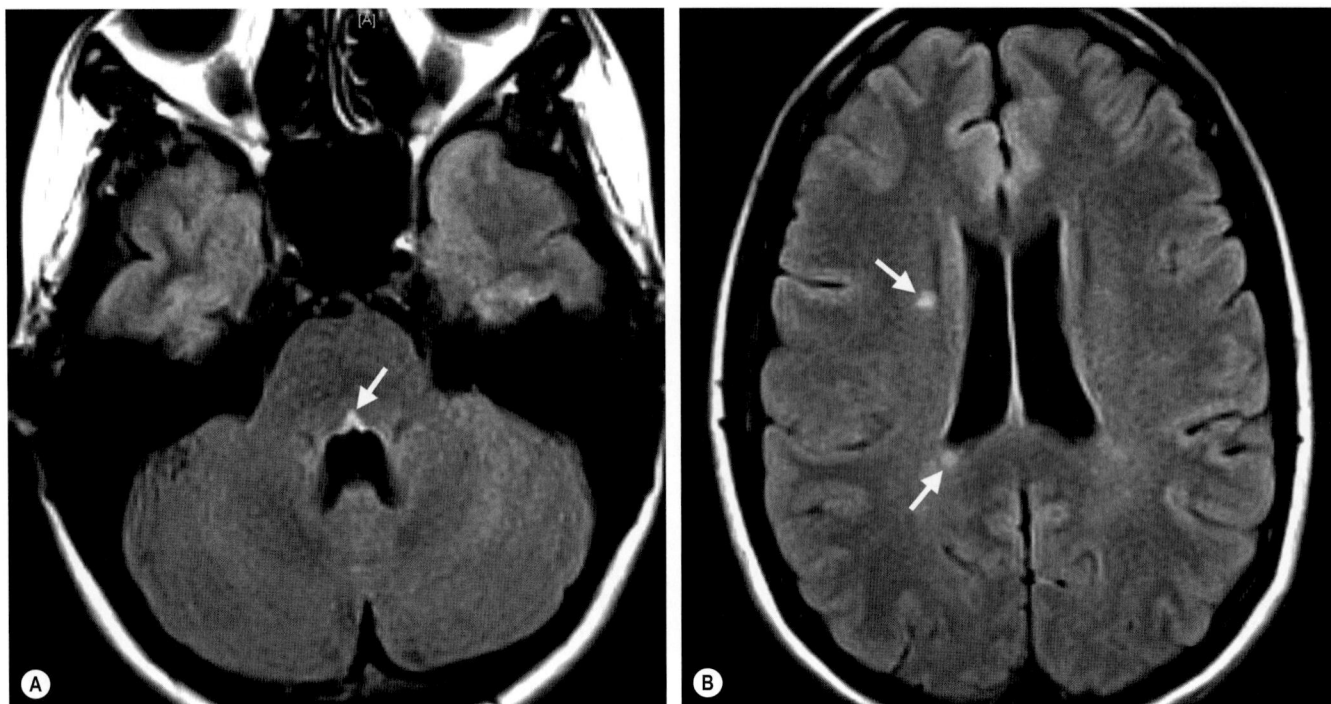

Figure 15–12. Axial FLAIR MR images in a woman with bilateral internuclear ophthalmoplegia (INO) due to demyelination. **A**. Lesion in the dorsal pons at the location of the medial longitudinal fasciculi (*arrow*). **B**. Two periventricular lesions (*arrows*) were demonstrated in more rostral images.

Video 15.3

mimic bilateral VIth nerve palsies. The distinction is important because convergence spasm (or spasm of the near reflex) is almost always indicative of a functional disorder.[56,57] Patients usually complain of double or blurry vision, and they often have other behaviors and symptoms which suggest a non-organic etiology. The hallmarks are pupillary constriction on attempted abduction and a variable esotropia (reflecting variable patient effort). Other features include normal abducting saccades, intact abduction during the oculocephalic maneuver or testing of monocular ductions, and resolution of the myopia following cycloplegia.[58] The miosis may resolve upon occlusion of the fellow eye by disrupting the binocular input necessary for convergence.[59]

Rarely, spasm of the near reflex may be seen in disease states such as metabolic encephalopathy,[60] Arnold–Chiari malformation, pituitary tumors, and trauma.[61] Treatment of the condition consists of cycloplegic eye drops (e.g., atropine) to inhibit accommodation, or weak minus lenses.[58] Other possible treatments, however, include opacification of the medial third of the lenses.[62] However, patient reassurance that no organic disease exists is often the best approach.[56] Convergence spasm should be distinguished from convergence retraction nystagmus or pseudoabducens palsy from pretectal lesions.

Convergence insufficiency

Patients with convergence insufficiency describe horizontal diplopia at near, typically after a period of reading. In a practical definition, patients with this condition are unable to maintain the esodeviation required for near tasks. Once an object is brought to within 10 cm of the bridge of their nose, affected patients are unable to converge. Medial rectus function is normal when ocular ductions are tested, but patients typically have an exodeviation worse at near. A common sequela of head trauma,[63] the condition may also be seen in association with dorsal midbrain lesions (Parinaud syndrome; see Chapter 16),[64] may be a decompensation of a long-standing exophoria, or may be idiopathic. The exact anatomical lesion which causes convergence insufficiency is unknown.

Convergence exercises such as "pencil push-ups," in which the patient is asked to focus on the pencil eraser as it is repeatedly brought close to the eyes, and base-out prisms, which forces convergence, can be tried. One randomized clinical trial in children demonstrated that office-based computerized vergence accommodative therapy with home reinforcement was superior to pencil push-ups.[65] However, these measures may be inadequate for many individuals, who may require either base in prisms for near tasks or strabismus surgery.

Divergence insufficiency

This ocular motility deficit is characterized by acquired horizontal diplopia at distance but not near, a comitant esophoria or esotropia at distance, motor fusion at near, and full ocular ductions without evidence of a VIth nerve palsy. The abnormality has been attributed to a disturbance of a poorly defined supranuclear "divergence center" in the brainstem. Divergence insufficiency is typically benign,[66] and affected patients are usually neurologically normal otherwise. Divergence insufficiency is seen most commonly in elderly individuals with vasculopathic risk factors. Nonspecific small vessel ischemic disease is a relatively common finding on magnetic resonance imaging (MRI) studies in such instances and is of uncertain significance.

However, since small bilateral VIth nerve palsies may mimic divergence insufficiency,[67] elevated intracranial pressure, and brainstem and skull-based lesions masses must be excluded with neuroimaging. Patients with pontine lesions associated with divergence insufficiency have been reported,[68–70] and in two of these discrete lesions in the unilateral tegmentum of the caudal pons were demonstrated,[70] suggesting that involvement of the nucleus reticularis tegmenti pontis might be responsible for this ocular motor disorder. Divergence insufficiency may also be a decompensation of an esophoria or alternatively result from an age-related loss of lateral rectus function from inferior displacement due to loss of orbital connective tissue.[71]

Patients can be treated extremely effectively with base out prisms or strabismus surgery.[72]

Pseudoabducens palsy

This entity is reviewed in detail in Chapter 16 because it often accompanies the dorsal midbrain syndrome or thalamic lesions.[73] Although the lateral rectus appears to be weak, oculocephalic maneuvers demonstrate full horizontal ductions. The esotropia is usually variable, and may represent excess convergence tone.

Skew deviation

Skew deviation refers to a vertical misalignment of the eyes that commonly occurs from acute brainstem lesions which disrupt prenuclear vestibular pathways to the IIIrd and IVth nerve nuclei.[74–76] Occasionally, skew deviation may also result from peripheral vestibular or cerebellar lesions.[77–82]

Symptoms and signs. Patients may complain of binocular vertical diplopia, sometimes with a torsional component. The presence of other neurologic symptoms and signs often helps to distinguish skew deviation from other causes of vertical misalignment such as IIIrd and IVth nerve palsies.[83] For example, a vertical deviation of the eyes with signs of pontomedullary dysfunction, such as ataxia, usually suggests a skew deviation is present.

Ocular-tilt reaction (OTR). The combination of skew deviation with ocular torsion and a head tilt is known as the ocular-tilt reaction (**Fig. 15–13**).[75] This triad of signs is typically observed with lesions of the lateral pontomedullary junction (**Fig. 15–14**) or the paramedian thalamic–mesencephalic region, and results from dysfunction of the utricular pathways that begin in the labyrinths and terminate in the rostral brainstem.[75,84,85] Although the exact neuroanatomic pathways that mediate the ocular-tilt reaction or its prime component, skew deviation, remain uncertain, the localizing value of skew deviation has evolved from clinical and experimental observation (**Table 15–3**).

Pathophysiology. It appears that both the utricular and the semicircular canal pathways that regulate vertical gaze synapse in the vestibular nuclei and cross the midline to ascend in the medial longitudinal fasciculus (**Fig. 15–15**).[75,84,85] There, the utricular pathway connects to the nuclei that activate the four vertically acting muscles, namely the superior rectus, superior oblique, inferior rectus, and inferior

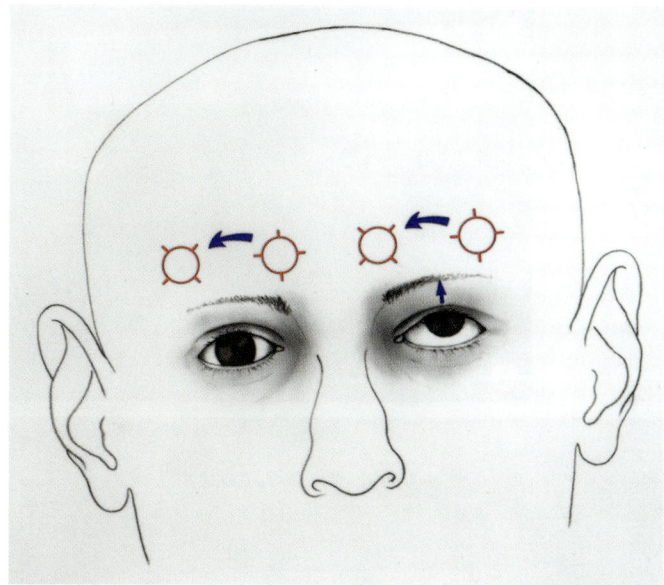

Figure 15–13. Diagram demonstrating the three components of the ocular tilt reaction (OTR): (1) right head tilt, (2) ocular counter-roll, and (3) skew deviation. Note that the eyes roll toward the hypotropic eye.

oblique. Remember that the superior rectus subnucleus and trochlear nucleus control the contralateral superior rectus and superior oblique muscles, respectively. Thus, a right utricular nerve lesion would result in a left hypertropia as a result of impaired action of the left inferior rectus muscle and the right superior rectus muscle. If the lesion occurs in the medial longitudinal fasciculus, the hypertropia will be ipsilateral unless lateral pontomedullary structures are also affected; in such a case, the hypertropia may be contralateral to the internuclear ophthalmoplegia.[85]

Skew deviation may also ensue following selective damage to the posterior or the anterior semicircular canal pathways.[85] For example, injury to the right posterior semicircular canal projections would lead to a left hypertropia and relative right eye excyclotorsion from impaired innervation to the left inferior rectus and right superior oblique muscles, respectively. Although both eyes are torted towards the hypotropic eye, the lower eye is usually more excyclorotated than the higher eye is incyclorotated; hence, the term relative excyclorotation.[83] Bilateral damage to the crossing posterior semicircular pathway projection in the dorsal medulla could lead to an alternating hypertropia (i.e., right hypertropia in right gaze from impaired action of the right inferior rectus muscle, and a left hypertropia in left gaze from disturbed function of the left inferior rectus muscle).[86,87] Patients who have skew deviation from interruption of the semicircular canal pathway often have associated vertical nystagmus. For instance, interruption of the posterior semicircular canal pathway leads to a skew deviation in association with downbeat nystagmus in one eye and a torsional nystagmus in the fellow eye.

Although brainstem strokes and tumors are the most common causes of skew deviation, this motility disturbance may be rarely observed as a false localizing sign of increased intracranial pressure including pseudotumor cerebri.[88,89]

Diagnosis. The hypertropia of a skew deviation may be comitant (deviation is the same in all positions of gaze) or

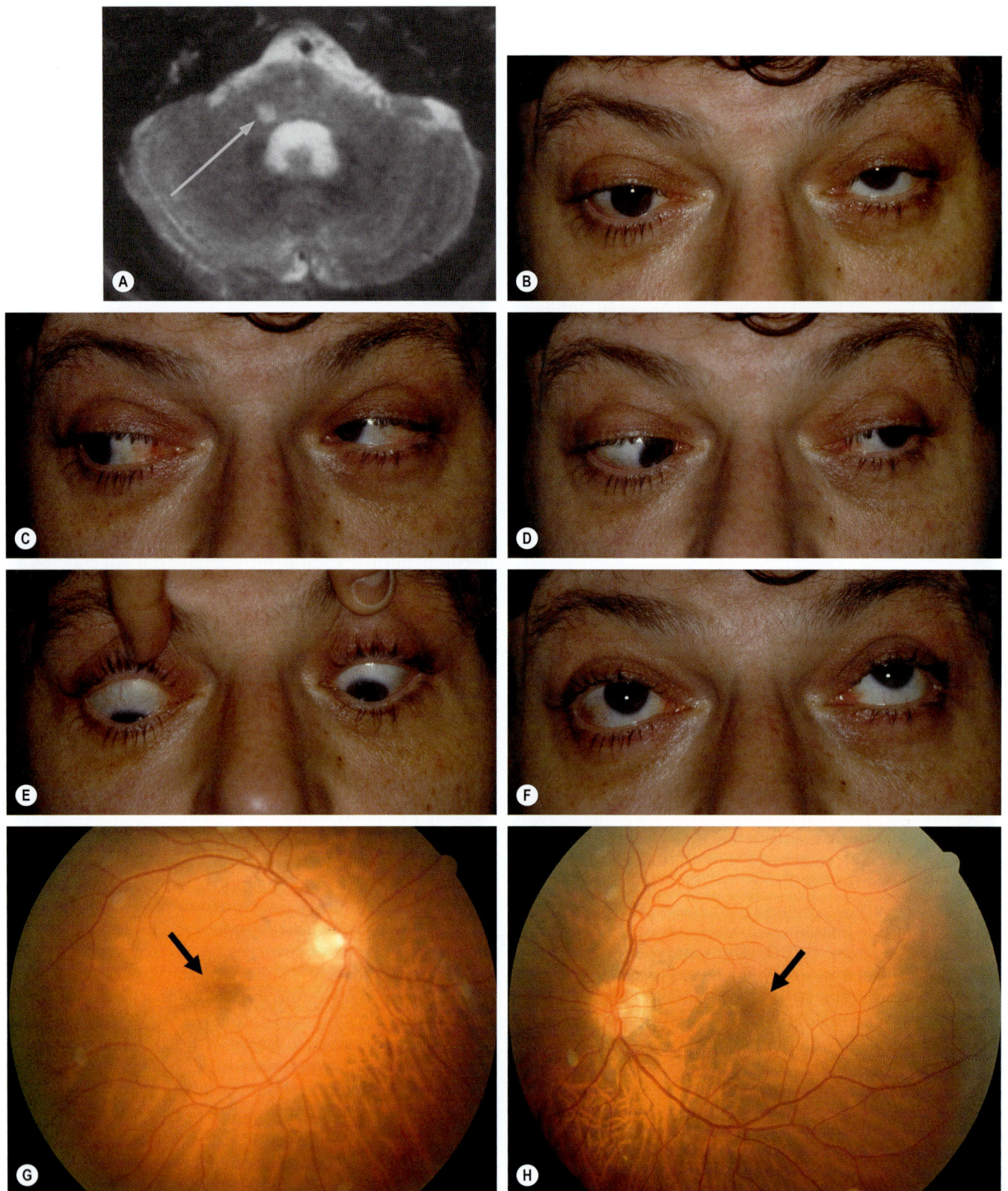

Figure 15–14. Pontomedullary lesion causing ocular tilt reaction. **A**. Axial T2-weighted MRI scan showing right lateral pontomedullary infarction (*arrow*). **B**. Left hypertropia in primary gaze, which was worse in right gaze (**C–F**). Excyclotorsion of the hypotropic right eye (**G**) (note downward displacement of macula (*arrow*) relative to the optic disc) and incyclotorsion of the hypertropic left eye (**H**) (note upward displacement of the macula (*arrow*), which normally lies below the horizontal meridian) were also present. (Courtesy of Stefania Bianchi, MD.)

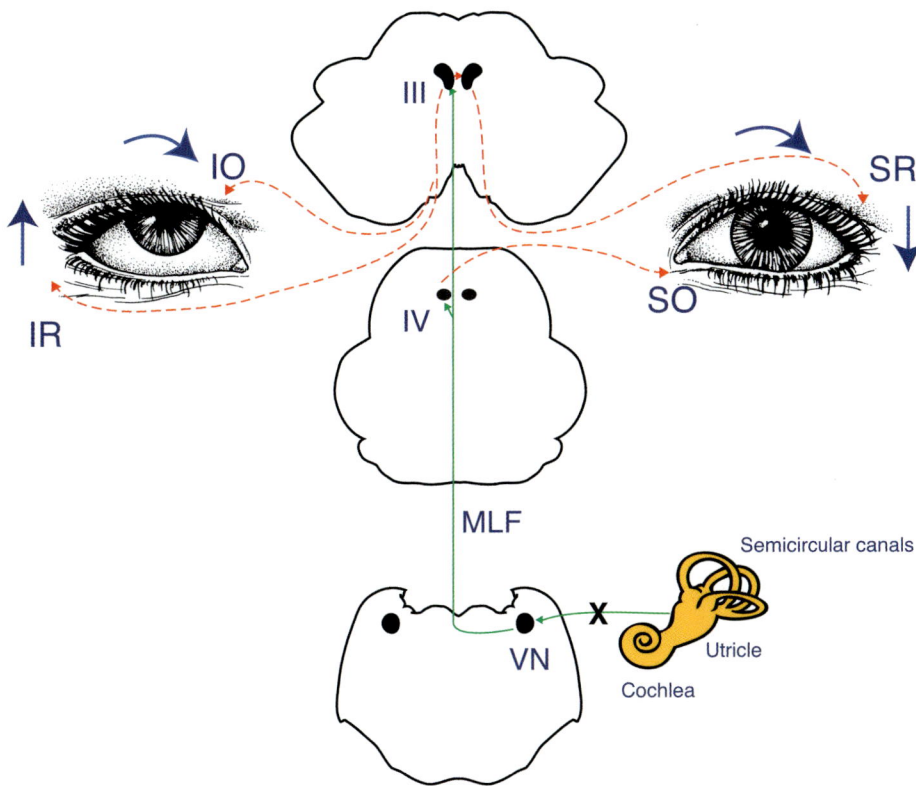

Figure 15–15. Diagram demonstrating the presumed projections of the utricular pathway for lateral head tilting. Note the utricular projections synapse in the vestibular nucleus (VN), which issues fibers that cross and ascend in the MLF to the subnuclei of the four vertically acting extraocular muscles. These subnuclei include the IVth nerve nucleus and the IIIrd nerve subnuclei controlling the superior rectus (SR), inferior rectus (IR), and inferior oblique (IO) and superior oblique (SO) muscles. Note that the IVth nerve nucleus and the superior rectus subnucleus innervate their respective muscles of the contralateral eye. For example, a lesion within the utricular connection to the (*left*) VN ("X", for instance) or the (*right*) MLF will produce a right hypertropia, a counter-roll of the eyes to the left (as shown), and a left head tilt. The SO is labeled in the lower part of the eye for the sake of simplicity.

Table 15–3 Localizing value of skew deviation

Lesion location	Type of skew	Associated signs
Lateral pontomedullary	Contralateral hypertropia	Ipsilateral excyclotorsion; ipsilateral facial numbness; ipsilateral Horner syndrome; lateropulsion
Midline cervicomedullary junction	Bilateral inferior rectus	Downbeat nystagmus
Medial longitudinal fasciculus	Ipsilateral hypertropia	Internuclear ophthalmoplegia
Rostral midbrain	Ipsilateral hypertropia	Vertical gaze palsy; conjugate cyclotorsion

noncomitant (deviation varies with gaze position). When a skew deviation is noncomitant, it may be difficult to distinguish from an ocular motor palsy or extraocular muscle weakness. A IVth nerve palsy is the motility disorder that may be the most difficult to distinguish from a skew deviation since both conditions may be associated with a positive head-tilt[83] or three-step test (see Fourth nerve palsies, below).[90] However, patients with skew deviation typically have binocular torsion as opposed to the excyclotorsion of one just eye seen in a IVth nerve palsy.[85,91] Furthermore, in skew deviation the hypertropic eye is usually incyclorotated and the hypotropic eye excyclorotated, while the affected hypertropic eye in a IVth nerve palsy is excyclorotated, and in an inferior oblique palsy the affected hypotropic eye is incyclorotated.[92] Torsion may be demonstrated by double Maddox rod testing (**Fig. 15–16**), fundus photography (see **Fig. 15–14**), indirect ophthalmoscopy, or measurement of the subjective visual vertical.[85,93] In addition, the supranuclear nature of the hyperdeviation associated with skew deviation may be evident during oculocephalic testing or forced eyelid closure (Bell's phenomenon).[83] Finally, the vertical deviation and torsion seen in skew deviation decreases when patients are supine compared with trochlear nerve palsy, which remains the same.[94]

Midbrain lesions involving the INC may also produce skew deviation with the hypertropic eye ipsilateral to the lesion. A full OTR may also ensue with midbrain lesions producing a conjugate counter-roll of the eyes toward the contralateral shoulder (**Fig. 15–17**).[95-97] The head tilt will be contralateral to the lesion as well. Alternating skew with lateral gaze may also be associated with midbrain lesions.[87]

Variations. Occasionally, irritative lesions of the midbrain will produce a paroxysmal skew deviation.[98-101] These patients have a contralateral hypertropia, ipsilateral head tilt, and a conjugate counter-roll of the eyes towards the ipsilateral shoulder. This triad replicates the eye findings observed with the electrical stimulation of the INC in animals.[98] One patient has been documented with skew deviation from ictal activity of the vestibular cortex.[102]

Alternating skew deviation in the primary position is an unusual eye movement disorder that may be observed with midbrain lesions. The hypertropia may switch sides over several minutes in an aperiodic or periodic manner.[103,104]

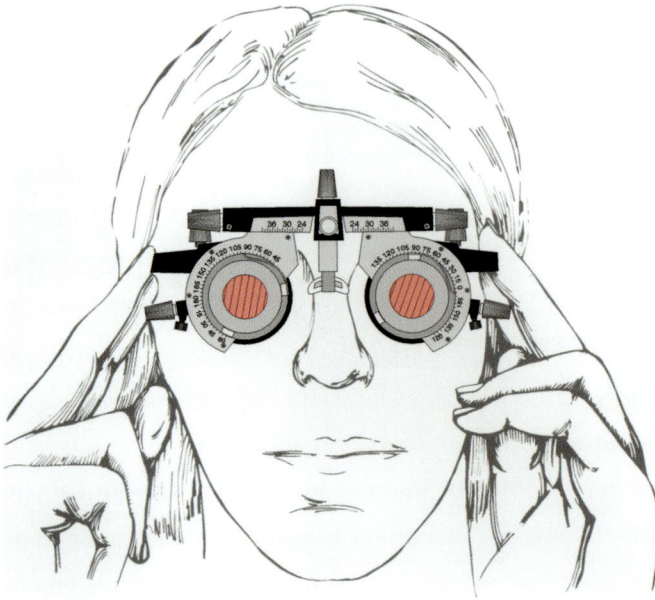

Figure 15–16. Drawing of double Maddox rod testing in a patient with a skew deviation (right hypertropia). Red Maddox rod lenses are placed over each eye in a trial frame, each at the 90° mark. As the patient is viewing a hand-held light at distance, two separate horizontal red lines will be seen, one from each eye. The patient is asked to align the two red lines so that they are parallel to each other and the floor by rotating the dials of the trial frame. In the example shown, the patient displayed asymmetric cyclotorsion of both eyes toward the left shoulder. In this case there was incyclotorsion of approximately 10° OD and excyclotorsion of approximately 15° OS.

Periodic alternating deviation may also coexist with periodic alternating nystagmus.

Acquired supranuclear monocular elevator palsy

This "double elevator palsy" is caused by a pretectal, supra-nuclear lesion.[105-108] Both superior rectus and inferior oblique function of one eye are affected by a unilateral lesion in the rostral mesencephalon. Such a lesion would disrupt the efferent fibers from the rostral interstitial nucleus of medial longitudinal fasciculus (riMLF) to the inferior oblique subnucleus and the contralateral superior rectus subnucleus, which innervates the superior rectus muscle contralateral to it (see **Fig. 16–18**). Thus a unilateral lesion produces a monocular elevation paresis. As the name of the condition implies, Bell's phenomena and the oculocephalic responses are intact in the affected eye. If reflex eye movements are not preserved with a monocular elevator palsy, one should consider a fascicular IIIrd nerve palsy or a lesion along the distal path of the IIIrd nerve including the orbit.

Third nerve palsies

As indicated earlier, a complete, isolated infranuclear IIIrd nerve palsy causes ipsilateral elevation, adduction, and depression weakness accompanied by abduction, hypode-viation, pupillary mydriasis, and ptosis (**Fig. 15–18**). The most feared cause of a IIIrd nerve palsy in adulthood is a posterior communicating artery aneurysm, which may com-press the IIIrd nerve within the subarachnoid space. In adults, the most common identifiable cause of acquired IIIrd nerve palsy is vascular insufficiency due to diabetes, hyper-tension, or atherosclerosis.[26] Less common causes of isolated

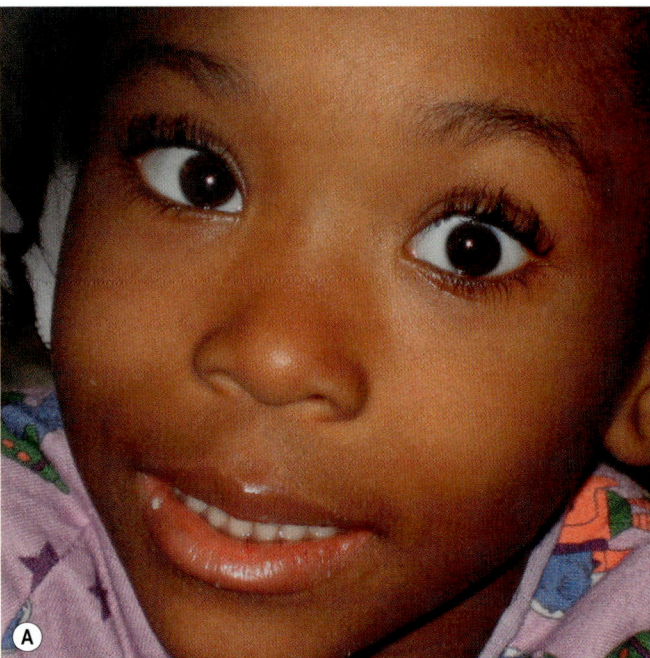

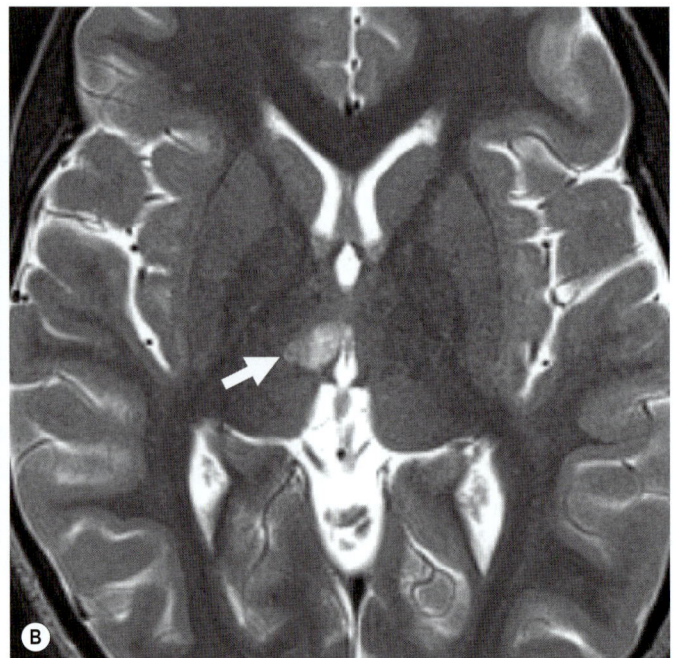

Video 15.

Figure 15–17. A. External photograph demonstrating a patient with an ocular tilt reaction (OTR) (large right hypertropia and left head tilt) due to a (**B**) right midbrain–thalamic infarction (*arrow*). The patient also had counter-rolling of the eyes toward the left shoulder on fundus examination.

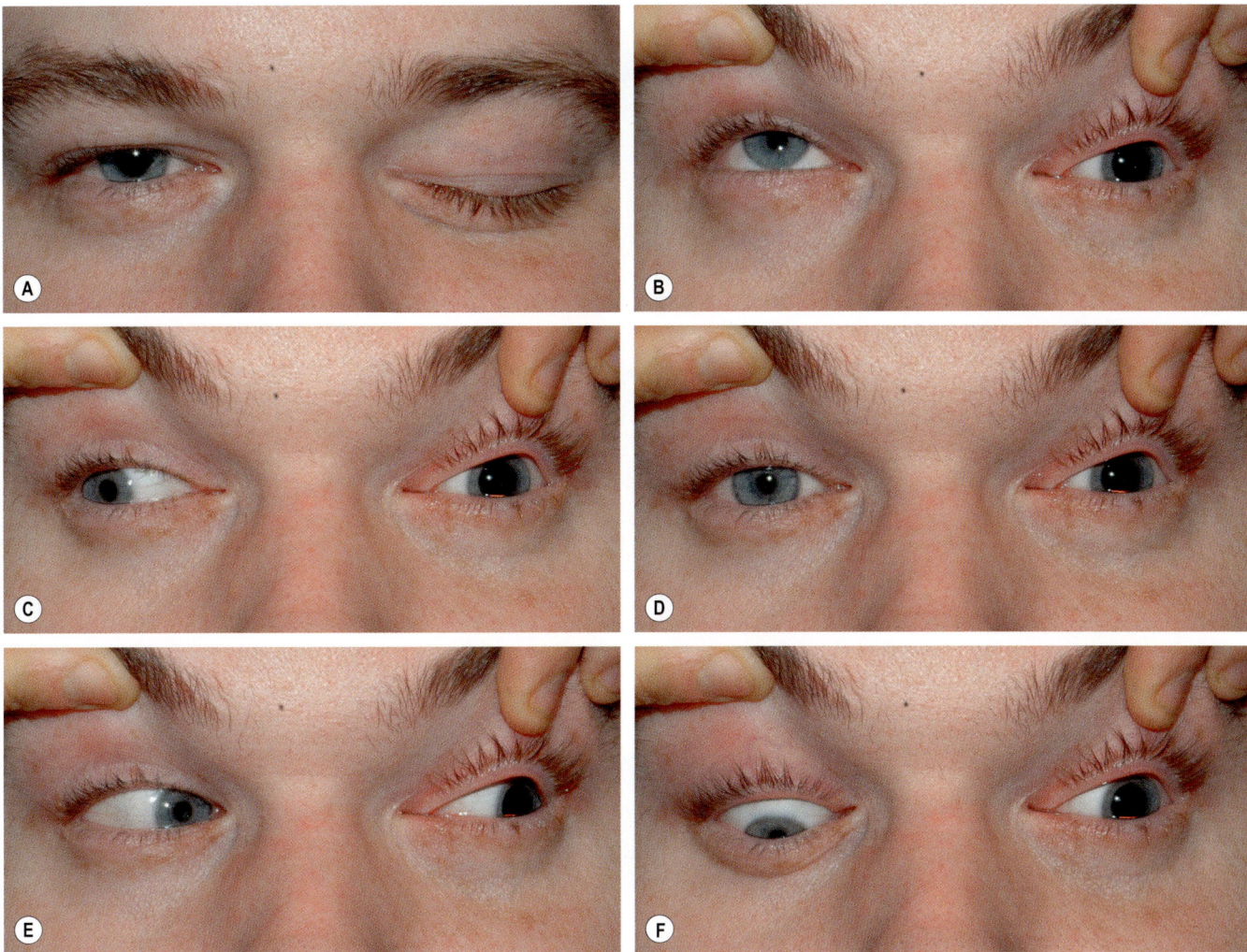

Figure 15–18. Complete pupil-involving left IIIrd nerve palsy due to a chondrosarcoma. The left eye has complete ptosis (**A**), defective elevation (**B**), absent adduction (**C**), a down and out position in primary gaze with a large unreactive pupil (**D**), intact abduction (**E**), and deficient downgaze (**F**).

IIIrd nerve palsies include trauma, meningitis, stroke, and mass lesion at the base of the skull. In children the most common cause of acquired IIIrd nerve palsy is trauma. This section will discuss other clinical features of IIIrd nerve palsies, then detail their various etiologies and workup in adults and children.

Other clinical features of third nerve palsies

Complete vs. incomplete (or partial). These terms refer to the extent of involvement of the eyelid and IIIrd nerve innervated extraocular muscles. These are nonlocalizing. Palsies of individual muscles can occur due to lesions at any level of the nerve.

Pupil involvement vs. sparing. If the pupil is mydriatic and less reactive to light than the pupil of the fellow eye, the pupil is said to be "involved." A normally reactive pupil which is the same size as the pupil of the fellow eye is "spared." These features are nonlocalizing.

Inferior vs. superior division. As alluded to earlier, the IIIrd nerve divides into two divisions in the anterior cavernous sinus, so divisional ocular paresis classically localizes to this region or to the posterior orbit. However, examples of fas-cicular[109,110] and subarachnoid[111,112] lesions causing involvement of IIIrd nerve inferior (**Fig. 15–19**) or superior division innervated muscles have been described.

Aberrant regeneration. Patients with traumatic or chronic compressive IIIrd nerve palsies may develop *aberrant regeneration, misdirection, or synkinesis*. Common abnormal patterns include lid elevation during adduction or depression of the eye (pseudo-Graefe phenomenon) (**Fig. 15–20**) or depression and miosis of a pupil unreactive to light during adduction (see **Fig. 13–12**).[113,114] Pupillary findings are discussed in more detail in Chapter 13. Less common patterns include defective vertical eye movements with retraction of the globe upon attempted vertical deviations, adduction of the eye during attempted vertical movement,[115] and transient synkinesis.[116,117]

Primary (spontaneous) and secondary (acquired) aberrant regeneration are usually considered separately because of their etiologic implications. The synkinesis is the first manifestation of IIIrd nerve dysfunction in primary aberrant regeneration. This type, manifesting as a ptotic eyelid which elevates in adduction or depression of the eye, is usually associated with expanding lesions in or around the cavernous sinus such as intracavernous meningiomas,[118–121]

Video 15.5

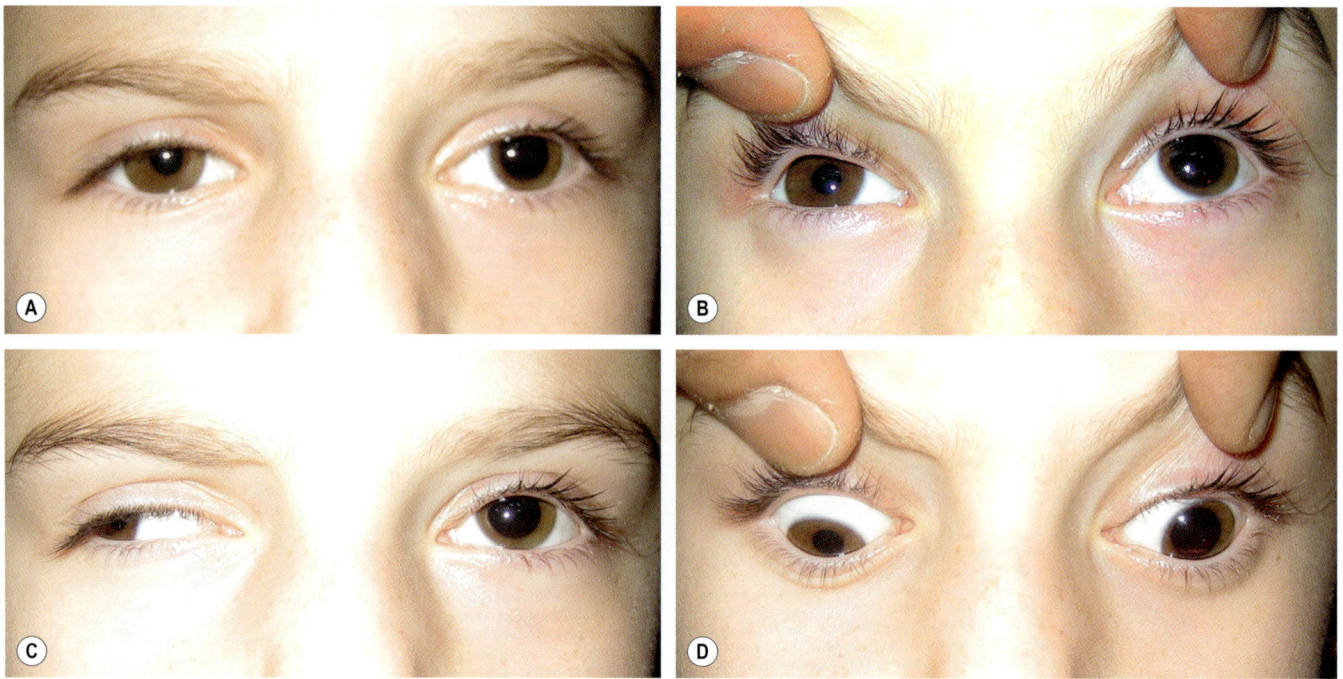

Figure 15–19. Inferior division left IIIrd nerve palsy. The left eye has an enlarged pupil but no ptosis (**A**) and intact upgaze (**B**), but defective adduction (**C**), and depression (**D**).

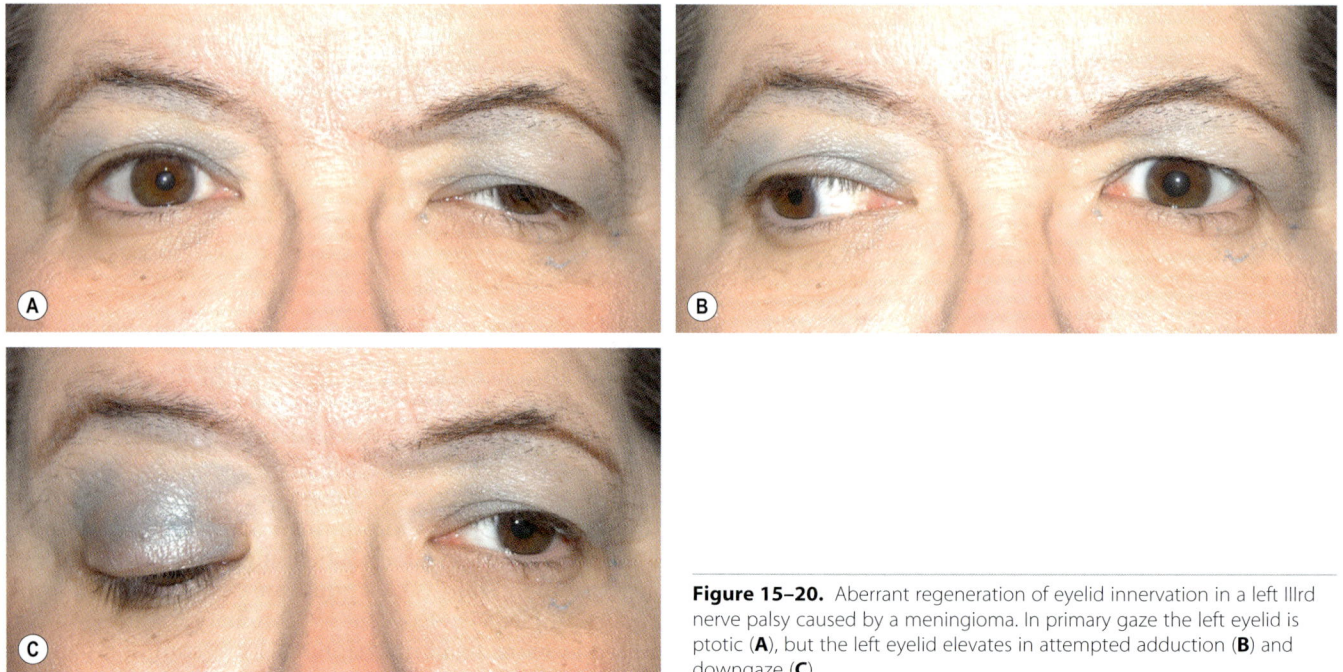

Figure 15–20. Aberrant regeneration of eyelid innervation in a left IIIrd nerve palsy caused by a meningioma. In primary gaze the left eyelid is ptotic (**A**), but the left eyelid elevates in attempted adduction (**B**) and downgaze (**C**).

aneurysms,[121-123] pituitary tumors,[115] and other extracavern-ous masses.[124,125] On the other hand, secondary aberrant regeneration occurs in the recovery phase several weeks after an acute IIIrd nerve palsy due to trauma,[126] ophthalmoplegic migraine,[121,127] pituitary apoplexy[117] (see **Fig. 13–12**), or inflammation,[116,128] for instance. Because aberrant regenera-tion after microvascular ischemic nerve palsies[129] or mid-brain infarction[130] is rare, in the absence of a history of trauma its presence should heighten suspicion for a com-pressive lesion.

In one purported mechanism, damaged, regenerating axons follow alternate pathways within the nerve sheath to innervate targets distinct from their original destination. Lid elevation in adduction would then be explained by misdirection of IIIrd nerve fibers for the medial rectus muscle incorrectly innervating the levator muscle. Similarly, miosis during adduction could be attributed to medial rectus fibers mistakenly innervating the pupillary sphincter. However, cases of spontaneous and transient synkinesis might argue against hardwired misdirection. Alternative

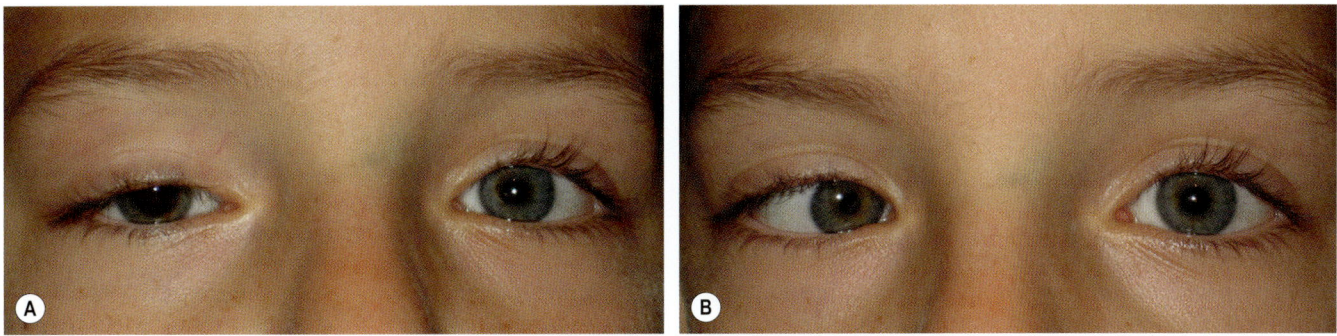

Figure 15–21. Cyclic spasms in a boy with a congenital right IIIrd nerve palsy. Periods of right eye ptosis, hypotropia, exotropia, and pupillary mydriasis (**A**), alternated with periods of right eyelid elevation, adduction, and pupillary miosis (**B**).

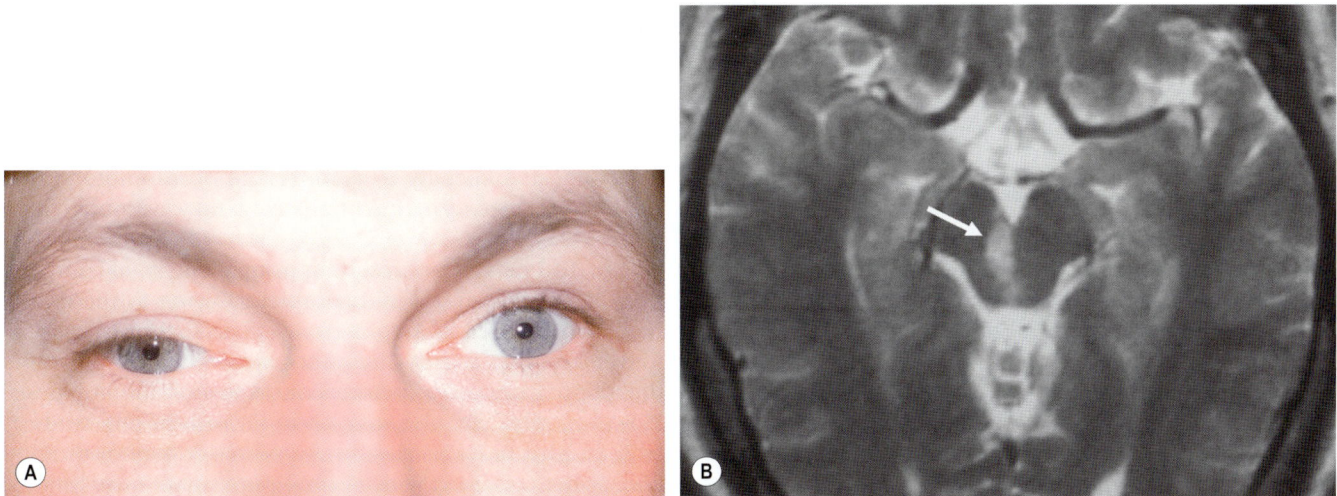

Figure 15–22. Fascicular right IIIrd nerve palsy (**A**) and contralateral ataxia (Claude syndrome) due to paramedian midbrain infarction (*arrow*) seen on T2-weighted axial MRI (**B**).

explanations include (1) ephaptic transmission, a cross-talk between adjacent injured and intact nerve fibers, and (2) central synaptic reorganization within the oculomotor subnuclei.[121,131]

Cyclic oculomotor spasms. In this eye movement disorder, a complete or IIIrd nerve palsy alternates with brief spasms of the IIIrd nerve innervated structures.[132] Often heralded by eyelid twitches,[133] the spastic phase is characterized by pupillary miosis, lid elevation, adduction, and depression but limited abduction of the eye (**Fig. 15–21**). The condition is usually unilateral, persists during sleep, and continues for the lifetime of the patient.[133] Most cases are seen in congenital IIIrd nerve palsies, but rarely they may be acquired.[134,135] Alternating phases of aberrant regeneration of the IIIrd nerve with an intermittent conduction block has been a proposed mechanism.[134]

Etiologies of IIIrd nerve palsies and their accompanying clinical features are discussed by location in the following sections:

Intra-axial lesions

Nuclear third nerve palsy. The classical unilateral lesion of the IIIrd nerve nucleus results in bilateral ptosis, worse ipsilaterally, ipsilateral mydriasis, ipsilateral palsy of the medial rectus, inferior rectus and inferior oblique muscles, and bilateral superior rectus palsies. However, bilateral ptosis with various combinations of oculomotor paresis have been described from nuclear IIIrd nerve lesions.[136–143] Other cases of nuclear IIIrd nerve palsies have been described without levator involvement,[144,145] with isolated inferior rectus palsy,[146–148] and with isolated contralateral superior rectus palsy.[149] Such patients without bilateral ptosis would be difficult to discern clinically from fascicular involvement only.

Fascicular third nerve palsy. Lesions of the midbrain tegmentum can affect the oculomotor nerve fascicles as they travel ventrally, and are often associated with "crossed" neurologic signs.[150] Involvement of the fascicle as it passes through the crossing dentatorubrothalamic fibers (from the superior cerebellar peduncle), just below and medial to the red nucleus, can produce an ipsilateral oculomotor palsy and contralateral ataxia (*Claude syndrome*) (**Fig. 15–22**).[151] A lesion of the cerebral peduncle results in ipsilateral oculomotor palsy and contralateral hemiparesis (*Weber syndrome*), and a larger process also involving the red nucleus can cause the same findings plus contralateral involuntary limb movements or tremor (*Benedikt syndrome*). Third nerve palsy accompanied by vertical gaze paresis, lid retraction, skew deviation, and convergence retraction saccades would be suggestive of dorsal midbrain process, as in the top of the basilar syndrome (see Chapter 16).[152] In this setting, emboli to the posterior cerebral arteries may also result in a homonymous hemianopsia and visual hallucinations. Secondary diencephalic lesions may cause additional memory disturbances, behavioral changes, and altered consciousness.

Fascicular oculomotor palsies may also be isolated,[153,154] and either pupil involvement or sparing may occur.[155-157] In incomplete oculomotor palsies, the pattern of ophthalmoplegia often reflects the topographical arrangement of the fibers to each extraocular muscle within the fascicle (see **Fig. 15–4**).[158-160] Divisional pareses may occur,[110,161] and, uncommonly, individual muscles may be affected.[162-164]

The usual cause of a nuclear or fascicular oculomotor palsy is infarction in the territory of a mesencephalic paramedian penetrating vessel arising from the proximal posterior cerebral artery,[165] but other etiologies include metastatic tumors,[166] vascular malformations,[167,168] abscesses,[169] cysts,[161] and multiple sclerosis.[148,170,171]

Subarachnoid processes

Uncal herniation. A IIIrd nerve palsy accompanied by altered mental status should suggest uncal herniation.[172] Ipsilateral pupillary dilation may be the first sign of transtentorial uncal herniation before other signs of IIIrd nerve paresis develop. In this setting, mechanisms for IIIrd nerve dysfunction include direct compression by the herniating uncus beneath the tentorial edge (**Fig. 15–23**), compression by the posterior cerebral artery or hippocampal gyrus, compression of the oculomotor complex in the midbrain, or displacement and kinking of the nerve over the clivus.[173] As the syndrome progresses with a decrease in level of consciousness, the IIIrd nerve palsy may become complete along with signs of ipsilateral hemiplegia and extensor plantar response (due to contralateral compression of the cerebral peduncle—Kernohan's notch syndrome).[174] Further clinical progression may be monitored by examining the opposite pupil, which initially may be midposition with a depressed light reaction, then slightly miotic, then finally dilated.[175] Transiently the pupils may acquire an oval shape.[176] Uncommonly in transtentorial herniation, the opposite pupil is paradoxically the first to dilate.[177]

Posterior communicating artery aneurysms. Within the subarachnoid space, posterior communicating artery (PCoA) aneurysms may compress the IIIrd nerve (**Fig. 15–24**), almost always causing pupillary dilatation. Aneurysms arising from the base of the PCoA as it emerges from the ICA are the second most common aneurysm in the anterior circle of Willis. In one study,[178] 34% of patients with a PCoA developed a IIIrd nerve palsy. However, greater than 90% of patients with PCoA aneurysms and subarachnoid hemorrhage present with symptoms of a IIIrd nerve palsy prior to rupture.[179] PCoA aneurysms and ICA aneurysms commonly project posterolaterally to compress the oculomotor nerve as it travels between the brainstem and cavernous sinus (**Fig. 15–25**).

The IIIrd nerve palsy resulting from aneurysmal compression is usually painful and complete. Owing to the dorsomedial location of the pupillomotor fibers in the oculomotor nerve bundle, aneurysmal compression often involves the pupil early, even before complete ophthalmoparesis. However, pupil sparing may occur,[180] and, in one study,[181] 14% of IIIrd nerve palsies due to posterior communicating aneurysms presented with normal pupils and partial motility deficits, but pupillary mydriasis developed within days in most of those cases. Rare oculomotor presentations of PCoA aneurysms include isolated ptosis,[182] ptosis and mydriasis,[183]

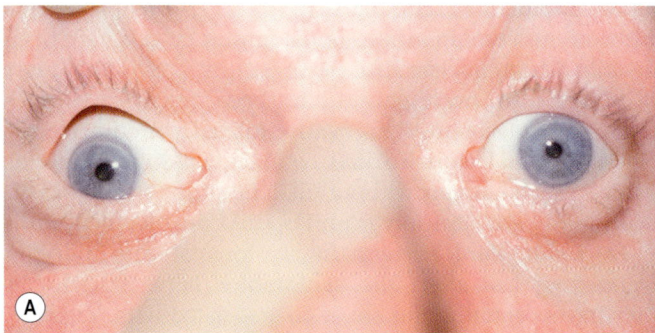

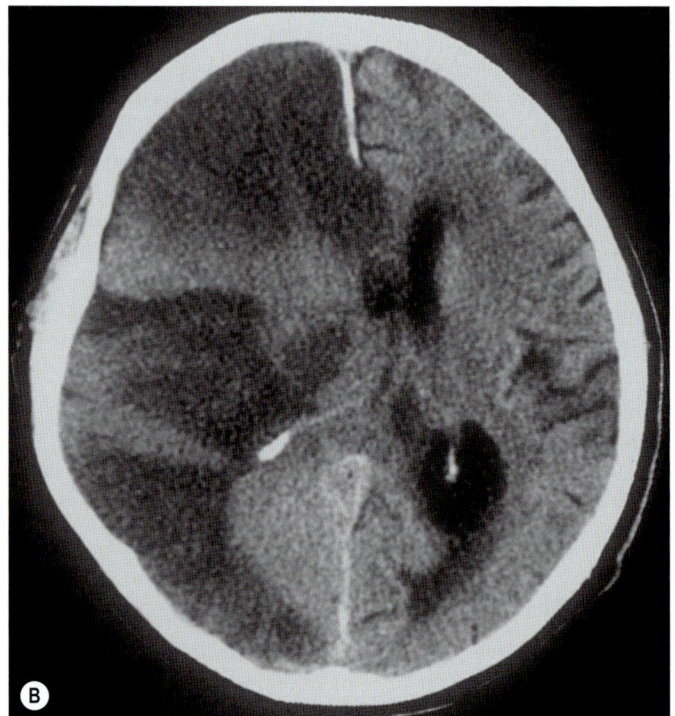

Figure 15–23. Third nerve palsy of the right eye in a comatose patient with uncal herniation. **A**. The right eye is exotropic and hypotropic, and the right pupil is larger and less reactive to light than the left. **B**. The IIIrd nerve palsy was caused by uncal transtentorial herniation in the setting of a large right hemispheric infarction with edema due to an internal carotid artery occlusion. (From Liu GT. Neurosurg Clin North Am 1999;10:579–586, with permission.)

pupillary light-near dissociation,[184] dorsal midbrain syndrome,[185] pupil sparing and aberrant regeneration,[186] and transient IIIrd nerve palsies.[187,188] Visual loss[189,190] may occur, and the pattern observed with PCoA aneurysms depends upon the anterior pathway structure which is compressed: optic nerve, chiasm, or tract.[189]

Treatment. Treatment of symptomatic PCoA aneurysms should not be unduly delayed, as bleeding and/or rebleeding

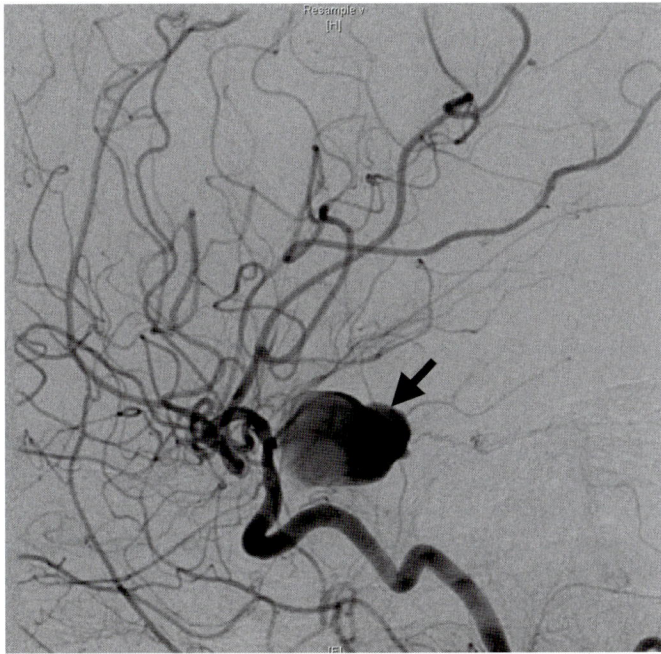

Figure 15–24. Large posterior communicating artery aneurysm (*arrow*) demonstrated on conventional angiography, lateral view. The patient presented with an acute, painful, pupil-involving complete IIIrd nerve palsy.

and death may occur when they are untreated. Treatment consists of surgical clipping, endovascular embolization, and less often carotid occlusion. The most significant complication of aneurysm surgery is ischemic stroke, due to either compromise of a dominant PCoA artery or interruption of circulation through adjacent vessels. Third nerve palsies can worsen after surgical repair due to aneurysm thrombosis or iatrogenic manipulation. Advances in endovascular approaches, particularly coil embolization, have resulted in a higher success rate and lower frequency of acute bleeding in the treatment of ruptured and unruptured aneurysms.[191,192]

After treatment of PCoA aneurysms, the recovery of the IIIrd nerve palsy is inconsistent and often slow.[193] Diplopia, residual ptosis, and occasionally photophobia are the main complaints, and aberrant regeneration is often seen.[194] Factors predicting a better prognosis for recovery of IIIrd nerve function include early treatment,[178] incomplete palsies,[195] younger age, and absence of diabetes.[196] Treatment with clipping and coiling have the same chance for recovery.[196]

Basilar artery aneurysms. Aneurysms of the basilar artery, trunk, and bifurcation are the most common aneurysm in the posterior fossa (**Fig. 15–25**).[197] The most frequent presentation is subarachnoid hemorrhage, but cranial nerve pareses are frequent, IIIrd and VIth nerve palsies being most common.[183,198] Patients with IIIrd or VIth nerve pareses may develop a concurrent crossed paralysis such as a Weber syndrome if the aneurysm injures the adjacent brainstem. Typically the IIIrd nerve palsies are pupil-involving, but pupil-sparing IIIrd nerve palsies in this setting have been reported.[199,200]

Other neurologic and neuro-ophthalmic signs may develop from basilar aneurysms due to brainstem

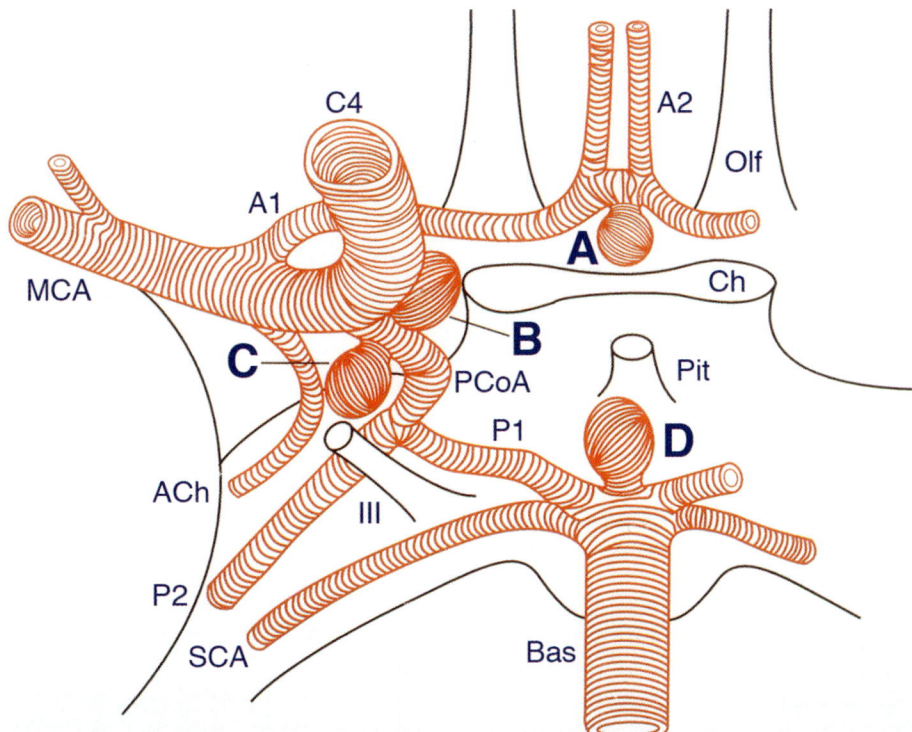

Figure 15–25. Drawing of the posterior communicating artery and other common aneurysms in the circle of Willis. **A**. Anterior communicating artery aneurysm. **B**. Internal carotid artery aneurysm. **C**. Posterior communicating artery (PCoA) aneurysm (note its proximity to the IIIrd nerve (III)). **D**. Basilar artery tip aneurysm. A1, A2, anterior cerebral artery segments; ACh, anterior choroidal artery; Bas, basilar artery; C4, internal carotid artery, supraclinoid portion; Ch, chiasm; MCA, middle cerebral artery; Olf, olfactory nerve; Pit, pituitary stalk; and P1, P2, posterior cerebral artery segments; SCA, superior cerebellar artery. (Courtesy of Dr. Jeffrey Bennett.)

compression or concurrent thromboembolic disease. Giant saccular or fusiform aneurysms may compress the adjacent midbrain or pons. Hemiparesis or other corticospinal tract signs may or may not be evident depending on the duration of the compression. Thrombus within the basilar aneurysm may obstruct flow or embolize to nearby perforating vessels, particularly at the basilar bifurcation.[152] Basilar artery insufficiency may result from midbasilar thrombosis. On rare occasions, giant fusiform aneurysms of the basilar artery may result in obstructive hydrocephalus due to aqueductal compression.

Other aneurysms. Posterior cerebral artery (PCA) aneurysms may result in IIIrd nerve palsies by compressing the oculomotor nerve as it travels between the posterior cerebral artery and superior cerebellar artery. Giant PCA aneurysms can compress the optic radiations or visual cortex, producing a contralateral homonymous hemianopsia.

Treatment. Therapy for posterior fossa aneurysms is either surgical or endovascular. Both treatments are complicated by significant morbidity and mortality due to occlusion of small perforating vessels or parent vessel thrombosis.[179] For instance, clipping of basilar tip aneurysms may cause infarction in paramedian mesencephalic–thalamic perforating territories. Surgical therapy is additionally complicated by cranial nerve palsies secondary to traction. The IIIrd nerve

palsy is most common, occurring in more than 60% of patients.[197] Despite the significant risk, surgical treatment is often warranted due to the even greater morbidity and mortality associated with progressive brainstem dysfunction and posterior fossa subarachnoid hemorrhage (SAH). If vessel occlusion can be tolerated in the vertebral or basilar artery, then the endovascular approach is often the safest. In certain cases of basilar artery dolicoectasia, endovascular occlusion is the only feasible approach.

Vasculopathic third nerve palsies. Ischemic (vasculopathic) IIIrd nerve palsies, associated with hypertension, diabetes, advanced age, atherosclerosis, smoking, and hypercholesterolemia,[201] are often preceded by orbital ache or pain and are characterized by pupillary sparing (**Fig. 15–26**).[202] In our experience, the pain can be rather severe, especially in younger patients. In fact, the presence or absence of pain cannot be used to distinguish aneurysmal from vasculopathic IIIrd nerve palsies. The symptoms and signs may progress over several days.[203]

Most cases are thought to have a peripheral lesion.[204] Presumably the IIIrd nerves develop ischemia and demyelination within the subarachnoid space[205] or cavernous sinus,[16] but there may also be a small infarction of the nerve within the mesencephalon.[206] The pupil sparing in peripheral cases is attributed to the location of the pupillary fibers on the

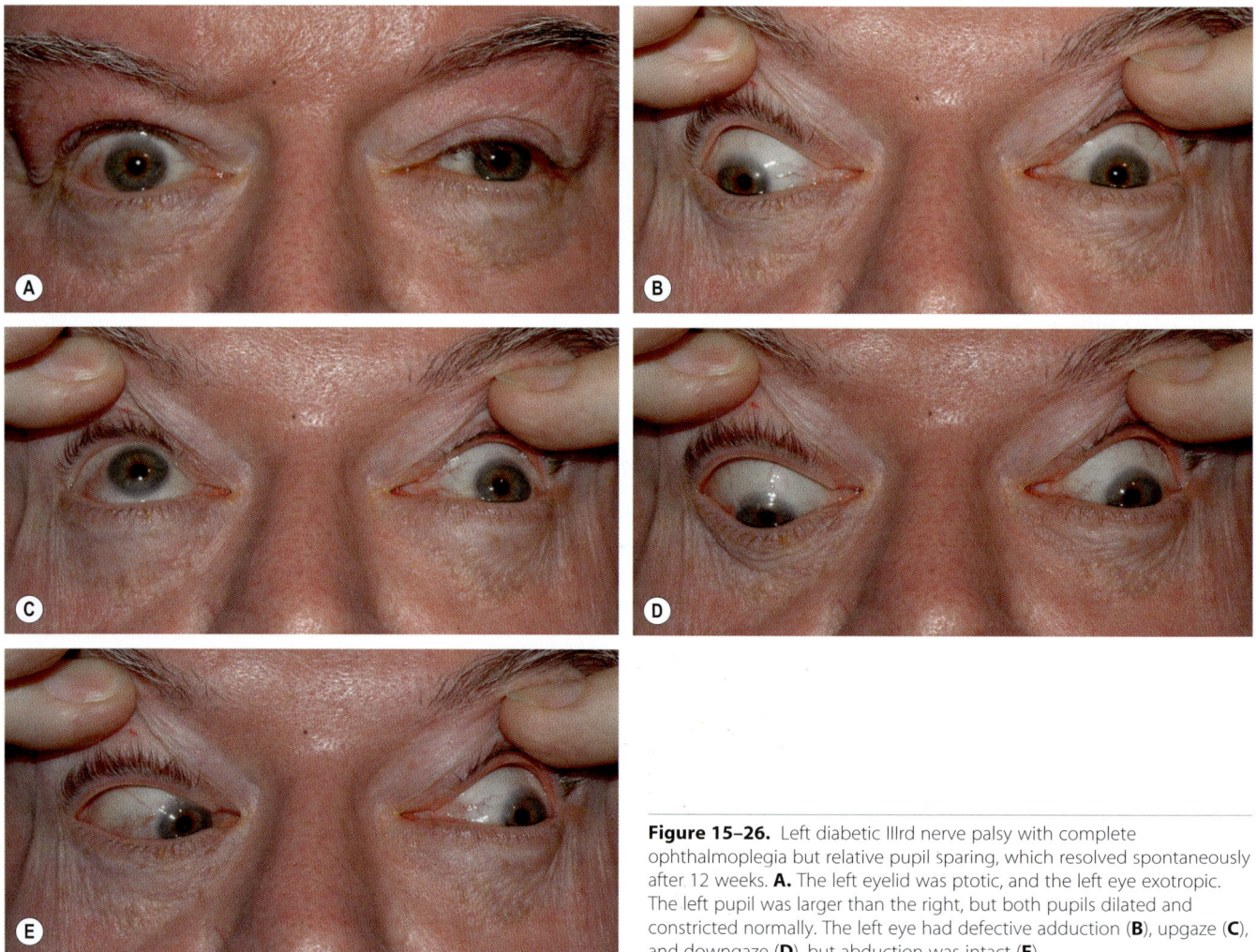

Figure 15–26. Left diabetic IIIrd nerve palsy with complete ophthalmoplegia but relative pupil sparing, which resolved spontaneously after 12 weeks. **A.** The left eyelid was ptotic, and the left eye exotropic. The left pupil was larger than the right, but both pupils dilated and constricted normally. The left eye had defective adduction (**B**), upgaze (**C**), and downgaze (**D**), but abduction was intact (**E**).

outside of the IIIrd nerve in areas less vulnerable to vascular insufficiency. However, some studies have suggested that minor pupillary involvement (less than 2 mm of anisocoria) may occur in as many as 38% of patients.[207] The pupil is rarely dilated and unreactive. The pain may be due to ischemia of trigeminal fibers within or around the oculomotor nerve,[208] but this has not been confirmed. Most patients with vasculopathic oculomotor palsies recover spontaneously within 8–12 weeks.[209] Rarely, vasculopathic IIIrd nerve palsies may be seen in combination with IVth, VIth, and VIIth nerve palsies.[210] Other responsible etiologies include vasculitis due to giant cell arteritis,[211–213] systemic lupus erythematosus,[214] and herpes zoster. There is no evidence that antiplatelet agents prevent ischemic oculomotor palsies.[215]

Trauma. Third nerve palsies due to trauma are typically caused by severe blows to the head,[63] often due to a motor vehicle accident.[216] The peripheral portion of the nerve may be damaged secondary to traction at the skull base or by an orbital or base of skull fracture. Alternatively, the nuclear complex or fascicle may be affected by brainstem shearing or hemorrhage.[217,218] Alternative causes include penetrating orbital or intracranial trauma or iatrogenic trauma during removal of suprasellar or posterior fossa masses.[219] Some oculomotor palsies from minor trauma are harbingers of an underlying aneurysm or mass lesion.[220,221] The prognosis for recovery of function in most cases of traumatic IIIrd nerve palsies is very good, but often with evidence of aberrant regeneration.

Primary tumors of the oculomotor nerves

Neurinomas and schwannomas. Stable or slowly progressive oculomotor palsies may be caused by tumors derived from the Schwann cells surrounding the extra-axial portion of the IIIrd nerve.[222,223] Tumor types include neurinomas, neurofibromas, neurilemmomas, and schwannomas.[224] Neuroimaging typically reveals an enhancing, thickened IIIrd nerve in the subarachnoid space or cavernous sinus,[225] but enlargement to several centimeters with mass effect can occur.[226,227] The best management of these cases is not certain. Because of their benign histology, complete removal is not necessary (though it has been done[228]) unless the lesions become large enough to compress surrounding structures. It is unclear whether radiation therapy is useful.

Others neoplasms. Uncommon considerations include primary neoplasms of the oculomotor nerve such as malignant meningioma[229] and primary glioblastoma multiforme.[230]

Other causes of third nerve palsies. Base of skull neoplasms, infectious disorders, and inflammatory disorders are discussed below in the section on combined ocular motor palsies. Less common causes include sinus mucoceles,[231] carotid insufficiency,[17,232,233] and intraneural cavernous hemangioma.[234]

Diagnostic evaluation of adults with acquired third nerve palsies

Although controversial, we believe that all patients with acute IIIrd nerve palsies should have neuroimaging and directed laboratory evaluation. Alternative guidelines for observing some affected patients have been based upon the patient's age, pupil involvement, and completeness of the motility deficit.[235,236] However, in our experience conservative observation may miss an underlying responsible vascular process or mass lesion.[237] Even isolated, *complete pupil-sparing* IIIrd nerve palsies can be caused by small infarcts in the mesencephalon and compressive lesions, so we have lowered our threshold to scan patients with isolated ocular motor palsies early in their course.

In adults with acquired, isolated IIIrd nerve palsies, particularly those which are pupil involving, a posterior communicating artery aneurysm should be excluded emergently. In this situation it is often useful to obtain an emergent computed tomography (CT) or MRI scan before proceeding with angiography since other compressive or infiltrative lesions may be found, eliminating the need for an invasive procedure. However, if the scan cannot be obtained immediately, we would proceed directly to angiography. If the scan is negative, even if it includes MR- or CT-angiography, conventional angiography may still be necessary to exclude an aneurysm.[238] Patients with IIIrd nerve palsy and posterior communicating artery aneurysms measuring 5–6 mm have been missed by MR-angiography.[239] Although MR-[236] and CT-angiographic techniques[240–243] continue to improve in their ability to detect small aneurysms, we are still reluctant to depend entirely on these noninvasive modalities. This is particularly true when the clinical suspicion remains high for the presence of an aneurysm. We still see patients with aneurysms missed either by poor resolution of noninvasive techniques or because the radiologist fails to detect the aneurysm on the scan.

In patients with normal neuroimaging and presumed vasculopathic IIIrd nerve palsies, those without identified vascular risk factors should have their blood pressure and fasting glucose, lipids, and cholesterol measured.

Processes which may mimic isolated *pupil-sparing* IIIrd nerve palsies in adults include myasthenia gravis, thyroid eye disease, and giant cell arteritis (due to muscle ischemia). When these disorders are considered, an edrophonium test, thyroid function tests, orbital neuroimaging, erythrocyte sedimentation rate, and C-reactive protein may be helpful.

We also have a low threshold for neuroimaging in patients with traumatic ocular motor palsies, even when isolated. These individuals may have a pseudoaneurysm or posteriorly draining cavernous sinus fistula (see below). In the setting of minor trauma, an underlying aneurysm or mass lesion should be excluded.[221] Extraocular muscle entrapment resulting from orbital wall fracture may mimic an oculomotor palsy.

Meningeal processes should also be considered in patients with oculomotor palsies, especially when they occur bilaterally or in combination, and when other cranial nerves or nerve roots are involved. MRI with gadolinium may disclose meningeal enhancement. In such instances, cerebrospinal fluid (CSF) examination, including cultures and cytology, should be performed to exclude acute bacterial and chronic fungal meningitis, tuberculosis, syphilis, Lyme, sarcoidosis, and carcinomatous or lymphomatous meningitis. In oculomotor palsies due to Guillain–Barré syndrome, the Fisher variant, or chronic inflammatory demyelinating polyneuropathy, the CSF protein should be elevated.

Management of third nerve palsy

The management of patients with IIIrd nerve dysfunction is the most complicated of all forms of paretic strabismus. This results from the potential involvement of four muscles and a complex pattern of extraocular muscle dysfunction. All decisions concerning the management of patients with IIIrd nerve palsy are divided into those which are recommended acutely and those recommended chronically when there is a fixed deficit.

As with other patients with the acute onset of double vision, after a diagnosis has been established, monocular occlusion and prisms can be used. In certain cases botulinum toxin can be injected into the lateral rectus muscle thereby eliminating the horizontal deviation and alleviating diplopia (occasionally with the aid of vertical prisms). Photophobia secondary to persistent pupillary dilation can be ameliorated with pharmacologic miosis or tinted lenses.

Once the palsy has been determined to be chronic and measurements have been stable for at least 6 months (preferably 12 months), various surgical strategies can be used to attempt to achieve realignment in the primary position and occasionally a useful field of single binocular vision.[244] In the setting of complete IIIrd nerve palsy, only realignment in the primary position can be hoped for. The surgeon must also consider the primary position ptosis. Many authorities feel that in the setting of complete ptosis, repair of the extraocular muscle alignment is not indicated. Furthermore, if eyelid elevation is defective and ptosis correction is attempted, the risk of corneal exposure is significant, particularly if supraduction is limited. Patients must be warned that, although there may be significant cosmetic benefit from realignment of the eyes, the potential for more disabling diplopia exists as the images are brought closer together. At this point an occlusive contact lens can be used to achieve a reasonable cosmetic and functional result.

Considerations in children with third nerve palsies[245]

Third nerve palsies in childhood may be congenital or acquired (**Table 15–4**). Almost every pediatric series has shown that the most common cause of an acquired IIIrd nerve palsy in this age group is trauma.[29,245–251] Neoplasms, inflammatory disorders, and ophthalmoplegic migraine should also be considered. Isolated IIIrd nerve palsies due to posterior communicating aneurysms and vasculopathic causes are rare in children.[252]

Congenital third nerve palsies. In Miller's series[246] of isolated IIIrd nerve palsies in pediatric patients, 43% were congenital in origin (**Fig. 15–27**). Most had pupillary involvement, aberrant regeneration, and amblyopia, and some went on to develop the phenomenon of oculomotor paresis with cyclic spasms. Forty percent of IIIrd nerve palsies in Harley's series[247] were also congenital, but in other studies[248,249] and in the Children's Hospital of Philadelphia (CHOP) series, they were seen less frequently. Monocular elevator palsies were grouped as congenital IIIrd nerve palsies in some series.[247]

Prior to the advent of modern neuroimaging, in most cases the responsible lesion was felt to be peripheral, due to birth trauma (skull molding) for instance, as suggested by the isolated nature of the IIIrd nerve palsy and the high

Table 15–4 Etiologies of **IIIrd** nerve palsies in children. When two figures are given, the first number refers to the number of isolated IIIrd nerve palsies in that category, while the number in parentheses refers to the number of patients seen with a IIIrd nerve palsy combined with a IVth or VIth nerve palsy or both. The CHOP series represents IIIrd nerve palsies seen by the authors at the Children's Hospital of Philadelphia during a 13 year period.[†]

	Miller[246] 1977 (1951–76)	Harley[247] 1980 (1968–79)	Keith[248] 1987 (1974–85)	Ing[249] 1992 (1970–91)	Kodsi[250] 1992 (1966–88)	Schumacher-Feero[251] 1999 (1981–96)	CHOP 2010 (1993–2006)
Congenital	13	15	8	8/(3)	Not included	20	17/(2)
Trauma	6	4	7	20/(11)	14	15	24/(13)
Neoplasm	3	3	1	1/(1)	5	6	17/(6)
Inflammatory/ infectious	4	3	6	6/(1)	1	3	9/(6)
Migraine	2	3	1	2	3		2
Aneurysm	2	0	0	0	0		1/(1)
Surgical	0	0	0	0	3		7
Idiopathic	0	0	4	1	6	1	3
Other	2	4	1	0	3	4	11/(2)*
Total	32	32	28	38/(16)	35	49	91/(30)

*Mesencephalic arteriovenous malformation, hydrocephalus, e.g.
[†]Tabulated by N. Mahoney, MD.

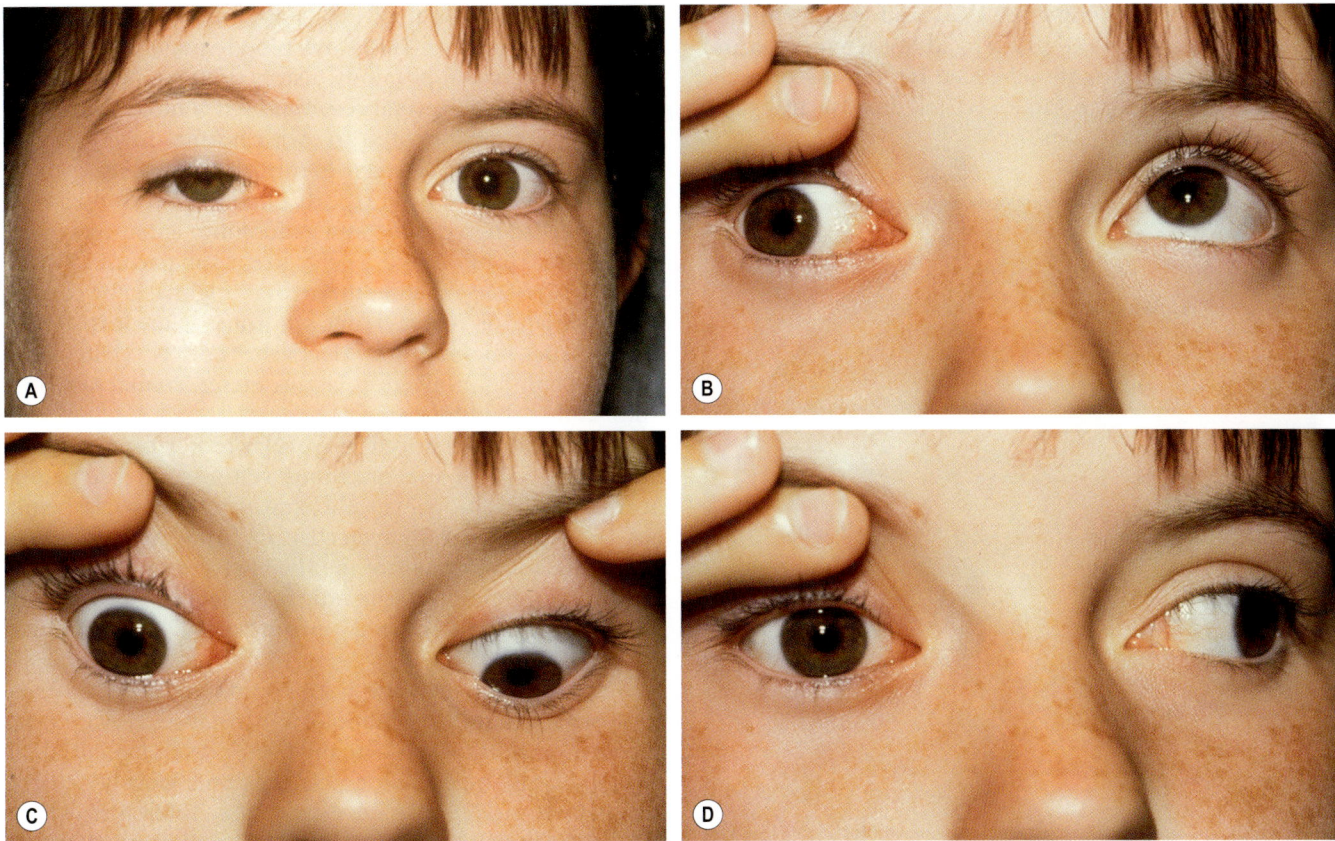

Figure 15–27. Pupil-sparing congenital right IIIrd nerve palsy. **A**. Primary gaze with right ptosis and head turn. Upgaze (**B**), downgaze (**C**), and adduction (**D**) were defective.

frequency of aberrant regeneration.[253] However, Balkan and Hoyt[254] reported 10 patients with congenital IIIrd nerve palsies, of whom four had focal neurologic abnormalities (e.g., hemiparesis) and two developmental delay. They and subsequent authors[255–257] suggested that, in some instances, congenital IIIrd nerve palsies may result from brainstem injury or reflect more widespread neurologic damage. Indeed, various autopsy studies have demonstrated aplasia of the ocular motor nuclei[258] or malformation of the midbrain,[259] reflective of an in utero insult to the central nervous system. MRIs can readily confirm midbrain damage in some cases.[256,260,261]

Miscellaneous common acquired etiologies

Inflammatory (including infections). Pneumococcal and *Haemophilus influenzae* meningitis have been associated with IIIrd nerve palsies in children.[246,249] In addition, in the CHOP series an isolated IIIrd nerve palsy was caused by tuberculous meningitis, and combined palsies were seen in association with Lyme meningitis[262] and Miller Fisher syndrome. A para-infectious IIIrd nerve palsy in a young child with cisternal nerve enhancement on MRI has been reported.[263] Rarely Tolosa–Hunt syndrome occurs in childhood[264,265] and can mimic ophthalmoplegic migraine (see below).[266]

Neoplasms. Posterior fossa tumors occur more frequently in children than in adults. However, these neoplasms tend to affect the pons and medulla, causing VIth nerve palsies more commonly (see below). When tumor-related IIIrd

nerve palsies occur, lesions affecting the midbrain (e.g., astrocytomas or higher grade gliomas),[267] orbit, orbital apex (e.g., rhabdomyosarcomas[268,269]), and leptomeninges may be implicated.[246,247] Schwannomas, neurinomas, and meningiomas of the oculomotor nerve may also be seen in childhood, especially in patients with neurofibromatosis type 2[270,271] (**Fig. 15–28**).

Ophthalmoplegic migraine. In children, IIIrd nerve palsies can accompany headaches in so-called ophthalmoplegic migraine (**Fig. 15–29**). Any ocular motor nerve can be involved, but isolated IIIrd nerve paresis is by far the most common, occurring in approximately 95% of cases. Sixth nerve palsies are the next most common, but IVth nerve palsies are hardly ever seen.[272] The IIIrd nerve palsy in ophthalmoplegic migraine is usually pupil involving, and complete resolution over weeks is the rule. However, aberrant regeneration can occur in some instances,[127] and, after multiple attacks, the motility deficits may heal only incompletely. We have a seen a child who became progressively more exotropic with each attack, which occurred yearly for 3 years.

Ophthalmoplegic migraine is an uncommon condition. The disorder was found in only 0.1% of children with migraine seen over an 18 year period in one institution,[273] and in only 8 of 5000 migraineurs in another study.[274] The first attack usually occurs before the child is 10 years of age, sometimes in infancy,[275,276] and uncommonly after age 20. Ipsilateral headache or periorbital pain usually precedes the ophthalmoparesis, sometimes by days, and young children often exhibit irritability and pallor in addition to nausea and vomiting.[277] Attacks, usually separated by months or years, are almost always in the same eye and involve the same ocular motor nerve each time.

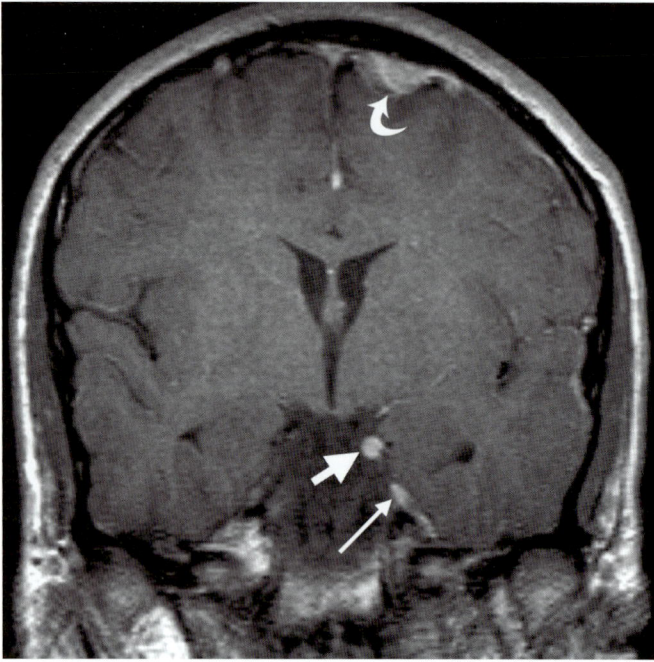

Figure 15–28. Gadolinium-enhanced coronal T1-weighted MRI in a child with neurofibromatosis type 2 and schwannomas of the oculomotor nerve (*short, thick arrow*) and trigeminal nerve (*thin arrow*) and a convexity meningioma (*curved arrow*).

The diagnosis is one of exclusion, following neuroimaging, lumbar puncture (LP), and blood studies, but is suggested by a personal or family history of migraine. Once the individual has had several recurrent, self-limited IIIrd nerve palsies over a period of years, with normal investigations and normal health between events, the diagnosis is more obvious. There have been reports of patients with migraine, a painful IIIrd nerve palsy, and gadolinium enhancement of the proximal portion of the nerve in the subarachnoid space (**Fig. 15–30**).[278-283] Whether these cases might also be considered a variant of Tolosa–Hunt syndrome is unclear. Nevertheless, the International Headache Society (IHS) now classifies ophthalmoplegic migraine under "cranial neuropathies" rather than migraine.[284]

Etiology. Compression of the ocular motor nerves against the lateral wall of the cavernous sinus by an edematous or dilated cavernous carotid and IIIrd nerve ischemia has been proposed as a mechanism. However, given the associated enhancement of the IIIrd nerve found frequently on MRI, ophthalmoplegic migraine is now thought to be a recurrent peripheral inflammatory demyelinating disorder.[285,286]

Treatment. Patients have been treated with ergotamines, corticosteroids, and propranolol for instance. However, no abortive medication has actually been proven beneficial, as most patients' oculomotor palsies spontaneously resolve. Prophylaxis may not be ideal in young children in whom the attacks may be separated by months or years. There are too few cases to study any drug's efficacy formally. One approach is to treat the headache symptomatically, allow the motility deficit to improve spontaneously, and avoid prophylactic therapy.

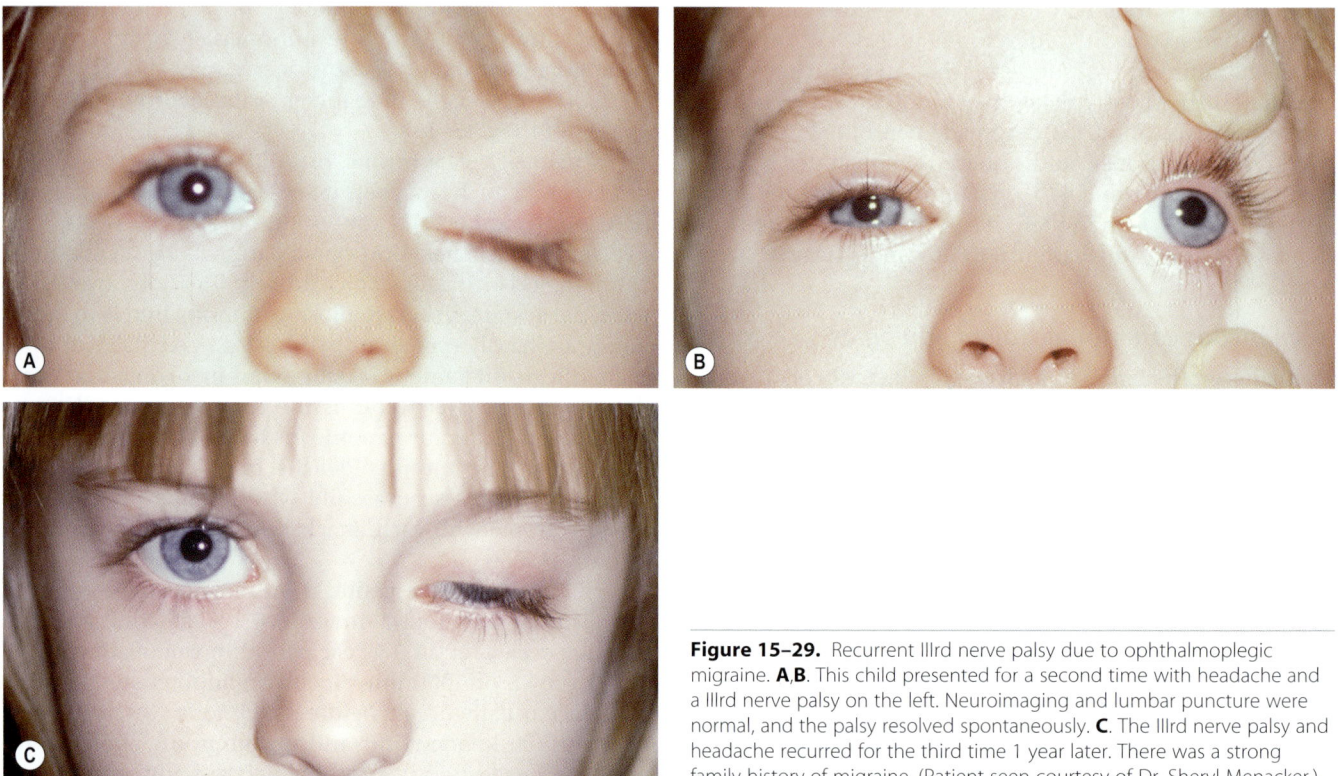

Figure 15–29. Recurrent IIIrd nerve palsy due to ophthalmoplegic migraine. **A,B**. This child presented for a second time with headache and a IIIrd nerve palsy on the left. Neuroimaging and lumbar puncture were normal, and the palsy resolved spontaneously. **C**. The IIIrd nerve palsy and headache recurred for the third time 1 year later. There was a strong family history of migraine. (Patient seen courtesy of Dr. Sheryl Menacker.)

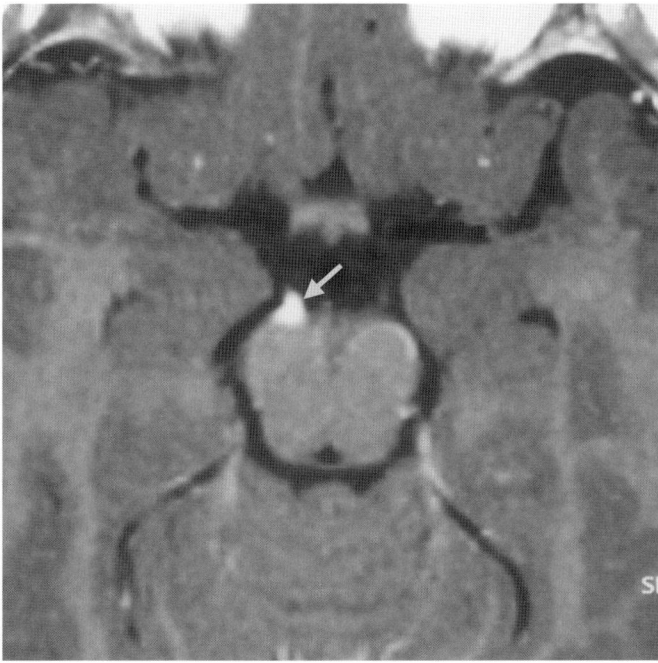

Figure 15–30. Axial T1-weighted MRI with gadolinium in a child with ophthalmoplegic migraine, demonstrating enhancement of the right IIIrd nerve (*arrow*).

Miscellaneous uncommon acquired etiologies

Aneurysms. Intracranial aneurysms are uncommon in childhood, thus isolated IIIrd nerve palsies due to posterior communicating aneurysms are extraordinarily infrequent in this age group as well. In the pediatric series[246–250] only two such patients, one aged 16 and one aged 17, were reported by Miller.[246] Younger patients have been the subject of single case reports by Gabianelli et al. (14 years old),[287] Wolin and Saunders (11 years old),[288] Mehkri et al. (10 years old),[289] Branley et al. (7 years old),[290] and Ebner (6 years old).[291] The first two had CT scans that missed the posterior communicating aneurysm, which was later confirmed on conventional angiography.

Third nerve palsies due to other intracranial aneurysms are even more rare. Fox,[292] in his editorial accompanying the article by Gabianelli et al.,[287] mentioned a 6-year-old child with a IIIrd nerve palsy due to a giant cavernous carotid aneurysm. A 4-year-old child with bilateral IIIrd nerve palsies owing to bilateral giant saccular cavernous carotid artery aneurysms has been reported.[293] We have seen a 5-year-old boy who presented with a sudden IIIrd, IVth, and VIth nerve palsy and optic neuropathy (orbital apex syndrome) due to a similar aneurysm, which was embolized. A 10-month-old child developed an isolated adduction deficit 7 days prior to fatal rupture of a congenital distal basilar artery aneurysm.[294] A IIIrd nerve palsy in a child due to a superior cerebellar artery aneurysm has been reported.[295] A 2-year-old child developed a IIIrd nerve palsy in association with a posterior cerebral artery aneurysm.[296] We have seen an 8-month-old infant with an acquired IIIrd nerve palsy due to a partially thrombosed aneurysm of the left internal carotid artery.[297] A brain MRI and MR-angiography were sufficient to detect the aneurysm.

Table 15–5 Pediatric **IIIrd** nerve palsies: suggested workup

1. Congenital
   a Careful neurological examination
   b MRI of the brain

2. Acquired
   a Exclude history of trauma or migraine
   b MRI and MR-angiography
   c Consider lumbar puncture, if the neuroimaging is negative
   d If MRI and LP negative, consider ophthalmoplegic migraine
   e If MRI and LP negative in a patient 10 years of age or above, consider conventional angiography

MRI, magnetic resonance imaging; MR-angiography, magnetic resonance angiography; LP, lumbar puncture.

Diabetes. For unclear reasons, diabetic cranial mononeuropathies are very rare in children. Grunt et al.[298] reported three such patients, but each had features which were atypical. A 12-year-old boy had a purported VIth nerve palsy, but an ophthalmologist diagnosed hyperopia with accommodative esotropia, and this coincided with temporary hyperglycemia. The "left internal strabismus" in this patient improved when the refractive error and insulin requirement resolved. The second patient was a 13-year-old child with a complete, pupil-sparing IIIrd nerve palsy, which did not resolve fully after 21 months of follow-up. The third patient was an 11-year-old child with a partial, pupil-involving IIIrd nerve palsy which lasted 16 months until strabismus surgery was performed.

Diagnostic evaluation in children with third nerve palsies. One suggested approach is outlined in **Table 15–5**. In children with congenital IIIrd nerve palsies present since birth, a careful neurologic examination should be performed, looking for other associated neurologic abnormalities. Then an MRI of the brain should be ordered to exclude congenital brain malformations.

When the IIIrd nerve palsy is acquired, a history of trauma or migraine should be excluded. In all acquired cases, MRI and CT- or MR-angiography should be performed, looking for mesencephalic, cavernous sinus, or orbital lesions, and to exclude an aneurysm. We disagree that some children with acquired, isolated IIIrd nerve palsies can be watched conservatively.[299] If the neuroimaging is negative and the child is ill-appearing or has a fever or stiff neck, a LP should be performed to exclude meningitis. If the MRI and LP are negative, a diagnosis of ophthalmoplegic migraine can be entertained. Finally, if the MRI and LP are negative in a patient 10 years of age or above, practitioners should consider conventional angiography to exclude a posterior communicating aneurysm.[245]

Fourth nerve palsies

Patients with superior oblique paresis complain of vertical diplopia, often with a torsional component, and they have an ipsilateral hypertropia worse on contraversive (contralateral conjugate) horizontal gaze and ipsilateral head tilt (Parks' three-step test, best demonstrated with alternate

Video 15.7

515

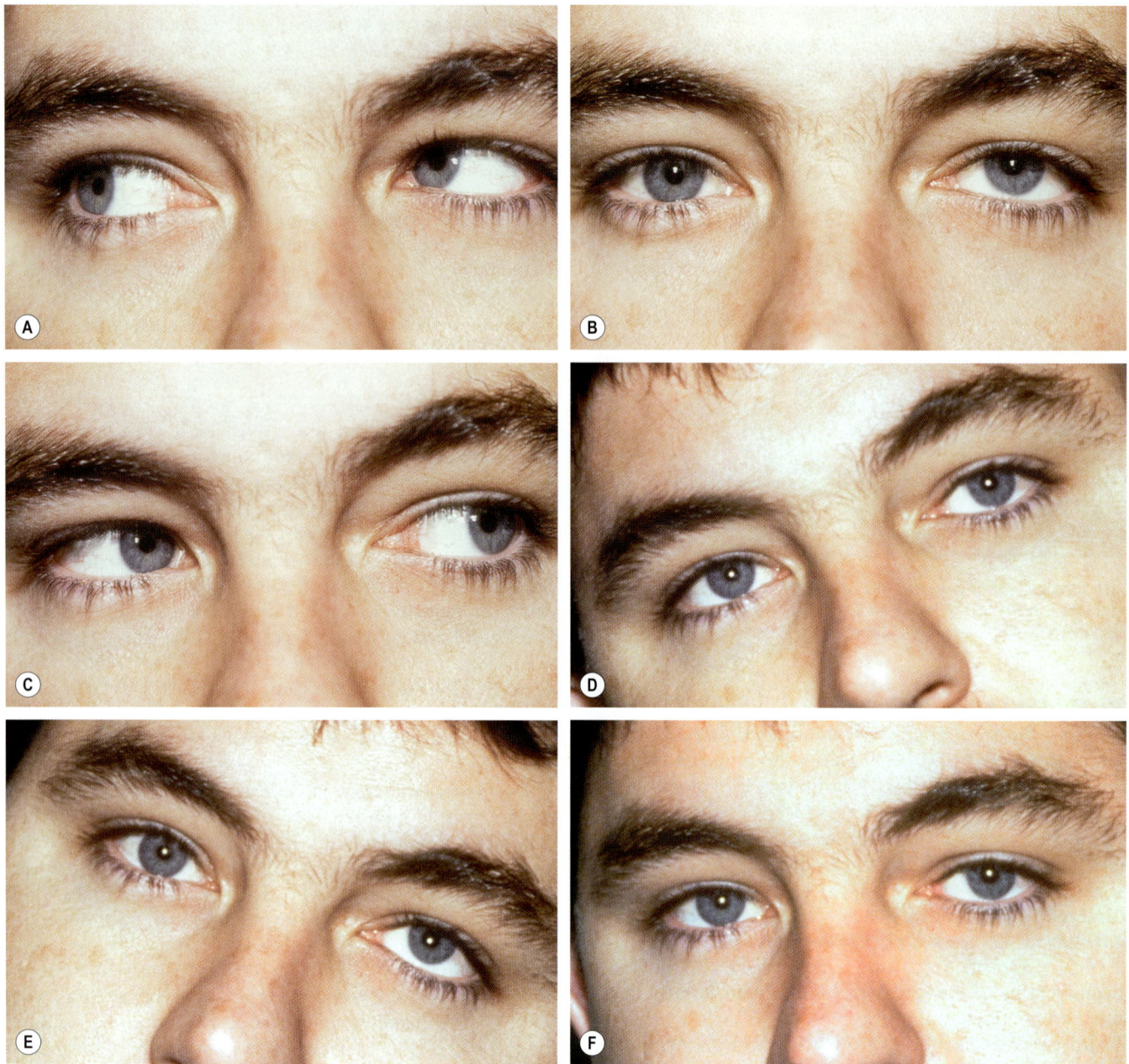

Figure 15–31. Traumatic left IVth nerve palsy, three-step test. **A**. Right gaze. **B**. Primary gaze. **C**. Left gaze. **D**. Right head tilt. **E**. Left head tilt. **F**. Preference for a right head turn (left gaze) and right head tilt, which minimizes the patient's vertical diplopia. *Step 1:* which eye is hypertropic (*left*; see B); *Step 2:* is the hypertropia worse in left or right gaze (*right*; see A vs. C); *Step 3:* is the hypertropia worse in left or right head tilt (*left*; see E vs. D). The *left* hypertropia, which is worse in *right* gaze and *left* head tilt, is consistent with weakness of the left superior oblique muscle. (From Liu GI. Disorders of the eyes and eyelids: disorders of eye movements. In Samuels MA, Feske S (eds): The Office Practice of Neurology, p 54. New York, Churchill Livingstone, 1996, with permission.)

cover or Maddox rod testing) (**Fig. 15-31**). In some instances the superior oblique weakness is evident on testing of ductions (**Fig. 15-32**), but more commonly alternate cover or Maddox rod testing is necessary to document the misalignment. Excyclotorsion of the involved eye may be documented using double Maddox rods.[300] Head tilt towards the contralateral shoulder is usually seen (**Fig. 15-32**). One can occasionally elicit which IVth nerve is affected by asking the patient to look at a horizontal straight edge such as a door, projector screen, or pen. If the patient sees two images, they can be asked to describe how they intersect. A patient with a unilateral IVth nerve palsy will see a horizon-

tal line and a tilted line below it, intersecting on the side of the abnormal eye ("the arrow points to the affected IVth nerve").

Trauma is one of the most common causes of acquired IVth nerve palsies (**Table 15-2**).[26,301–303] Traumatic IVth nerve palsies have been attributed to damage to the posterior decussation (anterior medullary vellum) due to its close anatomic relationship with the tentorium. Contusions in this area may be seen on neuroimaging. This is the likely explanation for the high incidence of bilateral IVth nerve palsies in trauma. Alternatively, hemorrhages of the IVth nerve more laterally at the tentorial edge have been docu-

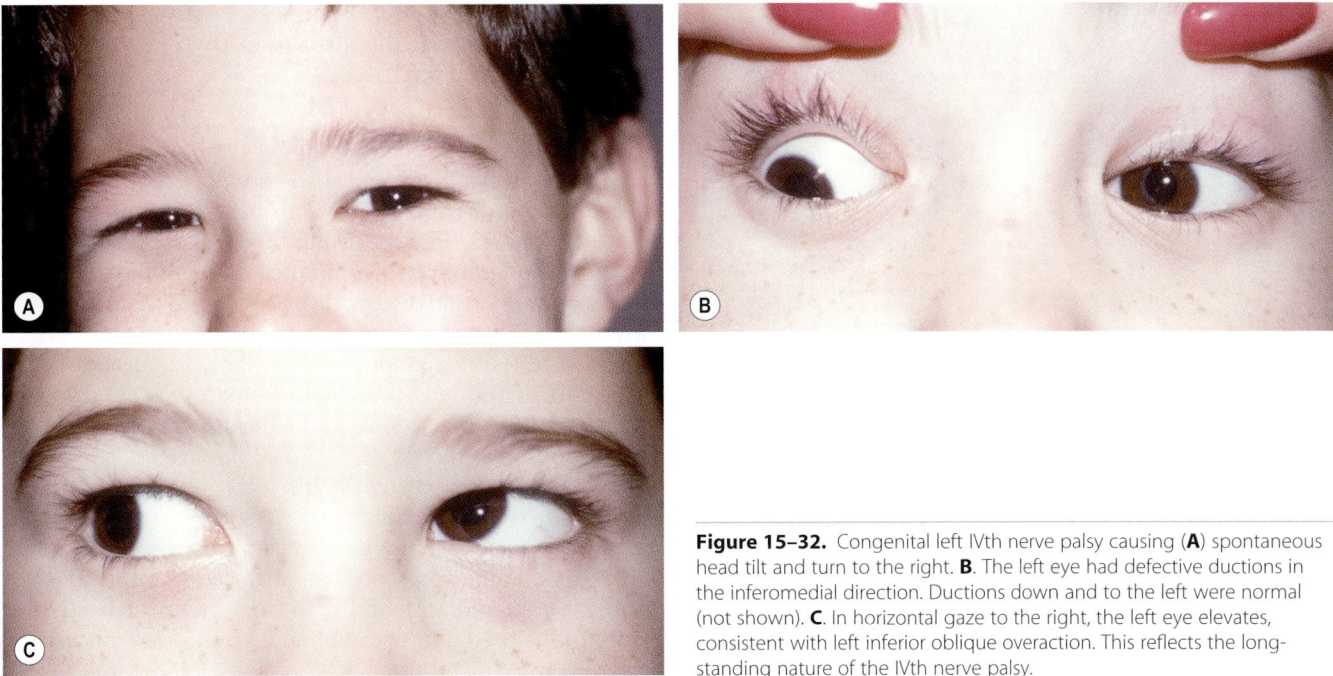

Figure 15–32. Congenital left IVth nerve palsy causing (**A**) spontaneous head tilt and turn to the right. **B**. The left eye had defective ductions in the inferomedial direction. Ductions down and to the left were normal (not shown). **C**. In horizontal gaze to the right, the left eye elevates, consistent with left inferior oblique overaction. This reflects the long-standing nature of the IVth nerve palsy.

mented.[304] In addition, skull base fractures may be responsible for traumatic IVth nerve palsies.

Decompensated congenital IVth nerve palsies are also common, and are discussed in more detail below. Ischemic IVth nerve palsies should be considered when an individual over 50 with vasculopathic risk factors develops vertical diplopia and periorbital ache. In such cases the prognosis for spontaneous recovery is excellent. Aneurysmal causes of IVth nerve palsies[305] are much less common than in IIIrd nerve weakness. Other less frequent causes of IVth nerve palsies include compressive[306] and infiltrative[307] neoplasms, meningitis, multiple sclerosis,[171,308] posterior midbrain hemorrhages[309,310] and strokes[311,312] (**Fig. 15–33**), vascular malformation,[313] giant cell arteritis,[314] schwannomas and neurinomas,[224,226,315–317] and anterior temporal lobectomy for epilepsy.[318]

Occasionally IVth nerve palsies are accompanied by other neurologic signs that aid in localization. For instance, a IVth nerve palsy accompanied by a contralateral Horner syndrome would localize to the dorsal pontomesencephalic junction (see **Fig. 13–22**).[319] A IVth nerve palsy with contralateral dysmetria suggests a lesion involving the superior cerebellar peduncle,[320] while one accompanied by contralateral internuclear ophthalmoplegia localizes to the proximal fascicle and MLF.[321]

Decompensated congenital fourth nerve palsies. Most of these patients present with head tilt or insidious onset of intermittent vertical double vision or focusing difficulty. A large hypertropia in adduction of the affected eye is sometimes noticed by the patient or family members. Complaints of torsion are less than in cases of acquired IVth nerve palsies. Additionally overaction of the ipsilateral inferior oblique muscle in adduction is usually evident on examination (**Fig. 15–32**). Some authors[302] prefer to call these palsies "cryptogenic" or "idiopathic" because the etiology is unclear. The congenital nature of the lesion is presumed, based upon

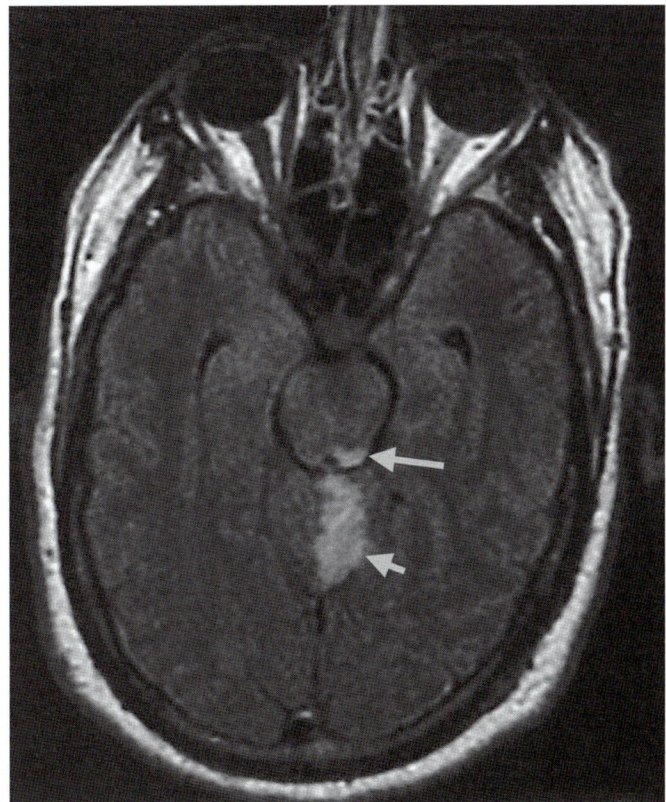

Figure 15–33. Axial FLAIR MRI demonstrating an infarction of the left posterior mesencephalon (*long arrow*) and cerebellum (*short arrow*) in a patient with a right "nuclear" IVth nerve palsy.

the often long-standing head tilt, as evidenced by review of old photographs and a family member's report, and the absence of an inciting event. Evidence of chronicity includes overaction of the ipsilateral inferior oblique muscle and a large vertical fusional amplitude. The latter refers to the

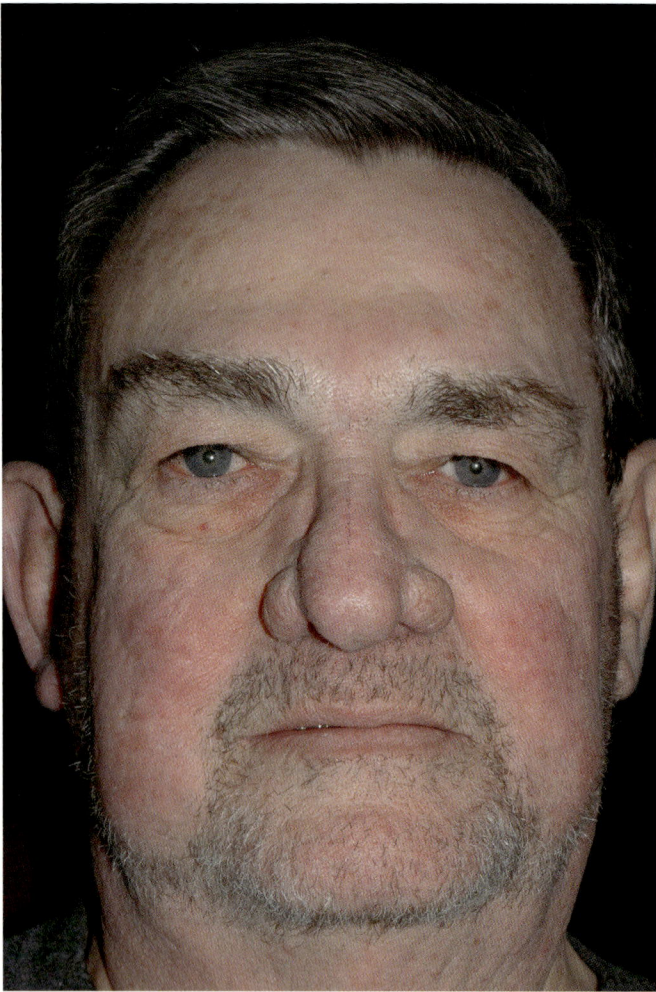

Figure 15–34. Facial asymmetry in a patient with a decompensated right congenital IVth nerve palsy. In addition to the right hypertropia (see the corneal light reflex in the bottom of the right pupil), note the right eye is set higher in the skull than the left.

patient's ability to fuse vertically separated images despite the placement of progressively large amounts of vertical prism over one eye. Facial asymmetries are also frequently associated with the long-standing head tilt (**Fig. 15–34**).[322]

Proposed etiologies for congenital IVth nerve palsies include hypoplasia or aplasia of the IVth nerve nucleus, birth trauma to the IVth nerve or superior oblique muscle, anomalous insertion of the muscle, muscle fibrosis, fibrous adhesions,[302] or structural abnormalities of the superior oblique tendon.[323] Usually congenital cases are sporadic. However, familial cases[324–326] and those associated with central nervous system abnormalities[327] have been reported. Decompensated congenital IVth nerve palsies are likely the result of progressive breakdown in vertical fusional capability rather than progression of IVth nerve weakness.[302]

Diagnostic evaluation of adults with acquired fourth nerve palsies

Without a history or clinical features of a long-standing decompensated congenital palsy, patients with IVth nerve palsies should undergo neuroimaging to exclude an intra-

cranial process. In addition, mimickers such as myasthenia gravis, thyroid-associated ophthalmopathy, and skew deviation should be excluded.

Management of fourth nerve palsy

Some patients can be treated with base down prism over the affected eye, and usually press-on Fresnel prisms are used before permanent ones are ground into the lenses. However the excyclotorsion and incomitancy of the deviation leave many patients unsatisfied with prisms. Others, particularly those with ischemic palsies, in whom recovery is expected, can occlude (with opaque or black tape, for instance) the lower half of the lens over the affected eye. This provides occlusion of the affected eye in the direction of action of the superior oblique muscle.

Patients with persistent IVth nerve palsies who are unsatisfied with prisms or patching may require strabismus surgery. The decision to intervene surgically is based on the presence of increasing symptoms of double vision, and an inability to carry on normal activities combined with stable measurements over a several month period.

Fourth nerve palsies in children

Fourth nerve palsies are less common in childhood than IIIrd and VIth nerve palsies. This is perhaps in part due to the fact that minor superior oblique paresis is harder to detect in younger children, especially when the IIIrd nerve is already involved. In Harley's[247] and Kodsi and Younge's[250] series, trauma was the most common cause of an acquired IVth nerve palsy (**Table 15–6**). However, in Harley's[247] and the CHOP series, congenital or decompensated congenital IVth nerve palsies were the most common of all cases.

Diagnostic evaluation in children with fourth nerve palsies. If the IVth nerve palsy is consistent with an isolated, decompensated congenital one, then no workup is necessary. Otherwise, head trauma and evidence for a posterior fossa mass should be excluded. If the etiology is unclear, an MRI can be performed, with attention to the posterior midbrain, cavernous sinus, and orbit. In children with a normal MRI but with a fever or stiff neck, a LP should be performed to exclude meningitis.

Sixth nerve palsies

Patients with a lateral rectus palsy complain of binocular horizontal double vision worse on ipsiversive gaze and at distance. In many cases the limitation of abduction is evident (**Fig. 15–35**), but, in more subtle instances, alternate cover or Maddox rod testing would confirm an esotropia largest on ipsiversive gaze.

Nuclear/fascicular. A lesion in the region of the VIth nerve nucleus would result in an ipsiversive conjugate gaze palsy and ipsilateral facial weakness (facial colliculus syndrome; see Chapters 14 and 16 and **Fig. 16–5**).[328,329] A lesion of the caudal ventral pons involving the abducens fascicle and corticospinal tract would result in a lateral rectus palsy and a contralateral hemiparesis (*Raymond syndrome*). However, iso-

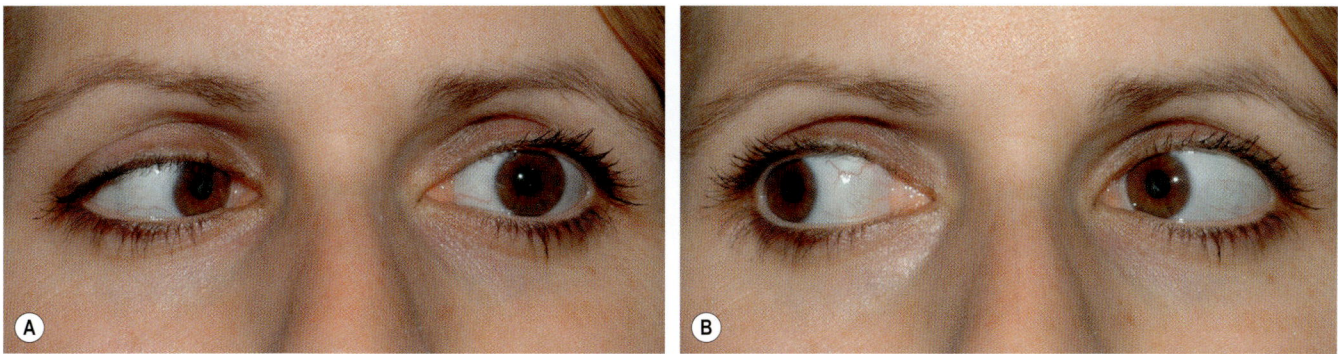

Figure 15–35. A. Idiopathic left VIth nerve palsy causing left lateral rectus weakness and limitation of abduction in a young adult. **B**. Conjugate gaze to the right is normal. MRI and acetylcholine receptor antibody testing were normal, and the eye movement abnormality spontaneously resolved.

Table 15–6 Etiologies of **IVth** nerve palsies in children. When two figures are given, the first number refers to the number of isolated IVth nerve palsies in that category, while the number in parentheses refers to the total of IVth nerve palsies combined with a IIIrd or VIth nerve palsy or both. The CHOP series represents IVth nerve palsies seen by the authors at the Children's Hospital of Philadelphia during a 13 year period.[†]

	Harley[247] 1980 (1968–79)	Kodsi[250] 1992 (1966–88)	CHOP 2010 (1993–2006)
Congenital	12	Not included	28
Trauma	5	7	3/(4)
Neoplasm	0	1	1/(3)
Inflammatory	1	1	1/(3)
Surgical	0	1	2
Idiopathic	0	4	0
Other	0	5	2/(1)*
Total	18	19	37/(11)

*Elevated intracranial pressure, cavernous–carotid aneurysm.
[†]Tabulated by N. Mahoney, MD.

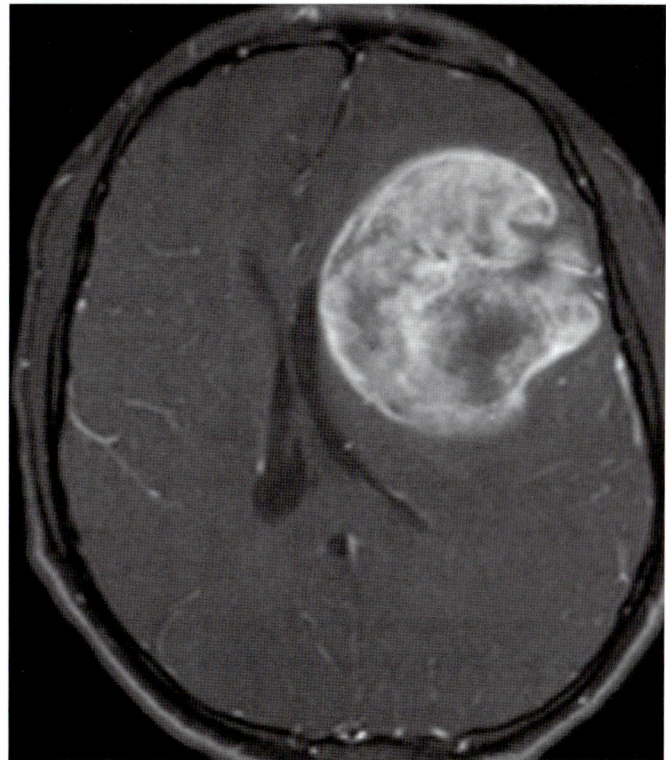

Figure 15–36. Axial T1-weighted MRI with gadolinium demonstrating a large left frontal glioblastoma with severe mass effect. The patient had papilledema and a VIth nerve palsy resulting from elevated intracranial pressure.

lated VIth nerve palsies due to pontine lesions may be seen in hypertension[330] or diabetes.[331] Embolic or thrombotic occlusion of paramedian penetrating branches of the basilar artery is the usual cause for disturbances in these areas, but multiple sclerosis,[171,332,333] vascular malformations, and metastases should also be considered.

Subarachnoid/base of skull. The VIth nerve, as it climbs along the clivus then over the petrous apex, is vulnerable to injury during downward brainstem shifts resulting from supratentorial masses ("false localizing sign"). Changes in intracranial pressure that occur in pseudotumor cerebri, supratentorial masses (**Fig. 15–36**), or hydrocephalus (intracranial hypertension) or after LP,[334] myelography,[335] or CSF leak[336] (intracranial hypotension) may also cause VIth nerve palsies. These tend to resolve within days or weeks after the intracranial pressure is normalized.

Skull base neoplasms such as meningiomas and chordomas (see below) are common causes of chronic isolated VIth nerve palsies.[337,338] Sixth nerve palsies in this setting may sometimes improve spontaneously and therefore mimic inflammatory and ischemic palsies.[339] A patient with an isolated acute VIth nerve palsy has been reported in association with pituitary apoplexy.[340] Since the parasympathetic fibers of the facial nerve travel along the floor of the middle cranial fossa on their way to supply the ipsilateral lacrimal gland, a patient with a VIth nerve palsy and ipsilateral dry eye may be harboring a mass in this region.

Otherwise, the same infectious and inflammatory processes in the subarachnoid space which affect the IIIrd nerve can also cause a VIth nerve palsy. Similarly, trauma and ischemia can lead to VIth nerve palsies. As with other traumatic ocular motor palsies, the trauma tends to be severe and accompanied by skull fractures (**Fig. 15–37**). The prognosis for spontaneous improvement within weeks or months

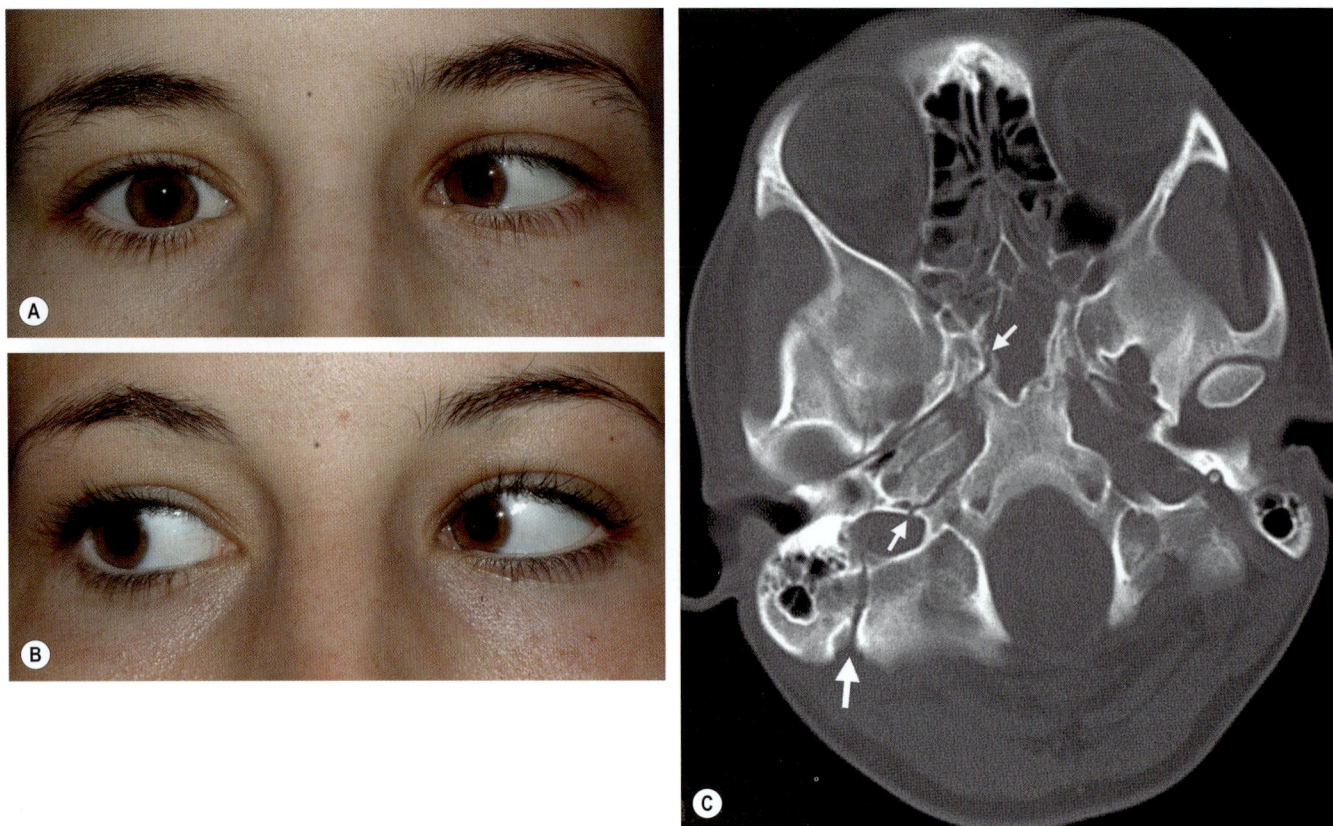

Figure 15–37. **A**. Traumatic right VIth nerve palsy following a motor vehicle accident and severe head injury. **B**. By 3 months later the VIth nerve palsy had spontaneously resolved. **C**. CT scan, bone windows, demonstrating multiple skull base fractures (*arrows*).

Video 15.8

is excellent,[341] but patients with complete palsies at presentation have a poorer chance for recovery.[342] Ischemic VIth nerve palsies are typically painful, of relatively sudden onset, and resolve within three months. Benign, idiopathic VIth nerve palsies which spontaneously resolve in young adults are also well recognized (see **Fig. 15–35**).[343,344] Guillain–Barré syndrome, Miller Fisher syndrome, and Gradenigo syndrome[345] should also be in the differential diagnosis of VIth nerve palsies. Other less common causes include schwannomas,[346] giant cell arteritis,[314] and compression of the VIth nerve by dolichoectatic basilar,[347] vertebral,[348] or carotid[349] arteries.

Diagnostic evaluation in adults with acquired sixth nerve palsies

As in adults with other acquired ocular motor palsies, we prefer to image those with acquired VIth nerve palsies to exclude intracranial processes.[237] In younger adults, neuroimaging is particularly important because of the relatively higher risk for neoplasms in this age group.[343,350] Serologies, including those for syphilis and Lyme disease, as well as a sedimentation rate to exclude giant cell arteritis, may be performed. LP may be necessary when infectious, carcinomatous, or lymphomatous meningitis are suspected.

Management of sixth nerve palsies

Once again, the options that exist acutely include occlusion and press-on Fresnel prisms. Base out prisms can be used to

significantly reduce the head turn while the patient is being followed for recovery. Alternatively, opaque tape can be placed over the temporal half of the lens over the affected eye. This occludes the affected eye in the direction of the lateral rectus palsy. In addition, botulinum injections to the ipsilateral medial rectus muscle can be very helpful in restoring a field of single binocular vision and potentially reducing the risk of medial rectus contracture. However, botulinum toxin injections may be limited by the side-effect of ptosis and the need for repeated injections. Once the VIth nerve palsy has been followed for 6–12 months without recovery, then patients can be offered strabismus surgery.

Sixth nerve palsies in children (acquired)

In three pediatric series,[247,250,351] trauma was the most common cause of an acquired VIth nerve palsy. In Robertson et al.'s,[352] Aroichane and Repka's,[353] and the CHOP series,[354] neoplasms were the most frequent cause. Thus, accounting for the results from all series, the most common cause of acquired, nontraumatic VIth nerve palsy is a tumor (**Table 15–7**). Separating VIth nerve palsies by etiology is often difficult because of the considerable overlap: trauma, neoplasms, and meningitis can be associated with elevated intracranial pressure or hydrocephalus, which by themselves are independent causes of VIth nerve palsies.

Neoplasms. In contrast to adult brain tumors, the majority of which are supratentorial, 45–60% of childhood brain neoplasms occur in the posterior fossa.[355] These lesions, such

Table 15-7 Etiologies of **VIth** nerve palsies in children. When two figures are given, the first number refers to the number of isolated VIth nerve palsies in that category, while the number in parentheses refers to the total of isolated and combined (VIth plus IIIrd or IVth nerve palsies or both) palsies. The CHOP series represents VIth nerve palsies seen by the authors at the Children's Hospital of Philadelphia during a 13 year period.[†]

	Robertson[352] 1970 (1952–64)	Harley[247] 1980 (1968–79)	Afifi[351] 1992 (1966–88)	Kodsi[250] 1992 (1966–88)	Aroichane[353] 1995 (1985–93) (age < 7)	CHOP 2010 (1993–2006)
Congenital	Not included	5	17	Not included	Not included	10/(2)
Trauma	26	21	37	37	12	23/(13)
Neoplasm	52	17	25	18	21	58/(6)
Surgical						34
Inflammatory/ infectious	23	8	13	5	4	23/(6)
Increased ICP (nontumor)	15	3	17	2	15	25/(1)
Idiopathic	12	4	14	13	3	26
Other	5	4	9	13	9	11/(2)*
Total	133	62	132	88	64	210/(30)

*For example, basilar artery thrombosis, vertebral artery dissection, and cavernous–carotid aneurysm.
[†]Tabulated by N. Mahoney, MD.
ICP, intracranial pressure.

as medulloblastomas, ependymomas, and pontine gliomas (**Fig. 15-38**), tend to compromise midline structures in the dorsal pons and pontine tegmentum, resulting not infrequently with gaze palsies and VIth nerve palsies. Fourth ventricular compression, resulting in noncommunicating hydrocephalus, is also common and is another cause of VIth nerve palsies. Ataxia and nystagmus, due to cerebellar or cerebellar pathway interference, are also frequently seen.

Inflammatory. Several reports[356–362] have described a benign isolated VIth nerve palsy in childhood (**Fig. 15-39**). The patients tend to be otherwise healthy with an antecedent viral or febrile illness, or recent history of immunization. The VIth nerve palsy lasts for weeks or months, spontaneously resolves, and can recur. Many of these patients,[356,357] however, were seen prior to the widespread use of MRI, which might have detected demyelination (in acute disseminated encephalomyelitis (ADEM) or multiple sclerosis, for example). In addition, many reported patients did not have LPs to exclude meningitis.[356,360,362] Benign VIth nerve palsy in childhood is a diagnosis of exclusion following normal neuroimaging and CSF examination. Recurrences, sometimes multiple, may occur in as many as one-third of affected children.[363,364]

Acquired comitant esotropia. *Comitant esotropia does not exclude a neurologic process*. In comitant esotropias the angle of ocular misalignment is unchanged regardless of the direction of gaze.[365] Comitant esotropias may be mistaken for bilateral VIth nerve palsies. Some authors[366] suggested that comitant esotropias, in contrast to incomitant esodeviations, are benign and do not warrant further neurologic investigation. However, several other reports[367–370] have established that brain tumors and other intracranial processes in pediatric patients may in fact present with comitant esotropias.

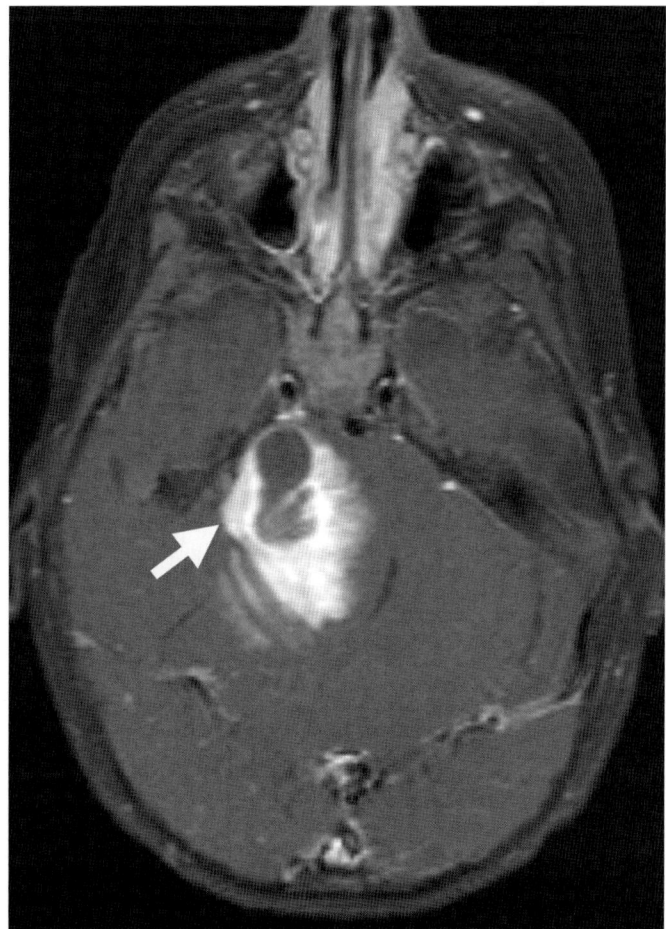

Figure 15-38. Pontine fibrillary astrocytoma associated with a right VIth nerve palsy. Axial MRI shows an enhancing mass (*arrow*) involving the right pons.

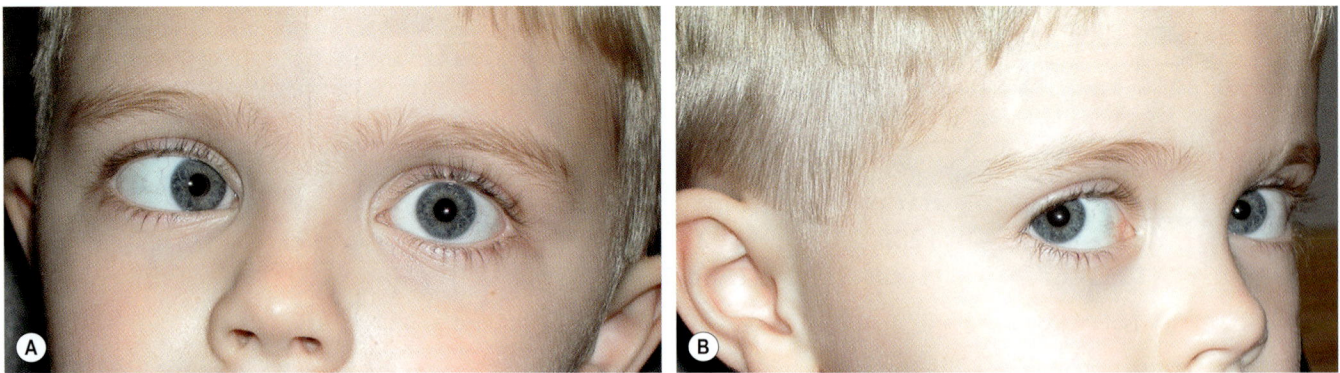

Figure 15–39. Benign VIth nerve palsy in childhood. **A**. Acquired left abduction deficit. **B**. Normal right gaze. Neuroimaging was normal, and the child was otherwise well. He experienced full recovery several weeks later.

The topic has been discussed in reviews by experts.[371,372] Acquired comitant esotropias in childhood have been reported in association with cerebellar astrocytomas,[368,369,373] medulloblastomas,[368] pontine gliomas,[368,374] and Chiari I malformation.[367,375–377] In cases due to Chiari I malformation, suboccipital decompression often leads to resolution of the esotropia.[378,379]

This finding appears to be primarily a pediatric phenomenon, and may not be as uncommon as previously suggested.[368] Of 30 children seen at CHOP with an acquired esodeviation associated with a neurologic insult, 12 (40%) had comitant measurements.[380] However, rarely is comitant esotropia the sole manifestation of an intracranial abnormality. Most patients will still have accompanying signs and symptoms of either elevated intracranial pressure (papilledema, headache, nausea or vomiting, or enlarging head size) or brainstem or cerebellar involvement (nystagmus, ataxia, hemiparesis, gait imbalance, dysarthria, or Parinaud syndrome).

Several authors have reviewed the possible mechanisms for comitant esotropia in the setting of neurologic disease. Lennerstrand,[381] Hoyt and Good,[372] and Ciancia[371] reasoned that comitant strabismus might result from injury to supranuclear mesencephalic structures which control vergence eye movements. Others have ascribed infranuclear insults. Flynn[382] described a child who presented with an acute onset comitant esotropia who weeks later developed VIth and VIIth nerve palsies as a manifestation of a pontine glioma. Jampolsky[383] and Kirkham et al.[67] suggested that acquired esotropia and divergence paralysis may result from varying degrees of bilateral VIth nerve paresis. Spread of comitance is another proposed mechanism.[357]

Cyclic esotropia. This rare ocular motility disorder is characterized by 48–96 hour cycles of esotropia and orthophoria or microstrabismus.[384] Usually idiopathic, cyclic esotropia may also be associated with intracranial tumors and epilepsy.[385] The cause is uncertain.

Suggested workup in pediatric acquired sixth nerve palsies. One suggested approach is given in **Table 15–8**. Because of the risk of an underlying neoplasm, even in isolated cases, in the absence of trauma an MRI with and without gadolinium, looking particularly for a posterior fossa lesion, is recommended. The diagnosis of a benign childhood VIth nerve palsy is one of exclusion.

Table 15–8 Pediatric **VIth** nerve palsies: suggested workup

1. Congenital
   a Consider Duane's retraction and Möbius syndromes
2. Acquired
   a Exclude history of trauma
   b MRI with and without gadolinium, looking particularly for a posterior fossa lesion
   c Consider LP, if the neuroimaging is negative, to exclude meningitis and to measure the CSF opening pressure
   d If MRI and LP negative, consider the diagnosis of a benign childhood VIth nerve palsy

MRI, magnetic resonance imaging; LP, lumbar puncture, CSF, cerebrospinal fluid.

Sixth nerve palsies in children (congenital)

The vast majority of children born with defective VIth nerve function have Duane's retraction syndrome. Less likely causes are Möbius syndrome or a nonsyndromic isolated congenital VIth nerve palsy.

Duane's retraction syndrome. This condition is characterized by the paradoxical co-contraction of the ipsilateral medial and lateral rectus muscles, which are normally antagonistic and customarily innervated by the IIIrd and VIth nerves, respectively.[386] Based on electromyographic recordings from the extraocular muscles of affected patients, Huber[387] classified cases into three types. *Narrowing of the palpebral fissure and retraction of the globe in attempted adduction are common to all.* Fissure narrowing is likely secondary to decreased levator firing in adduction.

1. Type I. *Abduction is impaired, but adduction is either normal or only slightly defective.* While the lateral rectus muscle does not contract during attempted abduction, both the medial and the lateral rectus muscles fire during adduction, thus producing the globe retraction (**Fig. 15–40**). Type I is the most common pattern of the three. Despite complete abduction deficits, most patients with type I are usually orthotropic in primary gaze. This feature distinguishes adults with Duane syndrome from those with acquired VIth nerve palsies, who are characteristically esotropic.

2. Type II. *Abduction is normal, but adduction is impaired.* Lateral rectus contraction in abduction is normal, but

Video 15

Video 15

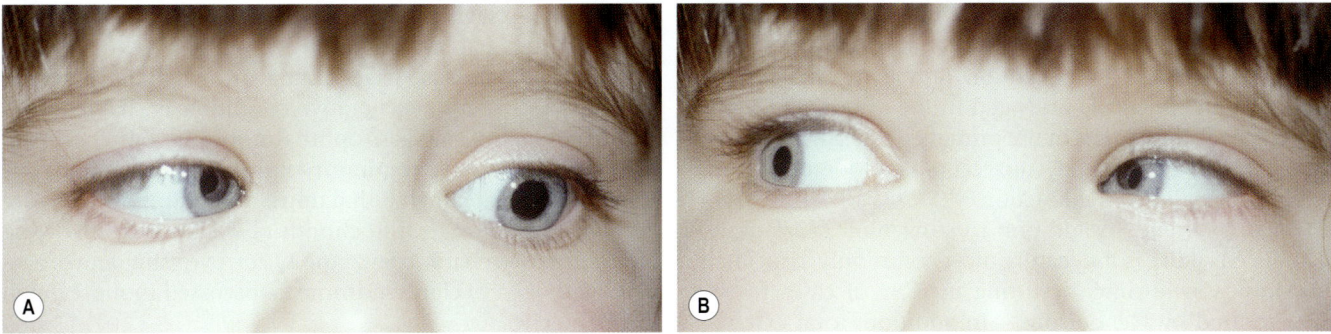

Figure 15–40. Duane's retraction syndrome type I. **A.** Left abduction deficit. **B.** In right gaze, globe retraction and fissure narrowing of the left eye are seen.

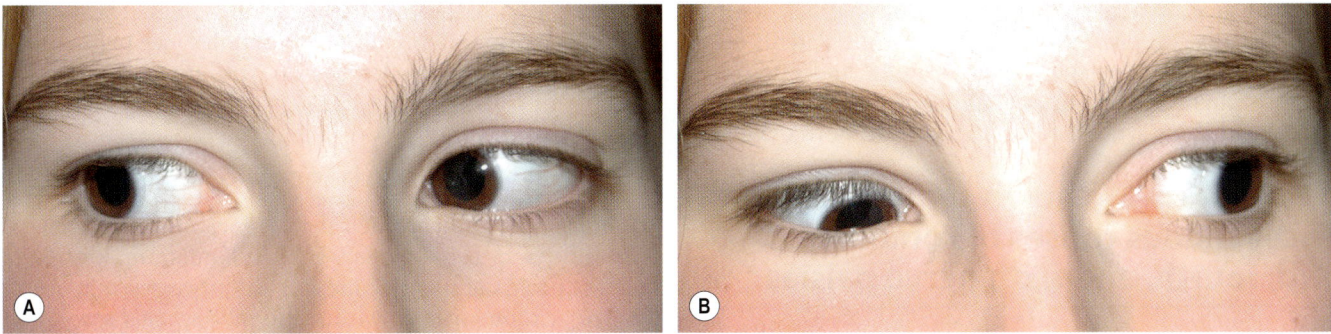

Figure 15–41. Duane's retraction syndrome type II. **A.** Normal right gaze. **B.** In left gaze, an adduction deficit, downshoot, globe retraction, and fissure narrowing of the right eye are seen.

the muscle also inappropriately contracts in attempted adduction, producing defective adduction and globe retraction (**Fig. 15–41**).

3. Type III. *Both abduction and adduction are defective.* The lateral and medial rectus muscles both contract in abduction and adduction, thus limiting motion of the eye in either direction. Clinically this pattern may be hard to distinguish from type I.

Other common features include upshoot or downshoot of the eye in adduction, and A-, V-, or X-pattern ocular deviations. Most patients preserve binocularity because they are orthotropic in primary gaze, but a minority of individuals adapt a compensatory head turn to achieve binocularity. In one meta-analysis,[388] there was a female preponderance (58%) and left eye (59%) predilection. Twenty-three percent of patients had just the right eye affected, while 18% had bilateral involvement. Other anomalous innervation phenomena, such as Marcus–Gunn jaw wink and paradoxical–gustatory–lacrimal reflex ("crocodile tears"), have been reported in association with Duane's retraction syndrome.[388]

Pathologic studies published by Miller and colleagues[389,390] have provided enormous insight into the neural substrate of Duane's retraction syndrome by confirming brainstem abnormalities and the anomalous innervation of the lateral rectus muscle. In their report of a patient with Duane's type I,[390] the VIth nerve was absent, the VIth nerve nucleus was hypoplastic, and branches of the inferior division of the oculomotor (IIIrd) nerve supplied the lateral rectus muscle. Within the hypoplastic nucleus, the VIth nerve interneurons,

which connect with the contralateral medial rectus subnucleus via the medial longitudinal fasciculus to mediate conjugate gaze, were presumably spared. In a patient with Duane's type III,[389] both VIth nerves and their nuclei were absent, and the lateral recti were innervated by branches from the oculomotor nerves. Consistent with these findings, MRI studies of patients with Duane's type I have demonstrated absence of the ipsilateral VIth nerve.[391–393] In addition, orbital imaging may show a normal ipsilateral lateral rectus muscle,[394] in contrast to a denervated atrophic muscle seen in a chronic VIth nerve palsy. Families with linkage at chromosome 2q31 have been identified,[395] and mutations on this chromosome have been discovered in CHN1, a gene that encodes for α_2-chimaerin, a signaling protein which may have a role in ocular motor axon pathfinding.[396]

Duane's retraction syndrome usually occurs sporadically, but rarely cases are familial as just alluded to.[397] Occasionally Duane syndrome is also associated with systemic anomalies.[388] Wildervanck (cervico-oculo-acoustic) syndrome consists of Duane syndrome, Klippel–Feil spinal anomaly, and sensorineural deafness.[398] Duane syndrome and congenital thenar hypoplasia comprise Okihiro syndrome. Duane syndrome may also be seen together with Goldenhar syndrome, which consists of epibulbar dermoids, conjunctival lipodermoids, upper lid colobomas, inner and external ear malformations (preauricular skin tags), facial hypoplasia, and cervical spine anomalies. Unusual associations with chromosomal abnormalities,[399] thalidomide embryopathy,[400] and intracranial lesions have also been reported.[401,402] Orbital blow-out fractures with medial rectus entrapment or orbital metastases may mimic Duane syndrome.[403]

Treatment. Since most patients with Duane syndrome have no primary position misalignment and no head turn, they usually require no intervention. Strabismus surgery, the mainstay of treatment, is indicated in the minority of cases with ocular misalignment in the primary position, an abnormal head turn, cosmetically unacceptable globe retraction, or vertical deviation on adduction.[388,404,405]

Möbius syndrome. In addition to congenital facial diplegia, abducens palsy is the feature most commonly associated with Möbius syndrome, occurring in 82% of cases in the series reported by Henderson.[406] In addition, total external ophthalmoplegia was present in 25% of the cases in this series, oculomotor palsy in 21%, and bilateral ptosis in 10%. The abducens weakness is almost always bilateral, but of varying degree. When the lateral rectus palsy is severe, there is usually complete conjugate gaze paresis. Parents may not notice the facial weakness if it is subtle, and often the child is brought to medical attention solely because of an esotropia. Möbius syndrome is discussed in more detail in Chapter 14.

Miscellaneous causes of combined third, fourth, and sixth nerve palsies

The differential diagnosis of any combination of IIIrd, IVth, and VIth nerve palsies is broad and includes brainstem, subarachnoid, base of skull, cavernous sinus, and orbital processes. Often the lesion can be localized and diagnosis made based upon the history and examination, but in many instances neuroimaging is required, especially for its etiology.

Brainstem

Motor neuron diseases. Amyotrophic lateral sclerosis (Lou Gehrig disease) is a degenerative disorder of corticobulbar and spinal tracts (upper motor neurons) and lower cranial nerves in the brainstem and anterior horn cells in the spinal cord (lower motor neurons). Patients are easily recognized by their dysphagia, dysarthria, requirement for respiratory support, weakness, muscular atrophy, fasciculations, hyperreflexia, and extensor plantar responses. In most instances, clinically the eye movements are spared. However, pathologically minor changes in the ocular motor nuclei may be seen.[407] Rarely, supranuclear eye movement disorders may be observed, and in late-stage patients whose course is artificially prolonged by long-term respiratory support, some may develop complete external ophthalmoplegia (see also Chapter 16).

In other motor neuron diseases and spinal muscular atrophies, the eye movements and ocular motor nuclei are also usually spared. However, rare exceptions have been reported.[408–411]

Wernicke's encephalopathy. Wernicke disease may present with ophthalmoplegia, nystagmus, altered mental status, and ataxia. These findings result from localized hemorrhagic necrosis of the midbrain and thalamus. This diagnosis should be considered in all ocular motor palsies as administration of thiamine may rapidly reverse the ophthalmoplegia and be life-saving. There is a more detailed discussion of this entity in Chapter 16.

Leigh syndrome. Also termed subacute necrotizing encephalopathy, this neurodegenerative condition is characterized by mental status changes, ophthalmoplegia, optic atrophy, ataxia, dystonia, and respiratory failure. Typical lesions are seen in the basal ganglia, thalamus, and brainstem, and are thought to be due to mitochondrial dysfunction involving the respiratory chain, coenzyme Q, or pyruvate dehydrogenase complex.[412] Leigh syndrome is discussed in more detail in Chapter 16.

Bickerstaff's encephalitis. Bickerstaff's brainstem encephalitis is a monophasic disease process typically proceeded by an infection or immunization. The disorder is characterized by stupor, ophthalmoparesis, ataxia, and brisk reflexes, and CSF pleocytosis and anti-GQ1b antibodies (see below) may be observed. Brainstem lesions on MRI are seen only in a minority of patients.[413]

Subarachnoid disturbances

Acute bacterial and chronic fungal, tuberculous, spirochetal (syphilitic and Lyme *Borrelia*),[414] and inflammatory (e.g., sarcoid, pachymeningitis) meningitic processes may affect the ocular motor nerves within the *subarachnoid space*, and other cranial nerves may be involved. Carcinomatous[415,416] or lymphomatous[417–419] meningitis may produce a similar clinical picture, sometimes accompanied by radicular signs and symptoms indicating more widespread meningeal involvement. Lymphoma may also directly invade the endoneurium of the cranial nerves.[420,421] The ocular motor nerves can be involved in Guillain–Barré syndrome, Miller Fisher syndrome (ophthalmoparesis, ataxia, and areflexia), and chronic inflammatory demyelinating polyneuropathy,[422–424] usually in the setting of systemic weakness. These conditions are discussed in detail in Chapter 14. Cerebrospinal fluid examination with cytology is essential for diagnosing and sorting out these infectious, neoplastic, and inflammatory disorders.

Anti-GQ1b antibody syndrome. In addition to Bickerstaff's brainstem encephalitis, elevated anti-GQ$_1$b antibody titers may also be found in patients with isolated acute ophthalmoparesis,[425,426] Miller Fisher syndrome, and in patients with Gullain–Barré syndrome and ophthalmoparesis.[427] These antibodies may also be observed in some patients with chronic[428] ophthalmoparesis of unknown etiology.

The anti-GQ$_1$b antibodies strongly stain the paranodal regions of the ocular motor nerves and have been found to inhibit acetylcholine release and neurite regrowth and may be cytotoxic to neurons.[429,430] There is a consensus that Miller Fisher syndrome and Bickerstaff's brainstem encephalitis represent a spectrum of a similar disease process.[431] Both of these entities share the anti-GQ$_1$b antibodies and are self-limited disorders.

Base of skull lesions

A combination of ocular motor nerve palsies may be due to skull base metastases[432] or primary skull base tumors such as sphenoid wing or clival meningiomas, chordomas, and chondrosarcomas. Metastatic tumors in this area typically derive from lung, breast, or prostate primary neoplasms.

Sphenoid wing meningiomas. The typical clinical presentation of a sphenoid wing meningioma is ipsilateral ophthalmoplegia, proptosis, and hyperostosis of the temporal bone. Frequently the anterior and middle cranial fossae as well as the zygomatic fossa are involved. Because of their relative lateral location, optic neuropathy is usually only a feature of large lesions. Surgical removal is often recommended.[433]

Clival meningiomas. Meningiomas can develop primarily in the area of the clivus in the region of the sphenoid and occipital bones. These benign, slow-growing tumors can present with a variety of ophthalmic or neurologic symptoms depending on whether their initial involvement is of the cranial nerves entering the cavernous sinus or compression of the brainstem or cerebellum. Patients can also present with signs and symptoms of increased intracranial pressure when CSF outflow is affected. Thus, papilledema as well as cranial nerve abnormalities such as ocular motor palsies, facial palsy, and trigeminal nerve dysfunction can be seen.[434] The most common initial symptom is headache followed by visual symptoms, gait disturbances, and trouble hearing.

The diagnosis of a clival meningioma is suggested based on neuroimaging studies when patients present with the symptoms outlined above. Meningiomas need to be differentiated radiographically from chordomas and chondrosarcomas also occurring in this region. The absence of extensive bony destruction (common in chordoma and chondrosarcoma) and diffuse and smooth gadolinium enhancement (present in meningioma and more irregular in chordoma and chondrosarcoma) are the best way to differentiate these tumors. The treatment involves surgical removal, which is rarely complete and can cause cranial nerve damage.[435] Depending on the clinical situation and the presence of residual tumor, adjunctive radiation therapy can be used.[436]

Chordomas. Chordomas are rare neoplasms that arise from the embryologic notochord, the foundation upon which the axial skeleton is formed. Ultimately, during embryology the notochord begins to involute and remains only in the intervertebral cartilaginous discs as the nucleus pulposus. It is from this tissue and/or remnants or ectopic fragments of notochord remaining in the bones of the base of the skull from which chordomas arise. About 50% occur in the sacrococcygeal region and about 35% develop in the base of the skull, usually near the clivus.[437] Intracranial chordomas can become symptomatic at any age. Although the tumors grow very slowly, they are locally invasive and destroy bone and infiltrate tissue. Histopathologically, chordomas appear to have physaliphorous or bubble-like appearance to the cytoplasm.

Because they tend to originate in clivus, chordomas most commonly present with either unilateral or bilateral VIth nerve palsies.[438] Other associated findings may include ipsilateral facial weakness and trigeminal nerve dysfunction. Patients also complain of headache. Rarely they extend superiorly to affect the anterior visual pathways and cause optic neuropathy.[438] Chordomas should be considered in the differential diagnosis of any patient with chronic unilateral or bilateral VIth nerve palsy with or without remitting symptoms.[338,438] Radiographically, a cystic, lobulated mass with

evidence of bone erosion and destruction seen on CT or MRI is characteristic.[439] Biopsy can confirm the diagnosis. Some authors have recommended radical resection.[440] After tumor removal, most patients are treated with radiation therapy, but recurrences are common.[440,441]

Chondrosarcomas. Chondrosarcomas, which are also relatively rare tumors, arise from cartilage in bone. These generally are adult tumors and can occur in both the extremities and the base of the skull. When they arise in the base of the skull, they tend to produce cranial nerve palsies in the cavernous sinus area (**Fig. 15–42**). Sixth nerve palsies are common, although patients can present with IIIrd, Vth, and VIIth nerve dysfunction as well, and multiple cranial nerve palsies are not uncommon.[438] Radiographically, they must be differentiated from nasopharyngeal carcinomas, chordomas, and meningiomas. When they arise around the tuberculum sella or the paranasal sinuses, they may invade the orbit, sometimes with optic neuropathy. The tumors are composed of undifferentiated mesenchymal cells surrounded by cartilage of varying levels of maturity with foci of immature chondrocytes. The most effective treatment is widespread surgical excision followed by radiation therapy.[442] Many of these tumors can demonstrate cellular atypia and behave aggressively with recurrence and local invasion. Patients with Ollier disease (multiple skeletal enchondromas) and Maffucci syndrome (multiple enchondromas associated with subcutaneous hemangiomas) may develop skull base chondrosarcomas as a delayed consequence of these disorders. We have seen three such patients who presented with VIth nerve palsies.[443]

Cavernous sinus disturbances

Cavernous sinus involvement is suggested by any combination of unilateral IIIrd, IVth, or VIth nerve dysfunction accompanied by hypesthesia of the forehead, cornea, or cheek due to involvement of V1 or V2, or by a Horner syndrome, owing to oculosympathetic disruption. Complete interruption of all three ocular motor nerves would result in total ophthalmoplegia, ptosis, and mydriasis. Most cavernous sinus disturbances are due to mass lesions.

Symptoms of cavernous sinus disease. Patients with cavernous sinus lesions may present with double vision, pupillary abnormalities, facial sensory loss, or orbital signs and symptoms. Pain may be referred to the orbit or supraorbital region by direct involvement of the trigeminal nerve or structures innervated by this nerve.

Other signs of cavernous sinus disease. The features of a complete cavernous sinus syndrome were alluded to in the first paragraph of this section. Less prominent characteristics of incomplete lesions are:

1. *Isolated cranial nerve palsies.* Commonly, only one or two of the nerves within the cavernous sinus are involved, and chronic isolated ocular motor palsies referable to this region are not rare.
2. *Alternating anisocoria.* Simultaneous oculoparasympathetic and sympathetic disruption within the cavernous sinus may result in the unusual clinical syndrome of "alternating anisocoria." In the light, the pupil on the affected side is larger than its fellow normal

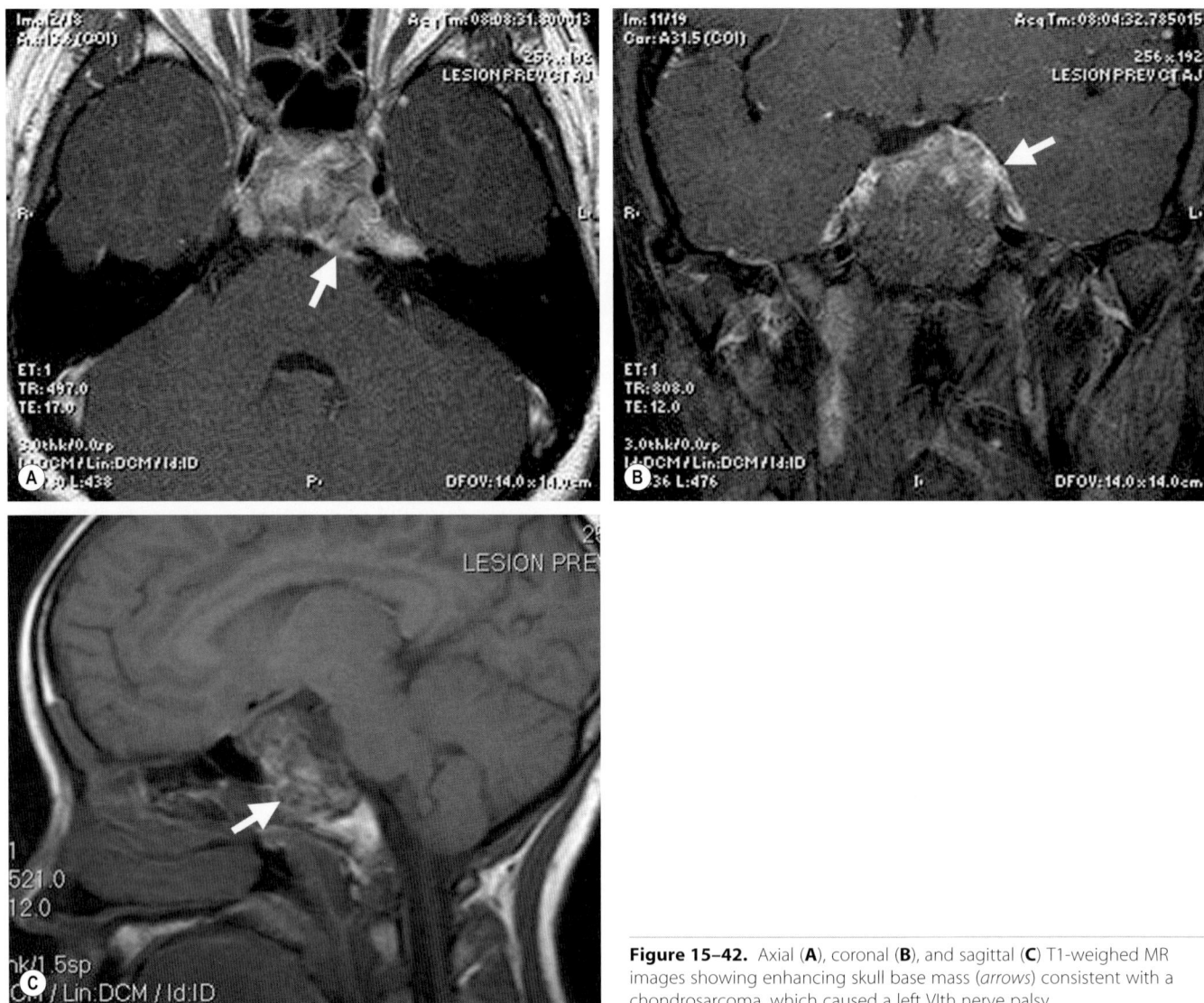

Figure 15–42. Axial (**A**), coronal (**B**), and sagittal (**C**) T1-weighed MR images showing enhancing skull base mass (*arrows*) consistent with a chondrosarcoma, which caused a left VIth nerve palsy.

eye, but in the dark the affected pupil may actually become smaller because of poor sympathetic tone.

3. *Pupillary sparing.* Third nerve palsies of cavernous sinus origin can spare pupillary function. Pupil sparing in cavernous sinus lesions may be explained by the typically slow growth of tumors in this region. One must also consider the possibility of pseudopupillary sparing, which results when the pupillary signs of IIIrd nerve dysfunction are masked by a concurrent Horner syndrome or aberrant regeneration of the IIIrd nerve.

4. *Divisional third nerve paresis.* Because the IIIrd nerve anatomically separates into superior and inferior divisions in the anterior cavernous sinus, a divisional paresis suggests a lesion in this region or anterior to it. However, this guideline has frequent exceptions, as a divisional IIIrd nerve palsy may occur anywhere posterior to this region, including the brainstem.[110]

5. *Aberrant regeneration of the third nerve.* Misdirection phenomena (see Third nerve palsies, above) may occur with cavernous sinus masses such as a meningioma (**Fig. 15–43**).[118]

6. *Ipsilateral Horner syndrome and abducens palsy.* This combination of findings results from a lesion involving both the VIth nerve and oculosympathetic fibers, where they co-mingle within the cavernous sinus.[444]

7. *Orbital signs.* Proptosis, periorbital swelling, chemosis, and conjunctival injection may occur when cavernous sinus lesions block orbital drainage and venous return.

Neuroimaging. MRI, with thin-section coronal slices through the cavernous sinus region, with and without gadolinium, is the imaging procedure of choice in this setting. When aneurysms are suspected, a CT- or MR-angiogram should also be ordered.

Differential diagnosis. Pathologic processes in this region may arise from surrounding dural walls, contiguous sites, or remote foci.[445] The differential diagnosis of cavernous sinus lesions includes neoplasms, trauma, Tolosa–Hunt syndrome, infection, septic cavernous sinus thrombosis, carotid–cavernous sinus fistulas, and intracavernous aneurysms. In one large series,[446] neoplasms were the most common cause of a cavernous sinus syndrome.

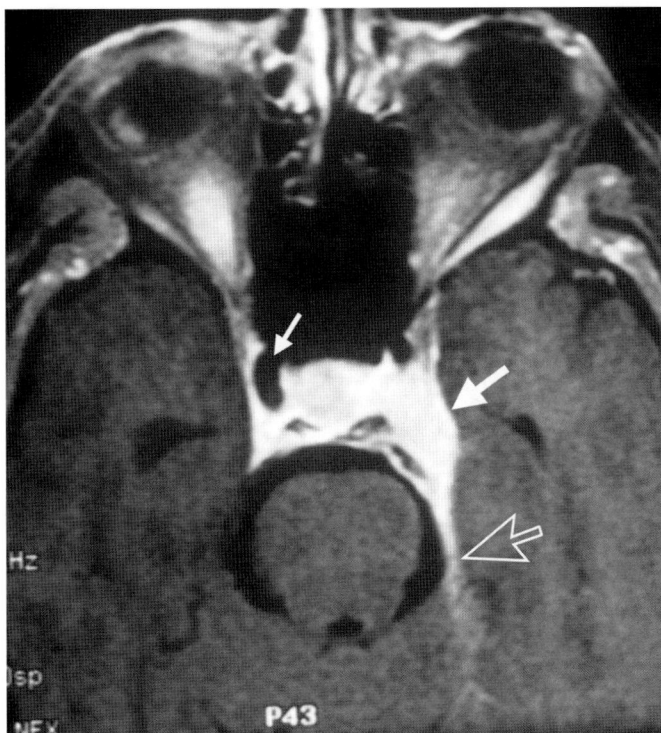

Figure 15–43. Cavernous sinus meningioma. This axial MRI scan demonstrates an enhancing mass involving the left cavernous sinus (*large solid arrow*) with a characteristic dural tail (*large open arrow*). The normal flow void of the intracavernous carotid artery on the right (*small arrow*) cannot be seen on the left. The patient presented with mild left proptosis and a partial left IIIrd nerve palsy. Two years later she developed aberrant regeneration of the eyelid.

Some cavernous sinus disturbances can be attributed to its anatomic features. Sellar masses (see Chapter 7), if large enough, may compress cavernous sinus structures, and the clinical scenario of acute headache, visual loss, and ophthalmoplegia should suggest pituitary apoplexy. The nerves within the cavernous sinus rarely give rise to primary tumors such as a neuroma of the Vth nerve. The trigeminal nerve may also serve as a conduit to the cavernous sinus for basal cell and squamous cell tumors arising from the face, head, and neck.[447] In a similar fashion, valveless veins of the face may spread infection from the skin to this region and ultimately lead to thrombosis of the cavernous sinus. The sphenoid sinus and nasopharynx lie inferiorly and medially to each cavernous sinus so that tumors and infections of these regions readily gain access to the cavernous sinus. The remainder of this section will discuss some of the common entities in this region.

Neoplasms. A variety of neoplasms may involve the cavernous sinus including meningiomas, neuromas, chordomas, chondrosarcomas, nasopharyngeal carcinomas, lymphoma, plasmacytoma, pituitary adenoma, and metastatic disease. A complete discussion of these tumors is beyond the scope of this chapter, but some of the more important and common tumors will be reviewed. Some were discussed above.

Nasopharyngeal tumors. Nasopharyngeal tumors may present as serous otitis media, nasal obstruction, atypical facial pain, recurrent epistaxis, or as a chronic isolated VIth nerve palsy.[448] The tumors either erode the skull base or enter the cavernous sinus through the foramen ovale or lacerum.[449] Approximately 20% of nasopharyngeal tumors may present as a cavernous sinus syndrome. Fifth nerve dysfunction followed closely by impairment of the ocular motor nerves are the major ophthalmic findings.

Pituitary tumors. Although there is frequent radiographic involvement of the cavernous sinus in pituitary adenomas, only rarely is there resultant chronic ocular motor dysfunction.[450,451] Importantly, the rapid onset of bilateral complete ophthalmoplegia and headache should suggest the possibility of pituitary apoplexy and neuroimaging studies should be obtained emergently. The clinical presentation of pituitary apoplexy may be confused with subarachnoid hemorrhage and bacterial meningitis. The administration of corticosteroids in this situation may be life-saving in order to prevent an Addisonian crisis. Pituitary adenomas and apoplexy are discussed in more detail in Chapter 7.

Tumors involving the trigeminal nerve. Trigeminal neuromas and schwannomas typically begin in the region of the gasserian ganglion and manifest clinically with complaints of altered facial sensation or facial pain.[452] Rarely, these tumors may present as a chronic isolated VIth nerve palsy without signs of Vth nerve dysfunction.[453]

Occasionally, tumors of the skin such as basal cell carcinoma and squamous cell carcinoma travel perineurally along branches of the Vth nerve to gain access to the cavernous sinus and orbital apex, causing ophthalmoplegia.[447,454] Facial nerve palsies are also frequent.[455] Remote tumor spread may present clinically years after the original skin lesion was removed.[456] Palliative radiation may be used, but the prognosis is poor.[457]

Cavernous sinus meningiomas. Meningiomas arising from the dural walls of the cavernous sinus represent one of the most frequent tumors of this area (**Fig. 15–43**). Cavernous sinus meningiomas typically present with painless, slowly progressive ocular motor palsies or a IIIrd nerve palsy with aberrant regeneration. Rarely, spontaneously resolving ocular motor palsies may occur.[458] Their MRI appearance is characteristic, as they are typically isointense with brain but enhance with gadolinium. A dural tail is often present. They may also encase the cavernous carotid, often leading to vascular narrowing.[459] Since these tumors may grow slowly, surgery or radiotherapy is usually not indicated until vital structures such as the brainstem or visual pathways are compromised. Many patients with stable diplopia that can be treated with prisms may be followed clinically and radiographically.[460] Alternatively, some authors have recommended total[461,462] or subtotal[459,463,464] resection, but the morbidity, including internal carotid or middle cerebral artery infarction, ocular motor palsies, and trigeminal nerve dysfunction associated with neurosurgery of these tumors can be high. Perioperative deaths can also occur.[461,465] Partial resection may be followed by adjunctive radiotherapy.[466–468]

Lymphoma. Lymphomatous involvement of the cavernous sinus may cause painful or painless ophthalmoplegia.[469,470]

Metastases. Breast, lung, and prostate cancer are well-recognized primary neoplasms which can metastasize to the cavernous sinus.[471] The ophthalmoplegia is frequently rapidly progressive.

Inflammatory disorders. Idiopathic granulomatous inflammation of the superior orbital fissure or cavernous sinus is known as the Tolosa–Hunt syndrome. Steroid-responsive painful ophthalmoplegia is the hallmark of this condition. The IIIrd nerve is the most commonly affected cranial nerve followed by the VIth, Vth, and IVth nerves.[472] Proptosis and optic nerve dysfunction is seen in approximately 20–30% of cases.[472] Based on limited anatomic studies, idiopathic orbital inflammatory syndrome and the Tolosa–Hunt syndrome appear to represent a similar pathologic process.

Since there are many causes of painful ophthalmoplegia, diagnosis of this syndrome should be one of exclusion. MRI in Tolosa–Hunt syndrome typically demonstrates enlargement and enhancement of the cavernous sinus, sometimes with extension into the orbital apex.[473] Imaging is also helpful in delineating other parasellar disease processes such as neoplasms and infections although oftentimes the distinction is difficult to make.[474] A rapid response to corticosteroids is characteristic but recurrence is not uncommon as steroids are tapered. Corticosteroids may have to be tapered over months, but steroid dependence should raise the suspicion of an alternative diagnosis such as lymphoma and a biopsy should be considered. Systemic lupus erythematosus should also be excluded with serologic testing.[475,476] Furthermore, a human immunodeficiency virus-positive patient with painful ophthalmoplegia was found to have an eosinophilic granuloma in the superior orbital fissure region.[477]

Herpes zoster ophthalmicus may also be associated with complete ophthalmoplegia or isolated ocular motor palsy resulting from a secondary vasculitis or direct inflammatory infiltration of the nerves and extraocular muscles. Although antiviral agents may be given to affected patients, most have resolution of the ocular motor palsy within 1 year.[478]

Cavernous sinus thrombosis. Prompt recognition of septic thrombosis of the cavernous sinus, a potentially life-threatening disorder, is essential. Patients present with fever, periorbital pain, swelling, and proptosis.[479] The abducens nerve is frequently affected first, but complete ophthalmoplegia may rapidly ensue.[479] Vision may be impaired as a result of arterial occlusion or emboli, venous congestion, increased intraocular pressure, or corneal exposure.[480,481] Staphylococcal and streptococcal organisms are the most frequent pathogens.[479] These organisms may gain entry through several routes, but most often invade the cavernous sinus by traversing the valveless veins of the face, teeth, middle ear, and neck. Direct spread of infection from the maxillary and sphenoid sinuses are alternative routes in patients with sinusitis.[479] Within several days of onset, the infection may reach the contralateral cavernous sinus and further dispersal may lead to meningitis or cerebral infarction by compromising the cavernous carotid artery. Uncommonly, extension to other venous sinuses, such as the lateral, sigmoid, and inferior sagittal sinuses, may occur.[482]

Most patients will have an elevated white blood count and positive blood cultures. Thirty-five percent of patients have changes in their cerebrospinal fluid consistent with bacterial meningitis (i.e., neutrophilic pleocytosis, elevated protein, and low glucose).[479] MRI is the preferred study to demonstrate thrombosis of the cavernous sinus (**Fig. 15–44**).[483]

After cultures have been collected, intravenous antibiotics should be administered at once. Antibiotic coverage is dependent upon the source of the infection but therapy against penicillinase-resistant *Staphylococcus* and anaerobes is essential.[479] Anticoagulation of patients with septic cavernous sinus thrombosis remains controversial,[484] but is still often recommended.[485,486] Surgery, if necessary, is reserved for drainage of the primary focus of infection.

Fungal infections. Mucormycosis and rarely aspergillosis may rapidly spread from the sinuses to the cavernous sinus and orbit,[487] and immunocompromised individuals such as those with diabetes or the elderly are susceptible. Mucormycosis, which requires a rich source of iron to grow effectively, may occur in patients taking iron-chelating agents. These organisms have a propensity to invade blood vessels.[488] Visual loss from central retinal or ophthalmic artery occlusion is not uncommon. Spread of infection to the cavernous

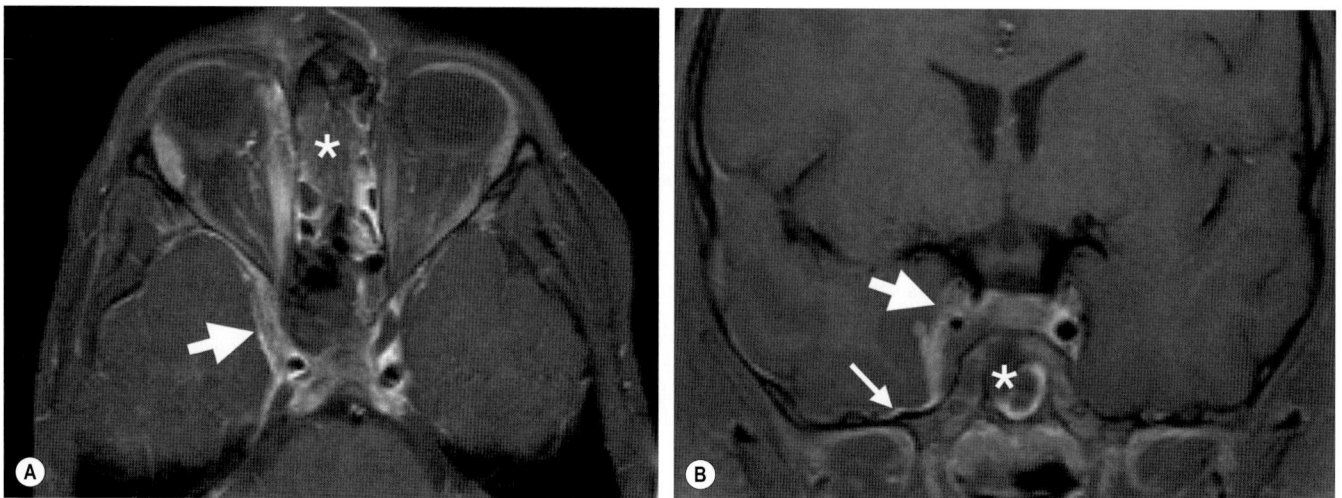

Figure 15–44. T1-weighted MR images (**A**, axial, **B**, coronal) show widening and enhancement of the right cavernous sinus (*thick arrows*) and dural enhancement (*thin arrow*), consistent with cavernous sinus thrombosis related to ethmoid sinusitis (*asterisk*).

carotid is heralded by the acute onset of a contralateral hemiparesis. Magnetic resonance studies are most useful in delineating the extent of the pathologic process. The diagnosis may be established by biopsy and drainage of infected areas. Treatment usually consists of intravenous amphotericin and surgical debridement. The amount of debridement is often dependent on the degree of visual loss and the extent of the infectious process.[488] Those patients with preserved visual acuity and disease limited to the orbital structures and sinuses may be spared an exenteration without altering outcome.[489]

High-flow (direct) carotid–cavernous fistulas. Carotid–cavernous fistulas (CCFs) are communications between the intracavernous carotid artery and the surrounding cavernous sinus. Several different classification schemes have been proposed and generally divide these CCFs based on their etiology, rate of flow, and source of feeder vessels.

The most important of these is the high-flow, direct CCF. In the majority of cases (80%) direct CCFs result from trauma and much less commonly arise spontaneously.[179,490] The neuro-ophthalmic presentation of these direct CCFs is generally dramatic and results from the reversal of blood flow in the orbital and ocular venous drainage. Usually there is an endothelized, single tear in the carotid wall.[491] These *direct*, high-flow fistulas are termed type A.[492]

Types B, C, and D fistulas are all low-flow, *indirect* communications between branches of the internal or external carotid artery within the dura of the cavernous sinus. These have also been grouped as dural CCFs or dural arteriovenous malformations (DAVMs). They generally arise spontaneously and have a lower flow and more insidious presentation than the direct CCFs. Type B fistulas are supplied by small branches of the cavernous carotid artery, type C by dural branches of the external carotid, and type D by a combination of external and internal carotid artery branches. The diagnosis of CCFs (and DAVMs) is suggested by the typical constellation of symptoms and signs (**Table 15–9**). Neuroradiologic confirmation of the diagnosis is based on orbital ultrasound, MRI, MR-angiography, and conventional angiographic findings. Treatment generally involves embolization.

This section will detail the diagnosis and management of high-flow CCFs, while a review of low-flow CCFs follows in the next section.

Traumatic direct CCFs. The majority of direct CCFs result from head trauma, which is usually severe following motor vehicle accidents, sports injuries, and falls.[179,490,493] Traumatic CCFs can present at the time of the injury or may be delayed in onset for days or weeks. Penetrating injuries such as stab wounds that enter the cavernous sinus through the superior orbital fissure can result in CCFs.[493] "Traumatic" CCFs can also result from iatrogenic injury to the carotid artery. This has been seen in the setting of carotid endarterectomy surgery, endovascular procedures, and as a complication of transsphenoidal pituitary surgery, otolaryngologic surgery, and in procedures directed at the gasserian ganglion for the treatment of trigeminal neuralgia.[494–496]

Spontaneous direct CCFs. Spontaneous, high-flow, direct CCFs arise in two different settings: (1) rupture of a preexisting cavernous sinus aneurysm (see below) or (2) a defective

Table 15–9 Ocular signs and symptoms in carotid–cavernous fistulas and dural arteriovenous malformations of the cavernous sinus. (Reproduced with permission from Bennett J, Volpe NJ, Liu GT, Galetta SL. Neurovascular neuro-ophthalmology. In: Jakobiec FA, Albert D (eds.): Principles of Ophthalmology, pp 4238–74. Philadelphia, W.B. Saunders, 1999.)

Symptoms
  Headache/orbital pain
  Proptosis
  Red eye
  Blurred vision
  Double vision
  Bruit

Signs
  Proptosis
  Orbital congestions
  Conjunctival chemosis
  Arterialization of episcleral vessels
  Increased intraocular pressure
  Venous stasis retinopathy
  Ophthalmoplegia
  Bruit
  Visual loss

vessel wall that may complicate a connective tissue disorder such as fibromuscular dysplasia,[497] Ehlers–Danlos syndrome,[498] and pseudoxanthoma elasticum.[499] However, in many instances an underlying cause cannot be found.[500]

Clinical presentation. Clinical findings in patients with high-flow direct CCFs result from arterialization of draining orbital veins by anterior blood flow from the cavernous carotid artery (**Table 15–9**). Usually this involves the eye and orbit ipsilateral to the fistula. However, the presentation can vary significantly and can include a silent orbital presentation particularly when the CCF drains posteriorly. Bilateral orbital signs can also develop depending upon the patency of the venous connections between the two cavernous sinuses.

Symptoms. Symptom onset is usually abrupt and may be rapidly progressive. Occasionally, the symptoms and signs that resulted from the traumatic injury (proptosis or cranial nerve palsy) may obscure those from the CCF. The most common complaints offered by patients with CCF include subjective bruit (80%), visual blur (59%), headache (53%), diplopia (53%), and ocular or orbital pain (35%).[179,493] Patients may describe a whooshing or swishing that is synchronous with the pulse. Headache may result from distension of the dura or trigeminal nerve compression. They or others may notice proptosis or a red eye.

Signs. The clinical signs correlate with the symptoms and include pulsatile exophthalmos, arterialization of conjunctival vessels, eyelid swelling, conjunctival chemosis, elevated (often pulsatile) intraocular pressure, restrictive ocular motility disturbances and cranial neuropathies, optic disc swelling, and venous stasis retinopathy. The bruit that is audible to the patient is usually also audible to the examiner, although not always. The best method for listening is with the bell of the stethoscope over the closed eyelid. In posterior draining fistulas the bruit may be detected over the area of the mastoid. The bruit is classically described as disappearing with ipsilateral carotid compression although this is neither a commonly performed nor recommended diagnostic maneuver.

Proptosis results from congestion of orbital tissues and displacement of the globe by the dilated superior ophthalmic vein. Ocular pulsation may be visible as well as palpable and results from transmission of the arterial pulse to the dilated ophthalmic veins and globe. The absence of globe pulsation may reflect thrombosis of the ophthalmic veins. Abnormalities in the ocular pulse may be suggested by wide to and fro movements of the Myers rings during applanation tonometry.

Arterialization of conjunctival and episcleral vessels results from blood forced into the orbital veins and subsequently into the conjunctival veins. The arterialization pattern may be diffuse or can be localized to one or two vessels. The vessels have a corkscrew appearance and this tortuosity and dilation extends all the way to the limbus (**Fig. 15–45**). These vessels can occasionally bleed profusely. Massive proptosis can lead to impaired corneal coverage and exposure. Exposure of the cornea (and conjunctiva) may lead to infectious ulceration if adequate lubrication is not used. This may be aggravated by corneal hypesthesia, which can occur secondary to trigeminal nerve dysfunction.

Increased intraocular pressure and glaucoma result from arterialization of episcleral vessels with elevation of episcleral venous pressure and blood forced into Schlemm's canal. This blood can be seen on gonioscopy. Ultimately intraocular pressure rises with this increase in episcleral venous pressure. Optic nerve damage ensues and glaucomatous optic neuropathy can occur in 20% of patients with untreated CCFs.[179] Rarely intraocular pressure rise is precipitous and may result in central retinal artery occlusion.[179] Other mechanisms responsible for the development of glaucoma include elevation of orbital pressure secondary to venous stasis and edema, anterior segment neovascularization and secondary rubeotic glaucoma,[501] and secondary angle closure from congestion of the choroid and a forward shift of the lens iris diaphragm.

Double vision from ocular misalignment occurs frequently. Isolated abduction deficits are quite common and presumably result from VIth nerve dysfunction in the majority of patients (50–85% of all patients with CCFs).[496] The VIth nerve is the most vulnerable because it floats freely adjacent to the lateral aspect of the carotid artery, while the IIIrd and IVth nerves are enveloped by dura in the lateral wall of the sinus. However, ocular motor dysfunction from the initial head trauma may be difficult to distinguish from the deficit acquired with the CCF. The oculomotor palsies may result from compression by the fistula or from ischemia due to altered blood flow in the vasa nervorum. These cranial nerve palsies can develop at any time after the fistula forms. Many patients describe pain in the first or even second division of the trigeminal nerve, resulting from compression of the ophthalmic or maxillary divisions of the Vth nerve in the cavernous sinus.

Other patients develop double vision as a result of restrictive myopathy secondary to orbital congestion. The eye muscles are enlarged and double vision is coincident with the development of proptosis. In many patients a combination of neurogenic and myopathic eye movement dysfunction occurs. Forced duction testing with forceps should not be used because of the risk of bleeding from arterialized conjunctival and episcleral vessels.

Vision loss can result from a variety of trauma- or fistula-related causes (**Table 15–10**). In Kupersmith's series[179] of 95 cases of traumatic CCFs the most common causes of vision

Table 15–10 Etiologies of visual loss due to carotid–cavernous fistulas (CCFs)

Venous stasis retinopathy
Ischemic optic neuropathy
Glaucoma
Choroidal effusions
Corneal ulcerations and perforation
Retinal vascular occlusion
Retrobulbar optic neuropathy (compressive vs. vascular steal)
Retrobulbar ischemia

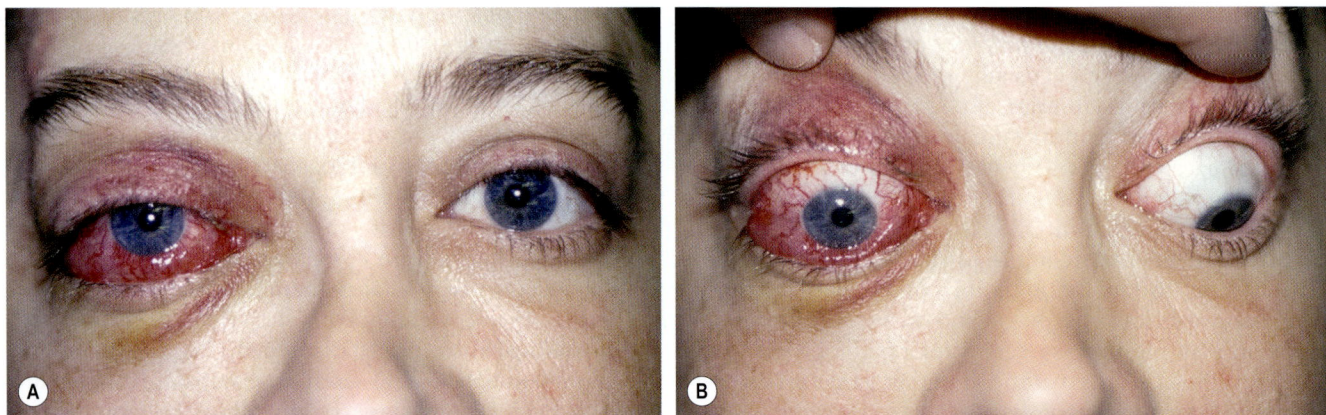

Figure 15–45. External appearance of a woman with a traumatic, high-flow, direct carotid–cavernous fistulas on the right. **A.** Proptosis, chemosis, arterialization of scleral and eyelid vessels, and periorbital swelling are seen. **B.** She had almost complete ophthalmoplegia of the right eye, including defective infraduction. Corkscrew scleral vessels are seen.

loss included traumatic optic neuropathy (five patients), postsurgical optic neuropathy (two patients), venous hypoxic retinopathy (three patients), globe injury (three patients), corneal ulceration and perforation (one patient), and central retinal artery occlusion secondary to elevated intraocular pressure (one patient). In four patients he also recognized a reversible retrobulbar optic neuropathy which was believed to result from either compression by the superior ophthalmic vein or a vascular steal phenomenon. Other causes of vision loss include anterior ischemic optic neuropathy, compressive optic neuropathy from an extended cavernous sinus, and retrobulbar ischemia.[501,502] Ophthalmoscopically, most patients show nonspecific findings of venous stasis retinopathy with distended retinal veins and intraretinal hemorrhages. Many patients have mild disc swelling as well. Choroidal detachment as an initial manifestation of direct CCF has also been noted.[503]

Diagnostic evaluation. A high-flow, direct CCF is usually suggested on clinical grounds in patients with or without a recent history of trauma that suddenly develop a bruit, proptosis, and a red eye. The clinical suspicion can be confirmed by diagnostic testing, which can include pneumotonometry, orbital ultrasound, color Doppler ultrasound, and neuroimaging with MRI, MR-angiography, and conventional angiography. Pneumotonometry may be used to document wide pulse pressures.[504] Orbital ultrasound can be used to document enlarged superior ophthalmic veins and extraocular muscles. A-scan ultrasound can also demonstrate rapid echo spikes within the superior ophthalmic vein when done in real time.[505] Color Doppler ultrasound can document reversal of flow in the superior ophthalmic vein with high flow. CT and MRI can similarly document enlargement of the orbital veins, eye muscles, and cavernous sinus.

Formal cerebral angiography is usually required to document the extent and location of feeding vessels. Selected injections of both internal and external carotid arteries are necessary.[179,493,506] Angiography will also help to define the other characteristics of the CCF including the presence of pseudoaneurysms, venous drainage pattern, and whether cavernous sinus thrombosis is present.[179,507]

Course and treatment. Nearly all high-flow direct CCFs require treatment. This is in contrast to the low-flow dural fistulas (types B–D, DAVMs), which can often be followed and may close spontaneously (see below). In direct CCFs which are left untreated, there is significant risk for serious vision loss secondary to corneal exposure, glaucoma, and venous stasis. Double vision may also linger as a chronic problem in untreated patients. Prior to definitive therapy of the CCF, its secondary manifestations such as glaucoma and exposure should be treated.

Approximately 20% of CCFs require emergency endovascular treatment because of vision compromise, rapid elevation of intraocular pressure, or bleeding (epistaxis or intracranial bleeding).[179] Surgical therapy of CCFs, such as ligating the common or internal carotid arteries, has been replaced by transvenous or transarterial endovascular obliteration. Transarterial occlusion with platinum coils or liquid embolic material such as cyanoacrylate is the treatment of choice.[508] The technique entails introducing a flow-directed catheter through the femoral artery then floating it into the venous side of the CCF. Detachable balloons are no longer used in the USA, but are still used elsewhere. Endovascular treatment preserves carotid artery patency and is successful in 59–88% of patients.[179,493,509,510] The remainder of the patients in these series were for the most part treated successfully with carotid occlusion.

Transvenous embolization can be performed through the femoral vein or through the orbit or venous sinuses. The latter approach is generally reserved for cases in which the transarterial approach failed or is not possible because of carotid anatomy or occlusion from the previous trauma.[511,512]

Complications of treatment. Complications include pseudoaneurysm formation from cavernous sinus filling and ocular motor palsies. Stroke from errant embolic material is rare.

Prognosis. With successful closure of a direct CCF, prognosis for virtually full recovery is excellent. The closure of the shunt is associated with immediate resolution of the bruit. Intraocular pressure elevation generally resolves within 2 days. Recurrence of the bruit or persistent elevated intraocular pressure strongly suggest that the fistula has recurred or was inadequately treated. Visual field defects that resulted from persistent elevated intraocular pressure tend not to improve. Orbital congestion and ophthalmoparesis generally take 1–4 weeks to resolve.[179,513]

Low-flow carotid–cavernous fistulas (dural arteriovenous malformations). DAVMs are abnormal communications between the arteries that supply the dura mater and the intracranial venous sinuses (**Fig. 15–46**). Although most DAVMs are acquired arteriovenous shunts, some may represent congenital lesions. They most likely develop from pre-existing microscopic communications between arteries and veins in the dura in the area near the venous sinuses. A second insult such as trauma or thrombosis then leads to conversion to a DAVM.

In Kupersmith's series,[179] 68% of the patients seen with shunts in the area of the cavernous sinus had low-flow DAVMs. There is considerable overlap in the symptomatology of DAVMs in the cavernous sinus region and direct CCFs since they both result in arterialization of the orbital venous drainage system (**Table 15–9**). The two arteries most commonly associated with DAVMs in the cavernous sinus region are meningeal branches of the cavernous carotid artery: the meningohypophyseal trunk and the artery of the inferior cavernous sinus.[492] The dorsal meningeal artery arises from the meningohypophyseal trunk and supplies the dura in the region of the clivus and is the most commonly involved artery in the formation of DAVMs. In this region, branches off the dorsal meningeal artery may anastomose with the external carotid artery. The meningeal branches of the external carotid artery in this region include the internal maxillary, ascending pharyngeal, and occipital arteries. The middle meningeal artery arises from the internal maxillary artery and supplies the dura in the region of the foramen ovale and foramen spinosum. In this area, there may be anastomoses with branches from the artery of the inferior cavernous sinus.

Clinical presentation. DAVMs in the region of the cavernous sinus are most often seen in woman over age 50 or in association with pregnancy, systemic hypertension,

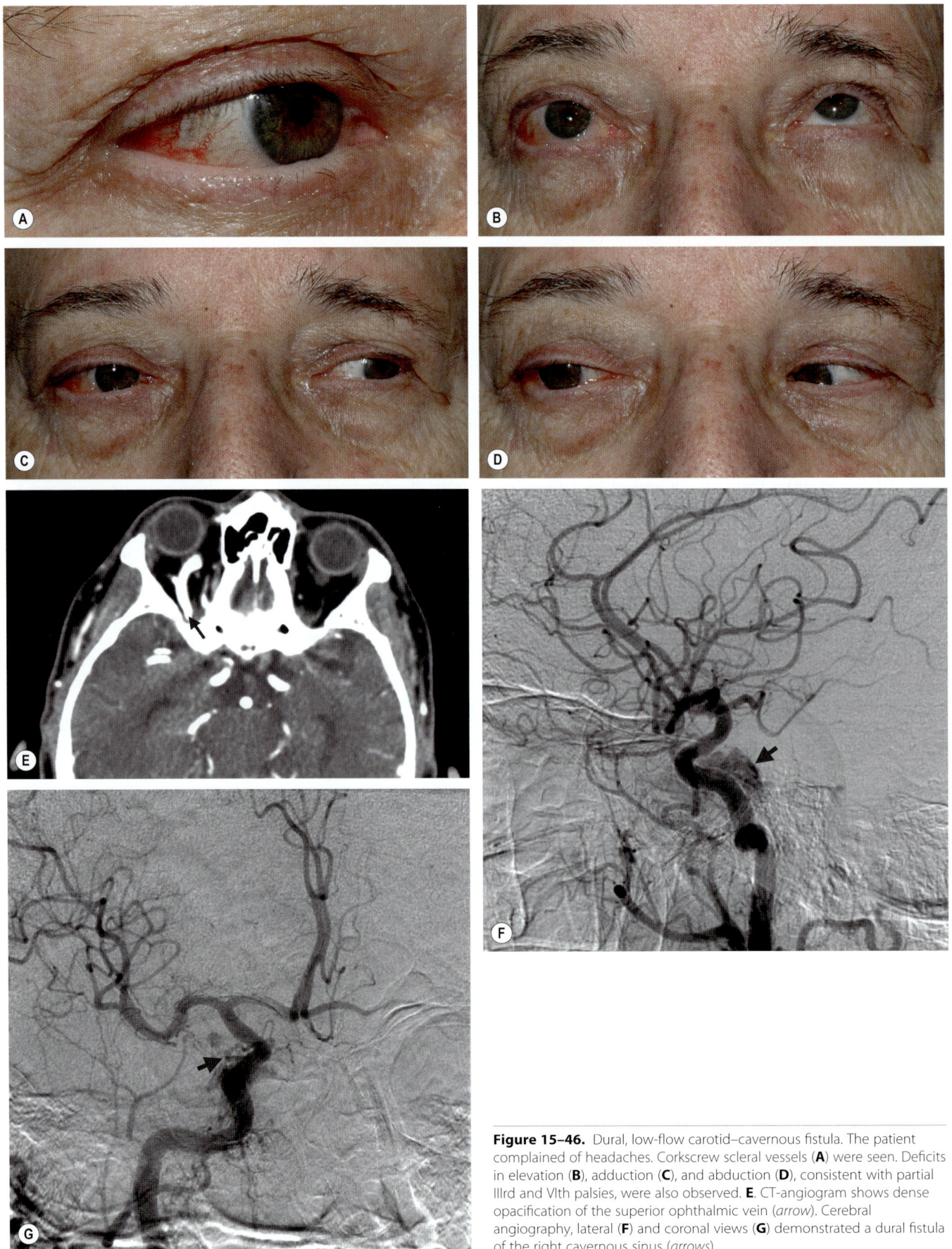

Figure 15–46. Dural, low-flow carotid–cavernous fistula. The patient complained of headaches. Corkscrew scleral vessels (**A**) were seen. Deficits in elevation (**B**), adduction (**C**), and abduction (**D**), consistent with partial IIIrd and VIth palsies, were also observed. **E**. CT-angiogram shows dense opacification of the superior ophthalmic vein (*arrow*). Cerebral angiography, lateral (**F**) and coronal views (**G**) demonstrated a dural fistula of the right cavernous sinus (*arrows*).

Ehlers–Danlos syndrome, and minor trauma. As with direct CCFs, DAVMs in the region of the cavernous sinus produce symptoms based on the rate of flow and pattern of venous drainage. Patients with posterior drainage into the petrosal sinus or basilar venous plexus would not be expected to have orbital symptoms. In fact, DAVMs draining posteriorly into the inferior petrosal sinus may cause no externally visible abnormalities (so-called "white-eyed shunt"). However, patients with posteriorly draining DAVMs in this region have also been reported to present with cranial nerve palsies including IIIrd, IVth, Vth, VIth, and VIIth nerve palsies.[514–519]

Ocular and orbital symptoms in patients with anteriorly draining DAVMs include proptosis, arterialization of conjunctival vessels, elevated intraocular pressure, oculomotor palsies, ptosis, bruit, venous stasis retinopathy, visual field defect, pain, chemosis and lid swelling (**Table 15–9**).[520] Because the onset of all of these symptoms is not explosive, there is often a delay in diagnosis with patients often treated for "nonspecific" red eye with antibiotics or steroids. Bruits are less commonly reported by patients and auscultated by examiners in patients with DAVMs as opposed to direct CCFs. Pain is infrequent and usually mild. The arterialized loops of episcleral and conjunctival vessels have a characteristic appearance called "limbal loops" in which vessels have an acute angulation near the limbus.[521] Like CCFs, patients often develop intraocular pressure elevation and glaucomatous visual field defects as a result of episcleral venous pressure elevation.[522–525] Glaucoma is treated the same way as it is in the case of direct CCFs, temporarily with topical and oral medications and definitively with closure of the DAVM and correction of the abnormal venous congestion.[525]

Proptosis, chemosis, and lid swelling are manifestations of elevated orbital venous pressure. These findings are more mild than with direct CCFs and generally do not lead to sight-threatening complications such as exposure keratitis with ulceration. Common misdiagnoses in the setting of DAVM-induced orbital congestion include conjunctivitis, acute orbital inflammatory syndrome, and thyroid orbitopathy (see Chapter 18). Orbital congestion can paradoxically worsen (sometimes with treatment), as a result of thrombosis of the orbital veins with increased orbital venous stasis.[526] This worsening may be followed by improvement if the thrombosis propagates into the DAVM and closes the shunt. Treatment with corticosteroids during this transient worsening can help to reduce severe orbital congestion.

Posterior segment complications include venous stasis retinopathy, vitreous hemorrhage, proliferative retinopathy, disc swelling, ischemic optic neuropathy, and exudative retinal detachments.[179,526–530] Venous stasis retinopathy occurs in about 15% of patients and results most commonly in cases with ophthalmic vein thrombosis rather than from arterialization of the orbital vessels.[531] Vision loss occurs in about 20–30% of patients and is usually a sequela of venous stasis retinopathy, ischemic optic neuropathy, or uncontrolled glaucoma (**Table 15–10**).[500,532] Choroidal effusions may occur as well but are often small and peripheral. They can be recognized by ophthalmoscopy and by ultrasound. Larger choroidal effusions can be associated with rotation of

the ciliary body and movement of the lens iris diaphragm, resulting in angle closure glaucoma or anterior displacement of a posterior chamber lens.[179,500,525,532–534]

Eye movement abnormalities result from either congestion and hypoxia of the eye muscles or cranial nerve palsies. The VIth nerve is the most commonly affected, but IIIrd[515] and IVth nerve palsies[535] have been reported. After closure of the shunt, the prognosis for recovery of the eye movement abnormalities is good whether they are the result of myopathic or neuropathic processes. Patients rarely can develop cerebral dysfunction including seizures, infarct, or hemorrhages as a result of abnormal pial drainage into the cerebral hemispheres. This is more common when there is significant cavernous sinus thrombosis resulting from bilateral fistulas.[179]

Diagnostic evaluation. The diagnostic modalities utilized in this setting are similar to those used in direct CCFs. If symptoms are mild, the diagnosis may be established by clinical findings, ultrasonography, and neuroimaging. MRI scanning can show thrombosis of the cavernous sinus and superior ophthalmic vein. This thrombosis usually appears as a white hyperintensity on T1-weighted images.[179] MRI scan can also demonstrate signal decrease in the cavernous sinus on spin echo imaging due to rapid blood flow.[536] If treatment is planned then angiography should be performed as it may be therapeutic and feeder vessels must be identified. Angiography must be performed on both the internal and external carotid arteries bilaterally.

Treatment. The morbidity of these DAVMs is primarily ocular, as hemorrhage and life-threatening complications are quite rare. Some of these lesions will close either spontaneously, after air travel, or after angiography or manual compression of the carotid artery.[179,500,510,522,537,538] These conservative measures can be used in asymptomatic patients. However, treatment by embolization with liquid agents or coils is recommended for patients who have ophthalmic symptoms.[539] Ideally this is accomplished transvenously through the inferior petrosal sinus, pterygoid venous plexus, superior petrosal sinus, facial vein, or the superior ophthalmic vein.[508,540] Alternatively, particularly after transvenous attempts have failed, a trans-internal carotid procedure is necessary.[541] Rarely, direct surgery on the cavernous sinus with DAVM removal can be performed. Others have used radiation to treat extensive lesions not amenable to embolization or surgery.[500,542,543] Complications of treatment are uncommon and include incomplete closure, venous thrombosis, cranial nerve palsies from nutrient vessel thrombosis, and cerebral infarctions. Ocular symptoms generally begin to improve within days of treatment and are usually completely resolved within 6 months. Pneumotonometry can be used prior to and after embolization to follow patients and be certain closure is complete without recanalization.

Intracavernous aneurysm. Aneurysms of the cavernous–carotid artery predominately present with orbital pain and diplopia due to ocular motor palsies. Cavernous–carotid aneurysms are uncommon, accounting for only 2% of all intracranial aneurysms.[544] Among symptomatic, unruptured aneurysms, the proportion of cavernous–carotid lesions increases to 15%.[544] Cavernous–carotid aneurysms are rarely life-threatening because their rupture is contained by rigid

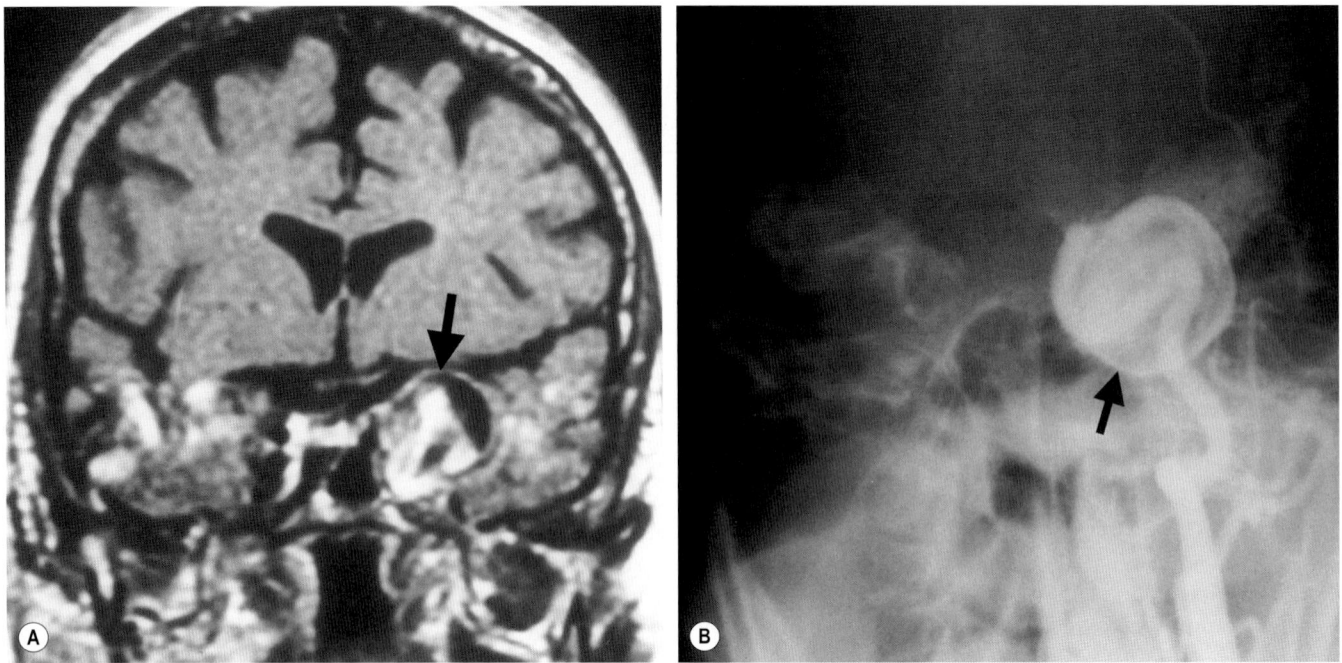

Figure 15–47. Cavernous carotid aneurysm. **A**. Coronal MRI demonstrates flow void (*arrow*) within left cavernous sinus. **B**. Angiography (coronal view) confirming large round aneurysm (*arrow*).

dural walls. Furthermore, owing to their extradural location, cavernous–carotid aneurysms rarely result in SAH, as aneurysmal rupture instead produces a cavernous–carotid fistula (see above).

Symptoms and signs. The frequency of involvement of the various cranial nerves with aneurysms in the cavernous sinus is dependent on their anatomic relationship to the carotid siphon. Cavernous aneurysms frequently involve the abducens nerve early due to its position lateral to the carotid artery within the cavernous sinus.[545] Oculomotor and ophthalmic (V1) involvement may also occur, but isolated IVth nerve palsies are rare.[179] Unlike posterior communicating aneurysms in which the pupil is usually dilated, a cavernous–carotid aneurysm may be associated with a pupil-sparing IIIrd nerve palsy. Pain in the distribution of V1 is the most common manifestation of early trigeminal nerve involvement,[546] as complete anesthesia arises only after chronic compression. Neurotrophic keratopathy is a significant complication of V1 compression, and patients complaining of visual blurring should receive a complete anterior segment examination. Additional causes of visual blurring include paralysis of accommodation from IIIrd nerve involvement and visual pathway impingement.

Visual loss secondary to anterior pathway compression is generally a late consequence of large aneurysmal expansion. The pattern of vision loss is dependent on the structure compressed. Anteromedial expansion results in optic nerve compression, while posteromedial expansion results in impingement on the optic chiasm. Proptosis, another late sequela of a cavernous aneurysm, occurs only after the enlarging mass has compromised venous drainage or compressed the globe by eroding through the posterior orbital wall.

Diagnostic imaging. The lesion is usually detected using MRI (**Fig. 15–47**). MR- or CT-angiography can be used to assess aneurysmal anatomy, luminal patency, and thrombus age. Cerebral angiography should be performed prior to treatment planning.

Treatment. Cavernous aneurysms in most patients, especially elderly ones, are not treated because of their relatively benign nature. However, treatment can be considered when ocular motor palsies or vision loss are progressive and debilitating or the orbital pain is intractable. With conservative therapy alone, 25–40% of patients will stabilize or improve.[179,547] Treatment options include ipsilateral carotid occlusion, surgical clipping, or endovascular embolization. Owing to the high morbidity and mortality of a surgical approach, treatment generally entails either carotid occlusion or endovascular therapy. A functional tolerance test can be performed prior to occlusion to test whether the patient can withstand permanent occlusion.[548] If neurologic symptoms result during a functional occlusion test, an extracranial–intracranial bypass may be indicated prior to definitive treatment.

Reconstructive endovascular procedures of cavernous aneurysms are often difficult.[549] Recently, excellent results were reported in a series of patients with cavernous lesions treated with electrolytically detachable coils.[550] Since cavernous aneurysms often lack a definitive neck, successful endovascular therapy often requires deconstructive embolization of the parent carotid artery.[551]

Prognosis. Following embolization or carotid occlusion, the pain and ophthalmoplegia of cavernous aneurysms improve in most cases. The timecourse of improvement is generally weeks to months. If compression of the anterior visual pathway has occurred, visual function stabilizes but

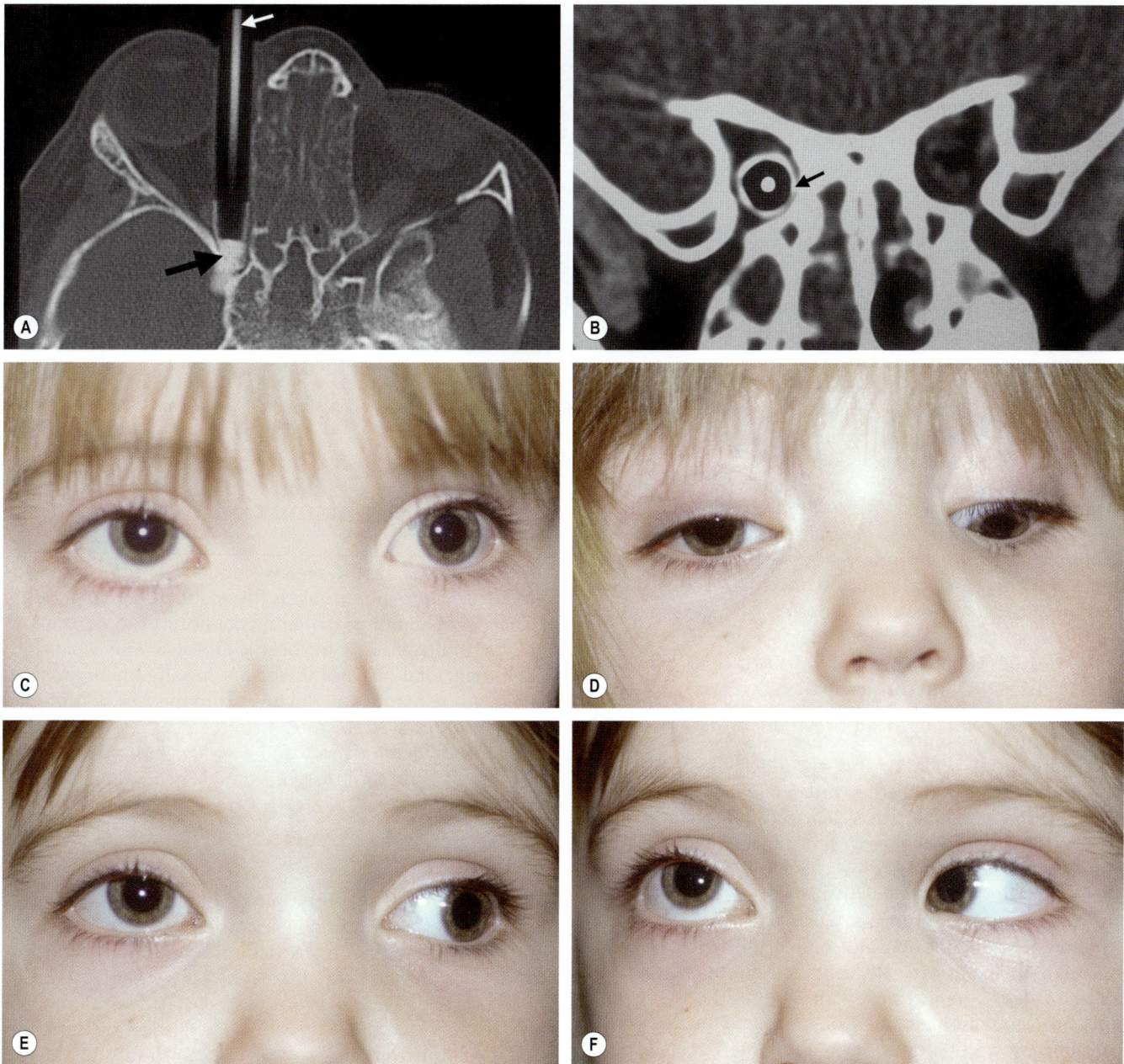

Figure 15–48. Orbital apex syndrome from a pencil in the orbit. This child had fallen, and a pencil (eraser end up) entered the orbit, medial to the medial rectus muscle. **A**. Orbital axial CT demonstrates the pencil eraser (*large arrow*) in the orbital apex and the rest of the pencil (*small arrow points to the pencil lead*) pushing the globe laterally. On fundus examination, indentation of the nasal retina was seen. **B**. Orbital coronal CT showing pencil (*arrow*) in orbital apex. The pencil was removed surgically without vascular complications. Postoperatively, the child had no light perception in the right eye from optic neuropathy; and ptosis and complete ophthalmoplegia of the right eye from IIIrd, IVth, and VIth nerve palsies (**C–F**). The ocular motor palsies resolved, but vision failed to recover.

rarely improves. In some cases, there is temporary worsening of symptoms after therapy due to sudden thrombosis and expansion of the aneurysm sac. If signs of aberrant regeneration are present prior to treatment, abnormalities in oculomotor nerve function generally persist.

Superior orbital fissure syndrome

Except for sparing of V2, lesions of the *superior orbital fissure* are clinically difficult to distinguish from those of the cavern-ous sinus, and the differential diagnosis is similar. The *orbital apex syndrome* consists of IIIrd, IVth, and VIth nerve paresis, V1 sensory loss, and optic neuropathy from cranial nerve II involvement (**Fig. 15–48**).

Congenital fibrosis syndromes

Patients with congenital fibrosis syndromes are born with nonprogressive ptosis and ophthalmoparesis. Because of severe strabismus or ptosis, binocular vision is usually

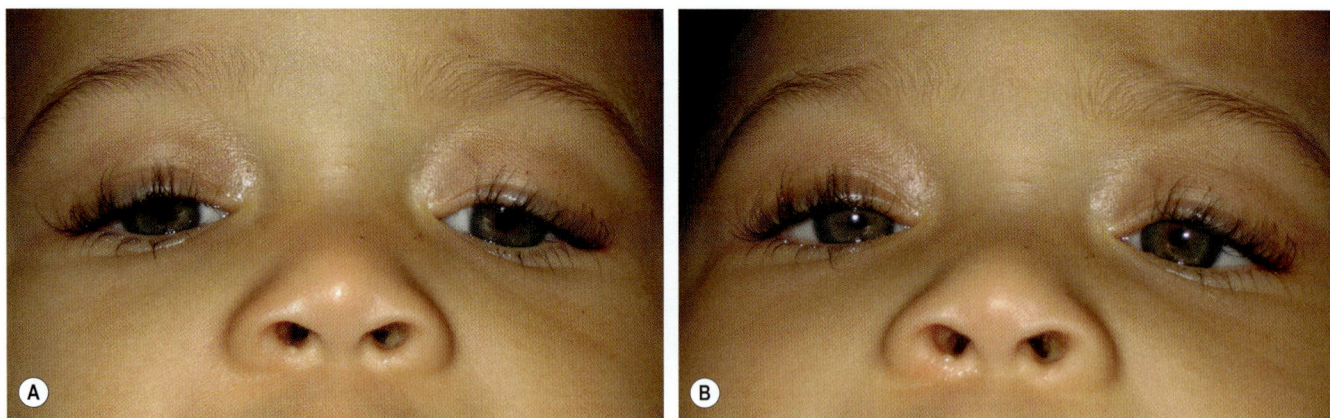

Figure 15–49. Congenital fibrosis syndrome (CFEOM1, K1F21A mutation). **A**. The child exhibited a chin-up posture because of bilateral ptosis and upgaze paresis. **B**. Convergence occurred in attempted upgaze. The child's father and paternal grandfather were similarly affected.

compromised, and amblyopia is common. Typically, affected patients are otherwise neurologically normal. Previously thought to result from primary fibrosis of the extraocular muscles, now they are considered congenital cranial dysinnervation disorders. Engle and colleagues[552–554] have mapped the genetic defect in the three major forms (congenital fibrosis of the extraocular muscles type 1 (CFEOM1), CFEOM2, CFEOM3 to chromosomes 12p11–q12, 11q13, and 16q24, respectively, and they have elucidated many of the genetic and pathophysiologic mechanisms.

Patients with CFEOM1, also called classic autosomal dominant CFEOM, typically have bilateral ptosis, downward pointed eyes, and supraduction deficits, often accompanied by convergence or divergence or other misinnervation phenomena in attempted upgaze (**Fig. 15–49**).[555,556] In a clinicopathologic study of a patient with CFEOM1, the superior division of the oculomotor nerve was absent, suggesting at least some of the abnormalities may result from defective congenital innervation of the extraocular muscles, analogous to Duane's retraction syndrome.[557] The syndrome results from mutations in the KIF21A gene, which encodes a kinesin motor protein responsible for anterograde axonal transport in neurons.[558] CFEOM1 can be associated with Marcus Gunn jaw winking.[559]

CFEOM2, an autosomal recessive syndrome, is characterized by bilateral ptosis, exotropia, and deficits in adduction, supraduction, and infraduction due to congenital bilateral absence of the IIIrd and IVth nerves.[560] Affected patients harbor a mutation in the PHOX2A/ARIX gene, which is a transcription factor thought to be essential in the formation of ocular motor neurons.[561,562]

CFEOM3 is also autosomal dominant and caused by mutations in the KIF21A gene. Affected patients have bilateral, sometimes asymmetric ptosis, exotropia, downward pointing eyes, and severe ophthalmoplegia.

Neuroimaging in the CFEOMs may demonstrate atrophy or increased width of the extraocular muscles.[560] Treatment, consisting of strabismus and ptosis surgery, is aimed at improving cosmesis, ocular alignment, and head position.

Childhood strabismus patterns

This section will briefly review childhood strabismus patterns, which may be mistaken for acquired ocular motility deficits. Long-standing eso- and exophorias can decompensate later in life, leading to chronic diplopia. The usual clues to the congenital onset of the ocular misalignment are their long-standing nature, full ductions, and the lack of diplopia. Other childhood strabismus patterns, such as congenital ocular motor nerve palsies and Duane syndrome, are discussed above, and Möbius syndrome is reviewed above and in Chapter 14.

Esotropia

Esotropia is the most common type of ocular misalignment in childhood, constituting at least half of cases in this age group.[563] The major categories of childhood esotropia include accommodative, infantile (congenital), acquired nonaccommodative, and esotropia associated with impaired sight (sensory esotropia).[365] Patients with these disturbances usually exhibit comitant esodeviations with full ductions.

Patients with accommodative esotropia, the most common cause of esotropia in childhood,[564] have moderate to severe hyperopia. They attempt to focus by accommodating, which is coupled with excessive convergence, so their esotropia improves with hyperopic correction (**Fig. 15–50**).[565] Accommodative esotropia usually presents insidiously although unusual cases following head or ocular trauma have been described.[566]

Nonaccommodative comitant esotropia may also be acquired suddenly in older children. Neuroimaging, while required in such cases, is usually normal.[567] In such children, if the esotropia persists, strabismus surgery is usually highly successful.[568]

Exotropia

Children with nonparalytic exotropia have a divergence of the eyes. Like in childhood esotropia, the deviation may be

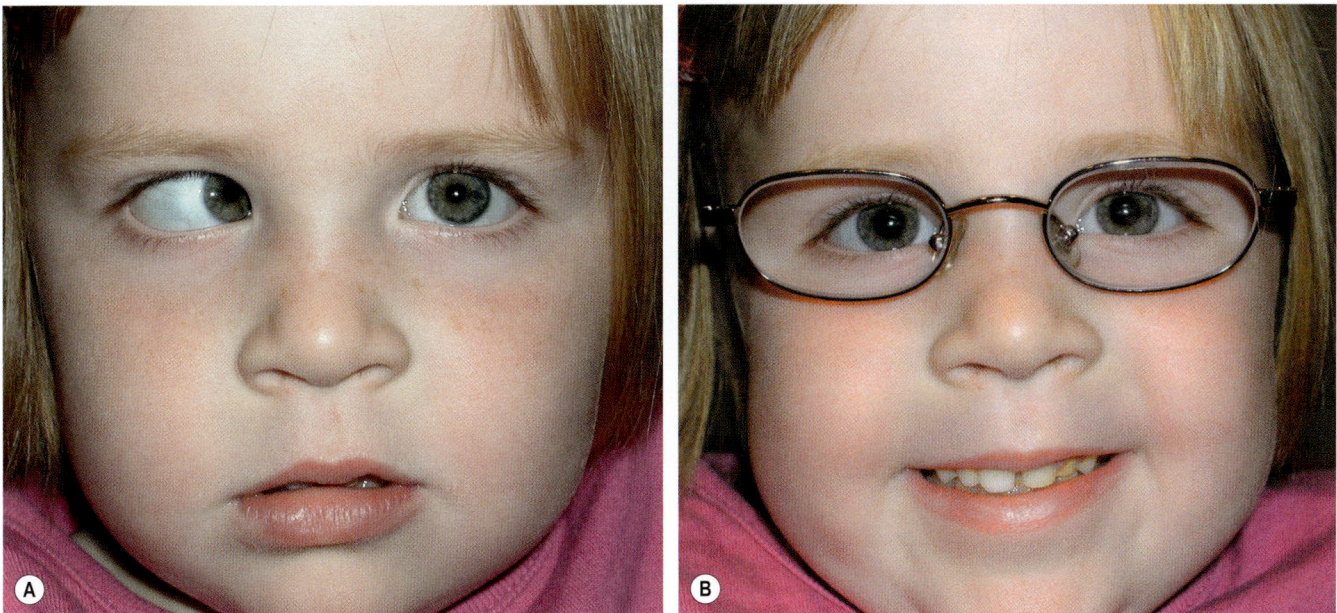

Figure 15–50. Accommodative esotropia. Large-angle esotropia (**A**) resolves with hyperopic spectacles (**B**).

intermittent or constant, ductions are normal, and the child may alternately fixate with either eye. In infants, exotropias tend to be more constant, while, in older children, intermittent exotropia with relatively good stereopsis is more commonly seen. When intermittent, fatigue or illness may worsen the exotropia.[569] Exotropia in childhood is associated with an increased prevalence of neurologic, ocular, and craniofacial abnormalities.[570]

Brown syndrome

This motility abnormality, also known as the "superior oblique tendon sheath syndrome," is characterized by a restriction of elevation of the eye in adduction and normal or near normal elevation in abduction (**Fig. 15–51**). The disorder can be distinguished clinically from an inferior oblique palsy by the presence of positive forced duction testing, the absence of superior oblique overaction, and, typically, normal alignment in primary gaze. Brown syndrome is attributed to a disturbance of free tendon movement through the trochlear pulley.[571] Patients may report an audible click or pop, discomfort, or pain upon attempted upgaze.

Although usually congenital, acquired cases of Brown syndrome may occur if the trochlea is affected by trauma, paranasal sinusitis, systemic inflammatory disease such as rheumatoid arthritis causing tenosynovitis,[572] or orbital lesions.[573,574] Some of the acquired cases may respond to anti-inflammatory agents such as corticosteroids. Congenital cases are usually observed, and oftentimes there is spontaneous resolution.[575] Strabismus surgery can be considered when there is a primary position hypotropia or abnormal head posture.

Dissociated vertical deviation (DVD)

During cover testing, in DVD the covered eye deviates upward and excyclorotates, then refixates when the occlu-

sion is removed. The fellow eye maintains fixation the entire time. The monocular upward drift may also occur spontaneously during periods of inattention. This dysmotility pattern contrasts to the vertical misalignment in skew or IVth nerve palsies, which is characterized by vertical drift and refixation movements of both eyes during cover testing.

DVD is usually associated with eso- or exotropias and nystagmus.[576–578] It may be mistaken for inferior oblique overaction. The mechanism is unknown, but is it is likely to be a supranuclear disturbance. Some authors have suggested that DVD is a disturbance or exaggeration of a normal vertical vergence eye movement.[579,580]

Synergistic divergence

In this miswiring phenomenon, both lateral rectus muscles contract when one eye is abducted.[581] This leads to a wall-eyed appearance. The exact anatomic substrate is unknown.

Trigemino-abducens synkinesis

This condition is also a congenital miswiring phenomenon and is characterized by ocular abduction leading to ipsilateral jaw deviation. Presumably fibers from the VIth nerve nucleus misinnervate masseter and pterygoid muscles,[582] which are normally supplied by the motor branch of the trigeminal nerve.

Orbital processes causing diplopia

Thyroid-associated ophthalmopathy

Restrictive thyroid myopathy due to thyroid-associated ophthalmopathy is one of the most common cause of diplopia in adults. The double vision is typically insidious and painless, often accompanied by complaints of eye irritation

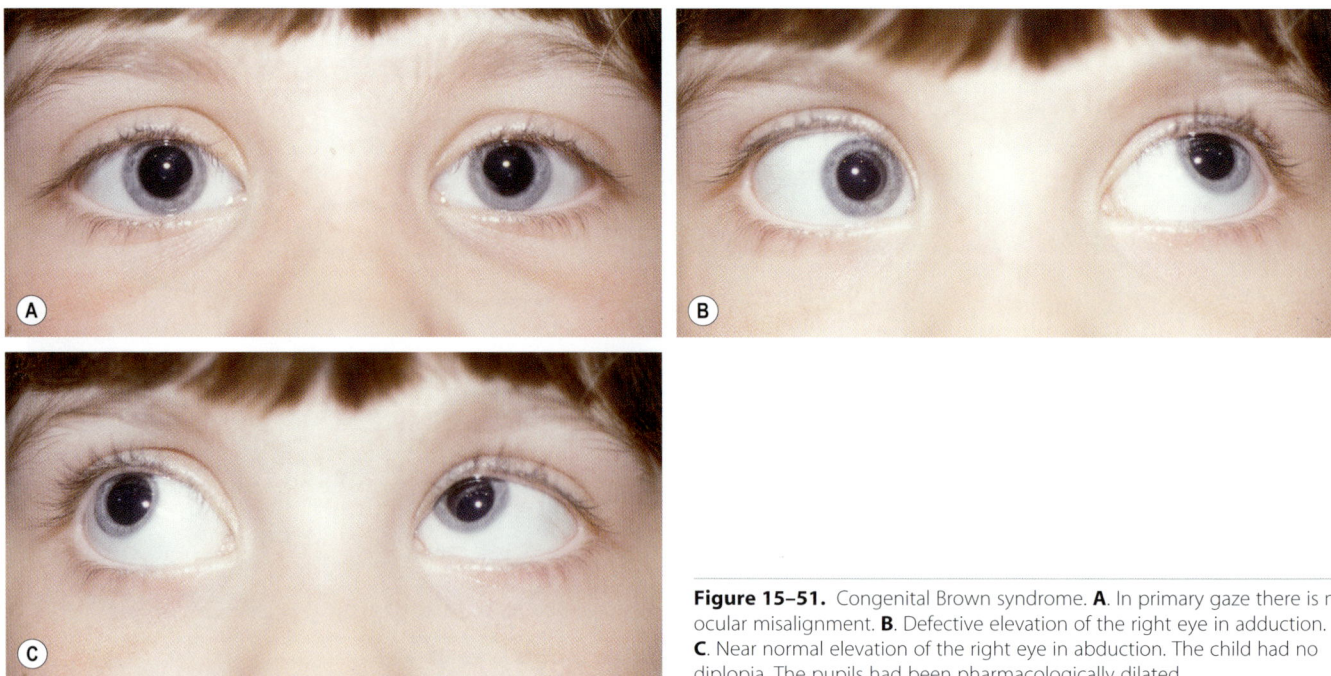

Figure 15–51. Congenital Brown syndrome. **A**. In primary gaze there is no ocular misalignment. **B**. Defective elevation of the right eye in adduction. **C**. Near normal elevation of the right eye in abduction. The child had no diplopia. The pupils had been pharmacologically dilated.

due to reduced tear film and decreased blink rate. One or both eyes may be proptotic with eyelid edema, lid retraction, and lagophthalmos (see Chapter 14). Restriction of ocular elevation with a positive forced duction test is characteristic of the disorder, but any muscle or combination may be involved. More occult presentations, particularly with isolated involvement of the inferior rectus, can closely mimic a contralateral IVth nerve palsy. Affected patients have either primary hyperthyroidism (Graves disease), primary hypothyroidism (e.g., Hashimoto's thyroiditis), or hypothyroidism due to treated hyperthyroidism. For unknown reasons, the extraocular muscles develop lymphocytic and plasmacytic infiltration with secondary production of acid mucopolysaccharides and fibrosis. Orbital echography or CT and MRI scanning of the orbits may demonstrate thickening of the extraocular muscles. The pathophysiology, diagnosis, and management of thyroid-associated ophthalmopathy are discussed in greater detail in Chapter 18.

Orbital inflammatory syndrome

Orbital myositis, with inflammation of muscles only, and *orbital pseudotumor*, with involvement of muscles and other contiguous structures, are characterized by painful double vision and restrictive ophthalmoplegia. Usually idiopathic but sometimes associated with systemic lupus erythematosus or Crohn disease, they probably represent the orbital versions of the Tolosa–Hunt syndrome. The pain and diplopia are usually responsive to oral corticosteroids. This condition is also discussed in more detail in Chapter 18.

Muscle infiltration

Isolated metastases to extraocular muscles are uncommon, but orbital metastasis from lung or breast carcinoma or lymphoma can involve the extraocular muscles.[583] CT or MRI usually reveals an orbital soft-tissue mass. The differential diagnosis of muscle infiltration is detailed in Chapter 18.

Neuromuscular junction

Myasthenia gravis

The extraocular muscles are involved in over 90% of patients with myasthenia gravis. Fifty percent present with motility abnormalities or ptosis only, and, of this group, half will remain "ocular myasthenics," while the other half will develop generalized symptoms, usually within 2 years. The diagnosis is supported by diurnal variation, fatigability, eyelid signs such as ptosis or Cogan's lid twitch (see Chapter 14), and the absence of pain. Any eye muscle can be affected, and the motility pattern may mimic a pupil-sparing IIIrd, IVth, or VIth nerve palsy, as well as supranuclear disturbances (see Chapter 16) such as a conjugate gaze palsy, internuclear ophthalmoplegia (**Fig. 15–52**), or one-and-a-half syndrome.[584–587] As a rule, the pupil is uninvolved. Resolution of appreciable ptosis or motility deficits following administration of intravenous edrophonium (Tensilon test) helps establish the diagnosis, but interpretation is more difficult with subtle ocular abnormalities. Acetylcholine receptor antibody levels, abnormal in half of patients with solely ocular myasthenia, and electromyography with repetitive stimulation and single-fiber studies are important complementary tests. Acetylcholinesterases usually fail to control the diplopia, which often requires the addition of corticosteroids. Myasthenia gravis is discussed in detail in Chapter 14.

Others

Eye muscle involvement is unusual in Lambert–Eaton myasthenic syndrome, although rarely patients may develop

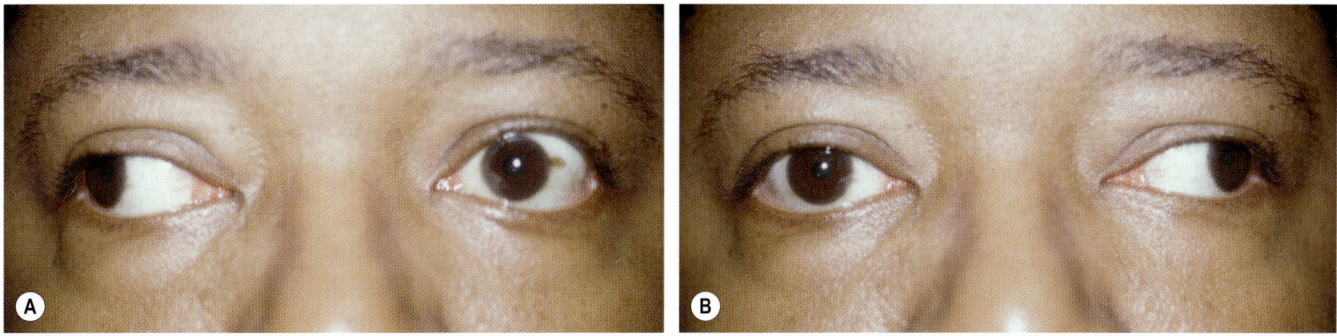

Figure 15–52. Pseudobilateral internuclear ophthalmoplegia in myasthenia gravis. The patient developed bilateral adduction weakness and abducting nystagmus. There was mild ptosis on the right. The motility disturbance and ptosis resolved with corticosteroids.

ptosis or minor transient motility disturbances. However, these patients do not typically have ocular misalignment on formal testing. Ocular motility and pupillary reactivity may be affected in botulism.

Primary ocular myopathies

Chronic progressive external ophthalmoplegia and Kearns–Sayre syndrome

Insidious, symmetric loss of eye movements, lack of diplopia, bilateral ptosis, and weakness of orbicularis oculi characterize "chronic progressive external ophthalmoplegia" (CPEO) due to mitochondrial dysfunction (external refers to extraocular muscles; internal refers to the pupillary sphincter). The Kearns–Sayre syndrome, typified by CPEO, pigmentary retinopathy, and cardiac conduction defects, is associated with mitochondrial DNA deletions. These conditions are reviewed in Chapter 14.

Other ocular myopathies

Patients with oculopharyngeal dystrophy and myotonic dystrophy, which are also discussed in Chapter 14, and myotubular myopathy, congenital fiber type disproportion, Bassen–Kornzweig syndrome (abetalipoproteinemia), Refsum disease, and multicore myopathy[588] may develop slowly progressive ptosis and ophthalmoparesis. Abnormal eye movements in Duchenne, Becker, and nemaline muscular dystrophies are exceptional.[589,590]

Extraocular muscle ischemia

Although uncommon, extraocular muscle ischemia due to giant cell arteritis (see Chapter 5) should be considered in any patient over 60 years of age with diplopia.[591] Ten to fifteen percent of patients with giant cell arteritis may have diplopia and unilateral ophthalmoplegia resulting from either ischemia of the extraocular muscles or ocular motor nerves.[592,593] In elderly individuals, symptoms of jaw claudication, headache, weight loss, and fever should be sought, and a sedimentation rate and C-reactive protein obtained. The double vision associated with giant cell arteritis

Table 15–11 Causes of double vision after cataract surgery

Monocular diplopia
Decentered or tilted intraocular lens
Cracked foldable intraocular lens
Irregular or high astigmatism from wound closure
Posterior capsule opacity or irregular opening
Iridectomy creating multiple "pupils"

Binocular diplopia
Iatrogenic anisophoria secondary to anisokonia or anisometropia from alteration of refractive error
Altered fusion secondary to surgical pupil changes
Extraocular muscle trauma from injection or bleeding:
  Needle or surgical trauma and anesthetic toxicity
    Fibrotic muscle with restrictive pattern
    Dysfunctional muscle with paretic pattern
  Trauma to an orbital nerve or extraocular muscle
Preexisting sensory exotropia prior to cataract surgery
Unmasking of alternative preexisting cause of misalignment not previously symptomatic because of poor vision in the eye with the cataract
Decentered intraocular lens with induced prism
Horror fusionis

may remit following the administration of high-dose corticosteroids.

Other miscellaneous causes of diplopia

Diplopia after cataract surgery

Patients with diplopia after cataract surgery represent a heterogeneous group of patients with symptoms arising for a variety of reasons (**Table 15–11**).[594] One study estimated the incidence to be as high as 2% of patients undergoing cataract surgery.[595] In our experience it occurs less frequently. Monocular diplopia, caused by an abnormality in the cornea, intraocular lens, or posterior capsule, should be excluded first. These should be apparent on examination, which should include keratometry and careful inspection of the lens and capsule through the dilated pupil.

Several etiologies of binocular diplopia following surgery, including optical, breakdown in fusion, neuropathic, and myopathic causes, can be considered. The position of the intraocular lens should be noted through the dilated pupil. Decentration of smaller intraocular lenses (optical zone less than 6 mm) and the presence of positioning holes can lead to optical aberrations.[596] Usually patients have to have at least 2 mm of decentration (usually vertically) to induce significant prismatic effect and resultant diplopia. The group of patients with optical causes of double vision after cataract surgery can be hard to recognize and characterize. The changes, which may be subtle such as induced anisometropia or altered brightness sense between the eyes, may still be sufficient to hinder fusion and induce diplopia.

Another set of patients with binocular diplopia lost their ability to fuse when binocular function was disrupted by a unilateral cataract. Intractable diplopia results when the cataract is removed, as the patient is unable to fuse or suppress the images. This syndrome is termed *horror fusionis*, an acquired disruption of central fusion.[597,598] Affected patients often resort to occlusion of one eye by either optical or mechanical means.

Most patients either have double vision from iatrogenic trauma (direct or secondary to anesthetic) to an extraocular muscle or nerve or had a pre-existing misalignment that was asymptomatic prior to cataract surgery because of reduced acuity in one eye or is now accentuated because of the improved image quality of the operated eye. In our experience, the most common diagnoses made in this setting include decompensated exotropia, decompensated congenital IVth nerve palsy, divergence insufficiency, and thyroid-associated ophthalmopathy. Some patients with poor vision from their cataract will develop a sensory exotropia. When the vision is cleared surgically the exotropia may persist and cause diplopia. This diplopia and sensory exotropia may spontaneously resolve over 6 months. Hence, we defer strabismus surgery for a least 6 months after cataract removal.

Other patients with pre-existing problems, such as thyroid-associated ophthalmopathy, will be recognized based on the characteristic examination findings such as proptosis and lid retraction and eye muscle enlargement on neuroimaging studies.[599] However, it often difficult to convince patients that their problem pre-existed the cataract surgery.

Patients with iatrogenic trauma to the extraocular muscles may have several different patterns of motility deficits and misalignment. Typically, the injury is produced by the periocular anesthetic injection.[600] This type of strabismus appears to result from a toxic effect of the local anesthetic or from direct trauma to the extraocular muscle.[601] Occasionally, the injection traumatizes the orbital nerves, ultimately producing strabismus. Previously it was thought that the bridle-suture used to hold the superior rectus muscle during cataract surgery was the culprit, but this seems to be less likely. Carlson and associates[602] were able to demonstrate that anesthetic injected directly into monkey extraocular muscles is capable of causing widespread damage to muscle fibers. This type of muscle injury can result in contracture, overaction, or paretic dysfunction, and therefore a variety of extraocular muscle dysfunction patterns have

been reported.[603] The most vulnerable muscle is the inferior rectus muscle, which can develop contracture after cataract surgery.[594,604,605] The resulting strabismus is very similar to that seen in patients with inferior rectus fibrosis from thyroid-associated ophthalmopathy. Patients develop a hypotropia with restriction of elevation in the affected eye. There may also be a "spring-like" overaction in downgaze. Similar contractures of the inferior oblique muscle have been described.[606] If the patient is seen acutely, a pattern of primary dysfunction or paresis may be evident before the muscle undergoes contractures.

Other patients may manifest with primary overaction of an extraocular muscle. This may result from myotoxicity of the antagonist muscle or may represent a component of the contracture phase of an injured muscle. A common scenario here again is primary inferior rectus dysfunction with superior rectus[607–609] or superior oblique[610] overaction. Most of these patients with overaction have patterns that simulate a mild contracture. The final group of patients have a primary paresis (usually of the inferior rectus muscle). These patients are recognized by the inability to depress the affected eye.[611] Patients with overaction or paresis should be able to benefit from strabismus surgery.

Hemifield slide phenomenon

Individuals with bitemporal hemianopias due to chiasmal disturbances may develop double vision from misalignment of noncorresponding nasal hemifields. This hemifield slide phenomenon is discussed in detail in Chapter 7. Vertical hemifield slide phenomenon has also been described in association with altitudinal visual field deficits.[612] This diagnosis should be considered in any patient with double vision who states that the two images slide in relation to one another. These patients may also complain of visual areas in which they cannot see.

Spontaneous extraocular muscle contractions

There are three conditions characterized by spontaneous extraocular muscle contractions: superior oblique myokymia, ocular neuromyotonia, and cyclic oculomotor spasms. The last was discussed above in the section on IIIrd nerve palsies.

Superior oblique myokymia. Intermittent, fine amplitude oscillatory contractions of a superior oblique muscle characterize this unusual eye movement disorder.[613,614] Patients are typically young adults, and they complain of monocular oscillopsia, often with vertical or torsional diplopia. The downward, intorting ocular oscillations are best seen with the slit lamp. Cover testing may reveal overaction of the affected superior oblique muscle. In the long-term follow-up in two series of patients,[615,616] recurrent spontaneous remissions and relapses were observed.

Usually unprovoked, superior oblique myokymia occasionally is associated with recovered IVth nerve palsies,[617] head trauma, and posterior fossa tumors.[618] As a result, some authors have attributed the myokymia to mild, usually subclinical IVth nerve injury, followed by axonal regeneration

Video 15

Video 17

and spontaneous discharging of trochlear motor neurons.[619,620] Defective supranuclear input to the IVth nerve nucleus has also been proposed.[616]

Frequently the symptoms are bothersome and uncomfortable enough to justify medical or surgical intervention. Medical therapy consists of carbamazepine,[621,622] propranolol,[623] or gabapentin.[624] Patients refractory to medical treatment may undergo superior oblique tenotomy, sometimes combined with inferior oblique tenectomy.[616] Some patients may benefit from microvascular decompression of the IVth nerve at the root exit zone.[625,626] Superior oblique myokymia is also discussed in Chapter 17.

Ocular neuromyotonia. In ocular neuromyotonia, tonic spasms of the muscles of an ocular motor nerve occur following sustained eccentric gaze. Affected patients complain of paroxysms of sustained diplopia for seconds or minutes. Some feel a pulling sensation in their orbit. The disorder is a delayed one, usually months or years following radiation for a sellar or parasellar tumor[627–629] or some other intracranial neoplasm.[630–632] Cases without antecedent radiation have also been reported in patients with spontaneous ocular neuromyotonia[633,634] and also in individuals with thyroid-associated orbitopathy,[635] carotid artery aneurysm,[636] cavernous sinus meningioma,[637] infectious cavernous sinus thrombosis,[638] midbrain–thalamic stroke,[639] and myelography with thorium dioxide.[632] The mechanism is thought to be related to unstable axonal membranes, ephaptic neural transmission, reorganization of the ocular motor nuclei following peripheral injury, or changes in neural activity following denervation.[633] Treatment usually consists of carbamazepine, which is thought to have membrane-stabilizing properties.

Ocular motility deficits in high (axial) myopia

Adults with unilateral or bilateral high myopia may develop an esotropia, abduction deficit, or vertical misalignment. Various explanations, including an elongated globe, tightness of the medial recti, decompensated esotropia, a heavy globe, lateral rectus abnormalities, (e.g. slipping inferiorly below the globe equator) and defective orbital connective tissues and muscle paths, have been proposed.[640–642]

Fixation switch diplopia

In adults with a history of childhood strabismus (e.g., eso- or exotropia), a change in refractive error of the dominant eye may lead to fixation with the nondominant eye. This may produce diplopia, but is managed by correcting the refractive error.[643]

Acute bilateral complete ophthalmoplegia

The differential diagnosis of an acute inability to move both eyes is narrow, and consists primarily of pituitary apoplexy, myasthenia gravis, botulism, Wernicke's encephalopathy, Guillain–Barré syndrome and Miller Fisher variant, and brainstem stroke or hemorrhage.[644–647] Distinguishing historical, examination, and diagnostic features of each are listed in **Table 15–12**. Less common causes, such as meningitis, phenytoin toxicity, and bilateral cavernous sinus masses or infection, should also be considered.[645]

Table 15–12 Common causes of acute bilateral ophthalmoparesis. (From Laskowitz D, Liu GT, Galetta SL. Acute visual loss and other disorders of the eyes. Neurol Clin N Am 1998:16:323–353, with permission).

Differential diagnosis	Associated symptoms and history	Signs	Ancillary diagnostic tests
Pituitary apoplexy	Severe headache, meningismus	Cranial nerve III, IV, VI, V1 or V2 involvement; visual loss may be present	MR imaging Lumbar puncture
Myasthenia gravis	Painless, fluctuates with fatigue, dysarthria	Pupil sparing, ptosis, with or without bulbar and generalized weakness	Edrophonium test, electrodiagnostic studies, anti-acetylcholine receptor antibody level
Botulism	May be associated with gastrointestinal symptoms: anorexia, nausea, vomiting	Dilated, unreactive pupils; bradycardia, constipation	Electrodiagnostic studies, serum bioassay
Wernicke's encephalopathy	History of alcohol abuse or malnutrition	Nystagmus, ataxia, confusional state, physical stigmata of long-term alcohol abuse	Improvement with thiamine
Guillain–Barré syndrome (Miller Fisher variant)	Preceding gastrointestinal or upper respiratory illness	Areflexia, ataxia, extremity weakness	Lumbar puncture, electrodiagnostic studies
Brainstem stroke	History of cardiac arrhythmia, vascular disease	Bilateral long tract signs, skew deviation	Magnetic resonance imaging

Video 15.14

References

1. Miller MJ, Mark LP, Ho KC, et al. Anatomic relationship of the oculomotor nuclear complex and medial longitudinal fasciculus in the midbrain. AJNR Am J Neuroradiol 1997;18:111–113.

2. Warwick R. Representation of the extra-ocular muscles in the oculomotor nuclei of the monkey. J Comp Neurol 1953;98:449–495.

3. Donzelli R, Marinkovic S, Brigante L, et al. The oculomotor nuclear complex in humans. Microanatomy and clinical significance. Surg Radiol Anat 1998;20:7–12.

4. Bienfang DC. Crossing axons in the third nerve nucleus. Invest Ophthalmol 1975;14:927–931.

5. Tubbs RS, Oakes WJ. Relationships of the cisternal segment of the trochlear nerve. J Neurosurg 1998;89:1015–1019.

6. Spektor S, Piontek E, Umansky F. Orbital venous drainage into the anterior cavernous sinus space: microanatomic relationships. Neurosurgery 1997;40:532–539.

7. Harris FS, Rhoton AL. Anatomy of the cavernous sinus, a microsurgical study. J Neurosurg 1976;45:169–180.

8. Taptas TN. The so-called cavernous sinus: a review of the controversy and its implications for neurosurgeons. Neurosurgery 1982;11:712–717.

9. Capo H, Kupersmith MJ, Berenstein A, et al. The clinical importance of the inferolateral trunk of the internal carotid artery. Neurosurgery 1991;28:733–738.

10. Tran-Dinh H. Cavernous branches of the internal carotid artery: anatomy and nomenclature. Neurosurgery 1987;20:205–210.

11. Umansky F, Nathan H. The lateral wall of the cavernous sinus with special reference to the nerves related to it. J Neurosurg 1982;56:228–234.

12. Striph GG, Burde RM. Abducens palsy and Horner's syndrome revisited. J Clin Neuroophthalmol 1988;8:13–17.

13. Porter JD, Baker RS, Ragusa RJ, et al. Extraocular muscles: basic and clinical aspects of structure and function. Surv Ophthalmol 1995;39:451–484.

14. Porter JD, Baker RS. Muscles of a different "color": the unusual properties of the extraocular muscles may predispose or protect them in neurogenic and myogenic disease. Neurology 1996;46:30–37.

15. Porter JD, Poukens V, Baker RS, et al. Structure-function correlations in the human medial rectus extraocular muscle pulleys. Invest Ophthalmol Vis Sci 1996;37:468–472.

16. Asbury AK, Aldredge H, Hershberg R, et al. Oculomotor palsy in diabetes mellitus: a clinico-pathological study. Brain 1970;93:555–566.

17. Balcer LJ, Galetta SL, Yousem DM, et al. Pupil-involving third nerve palsy and carotid stenosis: rapid recovery following endarterectomy. Ann Neurol 1997;41:273–276.

18. Marinkovic S, Gibo H. The neurovascular relationships and the blood supply of the oculomotor nerve: the microsurgical anatomy of its cisternal segment. Surg Neurol 1994;42:505–516.

19. Parkinson D. A surgical approach to the cavernous portion of the carotid artery: anatomical studies and case report. J Neurosurg 1965;23:474–483.

20. Cahill M, Bannigan J, Eustace P. Anatomy of the extraneural blood supply to the intracranial oculomotor nerve. Br J Ophthalmol 1996;80:177–181.

21. Marinkovic S, Gibo H, Zelic O, et al. The neurovascular relationships and the blood supply of the trochlear nerve: surgical anatomy of its cisternal segment. Neurosurgery 1996;38:161–169.

22. Brazis PW, Lee AG. Acquired binocular horizontal diplopia. Mayo Clinic Proc 1999;74:907–916.

23. Spector RH. Vertical diplopia. Surv Ophthalmol 1993;38:31–62.

24. Brazis PW, Lee AG. Binocular vertical diplopia. Mayo Clinic Proc 1998;73:55–66.

25. Wong AM, Tweed D, Sharpe JA. Vertical misalignment in unilateral sixth nerve palsy. Ophthalmology 2002;109:1315–1325.

26. Rush JA, Younge BR. Paralysis of cranial nerves III, IV, and VI. Arch Ophthalmol 1981;99:76–79.

27. Berlit P. Isolated and combined pareses of cranial nerves III, IV and VI. A retrospective study of 412 patients. J Neurol Sci 1991;103:10–15.

28. Richards DW, Jones FR, Younge BR. Causes and prognosis in 4,270 cases of paralysis of the oculomotor, trochlear, and abducens cranial nerves. Am J Ophthalmol 1992;113:489–496.

29. Holmes JM, Mutyala S, Maus TL, et al. Pediatric third, fourth, and sixth nerve palsies: a population-based study. Am J Ophthalmol 1999;127:388–392.

30. Newman NJ, Lambert SR. Botulinum toxin treatment of supranuclear ocular motility disorders. Neurology 1992;42:1391–1393.

31. Benegas NM, Egbert J, Engel WK, et al. Diplopia secondary to aniseikonia associated with macular disease. Arch Ophthalmol 1999;117:896–899.

32. Silverberg M, Schuler E, Veronneau-Troutman S, et al. Nonsurgical management of binocular diplopia induced by macular pathology. Arch Ophthalmol 1999;117:900–903.

33. Barton JJ. "Retinal diplopia" associated with macular wrinkling. Neurology 2004;63:925–927.

34. Foroozan R, Arnold AC. Diplopia after cataract surgery. Surv Ophthalmol 2005;50:81–84.

35. Leigh RJ, Zee DS. The Neurology of Eye Movements, 3rd edn, pp 502–510. New York, Oxford University Press, 1999.

36. Smith JL, David NJ. Internuclear ophthalmoplegia. Two new clinical signs. Neurology 1964;14:307–309.

37. Zee DS. Internuclear ophthalmoplegia: pathophysiology and diagnosis. Baillières Clin Neurol 1992;1:455–470.

38. Zwergal A, Cnyrim C, Arbusow V, et al. Unilateral INO is associated with ocular tilt reaction in pontomesencephalic lesions: INO plus. Neurology 2008;71:590–593.

39. Marshall RS, Sacco RL, Kreuger R, et al. Dissociated vertical nystagmus and internuclear ophthalmoplegia from a midbrain infarction. Arch Neurol 1991;48:1304–1305.

40. Dehaene I, Casselman JW, D'Hooghe M, et al. Unilateral internuclear ophthalmoplegia and ipsiversive torsional nystagmus. J Neurol 1996;243:461–464.

41. Cremer PD, Migliaccio AA, Halmagyi GM, et al. Vestibulo-ocular reflex pathways in internuclear ophthalmoplegia. Ann Neurol 1999;45:529–533.

42. Chen CM, Lin SH. Wall-eyed bilateral internuclear ophthalmoplegia from lesions at different levels in the brainstem. J Neuroophthalmol 2007;27:9–15.

43. Kim JS. Internuclear ophthalmoplegia as an isolated or predominant symptom of brainstem infarction. Neurology 2004;62:1491–1496.

44. Eggenberger ER, Desai NP, Kaufman DI, et al. Internuclear ophthalmoplegia after coronary artery catheterization and percutaneous transluminal coronary balloon angioplasty. J Neuroophthalmol 2000;20:123–126.

45. Eggenberger E, Golnik K, Lee A, et al. Prognosis of ischemic internuclear ophthalmoplegia. Ophthalmology 2002;109:1676–1678.

46. Chan JW. Isolated unilateral post-traumatic internuclear ophthalmoplegia. J Neuroophthalmol 2001;21:212–213.

47. Keane JR. Internuclear ophthalmoplegia: unusual causes in 114 of 410 patients. Arch Neurol 2005;62:714–717.

48. Galindo M, Pablos JL, Gomez-Reino JJ. Internuclear ophthalmoplegia in systemic lupus erythematosus. Semin Arthritis Rheum 1998;28:179–186.

49. Masai H, Kashii S, Kimura H, et al. Neuro-Behcet disease presenting with internuclear ophthalmoplegia. Am J Ophthalmol 1996;122:897–898.

50. Hughes TAT, Wiles CM, Hourihan M. Cervical radiculopathy and bilateral internuclear ophthalmoplegia caused by temporal arteritis. J Neurol Neurosurg Psychiatry 1994;57:764–765.

51. Arnold AC, Baloh RW, Yee RD, et al. Internuclear ophthalmoplegia in the Chiari type II malformation. Neurology 1990;40:1850–1854.

52. Hunnewell J, Miller NR. Bilateral internuclear ophthalmoplegia related to chronic toluene abuse. J Neuroophthalmol 1998;18:277–280.

53. Frohman EM, Zhang H, Kramer PD, et al. MRI characteristics of the MLF in MS patients with chronic internuclear ophthalmoparesis. Neurology 2001;57:762–768.

54. Silverman IE, Liu GT, Volpe NJ, et al. The crossed paralyses: the original brainstem syndromes of Millard-Gubler, Foville, Weber, and Raymond-Cestan. Arch Neurol 1995;52:635–638.

55. Thömke F, Hopf HC, Krämer G. Internuclear ophthalmoplegia of abduction: clinical and electrophysiological data on the existence of an abduction paresis of prenuclear origin. J Neurol Neurosurg Psychiatry 1992;55:105–111.

56. Griffin JF, Wray SH, Anderson DP. Misdiagnosis of spasm of the near reflex. Neurology 1976;26:1018–1020.

57. Keane JR. Neuro-ophthalmic signs and symptoms of hysteria. Neurology 1982;32:757–762.

58. Goldstein JH, Schneekloth BB. Spasm of the near reflex: a spectrum of anomalies. Surv Ophthalmol 1996;40:269–278.

59. Newman NJ, Lessell S. Pupillary dilatation with monocular occlusion as a sign of nonorganic oculomotor dysfunction. Am J Ophthalmol 1989;108:461–462.

60. Moster ML, Hoenig EM. Spasm of the near reflex associated with metabolic encephalopathy. Neurology 1989;38:150.

61. Dagi LR, Chrousos GA, Cogan DG. Spasm of the near reflex associated with organic disease. Am J Ophthalmol 1987;103:582–585.

62. Manor RS. Use of special glasses in treatment of spasm of near reflex. Ann Ophthalmol 1979;11:903–905.

63. Lepore FE. Disorders of ocular motility following head trauma. Arch Neurol 1995;52:924–926.

64. Ohtsuka K, Maeda S, Oguri N. Accommodation and convergence palsy caused by lesions in the bilateral rostral superior colliculus. Am J Ophthalmol 2002;133:425–427.

65. Convergence Insufficiency Treatment Trial Study Group. Randomized clinical trial of treatments for symptomatic convergence insufficiency in children. Arch Ophthalmol 2008;126:1336–1349.

66. Jacobson DM. Divergence insufficiency revisited. Natural history of idiopathic cases and neurologic associations. Arch Ophthalmol 2000;118:1237–1241.

67. Kirkham TH, Bird AC, Sanders MD. Divergence paralysis with raised intracranial pressure. Br J Ophthalmol 1972;56:776–782.

68. Schanzer B, Bordaberry M, Jeffery AR, et al. The child with divergence paresis. Surv Ophthalmol 1998;42:571–576.

69. Brown SM, Iacuone JJ. Intact sensory fusion in a child with divergence paresis caused by a pontine glioma. Am J Ophthalmol 1999;128:528–530.

70. Tsuda H, Ishikawa H, Koga N, et al. Magnetic resonance imaging findings in divergence paralysis. Neuroophthalmology 2006;30:59–62.

71. Rutar T, Demer JL. "Heavy eye" syndrome in the absence of high myopia: a connective tissue degeneration in elderly strabismic patients. J AAPOS 2009;13:36–44.

72. Wiggins RE, Baumgartner S. Diagnosis and management of divergence weakness in adults. Ophthalmology 1999;106:1353–1356.

73. Wiest G, Mallek R, Baumgartner C. Selective loss of vergence control secondary to bilateral paramedian thalamic infarction. Neurology 2000;54:1997–1999.

74. Keane JR. Ocular skew deviation. Arch Neurol 1975;32:185–190.

75. Brandt T, Dieterich M. Skew deviation with ocular torsion: a vestibular brainstem sign of topographic diagnostic value. Ann Neurol 1993;33:528–534.

76. Brodsky MC, Donahue SP, Vaphiades M, et al. Skew deviation revisited. Surv Ophthalmol 2006;51:105–128.

77. Halmagyi GM, Gresty MA, Gibson WPR. Ocular tilt reaction with peripheral vestibular lesion. Ann Neurol 1979;6:80–83.

78. Wolfe GI, Taylor CL, Flamm ES, et al. Ocular tilt reaction resulting from vestibuloacoustic nerve surgery. Neurosurgery 1993;32:417–421.

79. Safran AB, Vibert D, Issoua D, et al. Skew deviation after vestibular neuritis. Am J Ophthalmol 1994;118:238–245.

80. Zee DS. Considerations on the mechanisms of alternating skew deviation in patients with cerebellar lesions. J Vestib Res 1996;6:395–401.

81. Riordan-Eva P, Harcourt JP, Faldon M, et al. Skew deviation following vestibular nerve surgery. Ann Neurol 1997;41:94–99.

82. Wong AM, Sharpe JA. Cerebellar skew deviation and the torsional vestibuloocular reflex. Neurology 2005;65:412–419.

83. Galetta SL, Liu GT, Raps EC, et al. Cyclodeviation in skew deviation. Am J Ophthalmol 1994;118:509–514.

84. Dieterich M, Brandt T. Wallenberg's syndrome: lateralpulsion, cyclorotation, and subjective visual vertical in thirty-six patients. Ann Neurol 1992;31:399–408.

85. Brandt T, Dieterich M. Vestibular syndromes in the roll plane: topographic diagnosis from brainstem to cortex. Ann Neurol 1994;36:337–347.

86. Moster ML, Schatz NJ, Savino PJ, et al. Alternating skew on lateral gaze (bilateral abducting hypertropia). Ann Neurol 1988;23:190–192.

87. Keane JR. Alternating skew deviation: 47 patients. Neurology 1985;35:725–728.

88. Merikangas JR. Skew deviation in pseudotumor cerebri. Ann Neurol 1978;4:583.

89. Frohman LP, Kupersmith MJ. Reversible vertical ocular deviations associated with raised intracranial pressure. J Neuroophthalmol 1986;5:158–163.

90. Donahue SP, Lavin PJ, Hamed LM. Tonic ocular tilt reaction simulating a superior oblique palsy: diagnostic confusion with the 3-step test. Arch Ophthalmol 1999;117:347–352.

91. Trobe JD. Cyclodeviation in acquired vertical strabismus. Arch Ophthalmol 1984;102:717–720.

92. Donahue SP, Lavin PJ, Mohney B, et al. Skew deviation and inferior oblique palsy. Am J Ophthalmol 2001;132:751–756.

93. Donohue SP, Lavin PJ, Hamed L. Tonic ocular tilt reaction simulating a superior oblique palsy: diagnostic confusion with the 3 step test. Arch Ophthalmol 1999;117:347–352.

94. Parulekar MV, Dai S, Buncic JR, et al. Head position-dependent changes in ocular torsion and vertical misalignment in skew deviation. Arch Ophthalmol 2008;126:899–905.

95. Brandt T, Dieterich M. Pathological eye-head coordination in roll: tonic ocular tilt reaction in mesencephalic and medullary lesions. Brain 1987;110:649–666.

96. Halmagyi GM, Brandt T, Dieterich M, et al. Tonic contraversive ocular tilt reaction due to unilateral meso-diencephalic lesion. Neurology 1990;40:1503–1509.

97. Ohashi T, Fukushima K, Chin S, et al. Ocular tilt reaction with vertical eye movement palsy caused by localized unilateral midbrain lesion. J Neuroophthalmol 1998;18:40–42.

98. Westheimer G, Blair SM. The ocular tilt reaction: a brainstem oculomotor routine. Invest Ophthalmol 1975;14:833–839.

99. Rabinovitch HE, Shape JA, Sylvester TO. The ocular tilt reaction. A paroxysmal dyskinesia associated with elliptical nystagmus. Arch Ophthalmol 1977;95:1395–1398.

100. Hedges TR, Hoyt WF. Ocular tilt reaction due to an upper brainstem lesion: paroxysmal skew deviation, torsion, and oscillation of the eyes with head tilt. Ann Neurol 1982;11:537–540.

101. Lueck CJ, Hamlyn P, Crawford TJ, et al. A case of ocular tilt reaction and torsional nystagmus due to direct stimulation of the midbrain in man. Brain 1991;114:2069–2079.

102. Galimberti CA, Versino M, Sartori I, et al. Epileptic skew deviation. Neurology 1998;50:1469–1472.

103. Corbett JJ, Schatz NJ, Shults WT, et al. Slowly alternating skew deviation: description of a pretectal syndrome in three patients. Ann Neurol 1981;10:540–546.

104. Mitchell JM, Smith JL, Quencer RM. Periodic alternating skew deviation. J Clin Neuroophthalmol 1981;1:5–8.

105. Jampel RS, Fells P. Monocular elevation paresis caused by a central nervous system lesion. Arch Ophthalmol 1968;80:45–57.

106. Lessell S. Supranuclear paralysis of monocular elevation. Neurology 1975;25:1134–1136.

107. Ford CS, Schwartze GM, Weaver RG, et al. Monocular elevation paresis caused by an ipsilateral lesion. Neurology 1984;34:1264–1267.

108. Wiest G, Baumgartner C, Schnider P, et al. Monocular elevation paresis and contralateral downgaze paresis from unilateral mesodiencephalic infarction. J Neurol Neurosurg Psychiatry 1996;60:579–581.

109. Guy JR, Savino PJ, Schatz NJ, et al. Superior division paresis of the oculomotor nerve. Ophthalmology 1985;92:777–784.

110. Ksiazek SM, Repka MX, Maguire A, et al. Divisional oculomotor nerve paresis caused by intrinsic brainstem disease. Ann Neurol 1989;26:714–718.

111. Guy JR, Day AL. Intracranial aneurysms with superior division paresis of the oculomotor nerve. Ophthalmology 1989;96:1071–1076.

112. Bhatti MT, Eisenschenk S, Roper SN, et al. Superior divisional third cranial nerve paresis: clinical and anatomical observations of 2 unique cases. Arch Neurol 2006;63:771–776.

113. Czarnecki JSC, Thompson HS. The iris sphincter in aberrant regeneration of the third nerve. Arch Ophthalmol 1978;96:1606–1610.

114. Spector RH, Faria MA. Aberrant regeneration of the inferior division of the oculomotor nerve. Arch Neurol 1981;38:460–461.

115. Landau K. Discovering a dys-covering lid. Surv Ophthalmol 1997;42:87–91.

116. Sibony PA, Lessell S. Transient oculomotor synkinesis in temporal arteritis. Arch Neurol 1984;41:87–88.

117. Johnson LN, Pack WL. Transient oculomotor nerve misdirection in a case of pituitary tumor with hemorrhage [letter]. Arch Ophthalmol 1988;106:584–585.

118. Schatz NJ, Savino PJ, Corbett JJ. Primary aberrant oculomotor regeneration. A sign of intracavernous meningioma. Arch Neurol 1977;34:29–32.

119. Trobe JD, Glaser JS, Post JD. Meningiomas and aneurysms of the cavernous sinus. Neuro-ophthalmologic features. Arch Ophthalmol 1978;96:457–467.

120. Boghen D, Chartrand J-P, Laflamme P, et al. Primary aberrant third nerve regeneration. Ann Neurol 1979;6:415–418.

121. Lepore FE, Glaser JS. Misdirection revisited. A critical appraisal of acquired oculomotor nerve synkinesis. Arch Ophthalmol 1980;98:2206–2209.

122. Cox TA, Wurster JB, Godfrey WA. Primary aberrant oculomotor regeneration due to intracranial aneurysm. Arch Neurol 1979;36:570–571.

123. Carrasco JR, Savino PJ, Bilyk JR. Primary aberrant oculomotor nerve regeneration from a posterior communicating artery aneurysm. Arch Ophthalmol 2002;120:663–665.

124. Johnson LN, Kamper CA, Hepler RS, et al. Primary aberrant regeneration of the oculomotor nerve from presumed extracavernous neurilemmoma, meningioma, and asymmetric mammillary body. Neuroophthalmology 1989;9:227–232.

125. Varma R, Miller NR. Primary oculomotor nerve synkinesis caused by an extracavernous intradural aneurysm. Am J Ophthalmol 1994;118:83–87.

126. Keane JR. Bilateral aberrant regeneration of the third cranial nerve following trauma. J Neurosurg 1975;43:95–97.

127. O'Day J, Billson F, King J. Ophthalmoplegic migraine and aberrant regeneration of the oculomotor nerve. Br J Ophthalmol 1980;64:534–536.

128. Laguna JF, Smith MS. Aberrant regeneration in idiopathic oculomotor nerve palsy. J Neurosurg 1980;52:854–856.

129. Barr D, Kupersmith M, Turbin R, et al. Synkinesis following diabetic third nerve palsy. Arch Ophthalmol 2000;118:132–134.

130. Messé SR, Shin RK, Liu GT, et al. Oculomotor synkinesis following a midbrain stroke. Neurology 2001;57:1106–1107.

131. Sibony PA, Lessell S, Gittinger JW, Jr. Acquired oculomotor synkinesis. Surv Ophthalmol 1984;28:382–390.

132. Loewenfeld IE, Thompson HS. Oculomotor paresis with cyclic spasms. A critical review of the literature and a new case. Surv Ophthalmol 1975;20:81–124.

133. Susac JO, Smith JL. Cyclic oculomotor paralysis. Neurology 1974;24:24–27.

134. Bateman DE, Saunders M. Cyclic oculomotor palsy: description of a case and hypothesis of the mechanism. J Neurol Neurosurg Psychiatry 1983;46:451–453.

135. Miller NR, Lee AG. Adult-onset acquired oculomotor nerve paresis with cyclic spasms: relationship to ocular neuromyotonia. Am J Ophthalmol 2004;137:70–76.

136. Growdon JH, Winkler GF, Wray SH. Midbrain ptosis. A case with clinicopathologic correlation. Arch Neurol 1974;30:179–181.

137. Bogousslavsky J, Regli F, Ghika J, et al. Internuclear ophthalmoplegia, prenuclear paresis of contralateral superior rectus, and bilateral ptosis. J Neurol 1983;230:197–203.

138. Bogousslavsky J, Regli F. Nuclear and prenuclear syndromes of the oculomotor nerve. Neuroophthalmology 1983;3:211–216.

139. Biller J, Shapiro R, Evans LS, et al. Oculomotor nuclear complex infarction. Clinical and radiological correlation. Arch Neurol 1984;41:985–987.

140. Liu GT, Carrazana EJ, Charness ME. Unilateral oculomotor palsy and bilateral ptosis from paramedian midbrain infarction. Arch Neurol 1991;48:983–986.

141. Bengel D, Huffmann G. Oculomotor nuclear complex syndrome as a single sign of midbrain haemorrhage. Neuroophthalmology 1994;14:279–282.

142. Pratt DV, Orengo-Nania S, Horowitz BL, et al. Magnetic resonance imaging findings in a patient with nuclear oculomotor palsy. Arch Ophthalmol 1995;113:141–142.

143. Martin TJ, Corbett JJ, Babikian PV, et al. Bilateral ptosis due to mesencephalic lesions with relative preservation of ocular motility. J Neuroophthalmol 1996;16:258–263.

144. Keane JR, Zaias B, Itabashi HH. Levator sparing oculomotor nerve palsy caused by a solitary midbrain metastasis. Arch Neurol 1984;41:210–212.

145. Bryan JS, Hamed LM. Levator-sparing nuclear oculomotor palsy. J Clin Neuroophthalmol 1992;12:26–30.

146. Pusateri TJ, Sedwick LA, Margo CE. Isolated inferior rectus muscle palsy from solitary metastasis to the oculomotor nucleus. Arch Ophthalmol 1987;105:675–677.

147. Chou TM, Demer JM. Isolated inferior rectus palsy caused by a metastasis to the oculomotor nucleus. Am J Ophthalmol 1998;126:737–740.

148. Lee AG, Tang RA, Wong GG, et al. Isolated inferior rectus muscle palsy resulting from a nuclear third nerve lesion as the initial manifestation of multiple sclerosis. J Neuroophthalmol 2000;20:246–247.

149. Kwon JH, Kwon SU, Ahn HS, et al. Isolated superior rectus palsy due to contralateral midbrain infarction. Arch Neurol 2003;60:1633–1635.

150. Liu GT, Crenner CW, Logigian EL, et al. Midbrain syndromes of Benedikt, Claude, and Nothnagel: setting the record straight. Neurology 1992;42:1820–1822.

151. Seo SW, Heo JH, Lee KY, et al. Localization of Claude's syndrome. Neurology 2001;57:2304–2307.

152. Caplan LR. "Top of the basilar" syndrome. Neurology 1980;30:72–79.

153. Kim JS, Kang JK, Lee SA, et al. Isolated or predominant ocular motor nerve palsy as a manifestation of brain stem stroke. Stroke 1993;24:581–586.

154. Thömke F. Brainstem diseases causing isolated ocular motor nerve palsies. Neuroophthalmology 2002;28:53–67.

155. Nadeau SE, Trobe JD. Pupil sparing in oculomotor palsy: a brief review. Ann Neurol 1983;13:143–148.

156. Breen LA, Hopf HC, Farris BK, et al. Pupil-sparing oculomotor nerve palsy due to midbrain infarction. Arch Neurol 1991;48:105–106.

157. Kumar P, Ahmed I. Pupil-sparing oculomotor palsy due to midbrain infarction [letter]. Arch Neurol 1992;49:348.

158. Gauntt CD, Kashii S, Nagata I. Monocular elevation paresis caused by an oculomotor fascicular impairment. J Neuroophthalmol 1995;15:11–14.

159. Ksiazek SM, Slamovitz TL, Rosen CE, et al. Fascicular arrangement in partial oculomotor paresis. Am J Ophthalmol 1994;118:97–103.

160. Saeki N, Murai N, Sunami K. Midbrain tegmental lesions affecting or sparing the pupillary fibres. J Neurol Neurosurg Psychiatry 1996;61:401–406.

161. Eggenberger ER, Miller NR, Hoffman PN, et al. Mesencephalic ependymal cyst causing an inferior divisional paresis of the oculomotor nerve. Neurology 1993;43:2419–2420.

162. Castro O, Johnson LN, Mamourian AC. Isolated inferior oblique paresis from brain-stem infarction. Perspective on oculomotor fascicular organization in the ventral midbrain tegmentum. Arch Neurol 1990;47:235–237.

163. Tezer I, Dogulu CF, Kansu T. Isolated inferior rectus palsy as a result of paramedian thalamopeduncular infarction. J Neuroophthalmol 2000;20:154–155.

164. Lee DK, Kim JS. Isolated inferior rectus palsy due to midbrain infarction detected by diffusion-weighted MRI. Neurology 2006;66:1956–1957.

165. Bogousslavsky J, Maeder P, Regli F, et al. Pure midbrain infarction: clinical syndromes, MRI, and etiologic patterns. Neurology 1994;44:2032–2040.

166. Ishikawa H, Satoh H, Fujiwara M, et al. Oculomotor nerve palsy caused by lung cancer metastasis. Intern Med 1997;36:301–303.

167. Keane JR. Isolated brain-stem third nerve palsy. Arch Neurol 1988;45:813–814.

168. Getenet J-C, Vighetto A, Nighoghossian N, et al. Isolated bilateral third nerve palsy caused by a mesencephalic hematoma. Neurology 1994;44:981–982.

169. Traboulsi EI, Azar DT, Achram M, et al. Brainstem tuberculoma and isolated third nerve palsy. Neuroophthalmology 1985;5:43–45.

170. Newman NJ, Lessell SL. Isolated pupil-sparing third-nerve palsy as the presenting sign of multiple sclerosis. Arch Neurol 1990;47:817–818.

171. Thömke F, Lensch E, Ringel K, et al. Isolated cranial nerve palsies in multiple sclerosis. J Neurol Neurosurg Psychiatry 1997;63:682–685.

172. Liu GT. Coma. Neurosurg Clin N Am 1999;10:579–586.

173. Ropper AH, Cole D, Louis DN. Clinicopathologic correlation in a case of pupillary dilation from cerebral hemorrhage. Arch Neurol 1991;48:1166–1169.

174. Kole MK, Hysell SE. MRI correlate of Kernohan's notch. Neurology 2000;55:1751.

175. Ropper AH. The opposite pupil in herniation. Neurology 1990;40:1707–1709.

176. Fisher CM. Oval pupils. Arch Neurol 1980;37:502–503.

177. Chen R, Sahjpaul R, Del Maestro RF, et al. Initial enlargement of the opposite pupil as a false localising sign in intraparenchymal frontal haemorrhage. J Neurol Neurosurg Psychiatry 1994;57:1126–1128.

178. Soni SR. Aneurysms of the posterior communicating artery and oculomotor paresis. J Neurol Neurosurg Psychiatry 1974;37:475–484.

179. Kupersmith MJ. Neuro-vascular Neuroophthalmology. Berlin, Springer-Verlag, 1993.

180. Kasoff I, Kelly DL. Pupillary sparing oculomotor palsies with internal carotid-posterior communicating artery aneurysms. J Neurosurg 1975;42:713–717.

181. Kissel JT, Burde RM, Klingele TG, et al. Pupil-sparing oculomotor palsies with internal carotid-posterior communicating artery aneurysms. Ann Neurol 1983;13:149–154.

182. Good EF. Ptosis as the sole manifestation of compression of the oculomotor nerve by an aneurysm of the posterior communicating artery. J Clin Neuroophthalmol 1990;10:59–61.

183. Bartleson JD, Trautmann JC, Sundt TM. Minimal oculomotor nerve paresis secondary to unruptured intracranial aneurysm. Arch Neurol 1986;43:1015–1020.

184. Crompton JL, Moore CE. Painful third nerve palsy: how not to miss an intra-cranial aneurysm. Aust J Ophthalmol 1981;9:113–115.

185. Coppeto JR, Lessell S. Dorsal midbrain syndrome from giant aneurysm of the posterior fossa: report of two cases. Neurology 1983;33:732–736.

186. Grunwald L, Sund NJ, Volpe NJ. Pupillary sparing and aberrant regeneration in chronic third nerve palsy secondary to a posterior communicating artery aneurysm. Br J Ophthalmol 2008;92:715–716.

187. Greenspan BN, Reeves AG. Transient partial oculomotor nerve paresis with posterior communicating artery aneurysm. A case report. J Clin Neuroophthalmol 1990;10:56–58.

188. Foroozan R, Slamovits TL, Ksiazek SM, et al. Spontaneous resolution of aneurysmal third nerve palsy. J Neuroophthalmol 2002;22:211–214.

189. Peiris JB, Russel WR. Giant aneurysms of the carotid system presenting as visual field defect. J Neurol Neurosurg Psychiatry 1980;43:1053–1064.

190. Takahashi T, Kanatani I, Isayama Y, et al. Visual disturbance due to internal carotid aneurysm. Ann Ophthalmol 1983;13:1014–1024.

191. Brisman JL, Song JK, Newell DW. Cerebral aneurysms. N Engl J Med 2006;355:928–939.

192. Qureshi AI, Janardhan V, Hanel RA, et al. Comparison of endovascular and surgical treatments for intracranial aneurysms: an evidence-based review. Lancet Neurol 2007;6:816–825.

193. Fujiwara S, Fujii K, Nishio S, et al. Oculomotor nerve palsy in patients with cerebral aneurysms. Neurosurg Rev 1989;12:123–132.

194. Grayson MC, Soni SR, Spooner VA. Analysis of the recovery of third nerve function after direct surgical intervention for posterior communicating aneurysms. Br J Ophthalmol 1974;58:118–125.

195. Kyriakides T, Aziz TZ, Torrens MJ. Postoperative recovery of third nerve palsy due to posterior communicating aneurysms. Br J Neurosurg 1989;3:109–111.

196. Ahn JY, Han IB, Yoon PH, et al. Clipping vs coiling of posterior communicating artery aneurysms with third nerve palsy. Neurology 2006;66:121–123.

197. McKinna AJ. Eye signs in 61 cases of posterior fossa aneurysms: their diagnostic and prognostic value. Can J Ophthalmol 1983;18:3–6.

198. Boccardo M, Ruelle A, Banchero MA. Isolated oculomotor palsy caused by aneurysm of the basilar artery bifurcation. J Neurol 1986;233:61–62.

199. Lustbader JM, Miller NR. Painless, pupil-sparing but otherwise complete oculomotor nerve paresis caused by basilar artery aneurysm. Arch Ophthalmol 1988;106:583–584.

200. Ajtai B, Fine EJ, Lincoff N. Pupil-sparing, painless compression of the oculomotor nerve by expanding basilar artery aneurysm: a case of ocular pseudomyasthenia. Arch Neurol 2004;61:1448–1450.

201. Jacobson DM, McCanna TD, Layde PM. Risk factors for ischemic ocular motor nerve palsies. Arch Ophthalmol 1994;112:961–966.

202. Teuscher AU, Meienberg O. Ischaemic oculomotor nerve palsy. Clinical features and vascular risk factors in 23 patients. J Neurol 1985;232:144–149.

203. Jacobson DM, Broste SK. Early progression of ophthalmoplegia in patients with ischemic oculomotor nerve palsies. Arch Ophthalmol 1995;113:1535–1537.

204. Keane JR, Ahmadi J. Most diabetic third nerve palsies are peripheral. Neurology 1998;51:1510.

205. Weber RB, Daroff RB, Mackey EA. Pathology of oculomotor nerve palsy in diabetics. Neurology 1970;20:835–838.

206. Hopf HC, Gutmann L. Diabetic 3rd nerve palsy: evidence for a mesencephalic lesion. Neurology 1990;40:1041–1045.

207. Jacobson DM. Pupil involvement in patients with diabetes-associated oculomotor nerve palsy. Arch Ophthalmol 1998;116:723–727.

208. Bortolami R, D'Alessandro R, Manni E. The origin of pain in "ischemic-diabetic" third nerve palsy [letter]. Arch Neurol 1993;50:795.

209. Capó H, Warren F, Kupersmith MJ. Evolution of oculomotor nerve palsies. J Clin Neuroophthalmol 1992;12:21–25.

210. Eshbaugh CG, Siatkowski RM, Smith JL, et al. Simultaneous, multiple cranial neuropathies in diabetes mellitus. J Neuroophthalmol 1995;15:219–224.

211. Davies GE, Shakir RA. Giant cell arteritis presenting as oculomotor nerve palsy with pupillary dilation. Postgrad Med J 1994;70:298–299.

212. Bondenson J, Asman P. Giant cell arteritis presenting with oculomotor nerve palsy. Scand J Rheumatol 1997;26:327–328.

213. Lazaridis C, Torabi A, Cannon S. Bilateral third nerve palsy and temporal arteritis. Arch Neurol 2005;62:1766–1768.

214. Rosenstein ED, Sobelman J, Kramer N. Isolated, pupil-sparing third nerve palsy as initial manifestation of systemic lupus erythematosus. J Clin Neuroophthalmol 1989;9:285–288.

215. Johnson LN, Stetson SW, Krohel GB, et al. Aspirin use and the prevention of acute ischemic cranial nerve palsy. Am J Ophthalmol 2000;129:367–371.

216. Van Stavern GP, Biousse V, Lynn MJ, et al. Neuro-ophthalmic manifestations of head trauma. J Neuroophthalmol 2001;21:112–117.

217. Tognetti F, Godano U, Galassi E. Bilateral traumatic third nerve palsy. Surg Neurol 1988;29:120–124.

218. Balcer LJ, Galetta SL, Bagley LJ, et al. Localization of traumatic oculomotor nerve palsy to the midbrain exit site by magnetic resonance imaging. Am J Ophthalmol 1996;122:437–439.

219. Keane JR. Third-nerve palsy due to penetrating trauma. Neurology 1993;43:1523–1527.

220. Eyster EF, Hoyt WF, Wilson CB. Oculomotor palsy from minor head trauma. An initial sign of basal intracranial tumor. JAMA 1972;220:1083–1086.

221. Walter KA, Newman NJ, Lessell S. Oculomotor palsy from minor head trauma: initial sign of intracranial aneurysm. Neurology 1994;44:148–150.

222. Kansu T, Özcan OE, Ösdirim E, et al. Neurinoma of the oculomotor nerve. Case report. J Clin Neuroophthalmol 1982;2:271–272.

223. Egan RA, Thompson CR, MacCollin M, et al. Monocular elevator paresis in neurofibromatosis type 2. Neurology 2001;56:1222–1224.

224. Celli P, Ferrante L, Acqui M, et al. Neurinoma of the third, fourth, and sixth cranial nerves: a survey and report of a new fourth nerve case. Surg Neurol 1992;38:216–224.

225. Kadota T, Miyawaki Y, Nakagawa H, et al. MR imaging of oculomotor nerve neurilemmoma. Magn Reson Imaging 1993;11:1071–1075.

226. Leunda G, Vaquero J, Cabezydo J, et al. Schwannoma of the oculomotor nerves. Report of four cases. J Neurosurg 1982;1982:57.

227. Mehta VS, Singh RVP, Misra NK, et al. Schwannoma of the oculomotor nerve. Br J Neurosurg 1990;4:69–72.

228. Kaye-Wilson LG, Gibson R, Bell JE, et al. Oculomotor nerve neurinoma. Neuroophthalmology 1994;14:37–41.

229. Hart AJ, Allibone J, Casey AT, et al. Malignant meningioma of the oculomotor nerve without dural attachment. Case report and review of the literature. J Neurosurg 1998;88:1104–1106.

230. Reifenberger G, Bostrom J, Bettag M, et al. Primary glioblastoma multiforme of the oculomotor nerve. Case report. J Neurosurg 1996;84:1062–1066.

231. Ehrenpreis SJ, Biedlingmaier JF. Isolated third-nerve palsy associated with frontal sinus mucocele. J Neuroophthalmol 1995;15:105–108.

232. Wilson WB, Leavengood JM, Ringel SP, et al. Transient ocular motor paresis associated with acute internal carotid artery occlusion. Ann Neurol 1989;25:286–290.

233. Schievink WI, Mokri B, Garrity JA, et al. Ocular motor nerve palsies in spontaneous dissections of the cervical internal carotid artery. Neurology 1993;43:1938–1941.

234. Yamada T, Nishio S, Matsunaga M, et al. Cavernous haemangioma in the oculomotor nerve. A case report. J Neurol 1986;233:63–64.

235. Trobe JD. Third nerve palsy and the pupil. Footnotes to the rule. Arch Ophthalmol 1988;106:601–602.

236. Jacobson DM, Trobe JD. The emerging role of magnetic resonance angiography in the management of patients with third cranial nerve palsy. Am J Ophthalmol 1999;128:94–96.

237. Chou KL, Galetta SL, Liu GT, et al. Acute ocular motor mononeuropathies: prospective study of the roles of neuroimaging and clinical assessment. J Neurol Sci 2004;219:35–39.

238. Trobe JD. Searching for brain aneurysm in third cranial nerve palsy. J Neuroophthalmol 2009;29:171–173.

239. Keane JR, Ahmadi J. Third-nerve palsies and angiography. Arch Neurol 1991;48:470.

240. Lee AG, Hayman LA, Brazis PW. The evaluation of isolated third nerve palsy revisited: an update on the evolving role of magnetic resonance, computed tomography, and catheter angiography. Surv Ophthalmol 2002;47:137–157.

241. Vaphiades MS, Horton JA. MRA or CTA, that's the question. Surv Ophthalmol 2005;50:406–410.
242. Mathew MR, Teasdale E, McFadzean RM. Multidetector computed tomographic angiography in isolated third nerve palsy. Ophthalmology 2008;115:1411–1415.
243. Chaudhary N, Davagnanam I, Ansari SA, et al. Imaging of intracranial aneurysms causing isolated third cranial nerve palsy. J Neuroophthalmol 2009;29:238–244.
244. Noonan CP, O'Connor M. Surgical management of third nerve palsy. Br J Ophthalmol 1995;79:431–434.
245. Liu GT. Discussion of Mehkri IA, Awner S, Olitsky SE, et al. "Double vision in a child". Surv Ophthalmol 1999;44:45–52.
246. Miller NR. Solitary oculomotor nerve palsy in childhood. Am J Ophthalmol 1977;83:106–111.
247. Harley RD. Paralytic strabismus in children. Etiologic incidence and management of the third, fourth, and sixth nerve palsies. Ophthalmology 1980;87:24–43.
248. Keith CG. Oculomotor nerve palsy in childhood. Aust N Z J Ophthalmol 1987;15:181–184.
249. Ing EB, Sullivan TJ, Clarke MP, et al. Oculomotor nerve palsies in children. J Pediatr Ophthalmol Strabismus 1992;29:331–336.
250. Kodsi SR, Younge BR. Acquired oculomotor, trochlear, and abducent cranial nerve palsies in pediatric patients. Am J Ophthalmol 1992;114:568–574.
251. Schumacher-Feero LA, Yoo KW, Solari FM, et al. Third cranial nerve palsy in children. Am J Ophthalmol 1999;128:216–221.
252. Yang YC, Laws DE, Chandna A. The rules of third nerve palsy in children [letter]. Eye 1996;10:646–647.
253. Victor DI. The diagnosis of congenital unilateral third nerve palsy. Brain 1976;99:711–718.
254. Balkan R, Hoyt CS. Associated neurologic abnormalities in congenital third nerve palsies. Am J Ophthalmol 1984;97:315–319.
255. Good WV, Barkovich AJ, Nickel BL, et al. Bilateral congenital oculomotor nerve palsy in a child with brain anomalies. Am J Ophthalmol 1991;111:555–558.
256. Hamed LM. Associated neurologic and ophthalmologic findings in congenital oculomotor nerve palsy. Ophthalmology 1991;98:708–714.
257. Tsaloumas MD, Willshaw HE. Congenital oculomotor palsy: associated neurological and ophthalmological findings. Eye 1997;11:500–503.
258. Norman MG. Unilateral encephalomalacia in cranial nerve nuclei in neonates. Neurology 1974;24:378–380.
259. Routon MC, Expert-Bezançon MC, Bursztyn J, et al. Polymicrogyrie bioperculaire associée a une ophtalmoplégie congénitale par atteinte du noyau du nerf moteur oculaire commun. Rev Neurol 1994;150:363–369.
260. Prats JM, Monzon MJ, Zuazo E, et al. Congenital nuclear syndrome of oculomotor nerve. Pediatr Neurol 1993;9:476–478.
261. Lagrèze W-DA, Warner JEA, Zamani AA, et al. Mesencephalic clefts with associated eye movement disorders. Arch Ophthalmol 1996;114:429–432.
262. Savas R, Sommer A, Gueckel F, et al. Isolated oculomotor nerve paralysis in Lyme disease: MRI. Neuroradiology 1997;39:139–141.
263. Nazir SA, Murphy SA, Siatkowski RM. Recurrent para-infectious third nerve palsy with cisternal nerve enhancement on MRI [letter]. J Neuroophthalmol 2004;24:96–97.
264. Gordon N. Ophthalmoplegia in childhood. Dev Med Child Neurol 1994;36:370–374.
265. Zanus C, Furlan C, Costa P, et al. The Tolosa-Hunt syndrome in children: a case report. Cephalalgia 2009;29:1232–1237.
266. Kandt RS, Goldstein GW. Steroid-responsive ophthalmoplegia in a child. Diagnostic considerations. Arch Neurol 1985;42:589–591.
267. Barbas NR, Hedges TR, Schwenn M. Isolated oculomotor nerve palsy due to neoplasm in infancy. Neuroophthalmology 1995;15:157–160.
268. Mullaney PB, Nabi NU, Thorner P, et al. Ophthalmic involvement as a presenting feature of nonorbital childhood parameningeal embryonal rhabdomyosarcoma. Ophthalmology 2001;108:179–182.
269. Shindler KS, Liu GT, Womer RB. Long-term follow-up and prognosis of orbital apex syndrome resulting from nasopharyngeal rhabdomyosarcoma. Am J Ophthalmol 2005;140:236–241.
270. Piatt JH, Campbell GA, Oakes WJ. Papillary meningioma involving the oculomotor nerve in an infant. J Neurosurg 1986;64:808–812.
271. Norman AA, Farris BK, Siatkowski RM. Neuroma as a cause of oculomotor palsy in infancy and early childhood. J AAPOS 2001;5:9–12.
272. Troost BT. Ophthalmoplegic migraine. Biomed Pharmacother 1996;50:49–51.
273. Rust RS, Schutta HS. Ophthalmoplegic migraine [abstract]. Ann Neurol 1994;36:521.
274. Friedman AP, Harter DH, Merritt HH. Ophthalmoplegic migraine. Arch Neurol 1962;7:320–327.
275. Raymond LA, Tew J, Fogelson MH. Ophthalmoplegic migraine of early onset. J Pediatr 1977;90:1035–1036.
276. Robertson WC, Schnitzler ER. Ophthalmoplegic migraine in infancy. Pediatrics 1978;61:886–888.
277. Elser JM, Woody RC. Migraine headache in the infant and young child. Headache 1990;30:366–368.
278. Mark AS, Blake P, Atlas SW, et al. Gd-DTPA enhancement of the cisternal portion of the oculomotor nerve on MR imaging. AJNR Am J Neuroradiol 1992;13:1463–1470.
279. Stommel EW, Ward TN, Harris RD. MRI findings in a case of ophthalmoplegic migraine. Headache 1993;33:234–237.
280. Østergaard JR, Moller HU, Christensen T. Recurrent ophthalmoplegia in childhood: diagnostic and etiologic considerations. Cephalalgia 1996;16:276–279.
281. Wong V, Wong WC. Enhancement of oculomotor nerve: a diagnostic criterion for ophthalmoplegic migraine? Pediatr Neurol 1997;17:70–73.
282. O'Hara MA, Anderson RT, Brown D. Magnetic resonance imaging in ophthalmoplegic migraine of children. J AAPOS 2001;5:307–310.
283. Bharucha DX, Campbell TB, Valencia I, et al. MRI findings in pediatric ophthalmoplegic migraine: a case report and literature review. Pediatr Neurol 2007;37:59–63.
284. Headache Classification Subcommittee of the International Headache Society. The International Classification of Headache Disorders: 2nd edition. Cephalalgia 2004;24 (Suppl 1):9–160.
285. Lance JW, Zagami AS. Ophthalmoplegic migraine: a recurrent demyelinating neuropathy? Cephalalgia 2001;21:84–89.
286. Carlow TJ. Oculomotor ophthalmoplegic migraine: is it really migraine? J Neuroophthalmol 2002;22:215–221.
287. Gabianelli EB, Klingele TG, Burde RM. Acute oculomotor palsy in childhood. Is arteriography necessary? J Clin Neuroophthalmol 1989;9:33–36.
288. Wolin MJ, Saunders RA. Aneurysmal oculomotor nerve palsy in an 11-year-old boy. J Clin Neuroophthalmol 1992;12:178–180.
289. Mehkri IA, Awner S, Olitsky SE, et al. Double vision in a child. Surv Ophthalmol 1999;44:45–52.
290. Branley MG, Wright KW, Borchert MS. Third nerve palsy due to cerebral artery aneurysm in a child. Aust NZ J Ophthalmol 1992;20:137–140.
291. Ebner R. Angiography for IIIrd nerve palsy in children [letter]. J Clin Neuroophthalmol 1990;10:154–155.
292. Fox R. Angiography for third nerve palsy in children [editorial]. J Clin Neuroophthalmol 1989;9:37–38.
293. Cekirge S, Saatci I, Firat MM, et al. Bilateral cavernous carotid artery aneurysms in a 4-year-old child: endovascular treatment with mechanically detachable coils. Neuroradiology 1997;39:367–370.
294. DiMario FJ, Rorke LB. Transient oculomotor nerve paresis in congenital distal basilar artery aneurysm. Pediatr Neurol 1992;8:303–306.
295. Vincent FM, Zimmerman JE. Superior cerebellar artery aneurysm presenting as an oculomotor nerve palsy in a child. Neurosurgery 1980;6:661–664.
296. Huang LT, Shih TY, Lui CC. Posterior cerebral artery aneurysm in a two-year-old girl. J Formos Med Assoc 1996;95:170–172.
297. Tamhankar MA, Liu GT, Young TL, et al. Acquired, isolated third nerve palsies in infants with cerebrovascular malformations. Am J Ophthalmol 2004;138:484–486.
298. Grunt JA, Destro RL, Hamtil LW, et al. Ocular palsies in children with diabetes mellitus. Diabetes 1976;25:459–462.
299. Mizen TR, Burde RM, Klingele PG. Cryptogenic oculomotor nerve palsies in children. Am J Ophthalmol 1985;100:65–67.
300. Kraft SP, O'Reilly C, Quigley PL, et al. Cyclotorsion in unilateral and bilateral superior oblique paresis. J Pediatr Ophthalmol Strabismus 1993;30:361–367.
301. von Noorden GK, Murray E, Wong SY. Superior oblique paralysis: a review of 270 cases. Arch Ophthalmol 1986;104:1771–1776.
302. Mansour AM, Reinecke RD. Central trochlear palsy. Surv Ophthalmol 1986;30:279–297.
303. Keane JR. Fourth nerve palsy: historical review and study of 215 inpatients. Neurology 1993;43:2439–2443.
304. Hara N, Kan S, Simizu K. Localization of post-traumatic trochlear nerve palsy associated with hemorrhage at the subarachnoid space by magnetic resonance imaging. Am J Ophthalmol 2001;132:443–445.
305. Agostinis C, Caverni L, Moschini L, et al. Paralysis of fourth cranial nerve due to superior-cerebellar artery aneurysm. Neurology 1992;42:457–458.
306. Astle WF, Miller SJ. Bilateral fluctuating trochlear nerve palsy secondary to cerebellar astrocytoma. Can J Ophthalmol 1994;29:34–38.
307. Wilcsek GA, Francis IC, Egan CA, et al. Superior oblique palsy in a patient with a history of perineural spread from a periorbital squamous cell carcinoma. J Neuroophthalmol 2000;20:240–241.
308. Jacobson DM, Moster ML, Eggenberger ER, et al. Isolated trochlear nerve palsy in patients with multiple sclerosis. Neurology 1999;53:877–880.
309. Galetta SL, Balcer LJ. Isolated fourth nerve palsy from midbrain hemorrhage. Case report. J Neuroophthalmol 1998;18:204–205.
310. Thömke F, Ringel K. Isolated superior oblique palsies with brainstem lesions. Neurology 1999;53:682–685.
311. Keane JR. Tectal fourth nerve palsy due to infarction. Arch Neurol 2004;61:280.
312. Makki AA, Newman NJ. A trochlear stroke. Neurology 2005;65:1989.
313. Gonyea EF. Superior oblique palsy due to a midbrain vascular malformation. Neurology 1990;40:554–555.
314. Lotery A, Best J, Houston S. Occult giant cell (temporal) arteritis presenting with bilateral sixth and unilateral fourth nerve palsies [letter]. Eye 1998;12:1014–1016.
315. Santoreneos S, Hanieh A, Jorgensen RE. Trochlear nerve schwannomas occurring in patients without neurofibromatosis: case report and review of the literature. Neurosurgery 1997;41:282–287.
316. Feinberg AS, Newman NJ. Schwannoma in patients with isolated unilateral trochlear nerve palsy. Am J Ophthalmol 1999;127:183–188.
317. Elmalem VI, Younge BR, Biousse V, et al. Clinical course and prognosis of trochlear nerve schwannomas. Ophthalmology 2009;116:2011–2016.
318. Jacobson DM, Warner JJ, Ruggles KH. Transient trochlear nerve palsy following anterior temporal lobectomy for epilepsy. Neurology 1995;45:1465–1468.
319. Guy J, Day AL, Mickle JP, et al. Contralateral trochlear nerve paresis and ipsilateral Horner's syndrome. Am J Ophthalmol 1989;107:73–76.
320. Brazis PW. Localization of lesions of the trochlear nerve: diagnosis and localization-recent concepts. Mayo Clinic Proc 1993;68:501–509.
321. Vanooteghem P, Dehaene I, Van Zandycke M, et al. Combined trochlear nerve palsy and internuclear ophthalmoplegia. Arch Neurol 1992;49:108–109.
322. Greenberg MF, Pollard ZF. Ocular plagiocephaly: ocular torticollis with skull and facial asymmetry. Ophthalmology 2000;107:173–179.

323. Helveston EM, Krach D, Plager DA, et al. A new classification of superior oblique palsy based on congenital variations in the tendon. Ophthalmology 1992;99:1609–1615.

324. Astle WF, Rosenbaum AL. Familial congenital fourth cranial nerve palsy. Arch Ophthalmol 1985;103:532–535.

325. Harris DJ, Memmen JE, Katz NNK, et al. Familial congenital superior oblique palsy. Ophthalmology 1986;93:88–90.

326. Botelho PJ, Giangiacomo JG. Autosomal-dominant inheritance of congenital superior oblique palsy. Ophthalmology 1996;103:1508–1511.

327. Bale JF, Scott WE, Yuh W, et al. Congenital fourth nerve palsy and occult cranium bifidum. Pediatr Neurol 1988;4:320–321.

328. Pierrot-Deseilligny C, Goasguen J. Isolated abducens nucleus damage due to histiocytosis X. Electro-oculographic analysis and physiological deductions. Brain 1984;107:1019–1032.

329. Müri RM, Chermann JF, Cohen L, et al. Ocular motor consequences of damage to the abducens nucleus area in humans. J Neuroophthalmol 1996;16:191–195.

330. Donaldson D, Rosenberg NL. Infarction of abducens nerve fascicle as cause of isolated sixth nerve palsy related to hypertension. Neurology 1988;38:1654.

331. Fukutake T, Hirayama K. Isolated abducens nerve palsy from pontine infarction in a diabetic patient. Neurology 1992;42:2226.

332. Rose JW, Digre KB, Lynch SG, et al. Acute VIth cranial nerve dysfunction in multiple sclerosis. J Clin Neuroophthalmol 1992;12:17–20.

333. Sturzenegger M. Isolated sixth-nerve palsy as the presenting sign of multiple sclerosis. Neuroophthalmology 1994;14:43–48.

334. Thömke F, Mika-Grüttner A, Visbeck A, et al. The risk of abducens palsy after diagnostic lumbar puncture. Neurology 2000;54:768–769.

335. Bell JA, McIllwaine GG, O'Neill D. Iatrogenic lateral rectus palsies. A series of five postmyelographic cases. J Clin Neuroophthalmol 1994;14:205–209.

336. Berlit P, Berg-Dammer E, Kuehne D. Abducens nerve palsy in spontaneous intracranial hypotension. Neurology 1994;44:1552.

337. Currie J, Lubin JH, Lessell S. Chronic isolated abducens paresis from tumors at the base of the brain. Arch Neurol 1983;40:226–229.

338. Galetta SL, Smith JL. Chronic isolated sixth nerve palsies. Arch Neurol 1989;46:79–82.

339. Volpe NJ, Lessell S. Remitting sixth nerve palsy in skull base tumors. Arch Ophthalmol 1993;111:1391–1395.

340. Warwar RE, Bhullar SS, Pelstring RJ, et al. Sudden death from pituitary apoplexy in a patient presenting with an isolated sixth cranial nerve palsy. J Neuroophthalmol 2006;26:95–97.

341. Mutyala S, Holmes JM, Hodge DO, et al. Spontaneous recovery rate in traumatic sixth-nerve palsy. Am J Ophthalmol 1996;122:898–899.

342. Holmes JM, Beck RW, Kip KE, et al. Predictors of nonrecovery in acute traumatic sixth nerve palsy and paresis. Ophthalmology 2001;108:1457–1460.

343. Moster ML, Savino PJ, Sergott RC, et al. Isolated sixth-nerve palsies in younger adults. Arch Ophthalmol 1984;102:1328–1330.

344. Gilbert ME, Mizen T. Too young to…. Surv Ophthalmol 2006;51:520–524.

345. Davé AV, Diaz-Marchan PJ, Lee AG. Clinical and magnetic resonance imaging features of Gradenigo syndrome. Am J Ophthalmol 1997;124:568–570.

346. Nakamura M, Carvalho GA, Samii M. Abducens nerve schwannoma: a case report and review of the literature. Surg Neurol 2002;57:183–188; discussion 188–189.

347. Goldenberg-Cohen N, Miller NR. Noninvasive neuroimaging of basilar artery dolichoectasia in a patient with an isolated abducens nerve paresis. Am J Ophthalmol 2004;137:365–367.

348. Narai H, Manabe Y, Deguchi K, et al. Isolated abducens nerve palsy caused by vascular compression. Neurology 2000;55:453–454.

349. Neugebauer A, Kirsch A, Fricke J, et al. New onset of crossed eyes in an adult. Surv Ophthalmol 2001;45:335–344.

350. Peters GB, 3rd, Bakri SJ, Krohel GB. Cause and prognosis of nontraumatic sixth nerve palsies in young adults. Ophthalmology 2002;109:1925–1928.

351. Afifi AK, Bell WE, Menezes AH. Etiology of lateral rectus palsy in infancy and childhood. J Child Neurol 1992;7:295–299.

352. Robertson DM, Hines JD, Rucker CW. Acquired sixth-nerve paresis in children. Arch Ophthalmol 1970;83:574–579.

353. Aroichane M, Repka MX. Outcome of sixth nerve palsy or paresis in young children. J Pediatr Ophthalmol Strabismus 1995;32:152–156.

354. Lee MS, Galetta SL, Volpe NJ, et al. Sixth nerve palsies in children. Pediatr Neurol 1999;20:49–52.

355. Pollack IF. Brain tumors in children. N Engl J Med 1994;331:1500–1507.

356. Sternberg I, Ronen S, Arnon N. Recurrent isolated post febrile abducens nerve palsy. J Pediatr Ophthalmol Strabismus 1980;17:323–324.

357. Bixenman WW, von Noorden GK. Benign/recurrent VI nerve palsy in childhood. J Pediatr Ophthalmol Strabismus 1981;18:29–34.

358. Werner DB, Savino PJ, Schatz NJ. Benign recurrent sixth nerve palsies in childhood secondary to immunization or viral illness. Arch Ophthalmol 1983;101:607–608.

359. Boger WP, Puliafito CA, Magoon EH, et al. Recurrent isolated sixth nerve palsy in children. Ann Ophthalmol 1984;237–238, 240–244.

360. Sullivan SC. Benign recurrent isolated VI nerve palsy of childhood. Clin Pediatr 1985;24:160–161.

361. Cohen HA, Nussinovitch M, Ashkenazi A, et al. Benign abducens nerve palsy of childhood. Pediatr Neurol 1993;9.

362. Straussberg R, Cohen AH, Amir J, et al. Benign abducens palsy associated with EBV infection. J Pediatr Ophthalmol Strabismus 1993;30:60.

363. Yousuf SJ, Khan AO. Presenting features suggestive for later recurrence of idiopathic sixth nerve paresis in children. J AAPOS 2007;11:452–455.

364. Mahoney NR, Liu GT. Benign recurrent sixth (abducens) nerve palsies in children. Arch Dis Child 2009;94:394–396.

365. Parks MM, Wheeler MB. Concomitant esodeviations. In: Tasman W, Jaeger EA (eds): Duane's Clinical Ophthalmology, pp 1–14. Philadelphia, J. B. Lippincott, 1992.

366. Watson AP, Fielder AR. Sudden-onset squint. Dev Med Child Neurol 1987;29:207–211.

367. Bixenman WW, Laguna JF. Acquired esotropia as initial manifestation of Arnold-Chiari malformation. J Pediatr Ophthalmol Strabismus 1987;24:83–86.

368. Williams AS, Hoyt CS. Acute comitant esotropia in children with brain tumors. Arch Ophthalmol 1989;107:376–378.

369. Astle WF, Miller SJ. Acute comitant esotropia: a sign of intracranial disease. Can J Ophthalmol 1994;29:151–154.

370. Jaafar MS, Collins MLZ, Rabinowitz AI. Cerebellar astrocytoma presenting as acquired comitant esotropia at age 18 and 27 months [abstract]. J Pediatr Ophthalmol Strabismus 1995;32:63.

371. Ciancia AO. On infantile esotropia with nystagmus in abduction. J Pediatr Ophthalmol Strabismus 1995;32:280–288.

372. Hoyt CS, Good WV. Acute comitant esotropia: when is it a sign of serious neurologic disease? Br J Ophthalmol 1995;79:498–501.

373. Simon JW, Waldman JB, Couture KC. Cerebellar astrocytoma manifesting as isolated, comitant esotropia in childhood. Am J Ophthalmol 1996;121:584–586.

374. Gilbert ME, Meira D, Foroozan R, et al. Double vision worth a double take. Surv Ophthalmol 2006;51:587–591.

375. Passo M, Shults WT, Talbot T, et al. Acquired esotropia. A manifestation of Chiari I malformation. J Clin Neuroophthalmol 1984;4:151–154.

376. Lewis AR, Kline LB, Sharpe JA. Acquired esotropia due to Arnold-Chiari I malformation. J Neuroophthalmol 1996;16:49–54.

377. Weeks CL, Hamed LM. Treatment of acute comitant esotropia in Chiari I malformation. Ophthalmology 1999;106:2368–2371.

378. Biousse V, Newman NJ, Petermann SH, et al. Isolated comitant esotropia and Chiari I malformation. Am J Ophthalmol 2000;130:216–220.

379. Defoort-Dhellemmes S, Denion E, Arndt CF, et al. Resolution of acute acquired comitant esotropia after suboccipital decompression for Chiari I malformation. Am J Ophthalmol 2002;133:723–725.

380. Liu GT, Hertle RW, Quinn GE, et al. Comitant esodeviation due to neurologic insult in children. J Am Assoc Pediatr Ophthalmol Strab 1997;1:143–146.

381. Lennerstrand G. Central motor control in concomitant strabismus. Graefes Arch Clin Exp Ophthalmol 1988;226:172–174.

382. Flynn JT. Problems in strabismus management. In: Transactions New Orleans Academy of Ophthalmology, pp 456. New York, Raven Press, 1986.

383. Jampolsky A. Ocular divergence mechanisms. Trans Am Ophthalmol Soc 1970;68:756–762.

384. Parlato CJ, Nelson LB, Harley RD. Cyclic strabismus. Ann Ophthalmol 1983;15:1126–1129.

385. Pillai P, Dhand UK. Cyclic esotropia with central nervous system disease: report of two cases. J Pediatr Ophthalmol Strabismus 1987;24:237–241.

386. Duane A. Congenital deficiency of abduction, associated with impairment of adduction, retraction movements, contraction of the palpebral fissure and oblique movements of the eye. [Reprinted in abridged form in Arch Ophthalmol 1996 114:1255–1257]. Arch Ophthalmol 1905;34:133–159.

387. Huber A. Electrophysiology of the retraction syndromes. Br J Ophthalmol 1974;58:293–300.

388. DeRespinis PA, Caputo AR, Wagner RS, et al. Duane's retraction syndrome. Surv Ophthalmol 1993;38:257–288.

389. Hotchkiss MG, Miller NR, Clark AW, et al. Bilateral Duane's retraction syndrome. A clinical-pathologic case report. Arch Ophthalmol 1980;98:870–874.

390. Miller NR, Kiel SM, Green WR, et al. Unilateral Duane's retraction syndrome (type 1). Arch Ophthalmol 1982;100:1468–1472.

391. Parsa CF, Grant PE, Dillon WP, et al. Absence of the abducens nerve in Duane syndrome verified by magnetic resonance imaging. Am J Ophthalmol 1998;125:399–401.

392. Kim JH, Hwang JM. Presence of the abducens nerve according to the type of Duane's retraction syndrome. Ophthalmology 2005;112:109–113.

393. Demer JL, Ortube MC, Engle EC, et al. High-resolution magnetic resonance imaging demonstrates abnormalities of motor nerves and extraocular muscles in patients with neuropathic strabismus. J AAPOS 2006;10:135–142.

394. Kang NY, Demer JL. Comparison of orbital magnetic resonance imaging in Duane syndrome and abducens palsy. Am J Ophthalmol 2006;142:827–834.

395. Appukuttan B, Gillanders E, Juo SH, et al. Localization of a gene for Duane retraction syndrome to chromosome 2q31. Am J Hum Genet 1999;65:1639–1646.

396. Miyake N, Chilton J, Psatha M, et al. Human CHN1 mutations hyperactivate alpha2-chimaerin and cause Duane's retraction syndrome. Science 2008;321:839–843.

397. Chung M, Stout JT, Borchert MS. Clinical diversity of hereditary Duane's retraction syndrome. Ophthalmology 2000;107:500–503.

398. Brodsky MC, Fray KJ. Brainstem hypoplasia in the Wildervanck (cervico-oculo-acoustic) syndrome. Arch Ophthalmol 1998;116:383–385.

399. Chew CKS, Foster P, Hurst JA, et al. Duane's retraction syndrome associated with chromosome 4q27–31 segment deletion. Am J Ophthalmol 1995;119:807–809.

400. Miller MT, Strömland K. Ocular motility in thalidomide embryopathy. J Pediatr Ophthalmol Strabismus 1991;28:47–54.

401. Yamanouchi H, Iwasaki Y, Sugai K, et al. Duane retraction syndrome associated with Chiari I malformation. Pediatr Neurol 1993;9:327–329.

402. Brodsky MC, Boop FA. Fourth ventricular ependymoma in a child with Duane retraction syndrome. Pediatr Neurosurg 1997;26:157–159.

403. Duane TD, Schatz NJ, Caputo AR. Pseudo-Duane's retraction syndrome. Trans Am Ophthalmol Soc 1976;74:122–129.

404. Rogers GL, Bremer DL. Surgical treatment of the upshoot and downshoot in Duane's retraction syndrome. Ophthalmology 1984;91:1380–1383.

405. Pressman SH, Scott WE. Surgical treatment of Duane's syndrome. Ophthalmology 1986;93:29–38.

406. Henderson JL. The congenital facial diplegia syndrome: clinical features, pathology, and etiology. Brain 1939;62:381–403.

407. Okamoto K, Hirai S, Amari M, et al. Oculomotor nuclear pathology in amyotrophic lateral sclerosis. Acta Neuropathol 1993;85:458–462.

408. Gruber H, Zeitlhofer J, Prager J, et al. Complex oculomotor dysfunctions in Kugelberg-Welander disease. Neuroophthalmology 1983;3:125–128.

409. Sima AAF, Caplan M, D'Amato CJ, et al. Fulminant multiple system atrophy in a young adult presenting as motor neuron disease. Neurology 1993;43:2031–2035.

410. Hamano K, Tsukamoto H, Yazawa T, et al. Infantile progressive spinal muscular atrophy with ophthalmoplegia and pyramidal symptoms. Pediatr Neurol 1994;10:320–324.

411. Thurtell MJ, Pioro EP, Leigh RJ. Abnormal eye movements in Kennedy disease. Neurology 2009;72:1528–1530.

412. Finsterer J. Leigh and Leigh-like syndrome in children and adults. Pediatr Neurol 2008;39:223–235.

413. Odaka M, Yuki N, Yamada M, et al. Bickerstaff's brainstem encephalitis: clinical features of 62 cases and a subgroup associated with Guillain-Barré syndrome. Brain 2003;126:2279–2290.

414. Jordan K, Marino J, Damast M, et al. Bilateral oculomotor paralysis due to neurosyphilis. Ann Neurol 1978;3:90–93.

415. Balm M, Hammack J. Leptomeningeal carcinomatosis. Presenting features and prognostic factors. Arch Neurol 1996;53:626–632.

416. Oostenbrugge V, Twijnstra A. Presenting features and value of diagnostic procedures in leptomeningeal metastases. Neurology 1999;53:382–385.

417. Galetta SL, Sergott RC, Wells GB, et al. Spontaneous remission of a third-nerve palsy in meningeal lymphoma. Ann Neurol 1992;32:100–102.

418. Liu GT, Kay MD, Byrne GE, et al. Ophthalmoparesis due to Burkitt's lymphoma following cardiac transplantation. Neurology 1993;43:2147–2149.

419. Bhatti MT, Schmalfuss IM, Eskin TA. Isolated cranial nerve III palsy as the presenting manifestation of HIV-related large B-cell lymphoma: clinical, radiological and postmortem observations: report of a case and review of the literature. Surv Ophthalmol 2005;50:598–606.

420. Newman NJ. Multiple cranial neuropathies: presenting signs of systemic lymphoma. Surv Ophthalmol 1992;37:125–129.

421. Diaz-Arrastia R, Younger DS, Hair L, et al. Neurolymphomatosis: a clinicopathologic syndrome re-emerges. Neurology 1992;42:1136–1141.

422. Arroyo JG, Horton JC. Acute, painful, pupil-sparing third nerve palsy in chronic inflammatory demyelinating polyneuropathy. Neurology 1995;45:846–847.

423. Pieh C, Rossillion B, Heritier-Barras AC, et al. Isolated unilateral adduction deficit and ptosis as the presenting features of chronic inflammatory demyelinating polyradiculoneuropathy. J Neuroophthalmol 2002;22:92–94.

424. Alwan AA, Mejico LJ. Ophthalmoplegia, proptosis, and lid retraction caused by cranial nerve hypertrophy in chronic inflammatory demyelinating polyradiculoneuropathy. J Neuroophthalmol 2007;27:99–103.

425. Yuki N, Odaka M, Hirata K. Acute ophthalmoparesis (without ataxia) associated with anti-GQ1b IgG antibody: clinical features. Ophthalmology 2001;108:196–200.

426. Lee SH, Lim GH, Kim JS, et al. Acute ophthalmoplegia (without ataxia) associated with anti-GQ1b antibody. Neurology 2008;71:426–429.

427. Yuki N. Acute paresis of extraocular muscles associated with anti IgG anti GQ₁b antibody. Ann Neurol 1996;39:668–672.

428. Reddel SW, Barnett MH, Yan WX, et al. Chronic ophthalmoplegia with anti-GQ1b antibody. Neurology 2000;54:1000–1002.

429. Yuki N. Successful plasmapheresis in Bickerstaff's brainstem encephalitis associated with anti GQ₁b antibody. J Neurol Sci 1995;131:108–110.

430. Chiba A, Kusunoki S, Obata H, et al. Serum anti-GQ₁b antibody is associated with ophthalmoplegia in Miller Fisher syndrome and Guillain-Barré syndrome. Clinical and immunohistochemical studies. Neurology 1993;43:1911–1917.

431. Al-Din ASN. The nosological position of the ophthalmoplegia ataxia and areflexia syndrome: "The spectrum hypothesis". Acta Neurol Scand 1987;75:287–294.

432. Cullom ME, Savino PJ. Adenocarcinoma of the prostate presenting as a third nerve palsy. Neurology 1993;43:2146–2147.

433. Carrizo A, Basso A. Current surgical treatment for sphenoorbital meningiomas. Surg Neurol 1998;50:574–578.

434. Mayberg MR, Symon L. Meningiomas of the clivus and apical petrous bone. J Neurosurg 1986;65:160–167.

435. Spallone A, Makhmudov UB, Mukhamedjanov DJ, et al. Petroclival meningioma. An attempt to define the role of skull base approaches in their surgical management. Surg Neurol 1999;51:412–419.

436. Subach BR, Lunsford LD, Kondziolka D, et al. Management of petroclival meningiomas by stereotactic radiosurgery. Neurosurgery 1998;42:437–443.

437. Mindell ER. Current concept review: chordoma. J Bone Joint Surg 1981;63:501–505.

438. Volpe NJ, Liebsch NJ, Munzenrider JE, et al. Neuro-ophthalmologic findings in chordoma and chondrosarcoma of the skull base. Am J Ophthalmol 1993;115:97–104.

439. Sze G, Uichanco LS, Brant-Zawadzki MN, et al. Chordomas: MR imaging. Radiology 1988;166:187–191.

440. al-Mefty O, Borba LAB. Skull base chordomas: a management challenge. J Neurosurg 1997;86:182–189.

441. Austin Seymour M, Munzenrider J, Goitein M, et al. Fractionated proton radiation therapy of chordoma and low-grade chondrosarcoma of the base of the skull. J Neurosurg 1989;70:13–17.

442. Korten AGGC, ter Berg HJ, Spincemaille GH, et al. Intracranial chondrosarcoma: review of the literature and report of 15 cases. J Neurol Neurosurg Psychiatry 1998;65:88–92.

443. Balcer LJ, Galetta SL, Cornblath WT, et al. Neuro-ophthalmologic manifestations of Maffucci's syndrome and Ollier's disease. J Neuroophthalmol 1999;19:62–66.

444. Myles WM, Maxner CE. Localizing value of concurrent sixth nerve paresis and postganglionic Horner's syndrome. Can J Ophthalmol 1994;29:39–42.

445. Sheldon JJ, Tobias J, Soila K. MRI of the cavernous sinus. In: Smith JL, Katz R (eds): Neuroophthalmology Enters the Nineties, pp 67–90. Hialeah, Dutton Press, 1988.

446. Keane JR. Cavernous sinus syndrome. Analysis of 151 cases. Arch Neurol 1996;53:967–971.

447. Trobe JD, Hood I, Parsons JT, et al. Intracranial spread of squamous carcinoma along the trigeminal nerve. Arch Ophthalmol 1982;100:608–611.

448. Neel HB. Nasopharyngeal carcinoma. Otolaryngol Clin North Am 1985;18:479–490.

449. Chong VF, Fan YF, Khoo JB. Nasopharyngeal carcinoma with intracranial spread: CT and MR characteristics. J Comput Assist Tomogr 1996;20:563–569.

450. Trautmann JC, Laws ER. Visual status after transsphenoidal surgery at the Mayo Clinic, 1971–1982. Am J Ophthalmol 1983;96:200–208.

451. Wykes WN. Prolactinoma presenting with intermittent third nerve palsy. Br J Ophthalmol 1986;70:706–707.

452. Turgut M, Palaoglu S, Akpinar G, et al. Giant schwannoma of the trigeminal nerve misdiagnosed as maxillary sinusitis. A case report. S Afr J Surg 1997;35:131–133.

453. Del Priore LV, Miller NR. Trigeminal schwannoma as a cause of chronic, isolated sixth nerve palsy. Am J Ophthalmol 1989;108:726–729.

454. Alonso PE, Bescansa E, Salas J, et al. Perineural spread of cutaneous squamous cell carcinoma manifesting as ptosis and ophthalmoplegia (orbital apex syndrome). Br J Plast Surg 1995;48:564–568.

455. Clouston PD, Sharpe DM, Corbett AJ, et al. Perineural spread of cutaneous head and neck cancer. Its orbital and central neurologic complications. Arch Neurol 1990;47:73–77.

456. Catalano PJ, Sen C, Biller HF. Cranial neuropathy secondary to perineural spread of cutaneous malignancies. Am J Otol 1995;16:772–777.

457. McNab AA, Francis IC, Berger R, et al. Perineural spread of cutaneous squamous cell carcinoma via the orbit. Ophthalmology 1997;104:1457–1462.

458. Phillips PH, Newman NJ. Here today … gone tomorrow. Surv Ophthalmol 1997;41:354–356.

459. O'Sullivan MG, van Loveren HR, Tew JM. The surgical resectability of meningiomas of the cavernous sinus. Neurosurgery 1997;40:238–245.

460. Braunstein JB, Vick NA. Meningiomas: the decision not to operate. Neurology 1997;48:1459–1462.

461. DeMonte F, Smith HK, Al-Mefty O. Outcome of aggressive removal of cavernous sinus meningiomas. J Neurosurg 1994;81:245–251.

462. De Jesús O, Sekhar LN, Parikh HK, et al. Long-term follow-up of patients with meningiomas involving the cavernous sinus: recurrence, progression, and quality of life. Neurosurgery 1996;39:915–919.

463. Knosp E, Perneczky A, Koos WT, et al. Meningiomas of the space of the cavernous sinus. Neurosurgery 1996;38:434–442.

464. Klink DF, Sampath P, Miller NR, et al. Long-term visual outcome after nonradical microsurgery in patients with parasellar and cavernous sinus meningiomas. Am J Ophthalmol 2000;130:689.

465. Kim DK, Grieve J, Archer DJ, et al. Meningiomas in the region of the cavernous sinus: a review of 21 patients. Br J Neurosurg 1996;10:439–444.

466. Kurita H, Sasaki T, Kawamoto S, et al. Role of radiosurgery in the management of cavernous sinus meningiomas. Acta Neurol Scand 1997;96:297–304.

467. Pendl G, Schrottner O, Eustacchio S, et al. Cavernous sinus meningiomas: what is the strategy: upfront or adjuvant gamma knife surgery? Stereotact Funct Neurosurg 1998;70:33–40.

468. Chang SD, Adler JR, Jr., Martin DP. LINAC radiosurgery for cavernous sinus meningiomas. Stereotact Funct Neurosurg 1998;71:43–50.

469. Case Records of the Massachusetts General Hospital. Case 4-1993. A 73-year-old man with severe facial pain, visual loss, decreased ocular motility, and an orbital mass. N Engl J Med 1993;328:266–275.

470. Lee AG, Quick SJ, Liu GT, et al. A childhood cavernous conundrum. Surv Ophthalmol 2004;49:231–236.

471. Agarwal P, Sharma K, Gupta RK, et al. Acute bilateral ophthalmoplegia secondary to metastatic prostatic carcinoma. J Neuroophthalmol 1995;15:45–47.

472. Kline LB. The Tolosa-Hunt syndrome. Surv Ophthalmol 1982;27:79–95.

473. Kline LB, Hoyt WF. The Tolosa-Hunt syndrome. J Neurol Neurosurg Psychiatry 2001;71:577–582.

474. Odabasi Z, Gokcil Z, Atilla S, et al. The value of MRI in a case of Tolosa-Hunt syndrome. Clin Neurol Neurosurg 1997;99:151–154.

475. Evans OB, Lexow SS. Painful ophthalmoplegia in systemic lupus erythematosus. Ann Neurol 1978;4:584–585.

476. Dávalos A, Matías-Guiu J, Codina A. Painful ophthalmoplegia in systemic lupus erythematosus [letter]. J Neurol Neurosurg Psychiatry 1984;47:323–324.

477. Gross FJ, Waxman JS, Rosenblatt MA, et al. Eosinophilic granuloma of the cavernous sinus and orbital apex in an HIV positive patient. Ophthalmology 1989;96:462–467.

478. Marsh RJ, Dulley B, Kelly V. External ocular motor palsies in ophthalmic zoster: a review. Br J Ophthalmol 1977;61:677–682.

479. Dinubile MJ. Septic thrombosis of the cavernous sinus. Arch Neurol 1988;45:567–572.

480. Geggel HS, Isenberg SJ. Cavernous sinus thrombosis as a cause of unilateral blindness. Ann Ophthalmol 1982;14:569–574.

481. Gupta A, Jalali S, Bansal RV, et al. Anterior ischemic optic neuropathy and branch retinal artery occlusion in cavernous sinus thrombosis. J Clin Neuroophthalmol 1990;10:193–196.

482. Southwick FS, Richardson EP, Jr., Swartz MN. Septic thrombosis of the dural venous sinuses. Medicine 1986;65:82–106.

483. Igarashi H, Igarashi S, Fujio N, et al. Magnetic resonance imaging in the early diagnosis of cavernous sinus thrombosis. Ophthalmologica 1995;209:292–296.

484. Visudtibhan A, Visudiphan P, Chiemchanya S. Cavernous sinus thrombophlebitis in children. Pediatr Neurol 2001;24:123–127.

485. Levine SR, Twyman RE, Gilman S. The role of anticoagulation in cavernous sinus thrombosis. Neurology 1988;38:517–522.

486. Bhatia K, Jones NS. Septic cavernous sinus thrombosis secondary to sinusitis: are anticoagulants indicated? A review of the literature. J Laryngol Otol 2002;116:667–676.

487. Bienfang DC, Karluk D. Case records of the Massachusetts General Hospital. Weekly clinicopathological exercises. Case 9-2002. An 80-year-old woman with sudden unilateral blindness. N Engl J Med 2002;346:924–929.

488. Galetta SL, Wulc AE, Goldberg H, et al. Rhinocerebral mucormycosis: management and survival after carotid occlusion. Ann Neurol 1990;28:103–107.

489. Kohn R, Helper R. Management of limited rhino-orbital mucormycosis without exenteration. Ophthalmology 1985;92:1440–1444.

490. Fleishman JA, Garfinkel RA, Beck RW. Advances in the treatment of carotid cavernous fistula. Int Ophthalmol Clin 1986;26:301–311.

491. Parkinson D. Carotid cavernous fistulas. Direct repair with preservation of the carotid artery: technical note. J Neurosurg 1973;38:99–106.

492. Barrow DL, Spector RH, Braun IF, et al. Classification and treatment of spontaneous carotid-cavernous sinus fistulas. J Neurosurg 1985;62:248–256.

493. Lewis AI, Tomsick TA, Tew JM, Jr. Management of 100 consecutive direct carotid-cavernous fistulas: results of treatment with detachable balloons. Neurosurgery 1995;36:239–245.

494. Takahashi M, Killeffer F, Wilson G. Iatrogenic carotid cavernous fistulas: case report. J Neurosurg 1969;30:498–500.

495. Pedersen RA, Troost TB, Schramm VL. Carotid-cavernous sinus fistula after external ethmoid-sphenoid surgery. Arch Otolaryngol 1981;107:307–309.

496. Kupersmith MJ, Berenstein A, Flamm E, et al. Neuro-ophthalmologic abnormalities and intravascular therapy of traumatic carotid cavernous fistulas. Ophthalmology 1986;93:906–912.

497. Hieshima GB, Cahan LD, Mehringer CM, et al. Spontaneous arteriovenous fistulas of cerebral vessels in association with fibromuscular dysplasia. Neurosurgery 1986;18:454–458.

498. Chuman H, Trobe JD, Petty EM, et al. Spontaneous direct carotid-cavernous fistula in Ehlers-Danlos syndrome type IV: two case reports and a review of the literature. J Neuroophthalmol 2002;22:75–81.

499. Koo AH, Newton TH. Pseudoxanthoma elasticum associated with carotid rate mirable. Am J Roentgenol Radium Ther Nucl Med 1972;116:16–22.

500. Kupersmith MJ, Berenstein A, Choi IS, et al. Management of nontraumatic vascular shunts involving the cavernous sinus. Ophthalmology 1988;95:121–130.

501. Spencer WH, Thompson HS, Hoyt WF. Ischaemic ocular necrosis from carotid-cavernous fistula: pathology of stagnant anoxic "inflammation" in orbital and ocular tissues. Br J Ophthalmol 1973;57:145–152.

502. Hedges TR, Debrun G, Sokol S. Reversible optic neuropathy from carotid cavernous fistula. J Clin Neuroophthalmol 1985;5:37–40.

503. Berk AT, Ada E, Kir E, et al. Choroidal detachment associated with direct spontaneous carotid-cavernous sinus fistula. Ophthalmologica 1997;211:53–55.

504. Golnik KC, Miller NR. Diagnosis of cavernous sinus arteriovenous fistula by measurement of ocular pulse amplitude. Ophthalmology 1992;99:1146–1152.

505. Moster MR, Kennerdell JS. B-scan ultrasonic evaluation of dilated superior ophthalmic vein in orbital and retro-orbital arteriovenous anomalies. J Clin Neuroophthalmol 1983;3:105–198.

506. Debrun GM, Nauta HJ, Miller NR, et al. Combining the detachable balloon technique and surgery in imaging carotid cavernous fistulae. Surg Neurol 1989;32:3–10.

507. Barnwell SL, O'Neill OR. Endovascular therapy of carotid cavernous fistulas. Neurosurg Clin N Am 1994;5:485–495.

508. Gemmete JJ, Ansari SA, Gandhi DM. Endovascular techniques for treatment of carotid-cavernous fistula. J Neuroophthalmol 2009;29:62–71.

509. Kwan E, Heishima GB, Higashida RT, et al. Interventional neuroradiology in neuro-ophthalmology. J Clin Neuroophthalmol 1989;9:83–97.

510. Debrun GM, Vinuela F, Fox AJ, et al. Indications for treatment and classification of 132 carotid-cavernous fistulas. Neurosurgery 1988;22:285–289.

511. Halbach VV, Higashida RT, Hieshima GB, et al. Transvenous embolization of direct carotid cavernous fistulas. AJNR Am J Neuroradiol 1988;9:741–746.

512. Miller NR, Monsein LH, Debrun GM, et al. Treatment of carotid-cavernous sinus fistulas using a superior ophthalmic vein approach. J Neurosurg 1995;83:838–842.

513. Leonard TJ, Moseley IF, Sanders MD. Ophthalmoplegia in carotid cavernous sinus fistula. Br J Ophthalmol 1984;68:128–134.

514. Rizzo M, Bosch EP, Gross CE. Trigeminal sensory neuropathy due to dural external carotid-cavernous sinus fistula. Neurology 1982;32:89–91.

515. Hawke SHB, Mullie MA, Hoyt WF, et al. Painful oculomotor palsy due to dural-cavernous sinus shunt. Arch Neurol 1989;46:1252–1255.

516. Miyachi S, Negoro M, Handa T, et al. Dural carotid cavernous sinus fistula presenting as isolated oculomotor nerve palsy. Surg Neurol 1993;39:105–109.

517. Brazis PW, Capobianco DJ, Chang FLF, et al. Low flow dural arteriovenous shunt: another cause of "sinister" Tolosa-Hunt syndrome. Headache 1994;34:523–525.

518. Acierno MD, Trobe JD, Cornblath WT, et al. Painful oculomotor palsy caused by posterior-draining dural carotid cavernous fistulas. Arch Ophthalmol 1995;113:1045–1049.

519. Uehara T, Tabuchi M, Kawaguchi T, et al. Spontaneous dural carotid cavernous sinus fistula presenting isolated ophthalmoplegia: evaluation with MR angiography. Neurology 1998;50:814–816.

520. Stiebel-Kalish H, Setton A, Nimii Y, et al. Cavernous sinus dural arteriovenous malformations: patterns of venous drainage are related to clinical signs and symptoms. Ophthalmology 2002;109:1685–1691.

521. DeKeizer RJW. Spontaneous carotid-cavernous fistulas. The importance of the typical limbal vascular loops for the diagnosis, the recognition of glaucoma and the uses of conservative therapy in this condition. Doc Ophthalmol 1979;46:403–412.

522. Phelps CD, Thompson HS, Ossoinig KC. The diagnosis and prognosis of atypical carotid-cavernous fistula (red-eyed shunt syndrome). Am J Ophthalmol 1982;93:423–426.

523. Keltner JL, Gittinger JW, Miller NR, et al. A red eye and high intraocular pressure. Surv Ophthalmol 1986;31:328–336.

524. Keltner JL, Satterfield D, Dublin AB, et al. Dural and carotid cavernous sinus fistulas: diagnosis, management and complications. Ophthalmology 1987;94:1585–1600.

525. Fiore PM, Latina MA, Shingleton BJ, et al. The dural shunt syndrome. I. Management of glaucoma. Ophthalmology 1990;97:56–62.

526. Sergott RC, Grossman RI, Savino PJ, et al. The syndrome of paradoxical worsening of dural-cavernous sinus arteriovenous malformations. Ophthalmology 1987;94:205–212.

527. Harbison JW, Guerry D, Weisinger H. Dural arteriovenous fistula and spontaneous choroidal detachment: new cause of an old disease. Br J Ophthalmol 1978;62:483–490.

528. Jorgensen JS, Gutthoff RF. 24 cases of carotid cavernous fistulas: frequency, symptoms, diagnosis and treatment. Acta Ophthalmol 1985;63:67–71.

529. Brunette I, Boghen D. Central retinal vein occlusion complicating spontaneous carotid-cavernous fistula. Arch Ophthalmol 1987;105:464–465.

530. Garg SJ, Regillo CD, Aggarwal S, et al. Macular exudative retinal detachment in a patient with a dural cavernous sinus fistula. Arch Ophthalmol 2006;124:1201–1202.

531. Kupersmith MJ, Vargas EM, Warren F, et al. Venous obstruction as the cause of retinal/choroidal dysfunction associated with arteriovenous shunts in the cavernous sinus. J Neuroophthalmol 1996;16:1–6.

532. DeKeizer RJW. Spontaneous carotid cavernous fistulas. Neuroophthalmology 1981;2:35–46.

533. Fourman S. Acute closed-angle glaucoma after arteriovenous fistulas. Am J Ophthalmol 1989;107:156–159.

534. Harris GJ, Rice PR. Angle closure in carotid-cavernous fistula. Ophthalmology 1979;86:1521–1529.

535. Selky AK, Purvin VA. Isolated trochlear nerve palsy secondary to dural carotid-cavernous sinus fistula. J Neuroophthalmol 1994;14:52–54.

536. Hirabuki N, Miura T, Mitomo M, et al. MR imaging of dural arteriovenous malformations with ocular signs. Neuroradiology 1988;30:390–394.

537. Vinuela F, Fox AJ, Debrun GM, et al. Spontaneous carotid cavernous fistulas: clinical, radiological and therapeutic considerations. J Neurosurg 1984;60:976–984.

538. Luciani A, Houdart E, Mounayer C, et al. Spontaneous closure of dural arteriovenous fistulas: report of three cases and review of the literature. AJNR Am J Neuroradiol 2001;22:992–996.

539. Bhatia KD, Wang L, Parkinson RJ, et al. Successful treatment of six cases of indirect carotid-cavernous fistula with ethylene vinyl alcohol copolymer (Onyx) transvenous embolization. J Neuroophthalmol 2009;29:3–8.

540. Goldberg RA, Goldey SH, Duckwiler G, et al. Management of cavernous sinus-dural fistulas. Indications and techniques for primary embolization via the superior ophthalmic vein. Arch Ophthalmol 1996;114:707–714.

541. Gandhi D, Ansari SA, Cornblath WT. Successful transarterial embolization of a Barrow type D dural carotid-cavernous fistula with ethylene vinyl alcohol copolymer (Onyx). J Neuroophthalmol 2009;29:9–12.

542. Bito S, Hasegawa H, Fujiwara M, et al. Irradiation of spontaneous carotid-cavernous fistulas. Surg Neurol 1982;17:282–286.

543. Guo WY, Pan DH, Wu HM, et al. Radiosurgery as a treatment alternative for dural arteriovenous fistulas of the cavernous sinus. AJNR Am J Neuroradiol 1998;19:1081–1087.

544. Locksley HB. Natural history of subarachnoid hemorrhage, intracranial aneurysm and arteriovenous malformations. J Neurosurg 1966;25:219–239.

545. Barr HWR, Blackwood W, Meadows SP. Intracavernous carotid aneurysms a clinical pathological report. Brain 1971;94:607–622.

546. Hahn CD, Nicolle DA, Lownie SP, et al. Giant cavernous carotid aneurysms: clinical presentation in fifty-seven cases. J Neuroophthalmol 2000;20:253–258.

547. Linskey ME, Sekhar LN, Hirsch WL, Jr., et al. Aneurysms of the intracavernous carotid artery: natural history and indications for treatment. Neurosurgery 1990;26:933–937.

548. Berenstein A, Ransohoff J, Kupersmith M, et al. Endovascular treatment of giant aneurysms of the carotid and vertebral arteries. Functional investigation and embolization. Surg Neurol 1984;21:3–12.

549. Nelson PK, Levy D, Masters LT, et al. Neuro-endovascular management of intracranial aneurysms. Neuroimag Clin North Am 1997;7:739–762.

550. Halbach VV, Higashida RT, Dowd CF, et al. Cavernous internal carotid artery aneurysms treated with electrolytically detachable coils. J Neuroophthalmol 1997;17:231–239.

551. Kupersmith MT, Berenstein A, Choi IS, et al. Percutaneous transvascular treatment of giant carotid aneurysms: neuro-ophthalmologic findings. Neurology 1984;34:328–335.

552. Engle EC, Marondel I, Houtman WA, et al. Congenital fibrosis of the extraocular muscles (autosomal dominant congenital external ophthalmoplegia): genetic homogeneity, linkage refinement, and physical mapping on chromosome 12. Am J Hum Genet 1995;57:1086–1094.

553. Wang SM, Zwaan J, Mullaney PB, et al. Congenital fibrosis of the extraocular muscles type 2, an inherited exotropic strabismus fixus, maps to distal 11q13. Am J Hum Genet 1998;63:517–525.

554. Doherty EJ, Macy ME, Wang WM, et al. CFEOM3: a new extraocular congenital fibrosis syndrome that maps to 16q24.2-q24.3. Invest Ophthalmol Vis Sci 1999;40:1687–1694.

555. Brodsky MC. Hereditary external ophthalmoplegia, synergistic divergence, jaw winking, and oculocutaneous hypopigmentation. Ophthalmology 1998;105:717–725.

556. Kim JH, Hwang JM. Hypoplastic oculomotor nerve and absent abducens nerve in congenital fibrosis syndrome and synergistic divergence with magnetic resonance imaging. Ophthalmology 2005;112:728–732.

557. Engle EC, Goumnerov BC, McKeown CA, et al. Oculomotor nerve and muscle abnormalities in congenital fibrosis of the extraocular muscles. Ann Neurol 1997;41:314–325.

558. Engle EC. Oculomotility disorders arising from disruptions in brainstem motor neuron development. Arch Neurol 2007;64:633–637.

559. Yamada K, Hunter DG, Andrews C, et al. A novel KIF21A mutation in a patient with congenital fibrosis of the extraocular muscles and Marcus Gunn jaw-winking phenomenon. Arch Ophthalmol 2005;123:1254–1259.

560. Bosley TM, Oystreck DT, Robertson RL, et al. Neurological features of congenital fibrosis of the extraocular muscles type 2 with mutations in PHOX2A. Brain 2006;129:2363–2374.

561. Nakano M, Yamada K, Fain J, et al. Homozygous mutations in ARIX(PHOX2A) result in congenital fibrosis of the extraocular muscles type 2. Nat Genet 2001;29:315–320.

562. Yazdani A, Chung DC, Abbaszadegan MR, et al. A novel PHOX2A/ARIX mutation in an Iranian family with congenital fibrosis of extraocular muscles type 2 (CFEOM2). Am J Ophthalmol 2003;136:861–865.

563. Mohney BG. Common forms of childhood strabismus in an incidence cohort. Am J Ophthalmol 2007;144:465–467.

564. Greenberg AE, Mohney BG, Diehl NN, et al. Incidence and types of childhood esotropia: a population-based study. Ophthalmology 2007;114:170–174.

565. Donahue SP. Clinical practice. Pediatric strabismus. N Engl J Med 2007;356: 1040–1047.

566. Pollard ZF, Greenberg MF. 20 unusual presentations of accommodative esotropia. J AAPOS 2002;6:33–39.

567. Simon AL, Borchert M. Etiology and prognosis of acute, late-onset esotropia. Ophthalmology 1997;104:1348–1352.

568. Mohney BG. Acquired nonaccommodative esotropia in childhood. J AAPOS 2001;5: 85–89.

569. Nelson LB. Diagnosis and management of strabismus and amblyopia. Pediatr Clin N Am 1983;30:1003–1014.

570. Hunter DG, Ellis FJ. Prevalence of systemic and ocular disease in infantile exotropia. Comparison with infantile esotropia. Ophthalmology 1999;106:1951–1956.

571. Wilson ME, Eustis HS, Parks MM. Brown's syndrome. Surv Ophthalmol 1989;34:153–172.

572. Thorne JE, Volpe NJ, Liu GT. Magnetic resonance imaging of acquired Brown syndrome in a patient with psoriasis. Am J Ophthalmol 1999;127:233–234.

573. Pandey PK, Chaudhuri Z, Bhatia A. Extraocular muscle cysticercosis presenting as Brown syndrome. Am J Ophthalmol 2001;131:526–527.

574. Talebnejad MR, Lankaranian D, Warrian K, et al. Osteochondroma of the trochlea presenting as acquired Brown syndrome: a case report. J AAPOS 2007;11:305–306.

575. Gregersen E, Rindziunski E. Brown's syndrome. A longitudinal study of spontaneous course. Acta Ophthalmol 1993;71:371–376.

576. Helveston E. Dissociated vertical deviation: a clinical and laboratory study. Trans Am Ophthalmol Soc 1980;78:734–779.

577. Harcourt B, Mein J, Johnson F. Natural history and associations of dissociated vertical divergence. Trans Ophthal Soc UK 1980;100:495–497.

578. Noel LP, Parks MM. Dissociated vertical deviation: associated findings and results of surgical treatment. Can J Ophthalmol 1982;17:10–12.

579. Cheeseman EW, Guyton DL. Vertical fusional vergence. The key to dissociated vertical deviation. Arch Ophthalmol 1999;117:1188–1191.

580. Brodsky MC. Dissociated vertical divergence. A righting reflex gone wrong. Arch Ophthalmol 1999;117:1216–1222.

581. Freedman HL, Kushner BJ. Congenital ocular aberrant innervation: new concepts. J Pediatr Ophthalmol Strabismus 1997;34:10–16.

582. Lai T, Chen C, Selva D. Bilateral congenital trigemino-abducens synkinesis. Arch Ophthalmol 2003;121:1796–1797.

583. Lacey B, Chang W, Rootman J. Nonthyroid causes of extraocular muscle disease. Surv Ophthalmol 1999;44:187–213.

584. Glaser JS. Myasthenic pseudo-internuclear ophthalmoplegia. Arch Ophthalmol 1966;75:363–366.

585. Weinberg DA, Lesser RL, Vollmer TL. Ocular myasthenia: a protean disorder. Surv Ophthalmol 1994;39:169–210.

586. Schmidt D. Signs in ocular myasthenia and pseudomyasthenia. Differential diagnostic criteria. A clinical review. Neuroophthalmology 1995;15:21–58.

587. Bandini F, Faga D, Simonetti S. Ocular myasthenia mimicking a one-and-a-half syndrome. J Neuroophthalmol 2001;21:210–211.

588. Tein I, Haslam RHA, Rhead WJ, et al. Short-chain acyl-CoA dehydrogenase deficiency. A cause of ophthalmoplegia and multicore myopathy. Neurology 1999;52:366–372.

589. Scelsa SN, Simpson DM, Reichler BD, et al. Extraocular muscle involvement in Becker muscular dystrophy. Neurology 1996;46:564–566.

590. Wright RA, Plant GT, Landon DN, et al. Nemaline myopathy: an unusual cause of ophthalmoparesis. J Neuroophthalmol 1997;17:39–43.

591. Barricks ME, Traviesa DB, Glaser JS, et al. Ophthalmoplegia in cranial arteritis. Brain 1977;100:209–221.

592. Mehler MF, Rabinowich L. The clinical neuro-ophthalmologic spectrum of temporal arteritis. Am J Med 1988;85:839–843.

593. Hayreh SS, Podhajsky PA, Zimmerman B. Ocular manifestations of giant cell arteritis. Am J Ophthalmol 1998;125:509–520.

594. Hamed LM. Strabismus presenting after cataract surgery. Ophthalmology 1991;98: 247–252.

595. Wylie J, Henderson M, Doyle M, et al. Persistent binocular diplopia following cataract surgery: aetiology and management. Eye 1994;8:543–546.

596. McDonnell PJ, Spalton DJ, Falcon MG. Decentration of the posterior chamber lens implant: the effect of optic size on the incidence of visual aberrations. Eye 1990;4:132–137.

597. Pratt-Johnson JA, Tillson G. Intractable diplopia after vision restoration in unilateral cataract. Am J Ophthalmol 1989;107:23–26.

598. Sharkey JA, Sellar PW. Acquired central fusion disruption following cataract extraction. J Pediatr Ophthalmol Strabismus 1994;31:391–393.

599. Hamed LM, Lingua RW. Thyroid eye disease presenting after cataract surgery. J Pediatr Ophthalmol Strabismus 1990;27:10–15.

600. Johnson DA. Persistent vertical binocular diplopia after cataract surgery. Am J Ophthalmol 2001;132:831–835.

601. Rainin EA, Carlson BM. Postoperative diplopia and ptosis. A clinical hypothesis based on the myotoxicity of local anesthetics. Arch Ophthalmol 1985;103:1337–1339.

602. Carlson BM, Emerick S, Komorowski TE, et al. Extraocular muscle regeneration in primates. Local anesthetic-induced lesions. Ophthalmology 1992;99:582–589.

603. Spierer A, Schwalb E. Superior oblique muscle paresis after sub-Tenon's anesthesia for cataract surgery. J Cataract Refract Surg 1999;25:144–145.

604. Hamed LM, Mancuso A. Inferior rectus muscle contracture syndrome after retrobulbar anesthesia. Ophthalmology 1991;98:1506–1512.

605. Muñoz M. Inferior rectus muscle overaction after cataract extraction. Am J Ophthalmol 1994;118:664–666.

606. Hunter DG, Lam GC, Guyton DL. Inferior oblique muscle injury from local anesthesia for cataract surgery. Ophthalmology 1995;102:501–509.

607. Capó H, Guyton DL. Ipsilateral hypertropia after cataract surgery. Ophthalmology 1996;103:721–730.

608. Capó H, Roth E, Johnson T, et al. Vertical strabismus after cataract surgery. Ophthalmology 1996;103:918–921.

609. Kim JH, Hwang JM. Imaging of the superior rectus in superior rectus overaction after retrobulbar anesthesia. Ophthalmology 2006;113:1681–1684.

610. Phillips PH, Guyton DL, Hunter DG. Superior oblique overaction from local anesthesia for cataract surgery. J AAPOS 2001;5:329–332.

611. Esswein MB, von Noorden GK. Paresis of a vertical rectus muscle after cataract extraction. Am J Ophthalmol 1993;116:424–430.

612. Borchert MS, Lessell S, Hoyt WF. Hemifield slide diplopia from altitudinal visual field defects. J Neuroophthalmol 1996;16:107–109.

613. Hoyt WF, Keane JR. Superior oblique myokymia. Report and discussion on five cases of benign intermittent uniocular microtremor. Arch Ophthalmol 1970;84:461–467.

614. Thurston SE, Saul RF. Superior oblique myokymia: quantitative description of the eye movement. Neurology 1991;41:1679–1681.

615. Rosenberg ML, Glaser JS. Superior oblique myokymia. Ann Neurol 1983;13:667–669.

616. Brazis PW, Miller NR, Henderer JD, et al. The natural history and results of treatment of superior oblique myokymia. Arch Ophthalmol 1994;112:1063–1067.

617. Lee JP. Superior oblique myokymia. A possible etiologic factor. Arch Ophthalmol 1984;102:1178–1179.

618. Morrow M, Sharpe JA, Ranalli PJ. Superior oblique myokymia associated with a posterior fossa tumor: oculographic correlation with an idiopathic case. Neurology 1990;40:367–370.

619. Leigh RJ, Tomsak RL, Seidman SH, et al. Superior oblique myokymia: quantitative characteristics of the eye movements in three patients. Arch Ophthalmol 1991;109:1710–1713.

620. Mehta AM, Demer JL. Magnetic resonance imaging of the superior oblique muscle in superior oblique myokymia. J Pediatr Ophthalmol Strabismus 1994;31:378–383.

621. Susac JO, Smith JL, Schatz NJ. Superior oblique myokymia. Arch Neurol 1973;29:432–434.

622. Williams PE, Purvin VA, Kawasaki A. Superior oblique myokymia: efficacy of medical treatment. J AAPOS 2007;11:254–257.

623. Tyler TD, Ruiz RS. Propranolol in the treatment of superior oblique myokymia. Arch Ophthalmol 1990;108:175–186.

624. Deokule S, Burdon M, Matthews T. Superior oblique myokymia improved with gabapentin [letter]. J Neuroophthalmol 2004;24:95–96.

625. Samii M, Rosahl SK, Carvalho GA, et al. Microvascular decompression for superior oblique myokymia: first experience. Case report. J Neurosurg 1998;89:1020–1024.

626. Hashimoto M, Ohtsuka K, Suzuki Y, et al. Superior oblique myokymia caused by vascular compression. J Neuroophthalmol 2004;24:237–239.

627. Shults WT, Hoyt WF, Behrens M, et al. Ocular neuromyotonia: a clinical description of six patients. Arch Ophthalmol 1986;104:1028–1034.

628. Lessell S, Lessell I, Rizzo JF. Ocular neuromyotonia after radiation therapy. Am J Ophthalmol 1986;102:766–770.

629. Morrow MJ, Kao GW, Arnold AC. Bilateral ocular neuromyotonia: oculographic correlations. Neurology 1996;46:264–266.

630. Barroso L, Hoyt WF. Episodic exotropia from lateral rectus neuromyotonia — appearance and remission after radiation therapy for a thalamic glioma. J Pediatr Ophthalmol Strabismus 1993;30:56–57.

631. Haupert CL, Newman NJ. Ocular neuromyotonia 18 years after radiation therapy. Arch Ophthalmol 1997;115:1331–1332.

632. Yee RD, Purvin VA. Ocular neuromyotonia: three case reports with eye movement recordings. J Neuroophthalmol 1998;18:1–8.

633. Frohman EM, Zee DS. Ocular neuromyotonia: clinical features, physiological mechanisms, and response to therapy. Ann Neurol 1995;37:620–626.

634. Safran AB, Magistris M. Terminating attacks of ocular neuromyotonia. J Neuroophthalmol 1998;18:47–48.

635. Chung SM, Lee AG, Holds JB, et al. Ocular neuromyotonia in Graves dysthyroid orbitopathy. Arch Ophthalmol 1997;115:365–370.

636. Ezra E, Spalton D, Sanders MD, et al. Ocular neuromyotonia. Br J Ophthalmol 1996;80:350–355.

549

637. Jacob M, Vighetto A, Bernard M, et al. Ocular neuromyotonia secondary to a cavernous sinus meningioma. Neurology 2006;66:1598–1599.

638. Harrison AR, Wirtshafter JD. Ocular neuromyotonia in a patient with cavernous sinus thrombosis secondary to mucormycosis. Am J Ophthalmol 1997;124: 122–123.

639. Banks MC, Caruso PA, Lessell S. Midbrain-thalamic ocular neuromyotonia. Arch Ophthalmol 2005;123:118–119.

640. Aydin P, Kansu T, Sanac AS. High myopia causing bilateral abduction deficiency. J Clin Neuroophthalmol 1992;12:163–165.

641. Krzizok TH, Kaufman H, Traupe H. Elucidation of restrictive motility in high myopia by magnetic resonance imaging. Arch Ophthalmol 1997;115:1019–1027.

642. Krzizok TH, Schroeder BU. Measurement of recti eye muscle paths by magnetic resonance imaging in highly myopic and normal subjects. Invest Ophthalmol Vis Sci 1999;40:2554–2560.

643. Kushner BJ. Fixation switch diplopia. Arch Ophthalmol 1995;113:896–899.

644. Worthington JM, Halmagyi GM. Bilateral total ophthalmoplegia due to midbrain hematoma. Neurology 1996;46:1176.

645. Keane JR. Acute bilateral ophthalmoplegia: 60 cases. Neurology 1986;36:279–281.

646. Laskowitz D, Liu GT, Galetta SL. Acute visual loss and other disorders of the eyes. Neurol Clin N Am 1998;16:323–353.

647. Keane JR. Bilateral ocular paralysis: analysis of 31 inpatients. Arch Neurol 2007;64:178–180.

CHAPTER **16**

Eye movement disorders: conjugate gaze abnormalities

This chapter will cover eye movement disorders that are characterized by intact alignment, but the eyes have either restricted motility, move too slowly, or are misdirected. In neuro-ophthalmic terminology, these include horizontal and vertical conjugate gaze limitations, voluntary smooth pursuit and saccadic deficits, and involuntary conjugate gaze deviations.

These conditions tend to result from impaired supranuclear input upon the ocular motor nuclei. Thus, for the most part, third, fourth, and sixth nerve function, as well the oculocephalic and oculovestibular reflexes, are intact except in the situations noted. In contrast, the reader will find disorders in which the eyes tend to be misaligned are covered in Chapters 15 and 18. In Chapter 17, conditions characterized by excessive or inaccurate saccades are reviewed.

Types of conjugate eye movements

Definitions

The four major types of conjugate eye movements include saccades, pursuit, the vestibulo-ocular reflex, and optokinetic nystagmus (**Table 16–1**).[1] Because saccadic and pursuit abnormalities constitute the majority of the voluntary conjugate gaze abnormalities, they will be emphasized in this chapter, and their anatomy and physiology will be discussed in great detail. The vestibulo-ocular reflex and optokinetic nystagmus, deficits of which are typically not considered conjugate gaze abnormalities, will be alluded to throughout this chapter because of their close relationship with saccadic and pursuit function. However, they are discussed in more detail elsewhere (Chapter 17).

Saccades. Saccades are fast conjugate eye movements designed to refixate both foveas on a novel target (see **Fig. 2–27**). They have a peak velocity of up to 700 degrees per second.[2] There are several subtypes of saccades.[3] *Voluntary* saccades are intended eye movements toward a remembered target or during a search. *Reflexive* saccades occur in response to the sudden appearance of a new target in the retinal periphery or to a sudden noise. *Spontaneous* saccades, which may occur during speech or at rest during the darkness, have no particular goal. The saccadic system also supplements smooth pursuit by compensating for differences in target and foveal positions.[4]

Pursuit. On the other hand, smooth pursuit eye movements maintain both foveas conjugately on a slowly moving visual target (see **Fig. 2–26**). The goal of the pursuit system is to generate eye velocities which are similar to the target speed. Accurate pursuit can be achieved if the target is moving at less than 50 degrees per second.[2]

Vestibulo-ocular reflex. These eye movements stabilize a retinal image during head movement. The oculocephalic maneuver (see **Fig. 2–28**), elicited by moving the patient's head while asking him or her to maintain fixation, utilizes this reflex. Ice water irrigation of the ears (cold caloric testing) directly tests the vestibulo-ocular reflex (see **Fig. 2–41**).

Table 16–1 The five different types of eye movements and their supranuclear control. Saccades, pursuit, the vestibulo-ocular reflex, and optokinetic nystagmus are conjugate eye movements, while vergences are dysconjugate (e.g., convergence and divergence). All five types have as their final common output signals to the extraocular muscles from the third, fourth, and sixth nerve nuclei

Eye movement type	Purpose	Important supranuclear structure(s)	Important supranuclear structure receives major input from
1. Saccades	Rapid gaze shift	Omnipause neurons; Parapontine reticular formation (PPRF) Rostral interstitial nucleus of the medial longitudinal fasciculus (riMLF) Interstitial nucleus of Cajal (inC)	Cortical eye fields Superior colliculus
2. Pursuit	Follow a slowly moving object	Vestibular nuclei inC	Frontal and supplementary eye fields Occipito-temporal-parietal area (v5) Pontine nuclei Cerebellum
3. Vestibulo-ocular reflex	Coordinate eye position during head movements	Vestibular nuclei inC	Semicircular canals
4. Optokinetic nystagmus	Coordinate eye movements when environment moves	Vestibular nuclei	Occipito-parietal pursuit area and accessory optic nuclei
5. Vergence	Foveation	Pretectum; pons	? Cortex

Optokinetic nystagmus. A slow pursuit eye movement followed by a fast corrective saccade occurs when the surrounding visual field moves over the retina. Optokinetic nystagmus is readily seen at the bedside when small targets are moved in front of the patient's eyes (see **Fig. 2–30**).

Symptoms

Most patients with conjugate gaze abnormalities offer only vague visual complaints such as blurriness or dizziness.[5] Those with downgaze palsies may complain that they are unable to read or go down steps, but such patients are usually unaware that the problem stems from an inability to look down. Similarly, those with conjugate upgaze pareses might say they have trouble seeing bookshelves or other objects above eye level. We have seen a patient whose hydrocephalus manifested with difficulty playing basketball because he had trouble looking at the basket. Few actually complain that they are unable to look sideways or vertically although exceptions occur. Some are visually asymptomatic, and the ocular motility deficit is detected on examination.

Examination

Smooth pursuit can be tested at the bedside by having the patient follow a slowly moving target with both eyes. Optokinetic testing and suppression of the vestibulo-ocular reflex by visual fixation are two other ocular motor functions related to smooth pursuit eye movements. The relative speed and accuracy of saccades can be evaluated during refixation from eccentric gaze to a central target. Spontaneous saccades during the history-taking should also be observed. Chapter 2 also reviews these examination techniques, with figures, for testing conjugate gaze.

When pursuit is defective, it can either be slow, interrupted by catch-up saccades as in "saccadic pursuit," or limited. In such patients, pursuit of optokinetic targets may be slow and refixation saccades are absent. Failure of suppressing the vestibulo-ocular response may be evident when slippage of the eyes with corrective saccades occurs (**Fig. 2–29**).

Defective saccades are often characterized by slow velocities which cannot be mimicked by individuals with normal ocular motor systems. Some patients with defective saccades will use a compensatory head thrust in an attempt to shift gaze (see Ocular motor apraxia, below). When saccades are completely absent, a conjugate gaze palsy results. Sometimes the fast phase of optokinetic nystagmus is noted to be defective. The supranuclear nature of some pursuit and saccadic deficits can be proven by enhancing the ocular excursions with oculocephalic and vestibulo-ocular maneuvers.

The remainder of the neuro-ophthalmic and neurologic examinations should be used to screen for cortical deficits such as aphasia or hemianopia, and brain stem and cerebellar abnormalities such as facial palsies or incoordination. Finally, evidence of a degenerative process such as bradykinesia, tremor, or chorea, should be excluded.

Approach

One method for distinguishing supranuclear conjugate gaze disorders is to divide them into those that cause primarily horizontal versus vertical defects although there is considerable overlap (**Tables 16–2 to 16–5**). Those that are in the

Table 16–2 Etiologies of horizontal conjugate gaze deficits

Cortical lesions
  Frontal eye fields: saccades
  Occipito-parietal junction: pursuit
  Acquired ocular motor apraxia
Pontine lesions
  Paramedian pontine reticular formation
  Sixth nerve nucleus
  One-and-a-half syndrome
Other brain stem lesions
Congenital ocular motor apraxia
Other neurologic diseases
  Ataxia-telangiectasia*
  Inherited spinocerebellar ataxias*
  Multisystem atrophy
  Huntington disease
  Parkinson disease
  Corticobasal ganglionic degeneration
  Gaucher disease*
  Wernicke's encephalopathy and Leigh disease
Drugs

*Disorders whose ocular motility abnormality may mimic congenital ocular
  motor apraxia.

Table 16–3 Etiologies of abnormal horizontal conjugate
gaze deviations

Hemispheric lesions
  Frontal eye field
  Neglect, hemianopia
Seizures
Thalamic lesions
Brain stem lesions
  Pontine
  Medullary
Periodic alternating gaze deviation
  "Ping-pong" gaze

Table 16–4 Etiologies of vertical conjugate gaze deficits

Pretectal syndrome
  Paramedian midbrain-thalamic stroke
  Pineal region and thalamic masses
  Hydrocephalus
Midbrain downgaze paresis
Limitation of upgaze in elderly
Other neurologic disorders
  Progressive supranuclear palsy
  Niemann–Pick disease*
  Whipple disease
  Amyotrophic lateral sclerosis

*Disorders whose ocular motility abnormality may mimic congenital ocular
  motor apraxia.

Table 16–5 Etiologies of abnormal vertical conjugate
gaze deviations

Oculogyric crises
Ocular tics
Benign, tonic form in infancy
  Upward
  Downward
Pretectal syndrome

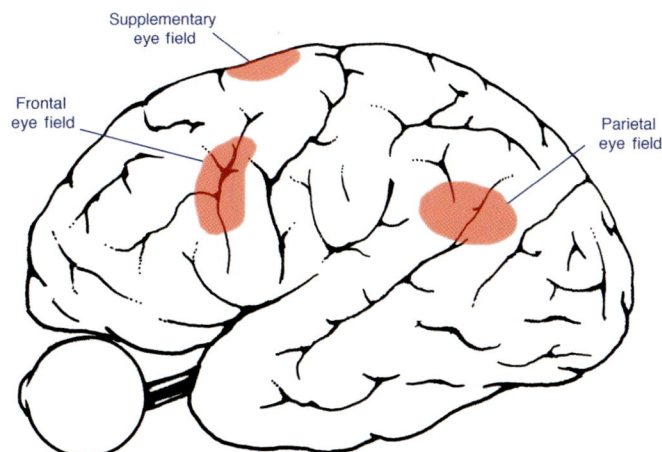

Figure 16–1. Drawing of the brain, lateral view of the left hemisphere, depicting the cortical areas which may generate saccades. These include the frontal, supplementary, and parietal eye fields.

and saccadic abnormalities are related, they are discussed below (Gaze deficits). When supranuclear gaze defects in all directions are present, the cause is often a degenerative neurologic disorder.

Horizontal conjugate gaze: neuroanatomy

Saccades

The major cortical control of horizontal saccadic eye movements, especially intentional ones, lies in the frontal eye fields (Brodmann area 8).[6] Each hemisphere has a frontal eye field located in the posterior portion of the second frontal gyrus and the adjacent part of the precentral gyrus and sulcus (**Fig. 16–1**). In one study[7] of awake patients evaluated with subdural electrodes for epilepsy surgery, electrical stimulation of the frontal eye fields caused contralateral horizontal conjugate eye movements in all patients. The ocular deviation was usually saccadic and accompanied by head versions. Two other cortical areas (**Fig. 16–1**) are capable of triggering other types of saccades: (1) the supplementary eye field in the supplementary motor area of the frontal lobe is important for generating saccades coordinated with head or body movements or motor programs involving several successive saccades[8,9] and (2) the parietal eye field, located in the posterior parietal cortex, is instrumental in producing reflexive saccades to visual targets.[3,10,11]

horizontal plane tend to localize to cerebral cortex or pontine lesions, while those that are in the vertical plane usually localize to midbrain disturbances. Then the type of disorder, such as a conjugate gaze limitation, smooth pursuit and saccadic deficit, or conjugate gaze deviation, should be determined. Since conjugate gaze limitations and smooth pursuit

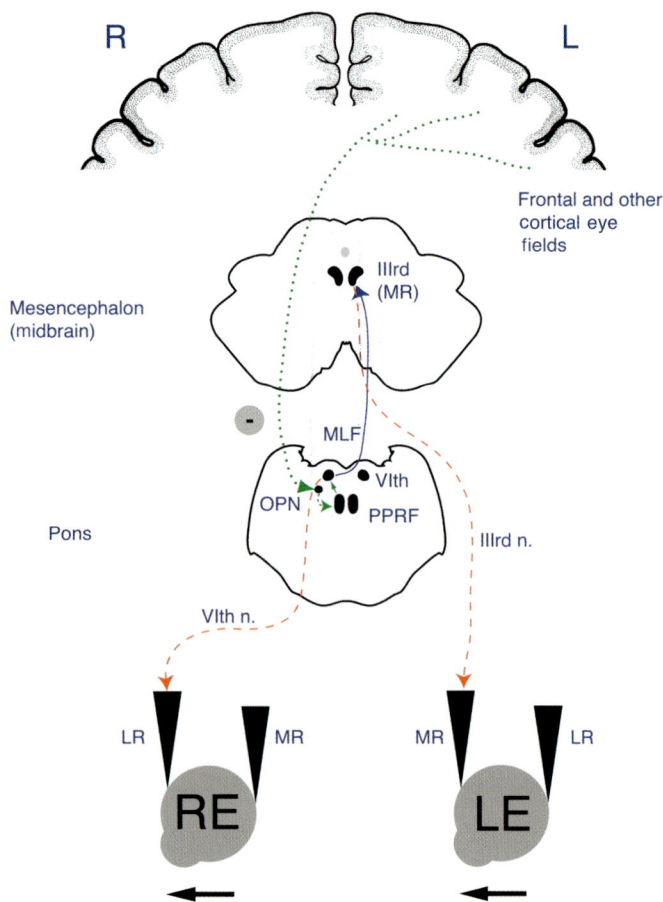

Figure 16–2. Generation of horizontal saccades. In this schematic drawing (ventral view), the pathways for a rightward saccade are depicted. The frontal and other cortical eye fields (see Fig. 16–1) from the left (L) hemisphere send fibers which decussate to inhibit the (R) omnipause neurons (OPN), which lie within the rootlets of the sixth nerve and between saccades tonically inhibits the paramedian pontine reticular formation (PPRF). Disinhibited burst neurons in the right PPRF excite cell bodies in the right sixth nerve (VIth) nucleus, which in turn innervates the ipsilateral lateral rectus (LR) muscle, which abducts the right eye (RE). Another set of neurons from the right sixth nerve nucleus cross the midline then ascend within the left medial longitudinal fasciculus (MLF). These reach the left medial rectus (MR) subnucleus in the oculomotor complex (IIIrd) in the midbrain, which issues third nerve neurons (IIIrd n.) that supply the left medial rectus muscle to adduct the left eye (LE).

Saccades are likely controlled by a neural network connecting these areas.[12,13]

These cortical areas mediating saccades send supranuclear fibers which decussate at the level of the oculomotor and trochlear nuclei before reaching the contralateral paramedian pontine reticular formation (PPRF) (**Fig. 16–2**).[14] Each PPRF also receives connections from the deep layer of the contralateral superior colliculus,[15] which may be involved in the selection of targets for foveation in retinotopic coordinates.[16,17] Located near the midline just ventral and rostral to each sixth nerve nucleus (see Chapter 15), each PPRF is the premotor center for generating horizontal saccadic eye movements. Between saccades, omnipause neurons in the nucleus raphe interpositus of the pons tonically inhibit the burst neurons in the PPRF and the rostral interstitial nucleus of the medial longitudinal fasciculus

in the midbrain (riMLF).[18,19] In one model, saccades are generated when signals from the supranuclear cortical and brain stem neurons inhibit the pontine omnipause neurons, allowing the burst neurons in the PPRF and riMLF to fire (**Fig. 16–2**).[17,20,21]

Each PPRF innervates the ipsilateral sixth nerve nucleus, which in turn innervates the ipsilateral lateral rectus muscle. The sixth nerve nucleus also supplies the interneurons which immediately cross the midline and then climb within the medial longitudinal fasciculus to reach the contralateral medial rectus subnucleus within the oculomotor complex in the midbrain (**Fig. 16–2**). The PPRF also sends fibers to the riMLF (see Vertical gaze, below). Thus, the PPRF primarily coordinates horizontal but also has an influence upon vertical eye movements.[5]

Information regarding eye position and maintenance of eccentric gaze is mediated by a neural integrator, consisting of neurons in the cerebellar flocculus, the perihypoglossal complex, and medial vestibular nuclei (also see Chapter 17). Following an eccentric saccade, viscoelastic forces in the orbit tend to drag the eye back into primary position. To counter this, neural integrator neurons modulate burst neuron activity in the PPRF and riMLF to maintain eccentric gaze.[22] The posterior vermis and the fastigial nuclei of the cerebellum are involved in the calibration of saccadic amplitude.[23]

Popular in detailed eye movement evaluations and as non-specific biomarkers (see below) in schizophrenia, for example,[24] *anti-saccades* are conjugate eye movements directed away from a visual stimulus. Individuals are shown a target in the periphery and instructed to look in the opposite direction. Anti-saccades require the suppression of reflexive saccades towards the target, and this inhibition is felt to be mediated by the dorsolateral prefrontal cortex.[10]

Smooth pursuit

Two descending parallel pathways mediate smooth pursuit (**Fig. 16–3**). In one, cortical signals arise from the occipito-temporal-parietal junction in Brodmann areas 19, 37, and 39 (area V5, see **Fig. 9–7b**), which are homologous to monkey areas MT (middle temporal) and MST (medial superior temporal).[25,26] Although areas 19, 37, and 39 are part of the dorsal stream, or magnocellular pathway, responsible for motion and spatial analysis of visual information (see Chapter 9), smooth pursuit is independent of motion detection and spatial attention.[27] The other pursuit pathway originates in the frontal lobes in the frontal and supplementary eye fields (see **Fig. 16–1**).[28–30]

These descending pathways for smooth pursuit then connect ipsilaterally with regions in the pons, the dorsolateral pontine nucleus (DLPN), and nucleus reticularis tegmenti pontis (NRTP). From these areas, a double decussation occurs, these regions innervating contralateral cerebellar structures such as the flocculus, paraflocculus, vermis, and fastigial nucleus, which in turn send inhibitory fibers via the inferior cerebellar peduncle to the medial vestibular nucleus, which then excites the contralateral sixth nerve nucleus (**Fig. 16–3**).[31] Note the smooth pursuit system is independent of the PPRF.[32–35]

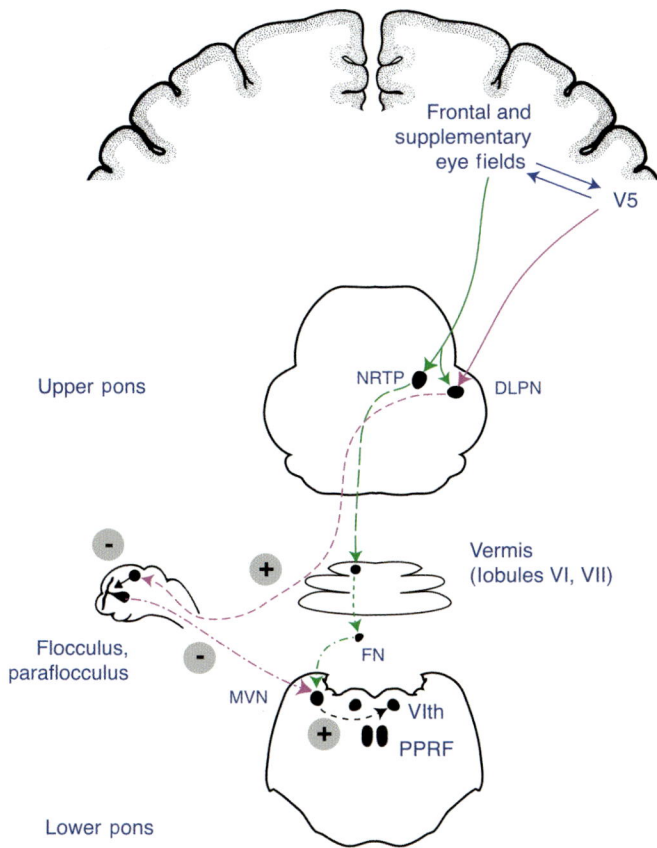

Figure 16–3. Parallel descending horizontal pursuit pathways from the frontal lobe and V5. Neurons from the frontal and supplementary eye fields (see Fig. 16–1) connect ipsilaterally to the dorsolateral pontine nucleus (DLPN) and nucleus reticularis tegmenti pontis (NRTP). V5 at the occipito-temporal-parietal lobe junction also sends fibers to the DLPN. A postulated double decussation of pursuit pathways in the brain stem and cerebellum then occurs. The first decussation consists of excitatory mossy fiber projections from the DLPN to granule cells, which excite basket cells and stellate cells in the contralateral cerebellar flocculus. The basket and stellate cells inhibit Purkinje cells, which in turn inhibit neurons in the medial vestibular nucleus (MVN). Fibers from the NRTP project to the vermis, which in turn connects to the fastigial nuclei (FN), which sends inhibitory axons to the MVN. The two inhibitory connections ultimately lead to activation of the MVN. The final common connection for both pathways is a second decussation consisting of excitatory projections from the MVN to the opposite abducens nucleus (VI), leading to ipsilateral gaze deviation (see Fig. 16–2).[32–35]

Vestibulo-ocular reflex and optokinetic nystagmus

Fibers mediating the vestibulo-ocular reflex arise from the vestibular nuclei, travel rostrally via the medial longitudinal fasiculus, pass through but do not synapse in the caudal portion of the PPRF, then finally arrive and synapse at the sixth nerve nucleus. The cerebellum is involved in the suppression of the vestibulo-ocular reflex. The generation of optokinetic nystagmus relies first upon cortical and subcortical areas which mediate smooth pursuit, then upon structures responsible for the generation of saccades as described above.[36]

The pathways for the vestibulo-ocular reflex and optokinetic nystagmus are discussed in more detail in Chapter 17.

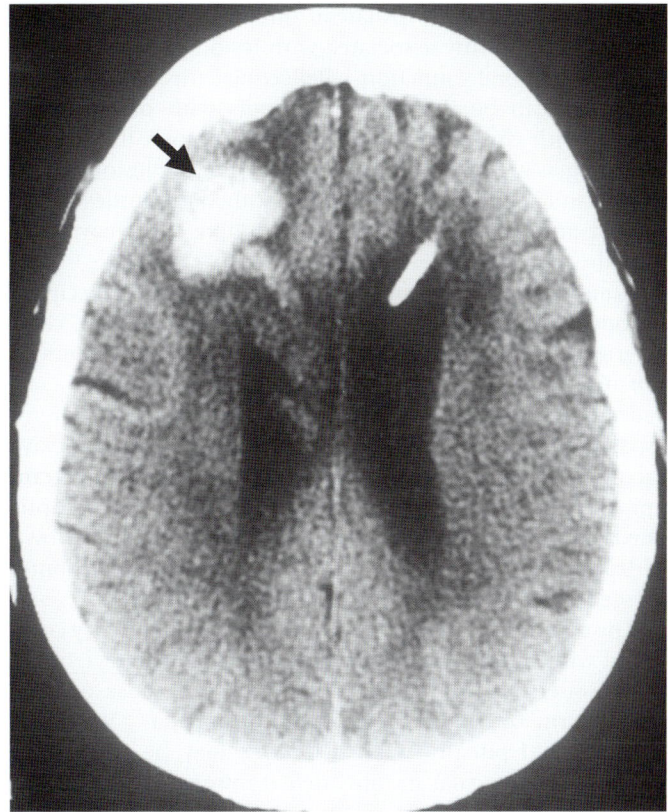

Figure 16–4. Axial CT scan of right frontal lobe hemorrhage (arrow), which caused difficulty with leftward saccades. A ventricular shunt is seen in the frontal horn of the left lateral ventricle.

Horizontal conjugate gaze deficits

Deficits caused by cortical lesions

Saccades. Unilateral frontal eye field lesions tend to cause contralateral saccadic eye movement impairment (**Fig. 16–4**).[37,38] Patients with lesions large enough to involve the adjoining motor cortex have a hemiparesis on the same side as the direction of the gaze paresis. Acutely, the eyes may be deviated ipsilaterally towards the lesion (see Gaze deviations, below), but this is usually only temporary.

Pursuit. Unilateral lesions within the occipito-temporal-parietal junction or the frontal and supplementary eye fields can cause a *directional* pursuit deficit, in which smooth pursuit of targets moving ipsilaterally towards the lesion is affected.[4,35,39] Directional deficits are independent of target position in space.[40] Less commonly, unilateral lesions in the occipito-temporal-parietal junction and in striate cortex may also cause *retinotopic* pursuit abnormalities of targets in the contralateral hemifield.[41,42] Retinotopic defects are location-dependent and uninfluenced by the direction of the target motion. Thus, in this situation, pursuit is abnormal in both directions in the contralateral hemifield. In a third type of pursuit defect, *craniotopic*, the patient cannot generate contralaterally directed pursuit eye movements past the midline of the head.[43] For instance, a patient with such a defect due to a left parietal lesion can pursue a rightward moving target only until the eyes reach midline.

In practice, cortical ipsilateral directional pursuit defects are most commonly associated with lesions at the occipito-parietal-temporal junction. Reflecting this, optokinetic responses can be defective in patients with parietal lobe lesions with contralateral hemianopia.[44] When the optokinetic targets are moved towards the side of the lesion, either the pursuit component is broken up, the amplitudes of the pursuit and saccades are smaller, or there is no corrective saccade.

Acquired ocular motor apraxia. Bilateral parieto-occipital lesions may lead to an acquired ocular motor apraxia, characterized by an absence or severe impairment of smooth pursuit, optokinetic responses, and visually guided saccades.[38] Because the eyes appear not to move, the term "spasm of fixation" has also been used. However, reflexive saccades may be preserved, justifying the use of the term apraxia. When ocular motor apraxia is combined with optic ataxia and simultanagnosia, the symptom complex is known as Balint syndrome, which is discussed in detail in Chapter 9 (see **Figs 9–9** and **9–10**).

The combination of bilateral parieto-occipital injury combined with bilateral lesions affecting both frontal eye fields, as in watershed ischemia for instance, can cause a more severe form of acquired ocular motor apraxia.[45] Voluntary saccades and pursuit in all directions may be completely paralyzed. The ocular motility deficit mimics the congenital type (see below), as patients may use a head thrust to aid refixation. In some cases reflexive saccades are also affected,[46] and in such instances the term ocular motor "paresis" may be preferred over "apraxia."[47]

Acquired ocular motor apraxia may also be seen in a number of progressive and inherited neurologic diseases (see **Table 16–2** and discussion below).

Deficits caused by pontine lesions

A lesion in the pons is the most common location for a brain stem disturbance that causes a horizontal gaze deficit, and there are frequently other accompanying signs. Pontine lesions are suggested when a conjugate gaze paresis is bilateral or accompanied by an internuclear ophthalmoplegia, ipsilateral facial paresis, contralateral hemiparesis, or skew deviation and when convergence and vertical eye movements are preserved.[48]

Conjugate gaze paresis. Two types of pontine lesions may result in a conjugate gaze paresis:

1. *Paramedian pontine reticular formation (PPRF).* Lesions restricted to the PPRF cause loss of all ipsilateral horizontal rapid eye movements such as voluntary and involuntary saccades and quick phases of nystagmus. Smooth pursuit and vestibulo-ocular reflexes may be spared in selective lesions of the rostral portion of the PPRF.[49]
2. *Sixth nerve nucleus.* A lesion of the sixth nerve nucleus, by damaging neurons innervating the ipsilateral lateral rectus muscle and the interneurons for the contralateral medial rectus, will cause an ipsilateral conjugate gaze palsy.[50] Because of the anatomical proximity of the genu of the facial nerve to the sixth nerve nucleus (see Chapters 14 and 15), a nuclear sixth nerve palsy is

often accompanied by ipsilateral facial weakness, as in the facial colliculus syndrome (**Fig. 16–5**).[51] All voluntary and reflexive ipsilateral conjugate eye movements are eliminated.[52,53]

Any combination of bilateral lesions affecting either the PPRF or sixth nerve nuclei will cause a bilateral conjugate gaze palsy (**Fig. 16–6**).

In patients with pontine horizontal gaze palsies who attempt to look in the direction of the palsy, an upward vertical or oblique movements of both eyes is often seen (**Fig. 16–5**). The misdirection or substitution movement may be explained by compensatory contraction or overaction of the obliquely acting extraocular muscles, but this is uncertain. In addition, some observers have documented abnormal oblique misdirection and slowing of vertical saccades in patients with lesions of the PPRF.[54,55] This finding, which is an inconsistent one,[49] has been attributed to disruption of the caudal PPRF's influence on the riMLF.[56]

One-and-a-half-syndrome. This highly localizing ocular motility disorder is characterized by a conjugate gaze palsy to one side accompanied by an ipsilateral internuclear ophthalmoplegia when the patient looks to the other side (**Fig. 16–7**). The name of the syndrome derives from the absence of conjugate eye movements in one direction and only preservation of abduction in the other direction.[57] In primary gaze the eyes may be exotropic, with lateral deviation of the eye with intact abduction. The association of one-and-a-half syndrome and exotropia has been termed paralytic pontine exotropia.[58] Convergence is often preserved.[59]

The one-and-a-half syndrome is caused by involvement of the PPRF or sixth nerve nucleus, causing the conjugate gaze paresis, combined with a lesion affecting the just crossed medial longitudinal fasciculus (MLF) (**Fig. 16–8**), which causes the internuclear ophthalmoplegia (see Chapter 15).[60,61] A lesion of the PPRF can be distinguished from one affecting the sixth nerve nucleus by the preservation of the oculocephalic or vestibulo-ocular responses in the former.[62]

Foville syndrome. A lesion in the caudal tegmental pons may cause a facial paralysis, conjugate gaze paresis, and contralateral hemiparesis by disrupting the fascicle of the VIIth nerve, the PPRF or VIth nerve nucleus, and the corticospinal tract, respectively. This localizing combination of findings, described by Foville,[63] is one of the crossed brain stem syndromes (see Chapter 15).[64]

Locked-in syndrome. Large bilateral lesions almost transecting the pons may cause a neurologic state characterized by quadriplegia, absence of horizontal eye movements, and mutism, but preservation of vertical eye movements, blinking, and consciousness. Patients in this "locked-in" state use these preserved functions to communicate, but they are often mistakenly diagnosed with coma. The area of the pons most commonly affected is the basis pontis, at the level of the sixth nerve nuclei.[65]

Defective smooth pursuit. Unilateral lesions of the dorsolateral pons have been associated with ipsilateral smooth pursuit deficits, without considerable abnormalities in

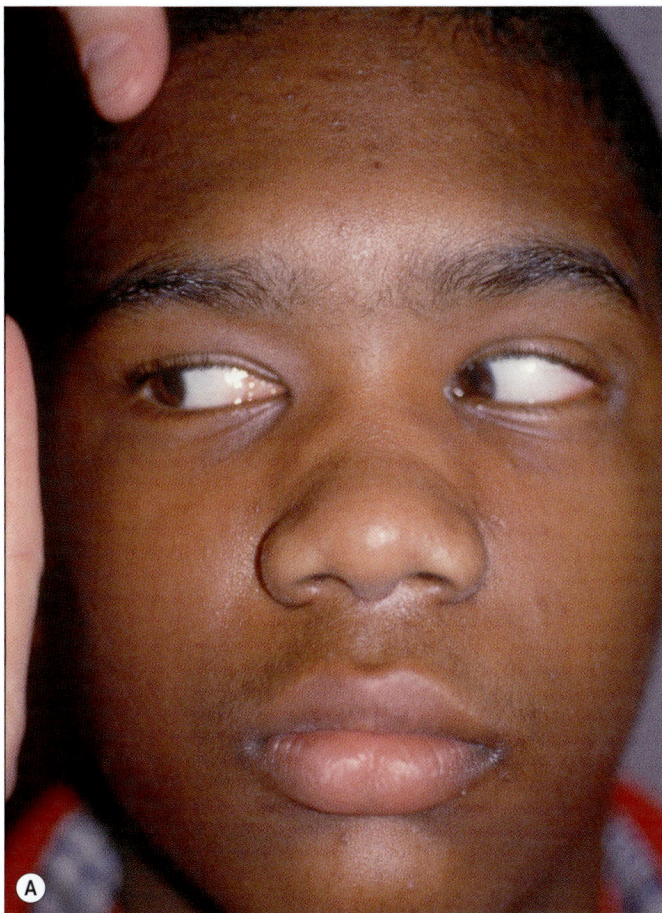

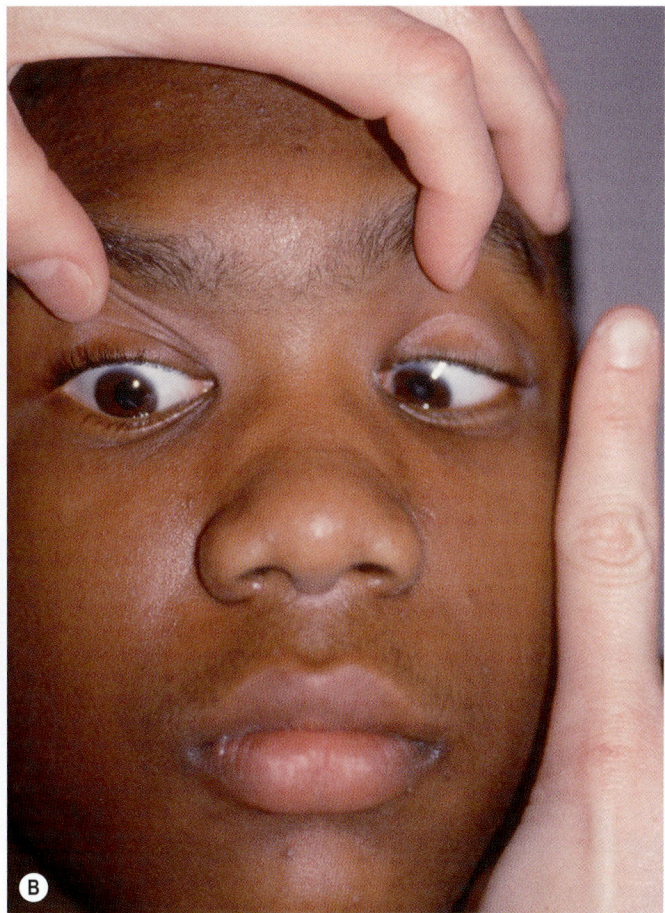

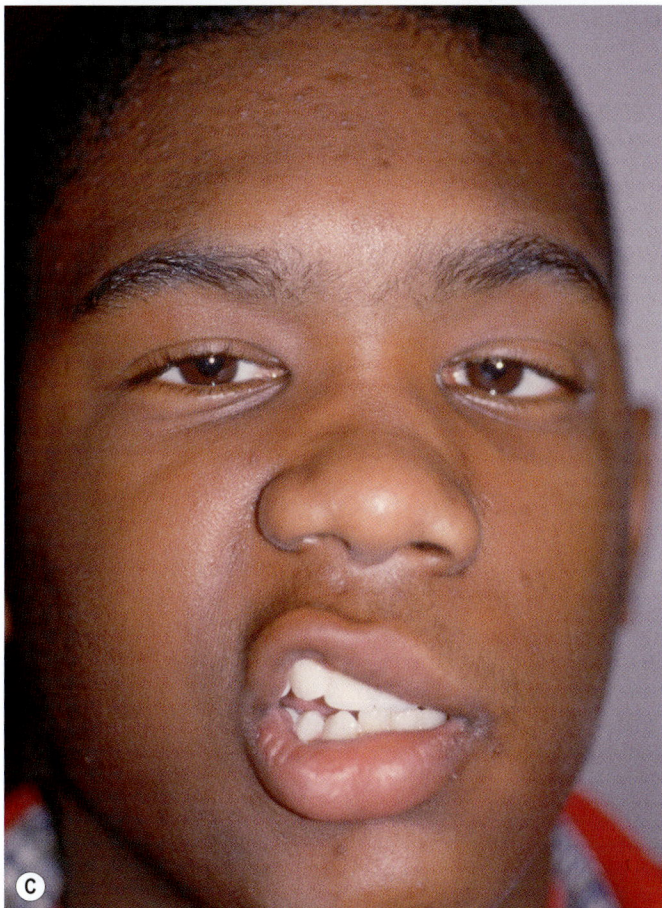

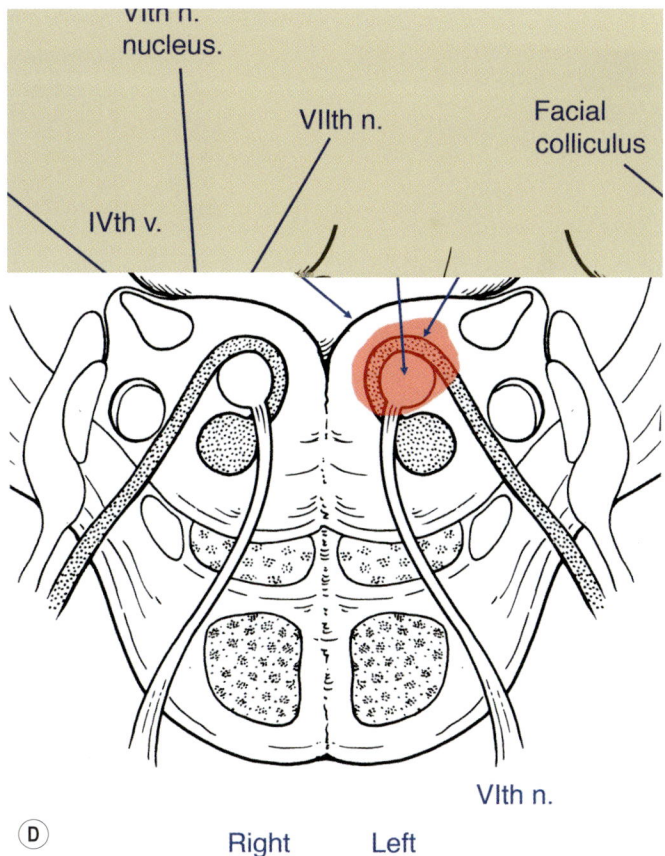

Figure 16–5. Left facial colliculus syndrome (peripheral VIIth n. palsy and nuclear VIth n. palsy causing ipsilateral facial and gaze paresis) due to radiation necrosis following treatment of a brain stem arteriovascular malformation. **A**. Normal gaze to the right. **B**. Defective gaze to the left. Note the eyes move downward in attempted leftward gaze. **C**. Left peripheral facial weakness. **D**. Drawing of location of the critical lesion (red area) in the left dorsal mid-pons (n., nerve; v., ventricle).

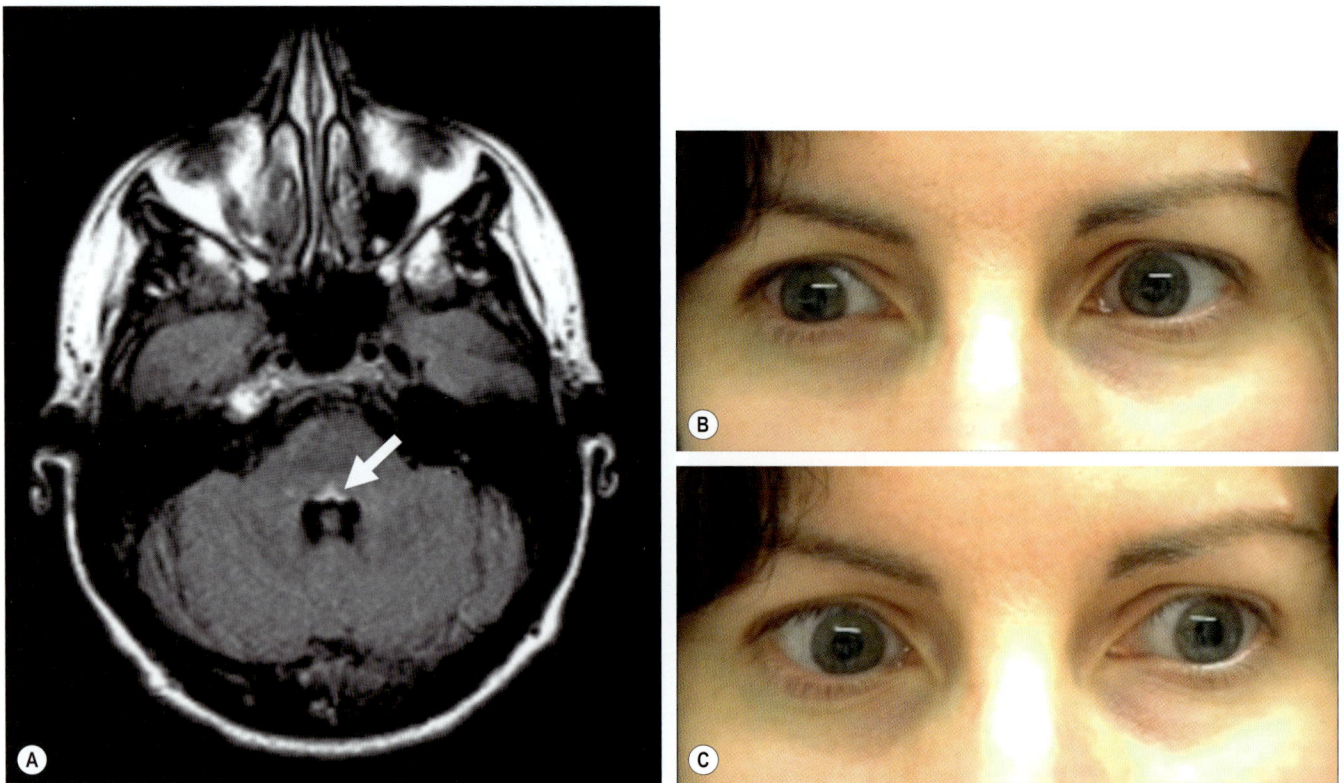

Figure 16–6. A. Dorsal pontine demyelination (arrow) in a patient with multiple sclerosis and bilateral horizontal gaze palsies from a lesion in the vicinity of the sixth nerve nuclei bilaterally. **B**. Attempted right gaze. **C**. Attempted left gaze. Adduction appears slightly worse than abduction in both directions, suggesting concomitant bilateral involvement of the medial longitudinal fasciculus (MLF). Courtesy of Dr. Clyde Markowitz.

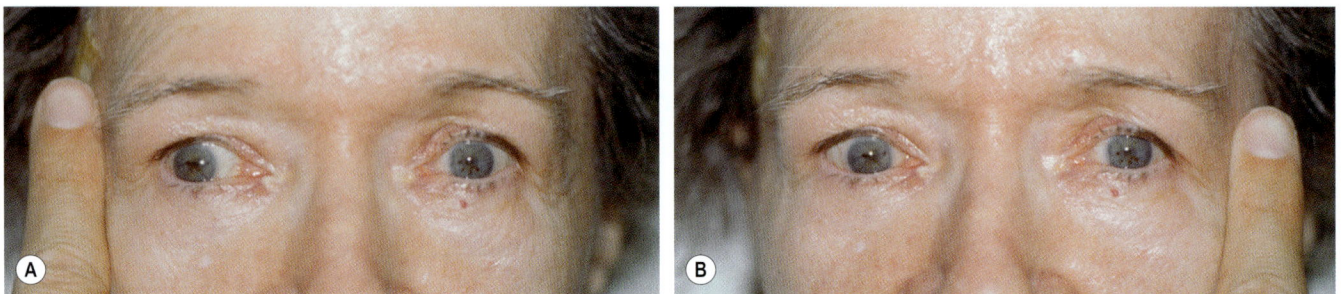

Figure 16–7. Left one-and-a-half syndrome due to left pontine infarction associated with giant cell arteritis. **A**. On attempted right gaze, the patient has a left internuclear ophthalmoplegia (defective adduction of the left eye and abducting nystagmus of the right eye). **B**. There is a conjugate gaze paresis on attempted left gaze, and neither eye can move past midline.

saccades or the vestibulo-ocular reflex.[32,35,66] These findings confirm the importance of pontine structures in the pathways for smooth pursuit described above (**Fig. 16–3**).

Etiology. In older adults the most frequent cause of a pontine horizontal gaze palsy is ischemia in the distribution of one of the pontine paramedian penetrating arteries arising from the basilar artery.[67] Atherosclerosis is by far the most common cause, but vasculitis due to giant cell arteritis,[68,69] for example, may be responsible. In younger adults, demyelinating processes such as multiple sclerosis are the most common etiology (see **Fig. 16–6**).[70] Other considerations in adults include hemorrhages due to hypertension, cavernous angiomas (**Fig. 16–9**), or trauma, for instance, as well as opportunistic infections.[71] Alcoholism

and overly rapid correction of hyponatremia may result in central pontine myelinolysis.[72,73]

In contrast, mid- and lower brain stem neoplasms such as pontine gliomas or medulloblastomas are the most common cause in children. Möbius syndrome (see Chapter 14), when it affects the sixth nerve nucleus, may cause horizontal conjugate gaze palsies.

Caution should be applied when diagnosing pontine lesions in this setting, because pontine horizontal gaze palsies can be mimicked by the Fisher variant of Guillain–Barré, myasthenia gravis, and thyroid eye disease. Thus, if neuroimaging is normal, these peripheral nerve, neuromuscular junction, and myopathic disorders should be excluded (see Chapters 14 and 18).

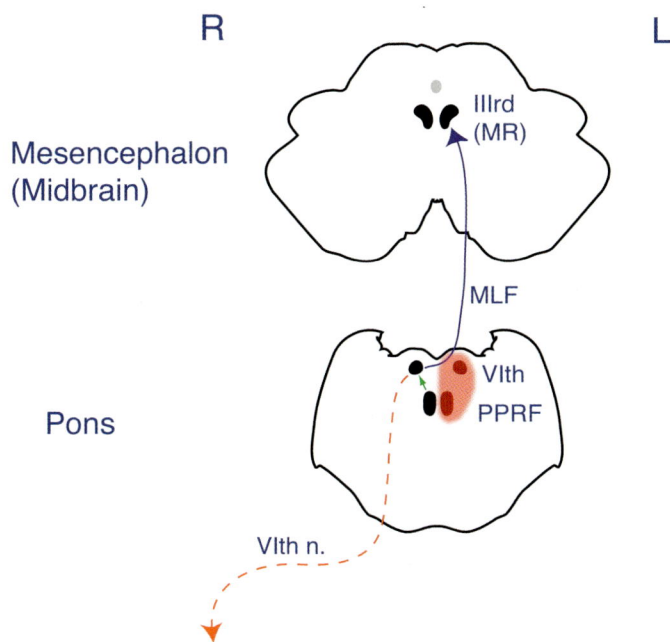

Figure 16–8. Schematic drawing of the lesion responsible for a left one-and-a-half syndrome (as in Fig. 16–7). This is caused by a lesion affecting the just crossed medial longitudinal fasciculus (MLF)—which contains fibers connecting the right VIth n. nucleus with the left medial rectus (MR) subnucleus in the IIIrd n. nuclear complex—leading to a left internuclear ophthalmoplegia (defecting adduction of the left eye), and both the left paramedian pontine reticular formation (PPRF) and the left VIth n. nucleus, either of which could cause defective conjugate gaze paresis to the left. Usually, because the VIth n. nucleus and the PPRF are in anatomical proximity, lesions which cause the one-and-a-half syndrome usually involve both.

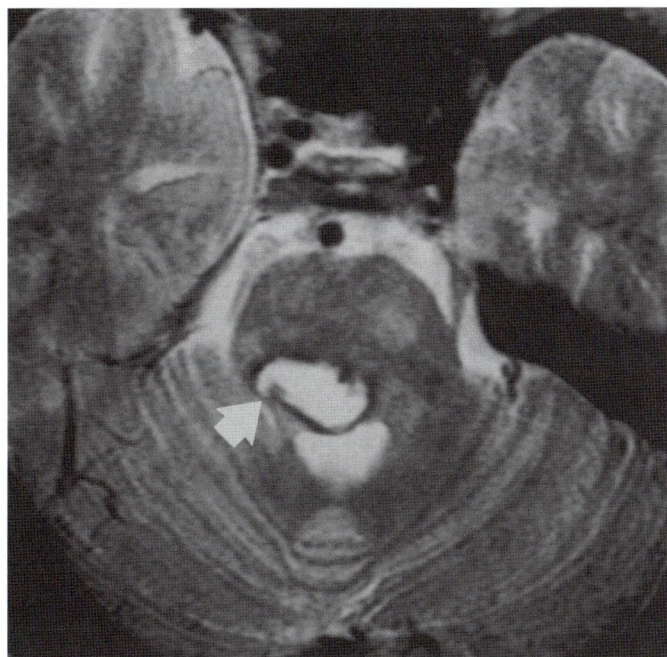

Figure 16–9. Cavernous angioma (arrow) of the pons associated with conjugate gaze deficits, demonstrated by high-resolution 4.0 Tesla MRI (TR = 5000, TE = 30, FOV = 22 cm, matrix = 512 × 256).

Horizontal gaze deficits caused by other posterior fossa lesions

Midbrain. Rarely conjugate horizontal saccades and pursuit may be abnormal following damage to the midbrain tegmentum.[74] Presumably the lesions affect descending horizontal gaze fibers destined for the PPRF. Zackon and Sharpe[75] reported two such patients, each with adduction paresis of the eye ipsilateral to the lesion accompanied by paresis of contralateral saccades in the fellow eye. These patients also exhibited conjugate paresis of ipsilateral smooth pursuit. Isolated lesions of the superior colliculi, which are also rare, may cause defective reflexive saccades.[76]

Medullary. Lateropulsion of saccades, characterized by overshoot of ipsilaterally directed saccades, undershoot of contralaterally directed saccades, and ipsilateral oblique trajectories during vertical refixation, is often a prominent ocular finding in lateral medullary lesions (see discussion of other neuro-ophthalmic complications of Wallenberg syndrome in Chapter 13).[77-80] Such patients also complain of body ipsipulsion, a sensation of the entire body being pulled towards the side of the lesion. Ipsilateral horizontal conjugate eye deviation may also occur, and is usually most obvious upon removal of visual fixation.[81-83] In other words, if the patient is asked to fixate straight ahead and close the eyes momentarily, the eyes may drift ipsilaterally.[84] As a result of this, upon eyelid opening a contralaterally directed refixation movement back to midline will then be seen (**Fig. 16–10**). Less commonly, an ipsilateral conjugate eye deviation is seen with eyelids open.[85,86]

Separate mechanisms may account for ipsipulsion of saccades and the conjugate eye deviation. However, each could result from damage to the inferior cerebellar peduncle and interruption of climbing fibers: (1) ipsipulsion of saccades from increased inhibition of the ipsilateral fastigial nucleus in the cerebellum and ultimately the contralateral PPRF and (2) conjugate gaze deviation either from increased inhibition of the ipsilateral vestibular nucleus or possibly from decreased tonic excitation of the contralateral PPRF.[86]

Lateral medullary lesions are also infrequently associated with difficulty pursuing contralaterally moving targets.[87] This deficit likely reflects damage to the vestibular nucleus. Ocular contrapulsion has been described in association with rostral medial medullary infarction.[88]

Cerebellar. Lesions in the cerebellum can cause saccadic overshoot and undershoot (dysmetria) as well as unsustained eccentric gaze with gaze-evoked nystagmus.[89] This results from damage to structures in the cerebellum responsible for the calibration of saccadic amplitude and gaze-holding, respectively (see above). Cerebellar hemispheric lesions tend to cause ipsilateral saccadic hypermetria (overshoot) and contralateral saccadic hypometria (undershoot). During attempted vertical saccades, there may be a contralaterally directed oblique drift (contrapulsion).[90] This is particularly true of lesions in the region of the superior cerebellar peduncle. Cerebellopontine angle tumors may cause an ipsilateral smooth pursuit defect if the vestibular nucleus, flocculus, or inferior cerebellar peduncle is involved.[87,91]

Familial horizontal gaze palsy and scoliosis. A rare autosomal recessive syndrome of horizontal gaze palsy and

Video 16.3

Video 16.4

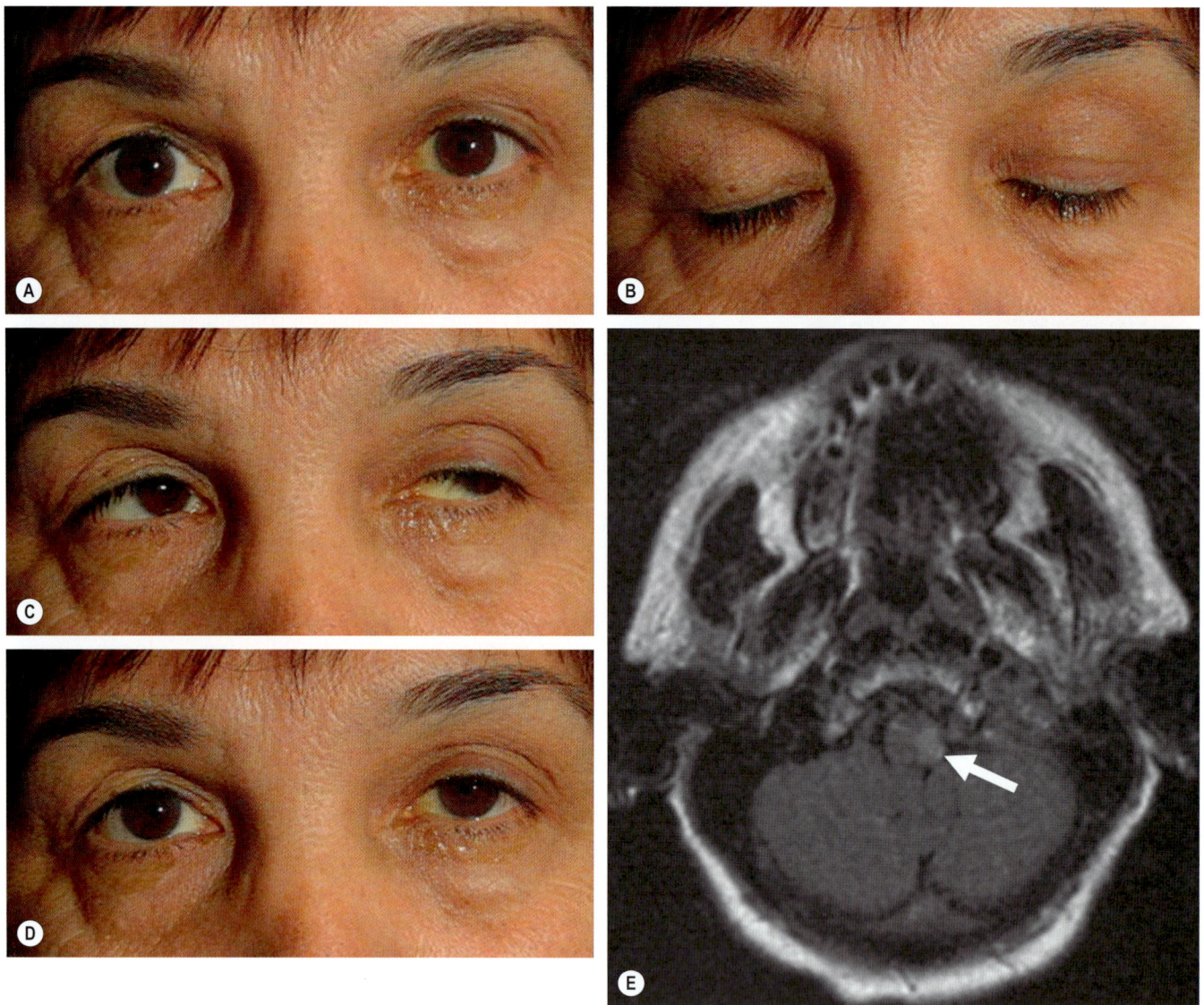

Figure 16–10. Ipsilateral conjugate gaze deviation in left Wallenberg syndrome. The patient has a residual left ptosis from Horner syndrome. **A**. At rest the patient is fixating on a target straight ahead; but in (**B**) with removal of fixation by closing the eyelids, the eyes deviate towards the side of the lesion; (**C**) the leftward deviation is noticeable immediately after the eyelids are reopened; (**D**) upon refixation the eyes move back to the midline; (**E**) axial FLAIR MRI demonstrating lateral medullary infarction (arrow).

progressive scolosis has also been described, and in most cases brain stem hypoplasia has been found on neuroimaging.[92,93] A responsible mutation of the ROBO3 gene on chromosome 11 has been identified, and congenital miswiring of the brain stem and spinal cord are suspected.[94,95]

Other horizontal gaze deficits

Saccadic palsy after cardiac surgery. Several patients with horizontal and vertical saccadic palsies have been reported as a complication of cardiac surgery, especially aortic valve replacement.[96–99] In most cases neuroimaging failed to disclose a responsible lesion in the cortex, brain stem, or cerebellum. Some authors have likened the ocular findings to those of progressive supranuclear palsy (see below).[100,101] Selective damage to the omnipause or excitatory burst neurons, superior colliculus, or cerebellum have been implicated,[97,102] but the exact cause is unknown.

Congenital ocular motor apraxia. In this ocular motility disorder of young children, infants may first appear to be blind or have decreased peripheral vision because they have defective or absence of horizontal saccades to novel visual stimuli. Quick phases of optokinetic nystagmus and the vestibulo-ocular reflex are also diminished, but smooth pursuit and vertical eye movements are usually preserved. At 5 or 6 months of age, when they achieve better head and neck control and can sit unassisted, they begin to use horizontal head thrusts to shift fixation (**Fig. 16–11**).[103] Often initiating the sequence with an eyelid blink, patients move their heads rapidly towards a new visual target.[104] Then the eyes slowly refixate. A final correction in head position sometimes then occurs, as the eyes are maintained on target using the vestibulo-ocular reflex.[105] Congenital ocular motor apraxia is almost always symmetric and bidirectional in the horizontal plane, but there have been exceptional asymmetric and vertical cases.[106,107] In many instances the

Video 16.5

Video 1

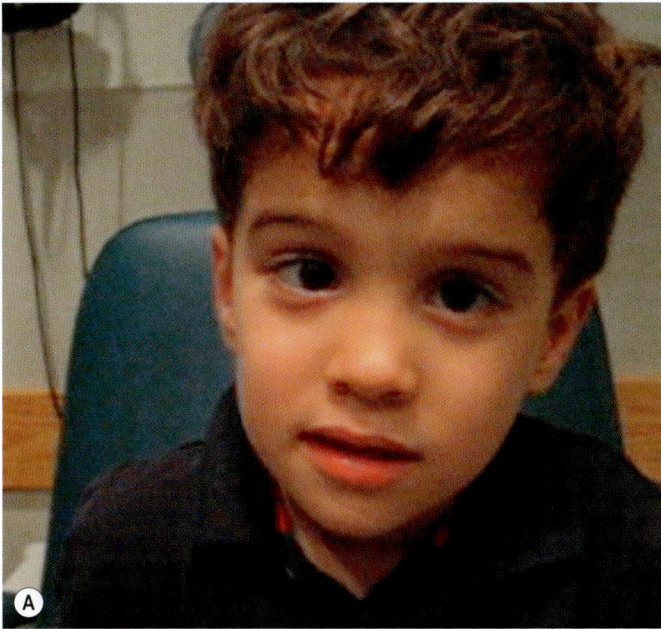

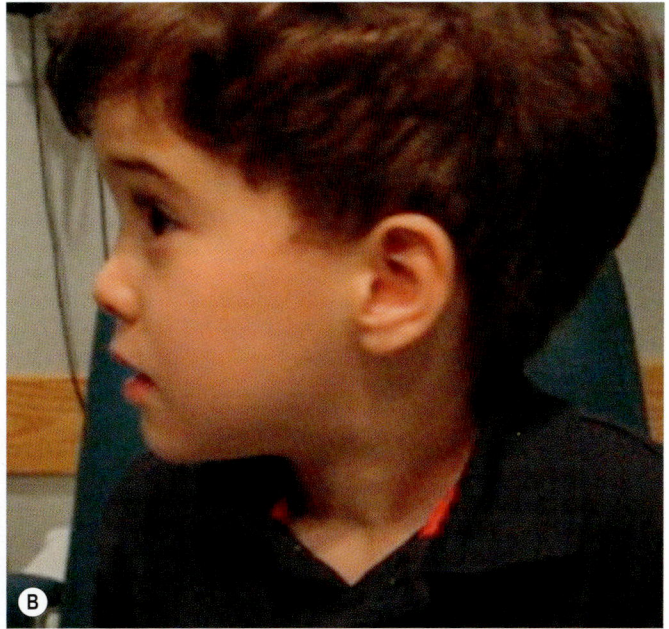

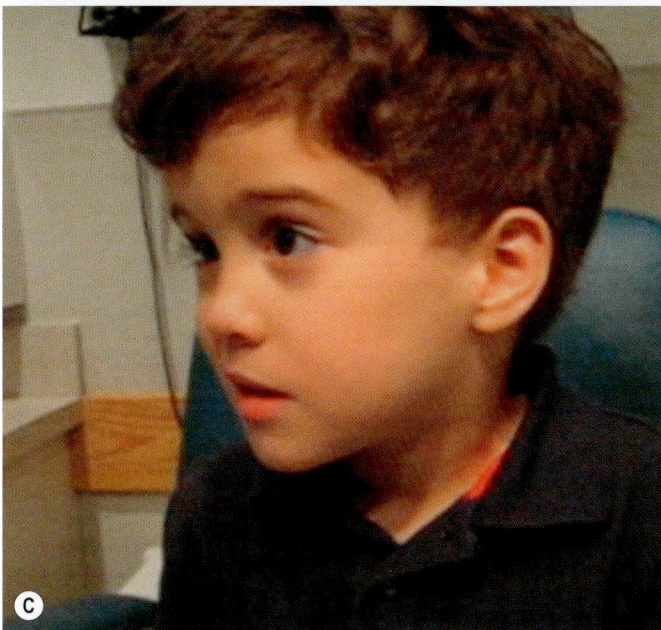

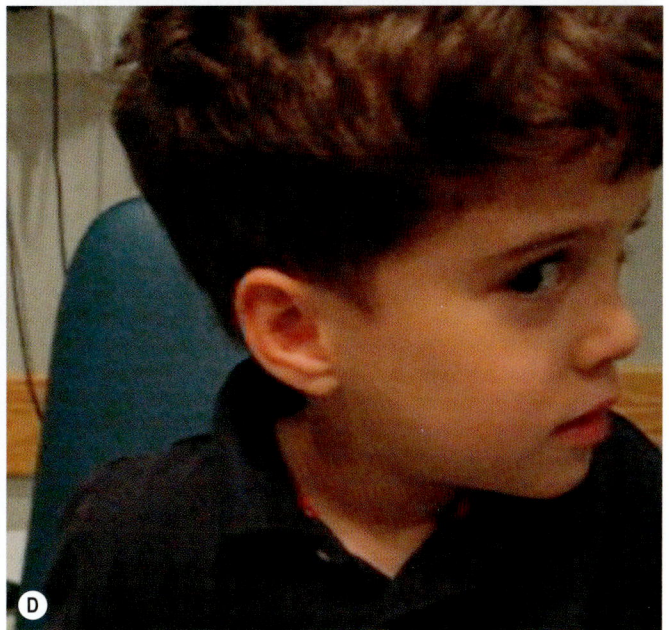

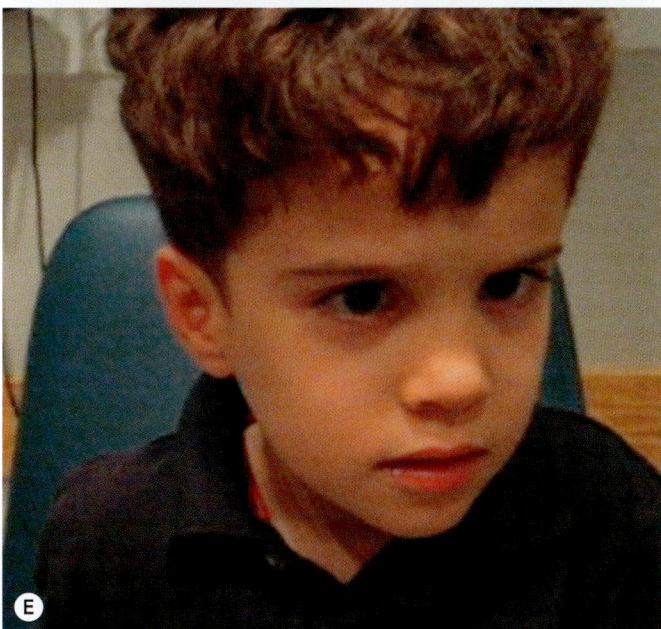

Figure 16–11. Child with idiopathic congenital ocular motor apraxia. **A**. Primary gaze. **B**. In attempted right lateral gaze to view a new target, the child thrusts his head past the target, then (**C**) the head position adjusts, and the eyes slowly refixate. (**D**) and (**E**) show similar head thrusting and head and eye repositioning in attempted left gaze to view another stimulus.

head thrusting and defective saccades spontaneously improve as the child gets older,[108] but the ocular motility disturbance may persist.[109] Because there are many causes (see below), the exact pathologic substrate is unclear although usually a defect in the saccadic system is implicated.

Two caveats regarding the use of the term "congenital ocular motor apraxia" should be made:

1. Because in some instances both voluntary and some reflexive saccades are defective, the term "apraxia," implying only voluntary saccades are affected, has been criticized. Other terms such as "congenital saccadic palsy"[110] and "intermittent horizontal saccade failure"[111] have been proposed. However, the term that Cogan[112] originally coined is unlikely to be supplanted, having already been heavily imbedded in the neuro-ophthalmic vernacular.

2. Although some authors[108,113] have applied the term "congenital" ocular motor apraxia in children of any age, we feel the term should be reserved only in those instances when the motility disorder is present in infancy.

Congenital ocular motor apraxia is observed in three main clinical situations:

a. In the "benign" or "idiopathic" variety of congenital ocular motor apraxia, neuroimaging is normal and there is no readily identifiable explanation for the disorder. Although the neurologic examination and intellect are usually normal, occasionally associated neurologic defects include hypotonia, motor and speech delay, and ataxia.[111,114] Many have infantile esotropia.[103] Familial cases have also been reported.[108,115,116] Parents should be informed that the afferent visual function of the affected child in this category is normal.[117]

b. Some patients with congenital ocular motor apraxia have a nonprogressive, noninherited structural abnormality of the brain, caused either by a developmental anomaly or by prenatal or perinatal insult.[118] These include: dysgenesis of the cerebellar vermis[119] or corpus callosum,[120,121] inferior vermian hypoplasia,[122] Dandy–Walker malformation (**Fig. 16–12**), gray matter heterotopias,[111] and perinatal ischemia.[106,107]

c. A variety of genetic disorders with multisystem involvement may present in infancy with congenital ocular motor apraxia.[105] These include Joubert syndrome (see Chapter 17),[123] Jeune syndrome (nephronophthisis, asphyxiating thoracic dystrophy, retinal degeneration, and ataxia),[124] and a subset of patients with Leber's congenital amaurosis, a retinal dystrophy.[125]

In contrast, we think the term "acquired" ocular motor apraxia is more appropriate when a similar disorder of head and eye coordination is seen in older children presenting with progressive, degenerative, or inherited metabolic neurologic diseases (see next section), for instance. The distinction may be difficult when children present with ocular

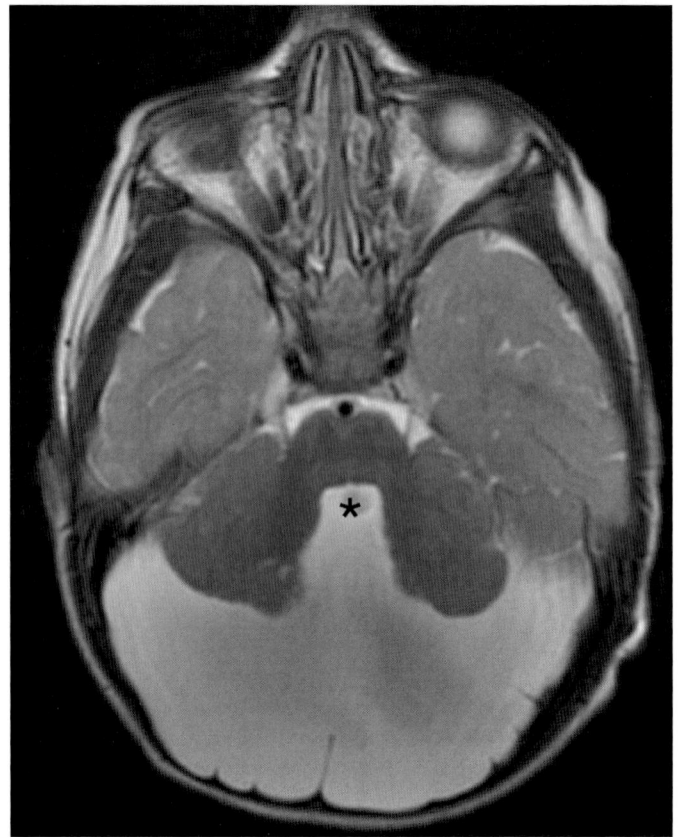

Figure 16–12. Dandy–Walker malformation associated with ocular motor apraxia. This T2-weighted axial MRI demonstrates the absence of the cerebellar vermis and cystic dilation of the fourth ventricle (asterisk).

motor apraxia at 6–12 months of age, at which time mild "congenital" and early "acquired" neurologic diseases may be confused.[126] However, some diagnostic guidelines include: (1) the voluntary ophthalmoparesis and head thrusts are almost always limited to the horizontal plane in congenital ocular motor apraxia and the acquired form due to Gaucher disease; (2) in contrast, the eye movement abnormalities and compensatory head movements are often in both the horizontal and vertical planes in ataxia telangiectasia and spinocerebellar ataxias; (3) they are primarily in the vertical plane in Niemann–Pick type C.

Other neurologic disorders associated with horizontal gaze deficits

Ataxia-telangiectasia (Louis-Bar syndrome). The cardinal clinical features of this childhood autosomal recessive phakomatosis are oculocutaneous nonhemorrhagic telangiectasias, cerebellar ataxia and dysarthria, multidirectional supranuclear ophthalmoparesis, and recurrent sinopulmonary infections.[127] The telangiectasias are seen most commonly in the bulbar conjunctiva. These can become more prominent with age and can also be observed on the earlobes, limbs, and trunk. Other skin lesions in this condition include follicular keratosis, seborrheic dermatitis, pigmentary disturbances, and secondary skin infections. Additionally, there is often dry coarse hair, vitiligo, and café au lait spots.[128]

Other neurologic features such as mental retardation, impassive facies, chorea, dystonia, and peripheral neuropathy can be observed.[129] Additional features include growth retardation, lymphoid hyperplasia, abnormally high rates of malignancy such as leukemia or breast cancer,[130,131] and elevated alpha-fetoprotein levels. The predisposition to infections and malignancy has been attributed to a high frequency of breaks in the loci on chromosome 11 containing a gene necessary for proper T- and B-cell function.[132,133] The gene codes for a putative DNA binding protein kinase called ATM,[134] which normally screens for DNA damage and activates DNA repair mechanisms.[135]

Most patients also have a supranuclear deficit in horizontal and vertical voluntary saccades and pursuit.[136,137] Reflexive saccades and the optokinetic quick phases may also be defective.[138] However, the oculocephalic and the slow phase of the vestibulo-ocular reflex are often preserved, so patients often exhibit head thrusts during attempted shifts of gaze similar to that seen in congenital ocular motor apraxia.[139] Fixation is sometimes also affected, as patients with ataxia-telangiectasia may exhibit abnormal saccadic intrusions such as square wave jerks or ocular flutter (see Chapter 17).[138,140] Strabismus, pursuit abnormalities, nystagmus, and accommodative insufficiency also may be seen.[141]

Imaging studies reveal diffuse cerebellar atrophy with marked involvement of the vermis and atrophy of the superior aspect of the cerebellar hemispheres.[142] The neuropathology of ataxia-telangiectasia consists of atrophy of the cerebellar cortex, particularly of the Purkinje cells. This is associated with the reduction in various neurotransmitters including glutamate and gamma-aminobutyric acid (GABA).

Treatment of patients with ataxia-telangiectasia is difficult. The prognosis for both quality and length of life past the late teens or twenties is poor. Because of the risk of infections and lymphoreticular malignancies, patients must be aware of the need for careful periodic examinations and the potential consequences of even minor infections.

Inherited spinocerebellar ataxias. These inherited diseases are divided into those which are autosomal dominant or recessive. Diseases with slow saccades or ophthalmoparesis in the dominantly inherited category include the spinocerebellar ataxias (SCA) types 1 (inherited olivopontocerebellar atrophy), 2, and 3 (Machado–Joseph disease), and 7.[143] A CAG trinucleotide repeat is responsible for each. Recessively inherited diseases with mild slowing of saccades include Friedreich ataxia[144] and the recently identified ataxia with oculomotor apraxia types 1 and 2.[145-147] The identification of the molecular basis of many of these disorders has allowed a genetic[148-151] rather than a phenomenologic[152] or pathologic classification.[152] Disease severity, including degree of saccadic abnormality, in many cases is related to the number of trinucleotide repeats.[153,154] **Table 16–6** highlights the inherited spinocerebellar ataxias with prominent slow saccades, including the localization of their genetic defects.

Patients with spinocerebellar ataxia usually exhibit dysmetria and gait ataxia, with some combination of absent tendon reflexes, defective proprioception, pyramidal (e.g., spasticity, hyperreflexia, and extensor plantar responses), and extrapyramidal (e.g., dystonia, parkinsonism) signs. Eye movement abnormalities are frequent and include gaze-evoked nystagmus, saccadic dysmetria, square-wave jerks, abnormal smooth pursuit, and inability to suppress the vestibulo-ocular response.[143,155,156] Saccades may be slow, and in severe cases patients lack voluntary saccades, use head thrusts, and have only preserved reflexive eye movements.[157,158] The slow eye movements and defective saccades have been attributed to degeneration of neurons in the PPRF[159,160] and the nucleus reticularis tegmenti pontis (NRTP).[161] Some subtypes (**Table 16–6**) have optic atrophy associated with progressive acuity, field, and color vision loss (see Chapter 5),[162] while others have macular or pigmentary retinal degeneration (see Chapter 4).[148,163] Magnetic resonance imaging typically shows some combination of cerebellar, pontine, and spinal cord atrophy.[164,165]

Multiple system atrophy. Diseases in this category are sporadic and nonhereditary. They are characterized clinically by parkinsonism, which is usually levodopa-unresponsive, autonomic failure, ataxia, and pyramidal signs. Three subtypes can be identified. First, noninherited olivopontocerebellar atrophy (OPCA), in which cerebellar signs predominate. Patients with this disorder may also have slow eye movements or an inability to initiate saccades in any direction.[166] Second, striatonigral degeneration, which is highlighted by parkinsonism, and sometimes by slow saccades and ophthalmoplegia. The pathologic hallmarks are loss of neurons and degeneration of the caudate nucleus and putamen, cerebellum, dentate nucleus, substantia nigra, inferior olivary nucleus, and intermediolateral columns of the spinal cord.[167] Third, Shy–Drager syndrome, which has no prominent eye movement features and has autonomic insufficiency as the primary abnormality.

Huntington disease. The principal clinical features of this neurodegenerative disease include progressive choreoathetosis, rigidity, and dystonia. The pathologic hallmark is atrophy of the caudate nucleus and putamen. The genetic basis is an abnormal CAG trinucleotide repeat expansion on chromosome 4p16.3.

Defective saccades in both horizontal and vertical directions have been documented in Huntington disease.[168] Slow saccades and difficulty in initiating saccades appear to be the most prominent eye movement deficits.[169-172] Patients also have increased distractability and unwanted saccades during attempted fixation as well as square-wave jerks (see Chapter 17).[173,174] Smooth pursuit can also be affected, but to a lesser extent.[175]

Parkinson disease. Parkinson disease is the second-most common neurodegenerative disorder following Alzheimer disease. It is characterized by parkinsonism—tremor, bradykinesia, rigidity, and postural instability—and is due to dopamine deficiency in striato-nigral pathways. Clinically, some patients exhibit saccadic pursuit in all directions of gaze. However, most patients with Parkinson disease do not exhibit any prominent eye movement abnormalities, distinguishing them from those with progressive supranuclear palsy. Abnormalities in saccades and pursuits may be found under experimental conditions.[176-178] Some of the ocular motility abnormalities are thought to reflect basal ganglia dysfunction and dopamine deficiency, as many[179,180] but not all[181] of these deficits have been shown to improve with levodopa therapy.

Table 16-6 Dominantly and recessively inherited cerebellar ataxias with slow saccades or ophthalmoparesis: genetic loci, and neuro-ophthalmic and neurologic features[148,149]

Name	Genetic locus	Slow saccades/ ophthalmoparesis	Optic atrophy	Retinal/macular degeneration	Other clinical features	References
Autosomal dominant						
SCA 1 (inherited OPCA, (formerly ADCA type I))	6p22–p23 with CAG repeats (ataxin 1 gene)	+	+	+/−		143,157,160,162,163,449,450
SCA 2 (formerly ADCA type I)	12q23–24 with CAG repeats (ataxin 2 gene)	+	−	−		143,158,450,451
SCA 3 (Machado–Joseph disease)	14q24.3–q32 with CAG repeats (ataxin 3 gene)	+ Vertical more than horizontal	−	Rare	Dystonia Amyotrophy Parkinsonism Facial fasciculations Lid retraction	143,450,452–458
SCA 7 (formerly ADCA type II)	3p14–21.1 with CAG repeats (ataxin 7 gene)	+	−	++ (defining feature; see Chapter 4 and Fig. 4–23)		148,459–461
Autosomal recessive						
Friedreich ataxia	9q13–q21.113 with GAA repeats (frataxin gene)	+/−	+/−	−	Areflexia in lower limbs Cardiomyopathy Diabetes mellitus	144,462,463
Ataxia with oculomotor apraxia (AOA) type 1	9p13.3 APTX (aprataxin gene)	+	−	−	Areflexia Peripheral neuropathy Elevated cholesterol, α-fetoprotein levels	147
Ataxia with oculomotor apraxia (AOA) type 2	9q34 SETX gene	+	−	−	Peripheral neuropathy, Elevated α-fetoprotein levels	145,146

Note: Patients with other autosomal dominant cerebellar ataxias, such as SCAs 4, 5, 6, 8, 10, and 12–17 and dentato-rubro-pallidoluysian atrophy (DRPLA) usually have normal or near-normal saccadic velocities, although saccades may be dysmetric and nystagmus is often present.[149,464–466] However, one kindred with DRPLA has been described with opsoclonus and nystagmus as prominent features.[467]
+, often present; +/−, occasionally present; −, often absent; ADCA, autosomal dominant cerebellar ataxia; CAG, CAG trinucleotide; GAA, GAA trinucleotide; OPCA, olivopontocerebellar atrophy; SCA, spinocerebellar ataxia. The ADCA types derive from Harding's[152] previous classification.

Corticobasal ganglionic degeneration. Corticobasal ganglionic degeneration is a rare, sporadic progressive neurodegenerative disease of the middle-aged or elderly.[182] It is characterized by clinical features which suggest both cortical and basal ganglionic dysfunction. These include dementia, levodopa-unresponsive parkinsonism, limb dystonia, ideomotor apraxia, hyperreflexia, cortical sensory loss, focal reflex myoclonus, and "alien limb" phenomena.[183,184] In the late stages of this disease, a supranuclear gaze paresis in all directions and eyelid opening apraxia (see Chapter 14) can be seen.[183,185,186] Although the clinical presentation may be confused with progressive supranuclear palsy (PSP), corticobasal ganglionic degeneration more commonly has asymmetric frontoparietal atrophy on neuroimaging, whereas patients with PSP more typically have midbrain atrophy.[187]

Pharmacologic therapies are largely ineffective.[188] The diagnosis can be confirmed only at autopsy, which typically demonstrates swollen, poorly staining (achromatic) neurons and degeneration of the cortex and substantia nigra.[183]

Gaucher disease. A lysosomal storage disorder, Gaucher disease is caused by decreased enzyme activity of glucocerebrosidase with resulting accumulation of a glycolipid, glucocerebroside, in macrophages. The glucocerebrosidase gene has been mapped to chromosome 1q21–31.[189] Anemia, thrombocytopenia, hepatosplenomegaly, infiltration of bone marrow with abnormal histiocytes, and fracture or aseptic necrosis of bone are common systemic features. In the infantile acute GD2 and later onset subacute GD3 forms, neurologic involvement is also seen, with a supranuclear horizontal gaze paresis as the most predominant feature.[190–192] Vertical eye movements are typically spared. Eye movements and head thrusts can mimic congenital ocular motor apraxia, but lateral movements of the eyes may be accompanied by an upward arcuate or looping excursion.[139]

Others. Horizontal saccadic failure has also been documented in association with other childhood neurodegenerative diseases such as Krabbe leukodystrophy, Pelizaeus Merzbacher disease, GM1 gangliosidosis, Refsum disease, and propionic acidemia.[193]

Ocular motor abnormalities as biologic markers. Interest has grown in the detection of abnormal eye movements, which are often subtle, as biologic markers in neuropsychiatric diseases in which abnormal ocular motility is not usually a prominent clinical finding.[22,171,172,194,195] For instance, patients with Alzheimer disease[196,197] and schizophrenia[22] may have abnormal anti-saccades. Smooth pursuit may also be abnormal in these patients[198,199] and their relatives.[200] These ocular motor abnormalities can offer insight into the abnormal neuronal circuitry and pharmacology of these disorders. However, their detection often requires eye movement recordings, they are rarely tested at the bedside, and are frequently too nonspecific to offer any diagnostic utility. Furthermore, in some cases they may be the result of neuropsychotropic medications.

Wernicke's encephalopathy. This disorder, due to a vitamin B₁ (thiamine) deficiency, is characterized clinically by a triad of eye movement abnormalities, gait ataxia, and encephalopathy. The full triad is present in only a minority of cases.[201]

In a large series of patients with Wernicke's encephalopathy,[202] 44% had conjugate gaze palsies. Typically the gaze palsy was horizontal, but sometimes vertical gaze was also affected. Vertical gaze abnormalities, which were usually upward, were rarely seen alone. Other prominent neuro-ophthalmic findings included nystagmus in 85%, lateral rectus palsies in 54%, and pupillary abnormalities in 19%.[202] Less frequent neuro-ophthalmic abnormalities include retinal hemorrhages, ptosis, and optic neuropathy.

Wernicke's encephalopathy is seen primarily in alcoholics and other malnourished individuals such as prisoners of war or women with hyperemesis gravidarum. Forced or involuntary starvation, cancer, gastric plication, and chronic renal dialysis are other associated conditions. Because thiamine is required for carbohydrate metabolism, Wernicke's encephalopathy can also be caused inadvertently in individuals with marginal thiamine stores who are given a carbohydrate (e.g., intravenous glucose) load.[203]

Characteristic neuropathologic findings include necrosis of nerves and myelin, hypertrophy and hyperplasia of small blood vessels, and pinpoint hemorrhages. These are typically located symmetrically in the mammillary bodies, superior cerebellar vermis, hypothalamus, thalamus, midbrain, and the ocular motor and vestibular nuclei.[203] The gaze abnormalities may be attributed to pathologic lesions affecting the sixth nerve nuclei, pretectal area, and periaqueductal gray matter. The nystagmus can be related to the damage to cerebellar and vestibular structures.[204] Neuroimaging typically reveals mamillary body and midline cerebellar signal changes or atrophy (**Fig. 16–13**).[205,206]

Following parenteral administration of 50–100 mg of thiamine in addition to receiving a balanced, high-caloric diet, patients often begin recovering from sixth nerve palsies and gaze deficits within 1–24 hours, and almost always within 1 week.[202] By 1 month these deficits usually resolve. However, many require several weeks for nystagmus, ataxia, and confusion to resolve. Improvement in the cognitive

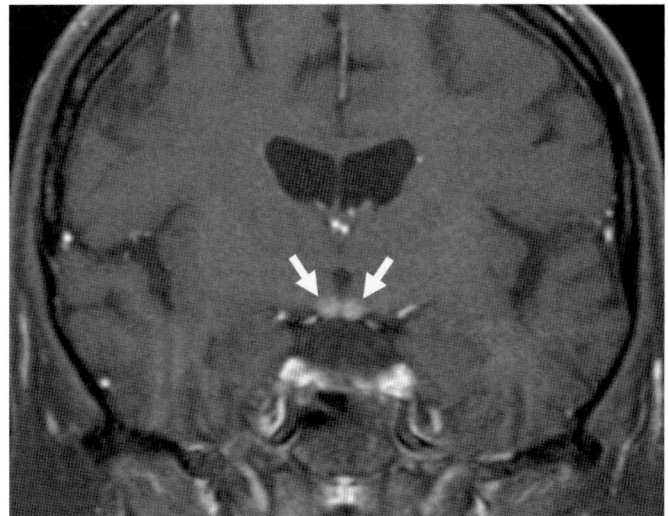

Figure 16–13. Wernicke's encephalopathy. This T1-weighted MRI with gadolinium shows contrast enhancement of the mamillary bodies (arrows) in a woman with ophthalmoplegia, memory loss, and behavioral changes following severe rapid weight loss. Her signs and symptoms improved rapidly with thiamine.

changes and ataxia is predictable. In addition, some patients develop Korsakoff's psychosis, characterized by retrograde and anterograde amnesia and confabulation, as long-term sequela.

Leigh syndrome (subacute necrotizing encephalomyelopathy). Abnormal conjugate and dysconjugate eye movements may be seen in this rare, invariably fatal disorder of young children. Psychomotor delay and hypotonia are typically the first manifestations, usually in the first year of life. Subsequent symptoms include abnormal eye movements, vision loss related to optic atrophy, ataxia, peripheral neuropathy, somnolence, deafness, movement disorders, spasticity, and respiratory difficulties.[207] Spasmus nutans has also been reported in association with Leigh syndrome.[208]

MRI characteristically demonstrates high-signal lesions in the basal ganglia. Pathologically, bilaterally symmetric necrotic lesions extend from the thalamus to the pons, but they also involve the inferior olives and posterior columns.[209] These abnormalities resemble those in Wernicke's encephalopathy and infantile beriberi.

Several biochemical and genetic defects affecting energy metabolism can lead to Leigh syndrome.[209] The more commonly identified ones are: a defect involving the pyruvate dehydrogenase complex, cytochrome oxidase deficiency, a T-to-G mutation at nucleotide 8993 in the mtDNA gene encoding ATPase 6 (the same mutation as in NARP syndrome; see Chapter 4),[210,211] and complex I deficiency.[212] Treatment in most cases is unsatisfactory.

Vitamin E deficiency. There are three major causes of vitamin E (alpha-tocopherol) deficiency: (1) abetalipoproteinemia (Bassen–Kornzweig disease), in which patients lack apolipoprotein B, which is essential for transporting fat-soluble vitamins; (2) malabsorption, due either to choles-tatic liver disease with resultant failure to secrete bile, cystic fibrosis, or bowel resection; and (3) familial isolated (autosomal recessive) vitamin E deficiency.[213] Slow saccades may be a feature of the first two causes, but not usually of the familial type.[214] Some exhibit dissociated eye movements, with slow but full abduction of one eye and fast but limited adduction of the other in attempted lateral gaze. Ocular motor palsies may occur, and we have seen aberrant regeneration of the third nerve in this condition. A pigmentary retinopathy may also be observed. Neurologically, patients with vitamin E deficiency may develop ataxia, long tract signs, proprioceptive loss, and areflexia, mimicking Friedreich ataxia.[215]

In suspected cases, serum vitamin E levels should be tested. In many instances vitamin E supplementation may halt or reverse the progression of ocular motor and neurologic symptoms.

Drugs. A number of drugs may impair smooth pursuit. These include phenytoin, barbiturates, carbamazepine, and lithium. Most drugs in toxic doses may cause a variety of ocular motor abnormalities when consciousness is decreased. At toxic levels the drugs mentioned above may cause complete ophthalmoplegia.

Abnormal horizontal conjugate gaze deviations

Stroke

Supratentorial. Acutely following a supratentorial infarction or hemorrhage, the eyes may be conjugately deviated ipsilaterally towards the lesion (**Figs 16–14** and **16–15**).[216] The

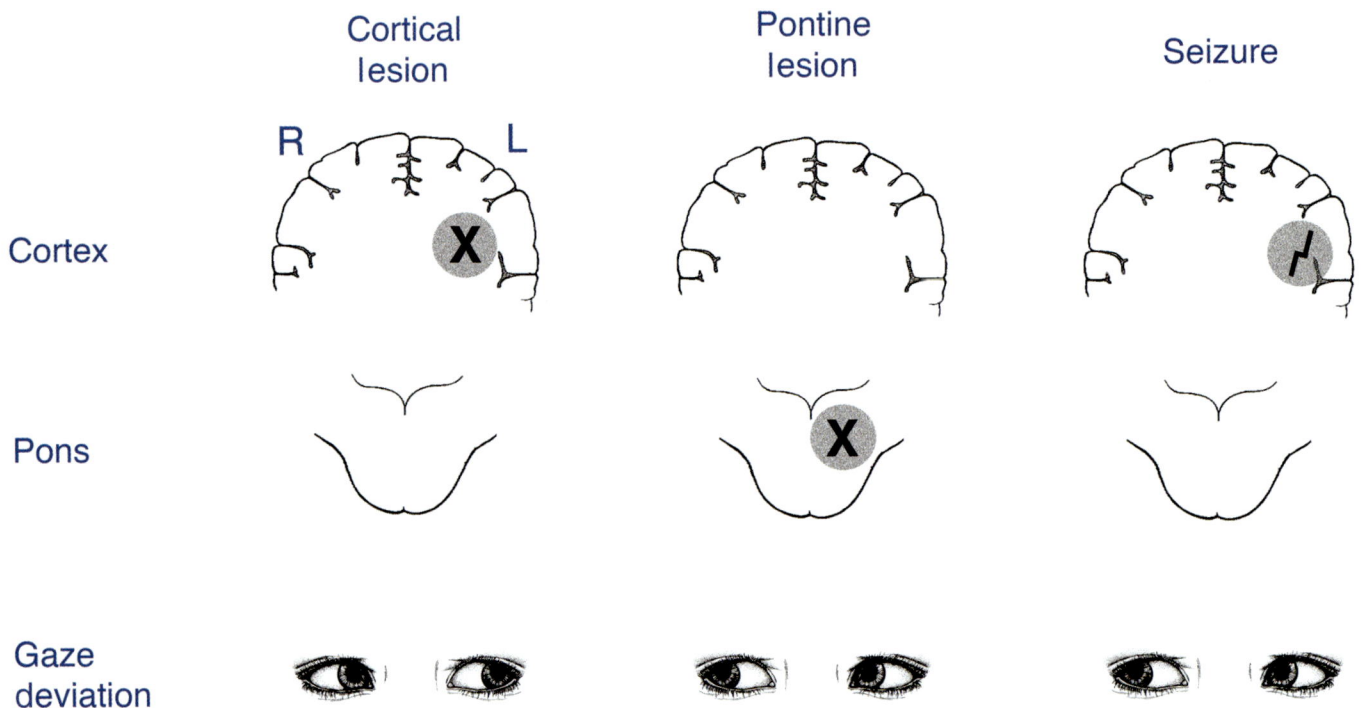

Figure 16–14. Common ipsilateral gaze deviations due to cerebral and pontine lesions and seizures. The eyes may deviate horizontally towards a cortical lesion, away from a pontine lesion, and away from a cortical seizure focus.

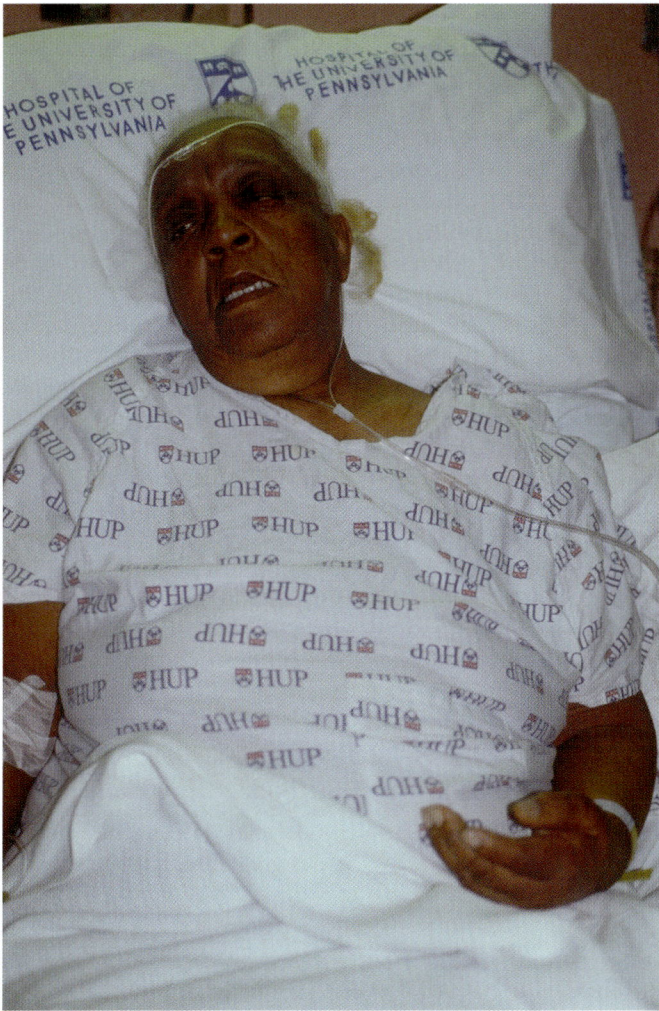

Figure 16–15. Right gaze preference in a patient with a right middle cerebral artery stroke, left homonymous hemianopia, left neglect, and left hemiparesis.

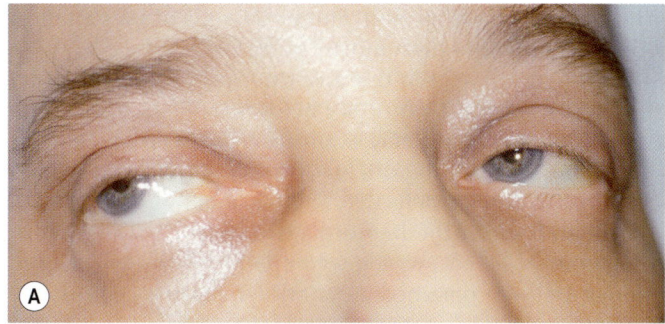

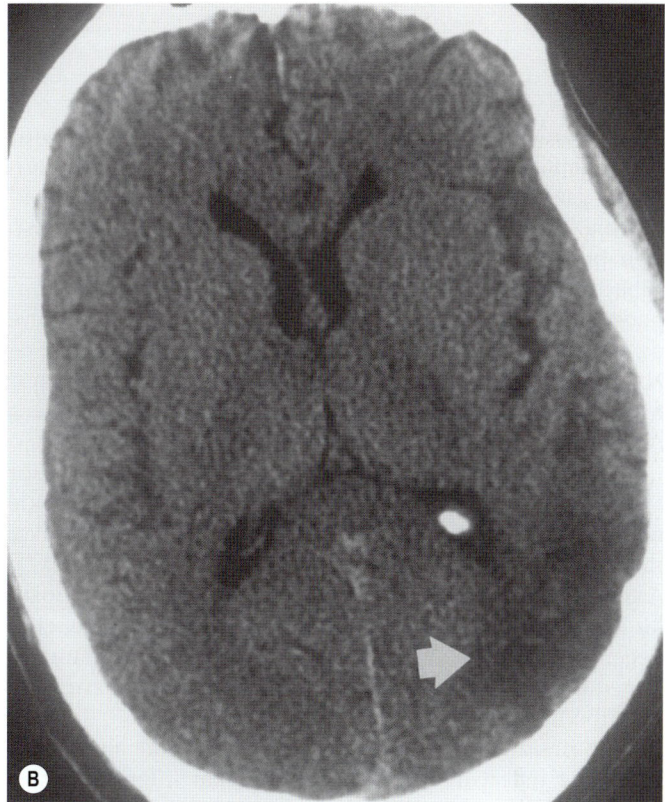

Figure 16–16. A. Right gaze deviation in a patient with seizures. **B**. CT scan reveals an old left middle cerebral infarction (arrow), which acted as a seizure focus.

eye deviation is often evident on neuroimaging,[217] and is more frequent and persistent with right hemispheric lesions.[218] This gaze deviation usually results either from impairment or neglect of the contralateral visual field[219] or from damage to ipsilateral fronto-pontine fibers descending from the FEF to the pons. The oculocephalic response is typically normal, but in the first few days it may be difficult to elicit.

Rarely, thalamic (see below) or frontoparietal hemorrhages may result in contralateral conjugate eye deviations.[220,221] Possible mechanisms include involvement or mass effect in the mesencephalon upon fronto-pontine fibers after they have crossed, irritative effects on the descending fibers (see below), or an interhemispheric smooth pursuit imbalance.[222]

Infratentorial. Unilateral pontine disturbances affecting the PPRF or sixth nerve nucleus may result in a contralateral gaze preference and ipsilateral gaze paresis (**Fig. 16–14**). As alluded to earlier, lateral medullary lesions may produce an ipsilateral gaze deviation. However, patients with lateral medullary lesions usually have full contralateral gaze but with hypometric saccadic eye movements.

Seizures

Ictal head and eye deviation are usually contralateral to a cortical seizure focus (**Figs 16–14** and **16–16**).[223] The diagnosis is usually obvious when there is hemibody twitching or loss of consciousness if the seizure activity generalizes. The gaze deviation may be nystagmoid, with a contralateral fast component followed by a slow drift of the eyes back towards midline.

Thalamic hemorrhages

Thalamic hemorrhages, which are usually the result of long-standing hypertension, are suggested by the sudden onset of headache and contralateral hemisensory loss and hemiparesis.[224] Large hemorrhages may cause a contralateral hemianopia (see **Fig. 8–29**). Depressed consciousness to the point of stupor or coma can occur, particularly when there is intraventricular extension. Stupor or coma at presentation is associated with a high mortality.[225]

Large hemorrhages in this area can cause both horizontal and vertical eye deviations (see below). Patients with severe hemianopia or neglect may exhibit an ipsilateral gaze preference. Contralateral saccades may be hypometric, and ipsilateral pursuit may be defective.[226] Occasionally the eyes may deviate away from the hemorrhage and towards the hemiparesis in so-called "wrong-way eyes."[57,227,228] This pattern mimics that of a paramedian pontine hemorrhage. Possible mechanisms were discussed above in the section on supratentorial lesions.

Periodic alternating gaze

This disorder is related to periodic alternating nystagmus (see Chapter 17), and consists of cycles of conjugate horizontal gaze deviation with compensatory contralateral head turning for 1–2 minutes, followed by a 10–15 second transition period with the eyes and head straight ahead, then subsequent gaze deviation to the opposite side with compensatory head turning for another 1–2 minutes. The eye deviation may be overcome by oculocephalic maneuvers. Nystagmus may be seen but is intermittent and not a major feature. Patients are typically awake although the pattern may be seen in comatose patients.[229]

In general, this motility pattern localizes to the posterior fossa. Reported underlying congenital conditions include hypoplasia of the cerebellar vermis as in Dandy–Walker malformation and Joubert syndrome (see Chapter 17), Arnold–Chiari malformations (downward cerebellar tonsillar herniation), occipital encephalocele, and spinocerebellar degeneration.[230] Acquired etiologies such as pontine damage, a medulloblastoma, and hepatic encephalopathy have been described.[229]

Like periodic alternating nystagmus, period alternating gaze may reflect damage to the cerebellar inferior vermis, including the uvula and nodulus.[230]

Ping-pong gaze. Also called short cycle periodic alternating gaze deviation, this ocular motility pattern has horizontal oscillation cycles of only 2.5–8 seconds.[231] The patient appears to be watching a ping-pong match. The side-to-side movements are usually smooth and sinusoidal, but a saccadic form has also been described.[232]

Ping-pong gaze is almost always seen in comatose or stuporous patients but implies the brain stem, especially the pons, is relatively intact. The responsible lesions are thought to disconnect the brain stem from cortical influences, which may hypothetically release oculovestibular generators. They are typically rostral midbrain-thalamic, bilateral basal ganglia, or bilateral hemispheric.[233-236] Cases associated with a cerebellar vermis hemorrhage[237] and bilateral cerebral peduncle infarctions have been reported.[238]

Vertical conjugate gaze: neuroanatomy

Crucial supranuclear structures mediating vertical gaze are located in the midbrain at the level of the *pretectum* (**Figs 16–17** and **16–18**). This term refers to the area in the mid-

brain immediately rostral to the tectum, another designation for the superior and inferior colliculi. The pretectum is also just rostral to the level of the third nerve and red nuclei. The two most important pretectal areas are the riMLF and interstitial nucleus of Cajal (inC).

Rostral interstitial nuclei of the medial longitudinal fasciculus (riMLF). At the pretectal level, in an area of the midbrain termed the mesencephalic reticular formation, up- and downward saccades are mediated by burst neurons within the paired paramedian riMLF (**Figs 16–17** and **16–18**).[239-242] These lie immediately above the rostral–medial portions of the red nuclei. The topographic separation of upgaze and downgaze burst and tonic neurons within each riMLF is uncertain in man.[243]

In the current view of vertical gaze control,[244,245] saccadic innervation is bilateral to the elevator muscles (the superior rectus and inferior oblique) (**Fig. 16–18A**), but only ipsilateral for downgaze (inferior rectus subnucleus and fourth nerve nucleus) (**Fig. 16–18B**). Projections for upgaze arising from the riMLF are no longer thought to cross in the posterior commissure, but rather bifurcate at the level of the third nerve nucleus. Each riMLF also contains neurons for ipsilateral torsional saccades. In addition, ascending projections to the riMLF arise from omnipause neurons in the pons.

The major clinicoanatomical implications of this arrangement are:

1. Unilateral lesions of an riMLF or its descending fibers will affect downward saccades greater than upward saccades. This is due to the duplication of riMLF input into the oculomotor subnuclei for upgaze but not downgaze.

2. Bilateral lesions of an riMLF or its descending fibers will result in a more severe defect of vertical saccades than that due to unilateral lesions. Again, downward saccades may be affected more than upward saccades.

3. A unilateral riMLF lesion may cause defective ipsitorsional quick phases with ipsilateral head tilting. For instance, in a left riMLF lesion there would be no quick extorsion of the left eye or intorsion of the right eye upon leftward head tilting. Therefore, torsional nystagmus may be evident in the opposite direction.

Interstitial nucleus of Cajal (inC). By coordinating signals from the saccadic burst neurons in the riMLF, vestibular projections (from the vestibular nuclei via the MLF), and descending pursuit fibers, the paired inC act as the neural integrator for vertical gaze and torsion.[244,245] They lie adjacent but dorsal and caudal to the riMLF (**Fig. 16–17**).[246] For upgaze, fibers from the inC cross via the posterior commissure, then connect to the contralateral superior rectus and inferior oblique subnuclei. For downgaze, fibers again travel across the posterior commissure, then innervate the contralateral inferior rectus subnucleus and fourth nerve nucleus (**Fig. 16–18**).

The major clinicoanatomical implications of this arrangement are:

1. Since the inC is considered a vertical and torsional integrator, lesions may produce vertical and torsional gaze-holding deficits.

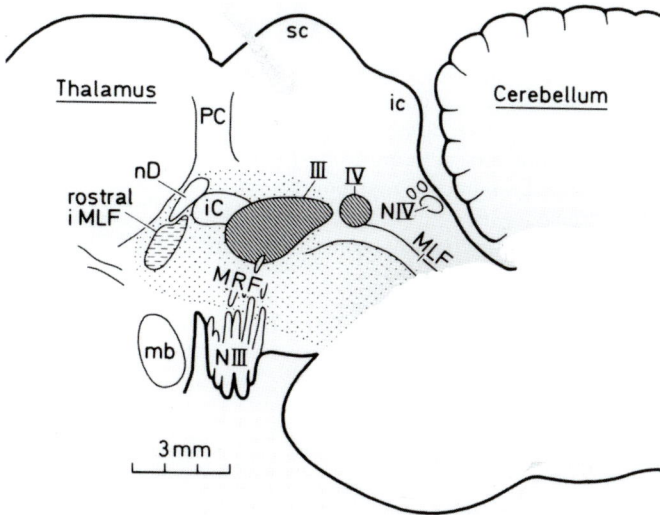

Figure 16–17. A schematic sagittal view of the upper brain stem, to demonstrate the anatomical localization of some structures involved in the generation of vertical eye movements. III, oculomotor nucleus; IV, trochlear nucleus; iC, interstitial nucleus of Cajal; ic, inferior colliculus; iMLF, (rostral) interstitial nucleus of the MLF; mb, mammillary body; MLF, medial longitudinal fasciculus; MRF, mesencephalic reticular formation; NIII, oculomotor nerve; NIV, trochlear nerve; NVII, facial nerve; nD, nucleus Darkschewitsch; PC, posterior commissure; sc, superior colliculus. (Adapted with permission from Büttner-Ennever JA. Anatomy of the ocular motor nuclei. In: Kennard C, Rose FC (eds): Physiological Aspects of Clinical Neuro-ophthalmology, p 203, Year Book, Chicago, 1988.)

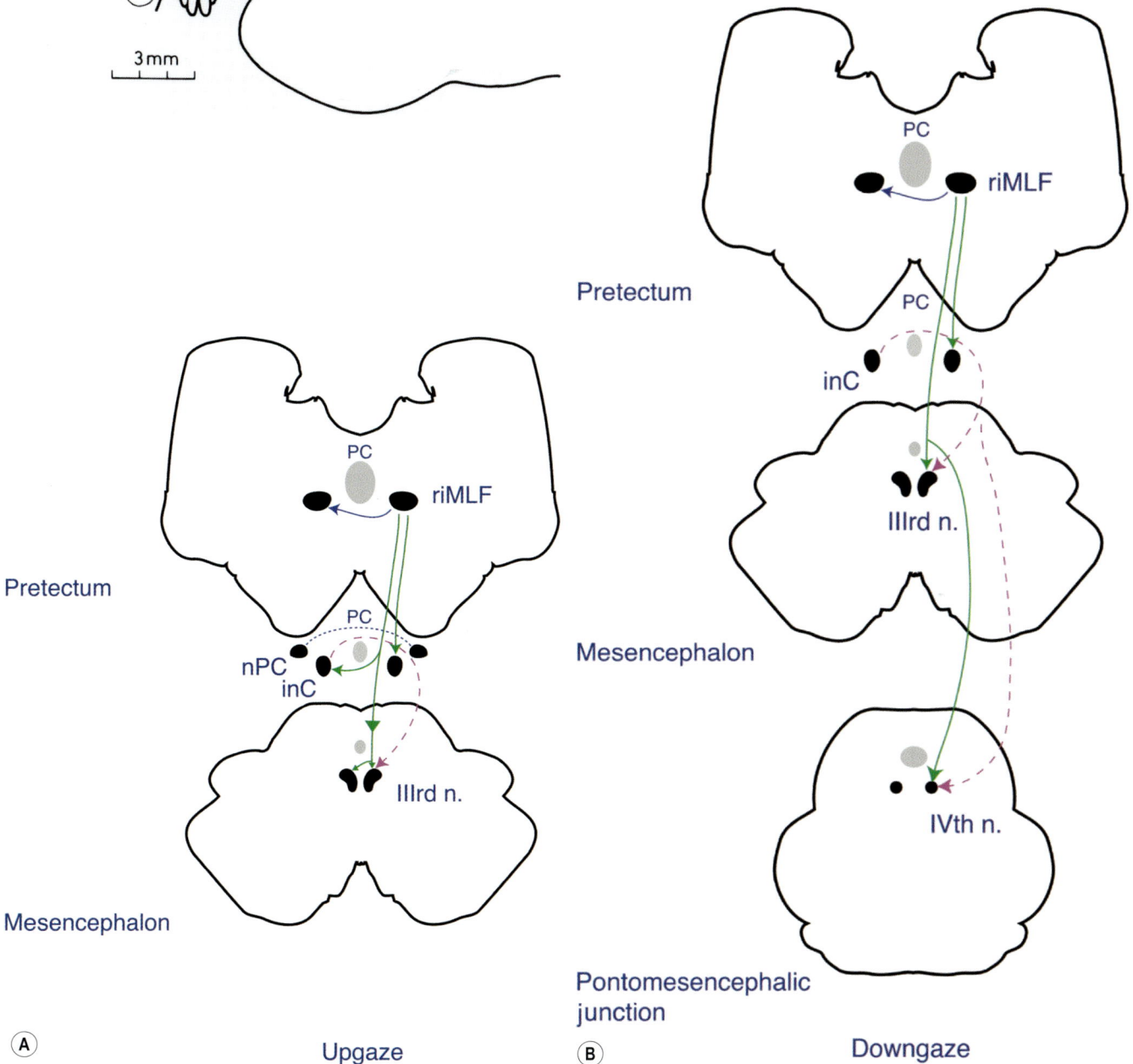

Figure 16–18. Major pathways subserving vertical eye movements.[244,245] For simplicity only fibers from one rostral interstitial nucleus of the medial longitudinal fasciculus (riMLF) and one interstitial nucleus of Cajal (inC) are shown on each side; the other riMLF and the other inC have identical, but mirror-image projections. **A**. *Upward eye movements*. Neurons from the riMLF, which contain burst neurons for vertical saccades, project ipsilaterally to the oculomotor nuclear complex. There fibers divide, with some crossing at this level, to innervate the superior rectus (SR) and inferior oblique (IO) subnuclei bilaterally. On the other hand, fibers from the inC, the neural integrator for vertical gaze, cross within the posterior commissure (PC) before reaching the contralateral oculomotor complex and the SR and IO subnuclei. The riMLF sends efferent fibers to both inCs. The nucleus of the posterior commissure (nPC) may also mediate upgaze through uncertain pathways. **B**. *Downward eye movements*. For downgaze, each riMLF supplies the ipsilateral inferior rectus subnucleus and the fourth nerve nucleus (IVth n.), which innervates the contralateral superior oblique muscle. Axons from the inC cross via the posterior commissure then innervate the contralateral inferior rectus subnucleus and fourth nerve nucleus.

2. Lesions to the inC or the afferents projecting to this nucleus may abolish the vertical vestibulo-ocular response,[1] while in contrast lesions solely of the riMLF tend not to affect it.

3. Destructive lesions of the inC are thought to be responsible for the ocular torsion and skew deviation seen in midbrain lesions. For instance, a lesion of the left inC may produce a left hypertropia, counter-roll of each eye toward the toward the right shoulder, and a right head tilt (see Chapter 15).

4. Lesions involving the projections of the inC in the posterior commissure are thought to produce vertical gaze abnormalities for all classes of eye movements. This is particularly true for upgaze.

5. Interestingly, the vertical saccades may be limited in their range of movement but their velocities will be normal with inC lesions.

Other supranuclear structures. In addition to the riMLF and inC, the nucleus of the posterior commissure (nPC) and M-group neurons likely aid in coordinating eyelid and vertical eye position (see Chapter 14) and also may play an important role in mediating upgaze. The role of the nucleus of Darkschewitsch in vertical eye movements is unclear.

There is considerable evidence in animals that the superior colliculus has a role in rapid gaze shifts, such as facilitating and inhibiting reflexive visually guided saccades. The function of the superior colliculus with regard to eye movements in man is probably similar but is less well understood, as isolated lesions of the superior colliculus are only rarely reported in humans.[76]

The cortical control of vertical eye movements is incompletely understood. Fibers from the frontal and supplementary eye fields mediating voluntary vertical saccades may pass through the thalamus before reaching the pretectum.[247] Reflexive vertical saccades may be mediated by axons arising from the parietal lobe.[248]

Vertical gaze limitations

Pretectal (Parinaud, dorsal midbrain) syndrome

This syndrome, the elements of which are listed in **Table 16–7**, is highlighted by supranuclear vertical upgaze paresis due to a dorsal midbrain disturbance (**Fig. 16–19**). The eponym is attributed to Henri Parinaud, an ophthalmologist who worked under Charcot at the Salpêtrière in Paris in the late 19th century[249] and wrote two landmark articles describing various types of conjugate gaze palsies and paralyses of convergence.[250,251]

More modern definitions of the syndrome have included pupillary and eyelid abnormalities, as well as convergence retraction nystagmus. For this reason, some authors such as Keane[252] have recommended using the anatomical term *pretectal syndrome*, but the term *dorsal midbrain syndrome* is also popular. Other names, such as Koeber–Salus–Elschnig sylvian aqueduct syndrome[253] and Nothnagel syndrome,[254,255] have been used but are less familiar.

Table 16–7 Elements of the pretectal (Parinaud) syndrome

Major components
  Supranuclear vertical gaze paresis
  Pupillary light–near dissociation
  Lid retraction (Collier's sign)
  Convergence–retraction nystagmus
Minor components
  Pseudo-abducens palsy (thalamic esotropia)
  Convergence insufficiency
  Accommodative insufficiency
Associated ocular motility deficits
  Skew deviation
  Third nerve palsy
  Internuclear ophthalmoplegia
  See-saw nystagmus

A lesion in the posterior commissure appears to be the one critical to producing the pretectal syndrome and all of the major elements.[256] The following sections describe the major and minor elements and some of the important disorders which commonly cause the pretectal syndrome.

Symptoms. Common neuro-ophthalmic complaints associated with the pretectal syndrome are difficulty looking up, diplopia, and blurred vision at near. Accompanying neurologic symptoms such as headache, nausea, and vomiting are suggestive of obstructive hydrocephalus. Acute pretectal neuro-ophthalmic symptoms in addition to ataxia or alteration in consciousness can occur in a midbrain infarction or thalamic hemorrhage.

Vertical upgaze paresis in the pretectal syndrome. The vertical gaze restriction in this syndrome results from involvement of the posterior commissure, inC, or the riMLF (**Figs 16–17** and **16–18**). Although vertical saccades and pursuit are both affected, the deficit of saccades is usually more prominent. Upgaze deficits may be seen alone or in combination with downgaze paresis, depending on the location of the involvement: lesions affecting the posterior commissure usually produce greater involvement of upgaze while those located more ventrally are usually associated with greater downgaze paresis.[240] Oculocephalic and oculovestibular maneuvers and attempted eye closure usually improve the vertical gaze limitation.[257] Lack of improvement by these measures frequently indicates coinvolvement of the third nerve nuclei or fascicles.

Other major elements of the pretectal syndrome

1. *Pupillary light–near dissociation.* The pupils are typically midposition (see **Fig. 13–9**), and they are poorly re active to light but more reactive to near (**Fig. 16–19D,E**). The pathophysiology is discussed in Chapter 13.

2. *Eyelid retraction (Collier's sign).* The eyelids may be elevated above the limbus in primary gaze (**Figs 16–19A** and **16–20A**). Sometimes there is also lid lag in downgaze. The involved pathways and mechanism are discussed in Chapter 14.

3. *Convergence retraction nystagmus.* Especially in attempted upward saccades, the eyes may jerk inward and into the globe (**Fig. 16–19C**). This type of nystagmus, which is

Video 13

Video 17

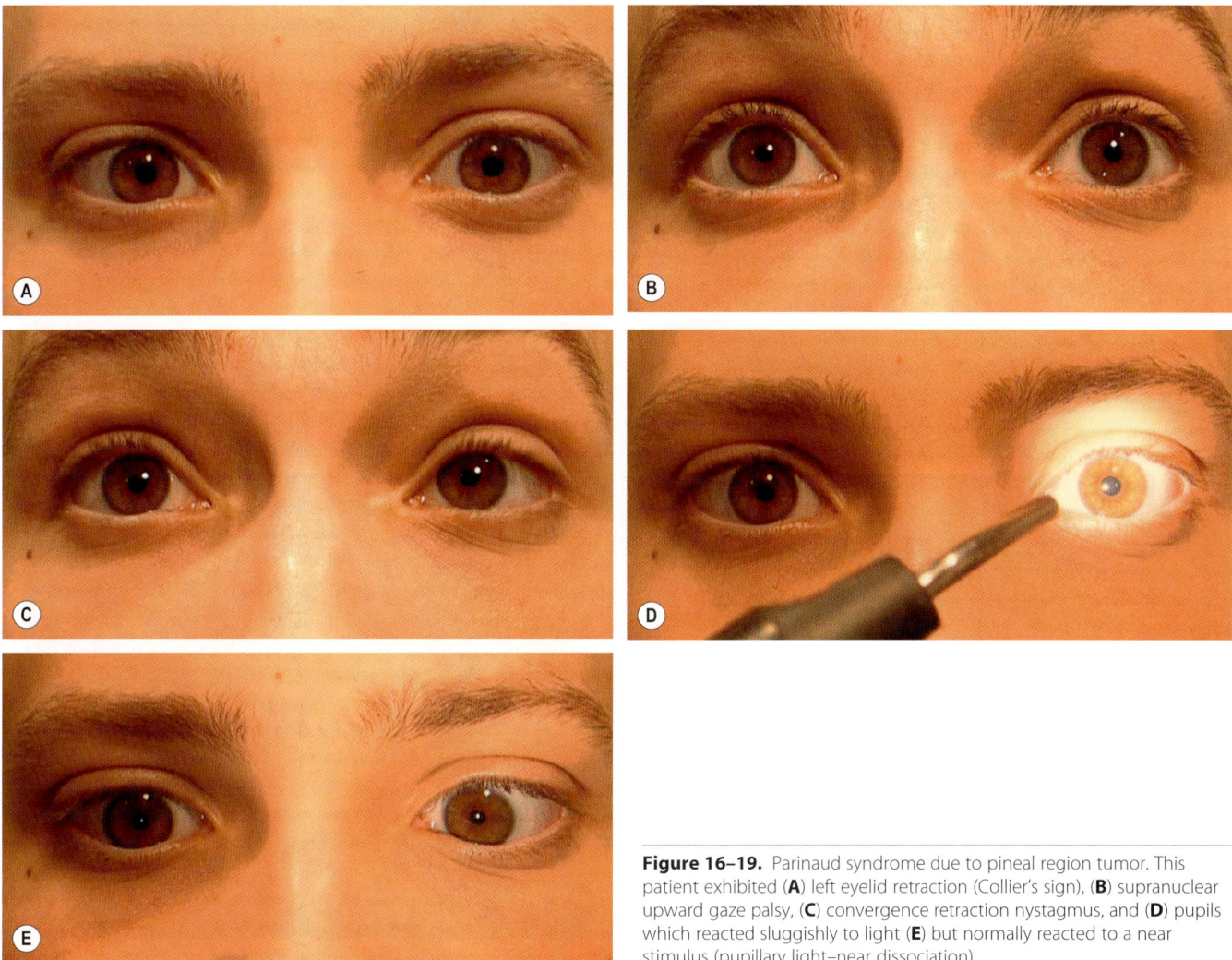

Figure 16–19. Parinaud syndrome due to pineal region tumor. This patient exhibited (**A**) left eyelid retraction (Collier's sign), (**B**) supranuclear upward gaze palsy, (**C**) convergence retraction nystagmus, and (**D**) pupils which reacted sluggishly to light (**E**) but normally reacted to a near stimulus (pupillary light–near dissociation).

reviewed in Chapter 17, is highly localizing to the pretectum.

Minor elements of the pretectal syndrome

1. *Pseudo-sixth nerve palsy*. Although the pons and sixth nerve may be spared, the eyes in patients with pretectal lesions may be esotropic (**Fig. 16–20B**).[258,259] One or both eyes may have an abduction deficit which is variable and easily overcome by horizontal oculocephalic movements. The "thalamic esotropia,"[260,261] associated with thalamic strokes and hemorrhages, is likely explained by pretectal involvement.[262] Like convergence retraction nystagmus, this ocular motility finding may in part reflect excess convergence tone as the pupils can be miotic. Other explanations include disruption in supranuclear fibers governing horizontal gaze, and fixation with the contralateral eye, which may have an adduction deficit due to an oculomotor palsy.[263]

2. *Convergence and accommodative insufficiency*. The critical structures for convergence (bilateral adduction) and accommodation lie in the midbrain and are reviewed in Chapter 13. Both functions are required for binocular viewing of near targets. Convergence insufficiency (see Chapter 15) causes horizontal binocular vision at near. Patients with accommodative insufficiency are unable to focus on near targets and may require the aid of plus lenses. We have seen young children with pineal region masses whose first complaints were diplopia and blurred vision at near.

Other associated ocular motility deficits

Skew deviation, see-saw nystagmus, third nerve palsy, and internuclear ophthalmoplegia. These ocular motility deficits may occur when the inC, the oculomotor nerve nucleus or fascicle, or medial longitudinal fasciculus, respectively, are disrupted by dorsal midbrain lesions which are large enough to affect the midbrain tegmentum. The skew may alternate sides,[264] or be part of an ocular tilt reaction.[265] They are discussed in great detail in Chapter 15. See-saw nystagmus, which may also be seen in this setting, is reviewed in Chapter 17.

Etiologies of the pretectal syndrome. Diagnostic considerations should be made in the context of the patient's age. In infants, obstructive hydrocephalus is the most common cause. In toddlers and other young children, pineal region masses are more common. In contrast, in adults, strokes and hemorrhages are the most frequent etiology.

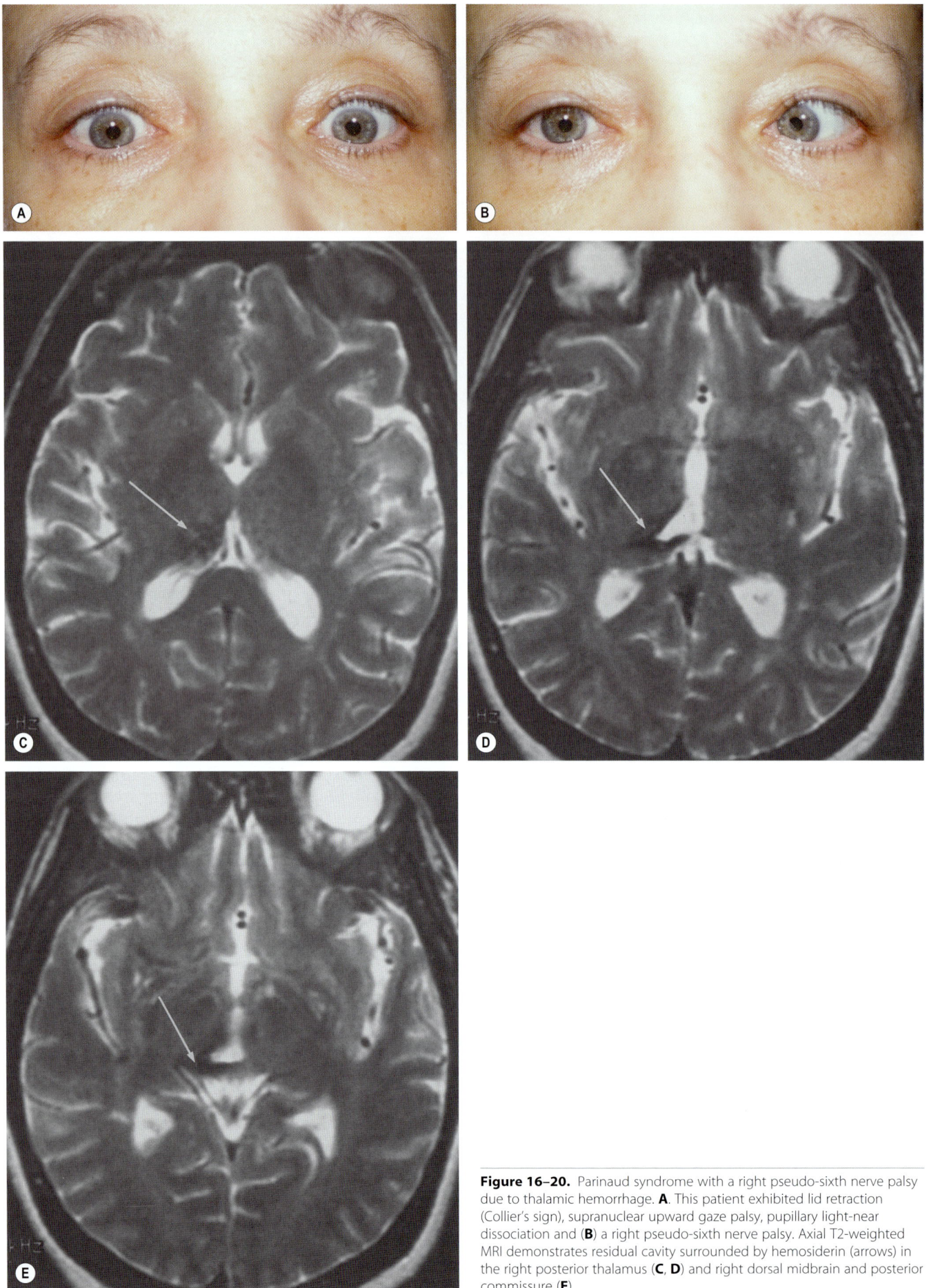

Figure 16–20. Parinaud syndrome with a right pseudo-sixth nerve palsy due to thalamic hemorrhage. **A**. This patient exhibited lid retraction (Collier's sign), supranuclear upward gaze palsy, pupillary light-near dissociation and (**B**) a right pseudo-sixth nerve palsy. Axial T2-weighted MRI demonstrates residual cavity surrounded by hemosiderin (arrows) in the right posterior thalamus (**C**, **D**) and right dorsal midbrain and posterior commissure (**E**).

Hydrocephalus. Pretectal signs and symptoms are frequently the first manifestations of obstructive (noncommunicating) hydrocephalus. The forced downward eye position in infants with hydrocephalus is said to mimic two setting suns. The mechanism is likely dilation of the third ventricle and of the rostral aqueduct, causing compression of pretectal structures.[266] Aqueductal dilation may also increase periaqueductal tissue water, which may decrease blood flow to structures in this area.[267] Ocular motor deficits usually resolve within days or weeks following ventricular decompression, but some patients are left with subtle permanent findings. Typical etiologies include congenital aqueductal stenosis or posterior fossa tumors causing fourth ventricular or aqueductal compression.

Pineal region tumors. Neoplasms in this region, when large enough, may compress the superior colliculi posteriorly and present with the pretectal syndrome. In most series,[268,269] about 90% of pineal region tumors presented with signs and symptoms due to increased intracranial pressure, such as papilledema, while about half presented with the pretectal syndrome (**Fig. 16–21**, and see **Fig. 13–9**).

One of the common neoplasms occurring in this region is a *germinoma*, which when isolated is associated with an excellent long-term outcome following radiation therapy. Treatment and presentation of germinomas, which also occur commonly in the sellar region, are discussed in Chapter 7. Less common germ cell tumor types occurring in the pineal region include embryonal cell, endodermal sinus, choriocarcinoma, and mature and immature teratomas.[270]

The other common tumor type in this area is a *pineal blastoma*, which is more highly malignant. They are also termed pineal primitive neuroectodermal tumors (PNET), similar in pathologic characteristics to medulloblastomas and supratentorial PNETs. These require surgical removal, exclusion of subarachnoid seeding, then in most instances radiation and chemotherapy. Pineal cytomas tend to occur

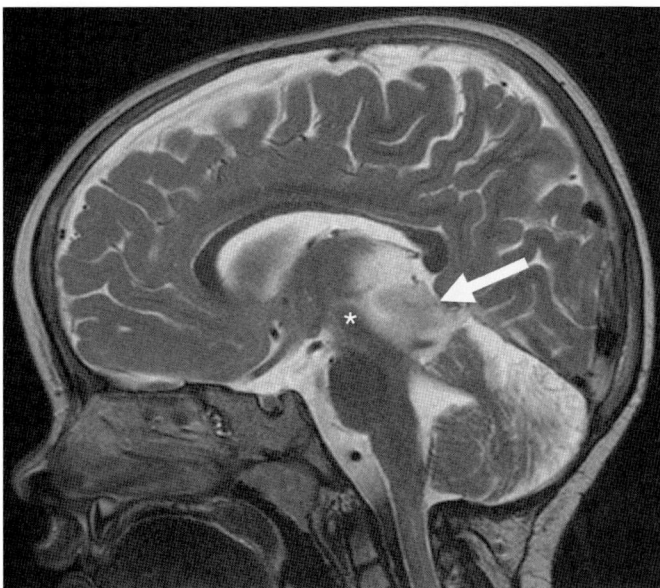

Figure 16–21. Pineal region tumor (arrow) associated with Parinaud syndrome. Note compression of the posterior portion of the midbrain (asterisk).

in older individuals and are usually more benign. Occasionally, aggressive atypical rhabdoid tumors are seen in this region as well.

Following surgical or radiotherapeutic decompression of pineal region tumors, most of the elements of Parinaud syndrome tend to resolve. The vertical gaze paresis usually resolves first, followed by improvement in the pupillary and eyelid abnormalities. Subtle convergence retraction nystagmus, provoked only by upward saccades, may be evident chronically in some patients. More prominent and persistent findings are typically the result of peritumoral radiation necrosis.

Pineal region cysts. Fluid-filled structures abutting the superior colliculi are usually asymptomatic.[271] They are often discovered incidentally in patients undergoing neuroimaging for other reasons such as headache. On MRI the cyst fluid, contained by a thin wall, is isointense or slightly hyperintense compared with cerebrospinal fluid (CSF). On CT, the cyst rim may contrast-enhance. They usually can be followed conservatively with serial examinations and neuroimaging. In only unusual instances the cysts are large enough to cause aqueductal compression and hydrocephalus. A case of hemorrhage into a pineal cyst associated with anticoagulation has been reported as a cause of "pineal apoplexy."[272]

Tectal gliomas. These relatively benign tumors usually surround the sylvian aqueduct and involve the superior collicular plate.[273] They are characterized pathologically as low-grade astrocytomas and radiographically on MRI by hyperintensity on T2-weighted images and gadolinium enhancement. Despite their location, they tend to be asymptomatic unless aqueductal compression and noncommunicating hydrocephalus occur. Consequently, the pretectal syndrome and signs and symptoms of elevated intracranial pressure such as headache, nausea, vomiting, and papilledema may be seen. The pretectal syndrome tends to be the result of the hydrocephalus and not of the tumor itself. Symptomatic tectal gliomas are usually treated with ventriculoperitoneal shunting to relieve the hydrocephalus, then serial examinations and radiographic observation of the neoplasm.[274] Surgery is usually not performed unless the lesions are exophytic, progressive, or appear to be higher grade,[275] when radiation or chemotherapy are also considered.

Paramedian midbrain/thalamic infarction. "Top of the basilar" strokes are associated with various combinations of oculomotor, behavioral, and motor findings.[258,276] The infarctions occur in the distribution of paramedian penetrating arteries arising from the proximal posterior cerebral arteries at the basilar bifurcation (P1 segments, or Percheron's basilar communicating arteries[277]) (see **Fig. 8–1**). The strokes can be unilateral, but because one paramedian artery may bifurcate and supply both sides of the mesencephalon and both thalami, often bilateral infarction at the two levels is seen (**Fig. 16–22**).[278] The infarctions sometimes take on a "butterfly" shape when viewed coronally. The etiology is typically vertebrobasilar atherosclerosis,[279] but emboli to the basilar bifurcation and proximal posterior cerebral arteries may also be responsible.[280]

When the lesions are ventral in the mesencephalon, fascicular third nerve palsies accompanied by contralateral

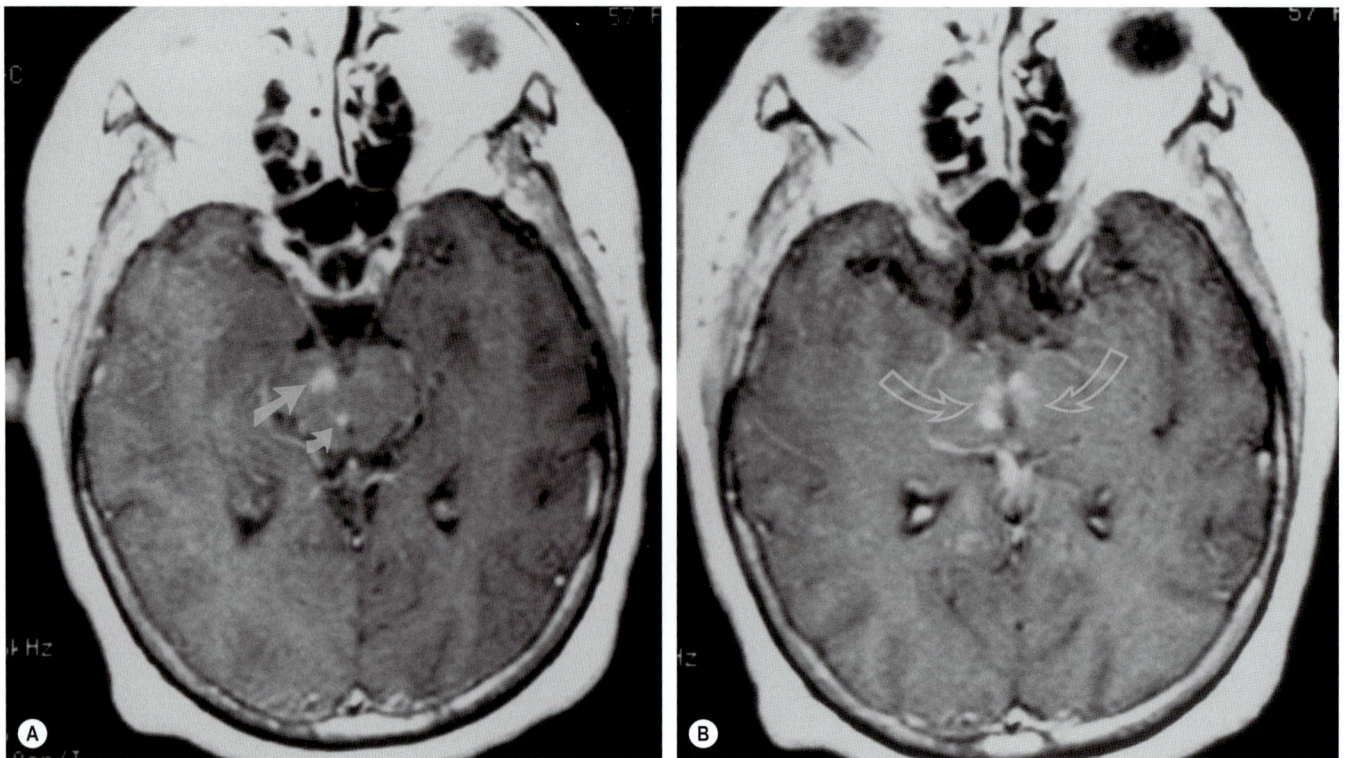

Figure 16–22. Top of the basilar infarction presenting with upgaze paresis and lethargy. **A**. Axial MRI with gadolinium through the midbrain demonstrating paramedian infarction of the ventral (large arrow) and dorsal (small arrow) mesencephalon. **B**. In the same patient, more rostral axial MRI showing bilateral mesial thalamic infarctions (arrows).

weakness or ataxia are seen (see Chapter 15). Rarely, peduncular hallucinations (Chapter 12) may also develop in ventral lesions. More dorsal infarction may affect the midbrain tegmentum and pretectum (**Fig. 16–22**).[281] These patients often exhibit nuclear and supranuclear vertical ocular motor disturbances and hypersomnolence due to disruption of the ascending reticular activating fibers and thalamic structures governing nonrapid eye movement (NREM) sleep.[282,283] Sensory deficits, aphasia, akinetic mutism, amnesia, and coma may also result from thalamic involvement.[284] If the proximal posterior cerebral artery is occluded, occipital lobe infarction leading to visual field defects (Chapter 8) and higher cortical visual disturbances (Chapter 9) may be seen.[258]

Thalamic hemorrhages. These lesions were discussed above in the section on horizontal gaze deviation. However, downward extension or hydrocephalus due to intraventricular extension of a thalamic hemorrhage may cause a pretectal syndrome.[226] In more severe cases the eyes may be esotropic and pointed downward, as if they were peering at the nose (**Fig. 16–23**).[285] The pupils tend to be small and sluggish or unreactive to light. The combination of a hemiparesis, sensory loss, hemianopia, or aphasia and pretectal syndrome is highly suggestive of a thalamic hemorrhage.

Thalamic tumors. The pretectal syndrome may result from thalamic tumors, usually gliomas, which extend below the tentorium to involve the upper midbrain.[286] Third ventricular compression may also lead to hydrocephalus and pretectal signs and symptoms on that basis.

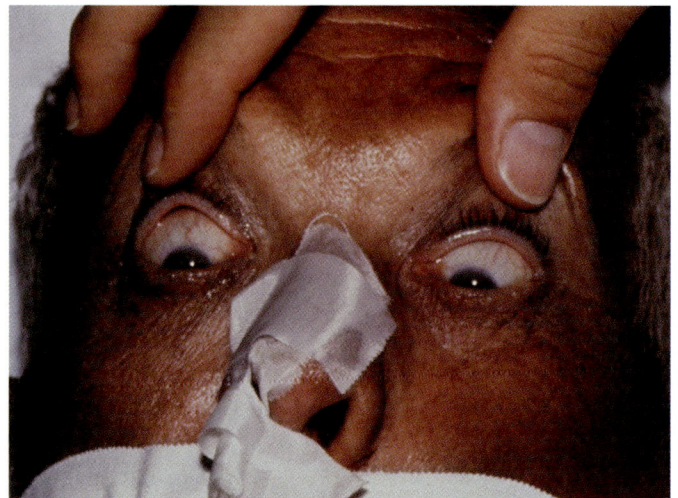

Figure 16–23. Severe downgaze deviation and stupor due to thalamic hemorrhage with intraventricular extension and hydrocephalus.

Infections. Tuberculomas and toxoplasmosis abscesses in the dorsal midbrain region should be considered, especially in immunocompromised patients such as those with acquired immunodeficiency syndrome (AIDS).[287,288] In Keane's series,[252] cysticercosis was one of the most frequent causes of dorsal midbrain syndrome. However, this likely reflected the prevalence of this infection in his patient population.

Other etiologies. A large variety of vascular, inflammatory, and compressive lesions have also been reported in association with the pretectal syndrome. These include transtentorial herniation,[289] arteriovenous malformations,[252] cavernous hemangiomas,[290,291] multiple sclerosis,[292–295] and posterior fossa aneurysms.[296]

Other mesencephalic vertical gaze deficits

Supranuclear downgaze paresis. Isolated downgaze paresis due to a midbrain lesion is much less common than isolated upgaze paresis or combined up- and downgaze paresis. Downgaze paresis may occur following damage in the mesencephalic reticular formation just dorsal and medial to the upper halves of the red nuclei.[240,297,298] Such lesions disrupt the efferents which emerge from the caudal–medial portions of the riMLF and head caudally towards the third and fourth nerve nuclei (see **Fig. 16–18**). As alluded to earlier, lesions producing prominent downgaze palsy are almost always bilateral,[286,297,299–301] but exceptional cases have been reported.[302]

The most common cause is a vascular insult involving a paramedian artery of the mesencephalon and thalamus.[303] However, degenerative disorders such as progressive supranuclear palsy (see below), and less commonly Huntington disease and pantothenate kinase-associated neurodegeneration (formerly Hallervorden–Spatz disease), should be considered.[304,305]

Vertical "one-and-a-half" syndrome. There are two variations of this ocular motility disorder, which borrow their label from their horizontal counterpart. In one of these vertical types, a monocular paresis of downgaze accompanied by a bilateral symmetric upgaze deficit can be caused by a unilateral thalamo-mesencephalic lesion.[306] The monocular downgaze deficit results either from disruption of the ipsilateral inferior rectus portion of the oculomotor fascicle or from an inferior rectus skew deviation (see Chapter 15). The upgaze paresis is due to involvement of either the (1) posterior commissure, resulting in a supranuclear vertical gaze paresis or the (2) oculomotor nucleus, which would lead to bilateral superior rectus weakness (see Chapter 15).

In another variation, there is a bilateral symmetric downgaze deficit accompanied by a monocular upgaze palsy. The downgaze paresis of saccades results from bilateral lesions in the mesencephalon affecting the downgaze efferents from the riMLF. The monocular upgaze deficit can be explained by disruption of the supranuclear fibers for upgaze of one eye (see supranuclear monocular elevator palsy, Chapter 15), by a superior rectus skew deviation, or by involvement of the fascicular fibers for the superior rectus and inferior oblique.[307]

Other neurologic disorders associated with vertical gaze deficits

Limited upgaze in elderly patients. Conjugate upgaze may be limited or reduced in otherwise normal elderly individuals.[308] Chamberlain[309] measured eye elevation in 367 normal volunteers aged 5–94. Those who were 5–14 years of age averaged 40.1 degrees of upward rotation, while those between 45 and 54 years averaged 30.4 degrees, and those aged 85–94 averaged 16.1 degrees. Downward rotations did not vary between age groups. The mechanism is unclear, but the deficits in many instances appear to be supranuclear.

Progressive supranuclear palsy. In 1963 and 1964, Steele, Richardson, and Olszewski[310–312] reported the clinical and pathologic findings of a neurodegenerative disorder to which there had previously been only vague reference in the literature. Clinically, their patients had progressive supranuclear ophthalmoparesis, pseudobulbar palsy, dysarthria, and rigidity of the neck and upper trunk. Pathologically, there were globose neurofibrillary tangles, neuronal loss, granulovacuolar degeneration, and gliosis in the basal ganglia, cerebellum, and mesencephalon. Richardson called the disorder progressive supranuclear palsy (PSP), although it is often referred to as the Steele–Richardson–Olszewski syndrome in honor of the individuals who crystallized the current understanding of its distinctive clinical and pathologic features.[313] Previous cases with similar clinical findings had been reported before their seminal reports, but in retrospect many of these had other diseases.[314,315] Today PSP is considered highly in the differential diagnosis of "parkinsonism plus."

Because neuro-ophthalmic signs and symptoms are so prominent in PSP, it is appropriate here to review the disorder in more detail.

Demographics. PSP is more common in elderly men than in women and uncommon before age 50.[316,317] Patients with PSP are less likely to have completed at least 12 years of school, suggesting that either poor early-life nutrition or occupational or residential toxic exposure are partly responsible.[318] Familial cases have been reported but are uncommon.[319,320]

Neuro-ophthalmic features. Eye movement abnormalities are eventually seen in the majority of patients with PSP. Affected patients may complain of blurred vision, trouble focusing, difficulty reading or looking down steps, eye pain, irritation, photophobia, or diplopia.[321] Because of their inability to look downward, patients with PSP can be "messy eaters."[322]

The clinical hallmark of PSP is a supranuclear vertical gaze paresis (**Fig. 16–24**), typically downward more than upward, which is usually evident within 3 years of symptom onset.[322] Often the oculocephalic maneuver is difficult to perform because of the nuchal rigidity. At first volitional vertical saccades are hypometric or slow,[323] but later they may become absent. In contrast to other saccadic disorders, head thrusting is generally not observed. Convergence is often impaired, and pursuit may be saccadic or "cogwheel."[324] As the disease progresses, horizontal gaze may become affected. The amplitude of quick phases of vestibular and optokinetic nystagmus may be diminished. In late, severe cases, some patients with PSP may develop an internuclear[325,326] or complete nuclear ophthalmoparesis.[327] However, autopsy-proven cases without eye movement deficits are well recognized.[328]

Other neuro-ophthalmic findings include horizontal square-wave jerks,[324] nystagmus, inability to suppress the vestibulo-ocular response (especially vertically), blepharospasm, and eyelid-opening apraxia.[321,328–330] Many have a characteristic facies with eyelid retraction, slow blink rate, and staring (**Fig. 16–24**).[331–333]

Video 16.7

Video 17.17

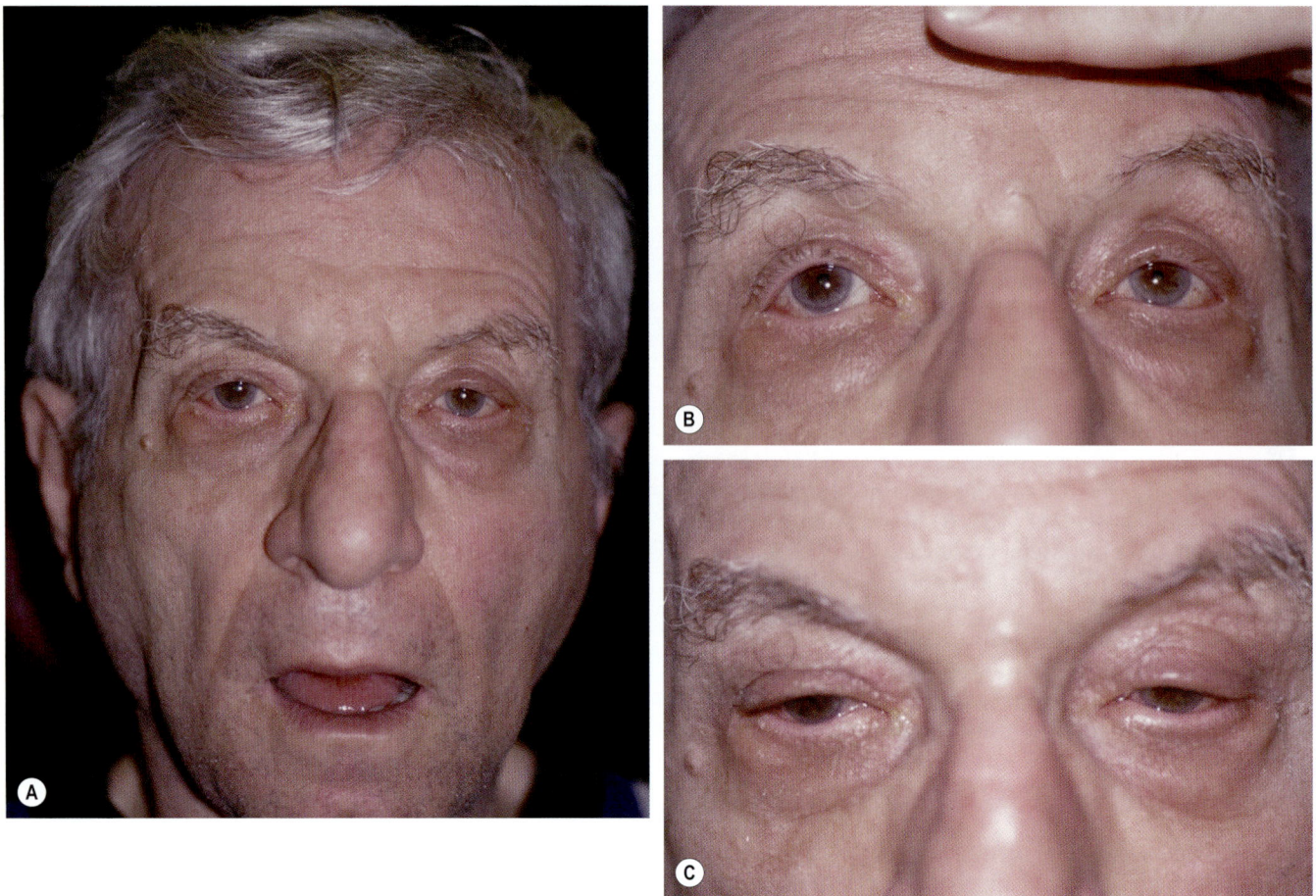

Figure 16–24. Patient with progressive supranuclear palsy. **A**. Characteristic stare. Defective (**B**) upgaze and (**C**) downgaze were also present.

Neurologic features. The most common initial neurologic complaints are postural instability and falling (often backwards), gait difficulty, dysarthria, and memory problems. Common behavioral features include apathy, disinhibition, depression, or withdrawal, but not irritability or agitation.[334]

On examination, parkinsonism is the most conspicuous finding and is characterized by bradykinesia and rigidity. Until patients with PSP develop the characteristic ocular motility findings, many are mistakenly given the diagnosis of Parkinson disease. However, in PSP, tremor is usually absent, and the rigidity is typically axial, affecting the neck and trunk, more than appendicular. Patients with PSP typically stand more upright than those with Parkinson disease, who often have a flexed posture. In PSP, limb dystonia[335] or apraxia[336] may also be observed. Cognitive impairment is most evident in tests sensitive to frontal lobe dysfunction, such as verbal fluency and motor sequencing.[337,338]

Table 16–8 summarizes criteria for the clinical diagnosis of PSP.[339,340] The combination of a supranuclear vertical gaze paresis plus postural instability and falling is highly suggestive of the diagnosis of PSP.[331,341] The ophthalmoplegia and gait, speech, and swallowing difficulty inexorably progress.[342,343] The median survival time in PSP is approximately 6 years following symptom onset, but it can range from 1 to 17 years.[344]

Pathologic features. The diagnosis of PSP can be established with certainty only at autopsy. PSP is characterized pathologically by atrophy predominantly of the subthalamic nucleus, the substantia nigra, and the globus pallidus.[345] Microscopically, gliosis, neuronal loss, and globose neurofibrillary tangles or neuropil threads are seen in these areas.[346] Other regions also involved include the striatum, periaqueductal gray, superior colliculi, oculomotor nuclei, red nuclei, locus ceruleus, pontine tegmentum, pontine nuclei, medulla, and cerebellar dentate nuclei.[331,346,347] Although the cerebral cortex may also be involved, the damage is typically less prominent.[348]

Within the neurofibrillary tangles, intraneuronal inclusions formed by aggregated tau protein are observed. Abnormal tau, a microtubule-associated protein, also accumulates in other neurodegenerative disorders such as Alzheimer and Pick diseases. PSP has been associated with the inheritance of a specific genotypes (A0/A0 and H1/H1) of the tau gene.[349–351] However, the tau genotype has no effect on onset, symptom severity, or survival.[352] In one study, truncated tau production in the CSF was found to be a reliable marker for PSP.

The supranuclear vertical gaze paresis can be explained by the presence of neurofibrillary tangles and neuronal damage to saccadic burst neurons in the riMLF.[332,353] The inC may also be involved.[354] Defective horizontal saccades may result

Table 16–8 Criteria for a clinical diagnosis of progressive supranuclear palsy[339,340]

Mandatory inclusionary criteria
  Onset at age 40 or later
  Progressive disease course
  Vertical supranuclear gaze palsy with downward gaze
    abnormalities
  Severe postural instability with unexplained falls

Supportive criteria
  Symmetric akinesia or rigidity, proximal more than distal
  Abnormal neck posture, especially retrocollis
  Poor or absent response of parkinsonism to levodopa therapy
  Early dysphagia and dysarthria
  Early onset of cognitive impairment including at least two of the
    following: apathy, impairment in abstract thought, decreased
    verbal fluency, utilization or imitation behavior, or frontal
    release signs

*Mandatory exclusionary criteria (and the disease for which the
  feature is more typical)*
  History of encephalitis (postencephalitic parkinsonism)
  Hallucinations (dementia with Lewy bodies)
  Early or prominent cerebellar signs (multisystem atrophy)
  Noniatrogenic dysautonomia (multisystem atrophy)
  Alien hand syndrome (corticobasal ganglionic degeneration)
  Early cortical dementia characterized by amnesia, aphasia, or
    agnosia (Alzheimer disease)
  Focal lesion on neurologic examination or neuroimaging
    (multi-infarct state)

Note these criteria are specific but not sensitive; they have a high positive predictive value. The diagnosis can be established with certainty only at autopsy, and even in retrospect some cases diagnosed post mortem will not have satisfied these criteria.

from cell loss in the PPRF,[355] while horizontal smooth pursuit impairment may be caused by damage in the nuclei of the basis pontis.[356] In one study, gaze palsy was associated pathologically with a decrease in neurons in the substantia nigra pars reticulata.[357] Damage to omnipause neurons in the nucleus raphe interpositus in the pons, leading to disinhibition of saccadic burst neurons, may be responsible for square-wave jerks and other saccadic intrusions.[358]

Neuroimaging. MRI early in the course of the disease may be normal. However, patients who have had PSP for years may exhibit putaminal hypointensity on T2-weighted images, representing iron deposition, and brain stem atrophy.[359,360] Focal midbrain atrophy, particularly of the superior colliculus, blurring ("smudging") of the margins of the substantia nigra, increased signal in the periaqueductal area, and atrophy of the superior cerebellar peduncles may also be seen.[187,361,362] When the midbrain is atrophied in PSP, on sagittal views on MR the brain stem is said to appear like the silhouette of a penguin (midbrain = head and beak; pons = body).[363,364] Diffusion-weighted MRI may demonstrate abnormal elevation in regional apparent diffusion coefficients (rADCs) in the basal ganglia.[365] MRI is also helpful in distinguishing patients with true PSP from those with PSP-like states due to multiple infarcts.[366,367]

Treatment. Although dopaminergic drugs such as levodopa, amantadine, bromocriptine or pergolide are generally unhelpful, a minority of patients may experience a transient mild to moderate benefit with these drugs.[327,368] However, the improvement is usually seen in the parkinsonism and bulbar signs, but not in ocular motility. Idazoxan, which increases norepinephrine transmission, was shown in a double-blind study to improve some aspects of motor function.[369]

Difficulty reading is a major complaint of patients with PSP because of their inability to look downward at their reading material and through their bifocal segment. Instructing such patients to bring reading materials to eye level may be the most practical advice, along with prescribing full-frame single-vision reading glasses for near.[321] Reading may also be complicated by convergence insufficiency, which can be ameliorated with base in prisms. Base-up prisms may be tried in patients with downgaze paresis to improve their awareness of objects below their eyes, but most find this too confusing.

Niemann–Pick disease. The Niemann–Pick disorders are autosomal recessive lysosomal storage conditions characterized by hepatosplenomegaly and progressive neurologic deterioration. The type C chronic neuronopathic form, one of the type II disorders in the more modern classification, typically presents with supranuclear vertical gaze paresis, mental and motor deterioration, ataxia, and visceromegaly.[370] The disorder has been mapped to chromosome 18q11–12 in most studied families. It is caused by a defect in intracellular mobilization and esterification of low-density lipoprotein (LDL)-derived cholesterol. Three subtypes of Niemann–Pick type C can be identified: (1) a rapidly progressive infantile form, (2) a juvenile form which occurs in previously healthy children, and (3) a slowly progressive form in adolescents and adults.[371,372] The bone marrow typically exhibits sea-blue histiocytes and foam cells. Cytochemical staining of cultured fibroblasts with filipine, which fluoresces after binding with unesterified cholesterol, may also be performed. Treatment, which is usually aimed at reducing cholesterol intake and administering cholesterol-lowering agents, is relatively ineffective.

The ocular motor disturbance, which occurs in about two-thirds of cases,[373] typically presents as a supranuclear downgaze saccadic paresis. This is followed by upgaze involvement, then results in extreme cases in a total vertical saccadic palsy.[374] Vertical pursuit movements as well as horizontal eye movements are usually preserved. Because of the characteristic phenotype, the designation DAF syndrome, for *d*owngaze paresis, *a*taxia, and *f*oam cells, has also been used.[139] A macular cherry-red spot, secondary to opacification of the nerve fiber layer, may also be seen.

Whipple disease. Central nervous system (CNS) involvement is a well-recognized complication of a multisystem chronic infection called Whipple disease, which is caused by the bacillus *Tropheryma whippelii*. In the brain there is a predilection for involvement of the periaqueductal gray matter, hypothalamus, hippocampus, cerebral cortex, basal ganglia, and cerebellum.[375]

A supranuclear vertical gaze paresis, in either up- or downgaze, is observed in approximately one-third of patients with CNS involvement.[376] When the vertical supranuclear gaze palsy is accompanied by dementia and a gait disturbance, Whipple disease may mimic progressive supra-nuclear palsy.[377] In a smaller proportion of patients, the supranuclear gaze paresis is both vertical and horizontal.[314] An isolated horizontal gaze paresis is usually not seen.

Oculomasticatory myorhythmia, characterized by pendular convergent–divergent nystagmus associated with rhythmic movements of the muscles of mastication, face, and extremities, is considered virtually pathognomonic (see also Chapter 17).[375,378] In a large meta-analysis of reported patients with Whipple's disease,[376] oculomasticatory myorhythmia was found always to occur with a supranuclear gaze paresis. Hypothalamic involvement may result in the syndrome of inappropriate antidiuretic hormone secretion (SIADH), insomnia, hypersomnia, and hyperphagia. Cognitive and psychiatric symptoms are also observed frequently.[376]

The most common symptoms in Whipple disease are gastrointestinal and include malabsorption, abdominal pain, weight loss, and diarrhea. Other systemic symptoms, such as pleuritis, lymphadenopathy, cardiac valvular lesions, fever, and arthritis, are often present.[379] CNS complications usually occur in association with systemic symptoms, but the latter may be absent in up to one-fifth of cases of CNS Whipple disease.[376] Rarely ocular involvement can occur and is characterized by uveitis, keratitis, vitreous hemorrhage, retinitis, or optic disc edema.[380,381]

The diagnosis is best established by small bowel biopsy or other samples of involved tissue and demonstration of *T. whippelii* DNA by polymerase chain reaction (PCR) testing.[352,379,382] Staining for period acid–Schiff (PAS)-positivity in macrophages, which can also be used, is not as sensitive or specific. Electron micrographic demonstration of the organism can be performed. *T. whippelii* is difficult to culture. Midbrain, hypothalamic, and temporal lobe hyperintensities may be seen on MRI,[383] and the spinal fluid analysis may reveal a pleocytosis and elevated protein. However, both neuroimaging and spinal fluid may also be normal.

Treatment with antibiotics such as intravenous trimethoprim–sulfamethoxazole or ceftriaxone[384] for 2 weeks followed by oral trimethoprim–sulfamethoxazole twice daily for 1 year is often effective.[385] Tetracycline and chloramphenicol have also been used.

Miscellaneous

Amyotrophic lateral sclerosis. Some reports[386–390] have suggested that supranuclear conjugate gaze rarely may be affected in amyotrophic lateral sclerosis (Lou Gehrig disease), even very early in its course. Slow saccades and pursuit in all directions, as well as vertical gaze palsies, were documented in one study.[388] In another,[390] neuropathologic examination in two patients with supranuclear upgaze paresis confirmed neuronal loss in the riMLF and periaqueductal gray and sparing of the third and fourth nerve nuclei. Amyotrophic lateral sclerosis, including third, fourth, and sixth cranial nerve involvement in this disorder, is also discussed in Chapter 15.

Other neuromuscular conditions. Subclinical defective saccades have been documented in myotonic dystrophy. It has been controversial whether the saccadic abnormalities in myotonic dystrophy are peripheral or central in origin.[391–395]

Saccades may also be defective in myasthenia gravis. These disorders are discussed in more detail in Chapter 14. Rare patients with mitochondrial disorders such as MELAS (mitochondrial encephalomyopathy, lactic acidosis, and stroke-like episodes; see Chapter 8) have been reported with slow horizontal saccades.[396]

Other basal ganglia disorders. Slow or limited saccades, particularly in upgaze, have been reported in Wilson disease.[397] We have also seen a patient with idiopathic calcification of the basal ganglia and dentate nuclei (Fahr disease) presenting with supranuclear ophthalmoparesis and parkinsonism, mimicking progressive supranuclear palsy.[398]

Paraneoplastic brain stem encephalitis. Ophthalmoparesis, of both nuclear and supranuclear origin, may be a manifestation of a paraneoplastic brain stem encephalitis. The anti-Hu antibody is the most commonly associated antibody and lung cancer is the most frequently found tumor.[399] An antibody known as anti-Ta has been associated with testicular cancer and ophthalmoparesis.[400,401]

Abnormal vertical conjugate gaze deviations

Oculogyric crises

Oculogyric crises are a dystonia of ocular muscles[402] characterized by dramatic involuntary conjugate deviation of the eyes.[403] The eyes usually inadvertently move straight upwards or up and to the left or right, and the position can change from crisis to crisis. Oculogyric crises are often associated with thought or emotional disturbances, are preceded by a brief stare, and last for hours.[404] However, they can occur without these features and last only a few seconds. Frequently they are accompanied by other dystonic or dyskinetic movements such as tongue protrusion, lip smacking, blepharospasm, choreoathetosis, anterocollis, and retrocollis.[405–407]

In the 1920s the French described crises (*crises oculogyres*) as complications of postencephalitic Parkinsonism,[403,408] but today they are usually acute or tardive extrapyramidal reactions to neuroleptics.[404–407,409–411] We have also seen oculogyric crisis with some of the newer agents such as aripiprazole. In addition to postencephalitic parkinsonism, oculogyric crises have been associated with other neurologic disorders such as Parkinson disease,[412] familial Parkinson–dementia syndrome,[413] dopa-responsive dystonia,[414] parkinsonism with basal ganglia calcifications (Fahr disease),[415] neurosyphilis, multiple sclerosis, ataxia-telangiectasia,[416] Rett syndrome,[417] Wilson disease,[418] cerebellar disease, trauma,[419] acute herpetic brain stem encephalitis,[420] a third ventricular cystic glioma,[421] paraneoplastic disease,[400] and striatocapsular infarction.[422,423] Besides neuroleptics, carbemazepine,[424,425] tetrabenazine,[426] gabapentin,[427] cetirazine,[428] and several other drugs[419] can also cause oculogyric crises.

The etiology of oculogyric crises is not certain. In postencephalitic patients, some authors believed they resulted from a release of supranuclear control of oculomotor centers as a result of injury to the corpus striatum or subthalamic nucleus.[403] Onuaguluchi[408] hypothesized they were due to

Video 17.13

an abnormal vestibulo-ocular reflex in the setting of brain stem lesions involving vestibular pathways. Leigh et al.[404] attributed the deviations to an incorrect efference copy of eye position. Based on the response to anticholinergic agents in neuroleptic-induced crises, they alternatively invoked a defect in mesencephalic vertical gaze-holding mechanisms normally dependent on balanced cholinergic and dopaminergic systems.[404] Another hypothesis explains oculogyric crises as a limbic–motor disorder.[419]

Treatment. Severe or painful oculogyric crises can be treated acutely with benztropine, 2 mg intramuscularly or intravenously, or diphenhydramine, 50 mg intramuscularly or intravenously.[419] A dose can be repeated in 30 minutes if there is no response. If these are unsuccessful, then diazepam, 5–10 mg intravenously, or lorazepam, 1 mg intramuscularly or intravenously, can be used. The underlying condition should be treated, or the offending drug removed or dosage lowered. Some patients with oculogyric crises owing to neuroleptic use may require short-term treatment with oral benztropine, 2–6 mg q.d., or oral trihexyphenidyl, 4–15 mg q.d., for 2 weeks following the acute episode.[419] One reported patient improved with vagus nerve stimulation.[429] Seizures should be excluded with an electroencephalogram (EEG).

Ocular tics

Brief dystonic eye rolling and torticollis, mimicking unsustained oculogyric crises, have also been described in tic disorders.[430,431] Benign ocular tics manifested by eye rolling, usually upward, are not infrequently seen in otherwise healthy children (**Fig. 16–25**). In these instances they are idiopathic and usually resolve spontaneously. Tourette syndrome is a tic disorder which is inherited, and children with this disorder have vocal tics and behavioral disturbances in addition to motor tics.[432] Typically an irresistible urge and an ability to suppress the eye movements precedes them. Ninety percent of patients with Tourette syndrome develop their first motor tic by age 10.[433] Isolated motor tics can also be secondary to drugs or basal ganglia injury ("acquired tourettism").[432] When bothersome, the tics may be treated

with dopamine antagonists. Eyelid tics are discussed in Chapter 14.

Benign tonic vertical gaze in infancy

Tonic up- or downward gaze in infants, lasting weeks to months, is well-recognized (**Fig. 16–26**).[434–438] The finding was seen in five of 242 healthy neonates in one study.[439] The gaze deviation is typically intermittent, lasting minutes, hours, or days.[440] Children can appear to have either a supranuclear gaze deficit or jerk nystagmus in the direction opposite to the gaze preference.[441] The eyes can easily be moved into a normal position by the oculocephalic maneuver. There are usually no central nervous system abnormalities. The course is usually benign with a gradual decrease in the frequency and duration of the episodes, and ultimately the children are normal within the first few months of age.[442,443] The mechanism is usually attributed to immaturity of either an ocular motor or a visual pathway: the vertical gaze centers in the midbrain, the vestibulo-ocular reflexes, or the afferent visual system.[436]

All patients should undergo a careful pediatric neurologic examination and neuroimaging. This is particularly important in those with tonic downgaze, in whom a pretectal syndrome due to hydrocephalus or a pineal region mass needs to be considered. An EEG should be performed to exclude seizure activity. Improvement with levodopa/carbidopa preparations has been reported. However, in most instances pharmacologic manipulations are not helpful and are usually unnecessary because of the self-limited nature of the disorder.

Acquired cases. A variation of this condition has been described in which some patients are normal at birth but develop the ocular motility disorder later in infancy.[444] The onset of the tonic gaze in some instances follows an intercurrent illness or vaccination. Some patients have similarly affected family members. The outcome in these acquired cases may be less sanguine, with some patients later exhibiting developmental delay, intellectual disability, language delay, and either persistent tonic vertical gaze or other eye

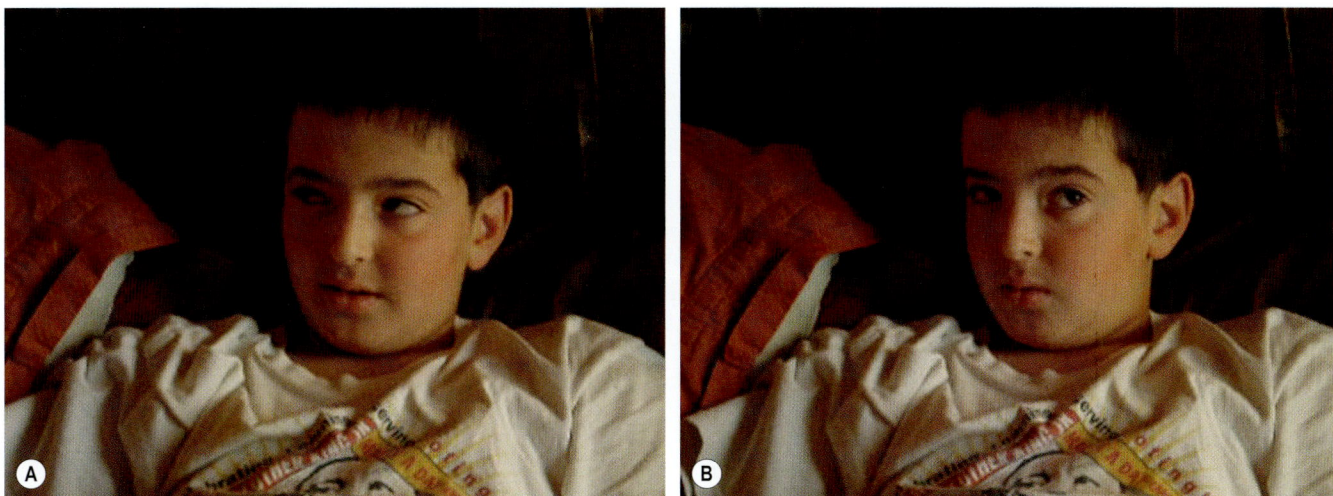

Figure 16–25. Benign ocular tics in an otherwise healthy boy. He developed brief episodes, each 1–2 seconds, of conjugate eye deviation either up and to the right (**A**) or up and to the left (**B**).

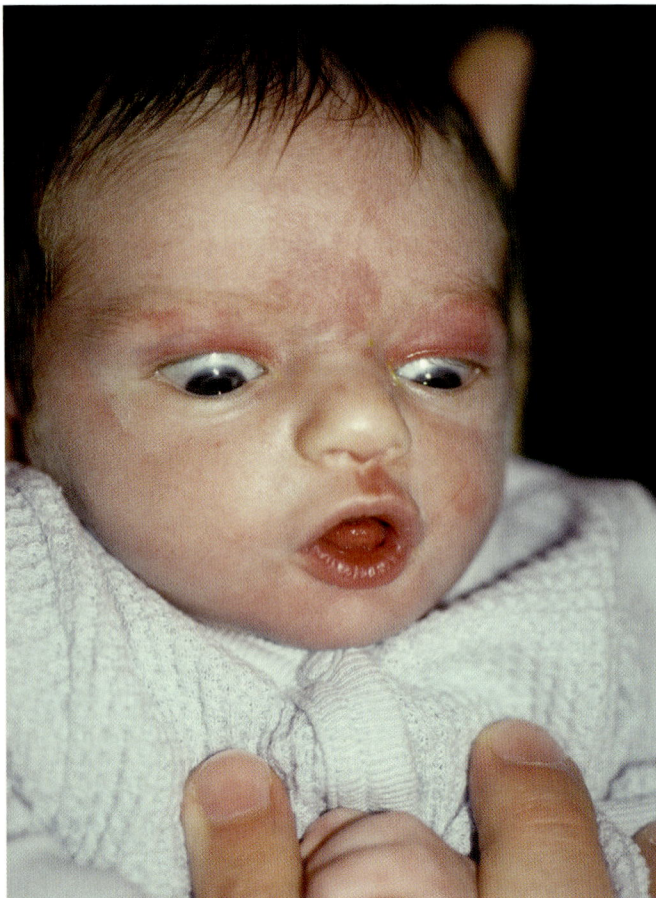

Figure 16–26. Ten-day-old infant exhibiting episodic tonic downward gaze, which was easily overcome by vertical oculocephalic movements. The workup was negative and the disorder spontaneously resolved by 4 months of age.

movement disorder.[445] The guarded prognosis may reflect the presence of a more widespread neurologic disorder.

Complete ophthalmoplegia

Most of the disorders which cause complete absence of eye movements are nuclear or infranuclear, affecting the oculo-motor nerves, neuromuscular junction, or extraocular muscles. However, some supranuclear disorders discussed in this chapter, when severe or in their end stages, may affect the ocular motor nuclei and therefore disrupt all voluntary and involuntary eye movements. These include Wernicke's encephalopathy, spinocerebellar ataxias, and progressive supranuclear palsy, for example. A list of disorders that cause complete ophthalmoplegia is in Chapter 15.

Coma

Conjugate gaze deviations and paresis during oculocephalic or vestibulo-ocular testing may be highly localizing in patients with coma.

Conjugate gaze deviations. The guidelines for considering etiologies according to those that cause horizontal versus

vertical gaze deviations apply here as well. For instance, a horizontal conjugate gaze deviation may be caused by an ipsilateral hemispheric lesion (**Figs 16–14** and **16–15**), contralateral pontine lesion, or contralateral hemispheric epileptic focus (**Figs 16–14** and **16–16**). Occasionally "wrong-way" eyes due to a contralateral hemispheric or thalamic hemorrhage should be considered. Fast cycle horizontal periodic alternating gaze, or "ping-pong" gaze, indicates an intact pons which is disconnected from bilateral hemispheric influences.

Eyes that are deviated downward suggest a dorsal midbrain or thalamic lesion such as an infarction, hemorrhage, or hydrocephalus. However, persistent downgaze has also been reported in patients with subarachnoid hemorrhage and hypoxic encephalopathy without pretectal lesions.[446,447] Tonic upgaze may be observed in anoxia, presumably due to diffuse injury to the cortex and cerebellum.[447,448] Inhibitory fibers from the cerebellum to the anterior semicircular canal projections are removed, resulting in tonic elevation of the eyes. After several weeks following the initial injury, downbeat nystagmus may evolve as the cortical inputs begin to recover. In general, the appearance of tonic upgaze after anoxic arrest is a poor prognostic sign for meaningful neurologic recovery.

Conjugate gaze paresis. An inability to move the eyes conjugately either by the oculocephalic maneuver or by cold caloric stimulation (see Chapter 2) is highly suggestive of an ipsilateral sixth nerve nucleus lesion in the pons, but a vestibular nerve or nucleus lesion should also be excluded. Defective vertical gaze during reflex testing implies a midbrain lesion involving the inC or oculomotor nuclei, fascicles, or nerves. Voluntary saccadic and pursuit function is obviously untestable in comatose patients.

Localization in coma is discussed further in Chapter 2.

References

1. Büttner-Ennever JA, Büttner U. Neuroanatomy of the ocular motor pathways. Baillières Clin Neurol 1992;1:263–287.
2. Sharpe JA. Neural control of ocular motor systems. In: Miller NR, Newman NJ (eds): Walsh and Hoyt's Clinical Neuro-ophthalmology, 4th edn, pp 1101–1167. Baltimore, Williams & Wilkins, 1998.
3. Pierrot-Deseilligny C, Rivaud S, Gaymard B, et al. Cortical control of saccades. Ann Neurol 1995;37:557–567.
4. Morrow MJ, Sharpe JA. Deficits of smooth-pursuit eye movement after unilateral frontal lobe lesions. Ann Neurol 1995;37:443–451.
5. Henn V. Pathophysiology of rapid eye movements in the horizontal, vertical and torsional directions. Baillières Clin Neurol 1992;1:373–391.
6. Pierrot-Deseilligny C, Gaymard B, Müri R, et al. Cerebral ocular motor signs. J Neurol 1997;244:65–70.
7. Godoy J, Lüders H, Dinner DS, et al. Versive eye movement elicited by cortical stimulation of the human brain. Neurology 1990;40:296–299.
8. Gaymard B, Pierrot-Deseilligny C, Rivaud S. Impairment of sequences of memory-guided saccades after supplementary motor area lesions. Ann Neurol 1990;28:622–626.
9. Gaymard B, Rivaud S, Pierrot-Deseilligny C. Role of the left and right supplementary motor areas in memory-guided saccade sequences. Ann Neurol 1993;34:404–406.
10. Pierrot-Deseilligny C, Muri RM, Ploner CJ, et al. Cortical control of ocular saccades in humans: a model for motricity. Prog Brain Res 2003;142:3–17.
11. McDowell JE, Dyckman KA, Austin BP, et al. Neurophysiology and neuroanatomy of reflexive and volitional saccades: evidence from studies of humans. Brain Cogn 2008;68:255–270.
12. Schall JD. Neural basis of saccade target selection. Rev Neurosci 1995;6:63–85.
13. Sharpe JA. Cortical control of eye movements. Curr Opin Neurol 1998;11:31–38.
14. Bender MB. Brain control of conjugate horizontal and vertical eye movements. A survey of the structural and functional correlates. Brain 1980;103:23–69.
15. Pierrot-Deseilligny C, Rivaud S, Penet C, et al. Latencies of visually guided saccades in unilateral hemispheric cerebral lesions. Ann Neurol 1987;21:138–148.

16. Munoz DP. Commentary: saccadic eye movements: overview of neural circuitry. Prog Brain Res 2002;140:89–96.

17. Ramat S, Leigh RJ, Zee DS, et al. What clinical disorders tell us about the neural control of saccadic eye movements. Brain 2007;130:10–35.

18. Horn AKE, Büttner-Ennever JA, Büttner U. Saccadic premotor neurons in the brainstem: functional neuroanatomy and clinical implications. Neuroophthalmology 1996;16:229–240.

19. Büttner-Ennever JA, Horn AKE. Anatomical substrates of oculomotor control. Curr Opin Neurobiol 1997;7:872–879.

20. Leigh RJ, Rottach KG, Das VE. Transforming sensory perceptions into motor commands: evidence from programming of eye movements. Ann N Y Acad Sci 1997;835:353–362.

21. Thurtell MJ, Tomsak RL, Leigh RJ. Disorders of saccades. Curr Neurol Neurosci Rep 2007;7:407–416.

22. Kennard C, Crawford TJ, Henderson L. A pathophysiological approach to saccadic eye movements in neurological and psychiatric disease [editorial]. J Neurol Neurosurg Psychiatr 1994;57:881–885.

23. Gaymard B, Rivaud S, Amarenco P, et al. Influence of visual information on cerebellar saccadic dysmetria. Ann Neurol 1994;35:108–112.

24. Ettinger U, Kumari V, Crawford TJ, et al. Smooth pursuit and antisaccade eye movements in siblings discordant for schizophrenia. J Psychiatr Res 2004;38:177–184.

25. Morrow MJ, Sharpe JA. Cerebral hemispheric localization of smooth pursuit asymmetry. Neurology 1990;40:284–292.

26. Nagel M, Sprenger A, Zapf S, et al. Parametric modulation of cortical activation during smooth pursuit with and without target blanking. an fMRI study. Neuroimage 2006;29:1319–1325.

27. Barton JJS, Sharpe JA, Raymond JE. Directional defects in pursuit and motion perception in humans with unilateral cerebral lesions. Brain 1996;119:1535–1550.

28. Petit L, Haxby JV. Functional anatomy of pursuit eye movements in humans as revealed by fMRI. J Neurophysiol 1999;81:463–471.

29. Krauzlis RJ. The control of voluntary eye movements: new perspectives. Neuroscientist 2005;11:124–137.

30. Lencer R, Trillenberg P. Neurophysiology and neuroanatomy of smooth pursuit in humans. Brain Cogn 2008;68:219–228.

31. Ohtsuka K, Enoki T. Transcranial magnetic stimulation over the posterior cerebellum during smooth pursuit eye movements in man. Brain 1998;121:429–435.

32. Johnston JL, Sharpe JA, Morrow MJ. Paresis of contralateral smooth pursuit and normal vestibular smooth eye movements after unilateral brainstem lesions. Ann Neurol 1992;31:495–502.

33. Fukushima K. Frontal cortical control of smooth-pursuit. Curr Opin Neurobiol 2003;13:647–654.

34. Thier P, Ilg UJ. The neural basis of smooth-pursuit eye movements. Curr Opin Neurobiol 2005;15:645–652.

35. Sharpe JA. Neurophysiology and neuroanatomy of smooth pursuit: lesion studies. Brain Cogn 2008;68:241–254.

36. Bucher SF, Dieterich M, Seelos KC, et al. Sensorimotor cerebral activation during optokinetic nystagmus. Neurology 1997;49:1370–1377.

37. Rivaud S, Müri RM, Gaymard B, et al. Eye movement disorders after frontal eye field lesions in humans. Exp Brain Res 1994;102:110–120.

38. Pierrot-Deseilligny C. Saccade and smooth-pursuit impairment after cerebral hemispheric lesions. Eur Neurol 1994;34:121–134.

39. Heide W, Kurzidim K, Kömpf D. Deficits of smooth pursuit eye movements after frontal and parietal lesions. Brain 1996;119:1951–1969.

40. Thurston SE, Leigh RJ, Crawford T, et al. Two distinct deficits of visual tracking caused by unilateral lesions of cerebral cortex in humans. Ann Neurol 1988;23:266–273.

41. Sharpe JA, Morrow MJ. Cerebral hemispheric smooth pursuit disorders. Acta Neurol Belg 1991;91:81–96.

42. Morrow MJ, Sharpe JA. Retinotopic and directional deficits of smooth pursuit initiation after posterior cerebral hemispheric lesions. Neurology 1993;43:595–603.

43. Morrow MJ. Craniotopic defects of smooth pursuit and saccadic eye movements. Neurology 1996;46:514–521.

44. Baloh RW, Yee RD, Honrubia V. Optokinetic nystagmus and parietal lobe lesions. Ann Neurol 1980;7:269–276.

45. Dehaene I, Lammens M. Paralysis of saccades and pursuit: clinicopathologic study. Neurology 1991;41:414–415.

46. Pierrot-Deseilligny C, Gautier J-C, Loron P. Acquired ocular motor apraxia due to bilateral frontoparietal infarcts. Ann Neurol 1988;23:65–70.

47. Sharpe JA, Johnston JL. Ocular motor paresis versus apraxia [letter]. Ann Neurol 1989;25:209–210.

48. Pierrot-Deseilligny C, Goasguen J, Chain F, et al. Pontine metastasis with dissociated bilateral horizontal gaze paresis. J Neurol Neurosurg Psychiatr 1984;47:159–164.

49. Baloh RW, Furman JM, Yee RD. Eye movements in patients with absent voluntary horizontal gaze. Ann Neurol 1985;17:283–286.

50. Hirose G, Furui K, Yoshioka A, et al. Unilateral conjugate gaze palsy due to a lesion of the abducens nucleus. J Clin Neuroophthalmol 1993;3:54–58.

51. Pierrot-Deseilligny C, Goasguen J. Isolated abducens nucleus damage due to histiocytosis X. Electro-oculographic analysis and physiological deductions. Brain 1984;107:1019–1032.

52. Müri RM, Chermann JF, Cohen L, et al. Ocular motor consequences of damage to the abducens nucleus area in humans. J Neuroophthalmol 1996;16:191–195.

53. Miller NR, Biousse V, Hwang T, et al. Isolated acquired unilateral horizontal gaze paresis from a putative lesion of the abducens nucleus. J Neuroophthalmol 2002;22:204–207.

54. Larmande P, Hénin D, Jan M, et al. Abnormal vertical eye movements in the locked-in syndrome. Ann Neurol 1982;11:100–102.

55. Johnston JL, Sharpe JA, Ranalli PJ, et al. Oblique misdirection and slowing of vertical saccades after unilateral lesions of the pontine tegmentum. Neurology 1993;43:2238–2244.

56. Hanson MR, Hamid MA, Tomsak RL, et al. Selective saccadic palsy caused by pontine lesions: clinical, physiological and pathological correlations. Ann Neurol 1986;20:209–217.

57. Fisher CM. Some neuro-ophthalmological observations. J Neurol Neurosurg Psychiatr 1967;30:383–392.

58. Sharpe JA, Rosenberg MA, Hoyt WF, et al. Paralytic pontine exotropia. A sign of acute unilateral pontine gaze palsy and internuclear ophthalmoplegia. Neurology 1974;24:1076–1081.

59. Pierrot-Deseilligny C, Chain F, Serdaru M, et al. The "one-and-a-half" syndrome. Electro-oculographic analyses of five cases with deductions about the physiological mechanisms of lateral gaze. Brain 1981;104:665–699.

60. Wall M, Wray SH. The one-and-a-half syndrome: a unilateral disorder of the pontine tegmentum: a study of 20 cases and review of the literature. Neurology 1983;33:971–980.

61. Bogousslavsky J, Miklossy J, Regli F, et al. One-and-a-half syndrome in ischaemic locked-in state: a clinico-pathological study. J Neurol Neurosurg Psychiatr 1984;47:927–935.

62. Deleu D, Solheid C, Michotte A, et al. Dissociated ipsilateral horizontal gaze palsy in one-and-a-half syndrome. Neurology 1988;38:1278–1280.

63. Foville A. Note sur une paralysie peu connue de certains muscles de l'oeil, et sa liaison avec quelques poins de l'anatomie et la physiologie de la protubérance annulaire. Bull Soc Anat Paris 1858;33:393–414.

64. Silverman IE, Liu GT, Volpe NJ, et al. The crossed paralyses: the original brainstem syndromes of Millard-Gubler, Foville, Weber, and Raymond-Cestan. Arch Neurol 1995;52:635–638.

65. Nordgren RE, Markesbery WR, Fukuda K, et al. Seven cases of cerebromedullospinal disconnection. The "locked in" syndrome. Neurology 1971;21:1140–1148.

66. Thier P, Bachor A, Faiss J, et al. Selective impairment of smooth-pursuit eye movements due to an ischemic lesion of the basal pons. Ann Neurol 1991;29:443–448.

67. Bassetti C, Bogousslavsky J, Barth A, et al. Isolated infarcts of the pons. Neurology 1996;46:165–175.

68. Galetta SL, Balcer LJ, Liu GT. Giant cell arteritis with unusual flow related neuro-ophthalmologic manifestations. Neurology 1997;49:1463–1465.

69. Eggenberger E. Eight-and-a-half syndrome: one-and-a-half syndrome plus cranial nerve VII palsy. J Neuroophthalmol 1998;18:114–116.

70. Tan E, Kansu T. Bilateral horizontal gaze palsy in multiple sclerosis. J Clin Neuroophthalmol 1990;10:124–127.

71. Hamed LF, Schatz NJ, Galetta SL. Brainstem ocular motility defects and AIDS. Am J Ophthalmol 1988;106:437–442.

72. Brunner JE, Redmond JM, Haggar AM, et al. Central pontine myelinolysis and pontine lesions after rapid correction of hyponatremia: a prospective magnetic resonance imaging study. Ann Neurol 1990;27:61–66.

73. Lampl C, Yazdi K. Central pontine myelinolysis. Eur Neurol 2002;47:3–10.

74. Chen CM, Wei JC, Huang TY. Mesencephalic bilateral horizontal gaze palsies. Neurology 2008;71:1039.

75. Zackon DH, Sharpe JA. Midbrain paresis of horizontal gaze. Ann Neurol 1984;16:495–504.

76. Pierrot-Deseilligny C, Rosa A, Masmoudi K, et al. Saccadic deficits after a unilateral lesion affecting the superior colliculus. J Neurol Neurosurg Psychiatr 1991;54:1106–1109.

77. Kommerell G, Hoyt WF. Lateropulsion of saccadic eye movements: electro-oculographic studies in a patient with Wallenberg's syndrome. Arch Neurol 1973;28:313–318.

78. Meyer KT, Baloh RW, Krohel GB, et al. Ocular lateropulsion. A sign of lateral medullary disease. Arch Ophthalmol 1980;98:1614–1616.

79. Kirkham TH, Guitton D, Gans M. Task dependent variations of ocular lateropulsion in Wallenberg's syndrome. Can J Neurol Sci 1981;8:21–26.

80. Waespe W, Wichmann W. Oculomotor disturbances during visual-vestibular interaction in Wallenberg's lateral medullary syndrome. Brain 1990;113:821–846.

81. Baloh RW, Yee RD, Honrubia V. Eye movements in patients with Wallenberg's syndrome. Ann N Y Acad Sci 1981;374:600–613.

82. Crevits L, vander Eecken H. Ocular lateropulsion in Wallenberg's syndrome: a prospective clinical study. Acta Neurol Scand 1982;65:219–222.

83. Estañol B, Lopez-Rios G. Neuro-otology of the lateral medullary infarct syndrome. Arch Neurol 1982;39:176–179.

84. Brazis PW. Ocular motor abnormalities in Wallenberg's lateral medullary syndrome. Mayo Clinic Proc 1992;67:365–368.

85. Hörnsten G. Wallenberg's syndrome. Part I. General symptomology, with special reference to visual disturbances and imbalance. Part II. Oculomotor and oculostatic disturbances. Acta Neurol Scand 1974;50:434–468.

86. Solomon D, Galetta SL, Liu GT. Possible mechanisms for horizontal gaze deviation and lateropulsion in the lateral medullary syndrome. J Neuroophthalmol 1995;15:26–30.

87. Furman JMR, Hurtt MR, Hirsch WL. Asymmetrical ocular pursuit with posterior fossa tumors. Ann Neurol 1991;30:208–211.

88. Kim JS, Moon SY, Kim KY, et al. Ocular contrapulsion in rostral medial medullary infarction. Neurology 2004;63:1325–1327.

89. Zee DS, Leigh RJ, Mathieu-Millaire F. Cerebellar control of ocular gaze stability. Ann Neurol 1980;7:37–40.

90. Ranalli PJ, Sharpe JA. Contrapulsion of saccades and ipsilateral ataxia: a unilateral disorder of the rostral cerebellum. Ann Neurol 1986;20:311–316.

91. Baloh RW, Konrad HR, Dirks D, et al. Cerebellar-pontine angle tumors. Results of quantitative vestibulo-ocular testing. Arch Neurol 1976;33:507–512.

92. Jen J, Coulin CJ, Bosley TM, et al. Familial horizontal gaze palsy with progressive scoliosis maps to chromosome 11q23–25. Neurology 2002;59:432–435.

93. Pieh C, Lengyel D, Neff A, et al. Brainstem hypoplasia in familial horizontal gaze palsy and scoliosis. Neurology 2002;59:462–463.

94. Bosley TM, Salih MA, Jen JC, et al. Neurologic features of horizontal gaze palsy and progressive scoliosis with mutations in ROBO3. Neurology 2005;64:1196–1203.

95. Abu-Amero KK, al Dhalaan H, al Zayed Z, et al. Five new consanguineous families with horizontal gaze palsy and progressive scoliosis and novel ROBO3 mutations. J Neurol Sci 2009;276:22–26.

96. Yee RD, Purvin VA. Acquired ocular motor apraxia after aortic surgery. Trans Am Ophthalmol Soc 2007;105:152–158; discussion 158–159.

97. Solomon D, Ramat S, Tomsak RL, et al. Saccadic palsy after cardiac surgery: characteristics and pathogenesis. Ann Neurol 2008;63:355–365.

98. Eggers SD, Moster ML, Cranmer K. Selective saccadic palsy after cardiac surgery. Neurology 2008;70:318–320.

99. Vaughan C, Samy H, Jain S. Selective saccadic palsy after cardiac surgery [letter]. Neurology 2008;71:1746; author reply 1746–1747.

100. Mokri B, Ahlskog JE, Fulgham JR, et al. Syndrome resembling PSP after surgical repair of ascending aorta dissection or aneurysm. Neurology 2004;62:971–973.

101. Bernat JL, Lukovits TG. Syndrome resembling PSP after surgical repair of ascending aorta dissection or aneurysm. Neurology 2004;63:1141–1142; author reply 1141–1142.

102. Solomon D, Ramat S, Leigh RJ, et al. A quick look at slow saccades after cardiac surgery: where is the lesion? Prog Brain Res 2008;171:587–590.

103. Tychsen L. Pediatric ocular motility disorders of neuro-ophthalmic significance. Ophthalmol Clin North Am 1991;4:615–643.

104. Zee DS, Yee RD, Singer HS. Congenital ocular motor apraxia. Brain 1977;100:581–599.

105. Gresty MA. Disorders of head-eye coordination. Baillières Clin Neurol 1992;1:317–343.

106. Hughes JL, O'Connor PS, Larsen PD, et al. Congenital vertical ocular motor apraxia. J Clin Neuroophthalmol 1985;5:153–157.

107. Ebner RB, Lopez L, Ochoa S, et al. Vertical ocular motor apraxia. Neurology 1990;40:712–713.

108. Prasad P, Nair S. Congenital ocular motor apraxia: sporadic and familial. Support for natural resolution. J Clin Neuroophthalmol 1994;14:102–104.

109. Cogan DG, Chu FU, Reingold RD, et al. A long-term follow up of congenital ocular motor apraxia: a case report. Neuroophthalmology 1980;1:145–147.

110. Daroff RB, Troost BT, Leigh RJ. Supranuclear disorders of eye movements. Clin Ophthalmol 1988;10:8–9.

111. Harris CM, Shawkat F, Russell-Eggitt I, et al. Intermittent horizontal saccade failure ("ocular motor apraxia") in children. Br J Ophthalmol 1996;80:151–158.

112. Cogan DG. A type of congenital ocular motor apraxia presenting with jerky head movements. Trans Am Acad Ophthalmol Otol 1952;56:853–862.

113. Eustace P, Beigi B, Bowell R, et al. Congenital ocular motor apraxia. Neuroophthalmology 1994;14:167–174.

114. Marr JE, Green SH, Willshaw HE. Neurodevelopmental implications of ocular motor apraxia. Dev Med Child Neurol 2005;47:815–819.

115. Narbona J, Crisci CD, Villa I. Familial congenital ocular motor apraxia and immune deficiency [letter]. Arch Neurol 1980;37:325.

116. Phillips PH, Brodsky MC, Henry PM. Congenital ocular motor apraxia with autosomal dominant inheritance. Am J Ophthalmol 2000;129:820–822.

117. Cassidy L, Taylor D, Harris C. Abnormal supranuclear eye movements in the child: a practical guide to examination and interpretation. Surv Ophthalmol 2000;44:479–506.

118. Kondo A, Saito Y, Floricel F, et al. Congenital ocular motor apraxia: clinical and neuroradiological findings, and long-term intellectual prognosis. Brain Dev 2007;29:431–438.

119. Whitsel EA, Castillo M, D'Cruz O. Cerebellar vermis and midbrain dysgenesis in oculomotor apraxia: MR findings. AJNR Am J Neuroradiol 1995;16(Suppl 4):831–834.

120. Fielder AR, Gresty MA, Dodd KL, et al. Congenital ocular motor apraxia. Trans Ophthalmol Soc UK 1986;105:589–598.

121. Borchert MS, Sadun AA, Sommers JD, et al. Congenital ocular motor apraxia in twins. J Clin Neuroophthalmol 1987;7:104–107.

122. Sargent MA, Poskitt KJ, Jan JE. Congenital ocular motor apraxia: imaging findings. AJNR Am J Neuroradiol 1997;18:1915–1922.

123. Lambert SR, Kriss A, Gresty M, et al. Joubert syndrome. Arch Ophthalmol 1989;107:709–713.

124. Donaldson MDC, Werner AA, Trompeter RS, et al. Familial juvenile nephronophthisis, Jeune's syndrome, and associated disorders. Arch Dis Child 1985;60:426–434.

125. Moore AT, Taylor SI. A syndrome of congenital retinal dystrophy and saccade palsy: a subset of Leber's amaurosis. Br J Ophthalmol 1984;68:421–431.

126. Zaret CR, Behrens MM, Eggers HM. Congenital ocular motor apraxia and brainstem tumor. Arch Ophthalmol 1980;98:328–330.

127. Bundey S. Clinical and genetic features of ataxia-telangiectasia. Int J Radiat Biol 1994;66:S23–S29.

128. Cohen LE, Tanner DJ, Schaefer HG, et al. Common and uncommon cutaneous findings in patients with ataxia-telangiectasia. J Am Acad Dermatol 1984;10:431–438.

129. Woods CG, Taylor AM. Ataxia telangiectasia in the British Isles: the clinical and laboratory features of 70 affected individuals. Q J Med 1992;82:169–179.

130. Swift M, Morrell D, Massey RB, et al. Incidence of cancer in 161 families affected by ataxia-telangiectasia. N Engl J Med 1991;32:1831–1836.

131. Bebb G, Glickman B, Gelmon K, et al. "AT risk" for breast cancer. Lancet 1997;349:1784–1785.

132. Case records of the Massachusetts General Hospital: Case 2–1987. N Engl J Med 1987;316:91–100.

133. Carbonari M, Cherchi M, Paganelli R, et al. Relative increase of T cells expressing the gamma/delta rather than the alpha/beta receptor in ataxia-telangiectasia. N Engl J Med 1990;322:73–76.

134. Hurko O. Recent advances in heritable ataxias [editorial]. Ann Neurol 1997;41:4–6.

135. Mavrou A, Tsangaris GT, Roma E, et al. The ATM gene and ataxia telangiectasia. Anticancer Res 2008;401–405.

136. Baloh RW, Yee RD, Boder E. Eye movements in ataxia telangiectasia. Neurology 1978;28:1099–1104.

137. Stell R, Bronstein AM, Plant GT, et al. Ataxia telangiectasia: a reappraisal of the ocular motor features and their value in the diagnosis of atypical cases. Mov Disord 1989;4:320–329.

138. Lewis RF, Lederman HM, Crawford TO. Ocular motor abnormalities in ataxia telangiectasia. Ann Neurol 1999;46:287–295.

139. Cogan DG, Chu FC, Reingold D, et al. Ocular motor signs in some metabolic diseases. Arch Ophthalmol 1981;99:1802–1808.

140. Shaikh AG, Marti S, Tarnutzer AA, et al. Gaze fixation deficits and their implication in ataxia-telangiectasia. J Neurol Neurosurg Psychiatry 2009;80:858–864.

141. Farr AK, Shalev B, Crawford TO, et al. Ocular manifestations of ataxia-telangiectasia. Am J Ophthalmol 2002;134:891–896.

142. Farina L, Uggetti C, Ottolini A, et al. Ataxia-telangiectasia: MR and CT findings. J Comput Assist Tomogr 1994;18:724–727.

143. Rivaud-Pechoux S, Durr A, Gaymard B, et al. Eye movement abnormalities correlate with genotype in autosomal dominant cerebellar ataxia type I. Ann Neurol 1998;43:297–302.

144. Fahey MC, Cremer PD, Aw ST, et al. Vestibular, saccadic and fixation abnormalities in genetically confirmed Friedreich ataxia. Brain 2008;131:1035–1045.

145. Criscuolo C, Chessa L, Di Giandomenico S, et al. Ataxia with oculomotor apraxia type 2: a clinical, pathologic, and genetic study. Neurology 2006;66:1207–1210.

146. Anheim M, Fleury MC, Franques J, et al. Clinical and molecular findings of ataxia with oculomotor apraxia type 2 in 4 families. Arch Neurol 2008;65:958–962.

147. D'Arrigo S, Riva D, Bulgheroni S, et al. Ataxia with oculomotor apraxia type 1 (AOA1): clinical and neuropsychological features in 2 new patients and differential diagnosis. J Child Neurol 2008;23:895–900.

148. Gouw LG, Digre KB, Harris CP, et al. Autosomal dominant cerebellar ataxia with retinal degeneration: clinical, neuropathic, and genetic analysis of a large kindred. Neurology 1994;44:1441–1447.

149. Rosenberg RN. Autosomal dominant cerebellar phenotypes: the genotype has settled the issue [editorial]. Neurology 1995;45:1–5.

150. Moseley Ml, Benzow KA, Schut LJ, et al. Incidence of dominant spinocerebellar and Friedreich triplet repeats among 361 ataxia families. Neurology 1998;51:1666–1671.

151. Martin JB. Molecular basis of the neurodegenerative disorders. N Engl J Med 1999;340:1970–1980.

152. Harding AE. Clinical feature and classification of inherited ataxias. Adv Neurol 1993;61:1–14.

153. Velazquez-Pérez L, Seifried C, Santos-Falcón N, et al. Saccade velocity is controlled by polyglutamine size in spinocerebellar ataxia 2. Ann Neurol 2004;56:444–447.

154. Schmitz-Hübsch T, Coudert M, Bauer P, et al. Spinocerebellar ataxia types 1, 2, 3, and 6: disease severity and nonataxia symptoms. Neurology 2008;71:982–989.

155. Baloh RW, Konrad HR, Honrubia V. Vestibulo-ocular function in patients with cerebellar atrophy. Neurology 1975;25:160–168.

156. Zee DS, Yee RD, Cogan DG, et al. Ocular motor abnormalities in hereditary cerebellar ataxia. Brain 1976;99:207–234.

157. Koeppen AH, Hans MB. Supranuclear ophthalmoplegia in olivopontocerebellar degeneration. Neurology 1976;26:764–768.

158. Wadia N, Pang J, Desai J, et al. A clinicogenetic analysis of six Indian spinocerebellar ataxia (SCA2) pedigrees. The significance of slow saccades in diagnosis. Brain 1998;121:2341–2355.

159. Zee DS, Optican LM, Cook JD, et al. Slow saccades in spinocerebellar degeneration. Arch Neurol 1976;33:243–251.

160. Murphy MJ, Goldblatt D. Slow eye movements with absent saccades, in a patient with hereditary ataxia. Arch Neurol 1977;34:191–195.

161. Rüb U, Bürk K, Schöls L, et al. Damage to the reticulotegmental nucleus of the pons in spinocerebellar ataxia type 1, 2, and 3. Neurology 2004;63:1258–1263.

162. Abe T, Abe K, Aoki M, et al. Ocular changes in patients with spinocerebellar degeneration and repeated trinucleotide expansion of spinocerebellar ataxia type 1 gene. Arch Ophthalmol 1997;115:231–236.

163. Colan RV, Snead OC, Ceballos R. Olivopontocerebellar atrophy in children: a report of seven cases in two families. Ann Neurol 1981;10:355–363.

164. Wüllner U, Klockgether T, Petersen D, et al. Magnetic resonance imaging in hereditary and idiopathic ataxia. Neurology 1993;43:318–325.

165. Ying SH, Choi SI, Perlman SL, et al. Pontine and cerebellar atrophy correlate with clinical disability in SCA2. Neurology 2006;66:424–426.

166. Lepore FE. Disorders of ocular motility in the olivopontocerebellar atrophies. Adv Neurol 1984;41:97–103.

167. Case records of the Massachusetts General Hospital: Case 30–1992. N Engl J Med 1992;327:261–268.

168. Starr A. A disorder of rapid eye movements in Huntington's chorea. Brain 1967;90:545–564.

169. Leigh RJ, Newman SA, Folstein SE, et al. Abnormal ocular motor control in Huntington's disease. Neurology 1983;33:1268–1275.

170. Lasker AG, Zee DS, Hain TC, et al. Saccades in Huntington's disease: slowing and dysmetria. Neurology 1988;38:427–431.

171. Blekher T, Johnson SA, Marshall J, et al. Saccades in presymptomatic and early stages of Huntington disease. Neurology 2006;67:394–399.

172. Golding CV, Danchaivijitr C, Hodgson TL, et al. Identification of an oculomotor biomarker of preclinical Huntington disease. Neurology 2006;67:485–487.

173. Lasker AG, Zee DS, Hain TC, et al. Saccades in Huntington's disease: initiation defects and distractibility. Neurology 1987;37:364–370.

174. Tian JR, Zee DS, Lasker AG, et al. Saccades in Huntington's disease: predictive tracking and interaction between release of fixation and initiation of saccades. Neurology 1991;41:875–881.

175. Lasker AG, Zee DS. Ocular motor abnormalities in Huntington's disease. Vision Res 1997;37:3639–3645.

176. White OB, Saint-Cyr JA, Tomlinson RD, et al. Ocular motor deficits in Parkinson's disease. II. Control of the saccadic and smooth pursuit systems. Brain 1983;106: 571–587.

177. Crawford TJ, Henderson L, Kennard C. Abnormalities of nonvisually guided eye movements in Parkinson's disease. Brain 1989;112:1573–1586.

178. Blekher T, Siemers E, Abel LA, et al. Eye movements in Parkinson's disease: before and after pallidotomy. Invest Ophthalmol Vis Sci 2000;41:2177–2183.

179. Gibson JM, Pimlott RM, Kennard C. Oculomotor and manual tracking in Parkinson's disease and the effect of treatment. J Neurol Neurosurg Psychiatr 1987;50:853–860.

180. Rascol O, Clanet M, Montastruc JL, et al. Abnormal ocular movements in Parkinson's disease: evidence for involvement of dopaminergic systems. Brain 1989;112:1193–1214.

181. Sharpe JA, Fletcher WA, Lang AE, et al. Smooth pursuit during dose related on-off fluctuations in Parkinson's disease. Neurology 1987;37:1389–1392.

182. Schneider JA, Watts RL, Gearing M. Corticobasal degeneration: neuropathologic and clinical heterogeneity. Neurology 1997;48:959–969.

183. Riley DE, Lang AE, Lewis A, et al. Cortical-basal ganglionic degeneration. Neurology 1990;40:1203–1212.

184. Grimes DA, Lang AE, Bergeron CB. Dementia as the most common presentation of cortical-basal ganglionic degeneration. Neurology 1999;53:1969–1974.

185. Gibb WRG, Luthert PJ, Marsden CD. Corticobasal degeneration. Brain 1989;112:1171–1192.

186. Vidailhet M, Rivaud S, Gouider-Khouja N, et al. Eye movements in Parkinsonian syndromes. Ann Neurol 1994;35:420–426.

187. Soliveri P, Monza D, Paridi D, et al. Cognitive and magnetic resonance imaging aspects of corticobasal degeneration and progressive supranuclear palsy. Neurology 1999;53: 502–507.

188. Kompoliti K, Goetz CG, Boeve BF, et al. Clinical presentation and pharmacological therapy in corticobasal degeneration. Arch Neurol 1998;55:957–961.

189. Tsuji S, Choudary PV, Martin BM, et al. A mutation in the human glucocerebrosidase gene in neuronopathic Gaucher's disease. N Engl J Med 1987;316:570–575.

190. Patterson MC, Horowitz M, Abel RB, et al. Isolated horizontal supranuclear gaze palsy as a marker of severe systemic involvement in Gaucher's disease. Neurology 1993;43: 1993–1997.

191. Bohlega S, Kambouris M, Shahid M, et al. Gaucher disease with oculomotor apraxia and cardiovascular calcification (Gaucher type IIIC). Neurology 2000;54:261–263.

192. Accardo AP, Pensiero S, Perissutti P. Saccadic analysis for early identification of neurological involvement in Gaucher disease. Ann N Y Acad Sci 2005;1039:503–507.

193. Shawkat FS, Kingsley D, Kendall B, et al. Neuroradiological and eye movement correlates in children with intermittent saccade failure: "ocular motor apraxia." Neuropediatrics 1995;26:298–305.

194. Abel LA, Levin S, Holzman PS. Abnormalities of smooth pursuit and saccadic control in schizophrenia and affective disorders. Vision Res 1992;32:1009–1014.

195. Clementz BA, Sweeney JA. Is eye movement dysfunction a biological marker for schizophrenia? A methodological review. Psychol Bull 1990;108:77–92.

196. Fletcher WA, Sharpe JA. Saccadic eye movement dysfunction in Alzheimer's disease. Ann Neurol 1986;20:464–471.

197. Currie J, Ramsden B, McArthur C, et al. Validation of a clinical antisaccadic eye movement test in the assessment of dementia. Arch Neurol 1991;48:644–648.

198. Hutton S, Kennard C. Oculomotor abnormalities in schizophrenia. A critical review. Neurology 1998;50:604–609.

199. Fletcher WA, Sharpe JA. Smooth pursuit dysfunction in Alzheimer's disease. Neurology 1988;38:272–277.

200. Thaker GK, Ross DE, Cassady SL, et al. Smooth pursuit eye movements to extraretinal motion signals: deficits in relative of patients with schizophrenia. Arch Gen Psychiatr 1998;55:830–836.

201. Charness ME, Simon RP, Greenberg DA. Ethanol and the nervous system. N Engl J Med 1989;321:442–454.

202. Victor M, Adams RD, Collins GH. The Wernicke-Korsakoff syndrome and related neurologic disorders due to alcoholism and malnutrition, 2nd edn, pp 17–21, 31–34, 114–116. Philadelphia, F.A. Davis, 1989.

203. Reuler JB, Girard DE, Cooney TG. Wernicke's encephalopathy. N Engl J Med 1985;312:1035–1039.

204. Furman JMR, Becker JT. Vestibular responses in Wernicke's encephalopathy. Ann Neurol 1989;26:669–674.

205. Charness ME, DeLaPaz RL. Mamillary body atrophy in Wernicke's encephalopathy: antemortem identification using magnetic resonance imaging. Ann Neurol 1987;22: 595–600.

206. Antunez E, Estruch R, Cardenal C, et al. Usefulness of CT and MRI imaging in the diagnosis of acute Wernicke's encephalopathy. AJR Am J Roentgenol 1998;171: 1131–1137.

207. Hayashi N, Geraghty MT, Green WR. Ocular histopathologic study of a patient with the T 8993-G point mutation in Leigh's syndrome. Ophthalmology 2000;107:1397–1402.

208. Sedwick LA, Burde RM, Hodges FJ. Leigh's subacute necrotizing encephalomyelopathy manifesting as spasmus nutans. Arch Ophthalmol 1984;102:1046–1048.

209. DiMauro S, De Vivo DC. Genetic heterogeneity in Leigh syndrome. Ann Neurol 1996;40:5–7.

210. Shoffner JM, Fernhoff PM, Krawiecki NS, et al. Subacute necrotizing encephalopathy: oxidative phosphorylation defects and the ATPase 6 point mutation. Neurology 1992;42:2168–2174.

211. Santorelli FM, Shanske S, Macaya A, et al. The mutation at nt 8993 of mitochondrial DNA is a common cause of Leigh's syndrome. Ann Neurol 1993;34:827–834.

212. Morris AAM, Leonard JV, Brown GK, et al. Deficiency of respiratory chain complex I is a common cause of Leigh disease. Ann Neurol 1996;40:25–30.

213. Kayden HJ. The neurologic syndrome of vitamin E deficiency: a significant cause of ataxia [editorial]. Neurology 1993;43:2167–2169.

214. Hamida MB, Belal S, Sirugo G, et al. Friedreich's ataxia phenotype not linked to chromosome 9 and associated with selective autosomal recessive vitamin E deficiency in two inbred Tunisian families. Neurology 1993;43:2179–2183.

215. Perkin GD, Murray-Lyon I. Neurology and the gastrointestinal system. J Neurol Neurosurg Psychiatry 1998;65:291–300.

216. Tijssen CC, van Gisbergen JAM, Schulte BPM. Conjugate eye deviation: side, site, and size of the hemispheric lesion. Neurology 1991;41:846–850.

217. Simon JE, Morgan SC, Pexman JH, et al. CT assessment of conjugate eye deviation in acute stroke. Neurology 2003;60:135–137.

218. Ringman JM, Saver JL, Woolson RF, et al. Hemispheric asymmetry of gaze deviation and relationship to neglect in acute stroke. Neurology 2005;65:1661–1662.

219. Fruhmann Berger M, Pross RD, Ilg UJ, et al. Deviation of eyes and head in acute cerebral stroke. BMC Neurol 2006;6:23.

220. Pessin MS, Adelman LS, Prager RJ, et al. "Wrong-way eyes" in supratentorial hemorrhage. Ann Neurol 1981;9:79–81.

221. Tijssen CC. Contralateral conjugate eye deviation in acute supratentorial lesions. Stroke 1994;25:1516–1519.

222. Sharpe JA, Bondar RL, Fletcher WA. Contralateral gaze deviation after frontal lobe haemorrhage. J Neurol Neurosurg Psychiatry 1985;48:86–88.

223. Kernan JC, Devinsky O, Luciano DJ, et al. Lateralizing significance of head and eye deviation in secondary generalized tonic-clonic seizures. Neurology 1993;43:1308–1310.

224. Kumral E, Kocaer T, Ertübey NÖ, et al. Thalamic hemorrhage. A prospective study of 100 patients. Stroke 1995;26:964–970.

225. Steinke W, Sacco RL, Mohr JP, et al. Thalamic stroke. Presentation and prognosis of infarcts and hemorrhages. Arch Neurol 1992;49:703–710.

226. Chung CS, Caplan LR, Han W, et al. Thalamic haemorrhage. Brain 1996;119:1873–1886.

227. Keane JR. Contralateral gaze deviation with supratentorial hemorrhage: three pathologically verified cases. Arch Neurol 1975;32:119–122.

228. Messe SR, Cucchiara BL. Wrong-way eyes with thalamic hemorrhage. Neurology 2003;60:1524.

229. Averbuch-Heller L, Meiner Z. Reversible periodic alternating gaze deviation in hepatic encephalopathy. Neurology 1995;45:191–192.

230. Legge RH, Weiss HS, Hedges TR, et al. Periodic alternating gaze deviation in infancy. Neurology 1992;42:1740–1743.

231. Ishikawa H, Ishikawa S, Mukuno K. Short-cycle periodic alternating (ping-pong) gaze. Neurology 1993;43:1067–1070.

232. Johkura K, Komiyama A, Tobita M, et al. Saccadic ping-pong gaze. J Neuroophthalmol 1998;18:43–46.

233. Stewart JD, Kirkham TH, Mathieson G. Periodic alternating gaze. Neurology 1979;29:222–224.

234. Masucci EF, Fabara JA, Saini N, et al. Periodic alternating ping-pong gaze. Ann Ophthalmol 1981;13:1123–1127.

235. Larmande P, Henin D, Jan M, et al. Periodic alternating gaze: electro-oculographic and anatomical observation of a new case. Neurosurgery 1982;10:263–265.

236. Diesing TS, Wijdicks EF. Ping-pong gaze in coma may not indicate persistent hemispheric damage. Neurology 2004;63:1537–1538.

237. Senelick RC. "Ping-pong" gaze: periodic alternating gaze deviation. Neurology 1976;26: 532–535.

238. Larmande P, Dongmo L, Limodin J, et al. Periodic alternating gaze: a case without any hemispheric lesion. Neurosurgery 1987;20:481–483.

239. Pasik P, Pasik T, Bender MB. The pretectal syndrome in monkeys. I. Disturbances of gaze and body posture. Brain 1969;92:521–534.

240. Pierrot-Deseilligny C, Chain F, Gray F, et al. Parinaud's syndrome. Electro-oculographic and anatomical analyses of six vascular cases with deductions about vertical gaze organization in the premotor structures. Brain 1982;105:667–696.

241. Büttner-Ennever JA, Büttner U, Cohen B, et al. Vertical gaze paralysis and the rostral interstitial nucleus of the medial longitudinal fasciculus. Brain 1982;105:125–149.

242. Hommel M, Bogousslavsky J. The spectrum of vertical gaze palsy following unilateral brainstem stroke. Neurology 1991;41:1229–1234.

243. Büttner U, Büttner-Ennever JA, Henn V. Vertical eye movement related unit activity in the rostral mesencephalic reticular formation of the alert monkey. Brain Res 1977;130: 239–252.

244. Bhidayasiri R, Plant GT, Leigh RJ. A hypothetical scheme for the brainstem control of vertical gaze. Neurology 2000;54:1985–1993.

245. Leigh RJ, Zee DS. The neurology of eye movements, 4th edn, pp 268–273. New York, Oxford University Press, 2006.

246. Horn AKE, Büttner-Ennever JA. Premotor neurons for vertical eye movements in the rostral mesencephalon of monkey and human: histologic identification by parvalbumin immunostaining. J Comp Neurol 1998;392:413–427.

247. Clark JM, Albers GW. Vertical gaze palsies from medial thalamic infarctions without midbrain involvement. Stroke 1995;26:1467–1470.

248. Kang JH, Sharpe JA. Dissociated palsy of vertical saccades: loss of voluntary and visually guided saccades with preservation of reflexive vestibular quick phases. J Neuroophthalmol 2008;28:97–103.

249. Ouvrier R. Henri Parinaud and his syndrome. Med J Aust 1993;158:711–714.

250. Parinaud H. Paralysie des mouvements associés des yeux. Arch Neurol 1883;5:145–172.

251. Parinaud H. Paralysis of the movement of convergence of the eyes. Brain 1886;9:330–341.

252. Keane JR. The pretectal syndrome: 206 patients. Neurology 1990;40:684–690.

253. Hatcher MA, Klintworth GK. The sylvian aqueduct syndrome. A clinicopathologic study. Arch Neurol 1966;15:215–222.

254. Nothnagel H. On the diagnosis of diseases of the corpora quadrigemina. Brain 1889;12:21–35.

255. Liu GT, Crenner CW, Logigian EL, et al. Midbrain syndromes of Benedikt, Claude, and Nothnagel: setting the record straight. Neurology 1992;42:1820–1822.

256. Keane JR, Davis RL. Pretectal syndrome with metastatic malignant melanoma to the posterior commissure. Am J Ophthalmol 1976;82:910–914.

257. Baloh RW, Furman JM, Yee RD. Dorsal midbrain syndrome: clinical and oculographic findings. Neurology 1985;35:54–60.

258. Caplan LR. "Top of the basilar" syndrome. Neurology 1980;30:72–79.

259. Pullicino P, Lincoff N, Truax BT. Abnormal vergence with upper brainstem infarcts: pseudoabducens palsy. Neurology 2000;55:352–358.

260. Hertle RW, Bienfang DC. Oculographic analysis of acute esotropia secondary to a thalamic hemorrhage. J Clin Neuroophthalmol 1990;10:21–26.

261. Gomez CR, Gomez SM, Selhorst JB. Acute thalamic esotropia. Neurology 1988;38:1759–1762.

262. Siatkowski RM, Schatz NJ, Sellitti TP, et al. Do thalamic lesions really cause vertical gaze palsies? J Clin Neuroophthalmol 1993;13:190–193.

263. Masdeu J, Brannegan R, Rosenberg M, et al. Pseudo-abducens palsy with midbrain lesions [abstract]. Ann Neurol 1980;8:103.

264. Corbett JJ, Schatz NJ, Shults WT, et al. Slowly alternating skew deviation: description of a pretectal syndrome in three patients. Ann Neurol 1981;10:540–546.

265. Hedges TR, Hoyt WF. Ocular tilt reaction due to an upper brainstem lesion: paroxysmal skew deviation, torsion, and oscillation of the eyes with head tilt. Ann Neurol 1982;11:537–540.

266. Swash M. Periaqueductal dysfunction (the sylvian aqueduct syndrome): a sign of hydrocephalus? J Neurol Neurosurg Psychiatr 1974;37:21–26.

267. Corbett JJ. Neuro-ophthalmologic complications of hydrocephalus and shunting procedures. Semin Neurol 1986;6:111–123.

268. Donat JF, Okazaki H, Gomez MR, et al. Pineal tumors: a 53-year experience. Arch Neurol 1978;35:736–740.

269. Cho B-K, Wang K-C, Nam D-H, et al. Pineal tumors: experience with 48 cases over 10 years. Childs Nervous System 1998;14:53–58.

270. Halperin EC, Constine LS, Tarbell NJ, et al. Supratentorial brain tumors except ependymoma; brain tumors in babies and very young children. In: Pediatric Radiation Oncology, 2nd edn, pp 40–89. New York, Raven Press, 1994.

271. Fetell MR, Bruce JN, Burke AM, et al. Non-neoplastic pineal cysts. Neurology 1991;41:1034–1040.

272. Apuzzo MLJ, Davey LM, Manuelidis EE. Pineal apoplexy associated with anticoagulant therapy. J Neurosurg 1976;45:223–226.

273. Squires LA, Allen JC, Abbott R, et al. Focal tectal tumors: management and prognosis. Neurology 1994;44:953–956.

274. May PL, Blaser SI, Hoffman HJ, et al. Benign intrinsic tectal "tumors" in children. J Neurosurg 1991;74:867–871.

275. Vandertop WP, Hoffman HJ, Drake JM, et al. Focal midbrain tumors in children. Neurosurgery 1992;31:186–194.

276. Segarra JM. Cerebral vascular disease and behavior. I. The syndrome of the mesencephalic artery (basilar artery bifurcation). Arch Neurol 1970;22:408–418.

277. Percheron G. Les artères du thalamus humain. II. Artères et territoires thalamiques paramédians de l'artère basilaire communicante. Rev Neurol (Paris) 1976;132:309–324.

278. Castaigne P, Lhermitte F, Buge A, et al. Paramedian thalamic and midbrain infarcts: clinical and neuropathological study. Ann Neurol 1981;10:127–148.

279. Sieben G, De Reuck J, Vander Eecken H. Thrombosis of the mesencephalic artery. A clinico-pathological study of two cases and its correlation with the arterial vascularisation. Acta Neurol Belg 1977;77:151–162.

280. Bogousslavsky J, Regli F, Uske A. Thalamic infarcts: clinical syndromes, etiology, and prognosis. Neurology 1988;38:837–848.

281. Tatemichi TK, Steinke W, Duncan C, et al. Paramedian thalamopeduncular infarction: clinical syndromes and magnetic resonance imaging. Ann Neurol 1992;32:162–171.

282. Beversdorf DQ, Jenkyn LR, Petrowski JT, et al. Vertical gaze paralysis and intermittent unresponsiveness in a patient with a thalamomesencephalic stroke. J Neuroophthalmol 1995;15:230–235.

283. Bassetti C, Mathis J, Gugger M, et al. Hypersomnia following paramedian thalamic stroke. Ann Neurol 1996;39:471–480.

284. Bogousslavsky J, Miklossy J, Deruaz JP, et al. Unilateral left paramedian infarction of the thalamus and midbrain: a clinico-pathological study. J Neurol Neurosurg Psychiatr 1986;49:686–694.

285. Walshe TM, Davis KR, Fisher CM. Thalamic hemorrhage: a computed tomographic-clinical correlation. Neurology 1977;27:217–222.

286. Christoff N. A clinicopathological study of vertical eye movements. Arch Neurol 1974;31:1–8.

287. Keane JR. Neuro-ophthalmologic signs of AIDS: 50 patients. Neurology 1991;41:841–845.

288. Hedges TR, Katz B, Slavin M. Ophthalmoplegia associated with AIDS. Surv Ophthalmol 1994;39:43–51.

289. Keane JR. Bilateral ocular motor signs after tentorial herniation in 25 patients. Arch Neurol 1986;43:806–807.

290. Sand JJ, Biller J, Corbett JJ, et al. Partial dorsal mesencephalic hemorrhages. Report of three cases. Neurology 1986;36:529–533.

291. Lee AG, Brown DG, Diaz PJ. Dorsal midbrain syndrome due to mesencephalic hemorrhage. Case report with serial imaging. J Neuroophthalmol 1996;16:281–285.

292. Slyman JF, Kline LB. Dorsal midbrain syndrome in multiple sclerosis. Neurology 1981;31:196–198.

293. Trend P, Youl BD, Sanders MD, et al. Vertical gaze palsy due to a resolving midbrain lesion [letter]. J Neurol Neurosurg Psychiatr 1990;53:708.

294. Quint DJ, Cornblath WT, Trobe JD. Multiple sclerosis presenting as Parinaud syndrome. AJNR Am J Neuroradiol 1993;14:1200–1202.

295. Lee WB, Berger JR, O'Halloran HS. Parinaud syndrome heralding MS. Neurology 2003;60:322.

296. Coppeto JR, Lessell S. Dorsal midbrain syndrome from giant aneurysm of the posterior fossa: report of two cases. Neurology 1983;33:732–736.

297. Trojanowski JQ, Wray SH. Vertical gaze ophthalmoplegia: selective paralysis of downgaze. Neurology 1980;30:605–610.

298. Jacobs L, Anderson PJ, Bender MB. The lesions producing paralysis of downward but not upward gaze. Arch Neurol 1973;28:319–323.

299. Halmagyi GM, Evans WA, Hallinan JM. Failure of downward gaze. The site and nature of the lesion. Arch Neurol 1978;35:22–26.

300. Trojanowski JQ, Lafontaine MH. Neuroanatomical correlates of selective downgaze paralysis. J Neurol Sci 1981;52:91–101.

301. Jacobs L, Heffner RR, Newman RP. Selective paralysis of downward gaze caused by bilateral lesions of the mesencephalic periaqueductal gray matter. Neurology 1985;35:516–521.

302. Alemdar M, Kamaci S, Budak F. Unilateral midbrain infarction causing upward and downward gaze palsy. J Neuroophthalmol 2006;26:173–176.

303. Green JP, Newman NJ, Winterkorn JS. Paralysis of downgaze in two patients with clinical-radiologic correlation. Arch Ophthalmol 1993;111:219–222.

304. Cogan DC. Paralysis of down-gaze. Arch Ophthalmol 1974;91:192–199.

305. Egan RA, Weleber RG, Hogarth P, et al. Neuro-ophthalmologic and electroretinographic findings in pantothenate kinase-associated neurodegeneration (formerly Hallervorden-Spatz syndrome). Am J Ophthalmol 2005;140:267–274.

306. Bogousslavsky J, Regli F. Upgaze palsy and monocular paresis of downward gaze from ipsilateral thalamo-mesencephalic infarction: a vertical "one-and-a-half" syndrome. J Neurol 1984;231:43–45.

307. Deleu D, Buisseret T, Ebinger G. Vertical one-and-a-half syndrome. Supranuclear downgaze paralysis with monocular elevation palsy. Arch Neurol 1989;46:1361–1363.

308. Clark RA, Isenberg SJ. The range of ocular movements decreases with aging. J AAPOS 2001;5:26–30.

309. Chamberlain W. Restriction in upward gaze with advancing age. Trans Am Ophthalmol Soc 1970;68:234–244.

310. Richardson JC, Steele J, Olszewski J. Supranuclear ophthalmoplegia, pseudobulbar palsy, nuchal dystonia and dementia: a clinical report on eight cases of "heterogeneous system degeneration". Trans Am Neurol Assoc 1963;88:25–29.

311. Olszewski J, Steele J, Richardson JC. Pathological report on six cases of "heterogeneous system degeneration". J Neuropathol Exp Neurol 1963;23:187–188.

312. Steele JC, Richardson JC, Olszewski J. Progressive supranuclear palsy. Arch Neurol 1964;10:333–359.

313. Williams DR, Lees AJ, Wherrett JR, et al. J. Clifford Richardson and 50 years of progressive supranuclear palsy. Neurology 2008;70:566–573.

314. Knox DL, Green WR, Troncoso JC, et al. Cerebral ocular Whipple's disease: a 62-year odyssey from death to diagnosis. Neurology 1995;45:617–625.

315. Siderowf AD, Galetta SL, Hurtig H, et al. Posey and Spiller and progressive supranuclear palsy: an incorrect attribution. Mov Disord 1998;13:170–174.

316. Bower JH, Maraganore DM, McDonnell SK, et al. Incidence of progressive supranuclear palsy and multiple system atrophy in Olmsted County, Minnesota, 1976 to 1990. Neurology 1997;49:1284–1288.

317. Nath U, Ben-Shlomo Y, Thomson RG, et al. The prevalence of progressive supranuclear palsy (Steele-Richardson-Olszewski syndrome) in the UK. Brain 2001;124:1438–1449.

318. Golbe LI, Rubin RS, Cody RP, et al. Follow-up study of risk factors in progressive supranuclear palsy. Neurology 1996;47:148–154.

319. David NJ, Mackey EA, Smith JL. Further observations in progressive supranuclear palsy. Neurology 1968;18:349–356.

320. Tetrud JW, Golbe LI, Forno LS, et al. Autopsy-proven progressive supranuclear palsy in two siblings. Neurology 1996;46:931–934.

321. Friedman DI, Jankovic J, McCrary JA. Neuro-ophthalmic findings in progressive supranuclear palsy. J Clin Neuroophthalmol 1992;12:104–109.

322. Jankovic J. Progressive supranuclear palsy. Clinical and pharmacologic update. Neurol Clin 1984;2:473–486.

323. Chu FC, Reingold DB, Cogan DG, et al. The eye movement disorders of progressive supranuclear palsy. Ophthalmology 1979;86:422–428.

324. Troost BT, Daroff RB. The ocular motor defects in progressive supranuclear palsy. Ann Neurol 1977;2:397–403.

325. Mastaglia FL, Grainger MR. Internuclear ophthalmoplegia in progressive supranuclear palsy. J Neurol Sci 1975;25:303–308.

326. Ushio M, Iwasaki S, Chihara Y, et al. Wall-eyed bilateral internuclear ophthalmoplegia in a patient with progressive supranuclear palsy. J Neuroophthalmol 2008;28:93–96.

327. Jackson JA, Jankovic J, Ford J. Progressive supranuclear palsy: clinical features and response to treatment in 16 patients. Ann Neurol 1983;13:273–278.

328. Duvoisin RC, Golbe LI, Lepore FE. Progressive supranuclear palsy. Can J Neurol Sci 1987;14:547–554.

329. Dehaene I. Apraxia of eyelid opening in progressive supranuclear palsy [letter]. Ann Neurol 1984;15:115–116.

330. Golbe LI, Davis PA, Lepore FE. Eyelid movement abnormalities in progressive supranuclear palsy. Mov Disord 1989;4:297–302.

331. Collins SJ, Ahlskog JE, Parisi JE, et al. Progressive supranuclear palsy: neuropathologically based diagnostic clinical criteria. J Neurol Neurosurg Psychiatry 1995;58:167–173.

332. Daniel SE, de Bruin VMS, Lees AJ, et al. The clinical and pathological spectrum of Steele-Richardson-Olszewski syndrome (progressive supranuclear palsy): a reappraisal. Brain 1995;118:759–770.

333. Romano S, Colosimo C. Procerus sign in progressive supranuclear palsy. Neurology 2001;57:1928.

334. Litvan I, Mega MS, Cummings JL, et al. Neuropsychiatric aspects of progressive supranuclear palsy. Neurology 1996;47:1184–1189.

335. Rafal RD, Friedman JH. Limb dystonia in progressive supranuclear palsy. Neurology 1987;37:1546–1549.

336. Soliveri P, Piacentini S, Girotti F. Limb apraxia in corticobasal degeneration and progressive supranuclear palsy. Neurology 2005;64:448–453.

337. Pillon B, Dubois B, Lhermitte F, et al. Heterogeneity of cognitive impairment in progressive supranuclear palsy, Parkinson's disease, and Alzheimer's disease. Neurology 1986;36:1179–1185.

338. Kaat LD, Boon AJ, Kamphorst W, et al. Frontal presentation in progressive supranuclear palsy. Neurology 2007;69:723–729.

339. Litvan I, Agid Y, Calne D, et al. Clinical research criteria for the diagnosis of progressive supranuclear palsy (Steele-Richardson-Olszewski syndrome): Report of the NINDS-SPSP International Workshop. Neurology 1996;47:1–9.

340. Litvan I, Agid Y, Jankovic J, et al. Accuracy of clinical criteria for the diagnosis of progressive supranuclear palsy (Steele-Richardson-Olszewski syndrome). Neurology 1996;46:922–930.

341. Litvan I, Campbell G, Mangone CA, et al. Which clinical features differentiate progressive supranuclear palsy (Steele-Richardson-Olszewski syndrome) from related disorders? A clinicopathological study. Brain 1997;120:65–74.

342. Goetz CG, Leurgans S, Lang AE, et al. Progression of gait, speech and swallowing deficits in progressive supranuclear palsy. Neurology 2003;60:917–922.

343. Nath U, Ben-Shlomo Y, Thomson RG, et al. Clinical features and natural history of progressive supranuclear palsy: a clinical cohort study. Neurology 2003;60:910–916.

344. Santacruz P, Uttl B, Litvan I, et al. Progressive supranuclear palsy. A survey of the disease course. Neurology 1998;50:1637–1647.

345. Case records of the Massachusetts General Hospital: Case 26–1997. N Engl J Med 1997;337:549–556.

346. Hauw J-J, Daniel SE, Dickson D, et al. Preliminary NINDS neuropathologic criteria for Steele-Richardson-Olszewski syndrome (progressive supranuclear palsy). Neurology 1994;44:2015–2019.

347. Kida M, Koo H, Grossniklaus HE, et al. Neuropathologic findings in progressive supranuclear palsy. A brief review with two additional case reports. J Clin Neuroophthalmol 1988;8:161–170.

348. Verny M, Duyckaerts C, Agid Y, et al. The significance of cortical pathology in progressive supranuclear palsy. Clinico-pathological data in 10 cases. Brain 1996;119:1123–1136.

349. Bennett P, Bonifati V, Bonuccelli U, et al. Direct genetic evidence for involvement of tau in progressive supranuclear palsy. Neurology 1998;51:982–985.

350. Oliva R, Tolosa E, Ezquerra M, et al. Significant changes in the tau A0 and A3 alleles in progressive supranuclear palsy and improved genotyping by silver detection. Arch Neurol 1998;55:1122–1124.

351. Hoenicka J, Pérez M, Pérez-Tur J, et al. The tau gene A0 allele and progressive supranuclear palsy. Neurology 1999;53:1219–1225.

352. Litvan I, Baker M, Hutton M. Tau genotype: no effect on onset, symptom severity, or survival in progressive supranuclear palsy. Neurology 2001;57:138–140.

353. Bhidayasiri R, Riley DE, Somers JT, et al. Pathophysiology of slow vertical saccades in progressive supranuclear palsy. Neurology 2001;57:2070–2077.

354. Juncos JL, Hirsch EC, Malessa S, et al. Mesencephalic cholinergic nuclei in progressive supranuclear palsy. Neurology 1991;41:25–30.

355. Malessa S, Hirsch EC, Cervera P, et al. Progressive supranuclear palsy: loss of choline-acetyltransferase-like immunoreactive neurons in the pontine reticular formation. Neurology 1991;41:1593–1597.

356. Malessa S, Gaymard B, Rivaud S, et al. Role of pontine nuclei damage in smooth pursuit impairment of progressive supranuclear palsy: a clinical-pathologic study. Neurology 1994;44:716–721.

357. Halliday GM, Hardman CD, Cordato NJ, et al. A role for the substantia nigra pars reticulata in the gaze palsy of progressive supranuclear palsy. Brain 2000;123 (Pt 4):724–732.

358. Revesz T, Sangha H, Daniel SE. The nucleus raphe interpositus in the Steele-Richardson-Olszewski syndrome (progressive supranuclear palsy). Brain 1996;119:1137–1143.

359. Stern MB, Braffman BH, Skolnick BE, et al. Magnetic resonance imaging in Parkinson's disease and parkinsonian syndromes. Neurology 1989;39:1524–1526.

360. Case records of the Massachusetts General Hospital: Case 46–1993. N Engl J Med 1993;329:1560–1567.

361. Savoiardo M, Strada L, Girotti F, et al. MR imaging in progressive supranuclear palsy and Shy-Drager syndrome. J Comput Assist Tomogr 1989;13:555–560.

362. Paviour DC, Price SL, Stevens JM, et al. Quantitative MRI measurement of superior cerebellar peduncle in progressive supranuclear palsy. Neurology 2005;64:675–679.

363. Oba H, Yagishita A, Terada H, et al. New and reliable MRI diagnosis for progressive supranuclear palsy. Neurology 2005;64:2050–2055.

364. Gröschel K, Kastrup A, Litvan I, et al. Penguins and hummingbirds: midbrain atrophy in progressive supranuclear palsy. Neurology 2006;66:949–950.

365. Seppi K, Schocke MF, Esterhammer R, et al. Diffusion-weighted imaging discriminates progressive supranuclear palsy from PD, but not from the Parkinson variant of multiple system atrophy. Neurology 2003;60:922–927.

366. Dubinsky RM, Jankovic J. Progressive supranuclear palsy and a multi-infarct state. Neurology 1987;37:570–576.

367. Josephs KA, Ishizawa T, Tsuboi Y, et al. A clinicopathological study of vascular progressive supranuclear palsy: a multi-infarct disorder presenting as progressive supranuclear palsy. Arch Neurol 2002;59:1597–1601.

368. Kompoliti K, Goetz CG, Litvan I, et al. Pharmacological therapy in progressive supranuclear palsy. Arch Neurol 1998;55:1099–1102.

369. Ghika J, Tennis M, Hoffman E, et al. Idazoxan treatment in progressive supranuclear palsy. Neurology 1991;41:986–991.

370. Higgins JJ, Patterson MC, Dambrosia JM, et al. A clinical staging classification for type C Niemann-Pick disease. Neurology 1992;42:2286–2290.

371. Hulette CM, Earl NL, Anthony DC, et al. Adult onset Niemann-Pick disease type C presenting with dementia and absent organomegaly. Clin Neuropathol 1992;11:293–297.

372. Lossos A, Schlesinger H, Okon E, et al. Adult-onset Niemann-Pick type C disease. Arch Neurol 1997;54:1536–1541.

373. van de Vlasakker CJW, Gabreëls FJM, Wijburg HC, et al. Clinical features of Niemann-Pick disease type C. An example of the delayed onset, slowly progressive phenotype and an overview of recent literature. Clin Neurol Neurosurg 1994;96:119–123.

374. Neville BGR, Lake BD, Stephens R, et al. A neurovisceral storage disease with vertical nuclear ophthalmoplegia and its relationship to Niemann-Pick disease: a report of nine patients. Brain 1973;96:97–120.

375. Simpson DA, Winslow R, Gargulinski RB, et al. Oculofacial-skeletal myorhythmia in central nervous system Whipple's disease: additional case and review of the literature. Mov Disord 1995;10:195–200.

376. Louis ED, Lynch T, Kaufmann P, et al. Diagnostic guidelines in central nervous system Whipple's disease. Ann Neurol 1996;40:561–568.

377. Amarenco P, Roullet E, Hannoun L, et al. Progressive supranuclear palsy as the sole manifestation of system Whipple's disease treated with perfloxacine [letter]. J Neurol Neurosurg Psychiatry 1991;54:1121–1122.

378. Schwartz MA, Selhorst JB, Ochs AL, et al. Oculomasticatory myorhythmia: a unique movement disorder occurring in Whipple's disease. Ann Neurol 1986;20:677–683.

379. Ramzan NN, Loftus E, Burgart LJ, et al. Diagnosis and monitoring of Whipple disease by polymerase chain reaction. Ann Intern Med 1997;126:520–527.

380. Rickman LS, Freeman WR, Green WR, et al. Brief report: uveitis caused by Tropheryma whippelii (Whipple's disease). N Engl J Med 1995;332:363–366.

381. Williams JG, Edward DP, Tessler HH, et al. Ocular manifestations of Whipple disease. An atypical presentation. Arch Ophthalmol 1998;116:1232–1234.

382. Lynch T, Odel J, Fredericks DN, et al. Polymerase chain reaction-based detection of Tropheryma whippelii in central nervous system Whipple's disease. Ann Neurol 1997;42:120–124.

383. Verhagen WIM, Huygen PLM, Dalman JE, et al. Whipple's disease and the central nervous system. A case report and a review of the literature. Clin Neurol Neurosurg 1996;98:299–304.

384. Adler CH, Galetta SL. Oculo-facial-skeletal myorhythmia in Whipple's disease: treatment with ceftriaxone. Ann Intern Med 1990;112:467–469.

385. Fenollar F, Puechal X, Raoult D. Whipple's disease. N Engl J Med 2007;356:55–66.

386. Kushner MJ, Parrish M, Burke A, et al. Nystagmus in motor neuron disease. Ann Neurol 1984;16:71–77.

387. Mizutani T, Sakamaki S, Tsuchiya N, et al. Amyotrophic lateral sclerosis with ophthalmoplegia and multisystem degeneration in patients on long-term use of respirators. Acta Neuropathol 1992;84:372–377.

388. Okuda B, Yamamoto T, Yamasaki M, et al. Motor neuron disease with slow eye movements and vertical gaze palsy. Acta Neurol Scand 1992;85:71–76.

389. Shaunak S, Orrell RW, O'Sullivan E, et al. Oculomotor function in amyotrophic lateral sclerosis: evidence for frontal impairment. Ann Neurol 1995;38:38–44.

390. Averbuch-Heller L, Helmchen C, Horn AKE, et al. Slow vertical saccades in motor neuron disease: correlation of structure and function. Ann Neurol 1998;44:641–648.

391. Verhagen WIM, ter Bruggen JP, Huygen PLM. Oculomotor, auditory, and vestibular responses in myotonic dystrophy. Arch Neurol 1992;49:954–960.

392. Anastasopoulos D, Kimmig H, Mergner T, et al. Abnormalities of ocular motility in myotonic dystrophy. Brain 1996;119:1923–1932.

393. Verhagen WI, Huygen PL. Abnormalities of ocular motility in myotonic dystrophy [letter]. Brain 1997;120:1907–1909.

394. Osanai R, Kinoshita M, Hirose K. Saccadic slowing in myotonic dystrophy and CTG repeat expansion. J Neurol 1998;245:674–680.

395. Versino M, Romani A, Bergamaschi R, et al. Eye movement abnormalities in myotonic dystrophy. Electroencephalogr Clin Neurophysiol 1998;109:184–190.

396. Gupta SR, Brigell M, Gujrati M, et al. Supranuclear eye movement dysfunction in mitochondrial myopathy with tRNA(LEU) mutation. J Neuroophthalmol 1995;15:20–25.

397. Kirkham TH, Kamin DF. Slow saccadic eye movements in Wilson's disease. J Neurol Neurosurg Psychiatr 1974;37:191–194.

398. Saver JL, Liu GT, Charness ME. Idiopathic striopallidodentate calcification with prominent abnormality of eye movement. J Neuroophthalmol 1994;14:29–33.

399. Crino PB, Galetta SL, Sater RA, et al. Clinicopathologic study of paraneoplastic brainstem encephalitis and ophthalmoparesis. J Neuroophthalmol 1996;16:44–48.

400. Bennett JL, Galetta SL, Frohman LP, et al. Neuro-ophthalmologic manifestations of a paraneoplastic syndrome and testicular carcinoma. Neurology 1999;52:864–867.

585

401. Voltz R, Gultekin SH, Rosenfeld MR, et al. A serologic marker of paraneoplastic limbic and brain-stem encephalitis in patients with testicular cancer. N Engl J Med 1999;340: 1788–1795.

402. Fahn S, Marsden CD, Calne DB. Classification and investigation of dystonia. In: Marsden CD, Fahn S (eds): Movement Disorders, 2nd edn, pp 332–358. London, Butterworths, 1987.

403. McCowan PK, Cook LC, Cantab BA. Oculogyric crises in chronic epidemic encephalitis. Brain 1928;51:285–309.

404. Leigh RJ, Foley JM, Remler BF, et al. Oculogyric crises: a syndrome of thought disorder and ocular deviation. Ann Neurol 1987;22:13–17.

405. Munetz MR. Oculogyric crises and tardive dyskinesia. Am J Psychiatr 1980;137:1628.

406. Nasrallah HA, Pappas NJ, Crowe RR. Oculogyric dystonia in tardive dyskinesia. Am J Psychiatr 1980;137:850–851.

407. FitzGerald PM, Jankovic J. Tardive oculogyric crises. Neurology 1989;39:1434–1437.

408. Onuaguluchi G. Crises in post-encephalitic parkinsonism. Brain 1961;84:395–414.

409. Dorevitch A. Neuroleptics as causes of oculogyric crises. Arch Neurol 1984;41:15–16.

410. Sachdev P. Tardive and chronically recurrent oculogyric crises. Mov Disord 1993;8:93–97.

411. Dave M. Tardive oculogyric crises with clozapine [letter]. J Clin Psychiatry 1994;55: 264–265.

412. Smith JL. Ocular signs of parkinsonism. J Neurosurg 1966;24:284–285.

413. Mata M, Dorovini-Zis K, Wilson M, et al. New form of familial Parkinson-dementia syndrome: clinical and pathologic findings. Neurology 1983;33:1439–1443.

414. Lamberti P, de Mari M, Iliceto G, et al. Effect of L-dopa on oculogyric crises in a case of dopa-responsive dystonia [letter]. Mov Disord 1993;8:236–237.

415. Kis B, Hedrich K, Kann M, et al. Oculogyric dystonic states in early-onset parkinsonism with basal ganglia calcifications. Neurology 2005;65:761.

416. Urra DG, Campos J, Ruiz PG, et al. Movement disorders in ataxia-telangiectasia: review of six patients. Neurology 1989;39(Suppl 1):321.

417. FitzGerald PM, Jankovic J, Glaze DG, et al. Extrapyramidal involvement in Rett's syndrome. Neurology 1990;40:293–295.

418. Lee MS, Kim YD, Lyoo CH. Oculogyric crisis as an initial manifestation of Wilson's disease. Neurology 1999;52:1714–1715.

419. Benjamin S. Oculogyric crisis. In: Joseph AB, Young RR (eds): Movement Disorders in Neurology and Neuropsychiatry, pp 111–122. Oxford, Blackwell, 1992.

420. Mastumura K, Sakuta M. Oculogyric crisis in acute herpetic brainstem encephalitis. J Neurol Neurosurg Psychiatr 1987;50:365–366.

421. Heimburger RF. Positional oculogyric crises. Case report. J Neurosurg 1988;69:951–953.

422. Liu GT, Carrazana EJ, Macklis JD, et al. Delayed oculogyric crises associated with striatocapsular infarction. J Clin Neuroophthalmol 1991;11:208–211.

423. Kim JS, Kim HK, Im JH, et al. Oculogyric crisis and abnormal magnetic resonance imaging signals in bilateral lentiform nuclei. Mov Disord 1996;11:756–758.

424. Berchou RC, Rodin EA. Carbamazepine-induce oculogyric crisis. Arch Neurol 1979;36: 522–523.

425. Gorman M, Barkley GL. Oculogyric crisis induced by carbamazepine. Epilepsia 1995;36: 1158–1160.

426. Burke RE, Reches A, Traub MM, et al. Tetrabenazine induces acute dystonic reactions. Ann Neurol 1985;17:200–202.

427. Reeves AL, So EL, Sharbrough FW, et al. Movement disorders associated with the use of gabapentin. Epilepsia 1996;37:988–990.

428. Fraunfelder FW, Fraunfelder FT. Oculogyric crisis in patients taking cetirizine. Am J Ophthalmol 2004;137:355–357.

429. Gatzonis SD, Georgaculias N, Singounas E, et al. Elimination of oxcarbazepine-induced oculogyric crisis following vagus nerve stimulation. Neurology 1999;52:1918–1919.

430. Frankel M, Cummings JL. Neuro-ophthalmic abnormalities in Tourette's syndrome: functional and anatomic implications. Neurology 1984;34:359–361.

431. Jankovic J, Stone L. Dystonic tics in patients with Tourette's syndrome. Mov Disord 1991;6:248–252.

432. Jankovic J, Rohaidy H. Motor, behavioral and pharmacologic findings in Tourette's syndrome. Can J Neurol Sci 1987;14:541–546.

433. Shapiro AK, Shapiro ES, Young JG, et al. Gilles de la Tourette Syndrome, 2nd edn, p 129. New York, Raven Press, 1988.

434. Ahn JC, Hoyt WF, Hoyt CS. Tonic upgaze in infancy. A report of three cases. Arch Ophthalmol 1989;107:57–58.

435. Echenne B, Rivier R. Benign paroxysmal tonic upward gaze. Pediatr Neurol 1992;8: 154–155.

436. Kleiman MD, DiMario FJ, Jr., Leconche DA, et al. Benign transient downward gaze in preterm infants. Pediatr Neurol 1994;10:313–316.

437. Ouvrier R, Billson F. Paroxysmal tonic upgaze of childhood: a review. Brain Dev 2005;27:185–188.

438. Wolsey DH, Warner JE. Paroxysmal tonic downgaze in two healthy infants. J Neuroophthalmol 2006;26:187–189.

439. Hoyt CS, Mousel DK, Weber AA. Transient supranuclear disturbances of gaze in healthy neonates. Am J Ophthalmol 1980;89:708–713.

440. Daroff RB, Hoyt WF. Supranuclear disorders of ocular control systems in man. In: Bach-y-Rita P, Collins CC, Hyde JE (eds): The Control of Eye Movements, pp 198–199. New York, Academic Press, 1971.

441. Goldblum TA, Effron LA. Upbeat nystagmus associated with tonic downward deviation in healthy neonates. J Pediatr Ophthalmol Strabismus 1994;31:334–335.

442. Miller VS, Packard AM. Paroxysmal downgaze in term newborn infants. J Child Neurol 1998;13:294–295.

443. Deonna T, Roulet E, Meyer HU. Benign paroxysmal tonic upgaze of childhood. Neuropediatrics 1990;21:213–214.

444. Campistol J, Prats JM, Garaizar C. Benign paroxysmal tonic upgaze of childhood with ataxia. A neuro-ophthalmological syndrome of familial origin? Dev Med Child Neurol 1993;35:436–439.

445. Hayman M, Harvey AS, Hopkins IJ, et al. Paroxysmal tonic upgaze: a reappraisal of outcome. Ann Neurol 1998;43:514–520.

446. Keane JR, Rawlinson DG, Lu AT. Sustained downgaze deviation: two cases without structural pretectal lesions. Neurology 1976;26:594–595.

447. Johkura K, Komiyama A, Kuroiwa Y. Vertical conjugate eye deviation in postresuscitation coma. Ann Neurol 2004;56:878–881.

448. Keane JR. Sustained upgaze in coma. Ann Neurol 1981;9:409–412.

449. Klostermann W, Zuhlke C, Heide W, et al. Slow saccades and other eye movement disorders in spinocerebellar atrophy type 1. J Neurol 1997;244:105–111.

450. Buttner N, Geschwind D, Jen JC, et al. Oculomotor phenotypes in autosomal dominant ataxias. Arch Neurol 1998;55:1353–1357.

451. Storey E, Forrest SM, Shaw JH, et al. Spinocerebellar ataxia type 2. Clinical features of a pedigree displaying prominent frontal-executive dysfunction. Arch Neurol 1999;56: 43–60.

452. Nakano KK, Dawson DM, Spence A. Machado disease: a hereditary ataxia in Portuguese emigrants to Massachusetts. Neurology 1972;22:49–55.

453. Woods BT, Schaumburg HH. Nigro-spino-dentatal degeneration with nuclear ophthalmoplegia: a unique and partially treatable clinicopathological entity. J Neurol Sci 1972;17:149–166.

454. Rosenberg RN, Nyhan WL, Bay C, et al. Autosomal dominant striatonigral degeneration. Neurology 1976;26:703–714.

455. Dawson DM, Feudo P, Zubick HH, et al. Electro-oculographic findings in Machado-Joseph disease. Neurology 1982;32:1272–1276.

456. Sudarsky L, Coutinho P. Machado-Joseph disease. Clin Neurosci 1995;3:17–22.

457. Isashiki Y, Kii Y, Ohba N, et al. Retinopathy associated with Machado–Joseph disease (spinocerebellar ataxia 3) with CAG trinucleotide repeat expansion. Am J Ophthalmol 2001;131:808–810.

458. Jardim LB, Pereira ML, Silveira I, et al. Neurologic findings in Machado-Joseph disease: relation with disease duration, subtypes, and (CAG)n. Arch Neurol 2001;58: 899–904.

459. Benomar A, Le Guern E, Dürr A, et al. Autosomal-dominant cerebellar ataxia with retinal degeneration (ADCA type II) is genetically different from ADCA type II. Ann Neurol 1994;35:439–444.

460. Morrow MJ, Zinn AB, Tucker T, et al. Maculopathy in spinocerebellar ataxia type 7. Neurology 1999;53:244.

461. Oh AK, Jacobson KM, Jen JC, et al. Slowing of voluntary and involuntary saccades: an early sign in spinocerebellar ataxia type 7. Ann Neurol 2001;49:801–804.

462. Dürr A, Cossee M, Agid Y, et al. Clinical and genetic abnormalities in patients with Friedreich's ataxia. N Engl J Med 1996;335:1169–1175.

463. Rosenberg RN. DNA-triplet repeats and neurologic disease [editorial]. N Engl J Med 1996;335:1222–1224.

464. Gomez CM, Thompson RM, Gammack JT, et al. Spinocerebellar ataxia type 6: gaze-evoked and vertical nystagmus, Purkinje cell degeneration, and variable age of onset. Ann Neurol 1997;42:933–950.

465. Evidente VG, Gwinn-Hardy KA, Caviness JN, et al. Hereditary ataxias. Mayo Clin Proc 2000;75:475–490.

466. Hübner J, Sprenger A, Klein C, et al. Eye movement abnormalities in spinocerebellar ataxia type 17 (SCA17). Neurology 2007;69:1160–1168.

467. Naito H, Oyanagi S. Familial myoclonus epilepsy and choreoathetosis: hereditary dentatorubral-pallidoluysian atrophy. Neurology 1982;32:798–807.

CHAPTER 17

Eye movement disorders: nystagmus and nystagmoid eye movements

Nystagmus is a rhythmic biphasic oscillation of the eyes. Since nystagmus results from a defect in the slow eye movement system, nystagmus always has a slow phase that initiates the ocular oscillation. Nystagmus should also be distinguished from other ocular oscillations or nystagmoid eye movements. These other ocular oscillations usually do not have a slow phase and often represent disorders of saccades. Characteristically, they interrupt foveal fixation, and although they can be distinguished clinically, some may be best characterized by eye movement recordings.[1]

This chapter will review the symptoms and examination of patients with nystagmus, and detail each of the important types of nystagmus and nystagmoid eye movements and their pathophysiology and management.

Nystagmus

Nystagmus may occur physiologically in response to environmental stimuli or from rotation of the body. More importantly, it may be a sign of central nervous system (CNS) dysfunction, peripheral vestibular disease, or visual loss. One method to organize the different types of nystagmus is to distinguish those cases with jerk properties from those with pendular waveforms and to consider the various types according to the patient's age (**Table 17–1**). In pendular nystagmus, the phases are of equal velocity and there are no corrective saccades. Jerk nystagmus has a slow phase followed by a rapid corrective phase in the opposite direction. Entities such as congenital nystagmus and spasmus nutans will more likely present in childhood.

By convention, the direction of jerk nystagmus is defined by its fast phase. Patients who have a slow phase to the left and a corrective phase to the right are said to have right-beating nystagmus. Frequently, jerk nystagmus will have a torsional or rotary component. This type of nystagmus is best described by whether it beats towards the patient's right or left shoulder (**Fig. 17–1**). Pendular nystagmus has no fast phase, so it is described as either vertical or horizontal. Occasionally, nystagmus results from a combination of vertical and horizontal phases to produce a circular, elliptical, or oblique waveform.

Most forms of nystagmus can be interpreted at the bedside. However, eye movement recordings can more accurately characterize the slow phases of nystagmus and define its underlying pathophysiologic substrate. For example, the slow phase velocity of vestibular nystagmus is linear, while congenital nystagmus displays an increasing slow phase velocity. Gaze paretic nystagmus usually has a declining slow phase velocity.[1]

Symptoms associated with nystagmus

The accompanying symptoms may be extremely helpful in discerning the various forms of nystagmus. Nystagmus may be asymptomatic or produce

Table 17–1 Grouping of nystagmus types by waveform and typical age at presentation

	Childhood	Any age
Jerk	Latent	Vestibular
		Peripheral and central
		Gaze-evoked
		Physiologic
		Pathologic
		Brun's
		Dissociated
		Periodic alternating (PAN)
		Downbeat
		Upbeat
		Convergence retraction
		Epileptic
		Drug-induced
		Optokinetic
		See-saw
Pendular	Spasmus nutans	Oculopalatal
	Monocular nystagmus due to visual deprivation/loss	Oculomasticatory myorhythmia
		See-saw
Either pendular and/or jerk in the same patient	Congenital	

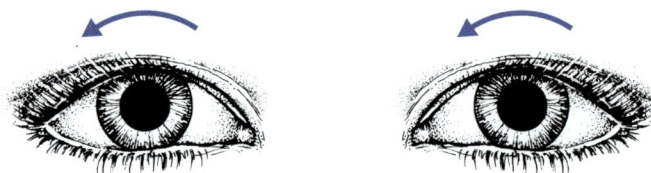

Figure 17–1. Diagram of torsional nystagmus. Nystagmus as demonstrated in this figure is described as beating toward the patient's right shoulder.

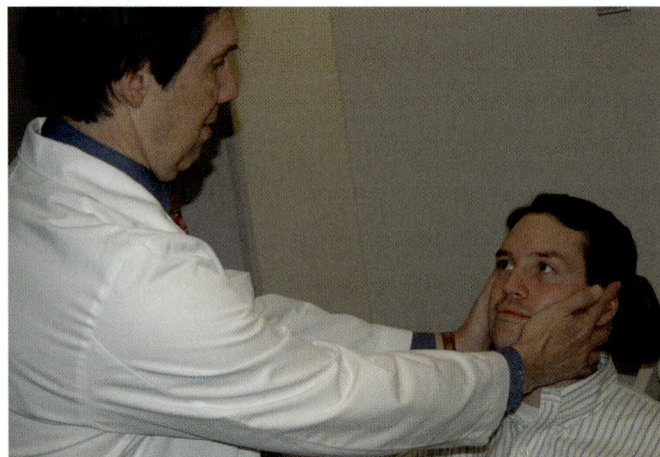

Figure 17–2. Testing of the vestibulo-ocular reflex. The patient's head is rotated quickly over short distances while the patient fixates on the examiner's nose. Patients with a decreased vestibulo-ocular reflex will show a catch-up saccade to maintain fixation.

a jumping of the visual environment called *oscillopsia*. A patient with acquired nystagmus often sees the visual environment moving in the direction of the fast phase. In contrast, patients with congenital nystagmus typically have a reduction in visual acuity without oscillopsia. Nausea and vomiting may accompany nystagmus and can be a prominent complaint of patients with peripheral vestibular disease. Symptoms such as diplopia, dysarthria, facial numbness, and dysphagia suggest a brain stem origin for the nystagmus. In contrast, hearing loss and tinnitus are more consistent with a peripheral vestibular cause.

Examination

The examination begins by observing the patient's eyes while they look straight ahead. Then the eyes are viewed in all positions of gaze. Smooth pursuit and saccadic eye movements are then evaluated (see Chapter 16). An abnormality of either the saccadic or the pursuit system suggests a central cause for the nystagmus. Ocular alignment should also be assessed. The vestibulo-ocular reflex may be tested by having

the patient focus on a distant object as the head is moved from side to side at 2 Hz. Alternatively, the patient focuses on the examiner's nose or finger as the examiner moves the patient's head quickly over very short distances (**Fig. 17–2**).[2] The appearance of nystagmus or a corrective saccade with this maneuver suggests a vestibular disorder.

Another useful bedside test is cancellation of the vestibulo-ocular reflex (see **Fig. 2–29**). In this test, patients focus on their outstretched thumb as they are rotated in a chair at low frequency. Normally, the eyes do not move during this maneuver. If the reflex is defective, fixation on the thumb is not maintained, the eyes drift, and nystagmus is generated. This is usually a sign of cerebellar or central vestibular dysfunction.

Occasionally, nystagmus is difficult to discern or is suppressed by fixation. Under these conditions, one eye is viewed with an ophthalmoscope. Simultaneously, the other eye is covered manually (**Fig. 17–3**). This procedure removes fixation, and the eye being viewed by the ophthalmoscope can be checked for nystagmus. It is helpful to remember that the disc moves in the direction opposite from the movement generated by the front of the eye. Therefore, if the disc is moving rapidly upward, the nystagmus direction is downbeat. Frenzel goggles, which contain high-plus lenses, also eliminate fixation and may provide magnification to help detect subtle forms of nystagmus (**Fig. 17–4**). Patients with perilymph fistulas may have nystagmus induced by a Valsalva maneuver or by replicating nose blowing.

In some patients, nystagmus may be evident only with provocative maneuvers. In the Dix–Hallpike maneuver

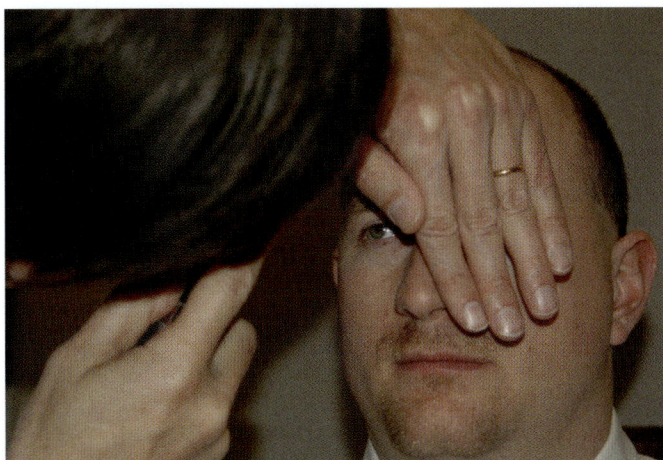

Figure 17–3. The examiner checks for nystagmus by viewing the eye with a direct ophthalmoscope and covering the other eye with his hand. This removes fixation.

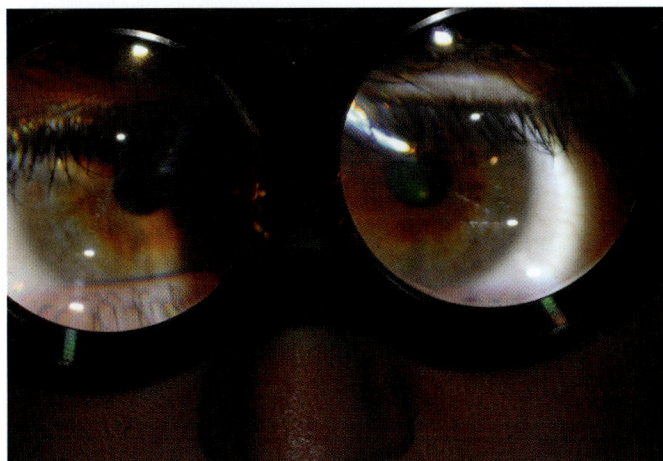

Figure 17–4. Frenzel goggles are lenses of high magnification that remove the patient's fixation and provide the examiner a large view of the patient's eyes. (Figure courtesy of Mark Moster, M.D.)

Table 17–2 Characteristics of nystagmus during the Dix–Hallpike maneuver in peripheral versus central positional vertigo

Findings	Peripheral	Central
Latency	Present	Absent
Duration	<1 minute	>1 minute
Fatigability	Yes	No
Nystagmus waveform	Upbeat and torsional	Pure torsional

Caloric stimulation is another method for provoking nystagmus. The test procedure itself is discussed in detail in Chapter 2 (see **Fig. 2–41**). Cold water injected into one ear produces a slow movement of the eyes toward the irrigated ear. There is a corrective phase toward the opposite direction in the awake and normal patient. By convention, nystagmus is named by its fast phase. Therefore, the consequence of canal irrigation with cold water may be remembered by the term "cows," which stands for cold–opposite and warm–same. This means when the right ear is irrigated with cold water, the fast phase of nystagmus should be to the left in a normal patient. In a comatose patient, just a slow phase or no response at all may be seen. Vertical eye movements in the comatose patient may be assessed by bilateral caloric stimulation. Cold water simultaneously injected into both ears produces a slow down phase and a corrective up phase. This might be remembered by the term "cuwd," which stands for cold–up and warm–down.

One can elicit some forms of nystagmus by asking patients to shake their head from side to side for 15 seconds. The appearance of nystagmus with this maneuver may aid localization. In a peripheral vestibular process, typically, the horizontal nystagmus will beat away from the injured ear. Nystagmus that beats vertically or ipsilaterally to the suspected lesion suggests a central vestibular process.[3]

Other findings in the neuro-ophthalmic or neurologic examination may aid in the diagnosis of patients with nystagmus or nystagmoid disorders. For instance, afferent visual function should be assessed carefully. Longstanding vision loss and pendular or jerk nystagmus suggests congenital sensory nystagmus. The examiner should be aware that in patients with congenital nystagmus, visual acuity should be tested with each eye separately then with both eyes open, in case there is latent nystagmus. The fundus exam might reveal a congenital optic disc abnormality, pigmentary retinopathy, or foveal hypoplasia (albinism) in congenital sensory nystagmus. Abnormalities in the cranial nerve examination, including hearing, should be excluded. Finally, motor and cerebellar dysfunction such as dysdiadokinesia or gait ataxia will suggest a central cause of the nystagmus. In addition, patients with peripheral vestibular disease may march in the direction of the affected ear with their eyes closed (*Fukuda stepping test*).

Pathophysiology of nystagmus

Nystagmus usually results from a defect in the slow eye movement system, which includes visual fixation, the vestibular system, smooth pursuit, vergence, and the

(Fig. 17–5 A,B), which is used to diagnose patients with positional vertigo, the patient sits on a table lengthwise. The patient is then brought backward, and the head is rotated 45 degrees to one side. The characteristics of the nystagmus, if present, may be helpful in differentiating central and peripheral forms of positional nystagmus. The examiner is interested in the nature of the nystagmus, its direction, its latency, and whether or not it fatigues (**Table 17–2**).

The optokinetic flag (see **Fig. 2–30**) may be helpful in the diagnosis of congenital nystagmus and convergence retraction nystagmus. Patients with congenital nystagmus may have a reversal of the normal response. For instance, the eyes usually follow then beat away from the direction of the moving tape. In some patients with congenital nystagmus, the eyes beat in the direction of the moving tape. Patients with a dorsal midbrain syndrome often display a characteristic eye movement abnormality, particularly in attempted upgaze, known as convergence retraction nystagmus. This nystagmus may be elicited by moving the optokinetic nystagmus (OKN) tape downward to induce upward saccades.

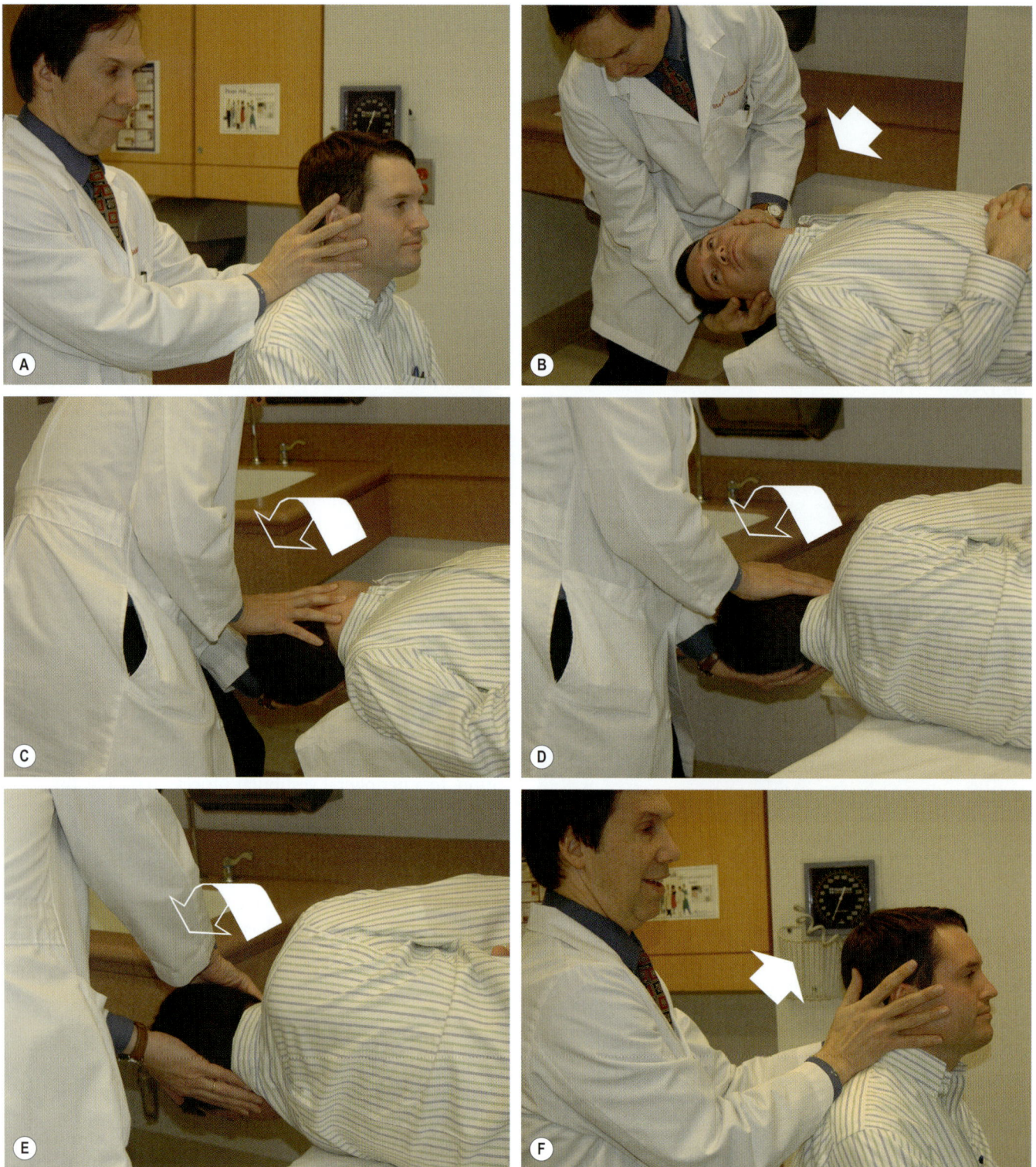

Figure 17–5. In the Dix–Hallpike maneuver, the patient is brought from the sitting position (**A**) to the head-hanging position at a 45-degree angle with the affected ear dependent (**B**). In a patient with benign positional vertigo (BPV), the eyes develop a torsional upbeating nystagmus (not shown) when the affected ear is dependent. The nystagmus may be more torsional in the dependent eye and more vertical in the higher eye.

In a patient with BPV affecting the right posterior semicircular canal, for example, the Dix-Hallpike maneuver is combined with steps C-F in the so-called *Epley maneuver*. After 30 seconds in the head-hanging position depicted in (**B**), the head is turned 90 degrees in the opposite direction so that the left ear is dependent (**C**). **D**. The patient is then placed on the left shoulder (the unaffected side). **E**. The patient's head is moved to the face down position for approximately 1–3 minutes. **F**. The patient is then rapidly brought upright again. The patient should remain upright for the next 48 hours, usually sleeping in a lounge chair.[79] If the patient is unable to sleep upright, the patient should be instructed not sleep on the affected ear for the next 7 days.

Table 17–3 Comparison of congenital nystagmus and spasmus nutans

Features	Congenital nystagmus	Spasmus nutans
Waveform	Mixed waveform (pendular and/or jerk); usually horizontal	Pendular; usually horizontal
Symmetry	Symmetric conjugate ocular oscillations	Monocular or asymmetric ocular oscillations
Amplitude	Low or high	Low
Frequency	Low	High
Other features	Horizontal in upgaze Null point	Head turn or tilt Head bobbing
Types	Motor (no vision loss) Sensory (vision loss)	Benign Suprasellar mass related Retina related
Onset	2–4 months	4–14 months
Course	Waveform may change	Benign type typically resolves by 5 years
Other ophthalmic findings	Esotropia, latent nystagmus in some cases	Amblyopia, refractive error

optokinetic and neural integrator pathways. Failure of visual fixation, imbalance in the vestibular system, or impairment of the gaze-holding mechanisms are the most common causes of nystagmus. Impaired visual fixation, due to disorders of the visual pathways for instance, may cause the eyes to drift from an object of regard and cause nystagmus.

The vestibular system allows images to remain steady on the fovea while the head is moving. Under normal conditions, the vestibulo-ocular reflex generates slow eye movements that are equal and in the opposite direction of the head movement. The vestibulo-ocular reflex pathway originates in the semicircular canals and synapses in the vestibular nuclei, ultimately connecting to the ocular motor nuclei and cerebellum. Peripheral vestibular nystagmus results from an imbalance of input from the semicircular canals. Complete unilateral loss of labyrinth function produces a mixed horizontal torsional nystagmus that may be suppressed by visual fixation. Central vestibular injury may produce downbeat, upbeat, or torsional nystagmus. This central vestibular nystagmus, typically results from injury to the vestibular nuclei or cerebellovestibular pathways.[1] The otoliths respond to linear acceleration of the head. Imbalance of the otoliths or their projections can cause any combination of torsional eye movements, skew deviation, and vertical nystagmus.

The neural integrator is a network of cells responsible for maintaining the eyes in eccentric gaze. When the system is defective, the eyes will drift back to the midline with a corrective fast phase. The cerebellar flocculus, the nucleus prepositus hypoglossi, and medial vestibular nucleus make up the neural integrator for horizontal gaze, for instance. A defect in this system is implicated in pathologic horizontal gaze-evoked nystagmus.

Types of nystagmus

In the following discussion of the various entities, those presenting predominantly in childhood will be reviewed first, then those without any particular age predilection will

be detailed afterwards (**Table 17–1**). In a young child with nystagmus, the most important distinction is between congenital nystagmus and spasmus nutans (**Table 17–3**).

Congenital nystagmus

Congenital (or "infantile") nystagmus is most frequently characterized by its early onset in life, symmetric and conjugate involvement of both eyes, a common pattern of mixed pendular and jerk waveforms, horizontal direction in upgaze, presence of a null point, and lack of oscillopsia. It does not localize to any particular lesion in the CNS, and it may be associated with either normal or reduced vision. Congenital nystagmus may be recognized rarely at birth but much more commonly arises in the second through fourth months of life when visual fixation normally develops.[4,5] Conjugate oscillations with several types of waveforms can be seen. Classically, congenital nystagmus is a horizontal nystagmus with a pendular waveform, but it may be rotary or rarely vertical in nature. Patients with congenital nystagmus may also demonstrate jerk properties, either in primary or in horizontal endgaze. In the jerk waveforms, the eyes drift during an increasing velocity slow phase, and a subsequent saccade brings the eyes back to foveation. A mixed waveform consisting of pendular nystagmus in primary and upgaze but jerk nystagmus in horizontal endgaze, right beating in right gaze and left beating in left gaze, is commonly seen and is unique to congenital nystagmus.

In addition, the waveform at onset in young infancy may differ from what is seen later in the same child at 1 year of age. In one recognized pattern, a young infant first exhibits a large amplitude but low-frequency strictly pendular eye oscillation, in so-called *triangular wave* nystagmus, named after the shape of the waveform. Then the eye movement disorder gradually converts to a smaller amplitude jerk nystagmus or the mixed pendular and jerk nystagmus described above some time before 1 year of life. The waveform progression reflects the maturation of the visual system.

Congenital nystagmus also is one of the few types of nystagmus that remains horizontal in vertical gaze. It is this

Video 17.1

Video 17.2

591

property that helps distinguish congenital nystagmus from gaze-evoked nystagmus. Other forms of nystagmus that remain horizontal in vertical gaze include peripheral vestibular nystagmus and periodic alternating nystagmus.

Adaptive mechanisms in patients with congenital nystagmus include preferring a head turn or tilt at an angle where the best vision and least amount of oscillopsia are achieved. In this *null point or position* of the eyes, the nystagmus is most diminished. In addition, convergence can dampen congenital nystagmus. In the most common example of the *nystagmus blockage syndrome*, an individual with congenital nystagmus, attempting to suppress it by converging, develops an esotropia with a head turn. Attempts at fixation may also exacerbate congenital nystagmus.

Despite the fact their eyes are almost constantly in motion, most patients with congenital nystagmus do not complain of oscillopsia. In congenital nystagmus, visual sampling occurs only during brief foveation periods, allowing optimal viewing of a visual target without a sense of motion despite the abnormal eye movement.[6,7] Many also have only slightly reduced visual acuities, especially when their visual pathways are normal. Explanations for these observations have included a reduced sensitivity to retinal image motion, adaptation to retinal image motion, information sampled only when the eyes are moving relatively slowly during the short foveation periods mentioned above, and the use of extra retinal information to cancel the effects of eye movements for review.[8] When oscillopia occurs later in life in a patient with congenital nystagmus, breakdown in motor or sensory status due to a decompensated strabismus, refractive error, return of an eccentric null position, or worsening of the underlying disorder of the visual pathways should be considered.[9]

A reverse optokinetic response may be seen in which the fast phase of the response abnormally moves in the same direction of the moving OKN tape.[10] In infants with horizontal nystagmus and apparent poor vision, the OKN tape can be moved vertically to elicit superimposed vertical eye movements. This would suggest potentially good vision.

Rarely patients with congenital nystagmus have alternating epochs of right then left beating nystagmus. This so-called congenital periodic alternating nystagmus can be observed in patients with albinism, but other patients with or without sensory deficits may also display this type of nystagmus.[11–13] In this form of congenital nystagmus, patients will adapt a slow back and forth head posture associated with the alternating null point.

Occasionally patients with congenital nystagmus may also exhibit head oscillations. Whether the head movements are an adaptive strategy to improve vision[14] or may represent an effect of a common disordered neural mechanism is unclear. In addition, strabismus and high refractive error, including astigmatism, are frequently associated with congenital nystagmus.

Etiology. In one approach to patients with congenital nystagmus, patients are subdivided into those with relatively normal vision (*congenital motor nystagmus*) versus those with vision loss (*congenital sensory nystagmus*). While likely an oversimplification discouraged by some experts,[15] this distinction is nevertheless extremely helpful in the clinic[16] for

both the physician and the patient's family for understanding the mechanism, deciding upon the evaluation, and predicting the visual outcome of a child with congenital nystagmus. The waveforms of the two types are indistinguishable at the bedside.

Congenital nystagmus may occur in isolation with relatively normal vision but completely normal fundus and neurological exams. These patients have *congenital motor nystagmus*, which may be considered to be an efferent pathway disorder, perhaps involving the ocular motor systems involved in visual fixation. Although usually sporadic, congenital motor nystagmus can be inherited in an autosomal-dominant, autosomal-recessive, or X-linked fashion.[17–19] Most such patients have nearly normal visual acuities which remain relatively stable over their lifetime.

However, many patients with congenital nystagmus have a component of afferent pathway dysfunction. Common causes of this *congenital sensory nystagmus* include congenital optic disc abnormalities such as optic nerve hypoplasia or atrophy, ocular albinism, retinal dystrophies such as congenital stationary night blindness or Leber's congenital amaurosis, or cataracts. Their visual prognosis depends on whether the underlying disorder is static or degenerative.

Multiple potential mechanisms of congenital nystagmus have been proposed. One theory posits that congenital nystagmus results from miswiring of the visual pathways or a maladaption to visual deprivation that leads to inadequate compensation for eye drifts. Recent theories also suggest that there are abnormalities of the extraocular muscle tendons enthesis (insertions) where they join the sclera. A decreased number and size of enthesial nerve endings, loss or fragmentation of perineurium, and narrowed vascular lumen have been observed in patients with congenital nystagmus. Enthesial nerve endings may be involved in monitoring eye position, so congenital nystagmus may be attributed to the presence of anomalous endings and a disturbance in ocular proprioception.[20,21]

Evaluation. The workup of a patient with congenital nystagmus requires a careful assessment of visual function and fundus appearance in order to establish whether the condition is sensory or motor. Paradoxic constriction of the pupils when the lights are turned off (see Chapter 13) suggests a retinal disorder. Transillumination of the iris, seen best with a slit lamp, or foveal hypoplasia would be consistent with ocular albinism. Children with congenital nystagmus require a careful refraction by a pediatric ophthalmologist.[22]

In most patients with congenital motor nystagmus, particularly when the child is developmentally normal, no further workup is necessary. These children can be followed conservatively. In those with congenital sensory nystagmus or when the examination alone is inconclusive, magnetic resonance imaging (MRI) of the brain, visual evoked responses, and electroretinography (ERG) are the laboratory tests that are most likely to provide useful diagnostic information.

Treatment. Treatment of congenital nystagmus first involves correction of any refractive error.[22] A recent study of patients with myopia and congenital nystagmus suggested that some patients will have improved visual foveation after laser refractive surgery when compared to best spectacle refraction.[23] Contact lenses may also dampen congenital nystagmus, presumably by enhancing sensory feedback and reducing the abnormal eye movements.[24,25]

Prism therapy may be used to shift the null point to the primary position or to induce convergence. Prisms may help to direct the line of sight toward primary gaze and thereby minimize abnormal head postures. In this situation, the prisms are oriented with the apices in the direction of the preferred gaze. This will move visualized objects toward the null point so the individual does not have to adopt a head turn. Base-out prisms can be used to induce convergence. If prism therapy fails, eye muscle surgery (Anderson–Kestenbaum procedure) may be performed to reposition the eyes and move the null point into the straight-ahead position.[26] In this procedure, for a patient with a face turn to the right (eyes shift to a null point in left gaze), the yoked muscles left lateral rectus and right medial rectus are weakened (recession) and left medial rectus and right lateral rectus muscles are strengthened (resection). Tenotomy, in which all four horizontal recti muscles are detached and then re-attached at their original site, has been associated with improved foveation times and improved vision.[27,28] Tenotomy coupled with strabismus surgery may be a particularly effective treatment to improve visual function in patients with congenital nystagmus and ocular misalignment.[29]

Recently, both memantine (40 mg/day) and gabapentin (2400 mg/day) were found to be effective in a randomized controlled trial of patients with congenital nystagmus. These agents improved visual acuity and foveation times in this type of nystagmus.[30] However, in our clinical experience, the response to these medications is mixed or limited by side effects.

Botulinum toxin has also been used in the therapy of congenital nystagmus, but its effect remains limited by its side effects of ptosis, double vision, and the need for repeat injections.[31,32]

Latent nystagmus

Latent nystagmus is a form of congenital nystagmus produced by unequal visual input into both eyes.[33] Most commonly observed when one eye is covered, in the uncovered eye the slow phase of this jerk nystagmus always beats toward the nose, while the fast phase beats in the direction of the uncovered eye (**Fig. 17–6**). The covered eye is moving conjugately. The alternating direction of this nystagmus with eye cover is characteristic of this entity. Latent nystagmus is also maximal in intensity when the uncovered eye is abducted and decreases when the eye is placed in adduction. These patients may fail routine eye tests because of the oscillopsia induced by the nystagmus during monocular testing. However, with both eyes open these patients may have much better vision. In the presence of latent nystagmus, methods of measuring monocular vision include fogging the other eye with high-plus lenses, testing with polarizing lenses, and using the red–green duochrome slide test.

Latent nystagmus is often a benign condition. It is usually unassociated with other neurologic abnormalities except patients with periventricular leukomalacia (PVL) seem more prone to developing latent nystagmus. Associated ophthalmologic abnormalities may include (1) congenital esotropia,

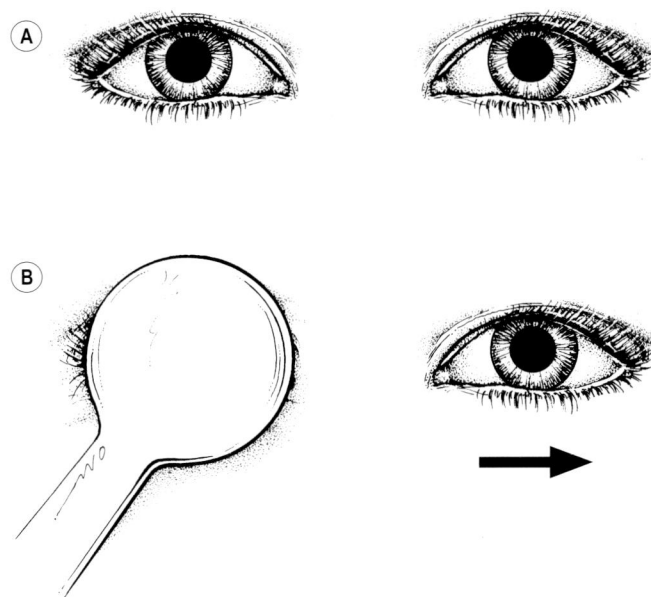

Figure 17–6. In latent nystagmus, with both eyes open (**A**) no abnormal eye movements may be evident. When one eye is covered (**B**), both eyes develop a jerk nystagmus with a fast phase towards the uncovered eye.

(2) congenital nystagmus, (3) dissociated vertical deviation, and (4) overaction of the inferior oblique muscle.[34] Latent nystagmus has a declining slow-phase waveform in distinction to the increasing slow-phase velocity characteristic of congenital nystagmus.[1] In *manifest* latent nystagmus, a process that reduces acuity in one eye, such as a cataract, uncorrected refractive error, or amblyopia, may cause latent nystagmus.

Latent nystagmus may be a form of peripheral nystagmus that is evoked by monocular viewing conditions.[33] In patients with congenital esotropia, there may be loss of binocularity in motion sensitive visual area V5 (see Chapter 9) and its connections to the pretectal area known as the nucleus of the optic tract (NOT).[33] Under monocular viewing conditions, the NOT is activated and latent nystagmus is generated. For example, covering the left eye of a patient with latent nystagmus will produce a stimulus from the right eye that activates the left nucleus of the optic tract. The NOT then activates the vestibular system to produce a leftward slow phase with corrective phase to the right. A similar vestibular response could be elicited with rotation of visual environment to the left or the body of a person to the right.

In general, latent nystagmus does not indicate a structural or progressive abnormality of the central nervous system. Neuroimaging is not indicated in latent nystagmus if the clinical examination shows the typical change in the direction of the waveform with occlusion, and there is no history of prematurity.

Spasmus nutans

Spasmus nutans is characterized by the triad of (1) torticollis, (2) head nodding (2–3 Hz), and (3) monocular or asymmetric nystagmus (**Table 17–3**).[35] The nystagmus is the hallmark, as both of the other features are not always present. The disorder usually starts between ages 4 and 14 months. The nystagmus may last between 1 and 2 years and typically

Video 17.3

Video 17.4

resolves clinically by 5 years. Spasmus nutans shows a pendular waveform of low amplitude and high frequency (up to 15 Hz).[36] However, the amplitude and frequency of the nystagmus may vary with gaze position. The nystagmus is often described as shimmering and horizontal, but it may be vertical, or rotary in nature. Rarely the nystagmus may be convergent.[37] Some patients may have subclinical nystagmus detected by eye movement recordings only.

Video 17.5

Spasmus nutans is usually a benign condition. However, there are a number of reports that document a similar nystagmus with parasellar and hypothalamic tumors[38–42] and retinal disorders. The nystagmus and head movements may be indistinguishable from idiopathic spasmus nutans, despite eye and head movement recordings.[43] The most common associated neoplasm is an optic pathway glioma. Patients who harbor tumors usually have other signs of afferent pathway dysfunction such as acuity loss, field defects or optic disc atrophy, or endocrinologic abnormalities including poor feeding or diencephalic syndrome (see Chapter 7). Spasmus nutans-like nystagmus and head movements have also been described in association with retinal diseases such as congenital stationary night blindness,[44,45] rod-cone or rod dystrophy,[46,47] or those associated with Bardet–Biedl syndrome[48] and spinocerebellar degenerations.[49] For unclear reasons, in demographic comparisons of patients with spasmus nutans and congenital nystagmus, the former is associated with lower socioeconomic status, parental drug and alcohol abuse, and Afro-American or Hispanic ethnicity.[50]

Evaluation and treatment. Patients with findings suggesting spasmus nutans should have a brain MRI to exclude a mass lesion. Some authors have suggested a more conservative approach,[51] but we believe that relying on an abnormal endocrinologic history or the presence of decreased vision or optic atrophy is problematic in young children, in whom the examination may be difficult. ERG to should be considered when subnormal vision, an abnormal fundus exam, paradoxic pupillary reaction, severe myopia, or photophobia suggest a retinal disorder.

Idiopathic spasmus nutans requires no specific treatment as the disorder usually spontaneously remits. However, careful follow-up by a pediatric ophthalmologist is mandatory as many children with idiopathic spasmus nutans will have amblyopia or strabismus in the eye with the nystagmus of greater amplitude.[52] Refractive errors are also common. In some patients, subclinical nystagmus may persist up to the age of 12.[35]

Monocular nystagmus and visual deprivation (Heimann–Bielschowsky phenomenon)

Children who develop severe visual loss in one eye may develop a slow monocular vertical oscillation of the eye known as the Heimann–Bielschowsky phenomenon.[53,54] It may appear years after visual loss and can resolve if vision is restored in the affected eye. Monocular pendular nystagmus has been reported as result of visual loss associated with a chiasmal glioma.[55] Therefore, acquired monocular pendular nystagmus in childhood should be evaluated with an MRI. Patients with the Heimann–Bielschowsky phenomenon usually have underlying optic nerve disease or amblyopia.[56]

Some adult patients with severe monocular visual loss can develop a similar slow (1–5 Hz) vertical pendular nystagmus in the affected eye, but this is much less common in this age group. Although the waveform is classically vertical, we have seen horizontal and elliptical oscillations in this situation. Again, we would recommend neuroimaging in such patients.

One report suggested that the vertical oscillations of the Heimann–Bielschowsky phenomenon can be reduced by gabapentin.[57]

Most of the nystagmus types described below that occur at any age (**Table 17–1**) are acquired forms of nystagmus. The one exception is physiologic endgaze nystagmus. The acquired types of nystagmus are usually best classified on the basis of waveform, either jerk or pendular, and this section will incorporate this distinction.[58] Acquired jerk nystagmus typically results from imbalance of the vestibular system or dysfunction of gaze holding, and it is often only observed in eccentric gaze.

Vestibular nystagmus

Vestibular nystagmus may result from dysfunction of the peripheral or central vestibular pathway. Conditions that involve the labyrinth, the vestibular nerve and its root entry zone may produce peripheral vestibular nystagmus. Unilateral peripheral vestibular lesions are quite common and usually produce a horizontal rotary nystagmus with a linear slow phase. The horizontal direction of vestibular nystagmus does not change with gaze position. Alexander's law describes the observation that the amplitude of the nystagmus usually increases when the eyes are moved in the direction of their fast phase.[59] In a peripheral vestibular lesion, the fast phase of the nystagmus is usually directed away from the side of a destructive lesion. One can remember this by recalling that cold water in the ear, which causes ipsilateral vestibular dysfunction, produces nystagmus to the opposite side ("cows") (see Chapter 2). For instance, a patient with left vestibular neuronitis will have a fast component to the right. Patients with peripheral vestibular lesions typically fall toward the side of their lesion or opposite the direction of their nystagmus.

In most instances, the various *peripheral* vestibular lesions described below are usually distinguished by the duration of the vertigo, the eye movement examination, and the accompanying signs on physical examination.

Labyrinthitis causes vertigo associated with hearing loss that lasts for days. The vertigo may recur weeks or months later.

Vestibular neuronitis is a similar condition but without the hearing loss. Both vestibular neuronitis and labyrinthitis may be caused by a variety of viruses, including Epstein–Barr, mumps, measles, and herpes. Treatment usually consists of corticosteroids.[60]

Ménière syndrome is characterized by attacks of vertigo that last hours. Patients often describe a fullness in their ear, tinnitus, and hearing loss. This disorder usually begins between the ages of 30 and 50 and may lead to progressive hearing loss. Patients who have a severe attack may suddenly fall to the ground. This event occurs without loss of consciousness and is known as *Tumarkin's crisis*.

Tullio phenomenon. In this condition, sounds such as a ringing telephone induce peripheral vestibular nystagmus or an ocular tilt reaction.[61] This phenomenon usually occurs in the setting of a superior semicircular canal dehiscence, perilymph fistula, or stapes footplate injury. These patients may also have vertigo and nystagmus that accompanies elevations in middle ear pressure (*Hennebert sign*) or intracranial pressure,[61] the latter by Valsalva maneuver for instance. Torsional nystagmus synchronous with their pulse can also occur.[62] CT scanning with 3D bone reconstructions of the semicircular canals may demonstrate the bony defect, a communication between the canal and intracranial space.

Migraine is another common cause of vertigo, but it remains under-recognized[63,64] (see Chapter 19 for additional discussion). The vertigo is typically episodic and can last minutes, hours, or days. During an attack of vertigo, many patients will have pathologic nystagmus, either spontaneous or positional or both, indicating both central and peripheral vestibular dysfunction.[65] In almost all cases, the nystagmus resolves between attacks. Attacks of migraine-related vertigo may be difficult to distinguish from those of *vestibular paroxysmia*, in which the events last just seconds to minutes.[66]

Benign positional vertigo (BPV) produces symptoms with changes in body position. This vertigo is short lived and usually lasts no more that 30–60 seconds.[67] It is very common for patients to experience this type of vertigo when they first lie down to go to bed or arise in the morning.

In BPV the nystagmus becomes mainly vertical when looking away from the affected ear and more rotatory when looking toward the involved ear. The pathophysiology of BPV is best explained by the canalolithiasis theory, which suggests that canal debris gravitates toward the cupula of the *posterior* semicircular canal to stimulate it.[67,68] Typically, benign positional vertigo is caused by calcium carbonate crystals (otoconia) that stimulate the hair cells of the affected semicircular canal. Since the posterior semicircular canal is the most inferior of the three semicircular canals, it is the most commonly affected. For instance, stimulation of the right *posterior* semicircular canal produces contraction of the right superior oblique and left inferior rectus muscles. This produces a slow downward phase of both eyes with a corrective upward phase. The fast corrective phase has a torsional component beating toward the stimulated or dependent ear.

The next most common variant of BPV involves dysfunction of the *horizontal* canal.[69,70] In these patients rotation to the affected ear produces an intense horizontal nystagmus beating toward the lower ear (*geotropic*, or gravity dependent). Some patients with both horizontal canals involved experience direction-changing nystagmus, depending upon which ear is lower. In another horizontal canal involved subtype, the nystagmus will beat toward the higher ear (*apogeotropic*, or away from gravity).

Least commonly, patients can experience *anterior* semicircular canal paroxysmal positional vertigo. These patients have a downbeat nystagmus with a torsional component toward the affected ear.[71]

It is important to distinguish peripheral causes of positional vertigo from those of central nervous system origin in the patient with acute vertigo and nystagmus. This may be best accomplished by recording the findings after placing the patient in the Dix–Hallpike or the head-hanging position (**Table 17-2**) (**Fig. 17-5A,B**).

Central causes. Occasionally, CNS vestibular dysfunction due to a brain stem lesion, for instance, will mimic the findings observed with peripheral vestibular disease.[72] Features that strongly suggest a central cause include (1) pure torsional nystagmus, particularly when fixation is removed, (2) asymmetric nystagmus between the two eyes, (3) vertical nystagmus in the primary position, and (4) nystagmus that changes direction in different gaze positions.

Video 17.6

Evaluation. When the diagnosis of vestibular disease remains poorly localized or defined, brain MRI, specialized recordings of eye movements (EOG, electro-oculography; or ENG, electronystagmography), with and without provocative maneuvers such as rotation and cold caloric irrigation, and audiograms to test hearing may be helpful.[73]

Treatment. If the cause of the vestibular nystagmus is BPV, a variety of therapeutic positioning techniques may be effective.[74,75] The Dix–Hallpike maneuver may be extended in the *Epley maneuver* (**Figs 17-5A–F**).[76–78] Alternatively, in the *Semont maneuver*, the patient moves from lying down on one side to lying down on the other. The Epley and the Semont maneuvers have a high degree of success, approximately 80%.[76,79] Treatment of the geotropic and apogeotropic forms of horizontal canal BPV involves rotating the patient 270 degrees in rapid steps of 90 degrees in the so-called *barbecue roll* (**Fig. 17-7**, **Table 17-4**).[80]

Patients who have cupulolithisis (debris attached to the cupula) rather than canalolithisis (debris free floating) may be refractory to the Epley maneuver. Furthermore, if the torsional component reverses direction (beats toward the healthy ear) during the second phase of the Epley maneuver, the treatment is also unlikely to be successful.[81] Patients with BPV who are refractory to the maneuver or have a recurrence may respond to self-treatment by doing the Epley maneuver at home.[82,83]

If the patient does not have BPV, then treatment depends on whether the patient suffers from acute or chronic vertigo. In patients with acute vertigo, it is reasonable to prescribe a vestibular suppressant such as diazepam for several days. Thereafter, vestibular adaptation exercises are prescribed for patients with chronic vertigo. Vestibular rehabilitation is the mainstay of therapy for those patients with chronic vertigo. Chronic use of vestibular suppressants is strongly discouraged, as they may delay adaptation and recovery.

Physiologic gaze-evoked nystagmus

Most normal individuals will have jerk nystagmus that fatigues with prolonged lateral gaze of about 30 degrees (**Table 17-5**). In extreme lateral gaze of 40 degrees, some normal patients will develop sustained physiologic nystagmus.[84] However, the amplitude of this nystagmus is usually less than 3 degrees, and it is symmetric in right and left gaze. Occasionally, physiologic nystagmus may be asymmetric between the two eyes. In this situation, it may be confused with the dissociated nystagmus that accompanies internuclear ophthalmoparesis.

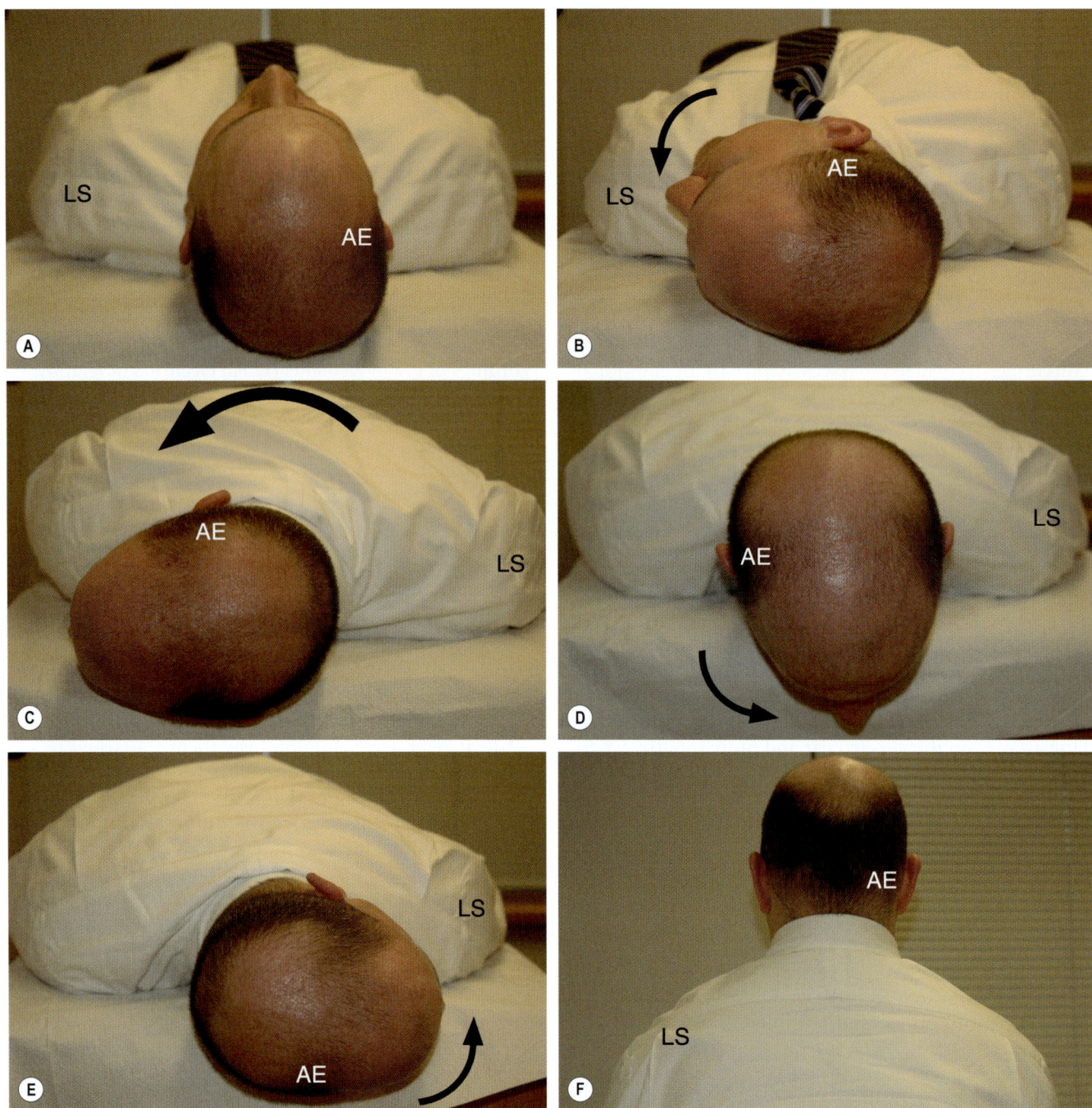

Figure 17–7. One method of treatment of the geotropic form of horizontal canal-benign positional vertigo.[80] In this example the right is the affected ear (AE). In contrast to the Dix–Hallpike and Epley maneuvers illustrated in Fig. 17–5, the patient starts in a supine position in this maneuver. The head positions should be held for 30 and 60 seconds. **A**. To start, the patient lies on his or her back with the head straight up. **B**. The patient turns the head towards the unaffected ear. **C**. The patient moves from a supine to a prone position while holding the position of the head in the same direction as B. **D**. The head is then rotated 90 degrees so that the patient looks toward the ground. **E**. The patient rotates the head another 90 degrees so that the affected ear is down. **F**. The patient sits up. LS, left shoulder.

Pathologic gaze-evoked nystagmus

Video 17.7

Defects in the neural integrator produce pathologic *gaze-evoked nystagmus*, which should be considered a gaze-holding nystagmus (**Table 17–5**). The neural integrator is the network of neurons required to hold the eyes in eccentric gaze. It converts eye velocity signals to position signals and sends commands to the oculomotor neurons to overcome the elastic forces that drive the eyes back toward the primary position. For horizontal eye movements, the medial vestibular nucleus, the nucleus prepositus hypoglossi, and cerebellar flocculus serve as the neural integrator. The interstitial nucleus of Cajal and paramedian tracts are the neural integrator for vertical eye movements. Gaze-evoked jerk nystagmus is pathologic when there is (1) an amplitude of greater than 4 degrees, (2) asymmetry in right and left gaze, or (3) exponential slow-phase velocity when the gaze angle is less than 40 degrees.[84]

Table 17–4 Diagnosis and treatment of benign positional vertigo

Affected canal	Type of nystagmus	Treatment
Right posterior canal	Upbeat, torsional to right shoulder	Epley maneuver, right ear down first
Right anterior canal	Downbeat, torsional to right shoulder	Epley maneuver, right ear down first
Right horizontal canal	Right-beating nystagmus with right ear down (geotropic), may have less intense left-beating nystagmus with left ear down	BBQ roll (90 degree rotations with left ear down first)
Right horizontal canal	Horizontal nystagmus beats toward uppermost ear (apogeotropic), nystagmus intensity greatest with left ear down*	1. Patient brought down toward right ear for 2 minutes, then: 2. Head rotated 45 degrees upward for 2 minutes, then: 3. BBQ roll (90-degree rotations toward left ear first)[264]

BBQ, barbecue roll; see Fig. 17–7.

*In the apogeotropic form the nystagmus will beat towards the uppermost ear regardless of which ear is down. In this form, the particles lie in the anterior portion of the horizontal canal. When the affected right ear is down, there is an inhibitory effect on the right horizontal canal. This leads to relative stimulation of the left vestibular nerve. Thus, the eyes are driven slowly to the right (down toward the floor) with a corrective phase to left (up to toward the unaffected ear or toward the ceiling). When the patient is placed with the left ear down, the right horizontal canal is stimulated. This will drive the eyes slowly toward the floor and a corrective phase toward the ceiling. The intensity of the nystagmus is always greater with an excitatory stimulus than an inhibitory stimulus. Thus, the nystagmus is greatest with the left ear down. However, the nystagmus will always be toward the uppermost ear in the apogeotropic form.

Table 17–5 Most common types of nystagmus in endgaze

Nystagmus features	Physiologic gaze evoked	Pathologic gaze evoked	Peripheral vestibular
Waveform	Horizontal usually, sometimes torsional	Horizontal and/or vertical	Horizontal rotary
Amplitude	Low, may be greater in abducting eye	High	Medium
Frequency	High	Low	High
Symmetry in gaze positions	Yes	Yes/no	No
Rebound nystagmus	No	Possible	No
Other neurologic signs	No	Possible	Hearing loss possible
Fatigue	Yes	No	No

Occasionally the term *gaze-paretic nystagmus* has been used in this setting. However, the term should be avoided since this type of nystagmus is not always associated with a true gaze palsy. In fact, nystagmus associated with a gaze palsy likely reflects associated injury to a component of the neural integrator.

When present in both horizontal and upgaze, gaze-evoked nystagmus usually signifies a toxic metabolic process. For instance, this pattern is seen in patients taking benzodiazepines, barbituates, or anticonvulsants (phenytoin and carbemazepine, for example, see drug-induced nystagmus, below).[85] When gaze-evoked nystagmus is asymmetric or present in only one direction, a structural lesion is suggested (i.e., stroke, demyelinating disease). Unilateral gaze-evoked nystagmus may indicate ipsilateral cerebellar or brainstem disease. Gaze-evoked nystagmus may also be observed contralateral to peripheral vestibular pathway damage. Gaze-evoked upbeat nystagmus commonly accompanies bilateral internuclear ophthalmoparesis.

A special form of gaze-evoked nystagmus known as *Brun's nystagmus* may be seen with cerebellopontine angle lesions.[86] Pathologic horizontal gaze-evoked nystagmus is typically observed when the patient gazes toward the side of the lesion and is probably produced by impaired connections from the cerebellar flocculus. Gaze away from the lesion is associated with the appearance of a high-frequency, low-amplitude horizontal-torsional nystagmus with the fast phase toward the side and shoulder contralateral to the lesion, reflective of vestibular dysfunction.

Dissociated nystagmus

When nystagmus is dissociated, the movements of the right and left eyes are in the same direction but the amplitudes are asymmetric. Dissociated nystagmus has been classically used to describe the eye findings associated with an internuclear ophthalmoplegia (INO, see Chapter 15 for more details). In this disorder, the abducting eye exhibits "nystagmus" with impaired adduction of the fellow eye. However, eye movements of the abducting eye may not represent a true nystagmus, but rather a series of saccades when the patient looks laterally. These abducting eye saccades may be an adaptive attempt by the brain to correct for the hypometric saccades of the weak medial rectus muscle.[87] Demyelination and brain stem stroke, resulting in disruption of the ipsilateral medial longitudinal fasciculus (MLF), are the most common causes of an INO. A pseudo-INO may be seen with myasthenia gravis and the Miller Fisher variant of GBS.

As will be discussed below, dissociated nystagmus may also be observed with the pendular nystagmus that occasionally complicates brain stem infarction and multiple sclerosis.

Rebound nystagmus

In this pathologic nystagmus, after the patient gazes eccentrically to the side for 10 seconds, then is asked to look straight ahead quickly, in primary gaze the eyes beat repeatedly in the direction of refixation. This finding usually indicates cerebellar pathway disease, and is usually accompanied by pathologic endgaze nystagmus. Rebound nystagmus usually beats away from the lesion. For instance, a patient with a right cerebellar lesion will have rebound nystagmus to the left when the eyes are brought back to the midline from eccentric right gaze.[88] Rebound nystagmus may represent the consequences of the brain trying to compensate for the centripetal drift of pathologic endgaze nystagmus.

Periodic alternating nystagmus (PAN)

Video 17.8

This rare type of nystagmus can be either acquired or congenital (as described above).[12] It typically changes direction approximately every 90 seconds with a rest period of 5–10 seconds. The hallmark of periodic alternating nystagmus is a shifting null point. PAN is sometimes seen with downbeat nystagmus, may remain horizontal even in vertical gaze, and may persist in sleep. PAN may be associated with a skew deviation similar to that seen with downbeat nystagmus. Even periodic skew deviation has been observed with PAN.[89] As an adaptive phenomenon, the patient may demonstrate alternating head turning and gaze deviation.[90]

Acquired PAN usually indicates a lesion of the cervicomedullary junction, particularly of the cerebellar nodulus or uvula.[91] Two reports documenting PAN in patients with isolated lesions of the cerebellar nodulus support this notion.[92,93] One was due to surgical resection of a tumor and the other a stroke.[92,93] PAN may also occur in multiple sclerosis,[94] trauma,[95] enlarged cisterna magna with Ménière's,[96] anticonvulsant use, Chiari I malformation, lithium therapy,[97] vision loss,[98] and cerebellar and spinocerebellar degenerations.

PAN presumably results from instability of the vestibular networks and a prolonged vestibular response with periodic cycles created by a normal vestibular repair mechanism.[93] Simply put, PAN may represent a state of vestibular overactivity related to the loss of cerebellar inhibition.

Baclofen, a GABA-B agonist, may ameliorate the acquired form of PAN (**Table 17–6**).[99,100] For patients with congenital PAN, surgical therapy may be appropriate.[13] Large horizontal recti resections have been effective.[12,95] One patient with PAN and visual loss related to vitreous hemorrhage had resolution of the nystagmus after vitrectomy.[98] Presumably this improvement was related to enhanced visual fixation.

Table 17–6 Pharmacologic treatment of nystagmus and nystagmoid eye movements

Nystagmus type	Effective medications
Periodic alternating nystagmus	Baclofen
Downbeat	3,4-diaminopyridine, 4-aminopyridine, clonazepam
See-saw nystagmus	Baclofen, clonazepam
Oculopalatal or acquired pendular nystagmus	Gabapentin, memantine, valproic acid, clonazepam
Opsoclonus	Corticosteroids, ACTH, IVIG, clonazepam
Superior oblique myokymia	Gabapentin, carbamazepine, propranolol
Oculomasticatory myorhythmia	Ceftriaxone
Congenital nystagmus	Gabapentin, memantine

ACTH, adrenocorticotropic hormone; IVIG, intravenous immunoglobulin.

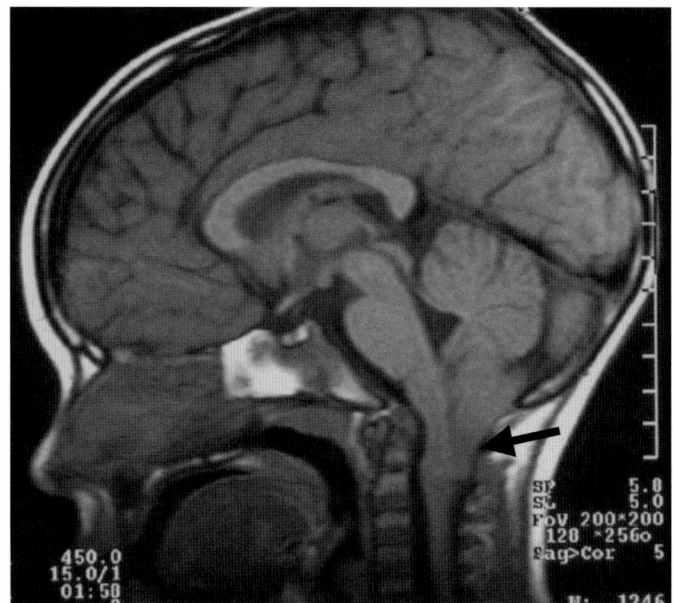

Figure 17–8. Chiari malformation type I. Sagittal T1-weighted MRI scan in a patient with downbeat nystagmus due to low-lying cerebellar tonsils (*arrow*).

Downbeat nystagmus

Video 17.

Downbeat nystagmus, a jerk nystagmus with an upward slow phase and downward fast phase, is often accentuated and therefore best seen in lateral gaze. Patients with downbeat nystagmus usually demonstrate downward pursuit abnormalities and an alternating hypertropia in lateral gaze.[101] With the latter, there will be a pattern that suggests bilateral inferior rectus skew deviation.

This type of nystagmus usually signifies a lesion of the cervicomedullary junction or cerebellar flocculus (Table 17–7). Common identifiable causes are Chiari type I malformations (**Fig. 17–8**), foramen magnum mass lesions, platybasia, and spinocerebellar degenerations.[102] Occasionally, downbeat nystagmus will be observed with midbrain lesions. Other causes to consider include hypomagnesemia,[103,104] thiamine or B_{12} deficiency, West Nile virus encephalomyelitis,[105] and phenytoin, carbamazepine, alcohol, lithium, and opiate toxicity.[106–110] Downbeat nystagmus has been reported in patients with antibodies to glutamic acid decarboxylase associated with stiff person syndrome and cerebellar dysfunction.[111,112] Congenital downbeat nystagmus has also been reported, and these patients may experience a spontaneous remission.[113]

In 30–40% of cases of acquired downbeat nystagmus, no cause is found despite standard anatomic MRI of the cervicomedullary junction region.[114] However, when more sophisticated neuroimaging techniques such as voxel-based morphometry are used,[115] small areas of atrophy in the lateral cerebellar hemispheres and vermis may be found. Functional MRI in such patients has shown reduced function in the parafloccular region and the pontomedullary area in the brain stem during downward eye movements.[115] This observation suggests that some patients with idiopathic downbeat nystagmus may have a primary degenerative disorder involving the cerebellum.

The final common mechanism for downbeat nystagmus appears to be an imbalance of the vertical semicircular canal pathways favoring the anterior canal (**Fig. 17–9**).[1] Unopposed input from the anterior semicircular canal will drive the eyes slowly upward. For instance, lesions of the cerebellar flocculus damage inhibitory projections to the anterior semicircular canal pathways.[116] In addition, lesions involving the dorsal medulla may selectively damage crossing information from the posterior semicircular canals or injure the gaze holding pathways traveling in the brain stem. Other proposed mechanisms of downbeat nystagmus include defects in the vertical smooth pursuit or neural integrator pathways or an imbalance in the otolith system.[117,118]

Treatment. Recent studies have suggested that the potassium channel blockers 3,4-diaminopyridine and 4-aminopyridine may suppress downbeat nystagmus.[119–122] Both of these drugs increase the firing rate of the Purkinje cells and thus may restore the inhibitory influence of the cerebellar cortex upon the anterior semicircular canals. 4-Aminopyridine may preferred over 3,4-diaminopyridine since the former crosses the blood–brain barrier more readily. Other drugs that may reduce downbeat nystagmus include clonazepam, gabapentin, baclofen, and intravenous scopolamine.[123–125] Since 3,4-diaminopyridine and 4-aminopyridine are not approved by the Food and Drug Administration (FDA) for nystagmus, clonazepam is often the first drug tried in the treatment of downbeat nystagmus.[126]

A small number of patients respond to prism therapy either to induce convergence or to deflect the perceived image upward.[1,127] The latter technique keeps the eyes out of

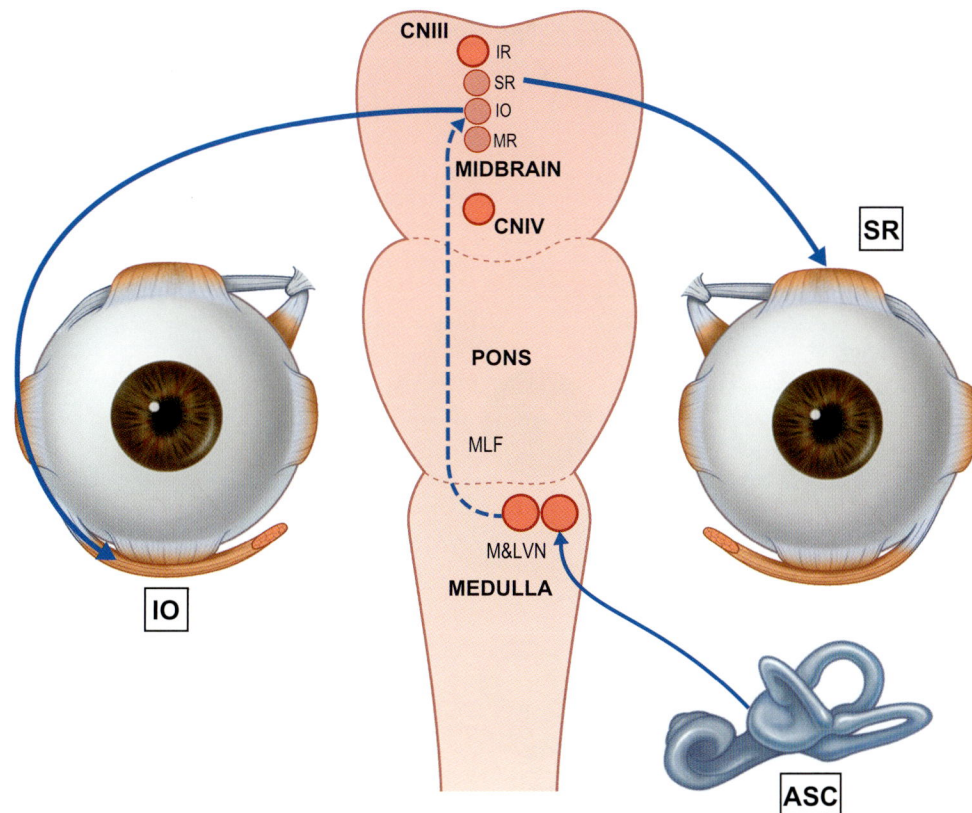

Figure 17–9. One mechanism for downbeat nystagmus. Unopposed input from anterior semicircular canal (ASC) pathways leads to a slow upward movement of eyes by activating the contralateral superior rectus (SR) and inferior oblique nuclei. M and LVN, medial and lateral vestibular nuclei; MLF, medial longitudinal fasciculus. (Figure courtesy of Lawrence Gray, O.D.)

downgaze, where downbeat nystagmus is usually maximal. Surgical decompression of a Chiari I malformation should be considered in selected patients with symptomatic downbeat nystagmus or progressive neurologic deficits.

Upbeat nystagmus

Upbeat nystagmus, which can be caused by lesions in the cerebellum, medulla, and midbrain, does not localize as exquisitely as downbeat nystagmus (**Table 17–7**). However, Daroff and Troost[128] have divided upbeat nystagmus into two types, each with characteristics providing some localizing value: (1) a coarse, large-amplitude nystagmus that increases in upgaze and that usually signifies a lesion in anterior vermis of the cerebellum; and (2) a small-amplitude (1–2 degrees) upbeat nystagmus in the primary position, which is usually caused by a medullary lesion. Upbeat nystagmus which become oblique in prolonged upgaze or which increases in downgaze also signifies a medullary process. Intercalatus nuclei,[129] medial,[130–133] and dorsal paramedial[134,135] lesions in the medulla may be responsible for upbeat nystagmus.

Upbeat nystagmus may also result from damage to connections from the anterior semicircular canal crossing in the ventral medulla and traveling through the brachium conjunctivum, thereby favoring pathways from the posterior semicircular canal (**Fig. 17–10**).[116,136–138] Finally, upbeat nystagmus may also occur with lesions of the midbrain and pons and commonly accompanies bilateral internuclear ophthalmoplegia (see Chapter 15).

Multiple sclerosis, infarction, cerebellar degeneration, and tumors are among the most common causes of upbeat nystagmus. Tobacco smoking has also been observed to produce upbeat nystagmus and horizontal square wave

Table 17–7 Localizing value of nystagmus patterns and nystagmoid eye movements

Type	Localization
Downbeat	Cervicomedullary junction, cerebellar flocculus
Periodic alternating	Cervicomedullary junction, cerebellar nodulus
Upbeat	Cerebellum, medulla, midbrain
Convergence retraction	Dorsal midbrain
See-saw	Parasellar, midbrain
Oculopalatal tremor (myoclonus)	Central tegmental tract
Oculomasticatory myorhythmia	Whipple's disease
Rebound	Cerebellum
Spasmus nutans	Exclude chiasmal glioma and craniopharyngioma
Brun's nystagmus*	Cerebellopontine angle

*Refers to ipsilateral gaze-evoked nystagmus and contralateral high-frequency, low-amplitude nystagmus of vestibular origin.

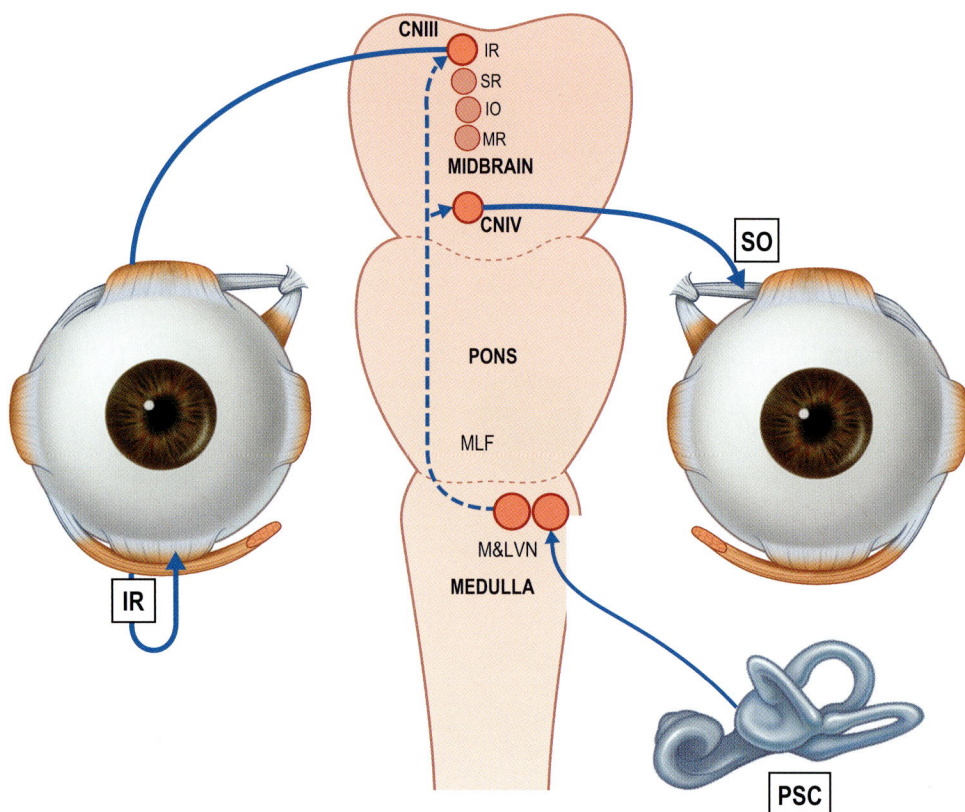

Figure 17–10. One mechanism for upbeat nystagmus. Unopposed input from posterior semicircular canal (PSC) pathways leads to slow downward movement of eyes by activating the contralateral inferior rectus (IR) and superior oblique (SO) nuclei. M and LVN, medial and lateral vestibular nuclei; MLF, medial longitudinal fasciculus. (Figure courtesy of Lawrence Gray, O.D.)

jerks.[139] Presumably, nicotine acts as a CNS excitatory neurotransmitter in this situation,[140] perhaps inducing an imbalance in the vestibulo-ocular reflex.[139] Transient upbeat nystagmus may be observed in healthy infants in the first few months of life. Treatment of upbeat nystagmus is similar to downbeat nystagmus and can include 4-aminopyridine, 3,4-diaminopyridine, or clonazepam.[126,141]

Pure torsional nystagmus

Nystagmus that is purely torsional is uncommon but usually signifies a central vestibular disorder. Patients often have an associated ocular tilt reaction (see Chapter 15). The torsional nystagmus usually beats toward the opposite shoulder in a medullary lesion. In midbrain lesions that involve the intersititial nucleus of Cajal, but spare the rostral interstitial nucleus of the medial longitudinal fasciculus (riMLF), patients will demonstrate a torsional nystagmus that beats toward the ipsilateral shoulder.[142]

Pendular nystagmus/other types

Pendular nystagmus occurs when the eyes move back and forth with equal velocity. There are only slow phases without a jerk or fast component. This type of nystagmus may be horizontal or vertical. Oblique, elliptical or circular pendular nystagmus may occur depending on how the vertical phase of nystagmus relates to the horizontal phase. Pendular nystagmus may also be dissociated, and this tends to occur when one eye has impaired visual function. One MRI study suggested that dysconjugate pendular nystagmus can also be produced by asymmetric brain stem damage.[143]

Acquired pendular nystagmus in adults is most often caused by multiple sclerosis and brain stem infarctions. It may be observed in patients with oculopalatal tremor (myoclonus) and as diagnostic feature of Whipple's disease (see below). Causes of pendular nystagmus more commonly seen in childhood, such as congenital nystagmus, spasmus nutans, and monocular nystagmus associated with visual loss, were discussed earlier in this chapter.

One explanation for the acquired pendular nystagmus seen in multiple sclerosis is an unstable neural integrator.[144] In one series of 37 patients with pendular nystagmus associated with multiple sclerosis, all patients had associated cerebellar dysfunction and optic neuropathy.[145] The most consistent lesion on MRI involved the dorsal pontine region. Patients with dissociated nystagmus often had the greatest nystagmus on the side with the more severe optic neuropathy.

Oculopalatal tremor (myoclonus). When pendular nystagmus occurs in combination with palatal tremor, the term *oculopalatal tremor* is used. There may also be rhythmic movements of the facial muscles, larynx, and diaphragm. The ocular oscillations are usually vertical or elliptical and may be dissociated. Oculopalatal tremor typically beats at a rate of 1–3 Hz. This nystagmus usually persists during sleep and exhibits a slower and more irregular waveform when compared to the pendular nystagmus of multiple sclerosis.[1] Ocular bobbing, gaze palsies, and internuclear ophthalmoplegia are other common motility findings associated with this nystagmus.

Oculopalatal tremor often follows the neurologic injury by several months. However, infrequently the pendular nystagmus may be apparent within 24 hours, and in rare cases there may be spontaneous remission.[146] Brain stem infarction and hemorrhage are common causes, but this nystagmus may be produced by any lesion that produces focal brain stem or cerebellar damage. The pathologic hallmark is olivary hypertrophy. Classically, interruption of connections between the red nucleus, inferior olive, and dentate nucleus (so-called Mollaret's triangle) has been implicated as the cause of oculopalatal tremor. Most cases of oculopalatal tremor involve the *central tegmental tract*, a pathway that connects the red nucleus and deep cerebellar nuclei projections to the inferior olive. Since the parapontine reticular formation lies near the central tegmental tract, oculopalatal myoclonus may subsequently develop in those patients who have a horizontal one-and-a-half syndrome (**Fig. 17–11**).[147] One proposed mechanism for the pendular nystagmus associated with oculopalatal tremor is the instability of the vertical neural integrator caused by injury to the descending paramedian tracts projecting to the dorsal part of the inferior olive.[146] Deafferentation of the olive may lead to synchronized firing of its neurons.[1] On the other hand metabolic studies have demonstrated increased activity of the inferior cerebellar vermis.[148] Valproic acid, gabapentin, and clonazepam may lessen the nystagmus.[149]

Rarely, oculopalatal tremor may also occur in the absence of an identifiable acute brain stem event.[150] These spontaneous cases may also be associated with progressive ataxia.[151–153]

Oculomasticatory myorhythmia. A rare pendular slow (1 Hz) convergence nystagmus may occur in association with slow rhythmic movements of the jaw and other muscles. This has been called *oculomasticatory myorhythmia* and it strongly suggests the diagnosis of Whipple's disease (see Chapter 16).[154,155] This nystagmus almost always occurs in association with a supranuclear ophthalmoparesis.

Other types. Pendular convergent divergent nystagmus at higher frequencies may be seen in patients with multiple sclerosis and brain stem stroke.[156] Elliptical pendular nystagmus together with upbeat nystagmus may also occur in Pelizaeus–Merzbacher disease,[157] a rare X-linked recessive neurodegenerative condition in young children caused by a deficiency in the proteolipid apoprotein PLP.[158] The disease primarily affects the CNS white matter, and pendular nystagmus accompanied by vision loss and optic atrophy may be the initial manifestations. Other childhood white matter disorders with a similar presentation include adrenoleukodystrophy (see Chapter 8) and Cockayne syndrome.[159]

Joubert syndrome. Pendular torsional, see-saw, and gaze-evoked nystagmus may be prominent features of Joubert syndrome.[160] This congenital, structural disorder is characterized by the symptom complex of developmental delay, hypotonia, truncal ataxia, episodic hypernea, and apnea in infancy,[161] and eye movement abnormalities such as nystagmus, impaired smooth pursuit and saccades, ocular motor apraxia, an inability to cancel the vestibulo-ocular reflex, and strabismus.[162,163] Other neuro-ophthalmic abnormalities include retinal dystrophy, chorioretinal coloboma,[164]

Video 17.6

Video 17.13

Video 17.11

Video 17.12

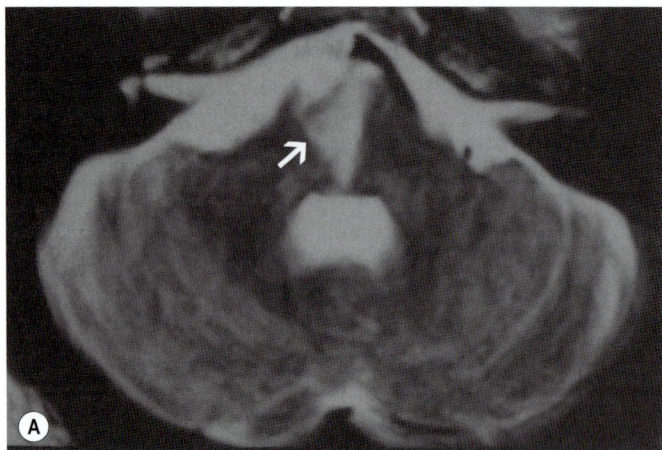

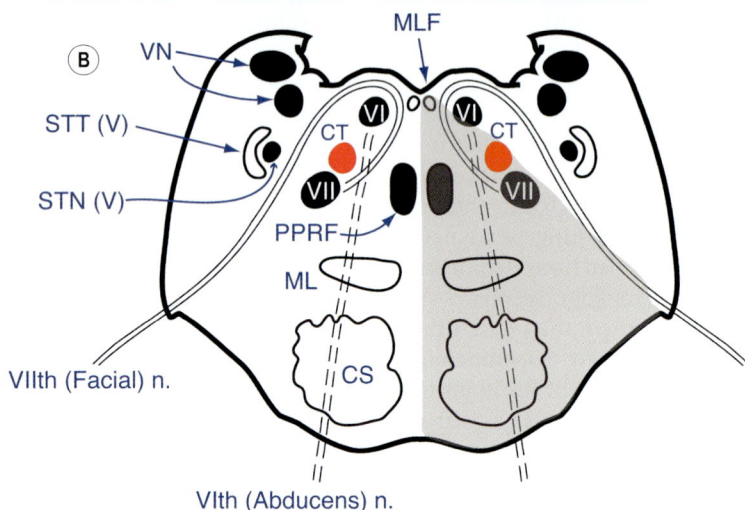

Figure 17–11. A. MRI scan from a patient with oculopalatal tremor and horizontal one-and-a-half syndrome (see Chapter 16) due to a high-signal wedge-shaped infarction (*arrow*) involving paramedian pontine structures. **B**. Diagram of axial section through the pons at the level of the sixth nerve nuclei to demonstrate the structures involved by the lesion in A (gray area). VI, sixth nerve; VII, seventh nerve; CT, central tegmental tract; CS, corticospinal tract; VN, vestibular nuclei; ML, medial lemniscus; MLF, medial longitudinal fasciculus; PPRF, parapontine reticular formation; STT (V), spinal trigeminal tract of the fifth nerve; STN (V), spinal trigeminal nucleus of the fifth nerve. Note the proximity of the central tegmental tract (CT) to the (PPRF).

ptosis,[165] and third nerve palsy. The unifying structural abnormality is dysgenesis or absence of the cerebellar vermis, creating the characteristic "molar tooth" sign with a deep interpeduncular fossa and thickened cerebellar peduncles seen radiographically (**Fig. 17–12**). In addition to the vermis abnormalities, neuropathologically multiple brain stem areas are also involved.[166] Mutations in the NPHP1, AHI1, and CEP290 genes have been found in some patients with Joubert syndrome, suggesting a disorder of the primary cilium.[167,168]

Treatment. No medicine or device can provide consistent, complete relief from pendular nystagmus.[126,169] However, some alleviation of oscillopsia and improvement in vision can occur with either gabapentin or memantine.[126,170–173] Both drugs are well tolerated and have proven to be effective in small studies. The other drugs to treat pendular nystagmus include anticholinergics, baclofen, valproic acid, clonazepam, carbamazepine, and scopolomine.[174] In one report, cannabis suppressed pendular nystagmus in a patient with multiple sclerosis.[175]

Prisms and other devices, such as a plus-sphere spectacle lens combined with a minus-sphere contact lens, may also be used in patients with acquired pendular nystagmus.[1,22,170] More invasive procedures may include strabismus surgery and botulinum toxin injections. Supramaximal vertical rectus muscle recessions can sufficiently limit the eye move-

ment to reduce symptomatic oscillopsia. In select cases, eye muscle surgery is used to move the eyes from their eccentric null point to the primary position. This will shift the null point to a more cosmetically acceptable position thus reducing associated head turn. Injecting botulinum toxin into the extraocular muscles or retrobulbar space may help a small number of patients disabled by oscillopsia but it is limited by the ptosis and double vision it produces. Typically, patients will have to patch the worse-seeing eye for comfort.[32,176] The need for repetitive injections is another detracting factor. Combined pharmacologic and surgical approaches may be used as well.[177]

Convergence retraction nystagmus (saccades)

This is a sign of pretectal dysfunction and may in part reflect excess convergence tone. It is not a true nystagmus because there is no slow phase, just opposing adducting saccades. A disorder of vergence has also been suggested.[178] Retraction results from cofiring of horizontally and vertically acting extraocular muscles. Convergence retraction saccades are elicited by having the patient look upward or by moving an OKN tape downward. Accompanying neurologic signs are usually present, including upgaze palsy, pupillary light-near dissociation, and eyelid retraction (see discussion on the Parinaud or pretectal syndrome in Chapter 16).

Video 17.1

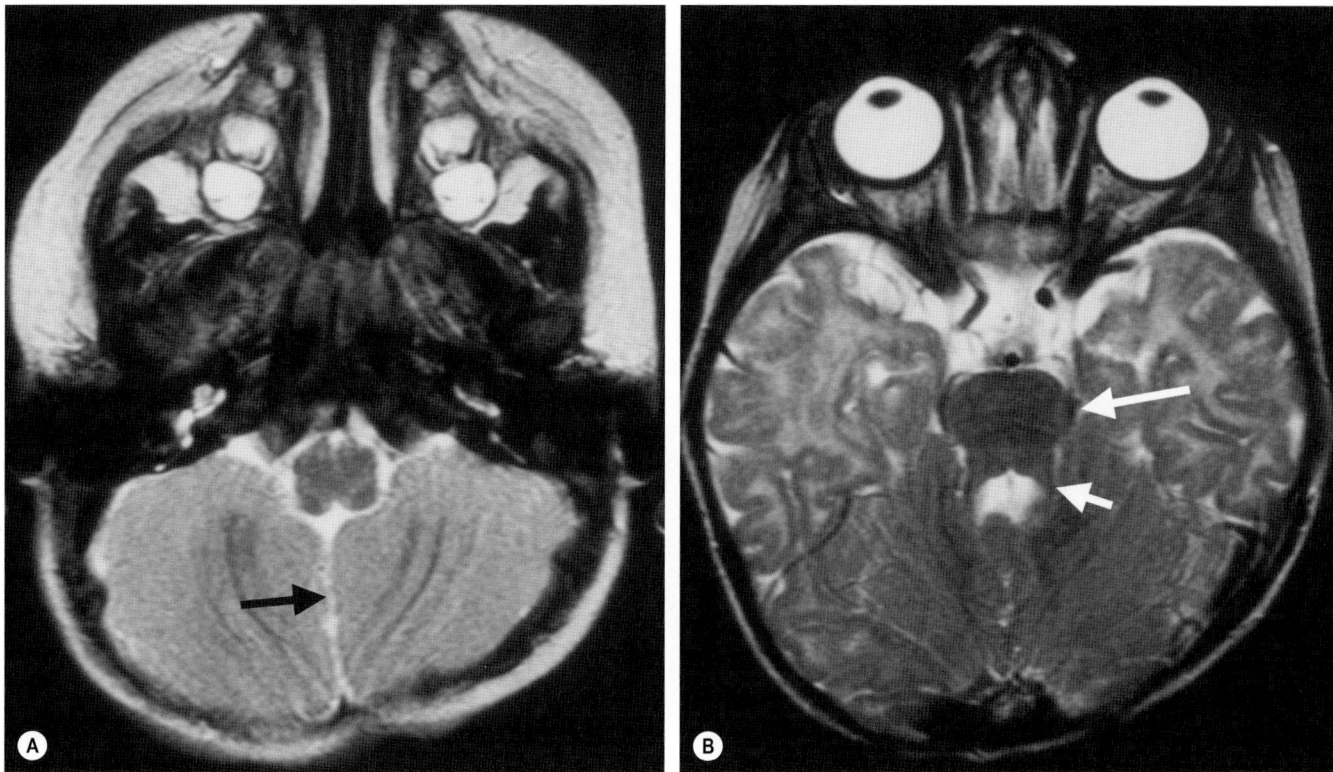

Figure 17–12. Joubert syndrome. Axial MRI scans of a child with pendular torsional nystagmus who was found to have (**A**) absence of the cerebellar vermis (*arrow*) and (**B**) stretching and thickening of the cerebellar peduncles (*small arrow*), producing a "molar tooth" appearance of the pontomesencephalon (*large arrow*).

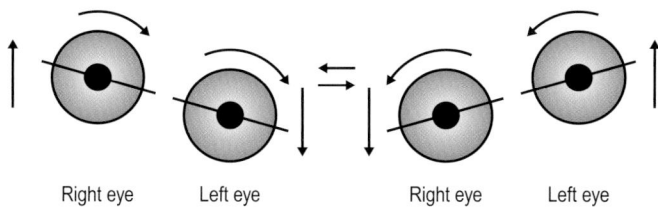

Figure 17–13. See-saw nystagmus. One eye depresses and extorts while the fellow eye elevates and intorts. The pattern alternates in a pendular or jerk fashion, simulating the motion of a see-saw.

Thyroid-associated ophthalmopathy may also produce eyelid retraction, and decreased upgaze. In rare instances, the globes may also retract, mimicking convergence retraction nystagmus. The absence of any pupillary abnormalities and the presence of exophthalmos, conjunctival injection, eyelid edema and positive forced ductions all should make the distinction relatively clear. Unfortunately, eyelid lag cannot be used as distinguishing feature since it may occur in both disorders (see Chapter 14).

See-saw nystagmus

This unusual nystagmus is highly localizing to the midbrain or parasellar region (Table 17–7), although there are many exceptions. See-saw nystagmus is characterized by the simultaneous pendular elevation and intorsion of one eye with the depression and extorsion of the other eye (**Fig. 17–13**).[179,180] To complete the see-saw cycle, the eye that was depressed and extorted will elevate and intort, and the eye that was elevated will fall and extort. Patients with *congenital see-saw nystagmus* may show no torsional component, or the elevating eye may extort while the falling eye intorts.

Some patients will display half of a see-saw cycle with a corrective quick phase. This has been called *hemi-* or *jerk see-saw nystagmus*.[181] It typically occurs from a unilateral mesodiencephalic lesion involving the interstitial nucleus of Cajal. The torsional nystagmus seen in midbrain lesions may beat either to the ipsilateral or contralateral shoulder.[142] Lesions affecting the interstitial nucleus of Cajal, but sparing the riMLF, produce a torsional nystagmus that beats towards the ipsilateral shoulder. For example, injury to the left interstitial nucleus of Cajal will result in a left hypertropia and counter-roll of the eyes toward the right shoulder. Then, if the left riMLF is intact, the eyes will show a corrective torsional movement towards the left shoulder. If the riMLF is involved, the nystagmus may beat contralesionally.[182]

Pendular see-saw nystagmus is usually caused by a sellar mass lesion (e.g., pituitary tumor, craniopharyngioma) (**Fig. 17–14**). It may abolished by removal of the offending mass. In addition, patients with visual loss alone may also have see-saw nystagmus,[183] and it may also be observed in patients with achiasma. The relationship between see-saw nystagmus and chiasmal visual loss is also discussed in Chapter 7. Joubert syndrome (see above) is also a well-recognized cause of this eye movement disorder.[160] Baclofen and clonazepam may help lessen see-saw nystagmus.[123,127]

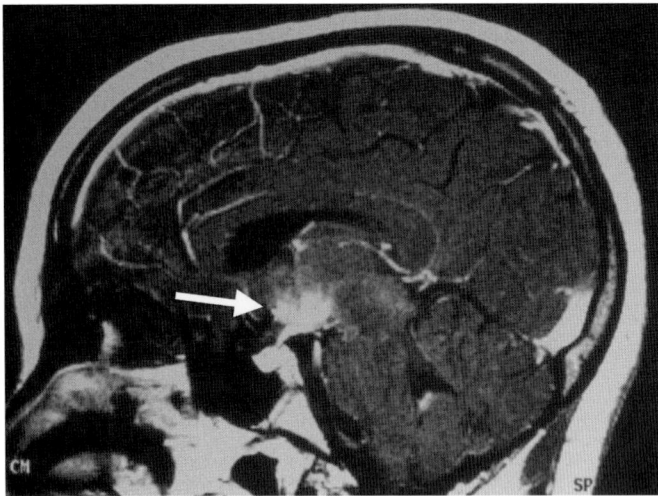

Figure 17–14. See-saw nystagmus. Gadolinium-enhanced T1-weighted sagittal MRI scan in a patient with see-saw nystagmus due to biopsy-proven granulomatous inflammation of the hypothalamus and chiasm (*arrow*), presumed to be sarcoidosis.

Voluntary nystagmus

Voluntary nystagmus is usually produced by individuals for amusement or by patients seeking secondary gain.[184] However, this nystagmus may also be seen in families.[185] A survey of a college age population revealed that 8% of students could produce voluntary nystagmus.[186] Most patients complain of decreased vision and oscillopsia. The nystagmus is recognized as a high-frequency, low-amplitude pendular oscillation that cannot be sustained. Eye movement recordings show the oscillations to be a series of rapidly alternating saccades, usually horizontal, with a frequency of 3–42 Hz.[187] Voluntary nystagmus usually occurs in bursts that last 5–10 seconds. Lid fluttering and squinting may accompany the ocular oscillation. Occasionally the strain in the patient's face may be observed as he or she tries to maintain the eye movements. The voluntary oscillations can be interrupted by having the patient pursue a target. Also, voluntary nystagmus disappears when the patient is distracted since significant concentration is required to generate it. By definition it can be "produced" by the patient, unlike all other nystagmoid movements which are involuntary.

Video 17.16

Convergence-evoked nystagmus

Convergence usually dampens nystagmus. However, in rare instances it may precipitate it. Both congenital and acquired nystagmus may be enhanced by convergence.[188] The congenital form may have conjugate oscillations, while the acquired form has disjunctive eye movements. Occasionally, upbeat nystagmus changes to downbeat with convergence. The pendular convergent nystagmus of Whipple's disease may be increased by convergence, and an acquired convergence-evoked pendular nystagmus in multiple sclerosis has been described.[189]

Lid nystagmus

The lids normally beat upward in patients with upbeat nystagmus. However, in some patients the amplitude of the lid movements is greater than that of the eye movements. Convergence may also precipitate lid nystagmus.[190] In general lid nystagmus has poor localizing value.[84] However, lid nystagmus initiated by lateral gaze has been associated with lateral medullary lesions.[191]

Epileptic nystagmus

Nystagmus may be induced by epileptic activity. Occasionally, nystagmus may be the only manifestation of a seizure, particularly in intensive care unit patients in whom nonconvulsive status epilepticus may be a concern. In most cases, the jerk horizontal nystagmus is directed away from the seizure focus.[192] There is a tendency for the epileptic focus to be located in the temporoparietal–occipital junction. The discharge frequency tends to be high, with a rate of approximately 10 per second. Rare types of ictal nystagmus are vertical, ipsilateral to the seizure focus, monocular,[193] and periodic alternating.[194] Clinicians should also be wary of voluntary nystagmus in patients with nonepileptic seizures.[184]

Drug- and alcohol-induced nystagmus

Drug-induced nystagmus is one of the most common forms of nystagmus. A variety of medications may produce nystagmus in the therapeutic range, including anticonvulsants, sedatives, barbiturates, and the phenothiazines.[85] Typically the nystagmus is present in horizontal endgaze and upgaze, but not downgaze. The nystagmus is symmetrical and usually does not fatigue. Rarely, drug-induced nystagmus is present in downgaze. In contrast, some medications, such as carbamazepine, phenytoin, and lithium, may produce a pure downbeat nystagmus.

Acute alcohol intoxication may produce a horizontal endgaze nystagmus known as positional alcohol nystagmus. Peripheral vestibular dysfunction resulting from the alcohol entering the cupula, rendering it lighter than the endolymph, is the purported "buoyancy" mechanism.[195] However, we cannot advocate the presence of nystagmus alone as a method to assess intoxication.[196] Clearly, the presence of physiologic nystagmus, congenital nystagmus, and the effects of other medications may fool the unwary observer.

Optokinetic nystagmus

When rotation of the head is sustained for more than a few seconds, the optokinetic system becomes active to permit fixation on stationary objects. It is an involuntary reflex, but may be suppressed if the stimulus is not full field and the patient decides to look above or below the moving target. At the bedside, the optokinetic response may be elicited by moving a striped tape in front of the patient (see **Fig. 2–30**). OKN is generated by pursuit of an object and a corrective saccade in the opposite direction to detect the next target. Both retinal and cerebral projections contribute to the optokinetic response, but it is the cerebral connections that are the most important in the adult patient.[197] The cerebral projections begin in area V5 (see Chapter 9), and parietal areas (PP) and connect to the nucleus of the optic tract and dorsolateral pontine nuclei. Ultimately these projections will reach the medial vestibular nucleus and from this area to the ocular motor nuclei.[1]

OKN may be helpful as a diagnostic tool to evaluate (1) visual function in infants with congenital nystagmus (using a vertical OKN) or central visual impairment (either absent or asymmetric); (2) a reverse OKN response characteristic of congenital nystagmus; (3) a deep parietal lesion causing a homonymous hemianopia (a reduced response is observed when the OKN tape is moved in the direction of a parietal lesion); (4) residual vision in a patient who claims complete blindness (an intact OKN response suggests vision is at least count fingers); (5) a subtle adduction weakness seen in internuclear ophthalmoparesis; (6) convergence retraction nystagmus (the OKN tape is taken downward to elicit this pretectal sign); (7) smooth pursuit and saccades; and (8) oculovestibular function.

As a research tool, OKN responses have been used as an objective estimation of visual acuity in patients with poor vision.[198,199] In addition, optokinetic nystagmus has been used as rehabilitative strategy in patients with right hemianopia and reading difficulty (hemianopic alexia), by improving their reading saccades towards the right.[200]

Nystagmoid eye movements

The eye movements discussed in this section are not pure forms of nystagmus. They are usually saccades that interrupt fixation. Alternatively, the ocular oscillations in this group have a fast phase followed by a slow phase. Ocular bobbing is an example of this type of eye movement.

Saccadic intrusions

Neurons in the pons and midbrain help generate the saccadic eye movements that allow the eyes to overcome the viscoelastic forces of the orbit. These neurons are called *burst neurons* and they reside in the paramedian pontine reticular formation for horizontal saccades and in the rostral interstitial nucleus of the medial longitudinal fasciculus for vertical saccades (see Chapter 16). The burst neurons are kept silent by a group of neurons called *pause cells* that reside in the paramedian pontine region. When a saccade is made, the pause cells are turned off by an inhibiting input from supranuclear structures. Many of the saccadic disorders described below are thought to be caused by pause cell dysfunction. However, pathologic confirmation of this theory is lacking. Inappropriate saccades (intrusions) may also result from disordered input to the burst neurons from other structures such as the superior colliculus, basal ganglia, or cerebellum.[1]

In order of increasing severity, square wave jerks, ocular dysmetria, macrosaccadic oscillations, and ocular flutter and opsoclonus represent the spectrum of saccadic intrusions.

Square wave jerks

These are horizontal back-to-back saccades that interrupt fixation (**Fig. 17–15**).[84] There are intersaccadic intervals of 200 msec each to help distinguish this saccadic disorder from ocular flutter. If the amplitude is greater than 5 degrees, the term *macrosquare wave jerk* is used. Square wave jerks may be seen in normal adults and children,[201] but more than 9 per minute is considered abnormal. Common causes of

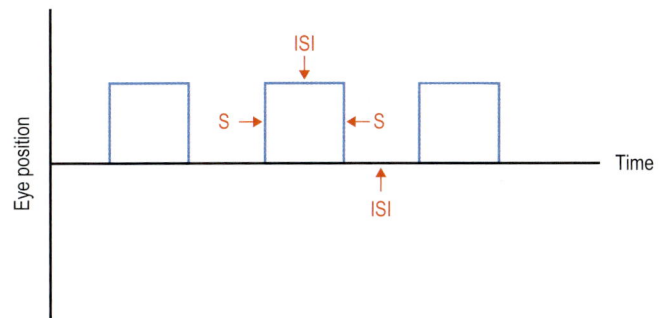

Figure 17–15. Square wave jerks. Eye movement recording (x-axis, time, y-axis, horizontal eye position) demonstrating back-to-back horizontal saccades separated by a 200-msec interval. S, saccade, ISI, intersaccadic interval.

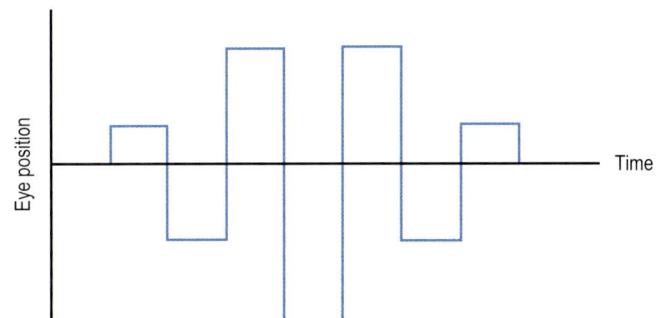

Figure 17–16. Macrosaccadic oscillations. Eye movement recording (x-axis, time, y-axis, horizontal eye position) demonstrating a crescendo–decrescendo pattern of saccades after the eyes attempt to return to fixation from eccentric gaze.

pathologic square wave jerks include cerebellar disease, schizophrenia, Parkinson's disease, and progressive supranuclear palsy.

Ocular dysmetria

This is a sign of cerebellar dysfunction similar to limb dysmetria. If upon refixation, the eyes overshoot the target and then saccade back to the intended fixation point, this is termed *saccadic hypermetria*. In *saccadic hypometria*, the eyes undershoot the target.

Macrosaccadic oscillations

These are horizontal saccades separated by 200-msec intervals that occur across the intended fixation point in a crescendo–decrescendo pattern (**Fig. 17–16**). They may have a large amplitude of 15–50 degrees.[202] They are felt to be an extreme form of saccadic dysmetria, characterized by eyes constantly overshooting the target.[1] Again, this a cerebellar eye sign that is most commonly observed in patients with multiple sclerosis.[84]

Opsoclonus and ocular flutter

Opsoclonus describes the dramatic occurrence of involuntary conjugate multidirectional saccades (saccadomania) that occur without an intersaccadic interval. The eye movement abnormality is often associated with eye blinking, facial twitching, myoclonus, and ataxia (Kinsbourne's "dancing eyes and dancing feet"). Ocular flutter, a related

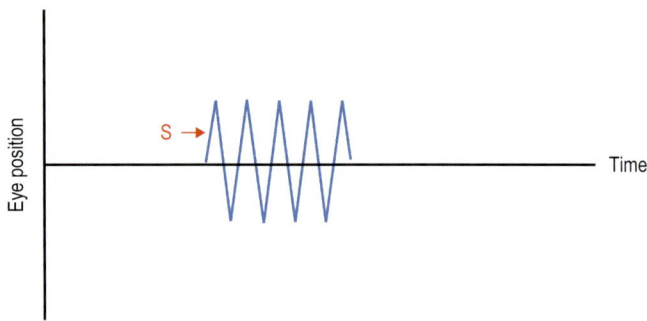

Figure 17–17. Ocular flutter. Eye movement recording (x-axis, time, y-axis, horizontal eye position) demonstrating spontaneous back-to-back horizontal saccades (S) without an intersaccadic interval. In contrast to square wave jerks (Fig. 17–15), there are no intersaccadic intervals.

Video 17.19

Video 17.20

Video 17.

disorder, refers to back-to-back horizontal saccades without an intersaccadic interval (**Fig. 17–17**). There is no vertical component in ocular flutter. The lack of an interval between the saccades distinguishes ocular flutter from square wave jerks. Ocular flutter has the same localizing value and differential diagnosis as opsoclonus. Reflecting saccadic dysfunction, ocular dysmetria is a common associated finding of both opsoclonus and ocular flutter. Saccadic oscillations very similar to ocular flutter and opsoclonus can rarely occur on a nonorganic basis.[203]

Paraneoplastic relationship with neuroblastoma. Fifty percent of children with opsoclonus (and ocular flutter) harbor a neuroblastoma, thus it is essential to exclude this tumor in any child with saccadomania. Conversely, only 2% with neuroblastoma have opsoclonus.[204] A complete screening protocol for neuroblastoma in a child with opsoclonus or ocular flutter would include (1) urine vanillylmandelic acid (VMA) and homovanillic acid (HVA) levels, (2) MRI of neck, chest, abdomen, and pelvis, and (3) metaiodobenzylguanidine (MIBG) whole-body scintigraphy if the MRI is unrevealing. The combination of MRI and MIBG may be necessary because false negative and positive results can occur with each in this setting.[205] There may also be cerebrospinal fluid pleocytosis. As in other paraneoplastic disorders, the underlying tumor may be found before, during, or after the eye abnormality occurs. In one report, the neuroblastoma was found 2 years after the presentation with opsoclonus.[206]

This condition can respond to tumor removal and adrenocorticotropic hormone (ACTH) or prednisone, sometimes in combination with immunomodulatory therapy such as intravenous gammaglobulin,[207] azathioprine, or rituximab[208] or plasmapheresis.[209,210] The response to these modalities suggests an autoimmune pathogenesis of opsoclonus associated with neuroblastoma.[211] In addition, expansion of certain B- and T-cell subsets in the CSF of affected patients have been found.[212] However, the immune hypothesis in this setting is unconfirmed, as no consistent antibody has been found,[213,214] and only a few patients with circulating antibodies, such as anti-Hu,[215] anti-neurofilament, and anti-Purkinje cell[216] have been identified. One in vitro study suggested the majority of children with opsoclonus myoclonus syndrome have circulating antibodies against the surface of cerebellar granular neurons.[217] Pathologic brain specimens have also either been normal or have shown Purkinje cell and granular cell loss with gliosis.[211]

Children with neuroblastoma and opsoclonus have a more favorable prognosis than those without opsoclonus. This may be due to immune surveillance, earlier tumor detection, or favorable tumor biology. Neuroblastomas associated with a poor prognosis often demonstrate amplification of the N-*myc* proto-oncogene, a feature almost always absent in patients with opsoclonus.[218] Furthermore, hyperdiploid neuroblastomas tend to have a lower-stage disease and longer survival than diploid tumors.[218]

Relapses and corticosteroid dependence are common in opsoclonus associated with neuroblastoma, and some children have long-term neurologic deficits.[219]

Other forms of opsoclonus in childhood. These include a benign, self-limited opsoclonus in neonates,[220,221] and opsoclonus associated with severe visual disturbances,[222] parainfectious cerebellitis, and encephalitis.[204] Like the paraneoplastic type, parainfectious opsoclonus myoclonus sometimes requires either ACTH or prednisone, and some children may still be left with some permanent neurologic abnormalities, including ataxia and defective cognition.[219] Therefore, in a complete workup of a child with opsoclonus, a head MRI and spinal fluid examination should be performed in addition to the neuroblastoma screen suggested above. In atypical cases, an electroencephalogram (EEG) is frequently considered to determine if the abnormal eye movement is epileptic in origin, but the yield is very low without other seizure-like symptoms such as change in mental status.[223]

Opsoclonus in adults. In adults, most commonly opsoclonus and ocular flutter may (1) be postinfectious, (2) be drug induced (e.g., amitriptyline, lithium, phenytoin, cocaine, organophosphates),[204,224,225] (3) occur as a remote effect of cancer,[226] or (4) result from encephalitis due to Lyme,[227] West Nile virus,[105,228,229] or other infections.[230-232] Associated tumors include small-cell lung (some cases with anti-Hu antibodies[233]), breast (with anti-Ri antibodies[234]), and gynecologic neoplasms.[235] Stroke, trauma, central nervous system tumors, or hyperosmolar nonketotic coma are other associations. Opsoclonus may also occur from cerebellar, brain stem,[236] or diffuse cerebral injury.

Postinfectious opsoclonus usually slowly improves, but recovery of paraneoplastic opsoclonus is more variable and depends upon whether the underlying tumor can be treated.[237-239] Both may be dampened by clonazepam, gabapentin, corticosteroids, or other immunosuppression such as gammaglobulin. Plasma exchange to remove immunoglobins may be effective in treating paraneoplastic opsoclonus.[240]

The exact etiology of opsoclonus remains uncertain, but impaired inhibition by the omnipause neurons or instability of the burst neurons have been proposed mechanisms. One leading hypothesis is that opsoclonus results from disinhibition of the cerebellar fastigial nucleus.[232,241]

Other nystagmoid eye movements

Superior oblique myokymia

Superior oblique myokymia, or microtremor, is a high-frequency monocular oscillation produced by spontaneous firing of one superior oblique muscle.[242-244] Patients often complain of intermittent episodes monocular vertical oscillopsia or vertical or torsional diplopia. The diagnosis is made by asking the patient to look into the field of action of the superior oblique muscle while the eye is observed with a slit lamp or the fundus with an ophthalmoscope.[245] Each episode is usually brief, lasting seconds, and occurs at irregular intervals.

This condition is usually idiopathic, but neuroimaging should be performed to exclude a midbrain lesion.[246] The mechanism of superior oblique myokymia is thought to result from phasic activity of the fourth nerve fascicles with resultant periodic contraction of the superior oblique muscle.[242] Recent evidence, however, suggests that the some cases may be produced by microvascular compression of the trunk (root exit zone) of the fourth nerve by branches of the superior cerebellar artery.[247-249]

Treatment. This disorder may spontaneously remit but gabapentin,[250] carbamazepine, baclofen, memantine,[251] or propranolol may be tried in resistant cases.[245,252] If symptoms persist and are disabling, one could consider tenectomy of the superior oblique muscle, in combination with recession or myectomy of the inferior oblique muscle. Alternatively, weakening of just the anterior portion of the superior oblique tendon may eliminate the superior oblique myokymia without affecting the vertical alignment of the eyes.[253] Microvascular decompression of the fourth nerve has also been used to alleviate superior oblique myokymia, but this procedure may result in a superior oblique palsy.[249,254]

Ocular bobbing

Ocular bobbing signifies brain stem dysfunction, and in many instances it reflects a pontine process.[255] It is an asynchronous eye movement disorder that begins with a quick conjugate down movement followed by a slow drift back to the midline. This sequence of fast then slow phases and its asynchrony distinguish ocular bobbing from vertical nystagmus.[256] Since ocular bobbing is commonly associated with pontine lesions, horizontal gaze palsies often coexist. A variety of lesions may produce ocular bobbing, including stroke, tumors, toxic-metabolic conditions, and inflammatory processes.[257,258] Ocular bobbing is usually associated with intra-axial brain stem disease; however, extra-axial brain stem compression may also produce this eye movement disorder.[259]

Variants of bobbing exist in which the eyes quickly move upward and then drift slowly downward (reverse bobbing). Some patients exhibit a downward slow phase with a quick upward correction (ocular dipping or inverse bobbing).[260] This eye movement disturbance may be seen in patients who suffered from status epilepticus, anoxic injury,[261,262] or paraneoplastic encephalitis.[263] Clearly, it is difficult to remember all the variants of bobbing and their names. Sometimes, it is more practical just to describe the bobbing phenomenon and recognize its significance as a brain stem sign.

References

1. Leigh RJ, Zee DS. The neurology of eye movements, 4th edn., pp 475–597. New York, Oxford Univ. Press, 2006.

2. Hain TC, Fetter M, Zee DS. Head-shaking nystagmus in patients with unilateral peripheral vestibular lesions. Am J Otolaryngol 1987;8:36–47.

3. Choi KD, Oh SY, Park SH, et al. Head-shaking nystagmus in lateral medullary infarction: patterns and possible mechanisms. Neurology 2007;68:1337–1344.

4. Gresty M, Page N, Barratt H. The differential diagnosis of congenital nystagmus. J Neurol Neurosurg Psychiatr 1984;47:936–942.

5. Gottlob I. Infantile nystagmus. Development documented by eye movement recordings. Invest Ophthalmol Vis Sci 1997;38:767–773.

6. Hertle RW, Dell'Osso LF. Clinical and ocular motor analysis of congenital nystagmus in infancy. JAAPOS 1999;3:70–79.

7. Hertle RW, Maldanado VK, Maybodi M, et al. Clinical and ocular motor analysis of the infantile nystagmus syndrome in the first 6 months of life. Br J Ophthalmol 2002;86:670–675.

8. Abadi RV, Bjerre A. Motor and sensory characteristics of infantile nystagmus. Br J Ophthalmol 2002;86:1152–1160.

9. Hertle RW, FitzGibbon EJ, Avallone JM, et al. Onset of oscillopsia after visual maturation in patients with congenital nystagmus. Ophthalmology 2001;108: 2301–2307; discussion 2307–2308.

10. Halmagyi GM, Gresty MA, Leech J. Reversed optokinetic nystagmus (OKN): mechanism and clinical significance. Ann Neurol 1980;7:429–435.

11. Abadi RV, Pascal E. Periodic alternating nystagmus in humans with albinism. Invest Ophthalmol Vis Sci 1994;35:4080–4086.

12. Gradstein L, Reinecke RD, Wizov SS, et al. Congenital periodic alternating nystagmus. Diagnosis and management. Ophthalmology 1997;104:918–929.

13. Shallo-Hoffmann J, Faldon M, Tusa RJ. The incidence and waveform characteristics of periodic alternating nystagmus in congenital nystagmus. Invest Ophthalmol Vis Sci 1999;40:2546–2553.

14. Brodsky MC, Wright KW. Infantile esotropia with nystagmus: a treatable cause of oscillatory head movements in children. Arch Ophthalmol 2007;125:1079–1081.

15. Dell'Osso LF, Hertle RW, Daroff RB. "Sensory" and "motor" nystagmus: erroneous and misleading terminology based on misinterpretation of David Cogan's observations. Arch Ophthalmol 2007;125:1559–1561.

16. Kupersmith MJ. Practical classification of nystagmus in the clinic [letter]. Arch Ophthalmol 2008;126:871–872.

17. Kerrison JB, Vagefi MR, Barmada MM, et al. Congenital motor nystagmus linked to Xq26-q27. Am J Hum Genet 1999;64:600–607.

18. Self JE, Shawkat F, Malpas CT, et al. Allelic variation of the FRMD7 gene in congenital idiopathic nystagmus. Arch Ophthalmol 2007;125:1255–1263.

19. Thomas S, Proudlock FA, Sarvananthan N, et al. Phenotypical characteristics of idiopathic infantile nystagmus with and without mutations in FRMD7. Brain 2008;131:1259–1267.

20. Optican LM, Zee DS. A hypothetical explanation of congenital nystagmus. Biol Cybern 1984;50:119–134.

21. Peng GH, Zhang C, Yang JC. Ultrastructural study of extraocular muscle in congenital nystagmus. Ophthalmologica 1998;212:1–4.

22. Hertle RW. Examination and refractive management of patients with nystagmus. Surv Ophthalmol 2000;45:215–222.

23. Mahler O, Hirsh A, Kremer I, et al. Laser in situ keratomileusis in myopic patients with congenital nystagmus. J Cataract Refract Surg 2006;32:464–467.

24. Leigh RJ, Dell'Osso LF, Yaniglos SS, et al. Oscillopsia, retinal image stabilization and congenital nystagmus. Invest Ophthalmol Vis Sci 1988;29:279–282.

25. Safran AB, Gambazzi Y. Congenital nystagmus: rebound phenomenon following removal of contact lenses. Br J Ophthalmol 1992;76:497–498.

26. Hertle RW, Anninger W, Yang D, et al. Effects of extraocular muscle surgery on 15 patients with oculo-cutaneous albinism (OCA) and infantile nystagmus syndrome (INS). Am J Ophthalmol 2004;138:978–987.

27. Hertle RW, Dell'Osso LF, FitzGibbon EJ, et al. Horizontal rectus tenotomy in patients with congenital nystagmus: results in 10 adults. Ophthalmology 2003;110:2097–2105.

28. Hertle RW, Dell'Osso LF, FitzGibbon EJ, et al. Horizontal rectus muscle tenotomy in children with infantile nystagmus syndrome: a pilot study. JAAPOS 2004;8:539–548.

29. Wang ZI, Dell'Osso LF, Tomsak RL, et al. Combining recessions (nystagmus and strabismus) with tenotomy improved visual function and decreased oscillopsia and diplopia in acquired downbeat nystagmus and in horizontal infantile nystagmus syndrome. JAAPOS 2007;11:135–141.

30. McLean R, Proudlock F, Thomas S, et al. Congenital nystagmus: randomized, controlled, double-masked trial of memantine/gabapentin. Ann Neurol 2007;61:130–138.

31. Carruthers J. The treatment of congenital nystagmus with Botox. J Pediatr Ophthalmol Strabismus 1995;32:306–308.

32. Tomsak RL, Remler BF, Averbuch-Heller L, et al. Unsatisfactory treatment of acquired nystagmus with retrobulbar injection of botulinum toxin. Am J Ophthalmol 1995;119:489–496.

33. Brodsky MC, Tusa RJ. Latent nystagmus: vestibular nystagmus with a twist. Arch Ophthalmol 2004;122:202–209.

34. Gresty MA, Metcalfe T, Timms C, et al. Neurology of latent nystagmus. Brain 1992;115:1303–1321.

35. Gottlob I, Wizov SS, Reinecke RD. Spasmus nutans. A long-term follow-up. Invest Ophthalmol Vis Sci 1995;36:2768–2771.

36. Weissman RM, Dell'Osso LF, Abel LA, et al. Spasmus nutans. A quantitative prospective study. Arch Ophthalmol 1987;105:525–528.

37. Massry GG, Bloom JN, Cruz OA. Convergence nystagmus associated with spasmus nutans. J Neuro-ophthalmol 1996;16:196–198.

38. Schulman JA, Shults WT, Jones JM. Monocular vertical nystagmus as an initial sign of chiasmal glioma. Am J Ophthalmol 1979;87:87–90.

39. Antony JH, Ouvrier RA, Wise G. Spasmus nutans. A mistaken identity. Arch Neurol 1980;37:373–375.

40. Lavery MA, O'Neill JF, Chu FC, et al. Acquired nystagmus in early childhood: a presenting sign of intracranial tumor. Ophthalmology 1984;91:425–435.

41. Farmer J, Hoyt CS. Monocular nystagmus in infancy and early childhood. Am J Ophthalmol 1984;98:504–509.

42. Kiblinger GD, Wallace BS, Hines M, et al. Spasmus nutans-like nystagmus is often associated with underlying ocular, intracranial, or systemic abnormalities. J Neuro-ophthalmol 2007;27:118–122.

43. Gottlob I, Zubcov A, Catalano RA, et al. Signs distinguishing spasmus nutans (with and without central nervous system lesions) from infantile nystagmus. Ophthalmology 1990;97:1166–1175.

44. Lambert SR, Newman NJ. Retinal disease masquerading as spasmus nutans. Neurology 1993;43:1607–1609.

45. Gottlob I, Wizov SS, Reinecke RD. Quantitative eye and head movement recordings of retinal disease mimicking spasmus nutans. Am J Ophthalmol 1995;119:374–376.

46. Smith DE, Fitzgerald K, Stass-Isern M, et al. Electroretinography is necessary for spasmus nutans diagnosis. Pediatr Neurol 2000;23:33–36.

47. Shawkat FS, Kriss A, Russell-Eggitt I, et al. Diagnosing children presenting with asymmetric pendular nystagmus. Dev Med Child Neurol 2001;43:622–627.

48. Gottlob I, Helbling A. Nystagmus mimicking spasmus nutans as the presenting sign of Bardet-Biedl syndrome. Am J Ophthalmol 1999;128:770–772.

49. Kalyanaraman K, Jagannathan K, Ramanujam RA, et al. Congenital head nodding and nystagmus with cerebellar degeneration. J Pediatr 1973;83:1023–1026.

50. Wizov SS, Reinecke RD, Bocarnea M, et al. A comparative demographic and socioeconomic study of spasmus nutans and infantile nystagmus. Am J Ophthalmol 2002;133:256–262.

51. Arnoldi KA, Tychsen L. Prevalence of intracranial lesions in children initially diagnosed with disconjugate nystagmus (spasmus nutans). J Ped Ophthalmol Strab 1995;32:296–301.

52. Young TL, Weis JR, Summers CG, et al. The association of strabismus, amblyopia, and refractive errors in spasmus nutans. Ophthalmology 1997;104:112–117.

53. Yee RD, Jelks GW, Baloh RW, et al. Uniocular nystagmus in monocular visual loss. Ophthalmology 1979;86:511–518.

54. Davey K, Kowal L, Friling R, et al. The Heimann-Bielschowsky phenomenon: dissociated vertical nystagmus. Aust NZ J Ophthalmol 1998;26:237–240.

55. King RA, Nelson LB, Wagner RS. Spasmus nutans. A benign clinical entity? Arch Ophthalmol 1986;104:1501–1504.

56. Smith JL, Flynn JT, Spiro HJ. Monocular vertical oscillations of amblyopia. The Heimann-Bielschowsky phenomenon. J Clin Neuro-ophthalmol 1982;2:85–91.

57. Rahman W, Proudlock F, Gottlob I. Oral gabapentin treatment for symptomatic Heimann-Bielschowsky phenomenon. Am J Ophthalmol 2006;141:221–222.

58. Stahl JS, Averbuch-Heller L, Leigh RJ. Acquired nystagmus. Arch Ophthalmol 2000;118:544–549.

59. Doslak MJ, Dell'Osso LF, Daroff RB. Alexander's law: a model and resulting study. Ann Otol Rhinol Laryngol 1982;91:316–322.

60. Strupp M, Zingler VC, Arbusow V, et al. Methylprednisolone, valacyclovir, or the combination for vestibular neuritis. N Engl J Med 2004;351:354–361.

61. Tilikete C, Krolak-Salmon P, Truy E, et al. Pulse-synchronous eye oscillations revealing bone superior canal dehiscence. Ann Neurol 2004;56:556–560.

62. Hain TC, Cherchi M. Pulse-synchronous torsional pendular nystagmus in unilateral superior canal dehiscence. Neurology 2008;70:1217–1218.

63. Cutrer FM, Baloh RW. Migraine-associated dizziness. Headache 1992;32:300–304.

64. Neuhauser HK, Radtke A, von Brevern M, et al. Migrainous vertigo: prevalence and impact on quality of life. Neurology 2006;67:1028–1033.

65. von Brevern M, Zeise D, Neuhauser H, et al. Acute migrainous vertigo: clinical and oculographic findings. Brain 2005;128:365–374.

66. Hüfner K, Barresi D, Glaser M, et al. Vestibular paroxysmia: diagnostic features and medical treatment. Neurology 2008;71:1006–1014.

67. Lanska DJ, Remler B. Benign paroxysmal positioning vertigo: classic descriptions, origins of the provocative positioning technique, and conceptual developments. Neurology 1997;48:1167–1177.

68. Furman JM, Cass SP. Benign paroxysmal positional vertigo. N Engl J Med 1999;341:1590–1596.

69. Baloh RW, Yue Q, Jacobson KM, et al. Persistent direction-changing positional nystagmus: Another variant of benign positional nystagmus? Neurology 1995;45:1297–1301.

70. Casani A, Giovanni V, Bruno F, et al. Positional vertigo and ageotropic bidirectional nystagmus. Laryngoscope 1997;107:807–813.

71. Jackson LE, Morgan B, Fletcher JC, Jr., et al. Anterior canal benign paroxysmal positional vertigo: an underappreciated entity. Otol Neurotol 2007;28:218–222.

72. Lee H, Sohn S-I, Cho Y-W, et al. Cerebellar infarction presenting as isolated vertigo. Neurology 2006;67:1178–1183.

73. Fife TD, Tusa RJ, Furman JM, et al. Assessment: vestibular testing techniques in adults and children: report of the Therapeutics and Technology Assessment Subcommittee of the American Academy of Neurology. Neurology 2000;55:1431–1441.

74. Troost BT, Patton JM. Exercise therapy for positional vertigo. Neurology 1992;42:1441–1444.

75. Brandt T, Steddin S, Daroff RB. Therapy for benign paroxysmal positioning vertigo, revisited. Neurology 1994;44:796–800.

76. Serafini G, Palmieri AMR, Simoncelli C. Benign paroxysmal positional vertigo of posterior semicircular canal: results in 160 cases treated with Semont's maneuver. Ann Otol Rhinol Laryngol 1996;105:770–775.

77. Katsarkas A. Paroxysmal positional vertigo: an overview and the deposits repositioning maneuver. Am J Otology 1995;16:725–730.

78. Fife TD, Iverson DJ, Lempert T, et al. Practice parameter: therapies for benign paroxysmal positional vertigo (an evidence-based review): report of the Quality

Standards Subcommittee of the American Academy of Neurology. Neurology 2008;70:2067–2074.

79. Epley JM. The canalith repositioning procedure: for treatment of benign paroxysmal positional vertigo. Otolaryngol Head Neck Surg 1992;107:399–404.

80. Lempert T, Wilck KT. A positional maneuver for treatment of horizontal canal benign positional vertigo. Laryngoscope 1996;106:476–478.

81. Oh HJ, Kim JS, Han BI, et al. Predicting a successful treatment in posterior canal benign paroxysmal positional vertigo. Neurology 2007;68:1219–1222.

82. Radtke A, von Brevern M, Tiel-Wilck K, et al. Self-treatment of benign paroxysmal positional vertigo: Semont maneuver vs Epley procedure. Neurology 2004;63:150–152.

83. Tanimoto H, Doi K, Katata K, et al. Self-treatment for benign paroxysmal positional vertigo of the posterior semicircular canal. Neurology 2005;65:1299–1300.

84. Dell'Osso LF, Daroff RB. Nystagmus and saccadic intrusions and oscillations. In: Glaser JS (ed): Neuro-ophthalmology, 3rd edn., pp 369–403. Philadelphia, Lippincott Williams & Wilkins, 1999.

85. Verrotti A, Manco R, Matricardi S, et al. Antiepileptic drugs and visual function. Pediatr Neurol 2007;36:353–360.

86. Croxson GR, Moffat DA, Baguley D. Bruns bidirectional nystagmus in cerebellopontine angle tumours. Clin Otolaryngol Allied Sci 1988;13:153–157.

87. Zee DS, Hain TC, Carl JR. Abduction nystagmus in internuclear ophthalmoplegia. Ann Neurol 1987;21:383–388.

88. Lin C-Y, Young Y-H. Clinical significance of rebound nystagmus. Laryngoscope 1999;109:1803–1805.

89. Lewis JM, Kline LB. Periodic alternating nystagmus associated with periodic alternating skew deviation. J Clin Neuro-ophthalmol 1983;3:115–117.

90. Kennard C, Barger G, Hoyt WF. The association of periodic alternating nystagmus with periodic alternating gaze. A case report. J Clin Neuro-ophthalmol 1981;1:191–193.

91. Waespe W, Cohen B, Raphan T. Dynamic modification of the vestibulo-ocular reflex by the nodulus and uvula. Science 1985;228:199–202.

92. Oh YM, Choi KD, Oh SY, et al. Periodic alternating nystagmus with circumscribed nodular lesion. Neurology 2006;67:399.

93. Jeong HS, Oh JY, Kim JS, et al. Periodic alternating nystagmus in isolated nodular infarction. Neurology 2007;68:956–957.

94. Matsumoto S, Ohyagi Y, Inoue I, et al. Periodic alternating nystagmus in a patient with MS. Neurology 2001;56:276–277.

95. Castillo IG, Reinecke RD, Sergott RC, et al. Surgical treatment of trauma-induced periodic alternating nystagmus. Ophthalmology 2004;111:180–183.

96. Chiu B, Hain TC. Periodic alternating nystagmus provoked by an attack of Meniere's disease. J Neuro-ophthalmol 2002;22:107–109.

97. Lee MS, Lessell S. Lithium-induced periodic alternating nystagmus. Neurology 2003;60:344.

98. Cross SA, Smith JL, Norton EWD. Periodic alternating nystagmus clearing after vitrectomy. J Clin Neuro-ophthalmol 1982;2:5–11.

99. Halmagyi GM, Rudge P, Gresty MA, et al. Treatment of periodic alternating nystagmus. Ann Neurol 1980;8:609–611.

100. Larmande P. Baclofen as a treatment for nystagmus [letter]. Ann Neurol 1982;11:213.

101. Zee DS, Friendlich AR, Robinson DA, et al. The mechanism of downbeat nystagmus. Arch Neurol 1974;30:227–237.

102. Halmagyi GM, Rudge P, Gresty M, et al. Downbeating nystagmus. A review of sixty-two cases. Arch Neurol 1983;40:777–784.

103. Saul RF, Selhorst JB. Downbeat nystagmus with magnesium depletion. Arch Neurol 1981;38:650–652.

104. Du Pasquier R, Vingerhoets F, Safran AB, et al. Periodic downbeat nystagmus. Neurology 1998;51:1478–1480.

105. Prasad S, Brown MJ, Galetta SL. Transient downbeat nystagmus from West Nile virus encephalomyelitis. Neurology 2006;66:1599–1600.

106. Alpert JN. Downbeat nystagmus due to anticonvulsant toxicity. Ann Neurol 1978;4:471–473.

107. Wheeler SD, Ramsay RE, Weiss J. Drug-induced downbeat nystagmus. Ann Neurol 1982;12:227–228.

108. Chrousos GA, Cowdry R, Schuelin M, et al. Two cases of downbeat nystagmus and oscillopsia associated with carbamazepine. Am J Ophthalmol 1987;103:221–224.

109. Halmagyi GM, Lessell I, Curthoys IS, et al. Lithium induced downbeat nystagmus. Am J Ophthalmol 1989;107:664–670.

110. Corbett JJ, Jacobson DM, Thompson HS, et al. Downbeating nystagmus and other ocular motor defects caused by lithium toxicity. Neurology 1989;39:481–487.

111. Ances BM, Dalmau JO, Tsai J, et al. Downbeating nystagmus and muscle spasms in a patient with glutamic-acid decarboxylase antibodies. Am J Ophthalmol 2005;140:142–144.

112. Eggenberger ER, Lee AG, Thomas M, et al. Neuro-ophthalmic findings in patients with the anti-GAD antibody syndrome. Neuro-ophthalmology 2006;30:1–6.

113. Brodsky MC. Congenital downbeat nystagmus. J Ped Ophthalmol Strab 1996;33:191–193.

114. Bronstein AM, Miller DH, Rudge P, et al. Downbeating nystagmus: case report with magnetic resonance imaging and neuro-otological findings. J Neurol Sci 1987;81:173–184.

115. Hüfner K, Stephan T, Kalla R, et al. Structural and functional MRIs disclose cerebellar pathologies in idiopathic downbeat nystagmus. Neurology 2007;69:1128–1135.

116. Pierrot-Deseilligny C, Milea D. Vertical nystagmus: clinical facts and hypotheses. Brain 2005;128:1237–1246.

117. Halmagyi GM, Leigh RJ. Upbeat about downbeat nystagmus [editorial]. Neurology 2004;63:606–607.

118. Glasauer S, von Lindeiner H, Siebold C, et al. Vertical vestibular responses to head impulses are symmetric in downbeat nystagmus. Neurology 2004;63:621–625.

119. Strupp M, Schuler O, Krafczyk S, et al. Treatment of downbeat nystagmus with 3,4-diaminopyridine: a placebo-controlled study. Neurology 2003;61:165–170.

120. Kalla R, Glasauer S, Schautzer F, et al. 4-aminopyridine improves downbeat nystagmus, smooth pursuit, and VOR gain. Neurology 2004;62:1228–1229.

121. Helmchen C, Sprenger A, Rambold H, et al. Effect of 3,4-diaminopyridine on the gravity dependence of ocular drift in downbeat nystagmus. Neurology 2004;63: 752–753.

122. Kalla R, Glasauer S, Büttner U, et al. 4-aminopyridine restores vertical and horizontal neural integrator function in downbeat nystagmus. Brain 2007;130:2441–2451.

123. Currie JN, Matsuo V. The use of clonazepam in the treatment of nystagmus induced oscillopsia. Ophthalmology 1986;93:924–932.

124. Dieterich M, Straube A, Brandt T, et al. The effects of baclofen and cholinergic drugs in upbeat and downbeat nystagmus. J Neurol Neurosurg Psychiatr 1991;54:627–632.

125. Young YH, Huang TW. Role of clonazepam in the treatment of idiopathic downbeat nystagmus. Laryngoscope 2001;111:1490–1493.

126. Straube A. Therapeutic considerations for eye movement disorders. Dev Ophthalmol 2007;40:175–192.

127. Carlow TJ. Medical treatment of nystagmus and ocular motor disorders. Int Ophthalmol Clin 1986;26:251–264.

128. Daroff RB, Troost BT. Upbeat nystagmus [letter]. JAMA 1973;225:312.

129. Ohkoshi N, Komatsu Y, Mizusawa H, et al. Primary position upbeat nystagmus increased on downward gaze: clinicopathologic study of a patient with multiple sclerosis. Neurology 1998;50:551–553.

130. Hirose G, Ogasawara T, Shirakawa T, et al. Primary position upbeat nystagmus due to unilateral medial medullary infarction. Ann Neurol 1998;43:403–406.

131. Choi KD, Jung DS, Park KP, et al. Bowtie and upbeat nystagmus evolving into hemi-seesaw nystagmus in medial medullary infarction: possible anatomic mechanisms. Neurology 2004;62:663–665.

132. Kim JS, Choi KD, Oh SY, et al. Medial medullary infarction: abnormal ocular motor findings. Neurology 2005;65:1294–1298.

133. Tilikete C, Hermier M, Pelisson D, et al. Saccadic lateropulsion and upbeat nystagmus: disorders of caudal medulla. Ann Neurol 2002;52:658–662.

134. Janssen JC, Larner AJ, Morris H, et al. Upbeat nystagmus: clinicoanatomical correlation. Journal of Neurology, Neurosurgery & Psychiatry 1998;65:380–381.

135. Munro NAR. The role of the nucleus intercalatus in vertical gaze holding [letter]. Journal of Neurology, Neurosurgery & Psychiatry 1999;66:552.

136. Keane JR, Itabashi HH. Upbeat nystagmus: clinicopathologic study of two patients. Neurology 1987;37:491–494.

137. Traccis S, Rosati G, Aiello I, et al. Upbeat nystagmus as an early sign of cerebellar astrocytoma. J Neurol 1989;1989:359–360.

138. Hirose G, Kawada J, Tsukada K, et al. Primary position upbeat nystagmus. J Neurol Sci 1991;105:159–167.

139. Pereira CB, Strupp M, Eggert T, et al. Nicotine-induced nystagmus: three-dimensional analysis and dependence on head position. Neurology 2000;55:1563–1566.

140. Sibony PA, Evinger C, Manning KA. Tobacco-induced primary-position upbeat nystagmus. Ann Neurol 1987;21:53–58.

141. Glasauer S, Kalla R, Buttner U, et al. 4-aminopyridine restores visual ocular motor function in upbeat nystagmus. J Neurol Neurosurg Psychiatry 2005;76:451–453.

142. Helmchen C, Rambold H, Kempermann U, et al. Localizing value of torsional nystagmus in small midbrain lesions. Neurology 2002;59:1956–1964.

143. Lopez LI, Bronstein AM, Gresty MA. Clinical and MRI correlates in 27 patients with acquired pendular nystagmus. Brain 1996;119:465–472.

144. Das VE, Oruganti P, Kramer PD, et al. Experimental tests of a neural-network model for ocular oscillations caused by disease of central myelin. Exp Brain Res 2000;133:189–197.

145. Barton JJ, Cox TA. Acquired pendular nystagmus in multiple sclerosis: clinical observations and the role of optic neuropathy. J Neurol Neurosurg Psychiatry 1993;56:262–267.

146. Kim JS, Moon SY, Choi KD, et al. Patterns of ocular oscillation in oculopalatal tremor: imaging correlations. Neurology 2007;68:1128–1135.

147. Wolin MJ, Trent RG, Lavin PJM. Oculopalatal myoclonus after the one-and-a-half syndrome with facial nerve palsy. Ophthalmology 1996;103:177–180.

148. Yakushiji Y, Otsubo R, Hayashi T, et al. Glucose utilization in the inferior cerebellar vermis and ocular myoclonus. Neurology 2006;67:131–133.

149. Lefkowitz D, Harpold G. Treatment of ocular myoclonus with valproic acid. Ann Neurol 1985;17:103–104.

150. Sperling MR, Herrmann C, Jr. Syndrome of palatal myoclonus and progressive ataxia: two cases with magnetic resonance imaging. Neurology 1985;35:1212–1214.

151. Deuschl G, Toro C, Valls-Sole J, et al. Symptomatic and essential palatal tremor. 1. Clinical, physiological and MRI analysis. Brain 1994;117 (Pt 4):775–788.

152. Eggenberger E, Cornblath W, Stewart DH. Oculopalatal tremor with tardive ataxia. J Neuro-ophthalmol 2001;21:83–86.

153. Brinar VV, Barun B, Zadro I, et al. Progressive ataxia and palatal tremor. Arch Neurol 2008;65:1248–1249.

154. Schwartz MA, Selhorst JB, Ochs AL, et al. Oculomasticatory myorhythmia: a unique movement disorder occurring in Whipple's disease. Ann Neurol 1986;20:677–683.

155. Louis ED, Lynch T, Kaufmann P, et al. Diagnostic guidelines in central nervous system Whipple's disease. Ann Neurol 1996;40:561–568.

156. Averbuch-Heller L, Zivotofsky AZ, Remler BF, et al. Convergent-divergent pendular nystagmus: possible role of the vergence system. Neurology 1995;45:509–515.

157. Trobe JD, Sharpe JA, Hirsh DK, et al. Nystagmus of Pelizaeus-Merzbacher disease. A magnetic search-coil study. Arch Neurol 1991;48:87–91.

158. Garbern J, Cambi F, Shy M, et al. The molecular pathogenesis of Pelizaeus-Merzbacher disease. Arch Neurol 1999;56:1210–1214.

159. Kori AA, Robin NH, Jacobs JB, et al. Pendular nystagmus in patients with peroxisomal assembly disorder. Arch Neurol 1998;55:554–558.

160. Lambert SR, Kriss A, Gresty M, et al. Joubert syndrome. Arch Ophthalmol 1989;107:709–713.

161. Joubert M, Eisenring J-J, Robb JP, et al. Familial agnesis of the cerebellar vermis. A syndrome of episodic hyperpnea, abnormal eye movements, ataxia, and retardation. Neurology 1969;19:813–825.

162. Maria BL, Hoang KB, Tusa RJ, et al. "Joubert syndrome" revisited: key ocular motor signs with magnetic resonance imaging correlation. J Child Neurol 1997;12:423–430.

163. Tusa RJ, Hove MT. Ocular and oculomotor signs in Joubert syndrome. J Child Neurol 1999;14:621–627.

164. Laverda AM, Saia OS, Drigo P, et al. Chorioretinal coloboma and Joubert syndrome: a nonrandom association. J Pediatr 1984;105:282–284.

165. Houdou S, Ohno K, Takashima S, et al. Joubert syndrome associated with unilateral ptosis and Leber congenital amaurosis. Pediatr Neurol 1986;2:102–105.

166. Yachnis AT, Rorke LB. Neuropathology of Joubert syndrome. J Child Neurol 1999;14:655–659; discussion 669–672.

167. Louie CM, Gleeson JG. Genetic basis of Joubert syndrome and related disorders of cerebellar development. Hum Mol Genet 2005;14 Spec No. 2:R235–242.

168. Parisi MA, Doherty D, Chance PF, et al. Joubert syndrome (and related disorders) (OMIM 213300). Eur J Hum Genet 2007;15:511–521.

169. Averbuch-Heller L, Leigh RJ. Medical treatments for abnormal eye movements: pharmacological, optical and immunological strategies. Aust NZ J Ophthalmol 1997;25:7–13.

170. Leigh RJ, Averbuch-Heller L, Tomsak RL, et al. Treatment of abnormal eye movements that impair vision: strategies based on current concepts of physiology and pharmacology. Ann Neurol 1994;36:129–141.

171. Stahl JS, Rottach KG, Averbuch-Heller L, et al. A pilot study of gabapentin as treatment for acquired nystagmus. Neuro-ophthalmology 1996;16:107–113.

172. Starck M, Albrecht H, Pöllmann W. Drug therapy for acquired pendular nystagmus in multiple sclerosis. J Neurol 1997;244:9–16.

173. Averbuch-Heller L, Tusa RJ, Fuhry L, et al. A double-blind controlled study of gabapentin and baclofen as treatment for acquired nystagmus. Ann Neurol 1997;41:818–825.

174. Barton JJ, Huaman AG, Sharpe JA. Muscarinic antagonists in the treatment of acquired pendular and downbeat nystagmus: a double-blind, randomized trial of three intravenous drugs. Ann Neurol 1994;35:319–325.

175. Schon F, Hart PE, Hodgson TL, et al. Suppression of pendular nystagmus by smoking cannabis in a patients with multiple sclerosis. Neurology 1999;53:2209–2210.

176. Repka MX, Savino PJ, Reinecke RD. Treatment of acquired nystagmus with botulinum neurotoxin A. Arch Ophthalmol 1994;112:1320–1324.

177. Jain S, Proudlock F, Constantinescu CS, et al. Combined pharmacologic and surgical approach to acquired nystagmus due to multiple sclerosis. Am J Ophthalmol 2002;134:780–782.

178. Rambold H, Kompf D, Helmchen C. Convergence retraction nystagmus: a disorder of vergence? Ann Neurol 2001;50:677–681.

179. Daroff RB. See-saw nystagmus. Neurology 1965;15:874–877.

180. Nakada T, Kwee IL. Seesaw nystagmus. Role of visuovestibular interaction in its pathogenesis. J Clin Neuro-ophthalmol 1988;8:171–177.

181. Halmagyi GM, Aw ST, Dehaene I. Jerk-waveform see-saw nystamus due to a unilateral meso-diencephalic lesion. Brain 1994;117:789–803.

182. Helmchen C, Glasauer S, Bartl K, et al. Contralesionally beating torsional nystagmus in a unilateral rostral midbrain lesion. Neurology 1996;47:482–486.

183. May EF, Truxal AR. Loss of vision alone may result in seesaw nystagmus. J Neuro-ophthalmol 1997;17:84–85.

184. Davis BJ. Voluntary nystagmus as a component of a nonepileptic seizure. Neurology 2000;55:1937.

185. Neppert B, Rambold H. Familial voluntary nystagmus. Strabismus 2006;14:115–119.

186. Zahn JR. Incidence and characterization of voluntary nystagmus. J Neurol Neurosurg Psychiatr 1978;41:617–623.

187. Shults WT, Stark L, Hoyt WF, et al. Normal saccadic structure of voluntary nystagmus. Arch Ophthalmol 1977;95:1399–1404.

188. Sharpe JA, Hoyt WF, Rosenberg MA. Convergence-evoked nystagmus. Arch Neurol 1975;32:191–194.

189. Barton JJS, Cox TA, Digre KB. Acquired convergence-evoked pendular nystagmus in multiple sclerosis. J Neuro-ophthalmol 1999;19:34–38.

190. Sanders MD, Hoyt WF, Daroff RB. Lid nystagmus evoked by ocular convergence: an ocular electromyographic study. J Neurol Neurosurg Psychiatr 1968;31:368–371.

191. Daroff RB, Hoyt WF, Sanders MD, et al. Gaze-evoked eyelid and ocular nystagmus inhibited by the near reflex: unusual ocular motor phenomena in a lateral medullary syndrome. J Neurol Neurosurg Psychiatr 1968;31:362–367.

192. Kaplan PW, Tusa RJ. Neurophysiologic and clinical correlations of epileptic nystagmus. Neurology 1993;43:2508–2514.

193. Grant AC, Jain V, Bose S. Epileptic monocular nystagmus. Neurology 2002;59:1438–1441.

194. Moster ML, Schnayder E. Epileptic periodic alternating nystagmus. J Neuro-ophthalmol 1998;18:292–293.

195. Fetter M, Haslwanter T, Bork M, et al. New insights into positional alcohol nystagmus using three-dimensional eye-movement analysis. Ann Neurol 1999;45:216–223.

196. Citek K, Ball B, Rutledge DA. Nystagmus testing in intoxicated individuals. Optometry 2003;74:695–710.

197. Dieterich M, Bucher SF, Seelos KC, et al. Horizontal or vertical optokinetic stimulation activates visual motion-sensitive, ocular motor and vestibular cortex areas with right hemispheric dominance. An fMRI study. Brain 1998;121:1479–1495.

198. Shin YJ, Park KH, Hwang JM, et al. Objective measurement of visual acuity by optokinetic response determination in patients with ocular diseases. Am J Ophthalmol 2006;141:327–332.

199. Wester ST, Rizzo JF, 3rd, Balkwill MD, et al. Optokinetic nystagmus as a measure of visual function in severely visually impaired patients. Invest Ophthalmol Vis Sci 2007;48:4542–4548.

200. Spitzyna GA, Wise RJ, McDonald SA, et al. Optokinetic therapy improves text reading in patients with hemianopic alexia: a controlled trial. Neurology 2007;68:1922–1930.

201. Salman MS, Sharpe JA, Lillakas L, et al. Square wave jerks in children and adolescents. Pediatr Neurol 2008;38:16–19.

202. Selhorst JB, Stark L, Ochs AL, et al. Disorders in cerebellar ocular motor control. II. Macrosaccadic oscillation. An oculographic, control system and clinico-anatomical analysis. Brain 1976;99:509–522.

203. Yee RD, Spiegel PH, Yamada T, et al. Voluntary saccadic oscillations, resembling ocular flutter and opsoclonus. J Neuro-ophthalmol 1994;14:95–101.

204. Pranzatelli MR. The neurobiology of the opsoclonus-myoclonus syndrome. Clin Neuropharm 1992;15:186–228.

205. McGarvey CK, Applegate K, Lee ND, et al. False-positive metaiodobenzylguanidine scan for neuroblastoma in a child with opsoclonus-myoclonus syndrome treated with adrenocorticotropic hormone (ACTH). J Child Neurol 2006;21:606–610.

206. Chang BH, Koch T, Hopkins K, et al. Neuroblastoma found in a 4-year-old after rituximab therapy for opsoclonus-myoclonus. Pediatr Neurol 2006;35:213–215.

207. Leen WG, Weemaes CM, Verbeek MM, et al. Rituximab and intravenous immunoglobulins for relapsing postinfectious opsoclonus-myoclonus syndrome. Pediatr Neurol 2008;39:213–217.

208. Pranzatelli MR, Tate ED, Travelstead AL, et al. Rituximab (anti-CD20) adjunctive therapy for opsoclonus-myoclonus syndrome. J Pediatr Hematol Oncol 2006;28:585–593.

209. Yiu VW, Kovithavongs T, McGonigle LF, et al. Plasmapheresis as an effective treatment for opsoclonus-myoclonus syndrome. Pediatr Neurol 2001;24:72–74.

210. Armstrong MB, Robertson PL, Castle VP. Delayed, recurrent opsoclonus-myoclonus syndrome responding to plasmapheresis. Pediatr Neurol 2005;33:365–367.

211. Pranzatelli MR. The immunopharmacology of the opsoclonus-myoclonus syndrome. Clin Neuropharm 1996;19:1–47.

212. Pranzatelli MR, Travelstead AL, Tate ED, et al. B- and T-cell markers in opsoclonus-myoclonus syndrome: immunophenotyping of CSF lymphocytes. Neurology 2004;62:1526–1532.

213. Bataller L, Rosenfeld MR, Graus F, et al. Autoantigen diversity in the opsoclonus-myoclonus syndrome. Ann Neurol 2003;53:347–353.

214. Posner JB. Paraneoplastic opsoclonus/myoclonus: B cells, T cells, both, or neither? [editorial]. Neurology 2004;62:1466–1467.

215. Fisher PG, Wechsler PG, Singer HS. Anti-Hu antibody in a neuroblastoma-associated paraneoplastic syndrome. Pediatr Neurol 1994;10:309–312.

216. Connolly AM, Pestronk A, Mehta S, et al. Serum autoantibodies in childhood opsoclonus-myoclonus syndrome: an analysis of antigenic targets in neural tissues. J Pediatr 1997;130:878–884.

217. Blaes F, Fuhlhuber V, Korfei M, et al. Surface-binding autoantibodies to cerebellar neurons in opsoclonus syndrome. Ann Neurol 2005;58:313–317.

218. Case records of the Massachusetts General Hospital: Case 27–1995. N Engl J Med 1995;333:579–586.

219. Hammer MS, Larsen MB, Stack CV. Outcome of children with opsoclonus-myoclonus regardless of etiology. Pediatr Neurol 1995;13:21–24.

220. Hoyt CS, Mousel DK, Weber AA. Transient supranuclear disturbances of gaze in healthy neonates. Am J Ophthalmol 1980;89:708–713.

221. Morad Y, Benyamini OG, Avni I. Benign opsoclonus in preterm infants. Pediatr Neurol 2004;31:275–278.

222. Bienfang DC. Opsoclonus in infancy. Arch Ophthalmol 1974;91:203–205.

223. Watemberg N, Lerman-Sagie T, Kramer U. Diagnostic yield of electroencephalograms in infants and young children with frequent paroxysmal eye movements. J Child Neurol 2008;23:620–623.

224. Scharf D. Opsoclonus-myoclonus following the intranasal usage of cocaine. J Neurol Neurosurg Psychiatry 1989;52:1447–1448.

225. Liang TW, Balcer LJ, Solomon D, et al. Supranuclear gaze palsy and opsoclonus after Diazinon poisoning. J Neurol Neurosurg Psychiatry 2003;74:677–679.

226. Darnell RB, Posner JB. Paraneoplastic syndromes involving the nervous system. N Engl J Med 2003;349:1543–1554.

227. Peter L, Jung J, Tilikete C, et al. Opsoclonus-myoclonus as a manifestation of Lyme disease. J Neurol Neurosurg Psychiatry 2006;77:1090–1091.

228. Khosla JS, Edelman MJ, Kennedy N, et al. West Nile virus presenting as opsoclonus-myoclonus cerebellar ataxia. Neurology 2005;64:1095.

229. Alshekhlee A, Sultan B, Chandar K. Opsoclonus persisting during sleep in West Nile encephalitis. Arch Neurol 2006;63:1324–1326.

230. Verma A, Brozman B. Opsoclonus-myoclonus syndrome following Epstein-Barr virus infection. Neurology 2002;58:1131–1132.

231. Candler PM, Dale RC, Griffin S, et al. Post-streptococcal opsoclonus-myoclonus syndrome associated with anti-neuroleukin antibodies. J Neurol Neurosurg Psychiatry 2006;77:507–512.

232. Wong A. An update on opsoclonus. Curr Opin Neurol 2007;20:25–31.

233. Hersh B, Dalmau J, Dangond F, et al. Paraneoplastic opsoclonus-myoclonus associated with anti-Hu antibody. Neurology 1994;44:1754–1755.

234. Luque FA, Furneaux HM, Ferziger R, et al. Anti-Ri: An antibody associated with paraneoplastic opsoclonus and breast cancer. Ann Neurol 1991;29:241–251.

235. Fitzpatrick AS, Gray OM, McConville J, et al. Opsoclonus-myoclonus syndrome associated with benign ovarian teratoma. Neurology 2008;70:1292–1293.

236. Schon F, Hodgson TL, Mort D, et al. Ocular flutter associated with a localized lesion in the paramedian pontine reticular formation. Ann Neurol 2001;50:413–416.

237. Bataller L, Graus F, Saiz A, et al. Clinical outcome in adult onset idiopathic or paraneoplastic opsoclonus-myoclonus. Brain 2001;124:437–443.

238. Hassan KA, Kalemkerian GP, Trobe JD. Long-term survival in paraneoplastic opsoclonus-myoclonus syndrome associated with small cell lung cancer. J Neuro-ophthalmol 2008;28:27–30.

239. Ko MW, Dalmau J, Galetta SL. Neuro-ophthalmologic manifestations of paraneoplastic syndromes. J Neuro-ophthalmol 2008;28:58–68.

240. Cher LM, Hochberg FH, Teruya J. Therapy for paraneoplastic neurologic syndromes in six patients with protein column immunoabsorption. Cancer 1995;75:1678–1683.

241. Helmchen C, Rambold H, Sprenger A, et al. Cerebellar activation in opsoclonus: an fMRI study. Neurology 2003;61:412–415.

242. Hoyt WF, Keane JR. Superior oblique myokymia. Report and discussion on five cases of benign intermittent uniocular microtremor. Arch Ophthalmol 1970;84:461–467.

243. Susac JO, Smith JL, Schatz NJ. Superior oblique myokymia. Arch Neurol 1973;29:432–434.

244. Suzuki Y, Washio N, Hashimoto M, et al. Three-dimensional eye movement analysis of superior oblique myokymia. Am J Ophthalmol 2003;135:563–565.

245. Rosenberg ML, Glaser JS. Superior oblique myokymia. Ann Neurol 1983;13:667–669.

246. Morrow M, Sharpe JA, Ranalli PJ. Superior oblique myokymia associated with a posterior fossa tumor: oculographic correlation with an idiopathic case. Neurology 1990;40:367–370.

247. Hashimoto M, Ohtsuka K, Hoyt WF. Vascular compression as a cause of superior oblique myokymia disclosed by thin-slice magnetic resonance imaging. Am J Ophthalmol 2001;131:676–677.

248. Yousry I, Dieterich M, Naidich TP, et al. Superior oblique myokymia: magnetic resonance imaging support for the neurovascular compression hypothesis. Ann Neurol 2002;51:361–368.

249. Hashimoto M, Ohtsuka K, Suzuki Y, et al. Superior oblique myokymia caused by vascular compression. J Neuro-ophthalmol 2004;24:237–239.

250. Tomsak RL, Kosmorsky GS, Leigh RJ. Gabapentin attenuates superior oblique myokymia. Am J Ophthalmol 2002;133:721–723.

251. Jain S, Farooq SJ, Gottlob I. Resolution of superior oblique myokymia with memantine. JAAPOS 2008;12:87–88.

252. Williams PE, Purvin VA, Kawasaki A. Superior oblique myokymia: efficacy of medical treatment. JAAPOS 2007;11:254–257.

253. Kosmorsky GS, Ellis BD, Fogt N, et al. Treatment of superior oblique myokymia utilizing the Harado-Ito procedure. J Neuro-ophthalmol 1995;15:142–146.

254. Scharwey K, Krzizok T, Samii M, et al. Remission of superior oblique myokymia after microvascular decompression. Ophthalmologica 2000;214:426–428.

255. Daroff RB, Waldman AL. Ocular bobbing. J Neurol Neurosurg Psychiatr 1965;28:375–377.

256. Susac JO, Hoyt WF, Daroff RB, et al. Clinical spectrum of ocular bobbing. J Neurol Neurosurg Psychiatr 1970;33:771–775.

257. Rai GS, Buxton-Thomas M, Scanlon M. Ocular bobbing in hepatic encephalopathy. Br J Clin Prac 1976;30:202–205.

258. Rudick R, Satran R, Eskin TA. Ocular bobbing in encephalitis. J Neurol Neurosurg Psychiatr 1981;44:441–443.

259. Finelli PF, McEntee WJ. Ocular bobbing with extra-axial haematoma of posterior fossa. J Neurol Neurosurg Psychiatr 1977;40:386–388.

260. Knobler RL, Somasundaram M, Schutta HS. Inverse ocular bobbing. Ann Neurol 1981;9:194–197.

261. Ropper AH. Ocular dipping in anoxic coma. Arch Neurol 1981;38:297–299.

262. Oh YM, Jeong SH, Kim JS. Ocular dipping and ping-pong gaze in hypoxic encephalopathy. Neurology 2007;68:222.

263. Shimazaki H, Morita M, Nakano I, et al. Inverse ocular bobbing in a patient with encephalitis associated with antibodies to the N-methyl-D-aspartate receptor. Arch Neurol 2008;65:1251.

264. Appiani GC, Catania G, Gagliardi M, et al. Repositioning maneuver for the treatment of the apogeotropic variant of horizontal canal benign paroxysmal positional vertigo. Otol Neurotol 2005;26:257–260.

CHAPTER **18**

Orbital disease in neuro-ophthalmology

Orbital disorders usually manifest with a unifying constellation of symptoms and signs that include proptosis, periocular swelling, blurred vision, and double vision. The presence of proptosis distinguishes diseases of the orbit from other neuro-ophthalmic conditions with similar symptomatology. The discussion below describes the relevant orbital anatomy and the typical signs and symptoms encountered in orbital disease. A review of orbital imaging techniques follows and emphasizes the advantages and disadvantages of each modality. Finally, the orbital entities frequently encountered in neuro-ophthalmic practice are analyzed.

Orbital anatomy

Familiarity with orbital anatomy is critical to understanding and recognizing the various conditions that are encountered. Several excellent texts and atlases are available[1-3] along with excellent review articles with correlation to radiographic studies.[4-7] The orbit contains a wide variety of tissue types including bone, periorbita, fibroadipose tissue, striated and smooth muscle, epithelial tissue of the lacrimal gland, the optic nerve, peripheral autonomic, sensory and motor nerves, the ciliary ganglion, arteries and veins, and finally cartilage in the trochlear of the superior oblique muscle. Although the orbit was traditionally thought not to contain lymphatics there is now considerable evidence to suggest that there are lymphatics in the orbital fat, lacrimal gland, and optic nerve sheath.[8-11]

A "functional" understanding of orbital anatomy and the interaction of all of these structures is grounded in the relationship of the various spaces within the 25–30 cc of the bony orbit.[12] These spaces include the globe and the space immediately around it (Tenon's space), the intraconal portion of the orbit (formed by the cone of the rectus muscles and containing the optic nerve), and the extraconal space (**Fig. 18–1**). There is also a potential space between the bone and the periorbita which is a common site for orbital involvement by paranasal sinus infections and tumors. Further division into the superior and inferior extraconal spaces is helpful as many conditions such as lymphoma and idiopathic orbital inflammatory syndrome have a predilection to develop in the superior and temporal orbit.

Bones of the orbit

The orbit is bound by portions of seven different bones (frontal, sphenoidal, zygomatic, lacrimal, maxillary, palatine, and ethmoidal), and they contribute variably to form the walls of the orbit (**Fig. 18–2, Table 18–1**). The ethmoidal bone contains the medially located and thin lamina papyracea, which is vulnerable both to fractures and to the passage of infection from the paranasal sinuses. The posterior border of the orbit is the optic canal, and the anterior extent is the orbital septum, which originates in the periorbita and blends into the connective tissue of the upper and lower eyelids.

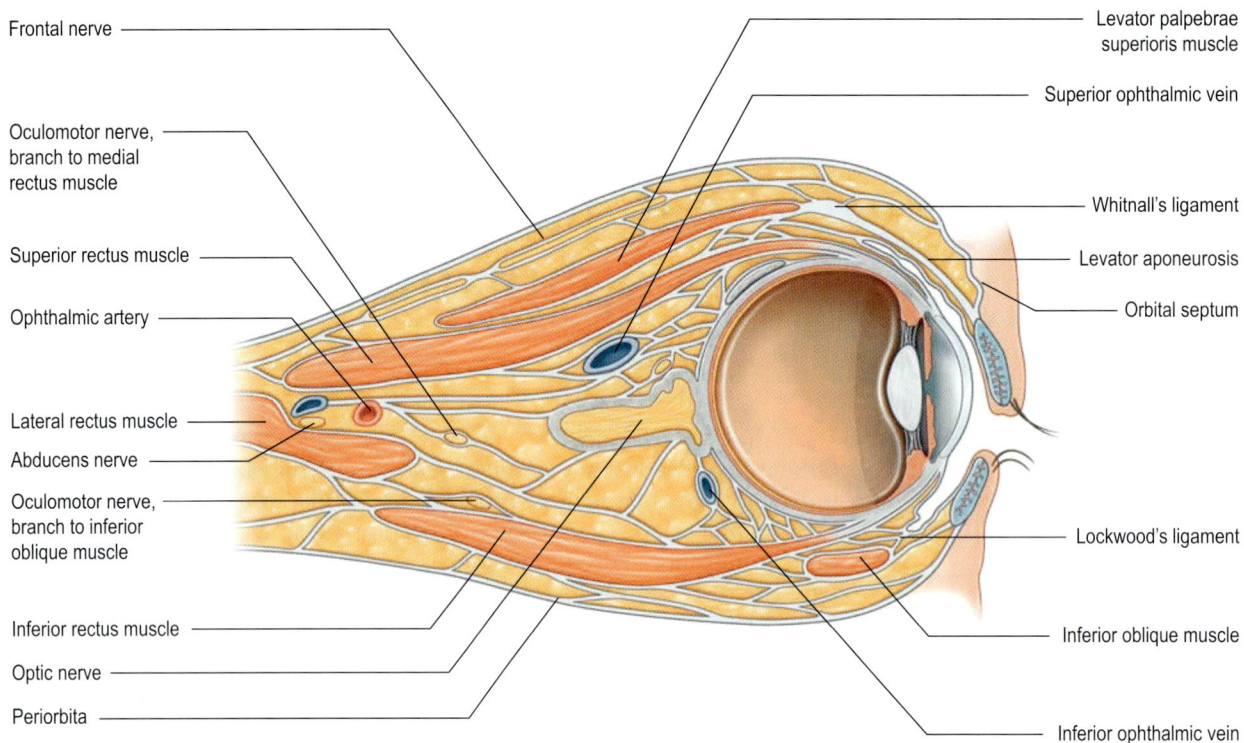

Figure 18–1. Sagittal section of the orbit demonstrating the various anatomic spaces and the orbital fascial system. The extraocular muscles and the intermuscular septae define the intraconal space. The extraconal space is outside of the muscle cone. Tenon's space is between Tenon's fascia (which surrounds the globe) and the globe. These spaces are often considered when developing a differential diagnosis of orbital lesions.

Table 18–1 Bones of the walls of the orbit

Orbital roof	Frontal bone Lesser wing of sphenoid
Lateral wall	Greater wing of sphenoid bone Zygomatic bone
Medial wall	Ethmoid bone Lacrimal bone Lesser wing of sphenoid Tip of maxilla
Orbital floor	Maxilla Zygomatic Palatine

There are three major bony openings into the orbit. The first is the optic canal through which passes the optic nerve, oculosympathetic nerves, and the ophthalmic artery. The second is the superior orbital fissure, formed by the greater and lesser wings of the sphenoid bone. The superior ophthalmic vein and the third, fourth, first (ophthalmic) division of the fifth, and sixth cranial nerves as well as some sympathetic nerves pass through the superior orbital fissure. Finally, the inferior orbital fissure is in the floor of the orbit, and through it passes the second (maxillary) branch of the fifth nerve, the inferior ophthalmic vein, heading into the pterygoid plexus, and branches of the sphenopalatine ganglion.

There are other important vascular foramina including openings in the medial orbital wall for the anterior and posterior ethmoidal arteries. The ethmoidal arteries are branches of the ophthalmic artery and supply the dura in the anterior cranial fossa and the nose. The anterior ethmoidal nerve, a branch of the nasociliary nerve, also passes through the anterior ethmoidal canal and supplies sensation to the tip of the nose and upper lip. This sensory branch of the first division of the fifth cranial nerve is the reason why the tip of the nose is often involved in herpes zoster ophthalmicus (Hutchinson's sign).

The bones of the orbit also contain important grooves and fossae. The infraorbital groove contains the infraorbital nerve, the terminal branch of the maxillary nerve, which exits the floor of the orbit through the infraorbital foramen to supply the sensation on the cheek and upper part of the jaw. The supraorbital nerve (a branch of the frontal nerve, which derives from the ophthalmic division of the fifth nerve) similarly reaches the skin of the forehead and frontal sinus through the supraorbital foramen or notch.[13] The trochlear fossa is located superomedially 5 mm from the anterior orbital rim. Here the cartilaginous trochlear (through which the tendon of the superior oblique passes) is attached. The lacrimal fossa is located superotemporally in the frontal bone.

The lateral wall of the orbit is thickest anteriorly and is the strongest of the orbital walls. In the most anterior portion of the lateral wall about 10–11 mm below the frontozygomatic suture is found the lateral orbital (Whitnall's) tubercle. This bony tubercle serves as the point of attachment of the levator aponeurosis, the suspensory (Lockwood's) ligament of the globe, the lateral palpebral ligament, and the check ligament of the lateral rectus muscle. The zygomatic canal is

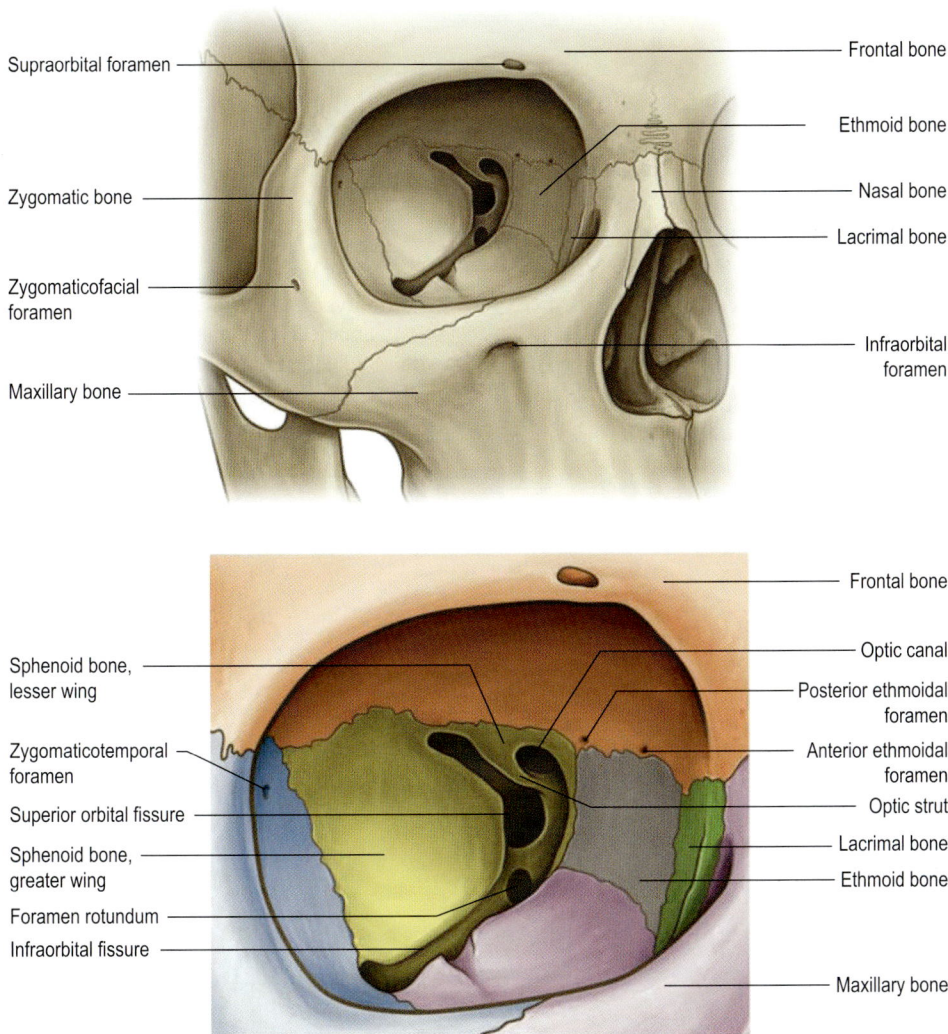

Figure 18–2. The bones, formina, and fissures of the left orbit. **A**. External views of the various bones that form the orbit. **B**. Higher-power view of the orbital apex of the left orbit. The greater and lesser wings of the sphenoid bone form the orbital apex. The superior orbital fissure, inferior orbital fissure, and optic canal can be seen.

posterior to the tubercle, and through it passes the zygomatic nerve, a proximal branch of the maxillary nerve. It divides in the orbit into the zygomaticotemporal and zygomaticofacial nerves, which supply the skin on the lateral portion of the forehead and cheek.

Vascular structures

The blood supply to the orbit derives from the ophthalmic artery, which is the first branch of the internal carotid artery after it pierces the dura of the cavernous sinus.[14,15] The artery enters the orbit inferiorly through the optic canal and then moves laterally between the optic nerve and lateral rectus, then superiorly and finally medially. Its terminal branches are the supratrochlear and dorsal nasal arteries. Some blood reaches the orbit through the facial, maxillary, and temporal branches of the external carotid artery. The branches of the ophthalmic artery (see **Fig. 4–1**), the structures they supply and their important external carotid artery anastomoses are summarized in **Table 18–2**.

The orbital veins are valveless. The superior ophthalmic vein and central retinal vein drain into the cavernous sinus.

The inferior orbital vein drains into the pterygoid plexus. Anterior venous drainage can also occur into the facial veins via the angular and inferior ophthalmic veins.

Extraocular muscles

The six extraocular muscles are striated with unique properties.[16] The four rectus muscles (each about 3–4 cm long) originate from the annulus of Zinn at the orbital apex, which is contiguous with the dura surrounding the optic nerve and the periorbita. In addition to their insertion on the globe there is increasing evidence for a second insertion in the connective tissue surrounding the muscle, creating a "pulley" which functions as a secondary origin for the rectus muscle action.[17–20] The levator palpebra also originates from the annulus of Zinn. The superior oblique originates just posterior to the annulus of Zinn and passes through the trochlear before turning posterolateral to insert on the globe under and posterior to the insertion of the superior rectus. The inferior oblique originates from the bone just posterolateral to the nasolacrimal fossa and travels posterolaterally under the inferior rectus (attached to inferior rectus by

Table 18–2 Branches of the ophthalmic artery, structures they supply, and important anastomoses[15]

Branch of ophthalmic artery	Structure(s) supplied	Important anastomoses with external carotid artery
Central retinal a.	Retina, optic nerve	
Lateral posterior ciliary a.	Choroid, optic nerve (20 short branches) Ciliary muscle, iris, anterior choroid (two long branches)	
Lacrimal a.	Lacrimal gland	With transverse facial, zygomatic, and frontal branches of superficial temporal aa. With middle meningeal a. from maxillary a.
Lateral muscular a.	Superior rectus, superior oblique, lateral rectus, and levator muscles Rectus muscles give off anterior ciliary aa. to anterior segment of eye	With orbital branches of infraorbital a., a branch of maxillary a.
Posterior ethmoid a. Supraorbital a. (together or separately)	Posterior ethmoid air cells Eyebrow, forehead Levator muscle	With lateral nasal a. from maxillary a.
Medial posterior ciliary a.	See lateral posterior ciliary a. above	
Muscular a.	Inferior rectus inferior oblique, and medial rectus muscles	
To areolar tissue	Areolar tissue	
Anterior ethmoid a.	Anterior ethmoid cells Frontal sinus Dura in anterior fossa Nose	With sphenopalatine a. from maxillary a.
Medial, inferior medial, and superior medial palpebral aa.	Eyelids	
Dorsal nasal (terminal) a.	Nose	With angular branch of facial a.
Supratrochlear a.	Superomedial orbit	

a, artery; aa, arteries.

Lockwood's ligament) to insert both into the connective tissue between it and the lateral rectus (its pulley or secondary origin[21]) and posteriorly on the globe in the region of the macula. The nerves innervating the rectus muscles enter them at the junction of the posterior and middle third of their bellies. These structures are discussed in more detail in Chapter 15.

Periorbita and septae

The periorbita is the periosteum of the orbital bones. It is only loosely adherent to the bones except where it is fixed at the anterior orbital rim, margins of fissures and canals, and the lacrimal crest. Posteriorly it is contiguous with the dura at the superior orbital fissure and optic nerve. The intraconal space is defined by the extraocular muscles and the intermuscular septa which are denser anteriorly and may be absent posteriorly.[22] Koornneef[23] has demonstrated that the anatomic distinction of the intraconal and extraconal spaces is more complex and that this division results from radial fibrovascular connective tissue septae which also attach the muscles to the periorbita. These septae separate the orbital fat into lobules. The orbital septum is the anterior

border of the orbit. It originates at the anterior orbital rim and superiorly fuses with the levator aponeurosis and inferiorly with the capsulopalpebral fascia.

Tenon's capsule is a layer of delicate connective tissue attached to the globe near the limbus. The capsule envelopes the globe, has fine posterior attachments to it, and separates it from the orbital fat. The extraocular muscles pierce the capsule anterior to the equator of the globe and are enveloped in a sleeve-like extension of the capsule. The muscles travel in the capsule for 7–10 mm, and the capsule gives off lateral extensions, forming the intermuscular membrane between the rectus muscles. Important attachments between rectus muscles and the surrounding connective tissue may serve as the functional origin for the each muscle.[18,19,21]

Ciliary ganglion

The ciliary ganglion, which is also discussed in Chapter 13 (see **Fig. 13–3**), lies in the posterior orbit between optic nerve and the lateral rectus muscle. The ganglion contains the synapses of the preganglionic parasympathetic fibers from the Edinger–Westphal nucleus of the third nerve and provides the postganglionic neurons destined for the ciliary body and pupillary sphincter. These fibers reach the ciliary ganglion with the oculomotor branch to the inferior oblique muscle. Postganglionic fibers reach the anterior portion of the globe via short posterior ciliary nerves. Sensory fibers from the ophthalmic division of the trigeminal nerve and postganglionic sympathetic fibers pass through the ciliary ganglion on their way to the globe but do not synapse there.

Lacrimal gland

The lacrimal gland sits in the lacrimal fossa and is separated from the globe by Tenon's capsule and orbital fat. The most lateral portion of the levator aponeurosis separates the lacrimal gland into the smaller palpebral and larger orbital lobes. Small portions of the palpebral lobe can be seen superolaterally upon eversion of the eyelid. The blood supply to the lacrimal gland derives from the lacrimal artery, a branch of the ophthalmic artery. Sensory innervation is from the ophthalmic division of the trigeminal nerve. Autonomic innervation is from parasympathetic fibers which synapse in the pterygopalatine ganglion and travel with the zygomatic branches of the maxillary division of the trigeminal nerve before reaching the lacrimal gland.

Neuro-ophthalmology of orbital disease

Symptoms

Patients with orbital disease present with a variety of symptoms including vision loss, double vision, swelling, ptosis, and proptosis. Most orbital disease is space occupying, and therefore the hallmark of orbital disease is proptosis or exophthalmos due to axial or forward displacement of the globe. Axial proptosis (**Fig. 18–3**) is usually caused by disease within the muscles or muscle cone while non-axial proptosis (displacement of the globe down, up or sideways in addition to forward) is usually caused by extraconal lesions. Although many patients may notice prominence of one eye or a widening of the palpebral fissure, others may have unrecognized moderate to severe proptosis. Lid retraction (sclera visible

between superior limbus and upper eyelid) is the hallmark of thyroid eye disease. Other causes of proptosis are generally not associated with lid retraction. In fact, superior orbital disease might also be associated with ptosis. Patients with orbital disease (particularly thyroid-associated ophthalmopathy (TAO) and idiopathic orbital inflammatory syndrome) also present with eyelid soft tissue swelling or conjunctival injection. Patients with orbital fractures or bone loss in association with sinus disease (see silent sinus syndrome discussion below) can present with enophthalmos or sinking back of the globe (**Fig. 18–3**). Here there may also be exaggeration of the superior sulcus adding to the "sunken appearance". Enophthalmos can also occur with processes associated with scarring of orbital tissue (e.g. metastatic breast cancer).

Double vision secondary to impaired eye movements is a frequent complaint. Double vision results from misalignment of the two eyes. Strabismus in this setting is usually non-comitant and results from a mechanical effect where the mass lesion or inflammatory process interferes with the movement of the eye directly or indirectly. Double vision can also result from extraocular muscle dysfunction by restricting the movement of the globe as in TAO. Lastly, diplopia can also result from cranial nerve (third, fourth, or sixth) dysfunction within the orbit or through invasion of the tumor into the cavernous sinus. Facial hypesthesia can result from involvement of the fifth cranial nerve or its branches in the orbit.

Slowly expanding benign orbital neoplasms may not cause any visual symptoms. However, optic nerve tumors (glioma and meningiomas) and large intraconal tumors frequently present with proptosis and decreased vision. Patients may describe a blur or recognize loss of visual field (see Chapter 5). A peculiar variation of transient monocular vision loss occurs in patients with orbital mass lesions, and is termed gaze-evoked amaurosis.[24–27] Vision darkens as the eye is moved and the optic nerve or central retinal artery is compressed by the mass lesion. Vision clears upon moving the eye back to the central position. However, gaze-evoked amaurosis has been described in association with a variety of other conditions, including intracranial lesions, vitreopapillary traction syndromes, orbital fractures, sinus disease,

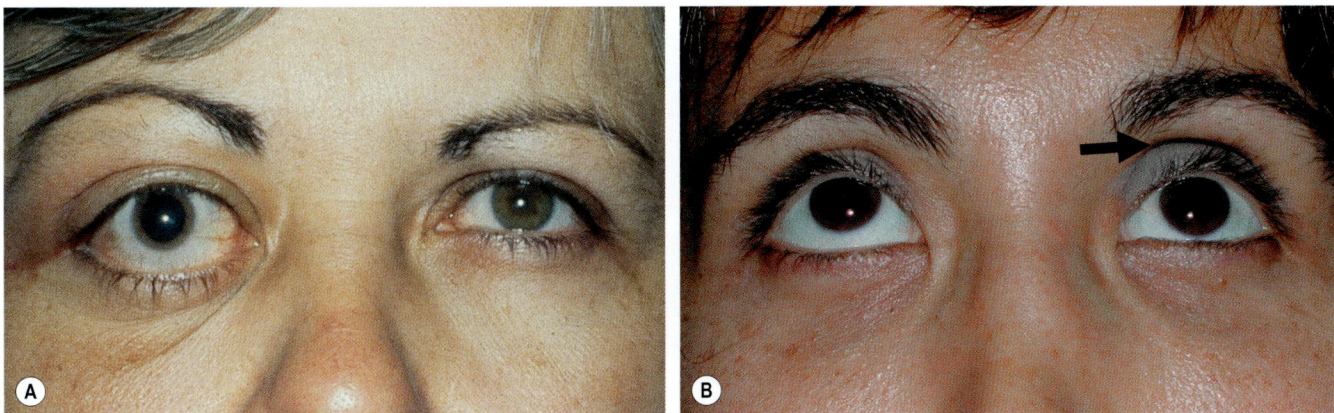

Figure 18–3. A. Patients with orbital disease present with axial proptosis (exophthalmos) as seen in the right eye of this patient. The right pupil has been pharmacologically dilated. **B**. Enophthalmos manifesting as exaggeration of the superior sulcus (arrow) and a sunken appearance to the eye can be seen with orbital processes that decrease the orbital volume such as fractures or those that cause scarring of orbital tissue (certain metastatic tumors).

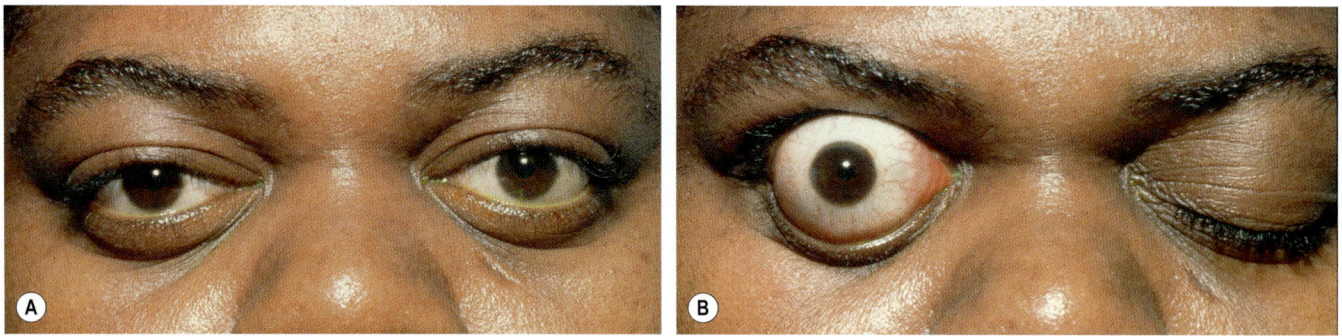

Figure 18–4. Patients with either shallow orbits (**A**) or on occasion with space-occupying lesions of the orbit can develop spontaneous proptosis. In this condition (**B**) the eye extends beyond the eyelids, which are trapped behind the globe. The globe can easily be pushed back into the orbit.

TAO, and elevated intracranial pressure.[28–33] Decreased vision can also result from direct compression of the optic nerve or from indentation of the globe by a mass lesion, compression of the optic nerve by enlarged eye muscles in TAO, or from an inflammatory perineuritis associated with idiopathic orbital inflammation. Rarely, individuals with shallow orbits or proptosis can develop spontaneous episodes in which the globe is trapped in front of the lids (**Fig. 18–4**). This can be associated with blurred and double vision and is easily reduced by gently pushing the globe posteriorly.

Examination

The details of formal neuro-ophthalmic examination have been described in Chapter 2. As with all patients, examination of patients with orbital disease begins with careful assessment of visual function including visual acuity, color vision, and visual fields. Beyond this, certain features of the examination of patients with orbital disease are unique and deserve review.

Examination overview. The external examination begins by assessing the outward appearance of the eye, looking for asymmetry, globe position, swelling, and abnormal eyelid position. Since lid retraction is often associated with lid lag, the patient is asked to look down. The lid is then observed to see if it "hangs up" abnormally. Since mass lesions can often be felt around the eye, particularly if they primarily involve the lacrimal gland, the orbit and globe should be palpated. At the same time the globe is retrodisplaced into the orbit and the presence of abnormal resistance or firmness, typical of most orbital disease, can be noted. Careful examination should be performed of the preauricular area and neck to look for evidence of abnormal adenopathy. The orbit can also be auscultated since bruits are present in some patients with arteriovenous malformations.

Proptosis can often be better appreciated if the patients are asked to tilt their head backward. Then the examiner looks from below, comparing the position of the eyes in relation to the brow or anterior orbital rim. Formal measurements of proptosis can be accomplished with various devices. The Hertel exophthalmometer is the combination of a scale and mirror (see **Fig. 2–36**) and is placed on the lateral orbital rims of the patient. The examiner can then determine the relative position of each globe compared to the lateral

orbital rim. Generally, the eyes are within 1–2 mm of each other, and any difference greater than that suggests either enophthalmos or exophthalmos. Serial measurements of proptosis with exophthalmometry are important in patients with active orbital disease to assess progression.

Optic disc findings. Initially, the optic nerve usually appears normal in patients presenting with orbital disease. Subsequently chronic low-grade compression of the intraorbital optic nerve can lead to atrophy of the optic nerve and disc pallor. However, some patients with optic nerve tumors, and rarely patients with other orbital tumors, may present with optic nerve head swelling. Swelling usually results from compression of the anterior half of the optic nerve, leading to impaired axonal transport. Lesions around the orbital apex usually do not cause optic disc swelling. As a rule, optic disc swelling is not associated with intracanalicular or intracranial tumors unless there is associated mass effect, elevated intracranial pressure, and resulting papilledema. Disc swelling secondary to a chronic compressive lesion is sometimes further characterized by the presence of collateral or shunt vessels. These abnormal vessels develop to shunt blood flow from the retinal to choroidal circulation, bypassing the chronically obstructed central retinal vein. Collateral vessels are a common feature of optic nerve sheath meningiomas and gliomas and are less commonly encountered with other causes of orbital disease.

Retinal findings. Retinal vascular changes are sometimes observed in patients with orbital disease. Venous engorgement or impending venous occlusion may be seen with optic nerve tumors, but is very rare in patients with neoplastic or inflammatory disease of the orbit. The most common fundus abnormality in patients with orbital mass lesions is choroidal (chorioretinal) folding. These have also been described in patients with TAO, inflammatory diseases of the sclera and orbit, and mucoceles.[34] The folding (**Fig. 18–5**) is the result of extrinsic compression of the globe, leading to flattening of the sclera and subsequent wrinkling or folding of the retina. The subsequent outer retinal folding follows corrugations in the choroid, Bruch's membrane, and retinal pigment epithelium.[35] This creates a highly characteristic ophthalmoscopic finding of parallel, alternating lines or folds most often seen in the posterior pole. The finding is easily confirmed on ocular coherence tomography, and the fluorescein angiographic pattern, first described by Norton,[36] has a diagnostic appearance of alternating light and dark

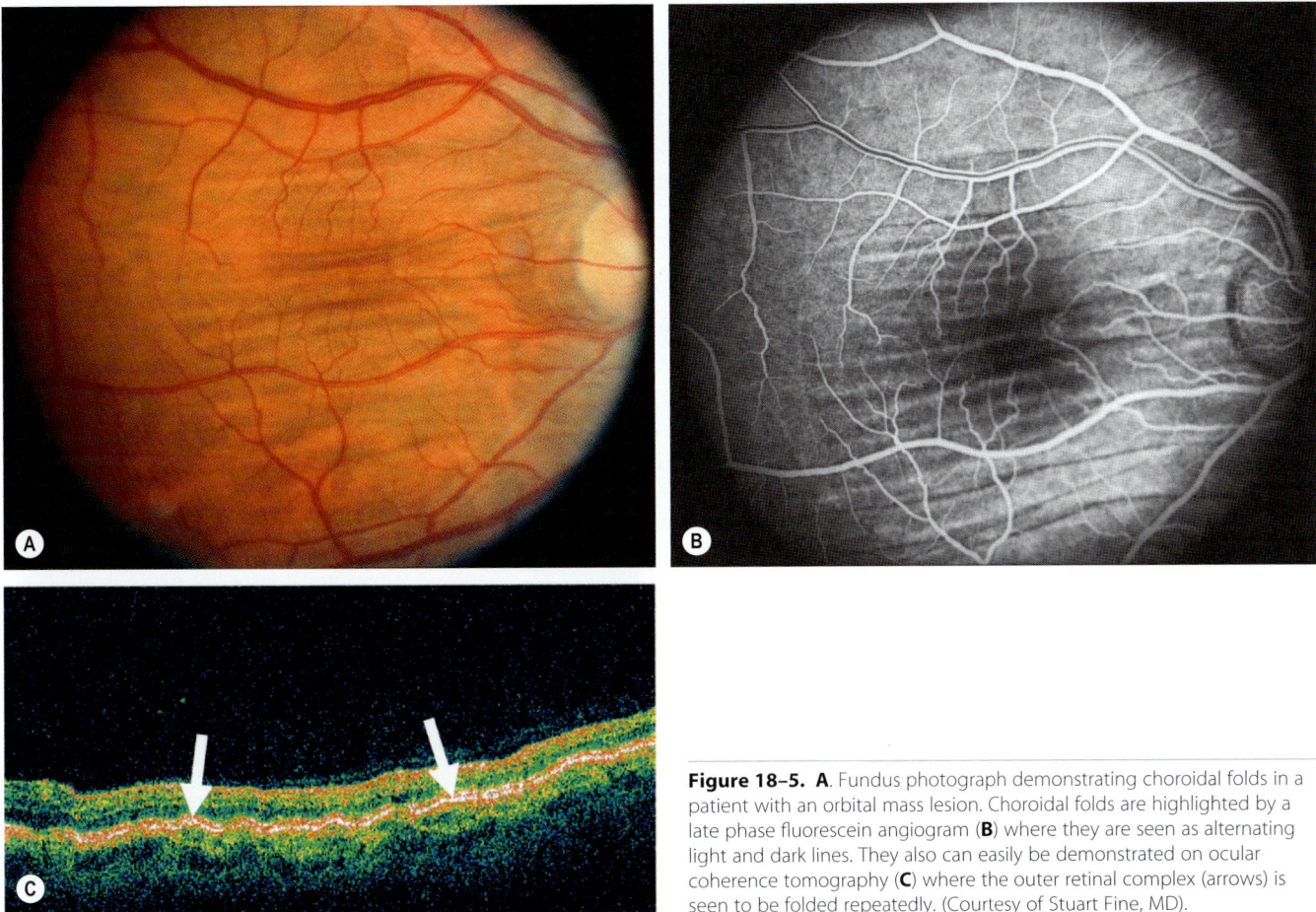

Figure 18–5. A. Fundus photograph demonstrating choroidal folds in a patient with an orbital mass lesion. Choroidal folds are highlighted by a late phase fluorescein angiogram (**B**) where they are seen as alternating light and dark lines. They also can easily be demonstrated on ocular coherence tomography (**C**) where the outer retinal complex (arrows) is seen to be folded repeatedly. (Courtesy of Stuart Fine, MD).

lines (**Fig. 18–5**). The recognition of choroidal folds demands investigation for orbital disease and globe compression, although they may also be secondary to hyperopia, hypotony, choroidal or retinal detachments, raised intracranial pressure, scleral buckles, subretinal neovascular membranes, and choroidal tumors. In many patients, and particularly in bilateral cases, choroidal folds are idiopathic.[37]

Retinal arterial abnormalities are uncommon. Rarely, occlusions of the retinal arteries can occur in association with acute trauma and retrobulbar hemorrhage or secondary to angioinvasive forms of mucormycosis or aspergillus. Exudative retinal detachments can be seen in patients with idiopathic orbital inflammatory syndrome.

Eye movement abnormalities. A mixed pattern of eye movement impairment is the hallmark of orbital disease and may reflect both muscle restriction and cranial nerve dysfunction. The speed of ocular ductions should be noted. For instance, if an eye moves quickly but abruptly stops, a restrictive process or mass lesion is suggested. When the movement is slow for the entire excursion it suggests a cranial nerve palsy rather than a restrictive process. Neurogenic and mechanical eye movement limitation may also be distinguished by performing forced duction and forced generation testing (see **Fig. 2–24**). In general, patients with orbital tumors will have a mixed pattern of eye movement limitation that does not fit clearly into the pattern of a single cranial nerve. For instance, if a patient can neither elevate nor abduct an eye, it is more likely the result of mass effect or restrictive myopathy than a combined partial-third and sixth nerve palsy.

Diagnostic orbital imaging

The diagnostic evaluation of orbital disease includes noninvasive imaging of the orbit either by echography (orbital ultrasound), computed tomography (CT scan), or magnetic resonance imaging (MRI scan). Each modality has advantages and disadvantages (**Table 18–3**), but the techniques are often complementary. Imaging studies may be non-diagnostic except for the unique patterns seen with thyroid eye disease and paraorbital sinus disease. However, taken in conjunction with the history and examination, a tentative diagnosis can usually be made.

Echography

Two types of analysis are used in orbital echography: amplitude mode (A-scan) and brightness mode (B-scan) (**Fig. 18–6**). Many different orbital disorders can be diagnosed and followed echographically.[38,39] An A-scan provides one-dimensional images and displays echoes as spikes. Elevated spike height implies increased echogenicity. The length between the transducer and the tissue is represented by the distance between spikes. An A-scan is commonly used to look for calcifications in the setting of optic nerve head drusen, to measure the size of lesions or of the extraocular

Table 18–3 Advantages and disadvantages of various imaging modalities of the orbit

Modality	Advantages	Disadvantages
Echography	Instant results Readily available Echogenicity helps determine lesion type Images globe 30 degree test Images eye muscles well	Requires skilled operator Does not image posterior orbit
Computed tomography (CT) scan	Available Affordable Evaluates bony changes Demonstrates calcification	Radiation exposure Inferior to MRI for soft tissue of the brain Poor imaging of cavernous sinus Lacks multiplanar reformatting capabilities of MRI
Magnetic resonance imaging (MRI) scan	Most machines surpass resolution of CT Exquisite soft tissue detail Demonstrates optic nerve enhancement Images cavernous sinus and orbital apex well No radiation Possible to perform magnetic resonance angiography Images wood foreign body Uniquely images melanin and hemosiderin	Does not image bone Expensive (cost of unit, slower, more technician time) Thicker sections Unwanted nonspecific data (white matter changes) Longer scan time Claustrophobia is prohibitive for some patients Incompatible with magnetic materials or pacemakers

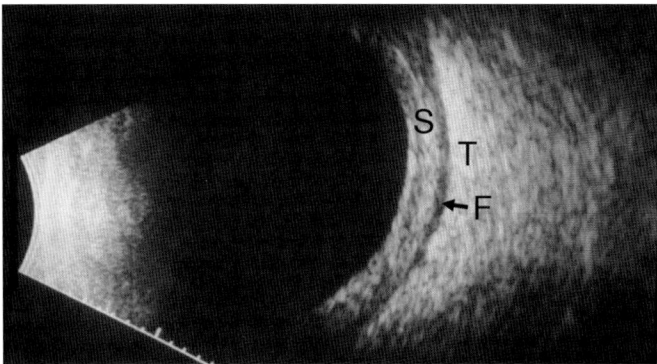

Figure 18–6. Orbital echography is an effective method for evaluating the posterior ocular layers as in this patient with posterior scleritis demonstrating thickening of the Tenon's (T) and scleral layer (S) with fluid (F) in the sub-Tenon space. Echography is also effectively used to characterize extraocular muscle enlargement.

muscles, and to determine the reflectivity (echogenicity) of a lesion or abnormal tissue. B-scan produces two-dimensional images of tissue sections, and images of the orbit are obtained along several different planes. An increase in the acoustic density of a tissue results in an increase in the brightness of the image. Fluid-filled structures (blood vessels, the globe, and cysts, for example) appear dark.

Echography is generally not used as the definitive study for orbital disease, although it has some particularly useful roles.[40,41] One example is posterior scleritis, a form of idiopathic orbital inflammatory syndrome, where a very typical finding of fluid in Tenon's space can be seen on echography (**Fig. 18–6**). Similarly, enlarged extraocular muscles of thyroid disease are easily demonstrated, and ultrasound can be also be used to quantify extraocular muscle thickness.[42]

In children, echography along with color Doppler imaging may be particularly helpful in identifying hemangiomas and dermoids.[43] In the evaluation of mass lesions, the nature of the mass lesion and its relation to the globe can be characterized. In addition, the internal reflectivity of a lesion, suggestive of a vascular or cystic nature, may be ascertained. Echography has been combined with color Doppler imaging to assess blood flow in the eye and orbit, particularly with vascular lesions.[44]

Computed tomography scan

Since bone, calcification, fat, and blood all have unique X-ray absorption patterns, CT scanning is a very effective technique for orbital imaging (**Fig. 18–7**).[4,7,45–47] In fact, the contrast of the surrounding orbital fat allows for excellent imaging of the soft tissues (muscles and optic nerve) of the orbit by CT scan. Specific absorption patterns can be highlighted ("windows") to emphasize bone, soft tissue, or blood.

CT images can be obtained in the axial, coronal, and sagittal planes and generally are done at 3 mm intervals. If necessary, CT scans of the orbit can have a 1 mm slice interval with good resolution. Axial and coronal images are obtained directly, and sagittal images are usually obtained by computer reformatting. Coronal images are often not included in regular studies and should be requested whenever ordering orbital CT scans. Occasionally patients will be unable to position for coronal images and reformatted views are necessary. Bone windows and blood windows are usually viewed as well, and contrast is reserved for evaluation of mass lesions or to evaluate for intracranial extension of orbital disease (MRI preferred, see below). Routine facial bone imaging is done with 5 mm axial and coronal cuts, and when

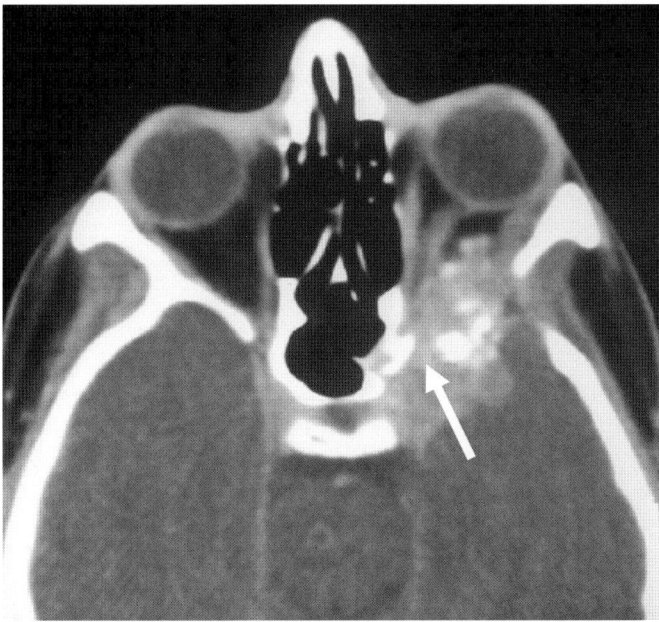

Figure 18–7. Axial computed tomography (CT) scan of a patient with meningioma demonstrating proptosis and bony destruction (arrow). CT scan is excellent for demonstrating both soft tissue and bony changes.

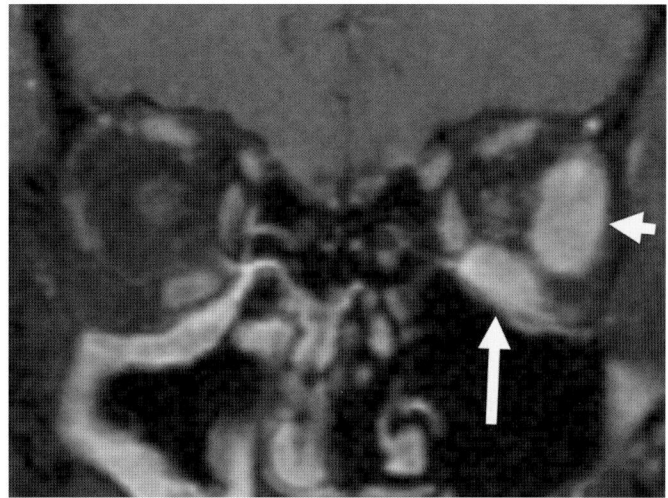

Figure 18–8. Coronal T1-weighted, gadolinium-enhanced, magnetic resonance imaging scan demonstrating enhancement and enlargement of the lateral (short arrow) and inferior rectus (long arrow) muscles and excellent delineation of the orbital soft tissues. The patient had idiopathic orbital inflammatory syndrome.

optic canal fractures are suspected, 1–3 mm coronal images should be obtained. In these cases, contrast is not utilized if bone and soft-tissue windows are viewed. Images are reformatted to produce three-dimensional, reconstructed views of the bony surface or deeper soft-tissue areas. These three-dimensional reconstructions are used for presurgical evaluation of facial fractures and for evaluation of the skull in children with craniosynostoses and other skull deformities and are not necessary in routine orbital imaging.

Magnetic resonance imaging (MRI scan). MRI is considered noninvasive because it does not utilize radiation. Instead a powerful magnetic field and radiofrequency (RF) pulses are used to create images. The images are created when the nuclei of atoms found within the various tissues align with the magnetic field and a RF pulse is applied. Most of the signals produced are from mobile protons of hydrogen atoms found within the water and lipids of tissues and protons which are immobile (bone) give no appreciable signal. Signals are received by RF receiver coils and can be reconstructed in the axial, coronal, or sagittal planes.

Prior to the advent of surface coils (receiver coils which wrap around the patient's face and eyes) and fat suppression techniques, CT was the preferred procedure for orbital imaging, even for the evaluation of soft tissue. However, MRI now offers many advantages over CT. MRI provides excellent images of the globe, orbit, and visual pathways and has become an invaluable tool in the diagnosis of pathologic lesions in the orbit and cavernous sinus. MRI provides excellent contrast resolution between soft tissues, and multiplanar imaging can be done without repositioning the patient (**Fig. 18–8**). As with CT, contrast agents are used (gadolinium) to highlight normal anatomy, show breakdown of the normal blood–brain barrier, identify inflammatory and mass lesions, and demonstrate vascularity. MRI gives very little information about bones and fractures. CT should

always be used when evaluating bony changes from tumors and in trauma. MRI scan times are considerably longer than CT. MRI is very sensitive to movement artifact (especially with surface coils), which can become significant when imaging the globe and orbit in uncooperative patients. MRI is contraindicated in patients with metallic objects in their eyes or head, cardiac pacemakers, or non-MR-compatible surgical clips.

Approach to the diagnosis of orbital disease

Clinical history

The time course over which pain, proptosis, blurred vision, and double vision develops often helps distinguish neoplastic disease from infectious and inflammatory disease. Patients with infectious or non-thyroid-associated inflammatory disease of the orbit generally have an acute course with symptom development over hours or days. In contrast, neoplastic conditions, including primary optic nerve tumors, usually evolve insidiously. The exceptions are with malignant tumors such as adenoid cystic carcinoma of the lacrimal gland, some metastatic tumors, and secondary orbital tumors extending from the paranasal sinuses.

Age

The patient's age group helps in the differential diagnosis of orbital disease. In the pediatric age group, congenital, developmental, and infectious lesions predominate. Fortunately, the majority of children with orbital disease will have a benign process.[48–53] Rhabdomyosarcoma is the most common malignant tumor of the orbit in children, while neuroblastoma and Ewing's sarcoma may metastasize to the orbit. In less developed countries, retinoblastoma spreading to the orbit is a common cause of proptosis.[54,55] Both idiopathic inflammatory disease of the orbit and TAO may occur in children, but are relatively infrequent entities. In adults, orbital cellulitis is less common, and thyroid eye disease becomes the most frequent cause of orbital dysfunction. Tumors of several different types may occur, with lymphoma being the most common.[56,57] In older adults, metastatic and secondary orbital tumors and dural sinus fistulas increase in frequency.

General physical findings

General physical findings are particularly important in several instances. In suspected TAO, the physical examination might show vital signs suggesting hyperthyroidism or hypothyroidism. Other patients may have a goiter. Any patient with an orbital mass lesion should have a careful examination for other signs of malignancy such as adenopathy that might be associated with systemic lymphoma or metastatic disease.

Imaging

Imaging will help localize the process and will often define an etiology. Although TAO may be diagnosed on clinical grounds, imaging is confirmatory and helps in staging and in determining whether the patient is at risk for vision loss. Patients with idiopathic orbital inflammatory disease should be imaged (echography, CT, or MRI) to aid in the differential diagnosis and determine disease extent at presentation. The vast majority of patients with orbital tumors will undergo neuroimaging with either CT scan or MRI scan. CT is the preferred modality in patients with a recent history of trauma and in patients in whom evaluation of bony changes is important. Both lytic lesions (malignant tumors) and hyperostosis (meningiomas or fibrous dysplasia) can be best demonstrated on CT. MRI has the distinct advantage over CT in terms of the details of soft tissue anatomy and abnormalities around the orbital apex and cavernous sinus. Both CT scan and MRI scanning will provide the necessary information to determine the relationship of an orbital mass lesion to the optic nerves, extraocular muscles, paranasal sinuses, and intracranial structures. Specific radiologic features for each of the various lesions are discussed below.

Neuro-ophthalmic examination

Although there is significant overlap in the examination findings of patients with each of the different forms of orbital disease and most cases are best qualified by diagnostic imaging studies, there are certain neuro-ophthalmologic examination features that help establish specific diagnoses (see examination section above). In general, the examiner must focus attention on identifying orbital disease. Externally the presence of swelling, chemosis, and hyperemia of the skin suggests an infectious or inflammatory process. Preseptal and orbital cellulitis are commonly associated with significant enough swelling to close the eye and create pseudoptosis. Idiopathic orbital inflammatory syndrome characteristically causes redness and swelling. The swelling of TAO is usually less acute but can be significant. Rarely, metastatic tumors and vascular lesions (with recent bleeding) can

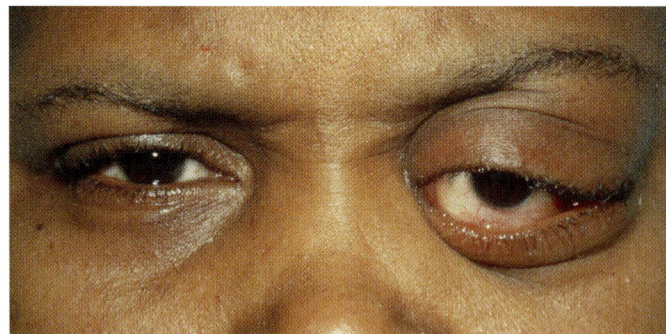

Figure 18–9. Non-axial (the globe is displaced downward in addition to outward) proptosis of the left eye and S-shaped deformity of the eyelid in a patient with an adenoid cystic carcinoma of the lacrimal gland.

present with acute swelling of the eyelid and periocular skin. The eyelid findings of lid retraction and lid lag are virtually diagnostic of TAO. Characteristic S-shaped deformity of the eyelid and non axial proptosis is present in patients with masses in and around the lacrimal gland (**Fig. 18–9**).

A mixed pattern eye movement abnormality, with positive forced ductions, is generally found on examination. Slowly expanding neoplasms can cause significant proptosis without motility restriction as opposed to TAO and myositis, which tend to restrict eye movements. The presence of optic nerve dysfunction with orbital signs suggests a primary optic nerve tumor, TAO, idiopathic orbital inflammation disease or a tumor of the sphenoid bone such as a meningioma. Other mass lesions and inflammatory diseases infrequently cause optic neuropathy.

Thyroid-associated ophthalmopathy

TAO is a self-limited, autoimmune condition usually occurring in association with hyperthyroidism. Historically a number of different terms have been used to label this condition including Graves orbitopathy, Graves ophthalmopathy, thyroid eye disease, thyroid orbitopathy, endocrine exophthalmos, malignant exophthalmos, and infiltrative ophthalmopathy. It is the most common orbital disorder in adults. In two separate series by orbital specialists, TAO constituted 32–47% of orbital disorders.[58,59] This percentage is different than the frequency of TAO in biopsy series,[60,61] since it rarely requires tissue confirmation to establish this clinical diagnosis. TAO should be considered in the neuro-ophthalmic differential diagnosis of double vision, particularly vertical double vision, and in any patient with orbital signs and symptoms.

Endocrine aspects of Graves disease

A negative feedback loop between the hypothalamus–anterior pituitary gland and the thyroid gland modulates thyroid function (see Chapter 7). The thyroid gland is composed of numerous tightly packed follicles invested in a rich capillary network. These follicles contain a rich proteinaceous colloid whose major component is thyroglobulin, the matrix protein in which thyroid hormones are synthesized. The hypothalamus secretes thyrotropin-releasing hormone (TRH), which in turn releases thyroid-stimulating hormone (TSH), a glycoprotein whose actions are mediated by cyclic adenosine monophosphate (cAMP). The TSH receptor on thyroid follicles is the site of action of autoantibodies which cause hyperthyroidism in Graves disease.[62-66] These antibodies are believed to be produced in the thyroid gland by clonally restricted B cells.[67,68] As well there may be an alteration in the organ-specific T-suppressor cells.[64-66] There is an extensive literature describing various environmentally triggered, immunogenetic events that lead to the development of Graves disease.[67,69-71]

Hormone production in the thyroid gland is followed by secretion of iodothyronines (T3 and T4). Most thyroid hormone is secreted as T4 and converted peripherally to T3. T4 is highly bound to thyroxin-binding globulin (TBG) and thyroxin-binding pre-albumin (TBPα). Thyrotoxicosis can result from overproduction of the hormone (true hyperthyroidism) or from inflammation-induced glandular hormone leakage. Graves disease or diffuse toxic goiter is the term used to describe a number of different conditions associated with elevated levels of thyroid hormones and associated ophthalmopathy and infiltrative dermatopathy.

Patients who develop hyperthyroidism present with a classic constellation of symptoms including nervousness, fatigue, weight loss, palpitations, heat intolerance, increased appetite, increased bowel movements, and sweating. Examination findings include tachycardia and a palpable goiter over which a thrill can often be felt. The laboratory abnormalities that accompany the presentation of Graves disease include elevated T3 and T4 levels, increased T3–T4 ratio, low TSH levels, thyrotropin receptor antibodies, antithyroid antibodies and abnormal T3 suppression tests. A low TSH level is believed to be the most sensitive indicator of thyroid dysfunction.[72-74]

Incidence and relationship of TAO to thyroid disease

Bartley et al.[75] reviewed the Mayo Clinic series within the Rochester Epidemiology project and identified 120 patients (103 women) with TAO in Olmsted county over a period of 15 years. The age-adjusted incidence rate for men was three cases per year per 100 000 people and for women 16 cases per year per 100 000 people. A bimodal age peak occurred in both sexes in the 40s and 60s with the peak in men occurring 5 years later than the peak in women. Endocrine dysfunction (most commonly Graves disease—autoimmune-induced hyperplasia of the thyroid gland associated with goiter and hyperthyroidism) developed in approximately 80–90% of patients found to have TAO. This endocrine dysfunction may manifest before, after, or concurrently with the ophthalmic findings.[76-80] However, many patients (35%) are diagnosed with TAO greater than 6 months after the diagnosis of hyperthyroidism. In the least common scenario, TAO precedes the endocrine dysfunction by more than 6 months (7%). Of all patients with hyperthyroidism, about 40% will develop clinical evidence of TAO at some time,[81] and the percentage is likely higher for subclinical disease found on orbital imaging. The disease is perhaps less common in Asian people[82,83] and black people from South Africa.[84]

Risk factors

The most potent risk factor for the development of TAO is hyperthyroidism, although there is a subset of patients who remain euthyroid. There may be other risk factors for the development of TAO, which include age, gender, smoking, and treatment of the hyperthyroid state with radioactive iodine. In several studies, smoking was shown to be a risk factor for the development and progression of TAO.[79,82,83,85-97] There is sufficient evidence to suggest that patients with hyperthyroidism or early TAO should be urged to stop smoking.[98]

TAO may also be more common and more severe in women with hyperthyroidism and in patients (particularly men) as they get older.[99] Although it remains a controversial issue, it appears that treatment of the hyperthyroid state with radioactive iodine is associated with new onset of TAO and exacerbations of TAO, perhaps associated with a sudden increase in autoantibodies.[86,100-102] This risk factor appears to be modified by the use of oral corticosteroids, which seem to reduce the risk of developing TAO and its progression to more severe stages in patients treated with radioactive iodine (see below).

Genetic predisposition

Graves disease and TAO occur in a population which is likely to be genetically at risk for an environmentally triggered autoimmune disease.[63,71,103-108] An immunogenetic predisposition is likely based on the increased incidence in certain human leukocyte antigen (HLA) (DR, B8, DQ3, and DW) types and recent genetic mapping of loci for Graves disease in some patients to chromosome 14.[105-112] This genetic localization to chromosome 14 is in the area of the gene for the TSH receptor, but to date there is significant genetic heterogeneity, and no mapping to the area of the HLA region has been found.[107,113,114] In current genetic models, the predisposition to autoimmune thyroid disease is thought to be multilocus and related to HLA genes and the TSH receptor gene.[115-118]

Pathophysiology

There is an extensive literature concerning the autoimmune mechanism of Graves disease and TAO.[119-126] It appears to be mediated by both humoral and cell-mediated immunity, although the cause, precise immunopathology, and the specific autoantigen that results in lymphocytic infiltration of the orbit are unknown.[126,127] The relationship between Graves disease and TAO may simply be a closely related organ-specific autoimmune condition with an antigenic similarity between orbital and thyroid tissues. Graves disease is likely to be mediated by an autoimmune process directed against a portion of the thyrotropin receptor.[128] These antibodies bind to the TSH receptor sites and increase the gland's activity. These thyrotropin receptor antibodies may stimulate the development of intracellular matrix proteins (glycosaminoglycans) in orbital fat and eye muscles. This subsequently leads to swelling of the orbital tissue and inflammation, then results in scarring. Activation of orbital fibroblasts seems also to play a role.[123,129]

Abnormal binding of the sera of patients with TAO to extraocular muscles in culture has been demonstrated.[130] However, the exact nature of the cross-reactive antigen in the orbital tissue is less clear and controversial, but it may be the thyrotropin receptor or a 64 kDa membrane antigen, tropomodulin.[131,132] A novel protein G2s (a portion of mito-chondrial succinate dehydrogenase) has been cloned and characterized and may be the best candidate for the cross-reactive antigen in eye muscle.[133] Other candidate antigens that have been characterized include the 67 kDa flavopro-tein (Fp) subunit of the enzyme succinate dehydrogenase, calsequestrin, a 63 kDa calcium-binding protein, and colla-gen XIII, a connective tissue antigen.[134–136] Wall and associ-ates[137–140] have postulated a two-stage process in which there is first autoantibodies and CD4 (helper) T cells which cross-react with eye muscle proteins leading to inflammation and swelling. The second stage involves a more cytotoxic stage in which there is inflammation and scarring of the muscles and orbital connective tissue secondary to released muscle membrane antigens during stage one. The antibodies to eye muscles may not be part of the pathogenesis but may develop subsequent to muscle damage by the cytotoxic T cells.[124,141] There may also be a direct effect of TSH receptor antibodies on orbital adipose cells stimulating adipogenesis and increased orbital fat volume. Alternatively antibodies to the insulin-like growth factor receptor may stimulate hyaluro-nan production, thus playing a key role in the development of inflammation.[124]

Pathology

The pathology of TAO reflects the above autoimmune inflammation. Infiltrating plasma cells, lymphocytes, and mast cells are seen. In addition there is deposition of hydrophilic glycosaminoglycans and collagen that are part of the scarring process. In acute stages, the changes are largely inflammatory. As the disease progresses there is more deposition of collagen and muscle degeneration. In the chronic inactive stage there is often fatty infiltration of the muscles.

Neuro-ophthalmic features of thyroid-associated ophthalmopathy

The clinical presentation of TAO is highly variable and has been divided and grouped in many different ways. Most classifications are artificial and do not reflect the step-wise progression that often characterizes TAO.

Symptoms. These include periocular soft tissue swelling (**Fig 18–10**), lid retraction, and bulging of the eyes. Some patients recognize and present with abnormal head postures or binocular double vision in upgaze or downgaze. Bartley and associates[142] reviewed their 120 patients and noted that 36 complained of pain, 20 patients had double vision, 25 patients had tearing, 19 patients had photophobia, and nine had "blurred" vision. Only two patients complained of decreased vision attributed to optic nerve dysfunction at presentation.[142] Thus, vision loss secondary to optic neu-ropathy is usually recognized while the patient is being monitored.

While discomfort, corneal irritation, foreign body sensa-tion, and "burning" are common complaints in patients with TAO, significant pain and pain on eye movements are unusual. In fact this is an important historical point to clarify in a patient with an acute orbital syndrome. The pres-ence of significant pain should point the examiner away

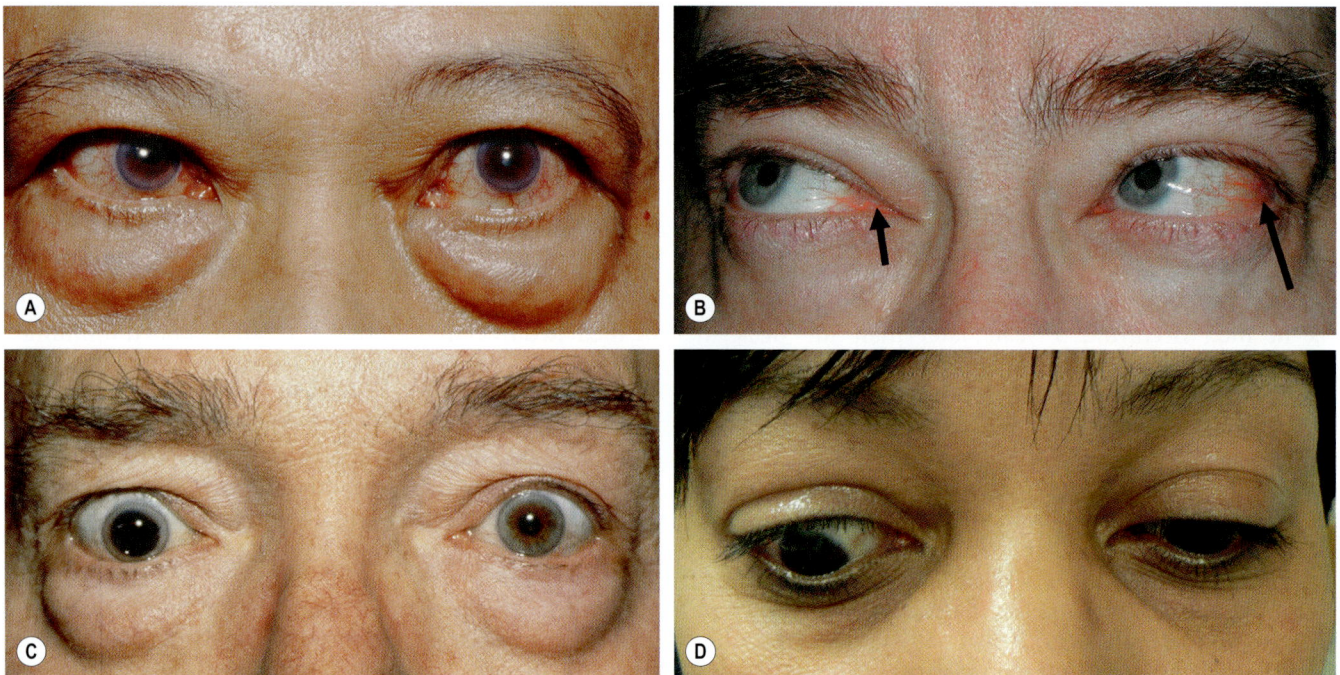

Figure 18–10. Typical appearance of thyroid-associated ophthalmopathy (TAO). **A**. Acute presentation. Proptosis as well as significant soft tissue swelling with fat herniation around the eyes and mild lid retraction are seen. In the acute phase (**B**) injection can be seen over the rectus muscle insertions (long arrow) and in the area of the caruncle (short arrow). **C**. Lid retraction with visible sclera between limbus and upper eyelid position is observed. The right pupil was pharmacologically dilated. **D**. Lid lag is common in TAO. The patient's right upper eyelid does not follow the globe in downgaze.

from TAO and towards idiopathic orbital inflammation, infections, and tumors. Similarly, the tempo of presentation is usually gradual as symptoms develop over weeks. Orbital symptoms developing over hours or even a few days are more consistent with other acute conditions, including infections and non-thyroid inflammatory conditions. The majority of patients with TAO will have bilateral signs and symptoms although asymmetric and even unilateral disease do occur.

Eyelid signs. The eyelid manifestations of TAO are virtually pathognomonic. Lid retraction, which is present if the upper eyelid rests above the superior corneal limbus, is evident in most patients with TAO (**Fig. 18–10**).[142] This likely results from local adhesion of the levator muscle to fixed orbital tissue.[143] Other postulated mechanisms include superior rectus overaction, secondary inferior rectus scarring, increased circulating sympathomimetics, and muscle hypertrophy. Although most patients with TAO have eyelid retraction, it is not always present (**Fig. 18–11**). Lid retraction can also be seen in patients with dorsal midbrain dysfunction, ptosis of the contralateral eyelid, use of sympathomimetic drugs, aberrant regeneration of the third nerve, previous retinal detachment surgery, and Guillain–Barré syndrome (see Chapter 14). Lid lag (persistent elevation of the upper eyelid in downgaze, **Fig. 18–10**) and lagophthalmos (inferior corneal exposure) are other common eyelid manifestations of TAO. Swelling and edema of the eyelids and periocular skin, dermatochalasis, and orbital fat herniation are also common (**Fig 18–10**). Periorbital swelling is typically worse in the morning after the patient sleeps, during which the eye is in a gravity-dependent position. Conjunctival chemosis and injection (particularly over the rectus muscle insertions) is often present (**Fig. 18–10**). Swelling and redness in the area of the caruncle is a particularly important sign of active TAO (**Fig. 18–10**). Occult TAO should be considered in the differential diagnosis of patients with dry eye.[144]

Proptosis. Axial proptosis is recognized in about two-thirds of patients with TAO.[142] The average normal measurement for the exophthalmometer in each eye is 17 mm, and in most patients is less than 22 mm. Any interocular difference greater than 2 mm is considered abnormal. The base used should be the same from exam to exam so that measurements from each visit can be compared.

Myopathy. The presentation of TAO-associated myopathy may be symptomatic (double vision or eye movement limitation) or asymptomatic (recognized on imaging studies). Patients may unknowingly and insidiously develop a chin-up posture because of ocular misalignment or restriction with fusion occurring more easily in downgaze. Muscle dysfunction usually begins gradually, may be intermittent and can occur without other evidence of significant inflammation. The inflammatory process has a peculiar predilection for the inferior and medial rectus muscles, and the restrictive myopathy results in the characteristic hypertropia and esotropia, respectively (**Fig. 18–12**). Involvement of the superior rectus is less frequent while lateral rectus involvement is rare.

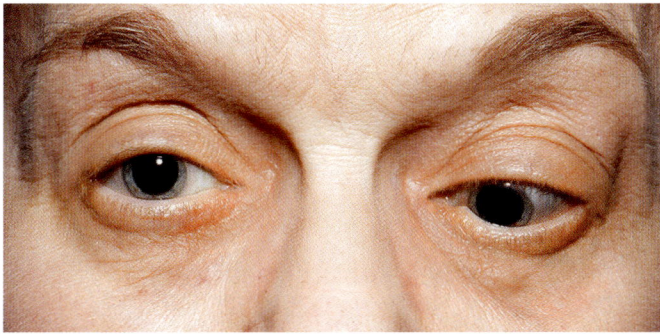

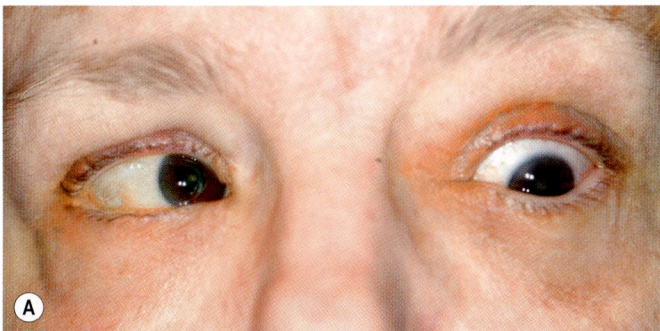

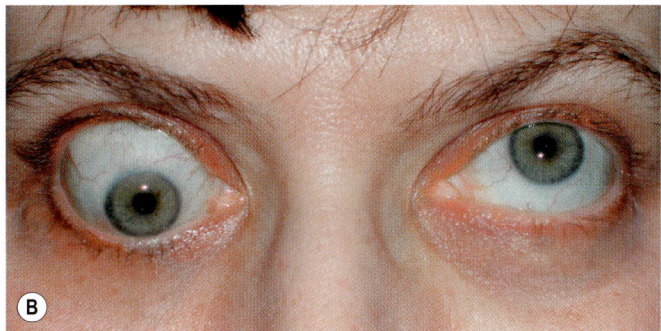

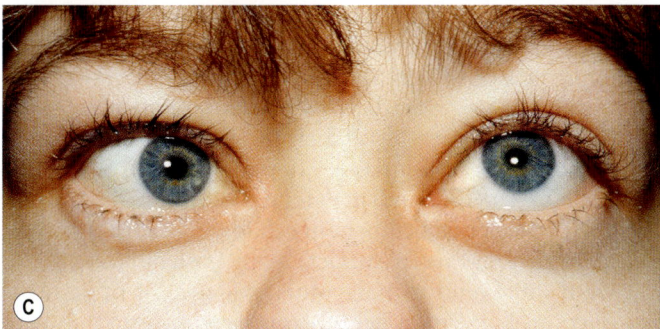

Figure 18–11. Thyroid-associated ophthalmopathy associated with left hypotropia and esotropia.

Figure 18–12. Restrictive eye movements in thyroid-associated ophthalmopathy. **A**. Most patients demonstrate limitation of elevation and abduction. Large hyperdeviations (**B**) with lid retraction on attempted upgaze and may be present significant asymmetry in eye muscle function. Patients with bilateral elevation deficits (**C**) can present with a chin up posture to lessen efforts to bring the eyes up to primary position.

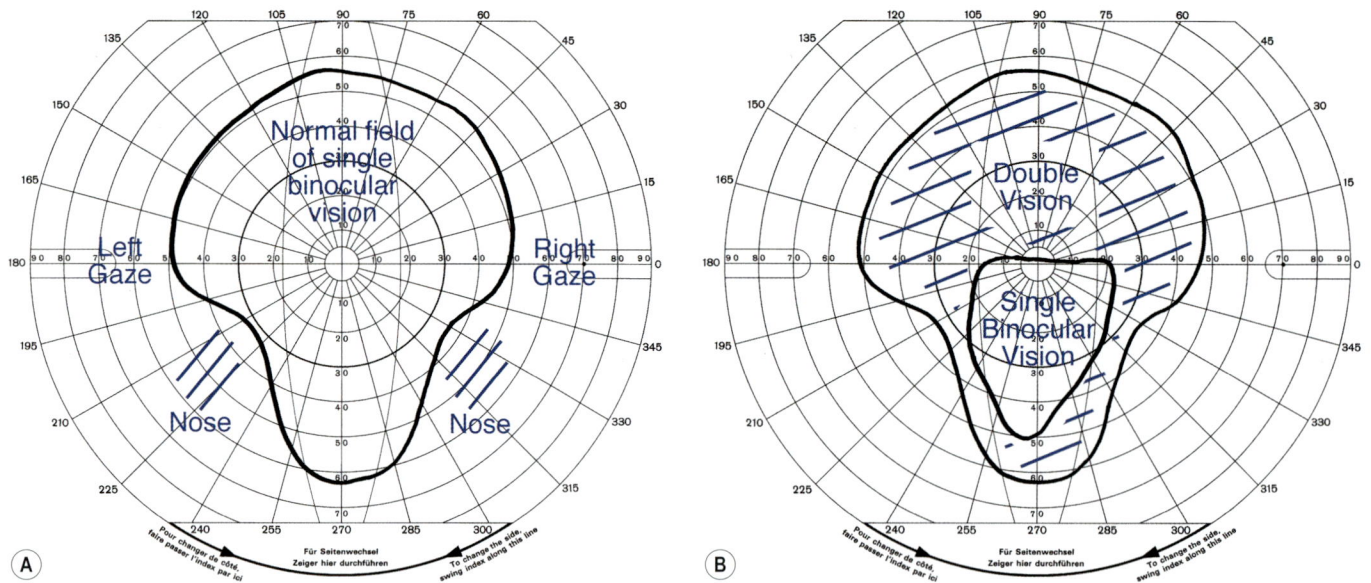

Figure 18–13. Diplopia visual fields are charted on the Goldmann perimeter and may be used to follow thyroid-associated ophthalmopathy (TAO) patients with diplopia. The patient is tested with both eyes open and asked to track the V4e stimulus and signal the perimetrist when diplopia develops. **A.** The normal field of single monocular vision is "skull" shaped and limited in down and lateral gazes by the nose. **B.** A patient with TAO demonstrating a reduced field of single monocular vision particularly in upgaze and lateral gaze.

Ocular ductions and alignment. Efforts have been made to measure eye movements in TAO, particularly for the purpose of classification within a grading system. Mourits and associates[145] suggested using a hand perimeter to measure the extent of ocular ductions. Although their method proved to be precise and reproducible, it is not wildly available, and in our opinion does not aid in the management of TAO-associated myopathy. Our preference is to grade eye movement limitations on a scale from –4 to +4 or in percentages (see Chapter 2) and to quantify ocular misalignments in all fields of gaze with prisms. "Diplopia visual fields" are also an effective method that can be used to quantify and follow patients with TAO-associated ocular misalignments. To perform this test a Goldmann perimeter is used, both eyes are left uncovered, and the head positioned in the center. The patient is asked to follow the stimulus and report when it becomes double. A field of single binocular vision is then charted (**Fig. 18–13**). Photographic documentation of the ocular ductions may also be helpful in following patients (**Fig. 18–12**).

Ocular cyclodeviations have also been described in TAO both spontaneously and as a complication of surgical treatment.[146,147] Involvement of the inferior rectus (without obvious eye movement limitations) can closely mimic the appearance of a contralateral superior oblique palsy.[148] Infiltrative TAO with restrictive myopathy is also associated with elevation of intraocular pressure on upgaze.[149,150] The significance of the pressure elevation is uncertain and is rarely used to make a diagnosis. Other causes of extraocular muscle dysfunction in patients with TAO include ocular neuromyotonia[151] and concurrent myasthenia gravis.[142,152,153]

Optic neuropathy. Optic neuropathy is the most feared complication from TAO. The incidence of visual loss is between 2% and 9% of all patients with TAO.[142,154–156] However, in patients with "severe" TAO requiring orbital

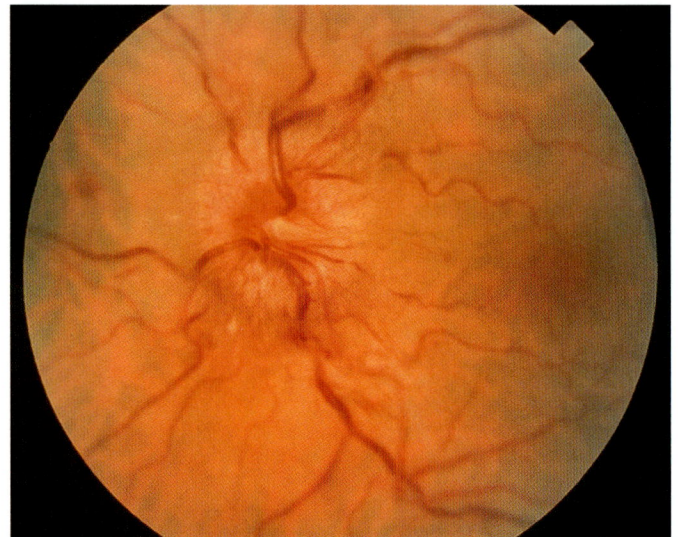

Figure 18–14. Acute optic nerve swelling in TA (thyroid-associated) ophthalmopathy. Some patients with compression of the optic nerve can develop disc edema in association with optic neuropathy.

decompression, optic neuropathy occurs in up to 50% of patients.[157–159] Vision loss from optic nerve dysfunction requires immediate management.

Neigel et al.[156] reported on the clinical profile of dysthyroid optic neuropathy in 58 (8.6%) patients out of 675 with TAO. About 20% of the patients present unilaterally. At the time of presentation roughly half the patients have normal appearing nerves, one-quarter showed pallor, and another quarter had swelling and hyperemia (**Fig. 18–14**).[160] About half the patients had acuity better than 20/40, but half were worse. In this and other studies, many patients were 20/20 but were still found to have other evidence of optic nerve dysfunction.[161,162] Visual field defects were measured in two-thirds of patients, and the most common defect types included paracentral scotomas, increased blind spots, nerve fiber defects, central or centrocecal defects, and generalized constriction.[156] Many patients can have relatively quiet and inactive appearing disease at the time of their presentation with optic neuropathy.[160] Persistent elevation of the intraocular pressure in patients with TAO may be associated with glaucomatous optic neuropathy, and this should be considered in the differential diagnosis of visual field defects in these patients.[163]

Apical crowding of the optic nerve by the enlarged extraocular muscles is the main mechanism of vision loss (**Fig. 18–15**).[158,161,162] Vision loss can also be associated with stretch or tenting of the optic nerve from severe proptosis (**Fig. 18–16**). Men with TAO seem to be a greater risk for the development of optic neuropathy. Advancing age, diabetes, the amount of restrictive strabismus as well as total volume of the extraocular muscles have all been reported as risk factors.[156,164,165]

Imaging in thyroid-associated ophthalmopathy

Noninvasive imaging of the orbit is the gold standard for the diagnosis of TAO. Echography, CT, and MRI may be used to confirm the diagnosis of TAO. The classic finding is enlargement of the extraocular muscle belly with relative sparing of the tendon (**Fig. 18–17**), although a small percentage of patients will demonstrate involvement of the tendon on CT or MRI.[166] Proptosis may also be recognized without extraocular muscle enlargement and presumably results from increased swelling and volume of the intraorbital fat. In addition, CT and MRI scans frequently demonstrate proptosis, enlargement of the lacrimal gland, and eyelid soft tissue swelling.[167–175] As expected, enlargement is most commonly seen in the inferior rectus and medial rectus but the lateral rectus can be involved (**Figs. 18–15, 18–16** and **18–17**). The disease is usually symmetric but cases of isolated muscle involvement and primarily lateral rectus involvement are

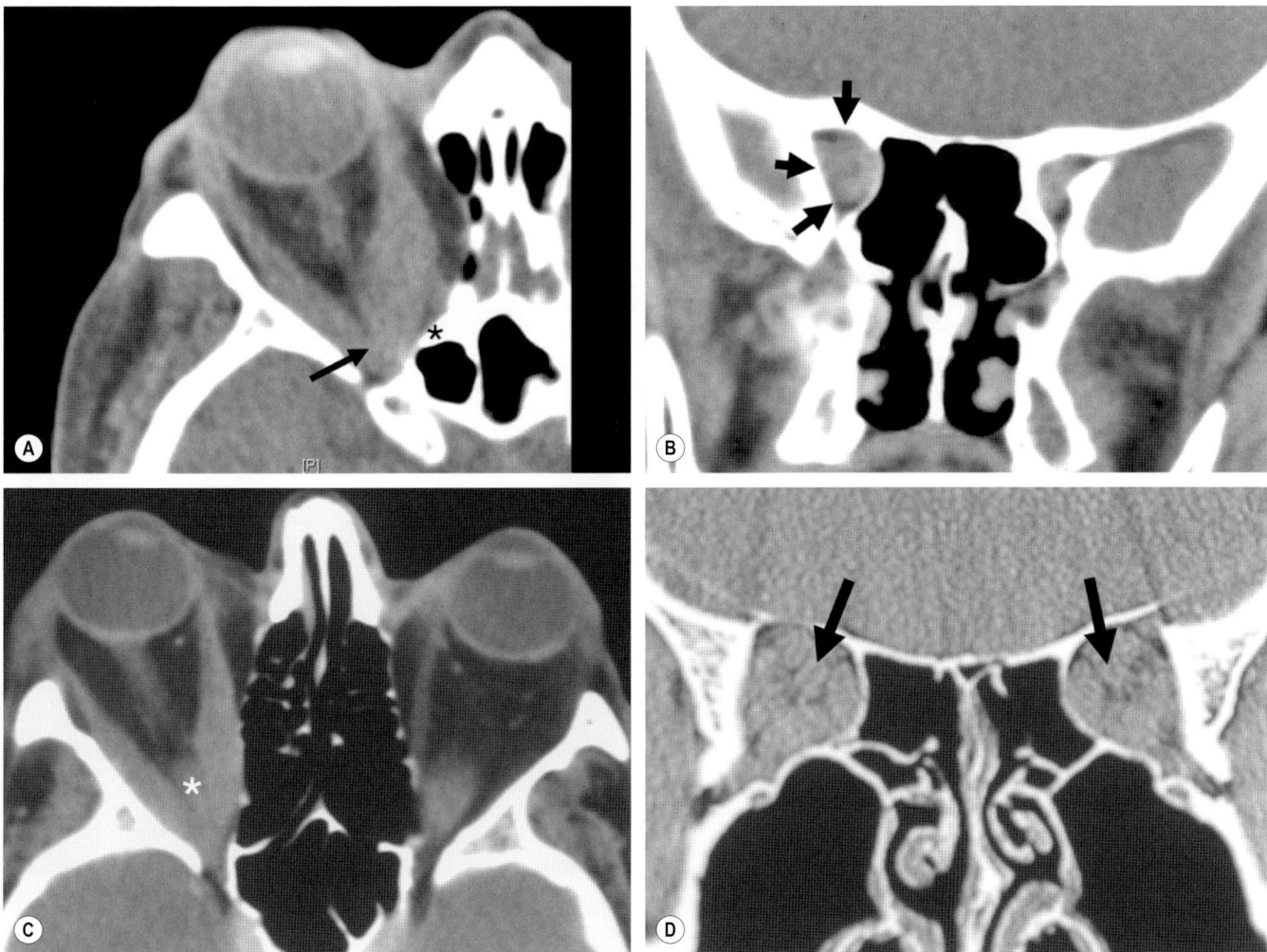

Figure 18–15. Orbital apex crowding in patients with thyroid-associated ophthalmopathy (TAO) and optic neuropathy. Patients with TAO should be screened with CT or MRI of the orbits and evaluated for crowding of the orbital apex on axial and coronal images. **A.** The enlarged medial rectus can be seen crowding and compressing the optic nerve (arrow) in the orbital apex. This patient has had a previous medial wall decompression but not complete decompression of the bone at the orbital apex (asterisk). On coronal CT scan (**B**) there is no distinction of the extraocular muscles (arrows) from the optic nerve indicating compression and contact of the muscles with the optic nerve. **C.** In another patient posterior fusiform enlargement of the medial rectus is seen crowding the orbital apex and compressing the optic nerve (asterisk). In a coronal image (**D**) the optic nerves (arrows) are difficult to distinguish from the surrounding enlarged extraocular muscles.

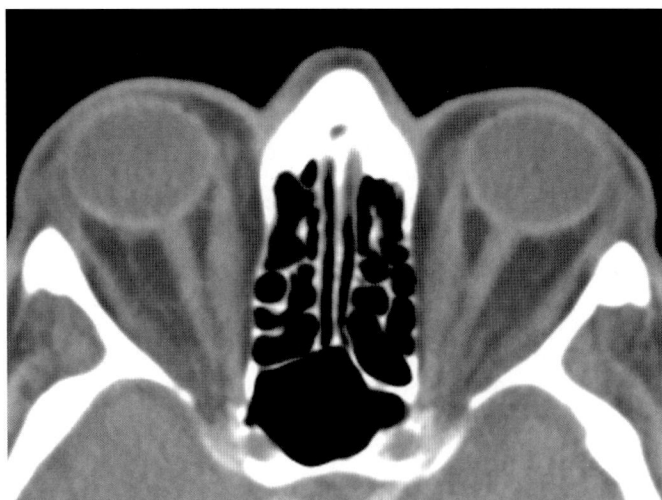

Figure 18–16. Tenting and stretching of the optic nerves in a patient with proptosis secondary to thyroid-associated ophthalmopathy and optic neuropathy. The optic nerves appear abnormally straightened secondary to orbital fat inflammation and proliferation.

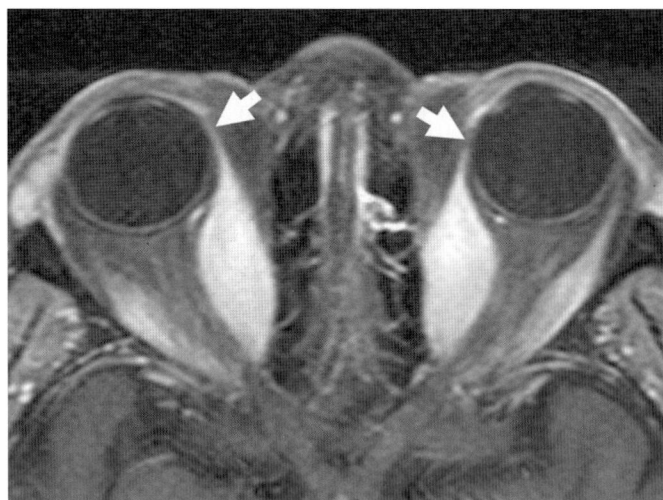

Figure 18–17. Axial T1-weighted gadolinium-enhanced MRI scan of a patient with thyroid-associated ophthalmopathy. Note the fusiform enlargement of the extraocular muscles with sparing of the tendonous insertions (arrows) which appear normal.

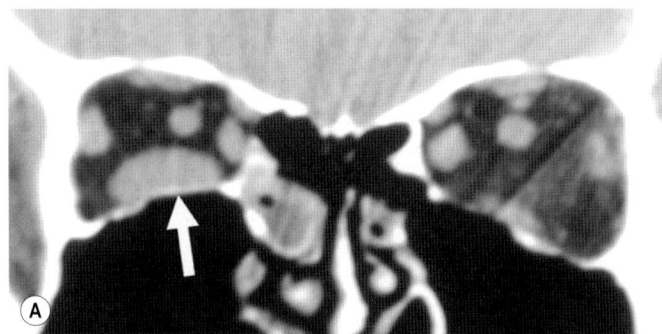

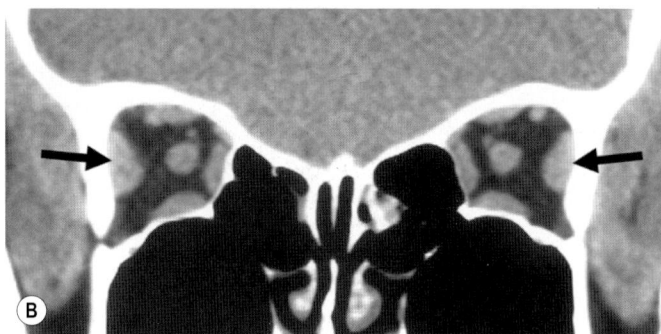

Figure 18–18. Atypical imaging findings (coronal CT scans) in thyroid-associated ophthalmopathy showing markedly asymmetric disease as in (**A**) which demonstrates primarily isolated involvement of the inferior rectus on the right side (arrow) and (**B**) enlargement of both lateral rectus muscles (arrows) in a patient presenting with an exotropia.

seen (**Fig. 18–18**). CT and MRI scans, unlike echography, provide excellent images of the orbital apex and usually document enlarged muscles surrounding and in contact with the optic nerve in patients with optic neuropathy (**Fig. 18–15**). Low-density areas may be noted in the muscle bellies and may represent collections of lymphocytes or glycosaminoglycan deposition. With chronic inactive disease larger low-density lesions can be seen within the muscles, owing to fatty infiltration (**Fig. 18–19**). Occasionally chronic medial rectus muscle enlargement can be associated with bone molding and bowing into the ethmoid sinus. CT scan can be used to monitor treatment.

MRI scanning of the orbit effectively images the orbital soft tissues, including enlarged extraocular muscles[168–172,176,177] and the orbital apex (**Figs. 18–17** and **18–19**), and may have a distinct advantage over CT scanning in assessing disease activity in addition to muscle size. The recommended MR sequence is STIR (short tau inversion recovery), which highlights the extraocular muscles, and peak signal intensity from the most inflamed muscle correlates well with clinical activity of the disease.[168–172] High water content can be detected with this sequence, presumably reflecting disease activity. This may be a method for following patients for radiographic

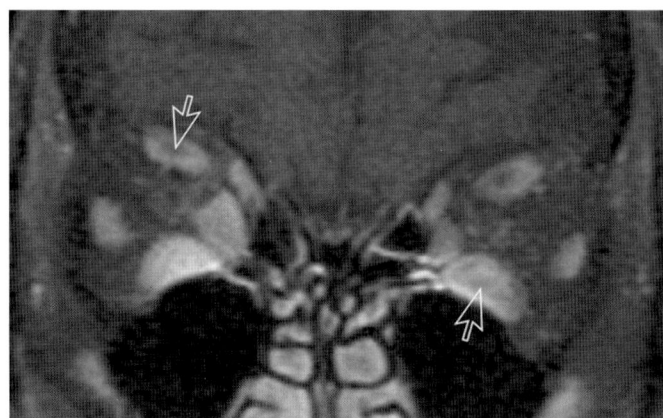

Figure 18–19. Coronal T1-weighted, fat suppressed, gadolinium-enhanced, MRI scan of a patient with thyroid-associated ophthalmopathy demonstrating lucencies (open arrows) in the extraocular muscles consistent with fatty infiltration.

evidence of persistent inflammation.[168–172,176,177] Studies measuring eye movements during cine MRI scanning have demonstrated normal movements early in the disease but confirmed the presence of restricted eye movements later in its course.[176]

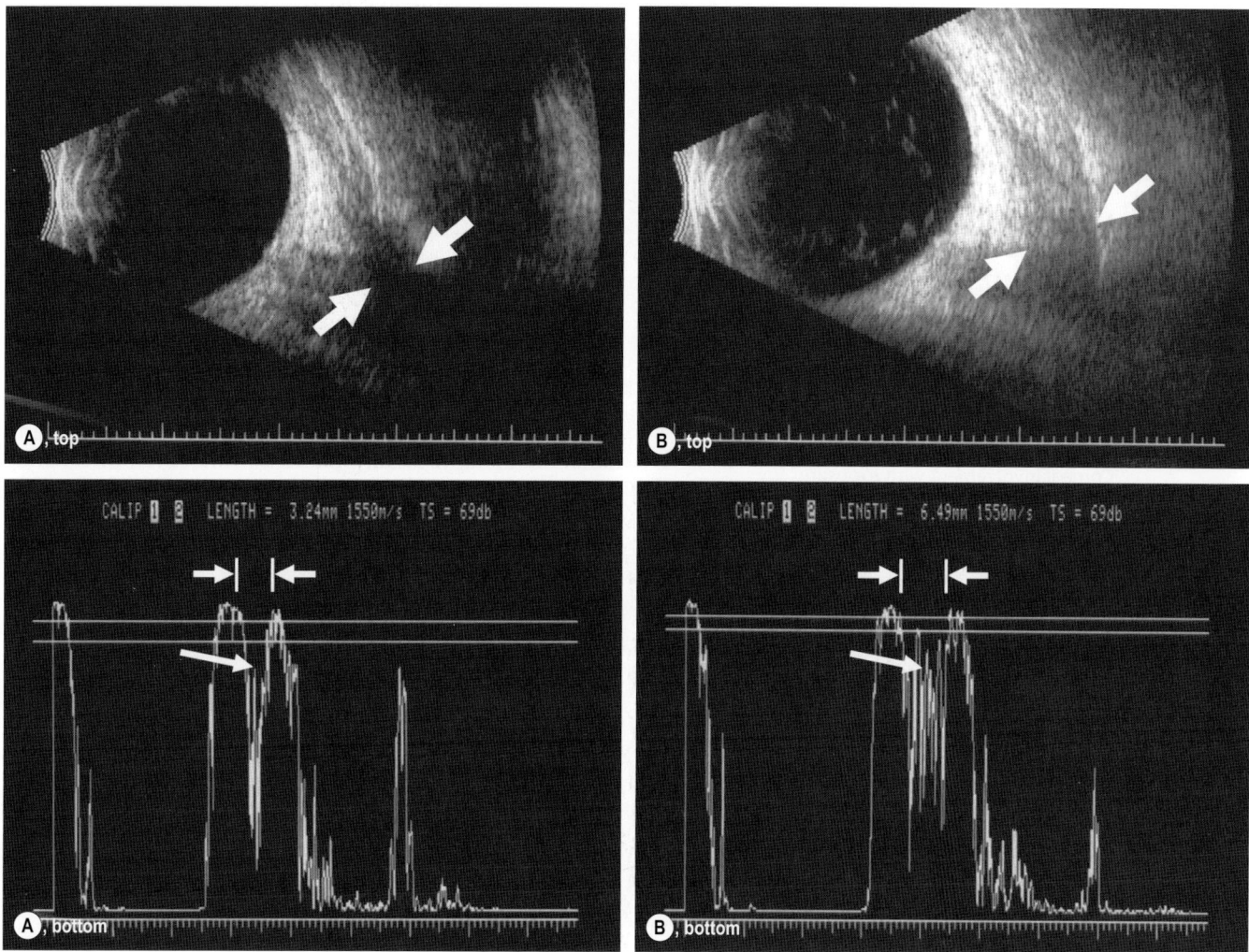

Figure 18–20. Orbital echography in a normal orbit and thyroid-associated ophthalmopathy (TAO). **A.** The normal appearance of an extraocular muscle on both A and B scan. The B scan (top) demonstrates normal muscle width (arrows). On the A scan (bottom) the white bars and small arrows delineate the limits of the muscle width, and there is low to medium muscle reflectivity (long arrow). In a patient with TAO (**B**) on B scan (top), the muscle belly (arrows) is enlarged. Simultaneous A scan (bottom) confirms an enlarged width of the extraocular muscle (denoted by white bars and small arrows) compared to normal, with numerous areas of high internal reflectivity (long arrow).

Echography has proven valuable in the office diagnosis of TAO.[38–40,42,169,178,179] Abnormal muscle size (A and B scan) and internal reflectivity (A scan) can be compared to normative data, and enlargement can be documented (**Fig. 18–20**).[180,181] The ability of echography to characterize muscle reflectivity in addition to enlargement is advantageous when trying to determine the etiology of an enlarged muscle. Echography was shown to be more sensitive than CT scan in detecting extraocular muscle enlargement and abnormal internal reflectivity secondary to separation of the muscle fibers,[40,178,179] and by demonstrating abnormal muscle reflectivity may be particularly useful in the evaluation of patients with double vision and minimal external signs of TAO.[179] However, echography may not be as efficacious as other imaging modalities for diagnosing orbital tumors.

Classification

Several different classification systems have been proposed for descriptive and clinical research studies of TAO. The so-called NOSPECS classification system was initially described by Werner (**Table 18–4**).[182,183] This classification system had been widely used in clinical research studies; however, not all patients progress through the seven classes as listed, and some have prominent features in the higher numbered classes without some of the milder signs. The NOSPECS classification system has been recently criticized because (a) its poor characterization of the condition with no indication of disease activity, marked underrepresentation of eyelid position, and overrepresentation of corneal problems; (b) it implies a continuous or stepladder progression of disease as a numbered classification system would suggest; (c) parts of it are subjective; and (d) the gradings within classes 3, 5, and 6 are poor.[184–186] More recently, the European Group on Graves Orbitopathy (EUGOGO), has proposed a more simplified system.[187] In this system patients are divided into three groups (**Table 18–5**), mild, moderate, and sight threatening. Along with clinical activity score these categories can used to guide the types and urgency of treatment.

Table 18–4 The NOSPECS classification of thyroid-associated ophthalmopathy[182,183]

Class	Clinical features
0	**N**o signs or symptoms
1	**O**nly signs such as lid retraction
2	**S**oft tissue periorbital swelling A–C: minimal to marked
3	**P**roptosis of the eyes A = 3–4 mm, B = 5–7 mm, C ≥ 8 mm
4	**E**xtraocular muscle involvement A = limitation B = evidence of restriction C = fixation of globe
5	**C**orneal involvement with exposure A = stippling B = ulceration C = clouding, necrosis, perforation
6	**S**ight loss secondary to optic neuropathy A = disc pale or swollen, 20/20–20/60, field defect B = same but vision 20/70–20/200, C = same but vision less than 20/200

Table 18–5 EUGOGO severity classification in thyroid-associated ophthalmopathy (TAO)[187]

Classification	Findings
Mild	Minor impact on daily life (not justifying steroid treatment) Minor (<2 mm) lid retraction Minor soft tissue swelling Less than 3 mm proptosis Transient or no diplopia Exposure symptoms responsive to lubricants
Moderate	Significant impact on daily life (which if active justifies steroid or surgical treatment) Greater than 3 mm or proptosis Diplopia
Sight threatening	TAO associated optic neuropathy Exposure keratitis warranting immediate intervention

Classification of TAO must be combined with some measure of the clinical activity of the disease when trying to make decisions about treatment. The Clinical Activity Score (CAS)[188-190] (**Table 18–6**) has been proposed to assess the degree of active inflammation, and accurate assessment of active disease will be critical when assessing different treatments in clinical trials. Patients can be considered to have mild, moderate, or severe periorbital swelling, with or without extraocular muscle dysfunction, and/or visual dysfunction secondary to compressive optic neuropathy or severe exposure. In this system patients with only mild or moderate symptoms are treated conservatively. Patients with

Table 18–6 Clinical Activity Score (CAS) in thyroid-associated ophthalmopathy.[188-190] A CAS score of ≥3/7 following signs and symptoms generally indicates active disease

Spontaneous retrobulbar pain
Pain on eye movement
Redness of the eyelids
Redness of the conjunctiva
Swelling of the eyelids
Inflammation of the caruncle or plica
Conjunctival edema

more debilitating symptoms of swelling and eye muscle involvement and a high CAS score are considered for more aggressive treatment, including systemic corticosteroids and radiation therapy. Finally patients with vision-threatening disease are treated emergently both medically (intravenous steroids) and with orbital decompression if necessary.

Treatment of TAO

The treatment of TAO is complex, often requiring a multidisciplinary approach which includes a neuro-ophthalmologist, orbital specialist and surgeon, radiation therapist, and endocrinologist. Fortunately most patients do well, and in fact three-quarters of patients require no or only supportive therapy. Most patients do not develop sight-threatening complications of double vision or optic neuropathy.[191] The disease usually runs a self-limited course of 18–36 months, and up to two-thirds of patients with TAO will improve spontaneously.[192]

Appropriate management is dependent on accurate assessment of the clinical findings at the time of presentation, including careful evaluation of visual function, eye movements, and orbital imaging. In patients with lid retraction and proptosis only, reassurance, ocular lubrication when exposure or ocular discomfort is present, elevation of the head of the bed to reduce dependency edema, and cessation of smoking are the only treatments recommended. Here it is important to emphasize to the patient that the condition tends to remit, and that ultimately cosmetic aspects of the disease can be addressed. These patients tend to be young, and when the disease is quiescent may choose to have orbital decompression or eyelid surgery to improve their appearance.

Infiltrative disease with myopathy and increased orbital congestion are indications for more aggressive forms of therapy to reduce symptoms and the likelihood of developing permanent dysfunction. Patients with double vision and no congestive signs are often treated conservatively with prisms or patching as needed. The two major options for those patients requiring more aggressive therapy are systemic corticosteroids and orbital radiation. With this in mind, a meta-analysis of the literature has been recently performed.[193]

Steroids and other medical therapies. As signs and symptoms of severe congestive orbitopathy increase, treatment should first consist of oral[194] (1–1.5 mg/kg prednisone daily) or intravenous corticosteroids (1 g methylprednisolone IV (intravenous) daily for 3–5 days). These doses are arbitrary and not based on any prospective data. Review of various clinical case series would suggest that intravenous steroids are slightly more effective and may be associated with fewer side-effects.[193] About two-thirds of patients will have reduction in their symptoms and swelling in about 1 week.[193,195] Although symptoms of congestion improve on steroids, only about one-third of patients show improvement of the eye movements. Intravenous steroids can be given in simple pulses or followed by oral steroids, which then can be slowly tapered by 10 mg per daily dose each week. If symptoms worsen then reinstituting the original successful dose and radiation therapy should be considered; however, the long-term use of recurrent doses of steroids is often associated with significant side-effects and should be avoided. In patients with more severe orbitopathy, or significant vision loss from compressive optic neuropathy, intravenous methylprednisolone is favored and has been shown to be effective.[88,196,197]

Other medical therapies, including plasmapheresis,[194,198] intravenous immunoglobulin,[199,200] intravenous somatostatin,[201] and rituximab[202,203] have been shown to be effective but have not assumed primary roles in the medical management of TAO. While not effective on its own, cyclosporine has been shown to be effective as a combined therapy with prednisone in patients who do not respond to either drug alone,[204] and octreotride long-acting repeatable (LAR), which initially was thought to be an effective treatment,[205] was found to be ineffective in a double-blind, placebo-controlled trial.[206]

As stated earlier, treatment of hyperthyroidism with radioactive iodine is associated with worsening of TAO. This deterioration may be lessened by the use of oral corticosteroids before and after the radioactive iodine treatment.[86,100,101,207] Bartalena and associates[100,101] found that 15% of patients treated with radioactive iodine alone developed or had worsening of TAO. In contrast, none of the patients treated with radioactive iodine and prednisone had progression of disease. Thus prednisone is recommended in all patients with active TAO undergoing treatment with radioactive iodine for hyperthyroidism. In addition, a prolonged period of hypothyroidism after treatment should also be avoided.[98,101] Steroids are not necessary in patients undergoing radioactive iodine treatment with no or inactive TAO. Some have recommended that radioactive iodine treatment be avoided in patients with active or severe TAO, and that medical therapy with antithyroid drugs be used instead.[207,208]

Radiation therapy. Radiotherapy for TAO has been reported to be effective in 70% of patients,[193–195,209] often taking several weeks (often with transient worsening requiring steroids) to take effect. Most patients considered for radiotherapy have congestive eye signs with diplopia or optic neuropathy. Several series have demonstrated favorable responses in patients treated with radiation with or without steroids.[193–195,197,209–214] However, Gorman and associates reported no long-term benefit of radiation in a prospective blinded study in which one orbit was radiated and the other left untreated.[215,216] This study has been criticized because some treated patients may have been in inactive phases of their disease. Other evidence suggests that radiation should not be considered as a last resort but more appropriately should be used early in the course of the disease in conjunction with steroid therapy in clinically active patients.[193]

The technique generally involves the use of 1500–2000 cGy in divided fractions over 10 days. Care is taken to irradiate only the posterior two-thirds of the orbit, thereby avoiding the globe. Radiation may be more effective than steroids in the treatment of optic neuropathy. In one study, only one of 29 patients treated with radiation for optic neuropathy required subsequent surgical decompression while six of 16 treated with steroids needed surgery.[217] Improvement in soft tissue swelling almost always occurs. MRI scanning has been used to monitor the positive effects of radiation treatment, as reduced signal in the eye muscles presumably correlates with lower water content.[213] Careful, quantitative measurements of eye movements often demonstrate some improvement, although this does not correlate with improvement in double vision.[218,219] Rootman[194] found that only 14% of his patients had recurrence of symptoms after radiotherapy. Complications of radiation therapy are rare although radiation retinopathy has been reported,[216,220] and a slight increase in the risk of secondary malignancy has been suggested.[221] The use of radiation therapy for TAO remains controversial and will remain so until a prospective trial is performed on patients with active disease.[193,216,222]

Surgery. Surgical treatment of TAO is indicated in two separate situations. The first is orbital decompression for sight-threatening disease secondary to severe exposure or optic neuropathy from orbital apex crowding. The second is the use of orbital decompression, eye muscle surgery, and eyelid surgery in the patient with quiescent disease who has double vision, exposure, or a significant cosmetic problem. Orbital decompression should not be used in the acute treatment of proptosis and swelling from TAO unless there is sight-threatening disease. Mechanical decompression of the orbit has been described in several large series and is safe and effective in improving visual function in patients with apex crowding secondary to TAO-associated myopathy[155,157,223–244] Removal of the orbital floor and medial wall (**Fig. 18–21**) using various approaches is the most common surgery performed. Mourits[238] and associates compared the coronal method to the inferomedial and the inferomedial plus lateral approach and found each to be equally effective in treating vision loss. Recently, endoscopic approaches have become popular as they appear to be equally effective and avoid external scarring.[229,233,235,239,241,244–247]

Regardless of the technique employed, successful treatment requires decompression of the orbital apex through removal of the apical portions of the orbital walls and opening or removing the periorbita (**Fig 18–21**). Visual improvement should be prompt and if vision fails to improve, the decompression was likely incomplete at the orbital apex. Severe vision loss preoperatively is associated with a worse prognosis postoperatively as only four of seven patients with less than 20/200 vision preoperatively attained visual acuity of 20/40 postoperatively in one series.[248] Significant improvement in nearly all parameters of the optic neuropathy including visual fields and optic disc swelling

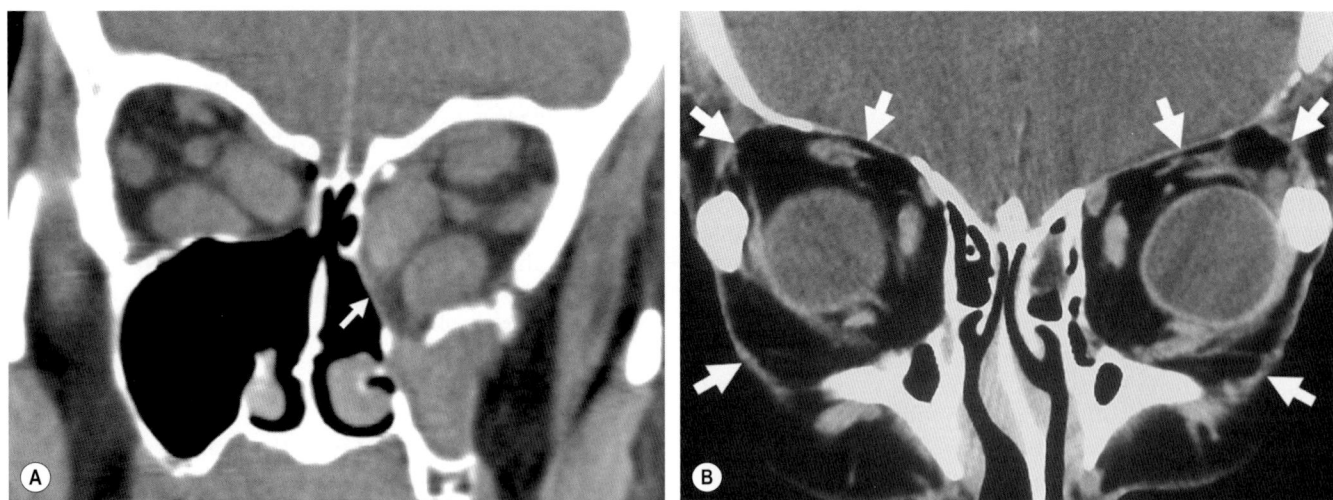

Figure 18–21. CT scan appearance of two patients after orbital decompression. **A**. The extraocular muscles are seen to fall into the maxillary sinus after removal of the medial wall (arrow) and the floor. **B**. Coronal CT scan of the orbits in a patient who had undergone four wall decompressions for proptosis and optic neuropathy. In this section portions of the superior and lateral walls of the orbit are missing (arrows). In this patient with pulsatile exophthalmos only dura and periorbita separate the orbit from brain.

occurs in most patients.[157] Patients also notice improvement in their congestive symptoms since the orbit is no longer under pressure. Most patients who undergo orbital decompression do so within 1 year from the onset of eye symptoms.[157] Double vision is present postoperatively in 33–63% of patients and may be worsened because of associated postoperative scarring.[158,159,223,224,248–251] Up to 70% of patients require one or two eye muscle surgeries to correct their double vision after orbital decompression.[157] Interestingly approximately 5% of patients experience improvement in their double vision after orbital decompression.[237,248,251]

Other indications for orbital decompression include severe orbital inflammation, the reduction of proptosis prior to eye muscle surgery, exposure, and steroid intolerance.[157] With increasing surgeon experience and successful results, orbital decompression is being performed more commonly for cosmetic reasons.[157,223,225,233–235,252] Reductions in proptosis of 4–5 mm may be achieved with good patient satisfaction. Further surgery may be performed for eyelid (many patients experience worsening of lid retraction) and eye muscle abnormalities. In one series of 15 patients with no preoperative double vision who underwent transantral orbital decompression primarily for cosmetic reasons, 11 (73%) developed double vision postoperatively, although no patient was dissatisfied with their surgical result.[225] A modified approach to orbital decompression for cosmetic purposes involves only removing orbital fat without bone removal.[224,253,254]

Eye muscle surgery for dysthyroid myopathy is often required to correct double vision. The strabismus may be more difficult to repair in the setting of previous orbital decompression when a large angle esotropia is present.[255,256] The goal is to establish a field of single vision that is as large as possible, including in primary position and downgaze. Rootman[194] found that 9% of his patients ultimately required eye muscle surgery. The most common misalignment is a combined esotropia and hypertropia, for which inferior rectus recession and/or medial rectus recessions either unilaterally or bilaterally are required (**Fig. 18–22**). Resections should be avoided. Adjustable sutures can be particularly helpful and we advocate their use when possible. A relaxed muscle technique has been described in which the detached muscle is sutured to the sclera at the point where the relaxed muscle rests freely on the globe.[257] The amount of correction increases when the disease only affects one muscle, which is more likely to be tethered. Surgery should not be performed until measurements have been stable for 6 months and a similar time has elapsed since the last intervention (radiation or decompression).[258] Intraoperative decision-making is always based on the results of forced duction testing, and the surgeon should be prepared to alter the plan particularly if the superior rectus is found to be tight. In cases with severe scarring, surgery and exposure of the muscle may be difficult. The initial surgical goal for hypertropias should be a slight undercorrection as a drift toward overcorrection occurs postoperatively.[258,259] About two-thirds of patients achieve a successful result of improved eye movements (**Fig. 18–23**) with single vision in the primary position and downgaze after a single operation.[149,257,260–262] However, undercorrections[263] as well as late overcorrections (particularly for inferior rectus recessions)[259] are common. It is not uncommon for patients to require multiple procedures.

Eyelid surgery is reserved as the last procedure performed (after decompression and muscle surgery), and usually entails lowering the upper eyelid and raising the lower eyelid. One common complication of strabismus surgery is lower eyelid retraction, and this is one reason why eyelid surgery should be deferred until after strabismus surgery. Procedures on the lower eyelid usually require detaching the capsulopalpebral fascia from the tarsus and inserting some type of spacer (sclera, hard palate, cartilage or fascia). The upper eyelid can be lowered by Müllerectomy or levator recession, and in many instances because of chronic swelling and fat herniation, this is combined with blepharoplasty.

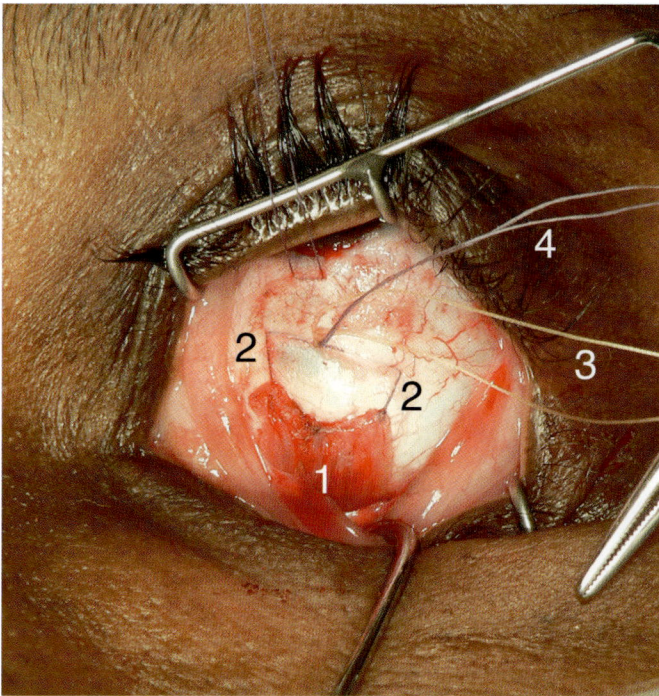

Figure 18–22. Extraocular muscle surgery for strabismus associated with thyroid-associated ophthalmopathy. Pictured is a left inferior rectus recession on an adjustable suture. This intraoperative photograph demonstrates an adjustable suture hang back technique. The inferior rectus (1) is seen to be hanging back from its original insertion attached at either end of the muscle insertion to a violet suture (2) that was placed prior to dissecting the muscle from its original insertion. The suture has been passed back through the original insertion. A noose suture (3) is placed tightly around the muscle suture (4) to hold the muscle in place until the patient can be examined while awake and based on examination findings the noose suture (3) can be moved to allow the distance (2) between the muscle (1) and the insertion to be altered thereby changing the amount of the recession and altering the ocular alignment. Once the muscle is in a satisfactory position the muscle suture (4) is tied permanently.

Course and outcome. The disease usually runs a course of 18 months to 3 years. There is some evidence that clinical activity correlates with thyroid-stimulating immunoglobulin (TSI) levels.[264,265] The symptoms may vary on a diurnal basis depending on the amount of venous and lymphatic drainage. Careful monitoring of the patient's endocrine status must be performed by an endocrinologist. We believe it is inadequate for the ophthalmologist or neurologist to order simply "thyroid function tests" and not involve the expertise of an endocrinologist. Bartley and associates[154] followed their cohort of 120 patients in Olmstead county for a median time of 10 years. Only two eyes had persistent vision loss from optic neuropathy (20/30 and 20/60). Seven patients had intermittent double vision and two other patients had constant double vision which was correctable by prisms. Twenty percent of the patients underwent at least one surgical procedure.[191] Many patients complained of persistent ocular discomfort which in most cases was the result of dry eyes. Although many patients (one-third) were unhappy with their appearance, with successful treatment functional impairment seems to be uncommon.[154]

Pediatric thyroid eye disease. Pediatric Graves disease or hyperthyroidism is not uncommon, and rarely may be associated with the development of TAO. Orbital signs and symptoms occur in about one-third to one-half of the patients[266–268] and the proptosis may be dramatic.[269] The incidence may be higher in countries where teenage smoking is more common.[266,267] Fortunately restrictive myopathy, exposure and optic neuropathy are rare in children.[269] Echography, CT scan and MRI scan have all demonstrated enlargement of the extraocular muscles in children, although motility for the most part remains normal.[268,269] The majority of children can be treated conservatively and orbital fat decompression has been reported to be helpful in reducing proptosis.

Idiopathic orbital inflammatory syndrome (orbital pseudotumor)

Patients with idiopathic orbital inflammatory syndrome (IOIS) are typified by their acute onset of proptosis and eyelid swelling associated with pain and double vision.[270] There is usually conjunctival swelling (chemosis) and injection (**Fig. 18–24**) and eyelid erythema similar to that seen with cellulitis is often present (**Fig. 18–25**), and there may be a violaceous injection over the muscle insertions. IOIS is usually distinguished from other causes of orbital disease (except infections and hemorrhages) by the rapidity of onset and discomfort. Symptoms result from a non-thyroid-related, non-infectious inflammation of the orbit characterized by polymorphous orbital infiltration of lymphocytes and plasma cells with varying amounts of fibrosis and mass effect.

IOIS is an umbrella term that applies to a heterogeneous group of presentations. It may be further subclassed according to the location of the inflammation within the orbit.[271] In this section, the pathogenesis and pathology of IOIS will be discussed, followed by a review of its classification, imaging, and treatment.

Pathogenesis

The cause of IOIS is unknown, and theories concerning pathogenesis include viral, allergic, and autoimmune mechanisms. Based on the lymphocytic nature of the infiltration, it is assumed to be an immune-mediated condition mediated by both B and T lymphocytes.[272] Whether it is a genetically predetermined autoimmune condition versus an environmentally triggered immune event is unclear. Other theories include aberrant wound healing and infection.[273] Several observations have been made to support an autoimmune inflammatory condition, although the significance of each is unclear. These include the identification of antibodies to eye muscle surface antigens in patients with IOIS;[274] reports of patients with upper respiratory tract infections prior to developing IOIS;[275–277] and the occasional association of IOIS with similar nonspecific inflammation of the paranasal sinuses.[278,279]

Differential diagnosis

IOIS-like presentations may occur with orbital inflammation due to systemic inflammatory conditions or vasculitis

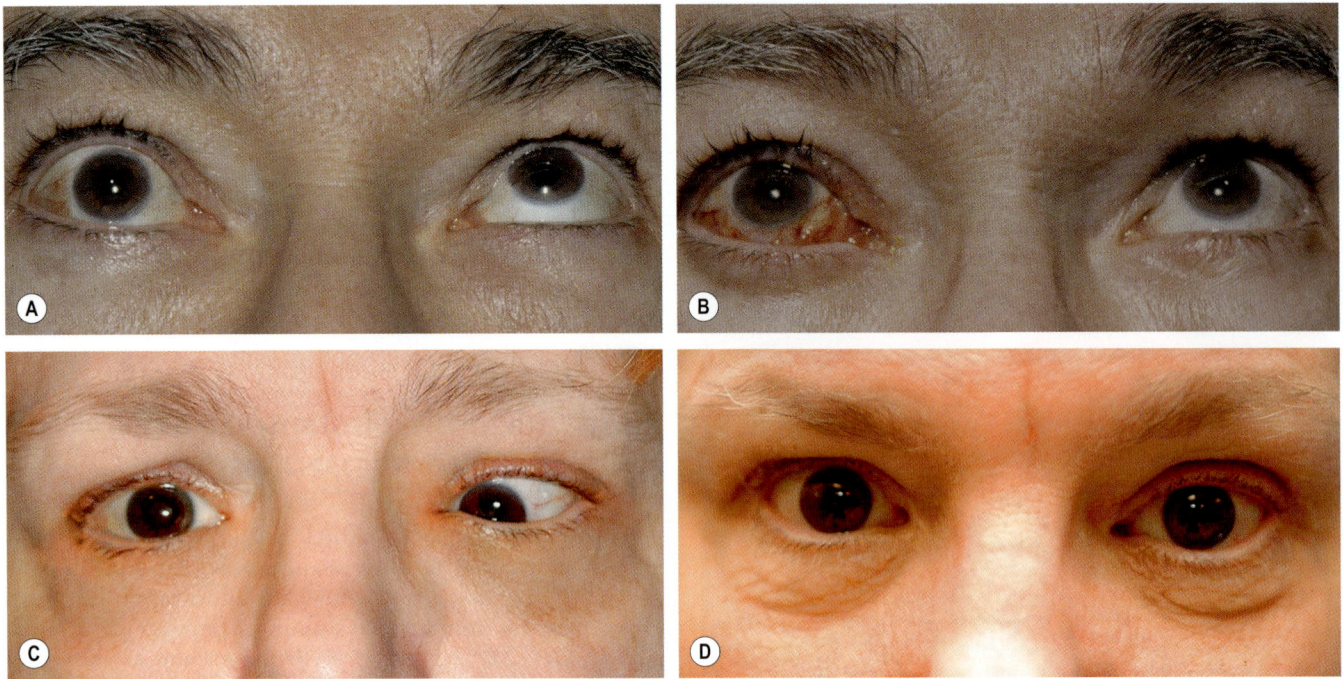

Figure 18–23. Improvement in ocular alignment after extraocular muscle surgery in two patients with thyroid-associated ophthalmopathy. **A.** Elevation deficit of the right eye improves (**B**) after inferior rectus recession. In another patient more severe eye movement limitation is associated with a large-angle esotropia and hypotropia (**C**) that improved (**D**) after medial rectus recession and inferior rectus recession on adjustable sutures along with a contralateral superior rectus recession.

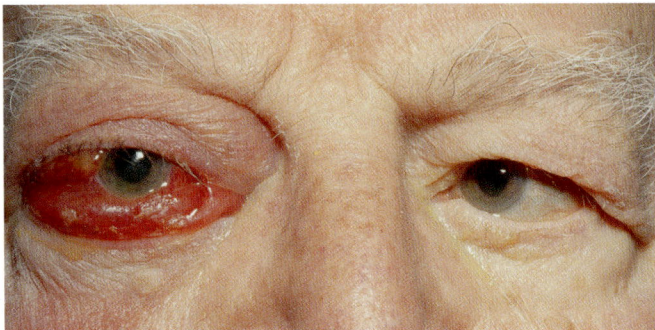

Figure 18–24. External appearance of posterior scleritis in a patient with idiopathic orbital inflammatory syndrome. Intense conjunctival injection and chemosis are seen.

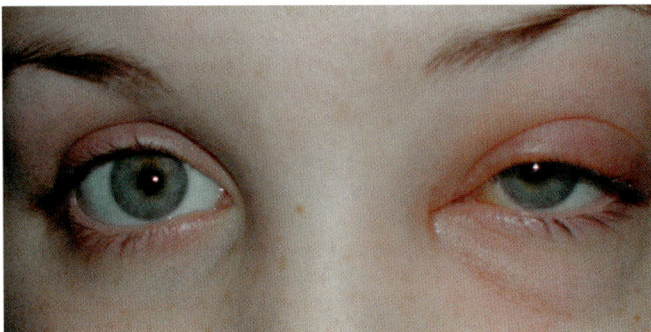

Figure 18–25. Clinical appearance of a patient with myositis in the setting of orbital inflammatory syndrome. Eyelid swelling and chemosis in addition to an esotropia are seen.

including temporal arteritis,[280] Wegener's granulomatosis,[281] polyarteritis nodosa, systemic lupus eythematosus,[282] gout, psoriatic and rheumatoid arthritis,[283] Behçet's,[284] syphilis, tuberculosis, sarcoidosis,[285] ulcerative colitis, and Crohn's disease.[286] Contrary to older theories concerning IOIS, it is no longer believed to be related to orbital reactive lymphoid hyperplasia (pseudolymphoma), or a lymphoid tumor. There is no apparent potential for malignant transformation.[273]

Pathology

Histologically, IOIS is characterized by lymphocyte, plasma cell, macrophage, and polymorphonuclear cell infiltration associated with a fibrovascular stroma. This inflammation eventually leads to fibrosis, but there should be no vasculitic features. More chronic forms of the disease are characterized by insidious development of fibrosis or desmoplasia leading to an apparent soft tissue mass, without an acute phase of cellular infiltration. Although there is significant overlap, some have suggested subgrouping IOIS pathologically into lymphoid, granulomatous,[287] and sclerosing varieties.[288] However, usually a more clinical and anatomic classification is preferred (see below).

Prevalence

IOIS is a relatively uncommon condition. In clinical series of patients presenting with orbital disease, patients with IOIS comprise between 6% and 8%.[58,59] It can occur at any age, with most patients presenting in middle life. There is no sex or race predilection.

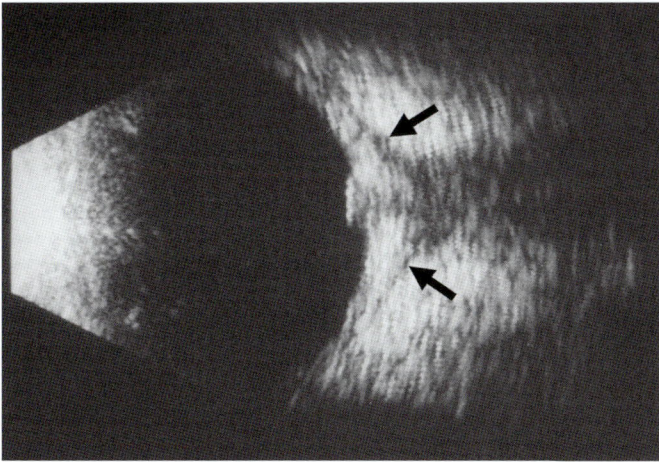

Figure 18–26. B-scan orbital echography of a patient with posterior scleritis. A "T" sign is seen secondary to a hypoechoic fluid filled (arrows) space in the Tenon's capsule.

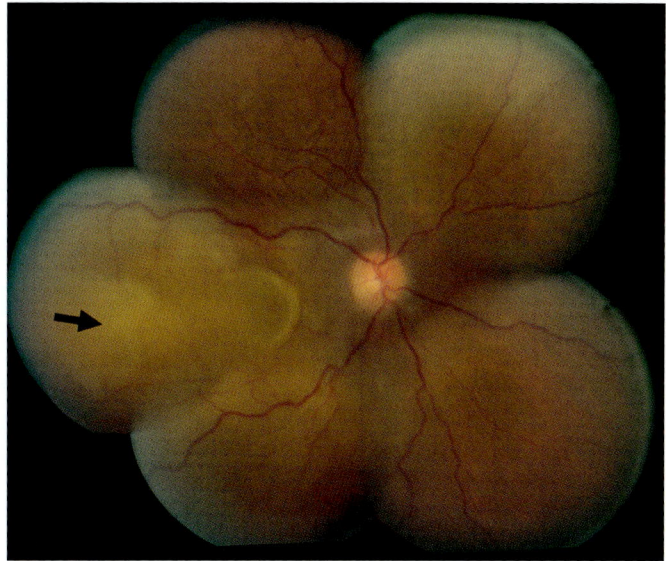

Figure 18–27. Exudative retinal detachment secondary to subretinal fluid in a patient with posterior scleritis. Yellow exudate (arrow) is seen under the macula in this patient presenting with eye pain and decreased vision.

Classification

Several different classifications schemes for IOIS have been described. Rootman and Nugent[289] have proposed a classification system which groups patients depending on the location of orbital involvement. Categories include anterior, diffuse, apical, lacrimal gland, and myositis. This system is helpful in understanding the highly variable clinical presentations of IOIS. For the purposes of neuro-ophthalmic differential diagnosis we find another related system helpful and consider patients with IOIS in six different categories: posterior scleritis, diffuse, myositis, dacryoadenitis, perineuritis, and finally sclerosing inflammation. This classification system allows for separating patients into categories that are unique with regards to their differential diagnosis, evaluation and treatment.

Posterior scleritis. This group of patients has inflammation focused on the eye wall and surrounding Tenon's capsule. Patients develop pain, proptosis, ptosis, lid swelling, chemosis and injection of the conjunctiva, and decreased vision. It occurs in all age groups but seems to be the most common form of IOIS to affect children.[290] Imaging reveals anterior ragged orbital inflammation, which involves the globe and is associated with retinochoroidal thickening.[289,291] Echography may demonstrate sclerotenonitis with edema or widening of Tenon's space (**Fig. 18–6**). This effusion at the neuro-ocular junction and doubling of the optic nerve shadow creates a specific echographic sign called the T-sign (**Fig. 18–26**). This form of IOIS may be characterized by ophthalmoscopic abnormalities including choroidal folds, exudative retinal detachment (**Fig. 18–27**), papillitis, and uveitis. Fluorescein angiographic abnormalities may include patchy choroidal infiltrates, exudative retinal detachments, and macular edema.[292] Treatment is with oral steroids, and their effect is usually prompt and dramatic. Glaucoma may complicate posterior scleritis. Mechanisms include choroidal effusion with anterior rotation of the lens iris diaphragm or uveitic glaucoma.

Diffuse inflammation. In the diffuse presentation, inflammation involves the entire orbit. Clinically patients have proptosis, eyelid swelling, ptosis, and occasionally extraocular muscle involvement and double vision. Papillitis and exudative retinal detachments may be present in this subgroup of patients as well. On imaging studies, the entire orbit is involved by the irregular infiltrate that often obscures normal orbital anatomy (**Fig. 18–28**). When orbital inflammation primarily involves the orbital apex (often subcategorized as "posterior IOIS") there may be a disproportionate amount of visual and eye movement dysfunction[289] and intracranial extension can occur.[293] Pupillary defects (internal ophthalmoplegia) have also been described with posterior orbital involvement, presumably due to disruption of the ciliary ganglion or third nerve.[294]

Myositis. Patients with myositis have a clinical presentation dominated by symptoms of double vision and pain on eye movements. Ptosis and eyelid swelling are common, and chemosis and conjunctival injection in the area overlying the inflamed muscle are prominent (**Fig. 18–25**).

Clinical distinction from TAO can usually be made based on the rapid development of myositis and its characteristic pain, eyelid findings, and diffuse involvement of the muscle and tendon on CT or MRI (**Fig. 18–29** and see **Tables 18–7** and **18–8** as well as discussion of other causes of enlarged eye muscles below). Orbital echography with A and B scan (**Fig. 18–30**) can be used to identify muscle enlargement with tendon involvement and low reflectivity consistent with edema. The most common muscles involved in Rootman et al.'s series[295] were the superior rectus/levator complex and the medial rectus, but any or multiple muscles may be involved. Involvement of the superior oblique with point tenderness over the superomedial aspect of the orbit has been described.[296]

Dacryoadenitis. Inflammation of the lacrimal gland occurs in a variety of circumstances including infection, infiltration by neoplasm, systemic inflammatory conditions, and finally nonspecific inflammation. In series reported by orbital specialists, dacryoadenitis was the most common form of

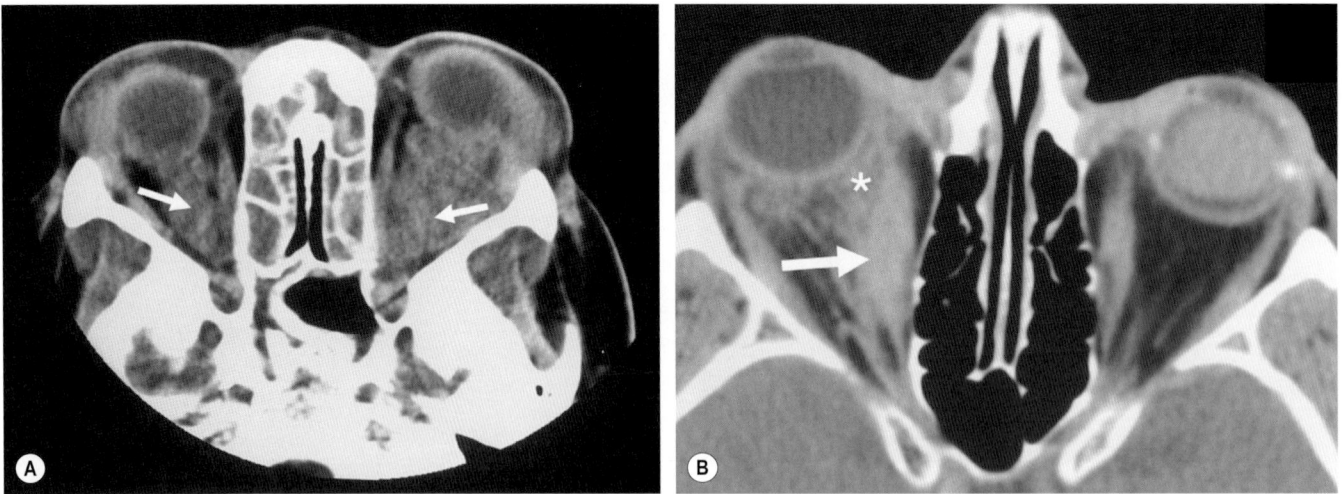

Figure 18–28. Orbital CT scan in patients with idiopathic orbital inflammatory syndrome. **A**. Heterogeneous contrast enhancement and soft tissue changes are seen diffusely in both orbits along with proptosis of the left globe. Infiltrative soft tissue lesions (arrows) are seen on both sides. **B**. In another patient abnormal signal intensity in the fat (asterisk) and enlargement of the medial rectus (arrow) are seen in the right orbit of this patient with idiopathic orbital inflammatory syndrome. The left eye has an unusual CT scan signal secondary to a silicone oil fill after vitrectomy.

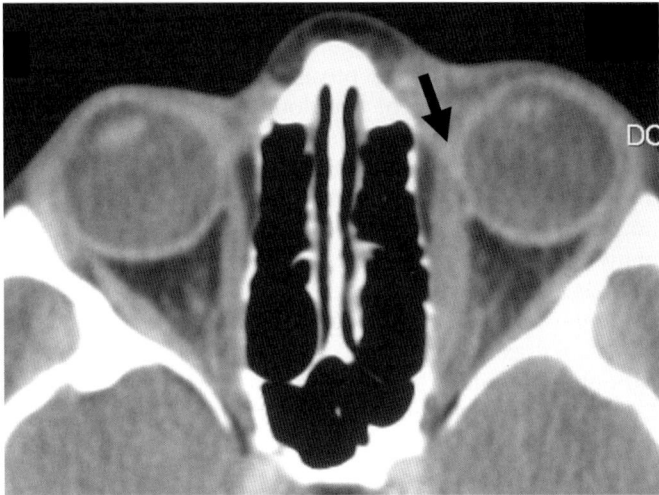

Figure 18–29. Axial CT scan of the same patient as in Fig. 18–25 demonstrating irregular thickening of the medial rectus muscle with involvement of the tendon (arrow). The patient was esotropic and had an abduction deficit of the left eye.

IOIS.[271] Pathologically these can be divided into categories which are specific (i.e. lymphoma, sarcoidosis) and nonspecific (IOIS, dacryoadenitis). Therefore biopsy of these lesions is often recommended.[295] In addition to the more typical acute and subacute varieties, there is a unique chronic (sometimes painless) presentation of IOIS involving the lacrimal gland.

Patients with dacryoadenitis typically develop pain and swelling and redness of the temporal portion of the eyelid. The lid acquires a characteristic S-shaped deformity. The globe may be displaced downward and inferiorly.[295] Bilateral presentation occurs occasionally. Elevation of the eyelid and inspection of the superotemporal area of the conjunctiva shows prominence of the secretory ducts and injection of the visible portions of the lacrimal gland. The superotemporal portion of the orbit may be exquisitely tender. Patients rarely have double vision or complain of decreased vision.

Imaging studies document the presence of an inflammatory mass lesion in the superotemporal orbit which is contiguous with the globe and generally does not involve other orbital tissues.

Perineuritis. The presence of optic neuropathy in association with nonspecific orbital inflammation is well-recognized and termed perineuritis.[291] Vision loss results from either optic nerve sheath inflammation or mass effect on the optic nerve. These patients can be difficult to distinguish from patients with optic neuritis but are often older, have spared central vision, and demonstrate enhancement of the sheath (**Fig. 18–31**) not the nerve itself.[297] Patients often develop optic disc edema and mild retinal venous obstruction. Sarcoid and syphilis are important alternative causes of perineuritis to consider. These must be excluded in patients with optic neuropathy and abnormal appearing optic nerve sheaths with enlargement and enhancement on neuroimaging.[298,300] Perineuritis is also discussed in Chapter 5.

Sclerosing orbital inflammation. Some patients with IOIS-like conditions develop a chronic scarring orbitopathy with exuberant desmoplastic reaction (fibroblastic proliferation with formation of dense fibrous connective tissue) and severe orbital dysfunction. This condition has been termed idiopathic sclerosing inflammation or sclerosing orbital pseudotumor.[288,301-309] This chronic sclerosing variant can be characterized by relentless loss of vision from optic nerve dysfunction and thickening (**Fig. 18–32**) and involvement of the extraocular muscles, leading to double vision. The onset is more insidious, occurs at any age (including young children)[303,310] and often simulates a tumor. There is a predilection for the lateral and superior quadrants of the orbit.[303] Patients develop pain and double vision along with proptosis. Patients can also present with isolated paresthesias in the trigeminal distribution.[305] Desmoplastic reaction around the optic nerve or elsewhere in the orbit can produce a radiographic picture that mimics a primary optic nerve tumor (**Fig. 18–33**). The compressive inflammatory mass may result in a venous obstructive appearance on ophthalmoscopy. (**Fig. 18–33**).

Table 18–7 Clinical distinction of thyroid-associated orbitopathy from idiopathic orbital inflammation

Feature	Thyroid	Idiopathic orbital inflammation
Pain	No pain or mild	More severe; worse on eye movement
Laterality	Most commonly bilateral Some asymmetry	Almost always unilateral
Onset	Gradual, subacute	Acute (hours or days)
Vision	Usually good unless orbital apex compromised	Impaired with posterior scleritis, perineuritis, and optic neuritis
Eye movement	Restrictive	Impaired in field of inflamed muscle
Eyelid	Retraction	Ptosis
Imaging	Multiple muscles enlarged; regular borders and tendon sparing; does not extend to fat	Multiple muscles enlarged with irregular borders and extension to the orbital fat, enhancement around globe
Response to steroids	Slow and moderate	Immediate and often complete

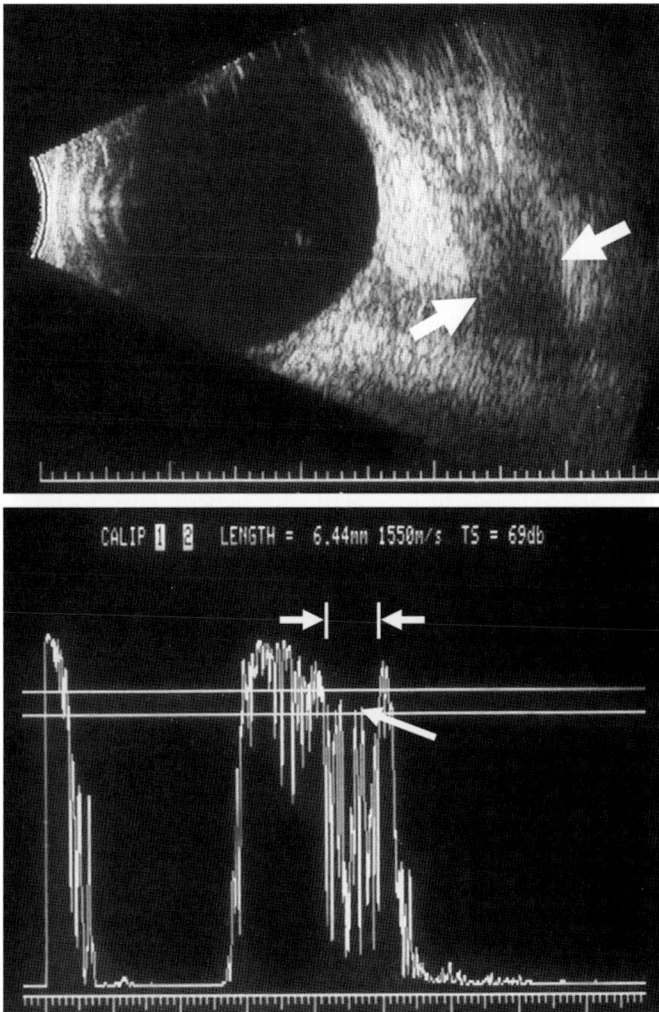

Figure 18–30. Orbital echography in myositis. B scan echography (top) demonstrating enlarged extraocular muscle (arrows) with involvement of the tendon. Corresponding A scan (bottom) showing increased width of the muscle (arrows pointing to the lines indicate muscle width) and moderate internal reflectivity (long arrow). For normal appearance of extraocular muscle on echography see Fig. 18–20A.

Table 18–8 Differential diagnosis of enlarged extraocular muscles

Thyroid-associated ophthalmopathy
Idiopathic orbital inflammatory syndrome with myositis
Lymphoma
Metastatic tumors
Acromegaly
Trichinosis
Carotid-cavernous fistula
Sarcoidosis
Wegener's granulomatosis
Rhabdomyosarcoma
Amyloidosis

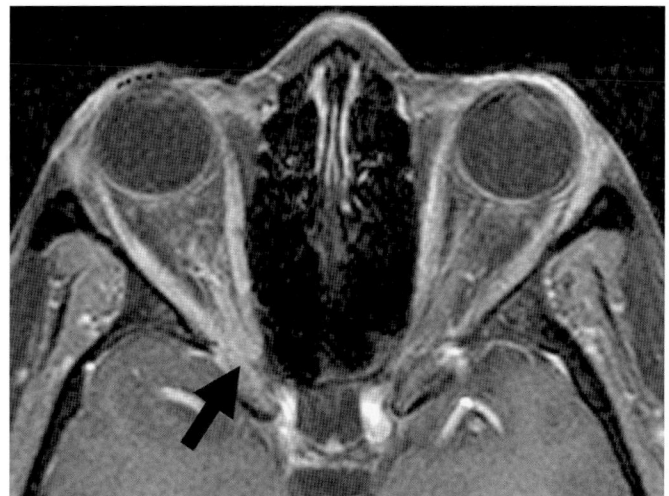

Figure 18–31. Axial T1-weighted, fat suppressed, gadolinium-enhanced MRI scan in a patient with optic nerve dysfunction and perineuritis in the setting of orbital inflammatory syndrome. Enhancement of the nerve sheath (arrow) is seen in the right posterior orbit.

The defining feature histopathologically is the dense desmoplastic reaction with scarring (collagen deposition) and only scant inflammatory infiltrates. These cases may respond poorly to treatment and may be the most common subtype of idiopathic orbital inflammation to erode bone and extend intracranially.[303,311–315] Patients may respond early to steroids but often have a relentless course regardless of treatment and many require second-line immunosuppressive agents.[303] Fourteen of 16 patients in Rootman et al.'s series[308] experienced permanent dysfunction in the form of either optic neuropathy or muscle restriction. Early and more aggressive treatment may be more successful.[303] Since this type of chronic scarring is unusual in other cases of appropriately treated IOIS, it is likely that orbital idiopathic sclerosing inflammation is a distinct clinical entity.[308] It is possible that this is a manifestation of a multifocal fibrosclerotic process, as patients who simultaneously developed retroperitoneal or mediastinal fibrosis have been described.[316–318]

Pediatric IOIS

IOIS occurs at any age. In Rootman's[59] series IOIS was the cause of orbital disease in 13/241 (5%) pediatric patients seen. Pediatric patients may have the diffuse or anterior forms of IOIS, posterior scleritis, uveitis and disc swelling. Ptosis is more prominent than in adults and in one series proptosis was less prominent than in adult cases.[319] In the pediatric population, the disorder is frequently bilateral even without a predisposing systemic condition. However, we have also seen several instances of isolated myositis. Diagnostic testing may show elevated erythrocyte sedimentation rate (ESR), eosinophilia, and cerebrospinal fluid (CSF) pleocytosis.[290]

Imaging

The diagnosis of IOIS is a clinical one but is usually confirmed by imaging studies of the orbit. These typically reveal an area of primary inflammation surrounded by an irregular margin, but findings can be subtle and enhancement can be masked by high signal intensity from fat.[320] Fat-suppressed images with contrast are the most likely to reveal an abnormality. This irregular infiltrate may involve all of the soft tissues of the orbit including Tenon's capsule, the optic nerve, the orbital fat, and the extraocular muscles. In one series of 21 patients, the most commonly identified CT features were contrast enhancement, fat infiltration, proptosis and muscle enlargement (**Fig. 18–28**).[321] MRI has also been shown to be helpful in the diagnosis of IOIS. In one series of 10 patients, IOIS lesions were found to be hypointense to fat and isointense to muscle on T1-weighted images. On T2-weighted images the lesions were isointense or only minimally hyperintense to fat in nine of 10 cases; in one case, the enlarged muscle was markedly hyperintense to fat.[322]

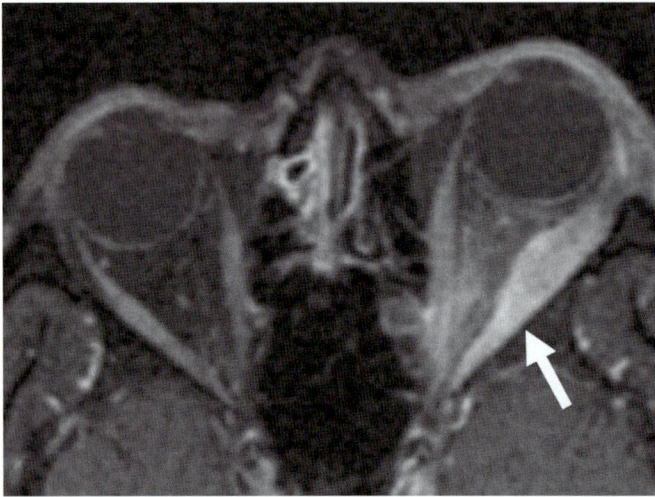

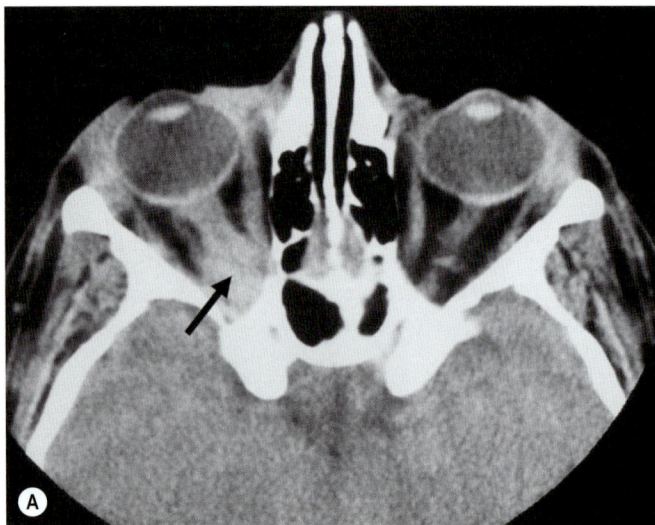

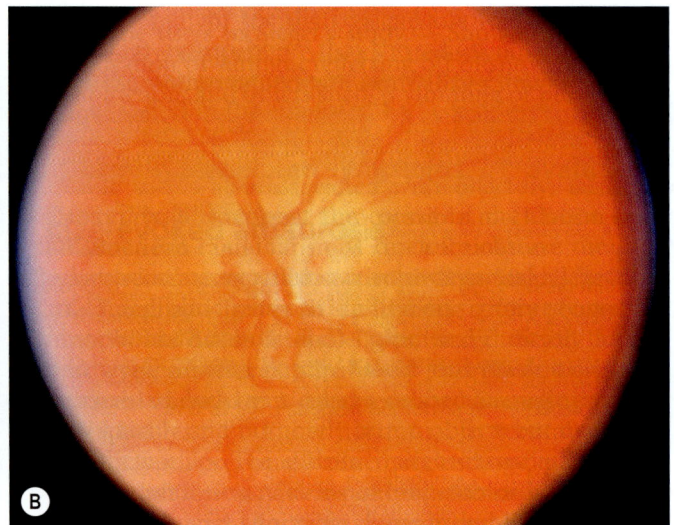

Figure 18–32. Axial T1-weighted, gadolinium-enhanced, fat suppressed orbital MRI scan in a patient with sclerosing orbital inflammation causing irregular thickening of the left lateral rectus (arrow). Mild enhancement of the surrounding fat is seen as well. The corresponding coronal image is depicted in Fig. 18–10.

Figure 18–33. **A**. Axial, contrast-enhanced, CT scan revealing a thickened and enhancing optic nerve (arrow) in a patient with sclerosing orbital inflammatory syndrome. **B**. In the same patient, fundus findings of optic nerve head swelling and intraretinal hemorrhages consistent with retinal vein occlusion were noted.

This pattern was felt to distinguish IOIS from orbital metastases, infections, and hematomas. Therefore it appears that MRI adds significantly to the diagnostic evaluation of patients with IOIS. T2-weighted fat-suppressed images can also be used to identify active inflammation in the extraocular muscle in patients being followed on treatment,[323] and diffusion-weighted images may be particularly helpful in distinguishing IOIS from lymphoma and orbital cellulitis.[324] In patients with likely myositis or posterior scleritis orbital echography with combined A and B scan can be very helpful in identifying abnormal muscle swelling or thickening of the ocular coats with sub-Tenon's fluid (**Figs. 18–6** and **18–30**).

Other diagnostic studies

Biopsy is usually deferred unless the inflammation is recurrent, atypical in appearance, or primarily involves the lacrimal gland. It is reasonable to perform a systemic workup to screen for other systemic inflammatory conditions, although this is almost always negative. Blood work should include syphilis serologies, antineutrophilic cytoplasmic antibodies (ANCA), antinuclear antibodies, and an angiotensin-converting enzyme (ACE), and a chest imaging for hilar adenopathy should be performed. In patients with a history of malignancy the possibility of metastatic disease to the orbit must be carefully considered, and the threshold for biopsy should be low.

Treatment

Treatment is initiated immediately after the clinical diagnosis is suspected and imaging studies support the diagnosis of IOIS. Treatment with corticosteroids (60–100 mg of prednisone) is usually both therapeutic and diagnostic. Most patients with IOIS will have a dramatic response within days of treatment although recurrences and refractory cases are common.[270,271,325] The course of steroids and a slow taper usually needs to be extended for several months. Nonsteroidal anti-inflammatory drugs may be helpful during the steroid taper but occasionally are useful as a primary treatment. Nonsteroidals may be most effective when the inflammatory burden is low and in select patients, such as those with diabetes, who tolerate steroids poorly.

A poor response to steroids should lead to consideration of alternative diagnoses, and then biopsy is often required.[326] Similarly, if the disease recurs after a slow steroid taper, then biopsy is also recommended. Alternative immunosuppressive therapies including cyclophosphamide,[307] cyclosporine,[327,328] and methotrexate[329] as well as intravenous immunogobulin[330] have been successfully used as adjunctive therapies to prednisone. Recently a series of patients has been reported that were successfully treated with the antibodies (infliximab and daclizumab) to tumor necrosis factor (TNF).[331–334]

In patients with refractory inflammation, recurrences, contraindications to systemic steroids, or the sclerosing variety of IOIS, radiation therapy to the orbit is an alternative treatment.[288,308,311,335–337] The dosage is between 1000 and 3000 cGy in 10 divided fractions, and complications are rare.[271,303,338] Lanciano and associates[336] report their experience with 23 patients who had either relapsed on steroids or had poor initial response and found nearly 90% of patients had an initial response to 2000 cGy. Two-thirds of the patients remained in complete remission, and three others were controlled with short courses of oral steroids after radiation. Three of five patients with decreased vision from optic neuropathy improved with radiation treatment.

Other inflammatory orbital conditions

Granulomatous orbital inflammation

Some patients have a non-infectious, granulomatous orbital inflammation. These patients often present with mild (compared to the more painful and acute IOIS) inflammatory symptoms with a palpable mass lesion.[295] In such cases, an extensive systemic evaluation for granulomatous disease is indicated. However, in some cases the orbital disease is the sole location of involvement.

Sarcoidosis

Sarcoidosis is a well-characterized systemic granulomatous disorder affecting multiple organ syndromes. Sarcoidosis is also important in the differential diagnosis of lacrimal gland enlargement and perineuritis. Fortunately, orbital involvement is uncommon in sarcoidosis. However, sarcoidosis may present with either focal or diffuse extraocular muscle enlargement along with proptosis and pain,[339–341] a soft tissue mass lesion, or as a lesion arising from contiguous bony involvement. Sarcoidosis is discussed in further detail in Chapters 5 and 7.

Wegener's granulomatosis

The classic clinical triad of this systemic inflammatory condition includes necrotizing granulomas of the upper and lower respiratory tract, necrotizing vasculitis of the lung, and glomerulonephritis. Wegener's is believed to be a T-cell-mediated condition and is characterized pathologically by granulomatous inflammation and necrotizing vasculitis. Patients usually present in the fifth decade with pneumonitis, sinusitis, and renal involvement.

Ophthalmic manifestations occur in 50–60% of patients with Wegener's granulomatosis and involves the orbit in about one-quarter of those with eye findings.[342,343] However, some patients will have a limited form in which the orbital and sinus involvement predominates.[344–346] Adjacent bony destruction may complicate the sinus disease and produce a saddle-nose, fistulas, and orbital extension. Approximately 40–50% of patients develop ocular manifestations including scleritis and episcleritis, uveitis, peripheral corneal ulceration, and occasionally conjunctival or retinal involvement.[295] The clinical presentation is variable, ranging from mild indolent inflammation to a more explosive inflammatory picture with proptosis, chemosis, optic nerve swelling, and decreased vision. Isolated myositis may occur as well.[347] These findings may necessitate orbital decompression. The diagnosis of Wegener's may be established by biopsy of the affected area. In some patients it is reasonable to treat the patient on the basis of a positive ANCA titer and appropriate clinical findings.

Neurological involvement in Wegener's occurs in about one-third of patients.[348] The most common findings include peripheral neuropathy, cranial neuropathy, ophthalmoplegia, stroke, seizure, and cerebritis.[348] Treatment of Wegener's usually requires long-term therapy with corticosteroids and immunosuppressant drugs such as methotrexate, cyclophosphamide, or rituximab.[349]

Polyarteritis nodosa

Patients with polyarteritis nodosa may occasionally present with orbital involvement.[350] This condition results from a vasculitis of medium and small arteries. The disorder may be segmental, and is characterized by inflammation and fibrinoid necrosis. The major sites of involvement are the kidney, heart, liver, and gastrointestinal tract. The condition shows a predilection for males in the second and fourth decade. Ophthalmic manifestations include retinal and choroidal ischemia related to vasculitis changes. Rarely patients may present with a nonspecific orbital inflammatory syndrome and proptosis in the absence of systemic symptoms.

Histiocytic disorders

A distinct group of histiocytic orbital inflammation is well recognized and includes eosinophilic granuloma (histiocytosis-X), juvenile xanthogranuloma, Erdheim–Chester disease, and necrobiotic xanthogranuloma. Erdheim–Chester disease is a systemic xanthogranulomatous disorder that affects bones and viscera, and bilateral diffuse orbital involvement has been described. The classic histologic features included Touton giant cells and a mixture of lymphocytes and plasma cells. Some of these entities are discussed further in Chapter 7.

Other causes of enlarged extraocular muscles

The vast majority of patients with enlarged extraocular muscles have either TAO or IOIS. However, there are several other causes of enlarged EOMs (**Table 18–8**). The clinical presentation often provides enough information to distinguish the various entities. However, significant overlap does exist. Radiographic features of the various causes of extraocular muscle enlargement have been reviewed.[174,351]

Patients with dural arteriovenous fistulas may have a clinical presentation very similar to IOIS with acute proptosis, conjunctival injection, chemosis, and enlarged muscles (**Fig. 18–34**). These patients generally have less pain than IOIS patients and have the characteristic arteriolized conjunctival vessels with elevation of intraocular pressure. An enlarged superior ophthalmic vein is diagnostic of blood flow reversal in the orbit and muscle enlargement is usually fusiform. These fistulas are discussed in more detail in Chapter 15.

Metastatic tumors to the extraocular muscles may present with an acute onset of proptosis, double vision, and enlarged muscles on neuroimaging studies (see below). The pain is usually less severe than IOIS, and only one muscle may be enlarged. The involved muscle may appear lumpy or irregular on neuroimaging studies.[352,353] Orbital lymphoid tumors usually involve the orbit diffusely but may be confined to a single extraocular muscle.[354,355]

Trichinosis may produce a myositis with enlarged extraocular muscles. The infection results from the ingestion of the *Trichinella spiralis* found in uncooked meat. Patients typically manifest with gastrointestinal complaints followed by myalgias, fever, periorbital pain, and chemosis of the conjunctiva.[356-358] Patients may develop proptosis and double vision.[356-358] Amyloid deposition in the orbit and acromegaly may also result in diffuse fusiform enlargement of the extraocular muscles.[174,351,359,360]

Orbital tumors and other orbital masses

Frequency of various orbital tumors

The proportion of orbital lesions which are neoplastic depends on the type of study (e.g. clinical, pathologic, or radiographic) and whether the patients are children or adults.[48,52,58-61,361-365] In most series, inflammatory diseases (thyroid and idiopathic orbital inflammatory syndrome) make up about one-third to a half of patients. This fraction is lower in pathologic studies since TAO is rarely biopsied. In Rootman's series[59] of 1409 patients, 22.3% had neoplastic lesions.

The most common orbital mass lesions are neurogenic tumors (gliomas, meningiomas, and schwannomas), cystic lesions (dermoids), vascular lesions (cavernous hemangioma), lymphoproliferative lesions (lymphomas), and finally secondary tumors (metastatic and contiguous spread). A survey of a cancer registry found lymphoma to be the most common malignancy.[57] In children, congenital and development lesions with cysts and vascular lesions make up 40% of the cases.[52] A familiarity with the most common causes of orbital space-occupying mass lesions is helpful when considering differential diagnoses.

Orbital lymphoma

Orbital lymphomas have been increasingly recognized,[362-364] and in one series represented 55% of the orbital tumors.[57] Orbital lymphoma may be primary, when it arises and is localized to the orbit, or secondary as a manifestation of a systemic lymphoma. The clinical and radiographic presentations are the same in both situations. Orbital lymphoma can be difficult to distinguish from IOIS both clinically and radiographically, but lymphomas are more likely to present with a mass lesion and less likely to have associated pain and eyelid swelling.[366] The orbital lesions tend to grow slowly and conform to the orbital tissues (**Fig. 18–35**). The lesions are painless and may be recognized only after producing noticeable proptosis, double vision, or a palpable mass which often involves the lacrimal gland. A visible subconjunctival component or "salmon patch" may be present (**Fig. 18–36**). On orbital imaging, lymphoma lesions are generally well defined and almost always demonstrate a characteristic of "molding" to the orbital tissue and globe (**Fig. 18–35**). Idiopathic orbital inflammation may also have

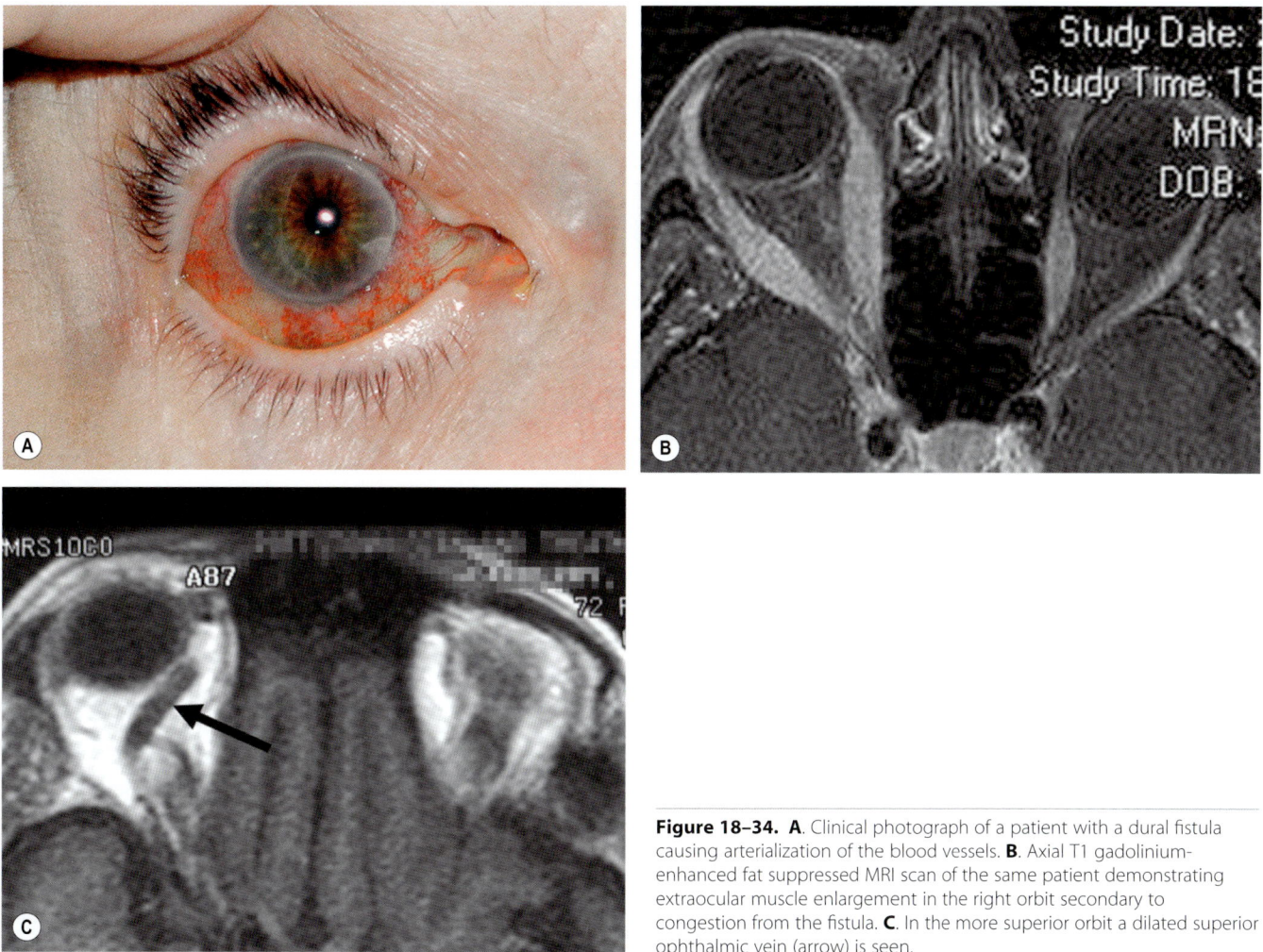

Figure 18–34. A. Clinical photograph of a patient with a dural fistula causing arterialization of the blood vessels. **B**. Axial T1 gadolinium-enhanced fat suppressed MRI scan of the same patient demonstrating extraocular muscle enlargement in the right orbit secondary to congestion from the fistula. **C**. In the more superior orbit a dilated superior ophthalmic vein (arrow) is seen.

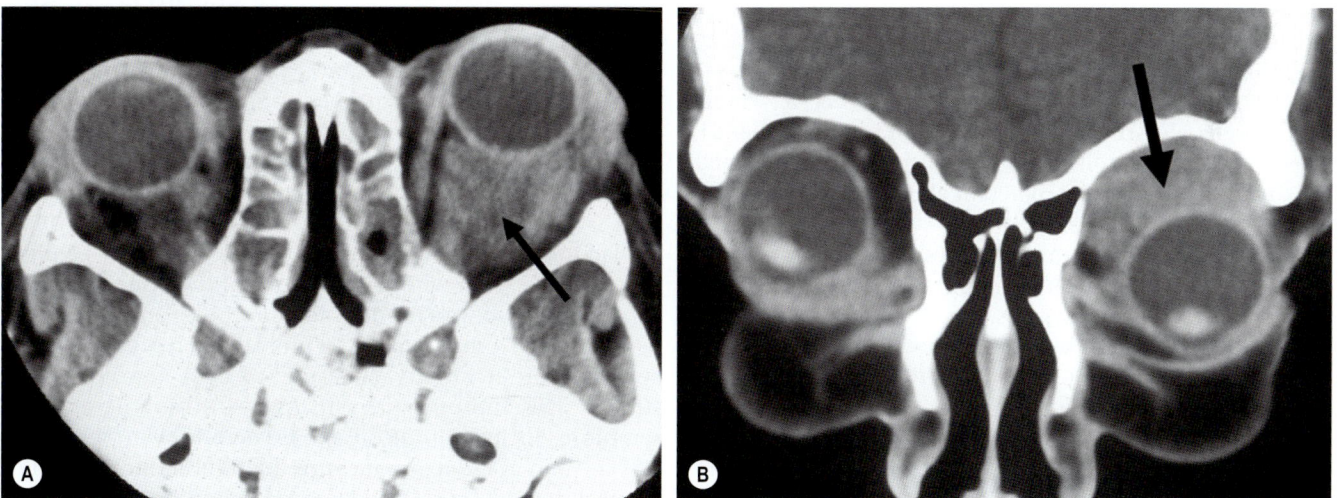

Figure 18–35. A. Axial CT scan of a patient with orbital lymphoma on the left side. An extensive soft tissue mass (arrow) is seen to surround but not indent the left globe. In another patient (**B**) a coronal CT scan similarly reveals a large soft tissue mass (arrow) which seems to surround the globe without indenting it.

a similar appearance (**Fig. 18–28**).[366] There are usually no bony changes.

When neuroimaging suggests a lymphoma, a systemic evaluation is indicated. The orbital mass may be biopsied, as it is often an accessible anterior lesion. The biopsy tissue should be examined by light microscopy and immunohisto-chemistry. If the orbital lesion is isolated, it is treated with local irradiation.[367–375] Ocular adnexal mucosa associated lymphoid tissue (MALT) lymphomas have a more indolent course and may not require as aggressive treatment.[372,374,376]

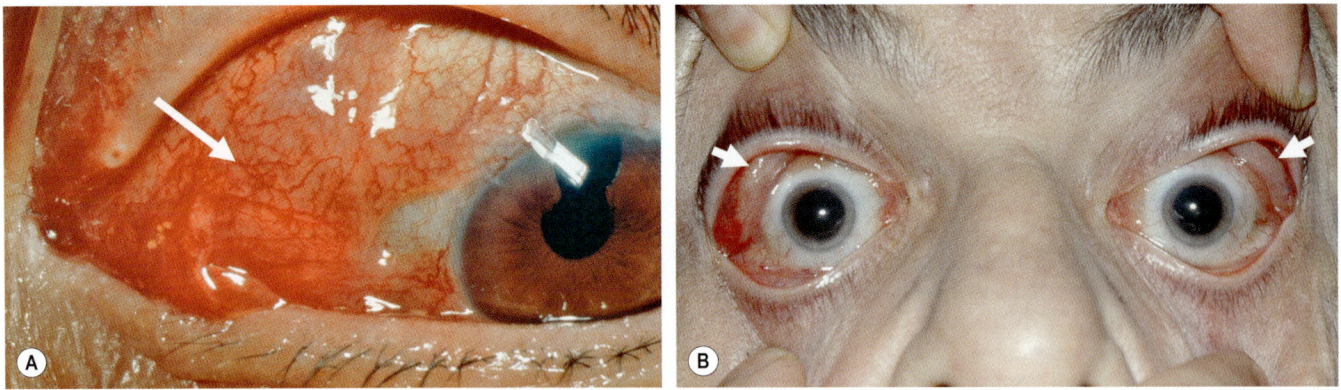

Figure 18–36. Clinical photographs of patients with orbital lymphoma that in one patient (**A**) extended into the subconjunctival space and presented as a fleshy, pink subconjunctival lesion (arrow) and in another patient (**B**) caused enlargement of both lacrimal glands (arrows).

If there is evidence of multiorgan involvement with lymphoma, then systemic protocols using chemotherapy are used. A small percentage of patients with localized orbital disease will develop systemic lymphoma.

Plasma cell tumors may manifest like lymphoproliferative lesions. Multiple myeloma of the orbit may present with proptosis or double vision.[377–380] The infiltrate usually affects the lacrimal gland, orbital fat, and muscles, and unlike lymphoma it is often associated with pain. Systemic evaluation for multiple myeloma is necessary, and if negative patients must be monitored closely for its development.

Neurogenic tumors

Most orbital peripheral nerve sheath tumors, such as schwannomas and neurofibromas, originate from the sensory branches of the first division of the trigeminal nerve. Unlike the optic nerve, the peripheral nerves contain an outer sheath called an epineurium, and are further divided into bundles by perineural cells possessing both contractile and undulating properties. Within each of the perineural compartments are located supportive Schwann cells. These Schwann cells give rise to the most common (peripheral) nerve tumors of the orbit called schwannomas or neurilemomas. In all, schwannomas represent about 1% of all orbital tumors.[59–61,364]

Schwannomas most commonly present in the second to fourth decades with a history of proptosis that extends over a period of several months or years.[381–384] Rarely, patients manifest with vision loss because of crowding of the orbital apex and optic nerve compression. In this setting, their presentation is not unlike other benign, well-circumscribed, rounded, slow-growing, orbital masses. In fact, schwannomas are very similar to cavernous hemangiomas in their presentation with the insidious onset of well-tolerated proptosis. On CT and MRI scans, schwannomas may be difficult to distinguish from primary optic nerve tumors, and this distinction should be made prior to surgical excision. Neuroradiographic features include a well-defined lesion which is isointense with the brain and enhances with gadolinium. They appear radiographically similar to cavernous hemangiomas, fibrous histiocytomas, and hemangiopericytomas. When treatment is indicated it requires surgical resection.[385]

Patients with an orbital plexiform neurofibroma due to neurofibromatosis type 1 (NF-1) may manifest with proptosis and massive overgrowth of the eyelid skin. A characteristic S-shaped deformity of the upper eyelid may be seen. Multiple isolated neurofibromas, café au lait spots, iris Lisch nodules, optic pathway gliomas (see Chapters 5 and 7), or a family history of neurofibromatosis should suggest the diagnosis of NF-1. The plexiform neurofibroma has a diagnostic appearance of infiltrating cords of cells that are non-encapsulated. Whether neurofibromas are truly schwannomas is a matter of debate as they often contain histologic features of perineural cells and fibroblasts.

Lacrimal tumors

Lacrimal tumors are relatively rare. About one-half of lacrimal gland masses are ultimately proven to be inflammatory (see discussion above on dacryoadenitis). About half of the tumors of the lacrimal gland are epithelial in nature; of these approximately half are benign and half are malignant.[59,386–388] The typical clinical presentation is characterized by deformity of the upper eyelid contour (S-shaped), fullness of the upper eyelid, and downward and nasal displacement of the globe. Mass lesions may be palpated in the superior sulcus at the lateral portion of the upper eyelid. CT scan is important to evaluate bony changes. Excavation of the lacrimal fossa or bony erosion is characteristic of a pleomorphic adenoma while lytic lesions of the bone characterize adenocystic carcinoma. Pleomorphic adenomas (or benign mixed tumors) of the lacrimal gland represent benign epithelial proliferations characterized by a myxoid fibrous stroma. This tumor usually manifests in middle age and symptoms include proptosis and lid deformity evolving over 1 year. With accurate preoperative identification, the goal of surgical therapy (usually via lateral orbitotomy) is complete excisional biopsy, otherwise there is risk of recurrence with orbital dysfunction and also increased risk of malignant transformation.[389] Adenoid cystic carcinoma of the lacrimal gland is the most common malignant lesion to arise in this area. The clinical presentation is characterized by a mass lesion, non-axial proptosis (**Fig. 18–9**) and neuropathic pain from perineural invasion. Unlike inflammatory lesions of the lacrimal gland, the eye is usually white and quiet, and the pain is not exacerbated by eye movements. Unfortunately only about 70% of all patients with adenoid cystic carcinoma are alive at 5 years.[390,391] The major cause of morbidity and mortality is intracranial invasion, which is facilitated by the perineural spread of the tumor. Surgical exenteration, or removal of all orbital contents, is the recommended therapy with or without postoperative radiation for this type of tumor.[390,391] Even with the most radical surgery and radiation the disease-free survival rate does not improve.

Metastatic tumors

The orbit is the second most common site for metastatic disease to the eye and its adnexa, with the uveal tract involved most frequently. Breast cancer is the most common primary tumor.[353,364,392,393] The incidence of metastatic tumors as the cause of orbital disease ranges in various series from 1% to 3%.[59,61,362–364] The prognosis for survival in patients with metastatic orbital tumors is uniformly poor, and few patients survive for more than 1 year. Using modern combined modalities of therapy, patient survival may be prolonged. However, most treatment is only palliative. Prompt recognition of this condition may help in the detection of an unrecognized primary systemic malignancy and allow for early treatment.

The clinical presentation of metastatic tumors is variable, but there are certain recurrent themes. Patients frequently complain of diplopia, ptosis, proptosis, eyelid swelling, and pain.[394–396] Most important is the relative abruptness and disproportionate amount of symptoms that these lesions cause compared with other space-occupying orbital lesions. Double vision is often an early manifestation of metastatic disease. This compares with primary orbital tumors, which are generally better compensated because of their more insidious evolution. Other commonly reported symptoms include a palpable mass and decreased vision. The most common signs include exophthalmos, noncomitant eye deviation, conjunctival injection, palpable mass, subnormal visual acuity, disc edema, choroidal folds, and enophthalmos. Metastatic breast carcinoma often causes enophthalmos secondary to contraction induced by the scirrhous nature of the tumor.[397]

At the time of diagnosis, metastatic tumors are usually characterized by unencapsulated tumor growth with diffuse involvement of the orbital structures (**Fig. 18–37**). Tumor emboli may lodge in muscle, fat, or bone. In clinical studies in which tumor localization can be accomplished by high-resolution CT scanning, the bone and fat are involved twice as often as the muscle.[394,395] Capone and Slamovits[352] found that 16 cases arose from the breast, and that six cases arose from melanoma in their literature review of 31 cases of metastatic tumors to the extraocular muscles. The lesions may be isolated and solitary (**Fig. 18–38**)[398] or involve the muscle(s) diffusely. Healy[399] reviewed 22 cases of orbital metastases evaluated by CT scan; two-thirds of these patients had some evidence of adjacent bone destruction, 60% of lesions were extraconal, 20% were intraconal, and 20% were both (**Fig. 18–39**). Enhancement was seen in all cases examined with contrast. Interestingly, two-thirds of patients had evidence of intracranial disease, either by direct extension or discrete metastases (**Fig. 18–40**).[399] Goldberg and Rootman[394]

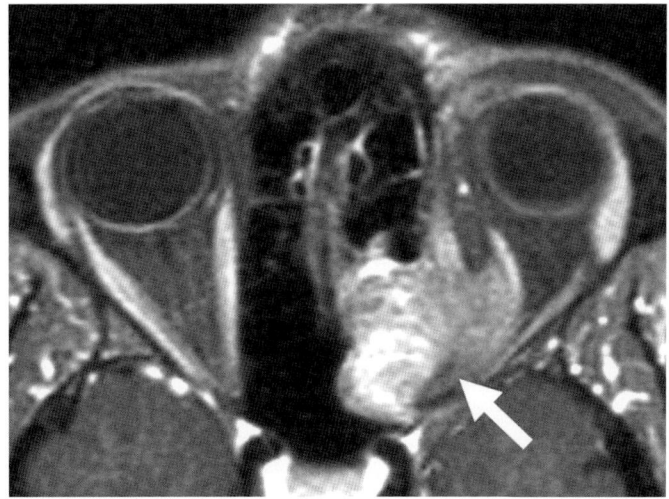

Figure 18–37. Axial T1-weighted, gadolinium enhanced MRI scan demonstrating orbital apex invasion (arrow) by a metastatic Ewing's sarcoma to the ethmoid sinus. The patient presented with a retrobulbar optic neuropathy and pain on eye movements that was initially thought to be due to optic neuritis. (Courtesy of Mark Moster, MD).

examined the spectrum of CT scan features reported in the literature and found that a mass lesion (**Fig. 18–39**) and tumor involving bone were the most common CT scan findings. Breast carcinoma most frequently involves the fat initially (**Fig. 18–41**) and can cause a unique presentation of enophthalmos and double vision, and prostate carcinoma has a strong predilection for bone.

The mainstay of treatment for metastatic tumors is radiotherapy but despite this there is often relentless tumor growth (**Fig. 18–40**). Most patients do not have radiation sequelae, which normally occur in a time frame beyond the average survival of these patients.

Secondary orbital tumors

Secondary orbital tumors involve the orbit by direct extension. They arise in any of the adjacent structures including the sinuses and nasopharynx, the meninges and brain, the eye, the conjunctiva and lids, and the lacrimal sac. Secondary tumors are a common cause of orbital disease and unfortunately the most common setting in which patients require exenteration.

The majority of secondary neoplasms arise from the paranasal sinus cavities.[59] Many patients with sinus tumors have signs and symptoms related to the eye or orbit. The primary mode of extension of sinus tumors to the orbit is direct extension. This may occur by bone erosion, extension through pre-existing bone canals, or extension along normal neurovascular bundles.[400] The maxillary sinus is the most common origin of these secondary orbital tumors. Only thin bone separates the inferior orbital fissure from the mucosa of the sinus.[400] The sinus tumors invading the orbit can be benign or malignant. Malignant lesions include squamous cell cancers and esthesioneuroblastoma.[401,402] Benign lesions include inverting papilloma, osteomas, juvenile angiofibroma, and unusual neuroectodermal tumors. Although mucoceles (see below) are typically unassociated with malignancy, Weaver and Bartley[403] reported seven patients in

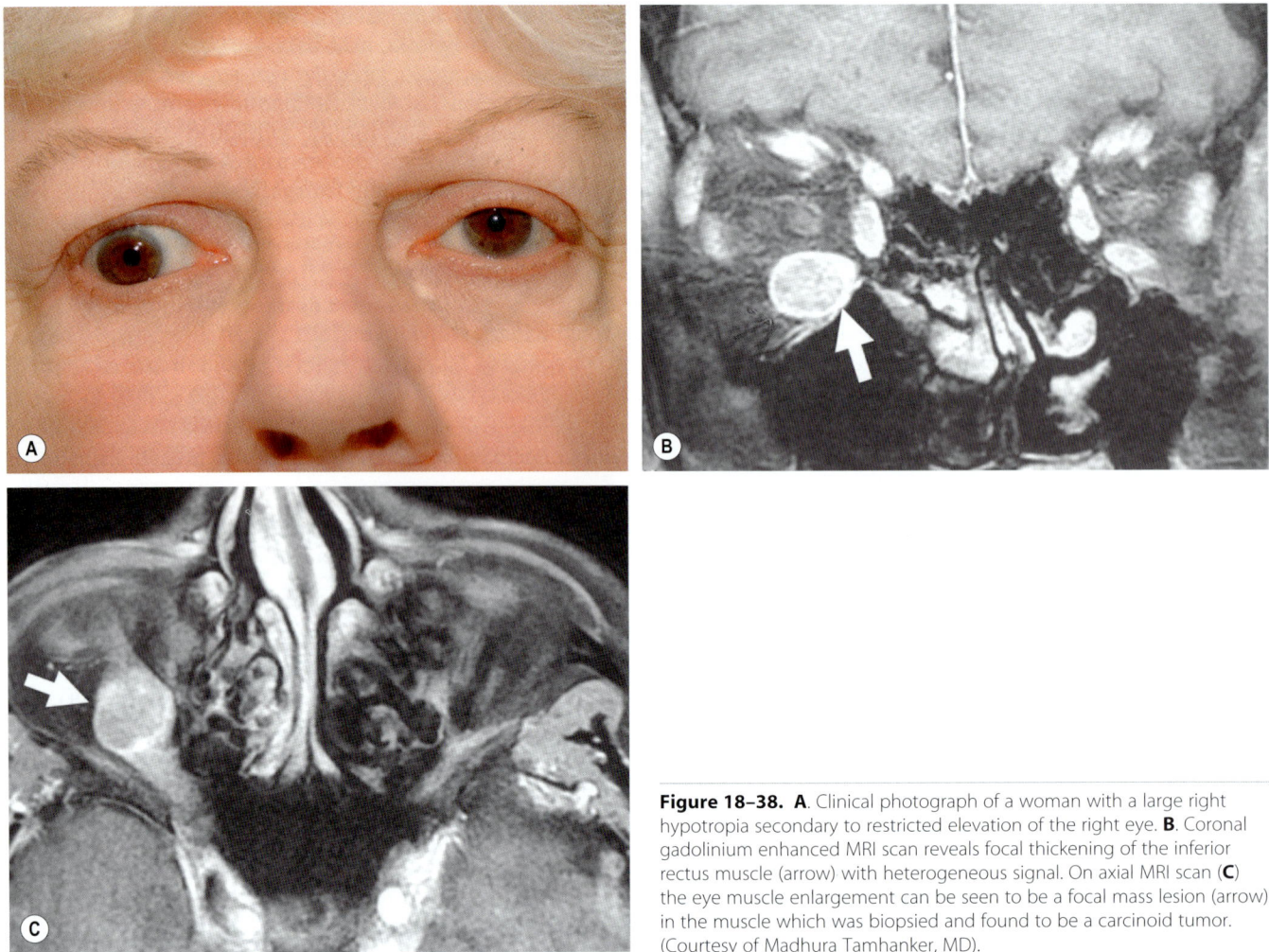

Figure 18–38. A. Clinical photograph of a woman with a large right hypotropia secondary to restricted elevation of the right eye. **B**. Coronal gadolinium enhanced MRI scan reveals focal thickening of the inferior rectus muscle (arrow) with heterogeneous signal. On axial MRI scan (**C**) the eye muscle enlargement can be seen to be a focal mass lesion (arrow) in the muscle which was biopsied and found to be a carcinoid tumor. (Courtesy of Madhura Tamhanker, MD).

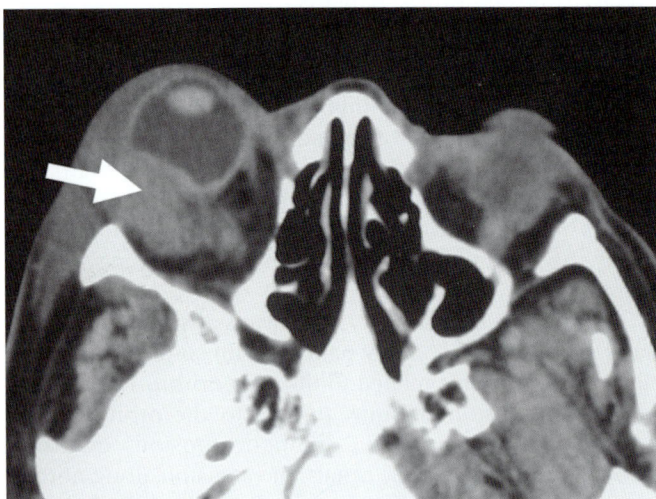

Figure 18–39. Axial CT scan of another patient with metastatic carcinoid. A soft tissue lesion (arrow) in the lateral orbit is seen which unlike lymphoma clearly indents the eye. On fundus exam the patient had choroidal folds.

whom a malignancy was found incidentally in association with the mucocele at the time of surgery.

The overall prognosis for these patients is poor, and the treatment is usually palliative. Surgical approaches can often be designed to spare the globe and not affect prognosis

although exenteration is often required.[404–407] In general, patients with sinus tumors have a 5 year survival rate as high as 74%, but in those with orbital involvement the rate is 25% even when a combination of radiation and radical surgery is used.[400] This difference in survival reflects a more advanced disease state when the orbit is involved. In many cases, these tumors may only be partially excised at initial surgery. They produce persistent morbidity through local invasion and metastasize only at a very late stage. Distant spread to lymph nodes and the lung is most common. Disease that is limited to regional nodes may be curable in certain cases with combined surgery and radiation therapy.

Orbital extension of intracranial tumors

Orbital involvement by intracranial tumors is rare. This mainly occurs with meningiomas, particularly those involving the sphenoid bone. Meningiomas may extend along the lateral orbital wall and posterior orbit, causing proptosis and lid swelling. If the tumor grows medially or along the lesser wing of the sphenoid, these tumors may involve the posterior orbit structures, producing ophthalmoplegia and visual loss with only minimal proptosis.

High-grade astrocytomas of the frontal lobe may invade the orbital roof. Clivus tumors including chordoma have

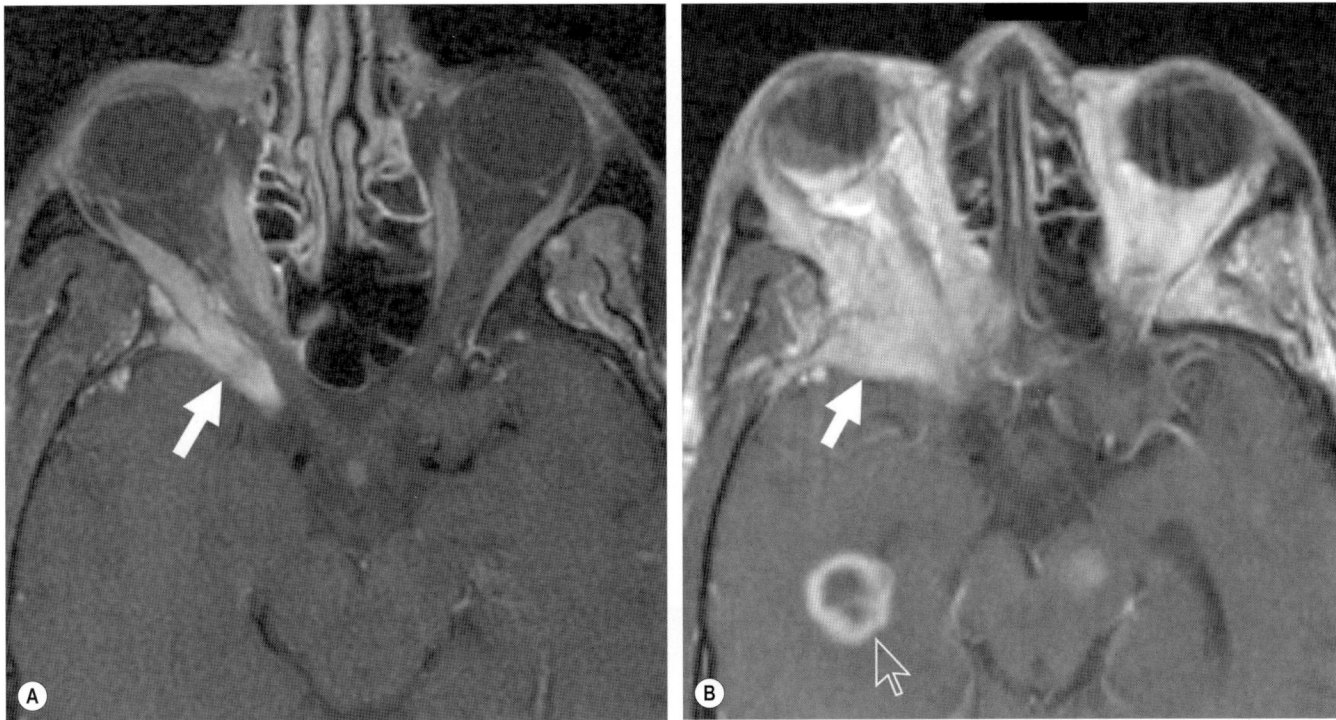

Figure 18–40. Axial T1-weighted, gadolinium enhanced MRI scans of a patient with metastatic adenoid cystic carcinoma to the right orbit. **A**. An enhancing mass lesion (arrow) is seen at the orbital apex and also involves the medial and lateral rectus muscles which are thickened. One year later (**B**) despite attempts at treatment the lesion is seen to have grown extensively to involve more of the orbital tissue with increased size and enhancement (arrow), muscle enlargement and proptosis. A new and separate metastatic focus is seen as a ring enhancing lesion in the right temporal lobe (open arrow).

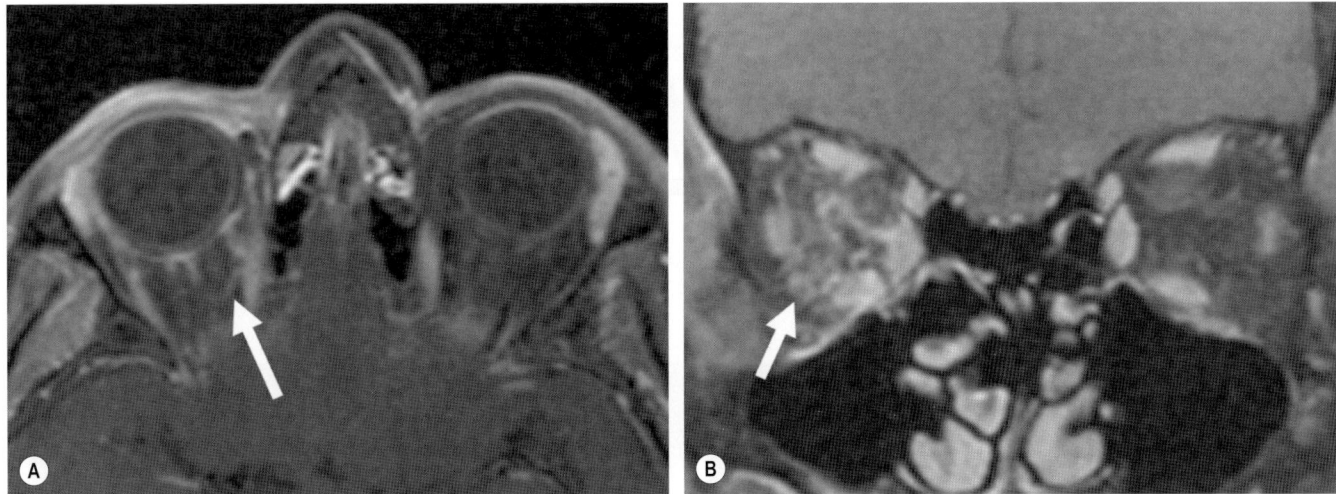

Figure 18–41. Axial MRI scan of a patient presenting with double vision and enophthalmos secondary to metastatic breast cancer. **A**. On the axial T1-weighted gadolinium-enhanced, fat suppressed study, irregular enhancement (arrow) and signal is seen throughout the right orbit. **B**. This is also seen on the coronal images (arrow). (Courtesy of Mark Moster, MD)

also been reported to extend into the orbit.[408-410] Typically, proptosis occurs late and is a manifestation of advanced disease. Other tumors occurring in the region of the sella and the base of the skull may also invade the orbit. Pituitary tumors and craniopharyngiomas only very rarely invade the orbit and cause proptosis. Orbital involvement may also occur with the extension of meningeal tumors, through the subarachnoid space and along the optic nerve sheath.

Vascular tumors

Cavernous hemangiomas are the most common vascular tumors of the orbit. They manifest insidiously with proptosis and double vision.[411-413] Blurred vision may result from a hyperopic shift from compression and shortening of the globe. Most patients become symptomatic in the second to fourth decade.[411-414] Cavernous hemangiomas are usually solitary and arise in the intraconal space. Imaging studies reveal a well-circumscribed, variably enhancing lesion (**Fig. 18–42**).[415] They are usually well defined, lobulated purplish lesions composed of a large number of spaces of variable size containing blood. Compression and displacement of the optic nerve can occur (**Fig. 18–42**). Lesions can contain thrombus or be calcified. Like intracranial cavernous hemangiomas, there usually is no large feeding vessel. The lesions are relatively easily excised via a lateral orbitotomy, do not recur, and have no potential to extend intracranially.[411–414]

Lymphangiomas of the orbit are congenital benign vascular tumors that contain venous and lymphatic channels.[363,364,416,417] They can present as a mass lesion (often in the superior and nasal portions of the orbit) (**Fig. 18–43**) insidiously, acutely due to spontaneous bleeding ("chocolate cysts"), or in association with upper respiratory tract infections. Lesions are typically hypointense on T1-weighted images, hyperintense on T2-weighted images and fluid levels and septations can be seen (**Fig. 18–43**). Most lymphangi-

omas are followed by observation for growth based on clinical exam and imaging. Treatment is indicated when optic neuropathy, corneal exposure problems or glaucoma occur. Resection is difficult and always incomplete so should be avoided unless absolutely necessary.

Venous angiomas may occur in the orbit and are often called varices. The clinical syndrome is usually characterized by intermittent filling and emptying of the varix, resulting in variable proptosis. Eye bulging in a crying infant, proptosis during Valsalva maneuver, or orbital ecchymoses should raise this diagnostic possibility. Lesions can be identified by CT or MR scanning, with and without raising intravenous pressure, and may be followed by orbital venography. Surgical intervention is recommended only for sight threatening lesions or progressive proptosis causing cosmetic disfiguration.

Hemangioblastomas in the orbit usually arise in or adjacent to the optic nerve sheath in patients with von Hippel–Lindau

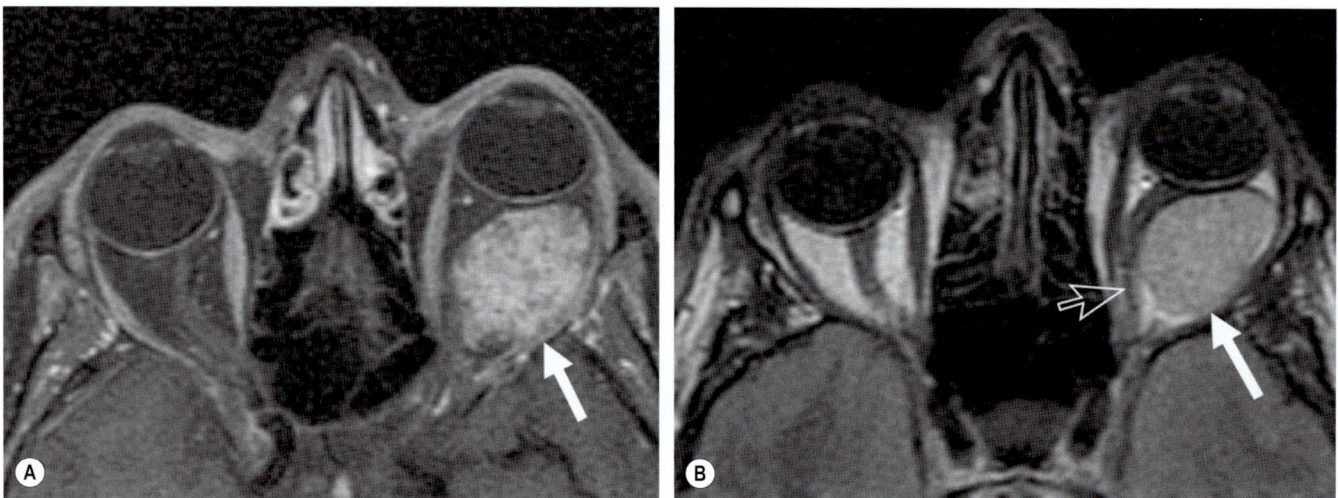

Figure 18–42. Axial T1-weighted gadolinium enhanced MRI scans in a patient with large cavernous hemangioma of the orbit and progressive vision loss. **A**. Fat-suppressed image shows the lesion (arrow) to demonstrate heterogeneous enhancement and signal pattern and to be in the intraconal space. In a non-fat-suppressed view (**B**) the lesion (arrow) compresses the optic nerve (open arrow). This patient presented with progressive vision loss.

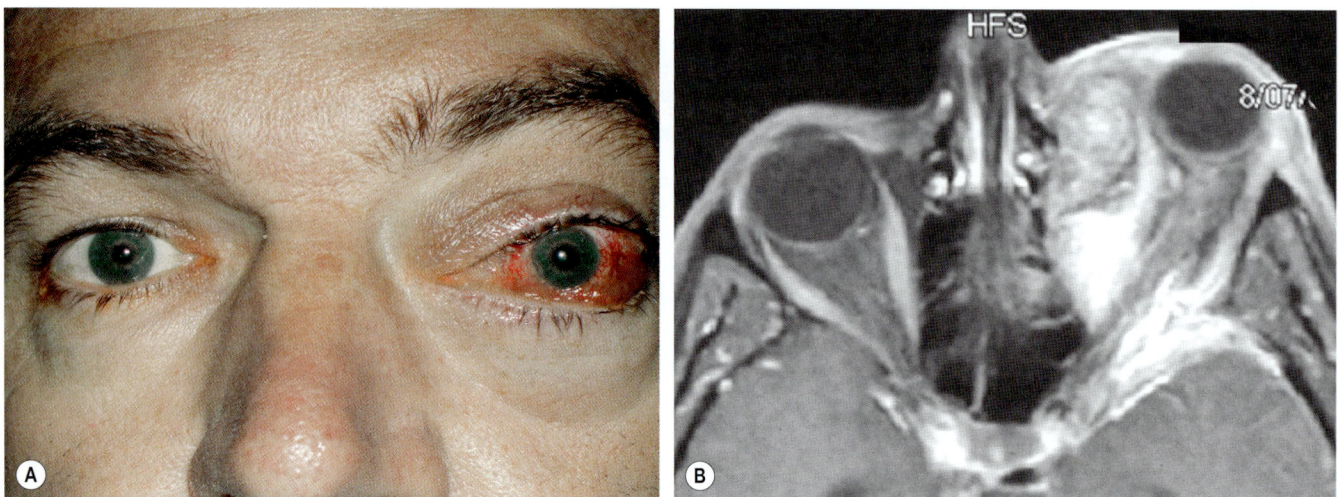

Figure 18–43. **A**. Proptosis, eyelid swelling and injection of the left eye secondary to recent bleeding in an orbital lymphangioma. **B**. Axial, T1-weighted, gadolinium-enhanced MRI scan of the same patient demonstrating a large heterogeneous enhancing lesion throughout the medial orbit.

disease.[418–420] Patients may manifest with vision loss and proptosis from the effects of an orbital mass lesion.

Because *hemangiopericytomas* are tumors that arise from pericytes of blood vessels, they can arise anywhere in the body where blood vessels are located, including the orbit. Rarely, they arise in the area of the occipital lobe and may present with homonymous hemianopia. In the orbit they may manifest with diplopia, proptosis and choroidal folds.[421,422] These tumors usually arise outside of the muscle cone, and patients develop vision loss as a manifestation of compression of the optic nerve. The diagnosis is rarely made preoperatively. Up to one-third of these lesions recur and some metastasize. therefore, successful treatment is greatly enhanced by the completeness of the excision.[421,422] Clinical and histopathologic overlap occurs with solitary fibrous tumor of the orbit.[423,424]

Pediatric orbital tumors

Congenital tumors and infectious processes are the most common causes of orbital disease in children. However, the types of orbital lesions in children vary among reported series.[48,52,59,364] Certain patterns are clear in a meta-analysis of these reports. Most children with proptosis have benign conditions that are infectious, inflammatory, or neoplastic. The benign tumors are commonly dermoids and vascular tumors (particularly capillary hemangiomas). The most common malignant tumors to involve the orbit in children are rhabdomyosarcoma and metastatic tumors including neuroblastoma and Ewing's sarcoma. The orbit is also occasionally involved by extension of intraocular retinoblastoma, leukemia, or lymphoma. The benign congenital cystic lesions such as dermoid tumors, as well as the common congenital vascular tumors (capillary hemangioma) often present with isolated orbital findings and rarely manifest with intracranial abnormalities.

Rhabdomyosarcoma is the most common orbital malignancy in children and is also the most common soft tissue tumor of childhood. Dramatic improvement in the survival of patients treated promptly with appropriate chemotherapy and radiotherapy has made the early diagnosis of rhabdomyosarcoma of the orbit critical. Patients with localized orbital disease enjoy a 90% chance for survival after successful chemo- and radiotherapy. Extension of rhabdomyosarcoma into the paranasal sinuses is not uncommon, although intracranial extension is quite rare. Nevertheless, staging of patients with rhabdomyosarcoma should include lumbar puncture to rule out central nervous system metastases.

Metastatic orbital tumors in children are distinct from those seen in adults. In children, tumors almost exclusively travel to the bony orbit. Soft tissue and ocular metastases as seen in adults are extremely rare. Neuroblastoma arises from primitive neuroblastic tissue and is the most common tumor to metastasize to the orbit in children. This tumor is second only to rhabdomyosarcoma as the most frequent malignant tumor of the orbit. The adrenal medulla is the most common primary site. Musarella and co-workers[425] found that 20% of children with neuroblastoma developed orbital metastases and typically present with either proptosis or ecchymoses.

This occurs because these tumors grow so rapidly and outstrip their blood supply. On CT scan, the temporal orbit (zygomatic bone) frequently demonstrates lytic bone destruction. Disc swelling may be evident because of optic nerve compression or from simultaneous intracranial involvement and elevated intracranial pressure. Diagnosis is established through a series of noninvasive tests including imaging studies of the head and orbit, chest, and abdomen, and analysis of urinary catecholamines. Treatment consists of removal of the primary tumor followed by radiation and chemotherapy.

Fibrous dysplasia

Fibrous dysplasia is a benign bone condition in which normal bone is replaced by immature bone and osteoid in a cellular fibrous matrix. In Rootman's[59] series of 1409 patients, nine patients had fibrous dysplasia. The associated expansion of the bone may be associated with swelling, disfigurement, and pain. When the orbital bones are involved, proptosis, decreased vision, and double vision may occur. In some patients, the abnormal bone growth occurs in one site and is termed monostotic. In other patients, multiple sites are involved (polyostotic). The McCune–Albright syndrome is characterized by polyostotic fibrous dysplasia, skin rash, and endocrine abnormalities. Fibrous dysplasia involves the craniofacial bones in about 20% of patients and is usually thought to be a disease of children and adolescents. However, it may also present in adults.[426,427]

The clinical syndrome of fibrous dysplasia evolves as the bones enlarge, and the globe is displaced (dystopia).[426–431] If the bones of the optic canal are involved and narrowed, vision loss from optic neuropathy can ensue.[426,432–435] Pain, proptosis, and globe displacement are the most common manifestations.[436] In Rootman et al.'s series,[436] the frontal bone was the most frequently involved orbital bone, although in Katz and Nerad's[426] series the maxilla was the most commonly involved. Fibrous dysplasia has a virtually diagnostic appearance on CT scan with the bone taking on a homogeneous, dense, ground glass appearance (**Fig. 18–44**).[426,437] Many patients show a Paget-like appearance with alternating areas of lucency and increased density.[426] Features on MRI scan include low to intermediate signal intensity on spin echo sequences and most lesions demonstrate moderate enhancement.[438,439] Distinction of fibrous dysplasia from meningioma may occasionally be difficult on CT scan, but MRI scan will usually discriminate the two entities.[426,438,439]

Management of patients is directed at improving the craniofacial abnormality and resulting facial deformity through surgical debulking (complete surgical resection is impossible). Surgical treatments for globe malposition are generally successful.[428] Radiation is not usually employed because of the potential increased risk of malignant degeneration. Craniofacial surgical teams have been increasingly successful with more than 60% of patients having a good cosmetic result at 1 year.[431]

Vision loss is a frequent complication of fibrous dysplasia involving the skull. Osguthorpe and Gudeman[430] identified

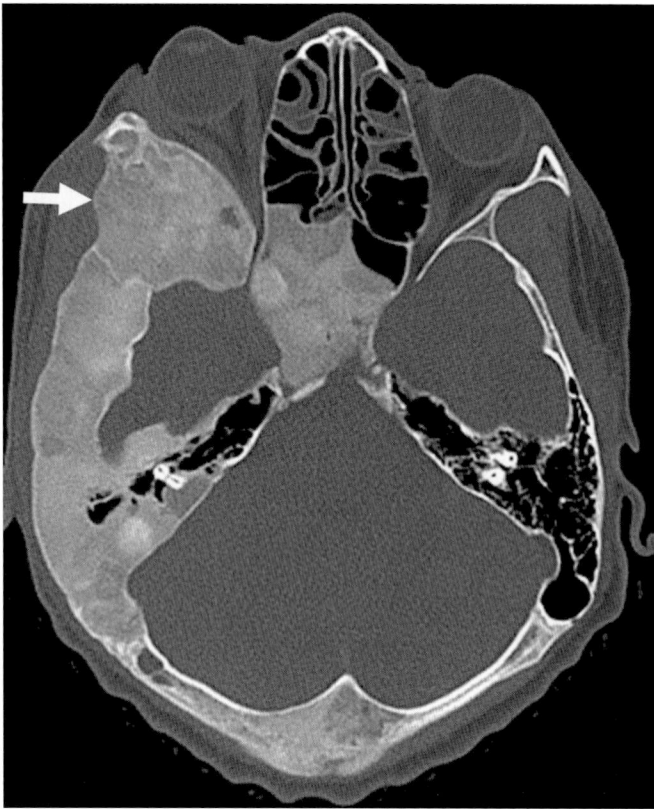

Figure 18–44. Axial CT scan, bone window, of a patient with fibrous dysplasia of the right sphenoid and temporal bones and clivus. The abnormal bone (arrow) has a thickened, ground glass appearance. The patient had severe proptosis of the right eye but no clinical evidence of optic neuropathy.

30 cases of monocular or binocular vision loss in the literature between 1965 and 1987. In Katz and Nerad's[426] series of 20 patients four were identified with vision loss and they emphasized that conditions associated with the bony abnormality such as mucoceles, hemorrhage, and aneurysmal bone cysts were the cause for the vision loss as opposed to actual bony narrowing of the optic canal by the fibrous dysplasia. Patients with vision loss from compressive optic neuropathy have been successfully treated with steroids,[435] and surgical decompression of the orbital apex and optic canal.[428,432,434,440] Blindness has also been described as a complication of prophylactic canal decompression in fibrous dysplasia.[441] Often, the process spontaneously arrests with no further bone growth. Thus, conservative therapy and observation are often employed,[429,433] particularly when there is no or minimal visual impairment even though radiographically the optic nerve appears compromised.[442] Surgical decompression is considered, however, when clinical evidence of progressive optic neuropathy (acuity, visual field, or color vision loss) occurs.

Orbital infections

Infections of the orbit are both potentially sight and life-threatening conditions that demand prompt recognition and therapeutic intervention. The spectrum of orbital infec-

tious disease is wide and ranges from acute, bacterial infections to more insidious processes due to fungi, for instance. Various bacteria have been reported to cause infectious orbital cellulitis, and the clinical setting may help determine the etiologic agent (pediatric, history of trauma, recent surgery). Anatomy also plays an important role in the genesis of orbital infection. Since the paranasal sinuses structurally represent walls of the orbit, infectious processes in the sinuses are a frequent cause of orbital cellulitis. Organisms may also gain entry into the orbit by traveling through the valveless veins of the face, teeth, and neck. The orbital septum is an effective barrier to the spread of infection. Thus, it is unusual for infections involving the eyelids (without penetrating trauma) to extend into the orbit.

Orbital infections may be characterized as being preseptal or postseptal. Preseptal cellulitis is usually characterized by isolated eyelid swelling, tenderness, and induration, but the patient remains free of any inflammatory changes in the orbit or eye movement limitations. Postseptal infections or orbital cellulitis are characterized by similar external eyelid changes in association with proptosis, eye movement limitations, and occasionally vision loss (**Fig. 18–45**). Patients with a subperiosteal abscess may have a relatively benign orbital examination with eyelid edema as sole manifestation of the infectious process.[443]

Clinical presentation

Presentation in children with an orbital infection is relatively common and characterized by pain, redness, fever, and an elevation of the white blood cell count. Sinus disease is common, and the ethmoid sinus is the most frequently involved.[444] A purple hue to the skin is sometimes seen in *hemophilus* infections. *Staphylococcus aureus*, streptococcus species, and *Hemophilus influenzae* are the most commonly encountered pathogenic organisms,[445,446] and methicillin-resistant cellulitis is occurring with increased frequency.[447] Evaluation of patients with suspected orbital cellulitis begins with imaging studies (usually CT scan, **Fig. 18–45**), measurement of body temperature, blood cultures, and a blood white count. Therapy is directed at the infection and includes intravenous antibiotics in addition to surgical drainage when necessary. Antibiotic coverage should include therapy against penicillinase-resistant staphylococcus and anaerobes. Ominous signs include loss of vision or worsening of proptosis, which could indicate either abscess compression of the optic nerve or extension of the infection into the cavernous sinus with resulting cavernous sinus thrombosis. Such cases with posterior orbital extension or cavernous sinus involvement may require more aggressive therapy.[448]

Mucoceles

Paranasal sinus mucoceles are cystic, expanding lesions that can arise in any of the paranasal sinuses (frontal and ethmoid most commonly). They can eventually erode bone and extend into the orbit (**Fig. 18–46**) or intracranially. The presentation is more like a mass lesion than an infection although more accelerated presentations can occur. Patients develop non-axial proptosis and double vision. Treatment is usually with endoscopic sinus surgery.[449]

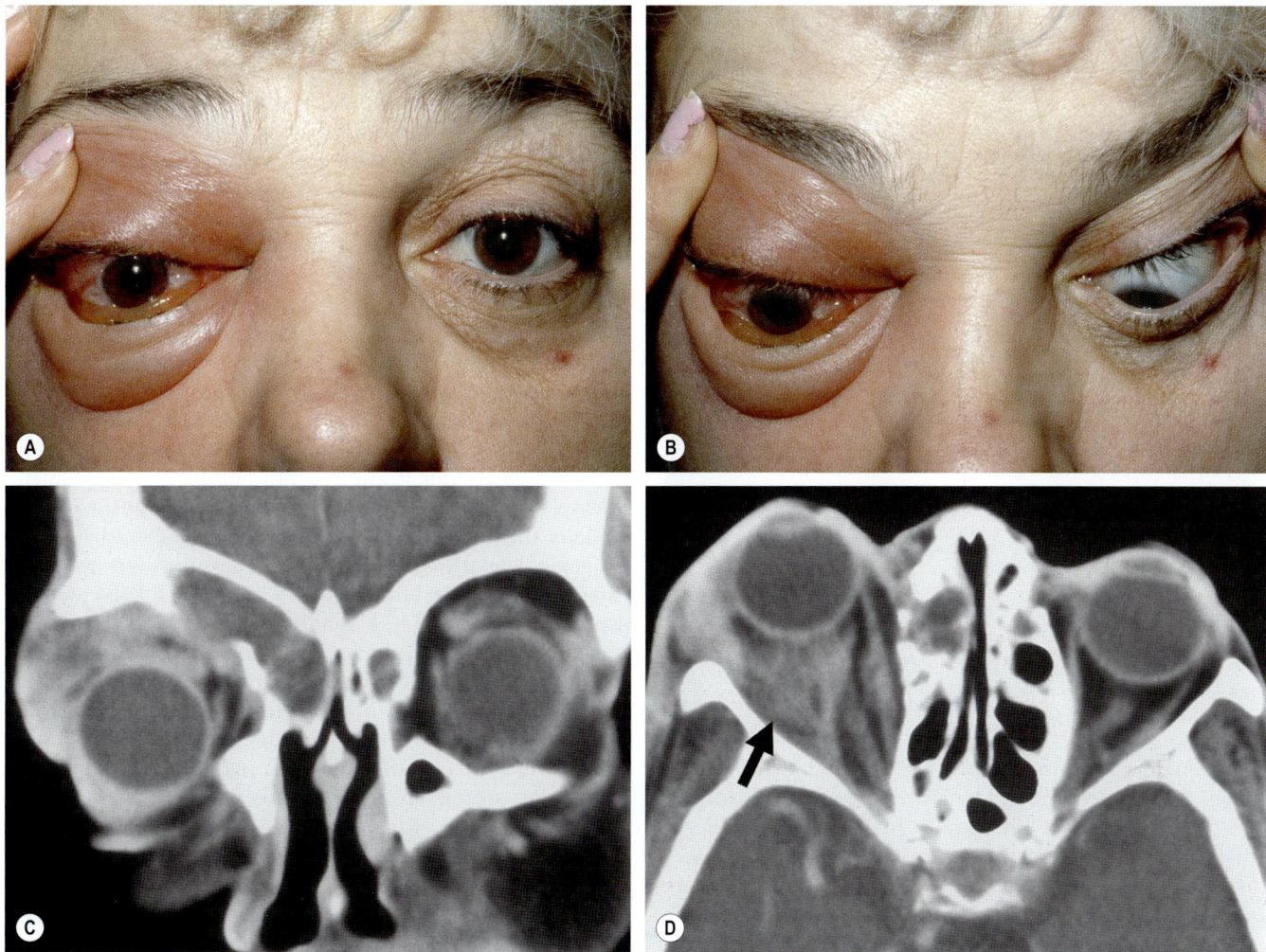

Figure 18–45. Orbital cellulitis in two patients. **A**. This patient has marked proptosis, eyelid swelling and chemosis secondary to orbital cellulitis. On attempted downgaze (**B**) the eye does not depress fully. Impaired eye movements almost always accompany orbital cellulitis but are rarely seen with preseptal cellulitis. In another patient (**C**) a coronal CT scan reveals an extensive enhancing lesion due to orbital cellulitis. The corresponding axial images (**D**) show the extent of the infectious infiltrate (arrow) (Courtesy of Scott Goldstein, MD).

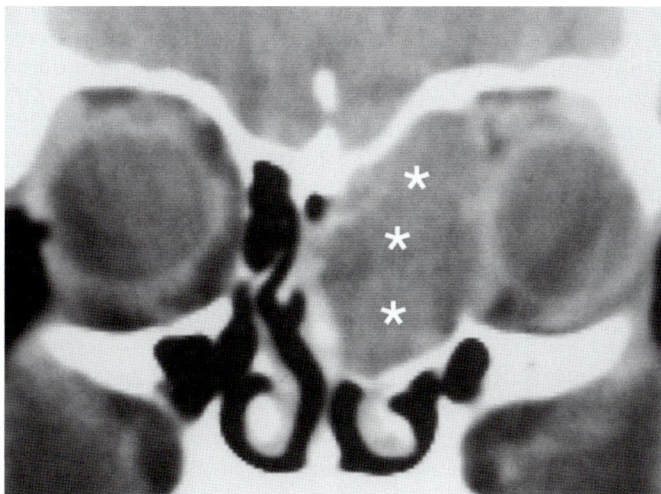

Figure 18–46. Coronal CT scan of an ethmoid sinus mucocele (asterisks) which appears as a cystic mass invading the left orbit.

Silent sinus syndrome

The silent sinus syndrome (or chronic maxillary atelectasis) consists of the painless onset of enophthalmos and vertical double vision worse in upgaze secondary to resorption of the bone of the orbital floor by chronic maxillary sinusitis.[450–456] Patients can present with insidious onset of enophthalmos with an exaggerated superior sulcus (**Fig. 18–3b**) and double vision. Occasionally there can be a more precipitous presentation if the floor of the orbit gives away more suddenly.[451] CT scan shows absence of the orbital floor with orbital contents bowing into the maxillary sinus (**Fig. 18–47**). Treatment is by surgical rebuilding of the orbital floor.

Fungal infections

Unlike patients with bacterial infections, fungal infections tend to occur in patients who are debilitated or immunocompromised. Both mucormycosis and aspergillus may spread from the sinus to the orbit. Isolated examples of even more obscure fungi such as blastomyces and sporothorix may be occasionally be encountered in the orbit.[457]

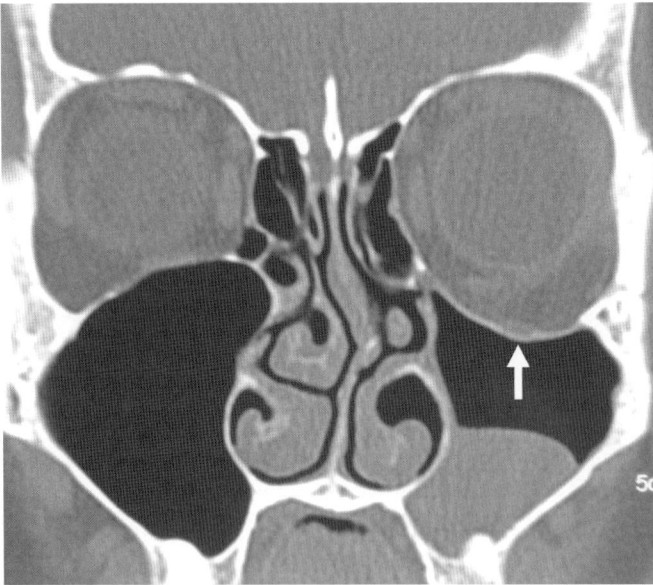

Figure 18–47. Coronal CT scan of a patient with silent sinus syndrome of the left orbit. Chronic inflammation of the maxillary sinus has eroded the floor of the left orbit (arrow) which has an abnormal concave appearance compared to the other side. This erosion alone can lead to enophthalmos and vertical strabismus. This CT scan corresponds to the clinical photograph of the patient depicted in Fig. 18–3b.

Phycomycosis (mucormycosis). Infections with the phycomycetes may involve the lungs, gastrointestinal tract, or the rhino-orbital structures. The rhino-orbital infection typically begins in the nose and spreads through the maxillary and ethmoid sinuses into the orbit.[458-463] However, occasionally there will be no obvious sinus lesion. The organism spreads by invading blood vessel walls and may produce necrosis, thrombosis, and ultimately infarction of the involved orbital tissues.[464] Most patients who develop mucormycosis have a predisposing risk factor such as diabetes, leukemia, lymphoma, septicemia, or burns.

Symptoms may include pain, fever, headache, reduced acuity, double vision, facial numbness, and sometimes a seropurulent discharge from the nose.[460] On examination of involved tissues, a black eschar characterized by necrosis and dark discoloration is frequently noted. However, the eschar is usually a late finding, and its absence does not exclude the diagnosis of mucormycosis. Many affected patients present with an orbital apex syndrome with both internal and external ophthalmoplegia, optic neuropathy, ptosis, and sensory loss in the trigeminal distribution.[459,460,464-467] Most cases are unilateral, but bilateral cases are well recognized. Orbital infarction syndrome can occur as a complication of mucormycosis because of its angioinvasive nature. Infarction of the orbit can also occur as a consequence of carotid occlusion, aneurysm or dissection, sickle cell disease, temporal arteritis, or as a complication of craniotomy.[468-471]

Neuroimaging studies typically reveal inflammatory disease in the sinuses and the orbits. Both blood and CSF cultures are seldom positive. The diagnosis of mucormycosis is best established by a biopsy demonstration of non-septate hyphae branching at 90-degree angles.

Treatment must be initiated promptly and usually requires both surgical and medical approaches. Complete excision of necrotic tissue is necessary and antifungal agents are started. However, many patients may be treated without orbital exenteration, particularly those with preserved visual acuity.[459-461,472] Amphotericin is the first-line drug but supplemental use of ketoconazole has also been suggested. Simultaneously the medical team must correct any metabolic acidosis or underlying bacterial infection. Ultimately, the extensive and aggressive debridement may require reconstructive efforts in the future. Mortality rates are in the range of 15–35%, and the prognosis seems to be dependent on prompt recognition.[459-461,464,472] Those individuals treated successfully have usually been diagnosed within 4 days of symptom onset.[461] Spread to brain and intracranial vascular structures in so-called angioinvasive rhino-orbital-cerebral mucormycosis, which is frequently associated with cerebral infarction, has an extremely high mortality rate.

Aspergillosis. This is another ubiquitous fungal organism that spreads to the orbits from the paranasal sinuses. Occasionally the organism affects immunocompetent hosts, but in general, patients are immunocompromised to some extent at the time of diagnosis.[473] Orbital involvement in aspergillosis occurs as a manifestation of a disseminated infection with widespread necrotizing angiitis from microscopic fungus invasion of small vessels. Endophthalmitis may occasionally occur in this setting. Infections tend to be more indolent than patients with mucormycosis. Despite this slower course, patients with orbital aspergillus may still lose vision or die from their infection. A patient with a steroid-responsive optic neuropathy was ultimately found to have aspergillosis as the primary cause of the problem and succumbed to the illness.[467,474-476]

Patients usually present with orbital signs of progressive exophthalmos and a chronic inflammation of the sinuses. Occasionally patients manifest with vision loss and the diagnosis is dependent upon a biopsy that reflects dichotomously branching septated hyphae. Treatment, as with mucormycosis, requires wide surgical debridement in conjunction with systemic amphotericin alone or in combination with other anti-fungal agents. Mortality, unfortunately, is high, and successful treatment again requires prompt recognition of the condition.

Allergic fungal sinusitis. Allergic fungal sinusitis (AFS) is a type of paranasal sinus mycosis encountered in patients with chronic sinusitis.[477-484] Unlike other forms of paranasal mycosis, AFS is a noninvasive form of sinusitis, and therefore requires a different approach to treatment. AFS typically occurs in immunocompetent hosts with a history of nasal polyposis and chronic sinusitis. Patients are frequently atopic and may have peripheral eosinophilia. Presenting symptoms include nasal obstruction, pain, rhinorrhea, visual loss, diplopia, proptosis, cranial nerve palsy, facial deformity and patients may produce a thick green or brown mucus.[477-484]

In one series, 17% of patients presented with orbital symptoms.[480] Radiographic studies typically show involvement of multiple sinuses with bone erosion or remodeling. The inflamed mucosa exhibits increased signal intensity on T2-weighted MRI images. Histopathologically there are embedded eosinophils, Charcot–Leyden crystals, and extramucosal fungal hyphae. The offending organisms are the dematiaceous fungi such as *Bipolaris*, *Exserohilum*, *Curvularia*, *Alternaria*, and *Aspergillus* species.[483] Unlike in patients with invasive sino-orbital mycoses that require more aggressive debridement, treatment in AFS includes debridement of just fungal debris, aeration of the involved sinuses, and systemic and topical steroids.[483] The role of topical antifugal agents has not yet been clarified.

Orbital trauma

Patients with craniofacial trauma commonly present for ophthalmic or neuro-ophthalmic evaluation, both in the acute and the resolution phases. Patients usually are evaluated in a compromised state, secondary to associated cranial injuries. Therefore, historical and examination information may be limited. Patients may also have significant proptosis and orbital soft tissue swelling that limit the initial evaluation. Exclusion of a ruptured globe or a significant retrobulbar hemorrhage (**Fig. 18–48**) requiring decompression is

critical in the early phases of evaluation. Recognition and treatment of traumatic optic nerve injuries may improve the ultimate prognosis in this condition (see Chapter 5). Radiographic imaging in the acute setting is critical to determine the extent of orbital injury and involvement of the extraocular muscles. Important features to evaluate include bony fractures, the degree and direction of bone displacement, soft tissue injury or abnormal globe contour, retrobulbar hemorrhage (**Fig. 18–48**), and the presence of air or foreign body in the orbit. CT scan is the imaging modality of choice and should include bony windows in both the axial and coronal planes. Occasionally MRI is helpful in the identification of traumatic optic nerve sheath hemorrhages or in the characterization of soft tissue swelling.

Orbital "blowout" or floor fractures are common after facial trauma. There may be obvious external evidence of trauma but in some blowout fractures the external appearance will be relatively normal (**Fig. 18–49**). Palpation of the bony orbital rim is necessary to exclude step-off fractures and

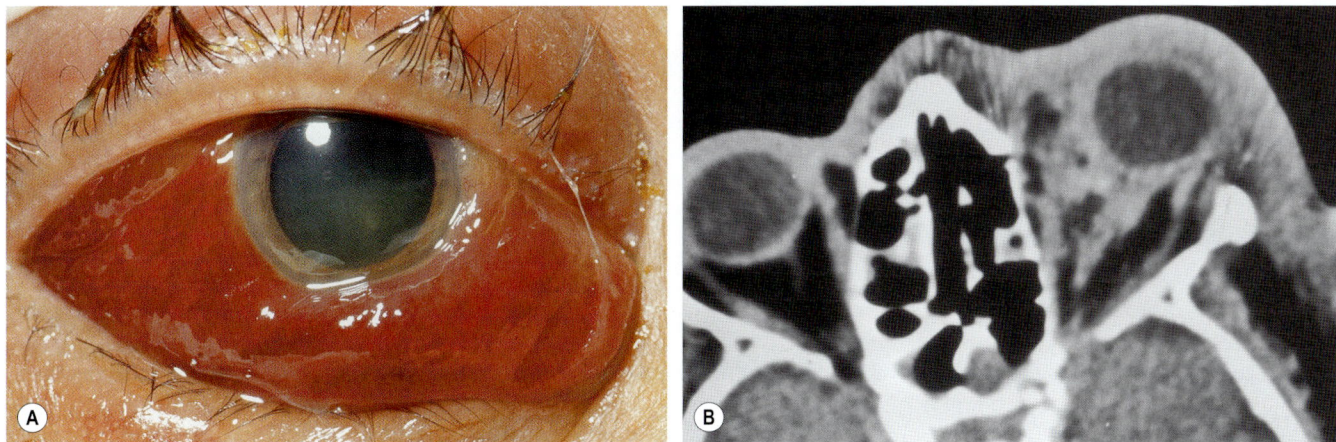

Figure 18–48. A. Clinical photograph of extensive subconjunctival hemorrhage in a patient with retrobulbar hemorrhage. The pupil has been pharmacologically dilated. In another patient (**B**) on axial CT scan massive left proptosis and blood within the left orbit and the retrobulbar space are demonstrated secondary to retrobulbar hemorrhage after trauma.

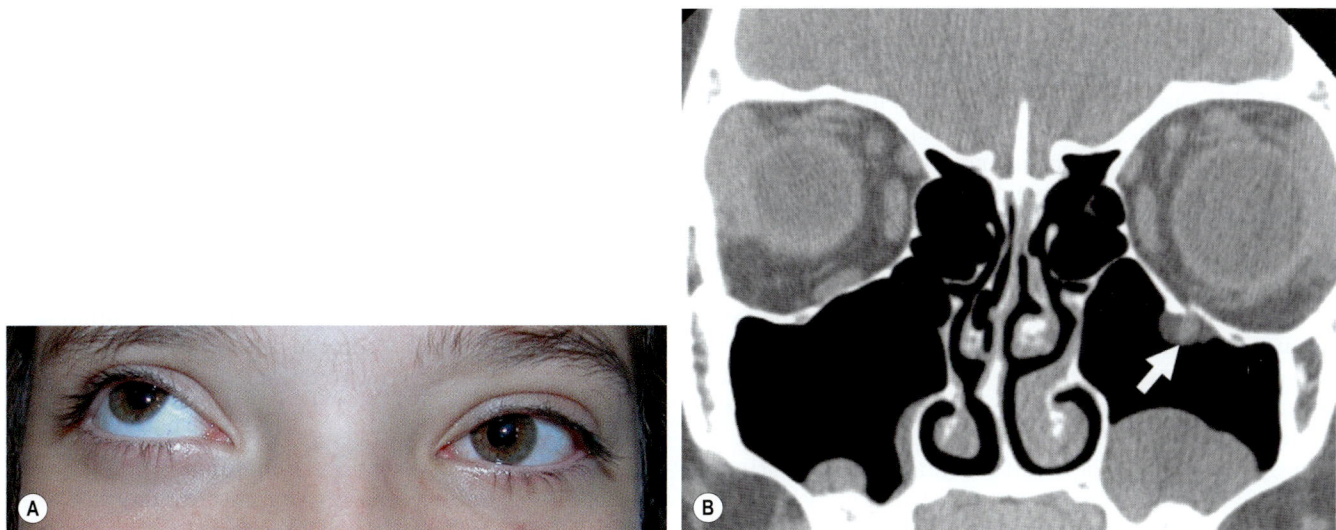

Figure 18–49. A. Clinical photograph of a patient with an elevation deficit of the left eye after blunt trauma. Despite no obvious external signs of trauma, elevation was markedly impaired and CT scan (**B**) demonstrated a "trap door" inferior floor fracture restricting the inferior rectus (arrow) which prevented the eye from elevating. (Courtesy of William Katowitz, MD).

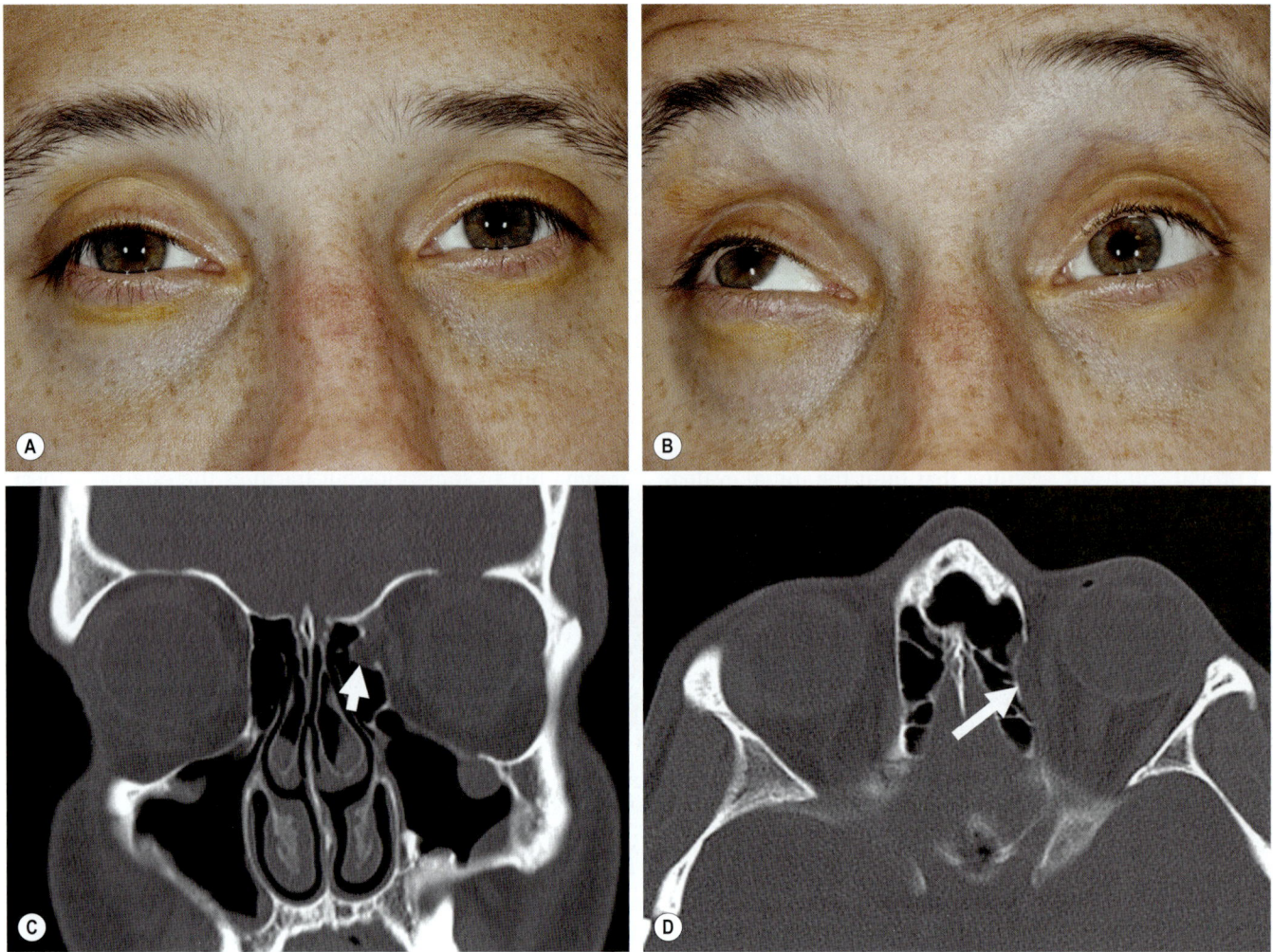

Figure 18–50. Clinical photograph (**A**) of a patient after orbital trauma. There is good ocular alignment in the primary position. However, in attempted elevation while in adduction (**B**) the left eye fails to elevate. On a coronal CT image (**C**) the superior oblique and surrounding soft tissue is seen to extend into the area of an ethmoidal fracture (arrow). Axial CT scan (**D**) shows how this causes an abnormal trajectory of the superior oblique muscle (arrow), resulting in impaired movement of the superior oblique tendon (acquired Brown syndrome).

to identify areas of reduced sensation. The measurement of the globe position to rule out enophthalmos or proptosis by exophthalmometry should be performed. Limited eye movements from entrapment (**Fig. 18–49**) should be distinguished from cranial nerve palsies through the use of forced duction testing. Other facial fractures important in craniofacial trauma include those involving the frontal bone since their presence may suggest brain involvement or affect the trochlear or the function of the superior oblique muscle (**Fig. 18–50**). Nasal ethmoidal fractures can present with telecanthus and lacrimal injury. Zygomatic fractures are important as they may involve the lateral rectus muscle and impair eye movements. Some orbital injuries can be associated with traumatic nerve damage causing isolated muscle palsies or actual trauma to the muscle causing a hematoma or traumatic rupture (**Fig. 18–51**).

The appropriate management of orbital blowout fractures remains a controversial issue, particularly in the early stages. Some favor early surgical intervention to restore orbital volume and anatomic relationships. Most agree that early surgical intervention for blowout fractures is indicated in patients with symptomatic diplopia and positive forced duc-

tions, particularly when there is CT scan evidence of soft tissue or muscle entrapment and no improvement over the first 7–14 days. If the fracture is not repaired and entrapment persists, the patient can be left with chronic eye movement limitation and diplopia (**Fig. 18–52**). Similarly, early enophthalmos of greater than 3 mm or significant globe ptosis or inferior displacement are important indications for orbital surgery. Early surgery is indicated in patients with extensive fractures in whom subsequent enophthalmos is almost certain.

However, it is clear that conservative management in patients with full eye movements, no soft tissue entrapment on CT scan, only small fractures, and minimal enophthalmos is a reasonable course. Such patients require no further surgery and will not develop more significant cosmetic or eye muscle abnormality.

The repair of orbital fractures usually involves surgery on the floor of the orbit, either through the eyelid or transconjunctivally. The fractures are identified under the periorbita and soft tissue is released. Some type of material is then used to bridge the orbital floor defect and to allow for restoration of normal soft tissue position. Both autogenous tissue such

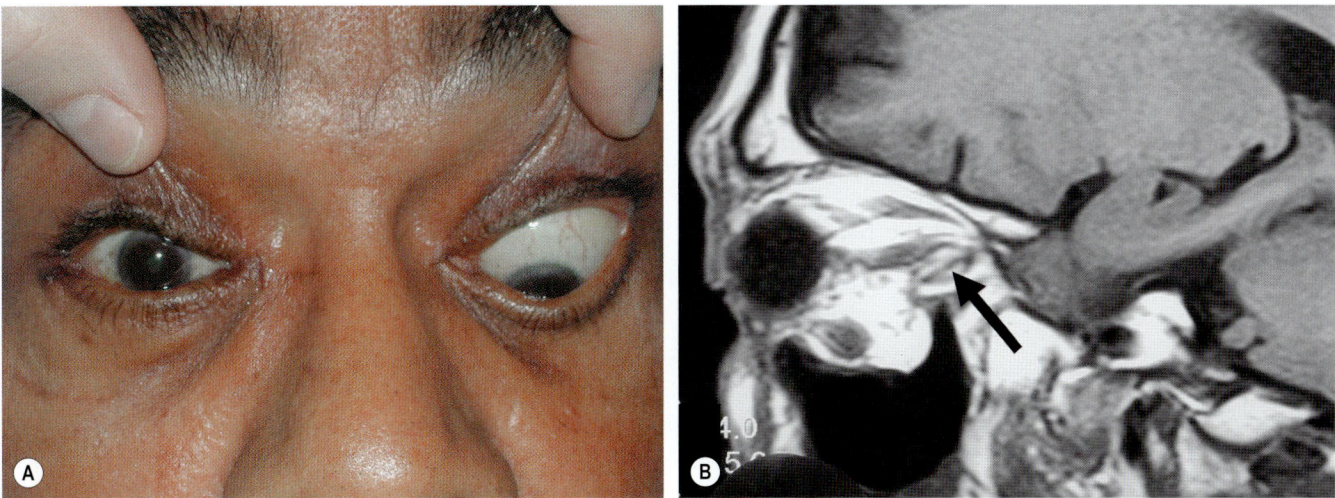

Figure 18–51. A. Impaired downgaze of the right eye in a patient after blunt trauma to the orbit. **B**. On a sagittal T1-weighted MRI scan the right inferior rectus has been ruptured (arrow).

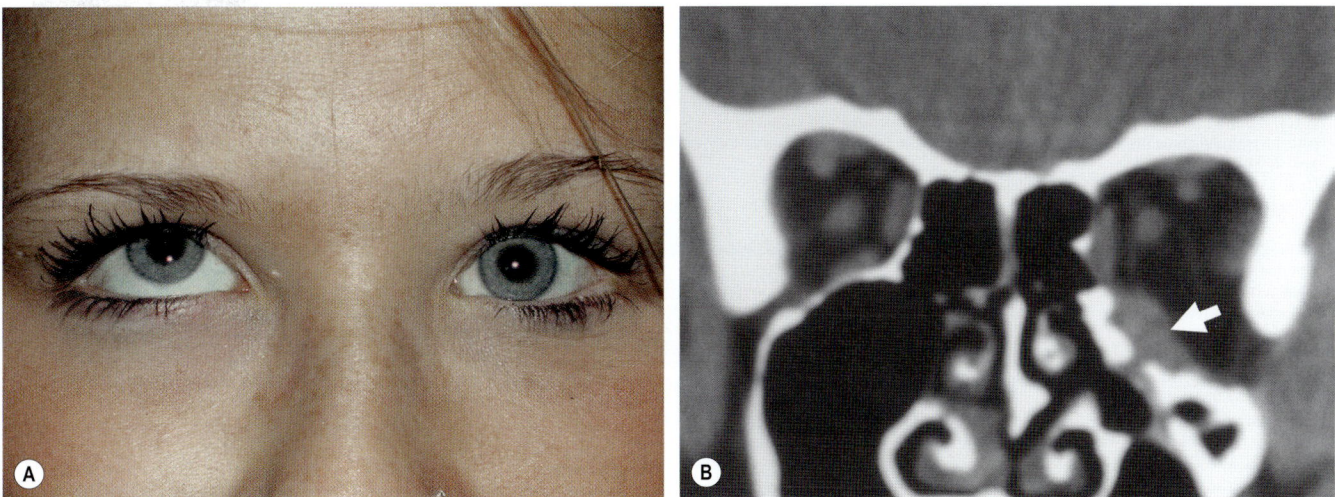

Figure 18–52. A. Clinical photograph of a patient with a distant history of orbital trauma complaining of chronic double vision. Elevation deficit of the left eye is seen and on coronal CT scan (**B**) scarring of the inferior rectus (arrow) is seen adjacent to an old orbital fracture.

as harvested graft material in the form of bone and alloplastic materials may be used. Most favor inert alloplastic materials which are available in many different forms, including porous polyethylene and metal alloys.

Orbital surgery

In addition to the decompression procedure for TAO and optic nerve sheath fenestration, orbitotomy is performed for biopsy and removal of mass lesions. The specific surgical approach is guided by the location of the lesion and can be grouped broadly as anterior, lateral, and superior.[485–488] A combination approach is occasionally used, requiring the cooperation of otolaryngologists, neurosurgeons, and reconstructive surgeons. The anterior approach is the most frequently employed and incisions may be made either transconjunctivally or through the skin. This technique may involve surgery through the orbital septum or can be extraperiosteal. This technique can be used to biopsy lesions

anywhere in the orbit and to remove palpable mass lesions. The retrobulbar space may be accessed through a conjunctival incision with temporary displacement of the medial rectus muscle. This technique is particularly useful for optic nerve sheath fenestration. The anterior extraperiosteal approach is particularly useful for lesions that are based in or involve the bone or sinuses.

Lateral orbitotomy allows access to the retrobulbar space and involves a lateral and sub-brow skin incision with removal of portions of the lateral wall of the orbit and zygomatic arch. In the superior approaches the orbit is accessed through a frontal or frontotemporal craniotomy. The superior procedures are usually necessary for removal of orbital apex lesions or lesions that involve the optic canal and intracranial contents. The procedure allows for en bloc excision of the roof and lateral wall of the orbit and provides a wide view of the orbit and the adjacent intracranial structures. If removal of the optic nerve is planned, the canal must be unroofed and the annulus of Zinn incised.

Some malignant tumors of the orbit threaten to extend beyond the orbit and require exenteration. This definitive procedure involves removal of the entire orbital contents. When the eyelids are also removed, this is called superexenteration. With malignant lacrimal gland tumors that involve bone, exenteration may include removal of involved portions of bone. Exenteration is also used in the surgical management of malignant tumors of the paranasal sinus and nasopharynx that extend into the orbit.

References

1. Beard C, Quickert MH. Anatomy of the Orbit (A dissection manual). Birmingham, Aesculapius Publishing Company, 1969.
2. Doxanas MT, Anderson RL. Clinical Orbital Anatomy. Baltimore, Williams and Wilkins, 1984.
3. Jakobiec FA. Ocular Anatomy, Embryology and Teratology. Philadelphia, Harper & Row, 1982.
4. Aviv RI, Casselman J. Orbital imaging: Part 1. Normal anatomy. Clin Radiol 2005;60:279–287.
5. Langer BG, Mafee MF, Pollack S, et al. MRI of the normal orbit and optic pathway. Radiol Clin North Am 1987;25:429–446.
6. Rhoton AL, Jr. The orbit. Neurosurgery 2002;51:S303–334.
7. Zonneveld FW, Koornneef L, Hillen B, et al. Normal direct multiplanar CT anatomy of the orbit with correlative anatomic cryosections. Radiol Clin North Am 1987;25: 381–407.
8. Dickinson AJ, Gausas RE. Orbital lymphatics: do they exist? Eye 2006;20:1145–1148.
9. Fogt F, Zimmerman RL, Daly T, et al. Observation of lymphatic vessels in orbital fat of patients with inflammatory conditions: a form fruste of lymphangiogenesis? Int J Mol Med 2004;13:681–683.
10. Gausas RE, Daly T, Fogt F. D2–40 expression demonstrates lymphatic vessel characteristics in the dural portion of the optic nerve sheath. Ophthal Plast Reconstr Surg 2007;23:32–36.
11. Gausas RE, Gonnering RS, Lemke BN, et al. Identification of human orbital lymphatics. Ophthal Plast Reconstr Surg 1999;15:252–259.
12. Jakobiec FA, Iwamoto T. Ocular adnexa: introduction to the lids, conjunctiva and orbit. In: Jakobiec FA (ed). Ocular Anatomy, Embryology and Teratology, pp 677–732. Philadelphia, Harper & Row, 1982.
13. Liu GT. Anatomy and physiology of the trigeminal nerve. In: Miller NR, Newman NJ (eds). Walsh and Hoyt's Clinical Neuro-ophthalmology, 5th edn, pp 1595–1648. Baltimore, Williams and Wilkins, 1998.
14. Bergen MP. Spatial aspects of the orbital vascular system. In: Jakobiec FA (ed). Ocular Anatomy, Embryology and Teratology, pp 859–868. Philadelphia, Harper & Row, 1982.
15. Hayreh SS. Arteries of the Orbit in the Human Being. Br J Surg 1963;50:938–953.
16. Eggers HM. Functional anatomy of the extraocular muscles. In: Jakobiec FA (ed). Ocular Anatomy, Embryology and Teratology, pp. 783–834. Philadelphia, Harper & Row, 1982.
17. Clark RA, Miller JM, Demer JL. Location and stability of rectus muscle pulleys. Muscle paths as a function of gaze. Invest Ophthalmol Vis Sci 1997;38:227–240.
18. Demer JL, Miller JM, Poukens V, et al. Evidence for fibromuscular pulleys of the recti extraocular muscles. Invest Ophthalmol Vis Sci 1995;36:1125–1136.
19. Demer JL, Oh SY, Poukens V. Evidence for active control of rectus extraocular muscle pulleys. Invest Ophthalmol Vis Sci 2000;41:1280–1290.
20. Jiang L, Demer JL. Magnetic resonance imaging of the functional anatomy of the inferior rectus muscle in superior oblique muscle palsy. Ophthalmology 2008;115: 2079–2086.
21. Demer JL, Oh SY, Clark RA, et al. Evidence for a pulley of the inferior oblique muscle. Invest Ophthalmol Vis Sci 2003;44:3856–3865.
22. Greiner JV, Covington HI, Allansmith MR. The human limbus. A scanning electron microscopic study. Arch Ophthalmol 1979;97:1159–1165.
23. Koornneef L. Orbital septa: anatomy and function. Ophthalmology 1979;86:876–880.
24. Bradbury PG, Levy IS, McDonald WI. Transient uniocular visual loss on deviation of the eye in association with intraorbital tumours. J Neurol Neurosurg Psychiatry 1987;50: 615–619.
25. Danesh-Meyer HV, Savino PJ, Bilyk JR, et al. Gaze-evoked amaurosis produced by intraorbital buckshot pellet. Ophthalmology 2001;108:201–206.
26. Segal S, Salyani A, DeAngelis DD. Gaze-evoked amaurosis secondary to an intraorbital foreign body. Can J Ophthalmol 2007;42:147–148.
27. Tsai RK, Chen JY, Wang HZ. Gaze-evoked amaurosis caused by intraconal cavernous hemangioma: a case report. Kaohsiung J Med Sci 1997;13:324–327.
28. Bremner FD, Sanders MD, Stanford MR. Gaze evoked amaurosis in dysthyroid orbitopathy. Br J Ophthalmol 1999;83:501.
29. Katz B, Hoyt WF. Gaze-evoked amaurosis from vitreopapillary traction. Am J Ophthalmol 2005;139:631–637.
30. O'Duffy D, James B, Elston J. Idiopathic intracranial hypertension presenting with gaze-evoked amaurosis. Acta Ophthalmol Scand 1998;76:119–120.
31. Otto CS, Coppit GL, Mazzoli RA, et al. Gaze-evoked amaurosis: a report of five cases. Ophthalmology 2003;110:322–326.
32. Pascual J, Combarros O, Berciano J. Gaze-evoked amaurosis in pseudotumor cerebri. Neurology 1988;38:1654–1655.
33. Sivak-Callcott J, Carpenter JS, Rosen CL, et al. Gaze-evoked amaurosis associated with an intracranial aneurysm. Arch Ophthalmol 2004;122:1404–1406.
34. De-LaPaz MA, Boniuk M. Fundus manifestations of orbital disease and treatment of orbital disease. Surv Ophthalmol 1995;40:3–21.
35. Newell FW. Choridal folds. Am J Ophthalmol 1973;75:930–942.
36. Norton EWD. A characteristic fluorescein angiographic appearance in choroidal folds. Proc Roy Soc Med 1969;62:119–128.
37. Leahey AB, Brucker AJ, Wyszynski RE, et al. Chorioretinal folds. A comparison of unilateral and bilateral cases. Arch Ophthalmol 1993;111:357–359.
38. Byrne SF. Standardized echography in the differentiation of orbital lesions. Surv Ophthalmol 1984;29:226–228.
39. Byrne SF. Standardized echography of the eye and orbit. Neuroradiology 1986;28:618–640.
40. Dallow RL. Evaluation of unilateral exophthalmos with ultrasonography: analysis of 258 consecutive cases. Laryngoscope 1975;85:1905–1919.
41. Dallow RL, Momose KJ, Weber AL, et al. Comparison of ultrasonography, computerized tomography (EMI scan), and radiographic techniques in evaluation of exophthalmos. Trans Amer Acad Ophthal Otolaryngol 1976;81:305–322.
42. Byrne SF, Gendron EK, Glaser JS, et al. Diameter of normal extraocular recti muscles with echography. Am J Ophthalmol 1991;112:706–713.
43. Neudorfer M, Leibovitch I, Stolovitch C, et al. Intraorbital and periorbital tumors in children—value of ultrasound and color Doppler imaging in the differential diagnosis. Am J Ophthalmol 2004;137:1065–1072.
44. Williamson TH, Harris A. Color Doppler ultrasound imaging of the eye and orbit. Surv Ophthalmol 1996;40:255–267.
45. Hilal SK. Computed tomography of the orbit. Ophthalmology 1979;86:864–870.
46. Hodes BL, Weinberg P. A combined approach for the diagnosis of orbital disease. Computed tomography and standardized A-scan echography. Arch Ophthalmol 1977;95:781–788.
47. Hunsaker JN, Anderson RE, Van DH, et al. A comparison of computed tomographic techniques in the diagnosis of Graves' ophthalmopathy. Ophthalmic Surgery 1979;10:34–40.
48. Bullock JD, Goldberg SH, Rakes SM. Orbital tumors in children. Oph Plas Reconstr Surg 1989;5:13–16.
49. Grossniklaus HE, Lass JH, Abramowsky CR, et al. Childhood orbital pseudotumor. Ann Ophthalmol 1985;17:372–377.
50. Gunalp I, Gunduz K. Pediatric orbital tumors in Turkey. Ophthal Plast Reconstr Surg 1995;11:193–199.
51. Haik BG, Ellsworth RM. Pediatric orbital tumors. Trans New Orleans Acad Ophthalmol 1986;109.
52. Kodsi SR, Shetlar DJ, Campbell RJ, et al. A review of 340 orbital tumors in children during a 60-year period. Am J Ophthalmol 1994;117:177–182.
53. Volpe NJ, Jakobiec FA. Pediatric orbital tumors. Int Ophthalmol Clin 1992;32:201–221.
54. Bajaj MS, Pushker N, Chaturvedi A, et al. Orbital space-occupying lesions in Indian children. J Pediatr Ophthalmol Strabismus 2007;44:106–111.
55. Bakhshi S, Singh P, Chawla N. Malignant childhood proptosis: study of 104 cases. J Pediatr Hematol Oncol 2008;30:73–76.
56. Demirci H, Shields CL, Karatza EC, et al. Orbital lymphoproliferative tumors: analysis of clinical features and systemic involvement in 160 cases. Ophthalmology 2008;115:1626–1631, 1631, e1621–1623.
57. Margo CE, Mulla ZD. Malignant tumors of the orbit. Analysis of the Florida Cancer Registry. Ophthalmology 1998;105:185–190.
58. Dallow RL, Pratt SG. Approach to orbital disorders and frequency of disease occcurence. In: Albert DM, Jakobiec FA (eds). Principles and Practice of Ophthalmology, pp 1881–1890. Philadelphia, W.B. Saunders, 1994.
59. Rootman J. Frequency and differential diagnosis of orbital disease. In: Rootman J (ed). Diseases of the Orbit: A Multidisciplinary Approach, pp 119–139. Philadelphia, J.B. Lippincott, 1988.
60. Kennedy RE. An evaluation of 820 orbital cases. Trans Am Ophthalmol Soc 1984;82: 134–157.
61. Shields JA, Bakewell B, Augsburger JJ, et al. Classification and incidence of space-occupying lesions of the orbit. A survey of 645 biopsies. Arch Ophthalmol 1984;102: 1606–1611.
62. Brand OJ, Barrett JC, Simmonds MJ, et al. Association of the thyroid stimulating hormone receptor gene (TSHR) with Graves' disease. Hum Mol Genet 2009;18: 1704–1713.
63. Dechairo BM, Zabaneh D, Collins J, et al. Association of the TSHR gene with Graves' disease: the first disease specific locus. Eur J Hum Genet 2005;13:1223–1230.
64. Volpe R. Immunological aspects of autoimmune thyroid disease. Prog Clin Biol Res 1981;74:1–27.
65. Volpe R. Autoimmune thyroid disease—a perspective. Mol Biol Med 1986;3:25–51.
66. Volpe R. Immunoregulation in autoimmune thyroid disease [editorial]. N Engl J Med 1987;316:44–46.
67. Weetman AP. Cellular immune responses in autoimmune thyroid disease. Clin Endocrinol (Oxf) 2004;61:405–413.
68. Weetman AP, Yateman ME, Ealey PA, et al. Thyroid-stimulating antibody activity between different immunoglobulin G subclasses. J Clin Invest 1990;86:723–727.
69. Char DH. Normal thyroid gland and mechanisms of hyperthyroidism. In: Throid Eye Disease, 3rd edn, pp 5–23. Boston, Butterworth-Heinemann, 1997.
70. Weetman AP. Graves' disease. N Engl J Med 2000;343:1236–1248.
71. Weetman AP. The genetics of autoimmune thyroid disease. Horm Metab Res 2009;41: 421–425.

72. Brent GA. Clinical practice. Graves' disease. N Engl J Med 2008;358:2594–2605.

73. Helfand M, Redfern CC. Clinical guideline, part 2. Screening for thyroid disease: an update. American College of Physicians [see comments]. Ann Intern Med 1998;129: 144–158.

74. Spencer CA, Schwarzbein D, Guttler RB, et al. Thyrotropin (TSH)-releasing hormone stimulation test responses employing-third and fourth generation TSH assays. J Clin Endocrinol Metab 1993;76:494–498.

75. Bartley GB, Fatourechi V, Kadrmas EF, et al. The incidence of Graves' ophthalmopathy in Olmsted County, Minnesota. Am J Ophthalmol 1995;120:511–517.

76. Bartley GB, Fatourechi V, Kadrmas EF, et al. Chronology of Graves' ophthalmopathy in an incidence cohort. Am J Ophthalmol 1996;121:426–434.

77. El-Kaissi S, Frauman AG, Wall JR. Thyroid-associated ophthalmopathy: a practical guide to classification, natural history and management. Intern Med J 2004;34:482–491.

78. Marcocci C, Bartalena L, Bogazzi F, et al. Studies on the occurrence of ophthalmopathy in Graves' disease. Acta Endocrinol (Copenh) 1989;120:473–478.

79. Wiersinga WM, Bartalena L. Epidemiology and prevention of Graves' ophthalmopathy. Thyroid 2002;12:855–860.

80. Wiersinga WM, Smit T, van der Gaag R, et al. Temporal relationship between onset of Graves' ophthalmopathy and onset of thyroidal Graves' disease. J Endocrinol Invest 1988;11:615–619.

81. Sridama V, DeGroot LJ. Treatment of Graves' disease and the course of ophthalmopathy. Am J Med 1989;87:70–73.

82. Lim SL, Lim AK, Mumtaz M, et al. Prevalence, risk factors, and clinical features of thyroid-associated ophthalmopathy in multiethnic Malaysian patients with Graves' disease. Thyroid 2008;18:1297–1301.

83. Tellez M, Cooper J, Edmonds C. Graves' ophthalmopathy in relation to cigarette smoking and ethnic origin. Clin Endocrinol (Oxf) 1992;36:291–294.

84. Joffe B, Gunji K, Panz V, et al. Thyroid-associated ophthalmopathy in black South African patients with Graves' disease: relationship to antiflavoprotein antibodies. Thyroid 1998;8:1023–1027.

85. Bartalena L, Martino E, Marcocci C, et al. More on smoking habits and Graves' ophthalmopathy. J Endocrinol Invest 1989;12:733–737.

86. Kung AW, Yau CC, Cheng A. The incidence of ophthalmopathy after radioiodine therapy for Graves' disease: prognostic factors and the role of methimazole. J Clin Endocrinol Metab 1994;79:542–546.

87. Prummel MF, Wiersinga WM. Smoking and risk of Graves' disease. JAMA 1993;269: 479–482.

88. Tagami T, Tanaka K, Sugawa H, et al. High-dose intravenous steroid pulse therapy in thyroid-associated ophthalmopathy. Endocr J 1996;43:689–699.

89. Tallstedt L, Lundell G, Taube A. Graves' ophthalmopathy and tobacco smoking. Acta Endocrinol (Copenh) 1993;129:147–150.

90. Winsa B, Mandahl A, Karlsson FA. Graves' disease, endocrine ophthalmopathy and smoking. Acta Endocrinol (Copenh) 1993;128:156–160.

91. Vestergaard P. Smoking and thyroid disorders: a meta-analysis. Eur J Endocrinol 2002;146:153–161.

92. Thornton J, Kelly SP, Harrison RA, et al. Cigarette smoking and thyroid eye disease: a systematic review. Eye 2007;21:1135–1145.

93. Manji N, Carr-Smith JD, Boelaert K, et al. Influences of age, gender, smoking, and family history on autoimmune thyroid disease phenotype. J Clin Endocrinol Metab 2006;91:4873–4880.

94. Krassas GE, Wiersinga W. Smoking and autoimmune thyroid disease: the plot thickens. Eur J Endocrinol 2006;154:777–780.

95. Eckstein A, Quadbeck B, Mueller G, et al. Impact of smoking on the response to treatment of thyroid associated ophthalmopathy. Br J Ophthalmol 2003;87:773–776.

96. Cawood TJ, Moriarty P, O'Farrelly C, et al. Smoking and thyroid-associated ophthalmopathy: a novel explanation of the biological link. J Clin Endocrinol Metab 2007;92:59–64.

97. Bartalena L, Bogazzi F, Tanda ML, et al. Cigarette smoking and the thyroid. Eur J Endocrinol 1995;133:507–512.

98. Bartalena L, Baldeschi L, Dickinson AJ, et al. Consensus statement of the European group on Graves' orbitopathy (EUGOGO) on management of Graves' orbitopathy. Thyroid 2008;18:333–346.

99. Perros P, Crombie AL, Matthews JN, et al. Age and gender influence the severity of thyroid-associated ophthalmopathy: a study of 101 patients attending a combined thyroid-eye clinic. Clin Endocrinol (Oxf) 1993;38:367–372.

100. Bartalena L, Marcocci C, Bogazzi F, et al. Relation between therapy for hyperthyroidism and the course of Graves' ophthalmopathy. N Engl J Med 1998;338:73–78.

101. Bartalena L, Marcocci C, Bogazzi F, et al. Use of corticosteroids to prevent progression of Graves' ophthalmopathy after radioiodine therapy for hyperthyroidism. N Engl J Med 1989;321:1349–1352.

102. Tallstedt L, Lundell G, Torring O, et al. Occurrence of ophthalmopathy after treatment for Graves' hyperthyroidism. The Thyroid Study Group [see comments]. N Engl J Med 1992;326:1733–1738.

103. Farid NR, Balazs C. The genetics of thyroid associated ophthalmopathy. Thyroid 1998;8:407–409.

104. Kendall Taylor P. The pathogenesis of Graves' ophthalmopathy. Clin Endocrinol Metab 1985;14:331–349.

105. Ofosu MH, Dunston G, Henry L, et al. HLA-DQ3 is associated with Graves' disease in African-Americans. Immunol Invest 1996;25:103–110.

106. Yanagawa T, DeGroot LJ. HLA class II associations in African-American female patients with Graves' disease. Thyroid 1996;6:37–39.

107. Tomer Y, Barbesino G, Keddache M, et al. Mapping of a major susceptibility locus for Graves' disease (GD-1) to chromosome 14q31. J Clin Endocrinol Metab 1997;82: 1645–1648.

108. Faure GC, Bensoussan Lejzerowicz D, Bene MC, et al. Coexpression of CD40 and class II antigen HLA-DR in Graves' disease thyroid epithelial cells. Clin Immunol Immunopathol 1997;84:212–215.

109. Barlow AB, Wheatcroft N, Watson P, et al. Association of HLA-DQA1*0501 with Graves' disease in English Caucasian men and women. Clin Endocrinol (Oxf) 1996;44:73–77.

110. Donner H, Rau H, Walfish PG, et al. CTLA4 alanine-17 confers genetic susceptibility to Graves' disease and to type 1 diabetes mellitus. J Clin Endocrinol Metab 1997;82:143–146.

111. Mariotti S, Chiovato L, Vitti P, et al. Recent advances in the understanding of humoral and cellular mechanisms implicated in thyroid autoimmune disorders. Clin Immunol Immunopathol 1989;50:S73–84.

112. Sergott RC, Felberg NT, Savino PJ, et al. Association of HLA antigen BW35 with severe Graves' ophthalmopathy. Invest Ophthalmol Vis Sci 1983;24:124–127.

113. Tomer Y, Barbesino G, Greenberg DA, et al. Linkage analysis of candidate genes in autoimmune thyroid disease. III. Detailed analysis of chromosome 14 localizes Graves' disease-1 (GD-1) close to multinodular goiter-1 (MNG-1). International Consortium for the Genetics of Autoimmune Thyroid Disease. J Clin Endocrinol Metab 1998;83:4321–4327.

114. Tomer Y, Barbesino G, Greenberg DA, et al. Mapping the major susceptibility loci for familial Graves' and Hashimoto's diseases: evidence for genetic heterogeneity and gene interactions. J Clin Endocrinol Metab 1999;84:4656–4664.

115. Davies TF, Greenberg D, Tomer Y. The genetics of the autoimmune thyroid diseases. Ann Endocrinol (Paris) 2003;64:28–30.

116. Levin L, Ban Y, Concepcion E, et al. Analysis of HLA genes in families with autoimmune diabetes and thyroiditis. Hum Immunol 2004;65:640–647.

117. Vieland VJ, Huang Y, Bartlett C, et al. A multilocus model of the genetic architecture of autoimmune thyroid disorder, with clinical implications. Am J Hum Genet 2008;82:1349–1356.

118. Yin X, Latif R, Bahn R, et al. Influence of the TSH receptor gene on susceptibility to Graves' disease and Graves' ophthalmopathy. Thyroid 2008;18:1201–1206.

119. Douglas RS, Gianoukakis AG, Goldberg RA, et al. Circulating mononuclear cells from euthyroid patients with thyroid-associated ophthalmopathy exhibit characteristic phenotypes. Clin Exp Immunol 2007;148:64–71.

120. Gianoukakis AG, Khadavi N, Smith TJ. Cytokines, Graves' disease, and thyroid-associated ophthalmopathy. Thyroid 2008;18:953–958.

121. Gianoukakis AG, Smith TJ. Recent insights into the pathogenesis and management of thyroid-associated ophthalmopathy. Curr Opin Endocrinol Diabetes Obes 2008;15: 446–452.

122. Heufelder AE, Joba W. Thyroid-associated eye disease. Strabismus 2000;8:101–111.

123. Hwang CJ, Afifiyan N, Sand D, et al. Orbital fibroblasts from patients with thyroid-associated ophthalmopathy overexpress CD40: CD154 hyperinduces IL-6, IL-8, and MCP-1. Invest Ophthalmol Vis Sci 2009;50:2262–2268.

124. Khoo TK, Bahn RS. Pathogenesis of Graves' ophthalmopathy: the role of autoantibodies. Thyroid 2007;17:1013–1018.

125. Lehmann GM, Feldon SE, Smith TJ. Immune mechanisms in thyroid eye disease. Thyroid 2008;18:959–965.

126. Smith TJ, Tsai CC, Shih MJ, et al. Unique attributes of orbital fibroblasts and global alterations in IGF-1 receptor signaling could explain thyroid-associated ophthalmopathy. Thyroid 2008;18:983–988.

127. Weetman AP, Fells P, Shine B. T and B cell reactivity to extraocular and skeletal muscle in Graves' ophthalmopathy. Br J Ophthalmol 1989;73:323–327.

128. Baker JR, Jr. Autoimmune endocrine disease. JAMA 1997;278:1931–1937.

129. Perros P, Kendall Taylor P. The pathogenesis of thyroid-associated ophthalmopathy. J Endocrinol 1989;122:619–624.

130. Perros P, Kendall Taylor P. Antibodies to orbital tissues in thyroid-associated ophthalmopathy. Acta Endocrinol Copenh 1992;126:137–142.

131. Heufelder AE. Pathogenesis of Graves' ophthalmopathy: recent controversies and progress. Eur J Endocrinol 1995;132:532–541.

132. Kubota S, Gunji K, Stolarski C, et al. Reevaluation of the prevalences of serum autoantibodies reactive with "64-kd eye muscle proteins" in patients with thyroid-associated ophthalmopathy. Thyroid 1998;8:175–179.

133. Gunji K, Kubota S, Swanson J, et al. Role of the eye muscles in thyroid eye disease: identification of the principal autoantigens. Thyroid 1998;8:553–556.

134. Gopinath B, Ma G, Wall JR. Eye signs and serum eye muscle and collagen XIII antibodies in patients with transient and progressive thyroiditis. Thyroid 2007;17: 1123–1129.

135. Gopinath B, Musselman R, Adams CL, et al. Study of serum antibodies against three eye muscle antigens and the connective tissue antigen collagen XIII in patients with Graves' disease with and without ophthalmopathy: correlation with clinical features. Thyroid 2006;16:967–974.

136. Gopinath B, Musselman R, Beard N, et al. Antibodies targeting the calcium binding skeletal muscle protein calsequestrin are specific markers of ophthalmopathy and sensitive indicators of ocular myopathy in patients with Graves' disease. Clin Exp Immunol 2006;145:56–62.

137. Wall J, Barsouk A, Stolarski C, et al. Serum antibodies reactive with eye muscle antigens and the TSH receptor in a euthyroid subject who developed ophthalmopathy and Graves' hyperthyroidism. Thyroid 1996;6:353–358.

138. Wall J, Kennerdell JS. Progress in thyroid-associated ophthalmopathy. Autoimmunity 1995;22:191–195.

139. Wall JR, Bernard N, Boucher A, et al. Pathogenesis of thyroid-associated ophthalmopathy: an autoimmune disorder of the eye muscle associated with Graves' hyperthyroidism and Hashimoto's thyroiditis. Clin Immunol Immunopathol 1993;68: 1–8.

140. Wall JR, Salvi M, Bernard NF, et al. Thyroid-associated ophthalmopathy—a model for the association of organ-specific autoimmune disorders. Immunol Today 1991;12: 150–153.

141. Mizokami T, Salvi M, Wall JR. Eye muscle antibodies in Graves' ophthalmopathy: pathogenic or secondary epiphenomenon? J Endocrinol Invest 2004;27:221–229.

142. Bartley GB, Fatourechi V, Kadrmas EF, et al. Clinical features of Graves' ophthalmopathy in an incidence cohort. Am J Ophthalmol 1996;121:284–290.

143. Feldon SE, Levin L. Graves' ophthalmopathy: V. Aetiology of upper eyelid retraction in Graves' ophthalmopathy. Br J Ophthalmol 1990;74:484–485.

144. Gupta A, Sadeghi PB, Akpek EK. Occult thyroid eye disease in patients presenting with dry eye symptoms. Am J Ophthalmol 2009;147:919–923.

145. Mourits MP, Prummel MF, Wiersinga WM, et al. Measuring eye movements in Graves ophthalmopathy. Ophthalmology 1994;101:1341–1346.

146. Garrity JA, Saggau DD, Gorman CA, et al. Torsional diplopia after transantral orbital decompression and extraocular muscle surgery associated with Graves' orbitopathy. Am J Ophthalmol 1992;113:363–373.

147. Trobe JD. Cyclodeviation in acquired vertical strabismus. Arch Ophthalmol 1984;102:717–720.

148. Chen VM, Dagi LR. Ocular misalignment in Graves disease may mimic that of superior oblique palsy. J Neuroophthalmol 2008;28:302–304.

149. Scott WE, Thalacker JA. Diagnosis and treatment of thyroid myopathy. Ophthalmology 1981;88:493–498.

150. Spierer A, Eisenstein Z. The role of increased intraocular pressure on upgaze in the assessment of Graves ophthalmopathy. Ophthalmology 1991;98:1491–1494.

151. Chung SM, Lee AG, Holds JB, et al. Ocular neuromyotonia in Graves dysthyroid orbitopathy. Arch Ophthalmol 1997;115:365–370.

152. Jacobson DM. Acetylcholine receptor antibodies in patients with Graves' ophthalmopathy. J Neuroophthalmol 1995;15:166–170.

153. Vargas ME, Warren FA, Kupersmith MJ. Exotropia as a sign of myasthenia gravis in dysthyroid ophthalmopathy. Br J Ophthalmol 1993;77:822–823.

154. Bartley GB, Fatourechi V, Kadrmas EF, et al. Long-term follow-up of Graves ophthalmopathy in an incidence cohort. Ophthalmology 1996;103:958–962.

155. Ben Simon GJ, Syed HM, Douglas R, et al. Clinical manifestations and treatment outcome of optic neuropathy in thyroid-related orbitopathy. Ophthalmic Surg Lasers Imaging 2006;37:284–290.

156. Neigel JM, Rootman J, Belkin RI, et al. Dysthyroid optic neuropathy. The crowded orbital apex syndrome. Ophthalmology 1988;95:1515–1521.

157. Garrity JA, Fatourechi V, Bergstralh EJ, et al. Results of transantral orbital decompression in 428 patients with severe Graves' ophthalmopathy. Am J Ophthalmol 1993;116:533–547.

158. Goh MS, McNab AA. Orbital decompression in Graves' orbitopathy: efficacy and safety. Intern Med J 2005;35:586–591.

159. Paridaens D, Lie A, Grootendorst RJ, et al. Efficacy and side effects of "swinging eyelid" orbital decompression in Graves' orbitopathy: a proposal for standardized evaluation of diplopia. Eye 2006;20:154–162.

160. McKeag D, Lane C, Lazarus JH, et al. Clinical features of dysthyroid optic neuropathy: a European Group on Graves' Orbitopathy (EUGOGO) survey. Br J Ophthalmol 2007;91:455–458.

161. Kennerdell JS, Rosenbaum AE, El-Hoshy MH. Apical optic nerve compression of dysthyroid optic neuropathy on computed tomography. Arch Ophthalmol 1981;99:807–809.

162. Trobe JD, Glaser JS, Laflamme P. Dysthyroid optic neuropathy: clinical profile and rationale for management. Arch Ophthalmol 1978;96:1199–1209.

163. Cockerham KP, Pal C, Jani B, et al. The prevalence and implications of ocular hypertension and glaucoma in thyroid-associated orbitopathy. Ophthalmology 1997;104:914–917.

164. Feldon SE, Lee CP, Muramatsu SK, et al. Quantitative computed tomography of Graves' ophthalmopathy. Extraocular muscle and orbital fat in development of optic neuropathy. Arch Ophthalmol 1985;103:213–215.

165. Feldon SE, Muramatsu S, Weiner JM. Clinical classification of Graves' ophthalmopathy. Identification of risk factors for optic neuropathy. Arch Ophthalmol 1984;102:1469–1472.

166. Ben Simon GJ, Syed HM, Douglas R, et al. Extraocular muscle enlargement with tendon involvement in thyroid-associated orbitopathy. Am J Ophthalmol 2004;137:1145–1147.

167. Enzmann DR, Donaldson SS, Kriss JP. Appearance of Graves' disease on orbital computed tomography. J Comput Assist Tomogr 1979;3:815–819.

168. Hoh HB, Laitt RD, Wakeley C, et al. The STIR sequence MRI in the assessment of extraocular muscles in thyroid eye disease. Eye 1994;8:506–510.

169. Lennerstrand G, Tian S, Isberg B, et al. Magnetic resonance imaging and ultrasound measurements of extraocular muscles in thyroid-associated ophthalmopathy at different stages of the disease. Acta Ophthalmol Scand 2007;85:192–201.

170. Mayer E, Herdman G, Burnett C, et al. Serial STIR magnetic resonance imaging correlates with clinical score of activity in thyroid disease. Eye 2001;15:313–318.

171. Mayer EJ, Fox DL, Herdman G, et al. Signal intensity, clinical activity and cross-sectional areas on MRI scans in thyroid eye disease. Eur J Radiol 2005;56:20–24.

172. Nishida Y, Tian S, Isberg B, et al. MRI measurements of orbital tissues in dysthyroid ophthalmopathy. Graefes Arch Clin Exp Ophthalmol 2001;239:824–831.

173. Nugent RA, Belkin RI, Neigel JM, et al. Graves orbitopathy: correlation of CT and clinical findings. Radiology 1990;177:675–682.

174. Rothfus WE, Curtin HD. Extraocular muscle enlargement: a CT review. Radiology 1984;151:677–681.

175. Trokel SL, Jakobiec FA. Correlation of CT scanning and pathologic features of ophthalmic Graves' disease. Ophthalmology 1981;88:553–564.

176. Bailey CC, Kabala J, Laitt R, et al. Magnetic resonance imaging in thyroid eye disease. Eye 1996;10:617–619.

177. Hiromatsu Y, Kojima K, Ishisaka N, et al. Role of magnetic resonance imaging in thyroid-associated ophthalmopathy: its predictive value for therapeutic outcome of immunosuppressive therapy. Thyroid 1992;2:299–305.

178. Holt JE, O'Connor PS, Douglas JP, et al. Extraocular muscle size comparison using standardized A-scan echography and computerized tomography scan measurements. Ophthalmology 1985;92:1351–1355.

179. Volpe NJ, Sbarbaro JA, Gendron Livingston K, et al. Occult thyroid eye disease in patients with unexplained ocular misalignment identified by standardized orbital echography. Am J Ophthalmol 2006;142:75–81.

180. Delint PJ, Mourits MP, Kerlen CH, et al. B-scan ultrasonography in Graves' orbitopathy. Doc Ophthalmol 1993;85:1–4.

181. Shammas HJ, Minckler DS, Ogden C. Ultrasound in early thyroid orbitopathy. Arch Ophthalmol 1980;98:277–279.

182. Werner SC. Modification of the classification of the eye changes of Graves' disease. Am J Ophthalmol 1977;83:725–727.

183. Werner SC. Modification of the classification of the eye changes of Graves' disease: recommendations of the Ad Hoc Committee of the American Thyroid Association [letter]. J Clin Endocrinol Metab 1977;44:203–204.

184. Bartley GB, Gorman CA. Diagnostic criteria for Graves' ophthalmopathy. Am J Ophthalmol 1995;119:792–795.

185. Frueh BR. Why the NOSPECS classification of Graves' eye disease should be abandoned, with suggestions for the characterization of this disease. Thyroid 1992;2:85–88.

186. Van Dyk HJ. Orbital Graves' disease. A modification of the "NO SPECS" classification. Ophthalmology 1981;88:479–483.

187. Bartalena L, Baldeschi L, Dickinson A, et al. Consensus statement of the European Group on Graves' orbitopathy (EUGOGO) on management of GO. Eur J Endocrinol 2008;158:273–285.

188. Mourits MP, Koornneef L, Wiersinga WM, et al. Clinical criteria for the assessment of disease activity in Graves' ophthalmopathy: a novel approach. Br J Ophthalmol 1989;73:639–644.

189. Mourits MP, Prummel MF, Wiersinga WM, et al. Clinical activity score as a guide in the management of patients with Graves' ophthalmopathy. Clin Endocrinol (Oxf) 1997;47:9–14.

190. Wiersinga WM, Perros P, Kahaly GJ, et al. Clinical assessment of patients with Graves' orbitopathy: the European Group on Graves' Orbitopathy recommendations to generalists, specialists and clinical researchers. Eur J Endocrinol 2006;155:387–389.

191. Bartley GB, Fatourechi V, Kadrmas EF, et al. The treatment of Graves' ophthalmopathy in an incidence cohort. Am J Ophthalmol 1996;121:200–206.

192. Perros P, Crombie AL, Kendall Taylor P. Natural history of thyroid associated ophthalmopathy. Clin Endocrinol (Oxf) 1995;42:45–50.

193. Zoumalan CI, Cockerham KP, Turbin RE, et al. Efficacy of corticosteroids and external beam radiation in the management of moderate to severe thyroid eye disease. J Neuroophthalmol 2007;27:205–214.

194. Rootman J. Graves' orbitopathy. In: Rootman J (ed). Disease of the Orbit: A Multidisciplinary Approach, pp 241–280. Philadelphia, J.B. Lippincott, 1988.

195. Wiersinga WM, Smit T, Schuster Uittenhoeve AL, et al. Therapeutic outcome of prednisone medication and of orbital irradiation in patients with Graves' ophthalmopathy. Ophthalmologica 1988;197:75–84.

196. Kendall Taylor P, Crombie AL, Stephenson AM, et al. Intravenous methylprednisolone in the treatment of Graves' ophthalmopathy. BMJ 1988;297:1574–1578.

197. Koshiyama H, Koh T, Fujiwara K, et al. Therapy of Graves' ophthalmopathy with intravenous high-dose steroid followed by orbital irradiation. Thyroid 1994;4:409–413.

198. Atabay C, Schrooyen M, Zhang ZG, et al. Use of eye muscle antibody measurements to monitor response to plasmapheresis in patients with thyroid-associated ophthalmopathy. J Endocrinol Invest 1993;16:669–674.

199. Baschieri L, Antonelli A, Nardi S, et al. Intravenous immunoglobulin versus corticosteroid in treatment of Graves' ophthalmopathy. Thyroid 1997;7:579–585.

200. Kahaly G, Pitz S, Muller Forell W, et al. Randomized trial of intravenous immunoglobulins versus prednisolone in Graves' ophthalmopathy. Clin Exp Immunol 1996;106:197–202.

201. Kung AW, Michon J, Tai KS, et al. The effect of somatostatin versus corticosteroid in the treatment of Graves' ophthalmopathy. Thyroid 1996;6:381–384.

202. Salvi M, Vannucchi G, Campi I, et al. Treatment of Graves' disease and associated ophthalmopathy with the anti-CD20 monoclonal antibody rituximab: an open study. Eur J Endocrinol 2007;156:33–40

203. Salvi M, Vannucchi G, Campi I, et al. Efficacy of rituximab treatment for thyroid-associated ophthalmopathy as a result of intraorbital B-cell depletion in one patient unresponsive to steroid immunosuppression. Eur J Endocrinol 2006;154:511–517.

204. Prummel MF, Mourits MP, Berghout A, et al. Prednisone and cyclosporine in the treatment of severe Graves' ophthalmopathy. N Engl J Med 1989;321:1353–1359.

205. Krassas GE. Somatostatin analogs: a new tool for the management of Graves' ophthalmopathy. J Endocrinol Invest 2004;27:281–287.

206. Dickinson AJ, Vaidya B, Miller M, et al. Double-blind, placebo-controlled trial of octreotide long-acting repeatable (LAR) in thyroid-associated ophthalmopathy. J Clin Endocrinol Metab 2004;89:5910–5915.

207. Tallstedt L, Lundell G. Radioiodine treatment, ablation, and ophthalmopathy: a balanced perspective. Thyroid 1997;7:241–245.

208. Prummel MF, Wiersinga WM. Medical management of Graves' ophthalmopathy. Thyroid 1995;5:231–234.

209. Hurbli T, Char DH, Harris J, et al. Radiation therapy for thyroid eye diseases. Am J Ophthalmol 1985;99:633–637.

210. Bartalena L, Marcocci C, Chiovato L, et al. Orbital cobalt irradiation combined with systemic corticosteroids for Graves' ophthalmopathy: comparison with systemic corticosteroids alone. J Clin Endocrinol Metab 1983;56:1139–1144.

211. Lloyd WCd, Leone CR, Jr. Supervoltage orbital radiotherapy in 36 cases of Graves' disease. Am J Ophthalmol 1992;113:374–380.

212. Marcocci C, Bartalena L, Panicucci M, et al. Orbital cobalt irradiation combined with retrobulbar or systemic corticosteroids for Graves' ophthalmopathy: a comparative study. Clin Endocrinol (Oxf) 1987;27:33–42.

213. Nakahara H, Noguchi S, Murakami N, et al. Graves ophthalmopathy: MR evaluation of 10-Gy versus 24-Gy irradiation combined with systemic corticosteroids. Radiology 1995;196:857–862.

214. Palmer D, Greenberg P, Cornell P, et al. Radiation therapy for Graves' ophthalmopathy: a retrospective analysis. Int J Radiat Oncol Biol Phys 1987;13:1815–1820.

215. Gorman CA, Garrity JA, Fatourechi V, et al. A prospective, randomized, double-blind, placebo-controlled study of orbital radiotherapy for Graves' ophthalmopathy. Ophthalmology 2001;108:1523–1534.

216. Gorman CA, Garrity JA, Fatourechi V, et al. The aftermath of orbital radiotherapy for graves' ophthalmopathy. Ophthalmology 2002;109:2100–2107.

217. Kazim M, Trokel S, Moore S. Treatment of acute Graves orbitopathy. Ophthalmology 1991;98:1443–1448.

218. Ferris JD, Dawson EL, Plowman N, et al. Radiotherapy in thyroid eye disease: the effect on the field of binocular single vision. J AAPOS 2002;6:71–76.

219. Wilson WB, Prochoda M. Radiotherapy for thyroid orbitopathy. Effects on extraocular muscle balance. Arch Ophthalmol 1995;113:1420–1425.

220. Miller ML, Goldberg SH, Bullock JD. Radiation retinopathy after standard radiotherapy for thyroid-related ophthalmopathy [letter]. Am J Ophthalmol 1991;112:600–601.

221. Akmansu M, Dirican B, Bora H, et al. The risk of radiation-induced carcinogenesis after external beam radiotherapy of Graves' orbitopathy. Ophthalmic Res 2003;35:150–153.

222. Bradley EA, Gower EW, Bradley DJ, et al. Orbital radiation for graves ophthalmopathy: a report by the American Academy of Ophthalmology. Ophthalmology 2008;115:398–409.

223. Chang EL, Bernardino CR, Rubin PA. Transcaruncular orbital decompression for management of compressive optic neuropathy in thyroid-related orbitopathy. Plast Reconstr Surg 2003;112:739–747.

224. Chiarelli AG, De Min V, Saetti R, et al. Surgical management of thyroid orbitopathy. J Plast Reconstr Aesthet Surg 2008.

225. Fatourechi V, Garrity JA, Bartley GB, et al. Graves ophthalmopathy. Results of transantral orbital decompression performed primarily for cosmetic indications. Ophthalmology 1994;101:938–942.

226. Fells P. Orbital decompression for severe dysthyroid eye disease. Br J Ophthalmol 1987;71:107–111.

227. Girod DA, Orcutt JC, Cummings CW. Orbital decompression for preservation of vision in Graves' ophthalmopathy. Arch Otolaryngol Head Neck Surg 1993;119:229–233.

228. Goldberg RA, Weinberg DA, Shorr N, et al. Maximal, three-wall, orbital decompression through a coronal approach. Ophthalmic Surg Lasers 1997;28:832–843.

229. Graham SM, Carter KD. Combined-approach orbital decompression for thyroid-related orbitopathy. Clin Otolaryngol Allied Sci 1999;24:109–113.

230. Hutchison BM, Kyle PM. Long-term visual outcome following orbital decompression for dysthyroid eye disease. Eye 1995;9:578–581.

231. Jernfors M, Valimaki MJ, Setala K, et al. Efficacy and safety of orbital decompression in treatment of thyroid-associated ophthalmopathy: long-term follow-up of 78 patients. Clin Endocrinol (Oxf) 2007;67:101–107.

232. Kennerdell JS, Maroon JC. An orbital decompression for severe dysthyroid exophthalmos. Ophthalmology 1982;89:467–472.

233. Lima WT, Perches M, Valera FC, et al. Orbital endoscopic decompression in Graves ophthalmopathy. Braz J Otorhinolaryngol 2006;72:283–287.

234. Lyons CJ, Rootman J. Orbital decompression for disfiguring exophthalmos in thyroid orbitopathy. Ophthalmology 1994;101:223–230.

235. Malik R, Cormack G, MacEwen C, et al. Endoscopic orbital decompression for dyscosmetic thyroid eye disease. J Laryngol Otol 2008;122:593–597.

236. Maroon JC, Kennerdell JS. Radical orbital decompression for severe dysthyroid exophthalmos. J Neurosurg 1982;56:260–266.

237. McNab AA. Orbital decompression for thyroid orbitopathy. Aust N Z J Ophthalmol 1997;25:55–61.

238. Mourits MP, Koornneef L, Wiersinga WM, et al. Orbital decompression for Graves' ophthalmopathy by inferomedial, by inferomedial plus lateral, and by coronal approach. Ophthalmology 1990;97:636–641.

239. Neugebauer A, Nishino K, Neugebauer P, et al. Effects of bilateral orbital decompression by an endoscopic endonasal approach in dysthyroid orbitopathy. Br J Ophthalmol 1996;80:58–62.

240. Schaefer SD, Merritt JH, Close LG. Orbital decompression for optic neuropathy secondary to thyroid eye disease. Laryngoscope 1988;98:712–716.

241. Silver RD, Harrison AR, Goding GS. Combined endoscopic medial and external lateral orbital decompression for progressive thyroid eye disease. Otolaryngol Head Neck Surg 2006;134:260–266.

242. Stannard L, Slater RM, Leatherbarrow B. Orbital decompression surgery for thyroid eye disease: implications for anaesthesia. Eur J Anaesthesiol 2006;23:183–189.

243. Tallstedt L, Papatziamos G, Lundblad L, et al. Results of transantral orbital decompression in patients with thyroid-associated ophthalmopathy. Acta Ophthalmol Scand 2000;78:206–210.

244. Tang IP, Prepageran N, Subrayan V, et al. Endoscopic orbital decompression for optic neuropathy in thyroid ophthalmopathy. Med J Malaysia 2008;63:337–338.

245. Khan JA, Wagner DV, Tiojanco JK, et al. Combined transconjunctival and external approach for endoscopic orbital apex decompression in Graves' disease. Laryngoscope 1995;105:203–206.

246. Metson R, Dallow RL, Shore JW. Endoscopic orbital decompression. Laryngoscope 1994;104:950–957.

247. Metson R, Shore JW, Gliklich RE, et al. Endoscopic orbital decompression under local anesthesia. Otolaryngol Head Neck Surg 1995;113:661–667.

248. Carter KD, Frueh BR, Hessburg TP, et al. Long-term efficacy of orbital decompression for compressive optic neuropathy of Graves' eye disease. Ophthalmology 1991;98:1435–1442.

249. DeSanto LW. The total rehabilitation of Graves' ophthalmopathy. Laryngoscope 1980;90:1652–1678.

250. Roncevic R. Correction of exophthalmos and eyelid deformities in patients with severe thyroid ophthalmopathy. J Craniofac Surg 2008;19:628–636.

251. Shorr N, Neuhaus RW, Baylis HI. Ocular motility problems after orbital decompression for dysthyroid ophthalmopathy. Ophthalmology 1982;89:323–328.

252. Shorr N, Seiff SR. The four stages of surgical rehabilitation of the patient with dysthyroid ophthalmopathy. Ophthalmology 1986;93:476–483.

253. Trokel S, Kazim M, Moore S. Orbital fat removal. Decompression for Graves orbitopathy. Ophthalmology 1993;100:674–682.

254. Ben Simon GJ, Schwarcz RM, Mansury AM, et al. Minimally invasive orbital decompression: local anesthesia and hand-carved bone. Arch Ophthalmol 2005;123:1671–1675.

255. Gilbert J, Dailey RA, Christensen LE. Characteristics and outcomes of strabismus surgery after orbital decompression for thyroid eye disease. J AAPOS 2005;9:26–30.

256. Ruttum MS. Effect of prior orbital decompression on outcome of strabismus surgery in patients with thyroid ophthalmopathy. J AAPOS 2000;4:102–105.

257. Dal Canto AJ, Crowe S, Perry JD, et al. Intraoperative relaxed muscle positioning technique for strabismus repair in thyroid eye disease. Ophthalmology 2006;113:2324–2330.

258. Fells P, Kousoulides L, Pappa A, et al. Extraocular muscle problems in thyroid eye disease. Eye 1994;8:497–505.

259. Sprunger DT, Helveston EM. Progressive overcorrection after inferior rectus recession. J Pediatr Ophthalmol Strabismus 1993;30:145–148.

260. Bok C, Hidalgo C, Morax S. [Surgical management of diplopia in dysthyroid orbitopathy]. J Fr Ophtalmol 2007;30:390–396.

261. Evans D, Kennerdell JS. Extraocular muscle surgery for dysthyroid myopathy. Am J Ophthalmol 1983;95:767–771.

262. Pitchon EM, Klainguti G. [Surgical treatment of diplopia in Graves' orbitopathy]. Klin Monatsbl Augenheilkd 2007;224:331–333.

263. Mocan MC, Ament C, Azar NF. The characteristics and surgical outcomes of medial rectus recessions in Graves' ophthalmopathy. J Pediatr Ophthalmol Strabismus 2007;44:93–100; quiz 118–109.

264. Dragan LR, Seiff SR, Lee DC. Longitudinal correlation of thyroid-stimulating immunoglobulin with clinical activity of disease in thyroid-associated orbitopathy. Ophthal Plast Reconstr Surg 2006;22:13–19.

265. Gerding MN, van der Meer JW, Broenink M, et al. Association of thyrotrophin receptor antibodies with the clinical features of Graves' ophthalmopathy. Clin Endocrinol (Oxf) 2000;52:267–271.

266. Krassas GE, Gogakos A. Thyroid-associated ophthalmopathy in juvenile Graves' disease—clinical, endocrine and therapeutic aspects. J Pediatr Endocrinol Metab 2006;19:1193–1206.

267. Krassas GE, Segni M, Wiersinga WM. Childhood Graves' ophthalmopathy: results of a European questionnaire study. Eur J Endocrinol 2005;153:515–521.

268. Young LA. Dysthyroid ophthalmopathy in children. J Pediatr Ophthalmol Strabismus 1979;16:105–107.

269. Liu GT, Heher KL, Katowitz JA, et al. Prominent proptosis in childhood thyroid eye disease. Ophthalmology 1996;103:779–784.

270. Swamy BN, McCluskey P, Nemet A, et al. Idiopathic orbital inflammatory syndrome: clinical features and treatment outcomes. Br J Ophthalmol 2007;91:1667–1670.

271. Yuen SJ, Rubin PA. Idiopathic orbital inflammation: distribution, clinical features, and treatment outcome. Arch Ophthalmol 2003;121:491–499.

272. Jakobiec FA, Lefkowitch J, Knowles DM. B- and T-lymphocytes in ocular disease. Ophthalmology 1984;91:635–654.

273. Mombaerts I, Goldschmeding R, Schlingemann RO, et al. What is orbital pseudotumor? Surv Ophthalmol 1996;41:66–78.

274. Atabay C, Tyutyunikov A, Scalise D, et al. Serum antibodies reactive with eye muscle membrane antigens are detected in patients with nonspecific orbital inflammation. Ophthalmology 1995;102:145–153.

275. Ludwig I, Tomsak RL. Acute recurrent orbital myositis. J Clin Neuroophthalmol 1983;3:41–47.

276. Purcell JJ, Jr., Taulbee WA. Orbital myositis after upper respiratory tract infection. Arch Ophthalmol 1981;99:437–438.

277. Slavin ML, Glaser JS. Idiopathic orbital myositis: report of six cases. Arch Ophthalmol 1982;100:1261–1265.

278. Eshaghian J, Anderson RL. Sinus involvement in inflammatory orbital pseudotumor. Arch Ophthalmol 1981;99:627–630.

279. Pillai P, Saini JS. Bilateral sino-orbital pseudotumour. Can J Ophthalmol 1988;23:177–180.

280. Islam N, Asaria R, Plant GT, et al. Giant cell arteritis mimicking idiopathic orbital inflammatory disease. Eur J Ophthalmol 2003;13:392–394.

281. Kiratli H, Sekeroglu MA, Soylemezoglu F. Unilateral dacryoadenitis as the sole presenting sign of Wegener's granulomatosis. Orbit 2008;27:157–160.

282. Amirlak I, Narchi H. Isolated orbital pseudotumor as the presenting sign of systemic lupus erythematosus. J Pediatr Ophthalmol Strabismus 2008;45:51–54.

283. Nabili S, McCarey DW, Browne B, et al. A case of orbital myositis associated with rheumatoid arthritis. Ann Rheum Dis 2002;61:938–939.

284. Hammami S, Yahia SB, Mahjoub S, et al. Orbital inflammation associated with Behcet's disease. Clin Experiment Ophthalmol 2006;34:188–190.

285. Peterson EA, Hymas DC, Pratt DV, et al. Sarcoidosis with orbital tumor outside the lacrimal gland: initial manifestation in 2 elderly white women. Arch Ophthalmol 1998;116:804–806.

286. Ramalho J, Castillo M. Imaging of orbital myositis in Crohn's disease. Clin Imaging 2008;32:227–229.

287. Mombaerts I, Schlingemann RO, Goldschmeding R, et al. Idiopathic granulomatous orbital inflammation. Ophthalmology 1996;103:2135–2141.

288. Fujii H, Fujisada H, Kondo T, et al. Orbital pseudotumor: histopathological classification and treatment. Ophthalmologica 1985;190:230–242.

289. Rootman J, Nugent R. The classification and management of acute orbital pseudotumors. Ophthalmology 1982;89:1040–1048.

290. Mottow Lippa L, Jakobiec FA, Smith M. Idiopathic inflammatory orbital pseudotumor in childhood. II. Results of diagnostic tests and biopsies. Ophthalmology 1981;88:565–574.

291. Kennerdell JS, Dresner SC. The nonspecific orbital inflammatory syndromes. Surv Ophthalmol 1984;29:93–103.

292. Benson WE. Posterior scleritis. Surv Ophthalmol 1988;32:297–316.

293. Mahr MA, Salomao DR, Garrity JA. Inflammatory orbital pseudotumor with extension beyond the orbit. Am J Ophthalmol 2004;138:396–400.

294. Ohtsuka K, Hashimoto M, Miura M, et al. Posterior scleritis with optic perineuritis and internal ophthalmoplegia [letter]. Br J Ophthalmol 1997;81:514.

295. Rootman J, Robertson W, Lapointe JS. Inflammatory diseases. In: Rootman J (ed). Diseases of the Orbit: A Multidiscipilinary Approach, pp 143–204. Philadelphia, J.B. Lippinicott, 1988.

296. Tychsen L, Tse DT, Ossoinig K, et al. Trochleitis with superior oblique myositis. Ophthalmology 1984;91:1075–1079.

297. Purvin V, Kawasaki A, Jacobson DM. Optic perineuritis: clinical and radiographic features. Arch Ophthalmol 2001;119:1299–1306.

298. Frohman L, Wolansky L. Magnetic resonance imaging of syphilitic optic neuritis/perineuritis. J Neuroophthalmol 1997;17:57–59.

299. Rush JA, Ryan EJ. Syphilitic optic perineuritis. Am J Ophthalmol 1981;91:404–406.

300. Toshniwal P. Optic perineuritis with secondary syphilis. J Clin Neuroophthalmol 1987;7:6–10.

301. Abramovitz JN, Kasdon DL, Sutula F, et al. Sclerosing orbital pseudotumor. Neurosurgery 1983;12:463–468.

302. Cervellini P, Volpin L, Curri D, et al. Sclerosing orbital pseudotumor. Ophthalmologica 1986;193:39–44.

303. Hsuan JD, Selva D, McNab AA. Idiopathic sclerosing orbital inflammation. Arch Ophthalmol 2006;124:1244–1250.

304. Kennerdell JS. The management of sclerosing nonspecific orbital inflammation. Ophthalmic Surg 1991;22:512–518.

305. Khine AA, Prabhakaran VC, Selva D. Idiopathic sclerosing orbital inflammation: two cases presenting with paresthesia. Ophthal Plast Reconstr Surg 2009;25:65–67.

306. McCarthy JM, White VA, Harris G, et al. Idiopathic sclerosing inflammation of the orbit: immunohistologic analysis and comparison with retroperitoneal fibrosis. Mod Pathol 1993;6:581–587.

307. Paris GL, Waltuch GF, Egbert PR. Treatment of refractory orbital pseudotumors with pulsed chemotherapy. Ophthal Plast Reconstr Surg 1990;6:96–101.

308. Rootman J, McCarthy M, White V, et al. Idiopathic sclerosing inflammation of the orbit. A distinct clinicopathologic entity. Ophthalmology 1994;101:570–584.

309. Weissler MC, Miller E, Fortune MA. Sclerosing orbital pseudotumor: a unique clinicopathologic entity. Ann Otol Rhinol Laryngol 1989;98:496–501.

310. Brannan PA, Kersten RC, Kulwin DR. Sclerosing idiopathic orbital inflammation. J Pediatr Ophthalmol Strabismus 2006;43:183–184.

311. de Jesus O, Inserni JA, Gonzalez A, et al. Idiopathic orbital inflammation with intracranial extension. Case report. J Neurosurg 1996;85:510–513.

312. Frohman LP, Kupersmith MJ, Lang J, et al. Intracranial extension and bone destruction in orbital pseudotumor. Arch Ophthalmol 1986;104:380–384.

313. Kaye AH, Hahn JF, Craciun A, et al. Intracranial extension of inflammatory pseudotumor of the orbit. Case report. J Neurosurg 1984;60:625–629.

314. Nishi T, Saito Y, Watanabe K, et al. Intracranial extension of an orbital pseudotumor accompanied by internal carotid artery occlusion—case report. Neurol Med Chir Tokyo 1992;32:758–761.

315. Noble SC, Chandler WF, Lloyd RV. Intracranial extension of orbital pseudotumor: a case report. Neurosurgery 1986;18:798–801.

316. Berger JR, Snodgrass S, Glaser J, et al. Multifocal fibrosclerosis with hypertrophic intracranial pachymeningitis. Neurology 1989;39:1345–1349.

317. Brazier DJ, Sanders MD. Multifocal fibrosclerosis associated with suprasellar and macular lesions. Br J Ophthalmol 1983;67:292–296.

318. Richards AB, Shalka HW, Roberts FJ, et al. Pseudotumor of the orbit and retroperitoneal fibrosis. A form of multifocal fibrosclerosis. Arch Ophthalmol 1980;98:1617–1620.

319. Yan J, Qiu H, Wu Z, et al. Idiopathic orbital inflammatory pseudotumor in Chinese children. Orbit 2006;25:1–4.

320. Hardman JA, Halpin SF, Mars S, et al. MRI of idiopathic orbital inflammatory syndrome using fat saturation and Gd-DTPA. Neuroradiology 1995;37:475–478.

321. Flanders AE, Mafee MF, Rao VM, et al. CT characteristics of orbital pseudotumors and other orbital inflammatory processes. J Comput Assist Tomogr 1989;13:40–47.

322. Atlas SW, Grossman RI, Savino PJ, et al. Surface-coil MR of orbital pseudotumor. AJR Am J Roentgenol 1987;148:803–808.

323. Kubota T, Kano H. Assessment of inflammation in idiopathic orbital myositis with fat-suppressed T2-weighted magnetic resonance imaging. Am J Ophthalmol 2007;143:718–722.

324. Kapur R, Sepahdari AR, Mafee MF, et al. MR imaging of orbital inflammatory syndrome, orbital cellulitis, and orbital lymphoid lesions: the role of diffusion-weighted imaging. AJNR Am J Neuroradiol 2009;30:64–70.

325. Mombaerts I, Schlingemann RO, Goldschmeding R, et al. Are systemic corticosteroids useful in the management of orbital pseudotumors [see comments]? Ophthalmology 1996;103:521–528.

326. Leone CR, Jr., Lloyd WC. Treatment protocol for orbital inflammatory disease. Ophthalmology 1985;92:1325–1331.

327. Bielory L, Frohman LP. Low-dose cyclosporine therapy of granulomatous optic neuropathy and orbitopathy. Ophthalmology 1991;98:1732–1736.

328. Diaz Llopis M, Menezo JL. Idiopathic inflammatory orbital pseudotumor and low-dose cyclosporine. Am J Ophthalmol 1989;107:547–548.

329. Smith JR, Rosenbaum JT. A role for methotrexate in the management of non-infectious orbital inflammatory disease. Br J Ophthalmol 2001;85:1220–1224.

330. Symon Z, Schneebaum N, Eyal A, et al. Successful intravenous immunoglobulin therapy for resistant inflammatory pseudotumor of the orbit. Thyroid 2005;15:398–399.

331. Garcia-Pous M, Hernandez-Garfella ML, Diaz-Llopis M. Treatment of chronic orbital myositis with daclizumab. Can J Ophthalmol 2007;42:156–157.

332. Garrity JA, Coleman AW, Matteson EL, et al. Treatment of recalcitrant idiopathic orbital inflammation (chronic orbital myositis) with infliximab. Am J Ophthalmol 2004;138:925–930.

333. Kapadia MK, Rubin PA. The emerging use of TNF-alpha inhibitors in orbital inflammatory disease. Int Ophthalmol Clin 2006;46:165–181.

334. Miquel T, Abad S, Badelon I, et al. Successful treatment of idiopathic orbital inflammation with infliximab: an alternative to conventional steroid-sparing agents. Ophthal Plast Reconstr Surg 2008;24:415–417.

335. Donaldson SS, McDougall IR, Egbert PR, et al. Treatment of orbital pseudotumor (idiopathic orbital inflammation) by radiation therapy. Int J Radiat Oncol Biol Phys 1980;6:79–86.

336. Lanciano R, Fowble B, Sergott RC, et al. The results of radiotherapy for orbital pseudotumor. Int J Radiat Oncol Biol Phys 1990;18:407–411.

337. Sergott RC, Glaser JS, Charyulu K. Radiotherapy for idiopathic inflammatory orbital pseudotumor. Indications and results. Arch Ophthalmol 1981;99:853–856.

338. Isobe K, Uno T, Kawakami H, et al. Radiation therapy for idiopathic orbital myositis: two case reports and literature review. Radiat Med 2004;22:429–431.

339. Cornblath WT, Elner V, Rolfe M. Extraocular muscle involvement in sarcoidosis [see comments]. Ophthalmology 1993;100:501–505.

340. Patel AS, Kelman SE, Duncan GW, et al. Painless diplopia caused by extraocular muscle sarcoid [letter]. Arch Ophthalmol 1994;112:879–880.

341. Simon EM, Zoarski GH, Rothman MI, et al. Systemic sarcoidosis with bilateral orbital involvement: MR findings. AJNR Am J Neuroradiol 1998;19:336–337.

342. Pakrou N, Selva D, Leibovitch I. Wegener's granulomatosis: ophthalmic manifestations and management. Semin Arthritis Rheum 2006;35:284–292.

343. Sadiq SA, Jennings CR, Jones NS, et al. Wegener's granulomatosis: the ocular manifestations revisited. Orbit 2000;19:253–261.

344. Diamond JP, Bloom PA, Ragge N, et al. Localised Wegener's granulomatosis presenting as an orbital pseudotumour with extension into the posterior cranial fossa. Eur J Ophthalmol 1993;3:143–146.

345. Duncker G, Nolle B, Asmus R, et al. Orbital involvement in Wegener's granulomatosis. Adv Exp Med Biol 1993;336:315–317.

346. Parelhoff ES, Chavis RM, Friendly DS. Wegener's granulomatosis presenting as orbital pseudotumor in children. J Pediatr Ophthalmol Strabismus 1985;22:100–104.

347. Salam A, Meligonis G, Malhotra R. Superior oblique myositis as an early feature of orbital Wegener's granulomatosis. Orbit 2008;27:203–206.

348. Nishino H, Rubino FA, DeRemee RA, et al. Neurological involvement in Wegener's granulomatosis: an analysis of 324 consecutive patients at the Mayo Clinic. Ann Neurol 1993;33:4–9.

349. Seo P, Specks U, Keogh KA. Efficacy of rituximab in limited Wegener's granulomatosis with refractory granulomatous manifestations. J Rheumatol 2008;35:2017–2023.

350. Koike R, Yamada M, Matsunaga T, et al. Polyarteritis nodosa (PN) complicated with unilateral exophthalmos. Intern Med 1993;32:232–236.

351. Patrinely JR, Osborn AG, Anderson RL, et al. Computed tomographic features of nonthyroid extraocular muscle enlargement. Ophthalmology 1989;96:1038–1047.

352. Capone A, Jr., Slamovits TL. Discrete metastasis of solid tumors to extraocular muscles. Arch Ophthalmol 1990;108:237–243.

353. Slamovits TL, Burde RM. Bumpy muscles. Surv Ophthalmol 1988;33:189–199.

354. Hornblass A, Jakobiec FA, Reifler DM, et al. Orbital lymphoid tumors located predominantly within extraocular muscles. Ophthalmology 1987;94:688–697.

355. Izambart C, Robert PY, Petellat F, et al. Extraocular muscle involvement in marginal zone B-cell lymphomas of the orbit. Orbit 2008;27:345–349.

356. Behrens Baumann W, Freissler G. Computed tomographic appearance of extraocular muscle calcification in a patient with seropositive trichinosis [letter]. Am J Ophthalmol 1990;110:709–710.

357. Nicol JL, Massin M, Ullern M. [A case of bilateral exophthalmos disclosing trichinosis]. Bull Soc Ophtalmol Fr 1987;87:577–578, 581–573.

358. Pasco M. [Ocular manifestations of trichinosis. Considerations on an epidemic of trichinosis]. Bull Mem Soc Fr Ophtalmol 1986;97:74–76.

359. Katz B, Leja S, Melles RB, et al. Amyloid ophthalmoplegia. Ophthalmoparesis secondary to primary systemic amyloidosis. J Clin Neuroophthalmol 1989;9:39–42.

360. Zafar A, Jordan DR. Enlarged extraocular muscles as the presenting feature of acromegaly. Ophthal Plast Reconstr Surg 2004;20:334–336.

361. Demirci H, Shields CL, Shields JA, et al. Orbital tumors in the older adult population. Ophthalmology 2002;109:243–248.

362. He Y, Song G, Ding Y. Histopathologic classification of 3 476 orbital diseases. Zhonghua Yan Ke Za Zhi 2002;38:396–398.

363. Ohtsuka K, Hashimoto M, Suzuki Y. A review of 244 orbital tumors in Japanese patients during a 21-year period: origins and locations. Jpn J Ophthalmol 2005;49:49–55.

364. Shields JA, Shields CL, Scartozzi R. Survey of 1264 patients with orbital tumors and simulating lesions: the 2002 Montgomery Lecture, part 1. Ophthalmology 2004;111: 997–1008.

365. Wende S, Aulich A, Nover A, et al. Computed tomography or orbital lesions. A cooperative study of 210 cases. Neuroradiology 1977;13:123–134.

366. Yan J, Wu Z, Li Y. The differentiation of idiopathic inflammatory pseudotumor from lymphoid tumors of orbit: analysis of 319 cases. Orbit 2004;23:245–254.

367. Chino K, Tanyi JA, Stea B. Stereotactic radiotherapy for unilateral orbital lymphoma and orbital pseudo-tumors: a planning study. Med Dosim 2009;34:57–62.

368. Goyal S, Cohler A, Camporeale J, et al. Intensity-modulated radiation therapy for orbital lymphoma. Radiat Med 2008;26:573–581.

369. Liao SL, Kao SC, Hou PK, et al. Results of radiotherapy for orbital and adnexal lymphoma. Orbit 2002;21:117–123.

370. Reddy EK, Bhatia P, Evans RG. Primary orbital lymphomas. Int J Radiat Oncol Biol Phys 1988;15:1239–1241.

371. Schick U, Lermen O, Unsold R, et al. Treatment of primary orbital lymphomas. Eur J Haematol 2004;72:186–192.

372. Suh CO, Shim SJ, Lee SW, et al. Orbital marginal zone B-cell lymphoma of MALT: radiotherapy results and clinical behavior. Int J Radiat Oncol Biol Phys 2006;65:228–233.

373. Yadav BS, Sharma SC. Orbital lymphoma: role of radiation. Indian J Ophthalmol 2009;57:91–97.

374. Yamashita H, Nakagawa K, Asari T, et al. Radiotherapy for 41 patients with stages I and II MALT lymphoma: a retrospective study. Radiother Oncol 2008;87:412–417.

375. Zhou P, Ng AK, Silver B, et al. Radiation therapy for orbital lymphoma. Int J Radiat Oncol Biol Phys 2005;63:866–871.

376. Tanimoto K, Kaneko A, Suzuki S, et al. Primary ocular adnexal MALT lymphoma: a long-term follow-up study of 114 patients. Jpn J Clin Oncol 2007;37:337–344.

377. Gonul E, Izci Y, Sefali M, et al. Orbital manifestation of multiple myeloma: case report. Minim Invasive Neurosurg 2001;44:172–174.

378. Knecht P, Schuler R, Chaloupka K. Rapid progressive extramedullary plasmacytoma in the orbit. Klin Monatsbl Augenheilkd 2008;225:514–516.

379. Rawlings NG, Brownstein S, Robinson JW, et al. Solitary osseous plasmacytoma of the orbit with amyloidosis. Ophthal Plast Reconstr Surg 2007;23:79–80.

380. Sen S, Kashyap S, Betharia S. Primary orbital plasmacytoma: a case report. Orbit 2003;22:317–319.

381. Cantore G, Ciappetta P, Raco A, et al. Orbital schwannomas: report of nine cases and review of the literature. Neurosurgery 1986;19:583–588.

382. Gunalp I, Gunduz K, Duruk K, et al. Neurogenic tumors of the orbit. Jpn J Ophthalmol 1994;38:185–190.

383. Konrad EA, Thiel HJ. Schwannoma of the orbit. Ophthalmologica 1984;188:118–127.

384. Rootman J, Goldberg C, Robertson W. Primary orbital schwannomas. Br J Ophthalmol 1982;66:194–204.

385. Schick U, Bleyen J, Hassler W. Treatment of orbital schwannomas and neurofibromas. Br J Neurosurg 2003;17:541–545.

386. Ni C, Cheng SC, Dryja TP, et al. Lacrimal gland tumors: a clinicopathological analysis of 160 cases. Int Ophthalmol Clin 1982;22:99–120.

387. Wright JE, Rose GE, Garner A. Primary malignant neoplasms of the lacrimal gland [see comments]. Br J Ophthalmol 1992;76:401–407.

388. Wright JE, Stewart WB, Krohel GB. Clinical presentation and management of lacrimal gland tumours. Br J Ophthalmol 1979;63:600–606.

389. Stewart WB, Krohel GB, Wright JE. Lacrimal gland and fossa lesions: an approach to diagnosis and management. Ophthalmology 1979;86:886–895.

390. Ahmad SM, Esmaeli B, Williams M, et al. American Joint Committee on Cancer Classification predicts outcome of patients with lacrimal gland adenoid cystic carcinoma. Ophthalmology 2009;116:1210–1215.

391. Gamel JW, Font RL. Adenoid cystic carcinoma of the lacrimal gland: the clinical significance of a basaloid histologic pattern. Hum Pathol 1982;13:219–225.

392. Fahmy P, Heegaard S, Jensen OA, et al. Metastases in the ophthalmic region in Denmark 1969–98. A histopathological study. Acta Ophthalmol Scand 2003;81:47–50.

393. Wickremasinghe S, Dansingani KK, Tranos P, et al. Ocular presentations of breast cancer. Acta Ophthalmol Scand 2007;85:133–142.

394. Goldberg RA, Rootman J. Clinical characteristics of metastatic orbital tumors. Ophthalmology 1990;97:620–624.

395. Goldberg RA, Rootman J, Cline RA. Tumors metastatic to the orbit: a changing picture. Surv Ophthalmol 1990;35:1–24.

396. Gunalp I, Gunduz K. Metastatic orbital tumors. Jpn J Ophthalmol 1995;39:65–70.

397. Cline RA, Rootman J. Enophthalmos: a clinical review. Ophthalmology 1984;91:229–237.

398. Kiratli H, Yilmaz PT, Yildiz ZI. Metastatic atypical carcinoid tumor of the inferior rectus muscle. Ophthal Plast Reconstr Surg 2008;24:482–484.

399. Healy JF. Computed tomographic evaluation of metastases to the orbit. Ann Ophthalmol 1983;15:1026–1029.

400. Johnson TE, Tabbara KF, Weatherhead RG, et al. Secondary squamous cell carcinoma of the orbit. Arch Ophthalmol 1997;115:75–78.

401. Oskouian RJ, Jr., Jane JA, Sr., Dumont AS, et al. Esthesioneuroblastoma: clinical presentation, radiological, and pathological features, treatment, review of the literature, and the University of Virginia experience. Neurosurg Focus 2002;12:e4.

402. Tramacere F, Bambace S, De Luca MC, et al. Esthesioneuroblastoma treated with external radiotherapy. Case report. Acta Otorhinolaryngol Ital 2008;28:215–217.

403. Weaver DT, Bartley GB. Malignant neoplasia of the paranasal sinuses associated with mucocele. Ophthalmology 1991;98:342–346.

404. Imola MJ, Schramm VL, Jr. Orbital preservation in surgical management of sinonasal malignancy. Laryngoscope 2002;112:1357–1365.

405. McCary WS, Levine PA. Management of the eye in the treatment of sinonasal cancers. Otolaryngol Clin North Am 1995;28:1231–1238.

406. McCary WS, Levine PA, Cantrell RW. Preservation of the eye in the treatment of sinonasal malignant neoplasms with orbital involvement. A confirmation of the original treatise. Arch Otolaryngol Head Neck Surg 1996;122:657–659.

407. Suarez C, Ferlito A, Lund VJ, et al. Management of the orbit in malignant sinonasal tumors. Head Neck 2008;30:242–250.

408. Ferry AP, Haddad HM, Goldman JL. Orbital invasion by an intracranial chordoma. Am J Ophthalmol 1981;92:7–12.

409. Gunalp I, Gunduz K. Secondary orbital tumors. Ophthal Plast Reconstr Surg 1997;13: 31–35.

410. Vidor I, Sivak-Callcott JA, Rosen CL, et al. Chordoma of the anterior cranial fossa and ethmoids with orbital involvement. Orbit 2008;27:444–450.

411. Scheuerle AF, Steiner HH, Kolling G, et al. Treatment and long-term outcome of patients with orbital cavernomas. Am J Ophthalmol 2004;138:237–244.

412. Schick U, Dott U, Hassler W. Surgical treatment of orbital cavernomas. Surg Neurol 2003;60:234–244; discussion 244.

413. Yan J, Wu Z. Cavernous hemangioma of the orbit: analysis of 214 cases. Orbit 2004;23:33–40.

414. Yamasaki T, Handa H, Yamashita J, et al. Intracranial and orbital cavernous angiomas. A review of 30 cases. J Neurosurg 1986;64:197–208.

415. Ohtsuka K, Hashimoto M, Akiba H. Serial dynamic magnetic resonance imaging of orbital cavernous hemangioma. Am J Ophthalmol 1997;123:396–398.

416. Bilaniuk LT. Vascular lesions of the orbit in children. Neuroimaging Clin N Am 2005;15:107–120.

417. Harris GJ. Orbital vascular malformations: a consensus statement on terminology and its clinical implications. Orbital Society. Am J Ophthalmol 1999;127:453–455.

418. In S, Miyagi J, Kojho N, et al. Intraorbital optic nerve hemangioblastoma with von Hippel-Lindau disease. Case report. J Neurosurg 1982;56:426–429.

419. Kerr DJ, Scheithauer BW, Miller GM, et al. Hemangioblastoma of the optic nerve: case report. Neurosurgery 1995;36:573–580.

420. Nerad JA, Kersten RC, Anderson RL. Hemangioblastoma of the optic nerve. Report of a case and review of literature. Ophthalmology 1988;95:398–402.

421. Karcioglu ZA, Nasr AM, Haik BG. Orbital hemangiopericytoma: clinical and morphologic features. Am J Ophthalmol 1997;124:661–672.

422. Kikuchi K, Kowada M, Sageshima M. Orbital hemangiopericytoma: CT, MR, and angiographic findings. Comput Med Imaging Graph 1994;18:217–222.

423. Bernardini FP, de Conciliis C, Schneider S, et al. Solitary fibrous tumor of the orbit: is it rare? Report of a case series and review of the literature. Ophthalmology 2003;110:1442–1448.

424. O'Donovan DA, Bilbao JM, Fazl M, et al. Solitary fibrous tumor of the orbit. J Craniofac Surg 2002;13:641–644.

425. Musarella MA, Chan HS, DeBoer G, et al. Ocular involvement in neuroblastoma: prognostic implications. Ophthalmology 1984;91:936–940.

426. Katz BJ, Nerad JA. Ophthalmic manifestations of fibrous dysplasia. A disease of children and adults. Ophthalmology 1998;105:2207–2215.

427. Bibby K, McFadzean R. Fibrous dysplasia of the orbit. Br J Ophthalmol 1994;78:266–270.

428. Yavuzer R, Bone H, Jackson IT. Fronto-orbital fibrous dysplasia. Orbit 2000;19:119–128.

429. Tabrizi R, Ozkan BT. Craniofacial fibrous dysplasia of orbit. J Craniofac Surg 2008;19: 1532–1537.

430. Osguthorpe JD, Gudeman SK. Orbital complications of fibrous dysplasia. Otolaryngol Head Neck Surg 1987;97:403–405.

431. Moore AT, Buncic JR, Munro IR. Fibrous dysplasia of the orbit in childhood. Clinical features and management. Ophthalmology 1985;92:12–20.

432. Seiff SR. Optic nerve decompression in fibrous dysplasia: indications, efficacy, and safety [letter]. Plast Reconstr Surg 1997;100:1611–1612.

433. Cruz AA, Constanzi M, de Castro FA, et al. Apical involvement with fibrous dysplasia: implications for vision. Ophthal Plast Reconstr Surg 2007;23:450–454.

434. Chen YR, Breidahl A, Chang CN. Optic nerve decompression in fibrous dysplasia: indications, efficacy, and safety. Plast Reconstr Surg 1997;99:22–30.

435. Arroyo JG, Lessell S, Montgomery WW. Steroid-induced visual recovery in fibrous dysplasia. J Clin Neuroophthalmol 1991;11:259–261.

436. Rootman J, Kemp E, Lapointe JS. Orbital tumors originating in bone. In: Rootman J, ed. Diseases of the Orbit: A multidisciplinary approach, pp 354–379. Philadelphia, J.B. Lippincott, 1988.

437. Chen YR, Wong FH, Hsueh C, et al. Computed tomography characteristics of non-syndromic craniofacial fibrous dysplasia. Chang Gung Med J 2002;25:1–8.

438. Casselman JW, De Jonge I, Neyt L, et al. MRI in craniofacial fibrous dysplasia. Neuroradiology 1993;35:234–237.

439. Faul S, Link J, Behrendt S, et al. MRI features of craniofacial fibrous dysplasia. Orbit 1998;17:125–132.

440. Weisman JS, Hepler RS, Vinters HV. Reversible visual loss caused by fibrous dysplasia. Am J Ophthalmol 1990;110:244–249.

441. Edelstein C, Goldberg RA, Rubino G. Unilateral blindness after ipsilateral prophylactic transcranial optic canal decompression for fibrous dysplasia. Am J Ophthalmol 1998;126:469–471.

442. Lee JS, FitzGibbon E, Butman JA, et al. Normal vision despite narrowing of the optic canal in fibrous dysplasia. N Engl J Med 2002;347:1670–1676.

443. Rubin SE, Slavin ML, Rubin LG. Eyelid swelling and erythema as the only signs of subperiosteal abscess. Br J Ophthalmol 1989;73:576–578.

444. Hornblass A, Herschorn BJ, Stern K, et al. Orbital abscess. Surv Ophthalmol 1984;29:169–178.

445. Donahue SP, Schwartz G. Preseptal and orbital cellulitis in childhood. A changing microbiologic spectrum. Ophthalmology 1998;105:1902–1905.

446. Weiss A, Friendly D, Eglin K, et al. Bacterial periorbital and orbital cellulitis in childhood. Ophthalmology 1983;90:195–203.

447. Blomquist PH. Methicillin-resistant *Staphylococcus aureus* infections of the eye and orbit (an American Ophthalmological Society thesis). Trans Am Ophthalmol Soc 2006;104:322–345.

448. Slavin ML, Glaser JS. Acute severe irreversible visual loss with sphenoethmoiditis-'posterior' orbital cellulitis. Arch Ophthalmol 1987;105:345–348.

449. Khong JJ, Malhotra R, Wormald PJ, et al. Endoscopic sinus surgery for paranasal sinus mucocoele with orbital involvement. Eye 2004;18:877–881.

450. Baujat B, Derbez R, Rossarie R, et al. Silent sinus syndrome: a mechanical theory. Orbit 2006;25:145–148.

451. Bossolesi P, Autelitano L, Brusati R, et al. The silent sinus syndrome: diagnosis and surgical treatment. Rhinology 2008;46:308–316.

452. Brandt MG, Wright ED. The silent sinus syndrome is a form of chronic maxillary atelectasis: a systematic review of all reported cases. Am J Rhinol 2008;22:68–73.

453. Gomez J, Villafane FG, Palacios E. Enophthalmos in silent sinus syndrome. Ear Nose Throat J 2008;87:496–498.

454. Hamedani M, Pournaras JA, Goldblum D. Diagnosis and management of enophthalmos. Surv Ophthalmol 2007;52:457–473.

455. Langer PD, Patel BC, Anderson RL. Silent sinus syndrome. Ophthalmology 1994;101:1763–1764.

456. Soparkar CN, Patrinely JR, Cuaycong MJ, et al. The silent sinus syndrome. A cause of spontaneous enophthalmos. Ophthalmology 1994;101:772–778.

457. Gutierrez Diaz A, del Palacio Hernanz A, Larregla S, et al. Orbital phycomycosis. Ophthalmologica 1981;182:165–170.

458. Ameen M, Arenas R, Martinez-Luna E, et al. The emergence of mucormycosis as an important opportunistic fungal infection: five cases presenting to a tertiary referral center for mycology. Int J Dermatol 2007;46:380–384.

459. Bhansali A, Bhadada S, Sharma A, et al. Presentation and outcome of rhino-orbital-cerebral mucormycosis in patients with diabetes. Postgrad Med J 2004;80:670–674.

460. Ferry AP, Abedi S. Diagnosis and management of rhino-orbitocerebral mucormycosis (phycomycosis). A report of 16 personally observed cases. Ophthalmology 1983;90:1096–1104.

461. Kohn R, Hepler R. Management of limited rhino-orbital mucormycosis without exenteration. Ophthalmology 1985;92:1440–1444.

462. Peterson KL, Wang M, Canalis RF, et al. Rhinocerebral mucormycosis: evolution of the disease and treatment options. Laryngoscope 1997;107:855–862.

463. Schwartze GM, Kilgo GR, Ford CS. Internal ophthalmoplegia resulting from acute orbital phycomycosis. J Clin Neuroophthalmol 1984;4:105–108.

464. Bray WH, Giangiacomo J, Ide CH. Orbital apex syndrome. Surv Ophthalmol 1987;32:136–140.

465. Balch K, Phillips PH, Newman NJ. Painless orbital apex syndrome from mucormycosis. J Neuroophthalmol 1997;17:178–182.

466. Bodenstein NP, McIntosh WA, Vlantis AC, et al. Clinical signs of orbital ischemia in rhino-orbitocerebral mucormycosis. Laryngoscope 1993;103:1357–1361.

467. Mauriello JA, Jr., Yepez N, Mostafavi R, et al. Invasive rhinosino-orbital aspergillosis with precipitous visual loss. Can J Ophthalmol 1995;30:124–130.

468. Wiroteurairueng T, Poungvarin N. Orbital infarction syndrome in nephrotic syndrome patient with extensive carotid arteries occlusion. J Med Assoc Thai 2007;90:2499–2505.

469. Maier P, Feltgen N, Lagreze WA. Bilateral orbital infarction syndrome after bifrontal craniotomy. Arch Ophthalmol 2007;125:422–423.

470. Yang SW, Kim SY, Chung J, et al. Two cases of orbital infarction syndrome. Korean J Ophthalmol 2000;14:107–111.

471. Borruat FX, Bogousslavsky J, Uffer S, et al. Orbital infarction syndrome. Ophthalmology 1993;100:562–568.

472. Hargrove RN, Wesley RE, Klippenstein KA, et al. Indications for orbital exenteration in mucormycosis. Ophthal Plast Reconstr Surg 2006;22:286–291.

473. Dortzbach RK, Segrest DR. Orbital aspergillosis. Ophthalmic Surg 1983;14:240–244.

474. Kronish JW, Johnson TE, Gilberg SM, et al. Orbital infections in patients with human immunodeficiency virus infection. Ophthalmology 1996;103:1483–1492.

475. Levin LA, Avery R, Shore JW, et al. The spectrum of orbital aspergillosis: a clinicopathological review. Surv Ophthalmol 1996;41:142–154.

476. Spoor TC, Hartel WC, Harding S, et al. Aspergillosis presenting as a corticosteroid-responsive optic neuropathy. J Clin Neuroophthalmol 1982;2:103–107.

477. Adam RD, Paquin ML, Petersen EA, et al. Phaeohyphomycosis caused by the fungal genera *Bipolaris* and *Exserohilum*. A report of 9 cases and review of the literature. Medicine Baltimore 1986;65:203–217.

478. Brummund W, Kurup VP, Harris GJ, et al. Allergic sino-orbital mycosis. A clinical and immunologic study. JAMA 1986;256:3249–3253.

479. Chang WJ, Shields CL, Shields JA, et al. Bilateral orbital involvement with massive allergic fungal sinusitis [letter]. Arch Ophthalmol 1996;114:767–768.

480. Cody DTI, Neel HBI, Ferreiro JA, et al. Allergic fungal sinusitis: the Mayo Clinic experience. Laryngoscope 1994;104:1074–1079.

481. Dunlop IS, Billson FA. Visual failure in allergic aspergillus sinusitis: case report. Br J Ophthalmol 1988;72:127–130.

482. Jacobson M, Galetta SL, Atlas SW, et al. Bipolaris-induced orbital cellulitis. J Clin Neuroophthalmol 1992;12:250–256.

483. Klapper SR, Lee AG, Patrinely JR, et al. Orbital involvement in allergic fungal sinusitis. Ophthalmology 1997;104:2094–2100.

484. Perry HD, Donnenfeld ED, Grossman GA, et al. Retained *Aspergillus*-contaminated contact lens inducing conjunctival mass and keratoconjunctivitis in an immunocompetent patient. CLAO J 1998;24:57–58.

485. Kennerdell JS, Maroon JC. Microsurgical approach to intraorbital tumors. Technique and instrumentation. Arch Ophthalmol 1976;94:1333–1336.

486. Kennerdell JS, Maroon JC, Malton ML. Surgical approaches to orbital tumors. Clin Plast Surg 1988:82.

487. Maroon JC, Kennerdell JS. Microsurgical approach to orbital tumors. Clin Neurosurg 1979;26:479–489.

488. Maroon JC, Kennerdell JS. Surgical approaches to the orbit. Indications and techniques. 1984;60:1226–1235.

Part **Four**

Other topics

CHAPTER **19**

Headache, facial pain, and disorders of facial sensation

Headache is a nearly universal experience as over 90% of individuals have noted at least one headache during their lifetime.[1] Since the eye receives a rich innervation from the trigeminal nerve, it is not surprising that many headache syndromes are associated with pain concentrated around the eye. Furthermore, many of the primary headache syndromes such as migraine and cluster headaches have prominent neuro-ophthalmic signs and symptoms. As such, the reader should become familiar with the many types of headache, facial pains, and disorders of facial sensation.

Headache

Approach

History. The cause of the patient's headache is usually established from the history. Important features include the frequency, location, laterality, mode of onset, duration, nature of the headache (throbbing, aching, pressure, dull or sharp), and the presence of accompanying symptoms along with precipitating and alleviating factors. Visual aura is highly suggestive of a migraine disturbance. Although nonspecific, photophobia, phonophobia, osmophobia, and gastrointestinal symptoms may also help to discriminate migraine from other causes of headache. Naturally, the patient's medical and psychiatric history and medication list provide essential information.

Classification. It is useful to classify headaches into those that are primary (or without specific cause) and those with an organic cause. Migraine, tension-type, and cluster headaches (and other trigeminal autonomic cephalgias) are the most common forms of primary headache. The International Headache Society (IHS) has established diagnostic criteria for a variety of headache disorders to provide uniformity in classification **(Tables 19–1 to 19–4)**.[2]

These guidelines were primarily created for the purpose of collecting epidemiologic and clinical trial data and may not always be practical for use in the clinical setting. Diagnostic difficulty occurs in patients with multiple headache syndromes and from the fact that headache characteristics may change over time. In addition, the restrictive IHS requirements for a minimum number of headaches with a certain duration may exclude many individuals who likely do have that headache type.

"Red-flag" headache characteristics that suggest a more ominous underlying cause are listed in **Table 19–5**. These types of headaches require more aggressive evaluation, including neuroimaging and possibly lumbar puncture.[3]

Migraine

Because it is such a common disorder, migraine will be discussed first. This section will review the epidemiology, genetic and clinical factors, pathophysiology, and treatment of migraine.

Table 19–1 International Headache Society (IHS) criteria for migraine without aura[2]

A	Five attacks fulfilling criteria B–D
B	Headache lasting 4–72 hours (untreated or unsuccessfully treated)
C	Headache has two of the following characteristics: 1. Unilateral location 2. Pulsating quality 3. Moderate to severe intensity 4. Aggravation by walking stairs or similar routine physical activity
D	During headache at least one of the following: 1. Nausea or vomiting 2. Photophobia or phonophobia
E	Not attributed to another disorder

Table 19–2 International Headache Society (IHS) criteria for typical migraine with aura[2]

A	At least two attacks fulfilling criteria B–D
B	Aura consisting of at least one of the following, but no motor weakness: 1. Fully reversible visual symptoms including positive features (e.g., flickering lights, spots or lines) and/or negative features (i.e., loss of vision) 2. Fully reversible sensory symptoms including positive features (i.e., pins and needles) and/or negative features (i.e., numbness) 3. Fully reversible dysphasic speech disturbance
C	At least two of the following: 1. Homonymous visual symptoms and/or unilateral sensory symptoms 2. At least one aura symptom develops gradually over ≥5 minutes and/or different aura symptoms occur in succession over ≥5 minutes 3. Each symptoms lasts ≥5 minutes and ≤60 minutes
D	Headache fulfilling criteria B–D for *Migraine without aura* (Table 19–1) begins during the aura or follows aura within 60 minutes
E	Not attributed to another disorder

Table 19–3 International Headache Society (IHS) Criteria for Frequent Episodic Tension Headaches[2]

A	At least 10 previous headaches episodes filling criteria B–D listed below; number of days with such headaches: fewer than 180 per year or fewer than 15 per month for at least 3 months
B	Headache lasting from 30 minutes to 7 days
C	At least two of the following pain characteristics: 1. Pressure/tightening (nonpulsating) quality 2. Mild or moderate intensity 3. Bilateral location 4. No aggravation with routine physical activity
D	Both of the following: 1. No nausea or vomiting 2. Photophobia and phonophobia are absent, or one but not the other is present
E	Not attributed to another disorder

Table 19–4 International Headache Society (IHS) Criteria for Cluster Headaches[2]

A	At least five attacks fulfilling criteria B–D
B	Severe unilateral orbital, supraorbital, and/or temporal pain lasting 15–180 minutes untreated
C	Headache associated with at least one of the following signs, which have to be present on the painful side: 1. Conjunctival injection and/or lacrimation 2. Nasal congestion and/or rhinorrhea 3. Eyelid edema 4. Forehead and facial sweating 5. Miosis and/or ptosis 6. A sense of restlessness or agitation
D	Frequency of attacks: from one to eight per day
E	Not attributed to another disorder

Table 19–5 Features of headache that suggest an ominous cause[3]

Abrupt onset
Association with fever, coughing, straining or sexual activity
Change with position or exertion
Focal neurological symptoms or signs
Onset after the fourth decade
Onset during pregnancy or postpartum
Papilledema
Progressive worsening
Underlying disorder such as cancer or HIV disease

Epidemiology

Approximately 18% of women and 6% of men endure recurrent headache classified as migraine.[4,5] Migraine prevalence is highest among 30–50-year-olds, with more white than black people and with an inverse relationship to income.[4] In one population study, approximately 90% of patients with migraine reported some disability associated with their headache, and one half had severe disability.[4] In fact, patients with migraine may lose several days of work per year related to headache.[6,7] Despite the high frequency of disability associated with migraine, many patients do not seek medical attention for their headache.[8] Most of these patients rely on over-the-counter medications and the majority are probably inadequately treated.[5] A subgroup of patients with episodic migraine may develop a chronic disease state, formerly termed *transformed migraine*, but now called *chronic migraine*,[9–11] characterized by 15 or more headaches per month.

A variety of neurologic and psychiatric disorders may also have an association with migraine.[12] According to one study, epilepsy patients have twice the risk of developing migraine as those without seizures.[13] There is a higher incidence of stroke in patients with migraine, particularly in those with aura.[14] Silent posterior circulation infarcts, particularly in the cerebellum, have been documented in migraine patients.[15,16] Nonspecific deep white matter lesions demonstrated best on magnetic resonance imaging (MRI) are commonly seen,[15,17] but their exact pathogenesis is unclear. A variety of affective disorders are related to migraine, including depression, manic depressive illness, and panic disorder. Co-sensitization may explain the association of chronic migraine with depression and anxiety.[18]

Genetic factors. A genetic basis for migraine has been long suggested by the observation that 70% to 90% of migraine patients have a positive family history.[19] In fact, migraine has been linked to both chromosomes 1 and 19.[20] Joutel and colleagues[21,22] have linked familial hemiplegic migraine to chromosome 19. Evidence suggests that the defective gene encodes for a voltage-dependent P-type calcium channel.[23] A link to chromosome 19 has also been established for the entity known as CADASIL (cerebral autosomal dominant arteriopathy with subcortical infarcts and leukoencephalopathy). This is an autosomal dominant arteriopathy characterized by leukoencephalopathy, subcortical infarction, and migraines. Other studies of familial hemiplegic migraine also suggest a link to chromosome 1 and a defect in calcium and potassium channels.[24,25] Thus, accumulating data suggest that migraine in some instances may be a channelopathy, a condition that ultimately leads to neuronal hyperexcitability.

Pathophysiology

Pain-sensitive structures of the head and face include the skin and blood vessels of the scalp, the dura, the venous sinuses, the arteries, and the sensory fibers of the fifth, ninth, and tenth nerves. Although the precise mechanism of migraine remains uncertain, evidence suggests an important role for the trigeminal vascular projections and the neurochemical serotonin. The trigeminal nerve has terminals on the pial and dural blood vessels that release a variety of vasoactive neuropeptides, including substance P, neurokinin A, and calcitonin gene-related peptide (CGRP). Release of these neuromediators produces sterile neurogenic inflammation by dilating meningeal blood vessels and increasing vascular permeability. Sumatriptan and dihydroergotamine (DHE) act on presynaptic $5\text{-}HT_1D$ receptors to block the release of these neuroactive peptides and $5HT_1B$ receptors to selectively constrict dilated meningeal vessels. In addition, $5HT_1B/D$ agonists such as the triptans that cross the blood–brain barrier may also block neurons of the trigeminal nucleus caudalis within the medulla.

Further evidence for the involvement of brain stem structures is supported by positron emission tomography studies that show increased blood flow in the reticular activating formation during the migraine episode.[26] The median raphe nucleus and the periaqueductal gray matter along with the locus ceruleus are regions thought to be activated during a migraine attack. In addition, activated parasympathetic projections from the superior salivatory nucleus may produce vasodilation of meningeal vessels.

Mechanism of migraine aura. Classic explanations for migraine attributed the aura to vasoconstriction and the headache to vasodilation. However, more contemporary theories suggest otherwise.[27] For instance, blood flow studies have demonstrated reduced flow preceding the onset of the aura but continuing into the headache phase.[28] Thus the headache occurred during a period of vasoconstriction. Currently the aura of migraine is thought to be related to the concept of spreading depression. This idea of cortical depression was promulgated by Leão,[29,30] who demonstrated that electrical depression moved over the cortex at a rate of 2–3 mm per minute. The observation of Leão was supported by Lashley,[31] who calculated his own aura progressing over the visual cortex at the same rate of 2–3 mm per minute. Although blood flow reduction spreads over the cortex at this rate, it now is believed to be a secondary event triggered by a primary neurogenic process. Modern imaging techniques such as perfusion-weighted imaging,[32] positron-emission tomography,[33] magnetoencephalography,[34] and functional MRI[35,36] have supported the notion of cortical spreading of oligemia and neuronal depression.

Lance[37] proposed that the neuroadrenergic locus ceruleus, which diffusely projects to the cerebral cortex, may be one neural network involved in the generation of migraine aura. Activation of the locus ceruleus has also been implicated in the development of photophobia and phonophobia. Ultimately, the locus ceruleus and the spinal nucleus of the trigeminal nerve are influenced by the cortex and other higher structures. Functional MRI studies[38,39] have suggested that the red nucleus and substantia nigra may also be involved in this neural network. Spreading depression may release a variety of substances in the cortex such as potassium, hydrogen, and nitric oxide that leak into the extracellular space and activate perivascular trigeminal nerve endings. How aura and headache are related mechanistically is still uncertain.[40]

Integrated theory. At this time, the precise pathophysiology of migraine remains uncertain,[41] but a cascade of events seems likely. In summary, migraine appears to be initiated by hyperexcitability of cortical and brain stem neurons (**Fig. 19–1**). The overactivation of these neurons may be the result of an underlying channelopathy seen in genetically predisposed individuals.[42] Presumably, these hyperexcitable neurons are responsible for activating portions of the cortex (aura) and meningeal vessels (pain). The firing of these hyperexcitable neurons may be influenced by internal and external factors such as hormonal balance, foodstuffs, stress, and sleep deprivation. The different symptoms observed in migraine probably reflect differential activation of cortical, brain stem, and vascular structures.

In some patients, the migraine process persists and central sensitization occurs.[43,44] Continued peripheral sensory input can lead to sensitization of central (second order) trigeminovascular neurons and third-order neurons in the thalamus. At this point, the centrally based pain neurons may continue to propagate pain impulses even in the absence of further input from the peripheral trigeminal neurons. Clinically, the patient may develop cutaneous allodynia, during which normally non-painful tactile stimuli become painful. Patients with cutaneous allodynia may experience localized pain with routine activities such as wearing eyeglasses, combing hair, wearing contact lenses, lying on a pillow, or taking a shower.[45,46] In this stage, the patient's pain may be refractory to triptan therapy.[44] It has also been suggested that

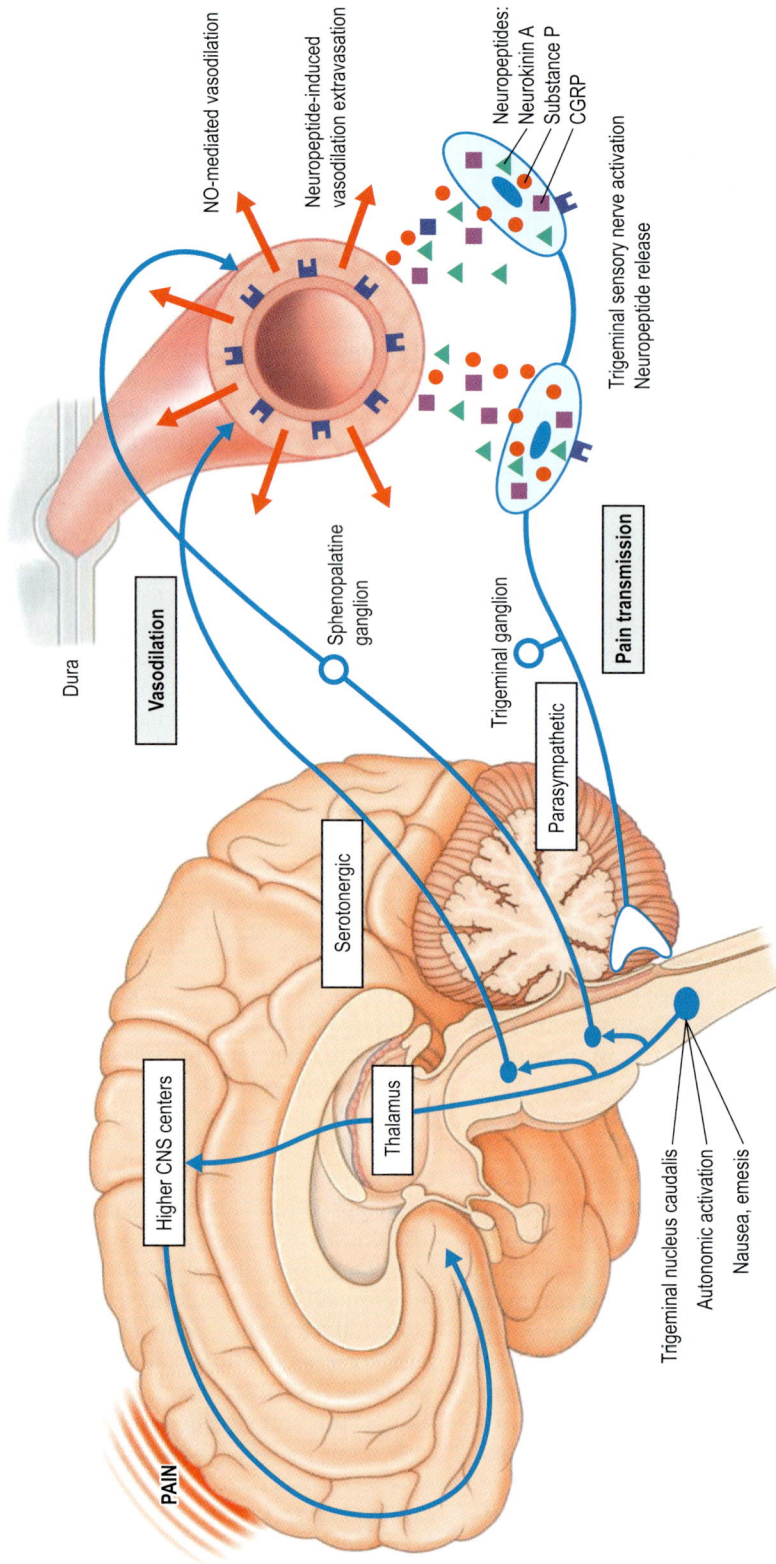

Figure 19–1. Trigeminal vascular theory of migraine headaches. Cortical hyperexcitable neurons, perhaps with an additional influence from brain stem structures, leads to activation of the trigeminovascular system. Signals reach the trigeminal nucleus caudalis in the brain stem, which in turn signals the thalamus, which in turn signals cortical regions, leading to the conscious sensation of headache and pain. Note activation of the trigeminal nerve afferents lead to neuropeptide release and vasodilation of dural blood vessels, which in turn leads to release of more neuropeptides, perpetuating the cycle.

Labels in figure:

NO-mediated vasodilation

Neuropeptide-induced vasodilation extravasation

Neuropeptides:
Neurokinin A
Substance P
CGRP

Trigeminal sensory nerve activation
Neuropeptide release

Dura

Vasodilation

Sphenopalatine ganglion

Trigeminal ganglion

Pain transmission

Parasympathetic

Serotonergic

Higher CNS centers

Thalamus

Trigeminal nucleus caudalis
Autonomic activation
Nausea, emesis

PAIN

chronic (transformed) migraine may result from repeated episodes of cutaneous allodynia.[47]

Symptoms and signs

As alluded to earlier, a variety of factors may provoke migraine, including menstruation, change in sleep patterns, hunger, stress, certain foods, odors, and even the type of lighting. Hours to days before the onset of migraine, the patient may experience prodromal symptoms manifesting as mood swings, food cravings, anorexia, fluid retention, or urinary frequency.

Headache. The headache of migraine is usually unilateral, throbbing, and of moderate severity (**Table 19–1**). It may start any time of the day or night, but has a tendency to start in the morning. The onset is usually gradual, and it is this feature that helps to distinguish migraine from a more ominous cause such as a subarachnoid hemorrhage. Migraine headaches usually last several hours, and may be exacerbated by physical activity. The headache may pass through stages ranging from mild to severe. A variety of symptoms may accompany the headache, including photophobia, phonophobia, osmophobia, nausea, vomiting, and autonomic symptoms (**Table 19–1**). Patients may also become irritable, anxious, or depressed during the headache phase.

Aura. The aura of migraine usually begins before the headache phase, but occasionally it will occur simultaneously or follow it (**Table 19–2**). Approximately one-third of migraine patients experience an aura.[48] The most characteristic aura is visual, but sensory dysfunction may also occur. The visual symptoms typically build up over several minutes and resolve by 20–40 minutes. Occasionally, the aura will extend to 60 minutes. Some patients will have recurrent auras during the day. Most patients are unable to determine whether the phenomenon occurred in one or both eyes. In fact, the vast majority of patients believe a hemifield disturbance occurred in one eye. Although fortification scotomas are the most characteristic visual disturbance, the patient may also complain of bright flashing lights or distorted vision. Some patients describe the sensation as if they were looking through clouded or prismatic glass. Classically, an arc of flashing zigzag light starts in the paracentral area of one hemifield and expands peripherally. As the wave of visual disturbance travels across the visual field it may rotate or undulate. Other patients will experience tunnel vision or a disturbance in both hemifields. Unusual disturbances of vision may occur, such as palinopsia (perseveration of visual images) or the Alice in Wonderland syndrome. In the latter, the patient may appreciate objects as overly large, small, or distorted. Rare patients may experience persistent positive visual phenomena.[49] In these patients, neuroimaging does not show any evidence of infarction, and the aura symptoms persist beyond one week. The various types of positive migraine visual aura are discussed in more detail and with figures in Chapter 12, and the negative visual auras (vision loss) in Chapter 10.

Sensory disturbance may include paresthesias, dysesthesias, numbness or hyperesthesia. It is not unusual for the sensory symptoms to follow the headache. Classically, the sensory symptoms begin in the fingertips and march up the arm and into the perioral area. Sensory auras are most convincingly migraine when they have been preceded by a classic visual aura. Aphasic and motor auras are uncommon, but their initial occurrence should prompt investigation for transient cerebral ischemia.

Interictal heightened visual sensitivity

Even between episodes of headache, migraine patients may have a heightened sensitivity to bright lights, glare, and other visual stimuli.[50] Patients may also complain of sensitivity to flickering lights (e.g., strobe and fluorescent), patterned stimuli,[51] moving objects,[52] and supermarket aisles (visual vertigo).[53] These visual stimuli may cause migraine headaches,[54,55] perhaps in part by lowering trigeminal and cervical pain thresholds.[56] Migraine patients may also have impaired inhibitory subcortical function that normally suppresses glare-induced pain.[57] Alternative explanations include primary visual cortex[58] and V5 hypersensitivity[59] or reduced inhibition by extrastriate structures.[60] Detailed psychophysical[61-67] and electrophysiologic studies[68,69] have also demonstrated that interictal visual function may be subtly altered in patients with migraine.

Migraine subtypes

Complicated migraine

The term *complicated migraine* refers to a permanent neurologic deficit whether it is visual, motor, or sensory in origin. In these patients, MRI may demonstrate the cerebral ischemic changes that typically occur in the occipital–parietal regions (**Fig. 19–2**).

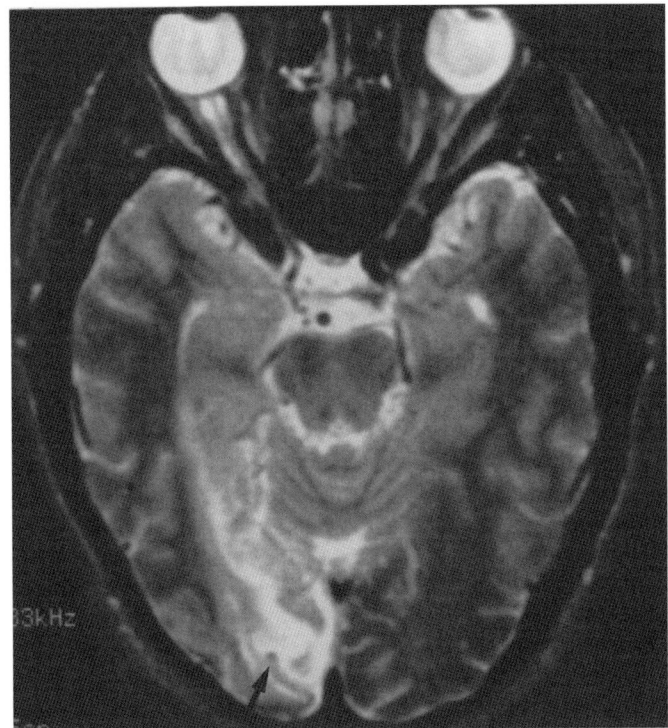

Figure 19–2. T2-weighted axial image in a patient with migrainous infarction, demonstrating high signal abnormality (arrow) in the right occipital lobe.

There is no effective therapy for evolving complicated migraine. We treat suspected complicated migraine with high-dose intravenous methylprednisolone and hydration. Triptan medications should be avoided because of their vasoconstrictive properties. Sublingual calcium channel blockers may help reduce vasospasm, but this beneficial effect must be weighed against their propensity to lower blood pressure.

Retinal migraine

These events typically occur in one eye. Unlike the migraine patient with occipital auras, the patient with retinal migraine frequently experiences a negative visual phenomenon described as a graying or blackout of vision. The pattern of visual loss is often described as a tunnel, but may be altitudinal or quadrantic in nature.[70] The diagnosis of retinal migraine is often one of exclusion, and it has been suggested that migraine is only a rare cause of transient or permanent visual loss.[71]

Observers have occasionally noted constriction of the retinal arterioles and venules during an attack (**Fig. 19–3**).[72]

During these episodes, the retina will transiently lose its orange color. It seems likely that retinal changes are primarily induced by local vascular changes.[73] Rarely, patients have permanent visual loss as the result of retinal or optic nerve damage (**Table 19–6**).[74]

The evaluation of retinal migraine patients usually consists of noninvasive studies of the carotid arteries, and checking for antiphospholipid antibodies. In some patients, echocardiography and a hypercoagulable workup are needed

Table 19–6 Ocular complications of migraine (very rare)

Anterior ischemic optic neuropathy
Central retinal artery occlusion
Branch retinal artery occlusion
Central retinal vein occlusion
Retinal hemorrhage
Vitreous hemorrhage
Retinal pigment changes
Central serous chorioretinopathy

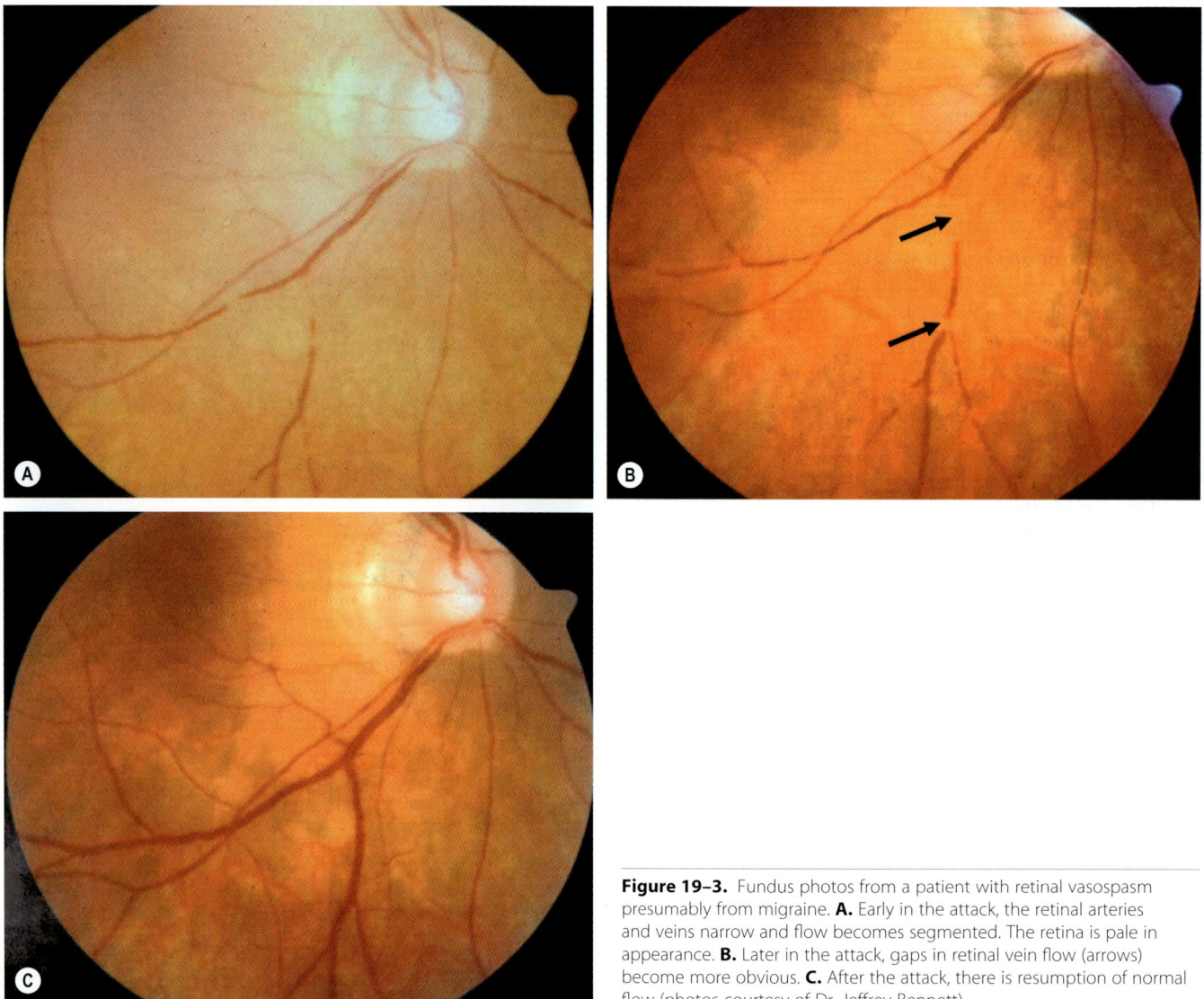

Figure 19–3. Fundus photos from a patient with retinal vasospasm presumably from migraine. **A.** Early in the attack, the retinal arteries and veins narrow and flow becomes segmented. The retina is pale in appearance. **B.** Later in the attack, gaps in retinal vein flow (arrows) become more obvious. **C.** After the attack, there is resumption of normal flow (photos courtesy of Dr. Jeffrey Bennett).

to exclude a non-migrainous cause. Calcium blockers have been particularly effective for these patients.[75] Occasionally, one aspirin a day will also reduce the frequency of retinal migraine.

This entity and other types of transient visual loss in migraine are also discussed in Chapter 10.

Ophthalmoplegic "migraine"

This rare disorder usually begins before the age of 10 in the patient with an otherwise typical migraine pattern. The ophthalmoplegia usually follows the headache by several days but occasionally it will occur simultaneously or precede it. The most common motility disturbance is a third nerve palsy, and the pupil is involved in about 50% of such patients.[76] Rarely, fourth and sixth nerve palsies or a combination of ocular motor palsies may be a manifestation of migraine. Clearly, other causes of a cavernous sinus syndrome need to be excluded fully in such situations. The ophthalmoparesis usually resolves after 1–4 weeks. After several episodes, a partial palsy may persist.

In patients under the age of 10, MRI should suffice to exclude most serious conditions when a pupil involving third nerve palsy is present. In the majority of patients with ophthalmoplegic migraine, transient third nerve enhancement is observed.[76] However, above age 10, an aneurysm is an increasing concern and should be excluded.

The cause of the ophthalmoparesis in migraine is uncertain and some have questioned whether this disorder should be classified under the rubric of migraine. The disorder is thought to be a recurrent inflammatory cranial neuropathy.[2,77] Other possibilities include microvascular occlusion, swelling of the intracavernous carotid, or microhemorrhages from a cavernous malformation intrinsic to the third nerve. We typically use a short course of oral prednisone in these patients. There is no solid evidence that preventive therapy alters the course of this disorder.

This entity is also discussed in further detail in Chapter 15.

Benign episodic mydriasis

Rarely, a dilated pupil may be a manifestation of migraine, and other signs of a third nerve palsy such as ptosis or ophthalmoparesis are absent. Angle-closure glaucoma should be excluded.[78] This entity is discussed in more detail in Chapter 13.

Basilar (Bickerstaff) migraine

These patients may experience transient symptoms of posterior circulation insufficiency, including visual field defects, vertigo, nystagmus, ataxia, impaired hearing, dysarthria, and motor and sensory symptoms.[79,80] Some patients may have an alteration of consciousness, presumably from involvement of the reticular activating system.[81] This disorder usually occurs in young women. This form of migraine may be the cause of episodic vertigo seen in young children. These patients may be more sensitive to the vasoconstrictive effects of triptan medication. As such, the triptan compounds are contraindicated in these groups of patients. Unfortunately, solid data regarding this important issue are lacking.

Hemiplegic migraine

This disorder usually occurs early in life as a prelude to headache. This disorder has a male predominance and may be familial. The hemiplegia usually lasts less than 1 hour, but it may persist for several days. Like the sensory aura, the headache may precede the hemiplegia. Recently, familial hemiplegic migraine has been linked to chromosome 19 and less frequently to chromosome 1. The genetic defect in familial hemiplegia appears to result from a defect in the calcium channel.[23] Likewise, these patients may be overly sensitive to the triptan compounds and their use in this subgroup of patients should be avoided until further data are available.

Migrainous vertigo

Patients with migraine commonly have vertigo as an associated symptom.[82] In some patients, however, episodic vertigo may be the only complaint. Confusion may exist with Ménière's disease, and in fact, the two entities may co-exist. Although phonophobia is another common symptom in migraine, a small percentage of patients may experience acute permanent hearing loss. The episodes of vertigo may begin abruptly, last from seconds to days, and can be extremely severe.[83] It is quite common for them to occur without headache. These patients may also experience a variety of abnormalities on vestibular testing, including caloric paresis, spontaneous nystagmus, positional nystagmus, and abnormal rotary-chair testing.[84,85] Patients may have nystagmus that can suggest either a central or peripheral vestibular disorder.[86–88] Baloh[89] has proposed that such patients may have a defective calcium channel manifesting within the inner ear and brain. The treatment is similar to that for other forms of migraine in terms of prophylactic and abortive therapies.

Migraine in women

Menstrual migraine. Migraine associated with menses is extremely common in women, and its pathogenesis is thought to be due to a fall in serum estrogen levels contemporaneous with the onset of bleeding. Many women can predict their headache occurrence in relationship to the onset of menses. These migraines tend to be more severe, longer lasting, and more difficult to treat than nonmenstrual migraines. In addition, usually they are unassociated with auras.

Migraine in pregnancy. While some women suffer from worsening of their migraine headaches during pregnancy, others, for unclear reasons, enjoy vast improvement. Most prophylactic and abortive migraine medications except acetaminophen are contraindicated in pregnancy.

Oral contraceptives and stroke in migraine. Controversy surrounds the use of oral contraceptive medication in women who suffer from migraine with aura. Migraine with aura itself may increase the risk of ischemic stroke in women of childbearing age,[90] and in some studies the use of oral contraceptives enhanced this risk.[91–94] However, the absolute risk is still low.[95] Nevertheless, we often discourage the use of oral contraceptives in patients with refractory migraine with aura. The risk of stroke may be most significant in female migraineurs who are over the age of 35, use contraceptives, and smoke cigarettes.

Diagnostic testing in a patient with suspected migraine

Visual fields should be assessed in all new patients with suspected migraine visual aura to exclude field defects. A homonymous defect, for instance, would suggest alternative diagnoses such as release hallucinations or seizures due to a neoplasm.

If the patient has a long history of typical migraine and a normal examination, it may be reasonable to defer neuroimaging. However, we have a low threshold for performing MRI in most patients because there are many causes of headache, and several organic disorders may mimic or even trigger migraine. This is particularly true in patients with new onset of symptoms in middle age, atypical features, or marked increase in frequency of headache (**Table 19–5**). Routine blood work is often unhelpful in young patients, but a sedimentation rate is extremely important in elderly patients with transient loss of vision or headache to help exclude temporal arteritis. Lumbar puncture, almost always following neuroimaging, is an important test when suspecting a diagnosis of subarachnoid hemorrhage, meningitis, or pseudotumor cerebri.

Treatment

Migraine treatment depends on the frequency, duration, and intensity of the pain. Symptomatic or abortive treatment alone is recommended when the attacks occur less than twice a week and are short lived (**Table 19–7**). Prophylactic or preventive therapy should be added when the headaches are more frequent or disabling enough to affect the patient's occupation or social activities. Many patients with frequent migraine are treated with a combination of preventive and abortive therapies.

Abortive therapy

Mild to moderate headaches. There are many patients who find relief with acetaminophen, nonsteroidal anti-inflammatory drugs (NSAIDs), or aspirin. Many of these patients do not seek medical attention. In fact, the non-prescription combination of acetaminophen, aspirin, and caffeine may be quite effective. In one study, pain intensity was reduced to mild or none in 59.3% of treated patients compared with 32.8% of placebo patients, 2 hours after the dose.[96] NSAIDs are very beneficial for patients with occasional headaches. NSAIDs are also very helpful for the brief lancinating pain which lasts seconds and plagues certain migraine patients. These pains are referred to as ice-pick-like (idiopathic stabbing pain) and may occur over the scalp, particularly over the temporal regions.

Other options for abortive therapy in patients with mild to moderate headache include butorphanol nasal spray, an isometheptene–dichloralphenazone–acetaminophen combination, and a butalbital–caffeine–acetaminophen combination. We use the butalbital–caffeine–acetaminophen combination cautiously because of its high abuse potential and its tendency to produce rebound headaches if used frequently. Butorphanol nasal spray is a mixed opiate agonist–antagonist. The dose is one spray in one nostril, which may

Table 19–7 Pharmacologic abortive therapy in migraine, including initial dosages and route of administration

	Dose	Route
Triptan medications		
Fast acting, non-oral		
Sumatriptan	20 mg	IN
Sumatriptan	4 mg, 6 mg	SQ
Zolmitriptan	5 mg	IN
Intermediate acting, oral		
Sumatriptan	25 mg, 50 mg, 100 mg	PO
Sumatriptan/Naproxen	85 mg/500 mg	PO
Rizatriptan	5 mg, 10 mg	PO, MLT
Zolmitriptan	2.5 mg, 5.0 mg	PO
Eletriptan	20 mg, 40 mg	PO
Almotriptan	6.25 mg, 12.5 mg	PO
Slower onset, longer acting		
Frovatriptan	2.5 mg	PO
Naratriptan	2.5 mg	PO
Nonsteroidal anti-inflammatory drugs (NSAIDs)		
Naproxyn	375 mg, 500 mg	PO
Indomethacin	75 mg	SR
Ketoralac	10 mg	PO
Antiemetics		
Droperidol	2.5 mg	IV
Prochlorperazine	2–10 mg	IV
Metoclopramide	10 mg	PO, IV
Corticosteroids		
Prednisone	60 mg	PO
Methylprednisolone	60–1000 mg	IV
Miscellaneous		
Butorphanol	1 spray	IN
Butalbital, caffeine, and acetaminophen preparation	1–2 pills	PO
Isometheptene mucate	1–2 capsules	PO
Dihydroergotamine	0.5–1 mg	IV
	2 mg	IN
Ergotamine	2 mg	SL

IN, intranasal; IV, intravenous; PO, oral; SQ, subcutaneous; SR, sustained release; SL, sublingual.

be repeated in 1 hour if pain relief is inadequate. However, the abuse potential of butorphanol is high, which limits its routine use. Intranasal lidocaine (4% soln, 0.5-ml dose) may also abort migraine headaches although recurrence is a problem with this drug.[97]

For some patients, the migraine begins as a mild headache with subsequent progression to a moderate or severe migraine. In this situation, it is best to recommend the early initiation of a triptan medication.[98–100] Therapy is most effective in the early headache stages before cutaneous allodynia ensues.[44]

Moderate to severe headache. For patients with moderate to severe pain, the options for therapy are also numerous. However, the triptans (5HT$_1$B/D serotonin agonists), which are migraine-specific medications, are the most widely used for such patients. The decision of which triptan to select largely depends on the rapidity and the length of the migraine headache as well as the presence of nausea and vomiting (**Table 19–7**). If the headache onset is between 15 and 45 minutes, and the patient is not severely nauseous or vomiting, one of the faster onset oral triptans (sumatriptan, zolmitriptan, eletriptan, almotriptan or rizatriptan) is an excellent option.[101] Rizatriptan (5–10 mg) comes in a wafer form, providing an alternative route of oral administration, even though its absorption is still primarily in the gastrointestinal tract. The wafer contains aspartame, so it may have limited use in patients who have their headache triggered by this artificial substance. Rizatriptan also interacts with propranolol, requiring the physician to half the dose of rizatriptan with concurrent use. However, rizatriptan 10 mg has a slight benefit over 100 mg of oral sumatriptan in terms of headache relief at 2 hours and sustained freedom from pain.[48,102] Because many patients were combining a triptan with a NSAID, sumatriptan together with napoxen is now also available in a single tablet.[103–105] Oral triptans may be taken at the onset of the aura. For unclear reasons, some patients seem to respond better to one triptan than to the others, and a trial and error approach among this group of triptans may be required.

In individuals with either rapid-onset migraine or severe nausea or vomiting precluding oral tablet use, subcutaneous (sumatriptan) and intranasal (sumatriptan or zolmitriptan) preparations are important alternative routes of triptan administration. Patients should be advised to take the subcutaneous or intranasal triptan preparation at the headache onset. Patients using the nasal form of triptans should be instructed to tilt their head forward during administration. This technique reduces the amount of the drug delivered to the gastrointestinal tract and helps eliminate some of the bitter taste. Since both of these routes of administration are quick, they may not be effective as oral preparations during the aura phase.

Patients with headaches with less rapid onset (over hours) and longer duration (days) and in whom recurrence is a problem may benefit from the triptans with slower onset and longer half lives (naratriptan or frovatriptan).[106] Since menstrual migraine has these characteristics, these triptans are often used in such patients.

Oral sumatriptan may not be as effective in children as in adults; however, studies to date have been relatively small.[107,108] Intranasal sumatriptan, zolmitriptan, or almotriptan may provide a reasonable option for children or adolescents with acute migraine.[109,110] Almotriptan has been approved for use in adolescents.

It should be noted that the amount of triptan that can be used in a 24-hour period is limited. For instance, the maximum single dose of oral sumatriptan is 100 mg and the dosage taken over 24 hours should not exceed 200 mg. Triptan contraindications include coronary artery disease, Prinzmetal's angina, poorly controlled hypertension, cerebrovascular disease, hemiplegic or basilar migraine, pregnancy, and use of an ergot-containing compound or monoamine oxidase inhibitors within the previous 24 hours. Serious cerebro- and cardiovascular side-effects are extremely rare.[111] Both electrocardiography and positron emission tomography perfusion studies suggest that most cases of chest pain associated with the triptans are not cardiac related.[112,113] Triptans are relatively contraindicated in individuals taking selective serotonin reuptake inhibitors (SSRIs) because of the risk of serotonin syndrome. However, this side-effect, characterized by tachycardia, hypertension, and hyperthermia, is extremely rare in our experience. The main side-effects of the oral triptans are paresthesias, fatigue, and dizziness.

Other treatment options for moderate to severe migraine include intranasal DHE and dopamine receptor antagonists. Haloperidol, droperidol, prochlorperazine, chlorpromazine, and metoclopramide may be effective in treating acute migraine, particularly in patients with nausea and vomiting.[114] In addition, an oral CGRP receptor antagonist has been investigated as a novel acute treatment for migraine.[115]

Currently there is no effective treatment for aborting the visual aura of migraine. Observation is usually the safest approach. In cases where it is suspected that migrainous infarction is about to evolve, one may try 10 mg of nifedipine sublingually, keeping in mind that hypotension is a possible side-effect. Inhaled amyl nitrate and isoproterenol are alternatives but the efficacy of all these regimens are unproven.

Severe migraine headache in the emergency department. For the patient with severe pain and nausea, the following regimens may be tried:

1. Subcutaneous sumatriptan.
2. Intramuscular ketorolac 30–60 mg. Prochlorperazine 10 mg could also be given before the ketorolac to lessen nausea.
3. Intravenous dihydroergotamine. Prochlorperazine 10 mg is combined with 1 mg of dihydroergotamine. One half of the solution is given intravenously over 1–2 minutes. If chest pain ensues, the drug is discontinued. If there is no response, the remaining solution is administered in 15–20 minutes. In rare cases of refractory migraine, dihydroergotamine 0.5–1 mg may be given every 8 hours for 3 days.
4. Intravenous prochlorperazine 10 mg. Boluses of 2 mg are given every 5 minutes until the headache abates or a total of 10 mg is given. When one administers prochlorperazine, it is important that the patient does not drive home alone because of its sedative effect. Intravenous hydration is also a very effective adjunct as most patients with severe acute migraine have become dehydrated. Droperidol 2.5 mg IV every hour to a maximum of 10 mg can also be tried.[116] Premedication with 1 mg of benztropine mesylate may help eliminate some of the side-effects of this regimen.
5. Intravenous valproic acid 10 mg/kg over 60 minutes.
6. Intravenous methylprednisolone or in prolonged migraine, dexamethasone.[117]

Preventive therapy

Preventive (prophylactic) therapy is indicated when headaches occur more than once or twice a week or produce significant disability, or when symptomatic therapy fails (**Table 19–8**). The goal of prophylaxis is to reduce or eliminate the need for acute therapy. Even if preventive therapy is not completely effective, it may render acute therapy more

Table 19–8 Pharmacologic preventative therapy in migraine, including oral daily dosages

Beta blockers	Dose
Propranolol	60–300 mg LA
Nadolol	40–160 mg
Metoprolol	50–200 mg
Atenolol	50–200 mg
Timolol	20–30 mg
Calcium channel blockers	
Verapamil	120–480 mg SR
Nifedipine	30–90 mg
Amlodipine	2.5–10 mg
Antidepressants	
Nortriptyline	10–150 mg
Amitriptyline	25–150 mg
Doxepin	75–300 mg
Fluoxetine	20–80 mg
Sertraline	50–100 mg
Duloxetine	20–60 mg
Venlafaxine	75–225 mg
Anticonvulsants	
Valproic acid	500–2000 mg
Gabapentin	300–3600 mg
Topiramate	25–300 mg (slow titration)
Lamotrigine	50–300 mg (slow titration)
Zonisamide	25–300 mg (slow titration)
Pregabalin	150–600 mg
Other	
Lithium	600–1800 mg
Methysergide	2 mg three times per day
Riboflavin	400 mg
Coenzyme Q10	150–300 mg
Botulinum toxin	Usually 100 units

SR, sustained release; LA, long-acting.

efficacious and lessen the risk of rebound headaches. Elimination of triggering factors such as certain foodstuffs, smoking, or alcohol (red wine, particularly) may also contribute to the effect of preventive therapy. Culprit foods include chocolate, cheeses, and nuts. We usually try to tailor preventive therapy to meet the individual needs of the patient. For instance, patients who are depressed may fare better with an antidepressant like nortriptyline, while other patients with mood swings might benefit from valproic acid. Propranolol may be best for patients with hypertension. Topiramate can be used in individuals interested in losing weight. The medications most frequently used to prevent migraine headaches include (1) beta-blockers, (2) calcium channel blockers, (3) anti-depressants, and (4) anticonvulsants.

Beta-blockers. Most of these drugs have to be administered for at least a month to assess their efficacy. Beta-blockers are often used as first-line agents and have an efficacy in the range of 60% to 80%.[118] Propranolol 60 mg LA (long-acting) is the usual starting dose, and patients are instructed to increase the dose to 120 mg LA after 7 days if the initial 60-mg dose is well tolerated. Thereafter, the dosage can be raised in 60-mg increments per week up to 300 mg a day. Occasionally, patients will not respond to propranolol but will to other beta-blockers such as metoprolol or atenolol. Side-effects of beta-blockers include congestive heart failure, asthma, hypotension, bradycardia, and depression. Men may suffer reversible impotence. If the patient is headache free for 6–12 months, a taper of the beta-blocker over several weeks can be attempted.

Calcium channel blockers. Calcium channel blockers are also an excellent choice for prophylactic therapy,[119] particularly in patients with migraine with aura and hemiplegic migraine. One of their main advantages is their limited side-effects in most patients. Constipation, arrhythmias, heart failure, and hypotension are among the most common side-effects. Verapamil is an excellent choice in this category. The initial dose is usually 120 mg SR (sustained release), which can be increased by 120-mg SR increments as necessary. Most patients respond by 360 mg, but occasionally 480 mg a day is necessary. Verapamil works in 60–70% of patients with migraine. It is recommended that the patient on verapamil have a baseline electrocardiogram and another check every 6 months. In one study of patients with cluster headache on verapamil, 18% of patients had a potentially serious cardiac rhythm disturbance.[120] Amlodipine is another good alternative, and doses of 2.5–5.0 mg are usually sufficient.

Antidepressants. Antidepressants are also highly effective, particularly when patients have sleeping problems, depressive symptoms, or a combination of migraine and tension-type headaches. Amitriptyline and nortriptyline seem to be the most effective in this category, although some patients may respond to fluoxetine, nefazodone hydrochloride, sertraline hydrochloride, venlafaxine hydrochloride, duloxetine and desipramine. It is those compounds that block norepinephrine uptake that seem to be the most effective. Nortriptyline is typically chosen over amitriptyline because the latter has more anticholinergic side-effects. In addition, these compounds produce dry mouth, constipation, urinary retention, tachycardia, and weight gain. Nortriptyline is started at either 10 or 25 mg, depending on the size and age of the patient. From there, the dosage can be increased as necessary, typically each week until a balance between efficacy and side-effects is achieved. Most patients, if they are going to respond to nortriptyline, they will do so by 50 mg a day.

Anticonvulsant drugs. The anticonvulsant drugs, in particular the newer ones, have proven to be relatively effective in the prevention of migraine.[121,122] Many patients find topiramate extremely effective,[123,124] although some find the cognitive side-effects intolerable. The initial dose can be 25 mg per day, then the dosage should be built up slowly over weeks (25 mg/week) to reduce the risk of cognitive side-effects, which are more likely to occur with rapid dose escalations and at doses higher than 200 mg/day. Many patients benefit from the associated appetite suppression and weight loss, but untoward side-effects include memory and language difficulty, paresthesias, kidney stones, glaucoma, and myopia. Zonisamide, a related drug, may be used in similar doses if the side-effects of topiramate are not tolerated or if a once a day regimen is desired.

Gabapentin has been effective in the treatment of both migraine and chronic daily headache.[125] High doses of gabapentin in the 2400–3600 mg per day range may be necessary to achieve a beneficial effect, but lower doses may also work in the occasional patient. Pregabalin and lamotrigine have also been successful in the treatment of migraine headaches. Older anticonvulsants such as carbamazepine and phenytoin may also be used but with more variable success.

Valproic acid may also used as a preventive treatment for migraine. The dose may be started at 125 mg twice a day and slowly increased to 500–1000 mg per day in divided doses. Patients often do not require large doses for a therapeutic effect. The side-effects of valproate, nausea, alopecia, tremor, and weight gain, usually limit the use of this agent as a primary preventive therapy. Hepatotoxicity is a concern, particularly in young children on multiple medications. Since valproic acid is teratogenic and associated with a 1% risk of neural tube defects, this drug needs to be used with caution in women of childbearing age. They should be advised of the risk and use appropriate contraception. The anticonvulsant drugs may be best utilized in patients with cardiac disease or mood disorders, or in those with concerns regarding exercise intolerance.

Miscellaneous prophylactic medications. Riboflavin in high doses (400 mg per day) may be effective in migraine prevention. Riboflavin may enhance a deficient mitochondrial energy reserve, a potential factor in the genesis of migraine.[126] Magnesium deficiency in the brain has also been suggested as a potential mechanism of migraine. Unfortunately, magnesium supplementation has not been convincingly effective.[127] Coenzyme Q10 in doses of 150–300 mg may be tried in patients reluctant to take more conventional preventive treatment.[128] *Petasites* extract (butterbur) has also been used.[129] Small studies have suggested botulinum injections in the frontal and neck areas can effectively prevent migraine,[130] but larger placebo-controlled trials have been unconvincing.[131]

Short-term continuous use of oral sumatriptan, frovatriptan, or naratriptan may be effective in preventing menstrual migraine.[132–134] One regimen used 25 mg of sumatriptan three times per day for a total of 5 days.[135] Transdermal estrogen, continuous contraception (ethinyl estradiol and levonorgestrel), and NSAIDS also may be used as prophylaxis for menstrual-related migraine.[136] Cyproheptadine is frequently used as migraine prophylaxis in children. NSAIDs are very beneficial prophylactically for patients with orgasmic migraine (coital headache).

Non-traditional treatments. Relaxation training, biofeedback, and cognitive–behavioral therapy may be helpful for some patients.[137] Although anecdotally acupuncture may be effective, confirming evidence for recommending its use is lacking.[138]

Some studies have suggested that percutaneous closure of patent foramen ovales in patients with migraine reduces their headache frequency.[139,140] The mechanism for this improvement is unclear but may be related to decreasing microemboli. However, randomized clinical trials have failed to prove this treatment effect.

The use of transmagnetic stimulation and occipital nerve stimulation in migraine treatment has also been suggested, but their benefit also remains unproven.

Acephalgic migraine

Patients with migraine may have transient neurologic events without headache. When these events occur in patients over the age of 40, concern over the possibility of a transient ischemic attack (TIA) is raised. In any age group, seizures may also be considered. Fortunately, there are some features that may differentiate these disorders. The migraine aura has a characteristic buildup of scintillations. The episodes may occur in a flurry and tend to last longer than a typical TIA. Patients often have a remote history of migraine headaches. Some even have mild accompanying discomfort but do not think it is important to report it. The intensity of their headache is often not as severe as it was previously.

In a relatively young patient with visual aura without headache, but with a previous history of migraine, further testing may not be necessary. However, in patients over age 40, the new onset of acephalgic migraine is a diagnosis of exclusion. Workup would include neuroimaging to exclude a structural lesion of the occipital cortex such as an arteriovenous malformation or meningioma and to check for ischemic changes. In some instances electroencephalography can be performed to rule out an irritative lesion. When the aura is characterized by visual loss, cardiac emboli, carotid insufficiency, and hypercoagulable states should also be considered.

Treatment of acephalgic migraine. If tolerated, 325 mg of aspirin per day may be given, particularly in elderly individuals in whom the diagnosis may not be certain. It may lessen acephalgic migraine episodes and help prevent stroke in case the events were in fact TIAs. In patients in whom aspirin is ineffective or not tolerated, calcium channel blockers such as verapamil, 120–360 mg (SR) per day, can be considered for those with recurrent disabling episodes. In many instances, patients are reassured knowing that their visual episodes are migrainous and benign, and choose to eschew pharmacologic treatment.

Other headache types

Chronic daily headache

This is not a diagnosis per se, but a category of headaches including for instance chronic migraine (described above), chronic tension-type headaches, hemicrania continua, new daily persistent headache, and post-traumatic headaches.[2] Affected patients have headaches for 15 or more days per month, and the majority have a element of medication overuse headache.

Tension-type headaches

Tension headaches are probably a continuum of migraine headaches. The pain is mild to moderate in intensity and is often described as pressure or tightness. There is no aura, nausea, or vomiting, and the headaches are usually not aggravated by exercise (**Table 19–3**). Photophobia and phonophobia are rarely present. The location of the headache is often bilateral. Common locations for tension headaches are over the eyes, on top of the head, over the temples, and over the occipital region. These patients often have tender spots over the shoulder girdle muscles. Most tension headaches are episodic. However, some patients have chronic tension-type headaches and are without pain-free intervals.

Many patients with chronic daily tension headaches have a history of migraine. In fact, migraine episodes may periodically occur in such patients. A significant proportion of this patient population has concurrent depression. In patients with tension headache, one also has to be aware of the possibility of secondary headache disorders or rebound headaches from analgesic overuse (see below).

Treatment. Patients with tension headaches, particularly those with chronic daily headaches, pose a therapeutic challenge. The abortive and prophylactic medications used to treat migraine may be tried in patients with tension headaches. The antidepressants nortriptyline and amitriptyline may be the first-line agents for these patients, and topiramate may also be effective. It is important to make sure that patients with tension headaches do not have temporomandibular joint dysfunction or sinus disease before committing them to preventive therapy. Some tension headache patients do not respond to medication and may benefit from alternative therapies, including stretching exercises, meditation, and acupuncture. Botulinum toxin injected into the frontal and occipital muscles may be used in refractory tension headache.[141]

Medication overuse headache

These type of headaches share similar clinical characteristics with tension headaches as described above. However, there is the complicating history of long-standing misuse of headache medications. Although rebound headache is classically associated with overuse of narcotics (taken 10 days a month or more) or other over-the-counter analgesics (taken 15 days a month or more),[2] this phenomenon also may be observed to a lesser degree with triptan and ergot overuse.[142]

Treatment. In this condition, it is important to taper the overused medication. If not already contributing to the problem, NSAIDs or a short course of corticosteroids may help ameliorate some of the patient's symptoms. If outpatient detoxification fails, inpatient management may be necessary. Intravenous dihydroergotamine 1 mg combined with 10 mg of intravenous metoclopramide every 8 hours for 3–5 days is one effective regimen to treat analgesic overuse.

Cluster headache

Cluster headache is a severe unilateral headache disorder that predominantly occurs in men (**Table 19–4**).[143] These headaches occur in clusters or on a daily basis for weeks to months. Although most cluster headaches are usually episodic, in a small minority of patients they are chronic and without remission. Cluster headaches are often severe and may awaken a patient from sleep. They typically occur over the periorbital region and are often associated with rhinorrhea and tearing. Alcohol is a common trigger. The attacks are much shorter than migraine, lasting 1/2 hour to 3 hours. There is often no nausea or vomiting; aura is rare but can occur.[144] Many patients will develop signs of a Horner syndrome. Occasionally, only ptosis or miosis will be present.

After several attacks, a permanent Horner syndrome may ensue. In contrast to the migraine patient who desires sleep, the cluster headache patient cannot stand still. The headache is so severe that some patients literally run around the room screaming, and some patients even contemplate suicide. In between the attacks, some patients will suffer typical migraine headaches.

The major entity to exclude in a patient with a painful Horner syndrome is a carotid dissection (see Chapter 13 for further discussion). Other entities that may mimic cluster headaches include arteriovenous malformation,[145] brain stem compression by tumor,[146] vertebral artery aneurysm,[147] cavernous carotid artery aneurysms,[148] sinusitis, temporal arteritis, the Tolosa–Hunt syndrome, orbital myositis,[149] and pituitary tumors.[150] In patients presenting with a painful Horner syndrome, MRI of the neck, including axial T1-weighted images and angiographic sequences, is recommended to exclude carotid dissection.

Treatment. The treatment of acute cluster attack may be difficult. Emergently, the following regimens may be tried:

1. 100% oxygen therapy via a face mask for 10 minutes.
2. Subcutaneous or intranasal sumatriptan.
3. Intranasal or intravenous dihydroergotamine.
4. Intranasal lidocaine 4%.
5. Corticosteroids (2-week prednisone taper).

Corticosteroids often take hours to begin to work. However, they may be useful in transition to other preventive therapies in cluster headache patients. The two most effective preventive therapies are lithium and verapamil.[151] Other options include methylsergide and twice-daily ergotamine therapy. Methylsergide should not be used for more than 3 months at a time because of the rare complication of retroperitoneal fibrosis. Indomethacin may provide benefit to certain patients, and valproic acid may also provide effective prophylaxis. The newer anticonvulsants such as gabapentin, pregabalin, topiramate, and lamotrigine may also be tried.

Occasionally, patients are refractory to monotherapy, and combination therapy may be necessary. Verapamil and lithium are usually tried together first. Valproate and verapamil is another effective combination.

Rarely, patients may require intravenous dihydroergotamine every 8 hours to break the cluster bout. If all medical therapy fails and headaches are strictly unilateral, then radiofrequency thermocoagulation of the gasserian ganglia[152] or trigeminal nerve section[153] may be tried. However, the resultant corneal and trigeminal anesthesia may lead to its own set of complications, and the procedures are not always effective.[154] Intractable cluster headaches have also been treated by deep hypothalmic and occipital nerve stimulation.[155,156]

Paroxysmal hemicrania and hemicrania continua

Paroxysmal hemicrania refers to a headache syndrome characterized by brief episodes of unilateral pain lasting 2–45 minutes. The pain tends to occur over the orbital and temporal regions. Patients often experience multiple attacks a day and some have 40–50 attacks in a 24-hour period.[157] The pain is typically associated with autonomic dysfunction such as conjunctival injection, lacrimation, nasal congestion, ptosis, and eyelid edema. There are many similarities between paroxysmal hemicrania and cluster headache. However, paroxysmal hemicrania is distinguished by its female predominance, shorter duration, and exquisite response to indomethacin.[158] Although indomethacin is the treatment of choice for paroxysmal hemicrania, other patients may respond to verapamil, acetazolamide, or other NSAIDs. Some patients with paroxysmal hemicrania will have superimposed mild and dull hemicranial discomfort between episodes.

Headaches which are similar in quality but continuous are termed *hemicrania continua*.[159,160] These headaches are also responsive to indomethacin.[161]

SUNCT syndrome

The acronym for this syndrome stands for "short-lasting, unilateral, neuralgiform headache with conjunctival injection, and tearing." Patients may experience hundreds of attacks a day lasting 5–240 seconds.[2] This rare condition is similar to the paroxysmal hemicranias, but is distinguished by less severe pain, more marked autonomic activation, and unresponsiveness to indomethacin.[157,162] Carbamazepine, lamotrigine,[163] gabapentin, and topiramate[164] can be used prophylactically. Like cluster headaches, SUNCT syndrome may be mimicked by pituitary tumors[165] and posterior fossa lesions.[166]

Ice pick headache (idiopathic stabbing headache)

Some patients experience sudden stabbing pain that may be described as like being stabbed with an ice pick.[157] The pain is often located in the temple region but the occipital area may also be involved. The pain often lasts seconds, but may persist for minutes. Many patients have underlying migraine or tension headaches. The pain may occur several times a day and may awaken the patient from sleep. Occasionally, the examiner can palpate the area and elicit the pain. The pain of a corneal erosion may be brief and present upon awakening and should be carefully considered in the patient with stabbing pain concentrated around the eye. Patients with stabbing pain respond best to indomethacin or other NSAIDs.

Cough headache

Patients with cough headache may be divided into two broad groups. First, cough-induced headaches may be associated with an intracranial lesion. The posterior fossa is the most frequent location for a lesion producing cough headache. An Arnold–Chiari malformation is a relatively common cause, but tumors and subdural hematomas are other reported causes.

Patients in the second group with cough-induced headache have no detectable intracranial lesions despite extensive investigation. These patients often respond to a course of indomethacin or other NSAID.

Thunderclap headache

Thunderclap headache is a term used to describe a sudden and severe headache. Although controversy exists regarding the significance of such a headache, we believe an intracerebral hemorrhage or even an unruptured aneurysm has to be strongly considered. Raps et al.[167] concluded that thunderclap headache may be induced by a variety of mechanisms, including thrombosis of the aneurysm, expansion of the aneurysm, or intramural hemorrhage. Some patients with thunderclap headache have no identifiable cause. Patients with thunderclap headache should be evaluated with emergent computed tomography (CT) and lumbar puncture. If both are negative, and the suspicion remains high for an unruptured aneurysm, CT or MR angiography should be performed.

Greater occipital neuralgia

Some patients experience episodic pain in the greater occipital region. Occasionally the pain will radiate forward toward the ipsilateral eye. The pain usually only lasts seconds, but may recur frequently during the day. The patient typically has pain and tenderness at the point where the greater occipital nerve pierces the tendinous insertion of the splenius capitis muscle at the skull base. Many patients have superimposed tension and migraine headaches.

Treatment with local injection of lidocaine has a high success rate. Occasionally repeated injections are necessary to break the cycle. If patients do not respond or are reluctant to have a local lidocaine injection, NSAIDS, carbamazepine, gabapentin, a soft cervical collar at night, or a short course of corticosteroids may be tried.

Hypnic headache

Elderly patients may experience headaches shortly after falling asleep.[168] The headache is throbbing and global in location. These headaches are short lived and usually resolve within an hour. This disorder is also recognized in young patients and may be unilateral. Lithium may prevent the headaches, but the side-effects of this medication in the elderly population may limit its use.

Carotid dissection

Patients with acute carotid dissection may develop throbbing pain over the periorbital area. Many patients will have accompanying neurologic signs such as a Horner syndrome or contralateral weakness or numbness. A patient with an isolated painful Horner syndrome should be considered to have a carotid dissection until proven otherwise. Other clinical manifestations, radiographic features, and management of this condition are discussed in detail in Chapter 13.

Temporal arteritis

The headache of temporal arteritis is often described as an ache concentrated over the temporal arteries.[169] The pain rarely can be severe and the area exquisitely sensitive to touch. Although the pain is often concentrated over the temporal region, it may occur over any portion of the head. The pain of giant cell arteritis typically abates within days of starting corticosteroids. This condition, particularly with regard to visual loss, pathophysiology, and management, is reviewed in Chapter 5.

Posttraumatic headache

Mild to moderate headaches are common after head injury. Patients may or may not have experienced a loss of consciousness. Typically, the headache is one of many symptoms that accompany the posttraumatic syndrome. Vertigo, irritability, concentration difficulty, and short-term memory loss are other frequent complaints. The posttraumatic headache may simulate tension headaches or migraine headaches. The headache may improve spontaneously or persist indefinitely. The IHS criteria require the onset of the headache within 7 days after the injury or upon return of consciousness.[2] Migraine, common daily headache, and cluster may follow mild head trauma. Posttraumatic headaches may last for several years, regardless of financial compensation issues. If tolerated, antidepressant compounds may reduce some of the symptoms. Other prophylactic headache medications such as propranolol, verapamil, topiramate, and valproic acid may also be tried with variable success.

Glossopharyngeal neuralgia

Patients with glossopharyngeal neuralgia experience pain in the pharynx and base of the tongue. The pain may be triggered by swallowing, coughing, or talking. Like trigeminal neuralgia, the pain is usually sharp, stabbing, or lacinating. The condition is usually idiopathic but mass lesions should be carefully considered. Most cases result from compression by a dolichoectatic artery or venous structure. Treatment of glossopharyngeal neuralgia is similar to trigeminal neuralgia and includes anticonvulsants, antidepressants, and baclofen therapy. If medical therapy fails, the glossopharyngeal nerve may be thermocoagulated. Other patients may benefit from microvascular decompression.

Intracranial hypotension

Headache is a prominent symptom of patients suffering from intracranial hypotension, also termed cerebrospinal fluid (CSF) hypovolemia syndrome.[170,171] Patients may have associated nausea, vomiting, tinnitus, and photophobia. The hallmark feature of this disorder is pain aggravated by an upright posture.[172] Some patients will develop unilateral or bilateral sixth nerve palsies resulting from the traction on these nerves as the brain sinks downward from the intracranial hypotension. Rarely, patients may complain of transient visual obscurations or blurred vision, and binasal field defects have been documented.[173] The downward displacement of the brain is frequently evident on sagittal MRI, and diffuse meningeal enhancement is often present (**Fig. 19–4A,B**).[174–176] If severe, bilateral subdural hematomas or organized hygromas (**Fig. 19–4C**) may develop.

Of course, most commonly the cause of intracranial hypotension is iatrogenic, induced by lumbar puncture, spinal anesthesia, or shunting.[177,178] Other causes of intracranial hypotension include traumatic injury, particularly those that lead to CSF rhinorrhea. Other traumatic causes include weight-lifting, yoga stretching, and straining.[179] Spontaneous intracranial hypotension may also occur when there is a spontaneous tear of the dura, especially along a spinal nerve root sleeve.[172] The source of the CSF leak may be established with radionuclide cisternography or metrizamide myelography. In our experience, these tests have a low diagnostic yield.

Even if no source of CSF leak is found, patients may still respond to blood patching.[172,180,181] If the source of the CSF leak is found, it should be repaired, if possible. Other nonspecific treatment measures include bedrest, caffeine, volume expansion, corticosteroids, and the use of an abdominal binder. In refractory cases, intrathecal saline solution may be tried. Some anecdotal success using theophylline has been reported in refractory cases.[172]

Intracranial hypertension without papilledema

A small group of patients with chronic daily headaches may have raised intracranial pressure without evidence of papilledema. These patients may be distinguished from other patients with chronic daily headaches by a high frequency of pulsatile tinnitus and obesity. Unfortunately, therapies aimed at lowering the increased intracranial pressure may not reduce the headaches. Intracranial hypertension without and with papilledema is discussed in more detail in Chapter 6.

Headaches and ocular diseases

A variety of ocular conditions may be associated with eye or periorbital pain. Headaches of ocular origin are often accompanied by other eye signs such as conjunctival or scleral injection. The frequency and intensity of the pain is often dependent on the ocular structure affected.

Corneal diseases

Among the most common causes of periorbital discomfort is dry eyes. These patients complain of a gritty, achy, or burning sensation. They may have associated dry mouth and Sjögren syndrome. The diagnosis of dry eyes is established during the slit-lamp examination for a quick breakup of the tear film or punctate corneal epithelial defect or by performing the Schirmer test. An abnormal Schirmer test occurs when there is less than 15 mm of strip wetting at 5 minutes. The dry eye syndrome may be treated with lubricants or artificial tears. Dry eye as a cause of transient visual loss is discussed in Chapter 10.

Severe pain and foreign body sensation in one eye upon awakening suggests the possibility of recurrent corneal erosion. Slit-lamp examination can confirm a corneal epithelial defect. Corneal erosion may occur on an idiopathic basis, after previous corneal abrasion, or in association with a corneal dystrophy.

Intraocular causes

Scleritis, iritis, and uveitis may be associated with severe eye pain. The pain may be referred to other regions of the face, but most often is concentrated over the eye. The eye may be exquisitely tender to palpation in this situation and photophobia is universal.

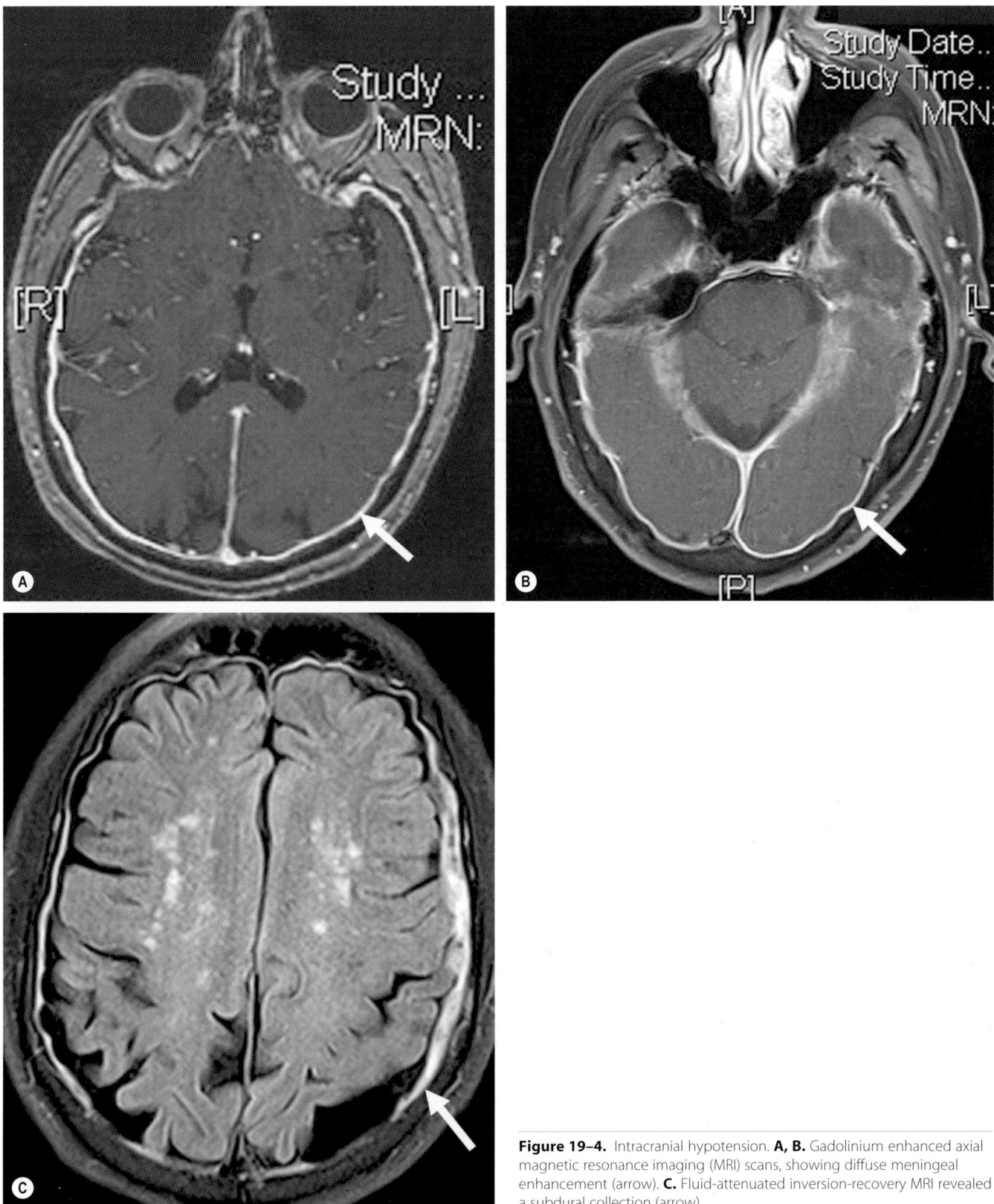

Figure 19–4. Intracranial hypotension. **A, B.** Gadolinium enhanced axial magnetic resonance imaging (MRI) scans, showing diffuse meningeal enhancement (arrow). **C.** Fluid-attenuated inversion-recovery MRI revealed a subdural collection (arrow).

Angle-closure glaucoma may be associated with variable pain, ranging from virtually none to severe. The patient's pain may be triggered by walking into a dark room or from pupillary dilation. The pain may be throbbing and associated with nausea and vomiting. As such, patients with angle-closure glaucoma may be misdiagnosed with migraine.[78] Since the patients may have associated visual loss, temporal arteritis may also be confused with angle-closure glaucoma. The patient with angle-closure glaucoma often has a red eye and a cloudy cornea during the episode. The diagnosis of

Optic nerve diseases

Nearly 90% of patients with optic neuritis have periocular pain. In fact, the absence of pain in such a situation raises the possibility of an alternative cause. The pain of optic neuritis usually occurs upon eye movements and the eye may be tender, but in some patients it manifests as a dull periocular ache. Although pain has been described with non-arteritic anterior ischemic optic neuropathy (AION),[182] alternatively arteritic AION should be strongly considered until proven otherwise. Pain on eye movement may also accompany orbital myositis or idiopathic inflammatory orbital pseudotumor.

Eye strain

Many patients attribute their headaches to eye strain. However, eye strain is a relatively uncommon cause of headaches presenting to a physician. Pain is often described as aching and is relieved by resting or not reading. The pain often begins over the brow and may spread to other scalp muscles. Often, an uncorrected hyperopic refractive error or an ocular motility problem such as convergence insufficiency is found in patients with headaches related to eye strain. Some patients will have eye strain while getting adjusted to a new pair of glasses.

Photophobia

Pain produced by a bright light is known as photophobia. The pain is transmitted to the brain stem from the ophthalmic division of the trigeminal nerve. As discussed above, migraine may be associated with photophobia both ictally and interictally. Unfortunately, some patients with migraine may have prolonged unexplained photophobia. Photophobia may also be a symptom of meningeal irritation, and such a possibility should always be carefully considered in patients with light sensitivity. A variety of ocular inflammatory disorders may also be associated with photophobia. Rarely, photophobia is a symptom of a lesion of the chiasm, retrochiasmal visual pathways, or thalamus.[183–185] However, many patients have no clear cause for their photophobia. Tinted glasses or lenses that block ultraviolet ray transmission may help relief the discomfort of photophobia.

Primary trochlear headache

Patients affected with this condition complain of pain localized to the superior nasal portion of the orbit due to inflammation in the trochlear region.[186,187] Orbital imaging should be performed to exclude an orbital mass, and systemic causes such as rheumatoid arthritis, systemic lupus erythematosus, and psoriasis should be considered. Treatment recommendations include local lidocaine injections, oral corticosteroids, and NSAIDs.

Miscellaneous

Table 19–9 outlines some other causes of headache not reviewed in the text.

Facial pain and disorders of facial sensation

Approach

Many patients with facial pain will suffer from migraine or local conditions such as sinusitis or dental disease. However, a group of patients with facial pain will have sensory or motor dysfunction within the trigeminal nerve distribution. Trigeminal nerve dysfunction commonly manifests with sensory changes such as paresthesias, dysesthesias, or anesthesia. Other patients complain of paroxysmal or chronic facial pain.

Understanding the nature of the patient's complaint is often critical in establishing a proper diagnosis. For example, the lancinating, excruciating pain of trigeminal neuralgia

Table 19–9 The differential diagnosis of other miscellaneous headache disorders and their clinical features

Entity	Onset	Location	Pain characteristics	Duration	Associated symptoms	Diagnostic evaluation
Subarachnoid hemorrhage	Acute	Global, occipital	Worst ever	Brief or prolonged	Meningismus	CT, LP
Brain tumor	Subacute	Focal	Dull pressure	Prolonged	Focal signs	Brain MRI
Painful eye movements	Acute	Retrobulbar	Sharp	Days	Optic neuritis—reduced vision / Myositis—ptosis, diplopia	Orbit MRI
Hypertension	Acute	Frontal, occipital	Throbbing	Brief	Focal signs suggest hemorrhage	Consider CT
Pseudotumor cerebri	Subacute	Bifrontal	Dull or throbbing	Prolonged	Pulsatile tinnitus, papilledema, transient visual obscuration	Neuroimaging, then LP
Meningitis	Acute or chronic	Neck	Throbbing severe	Brief or prolonged	Fever, meningismus	LP

CT, computed tomography; MRI, magnetic resonance imaging; LP, lumbar puncture.

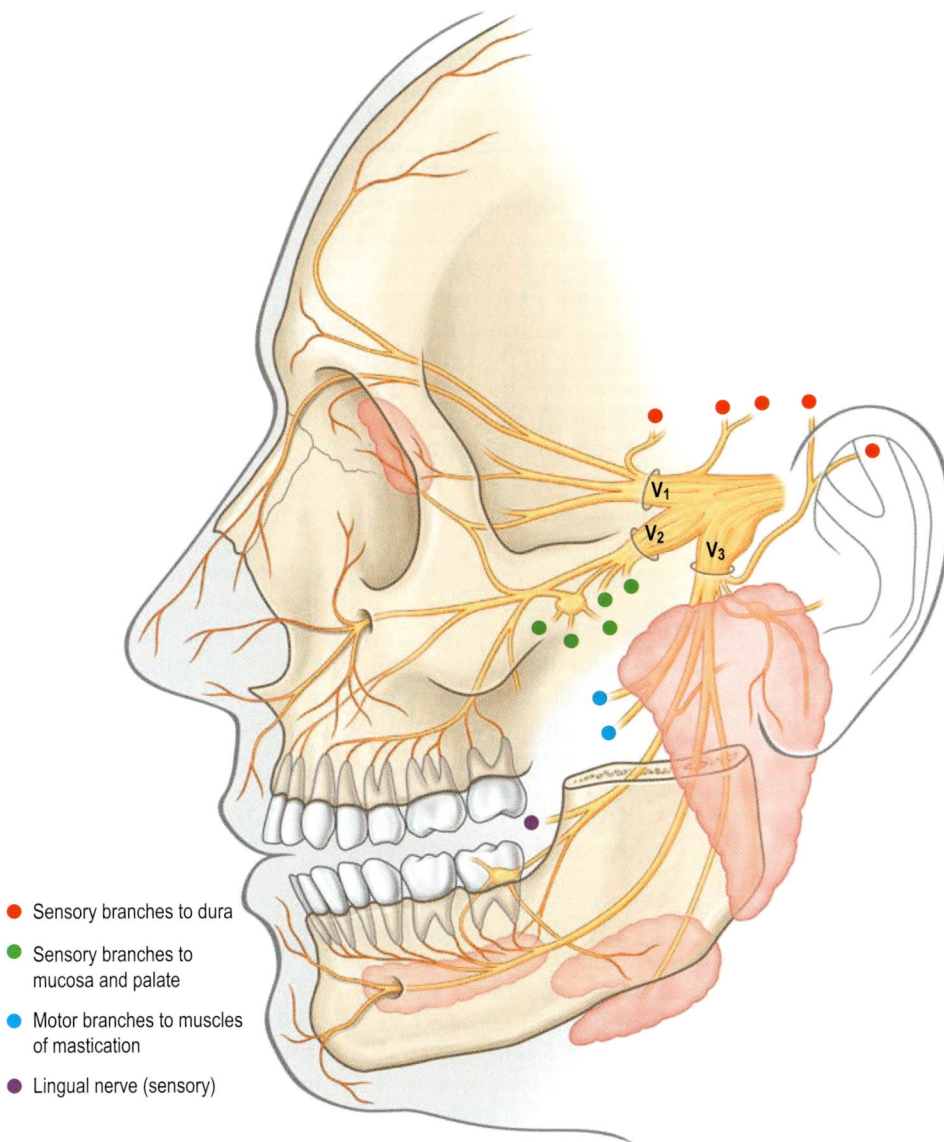

● Sensory branches to dura

● Sensory branches to mucosa and palate

● Motor branches to muscles of mastication

● Lingual nerve (sensory)

Figure 19–5. The peripheral sensory and motor branches of the trigeminal nerve.

must be distinguished from the more tolerable yet disturbing paresthesias of trigeminal sensory neuropathy. The temporal profile of symptom onset often provides invaluable diagnostic clues. For instance, sudden complaints of sensory loss, paresthesias, or motor dysfunction in the face are consistent with vascular, traumatic, or demyelinating processes, whereas similar complaints developing over weeks to months are more suggestive of neoplastic or infiltrative processes.

Neuroanatomy

The trigeminal nerve is a mixed nerve conveying both sensory input from and motor information to the face.[188] Sensory neurons of the trigeminal fibers V_1 to V_3 lie in the gasserian ganglion, which is embedded in the temporal bone within the middle cranial fossa. The dura-lined cavity in the middle cranial fossa that surrounds the gasserian ganglion and its branches as they exit into the petrous temporal bone is

known as Meckel's cave. From the gasserian ganglion, three trigeminal divisions proceed forward and exit from distinct skull-base foramina: V_1 exits the superior orbital fissure, V_2 via foramen rotundum, and V_3 via the foramen ovale (**Fig. 19–5**).

The *ophthalmic division* (V_1) is entirely sensory, and its branches innervate the orbit and the eye (lacrimal and nasociliary branches), upper eyelid, forehead and nose (frontal branches), nasal cavity, and nasal sinus (nasociliary branches) (**Fig. 19–6**). V_1 passes within the cavernous sinus, where it lies inferolateral to the oculomotor, trochlear, and abducens nerves. From the cavernous sinus, V_1 extends through the superior orbital fissure in association with the ocular motor nerves before dividing into lacrimal, frontal, and nasociliary nerves. Cutaneous fibers reach the skin via the supraorbital foramen along the ridge of the brow (**Fig. 19–6**). V_1 sensory fibers provide afferents for the corneal reflex. Smaller tentorial and dural branches innervate the tentorium and dura mater. The trigeminal system also pro-

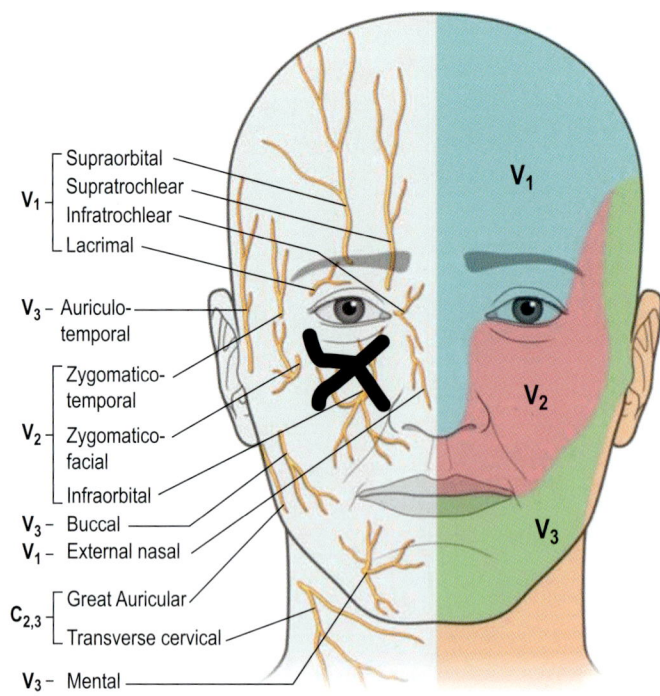

Figure 19–6. Sensory innervation of the face and scalp.

vides inputs to the intracranial vessels (trigeminovascular system) that are considered important in the pathogenesis of migraine (see earlier discussion of migraine pathophysiology). Autonomic fibers that originate from the facial nerve run with the lacrimal nerve of V_1 to innervate the lacrimal gland.

The *maxillary division* (V_2) is also completely sensory and innervates the skin of the cheek, upper lip, maxillary sinus, nasopharynx, soft and hard palate, and upper teeth. A small meningeal branch follows the middle meningeal artery and supplies dura. These fibers leave the gasserian ganglion and run inferior within the cavernous sinus before exiting the foramen rotundum. V_2 axons pass through the pterygopalatine fossa to exit the infraorbital foramen. The cutaneous branches of V_2 include the zygomaticotemporal, zygomaticofacial, and infraorbital nerves (**Fig. 19–6**). Branches innervating the nasopharynx and maxillary sinus include the greater and lesser palatine nerves, the nasopalatine nerves, and pharyngeal nerve. V_2 also supplies innervation to the upper teeth, maxillary sinus, and palate via the anterior, middle, and posterior superior alveolar nerves, respectively. Autonomic fibers that originate in the facial nerve (superior salivatory) nuclei accompany V_2 branches and make up the superficial petrosal nerve. Superficial petrosal nerve fibers synapse within the pterygopalatine ganglion and provide parasympathetic input to the lacrimal, nasal, and palatine glands. Fibers of the superficial petrosal nerve join the deep petrosal nerve to form the nerve of the pterygoid canal. The deep petrosal nerve is a branch of the internal carotid plexus and carries postganglionic sympathetic fibers from the superior cervical ganglion to the lacrimal glands.

The *mandibular division* (V_3) carries both sensory fibers from and motor axons to the lower face. V_3 axons leave the gasserian ganglion posterior to the cavernous sinus and exit the skull base via the foramen ovale. The fibers ramify

through the deep face lateral to the middle pterygoid muscles then divide into branches that provide sensation to the skin around the mandible, chin, and ear (lingual, auriculotemporal, and mental branches), mucosa around the inner cheek (buccal branch), lower teeth (inferior alveolar nerve), and dura (meningeal branch) (**Figs 19–5 and 19–6**). Parasympathetic fibers synapse within the otic and submandibular ganglia and project to the submandibular and parotid glands, respectively.

Central projections. Proximal connections of the primary sensory neurons travel within the trigeminal root before synapsing in the brain stem in three sensory subnuclei that extend from the cervical spine to the pontomesencephalic junction. These include (1) the spinal (descending) trigeminal tract and nucleus, which is organized rostrally–caudally to receive fibers responsible for pain perception on the face from the inside out in an "onion-skin" fashion; (2) the principal sensory nucleus, which governs tactile sensation on the face; and (3) the mesencephalic nucleus, which mediates proprioception for V_3-innervated muscles. Neurons from these nuclei primarily cross and head rostrally within the ventral trigeminothalmic tract before reaching the ventral posteromedial nucleus of the thalamus. From there, thalamic neurons project to the facial portion of the somatosensory cortex.

Clinical syndromes causing face pain and sensory loss

Lesions involving the proximal portion of the trigeminal system usually present no diagnostic problem as concomitant neurologic features usually help in localization. For instance, thalamic lesions usually cause facial and ipsilateral hemibody numbness together. In Wallenberg's lateral medullary syndrome, the facial anesthesia is contralateral to the hemibody sensory loss.[189] Syringobulbia (**Fig. 19–7**), which can affect the nucleus of the spinal tract in the medulla, might cause ipsilateral facial anesthesia, tongue fasciculations, and weakness and atrophy of upper extremity muscles. Cavernous sinus and superior orbital fissure disturbances (see Chapter 15) and orbital apex lesions (see Chapter 18) will be characterized by concomitant ocular motor palsies or Horner syndrome.

The rest of this section will focus on the more diagnostically challenging conditions that might present with isolated facial pain or sensory loss in the trigeminal distribution.

Isolated trigeminal neuropathy

A benign, self-limited trigeminal neuropathy may be seen 7–21 days after a nonspecific viral illness or upper respiratory infection, similar to the postinfectious cranial neuropathy affecting the abducens, facial, or hypoglossal nerves. Diagnostic evaluations are unremarkable or can demonstrate a mild CSF pleocytosis. Symptoms usually resolve within several weeks.[190] It is unclear whether these postinfectious neuropathies result from brain stem, gasserian ganglion, or peripheral nerve dysfunction.

Trigeminal sensory neuropathy may also occur in association with connective tissue disorders such as Sjögren syndrome, systemic sclerosis, and systemic lupus

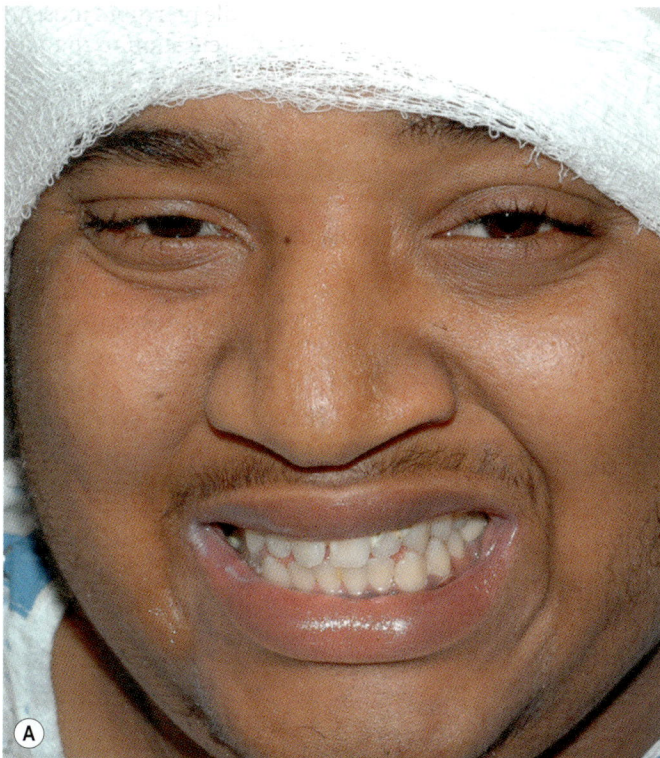

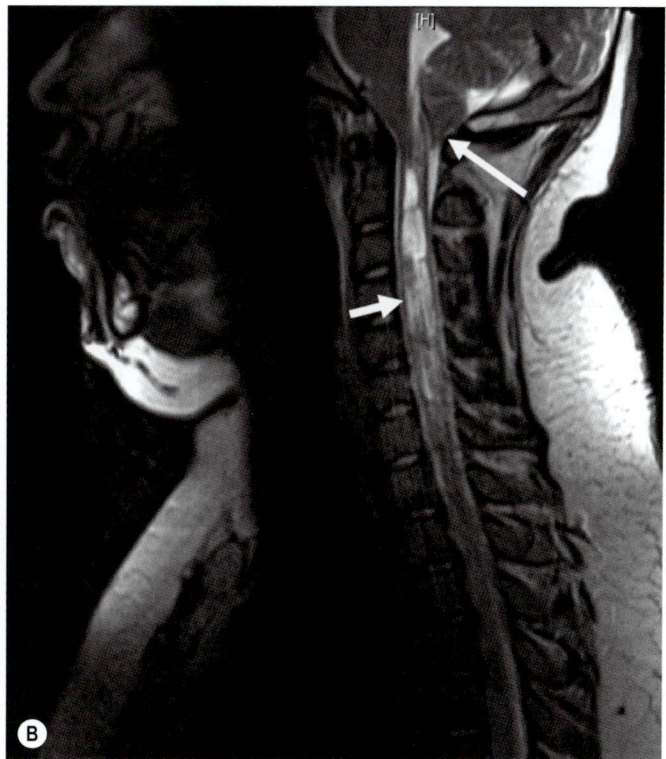

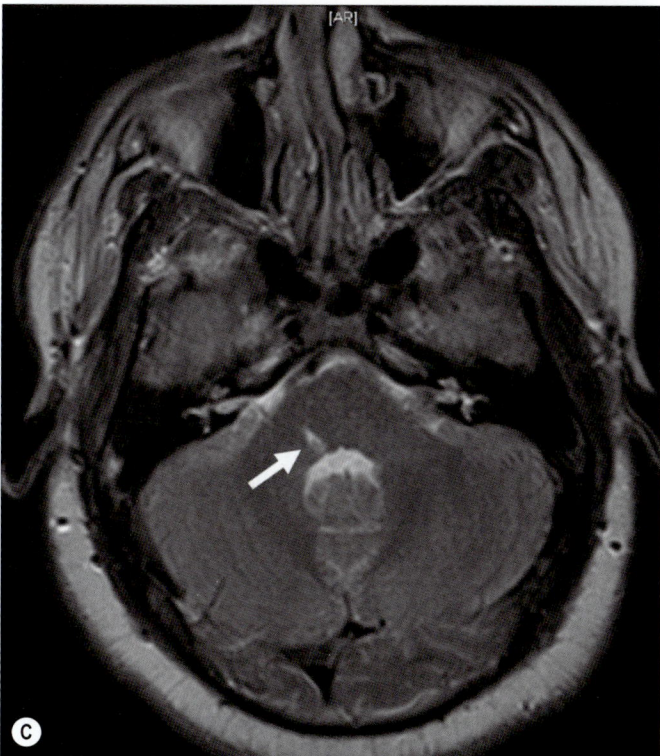

Figure 19–7. Trigeminal neuropathy due to syringomyelia. **A.** The patient had right facial numbness, right facial weakness, right Horner syndrome, and horizontal end-gaze nystagmus. **B.** Sagittal T2-weighted magnetic resonance imaging (MRI) of the cervical region revealed a multilevel cavity (short arrow) within the spinal cord, consistent with a syrinx, and a related Chiari malfomation (longer arrow). **C.** Axial T2-weighted MRI through the pons demonstrating rostral extent of the syrinx (arrow) in the region of the principle sensory nucleus of V.

erythematosus.[191] On the basis of radiographic and electrophysiologic studies, the gasserian ganglion has been suggested as the site of injury in such cases.[192] A variety of other conditions may also produce a trigeminal sensory neuropathy, such as tuberculosis, syphilis, Lyme disease, and granulomas.[193,194] Likewise, neoplasms of the middle cranial fossa, such as schwannomas and meningiomas, may produce trigeminal sensory dysfunction.[195] In young patients with facial sensory loss and lancinating pain, a central demyelinating process should be considered. Occasionally, such a symptom may be a manifestation of multiple sclerosis.[196]

Facial paresthesias in the V_1 to V_3 distributions may occur in patients with peripheral nerve disorders such as the Guillain–Barré syndrome, diabetes, hereditary sensory-motor neuropathy,[197] and chronic inflammatory demyelinating polyneuropathy. Compressive or infiltrative conditions affecting the peripheral nerve branches may also produce circumscribed sensory loss.

Numb chin syndrome (mental neuropathy)

The numb chin syndrome typically results from a bony lesion affecting the mental foramen, through which V_3 passes to innervate the chin and mandible.[198,199] Patients often complain of numbness of chin that spreads to the lower lip but respects the midline. The numb chin syndrome is an ominous sign that may be produced by a variety of mass lesions, including metastatic lung, breast, and prostate carcinoma.[200,201] Lymphoma, particularly of the non-Hodgkin's type, may also be responsible for this syndrome. Primary bony malignancies such as osteosarcoma, fibrosarcoma, and plasmacytoma are other considerations. Development of the numb chin syndrome in a patient previously treated for cancer may signal a recurrence. Nonmalignant causes include granulomatous processes, collagen vascular disorders, trauma, periodontal disease, bony cysts, focal idiopathic osteolysis (Gorham's disease), and sickle cell disease.

The numb cheek syndrome is a variant of the numb chin syndrome and results from a bony lesion involving the infraorbital foramen and the trigeminal branch V_2.[202] Patients with the numb chin or cheek syndrome require an aggressive evaluation. Careful examination of the oropharynx, dentition, and skin of the face should be performed. CT through the mandible with bone windows is the test of choice. Bone scans can occasionally be helpful when the CT scan is negative. A search for occult malignancy may be necessary to include CT of the chest and abdomen, prostate-specific antigen, and even bone marrow biopsy. Since brain stem lesions or carcinomatous meningitis may also cause focal trigeminal dysfunction, brain MRI and a lumbar puncture for cytology may be necessary.

Neurotrophic cornea (neuroparalytic keratopathy)

By mediating the sensory limb of the corneal reflex, the trigeminal nerve plays a role in protecting the cornea from foreign bodies. In addition, the trigeminal system is important for reflex tearing and maintaining the integrity and function of the cornea, particularly the epithelium.[203] Thus, trophic or degenerative corneal changes can occur when the cornea is denervated from lesions of the trigeminal nerve, ganglion, or tract. In neuro-ophthalmic settings, the cause is usually iatrogenic in the setting of surgery in or near the cerebellopontine angle or after trigeminal rhizotomy.[188] Neurotrophic corneal damage ranges from mild keratopathy to widespread damage, melting, and ulceration, which can lead to secondary infection and perforation. The condition can be difficult to manage, particularly when concomitant seventh nerve injury reduces eyelid closure. Topical artificial tears or ointments can be used in mild cases, but more severely affected patients may require tarsorrhaphy to preserve the eye.

Trigeminal neuralgia

Trigeminal neuralgia (tic douloureux) describes a brief lancinating, electric shock-like pain that occurs in the distribution of the trigeminal nerve. The pain is often triggered by chewing, speaking, or simply touching the affected area. Most cases are idiopathic with a tendency to occur in the middle-aged or elderly population. The pain typically occurs in the second and third trigeminal divisions, lasts seconds to 2 minutes, and may recur several times a day.[204] Most cases are believed to result from compression of the trigeminal nerve root by a dolichoectatic superior cerebellar artery or an adjacent venous structure. Other causes include posterior fossa mass lesions,[205] pontine demyelination in multiple sclerosis,[206] pontine infarction,[207] and dental disease. Focal demyelination of axons occurs in the area of compression or injury, and this is thought to allow ectopic generation of spontaneous impulses and ephaptic conduction to adjacent fibers.[208,209] In cases with a structural cause, one can usually detect an area of numbness in the trigeminal territory to distinguish them from idiopathic cases. Patients with multiple sclerosis also have an increased frequency of bilateral trigeminal neuralgia.[210] In patients with a new clinical diagnosis of trigeminal neuralgia, an MRI of the brain should be performed to exclude an underlying posterior fossa lesion.

Treatment. Many patients respond to carbamazepine, oxcarbazepine, phenytoin, gabapentin, pregabalin, baclofen, lamotrigine, or tricyclic antidepressants.[211-213] Sometimes trigeminal neuralgia may spontaneously remit. Acupuncture may help in others. Patients who do not respond to medical therapy may be offered trigeminal nerve root or ganglion destruction. Glycerol injection,[214] radiofrequency thermocoagulation, and balloon occlusion are percutaneous methods that can be considered.

In certain centers, microvascular decompression of the trigeminal nerve (Fig. 19–8) is the preferred surgical method because it tends to spare facial sensation and has an 80% to 90% chance of producing immediate relief.[215] Long-term outcome is also excellent as approximately 70% of patients will remain pain free 10 years later.[216] Major complications of microvascular surgery are low, but in one series included brain stem stroke (0.1%), hearing loss (1%), and abducens or trochlear nerve palsies (1%).[216]

Gamma knife radiosurgery of the trigeminal nerve is also being used in some centers.[217] Studies show excellent short-term results, with 70–80% of patients experiencing improvement or complete resolution of their pain.[218,219] The mechanism of action of radiosurgery in trigeminal neuralgia is unclear, but it may reduce ephaptic transmission.[220] Complications are low, but 5–10% of patients may experience increased facial numbness or paresthesias.[218]

In our practice, patients with trigeminal neuralgia are first offered medical therapy with a trial of at least two drugs.[221] When this fails, either gamma knife radiosurgery or microvascular decompression to healthy patients able to withstand surgery is offered.[217]

Herpes zoster ophthalmicus

Herpes zoster ophthalmicus results when the varicella zoster virus (VZV) lying dormant in the gasserian ganglion reactivates and spreads to the face along the V_1 dermatome. The infection is primarily observed in older patients, but young

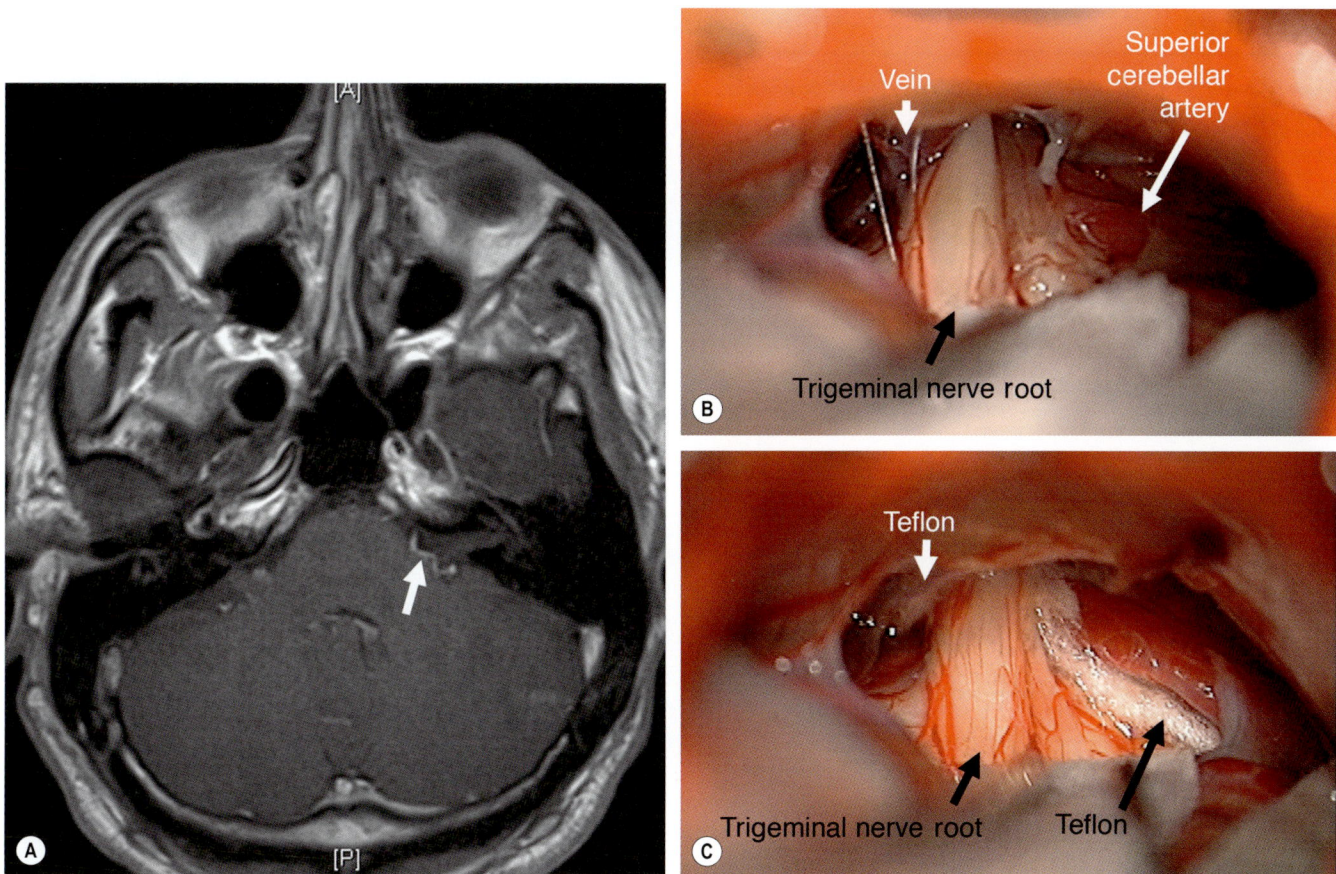

Figure 19–8. Neuroimaging and surgery in a patient with trigeminal neuralgia due to vascular compression. **A.** Axial T1-weighted magnetic resonance imaging (MRI) scan with gadolinium demonstrating a vascular loop (arrow), either the left superior cerebellar artery or a nearby vein, adjacent to the root entry zone of the left trigeminal nerve. Courtesy of Dr. Sashank Prasad. **B.** Intra-operative photographs of a microvascular decompression of the trigeminal nerve root. The trigeminal nerve root was abutted by the superior cerebellar artery and an overlying vein. A left suboccipital approach was used. **C.** Teflon was placed between the trigeminal nerve root and the artery and vein. Operative photos courtesy Dr. Eric Zager and Dr. Neil Malhotra.

patients, particularly those who are immunocompromised, may also experience this unpleasant condition. Both neuropathic pain and pain secondary to eye findings can occur. The neuralgic pain of herpes zoster ophthalmicus may begin a week before the onset of the rash. In some cases the rash never appears. The pain, which is often described as aching or burning, may be quite severe but usually resolves in several weeks. Eye involvement commonly includes keratitis and uveitis, and rarely optic neuritis and ocular motor palsies. Standard treatment for herpes zoster ophthalmicus includes oral antiviral therapy.[222] Prevention may be the best treatment, as vaccination to boost immunity to the VZV and reduce the risk of herpes zoster is recommended for patients older than 60.[223,224]

Postherpetic neuralgia. The pain of herpes zoster ophthalmicus may evolve directly into postherpetic neuralgia, but some patients have a grace period of several weeks. Postherpetic pain can be unrelenting and is often described as aching, burning, or boring in nature. In the affected dermatome, the patient may have an area of increased or decreased sensation. Postherpetic neuralgia may improve over months, or unfortunately, the pain may persist indefinitely.

Treatment of postherpetic neuralgia can be extremely difficult. It is always reasonable to give the patient a trial of antiviral therapy for either the acute infection or the postherpetic phase. Early in the infection, corticosteroids may be helpful to reduce the acute pain and possibly abort the delayed neuralgia. Anticonvulsants (gabapentin and pregabalin), tricyclic antidepressants (e.g., nortriptyline), and lidocaine patches are reasonable options reducing postherpetic neuralgia.[225] Topical capsaicin also can be tried, but the patient has to be meticulous about avoiding cream in the eye. The medication sometimes intensifies the burning pain and cannot be tolerated. Acupuncture and biofeedback are some alternative approaches that occasionally work.

Atypical facial pain

There is a group of patients who have facial pain that defies classification. The pain tends to be deep and boring. It is separated from trigeminal neuralgia by its persistent nature and its tendency not to respect a single dermatome. Many patients relate their pain to prior surgery whether it be dental, sinus, or cosmetic in nature. Again, an underlying structural lesion needs to be carefully considered.

Treatment of atypical facial pain may be difficult. A variety of measures can be taken, with variable success. Trials of anticonvulsants and antidepressant compounds may be tried. Local nerve blocks usually only provide short-term relief. Alternative treatments, such as acupuncture, occasionally benefit the refractory patient. The pain may persist for years, but some patients have a spontaneous remission.

References

1. Linet MS, Stewart WF, Celentano DD. An epidemiologic study of headache among adolescents and young adults. JAMA 1989;261:2211–2216.

2. Headache Classification Subcommittee of the International Headache Society. The International Classification of Headache Disorders, 2nd edn. Cephalalgia 2004;24(Suppl 1):9–160.

3. Lipton RB, Bigal ME, Steiner TJ, et al. Classification of primary headaches. Neurology 2004;63:427–435.

4. Lipton RB, Stewart WF, Diamond S, et al. Prevalence and burden of migraine in the United States. Data from the American Migraine Study II. Headache 2001;41:646–657.

5. Diamond S, Bigal ME, Silberstein S, et al. Patterns of diagnosis and acute and preventive treatment for migraine in the United States. Results from the American Migraine Prevalence and Prevention study. Headache 2007;47:355–363.

6. Stewart WF, Lipton RB, Simon D. Work-related disability. Results from the American migraine study. Cephalalgia 1996;16:231–238.

7. Burton WN, Landy SH, Downs KE, et al. The impact of migraine and the effect of migraine treatment on workplace productivity in the United States and suggestions for future research. Mayo Clin Proc 2009;84:436–445.

8. Lipton RB, Scher AI, Kolodner K, et al. Migraine in the United States. Epidemiology and patterns of health care use. Neurology 2002;58:885–894.

9. Bigal ME, Lipton RB. Clinical course in migraine. Conceptualizing migraine transformation. Neurology 2008;71:848–855.

10. Bigal ME, Serrano D, Buse D, et al. Acute migraine medications and evolution from episodic to chronic migraine. A longitudinal population-based study. Headache 2008;48:1157–1168.

11. Bigal ME, Serrano D, Reed M, et al. Chronic migraine in the population. Burden, diagnosis, and satisfaction with treatment. Neurology 2008;71:559–566.

12. Saunders K, Merikangas K, Low NC, et al. Impact of comorbidity on headache-related disability. Neurology 2008;70:538–547.

13. Ottman R, Lipton RB. Cormorbidity of migraine and epilepsy. Neurology 1994;44: 2105–2110.

14. Welch KMA. Relationship of stroke and migraine. Neurology 1994;44(Suppl 7): S33–S36.

15. Kruit MC, van Buchem MA, Hofman PA, et al. Migraine as a risk factor for subclinical brain lesions. JAMA 2004;291:427–434.

16. Kruit MC, Launer LJ, Ferrari MD, et al. Infarcts in the posterior circulation territory in migraine. The population-based MRI CAMERA study. Brain 2005;128:2068–2077.

17. Swartz RH, Kern RZ. Migraine is associated with magnetic resonance imaging white matter abnormalities. A meta-analysis. Arch Neurol 2004;61:1366–1368.

18. Cady RK, Farmer K, Dexter JK. Co-sensitization of pain and psychiatric comorbidity in chronic daily headache. Curr Pain Headache Rep 2005:47–52.

19. Peroutka SJ, Howell TA. The genetic evaluation of migraine. clinical database requirements. In: Rose FC (ed.) Towards Migraine 2000, pp 34–48. Amsterdam, Elsevier Science, 1996.

20. Kors E, Haan J, Ferrari M. Migraine genetics. Curr Pain Headache Rep 2003;7:212–217.

21. Joutel A, Boussermg, Biousse V, et al. A gene for familial hemiplegic migraine maps to chromosome 19. Nature Genet 1993;5:40–45.

22. Ducros A, Denier C, Joutel A, et al. The clinical spectrum of familial hemiplegic migraine associated with mutations in a neuronal calcium channel. N Engl J Med 2001;345:17–24.

23. Ophoff RA, Terwindt GM, Vergouwe MN, et al. Familial hemiplegic migraine and episodic ataxia type 2 are caused by mutation in the calcium channel gene CACNLA4. Cell 1996;87:543–552.

24. Ducros A, Joutel A, Vahedi K, et al. Mapping of a second locus for familial hemiplegic migraine to 1q21-q23 and evidence of further heterogeneity. Ann Neurol 1997;42: 885–890.

25. Gardner K, Barmada MM, Ptacek LJ, et al. A new locus for hemiplegic migraine maps to chromosome 1q31. Neurology 1997;49:1231–1238.

26. Weiller C, May A, Limmroth V, et al. Brainstem activation in spontaneous human migraine attacks. Nature Medicine 1995;1:658–660.

27. Charles A. Advances in the basic and clinical science of migraine. Ann Neurol 2009;65:491–498.

28. Olesen J, Friberg L, Olsen TS, et al. Timing and topography of cerebral blood flow, aura, and headache during migraine attacks. Ann Neurol 1990;28:791–798.

29. Leão AAP. Spreading depression of activity in the cerebral cortex. J Neurophysiol 1944;7:359–390.

30. Teive HA, Kowacs PA, Maranhao Filho P, et al. Leao's cortical spreading depression. From experimental "artifact" to physiological principle. Neurology 2005;65:1455–1459.

31. Lashley KS. Patterns of cerebral integration indicated by the scotomas of migraine. Arch Neurol Psychiatry 1941;46:331–339.

32. Cutrer FM, Sorensen AG, Weisskoff RM, et al. Perfusion-weighted imaging defects during spontaneous migrainous aura. Ann Neurol 1998;43:25–31.

33. Woods RP, Iacoboni M, Mazziotta JC. Brief report. Bilateral spreading cerebral hypoperfusion during spontaneous migraine headache. N Engl J Med 1994;331:1689–1692.

34. Bowyer SM, Aurora KS, Moran JE, et al. Magnetoencephalographic fields from patients with spontaneous and induced migraine aura. Ann Neurol 2001;50:582–587.

35. Cao Y, Welch KM, Aurora S, et al. Functional MRI-BOLD of visually triggered headache in patients with migraine. Arch Neurol 1999;56:548–554.

36. Hadjikhani N, Sanchez Del Rio M, Wu O, et al. Mechanisms of migraine aura revealed by functional MRI in human visual cortex. Proc Natl Acad Sci U S A 2001;98:4687–4692.

37. Lance JW. Current concepts of migraine pathogenesis. Neurology 1993;43(Suppl 1): S11–S15.

38. Welch KM, Cao Y, Aurora S, et al. MRI of the occipital cortex, red nucleus, and substantia nigra during visual aura of migraine. Neurology 1998;51:1465–1469.

39. Cao Y, Aurora SK, Nagesh V, et al. Functional MRI-BOLD of brainstem structures during visually triggered migraine. Neurology 2002;59:72–74.

40. Spierings EL. The aura-headache connection in migraine. A historical analysis. Arch Neurol 2004;61:794–799.

41. Welch KM. Contemporary concepts of migraine pathogenesis. Neurology 2003;61:S2–8.

42. Rogawski MA. Common pathophysiologic mechanisms in migraine and epilepsy. Arch Neurol 2008;65:709–714.

43. Burstein R, Cutrer MF, Yarnitsky D. The development of cutaneous allodynia during a migraine attack clinical evidence for the sequential recruitment of spinal and supraspinal nociceptive neurons in migraine. Brain 2000;123:1703–1709.

44. Burstein R, Collins B, Jakubowski M. Defeating migraine pain with triptans. A race against the development of cutaneous allodynia. Ann Neurol 2004;55:19–26.

45. Mathew NT, Kailasam J, Seifert T. Clinical recognition of allodynia in migraine. Neurology 2004;63:848–852.

46. Lipton RB, Bigal ME, Ashina S, et al. Cutaneous allodynia in the migraine population. Ann Neurol 2008;63:148–158.

47. Lipton RB, Pan J. Is migraine a progressive brain disease? JAMA 2004;291:493–494.

48. Goadsby PJ, Lipton RB, Ferrari MD. Migraine—current understanding and treatment. N Engl J Med 2002;346:257–270.

49. Liu GT, Schatz NJ, Galetta SL, et al. Persistent positive visual phenomena in migraine. Neurology 1995;45:664–668.

50. Wray SH, Mijovic-Prelec D, Kosslyn SM. Visual processing in migraineurs. Brain 1995;118:25–35.

51. Harle DE, Evans BJ. The optometric correlates of migraine. Ophthalmic Physiol Opt 2004;24:369–383.

52. Shepherd AJ. Local and global motion after-effects are both enhanced in migraine, and the underlying mechanisms differ across cortical areas. Brain 2006;129:1833–1843.

53. Guerraz M, Yardley L, Bertholon P, et al. Visual vertigo. Symptom assessment, spatial orientation and postural control. Brain 2001;124:1646–1656.

54. Kowacs PA, Piovesan EJ, Werneck LC, et al. Headache related to a specific screen flickering frequency band. Cephalalgia 2004;24:408–410.

55. Harle DE, Shepherd AJ, Evans BJ. Visual stimuli are common triggers of migraine and are associated with pattern glare. Headache 2006;46:1431–1440.

56. Kowacs PA, Piovesan EJ, Werneck LC, et al. Influence of intense light stimulation on trigeminal and cervical pain perception thresholds. Cephalalgia 2001;21:184–188.

57. Drummond P. Photophobia and autonomic responses to facial pain in migraine. Brain 1997;120:1857–1864.

58. Mulleners WM, Chronicle EP, Palmer JE, et al. Visual cortex excitability in migraine with and without aura. Headache 2001;41:565–572.

59. Battelli L, Black KR, Wray SH. Transcranial magnetic stimulation of visual area V5 in migraine. Neurology 2002;58:1066–1069.

60. Mulleners WM, Chronicle EP, Palmer JE, et al. Suppression of perception in migraine. Evidence for reduced inhibition in the visual cortex. Neurology 2001;56:178–183.

61. Shepherd AJ. Visual contrast processing in migraine. Cephalalgia 2000;20:865–880.

62. McKendrick AM, Vingrys AJ, Badcock DR, et al. Visual dysfunction between migraine events. Invest Ophthalmol Vis Sci 2001;42:626–633.

63. McKendrick AM, Cioffi GA, Johnson CA. Short-wavelength sensitivity deficits in patients with migraine. Arch Ophthalmol 2002;120:154–161.

64. McKendrick AM, Badcock DR. Contrast-processing dysfunction in both magnocellular and parvocellular pathways in migraineurs with or without aura. Invest Ophthalmol Vis Sci 2003;44:442–448.

65. McKendrick AM, Badcock DR. An analysis of the factors associated with visual field deficits measured with flickering stimuli in-between migraine. Cephalalgia 2004;24: 389–397.

66. McKendrick AM, Badcock DR. Decreased visual field sensitivity measured 1 day, then 1 week, after migraine. Invest Ophthalmol Vis Sci 2004;45:1061–1070.

67. Shepherd AJ. Colour vision in migraine. Selective deficits for S-cone discriminations. Cephalalgia 2005;25:412–423.

68. Oelkers R, Grosser K, Lang E, et al. Visual evoked potentials in migraine patients. Alterations depend on pattern spatial frequency. Brain 1999;122:1147–1155.

69. Shibata K, Yamane K, Otuka K, et al. Abnormal visual processing in migraine with aura. A study of steady-state visual evoked potentials. J Neurol Sci 2008;271:119–126.

70. Hupp SL, Kline LB, Corbett JJ. Visual disturbances of migraine. Surv Ophthalmol 1989;33:221–236.

71. Hill DL, Daroff RB, Ducros A, et al. Most cases labeled as "retinal migraine" are not migraine. J Neuro-Ophthalmol 2007;27:3–8.

72. Burger SK, Saul RF, Selhorst JB, et al. Transient monocular blindness caused by vasospasm. N Engl J Med 1991;12:870–873.

73. Tomsak RL, Jergens PB. Benign recurrent transient monocular blindness. A possible variant of acephalgic migraine. Headache 1987;27:66–69.

74. Lewis RA, Vijayan N, Watson C, et al. Visual field loss in migraine. Ophthalmology 1989;96:321–326.

75. Winterkorn JMS, Kupersmith MJ, Wirtschafter JD, et al. Treatment of vasospastic amaurosis fugax with calcium channel blockers. N Engl J Med 1993;329:396–398.

76. Bharucha DX, Campbell TB, Valencia I, et al. MRI findings in pediatric ophthalmoplegic migraine: a case report and literature review. Pediatr Neurol 2007;37:59–63.

77. Carlow TJ. Oculomotor ophthalmoplegic migraine. Is it really migraine? J Neuroophthalmol 2002;22:215–221.

78. Shindler KS, Sankar PS, Volpe NJ, et al. Intermittent headaches as the presenting sign of subacute angle-closure glaucoma. Neurology 2005;65:757–758.
79. Bickerstaff ER. Basilar artery migraine. Lancet 1961;1:15–17.
80. Kirchmann M, Thomsen LL, Olesen J. Basilar-type migraine. Clinical, epidemiologic, and genetic features. Neurology 2006;66:880–886.
81. Troost BT. Migraine and other headaches. In: Glaser JS (ed). Neuro-ophthalmology, 2nd edn, pp 487–518. Philadelphia, J.B. Lippincott, 1990.
82. Neuhauser H, Leopold M, von Brevern M, et al. The interrelations of migraine, vertigo, and migrainous vertigo. Neurology 2001;56:436–441.
83. Dieterich M, Brandt T. Episodic vertigo related to migraine (90 cases). Vestibular migraine? J Neurol 1999;246:883–892.
84. Cutrer FM, Baloh RW. Migraine-associated dizziness. Headache 1992;32:300–304.
85. Johnson GD. Medical management of migraine-related dizziness and vertigo. Laryngoscope 1998;108(Jan. suppl):1–28.
86. von Brevern M, Radtke A, Clarke AH, et al. Migrainous vertigo presenting as episodic positional vertigo. Neurology 2004;62:469–472.
87. von Brevern M, Zeise D, Neuhauser H, et al. Acute migrainous vertigo. Clinical and oculographic findings. Brain 2005;128:365–374.
88. Oh SY, Seo MW, Kim YH, et al. Gaze-evoked and rebound nystagmus in a case of migrainous vertigo. J Neuroophthalmol 2009;29:26–28.
89. Baloh RW. Neurotology of migraine. Headache 1997;37:615–621.
90. Kurth T, Gaziano JM, Cook NR, et al. Migraine and risk of cardiovascular disease in women. JAMA 2006;296:283–291.
91. Tzourio C, Tehindrazanarivielo A, Iglesias S, et al. Case control study of migraine and risk of ischaemia stroke in young women. Br Med J 1995;310:830–833.
92. Carolei A, Marini C, De Matteis G. History of migraine and risk of cerebral ischaemia in young adults. The Italian National Research Council Study Group on stroke in the young. Lancet 1996;347:1503–1506.
93. Pettiti DB, Sidney S, Bernstein A. Stroke in users of low dose oral contraceptives. N Eng J Med 1996;335:8–15.
94. Chang CL, Donaghy M, Poulter N, et al. Migraine and stroke in young women. Case-control study. BMJ 1999;318:13–18.
95. Kurth T, Slomke MA, Kase CS, et al. Migraine, headache, and the risk of stroke in women. A prospective study. Neurology 2005;64:1020–1026.
96. Lipton RB, Stewart WF, Ryan RE, Jr., et al. Efficacy and safety of acetaminophen, aspirin, and caffeine in alleviating migraine headache pain. Three double-blind, randomized, placebo-controlled trials. Arch Neurol 1998;55:210–217.
97. Maizels M, Scott B, Cohen W, et al. Intranasal lidocaine for treatment of migraine. A randomized, double-blind, controlled trial. JAMA 1996;276:319–321.
98. Winner P, Mannix LK, Putnam DG, et al. Pain-free results with sumatriptan taken at the first sign of migraine pain: 2 randomized, double-blind, placebo-controlled studies. Mayo Clin Proc 2003;78:1214–1222.
99. Cady R, Elkind A, Goldstein J, et al. Randomized, placebo-controlled comparison of early use of frovatriptan in a migraine attack versus dosing after the headache has become moderate or severe. Curr Med Res Opin 2004;20:1465–1472.
100. Brandes JL, Kudrow D, Cady R, et al. Eletriptan in the early treatment of acute migraine. Influence of pain intensity and time of dosing. Cephalalgia 2005;25:735–742.
101. Mathew NT, Loder EW. Evaluating the triptans. Am J Med 2005;118(Suppl 1):28S–35S.
102. Ferrari MD, Roon KI, Lipton RB, et al. Oral triptans (serotonin 5-HT(1B/1D) agonists) in acute migraine treatment. A meta-analysis of 53 trials. Lancet 2001;358:1668–1675.
103. Winner P, Cady RK, Ruoff GE, et al. Twelve-month tolerability and safety of sumatriptan-naproxen sodium for the treatment of acute migraine. Mayo Clin Proc 2007;82:61–68.
104. Brandes JL, Kudrow D, Stark SR, et al. Sumatriptan-naproxen for acute treatment of migraine. A randomized trial. JAMA 2007;297:1443–1454.
105. Silberstein SD, Mannix LK, Goldstein J, et al. Multimechanistic (sumatriptan-naproxen) early intervention for the acute treatment of migraine. Neurology 2008;71:114–121.
106. Géraud G, Keywood C, Senard JM. Migraine headache recurrence. Relationship to clinical, pharmacological, and pharmacokinetic properties of triptans. Headache 2003;43:376–388.
107. Hamalainen ML, Hoppu K, Santavuori P. Sumatriptan for migraine attacks in children. A randomized placebo-controlled study. Do children with migraine respond to oral sumatriptan differently from adults? Neurology 1997;48:1100–1103.
108. Lewis D, Ashwal S, Hershey A, et al. Practice parameter. Pharmacological treatment of migraine headache in children and adolescents. Report of the American Academy of Neurology Quality Standards Subcommittee and the Practice Committee of the Child Neurology Society. Neurology 2004;63:2215–2224.
109. Ueberall MA, Wenzel D. Intranasal sumatriptan for the acute treatment of migraine in children. Neurology 1999;52:1507–1510.
110. Lewis DW, Winner P, Hershey AD, et al. Efficacy of zolmitriptan nasal spray in adolescent migraine. Pediatrics 2007;120:390–396.
111. Hall GC, Brown MM, Mo J, et al. Triptans in migraine. The risks of stroke, cardiovascular disease, and death in practice. Neurology 2004;62:563–568.
112. Lewis PJ, Barrington SF, Marsden PK, et al. A study of the effects of sumatriptan on myocardial perfusion in healthy female migraineurs using 13NH3 positron emission tomography. Neurology 1997;48:1542–1550.
113. MaassenVanDenBrink A, Reekers M, Bax WA, et al. Coronary side-effect potential of current and prospective antimigraine drugs. Circulation 1998;98:25–30.
114. Silberstein SD, Young WB, Mendizabal JE, et al. Acute migraine treatment with droperidol. A randomized, double-blind, placebo-controlled trial. Neurology 2003;60:315–321.
115. Ho TW, Mannix LK, Fan X, et al. Randomized controlled trial of an oral CGRP receptor antagonist, MK-0974, in acute treatment of migraine. Neurology 2008;70:1304–1312.
116. Wang SJ, Silberstein SD, Young WB. Droperidol treatment of status migrainosus and refractory migraine. Headache 1997;37:377–382.
117. Friedman BW, Greenwald P, Bania TC, et al. Randomized trial of IV dexamethasone for acute migraine in the emergency department. Neurology 2007;69:2038–2044.
118. Diamond S, Kudrow L, Stevens J, et al. Long term study of propranolol in the treatment of migraine. Headache 1982;22:268–271.
119. Jonsdottir M, Meyer JS, Rogers RL. Efficacy, side effects and tolerance compared during headache treatment with three different calcium blockers. Headache 1987;27:364–369.
120. Cohen AS, Matharu MS, Goadsby PJ. Electrocardiographic abnormalities in patients with cluster headache on verapamil therapy. Neurology 2007;69:668–675.
121. Cutrer FM. Antiepileptic drugs. How they work in headache. Headache 2001;41(Suppl 1):S3–10.
122. Mathew NT. Antiepileptic drugs in migraine prevention. Headache 2001;41(Suppl 1):S18–24.
123. Silberstein SD, Neto W, Schmitt J, et al. Topiramate in migraine prevention. Results of a large controlled trial. Arch Neurol 2004;61:490–495.
124. Brandes JL. Practical use of topiramate for migraine prevention. Headache 2005;45(Suppl 1):S66–73.
125. Mathew N. Gabapentin in migraine prophylaxis. Cephalalgia 1996;16:397.
126. Schoenen J, Jacquy J, Lenaerts M. Effectiveness of high-dose riboflavin in migraine prophylaxis. A randomized controlled trial. Neurology 1998;50:466–469.
127. Pfaffenrath V, Wessely P, Meyer C, et al. Magnesium in the prophylaxis of migraine. A double blind placebo controlled study. Cephalalgia 1996;16:436–440.
128. Sándor PS, Di Clemente L, Coppola G, et al. Efficacy of coenzyme Q10 in migraine prophylaxis. A randomized controlled trial. Neurology 2005;64:713–715.
129. Lipton RB, Gobel H, Einhaupl KM, et al. Petasites hybridus root (butterbur) is an effective preventive treatment for migraine. Neurology 2004;63:2240–2244.
130. Evers S, Vollmer-Haase J, Schwaag S, et al. Botulinum toxin A in the prophylactic treatment of migraine–a randomized, double-blind, placebo-controlled study. Cephalalgia 2004;24:838–843.
131. Naumann M, So Y, Argoff CE, et al. Assessment: Botulinum neurotoxin in the treatment of autonomic disorders and pain (an evidence-based review): report of the Therapeutics and Technology Assessment Subcommittee of the American Academy of Neurology. Neurology 2008;70:1707–1714.
132. Loder E. Prophylaxis of menstrual migraine with triptans. Problems and possibilities. Neurology 2002;59:1677–1681.
133. Silberstein SD, Elkind AH, Schreiber C, et al. A randomized trial of frovatriptan for the intermittent prevention of menstrual migraine. Neurology 2004;63:261–269.
134. Pringsheim T, Davenport WJ, Dodick D. Acute treatment and prevention of menstrually related migraine headache: evidence-based review. Neurology 2008;70:1555–1563.
135. Newman LC, Lipton RB, Lay CL, et al. A pilot study of oral sumatriptan as intermittent prophylaxis of menstruation-related migraine. Neurology 1998;51:307–308.
136. Boyle CA. Management of menstrual migraine. Neurology 1999;53(Suppl 1):S14–18.
137. Silberstein SD. Practice parameter: evidence-based guidelines for migraine headache (an evidence-based review). Report of the Quality Standards Subcommittee of the American Academy of Neurology. Neurology 2000;55:754–762.
138. Linde K, Streng A, Jurgens S, et al. Acupuncture for patients with migraine. A randomized controlled trial. JAMA 2005;293:2118–2125.
139. Schwerzmann M, Wiher S, Nedeltchev K, et al. Percutaneous closure of patent foramen ovale reduces the frequency of migraine attacks. Neurology 2004;62:1399–1401.
140. Post MC, Thijs V, Herroelen L, et al. Closure of a patent foramen ovale is associated with a decrease in prevalence of migraine. Neurology 2004;62:1439–1440.
141. Ashkenazi A, Silberstein S. Botulinum toxin type A for the treatment of headache. Why we say yes. Arch Neurol 2008;65:146–149.
142. Limmroth V, Katsarava Z, Fritsche G, et al. Features of medication overuse headache following overuse of different acute headache drugs. Neurology 2002;59:1011–1014.
143. Bahra A, May A, Goadsby PJ. Cluster headache. A prospective clinical study with diagnostic implications. Neurology 2002;58:354–361.
144. Silberstein SD, Niknam R, Rozen TD, et al. Cluster headache with aura. Neurology 2000;54:219–221.
145. Mani S, Deeter J. Arteriovenous malformation of the brain presenting as a cluster headache—a case report. Headache 1982;22:184–185.
146. Kuritzky A. Cluster headache-like pain caused by an upper cervical meningioma. Cephalalgia 1984;4:185–186.
147. West P, Todman D. Chronic cluster associated with a vertebral artery aneurysm. Headache 1991;31:210–212.
148. Koenigsberg AD, Solomon GD, Kosmorsky GO. Pseudoaneurysm within the cavernous sinus presenting as cluster headache. Headache 1994;34:111–113.
149. Lee MS, Lessell S. Orbital myositis posing as cluster headache. Arch Neurol 2002;59: 635–636.
150. Favier I, van Vliet JA, Roon KI, et al. Trigeminal autonomic cephalgias due to structural lesions: a review of 31 cases. Arch Neurol 2007;64:25–31.
151. Leone M, D'Amico D, Frediani F, et al. Verapamil in the prophylaxis of episodic cluster headache: a double-blind study versus placebo. Neurology 2000;54:1382–1385.
152. Mathew NT, Hurt W. Percutaneous radiofrequency trigeminal gangliorhizolysis in intractable cluster headache. Headache 1988;28:328–331.
153. Jarrar RG, Black DF, Dodick DW, et al. Outcome of trigeminal nerve section in the treatment of chronic cluster headache. Neurology 2003;60:1360–1362.
154. Matharu MS, Goadsby PJ. Persistence of attacks of cluster headache after trigeminal nerve root section. Brain 2002;125:976–984.
155. Magis D, Allena M, Bolla M, et al. Occipital nerve stimulation for drug-resistant chronic cluster headache: a prospective pilot study. Lancet Neurol 2007;6:314–321.
156. Burns B, Watkins L, Goadsby PJ. Treatment of intractable chronic cluster headache by occipital nerve stimulation in 14 patients. Neurology 2009;72:341–345.
157. Goadsby PJ, Lipton RB. A review of paroxysmal hemicranias, SUNCT syndrome and other short lasting headaches with autonomic feature, including new cases. Brain 1997;120:193–209.

158. Cittadini E, Matharu MS, Goadsby PJ. Paroxysmal hemicrania: a prospective clinical study of 31 cases. Brain 2008;131:1142–1155.

159. Peres MF, Silberstein SD, Nahmias S, et al. Hemicrania continua is not that rare. Neurology 2001;57:948–951.

160. Silberstein SD, Peres MF. Hemicrania continua. Arch Neurol 2002;59:1029–1030.

161. Klein JP, Kostina-O'Neil Y, Lesser RL. Neuro-ophthalmologic presentations of hemicrania continua. Am J Ophthalmol 2006;141:88–92.

162. Cohen AS, Matharu MS, Goadsby PJ. Short-lasting unilateral neuralgiform headache attacks with conjunctival injection and tearing (SUNCT) or cranial autonomic features (SUNA)–a prospective clinical study of SUNCT and SUNA. Brain 2006;129:2746–2760.

163. D'Andrea G, Granella F, Ghiotto N, et al. Lamotrigine in the treatment of SUNCT syndrome. Neurology 2001;57:1723–1725.

164. Matharu MS, Boes CJ, Goadsby PJ. SUNCT syndrome: prolonged attacks, refractoriness and response to topiramate. Neurology 2002;58:1307.

165. Rozen TD. Resolution of SUNCT after removal of a pituitary adenoma in mild acromegaly. Neurology 2006;67:724.

166. Blättler T, Capone Mori A, Boltshauser E, et al. Symptomatic SUNCT in an eleven-year-old girl. Neurology 2003;60:2012–2013.

167. Raps EC, Rogers JD, Galetta SL, et al. The clinical spectrum of unruptured intracranial aneurysms. Arch Neurol 1993;50:265–268.

168. Gould JD, Silberstein SD. Unilateral hypnic headache. A case study. Neurology 1997;49:1749–1751.

169. Brass SD, Durand ML, Stone JH, et al. Case records of the Massachusetts General Hospital. Case 36-2008. A 59-year-old man with chronic daily headache. N Engl J Med 2008;359:2267–2278.

170. Chung SJ, Kim JS, Lee MC. Syndrome of cerebral spinal fluid hypovolemia. Clinical and imaging features and outcome. Neurology 2000;55:1321–1327.

171. Miyazawa K, Shiga Y, Hasegawa T, et al. CSF hypovolemia vs intracranial hypotension in "spontaneous intracranial hypotension syndrome". Neurology 2003;60:941–947.

172. Rando TA, Fishman RA. Spontaneous intracranial hypotension. Report of two cases and review of literature. Neurology 1992;42:481–487.

173. Horton JC, Fishman RA. Neurovisual findings in the syndrome of spontaneous intracranial hyptension from dural cerebrospinal fluid leak. Ophthalmology 1994;101:244–251.

174. Pannullo SC, Reich JB, Krol G, et al. MRI changes in intracranial hypotension. Neurology 1993;43:919–926.

175. Krause I, Kornreich L, Waldman D, et al. MRI meningeal enhancement with intracranial hypotension caused by lumbar puncture. Pediatr Neurol 1997;16:163–165.

176. Mokri B. Spontaneous cerebrospinal fluid leaks. From intracranial hypotension to cerebrospinal fluid hypovolemia–evolution of a concept. Mayo Clinic Proc 1999;74:1113–1123.

177. Kosmorsky G. Spontaneous intracranial hypotension. A review. J Neuroophthalmol 1995;15:79–83.

178. Hochman MS, Naidich TP. Diffuse meningeal enhancement in patients with overdraining, long-standing ventricular shunts. Neurology 1999;52:406–409.

179. Schievink WI, Louy C. Precipitating factors of spontaneous spinal CSF leaks and intracranial hypotension. Neurology 2007;69:700–702.

180. Sencakova D, Mokri B, McClelland RL. The efficacy of epidural blood patch in spontaneous CSF leaks. Neurology 2001;57:1921–1923.

181. Berroir S, Loisel B, Ducros A, et al. Early epidural blood patch in spontaneous intracranial hypotension. Neurology 2004;63:1950–1951.

182. Swartz NG, Beck RW, Savino PJ, et al. Pain in anterior ischemic optic neuropathy. J Neuroophthalmol 1995;15:9–10.

183. Du Pasquier RA, Genoud D, Safran AB, et al. Monocular central dazzle after thalamic infarcts. J Neuroophthalmol 2000;20:97–99.

184. Kawasaki A, Purvin VA. Photophobia as the presenting visual symptom of chiasmal compression. J Neuroophthalmol 2002;22:3–8.

185. Kawasaki A, Borruat FX. Photophobia associated with a demyelinating lesion of the retrochiasmal visual pathway. Am J Ophthalmol 2006;142:854–856.

186. Yangüela J, Pareja JA, Lopez N, et al. Trochleitis and migraine headache. Neurology 2002;58:802–805.

187. Yangüela J, Sanchez-del-Rio M, Bueno A, et al. Primary trochlear headache. A new cephalgia generated and modulated on the trochlear region. Neurology 2004;62:1134–1140.

188. Liu GT. The trigeminal nerve and its central connections. In: Miller NR, Newman NJ, Biousse V, Kerrison JB (eds) Walsh and Hoyt's Clinical Neuro-ophthalmology, 6th edn, pp 1233–1274. Baltimore, Williams and Wilkins, 2005.

189. Kim JS. Pure lateral medullary infarction: clinical-radiological correlation of 130 acute, consecutive patients. Brain 2003;126:1864–1872.

190. Matoth I, Taustein I, Shapira Y. Idiopathic trigeminal sensory neuropathy in childhood. J Child Neurol 2001;16:623–625.

191. Lecky BRF, Hughes RAC, Murray NMF. Trigeminal sensory neuropathy. A study of 22 cases. Brain 1987;110:1463–1485.

192. Forster C, Brandt T, Hund E, et al. Trigeminal sensory neuropathy in connective tissue disease; evidence for the site of the lesion. Neurology 1996;46:270–271.

193. Arias M, Iglesisas A, Vila O, et al. MR imaging findings of neurosarcoidosis of the gasserian ganglion. An unusual presentation. Eur Radiol 2002;12:2723–2725.

194. Ahn JY, Kwon SO, Shin MS, et al. Chronic granulomatous neuritis in idiopathic trigeminal sensory neuropathy. Report of two cases. J Neurosurg 2002;96:585–588.

195. Al-Mefty O, Ayoubi S, Gaber E. Trigeminal schwannomas. Removal of dumbbell-shaped tumors through the expanded Meckel cave and outcomes of cranial nerve function. J Neurosurg 2002;96:453–463.

196. Nakashima I, Fujihara K, Kimpara T, et al. Linear pontine trigeminal root lesions in multiple sclerosis. Clinical and magnetic resonance imaging studies in 5 cases. Arch Neurol 2001;58:101–104.

197. Coffey RJ, Fromm GH. Familial trigeminal neuralgia and Charcot-Marie-Tooth neuropathy. Report of two families and review. Surg Neurol 1991;35:49–53.

198. Massey EW, Moore J, Schold SC. Mental neuropathy. Neurology 1981;31:1277–1281.

199. Brazis PW, Vogler JB, Shaw KE. The "numb cheek-lip lower lid" syndrome. Neurology 1991;41:327–328.

200. Lossos A, Siegal T. Numb chin syndrome in cancer patients. Etiology, response to treatment, and prognostic significance. Neurology 1992;42:1181–1184.

201. Laurencet FM, Anchisi S, Tullen E, et al. Mental neuropathy. Report of five cases and review of the literature. Crit Rev Oncol/Hematol 2000;34:71–79.

202. Campbell WW. The numb cheek syndrome. A sign of infraorbital neuropathy. Neurology 1986;36:421–423.

203. Bonini S, Rama P, Olzi D, et al. Neurotrophic keratitis. Eye 2003;17:989–995.

204. Bennetto L, Patel NK, Fuller G. Trigeminal neuralgia and its management. BMJ 2007;334:201–205.

205. Cheng TMW, Cascino TL, Onofrio BM. Comprehensive study of diagnosis and treatment of trigeminal neuralgia secondary to tumors. Neurology 1993;43:2298–2302.

206. Gass A, Kitchen N, MacManus DG, et al. Trigeminal neuralgia in patients with multiple sclerosis. Lesion localization with magnetic resonance imaging. Neurology 1997;49:1142–1144.

207. Iizuka O, Hosokai Y, Mori E. Trigeminal neuralgia due to pontine infarction. Neurology 2006;66:48.

208. Love S, Coakham HB. Trigeminal neuralgia. Pathology and pathogenesis. Brain 2001;124:2347–2360.

209. Devor M, Govrin-Lippmann R, Rappaport ZH. Mechanism of trigeminal neuralgia. An ultrastructural analysis of trigeminal root specimens obtained during microvascular decompression surgery. J Neurosurg 2002;96:532–543.

210. Hooge JP, Redekop WK. Trigeminal neuralgia in multiple sclerosis. Neurology 1995;45:1294–1296.

211. Sist T, Filadora V, Miner M, et al. Gabapentin for idiopathic trigeminal neuralgia. Report of two cases. Neurology 1997;48:1467–1471.

212. Jorns TP, Zakrzewska JM. Evidence-based approach to the medical management of trigeminal neuralgia. Br J Neurosurg 2007;21:253–261.

213. Gronseth G, Cruccu G, Alksne J, et al. Practice parameter. The diagnostic evaluation and treatment of trigeminal neuralgia (an evidence-based review). Report of the Quality Standards Subcommittee of the American Academy of Neurology and the European Federation of Neurological Societies. Neurology 2008;71:1183–1190.

214. Cappabianca P, Spaziante R, Graziussi G, et al. Percutaneous retrogasserian glycerol rhizolysis for treatment of trigeminal neuralgia. Technique and results in 191 patients. J Neurosci 1995;39:37–45.

215. Walchenbach R, Voormolen JHC. Surgical treatment for trigeminal neuralgia. We must have a direct, randomized comparison between decompression and thermocoagulation. Br Med J 1996;313:1027–1028.

216. Barker FG, Jannetta PJ, Bissonette DJ, et al. The long-term outcome of microvascular decompression for trigeminal neuralgia. N Engl J Med 1996;334:1077–1083.

217. Gorgulho AA, De Salles AA. Impact of radiosurgery on the surgical treatment of trigeminal neuralgia. Surg Neurol 2006;66:350–356.

218. Kondziolka D, Perez B, Flickinger JC, et al. Gamma knife radiosurgery for trigeminal neuralgia. Results and expectations. Arch Neurol 1998;55:1524–1529.

219. Young RF, Vermeulen SS, Grimm P, et al. Gamma knife radiosurgery for treatment of trigeminal neuralgia. Idiopathic and tumor related. Neurology 1997;48:608–614.

220. Tenser RB. Trigeminal neuralgia. Mechanisms of treatment. Neurology 1998;51:17–19.

221. Prasad S, Galetta S. Trigeminal neuralgia. Historical notes and current concepts. Neurologist 2009;15:87–94.

222. Opstelten W, Zaal MJ. Managing ophthalmic herpes zoster in primary care. BMJ 2005;331:147–151.

223. Liesegang TJ. Herpes zoster ophthalmicus natural history, risk factors, clinical presentation, and morbidity. Ophthalmology 2008;115:S3–12.

224. Sampathkumar P, Drage LA, Martin DP. Herpes zoster (shingles) and postherpetic neuralgia. Mayo Clin Proc 2009;84:274–280.

225. Dubinsky RM, Kabbani H, El-Chami Z, et al. Practice parameter. Treatment of postherpetic neuralgia. An evidence-based report of the Quality Standards Subcommittee of the American Academy of Neurology. Neurology 2004;63:959–965.

Index

Page numbers followed by *f* indicates figures; *t* indicates tables; *b* indicates boxes

tuberculum sellae meningiomas 267
tuberous sclerosis 34, 87–91, 91f–93f
Tullio phenomenon 595
"Tumbling Es" test 8–10, 10f
tumefactive multiple sclerosis 323–324
tumor necrosis 69
tumor necrosis factor-α-inhibitors 181
tumors
   see also neoplasms
   brain, in childhood disorders 212
   granular cell 279
   intracranial, orbital extension 642–643
   nasopharyngeal 527
   oculomotor nerves 511
   optic pathway 3
   orbital *see* orbital tumors
   paraneoplastic retinopathy 67
   pineal region 573, 573f
   pituitary 527
   see also pituitary adenomas
   pituitary apoplexy 259
   radiation-induced 282
   secondary 67, 641–642
   see also metastatic disease
   spinal cord 230
   thalamic 574
   trigeminal nerve, involving 527
   upbeat nystagmus 600–601

U

Uhthoff's phenomenon
   Leber's hereditary optic neuropathy 126
   optic neuritis 132
   transient visual loss 364, 372
ultrasound
   carotid disease 368–369, 368f
   papilledema 208
uncal herniation 508, 508f
unilateral vision loss, severe 381–383
unilateral visual hemi-inattention 349
upper motor neuron dysfunction 34
uveitis
   bilateral diffuse uveal melanocytic proliferation 70
   eye pain 674
   optic disc swelling associated with 144
   slit-lamp examination 110
   transient visual loss 364
   Vogt-Koyanagi-Harada syndrome 82–83

V

vagus nerve stimulation 579
valproate 672
valproic acid 602, 669–671
valvular disease 314
varicella zoster virus (VZV), acute retinal necrosis 85
vascular malformations, chiasm 270–271
vascular tumors, orbital 643–645
vasculitis 318–320
   giant cell arteritis 319
   primary CNS 318–319
   systemic 319–320
   systemic lupus erythematosus 85, 320
vasculopathic disease, risk factors 107
vasculopathic third nerve palsies 510–511, 510f
vaso-occlusive stroke 353
vasopressin 247
VDRL test, syphilis 148–149
venlafaxine hydrochloride 670
venography
   pseudotumor cerebri 220
   venous thrombosis/obstruction 226–227
venous angiomas 271, 644
venous thrombosis/obstruction 225–228, 226f
   neuroimaging 226–227
   presenting signs and symptoms 226
   treatment 228
   workup 227–228

ventriculoperitoneal (VP) shunting, pseudotumor cerebri 224
verapamil 670, 672
verbal memory, testing 31
vergences 24–26
vertebrobasilar disease, ischemic stroke 315
vertical conjugate gaze
   deviations 578–579
   limitations
      amyotropic lateral sclerosis 578
      basal ganglia disorders 578
      benign tonic vertical gaze in infancy 579–580, 580f
      neurologic disorders 575–578
      neuromuscular conditions 578
      Niemann–Pick disease 577
      ocular tics 579, 579f
      "one-and-a-half" syndrome 575
      paraneoplastic brainstem encephalitis 578
      Parinaud syndrome 570–575
      progressive supranuclear palsy *see* progressive supranuclear palsy
      supranuclear downgaze paresis 575
      Whipple disease 577–578
   neuroanatomy 568–570
vertical misalignment 24
vertigo, migrainous 667
very long-chain fatty acid (VLCFA) metabolism 327
vestibular disease, tilted and upside-down vision association 409
vestibular neuronitis 594
vestibular nystagmus 587, 594–595
vestibular paroxysmia 595
vestibular stimulation, visual neglect 350
vestibular-ocular reflex 551, 555, 588
vestibulo-ocular response (VOR) 24–26, 27f
Veterans Administration Cooperative Symptomatic Carotid Stenosis Trial 369–370
vigabatrin (anticonvulsant) 75–76
vinblastine 276
vincristine 70, 167, 276
vision loss
   see also blindness
   Charles Bonnet syndrome 402–403
   drusen, disc 125
   functional *see* functional visual loss
   hallucinations and illusions 400–403, 401t, 402f
      Charles Bonnet syndrome 402–403
      evaluation 403
      treatment 403
   "hysterical" 377–379
   in migraine 666
   moderate binocular 386
   moderate monocular 383–386
   optic neuropathies *see* optic neuropathies
   retinal disorders *see* retinal disorders
   severe unilateral 381–383
   transient *see* transient visual loss
visual acuity 7–10
   chiasmal disorders 239
   degree of vision, recording 8, 10f
   distance vision 7
   hallucinations and illusions 395
   moderate monocular vision loss, testing 384
   near vision 7
   in newborns 8–10
   optic nerve examination 107
   pinhole testing 7, 8f
   recording as fraction 7–8
   tilted disc anomaly, decreased in 118
visual association areas 41
visual evoked potentials, total blindness, testing for 381
visual field defects
   "clover leaf" 384–386, 387f–388f
   confrontation visual field assessment 14–15
   functional loss 386–390
   lateral geniculate nucleus 298
   occipital lobe/striate cortex 306–308
   optic radiations 301–302

optic tract 295
   paracentral 108, 389–390
visual field loss patterns 50–51
   ancillary testing 50–51
   chiasmal disorders 242–246, 242f–243f, 245f
   differential diagnosis 51
visual field testing 41–47
   advantages, disadvantages and most appropriate neuro-ophthalmic uses 42t
   chiasmal disorders 247
   in childhood disorders 42
   computerized static perimetry 45
   Goldmann kinetic perimetry 41, 45, 47f–48f
   higher cortical visual function disorders 340
   hill of vision concept 42, 43f–44f
   laser pointers, screening of visual field 15, 47, 50f
   papilledema 208–209
   pseudotumor cerebri 220
   tangent screen 41, 45–47, 50f
   threshold perimetry *see* threshold (static) perimetry, visual field testing
visual fields
   constricted 384–386, 385f
   diplopia 624
   disc drusen, effect on 124
   generalized constriction 108
   nonphysiologic constriction 384–386, 386f–388f
   optic nerve examination 108
   optic neuropathies, loss in 107
   pantomime 384–386
   pattern of loss *see* visual field loss pattern
   pituitary adenomas 253–254
   spiraling 384–386, 388f
   testing *see* visual field testing
   tilted disc anomaly 118
   tubular 384–386, 385f
visual form agnosia 344
visual imagery 352–353
visual neglect (hemi-inattention) 349–350
visual object agnosia 344
visual perseveration 408
visual word form area (VWFA) 342–343
visual-evoked potentials (VEPs)
   ischemic optic neuropathy 152
   optic neuritis 134
   retrochiasmal disorders, suspected 329
   visual loss pattern 50
visuomotor (optic) ataxia 352, 352f
vitamin A intoxication, pseudotumor cerebri 217
vitamin E deficiency/therapy 354, 566
vitreous abnormalities, transient visual loss 364
vitreous condensation, floaters 404
vitreous hemorrhage 10, 48
vitritis
   entoptic phenomena 404
   reduced visual acuity 10
   sarcoidosis 83–85
   swelling of optic nerve disc 113
Vogt-Koyanagi-Harada syndrome 82–83, 82f
voluntary nystagmus 604
von Hippel-Lindau (VHL) disease 91–93, 175–176

W

Wallenberg stroke 32–34
Wallenberg syndrome 432, 433f
warfarin 314, 369
Weber syndrome 507–508
Weber test, cranial nerve evaluation 32
Wegener's granulomatosis 79, 159, 637–638
Wernicke's encephalopathy 179, 524, 565–566, 565f
Westphal-Piltz reflex 443
WFS1 gene, Wolfram syndrome 129
Whipple disease 577–578
Whitnall's tubercle 612–613
Wilbrand's knee, chiasm 40–41, 45f, 239, 244–245